Brief Contents

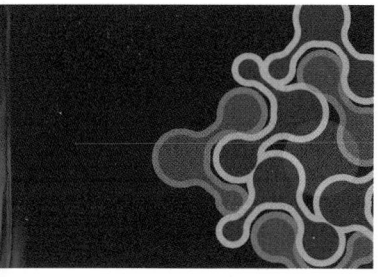

TIMBY'S INTRODUCTORY

Medical-Surgical Nursing

Loretta A. Donnelly-Moreno, DNP, RN, MSN
LVN/LPN Program Director
Nurse Faculty
Schreiner University
Kerrville, Texas

Brigitte Moseley, RN, MSN
Nursing Faculty
Vocational Nursing Program
Schreiner University
Kerrville, Texas

THIRTEENTH EDITION

Wolters Kluwer

Philadelphia • Baltimore • New York • London
Buenos Aires • Hong Kong • Sydney • Tokyo

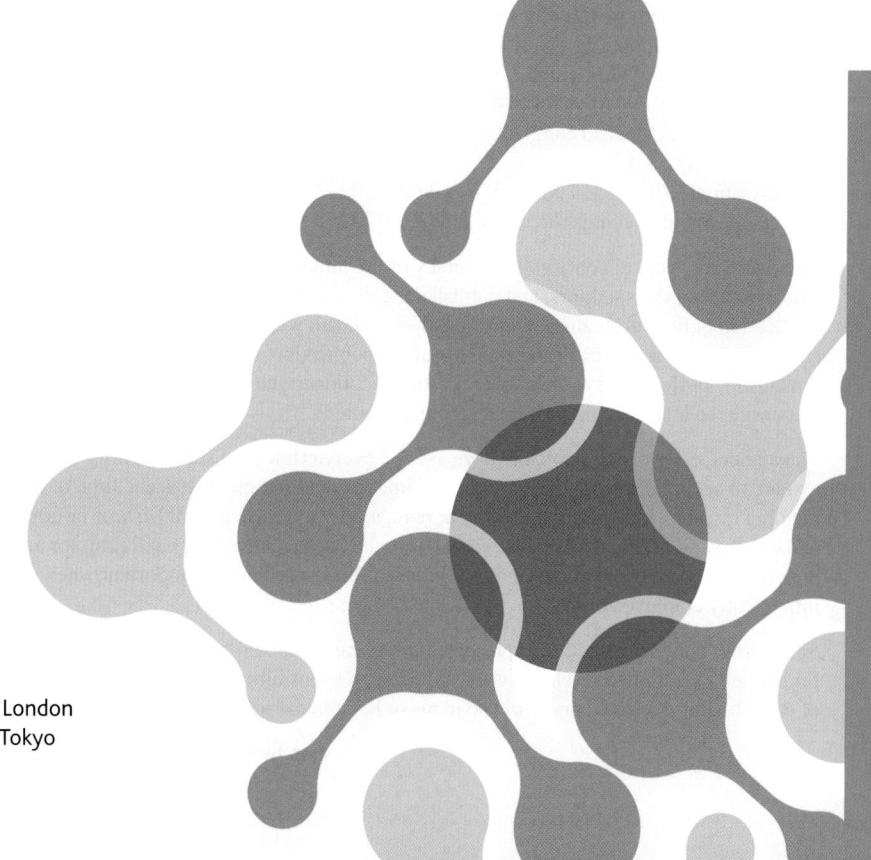

Vice President and Publisher: Julie K. Stegman
Senior Acquisitions Editor: Jonathan Joyce
Manager, Nursing Education and Practice Content: Jamie Blum
Associate Development Editor: Rebecca J. Rist
Editorial Coordinator: Sean Hanrahan
Marketing Manager: Brittany Clements
Editorial Assistant: Molly Kennedy
Design Manager: Stephen Druding
Art Director, Illustration: Jennifer Clements
Production Project Manager: Barton Dudlick
Manufacturing Coordinator: Margie Orzech-Zeranko
Prepress Vendor: S4Carlisle Publishing Services

Thirteenth Edition

9 8 7 6 5 4 3 2 1

Printed in Singapore

Library of Congress Cataloging-in-Publication Data

Names: Donnelly-Moreno, Loretta A. author. | Moseley, Brigitte, author. | Timby, Barbara Kuhn. Introductory medical-surgical nursing.
Title: Timby's introductory medical-surgical nursing / Loretta A. Donnelly-Moreno, Brigitte Moseley.
Description: Thirteenth edition. | Philadelphia: Wolters Kluwer Health, [2022] | Preceded by: Introductory medical-surgical nursing / Barbara K. Timby, Nancy E. Smith. Twelfth edition. Philadelphia: Wolters Kluwer, [2018]. | Includes bibliographical references and index.
Identifiers: LCCN 2021025073 | ISBN 9781975172237 (paperback)
Subjects: MESH: Medical-Surgical Nursing | Nursing Care | BISAC: MEDICAL / Nursing / LPN & LVN
Classification: LCC RT41 | NLM WY 150 | DDC 617/.0231—dc23
LC record available at https://lccn.loc.gov/2021025073

Care has been taken to confirm the accuracy of the information presented and to describe generally accepted practices. However, the authors, editors, and publisher are not responsible for errors or omissions or for any consequences from application of the information in this book and make no warranty, expressed or implied, with respect to the currency, completeness, or accuracy of the contents of the publication. Application of this information in a particular situation remains the professional responsibility of the practitioner; the clinical treatments described and recommended may not be considered absolute and universal recommendations.

The authors, editors, and publisher have exerted every effort to ensure that drug selection and dosage set forth in this text are in accordance with the current recommendations and practice at the time of publication. However, in view of ongoing research, changes in government regulations, and the constant flow of information relating to drug therapy and drug reactions, the reader is urged to check the package insert for each drug for any change in indications and dosage and for added warnings and precautions. This is particularly important when the recommended agent is a new or infrequently employed drug.

Some drugs and medical devices presented in this publication have Food and Drug Administration (FDA) clearance for limited use in restricted research settings. It is the responsibility of the health care provider to ascertain the FDA status of each drug or device planned for use in his or her clinical practice.

shop.lww.com

MKO721

This textbook is dedicated to all current and future nursing students in their quest to comprehend diseases and disorders that continue to plague the human body, and to learn how to care for them with understanding and compassion.

—LADM & BM

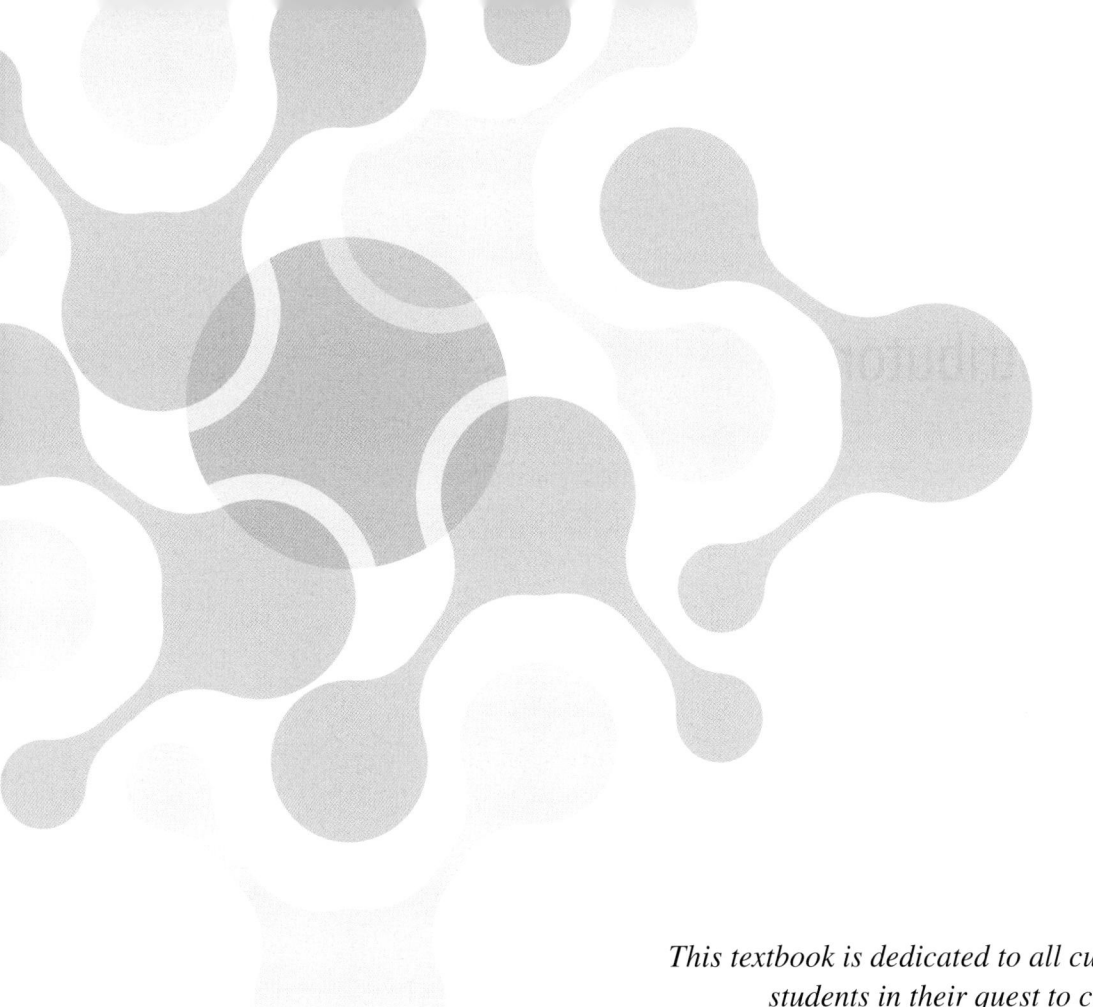

Contributor

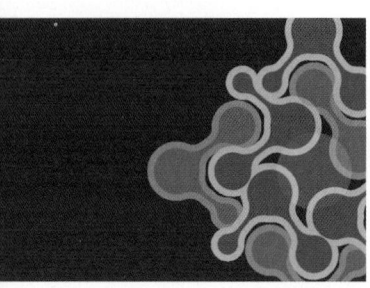

Rikke Sorensen, RN, BSN, MBA
Nursing Administrator
La Hacienda Treatment Center
Hunt, Texas

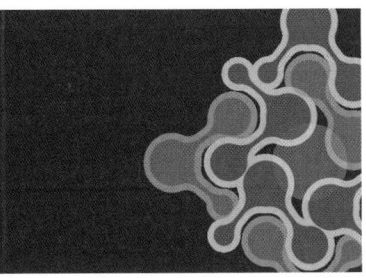

Features and Learning Tools

The 13th edition includes updated features that long-time users of *Timby's Introductory Medical-Surgical Nursing* love:

A **user-friendly design** along with **figures** of diseases, procedures, signs, symptoms, and normal-versus-abnormal comparisons helps visual learners understand the whole picture.

NCLEX-PN Review Questions found at the end of each chapter help the students understand how the National Council Licensure Examination for Practical Nurses (NCLEX-PN) examination relates to the chapter content they just read.

NCLEX-STYLE REVIEW QUESTIONS PrepU

1. A client with chronic illness always reports feeling great. What does this tell the nurse about the client?
1. The client is able to define health in a positive way.
2. The client is able to dismiss the chronic illness.
3. The client is able to engage in meaningful activities.
4. The client is able to put on a positive demeanor.

Words to Know listed at the beginning of each chapter along with the chapter **Learning Objectives** help focus student reading and identify important information to learn in each chapter.

Words To Know

capitation
client
diagnosis-related groups (DRGs)
disease
early detection
health
health care delivery system
health care team
health maintenance
health maintenance organization (HMO)
health promotion
holism
illness

Learning Objectives

On completion of this chapter, you will be able to:

1. Explain the concepts of health, holism, wellness, illness, disease, and the health–illness continuum.
2. Describe how clients with chronic illness may still be considered healthy.
3. Differentiate between health maintenance and health promotion.
4. Identify members of the health care team.
5. Describe three levels of care that the health care delivery system provides.
6. Describe problems related to access to health care.
7. Describe Medicare, Medicaid, and Medigap insurance.

New! Key Points were added at the end of each chapter. Important information is included in outline form to assist the reader with studying key information from each chapter.

KEY POINTS

- Definitions
  - *Health: state of complete physical, mental, and social well-being
  - Holism: viewing a person's health as a balance of body, mind, and spirit
  - Wellness: a constant and intentional effort to stay healthy
  - Illness: a state of being sick

Stop, Think, and Respond exercises encourage rapid recall and practical assimilation of contents. These questions are found in every chapter and require students to apply content as they read.

››› *Stop, Think, and Respond 1-1*

A homeless client who collapsed on the street is brought to the emergency room by the local police for treatment. Without knowing the actual diagnosis, what factors related to health and illness concepts may have contributed to this client's poor health?

Concept Mastery Alerts highlight and clarify fundamental nursing concepts to improve understanding of difficult topics that are identified by Misconception Alerts in Lippincott's Adaptive Learning Powered by PrepU, an adaptive quizzing platform. Data from hundreds of actual students using this program in medical-surgical courses across the United States identified common misconceptions for the authors to clarify in this feature.

> *Concept Mastery Alert*
>
> **Prevention QIs have to do with avoidable hospitalizations. Client safety QIs reflect quality of care within the hospital, including safety issues.**

Clinical Scenarios, related to Nursing Care Plans and Nursing Process sections, introduce the reader to a client's problem and include a critical thinking question to help students begin to think through each situation.

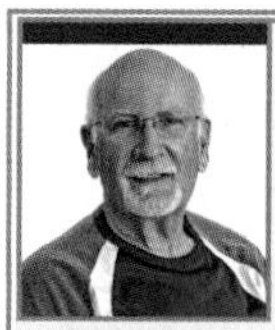

> **Clinical Scenario** An older client seeks medical attention, complaining of nausea and vomiting that has persisted for more than 24 hours. The client states that family members had similar symptoms several days ago. What issues are of concern for the nurse? (See the following Nursing Process section for dealing with clients experiencing nausea and vomiting.)

Nursing Care Plans provide an overview of nursing care (with rationales) for clients experiencing common conditions. Each Nursing Care Plan relates to the client introduced in the Clinical Scenario. (See Quick Reference to Nursing Care Plans on p. xviii.)

NURSING CARE PLAN 66-1 The Client With Burns

Assessment

- Assess vital signs.
- Look for evidence of inhalation injury.
- Determine the oxygen saturation and respiratory effort.
- Evaluate pain intensity.
- Determine the volume and characteristics of urine.
- Note the percentage and depth of burn.
- Auscultate bowel sounds.
- Assess for concurrent medical problems, and review the results of laboratory tests.

Depending on the extent and degree of burns, some or all of the following nursing diagnoses may apply. Diagnoses change as the client progresses through treatment and the stages of healing.

Nursing Diagnoses. **Ineffective Airway Clearance Risk** related to increased airway secretions; **Impaired Gas Exchange** related to edema of airway and inhalation of carbon

Expected Outcomes. (1) The airway will be patent. (2) Gas exchange will be adequate as evidenced by clear lung sounds, blood oxygen saturation (SpO_2) greater than 90%, and arterial oxygen pressure (PaO_2) greater than 80 mm Hg.

Interventions	Rationales
Monitor characteristics of respirations and lung sounds frequently.	*Frequent focused assessments of respiratory function facilitate early detection of compromised ventilation.*
Check respiratory rate before and after administering an opioid analgesic.	*Narcotic analgesics depress the respiratory center in the brain.*
Measure SpO_2 with a pulse oximeter or analyze arterial blood gas (ABG) results.	*The PaO_2 can be determined deductively from the SpO_2; an SpO_2 of 90% or greater suggests that the PaO_2 is at least 80 mm Hg. ABGs provide objective measurements of serum O_2, CO_2, and bicarbonate levels.*
Administer oxygen as prescribed.	*Supplemental oxygen increases the percentage of inhaled oxygen above that in room air.*
Suction the airway cautiously if edema is present.	*Suctioning removes accumulated secretions, but the trauma of catheter insertion can worsen edema.*
Facilitate ventilation with artificial airways, such as with an endotracheal tube and ventilator.	*An artificial airway and ventilator facilitate the maintenance of adequate gas exchange.*
Be prepared to assist with an escharotomy if there is a circumferential burn of the chest.	*An escharotomy releases constriction and allows greater chest expansion.*

Evaluation of Expected Outcome

Client breathes effortlessly and is well oxygenated.

Nursing Diagnosis: Hypovolemia related to volume loss

Expected Outcome. Nurse will monitor to detect, manage, and minimize hypovolemia.

Interventions	Rationales
Monitor vital signs every 15 minutes.	*Hypotension and tachycardia suggest impending shock.*
Measure intake and output hourly.	*Hourly measurements facilitate early detection of mismatches between fluid intake and output.*
Weigh the client daily at the same time with similar dressings.	*A loss of 2 lb in 24 hours suggests a 1-L deficit in fluid.*
Administer fluids according to the fluid resuscitation formula.	*A large volume of fluid is necessary to prevent hypovolemic shock.*
Report urine output of <50 mL/hour.	*Urine output <50 mL/hour suggests inadequate renal perfusion due to hypovolemia or other causes.*

Evaluation of Expected Outcome

Client does not experience hypovolemic shock.

Nursing Process sections also relate to a specific client introduced in the Clinical Scenario. These sections emphasize a nursing process approach to care and provide rationales in italics for all interventions.

NURSING PROCESS FOR THE CLIENT WITH NAUSEA AND VOMITING

Assessment

Obtain a complete medical, dietary, drug, and allergy history. In addition, compile a list of symptoms that occurred before and along with nausea and vomiting; how long the problem has existed; and the frequency, color, and amount of vomited material. List the foods and where the client has eaten in the past 24 hours. In addition, assess the general appearance, weight, and vital signs. Documenting intake and output and monitoring for signs of fluid volume deficit are additional essential assessment requirements (see Chapter 16).

Diagnosis, Planning, and Interventions

Hypovolemia: Related to prolonged vomiting and decreased intake of oral fluids
Expected Outcome: Fluid balance will be restored as evidenced by intake of 1500 to 3000 mL/day with similar fluid loss.

- Offer clear fluids in small amounts. *Slow introduction of fluids allows the client to develop tolerance and determine if they can advance the diet.*
- Recommend commercial over-the-counter beverages such as Gatorade. *Gatorade replaces fluids and electrolytes.*
- Inform the primary provider if urine output is below 500 mL/day or serum electrolyte levels are abnormal. *Such findings indicate severe dehydration and the need for IV replacement fluids.*
- Monitor weight daily. *Daily monitoring helps to determine trends in weight loss or gain.*
- Assess skin turgor and mucous membranes. *Decreased skin turgor and dry mucous membranes indicate dehydration.*

Malnutrition Risk: Related to nausea and vomiting
Expected Outcome: The client's nutritional status will be adequate as evidenced by maintenance of weight and normal electrolyte and blood values.

- When the client tolerates clear fluids, advance diet to full liquids, then to soft, bland foods, such as creamed soups, crackers, or toast. *Advancing diet slowly helps the client develop tolerance for fluids and food.*
- Collaborate with the dietitian to provide nutritional foods. *The dietitian can help create a plan that assists the client to increase caloric intake with foods that they can tolerate.*
- Discourage caffeinated or carbonated beverages. *Such drinks may decrease appetite and lead to early satiety.*

Evaluation of Expected Outcomes

The client has an oral intake of 2500 mL and an output of 2600 mL. Weight is maintained or restored to preillness level. Serum electrolyte levels and other laboratory test results are within normal limits.

Cancer of the Oral Cavity and Pharynx

Cancer cells undergo changes in structure and appearance. They multiply, eventually forming a colony of abnormal and dysfunctional cells (see Chapter 18). When cancer affects the oral cavity, cells in the lips, mouth, or pharynx undergo malignant changes. When cancers of the oral cavity are detected early, the rate of cure is fairly good.

Pathophysiology and Etiology

Development of oral cancers is linked to smoking (includes cigarettes, cigars, and pipes), smokeless tobacco, drinking alcohol in excess, and human papillomavirus (HPV). Lip cancer is associated with pipe smoking and prolonged exposure to wind and sun. Tobacco, in particular, increases the risk of oral cancer, but clients who use both tobacco and alcohol have an extreme risk of developing oral cancer. It is hypothesized that tobacco and alcohol have a synergistic effect, in that they increase the others' carcinogenic effect. It is believed that alcohol dehydrates the cell walls on the oral mucosa, increasing the ability of tobacco carcinogens to permeate these cells. Research on this phenomenon is ongoing (The Oral Cancer Foundation, 2020).

Evidence-Based Practice boxes include a Clinical Question, Evidence, and Nursing Implications to help students understand how research relates to current nursing practice.

Evidence-Based Practice 1-1

Nursing Care, Health Care Management, and Hospital Reimbursement

Clinical Question

How will nursing care in the future affect health care management and hospital reimbursement?

Evidence

The ACA established the "Hospital-Acquired Condition (HAC) Reduction Program." This program guides the secretary of Health and Human Services on the amount of reimbursement health care facilities receive based on quality measures. The amount of reduction in payment will depend on their ranking in the performance quartile. The HAC program scores on Research and Quality, Patient Safety Indicators, Central Line Infections, Surgical Site Infections, and Urinary Tract Infections. The health care facility scores are also published and become public record through the ACA (Quality Net, n.d.).

Nursing Implications

Employers will work within their health care facilities to improve in all categories through education and training. Nurses play a part in each of the quality measures listed above. Proper training, orientation, continuing education, providing quality care, and following policies and guidelines are part of the professional responsibility of the nurse. As part of the health care team, nurses have a large impact on the health care facility's success in this reduction program. Aiming the focus on evidence-based practice and nursing outcomes may greatly affect the outcomes of these reimbursements.

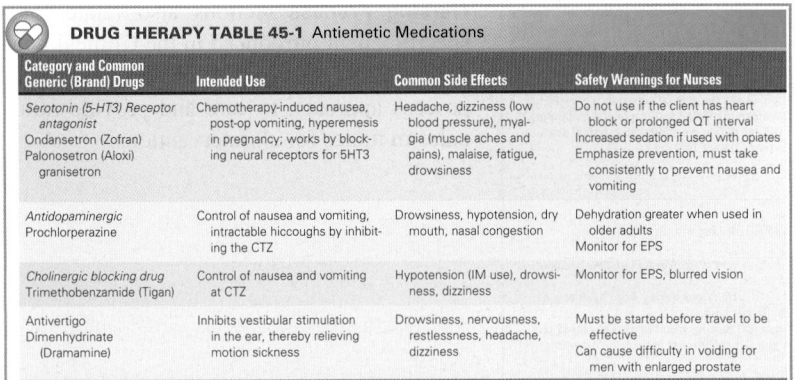

DRUG THERAPY TABLE 45-1 Antiemetic Medications

Category and Common Generic (Brand) Drugs	Intended Use	Common Side Effects	Safety Warnings for Nurses
Serotonin (5-HT3) Receptor antagonist Ondansetron (Zofran) Palonosetron (Aloxi) granisetron	Chemotherapy-induced nausea, post-op vomiting, hyperemesis in pregnancy; works by blocking neural receptors for 5HT3	Headache, dizziness (low blood pressure), myalgia (muscle aches and pains), malaise, fatigue, drowsiness	Do not use if the client has heart block or prolonged QT interval Increased sedation if used with opiates Emphasize prevention, must take consistently to prevent nausea and vomiting
Antidopaminergic Prochlorperazine	Control of nausea and vomiting, intractable hiccoughs by inhibiting the CTZ	Drowsiness, hypotension, dry mouth, nasal congestion	Dehydration greater when used in older adults Monitor for EPS
Cholinergic blocking drug Trimethobenzamide (Tigan)	Control of nausea and vomiting at CTZ	Hypotension (IM use), drowsiness, dizziness	Monitor for EPS, blurred vision
Antivertigo Dimenhydrinate (Dramamine)	Inhibits vestibular stimulation in the ear, thereby relieving motion sickness	Drowsiness, nervousness, restlessness, headache, dizziness	Must be started before travel to be effective Can cause difficulty in voiding for men with enlarged prostate

Updated Drug Therapy tables provide an overview of the major categories of drugs used for common conditions ensuring safe, effective practice.

NURSING GUIDELINES 45-1

Managing the Care of Clients With Anorexia

- Provide foods that the client likes during meals.
- Offer nourishing beverages (eggnog, milk shakes, and commercial concentrates such as *Ensure* or *Instant Breakfast*) as between-meal snacks.
- If the client is hospitalized or in another health care facility, encourage family members to bring favorite foods that can be refrigerated or reheated.
- Conduct a daily caloric count if necessary to determine total proteins and carbohydrates in the client's diet.
- Keep serving sizes and containers small to avoid overwhelming the client.
- Serve and keep hot foods hot and cold foods cold.
- Encourage eating in the company of others.
- Formulate a nutritional plan with the client and dietitian that promotes weight gain (approximately 600 calories per meal).
- If necessary, arrange for supplementation based on documented deficiencies in the client's intake.
- Consult the primary provider and dietitian in cases of prolonged anorexia.

Nursing Guidelines present essential information nurses need to perform specific nursing skills or to manage care for a client with a particular disorder.

Client and Family Teaching boxes present instructions and information the nurse can give to the client and family to help improve client outcomes.

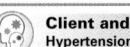

Client and Family Teaching 27-1
Hypertension

The nurse instructs as follows:

- Adhere to the treatment regimen even if you have few, if any, symptoms and feel well. Hypertension is a chronic condition requiring lifelong management and treatment.
- Learn to regularly monitor BP using a home sphygmomanometer or arrange for monitoring by a community agency that provides this service at no or low cost.
- Keep a log of BP measurements for follow-up visits.
- Comply with the treatment regimen involving diet, exercise, and drug therapy.
- Consult cookbooks published or endorsed by the American Heart Association, American Diabetes Association, or other reliable sources for "heart smart" recipes.
- Follow directions for medications; never increase, decrease, or omit a prescribed drug unless first conferring with the primary care provider.
- Report adverse effects from medications to the prescribing provider. Get medical approval before taking nonprescription drugs. Inform all primary providers and dentists of medications that you are taking.
- Avoid tobacco and beverages containing caffeine or alcohol unless permitted by the provider.

Gerontologic Considerations

- The components of blood change only slightly with age. RBCs become slightly less flexible and fewer in number. Lymphocytes also decrease in number, causing a decreased resistance to infection.
- Decreased renal perfusion can result in inadequate erythropoietin production, resulting in decreased RBC production.
- Cellular and humoral immunity are affected by age-related changes in the lymphatic system, including decreases in primary antibody, T-Cell and B-cell responses, and antibody production. This results in an increased susceptibility of older adults to infections and malignancies, and indication for recommended adult immunizations.
- The Schilling test may pose a problem in older adults if proper collection of the 24-hour specimen is not possible as a result of cognitive problems or urinary incontinence. Recent research indicates that gastric pH levels vary in older adults, requiring individual consideration of appropriateness of the Schilling test to detect B12 deficiencies for older adults. However, the full Schilling test is indicated if other causes are suspected.

Gerontologic Considerations are now located at the beginning of each chapter so that the student can incorporate these considerations into their thinking as they read the chapter. Students can reflect on current research and theory as they read and think about how pathophysiology, signs and symptoms, or nursing care differ for the older population.

Pharmacologic Considerations highlight special considerations nurses need to remember when administering or caring for clients receiving specific drugs.

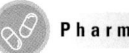

Pharmacologic Considerations

- Consult the primary provider for changes in drug orders if a client cannot retain a medication orally.

Nutrition Notes

The Client With Nausea

- The client should eat small meals and eat and drink slowly.
- Dry, salty foods, such as crackers and pretzels, may relieve nausea.
- Fried food, spicy food, and foods with strong odors should be avoided.
- Cold foods may be preferable to hot foods.

Nutrition Notes pinpoint key nutrition information for clients with certain types of conditions.

CRITICAL THINKING EXERCISES

1. Interview older clients to explore their understanding of the health care coverage including access to prescription drugs. Compare their knowledge with information available from the Medicare & You website at www.medicare.gov/publications.
2. Ask the nurse manager on your assigned clinical unit about the QIs the unit must provide data on and what impact they have had on client care.

Critical Thinking Exercises, at the end of each chapter, challenge students to apply the content they have read.

Preface

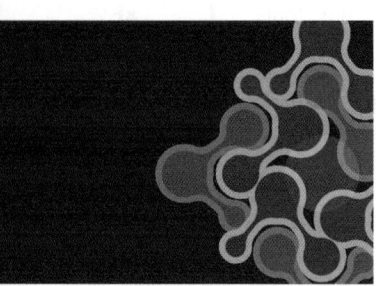

In today's changing health care environment, nurses continue to face many challenges and opportunities. *Timby's Introductory Medical-Surgical Nursing* provides the necessary information to help nurses meet these challenges and embrace expanding opportunities. The textbook addresses common adult disorders that are treated medically and surgically and also covers basic concepts student nurses need to know to care for clients with these disorders. Written at a level appropriate for the practical/vocational nursing student, this textbook provides comprehensive information about medical-surgical nursing that is easy to understand.

For the 13th edition, the textbook was revised and updated to reflect current medical and nursing practice. New to this edition are **Key Points** found at the end of each chapter. These important learning points from the chapter are presented in an outline of bulleted points that highlight important concepts for students to master. This edition continues to include methodology for planning nursing care. Each of the **Nursing Process** sections, **Nursing Care Plans**, is preceded by a **Client Scenario** to assist students in relating the plan of care to a specific client. Other highlights of this edition include **Evidence-Based Practice** boxes. Also updated in this edition are **Concept Mastery Alerts**, which clarify fundamental nursing concepts to improve the reader's understanding of potentially confusing topics, as identified by Misconception Alerts in Lippincott's Adaptive Learning Powered by PrepU. Data from thousands of actual students using this program in courses across the United States identified common misconceptions to be clarified in this new feature.

Information in this text is updated to include and discuss new goals for Healthy People 2030. Cultural awareness is brought to the forefront throughout the text, as well as specifics as discussed in Chapter 8. The worldwide pandemic related to Covid-19 is addressed in several areas, as it does affect nursing care throughout the world.

CLINICAL JUDGMENT

Clinical judgment is an important part of the nursing process. Clinical judgment allows an individual to think like a nurse in preparation for becoming a nurse. To achieve clinical judgment, the nurse must first obtain the knowledge, analyze the data provided, prioritize the information, determine which action should be taken first, take the needed actions, and then evaluate the outcomes and determine if the process needs to start again.

Clinical judgment is supported in this textbook in multiple areas, such as the Case Studies, Evidence-Based Practice, and the Stop, Think, and Respond sections. Reviewing, processing, and mastering this information will help one become more confident with clinical judgment skills.

ORGANIZATION OF THE TEXT

The 13th edition of *Timby's Introductory Medical-Surgical Nursing* continues to provide readability and clarity. Information is presented in a logical and informative manner with 72 chapters organized into 17 units.

- ***Unit 1*, Nursing Roles and Responsibilities,** includes foundational chapters covering concepts and trends in health care, nursing roles and settings, the nursing process (including mention of concept care mapping), interviewing and physical assessment, legal and ethical issues, and leadership and management.
- ***Unit 2*, Client Care Concerns,** explores areas in which nurses interact and work with clients to manage their health. Topics include nurse–client relationships, culture, complementary and alternative therapies, and end-of-life care.
- ***Unit 3*, Foundations of Medical-Surgical Nursing,** includes chapters on frequent and regular topics in medical-surgical nursing care. These include pain, infection, intravenous therapy, perioperative care, and disasters.
- ***Unit 4*, Caring for Clients With Multisystem Disorders,** includes chapters on fluid, electrolyte, and acid–base imbalances; shock; and cancer.
- ***Units 5 through 16*** present information on disorders according to body systems. Each unit begins with an introductory chapter that includes a general review of anatomy and physiology, a discussion of client assessment, and common diagnostic and laboratory tests that pertain to particular disorders.
- ***Unit 17*, Caring for Clients With Psychobiologic Disorders,** contains chapters on frequently encountered emotional and behavioral issues: anxiety disorders, mood disorders, eating disorders, chemical dependency, and dementia and thought disorders.

At the end of the textbook, Appendix A lists commonly used abbreviations and acronyms. A glossary provides a quick reference to definitions for Words to Know that appear throughout the textbook. Additional resources available on thePoint® include Appendix B that provides a convenient reference for laboratory values. You will also find a comprehensive listing of references and suggested readings, including general recommendations as well as unit-specific citations, that provide a streamlined guide to current literature about topics discussed in the textbook.

TEACHING AND LEARNING RESOURCES

The 13th edition of *Timby's Introductory Medical-Surgical Nursing* features a compelling and comprehensive complement of additional resources to help instructors teach and students learn.

Resources for Instructors on thePoint®

Tools to assist you with teaching your course are available upon adoption of this textbook at https://thePoint.lww.com/TimbyMS13e.

- **Test Generator**, completely revised for this edition by expert NCLEX-PN test writers, contains thousands of questions to help you in assessing your students' understanding of the material.
- **PowerPoint Presentations** provide an easy way for you to integrate the textbook with your students' classroom experience, either via slide shows or through handouts. Multiple-choice and true/false questions are integrated into the presentations to promote class participation and allow you to use i-clicker technology.
- An **Image Bank** lets you use the photographs and illustrations from this textbook in your PowerPoint slides or as you see fit in your course.
- **Pre-Lecture Quizzes** (and answers) are quick, knowledge-based assessments that allow you to check student reading.
- **Guided Lecture Notes** walk you through the chapters, objective by objective, and provide you with corresponding PowerPoint slide numbers.
- **Discussion Topics** (and suggested answers) can be used as conversation starters or in online discussion boards.
- **Assignments** (and suggested answers) include group, written, clinical, and web assignments.
- **Case Studies** with related questions (and suggested answers) give students an opportunity to apply their knowledge to a client case similar to one they might encounter in practice.
- **Answers to Questions in the Book** (Stop, Think, and Respond Exercises; Critical Thinking Exercises; and NCLEX-style Review Questions) are provided for each chapter. Instructors are free to share these with their students to enhance student self-learning.
- A **Sample Syllabus** provides guidance for structuring your medical-surgical nursing course.
- **Lesson Plans** provide you with a lesson outline that links key concepts back to PowerPoint slides; figures, tables, and features; and lists resources for in- and out-of-class activities.
- **Quality and Safety Education for Nurses (QSEN) map** links key competency knowledge, skills, and abilities (KSAs) to the textbook to ensure quality assurance.
- **Answer Key for the Workbook** supplies answers to the questions appearing in *Workbook for Timby's Introductory Medical-Surgical Nursing*, 13th edition, the accompanying for-sale workbook.

RESOURCES FOR STUDENTS ON thePoint®

Free resources are available on thePoint® to help students review material and become even more familiar with vital concepts. Students can access all these resources on using the codes printed in the front of their textbooks. Resources include:

- **Appendix B** from the textbook provides a convenient reference for laboratory values.
- **References and Suggested Readings**, including general recommendations as well as unit-specific citations, provide a streamlined guide to current literature about topics discussed in the textbook.
- **NCLEX-Style Chapter Review Questions**, now including more than 1400 questions, help students review important concepts and practice for NCLEX-PN examination.
- **Concepts in Action animations** bring physiologic and pathophysiologic concepts to life and enhance student learning.
- **Watch and Learn video clips** demonstrate specific skills to enhance student understanding of key nursing techniques.
- **Heart and breath sounds** demonstrate key differences in the sounds that nurses need to identify when examining patients.
- A **Spanish–English audio glossary** provides helpful terms and phrases for communicating with clients who speak Spanish.

STUDENT WORKBOOK

The *Workbook for Timby's Introductory Medical-Surgical Nursing*, 13th edition, complements the textbook and reinforces information students need to learn and is available for purchase. **Case Studies with critical thinking questions** are included in every unit that offer a unique way for students to relate to a particular client situation and think about the type of care needed. Other key activities in the workbook include **review exercises**, **application activities**, **NCLEX-style practice questions**, and images from the textbook for **labeling activities**. Answers to the workbook questions are provided to instructors on thePoint®.

LIPPINCOTT ® COURSEPOINT

Lippincott CoursePoint

Lippincott® CoursePoint is an integrated, digital curriculum solution for nursing education that provides a completely interactive and adaptive experience geared to help students understand, retain, and apply their course knowledge and be prepared for practice. The time-tested, easy-to-use, and trusted solution includes engaging learning tools, evidence-based practice, case studies, and in-depth reporting to meet students where they are in their learning, combined with the most trusted nursing education content on the market to help prepare students for practice. This easy-to-use digital learning solution of *Lippincott® CoursePoint*, combined with unmatched support, gives instructors and students everything they need for course and curriculum success!

Lippincott® CoursePoint includes:

- Engaging course content with a variety of learning tools to engage students of all learning styles
- Adaptive and personalized learning helps students learn the critical thinking and clinical judgment skills needed to help them become practice-ready nurses.
- Immediate, evidence-based, online nursing clinical decision support with Lippincott Advisor for Education
- Unparalleled reporting provides in-depth dashboards with several data points to track student progress and help identify strengths and weaknesses.

Unmatched support includes training coaches, product trainers, and nursing education consultants to help educators and students implement *Lippincott® CoursePoint* with ease.

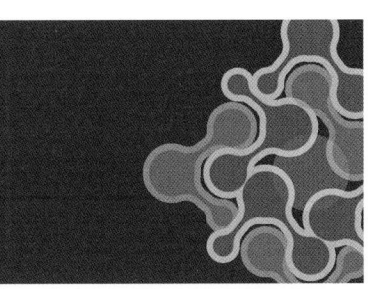

Acknowledgments

We the authors wish to thank all those who helped in the preparation of this edition. We remain grateful to the skilled and knowledgeable professionals at Wolters Kluwer. Although we never meet most of them, we appreciate their expert ability to keep us on track and in turn respond to our many requests and needs when this textbook was in production.

We hope that *Timby's Introductory Medical-Surgical Nursing*, 13th edition, provides the readers with the practical knowledge and skills to manage the nursing care of clients in today's changing health care environments. We also hope that our contributions provide students with similar joys and rewards that we have experienced in our nursing careers.

Loretta A. Donnelly-Moreno, DNP, RN, MSN
Brigitte Moseley, RN, MSN

Contents

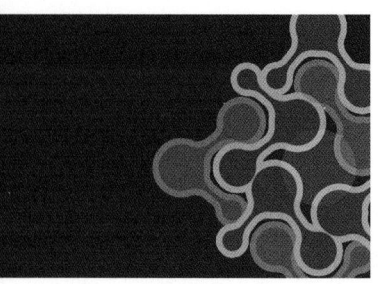

RESOURCES AVAILABLE ON thePoint®

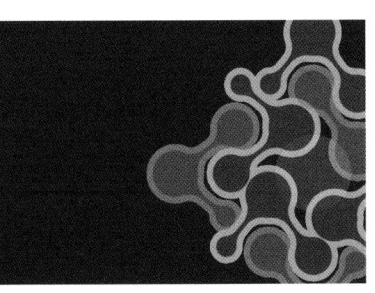

Quick Reference to Nursing Care Plans

UNIT 1
Nursing Roles and Responsibilities

1 Concepts and Trends in Health Care

Words To Know

capitation
client
diagnosis-related groups (DRGs)
disease
early detection
health
health care delivery system
health care team
health maintenance
health maintenance organization (HMO)
health promotion
holism
illness
illness prevention
integrated delivery systems (IDSs)
managed care organizations (MCOs)
Medigap insurance
morbidity
mortality
physician hospital organizations (PHOs)
point-of-service (POS)
preferred provider organization (PPO)
primary care
prospective payment system (PPS)
secondary care
tertiary care
unlicensed assistive personnel (UAP)
wellness

Learning Objectives

On completion of this chapter, you will be able to:

1. Explain the concepts of health, holism, wellness, illness, disease, and the health–illness continuum.
2. Describe how clients with chronic illness may still be considered healthy.
3. Differentiate between health maintenance and health promotion.
4. Identify members of the health care team.
5. Describe three levels of care that the health care delivery system provides.
6. Describe problems related to access to health care.
7. Describe Medicare, Medicaid, and Medigap insurance.
8. Explain how a prospective payment system (PPS) works.
9. Explain how the different types of managed care organizations (MCOs) work.
10. Discuss the difference between capitation and fee-for-service insurance.
11. Discuss the effects of cost-driven changes on health care.
12. Discuss methods for monitoring quality of care.
13. Describe national and worldwide health care campaigns designed to improve health care and health care outcomes.
14. Identify trends that influence future health care policy.

The roles of nurses in the health care delivery system are multiple and complex. Nurses collect data, diagnose human responses to health problems, plan and provide care, and evaluate outcomes of care. They work in various settings, adhering to facility policies and state nurse practice acts. Nurses educate clients, families, and staff. They manage resources and act as advocates for clients. In addition, they participate in disease prevention and health promotion activities for clients, families, and communities.

CONCEPTS RELATED TO HEALTH

Health and Wellness

The constitution of the World Health Organization (WHO, n.d., para. 1) defines **health** as "a state of complete physical, mental, and social well-being and not merely the absence of disease or infirmity." Although this definition of health is useful, it presents health and illness in absolute terms. If a person is not functioning optimally in every way, they are not healthy. It also implies that an infirmity negates the possibility of health. Nurses practice from the perspective of holism. **Holism** means viewing a person's health as a balance of body, mind, and spirit. Treating only the body will not necessarily restore optimal health. In addition to physical needs, nurses must also consider the client's psychological, sociocultural, developmental, and spiritual needs.

Wellness describes a state of being. It is a constant and intentional effort to stay healthy and achieve the highest potential for total well-being. It requires lifestyle choices that assist individuals to strive for and maintain a balance in their physical, occupational/leisure, environmental, intellectual, spiritual, and emotional/social domains. Activities and choices should help individuals to promote good physical self-care, prevent illness and injury, use their full intellectual potential, express appropriate emotions in response to changes and the behavior of others, manage stress, and maintain positive interpersonal relationships. As with health and illness, one's determination of a state of wellness is highly individual.

Illness and Disease

Theoretically, **illness** refers to a state of being sick. Illness may be viewed as catastrophic (sudden, traumatic), acute, chronic, or terminal. **Disease** refers to a pathologic condition of the body that presents with clinical signs and symptoms and changes in laboratory values. The term *disease* has related terminology and concepts. Table 1-1 provides a list of these terms with brief definitions.

The major difference between illness and disease is that illness is highly individual and personal, whereas disease is something more definitive and measurable. For example, a client with arthritis presents with distinct pathologic changes associated with the disease. A person, however, may or may not be ill with arthritis. The degrees of pain, suffering, and immobility vary with each person.

The Health–Illness Continuum

In contrast to definitions of health and illness, the health–illness continuum considers level of health, which continually changes for each person. The health–illness continuum illustrates this process of change, in which individuals face various states of health and illness, ranging from extremely good health to death (Fig. 1-1). Within this continuum, clients adapt physically, emotionally, and socially, enabling maintenance of comfort, stability, and self-expression. Therefore, clients with chronic illness can achieve a high

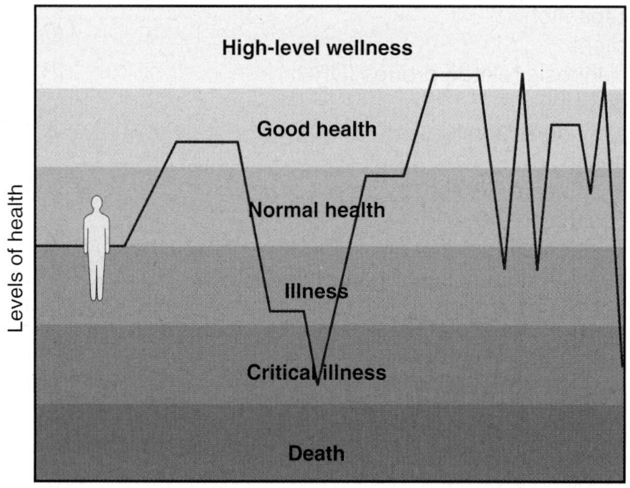

Figure 1-1 The health–illness continuum.

TABLE 1-1 Disease-Related Terminology

TERM	DEFINITION
Etiology	The cause of a disease
Incidence	The frequency of a particular disease in a specific population during a specific period
Morbidity	The number of sick persons with a particular disease in a specific population
Mortality	The death rate or the ratio of the number of deaths for a specific population
Pathophysiology	Study of how disease alters normal physiologic processes
Prevalence	The number of cases of a disease in a specific population during a specific period
Primary prevention	Prevention of the development of disease in a susceptible or potentially susceptible population; includes health promotion and immunization
Secondary prevention	Early diagnosis and treatment to shorten duration and severity of an illness, reduce contagion, and limit complications
Sign	Objective manifestation of a disease; can be seen, heard, measured, or felt
Symptom	Subjective manifestation of a disease or illness; what the client relates is happening
Tertiary prevention	Health care to limit the degree of disability or promote rehabilitation in chronic, irreversible diseases

level of wellness if they can experience a high quality of life within the limits of that illness. For example, physically disabled people are considered healthy if they are physiologically stable and engaged in personal and social activities that they find meaningful.

Health Maintenance and Promotion

Many people now believe they have control over their well-being and are taking more responsibility for their health status. **Health maintenance** refers to protecting one's current level of health by preventing illness or deterioration, such as by complying with medication regimens, being screened for diseases such as breast and colon cancers, or practicing safe sex. **Health promotion** refers to engaging in strategies to enhance health. Such strategies include eating a diet rich in fiber, complex carbohydrates, low in fat, and high in fruits and vegetables; exercising regularly; balancing work with leisure activities; and practicing stress-reduction techniques. **Illness prevention** involves identifying risk factors such as a family history of hypertension or diabetes and reducing the effects of risk factors on one's health. In addition, **early detection**, such as mammographies and colonoscopies, uses screening diagnostic tests and procedures to identify a disease process earlier, so that treatment may be initiated earlier and be more effective.

A **client** is an active partner in nursing care. Thus, the person receiving health care services no longer plays a passive, ill role but is an active purchaser of health care services. The use of the term *client* in this textbook reflects the attitude of personal responsibility for health. Clients may or may not be ill, but they take great responsibility for meeting their health maintenance and promotion needs and actively participate in treatment decisions regarding health restoration.

HEALTH CARE

Just as the concept of health has changed in recent decades, so, too, has the health care industry. Rapid advances in science and technology have contributed to the development of highly sophisticated methods for diagnosing and treating disease. At the same time, escalating health care costs have created difficult economic conditions and disparity in access to care and have led to shorter lengths of stays in hospitals. The health care system has grown to include multiple outpatient, short-term, and long-term care facilities, with care given by various providers.

Health Care Providers

The **health care team** consists of specially trained providers who work together to help clients meet their health care needs. The team includes primary providers, nurses, psychologists, pharmacists, dietitians, social workers, respiratory and physical therapists, occupational therapists, nursing assistants, technicians, and insurance company staff (Fig. 1-2). All members of this team collaborate on client issues (medical, social, and financial) to achieve the best possible outcomes.

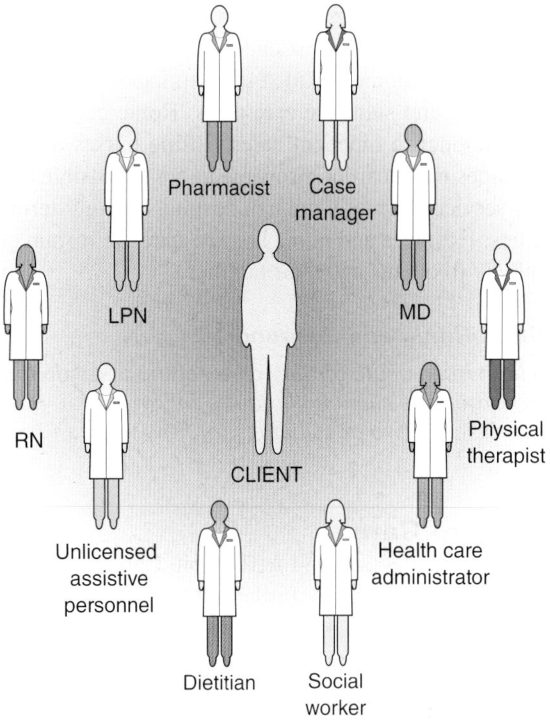

Figure 1-2 Members of the health care team.

>>> ***Stop, Think, and Respond 1-1***

A homeless client who collapsed on the street is brought to the emergency room by the local police for treatment. Without knowing the actual diagnosis, what factors related to health and illness concepts may have contributed to this client's poor health?

The Health Care Delivery System

The **health care delivery system** refers to the full range of services available to people seeking prevention, identification, treatment, or rehabilitation of health problems. The first resource person or agency that clients contact about a health need provides **primary care**. This initial contact is often with a family health care provider, internist, or nurse practitioner. Emphasis is on health promotion, preventive care, health education, early detection, and treatment. **Secondary care** includes referrals to facilities for additional testing such as cardiac catheterization, consultation, and diagnosis as well as emergency and acute care interventions. **Tertiary care** focuses more on complex medical and surgical interventions, cancer care, rehabilitative services, long-term care such as burn care, and palliative and hospice care.

In addition to their roles at the settings already mentioned, nurses provide care in a variety of other settings. Skilled nursing care occurs in facilities or units that offer prolonged health maintenance or rehabilitative services, such as long-term care or extended care facilities. Examples include nursing homes, skilled nursing facilities, rehabilitation centers, and subacute care units. Home care is an important adjunct to inpatient care; visiting nurses and home health aides make earlier discharge to home possible by providing services formerly done in hospitals or long-term care facilities. Hospices and home hospice care are resources for terminally ill clients and their families.

››› *Stop, Think, and Respond 1-2*

A client in an acute tertiary care setting is ready for discharge. This client will require follow-up for wound care. Discuss two possibilities for how this can be managed.

Access to Care

The Patient Protection and Affordable Care Act (PPACA; often shortened to the Affordable Care Act [ACA]) was passed in 2010. Also known as Health Care Reform or Obamacare, it is designed to provide affordable health care to U.S. citizens who previously had no access to health insurance. Prior to its passage, approximately 48.6 million Americans had no access to health care (15.7% of the population). The number of uninsured dropped to 10.9% in 2016, but as of 2019 it is 13.7% (Obamacare Facts, 2019). The overall goal of health care reform is to provide affordable health care to more U.S. citizens. Other goals are to reduce insurance company control of health care and to provide more assistance to senior citizens on fixed incomes. The controversy surrounding the PPACA has been overwhelming, and its future remains dependent on the current elected officials. Box 1-1 provides an overview of the PPACA.

FINANCING THE COSTS OF HEALTH CARE

Historically, private insurance, self-insurance systems, and Medicare paid for health care. Hospitals and approved providers received payment for what they charged; more charges meant more revenues. Thus, these plans had no incentives to control costs. Not only did charges escalate at an alarming rate, but abuse and fraudulent billing escalated as well. Disparities in access to health care coupled with its high costs prompted evaluation of spending in the entire health care industry. The 1990s was a decade of streamlining governmental payment systems and finding innovative approaches from private insurers and corporate health plans.

The 21st century has brought more reform and innovation in an attempt to trim health care costs. Currently, the United States ranks second globally (below Switzerland) in health care spending per capita. Despite higher health care spending, America's health outcomes are not any better than

BOX 1-1 Summary of the Patient Protection and Affordable Care Act (PPACA)

The PPACA ensures that all U.S. citizens and legal residents have access to quality, affordable health care. The PPACA contains nine titles, each addressing an essential component of reform:

- *Quality, affordable health care for all Americans*—include shared responsibility for health care (e.g., requirements for preventive care and immunizations), eliminate discriminatory practices (e.g., denial of coverage related to preexisting conditions), and increase dependent health care coverage up to 26 years of age
- *The role of public programs*—expand Medicaid eligibility, simplify enrollment methods, and establish a Federal Coordinated Health Care Office to integrate care under Medicare and Medicaid
- *Improving the quality and efficiency of health care*—link payment to quality outcomes in Medicare, encourage development of new client care models, and make improvements to Medicare programs
- *Prevention of chronic disease and improving public health*—implement methods to prevent chronic diseases and improve public health, increase access to clinical preventive services, and support innovative programs for public health
- *Health care workforce*—review and project future health care workforce needs, support workforce training needs, and support the current health care workforce to increase and enhance their training and education
- *Transparency and program integrity*—implement new requirements to provide information to the public on the health system and promote a newly invigorated set of requirements to combat fraud and abuse in public and private programs
- *Improve access to innovative medical therapies*—through the expansion of biologics price competition and innovation, it will make more affordable medicines for children and underserved communities
- *Community living assistance services and supports*—establish a new, voluntary, self-funded long-term care insurance program
- *Revenue provisions*—levy excise tax on high-cost employer-sponsored health coverage; increase transparency in employer reporting of value of health benefits; impose a manufacturer's fee on pharmaceutical, medical devices companies, and health insurance providers; and other provisions

Reauthorization of the Indian Health Care Improvement Act reauthorizes the provision and modernization of the Indian Health Care system for American Indians and Alaskan Natives

Adapted from Obamacare Facts. (2014, August 8). *Summary of provisions in the Patient Protection and Affordable Care Act.* http://obamacarefacts.com /summary-of-provisions-patient-protection-and-affordable-care-act/

those in other developed countries (Peter G. Peterson, Foundation, 2020). Financing health care remains a challenge as policy-makers attempt to reduce costs and yet provide quality care and prevent Americans from being devastated by overwhelming health care expenses. Many of the systems implemented in earlier decades remain. Health care reform has focused on extending current insurance programs while improving efficiency and expanding health promotion and illness prevention programs.

Government-Funded Health Care

In 1965, federal legislation created Medicare and Medicaid.

Medicare

Medicare is a federally run program financed primarily through employee payroll taxes. It covers individuals who are 65 years of age or older, permanently disabled workers of any age with specific disabilities, and persons with end-stage renal disease. According to the Centers for Medicare & Medicaid Services in 2019, Medicare has several parts:

- *Part A*—covers hospital care, skilled care, nursing home (if services other than custodial or long-term care are required), hospice, and home health services; may require participants to pay a monthly fee for this coverage if they did not pay Medicare taxes when they were working. All participants may have to pay copayments, coinsurance, and deductibles.
- *Part B*—covers medically necessary services such as physician services, outpatient care, home health services, and other selected services not covered under Part A, including preventive services; requires an annual deductible, and after the deductible is met, the participant pays 20% of the Medicare-approved amount of the service or a monthly premium unless the participant has other insurance.
- *Part C (Medicare Advantage Plan)*—includes Parts A (hospital insurance) and B (medical insurance) and sometimes Part D as well. Private insurance companies approved by Medicare manage these plans and may implement different premiums, copays, coinsurance, or deductibles.
- *Part D (Medicare Prescription Drug Coverage)*—helps to cover and possibly reduce prescription drug costs and protect against catastrophic drug expenses. Premiums vary depending on the plan manager and a person's income.

Clients on Social Security automatically participate in Part A, whereas the other parts are optional. Although Medicare is primarily for older Americans, it does not cover custodial or long-term care and limits coverage for health promotion and illness prevention. The increased costs of Medicare coupled with decreases in benefits make the program prohibitively expensive for many older adults. Those people with adequate resources may purchase private **Medigap insurance** policies to cover other expenditures such as copayments and deductibles. Box 1-2 highlights information that clients need regarding Medicare prescription drug plans.

BOX 1-2 Medicare Prescription Drug Coverage, 2020

Who is eligible for a Medicare prescription drug plan (PDP)?

Everyone can enroll in Medicare.

When does a client join?

The client must join when first eligible for Medicare or wait for the enrollment period and pay a late penalty fee. If a client is unable to do this themselves, Medicare will enroll that person.

What types of PDP plans are there?

- *Medicare PDP*
- Original Medicare PDP
- *Medicare Advantage Plan:* a plan for clients with Medicare Parts A, B, and D that includes prescription drug care; sometimes called MA-PDs

What needs to be considered when selecting a plan?

- Does the plan include the client's prescription drugs?
- What are the costs, such as premiums, deductibles, or copayments?
- Does the client's preferred pharmacy accept the plan?

From Medicare & You. (n.d.). https://www.medicare.gov/sites/default/files/2020-12/10050-Medicare-and-You_0.pdf

Medicaid

Medicaid programs are administered by each state in accordance with federal requirements and funded jointly by state and federal governments. Medicaid provides health coverage for individuals and families with limited incomes and resources. Mandatory benefits include:

- Inpatient and outpatient hospital services
- Screening, diagnostic, and treatment services
- Home health services
- Physician services
- Rural health clinic services
- Federally qualified health center services
- Laboratory and X-ray services
- Family planning services
- Nurse midwife services
- Certified pediatric and family nurse practitioner services
- Freestanding birth center services (when licensed or otherwise recognized by the state)
- Transportation to medical care
- Tobacco cessation counseling for pregnant women

There are optional benefits that vary from state to state, and they may include services such as clinic care; physical and occupational therapy; speech therapy; respiratory, podiatry, optometry, and dental care; and other such services.

The ACA created a national Medicaid minimum eligibility level of 133% of the federal poverty level ($26,200 for a family of four in 2020) for nearly all Americans under age 65. This part of the Medicaid eligibility expansion went into effect in 2014. As of January 2019, 37 states have expanded Medicaid coverage with federal support any time before this date (Medicare.gov, 2020).

Prospective Payment Systems

In 1983, Medicare implemented a **prospective payment system (PPS)** in an attempt to control costs. A PPS is a method of reimbursement in which health care providers receive payment for services based on a predetermined, fixed rate. The payment amount for a particular service is derived from the classification system of that service. One classification system for inpatient hospital services uses 467 **diagnosis-related groups (DRGs)** to group services for clients with similar diagnoses. For example, all clients receiving a hip, knee, or shoulder replacement fall into DRG, total joint replacement, and their surgeries are reimbursed at basically the same rate. Other classification systems may be used for other health care services. Private insurers may use DRGs or other classification systems for reimbursement.

PPSs are largely responsible for the marked decreases in hospital lengths of stay since the early 1980s. Possible premature discharge of clients and increased responsibility for family members who may be unable to provide adequate care has created much criticism of PPSs. These systems have also caused shifts in costs from clients with Medicare to those who have private insurance. Providers charge privately insured clients inflated amounts to make up for losses in Medicare revenues. In response to this cost shifting and other economic forces, insurers have challenged hospital charges aggressively, refused payment when hospital level of care is not provided, and shifted their clients into cost-containment reimbursement systems known as *managed care*.

Managed Care

Managed care organizations (MCOs) are insurers who carefully plan and closely supervise the distribution of health care services. Although it is a business venture that emphasizes costs of services and economic use of resources, managed care focuses on prevention as the best way to manage health care costs (Box 1-3). The two most common types of managed care systems are health maintenance organizations (HMOs) and preferred provider organizations (PPOs). Two other models—point-of-service (POS) plans and physician hospital organizations (PHOs)—are becoming more prominent.

BOX 1-3 Goals of Managed Care

- Use health care resources efficiently.
- Deliver high-quality care at a reasonable cost.
- Measure, monitor, and manage fiscal and client outcomes.
- Prevent illness through screening and health promotion activities.
- Provide client education to decrease risk of disease.
- Case manage clients with chronic illness to minimize number of hospitalizations.

Health Maintenance Organizations

A **health maintenance organization (HMO)** is a group insurance plan in which participants pay a preset, fixed fee in exchange for health care services. The fee is not based on the number of services provided but rather is projected to the number of participants and expected services. This type of financial management is referred to as **capitation**, which refers to the actual head or person count. Primary providers have an incentive to keep costs low because the fee paid to the primary providers remains the same regardless of the actual services or frequency of care provided. The financial stability of HMOs is based on their ability to keep members healthy and out of the hospital through periodic screening, health education, and preventive services. Participant fees cover all medical costs incurred and are paid regardless of whether members require health care services. If they do not require much high-cost care, providers make money; if members use many high-cost resources, providers lose money. This method of financing provides the strongest incentives for limiting use of expensive services and focusing health care on health maintenance and health promotion.

HMOs provide ambulatory, hospitalization, and home care services. Some HMOs have their own facilities; others use community agencies for services. Members of an HMO must receive authorization (referral) for secondary care, such as second opinions from specialists or diagnostic testing. If members obtain unauthorized care, they are responsible for the entire bill. In this way, HMOs serve as gatekeepers for health care services.

>>> *Stop, Think, and Respond 1-3*

An older client tells you that they receive Social Security benefits but is not clear about their Medicare benefits. What information would you provide to this client?

Preferred Provider Organizations

A **preferred provider organization (PPO)** operates on the principle that competition can control costs. Acting as agents for health insurance companies, PPOs create a community network of providers who are willing to discount their fees for service in exchange for a steady stream of referred customers. Consumers can lower their health care costs if they receive care from the preferred providers. If they select providers outside the network, they pay a higher percentage of the costs.

Point-of-Service Plans

Point-of-service (POS) allows clients the flexibility of using services out of network. Clients select a primary care physician within the group who then serves as the gatekeeper for other health care services. Clients can use health care providers in or out of the provider group; if they stay in the network they will get a higher benefit, if they choose to go out of network for services, they would be covered, but at a lower rate. The client also has the option to go to a specialized provider without a referral.

Physician Hospital Organizations

In **physician hospital organizations (PHOs)** the participating providers and the hospital develop contract terms and reimbursement levels and use those terms to negotiate with MCOs. The goals are to maintain high-quality service and contain costs while fostering group contracts, collaboration, and capitation.

BOX 1-4 Integrated Delivery Systems

Fully integrated health care delivery systems will provide the following:

- Wellness programs
- Preventive care
- Ambulatory care
- Outpatient diagnostic and laboratory services
- Emergency care
- General and tertiary hospital services
- Rehabilitation
- Long-term care
- Assisted living facilities
- Psychiatric care
- Home health care services
- Hospice care
- Outpatient pharmacies

CHANGES AND TRENDS IN HEALTH CARE

Effects of Cost-Driven Changes

Changes in reimbursement structures and practices have created a shift in economic and decision-making power from hospitals, nurses, and primary providers to insurers. Much concern and criticism accompany this shift as primary providers, nurses, other providers, and consumers find themselves unable to obtain or provide care free from the insurer's economic pressures. As a result of managed care's influence, hospitals have downsized, restructured, or sometimes closed. Consequently, many regions are left with fewer hospitals, higher nurse–client ratios, and higher client acuity levels on general medical–surgical units, skilled nursing facilities, long-term care facilities, and home health settings. Thus, many claim that profits posted by large insurance companies come at the expense of quality care and jobs of health care providers.

Changes in the health care industry have also affected employment for health care workers. Hospitals employ **unlicensed assistive personnel (UAP)** to perform some duties that practical and registered nurses once provided. Many are concerned that the use of UAPs will jeopardize quality of care. In addition, primary provider's income has decreased in recent years. This trend will most likely continue, partly because of the growth of nurse practitioners and physician assistants. The predicted decrease in income may lead to fewer men and women entering the medical profession. Rural areas already suffering with inadequate numbers of primary providers will not see an improvement in this situation.

These changes also may affect the client's experience and satisfaction with health care. A single episode of illness can involve negotiating for a referral, receiving testing at a site other than the hospital, staying a shorter time in the hospital, transferring to a skilled nursing facility, and obtaining outpatient rehabilitation and home health services. Although much effort is made to coordinate care, particularly by nurse case managers (see Chapter 2), this fragmentation forces clients to repeatedly build therapeutic relationships and may leave them unsure of who is in charge.

Cost-driven changes have had positive effects as well. In an attempt to reduce redundancy of health care services and increase economic leverage, hospitals and other health care facilities are forming networks known as **integrated delivery systems (IDSs**; Box 1-4). IDSs provide a full range of health care services with a goal of achieving highly coordinated and cost-effective care. Mandated shorter hospital stays may result in fewer nosocomial (acquired in the hospital) complications and a quicker return to self-care. Nurses have a greater ability to take an active role in advocating for high-quality, nurse-provided care. Nurses work in new and expanded positions in the health care industry (see Chapter 2). There is also increased attention to monitoring quality and best practices in health care.

Implementation of health care reform has many benefits but also raises many concerns. Paying for the reform is complicated and controversial. Tax credits for small businesses, increased health insurance premiums, high deductibles, and the requirement for most Americans to buy health insurance or face penalties will provide some of the revenues to pay for health care. Individuals and families may more easily qualify for subsidies and sliding scale tax breaks. Insurers will be monitored more closely and will no longer be able to impose inequities and disparities in health care coverage. Health care reform continues to be a major challenge for legislators, consumers, and taxpayers.

Measures of Quality of Care

Demand for evidence that hospitals and practitioners provide high-quality, cost-effective care comes from insurers, regulatory bodies such as The Joint Commission, and consumers. To meet this demand, hospitals form performance improvement committees. These groups or hospital departments also may be called *quality improvement* or *outcomes management committees*. These committees use standardized indicators to measure health care quality.

One example of standardized indicators is the quality indicators (QIs) provided by the Agency for Healthcare Research and Quality (AHRQ). These QIs can be used to measure health care quality at the federal, state, and local levels.

Although specifically for use by hospitals, similar tools for other health care organizations are used or are in process. The AHRQ uses hospital administrative data to highlight potential quality concerns, identify areas that need further study and investigation, and track changes over time. As of 2020, the AHRQ QIs consist of the following four modules:

- Prevention QIs are measures used with hospital inpatient discharge data to identify hospital admissions that could be avoided through high-quality outpatient care.
- Inpatient QIs, which reflect quality of care inside hospitals, include inpatient mortality for medical conditions and surgical procedures.
- Client safety QIs also reflect quality of care within hospitals, but focus on potentially avoidable complications and adverse events.
- Pediatric QIs are measures used with hospital inpatient data to determine quality of care inside hospitals and identify potentially avoidable hospitalizations among children.

Concept Mastery Alert

Prevention QIs have to do with avoidable hospitalizations. Client safety QIs reflect quality of care within the hospital, including safety issues.

In 2002, The Joint Commission established National Patient Safety Goals, which are updated annually. The goals were established in order for accredited organizations to address areas of concern related to client safety. The 2016 hospital safety goals are focused on the following:

- Identify clients correctly.
- Improve staff communication.
- Use medicines safely.
- Use alarms safely.
- Prevent infection.
- Identify client safety risks.
- Prevent mistakes in surgery.

The goals established by The Joint Commission form the foundation for an evaluation process so that health care organizations can measure, assess, and improve performance (The Joint Commission, 2020).

Other methods exist for determining quality of care. Client satisfaction surveys, quality-of-life questionnaires, functional assessment tools, number of hospital admissions per year for clients with chronic illnesses, and **morbidity** (complications) and **mortality** (deaths) rates are a few important measures assessed when examining quality (Evidence-Based Practice 1-1).

Future Trends and Goals for Health Care

The health care system will continue to respond to changes in the demographics and cultural diversity as well as to technological innovations and the impact of the shortage of nurses. In the United States, the number of people over 65 years of age is projected to be 78 million by 2030 (AARP, 2020). It is also predicted that 40% of the population in 2030 will belong to ethnic minority groups. Concern remains regarding the health of all Americans. Several initiatives are directed at promoting health and monitoring progress toward health goals and prevention of treatable problems as well as actual treatment of illness without complications. The Healthy People 2030 campaign provides an overall action plan to improve the health and quality of life for people living in the United States. The U.S. Department of Health and Human Services (2020) identified five overarching health goals, which include the following:

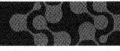

- Attain healthy, thriving lives and well-being, free of preventable disease, disability, injury, and premature death.
- Eliminate health disparities, achieve health equity, and attain health literacy to improve the health and well-being of all.
- Create social, physical, and economic environments that promote attaining full potential for health and well-being for all.
- Promote healthy development, healthy behaviors, and well-being across all life stages.
- Engage leadership, key constituents, and the public across multiple sectors to take action and design policies that improve the health and well-being of all.

Evidence-Based Practice 1-1

Nursing Care, Health Care Management, and Hospital Reimbursement

Clinical Question

How will nursing care in the future affect health care management and hospital reimbursement?

Evidence

The ACA established the "Hospital-Acquired Condition (HAC) Reduction Program." This program guides the secretary of Health and Human Services on the amount of reimbursement health care facilities receive based on quality measures. The amount of reduction in payment will depend on their ranking in the performance quartile. The HAC program scores on Research and Quality, Patient Safety Indicators, Central Line Infections, Surgical Site Infections, and Urinary Tract Infections. The health care facility scores are also published and become public record through the ACA (Quality Net, n.d.).

Nursing Implications

Employers will work within their health care facilities to improve in all categories through education and training. Nurses play a part in each of the quality measures listed above. Proper training, orientation, continuing education, providing quality care, and following policies and guidelines are part of the professional responsibility of the nurse. As part of the health care team, nurses have a large impact on the health care facility's success in this reduction program. Aiming the focus on evidence-based practice and nursing outcomes may greatly affect the outcomes of these reimbursements.

Reference

Quality Net. (n.d.). *Hospital-acquired condition (HAC) reduction program* (cms.gov). https://qualitynet.cms.gov/inpatient/hac/payment

TABLE 1-2 Healthy People 2030 Goals

OVERARCHING GOALS OF HEALTHY PEOPLE 2030	FOUNDATION MEASURES CATEGORY	MEASURES OF PROGRESS
Attain healthy, thriving lives and well-being, free of preventable disease, disability, injury, and premature death.	General Health Status	• Life expectancy • Healthy life expectancy • Physical and mental unhealthy days • Self-assessed health status • Limitation of activity • Chronic disease prevalence • International comparisons (*where available*)
Eliminate health disparities, achieve health equity, and attain health literacy to improve the health and well-being of all.	Disparities and Inequity	Disparities/inequity to be assessed by: • Race/ethnicity • Gender • Socioeconomic status • Disability status • Lesbian, gay, bisexual, and transgender status • Geography
Create social, physical, and economic environments that promote attaining full potential for health and well-being for all.	Social Determinants of Health	Determinants can include: • Social and economic factors • Natural and built environments • Policies and programs
Promote healthy development, healthy behaviors, and well-being across all life stages.	Health-Related Quality of Life and Well-Being	• Well-being/satisfaction • Physical, mental, and social health-related quality of life • Participation in common activities
Engage leadership, key constituents, and the public across multiple sectors to take action and design policies that improve the health and well-being of all.	Government Leadership—Actions and Policies	Government lead programs encouraged to provide easier access to healthier foods and healthy activities

From Healthy People 2030 Framework. (2020, October 8). *What is the Healthy People 2030 framework?* https://www.healthypeople.gov/2020/About-Healthy-People/Development-Healthy-People-2030/Framework

Table 1-2 provides a comprehensive methodology used to assess progress toward achievement of the five overarching health goals of Healthy People 2030.

U.S. Nutritional Strategies

Healthy People 2030 is a national effort to improve the health of Americans by providing recommendations to enhance nutrition and weight status. Other nutritional strategies include using the U.S. Department of Agriculture's MyPlate, referring to the nutrition labels on processed and packaged foods, and understanding standard definitions for the terms used on food labels.

Healthier Food Access

Healthy People 2030 aims to have an increased number of healthy food outlets, like farmer's markets, and displays of healthier foods by food retailers. Another objective is to promote availability and accessibility for people to use food as an incentive program for a healthier diet, including whole grains and fruits and vegetables.

Availability of Recreational Facilities

Where we live affects our health in multiple ways. Poor health measures are focused in neighborhoods that are most disadvantaged by society's social, economic, and housing inequities, which leads to a higher problem of chronic diseases.

Studies show that people who live close to recreational areas experience better mental health, *and* that frequency of exercise by adults and children and having fresh produce available are associated with healthier lifestyles.

Each of the indicators is tracked, measured, and reported on in a timely and regular basis. Data are provided from health care agencies at all levels to the National Center for Health Statistics. Progress reports are available quarterly and annually. A final report will be released in 2020 (Office of Disease Prevention and Health Promotion, 2016). As the 21st century progresses, economics, consumer satisfaction, effectiveness of traditional medical care, alternative medicine, disease prevalence, global emergence of drug-resistant organisms, and cultural diversity are forces that will influence the direction of worldwide health care. The continued effects of infectious diseases on global health, particularly in developing nations, and epidemics of cancer and other chronic diseases remain likely.

The United Nations Sustainable Developmental Goals build on the WHO's Millennium Developmental Goals (MDGs). The U.N. members want to achieve these goals by 2030 (Box 1-5).

In the midst of these dramatic changes and challenges, nurses must continue to provide safe, high-quality, cost-effective care to individuals, families, and communities. It is also imperative that nurses distinguish and communicate to clients the various choices that the clients may make about their health care.

BOX 1-5 United Nations Sustainable Development Goals

Goal 1: End poverty in all its forms everywhere.

Goal 2: End hunger, achieve food security and improved nutrition, and promote sustainable agriculture.

Goal 3: Ensure healthy lives and promote well-being for all at all ages.

Goal 4: Ensure inclusive and equitable quality education and promote lifelong learning opportunities for all.

Goal 5: Achieve gender equality and empower all women and girls.

Goal 6: Ensure availability and sustainable management of water and sanitation for all.

Goal 7: Ensure access to affordable, reliable, sustainable, and modern energy for all.

Goal 8: Promote sustained, inclusive, and sustainable economic growth, full and productive employment, and decent work for all.

Goal 9: Build resilient infrastructure, promote sustainable industrialization, and foster innovation.

Goal 10: Reduce inequality within and among countries.

Goal 11: Make cities and human settlements inclusive, safe, resilient, and sustainable.

Goal 12: Ensure sustainable consumption and production patterns.

Goal 13: Take urgent action to combat climate change and its impacts.

Goal 14: Conserve and sustainably use the oceans, seas, and marine resources.

Goal 15: Protect, restore, and promote sustainable use of terrestrial ecosystems, sustainably manage forests, combat desertification, and halt and reverse land degradation, and halt biodiversity loss.

Goal 16: Promote peaceful and inclusive societies for sustainable development, provide access to justice for all, and build effective, accountable, and inclusive institutions at all levels.

Goal 17: Strengthen the means of implementation and revitalize the global partnership for sustainable development.

From United Nations. (2015). *Sustainable Development Goals.* https://www.un.org/sustainabledevelopment/sustainable-development-goals/

KEY POINTS

- Definitions
  - *Health: state of complete physical, mental, and social well-being
  - Holism: viewing a person's health as a balance of body, mind, and spirit
  - Wellness: a constant and intentional effort to stay healthy
  - Illness: a state of being sick
  - Disease: refers to a pathologic condition of the body that presents with clinical signs and symptoms and changes in laboratory values
  - Health–illness continuum: level of health, which continually changes for each person
  - Health maintenance: refers to protecting one's current level of health by preventing illness or deterioration
  - Health promotion: refers to engaging in strategies to enhance health
- The health care team
  - Primary providers
  - Nurses
  - Psychologists
  - Pharmacists
  - Dietitians
  - Social workers
  - Respiratory therapists
  - Physical therapists
  - Occupational therapists
  - Nursing assistants
  - Technicians
  - Insurance company staff
- Three levels of care
  - Primary: person or agency that the clients contact about a health need
  - Secondary: referrals to facilities for additional testing such as cardiac catheterization, consultation, and diagnosis as well as emergency and acute care intervention
  - Tertiary: focuses more on complex medical and surgical interventions, and specialized services such as cancer care and rehabilitative services
- The PPACA (often shortened to the ACA) was passed in 2010. Also known as Health Care Reform or Obamacare, it is designed to provide affordable health care to U.S. citizens who previously had no access to health insurance.
- Medicare: a federally run program financed primarily through employee payroll taxes. It covers individuals who are 65 years of age or older, permanently disabled workers of any age with specific disabilities, and persons with end-stage renal disease.
- Medicaid: programs are administered by each state in accordance with federal requirements and funded jointly by state and federal governments. Medicaid provides health coverage for individuals and families with limited incomes and resources.
- Prospective payment system: a method of reimbursement in which health care providers receive payment for services based on a predetermined, fixed rate
- Managed care organizations:
  - HMO is a group insurance plan in which participants pay a preset, fixed fee in exchange for health care services.

- PPO operates on the principle that competition can control costs, consumers can lower their health care costs if they receive care from their preferred providers.
- POS organizations involve a network of providers, allow clients the flexibility of using services out of network.
- PHOs: the participating providers and the hospital develop contract terms and reimbursement levels and use those terms to negotiate with MCOs.

- AHRQ: These QIs can be used to measure health care quality at the federal, state, and local levels. The AHRQ uses hospital administrative data to highlight potential quality concerns, identify areas that need further study and investigation, and track changes over time.
- Healthy People 2030: campaign that provides an overall action plan to improve the health and quality of life for people living in the United States
- MDGs: developed by the WHO, consist of eight goals with measurable targets and clear deadlines to improving the lives of the world's poorest people
- Sustainable Developmental Goals: developed by the United Nations to address a better and more sustainable future for all

CRITICAL THINKING EXERCISES

1. Interview older clients to explore their understanding of the health care coverage including access to prescription drugs. Compare their knowledge with information available from the Medicare & You website at www.medicare.gov/publications.

2. Ask the nurse manager on your assigned clinical unit about the QIs the unit must provide data on and what impact they have had on client care.

NCLEX-STYLE REVIEW QUESTIONS PrepU

1. A client with chronic illness always reports feeling great. What does this tell the nurse about the client?
   1. The client is able to define health in a positive way.
   2. The client is able to dismiss the chronic illness.
   3. The client is able to engage in meaningful activities.
   4. The client is able to put on a positive demeanor.

2. The nurse is meeting with a group of clients to discuss health promotion activities in an effort to target poor lifestyle habits. Which of the following activities promotes health? Select all that apply.
   1. Engage in activities to manage stress.
   2. Exercise for 30 to 40 minutes five times a week.
   3. Increase fiber in the diet.
   4. Reduce caloric intake.
   5. Sleep at least 6 hours a night.

3. After a client has a physical examination, the health care provider orders blood tests and a consult with a neurologist. In a review of the client's new insurance plan, what type of service does a consultation fall under?
   1. Acute care
   2. Primary care
   3. Secondary care
   4. Tertiary care

4. A nurse is working with an adult client who is scheduled for an annual physical examination. The nurse explains that some screening diagnostic tests may be done, such as blood pressure, blood cholesterol, and an electrocardiogram. What comment by the client indicates an understanding of the purpose of screening tests?
   1. "I may need more tests depending on the results of the screening tests."
   2. "The doctor can prescribe medications based on these tests."
   3. "The tests determine if I have a serious illness."
   4. "You will be checking my blood pressure and taking blood."

5. Nurses provide care in a variety of settings. Which of the following is an example of a nurse providing care in a primary care setting?
   1. The nurse explains the need for follow-up postoperative physical therapy.
   2. The nurse gives a tetanus booster to a healthy 40-year-old.
   3. The nurse prepares a client for a colonoscopy procedure.
   4. The nurse teaches a client about the effects of anesthesia.

6. A licensed practical nurse (LPN) is employed at a primary provider's office that is part of an organization that provides client referrals to this practice. In exchange, the primary provider's office offers services at a reduced cost. What is this practice a part of?
   1. An HMO—health maintenance organization
   2. A PHO—physician hospital organization
   3. A PPO—preferred provider organization
   4. A PPS—prospective payment system

7. A group of nurses discussing the changes in the health care system agree that future changes will be most greatly influenced by some key factors. What do these include? Select all that apply.
   1. Advances in medical technology
   2. Aging of the population
   3. Increase in chronic health problems
   4. Level of education of clients
   5. Workforce shortages

8. An LPN is assigned to serve on their unit's quality improvement committee. Which of the following statements by the nurse manager is correct in explaining the primary purpose of this committee?
1. The purpose of the quality improvement committee is to audit client care based on standard measures.
2. The purpose of the quality improvement committee is to determine safe nurse–client ratios.
3. The purpose of the quality improvement committee is to develop systems to improve client care.
4. The purpose of the quality improvement committee is to establish standards of care.

WANT TO KNOW MORE? There are a wide variety of online resources available on thePoint to enhance learning and understanding of this chapter.

Go to **thePoint.lww.com/activate** and use the activation code found in the front of this text to unlock these online resources.

2 Settings and Models for Nursing Care

Words To Know

acuity
ambulatory care
assisted living facilities
boarding homes
case management
case method
congregate housing
functional nursing
home health care
nonprofit agencies
partnership model
primary care nursing
proprietary agencies
team nursing

Learning Objectives

On completion of this chapter, you will be able to:

1. Define nursing.
2. Describe the different roles of the licensed practical/vocational nurse (LPN/LVN) and registered nurse (RN).
3. List three ways to classify health care agencies in which nurses practice.
4. Describe the settings where nurses practice and the nurse's roles in each setting.
5. Compare nursing care delivery models.
6. Define case management and explain the nurse case manager's role.

Today's dynamic health care environment challenges traditional roles and responsibilities of health care providers and institutions. Clients and family members now manage, with the support of visiting nurses, conditions and treatments that were previously relegated to intensive care units (ICUs). Procedures that formerly required clients to stay in the hospital for at least 1 week may now be done on a short-stay unit (less than 24 hours). In many instances, insurance companies and case managers dictate choice of services, treatment options, and hospital lengths of stay, which were formerly determined by attending primary providers. No matter the setting or circumstances, current health care mandates that nurses provide high-quality nursing care wherever needed and function in both traditional and evolving roles.

NURSING CARE

Nursing is concerned with caring for individuals, families, or groups. Nurses not only care for clients when they are ill but also play a significant role in health education, illness prevention, and promotion. Nurses attend to client needs related to hygiene; activity; diet; the environment; medical treatment; and physical, emotional, and spiritual comfort.

Definitions of Nursing

Arriving at a clear and comprehensive definition of nursing is difficult. Florence Nightingale (1859, p. 75) described the role of the nurse as putting "the patient in the best condition for nature to act upon him." Virginia Henderson (1966), one of the first nursing theorists, envisioned the nurse's role as helping people (sick or well) to carry out those activities contributing to health, recovery, or a peaceful death that they would do for themselves if they had the necessary strength, will, or knowledge. Her definition also focused on regaining independence.

The American Nurses Association (ANA, 2017) defines nursing as the "protection, promotion, and optimization of health and abilities, prevention of illness and injury, facilitation of healing, alleviation of suffering through the diagnosis and treatment of human response, and advocacy in the care of individuals, families, groups, communities, and populations." Nursing responsibilities include the following:

- Performing physical examinations and writing health histories
- Providing health promotion, counseling, and education
- Administering medications, wound care, and numerous other personal interventions
- Interpreting client information and making critical decisions about needed actions
- Coordinating care in collaboration with a wide array of health care professionals
- Directing and supervising care delivered by other health care personnel such as licensed practical nurses (LPNs) and nurse aides or unlicensed assistive personnel (UAP), as defined in individual nurse practice acts (see Chapter 5)
- Conducting research in support of improved practice and client outcomes

Other definitions of nursing have endured throughout the nursing profession's history. Table 2-1 provides other definitions of nursing by selected theorists.

TABLE 2-1 Definitions of Nursing by Selected Theorists

THEORIST	DEFINITION
Florence Nightingale (1859)	Nurses alter the environment to put the client in the best condition for nature to act.
Virginia Henderson (1966)	Nurses assist clients to carry out those activities that they would perform unaided if they possessed the necessary strength, will, or knowledge.
Ernestine Wiedenbach (1964)	Nursing is a helping, nurturing, and caring service delivered sensitively with compassion, skill, and understanding.
Dorothea Orem (1980)	Nursing care is directed at restoring self-care abilities, which are activities that clients initiate on their own behalf in maintaining health, life, and well-being.
Imogene M. King (1981)	Nursing is the care of human beings; individuals and groups are viewed as open systems in continual interaction with the environment.
Sister Callista Roy (1976)	Nursing encourages clients to reach their highest level of functioning through adaptation.
Jean Watson (1988)	Nursing is the science of human caring to help patients reach their greatest potential.

››› *Stop, Think, and Respond 2-1*

Imogene M. King stated that clients are open systems in constant interaction with their environment. Compare King's definition with Virginia Henderson's. What is different? What is the same?

Nursing Roles

Nurses with different levels of education perform various care activities in diverse settings. The LPN/licensed vocational nurse (LVN) provides care to clients under the direction of a registered nurse (RN), advanced practice registered nurse (APRN), or primary provider in a structured health care setting. LPNs/LVNs care for clients with well-defined, common problems that often require a high level of technical competency and expertise. They frequently work in settings in which RN supervision is available but must be sought after the LPN/LVN determines the need to do so. The RN's role is more complex, involving the management and coordination of all the care provided to a group of clients. As health care delivery models continue to change, LPN/LVN and RN roles are likely to change as well.

SETTINGS AND TYPES OF NURSING CARE

Nursing care is provided in various settings, with many classifications of health care agencies. Health care agencies can be classified by length of stay (Table 2-2), ownership (Table 2-3), or type of care.

Although hospitals employ all levels of nurses in outpatient care areas (e.g., dialysis units, clinics, same-day surgery units, related diagnostic departments), inpatient units have been the traditional site for much of the nursing workforce. Trends in financing suggest that nursing care will rely less on hospital settings in the future. However, there is a great deal of interest in determining the best, most cost-effective methods and settings for providing care as well as meeting client needs. Client needs determine the setting for care.

TABLE 2-2 Health Care Institutions Classified by Length of Stay

LENGTH OF STAY	DESCRIPTION
In-and-out care	Contact with client is measured in minutes versus hours. Typical examples are office visits, emergency department visits, and therapy sessions.
Short stay	Provides care to clients who suffer from acute conditions or need treatments that require fewer than 24 hours of care and monitoring. Diagnostic tests or minimally invasive surgeries are examples.
Acute care	Traditionally occurs in hospitals where clients stay more than 24 hours but fewer than 30 days. Stays have been shortened since the advent of managed care and Diagnosis-Related Groups (see Chapter 1).
Long-term care	Provides care to residents for the remainder of their lives; care also includes services to clients with limited recovery needs, functional losses, chronic disease, mental illness, or major rehabilitation, which may range from 30 to 90 days.

Reprinted with permission from Stegen, A. J., & Sowerby, H. (2019). *Nursing in today's world: Trends, issues, and management* (11th ed., p. 182). Wolters Kluwer.

TABLE 2-3 Health Care Institutions Classified by Ownership

OWNERSHIP	DESCRIPTION
Government-owned or public facilities	Receive at least some tax support for costs and can be governed by federal, state, or local governments. Examples include veterans hospitals (federal), mental health facilities (state), and visiting nursing agencies (county).
Proprietary agencies	Often referred to as for-profit agencies. These facilities are owned and operated by corporate groups with investors and stockholders. Prominent examples include Humana Incorporated (full array of health care facilities) and Hillhaven Corporation (nursing homes).
Nonprofit agencies	Include facilities owned and operated by nonprofit groups, such as universities or religious organizations. The term *nonprofit* means that any income that exceeds operating and maintenance costs must be used for growth and development of the facility as opposed to distribution to stockholders.

The following sections discuss the various health care agencies according to the type of care.

Acute Care

The term **acuity** refers to the gravity and the degree to which a person's condition changes. Higher acuity refers to clients with severe illness whose condition changes rapidly. Generally, higher client acuity requires a greater need for highly skilled care. Clients with complicated or high-risk surgery, massive trauma, or critical illness will be cared for in an acute care hospital, where a high level of professional, skilled, and technological care is available. RNs are instrumental in caring for these clients.

Long-Term Acute Care

Clients who require long-term wound care or ventilator support or who have other conditions that are potentially unstable but do not have rapid changes may receive care in a long-term acute care facility (long-term acute care hospitals [LTACHs]). Generally, clients are discharged from ICUs, but still require a higher level of care than they would receive in a rehabilitation center or skilled care nursing facility. Often, these facilities are located in an acute care hospital but are licensed and funded independently. RNs manage client care.

Subacute Care

Subacute care or step-down beds provide an intermediate level of care for clients with requirements somewhere between that of the general unit and the ICU. The treatment plan requires frequent assessments and periodic review of client progress. Generally, clients are in these facilities for a brief period—up to 30 days. Some subacute units may have a longer length of stay—up to 90 days. RNs coordinate client care, and LPNs/LVNs provide and oversee care provided by UAPs.

Skilled Nursing Care

Skilled nursing care facilities and Acute Rehabilitation units provide skilled nursing and rehabilitative care to people who have the potential to regain function but need skilled observation and nursing care during an acute illness. Clients using these facilities may also require invasive procedures and therapies (e.g., tube feedings, intravenous fluids, and sterile dressing changes). An RN must be in charge of client care, although other health care providers, particularly LPNs/LVNs, participate in their care.

Intermediate Care Facilities

Intermediate care facilities (ICFs) are nursing homes that provide custodial care for people who cannot care for themselves because of mental or physical disabilities. Clients must meet specific criteria related to an inability to meet their own activities of daily living (ADLs). ICFs do not receive reimbursement from Medicare because they are not considered medical facilities. LPNs/LVNs and nursing assistants generally provide care under the supervision of RNs (Fig. 2-1).

Rehabilitation Care

Rehabilitation centers provide physical and occupational therapy to clients and families to help individuals regain as much independence with ADLs as possible. RNs are part of a multidisciplinary team that provides a full range of rehabilitative services.

Hospice Care

Hospices provide care for clients diagnosed with a terminal illness whose life expectancy is fewer than 6 months. Hospices allow terminally ill clients to live as fully as possible while managing pain, discomfort, and other symptoms. Hospice staffs, generally supervised by RNs, are specially trained to help families with the grief process. Medicare covers many of the services provided by hospice care.

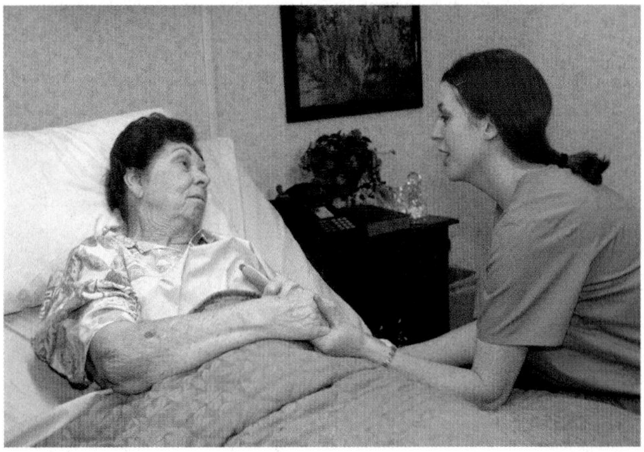

Figure 2-1 Licensed practical/vocational nurses (LPNs/LVNs) may provide care in intermediate care facilities for clients who cannot care for themselves.

Palliative Care

Palliative care is medical and related care provided to a client with a serious, life-threatening, or terminal illness. It is not intended to provide curative treatment but rather to manage symptoms, relieve pain and discomfort, improve quality of life, and meet the emotional, social, and spiritual needs of the client (Palliative Care, 2020).

Transitional Care

Transitional care refers to the coordination and continuity of health care during a movement from one health care setting to either another or to home. Transitional care assists the clients to transition between health care practitioners and settings as their condition and care needs change during the course of a chronic or acute illness.

Ambulatory Care

Ambulatory care is also referred to as outpatient care. Many settings qualify as outpatient settings: diagnostic centers, such as gastroenterology centers, day surgery centers, and medical treatment centers, such as those for specific therapies or dialysis. Clinics and primary care centers are also considered outpatient settings. Depending on the purpose of the outpatient setting, RNs and LPNs/LVNs may or may not play a prominent role.

Home Care

Cost containment measures in the last 20 years have resulted in the expansion of home health care services. **Home health care** addresses both long- and short-term health needs and can provide comprehensive services. Home health nurses provide specialized care, such as intravenous infusion of fluids, medications, and chemotherapy; hospice care; postcardiac surgery care; and care to ventilator-dependent clients (Fig. 2-2). RNs manage and coordinate the care clients receive and have a high level of competency in assessment skills, communication, teaching, management, and documentation abilities. The RN encourages clients and family members to develop self-care skills, with support from community resources. Box 2-1 lists other functions of the home health nurse. Besides nursing, home health care agencies provide many other services (Table 2-4).

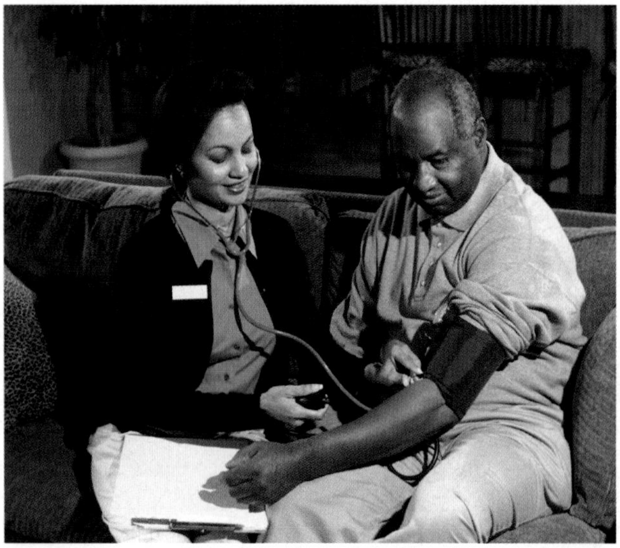

Figure 2-2 Home health nurses provide specialized care in the client's home.

BOX 2-1 Functions of the Home Health Care Nurse

- Plan, coordinate, and provide care in consultation with hospital personnel and primary provider.
- Teach client and family to perform procedures, monitor symptoms, administer medications, and report to primary provider.
- Assess client and consult with primary provider as needed.
- Evaluate the home environment for safety hazards, cleanliness, ability to safely store medication, family support, and adequacy of food supplies.
- Connect client and family with community resources.
- Advocate for the client when additional services are needed.
- Document care and teaching provided.
- Complete forms required for reimbursement.

Community Health Centers

Community health centers and local health departments provide a range of services to the districts, counties, or communities they serve. These agencies receive partial or complete funding from federal, state, and local governments. Community mental health centers are also part of this network. Neighborhood health clinics make health care more accessible, and when health facilities are more accessible, people are more likely to seek prompt treatment and reduce the need for acute care.

TABLE 2-4 Services Provided by Home Health Agencies

TYPE OF SERVICE	DESCRIPTION
Physical therapy	Therapist assesses the client's mobility after orthopedic surgery, injury, or stroke. They assess the need for assistive devices. Client must meet Medicare requirements to receive physical therapy.
Speech therapy	Therapist provides rehabilitation to clients with speech or swallowing disorders. Client must meet Medicare requirements.
Occupational therapy	Therapist assesses need for assistive devices to aid in activities of daily living and identify issues related to fine motor movements and muscle retraining.
Social services	Social worker meets with client and family to identify difficulties with managing illness at home and provides information about financial assistance and community services.
Home health aides	Aides provide personal care such as bathing and dressing and basic skills such as taking vital signs.
Homemakers	Homemakers clean, do laundry, and shop for groceries.

Alternative Health Care Settings

In addition to the community-based settings described previously, other facilities and services are available for seniors and adults with physical or mental disabilities. These individuals are relatively healthy and do not need extended care but may need some assistance with ADLs. The goal of alternative care facilities is to provide the least restrictive living arrangements while maintaining safety and quality. These facilities include congregate housing, boarding homes, assisted living facilities, or adult or senior day care centers.

Congregate housing provides independent living for seniors or disabled adults who need minimal to no assistance. There are freestanding apartments, private rooms, or both. Often, residents must meet certain qualifications and may have subsidized rent based on income. Some congregate housing centers may provide other services such as serving one or more meals per day in a common dining room and offering recreational activities. In general, congregate housing is affordable, but residents may not have any other resources to purchase extra services or goods. They are assured of appropriate housing but may lack the resources, ability, or opportunity to participate in outside activities.

Boarding homes usually are small homes with individual rooms where residents pay for room and board and minimal nursing services. Residents often share rooms. Boarding homes usually have a common dining area for all meals. Often, boarding homes also oversee employment for disabled adults and provide a stable environment for those who cannot live independently. In this type of setting, residents receive needed supervision but may relinquish some independence and privacy.

Assisted living facilities provide care to residents who require assistance with up to three ADLs. Residents maximize their independence in a setting that maintains their privacy and dignity. These facilities are not regulated as long-term care facilities are, and there is some concern that the quality of care is not at an appropriate level. The Joint Commission is developing a voluntary accreditation process for assisted living facilities to ensure consistency and quality of care. In many instances, this type of living arrangement is very expensive. Residents must provide a large, upfront investment and then a high monthly fee. The facility may or may not provide such services as housekeeping, laundry, transportation, and meals. Residents can, however, maintain a lifestyle more similar to that which they previously enjoyed. They also are more able to participate in decisions that affect their future care needs.

MODELS FOR NURSING CARE DELIVERY

Over the years, the delivery of nursing care has been structured in different ways. The structures or models of care used today may vary in different settings depending on client needs and cost of services.

Case Method

Nursing care was historically provided on a **case method** basis by which one nurse provided all the services that a particular client required. Although the nurse would accompany the client to the hospital if necessary, the nurse provided care in the home and performed many household duties as well. As times changed and care became more complex, this method became impractical, and different models for the hospital-based delivery of nursing care evolved. A modern version of the case method is private duty nursing.

Functional Nursing

Functional nursing, a task-oriented method, evolved during the 1930s. In functional nursing, distinct duties are assigned to specific personnel. For example, one nurse takes all the vital signs, someone else makes all the beds, a third nurse does all the dressing changes, and so on. Tasks are divided, and clients see several people during the shift. Although efficient, functional nursing fragments care and is confusing for clients.

Team Nursing

Team nursing emerged in the 1950s, partially in response to the fragmented care of functional nursing and to accommodate staff with varying levels of education and skill. In team nursing, teams made up of an RN team leader, other RNs, LPNs/LVNs, and nursing assistants provide care to a group of clients. The RN team leader directs the care provided by the RNs, LPNs/LVNs, and aides and works with them in various capacities. Team conferences allow for discussion and care planning (Evidence-Based Practice 2-1).

Total Client Care

Total client care refers to assignments in which a nurse assumes all the care for a small group of clients. This method focuses more on the client as a whole rather than the collection of nursing tasks that need to be accomplished. Total client care often is practiced in ICUs where nurses are assigned one or two clients.

Primary Care Nursing

In **primary care nursing**, an RN assumes 24-hour accountability for the client's care and has total responsibility for the nursing care of assigned clients during their shift. Secondary nurses carry out the plan of care in the primary nurse's absence. This approach, initiated in the 1970s, is expensive because it relies entirely on RNs. An advantage, however, is that the client has a caregiver who sees to all of their needs and who provides holistic and comprehensive care. Some settings, such as home care, still use this model effectively.

Partnership Models

An updated version of primary care and team nursing is referred to as **partnership models**. This method uses an RN partnered with one or more assistive personnel to care for a group of clients. The RN may work with an LPN/LVN and an assistant, a respiratory therapist and an assistant, or a similar combination of staff. The licensed and unlicensed

Evidence-Based Practice 2-1

Models for Nursing Care Delivery

Clinical Question

Is teamwork and collaboration important in the nursing profession for quality client care?

Evidence

In 2003, the Institute of Medicine developed quality and safety competencies for prelicensure and graduate nurses. These standards are implemented in nursing programs to improve the outcomes of quality nursing care in graduates. The number six competency developed was: Teamwork and Collaboration. QSEN defines this competency as "Function effectively within nursing and inter-professional teams, fostering open communication, mutual respect, and shared decision making to achieve quality client care" (QSEN, 2020a). Nurses advocate for improved communication that focuses on streamlining communication practices, such as implementing clinical rounds, safety huddles, staff meetings, and documentation systems that are congruent with electronic medical records systems (thenursespeak.com-blog).

Nursing Implications

The above QSEN competencies were implemented almost two decades ago and continued to be imbedded in many nursing programs. The future trends in health care call for collaboration and interdisciplinary relationships with health care team members. Nurses contribute to the health care team and bring many different attributes to the team to improve outcomes. As governing bodies and accreditation bodies of professions call for more collaboration in the health care disciplines, nurses must be able to acknowledge the importance of the collaboration and what their contribution is that they can bring to the team to strive for better client outcomes (QSEN, 2020b).

References

QSEN. (2020a). *Competencies.* http://qsen.org/competencies/

QSEN. (2020b). *Graduate KAS.* http://qsen.org/competencies/graduate-ksas/#teamwork_collaboration

A framework of nurses' responsibilities for quality health care—Exploration of content validity. https://www.collegianjournal.com/article/S1322-7696(19)30118-0/fulltext Practice 2-1.

assistants are cross-trained to do many functions formerly done by separate departments, such as drawing blood or obtaining electrocardiograms. The RN may have a role in resource management and may be held accountable for outcomes of nursing care such as skin breakdown (negative outcome) or early ambulation (positive outcome).

Case Management

Although it is not a model of primary nursing care, a new role and responsibility for nurses that affects delivery of care is case management. **Case management** maximizes fiscal outcomes without sacrificing quality through careful oversight of a client's health care. The person responsible for overseeing the client's care, usually an RN with a bachelor's or master's degree or another highly experienced health care provider, is called the *case manager* (Fig. 2-3).

In some specialized settings, a case manager may have a very specific group of clients, such as those with renal failure or diabetes. Insurance companies and hospitals employ case managers. A hospital-based case manager may have a

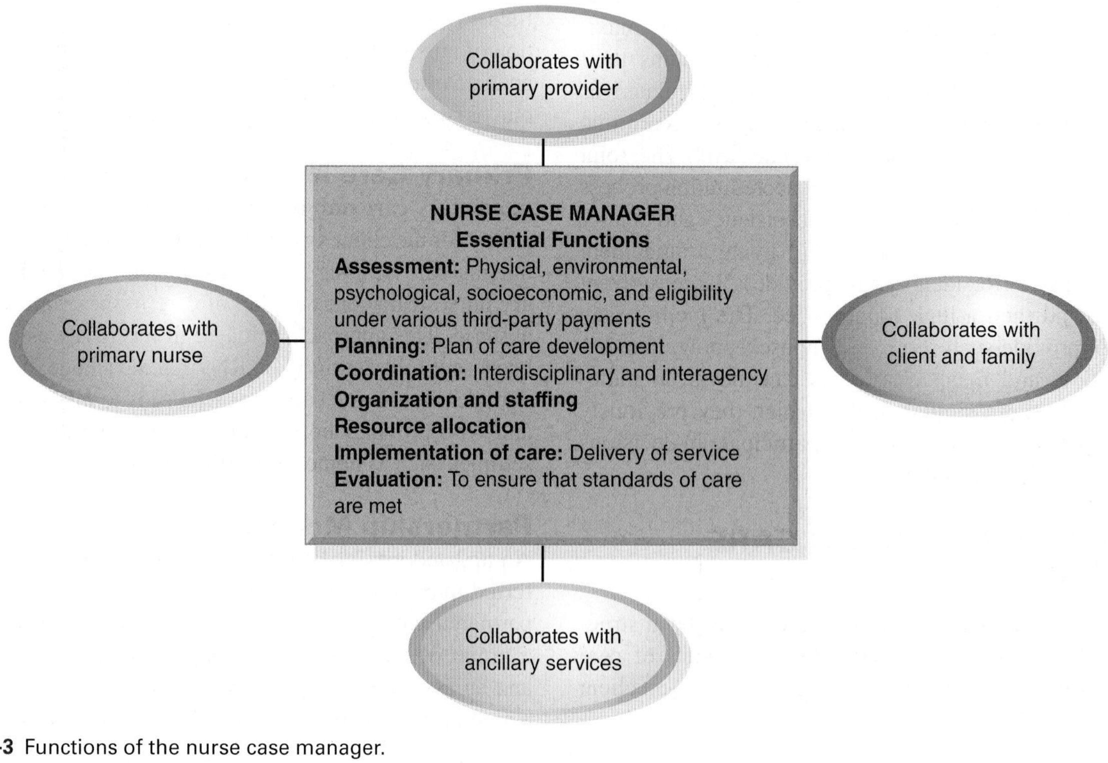

Figure 2-3 Functions of the nurse case manager.

caseload of 15 to 25 clients, depending on the acuity (degree of illness) of the clients. Not every client is aggressively case managed—only those who are sickest, experience complications, or have chronic illnesses that require more intensive case management. The case manager follows clients when they are scheduled for admission until the day of discharge. An insurance-based case manager often maintains contact with the client, especially one with a chronic illness, in the home. Regardless of the employer, case managers plan and coordinate the client's progress through the various phases of care to avoid delays, unnecessary diagnostic testing, and overuse of expensive resources. An important function of case managers is early, thorough discharge planning. Case managers often use tools such as clinical pathways (use of protocols to guide treatment and measure outcomes), practice guidelines, and standards of care to help them plan and coordinate care. Hospitals and insurance companies may develop their own or rely on published protocols for guidance. (A cautionary note: Experts using published research should develop all protocols.)

››› *Stop, Think, and Respond 2-2*

A 70-year-old client was admitted to the hospital with several chronic diagnoses, including diabetes, arthritis, and emphysema. The client tells you that they have a case manager, but they do not understand what that means. How would you explain the case manager's role to this client?

Along with the increase in responsibility, autonomy, and power, nurse case managers have increased accountability for financial and health outcomes of care. Many employers, particularly insurance companies, measure costs of services provided to the case manager's clients as a means of assessing their effectiveness. One of the complaints about case management—and its parent, managed care—is that the "bottom line" can become more important than quality. For this reason, and because they are in the best position to collect outcome data, case managers often are integral members of hospital- and insurance-based quality improvement programs.

KEY POINTS

- Nursing: the protection, promotion, and optimization of health and abilities; prevention of illness and injury; facilitation of healing; alleviation of suffering through the diagnosis and treatment of human response; and advocacy in the care of individuals, families, groups, communities, and populations
- Nurses LPN/LVN: provide care to clients under the direction of an RN—complex role involving the management and coordination of all the care provided to a group of clients
- Settings:
  - Acute care: complicated or critical illness will be cared for in an acute care hospital, where a high level of professional, skilled, and technological care is available
  - Long-term acute care: long-term wound care or ventilator support or who have other conditions that are potentially unstable but do not have rapid changes
  - Subacute care/step-down: provide an intermediate level of care for clients with requirements somewhere between that of the general unit and the ICU
  - Skilled nursing facilities: provide skilled nursing and rehabilitative care to people who have the potential to regain function but need skilled observation and nursing care during an acute illness
  - Intermediate care: nursing homes that provide custodial care for people who cannot care for themselves because of mental or physical disabilities
  - Rehabilitation care: provide physical and occupational therapy to clients and families to help individuals regain as much independence with ADLs as possible
  - Hospice: provide care for clients diagnosed with a terminal illness whose life expectancy is fewer than 6 months
  - Palliative care: not intended to provide curative treatment but rather to manage symptoms, relieve pain and discomfort, improve quality of life
  - Transitional care: refers to the coordination and continuity of health care during a movement from one health care setting to either another or to home
  - Ambulatory care or outpatient care: diagnostic centers, such as gastroenterology centers, day surgery centers, and medical treatment centers, such as those for specific therapies or dialysis, clinics and primary care centers are also considered outpatient settings
  - Home care: addresses both long- and short-term health needs and can provide comprehensive services
- Nursing care delivery models:
  - Functional nursing: distinct duties are assigned to specific personnel
  - Team nursing: teams made up of an RN team leader, other RNs, LPNs/LVNs, and nursing assistants provide care to a group of clients
  - Total client care refers to assignments in which a nurse assumes all the care for a small group of clients.
  - Primary care nursing: RN assumes 24-hour accountability for the client's care and has total responsibility for the nursing care of assigned clients during their shift.
  - Partnership nursing: partnered with one or more assistive personnel to care for a group of clients
  - Case management: responsible for overseeing the client's care

CRITICAL THINKING EXERCISES

1. How do you think nurses will practice in 2050?
2. What is your definition of nursing?
3. Discuss the pros and cons of case management for both the client and the nurse case manager.

NCLEX-STYLE REVIEW QUESTIONS PrepU

1. Definitions of nursing have changed as nursing has evolved. Responsibilities of nursing, as defined by the ANA, include which of the following? Select all that apply.
   1. Administer treatments to clients.
   2. Interpret client data.
   3. Perform a thorough assessment of assigned clients.
   4. Prescribe medications after assessing the client.
   5. Supervise the work of other health care providers.
2. Student nurses are reviewing nursing roles. A student is correct in stating that nurses not only care for people when they are ill but also are involved with which of the following? Select all that apply.
   1. Managing health finances
   2. Preventing illness
   3. Providing spiritual comfort
   4. Teaching clients self-care
   5. Transferring clients to other health care settings
3. A client who is recovering from a hip replacement requires further rehabilitation. The client is most likely to be transferred from an acute care facility to which of the following?
   1. An ambulatory care facility
   2. A subacute care facility
   3. An intermediate care facility
   4. A skilled care facility
4. A client is admitted to a same-day surgery facility for a liver biopsy. Which of the following statements best reflects the client's understanding of a stay at this facility?
   1. "I will be cared for by a technician following the procedure."
   2. "I will be here for a few hours to ensure there are no problems after the biopsy."
   3. "I will be transferred to a recovery room at the hospital after the test."
   4. "I will have the procedure and go home right after it is done."
5. Home health nurses care for clients in their homes. Which of the following best describes the service provided by home health nurses?
   1. Home health nurses have 24-hour accountability for the client's care.
   2. Home health nurses implement the plan of care in the primary nurse's absence.
   3. Home health nurses provide total care for a small group of clients.
   4. Home health nurses adapt care for a client's long- and short-term needs.
6. An older adult client lives alone and is having difficulty with preparing meals and taking care of personal needs, such as bathing, dressing, and toileting. The client's family members are not nearby and are concerned about the client's well-being. The home health nurse would be correct in recommending which of the following alternative health care settings for this client?
   1. Assisted living facility
   2. Boarding home
   3. Congregate housing
   4. Long-term care facility
7. The charge nurse on a skilled care unit in a nursing home reviews the evening assignments: the UAP will take all the vital signs and oversee client meals; the LPN will administer all oral medications and assist with treatments; the RN will do all treatments and any medications that are not oral. Which model of nursing care is this unit following?
   1. Case method nursing
   2. Functional nursing
   3. Primary nursing care
   4. Team nursing
8. The nurse explains to a group of nursing students that they will be providing care within a partnership model. Which of the following student statements best explains a partnership model?
   1. "Each staff person has assigned duties when caring for the clients on the entire unit."
   2. "The RN or LPN, working alone, is responsible for all of the care a small group of clients requires."
   3. "The RN team leader directs the care provided by other RNs, LPNs/LVNs, and UAPs."
   4. "The RN, with a UAP and other personnel, provides total care to a small group of clients."
9. Student nurses are discussing the role of a case manager. Which of the following student statements best describes the role of a case manager?
   1. "Case managers are hired by clients to ensure safe care while hospitalized."
   2. "Case managers have responsibility for the direct care of the client."
   3. "Case managers reduce fragmented care and promote continuity of care."
   4. "Case managers work to decrease primary provider visits."

WANT TO KNOW MORE? There are a wide variety of online resources available on thePoint to enhance learning and understanding of this chapter.

Go to **thePoint.lww.com/activate** and use the activation code found in the front of this text to unlock these online resources.

3

The Nursing Process

Words To Know

assessment
client database
clinical reasoning
collaborative problems
concept care mapping
critical thinking
documentation
evaluation
expected outcomes
health promotion nursing analysis
implementation
nursing analysis
nursing interventions
nursing process
planning
problem-focused nursing analysis
risk nursing analyses
syndrome nursing analyses

Learning Objectives

On completion of this chapter, you will be able to:

1. State the purpose of the nursing process.
2. Describe the five steps of the nursing process.
3. Define assessment.
4. Discuss the parts of a nursing diagnostic statement.
5. Differentiate types of nursing analysis.
6. Explain the five levels of human needs as identified by Maslow.
7. Clarify how nurses use the hierarchy of needs to establish nursing priorities.
8. Define expected outcomes.
9. Explain the implementation phase of the nursing process and its relationship with documentation.
10. Explain the purpose of evaluation.
11. Give reasons why expected outcomes may not be accomplished.
12. Explain critical thinking and clinical reasoning and the relevance to nursing process.
13. List characteristics of nurses who use clinical reasoning and critical thinking.
14. Describe concept care mapping as a method to think critically about client care needs.

Providing health care is a process of problem-solving. Clients present with multiple health care needs that the caregiver must approach in an organized, systematic manner to provide efficient and effective care. The purpose of the **nursing process** is to provide a systematic method for nurses to plan and implement client care to achieve desired outcomes. The nursing process for making clinical decisions grew from problem-solving techniques and the scientific process. It includes collecting information, identifying problems, developing an outcome-based plan, carrying out the plan, and evaluating the results. Other reasons for learning and using the nursing process include:

- Most states' nurse practice acts include the nursing process as part of practice standards.
- Nurse educators use the nursing process in the organizational structure of nursing curricula.
- The nursing process forms the basis for the National Council Licensure Examination (NCLEX) registered nurse (RN) and practical nurse (PN).

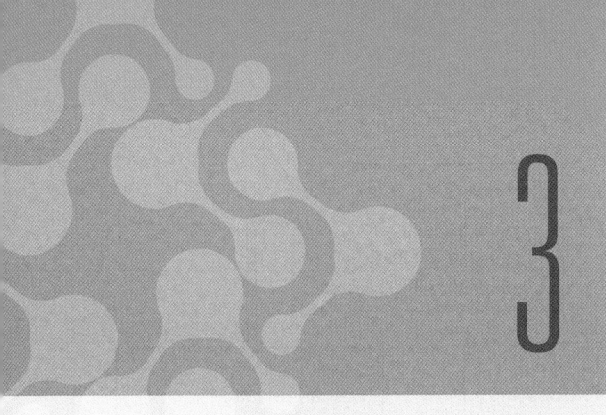

Learning the nursing process is essential to all nursing practice. The use of computerized and standardized nursing care plans may seem to negate the necessity to learn the nursing process. However, the nursing process changes as the client's status changes, and the nurse must review and update the care plans as needed. Computerized systems serve as a guide for problem-solving, not a substitute. Nursing process is about continuous action and thinking.

STEPS OF THE NURSING PROCESS

The nursing process begins when a client enters the health care system. It consists of five steps:

1. Assessment
2. Analysis (nursing)
3. Planning
4. Implementation
5. Evaluation

The nurse collects data (assessment), defines problems or needs (diagnosis/analysis), establishes outcomes and actions that will help achieve the overall goals (planning), puts the plan into action (implementation), and determines the client's responses to the care provided (evaluation). Figure 3-1 depicts these five steps in a dynamic, circular model, showing that each component is not only separate and distinct but also interrelated and continuous with the others. Table 3-1 compares the roles of the licensed practical nurse (LPN) and RN in each step of the nursing process.

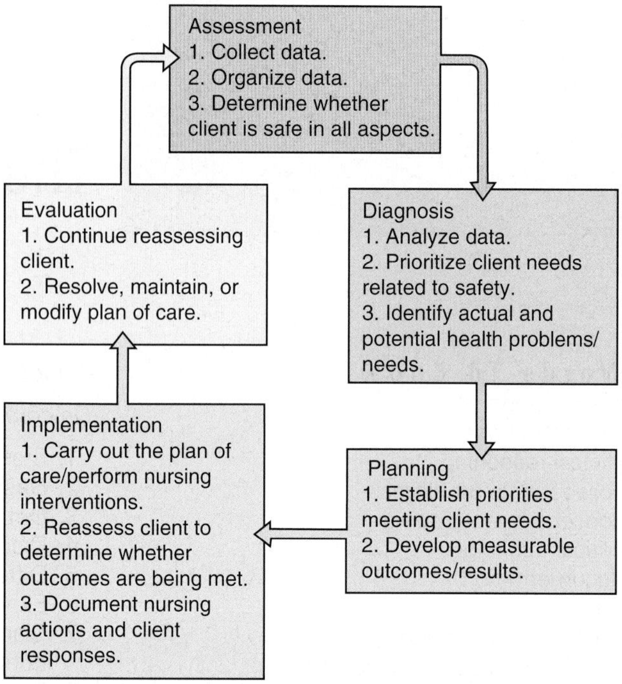

Figure 3-1 Steps in the nursing process.

Assessment

Assessment is the careful observation and evaluation of a client's health status. During assessment, the nurse collects information to determine abnormal function and risk factors that has an impact on a client's health status and safety. Not only is assessment the first step in the nursing process, but it is also an important, recurrent nursing activity that continues as long as a need for health care exists. During assessment, the nurse methodically obtains data about the client's health and illness. Chapter 4 describes the assessment process and data collection in greater detail.

The nurse documents the data in the medical record, which contributes to the client database. The **client database** includes all the information obtained from the medical

TABLE 3-1 Comparison of the Role of the Licensed Practical/Vocational Nurse (LPN/LVN) and Registered Nurse (RN) in the Nursing Process

NURSING PROCESS PHASE	ROLE OF LPN/LVN	ROLE OF RN
Assessment	• Gathers data • Performs assessment • Identifies client's strengths • Assures client is safe	• Gathers more extensive biopsychosocial data • Groups and analyzes data • Researches additional data needed • Identifies client resources • Validates client safety
Nursing analysis	• Does not establish nursing analysis but contributes to identifying the client's problems and understands analyses written by RN	• Uses clinical reasoning to determine nursing analysis(es) • Identifies problems and risks that require nursing management
Planning	• Contributes to development of care plans, including interventions and maintenance of client safety	• Establishes priorities • Sets short- and long-term client outcomes • Collaborates • Makes referrals for client needs that cannot be solely resolved by nursing actions
Implementation	• Provides basic therapeutic and preventive nursing measures • Provides client education • Records information	• Manages client care (performs and delegates) • Provides client and family teaching • Makes referrals • Records and exchanges information with health care team
Evaluation	• Evaluates effects of care given	• Evaluates effectiveness of overall plan • Analyzes new data • Modifies and redesigns plan • Collaborates with health care team members

and nursing history, physical examination (see Chapter 4), and diagnostic studies. Baseline data serve as a comparison for future signs and symptoms and provide a reference for determining whether a client's health is improving or worsening. Initial and ongoing assessment is essential to the provision of nursing care.

Nursing Diagnosis/Analysis

In establishing **nursing analysis**(es), the second phase of the nursing process, the nurse interprets data to identify and define health problems that independent or primary provider–prescribed nursing actions can prevent or solve. As in other phases of the nursing process, the nurse's role depends on their level of practice. LPN/licensed vocational nurses (LVNs) report information that suggests problem-focused or potential health problems. RNs examine and analyze the client database to formulate nursing diagnoses.

Nursing Diagnostic Statements

A diagnostic statement includes one to three parts: (1) the name, or label, of the problem; (2) the cause and related factors of the problem; and (3) the signs and symptoms, or data and defining characteristics that describe the problem. The name, or label, portion of the statement is linked to the cause with the phrase *related to*, and the data are linked to the name/label and cause by the phrase *as evidenced by*. The following is an example of a nursing diagnostic statement:

> *Constipation* (name of the problem) *related to decreased fluid intake*, *lack of dietary fiber* and *lack of exercise* (causes) *as evidenced by no bowel movement for the past 3 days*, *abdominal cramping*, and *straining to pass stools* (signs and symptoms).

Sometimes, the cause is explained in more depth using the term *secondary to*, as in *decreased fluid intake secondary to nausea*. Different types of analyses, as outlined in the following, also have different prefixes or stems.

Collaborative Problems

Collaborative problems denote complications with a physiologic origin and differ from nursing diagnoses, which address client responses to various circumstances and are managed by nursing interventions (Carpenito, 2014). Collaborative problems involve activities of nurses to monitor clients for the purpose of detecting physiologic changes or the onset of physiologic problems. Carpenito (2014) explains, "Nurses manage collaborative problems using physician-prescribed interventions and nursing-prescribed interventions to minimize the complications of the events" (p. 6). Carpenito recommends that collaborative problems be labeled as "*Risk for Complications (RC) of*" (p. 7), as in RC of pulmonary embolism. Nurses do not include related factors and supporting data when writing collaborative problem statements.

Planning

The third step of the nursing process is **planning**, which involves several steps: setting priorities, defining expected (desired) outcomes (goals), determining specific nursing interventions, and recording the plan of care. Respecting client right to participate in their health care is an important ethical principle. Actively involved clients are more committed to carrying out the plan and achieving the outcomes. Thus, nurses ensure that clients and families participate in care planning as much as possible. Nurses consult with clients about specific activities that are equally effective in achieving the outcomes.

For example, a woman client has a nursing analysis finding of malnutrition risk: receiving less than body needs related to poor appetite and medication side effects as evidenced by an intake of less than 1,000 calories/day and weight loss of 3 kg in 10 days. When planning care for this client, the nurse must talk with her about the importance of increased caloric intake and ways to accomplish it, including different types of foods, frequency of meals, and timing of medications. If the nurse simply decides to add certain high-calorie foods to the client's food tray, it is highly possible that the client will reject the foods because she may not like them.

Establishing Priorities

Some problems require immediate action, whereas others may not have high priority. The nurse prioritizes the client's multiple problems by first ranking the diagnoses that define the client's most important, serious, or immediate needs, followed by the remainder in descending order of importance. A framework that nurses frequently use when prioritizing client problems is the hierarchy of human needs developed by Maslow (1968). Maslow proposed five levels of needs that motivate human behavior and grouped them as follows, according to their significance:

1. Physiologic needs (first level)—breathing, food, water, sex, sleep, homeostasis, elimination
2. Safety and security needs (second level)—security of body, employment, resources, morality, family, health, property
3. Love and belonging needs (third level)—friendship, family, sexual intimacy
4. Esteem and self-esteem needs (fourth level)—self-esteem, confidence, achievement, respect of others, respect by others
5. Self-actualization needs (fifth level)—morality, creativity, spontaneity, problem-solving, lack of prejudice, acceptance of facts

The first-level needs, sometimes called "baseline survival needs," have the highest priority. These activities (such as eating, breathing, and drinking) sustain life. Maslow believed humans could not or would not seek to fulfill higher level needs until physiologic needs were satisfied. Thus, nurses must rank any problem that poses a threat to physiologic functioning first. For example, nursing diagnoses such as altered breathing pattern and dehydration demand the nurse's attention more than other analyses because these conditions may be life-threatening.

Nursing analyses such as acute anxiety or injury risk address the second-level needs of safety and security. Safety is an example of nursing analyses that apply to the third level of love and belonging needs. Examples of nursing analyses that affect the fourth level of esteem and self-esteem needs are coping impairment and situational low self-esteem. Psychosocial/spiritual needs is an example of nursing analyses that interfere with an individual's ability to achieve fifth-level, self-actualization needs.

Defining Expected Outcomes

Defining **expected outcomes** is an important part of the care planning process. The nurse includes the client and family in establishing outcomes. Outcomes are specific and realistic, so the client can attain them and not become frustrated, and measurable, so the nurse can reliably determine to what extent the client is meeting the goals.

The nurse determines client-centered outcomes from the nursing diagnoses so that the focus is on the treatments and results, as opposed to what the nurse hopes to achieve. For example, a nurse may desire the outcome that the client understands everything the nurse teaches. Instead, the outcome needs to focus on the essential care techniques for the client to master before leaving the health care facility. Thus, an appropriate outcome in this scenario would be, "Before discharge, the client will demonstrate clean technique when changing the dressing on their left calf wound."

Nursing outcomes are derived from the nursing diagnoses. In 1981, George T. Doran created the SMART framework in his paper, *There's a S.M.A.R.T. Way to Write Management's Goals and Objectives*. The SMART methodology helps you to construct clearly defined goals using five attributes (S.M.A.R.T., 1981):

S — Specific
M — Measurable
A — Agreed upon by all parties/Achievable
R — Realistic/Relevant
T — Time bound/Timely

As the nurse develops the expected outcomes, they should relate them directly to the nursing diagnoses and make them clear and specific. For example, if the nursing analysis is "injury risk related to left knee replacement surgery," an expected outcome is that "the client will ambulate with a walker to the nurse's station and back on the third postoperative day." Table 3-2 provides examples of client-centered outcomes for each type of nursing diagnosis.

In some settings, it may be necessary to identify short- and long-term outcomes. For example, in a rehabilitation center, clients may be involved in therapy for weeks or months. The expected outcomes need to reflect this length of treatment. In this situation, a short-term outcome is that "the client will ambulate 20 feet on the first postoperative day," whereas a long-term outcome is that "the client will ambulate with a walker by the end of 3 weeks."

Unlike nursing analyses that require client-centered outcomes, collaborative problems need nurse-centered outcomes because the nurse is managing situations that rely on primary provider and nursing interventions. The nurse-centered outcomes require collaborative nurse and primary provider interventions; for example, for ineffective airway clearance, the outcome would be that the nurse will monitor client secretions.

Determining Specific Interventions

The plan of care identifies interventions or actions for achieving the outcomes. Relieving the cause of the problem directs the interventions. If the cause cannot be fixed, such as in permanent injury, then the interventions focus on reducing consequences of the problem.

For example, if a client has the nursing analysis of "altered skin integrity related to the effects of pressure secondary to decreased mobility as evidenced by a 2-cm ulcer on the right heel," the nurse needs to identify measures directed at relieving pressure and its effects (decreased circulation). Such interventions would include elevating the heel off the bed to relieve pressure and having the client do ankle-pumping exercises to increase blood flow to the area. If the analysis is "feeding activities of daily living (ADL) deficit related to right hemiparesis (paralysis affecting one side of the body) secondary to stroke as evidenced by inability to grasp utensils," the nurse may provide utensils with large rubber grips to decrease the effects of the problem.

Recording the Plan of Care

Once the RN determines the interventions (sometimes referred to as *nursing orders*), they write the interventions in the written plan. **Nursing interventions** are specific nursing

TABLE 3-2 Examples of Expected Outcomes Derived From Nursing Diagnoses

NURSING ANALYSIS	EXPECTED OUTCOME
Ineffective airway clearance related to excessive secretions secondary to inflammation okay	The client will demonstrate optimal positioning to facilitate drainage of secretions on the day of admission.
Dehydration related to nausea and vomiting and increased loss of fluids and electrolytes from gastrointestinal tract	The client will maintain fluid balance as evidenced by total intake greater than or equal to 2500 mL, with output equal to intake or differing from intake by no more than 500 mL.
Disuse syndrome: injury risk related to mechanical immobilization	The client will demonstrate ability to turn with assistance, maintaining restrictions, by the second postoperative day.
RC of congestive heart failure	The nurse will monitor the client for shortness of breath, dyspnea on exertion, and orthopnea.

RC, Risk for Complications.

BOX 3-1 SMART Goal Setting Template

- **S**—What do I want to achieve? Be precise.
- **M**—How will I know when I have reached my goal? What are the metrics and milestones I need to hit along the way?
- **A**—Is this goal realistic for me? What support do I need to make sure I achieve my goal?
- **R**—Why is this goal worthwhile? Does it support the wider team and my other responsibilities?
- **T**—When do I want to achieve this goal? Write down a target date.

From Strickland, K. (2019, August 21). *SMART Goals in Nursing: 5 Examples. PeopleGoal*. https://www.peoplegoal.com/blog/smart-goals-in-nursing-examples. Reprinted with permission from PeopleGoal, Inc. https://www.peoplegoal.com.

directions such that all health care team members understand exactly what to do for the client (Box 3-1). People are likely to interpret an intervention, such as "encourage fluids," differently, which results in inconsistent care. In such cases, if outcomes are not met, determining whether the nursing measures themselves were ineffective or whether they were carried out ineffectively becomes difficult. A more appropriate nursing intervention is "give the client 30 mL of juice, water, tea, or milk every hour while awake." Interventions in the nursing care plan must also be compatible with the medical orders. For instance, if the primary provider has prescribed complete bed rest, a nursing order should not call for ambulation.

Many agencies have preprinted or computer-generated care plans that help identify nursing interventions for specific nursing or medical diagnoses. They save time by providing general suggestions for common conditions. The nurse selects appropriate interventions from the list, makes the orders specific for the individual client, and eliminates whatever is unnecessary. A complete plan of care provides a means to communicate to all shifts of nursing personnel. This communication establishes a basis for continuity of care.

Implementation

As the fourth step of the nursing process, **implementation** means carrying out the written plan of care, performing the interventions, monitoring the client's status, and assessing and reassessing the client before, during, and after treatments. Carrying out the plan involves the client and one or more members of the health care team. It may also include the client's family and the community. It requires that the nurse not only act but also think before acting. For example, the nurse looks for any changes in the client's condition, reviews the client's responses to changes or care, and determines whether changes need to be made in the plan of care.

An important element of implementation is **documentation**. Accurate and thorough documentation in the medical record serves a number of functions (Alfaro-LeFevre, 2014, p. 176, 177):

1. Communicates care
2. Shows trends and patterns in client status
3. Ensures that interventions are evidence based (time frames for medications, rationales for interventions)
4. Provides a foundation for evaluation, research, and quality improvement
5. Creates a legal document
6. Supplies validation for reimbursement

By law, nurses must document all nursing actions, observations, and client responses in a permanent record. This record of nursing actions should be a mirror image of the written plan of care. Appropriate documentation is essential in maintaining communication among members of the health care team and ensuring that nurses monitor the client's progress.

Evaluation

Evaluation, the fifth step of the nursing process, consists of assessment and review of the quality and suitability of care given and the client's responses to that care. During evaluation, nurses compare the actual outcomes with the expected outcomes. This process enables the nurse to revise the expected outcomes or select alternative plans of action when expected outcomes are not met. The nurse may reach one of several conclusions during evaluation:

- The outcome is achieved, the problem is solved, and the nursing interventions are discontinued.
- The outcome is not met, but progress is being made and the plan of care is continued or revised with minor changes.
- The outcome is not achieved, and the plan requires critical reevaluation and major revision.

A client's lack of progress may result from unrealistic expectations, incorrect analysis of the original problem, development of additional problems, ineffective nursing measures, or a premature target date. Once nurses identify the deficiency in the plan, they may implement a revision. See the sample Nursing Care Plan 3-1.

THE NURSING PROCESS AND CLINICAL REASONING/CRITICAL THINKING

The terms **clinical reasoning** and **critical thinking** are often interchangeable concepts. According to Alfaro-LeFevre (2014), **clinical reasoning** is "a specific term that refers to the assessment and management of patient problems at the point of care" (p. 4). **Critical thinking**, a broader term, is intentional, contemplative, and outcome-directed thinking. In nursing, clinical reasoning and critical thinking use nursing process, problem-solving, and the scientific method. Standards, policies, ethics codes, and laws guide thinking, assuring that safety and quality are integral components.

When caring for clients, nurses continually assess their needs and frequently confront situations that require multiple interventions. Developing good clinical reasoning skills makes nurses more efficient and effective at resolving these situations. This careful, deliberate, outcome-directed thinking has predictable features that nurses can practice and learn. One key feature is the ability to maintain a questioning attitude. "What information is relevant to this situation?"

NURSING CARE PLAN 3-1 Postoperative Abdominal Surgery Care

Assessment

- Check the client's abdominal dressing.
- Assess the Hemovac drain.
- Check the nasogastric tube.
- Assess the Foley catheter.
- Review the intravenous (IV) infusion rate.
- Assess the patient-controlled analgesia (PCA).
- Evaluate the IV insertion site.
- Take the client's vital signs.
- Determine the client's ability to ambulate.
- Assess the client's level of consciousness.
- Assess the client's pain.

Nursing Diagnosis. Ineffective airway clearance related to depressed respiratory function, pain, and bed rest

Expected Outcomes. (1) Client maintains a patent airway at all times. (2) Client's breath sounds remain clear.

Interventions	Rationales
Monitor breath sounds at least every 4 hours for 48 hours.	*Breath sounds with crackles and wheezes indicate retained secretions.*
Instruct client to deep breathe and cough every 2 hours.	*Lung expansion prevents atelectasis and keeps secretions cleared.*
Turn client at least every 2 hours.	*Turning promotes lung expansion and movement of secretions.*

Evaluation of Expected Outcomes

- Client's respirations are unlabored and regular.
- Client's bilateral breath sounds are clear.
- Client performs deep breathing and coughing exercises with coaching.
- Client turns every 2 hours with maximum assistance.

Collaborative Problem. RC of wound infection.

Expected Outcome. The nurse will minimize the client's potential for a wound infection.

Interventions	Rationales
Observe incision for signs and symptoms of infection.	*Redness, warmth, fever, or swelling indicates a wound infection.*
Monitor wound drainage, dressing, and Hemovac drain.	*Changes in wound drainage from serosanguinous to purulent indicate a wound infection.*
Maintain sterile technique for dressing changes.	*Sterile technique reduces potential for development of infection.*

Evaluation of Expected Outcomes

- Incision remains free of redness, warmth, and swelling.
- Drainage is decreased and serosanguinous.
- The nurse changes the dressing every 8 hours, with scant serosanguinous drainage on old dressings.

"What needs to be monitored now?" "What could contribute to a complication?" "Have the nursing interventions been effective?"

The use of the nursing process in nursing combines critical thinking and clinical reasoning with problem-solving methods. Nurses identify client problems and develop and implement plans of care with a logical, purposeful, and outcome-based method. The nursing process assists nurses to acquire clinical reasoning, critical thinking, and problem-solving skills because it entails scientific problem-solving in a systematic, client-centered, outcome-based way. It is also a dynamic continuous process. When thinking critically, nurses use specific cognitive skills to analyze, solve problems, and make decisions.

Nurses use critical thinking skills in all practice settings. Each client presents with unique and dynamic issues. The nurse considers all factors and interprets the information to focus on the most needed elements and make decisions relevant to the individual client's care. Developing critical thinking skills requires knowledge, practice, and experience. This text presents critical thinking exercises at the end of each chapter as well as "Stop, Think, and Respond" exercises in many chapters. These exercises encourage the reader to begin the process of critical analysis and interpretation as well as providing a foundation for clinical reasoning and critical decision-making.

>>> *Stop, Think, and Respond 3-1*

A do-not-resuscitate (DNR) order was just added to a terminally ill client's plan of care. Using critical thinking skills, what must the nurse consider when adapting the nursing care plan? What types of nursing diagnoses should the nurse consider adding to the care plan?

CONCEPT CARE MAPPING

Concept care mapping is an alternate to nursing care plans. It links important ideas about the care a client requires in a visual format that displays how ideas are linked and interrelated. It provides a means for students and nurses to consider all of the client's problems as a whole and then develop a plan to treat the problems. Specifically, a concept care map presents the client's medical and nursing diagnoses with the relevant clinical data. It assists the student to assess what is known about the client and determine what other information is needed.

KEY POINTS

- The nursing process: to provide a systematic method for nurses to plan and implement client care to achieve desired outcomes
- The five steps of the nursing process:
  - Assessment: careful observation and evaluation of a client's health status
  - Diagnosis (nursing) or analysis: reviewing data to identify and define health problems that independent or primary provider–prescribed nursing actions can prevent or solve
  - Planning: setting priorities, defining expected (desired) outcomes (goals), determining specific nursing interventions, and recording the plan of care
  - Implementation: carrying out the written plan of care, performing the interventions, monitoring the client's status, and assessing/reassessing the client before, during, and after treatments
  - Evaluation: assessing and reviewing of the quality and suitability of care given and the client's responses to that care, and compare the actual outcomes with the expected outcomes
- Nursing diagnostic statement:
  - The name, or label, of the problem
  - The cause and related factors of the problem
  - The signs and symptoms
- The five levels of human needs as identified by Maslow:
  - Physiological
  - Safety and security
  - Love and belonging
  - Esteem and self-esteem
  - Self-actualization
- Expected outcome evaluations:
  - The outcome is achieved, the problem is solved, and the nursing interventions are discontinued.
  - The outcome is not met, but progress is being made and the plan of care is continued or revised with minor changes. The outcome is not achieved, and the plan requires critical reevaluation and major revision.
- Critical thinking: intentional, contemplative, and outcome-directed thinking
- Clinical reasoning: a specific term that refers to the assessment and management of client problems at the point of care
- Concept care mapping: provides the means for students and nurses to consider all of the client's problems, both the medical and nursing diagnoses, and the care required to develop a plan to treat the problems

CRITICAL THINKING EXERCISES

1. List several reasons why including clients in care planning is important.
2. Explain the importance of the five steps of the nursing process. Give examples of what problems might arise if the nurse skips any steps.
3. Think of a client problem and a personal problem you encountered recently and refer to the characteristics of critical thinkers to determine which characteristics you demonstrated. Apply the other characteristics to the problems and discuss how the outcomes might have been different.
4. Take the following medical diagnosis and consider associated nursing analyses/problems that could be part of a nursing care plan.

NCLEX-STYLE REVIEW QUESTIONS PrepU

1. Which of the following is an appropriate role for the LPN/LVN related to nursing process?
   1. Analyze data on a client admitted for a surgical procedure.
   2. Collect data on a client who reported feeling nauseous.
   3. Make referrals for client follow-up care.
   4. Modify plan of care related to assessment data.
2. What is "malnutrition risk: Less than body requirements related to loss of appetite, difficulty swallowing, and side effects of chemotherapy" an example of?
   1. Health promotion nursing diagnosis
   2. Problem-focused diagnosis
   3. Risk nursing diagnosis
   4. Syndrome nursing diagnosis
3. Using Maslow's hierarchy of needs, arrange the following nursing analyses in order of highest priority to lowest priority.
   1. Anxiety
   2. Decreased cardiac output
   3. Disturbed body image
   4. Ineffective relationship
   5. Sleep deprivation
4. A nurse writes expected outcomes for one of the assigned clients. Which of the following is appropriate?
   1. Client will ask for pain medication.
   2. Client will be free of pain.
   3. Client will experience less pain.
   4. Client will report a pain level of less than 3 on a pain scale of 0 to 10.
5. Nursing analyses include nursing and collaborative problems. When determining care for a client, the nurse identifies which of the following as a collaborative problem?
   1. Altered health maintenance
   2. Hypoglycemia risk
   3. Constipation risk
   4. Urinary retention

6. A nurse stops to assist an adult individual involved in a motor vehicle accident. The victim was not wearing a seat belt and was thrown from the car. Of the following emergency measures, which one should the nurse perform first?
   1. Assess for signs of injuries.
   2. Check the victim's breathing.
   3. Cover the victim with a blanket.
   4. Move the victim to the curb.
7. Nurses frequently face client situations that require clinical reasoning. In the following scenarios, which nurse is using clinical reasoning skills?
   1. The nurse who is concerned about the dosage of an ordered medication but administers it anyway
   2. The nurse who makes rounds on their clients in the order of the rooms
   3. The nurse who places a seriously ill client near the nurse station
   4. The nurse who resets an IV pump without adequate instruction

WANT TO KNOW MORE? There are a wide variety of online resources available on thePoint to enhance learning and understanding of this chapter.

Go to **thePoint.lww.com/activate** and use the activation code found in the front of this text to unlock these online resources.

4 Interviewing and Physical Assessment

Words To Know

auscultation
chief complaint
closed questions
cultural history
focused assessment
functional assessment
head-to-toe method
inspection
objective data
open-ended questions
palpation
past health history
percussion
physical assessment
psychosocial history
subjective data
systems method

Learning Objectives

On completion of this chapter, you will be able to:

1. Explain the purpose of the interview and physical assessment.
2. Define subjective and objective data, symptoms, and signs.
3. Explain the three phases of the interview process.
4. Differentiate a systems method of assessment from a head-to-toe method of assessment.
5. Identify four assessment techniques.
6. Describe general assessment measures that all nurses can perform.

Assessment is the process of gathering information about a client's health (see Chapter 3). Through systematic assessment, the nurse identifies the client's

- current and past health status
- current and past functional status
- coping patterns
- health beliefs
- lifestyle and health practices
- relevant cultural practices
- risks for potential health problems
- responses to care
- nursing care needs
- referral needs

The nurse first assesses the client when they are admitted to the health care system. Findings from this comprehensive initial assessment establish a database that gives all team members relevant client information and becomes a yardstick for measuring effectiveness of care. The initial assessment consists of two parts: the interview and the physical assessment.

During the interview, the nurse gathers subjective data. **Subjective data** are statements the client makes about what they feel. When the client tells the nurse about nausea, pain, fear, bloating, or other feelings of discomfort, they are providing subjective data. These feelings of discomfort may be referred to as symptoms. During the physical assessment, the nurse gathers objective data. **Objective data** are facts obtained through observation, physical examination, and diagnostic testing. When the nurse assesses blood pressure or heart rate or examines results from urinalysis, they obtain objective data. When objective data are abnormal, they may be referred to as signs. Objective data often support the subjective data.

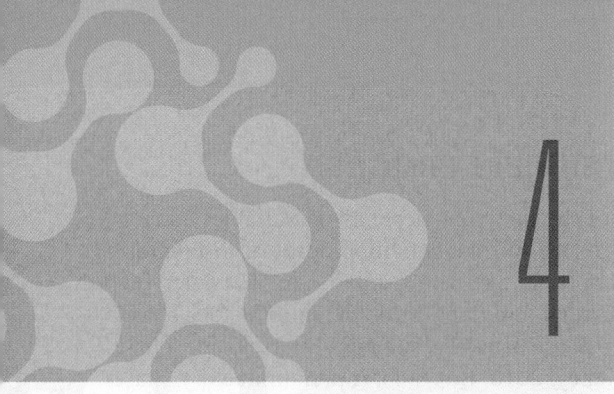

Gerontological Considerations

- When interviewing the older client, ask them to describe activities in a usual day. Also ask questions about family and social supports. Use this information as a foundation for other interview questions.
- In order to gain more complete information and to plan culturally appropriate care, the explanatory model of questioning is helpful. Ask the client to explain in their own words the nature of the problem, its duration, factors that have contributed to the problem, measures currently underway to help the problem, and what they believe will help resolve the problem.
- Ask about ability to perform activities of daily living (ADLs) and responsibilities such as shopping, cleaning, yard work, managing finances, and managing medications that must be fulfilled for independent living. If the client expresses difficulty with any ADL area, follow up to determine what resources are being used or may be needed to support independence.
- Older adults may take medications that are intended to counteract the effects of other medications or have changes in absorption, metabolism, and excretion. To identify polypharmacy or risk for interactions, ask how all medications and health care practices are used and at what time of day. Asking the client to bring all medications (prescription, over-the-counter [OTC], herbal) and to describe other nutritional or folk practices provides further information from which risks for medication interactions can be identified.
- When interviewing an older client, allow a friend or family caregiver to remain during the history if the client requests. This support person may serve as an additional resource for information.
- During the interview, use silence to allow more time for the client to respond to questions.
- Include in the interview questions regarding changes that may affect nutrition, such as taste, smell, swallowing, ability to obtain or prepare foods, fit of dentures, fit of clothing, and if meals are eaten alone or if mealtimes are shared with another person.
- Data obtained from the interview may need to be validated with family or significant others involved in the client's care.
- When performing a physical assessment for an older client, keep in mind:
  - Ascertain a baseline cognitive function level at onset of interviewing. The Mini-Cog is a quick and simple four-question method.
  - Ask what chronic condition may impact the assessment (e.g., arthritis may limit range of motion of a particular extremity).
  - Avoid tiring the client—allow rest periods if needed.
  - Keep the older client warm and away from drafts.
  - Be aware of privacy issues if the older client is hearing impaired.
  - Allow ample time for the client to respond to directions and to make position changes.
  - If possible, observe the client performing ADLs. Include an unaided "get-up-and-go" assessment of the client rising from a seated position and ambulating to assess ability.

THE INTERVIEW PROCESS

The length of the interview depends on variables such as the severity of the client's condition, level of discomfort, ability to cooperate, age, and mental state. The interview process is divided into three parts: the introductory phase, the working phase, and the summary and closing phase (Weber & Kelley, 2016; Box 4-1). A preintroductory phase involves reviewing any medical documents related to the client. This can assist the nurse to gather some information prior to meeting the client and perhaps help to establish rapport. The nurse also can be better prepared to talk with the client if they are aware of any physical deficits, hearing and/or visual impairments, or any cultural or age-related considerations.

Introductory Phase

The introductory phase establishes initial rapport with the client and family members and informs the client about the nurse's need to ask questions and gather information. When making introductions, the nurse should introduce themselves and include credentials (e.g., licensed practical/vocational nurses [LPN/LVN] or registered nurse [RN]), explain their role, and address the client by their surname. A private setting for the interview is essential to eliminate interruptions and maintain the client's confidentiality (Fig. 4-1). The nurse should explain that information obtained during the interview helps with planning care. They should tell the client that all information is kept confidential, although all members of the health care team share the data.

>>> *Stop, Think, and Respond 4-1*

Describe approaches you would use in the introductory phase for a client who is hearing- or vision-impaired.

BOX 4-1 Parts of the Interview

Introductory Phase

Establish rapport.
Explain the purpose of the interview.
Explain the types of questions that will be asked and reasons for taking notes or using a computer to record information.

Working Phase

Collect information related to demographic data, reason(s) for seeking care, history of present health concern(s), family history, review of body systems, health practices, and developmental level.

Summary and Closure Phase

Review information obtained and confirm problems and concerns.
Discuss any plans to resolve the health concern(s).
Ask client if there are any questions.

Adapted from Weber, J., & Kelley, J. (2016). *Health assessment in nursing* (6th ed.). Wolters Kluwer.

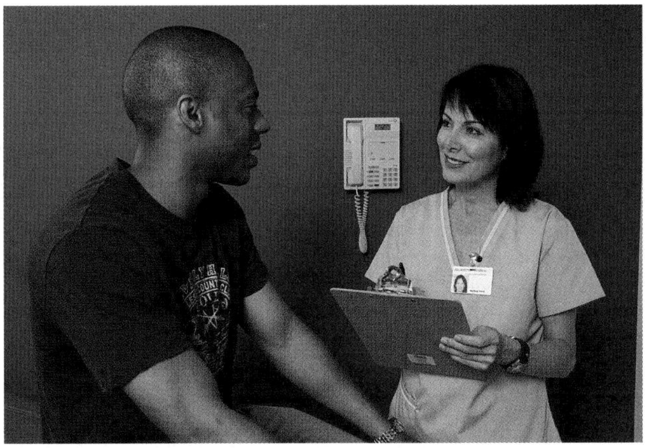

FIGURE 4-1 The nurse provides a relaxed and private atmosphere when conducting an interview.

Concept Mastery Alert

Interview

A client answers questions by the nurse during the *working phase* of the interview process. This is preceded by the *introductory phase*, when the nurse establishes rapport with the client and presents information about what the client can expect during the interview process.

Working Phase

During the working phase, the nurse asks the client questions to gather data for the client database. Good communication skills are essential. The nurse should avoid using medical terms. Questions are best phrased as **open-ended questions** that require discussion rather than **closed questions** that require only yes or no answers. Giving the client ample time to answer each question and maintaining frequent eye contact are important measures.

Many institutions have assessment forms that help ensure the database is complete. If the nurse asks the client to complete the assessment form, they should clarify information that the client gives during the interview. Many hospitals are using handheld or bedside computers to complete the database. Whether entering data on a computer or writing on a form, the nurse should connect with the client in a meaningful way and not focus entirely on the process of data entry.

Completing the database includes the following components (Box 4-2):

- Psychosocial and cultural history
- Chief complaint
- History of the present health concern
- Functional status—self-care ability
- Past health history
- Family health history
- Review of body systems for current health problems
- Lifestyle and health practices profile

It is unnecessary to discuss these topics in a specific pattern. The examiner can rearrange the order in which topics are discussed, digress from an established format if additional information seems pertinent, or omit areas that are not applicable.

Psychosocial and Cultural History

The **psychosocial history** and **cultural history** include the client's age, occupation, religious affiliation, cultural background and health beliefs (see Chapter 8), marital status, and home and working environments. Although some of this material may be found on the client's record, specific aspects may need further exploration. For example, if the client is a factory worker, then the examiner would ask if the client works around hazardous chemicals or if they experienced any job-related injuries.

Chief Complaint

The **chief complaint** is the current reason the client is seeking care. The purpose of asking the client about their primary health concern is to discover what the client perceives as the health problem that needs treatment. Recording information in the client's own words is best. For example, "I had a terrible pain in the right side of my stomach after I ate. I never had it so bad. The doctor said that maybe it's my gallbladder."

History of Present Health Concern

The nurse asks the client to describe all present problems, including the onset, frequency, and duration of symptoms. Asking for more detailed information about one body system or problem is called a **focused assessment** because it adds depth to the original data. For example, a client may reveal that they have experienced abdominal pain for the past several weeks. Further questioning then addresses what causes the pain, how long it lasts, what the quality of the pain is, and what makes it better or worse.

Functional Assessment

A **functional assessment** determines how well the client can manage ADLs. ADLs include self-care activities, such as walking moderate distances, bathing, and toileting, and instrumental activities, such as preparing meals, obtaining transportation, and dialing the telephone. This assessment component is particularly important when assessing older adults or physically challenged clients of any age.

Past Health History

The client's **past health history** includes identifying childhood diseases, previous injuries, major illnesses, prior hospitalizations, surgical procedures, and drug history. Obtaining this information is important because it may affect current care. When discussing the client's past medical problems, the nurse should ask the age at which the problem was diagnosed, treatments prescribed, and whether the problem still exists. Information about past surgeries includes types, when each was done, and whether recoveries were uneventful or accompanied by complications.

The nurse identifies any current and past use of prescription and nonprescription drugs or herbal products. They ask about the client's use of alcohol, tobacco, and/or other

BOX 4-2 Interview Guide

The interviewer establishes a database by asking the client questions about their health.

Psychosocial and Cultural History

Age; gender; marital status; number of children; occupation; highest level of education; religious affiliation; place of residence; country of origin; primary language; military service; date, location, and length of foreign travel or residence

Chief Complaint

Reason for seeking care; type, location, and severity of symptoms

History of Present Health Concern

Chronologic description of the onset, frequency, and duration of current symptoms; attempts at and outcomes of self-treatment; what the client thinks caused the problem; how the illness affects the client's life at home, at work, and socially

Functional Assessment

Ability to walk, get in and out of bed, bathe, dress, eat, and get to and from the bathroom; ability to drive, take public transportation, get groceries, or prepare meals

Past Health History

Childhood diseases, physical injuries, major illnesses, previous medical or psychiatric hospitalizations, surgical procedures, drug history, use of alcohol and tobacco, allergy history

Family Health History

Health problems among relatives living and deceased; longevity and cause of death among deceased blood relatives

Review of Body Systems for Current Health Problems

General. Usual weight, recent weight change, weakness, fatigue, fever

Skin. Rashes, lumps, sores, itching, dryness, color change, changes in hair or nails

Head. Headache, head injury

Eyes. Vision, glasses or contact lenses, last eye examination, pain, redness, excessive tearing, double vision, blurred vision, spots, specks, flashing lights, glaucoma, cataracts

Ears. Hearing, tinnitus, vertigo, earaches, infection, discharge, use of hearing aids

Nose and sinuses. Frequent colds; nasal stuffiness, discharge, or itching; hay fever; nosebleeds; sinus trouble

Mouth and throat. Condition of teeth and gums; bleeding gums; dentures, if any, and how they fit; last dental examination; sore tongue; dry mouth; frequent sore throats; hoarseness

Neck. Lumps; "swollen glands," goiter, pain or stiffness in the neck

Breasts. Lumps, pain or discomfort, nipple discharge, self-examination

Respiratory. Cough; sputum (color, quantity); hemoptysis, wheezing, asthma, bronchitis, emphysema, pneumonia, tuberculosis, pleurisy, last chest X-ray film

Cardiac. Heart trouble, high blood pressure, rheumatic fever, heart murmurs, chest pain or discomfort, palpitations, dyspnea, orthopnea, paroxysmal nocturnal dyspnea, edema, past electrocardiogram, or other heart test results

Gastrointestinal. Trouble swallowing, heartburn, appetite, nausea, vomiting, regurgitation, vomiting of blood, indigestion, frequency of bowel movements, color and size of stools, change in bowel habits, rectal bleeding or black tarry stools, hemorrhoids, constipation, diarrhea, abdominal pain, food intolerance, excessive belching or passing of gas, jaundice, liver or gallbladder trouble, hepatitis

Urinary. Frequency of urination, polyuria, nocturia, burning or pain on urination, hematuria, urgency, reduced caliber or force of the urinary stream, hesitancy, dribbling, incontinence, urinary infections, stones

Genital. Male: Hernias, discharge from or sores on the penis, testicular pain or masses, history of sexually transmitted diseases and their treatments, sexual preference, interest, function, satisfaction, and problems. *Female:* Age at menarche; regularity, frequency, and duration of periods; amount of bleeding; bleeding between periods or after intercourse; last menstrual period; dysmenorrhea; premenstrual tension; age at menopause; menopausal symptoms; postmenopausal bleeding. If the client was born before 1971, exposure to diethylstilbestrol from maternal use during pregnancy. Discharge, itching, sores, lumps, sexually transmitted diseases and their treatments. Number of pregnancies, deliveries, or abortions (spontaneous and induced); complications of pregnancy; birth control methods. Sexual preference, interest, function, satisfaction; any problems, including dyspareunia (painful intercourse)

Peripheral vascular. Intermittent claudication, leg cramps, varicose veins, past history of blood clots in the veins

Musculoskeletal. Muscle or joint pains, stiffness, arthritis, gout, backache. If present, describe location and symptoms (e.g., swelling, redness, pain, tenderness, stiffness, weakness, limitation of motion or activity)

Neurologic. Fainting, blackouts, seizures, weakness, paralysis, numbness or loss of sensation, tingling or "pins and needles," tremors or other involuntary movements

Hematologic/immunologic. Anemia, easy bruising or bleeding, past transfusions and any reactions to them, status for human immunodeficiency virus infection, autoimmune disorders

Endocrine. Thyroid trouble, heat or cold intolerance, excessive sweating, diabetes, excessive thirst or hunger, polyuria

Psychobiologic. Nervousness, tension, mood, memory

Lifestyle and Health Practices Profile

Social activities, relationships, values and belief system, education and work, stress levels and coping styles, and environment

Adapted from Bickley, L. S. (2016). *Bates' guide to physical examination and history taking* (12th ed.). Wolters Kluwer; Weber, J., & Kelley, J. (2016). *Health assessment in nursing* (6th ed.). Wolters Kluwer.

addictive drugs because these drugs can create or contribute to other health problems.

The nurse compiles a list of the client's allergies, including sensitivities to drugs, foods, and environmental substances. If the client has a drug allergy, then the drug and the client's reaction are described. Some clients confuse a drug's side effects with an allergic response. If the client or family cannot remember the name of the drug, then the nurse should try to identify it from another source, such as the prescribing primary provider, pharmacy, or past hospital records.

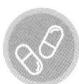

Pharmacologic Considerations

- When clients are encouraged to explain medication use in their own terms, you may discover how prescriptions are modified. For example, during the interview, you learn that an antihistamine pill prescribed for allergy relief is being used routinely as a sleep aid, taking advantage of the drowsiness side effect of the drug.

Family Health History

The family health history is important because many disorders are hereditary. The nurse asks if parents, siblings, and grandparents are living or deceased. If any blood relatives in the immediate family have passed away, then the nurse documents the causes of their deaths and the ages at which they died. The nurse identifies health problems that affect other living relatives.

Review of Body Systems for Current Health Problems

The nurse asks general questions about each body system to trigger the client's memory of inadvertently overlooked health problems. For example, when reviewing the gastrointestinal system, the nurse should ask if the client has a history of nausea, vomiting, food intolerance, bowel irregularity, stomach ulcer, changes in the color of stool, and similar questions that suggest a current or past health problem. Asking an exhaustive number of questions for each system may be unnecessary, but the review should include a few questions about each system. If the client affirms that a problem exists, the nurse asks more focused questions until they have obtained adequate data about the problem (Evidence-Based Practice 4-1).

Lifestyle and Health Practices Profile

An important focus of the interview is to determine how a client deals with their own health in terms of nutrition, exercise, medication and substance use, sleep and rest, and how the client generally engages in self-care activities. The nurse can discover how the client copes, what their support systems are, and any relevant environmental issues through using open-ended questions (Weber & Kelley, 2016).

SUMMARY AND CLOSING PHASE

An effective way of ending the interview is to summarize what occurred and thank the client for cooperating. Asking the client if they need more information provides an opportunity for the client to express concerns and ask questions. The nurse may also validate any problems or health care goals that the client discussed. The nurse can also ask if there is any information the nursing staff needs to ensure that the care is individualized and prioritized for the client. This gives the client and significant others an opportunity to share additional concerns and needs. It is also helpful for clients to feel that they have some control.

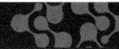

Evidence-Based Practice 4-1

Lifestyle and Health Practices Profile

Clinical Question

Should an older adult client with sudden symptoms of confusion be assessed for a urinary tract infection (UTI)?

Evidence

UTIs occur when bacteria enters the urethra and goes into the bladder. The infection can occur anywhere along the urinary tract. Older adults are at risk for UTIs due to some of the following: poor hygiene, urinary retention, diabetes, dementia, lower fluid intake, and incontinence (SeniorLiving, 2018). UTIs can cause sudden confusion or a more severe state of confusion in the older adult population or people already suffering from dementia. The client may present with a history of a sudden change in behavior that would include confusion, disorientation, falling, or agitated behavior (SeniorLiving, 2018).

Nursing Implications

Nurses are responsible for taking past, family, and current history to be included in the assessment of their clients. Having a client present with the symptoms mentioned above is critical for the nurse to document and report to the health care provider. Knowing that UTIs may cause the above symptoms will guide the nurse in taking a further history. The nurse may provide the appropriate client education, if diagnosis and treatment occur, on risks and prevention of UTIs.

Reference

SeniorLiving. (2018). *UTI's in the elderly*. Retrieved October 20, 2020 from https://www.seniorliving.org/health/uti/

THE PHYSICAL ASSESSMENT

The second part of the assessment process is the collection of objective data through a physical assessment. During the **physical assessment**, the nurse examines body structures and observes the client's physical appearance, mood, mental status, behaviors, and ability to interact. LPNs/LVNs participate in some aspects of the physical assessment but are generally limited by education and experience as well as scope of practice. Understanding the role of RNs, nurse practitioners, and primary providers is essential so that the LPN/LVN can provide explanations to the client and assist the other health care providers as they assess the client.

The physical assessment is conducted using one of two methods: the systems method or the head-to-toe method. The **systems method** approaches the examination by assessing each body system separately (Box 4-3). The **head-to-toe method** of assessment begins at the top of the body and progresses downward. Sometimes, health care providers use parts of both methods.

Assessment Techniques

There are four assessment techniques that the nurse or other health care provider performs during a physical assessment: inspection, palpation, percussion, and auscultation (Fig. 4-2).

BOX 4-3 Components of the Physical Assessment

Using inspection, palpation, percussion, and auscultation, the examiner assesses and records findings about the following attributes, body functions, and systems:

General Appraisal
Physical appearance, age, overall physical development, hygiene, grooming, posture, mobility, use of ambulatory devices, weight, height, and vital signs

Skin and Related Structures
Color, moisture, temperature, texture, turgor, skin integrity, rash, edema (swelling caused by the collection of fluid in the tissues), warts, moles, petechiae (hemorrhagic spots on the skin), distribution of body hair, condition and shape of fingernails and toenails

Head
Shape and size of head; texture, color, and distribution of hair

Eyes
External structures of the eyes (upper and lower lids, eyelashes, cornea, conjunctiva, sclera, iris, and pupil), pupil size and reaction to light, eye movement, anterior chambers of the eye, visual acuity

Lips and Mouth
Condition of the teeth and gums, oral cavity and mucous membranes, oral pharynx, tonsils, uvula

Ears
External ear (the earlobe, auricle, and surrounding tissues), tympanic membrane, hearing

Neck
Lymph nodes, thyroid, position of trachea, carotid arteries, neck veins

Thorax and Lungs
Shape of the chest, expansion, axilla (armpits), breathing patterns, respiratory rate and depth, use of accessory muscles, breath sounds

Breasts
Appearance, skin characteristics, nipples, presence of lumps or masses

Cardiovascular System
Radial pulse rate; apical pulse rate; heart sounds; blood pressure measurements in both arms while standing, sitting, and lying down; pedal pulses

Abdomen
Bowel sounds, tenderness, pain, muscle resistance or rigidity, masses, scars, hernia, liver size, spleen, kidneys, abdominal aorta

Anus and Rectum
Hemorrhoids, fissures, prostate gland in male clients, stool

Genitalia
Male: penis, scrotum, inguinal lymph nodes. *Female:* external genitalia (labia, clitoris, urethral orifice, and vaginal opening), internal structures (vaginal wall and the cervix), inguinal lymph nodes

Musculoskeletal System
Contour and size of joints, range of motion, muscle size and strength

Neurologic System
Level of consciousness; orientation; intellectual functioning; emotional state; speech patterns; short-term and long-term memory; perception of pain, heat, cold, light touch, and vibration; gait; reflexes; cranial nerves; muscle strength; movement; coordination; tendon reflexes; proprioception (or position awareness)

Inspection

Inspection is the systematic and thorough observation of the client and specific areas of the body (see Fig. 4-2A). The nurse (including the LPN/LVN who learns and practices inspection techniques) uses the senses of vision, smell, and hearing to inspect a client. Inspection includes examining the client for changes in skin color, temperature, or both; observing a wound for signs of healing or infection; or generally noting color, size, location, texture, symmetry, odors, and sounds. The technique of inspection includes the following measures (Weber, 2018):

- Expose the area being inspected while draping the rest of the client.
- Look before touching.
- Use adequate lighting.
- Provide a warm room for examination.

Palpation

Palpation is assessing the characteristics of an organ or body part by touching and feeling it with the hands or fingertips (see Fig. 4-2B). The process of palpation provides information about texture, temperature, moisture, motion, and consistency or firmness of structures (solid vs. fluid). Palpation detects abnormal conditions, such as enlarged organs, tumors, or fluid, in a cavity. When palpating, the nurse uses the fingertips to detect pulsations or to differentiate between surfaces, the surface of the palm to sense vibrations, and the back of the hand to determine temperature. Techniques for palpation include using first light and then deep palpation and palpating tender areas last (Weber, 2018). The LPN/LVN does some palpation for initial gathering of data, but generally the RN, nurse practitioner, or primary provider performs this assessment technique. The LPN/LVN assists the client to move or turn so that the examiner can more easily palpate a particular area on the client.

Percussion

Percussion is tapping a portion of the body to determine if there is tenderness or to elicit sounds that vary according to the density of underlying structures (see Fig. 4-2C). Table 4-1 provides a description of sounds that may be heard with percussion.

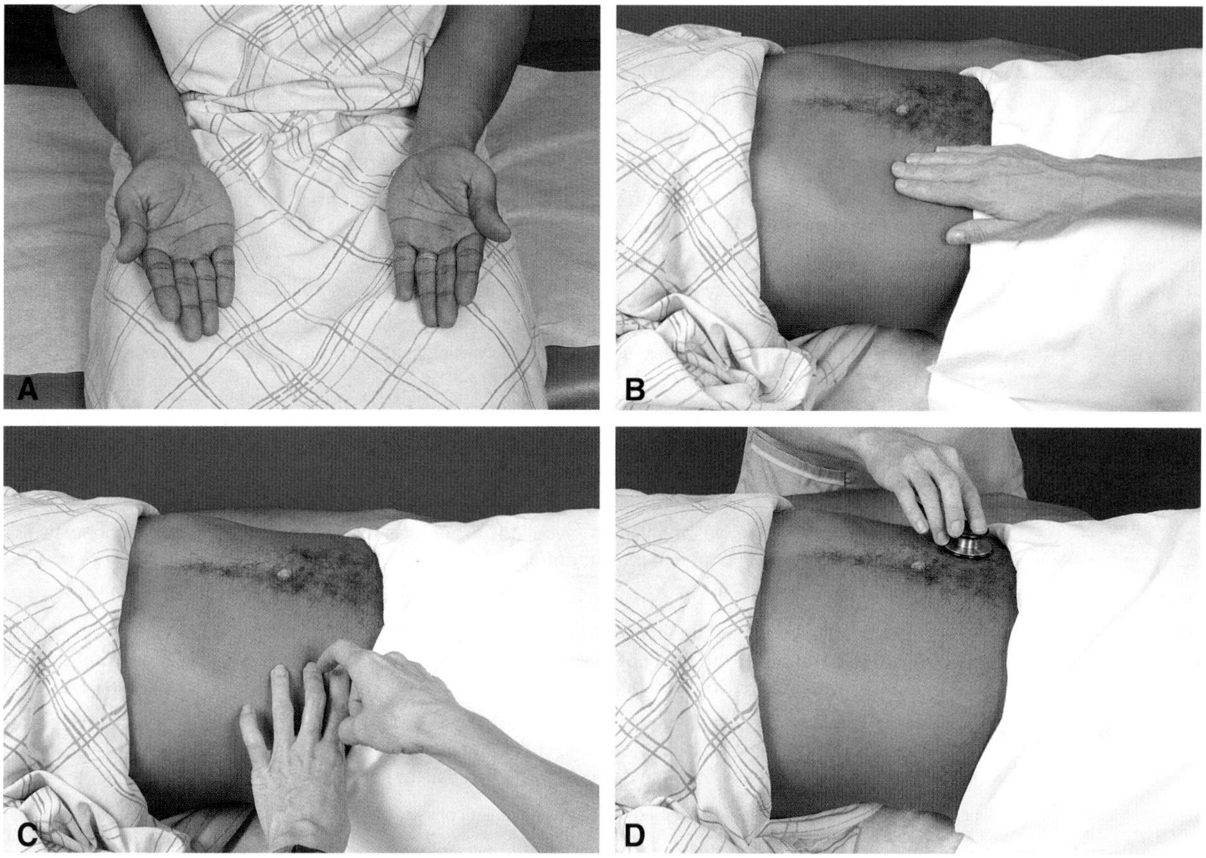

FIGURE 4-2 Assessment techniques: **(A)** inspection, **(B)** palpation, **(C)** percussion, and **(D)** auscultation.

TABLE 4-1 Sounds (Tones) Elicited by Percussion

SOUND	INTENSITY	PITCH	LENGTH	QUALITY	EXAMPLE OF ORIGIN
Resonance (heard over part air and part solid)	Loud	Low	Long	Hollow	Normal lung
Hyperresonance (heard over mostly air)	Very loud	Low	Long	Booming	Lung with emphysema
Tympany (heard over air)	Loud	High	Moderate	Drum-like	Puffed-out cheek, gastric bubble
Dullness (heard over more solid tissue)	Medium	Medium	Moderate	Thud-like	Diaphragm, pleural effusion, liver
Flatness (heard over very dense tissue)	Soft	High	Short	Flat	Muscle, bone, sternum, thigh

Reprinted with permission from Weber, J. (2014). *Nurse's handbook of health assessment* (8th ed., p. 51). Wolters Kluwer Health/Lippincott Williams & Wilkins.

The procedure for percussion is as follows:

1. Place the index or middle finger of the nondominant hand firmly on the surface to be percussed. Only the finger should have contact with skin surface. Raise the other fingers and heel of the hand off the surface.
2. Use quick, light, firm strikes with the tip of the middle finger of the dominant hand against the distal end of the nondominant finger. Use wrist motion to make tapping movements; keep forearm stable.
3. Deliver one to three taps and then move the nondominant finger to another area.

The technique of percussion requires practice and skill and is generally performed by nurse practitioners and primary providers. LPNs/LVNs assist the client to move or turn so that the examiner may more easily percuss a particular area on the client.

Auscultation

Auscultation means listening with a stethoscope for normal and abnormal sounds generated by organs and structures such as the heart, lungs, intestines, and major arteries (see Fig. 4-2D). When performing auscultation, nurses describe normal and abnormal sounds using descriptive terms such as high-pitched, low-pitched, harsh, blowing, crackling, loud, distant, and soft. They auscultate the lungs, heart, and abdomen.

Depending on the health care setting, LPNs/LVNs may auscultate breath and bowel sounds, but generally RNs, nurse practitioners, and primary providers perform this assessment technique. LPNs/LVNs assist the client to move or turn so that the examiner is able to auscultate the client more easily.

TABLE 4-2 Head-to-Toe Approach for Physical Assessments

ASSESSMENT AREA	DATA
General safety survey	**Assess:** Bed position, call bell positioning, emergency equipment, ambulatory devices, fall hazards
Vital signs	**Assess:** Temperature, pulse, respirations, blood pressure, oxygen saturation, pain assessment **Subjective data:** Have you had any pain in the last 12 hours? Are you having any pain now?
Mental status	**Assess:** Level of consciousness; orientation to person, place, and time; confusion assessment, if indicated **Subjective data:** What's the date today? Where are you?
Psychosocial	**Assess:** Client behavior and effect **Subjective data:** How do you feel today? How have you been coping with being in the hospital?
Head, eyes, ears, nose, throat, neck	**Assess:** Eyes, pupils, mouth, speech, carotid arteries, swallowing; facial color, moisture, lesions **Subjective data:** Do you wear glasses? Can I get your glasses for you? Do you use a hearing aid? Can I get your hearing aid for you?
Chest anterior/posterior	**Assess:** Chest color, moisture, lesions, quality of respirations (depth, effort, symmetry), heart sounds **Subjective data:** Have you been coughing? If yes: Is it a dry cough or have you been able to cough up sputum?
Abdomen	**Assess:** Abdomen color, moisture, lesions, bowel sounds. Inspect and lightly palpate for distension and pain/discomfort. **Subjective data:** When was the last time you ate? When was the last time you moved your bowels and/or urinated? What did your bowel movement/urine look like?
Upper and lower extremities	**Assess:** SCATTERS: **S**kin, **C**olor, **A**rteries, **T**emperature, **T**enderness, **E**dema, **R**efill, and **S**trength and Sensation
Activity	**Assess:** Client movement and ambulation **Subjective data:** Have you been out of bed? How much activity have you been able to do? Can you walk to the sink and back? Do you require assistance with toileting at this time?
Therapeutic devices	**Assess:** Peripheral and central venous access devices. Supplemental oxygen settings, pacemakers, cardiac monitor, urinary catheters, gastric tubes, chest tubes, dressings, braces, slings **Subjective data:** Are any of these devices giving you pain or concern?

Reprinted with permission from Haugh, K. H. (2015). Head-to-toe: Organizing your baseline patient physical assessment. *Nursing, 45*(12), 58–61. https://doi.org/10.1097/01.NURSE.0000473396.43930.9d.

Performing the Assessment

As stated earlier, in-depth physical assessment requires practice and skill. Nurse practitioners or primary providers perform many components of the physical assessment. The extent of the assessment performed by the LPN/LVN or RN depends on the nurse's skill, the client's condition, and facility practices. In any case, the nurse gives the client an examination gown or drape and maintains the client's privacy. They should ensure that there is adequate lighting in the examination area and gather all equipment, such as a penlight, stethoscope, and sphygmomanometer. Another important nursing measure is to maintain standard precautions (see Chapter 12). Table 4-2 provides a generic head-to-toe approach for physical assessments. Although it appears to be briefer, it is effective and efficient and promotes consistency.

Clients often feel anxiety, embarrassment, and fear when undergoing a physical examination. They are concerned about the findings and implications of those findings for their future well-being. Explaining what will happen helps the client prepare for the examination and assists in obtaining the most accurate information. The nurse should avoid showing surprise or concern at any findings to prevent increasing the client's anxiety level.

At the conclusion of the examination, the nurse allows the client to dress privately or helps the client dress if needed, helps the client get into a comfortable position, and asks if they have any questions. Finally, the nurse informs the client and family that data will be shared with the primary provider.

››› *Stop, Think, and Respond 4-2*

Refer to Table 3-1 and consider the role of the LPN when a client is having a physical assessment. For each aspect of the physical assessment, list one activity for the LPN.

KEY POINTS

- Interview and physical assessment:
  - Interview: the nurse gathers subjective data.
    - Subjective data are statements the client makes about what they feel. The client tells the nurse about nausea, pain, fear, bloating, or other feelings of discomfort.
  - Physical assessment: the nurse gathers objective data.
    - Objective data are facts obtained through observation, physical examination, and diagnostic testing.
- Three phases of the interview process:
  - Introductory phase
  - Working phase
  - Summary and closure phase
- Physical assessment database
  - Psychosocial and cultural history
  - Chief complaint
  - History of the present health concern
  - Functional status—self-care ability
  - Past health history

- Family health history
- Review of body systems for current health problems

- Lifestyle and health practices profile
  - Identify four assessment techniques:
    - Inspection
    - Palpation
    - Percussion
    - Auscultation
  - General assessment measures:
    - Ensure adequate lighting in the examination area
    - Gather all equipment, such as a penlight, stethoscope, and sphygmomanometer
    - Maintain standard precautions
    - Provides a head-to-toe approach for physical assessments

CRITICAL THINKING EXERCISES

1. How might you handle a situation in which a client's partner answers questions instead of the client? Role-play a possible nurse–client scenario.
2. How might room temperature, lighting, lack of privacy, or limited time affect the assessment of a client?
3. A client is admitted with the medical diagnosis of chronic obstructive lung disease. What focus assessment data might be essential?
4. A client admitted to a nursing facility is disoriented and confused. How might the assessment be different for this client?

NCLEX-STYLE REVIEW QUESTIONS PrepU

1. A nurse is obtaining information from a client as part of admission to the medical unit. Which of the following questions/statements is most likely to elicit more information from the client?
   1. "Do you have children living at home?"
   2. "How many packs of cigarettes do you smoke?"
   3. "Tell me why you are being admitted to the hospital."
   4. "What do you estimate is your daily beer consumption?"
2. The nurse is completing a health assessment on a newly admitted client. Which of the following documented findings is classified as subjective data? Select all that apply.
   1. "I have not had a bowel movement for 3 days."
   2. The client's blood pressure is 148/72 mm Hg.
   3. The client states that the pain is worse at night.
   4. The client voided 120 mL of dark yellow urine.
   5. The unlicensed assistive personnel (UAP) reports a temperature of 100°C.
3. A client recovering from abdominal surgery complains of feeling full and bloated after a clear liquid lunch. What type of assessment should the nurse conduct?
   1. Focus assessment
   2. Functional assessment
   3. Head-to-toe assessment
   4. Systems assessment
4. A nurse asking a client about family history is primarily interested in what aspect?
   1. The family's ability to provide emotional support
   2. The health and illnesses of close family members
   3. The location and proximity of family members
   4. The number and ages of the client's siblings
5. The nurse is preparing to interview a client who was just admitted. The client's partner mentions that the client is somewhat hard of hearing. What is the nurse's best approach when speaking with this client?
   1. The nurse asks the spouse to convey the questions to the client.
   2. The nurse faces the client and speaks slowly when asking questions.
   3. The nurse speaks loudly and sits near the client.
   4. The nurse uses a dry erase board to ask the required admission questions.
6. A student nurse is learning the process of physical examination. A nurse using palpation is most likely to detect which of the following findings?
   1. Abnormal body tenderness
   2. Abnormal lung sounds
   3. Abnormal organ size
   4. Abnormal skin color

WANT TO KNOW MORE? There are a wide variety of online resources available on thePoint to enhance learning and understanding of this chapter.

Go to **thePoint.lww.com/activate** and use the activation code found in the front of this text to unlock these online resources.

5 Legal and Ethical Issues

Words To Know

administrative law
advance directives
advocacy
anecdotal record
civil law
common law
constitutional law
criminal law
deontology
durable power of attorney (DPOA) for health care
duty
ethics
Good Samaritan laws
health care proxy
incident report
informed consent
intentional tort
laws
liability
living will
malpractice
negligence
never events
nurse practice acts
rights
risk management
sentinel events
serious reportable events (SREs)
standards of practice
state board of nursing
statute of limitations
statutory law
tort
tort law
unintentional torts
utilitarianism
values

Learning Objectives

On completion of this chapter, you will be able to:

1. Explain the difference between laws and ethics.
2. Categorize sources of U.S. law.
3. Differentiate intentional and unintentional torts.
4. Summarize negligence, malpractice, and liability.
5. Describe measures such as risk management that help limit a nurse's liability in malpractice suits.
6. Discuss the significance of sentinel events and never events, as they relate to client safety.
7. Describe procedures and regulations to protect client information.
8. Discuss informed consent, advance directives, and do-not-resuscitate orders.
9. Explain utilitarianism, deontology, duties, and rights.
10. Summarize the characteristics of ethical values.
11. Define six professional values.
12. Describe factors that affect health care ethics.
13. Explain an ethical decision-making model.

A system of laws and ethical beliefs helps to establish and maintain order and harmony within a society. **Laws** are written rules for conduct and actions. They are binding for all citizens and ensure the protection of rights. **Ethics** are moral principles and values that guide the behavior of honorable people. Ethical standards dictate the rightness or wrongness of human behavior. Box 5-1 highlights the differences between laws and ethics.

The health care delivery system affects and is affected by societal beliefs, values, and laws. It is accountable to society for maintaining established legal and ethical standards. In turn, legal and ethical situations that health care providers face also may become issues for society. Nurses today require a basic understanding of laws and ethics that may affect their practice. Issues related to competence, safety, optimal care, protecting client rights, and practicing according to professional standards of care are of most concern to nurses. This chapter provides an introduction to the legal and ethical dimensions of nursing practice.

LEGAL ISSUES IN NURSING PRACTICE

Federal and state legislation directly affects the health care industry. Laws and regulations that affect nursing practice and the safety of clients are essential for nurses to know.

BOX 5-1 Laws Versus Ethics

Laws
- Serve as rules of conduct
- Guide actions and interactions within a society
- Are regulated by authorized organizations and law officers

Ethics
- Deal with right and wrong
- Consider beliefs about morals and values
- Do not have a formal enforcement system

Gerontologic Considerations

■ Older adults often experience physical, emotional, or spiritual vulnerabilities that require assistance of health care providers. Federal and state laws regulate care provided in licensed health care facilities. These regulations address all aspects of care and include sanctions to ensure compliance.

■ The ability to give informed consent is an issue that arises every time an older adult is asked to agree to treatment or to execute an advance directive. Cognitive impairment does not automatically constitute incompetence. Older people with fluctuating cognitive status may retain sufficient ability to make some, if not all, of their health care decisions. For example, an older adult may be unable to decide to have a feeding tube but can appoint a daughter or son to make such decisions. Client and family education regarding anticipated disease trajectories may prompt discussion of client desires and designation of a trusted person to serve as the durable power of attorney (DPOA) for health care.

■ The aging process and presence of one or more chronic diseases may necessitate older adult reliance on the health care team to a greater extent than they may have in younger years. However, the older adult should always be considered as being central in care decisions rather than the recipient of care mandated by the health care team for the client. Planning with older adults and families to meet unique needs presents meaningful legal and ethical questions.

Sources of Law

Laws stem from several sources. Types of law discussed in this section include constitutional, statutory, administrative, common, criminal, and civil law.

Constitutional Law

Constitutional law is based on the constitution, which guarantees fundamental freedoms to all people in the United States. This type of law affects nurses in that it protects their basic rights, just as it protects the rights of clients. For example, freedom of speech and the right to privacy are rights that nurses and clients have as citizens of the United States.

Statutory Law

Statutory law is a law that any local, state, or federal legislative body enacts. These laws can significantly affect health care providers. For example, the "diagnosis-related group (DRG) law," described in Chapter 1, greatly influenced health care reimbursement and length of hospital stays.

Another example of statutory law is the nurse practice act in each state. **Nurse practice acts** define nursing practice and set standards for nurses in each state. These legal statutes regulate the practice of nursing to protect the health and safety of citizens. Although each state has its own nurse practice act, they all share common components:

- Define the scope of practice.
- Establish requirements for licensure and entry into practice.
- Create a board of nursing to oversee nursing practice.
- Identify legal titles for nurses, such as *registered nurse* (RN) and *licensed practical/vocational nurse* (LPN/LVN).
- Define the role and oversight of unlicensed assistive personnel (UAP), such as certified nurse aides (CNAs).
- Determine what constitutes grounds for disciplinary action.

Administrative Law

Statutory law empowers regulatory agencies to create and carry out the laws. These federal and regulatory agencies practice **administrative law**, the rules and regulations that concern the health, welfare, and safety of federal and state citizens. For example, the Occupational Safety and Health Administration (OSHA) is the federal agency that develops the rules and regulations governing workplace safety. State statutory law forms nurse practice acts, but the authority to regulate those acts is given to an administrative agency, usually called the state board of nursing.

The primary responsibility of a **state board of nursing** is to protect the public's health and well-being. Other responsibilities include reviewing and approving nursing education programs in the state, forming criteria for granting licensure, overseeing procedures for licensure examinations, issuing or transferring licenses, investigating complaints, and implementing disciplinary procedures.

Common Law

Common law, also known as judicial law, is based on earlier court decisions, judgments, and decrees. These earlier decisions set precedents for interpretation of laws. Common law evolved when courts began to present written decisions based on prior court cases. Stated another way, if one court has previously decided on a particular case and another court reviews a similar case, the second court will make the same decision, citing the precedent of the previous case. The court will make new rules if the precedent is outdated.

Criminal Law

Criminal law concerns offenses that violate the public's welfare. A crime is a violation of criminal law. There are two categories of offenses: (1) misdemeanors, which are minor offenses, and (2) felonies, which are serious offenses. Misdemeanors involving health care workers are similar to those for all citizens (e.g., driving violations). Examples of felonies involving health care workers include falsification of medical records, insurance fraud, and theft of narcotics. If an individual misrepresents themselves as a licensed nurse, this person commits the crime of practicing without a license.

Civil Law

Civil law applies to disputes that arise between individual citizens. Civil laws protect each individual's personal freedoms and property rights. Some civil laws include the right to be left alone, freedom from threats of injury, freedom from offensive contact, and freedom from character attacks. The plaintiff is the individual who brings a dispute to the court; the complaint is the formal written dispute and the restitution that the plaintiff seeks. The individual or party against whom the complaint is filed is the defendant. **Liability** means legal responsibility. If a client receives the wrong medication and is harmed as a result, the nurse is liable, or held responsible, for that harm.

Although there are various branches of civil law, tort law is most likely to affect nurses. **Tort law** is the body of law that governs breaches of duty owed by one person to another. A **duty** is an expected action based on moral or legal obligations. A **tort** is an injury that occurred because of another person's intentional or unintentional actions or failure to act. This injury can be physical, emotional, or financial. If the defendant is found to have breached their duty and that breach causes harm, they must pay restitution for damages. The types of torts that involve nurses are intentional and unintentional.

Intentional Torts

An **intentional tort** is a deliberate and willful act that infringes on another person's rights or property. Examples of intentional torts include assault, battery, false imprisonment, invasion of privacy, and defamation.

Assault and Battery. Assault is an act that involves a threat or attempt to do bodily harm. Types of assault include physical intimidation, verbal remarks, or gestures that lead the client to believe that force or injury may be forthcoming. For example, a nurse is frustrated because a client constantly turns on the call light. The nurse threatens to restrain the client's hands if they continue this action. This verbal threat constitutes assault. Battery is actual physical contact with another person without that person's consent. The contact can include touching a person's body, clothing, chair, or bed. A charge of battery can be made even if the contact did not cause physical harm to the individual.

To protect health care providers from being charged with assault and/or battery, clients sign a general permission for care and treatment at the time of admission (Fig. 5-1). They also sign a written consent before undergoing special tests, procedures, or surgery. A parent or guardian must provide consent if the client is a minor, mentally retarded, or mentally incompetent. In an emergency, health care providers can infer consent, meaning the law assumes that in life-threatening circumstances, clients would provide consent.

Nonconsensual physical contact sometimes is justified. When mentally ill or intoxicated clients are endangering their own safety and/or the safety of others, health care providers may use physical force to subdue them. The nurse must clearly document that the situation required the degree of restraint used. Excessive force never is appropriate when less force would have been just as effective. When recording these incidents, the nurse must document the behavior that resulted in the use of force and the client's response when the nurse tried lesser forms of restraint first. Health care facilities have specific requirements related to the use of physical and chemical restraints. Nurses need to adhere strictly to agency policies related to restraints.

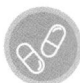

Pharmacologic Considerations

- Chemical restraints are drugs used to reduce movement or sedate a client, typically one who is unable to control their behavior. Antipsychotics (both first and second generations) and benzodiazepines are most commonly used as chemical restraints. Learn more about these drugs in Unit 17.

False Imprisonment. *False imprisonment* occurs when health care providers physically or chemically restrain an individual from leaving a health care institution. Mentally impaired, confused, or disoriented clients may be restrained if their safety or the safety of others is at risk. This confinement requires restraining orders, court-ordered commitments, or medical orders. A nurse, however, cannot detain a competent client who wishes to leave a hospital or long-term care facility before being discharged by the primary provider. If a client wishes to leave the facility against medical advice, they sign a form (Fig. 5-2) that releases the health care facility from responsibility.

The unnecessary or unprescribed application of physical or chemical restraints also creates potential liability for battery and false imprisonment. If the nurse must apply restraints and no current medical order exists, the best legal defense is to show just cause through accurate documentation. Because confined and restrained clients cannot protect themselves or meet their own needs, documentation must show that the nurse assessed the client frequently, offered fluids and nourishment, and provided an opportunity for bowel and bladder elimination. It is expected that the restraints will be discontinued when the client no longer poses a threat to self or others.

››› *Stop, Think, and Respond 5-1*

An older adult client refuses to take their medication for hypertension. The nurse informs them that if they do not take it, then their blood pressure will skyrocket, and they will have a stroke that may kill or disable them. The nurse also states that the client may need to be restrained so they will take their medication as ordered. Is the nurse threatening the client or providing important information?

Invasion of Privacy. The right to privacy means that persons have the right to expect that they and their property will be left alone. Failure to do so is an *invasion of privacy*. Nonmedical

CONSENT FOR TREATMENT

HEALTH AND MEDICAL CARE CONSENT: I give my consent to all healthcare services performed by the Medical Center, its employees, agents and affiliates, to provide such medical care (including evaluation, diagnostic procedures, medical treatment and telemedicine services) as may be deemed necessary and appropriate by my attending physician or surgeon, his/her assistants, or his/her designees. The Medical Center conducts training programs for health care professionals. These persons may be observing or participating in the Medical Center's treatment programs. They will be under the direct supervision of licensed professionals. I understand that I have the right to refuse to have trainers participated at any time, in my care. I also authorize any photographs and/or videos that may be made by my physician or care givers in order to facilitate my treatment at the Medical Center.

LEGAL RELATIONSHIP BETWEEN HOSPITAL AND PHYSICIAN: I understand that all the physicians furnishing services to me, including the emergency room physician, on-call physician, radiologist, pathologist, and anesthesiologist are independent practitioners and unless otherwise indicated, are not employees or agents of the Medical Center. I understand that my relationship with my treating physicians is initiated, continued, and/or changed by me and is at my discretion. These providers may bill separately for their services and may not be covered by your insurance.

RELEASE OF INFORMATION AND INSURANCE BENEFITS: I authorize the Medical Center and my physician to release my medical and/or financial records to individuals and entities as specified and the Notice of Privacy Practices and/or by federal and state law. I understand that the Medical Center may also release medical information about me to physicians or other health care providers who may be involved in my continued care. I understand that this authorization will remain in effect for twelve (12) months unless I revoke it, in writing. I understand that nay revocation will not be effective for disclosures necessary to effectuate payments for health care that has been provided.

ASSIGNMENT OF BENEFITS AND FINANCIAL RESPONSIBILITY: I authorize and assign direct payment of insurance benefits to the Medical Center and physicians involved in my care for all amounts due from my primary and/or supplemental insurance carrier(s). I understand and agree that I am financially responsible for payment of any charges which the insurance does not pay. I further understand, lacking timely payment by my insurance, I will be required to assume responsibility for payment of my account. If financial assistance is requested for payment of my account, I hereby give my permissions for investigation of my credit including a receipt of my consumer report from a consumer reporting agency. I understand that services are provided to me, the patient, and not my insurance company. I understand and agree that I am totally responsible for payment of all the Medical Center charges and the fees of other professional providers for care rendered to me at the Medical Center. If my bill in not pain in full thirty (30) days from the date the services are provided, I understand finance charges may be added at the rate of 1% per month, or 12% per year. I agree to be responsible for all attorney fees and court costs in collecting any sums due and owing for services rendered.

PERSONAL VALUABLES: I understand and agree that the Medical Center shall not be liable for loss or damage to personal property not deposited in the hospital safe. The Medical Center reserves the right to inventory items placed in the safe, to refuse to accept items, and to dispose of items after my discharge if unclaimed thirty (30) days after written notice is mailed to my last known address.

ACKNOWLEDGEMENTS:
________I acknowledge receipt of the Notice of Privacy Practiced on ________
________Patient Bill of Rights and Responsibilities given
________Medicare/Tricare Patient Rights and Responsibilities given

NO RESTRICTIONS
________The patient's name, facility location, and religious affiliation will be included in the Facility Directory

NAME, LOCATION, AND CONDITION RESTRICTION
________The patient's name, facility location, and condition will NOT be included in the Facility Directory
(a) If a relative, friend, or community clergy calls asking for the patient by name, they will be told "We have no information on that person."
(b) If flowers, gifts, or mail are delivered, they may be refused and returned

RELIGIOUS PREFERENCE RESTRICTION
________The patient's name, facility location, and religious affiliation will NOT appear on the Clergy Census
(a) Patient's name will not appear on the list that may be provided to community clergy, hospital trained volunteer, Eucharistic and lay ministers

RESTRICT BOTH
________The patient's name, facility location, condition, and religious affiliation will NOT be included in the Facility Directory or Clergy Census
(a) If a relative, friend, or community clergy calls asking for the patient by name, they will be told "We have no information on that person."
(b) If flowers, gifts, or mail are delivered, they may be refused and returned
(a) Patient's name will not appear on the list that may be provided to community clergy, hospital trained volunteer, Eucharistic and lay ministers

I have read this form and understand its contents. I have had an opportunity to ask questions, which have been answered to my satisfaction.

____
Patient Signature Date

____
Signature of Authorized Representative/Parent/Guardia Witness Date

Figure 5-1 Generic Hospital consent for treatment.

AGAINST MEDICAL ADVICE (AMA FORM)

This is to certify that I, ____,
a patient at ____ (fill in name of your hospital), at my own insistence and without the authority of and against the advice of my attending physician(s)
____, request to leave against medical advice.

The medical risks/benefits have been explained to me by a member of the medical staff and I understand those risks.

I hereby release the medical center, its administration, personnel, and my attending and/or resident physician(s) from any responsibility for all consequences which may result by my leaving under these circumstances.

MEDICAL RISKS

_____Death _____Additional pain and/or suffering

_____Risks to unborn fetus _____Permanent disability/disfigurement

_____Other:____
____
____

MEDICAL BENEFITS

_____History/physical examination, further additional testing and treatment as indicated.
_____Radiological imaging such as:
_____CAT scan _____x-rays _____ ultrasound (sonogram)

_____Laboratory testing _____ Potentional admission and/or follow-up
_____Medications as indicated for infection, pain, blood pressure, etc.
_____Other:____

Please return at any time for further testing or treatment.

Patient Signature__________________________ Date_________________

Physician Signature________________________ Date_________________

Witness ___________________________________ Date_________________

Figure 5-2 Example of a release form for leaving against medical advice.

torts of this nature generally include trespassing, illegal search and seizure, or wiretapping. Invasion of privacy also applies to releasing private information about a person, regardless of whether or not the information is true.

Examples of invasion of privacy in health care include photographing an individual without consent, revealing a client's name in a public report or research paper, and allowing unauthorized persons to observe a client during treatment or care. Health care providers protect a client's privacy by

- Obtaining a signed release for recognizable photographs for publications or presentations
- Using initials or code numbers instead of names in written reports or research papers
- Closing bedside curtains when giving personal care
- Obtaining a client's permission for a nursing student or other health care provider to observe treatment

Defamation. *Defamation* is an act that harms a person's reputation and good name. If a person orally utters a character attack in the presence of others, the action is called *slander*. If the damaging statement is written and read by others, it is called *libel*. Nurses must avoid offering unfounded or exaggerated negative opinions about clients, the expertise of primary providers, or other health care providers. Injury occurs because the derogatory remarks may mark a person's public image or keep potential clients from seeking the services of the defamed person. If a client accuses a nurse of defamation of character, the client must prove that there was malice, misuse of privileged information, and spoken or written untruths.

Nurses are at risk for defamation of character suits if they make negative comments in public areas (e.g., elevators, cafeterias) or assert opinions regarding a client's character in the medical record. Use of social media has escalated a nurse's risk of invading client privacy or defaming client and/or colleague character. ". . . increased access to communication through social media does not change the health care professional's responsibility to protect patient information" (National Council of State Boards of Nursing, 2012). In addition, posting any information about a client or colleague can lead to consequences, such as legal issues and job loss.

Unintentional Torts

Unintentional torts involve situations that result in injuries, although the person responsible did not mean to cause any harm. Types of unintentional torts involve negligence and malpractice.

Negligence describes the failure to act as a reasonable person would have acted in a similar situation. If harm results from the action or failure to take action, a person may sue that individual for negligence. For example, a homeowner fails to repair a broken step or warn a visitor to be careful. The visitor falls and suffers an injury. The jury decides if another reasonable, prudent person would have repaired the step and/or warned the visitor to be careful.

The law defines **malpractice** as professional negligence. It refers to harm resulting from a licensed person's actions or lack of action. A jury must determine whether the responsible person's conduct deviated from the standard expected of others with similar education and experience. Box 5-2 provides a summary of elements that must be demonstrated for malpractice claims.

BOX 5-2 Essential Elements of Malpractice in Nursing

- **Duty:** provide a safe environment
- **Breach of duty:** where the nurse failed in complying with policy
- **Damages:** injury, illness, pain, or other harm to the client
- **Causation:** a determination of cause and effect of harm

From Nurse Together. (2020). *The four elements of medical malpractice in nursing*. https://www.nursetogether.com/4-elements-medical-malpractice-nursing/

One determination of a nurse's duty to a client involves standards of practice. **Standards of practice** are guidelines that the nursing profession establishes for the knowledge, skills, and attitudes that are required for safe nursing practice (Table 5-1). These standards evolve as research and evidence change treatments, procedures, and practices. They provide a foundation for measuring quality of care. Nurses revise their methods of delivering care as standards evolve. The level of nurse accountability and responsibility is high as they provide care to their clients. Nurses have a duty to provide professional care that is up to date and meets current established standards. Unintentional tort law holds health care providers to a higher standard than that used in negligence cases. Factors that contribute to the increased number of malpractice suits against nurses include:

- Better informed consumers
- Delegation of more tasks to UAPs
- Early discharge of clients
- Errors that result in serious consequences
- Increased willingness of clients to bring suit
- Shortage of professional nurses
- Technological advances that require greater expertise

Rather than being held accountable for acting as an ordinary, reasonable layperson, the court will determine whether a nurse acted in a manner comparable with that of their peers. For example, if a client sustains a burn from warm soaks, the nurse who failed to check the water temperature could be found liable because they violated professional standards by not checking the temperature of the water before applying the soak to the skin. Published standards, the testimony of expert witnesses, written agency policies and procedures, *The Patient Care Partnership* (Box 5-3), and standardized care plans are examples of documents that establish professional standards of care (Fig. 5-3). These help familiarize the jury with the scope of a nurse's practice.

Measures to Limit Liability

Some measures protect nurses and other health care workers from litigation (lawsuits) or provide a foundation for legal defense. Good Samaritan laws, statutes of limitations,

TABLE 5-1 American Nurses Association Standards of Practice

NURSING PROCESS COMPONENT	STANDARD	EXAMPLES OF COMPETENCIES
1. Assessment	The registered nurse (RN) collects relevant data and information related to the health care consumer' health or the condition.	1. Arranges data collection based on the health care consumer's immediate condition or the expected needs of the health care consumer or condition. 2. Uses evidence-based assessment techniques, instruments, tools, available data, information, and knowledge pertinent to the situation to identify arrangements and variances.
2. Diagnosis	The RN evaluates the assessment data to determine actual or potential diagnoses, problems, and issues.	1. Arranges diagnoses, problems, and issues based on mutually established goals to meet the needs of the health care consumer across the health–illness range. 2. Documents diagnoses, problems, and issues in a manner that enables the purpose of the expected outcomes and plan.
3. Outcomes documentation	The RN recognizes expected outcomes for a plan individualized to the health care consumer or the condition.	1. Develops expected outcomes that enable coordination of care. 2. Identifies expected outcomes as measurable goals.
4. Planning	The RN creates a plan that prescribes strategies to achieve expected, measurable outcomes.	1. Creates an individualized, holistic, evidence-based plan in partnership with the health care consumer and interprofessional team. 2. Arranges elements of the plan based on the assessment of the health care consumer's level of risk and safety needs.
5. Implementation	The RN applies the identified plan of care.	1. Demonstrates caring behaviors to develop therapeutic relationships. 2. Documents information and any modifications, including changes or omissions, of the identified plan.
A. Coordination of treatment	The RN manages care delivery.	1. Manages the components of the plan. 2. Documents the organization of treatment.
B. Health teaching and health promotion	The RN employs strategies to promote health and a safe environment.	1. Uses feedback and evaluations for the health care consumer to determine the success of the employed plans. 2. Provides anticipatory guidance to health care consumers to promote health and prevent or reduce the risk of negative undesirable health outcomes.
6. Evaluation	The RN analyzes progress toward attainment of goals and outcomes.	1. Uses ongoing assessment data to modify the diagnoses, outcomes, plan, and implementation strategies. 2. Documents the outcomes of the evaluation.

From American Nurses Association. (2018). *Nursing: Scope and standards of nursing practice* (3rd ed.). Nursebooks.org.

principles regarding assumption of risk, documentation, risk management, anecdotal records, and liability insurance can limit or reduce a nurse's liability.

Good Samaritan Laws

Many states have enacted **Good Samaritan laws**, which provide legal immunity for rescuers who provide first aid to accident victims in an emergency. The law defines an emergency as one occurring outside a hospital, not in an emergency department.

None of the Good Samaritan laws provides absolute exemption from prosecution in the event of an injury. The law still holds paramedics, emergency medical technicians, primary providers, and other health care providers who stop to provide assistance to a higher standard of care because they have training above and beyond that of laypersons. In cases where there has been gross negligence (total disregard for another's safety), individuals may be charged with a criminal offense.

BOX 5-3 The Patient Care Partnership

In 2003, the American Hospital Association updated the Patients' Bill of Rights and renamed it *The Patient Care Partnership.* It outlines what clients may expect during a hospital stay, encouraging clients and/or their significant others to ask questions and voice their concerns.

Statute of Limitations

Each state establishes statutes of limitations related to civil laws. A **statute of limitations** is the designated time in which a person can file a lawsuit. The time usually is calculated from when the incident occurred. When the injured party is a minor, however, the statute of limitations sometimes does not commence until the victim reaches adulthood. Once the period expires, an injured party can no longer sue.

Assumption of Risk

If a client is forewarned of a potential hazard to their safety and chooses to ignore the warning, the court may hold the client responsible. For example, if the client objects to having the side rails up or lowers the rails independently, the nurse or health care facility may not be held fully accountable if an injury occurs. It is essential that the nurse document that they warned the client and that the client disregarded the

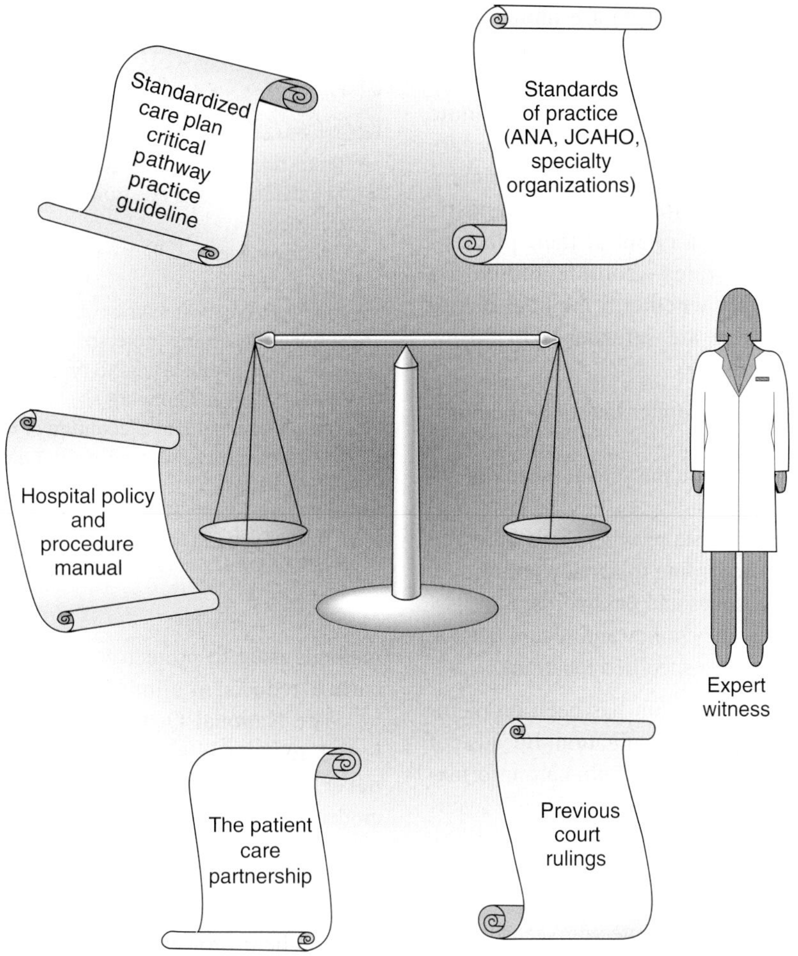

Figure 5-3 How the court establishes professional standards of care. ANA, American Nurses Association; JCAHO, Joint Commission on Accreditation of Healthcare Organizations.

warning. The same recommendation applies when nurses caution clients about ambulating only with assistance.

Documentation

A major component in limiting liability is accurate, thorough documentation. Nurses are held responsible or liable for information that they either include or exclude in reports and documentation. Each health care setting requires accurate and complete documentation. The medical record is a legal document and is used as evidence in court. Records must be timely, objective, accurate, complete, and legible. The quality of the documentation, including clarity and accurate spelling, can influence a jury's decision. Box 5-4 lists rules for legally safe documentation.

Records related to client care are essential to monitoring assessments, analysis of client data, plan of care, actions taken to treat the client, and evaluation of the client's responses to care. Each facility has its own method and process, but there is standardization in what is required, such as sequential documentation, actions taken based on assessment data, and adherence to agency policy regarding accuracy and correction of errors, use of approved abbreviations, and follow-up for client-related problems.

BOX 5-4 Rules for Legally Safe Documentation

- Follow agency procedures for written and/or electronic documentation.
- Document promptly.
- Write legibly, if not using electronic records.
- Document objectively, accurately, and concisely.
- Use only standard and accepted abbreviations.
- Correct errors according to agency policy. For electronic documentation, there are specific methods for correcting errors. For paper records, do not destroy or attempt to obliterate documentation. Using liquid erasing fluid, erasures, and heavy crossing out are not acceptable.
- Sign every entry, either electronically or as a written signature, depending on system used.
- Keep documentation free of criticism or complaints.
- Do not use statements that imply negligence. Do not indicate that an incident report was completed.
- Record the date of a return visit, cancellation, or missed appointments.
- Document all telephone conversations and follow-up instructions.

Electronic medical records (EMRs) are increasingly common and are mandated with health care reform. Advantages of EMRs are that they are clear, prevent errors through flagging of contraindicated orders, promote continuity of care, and can be shared within health care systems at the point of care. In other words, primary providers may access client hospital records, diagnostic tests, and the like when seeing a client at their place of practice. However, the same rules—confidentiality, accuracy, and timeliness—apply whether a medical record is written or electronic. There are safeguards to follow when using electronic records:

- Access client information in a manner that only the nurse and/or client can view it.
- Do not leave client information on the screen when not using the information.
- If printing client information, secure where it is kept and dispose of printed records according to agency policy.
- Maintain privacy of access codes and passwords.
- Use handheld devices per agency policy and secure them at all times (on your person or in a specified location).

The sharing of private information has been problematic for as long as there has been documentation. Because of problems related to unregulated use of health care information, the federal government implemented the Health Insurance Portability and Accountability Act (HIPAA) of 1996. The original purposes of this act include ensuring health insurance portability for people who change jobs, reducing health care fraud and abuse, guaranteeing security and privacy of health information, limiting exclusions for preexisting conditions, improving access to health insurance coverage for small employers, and enforcing standards for health information (Ellis & Hartley, 2012). In 2000, HIPAA added rules for the exchange of electronic information related to the administration of health care. Standardized electronic forms are now required for claims for health care services. The following year, HIPAA required that clients must consent to the use or disclosure of any information for treatment, payment, or health care procedures. In 2003, an amendment referred to as the *Privacy Rule* was enacted. The regulations have several major client protections, which are outlined in Box 5-5. Potential revisions expected in the next few years include "making changes that will make compliance less of a burden without negatively affecting patient privacy or decreasing the security of individuals' protected health information" (Hippa Updates, 2020).

Risk Management

Risk management, a concept developed by insurance companies, refers to the process of identifying and then reducing the costs of anticipated losses. Health care institutions that employ risk managers may use this term. The risk manager is responsible for reviewing all problems that occur at the workplace, identifying common elements, and then developing methods to reduce the risk of their occurrence. In addition, nurses must assess the client's environment and methods used to protect clients to assure that potential for harm is reduced or eliminated.

BOX 5-5 Overview of the Major Client Protections Provided by Health Insurance Portability and Accountability Act (HIPAA)

- Protection for the security of protected health information
- Standardization of electronic data interchange in health care transactions
- The privacy rule, which creates five individual client rights:
  - Right to notice of a covered entity's private practices
  - Right to request restrictions and confidential communications concerning protected health information
  - Right to obtain access to protected health information for inspection and copying
  - Right to obtain an accounting of certain disclosures
  - Right to request amendment of protected health information

From U.S. Department of Health and Human Services. (2003). *Summary of the HIPAA privacy rule*. Author.

The National Quality Forum (NQF) created a list referred to as the **serious reportable events (SREs)**, or **never events**—events that should never occur. The list includes events that are unambiguous (in other words are clearly identifiable and measurable), serious (resulting in death or significant disability), and usually preventable. There are seven identified categories: surgical, product or device, client protection, care management, environmental, radiologic, and criminal (Never Events, 2019). In addition, The Joint Commission requires the institutions that they accredit to investigate and report all **sentinel events**, which are unexpected events that result in death, or serious injury—both physical and psychological. Box 5-6 outlines categories used for improving client safety. Examples of occurrences that are considered sentinel events are listed in Box 5-7. The purpose is to increase accountability to the public, provide transparency and access to the performance of health care institutions, and outline proactive steps that are taken to prevent future occurrences.

BOX 5-6 Categories for Improving Patient Safety

Patient identification by two forms
Enhance communication between staff
Observe the five rights of medication administration
Use patient alarms safely
Practice infection control
Identify risks of patient safety
Practice enhanced safety measures in surgery

Based on The Joint Commission. (n.d.). *2020 Hospital National Patient Safety Goals*. https://www.jointcommission.org/-/media/tjc/documents/standards/national-patient-safety-goals/2020/simplified_2020-hap-npsgs-eff-july-final.pdf

BOX 5-7 Some Occurrences Considered Sentinel Events

- Surgery on the wrong body part
- Tubing and catheter misconnections
- Overdosing with commonly used anticoagulants
- Death resulting from a treatment-related or medication error
- Client suicide occurring in a setting in which around-the-clock care is provided
- Assault, rape, or homicide of patients or visitors perpetrated by staff, other patients, visitors, or intruders
- A maternal death
- Discharge of an infant to the wrong family
- Unprofessional provider behavior

Reprinted with permission from Ellis, J. R., & Hartley, C. L. (2012). *Nursing in today's world: Trends, issues & management* (10th ed., Display 10.2, p. 375). Wolters Kluwer Health/Lippincott Williams & Wilkins.

One of the primary tools of risk management is the **incident report** or event reporting form. Health care workers complete incident reports when they make or discover errors or when an event occurs that results in harm. The incident report identifies the nature of the incident (who, what, where, and when), witnesses, what actions were taken at the time, and the client's condition. The incident report is not intended to be a punitive tool but rather a means to collect data. It is factual and complete and does not include excuses for behaviors or actions. The nurse records the incident in the client's record but does not refer to the incident report because it is not part of the medical record.

Risk management also is a function of the individual nurse. Risk management for nurses includes steps that nurses take to reduce harm to clients and avoid litigation (Evidence-Based Practice 5-1). These steps include the following:

- Respecting legal boundaries of practice
- Following institutional procedures and policies
- Acknowledging personal strengths and weaknesses
- Seeking means of growth, education, and supervised experiences
- Discussing issues or problems with colleagues
- Evaluating proposed assignments and refusing to accept responsibilities for which one is not prepared
- Keeping knowledge and skills current
- Respecting client rights and developing rapport with clients
- Documenting client care accurately and thoroughly
- Working within the institution to develop and support management policies

Anecdotal Records

An **anecdotal record** is a handwritten, personal account of an incident made at the time of occurrence and updated as needed. Such records are not official but are useful in refreshing the nurse's memory. Anecdotal records may be used as evidence in court, particularly if testimony about the events that transpired is conflicting.

Evidence-Based Practice 5-1

Unintentional Torts

Clinical Question

What is the nurse's responsibility in the new era of social media and protecting client privacy?

Evidence

Social media is a way to communicate through internet websites such as Facebook, Twitter, and LinkedIn, to name a few. The use of this media has changed the way people, businesses, organizations, and the world communicate. Clients and families use the social media world to search for medical advice and support. Nurses have a responsibility to understand a safe and client-protected use of social media. Nurses should not post or share any client specific information through the form of social media. "The American Nurses Association (ANA) believes that protection of privacy and confidentiality is essential to maintaining the trusting relationship between healthcare providers and patients and integral to professional practice" (ANA, 2016).

Nursing Implications

Nurses are obligated to be professional and protect client privacy. Social media is very easy to use and readily accessible. This is sometimes challenging among the newer generations on chatting, blogging, and posting about their jobs, days, and clients. Nurses are not to compromise client privacy. They may use social media for personal use, but never to post client information. Nurses should be aware of the nurse practice act in the state they practice. The nurse practice act will describe their professional obligations.

References

American Nurses Association. (2016). *Position statement: Privacy and confidentiality.* https://www.nursingworld.org/practice-policy/nursing-excellence/official-position-statements

Liability Insurance

Today, all health care providers need liability or malpractice insurance. Liability insurance provides funds for attorney fees and damages awarded in malpractice lawsuits. All health care institutions carry liability insurance, and some may insure their employees. Nurses also should carry their own personal malpractice insurance, however; so they have a separate attorney working on their sole behalf. Because the damages sought in malpractice lawsuits are so high, the attorneys hired by health care institutions sometimes are more committed to defending the institution rather than the nurse against liability. There also have been instances in which health care facilities have countersued negligent nurses for reimbursement of damages.

Other Legal Issues

Some legal issues and regulations affect client care. Two prominent issues are informed consent and advance directives. Another issue involves do-not-resuscitate (DNR) orders.

Informed Consent

Informed consent is the voluntary permission granted by a client, or the client's assigned **DPOA for health care** (a person who legally may make medical decisions for a client) or **health care proxy**, for medical staff to perform an invasive procedure or surgery on the client. The primary provider obtains the informed consent and must inform the client of the following:

- Description of treatment, procedure, or surgery proposed
- Potential benefits
- Material risk involved
- Acceptable alternatives available
- Expected outcome(s)
- Consequences if treatment, procedure, or surgery is not done

Only competent adults may sign the informed consent form. If a person is not competent, a guardian or DPOA for health care may sign for the client. In an emergency, primary providers may invoke implied consent if the client cannot sign but is at high risk if a procedure is not done. The primary providers documents these facts in the medical record, and, in most facilities, another primary providers must verify the need for the emergency procedure.

Nurses may witness the client's signature on the consent form. The nurse must be certain that the client has the necessary information before signing. If it appears that the client is uncertain or lacks the appropriate information, the nurse must notify the primary provider. Sometimes, the nurse just needs to clarify the information and teach the client more about the procedure.

Advance Directives

The federal Patient Self-Determination Act (PSDA) of 1990 mandates that all federally funded health care facilities inform clients of their right to have and prepare advance directives. **Advance directives** provide an opportunity for clients to determine in advance their wishes regarding life-sustaining treatment and other medical care, so that their significant others will know what decisions clients desire. The two types of advance directives are the living will and DPOA for health care.

Living Will

A **living will** is a document that states a client's wishes regarding health care if they are terminally ill (Fig. 5-4). It is specific about what the client will accept and not accept for medical treatment if they are no longer competent or able to make medical decisions. The living will does not necessarily mean legal consent, but it does indicate the client's wishes. Many states provide a living will form, and there are many online sites that are easily accessed for living will forms.

Durable Power of Attorney for Health Care

A client may designate another person to be the DPOA for health care or health care proxy. This person has the authority to make health care decisions for the client if they are no longer competent or able to make these decisions. Although DPOA for health care forms are available in office supply stores, it is desirable to consult a lawyer when making these arrangements. The document may simply name the appointed person, or it may also include the client's preferences for end-of-life care.

Do-Not-Resuscitate Orders

Legally, nurses cannot act on a client's advance directive without a primary provider's order. DNR orders involve a written medical order for end-of-life instructions. If a DNR order is written, the client wishes to have no resuscitative action taken if they experience a cardiac arrest. Often, DNR instructions may be part of an advance directive, but when a client is in the hospital or other health care facility, there must be a written medical order for a "no code." Each facility should have a policy regarding DNR orders.

››› *Stop, Think, and Respond 5-2*

A primary provider tells the nurse that they informed the client about their lung biopsy scheduled for the following day, and the client needs to sign the form for the procedure to move forward. The doctor asks the nurse to take the form to the client for their signature. When the nurse asks the client if they understand what the lung biopsy will involve, the client states that after the biopsy, the spot on their lung will be gone. Should the nurse allow the client to sign the form at this time or take another action?

ETHICAL ISSUES IN NURSING PRACTICE

Nurses frequently encounter complex situations that require decisions based on determining not what is legally right or wrong but what is morally good or bad. Ethical issues do not have absolute answers. Conflicts may arise related to the desire to maintain the client's rights and yet uphold professional values and institutional policies.

For example, a mildly confused, older client has liver cancer but is expected to live at least several more months. The client eats and drinks some, but, overall, her intake is poor. Efforts to help the client drink and eat more have failed. The primary provider obtains consent from the client's DPOA for health care to place a feeding tube in the client. The primary provider asks the nurse to assist while the tube is placed. The client resists placement, and the nurse must restrain the client's hands to place the feeding tube. Because the client makes frequent attempts to remove the feeding tube, the restraints remain in place, with frequent checks by the nursing staff. In such a situation, knowing the ethically right course of action is difficult. The client receives better nutrition this way but must endure the discomfort of the tube and wrist restraints. What

Living will

If my attending physician and one other physician who examines me determine, to a reasonable degree of medical certainty and in accordance with reasonable medical standards, that I am in a terminal condition or in a permanently unconscious state, and if my attending physician determines that at that time I no longer am able to make informed decisions regarding the administration of life-sustaining treatment, and that, to a reasonable degree of medical certainty and in accordance with reasonable medical standards, there is no reasonable possibility that I will regain the capacity to make informed decisions regarding the administration of life-sustaining treatment, then I direct my attending physician to withhold or withdraw medical procedures, treatment, interventions, or other measures that serve principally to prolong the process of my dying, rather than diminish my pain or discomfort.

I have used the term "terminal condition" in this declaration to mean an irreversible, incurable, and untreatable condition caused by disease, illness, or injury from which, to a reasonable degree of medical certainty as determined in accordance with reasonable medical standards of my attending physician and one other physician who have examined me, both of the following apply:

1. There can be no recovery.
2. Death is likely to occur within a relatively short time if life-sustaining treatment is not administered.

I have used the term "permanently unconscious state" in this declaration to mean a state of permanent unconsciousness that, to a reasonable degree of medical certainty, is determined in accordance with reasonable medical standards by my attending physician and one other physician who have examined me, as characterized by both of the following:

1. I am irreversibly unaware of myself and my environment.
2. There is a total loss of cerebral cortical functioning, resulting in my having no capacity to experience pain or suffering.

Nutrition and hydration

I hereby authorize my attending physician to withhold or withdraw nutrition and hydration from me when I am in a permanent unconscious state if my attending physician and at least one other physician who have examined me determine, to a reasonable degree of medical certainty and in accordance with reasonable medical standards, that nutrition or hydration will not or no longer will serve to provide comfort to me or alleviate my pain.

____

[Sign here for withdrawal of nutrition or hydration]

I hereby designate [print name of person to decide] as the person who I wish my attending physician to notify at any time that life-sustaining treatment is to be withdrawn or withheld pursuant to this declaration.

____________________ ____________________

[Sign your name here] [Today's date]

Witness by:
[Living will person's name] voluntarily signed or directed another individual to sign this living will in the presence of the following who each attests that the declarant appears to be of sound mind and not under or subject to duress, fraud, or undue influence.

____

[First witness signs here]

____

[Second witness signs here]

Figure 5-4 Example of a living will. (Reprinted with permission from Ferrell, K. G. (2016). *Nurses' legal handbook* (6th ed.). Wolters Kluwer.)

are the benefits and harms of the feeding tube and the wrist restraints? Should the client be forced to accept a treatment that necessitates the use of physical restraints? In the following material, theories of ethical practice and an ethical decision-making model provide essential information to consider situations such as the one just described. Refer to Box 5-8 for definitions of terms related to ethics.

Theories of Ethics

Ethical theories provide a means to determine whether a particular action is good or bad. In nursing ethics, two systems or theories predominate: utilitarianism and deontology.

Utilitarianism

Utilitarianism, also referred to as *teleologic theory*, is an outcome-oriented approach for decision-making. There are

BOX 5-8 Terms Related to Ethics

Ethics: decisions regarding what is right and wrong; often a system that is used to protect the rights of individuals or groups
Code of ethics: standards of conduct and values as defined by a profession; forms the basis for ethical decision-making by a profession
Values: the ideals and beliefs held by an individual or group; usually influenced by family, society, and religion; greatly influence behavior
Morals: an individual's standards of right and wrong; formed in childhood; also influenced by family, society, and religion
Bioethics: ethical questions surrounding life and death questions and concerns regarding quality of life as it relates to advanced technology
Ethical dilemma: a situation in which an individual must choose between two undesirable alternatives; often involves examining rights and obligations of particular individuals; choice frequently defended

two important principles: "the greatest good for the greatest number" and "the end justifies the means." When individuals or groups use utilitarianism to make ethical decisions, they consider the consequences of their actions and make decisions that benefit the greatest number and harm the fewest. Furthermore, an action is not good or bad in and of itself. Instead, the consequences of the action (the end) determine whether the action (the means) was good or bad. Utilitarianism compels the individual or group to evaluate consequences. Theorists suggest that

- Consequences are good if they bring pleasure.
- The primary consideration is the outcome desired by those who are most affected.

Allocation of health care dollars provides an example of the use of utilitarianism. If a group is considering funding vaccines for many children or organ transplants for a few, the group will decide to give the money for the vaccines because a greater number will benefit.

Deontology

Another theory of ethics, **deontology**, argues that consequences are not the only important consideration in ethical dilemmas. Deontology states that duty is equally important. Duties are part of our understanding of the situations and relationships in which we find ourselves. We know intuitively that we must tell the truth, not harm someone, keep promises, return borrowed items, or help an injured person (Guido, 2014). We have an obligation to perform or avoid some actions, regardless of the consequences, because of our duties to others. For example, the deontologist would say that lying is never acceptable because it disregards one's duty to tell the truth. They would believe abortion is unethical because it violates the duty to respect and preserve life (Zerwekh & Garneau, 2015).

Implied in the concept of duties is the idea of rights. **Rights** are freedoms or actions to which individuals have a just moral or legal claim. Another individual is entitled to what we have a duty to provide. For example, a person has a right to have their belongings returned or to have promises kept. This concept is particularly important in nursing practice. Nurses have a professional duty to their clients, and those clients have a right to expect that the nurse will perform their duties.

The deontologic approach considers the rights of each person—a distinct advantage. A second advantage is that the obligation to duty and moral thinking is foremost, and thus, the decisions for similar situations are the same. Applying the deontologic method may be difficult, however, when the consequence of the decision can be harmful to an individual. For example, the decision to maintain life for all infants, regardless of the outcome, may be difficult when the infant is severely deformed and will require many invasive and expensive procedures to survive in a vegetative state.

Factors that Influence Ethical Decision-Making

Selecting a system for ethical decision-making should simplify the process; however, most nurses do not necessarily use one system or another. Other factors influence their decisions, not just knowledge of ethical theory.

Professional Values

Values are the beliefs that individuals find most meaningful. People acquire their values through societal norms, religious and cultural experiences, and life experiences. Although abstract, values become standards by which one conducts their life. Trustworthiness, honesty, reliability as a worker, and dedication are examples of values.

Professional values are principles intended to support the ethical conduct of the profession. Some of those values do not differ from personal values, whereas some may come from a person's professional education. Several professional values guide the decisions that nurses make: beneficence, nonmaleficence, autonomy, justice, fidelity, and veracity.

Beneficence

Beneficence is the duty to do good for the clients assigned to the nurse's care. This "good" includes technical competence and a humanistic, holistic approach. Stated another way, a nurse ought to prevent or remove harm and promote or do good. The nurse has a duty to remove wrist restraints whenever possible (removing a harm) and to help the client regain independence (promoting and doing good). The principle of beneficence directly supports the nurse's role of client advocacy. **Advocacy** is safeguarding client rights and supporting their interests. For example, if a client is being discharged before mastering a complicated dressing change, the nurse advocates for an additional day in the hospital or home health visits.

Nonmaleficence

Nonmaleficence is the duty to do no harm to the client. If a nurse fails to check an order for an unusually high dose of insulin and administers it, they have violated the principle of nonmaleficence. Sometimes, it is difficult to reconcile nonmaleficence with medical care because the choice of treatment may initially cause harm, even though the outcome is potentially good. For example, a client with colon cancer has a resection with a colostomy and endures the pain of surgery. In addition, the client undergoes unpleasant chemotherapy and radiation treatments. Although the client is harmed in many ways, the ultimate goal is for the client to be free of cancer. In these cases, the treatment still is ethically right because the intended effect is good and outweighs the bad effect. If the outcome is likely to be poor despite the treatment, what is ethically right may be difficult to determine.

Autonomy

Autonomy refers to a client's right to self-determination or the freedom to make choices without opposition. Nurses respect the client's right of autonomy even if the client's decision conflicts with the nurse's values. Through their advocacy role, nurses support client autonomy.

Justice

Justice is the duty to be fair to all people without prejudice, regardless of age, sex, race, sexual orientation, or other factors. The American Nurses Association Code of Ethics for Nurses has the principle of justice as its first statement. A conflict can occur if health care resources are limited or when fairness to one means discrimination to another.

Fidelity

Fidelity is the duty to maintain commitments of professional obligations and responsibilities. Such obligations and responsibilities are usually defined by nurse practice acts.

Veracity

Veracity is the duty to tell the truth. The nurse must provide factual information to the client so that they may exercise autonomy. There are potential conflicts if the family or primary provider withholds information from the client. The issues of beneficence and nonmaleficence can enter into this ethical conflict.

Legislative and Judicial Influences

Society's struggles with ethical issues result in legislative and judicial decisions that affect ethical decisions. For example, the issue of declaring death and removing life support has become more difficult with advances in technology. Often, there are examples in the news that highlight legislative and judicial involvement with decisions related to removal of life support and termination of tube feedings. Formerly, the loss of cardiac and respiratory function was the deciding factor in determining death. With greater abilities to maintain cardiac and respiratory function, however, society, through laws and judicial decisions, has redefined death. Definitions of death now encompass brain criteria, including lack of movements or breathing, absence of reflexes, a flat reading on an ECG, and unresponsiveness. Most states accept such criteria. The ethical issues for many nurses are related to their own beliefs about the dignity of life, harvesting of donor organs from an individual who is brain dead, and supporting the family members who may be asked to make decisions. The legality of brain death has removed some of the uncertainties for nurses regarding ethical issues.

Another topic that creates debate is physician-assisted suicide and euthanasia. Many people fear a prolonged and painful death. This has given rise to a movement for a legally sanctioned, medically assisted, peaceful death as an option for clients of sound mind with terminal illnesses. Nurses are committed to preserving life and also to maintaining quality of life. Nurse practice acts prohibit nurses from assisting clients to die; however, nurses have a unique understanding of client wishes and suffering. Some nurses may face dilemmas in advocating for their clients.

Influence of Technology

Developments in science and technology produce ethical issues that were unheard of even 10 years ago. Some examples include the following:

- Successful impregnation of a woman past menopause—some governments are considering age limitations for such procedures.
- Genetic engineering—such procedures may potentially harm humans, create a "perfect" being, or lead to discrimination.
- Cloning animals or humans or both—this raises difficult questions about the creation of life and individuality.
- Organ donation and stem cell research.

These advances, once in the realm of science fiction, now pose serious ethical dilemmas. Nurses definitely will play a key role in the decisions involved with these issues. They also will have particular problems if the need to promote science and progress obscures the nurse's duty to clients.

Health Care Reform

Cost control, shortened hospital stays, increased client acuity, and interest in alternative health care are factors that affect ethical decision-making. The discharge of clients to their homes when they are sicker and more vulnerable is of great concern. Issues related to the allocation of health care dollars to those who need it the most or who have the greatest potential to have a positive outcome also are ethically challenging. Nurses will face questions that make them examine their own values as they relate to providing quality care to clients and their families.

Ethical Decision-Making Process

Nurses use a problem-solving method (the nursing process) to provide care to clients. Health care providers use a similar problem-solving approach for ethical dilemmas. Nurses can use the following steps when making ethical decisions:

1. Obtain as much information as possible to understand the situation. Identify the problem and describe it. Determine what values are involved and whom the decision will affect. A statement of the dilemma (after considering all the data) helps define the issue as clearly as possible.
2. List all the possible options for solving the dilemma; this process is referred to as *brainstorming*. Do not determine the consequences at this point.
3. Examine the pros and cons of each option, foreseeing possible consequences from both a utilitarian and a deontologic approach. Consider the effects on the individual.
4. Make the decision and follow through on it.
5. Evaluate the decision in terms of effects and results.

››› *Stop, Think, and Respond 5-3*

A kidney becomes available for transplantation. The tissue matches that of an adolescent and a middle-aged client, both of whom need the organ. If you were responsible for deciding which client receives the kidney transplant, how would you decide?

Ethics Committees

Hospitals and other health care institutions often have ethics committees to help resolve ethical dilemmas and make decisions on a case-by-case basis. Ethics committees are composed of individuals with diverse backgrounds. They often include primary providers, nurses, clergy, social workers, and community members. Ethics committees establish guidelines and policies before an ethical dilemma develops. They also may be called on to act as an advocate for clients who no longer are mentally capable of making their own decisions. Ethics committees are a valuable resource for reviewing difficult cases and help ensure a careful and unbiased decision.

KEY POINTS

- Laws: are written rules for conduct and actions, for all citizens, ensuring the protection of rights
- Ethics: are moral principles and values that guide the behavior of honorable people, these ethical standards dictate the rightness or wrongness of human behavior
- Categories of U.S. law:
  - Constitutional law: is based on the constitution and guarantees fundamental freedoms to all people in the United States
  - Statutory law: is a law that any local, state, or federal legislative body enacts
  - Administrative law: the rules and regulations that concern the health, welfare, and safety of federal and state citizens
  - Common law: also known as judicial law, is based on earlier court decisions, judgments, and decrees
  - Criminal law: concerns offenses that violate the public's welfare
  - Civil law: applies to disputes that arise between individual citizens, it protects each individual's personal freedoms and property rights
- Intentional torts: is a deliberate and willful act that infringes on another person's rights or property
  - Unintentional torts involve situations that result in injuries, although the person responsible did not mean to cause any harm
- Negligence: the failure to act as a reasonable person would have acted in a similar situation
- Malpractice: professional negligence
- Sentinel events: are unexpected events that result in death or serious injury—both physical and psychological
- Never events: events that should never occur, events that are unambiguous, serious, and usually preventable
- HIPAA: national standards for the protection of individually identifiable health information by three types of covered entities: health plans, health care clearinghouses, and health care providers who conduct the standard health care transactions electronically
- Informed consent: is the voluntary permission granted by a client, or the client's assigned DPOA for health care or health care proxy, for medical staff to perform an invasive procedure or surgery on the client
- Advance directives: a client's wishes regarding life-sustaining treatment and other medical care so that their significant others will know what decisions clients desire
- DNR orders: orders written that the client wishes to have no resuscitative action taken if they experience a cardiac arrest
- Professional values: belief acquired values from societal norms, religious and cultural experiences, and life experiences. Values become standards by which one conducts their life.
- *Beneficence* is the duty to do good for the clients.
- *Nonmaleficence* is the duty to do no harm to the client.
- *Autonomy* refers to a client's right to self-determination or the freedom to make choices without opposition.
- *Justice* is the duty to be fair to all people without prejudice, regardless of age, sex, race, sexual orientation, or other factors.

- *Fidelity* is the duty to maintain commitments of professional obligations and responsibilities.
- *Veracity* is the duty to tell the truth.

CRITICAL THINKING EXERCISES

1. A confused client has attempted to get out of bed by climbing over the side rails. What actions would you take to protect yourself from being sued?
2. Consider the case of the client who needed to be restrained to receive tube feedings (presented earlier in this chapter). Discuss the ethical issues involved from the standpoint of values. Assess the situation from a utilitarian and a deontologic viewpoint using the ethical decision-making model. Do you think inserting the feeding tube and using wrist restraints were ethically good decisions?
3. You are caring for a woman client who had a hysterectomy 2 days ago. When you enter the room to administer her medications, the client's husband tells you that he has a history of high blood pressure and would like you to take his blood pressure and tell him if he needs to increase his blood pressure medication. What is your best response?
4. In the following situation, determine whether there are the necessary elements that could bring about a claim of malpractice. The LPN is working in a long-term care facility and is responsible for administering medications to 20 residents. One of the clients has a new order for a heart medication that the LPN is familiar with. The client thinks it may be a higher dose than usually ordered but does not have time to look it up and decides to give it because the primary provider who ordered it is reliable. Later that day, the client's blood pressure and pulse fall, and the client becomes unresponsive. The client is transferred to the hospital and is hospitalized for several days. It is later determined that the medication was transcribed incorrectly, and the client received twice the normal dose. The family is very unhappy and hires a lawyer.

NCLEX-STYLE REVIEW QUESTIONS PrepU

1. Two nursing students are reviewing laws that govern nursing practice. Which of the following statements best applies to nursing practice?
   1. Administrative law empowers state agencies to serve as regulators of statutory law.
   2. Civil law protects personal freedoms and property rights for all citizens.
   3. Common law is based on previous court decisions and impact future cases that are similar.
   4. Criminal law oversees unacceptable actions that include misdemeanors and felonies.
2. A friend shares with a nurse that the friend is engaged to be married. The nurse knows that the friend's fiancé has tested positive for the human immunodeficiency virus (HIV). What is the nurse's legal obligation?
   1. Advise the friend to postpone the marriage indefinitely.
   2. Inform the friend of the fiancé's HIV infectious status.
   3. Recommend that the friend be tested for HIV antibodies.
   4. Safeguard information in the fiancé's health history.
3. A practical nursing student works part-time as a UAP. The RN asks this UAP to catheterize a client because the RNs are tied up with other responsibilities. What determines if this student nurse/UAP can perform this procedure?
   1. The UAP may perform any function that requires technical competency.
   2. The UAP may perform any procedure delegated by the RN.
   3. The UAP may perform any skill that was learned in school.
   4. The UAP may perform any task included in the job description.
4. A nurse who witnesses a motor vehicle accident stops to provide emergency assistance to the injured motorists. What is most appropriate for the nurse to do to reduce the risk of liability?
   1. Avoid giving the accident victim any personal identification.
   2. Conceal the fact that they are a nurse.
   3. Let others at the scene provide direct care.
   4. Remain with the accident victim until paramedics arrive.
5. Several years ago, a client with an abdominal aortic aneurysm prepared an advance directive indicating that no heroic measures should be taken to sustain life. The primary provider wrote a "DNR" order on the medical record. Which nursing action is most appropriate if the client loses consciousness and remains unresponsive?
   1. Call the client's immediate next of kin.
   2. Call the local ambulance service.
   3. Have the client transferred to the hospital.
   4. Notify the client's attending primary provider.
6. The LPN/LVN tells the postoperative client to turn, take deep breaths, and cough every 2 hours. Which ethical value is the LPN/LVN using?
   1. Autonomy
   2. Beneficence
   3. Justice
   4. Veracity

7. Which of the following scenarios presents a potential ethical dilemma for the LPN?
   1. A client asks the nurse if there is improvement in their blood pressure results.
   2. A competent client has clearly written plans for end-of-life care.
   3. Family members request that their loved one be allowed to get up in a wheelchair.
   4. The primary provider orders a tube feeding for a terminally ill client.

WANT TO KNOW MORE? There are a wide variety of online resources available on thePoint to enhance learning and understanding of this chapter.

Go to **thePoint.lww.com/activate** and use the activation code found in the front of this text to unlock these online resources.

6 Leadership Roles and Management Functions

Words To Know
accountability
advocacy
authoritarian leadership
collaboration
delegation
democratic leadership
laissez-faire leadership
leadership
management
multicratic leadership
power
resource management
responsibility
supervision
time management

Learning Objectives

On completion of this chapter, you will be able to:

1. Differentiate between leadership and management.
2. Define three styles of leadership.
3. Outline the purpose of power in the leadership role.
4. Describe the role of the LPN/LVN in managing client care.
5. Distinguish delegation and supervision.
6. Compare responsibility and accountability.
7. Discuss problems that may occur with delegation and supervision.
8. Describe the role of the LPN/LVN in collaboration and advocacy.
9. Explain the role of the LPN/LVN in resource management.
10. Discuss methods to manage time effectively.

Licensed practical/vocational nurses (LPNs/LVNs), in their role of providing care to clients, must have skills in organizing client care, supervising care provided by unlicensed personnel, collaborating with other health care providers, managing time and resources, and being accountable for assigned client care. Although primarily educated to provide direct client care, LPNs/LVNs need a basic understanding of management and supervisory principles to function in leadership roles in various health care settings. This chapter provides an overview of theory related to leadership and management, with a focus on the role of the LPN/LVN in delegation and supervision.

LEADERSHIP AND MANAGEMENT

In many ways, leadership and management are interrelated concepts; discussing one is impossible without reference to the other. These terms, however, are not synonymous.

Leadership

Leadership involves qualities related to a person's character and behaviors as well as roles within a group or organization. It requires that a person have the ability to guide and influence another person, group, or both to think in a certain way, achieve common goals, or provide inspiration for change. Essential Qualities (2018) describes the eight essential qualities for a great leader:

- Sincere enthusiasm
- Integrity
- Great communication skills
- Loyalty
- Decisiveness

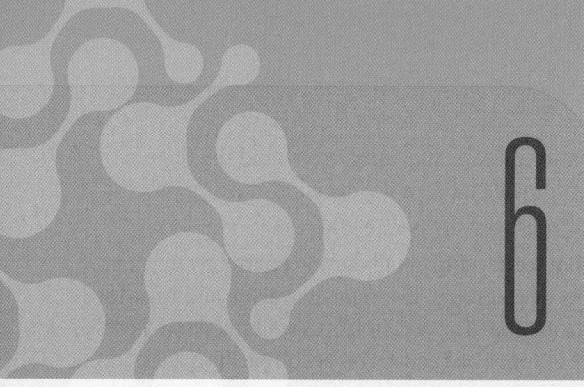

- Managerial competence
- Empowerment
- Charisma

Any health care provider has the potential to be a leader in terms of influencing a group or exercising power in a particular situation. Accordingly, LPNs/LVNs also may be leaders, informally or formally. For example, an LPN working on a medical–surgical unit may assume responsibility for organizing social events for fellow employees. A more formal leadership role would be acting as co-chairperson of the unit's staffing policy committee.

Management

Management works to guide a group of people working in an organization and coordinates their efforts toward the achievement of a common goal. The manager's overall goal is to manage and direct resources, which include workspace, supplies, equipment, budgetary concerns, and services. In addition, managers direct and coordinate the work of assigned employees. The basic functions of managers are (1) setting objectives, (2) organizing, (3) motivating the team, (4) devising systems of measurement, and (5) developing people (Career-development, n.d.). A key feature is the individual manager's responsibility and accountability for the achievement of duties.

The Relationship of Leadership and Management

To be effective, leaders and managers must possess certain qualities (Marquis & Huston, 2015):

- An ability to gain respect of others through competence and shared goals
- Expertise in communication skills, both oral and written
- A capacity to motivate others to achieve a particular purpose or accomplish goals

Ideally, a good manager is also a good leader, and a good leader is a good manager. In reality, some managers do not possess good leadership skills, and some leaders are ineffective managers. People can learn to be effective leaders and managers. Improving and developing skills through education and experience enhance a person's ability to lead and manage.

Integrated leaders/managers have traits that distinguish them from just leaders or managers:

- Thinking in the long term
- Seeing the big picture
- Influencing others outside their own group
- Emphasizing vision, values, and motivation
- Being politically astute
- Embracing change and modification

In addition, integrated leaders/managers set reasonable goals, think positively, and are willing to take risks.

Leadership Styles

Lewin (1951) identified three prevalent leadership styles that managers use, either consciously or unconsciously, to accomplish certain goals and tasks. These styles vary in the amount of control that the manager exerts and the degree of input that subordinates have in the decision-making process. The three styles include the following:

- **Authoritarian leadership** entails strong control by the manager over the work group. The manager gives and asks for little input from staff for decisions. Communication flows from top to bottom. The focus is on accomplishing tasks.
- **Democratic leadership** involves more participation in decision-making by the work group. Leaders with this style often see themselves as coworkers or colleagues, as opposed to superiors. Communication, compromise, and teamwork direct this type of style.
- **Laissez-faire leadership**, or permissive management, involves the least structure and control. The manager allows the work group to set goals, make decisions, and take responsibility for their own management.

Table 6-1 provides information about the advantages and disadvantages of the three leadership styles. Each style may be effective, depending on the particular situation. A good leader can determine which approach is best for a particular circumstance. **Multicratic or participative leadership** style combines the best of all styles, mediated by requirements of the situation at hand. The multicratic leader provides maximum structure when appropriate to the situation, asks for maximum group participation when needed, and gives support and encouragement to all members.

>>> *Stop, Think, and Respond 6-1*

A new LPN/LVN works on a long-term care unit where the nurse manager typically uses an autocratic style of leadership. What are the advantages and disadvantages of this style for the new LPN/LVN?

Power and Leadership

The leader/manager has the potential to provide guidance, direction, and support to coworkers. The leader/manager also exerts a certain power. **Power** is the ability to control, influence, or hold authority over an individual or group. People in leadership/management positions are in a position to exert power in an organization. If leadership is to be effective, a degree of power must support it.

Each type of power has a particular source or base (Table 6-2). The first type of power is *reward power*, which a person attains through the ability to grant favors or rewards. For example, organizational leaders have the ability to grant financial rewards or special favors.

Coercive or *punishment power* is the ability to threaten or punish someone who fails to meet expectations. In using such power, a manager may threaten undesirable schedules, denial of vacation time, or layoff if an employee is not compliant.

A manager exercises legitimate *power* through a designated position, which also may be referred to as *authority*. A manager has legitimate power by virtue of the management position.

TABLE 6-1 Advantages and Disadvantages of Leadership Styles

LEADERSHIP STYLE	ADVANTAGES	DISADVANTAGES
Authoritarian	Tasks are accomplished without questions. Communication is directive and flows downward. Lines of authority and policies are clear. Decisions are made quickly. Authoritarian leadership works best in bureaucracies and with employees who have limited education or training.	Subordinates have little input into decision-making or policy-making and receive little feedback or recognition. Staff members are not invested in management's goals. Leaders may create hostility and dependency. Work is highly controlled and dictated.
Democratic	Subordinates contribute to decision-making and policy-making. Staff members are invested in planning and accomplishing goals. Communication is mutual—back and forth. Employees receive regular feedback. Democratic leadership works well with competent and motivated employees.	Decisions may not occur in a timely way. Staff members may fail to acknowledge the manager's role. Employees do not recognize the need for urgent decisions that are made without staff input.
Laissez-faire	Coworkers can develop their own goals, make their own decisions, and take full responsibility for their actions. Managers provide support and freedom for employees. Subordinates perform at high levels because of their independence. Staff members share the process of making decisions for the group. Laissez-faire leadership works well with professional employees.	Employees receive little direction or guidance. Generally, decisions are not made because managers are unable or unwilling to make them. Staff members do not receive feedback regarding their performance. Communication is limited to memos. Change is rare.
Multicratic/participative	A multicratic approach combines the best aspects of the other leadership styles. Leader uses the style best suited for each situation.	New leaders must learn to employ the appropriate leadership style for each situation.

TABLE 6-2 Sources of Power

TYPE OF POWER	SOURCE OF POWER	EXAMPLE
Reward power	Ability to grant favors	Team leader making assignments
Coercive power	Fear	Head nurse scheduling vacations
Legitimate power	Position	Director of nursing
Expert power	Knowledge and skill	An LPN/LVN with 20 years' experience working on a medical unit
Referent power	Association with others	Shift supervisor
Informational power	Need for information to accomplish a goal	Merit raise information related to annual evaluations
Connection power	Nurses working together toward a goal	Nurses engaged in achieving a policy change
Motivational power	Nurses feeling stimulated to work toward a goal	Leader motivates nurses to participate in implementing a new system of documentation

LPN/LVN, licensed practical/vocational nurse.
Adapted from Stegen, A., & Sowerby, H., (2019). *Nursing in today's world: Trends, issues, and management* (11th ed.). Wolters Kluwer.

Expert power results from knowledge, expertise, or experience in a particular area. Managers typically possess expert power through education and work experience.

Referent power concerns the power a person has because of their association with others who are powerful. For example, society perceives that primary providers are powerful. A new primary provider may use this referent power to their advantage. Referent power may also be called *charismatic power*, referring to personal characteristics such as charisma, the way a person talks or acts, the people they associate with, or the organizations to which they belong.

Another type of power is *informational power*, which exists when a person has information that others need to accomplish certain goals. Examples may relate to budget preparation, planning for educational events, or making changes in an organization.

Connection power involves the use of networking or involving more than one person to work collaboratively toward a common goal. *Motivational power* refers to a leader's ability to create enthusiasm for a collaborative project or achievement of a common goal.

Leaders and managers may exercise power to accomplish assigned tasks. They also must have the authority or legitimate right to direct and guide work. A nurse in an authorized position (e.g., team leader, charge nurse) can exert power in a positive way.

THE LICENSED PRACTICAL/ VOCATIONAL NURSE AS LEADER/ MANAGER

Usually, managers are appointed to or hired for a specific management position. In health care, however, the term *manager* may be used more broadly, in that nurses manage the care of clients. This role involves overseeing the care that a client receives. Other health care providers may actually care for the clients. In acute care settings, registered nurses (RNs) are assigned to a group of clients. An LPN/LVN and certified nursing assistant (CNA) may work with the RN and be responsible for certain aspects of client care. The RN, as the manager of care, ensures that the LPN/LVN and CNA complete all assigned tasks, assess the clients, and evaluate the effects of nursing interventions.

In other health care settings, the role of the LPN/LVN may be extended. For example, in long-term care settings, LPN/LVNs may be team leaders and thus assigned to oversee the work of unlicensed assistive personnel (UAP). In medical offices, an LPN/LVN may be the office manager, coordinating certain aspects of the office work such as scheduling and coordinating work assignments. These roles require the LPN/LVN to delegate responsibility for certain tasks and then supervise the accomplishment of the work.

Primary Leadership and Management Functions

Primary functions of LPN/LVNs as leaders/managers include *delegation*, *supervision*, *responsibility*, and *accountability*.

Delegation

The National Council of State Boards of Nursing (NCSBN) and American Nurses Association (ANA) in joint statement guidelines maintain that the "delegation process is multifaceted, and it begins with the administrative level of the organization including determining nursing responsibilities that can be delegated, to whom, and what circumstances; developing delegation policies and procedures; periodically evaluating delegation processes; and promoting positive culture/ work environment" (Nursing Delegation, n.d.). The ability to guide, teach, and direct others is integral to the ability to delegate.

There are direct and indirect client care activities that may be delegated to UAPs. Direct care activities are those that assist clients to meet basic needs, including vital signs, weights, specimen collection, and ambulation. Indirect activities are more focused on environmental tasks, such as cleaning equipment, emptying trash or soiled linen receptacles, and delivering meal trays.

Nurses need to learn delegation skills. The NCSBN (2019, p. 4) identified the following five rights of delegation:

1. Right task
2. Right circumstances
3. Right person
4. Right direction/communication
5. Right supervision/evaluation

Evidence-Based Practice 6-1

Supervision

Clinical Question

Why is delegation an important part of nursing practice?

Evidence

In 2019, the ANA and NCSBN described delegation in nursing practice as nurses making a decision to direct another individual to perform a duty or task that nurses usually complete (NCSBN, 2019). Nurse practice acts vary from state to state. Some states allow LPNs to supervise and delegate, whereas others do not. RNs and LPNs practice at different levels and regulations. Delegation may be used with UAP; however, both RNs and LPNs must know their scope of practice in the state in which they are licensed to provide safe care.

Nursing Implications

Nurses are accountable for their practice. Delegation directs part of the responsibility of care to another person. However, the responsibility lies with the RN or LPN who has the authority to delegate. It is the RN's or LPN's responsibility to know the nurse practice act for the state in which they practice and make sure they are responsible and supervise the care being delegated. "Ignorance of the law is not an excuse to not follow the Nurse Practice Act. Nurses are responsible to know the details of the NPA in the states where they practice. Nurses can be held accountable when they, even mistakenly, violate NPA standards" (Registered Nursing, n.d.).

Reference

Registered Nursing. (n.d.). *How is the scope of practice determined for a nurse?* https://www.registerednursing.org/answers/how-scope-practice-determined/

National Council of State Boards of Nursing. (2019). *National guidelines for nursing delegation.* https://www.ncsbn.org/NGND-PosPaper_06.pdf

The five rights of delegation resemble the steps required for the nursing process:

- *Assess the situation*: know the client's needs, the skills of the UAPs, and the priorities. Match the UAPs' skills with the tasks to be completed (Evidence-Based Practice 6-1).
- *Plan actions*: identify the UAPs who will best handle the delegated tasks.
- *Implement the plan*: communicate expectations clearly to UAPs, including what they need to do, what to watch for, and potential problems.
- *Evaluate the results*: ensure that tasks are completed according to standards.

Box 6-1 provides tips for delegating successfully. Part of succeeding at delegating involves the process of supervision.

Supervision

Supervision involves making appropriate judgments about clinical assignments and delegation of tasks and then following up to see that tasks were effectively accomplished. Delegation and supervision are tightly connected because once a nurse has delegated a task, they are obligated to supervise

BOX 6-1 Tips for Delegating Successfully

- The employer must identify a nurse leader responsible for oversight of delegated responsibilities for the facility.
  - The designated nurse leader responsible for delegation must determine which nursing responsibilities may be delegated, to whom and under what circumstances.
  - Policies and procedures for delegation must be developed.
  - The employer/nurse leader must communicate information about delegation to the licensed nurses and UAP and educate them about what responsibilities can be delegated.
  - All delegates must demonstrate knowledge and competency on how to perform a delegated responsibility.
  - The nurse leader responsible for delegation must periodically evaluate the delegation process.
  - The employer/nurse leader must promote a positive culture and work environment for delegation.

National Guidelines for Nursing Delegation. https://www.ncsbn.org/NGND-PosPaper_06.pdf. Reprinted with permission from National Council of State Boards of Nursing.

the person assigned to that task. In reviewing the steps of delegation described in the previous section, supervision begins when the LPN/LVN implements the plan. The implementation step includes giving instructions about what needs to be done and when. The nurse must include any specific issues, such as telling the UAP that a client must complete morning care before going for physical therapy at 10 A.M. In addition, the nurse needs to tell the UAP about any potential problems, such as a client who may experience dizziness when getting up secondary to antihypertensive medications.

Supervision is also necessary throughout the implementation step. The LPN/LVN must check with UAPs during the shift to assess whether tasks are complete, what the outcome is, whether something has changed that may interfere with the work, or whether the UAP is having problems accomplishing the task safely.

The evaluation step of delegation also includes supervision of the UAP in that the LPN/LVN ensures that the client received the appropriate care, that the client's needs were met, and that problems were addressed. Providing feedback to UAPs is also important in terms of letting them know that they did a good job or asking questions about the client's response to the care provided.

Delegation and supervision imply that the people carrying out these functions assume responsibility and accountability for their actions as well as the actions of those to whom they delegate. The next section defines these concepts. See the Evidence-Based Practice 6-1.

Responsibility and Accountability

Responsibility is a duty or assignment related to a specific job. It means being obligated to perform certain activities and duties. When a person is responsible for something, they are required to ensure that the assignment or job is completed.

Accountability means being answerable for the consequences of one's actions or inactions. The term *liability* (see Chapter 5) is closely associated with accountability because of the legal implications. Tasks an LPN/LVN delegates to a UAP remain the responsibility of the LPN/LVN, who must ensure that the task is appropriate for the UAP and that the UAP has the knowledge and skills to complete the task. The LPN/LVN is accountable for determining whether the task is accomplished and if there are any issues associated with completing or not completing the task. In addition, the LPN/LVN is also accountable for evaluating the results of the tasks. The UAP is responsible for performing the actual task.

››› *Stop, Think, and Respond 6-2*

An LPN is the team leader for 20 clients on a long-term care unit. They delegate to an experienced UAP the task of feeding supper to an older client. When the UAP feeds this client, the client begins to cough and choke, aspirating some food. The client eventually develops pneumonia and must be hospitalized for 1 week. Who is responsible for this incident?

Challenges to Leading and Managing

LPNs/LVNs may experience some problems with delegation and supervision of tasks. In part, this is because LPNs/LVNs may not be well prepared for the role of team leader. Schools of practical/vocational nursing traditionally have focused primarily on the direct caregiver role. In turn, employers may not plan for LPNs/LVNs to be team leaders or other managers of care, but out of necessity place LPNs/LVNs in these roles. Other factors that may interfere with effective delegation and supervision are as follows:

- Reluctance to delegate from fear of overloading a coworker or the desire to do everything
- Inability to move out of the role of direct caregiver—"It is easier to do it myself"
- Miscommunication regarding specific directions and desired outcomes
- Desire to be liked by coworkers, which interferes with ability to delegate or supervise or both

In addition, LPNs/LVNs are not strictly supervisors, in that they do not have the authority to hire or fire. They may have responsibility for overseeing and directing the care that UAPs provide, but they do not have the responsibility for disciplining them.

Solutions for improving one's ability to delegate and direct UAPs include obtaining education for this role. In addition, LPNs/LVNs must focus on client care needs first. In this way, the LPN/LVN ensures that clients receive appropriate care and that tasks are carried out efficiently and in a caring manner. If an LPN/LVN remains responsible and accountable for their actions, it assists them in learning to delegate and direct responsibly.

Other Functions

Although LPNs/LVNs as team leaders have the primary responsibility of delegating tasks to UAPs, other functions are important for the LPN/LVN leader/manager. These functions include collaboration, advocacy, resource management, and time management.

Collaboration

Collaboration involves a team effort to achieve client care outcomes. Although RNs often direct collaborative efforts, LPNs/LVNs are responsible for directing the care of UAPs. As a team member and leader, LPNs/LVNs maintain open and effective communication with all team members. They also assist in solving problems related to client care. LPNs/LVNs may contribute to decisions about client care and unit activities by participating in client care conferences and unit meetings. Lastly, collaborative behavior for the LPN/LVN involves participating in the management of the unit by following the appropriate channels of communication and supporting the group in collaborative efforts.

Advocacy

Advocacy means promoting the cause of another person or organization. In health care, advocates support the needs of a client or organization. Nurses in general act on behalf of their clients. The *Code of Ethics for Nurses* (ANA, 2015, p. 9) states, "The nurse promotes, advocates for, and protects the rights, health, and safety of the patient." LPNs/LVNs function as client advocates by (Benyon, 2020):

- Ensuring safety
- Giving clients a voice
- Educating
- Protecting client's rights
- Double checking for errors
- Connecting clients to resources

Resource Management

Resource management, the responsibility of all who work in health care, means using resources, which include not only actual money but also supplies, equipment, buildings, and personnel, optimally. Nurses who provide direct care may not have a direct role in formulating budgets, but they are responsible for controlling the use of resources and recognizing when resources are inadequate. In addition, they must know the costs of resources and the importance of using cost-effective measures when caring for clients.

Many factors are related to the rising costs of health care (Box 6-2). In general, new technologies increase costs, which leads to the need for better facilities and, it is hoped, better outcomes for client care. Related costs are salaries for health care providers, newer and more expensive medications, and equipment. As a result of increased costs, health care providers are expected to be more cost conscious. Cost-conscious measures include prudent use of expensive supplies, knowledgeable operation of medical equipment, careful monitoring of clients to reduce potential complications and lengths of stay, heightened awareness of practicing measures that reduce costs, essential knowledge of all costs of caring for clients, and deliberate reduction of waste of limited resources.

A provision in the Patient Protection and Affordable Care Act has created a financial penalty for excessive unplanned readmissions within 30 days for clients with chronic obstructive lung disease (COPD), acute myocardial infarctions (AMIs), heart failure, pneumonia, or stroke, as well as surgical clients after coronary artery bypass graft (CABG) or hip/knee replacements. This program has the potential to increase costs and reduce revenues to hospitals. Nursing staff and other health care providers will be even more accountable for implementing and maintaining standards of care.

Acuity measures are frequently used by inpatient facilities to collect data that quantify costs of services. "Acuity . . . refers to the severity of the illness and the rapidity of change in the client, and thus the intensity of medical and nursing care and other therapies required" (Ellis & Hartley, 2012, p. 230). The acuity values or intensity measures may be used to determine staffing needs. Nurses frequently assign the points used for staffing decisions. In addition, the acuity measures may also be used for billing clients based on the required care. In any sense, the use of acuity measures has a direct impact on nurses and the management of resources.

Time Management

Time is an essential resource, particularly in today's fast-paced health care environment. **Time management** involves organizing time as well as delegating tasks to other personnel and essentially optimizing available time. Five basic steps for managing time are learn how to set priorities, be flexible and patient, cluster care, create the mental space to implement your time management skills by arriving early, and take a break when you need it (Time Management, 2018).

The onset of managed care increased the focus on efficiency and productivity. Making the most of one's time is an important skill that takes effort to achieve. Although, on chaotic days, it may seem that nothing works, those who are most effective at managing time will have the most success in accomplishing the work that needs to be done. New nurses usually need to learn to organize their time. The following techniques are useful in learning to manage time:

- Assess expectations for the shift. Do so in a chart that identifies specific periods (e.g., 30-minute increments). This can also be done after a shift to determine how one spent time that particular day and how it might help organize another shift.

BOX 6-2 Factors Involved in Rising Health Care Costs

- Price of new technology
- Construction of new facilities
- Higher survival rates leading to greater need for costly intensive or long-term care
- Growing population of the older adults requiring health care
- Increase in salaries for health care providers
- High costs of drugs and health-related equipment

Reprinted with permission from Ellis, J. R., & Hartley, C. L. (2012). *Nursing in today's world: Trends, issues & management* (10th ed., p. 226). Wolters Kluwer Health/Lippincott Williams & Wilkins.

- Use a worksheet to identify specific tasks and important assessments that need to be done for that particular shift. This works very well with multiple client assignments. Organize the worksheet according to each client. Many nurses refer to this as a "to-do" list or "brain sheet." They use the worksheet not only to identify tasks but also to write quick notes to jog their memories for further tasks or assessments.
- Prioritize tasks that need to be accomplished (Box 6-3). Reprioritize as needed.
- Write things down to remember later for documenting and reporting. Many nurses use their worksheet as a report sheet for the oncoming shift.
- Develop efficiency and the ability to multitask, which means engaging in more than one task at a time. For example, if a client requests pain medication and you need to assess their roommate's vital signs, bring the needed equipment as well as the pain medication.
- Delegate appropriate tasks to appropriate personnel.

Most people readily admit that they do not always make good use of their time and then have to scramble to complete tasks. Box 6-4 identifies some "time wasters." These essentially include an inability to plan, procrastination, chatting, allowing low-priority tasks to take precedence, inability to delegate appropriately, and difficulty saying "no." Assessing what wastes one's time is an important step in using time more effectively.

BOX 6-3 Criteria for Setting Priorities

1. Items critical to maintaining life: Think in terms of your cardiopulmonary resuscitation basics.
   - Essential assessment
   - Airway management
   - Breathing support
   - Circulation needs
   - Neurologic stability
2. Critical symptom management: What is important to the client?
   - Pain management
   - Relief of nausea
   - Relief of diarrhea
   - Relief of severe anxiety
3. Items needed to progress in health restoration: What orders has the primary provider written? What nursing plans have been developed?
   - Medication and fluid administration
   - Completing treatments
   - Preventing complications
   - Meeting nutritional needs
4. Items needed to move toward self-care
   - Teaching
   - Contacting referral needs
   - Meeting psychosocial needs
   - Creating comfort and feelings of well-being
   - Bathing
   - Changing linens

Adapted from Ellis, J. R., & Hartley, C. L. (2009). *Managing and coordinating nursing care* (5th ed.). Wolters Kluwer Health/Lippincott Williams & Wilkins.

BOX 6-4 Time Wasters

- Poor planning
- Inability to delegate
- Procrastination
- Socializing
- Unwillingness to say "no"
- Poor communication
- Inefficient use of time
- Failure to write things down
- Haste
- Repetitive paperwork
- Unclear direction
- Management by crisis

KEY POINTS

- Leadership: involves qualities related to a person's character and behaviors as well as roles within a group or organization. It requires that a person have the ability to guide and influence another person, group, or both to think in a certain way, achieve common goals, or provide inspiration for change
  - Authoritative: entails strong control by the manager over the work group
  - Democratic: involves more participation in decision-making by the work group
  - Laissez-faire (permissive management): involves the least structure and control; the manager allows the work group to set goals, make decisions, and take responsibility for their own management
  - Multicratic/participative: provides maximum structure when appropriate to the situation, asks for maximum group participation when needed, and gives support and encouragement to all members
- Management: ability to guide a group of people working in an organization and coordinates their efforts toward the achievement of a common goal
  - Five rights of delegation determine each person's ability and responsibility:
    1. Right task
    2. Right circumstances
    3. Right person
    4. Right direction/communication
    5. Right supervision/evaluation
  - Supervision: involves making appropriate judgments about clinical assignments and delegation of tasks and then following up to see that tasks were effectively accomplished
- Compare:
  - *Responsibility* is a duty or assignment related to a specific job, it means being obligated to perform certain activities and duties
  - *Accountability* means being answerable for the consequences of one's actions or inactions
  - *Colloboration* involves a team effort to achieve client care outcomes
  - *Advocacy* means promoting the cause of another person or organization

- Managing time effectively: time management is an essential resource, particularly in today's fast-paced health care environment, it involves organizing time as well as delegating tasks to other personnel and essentially optimizing available time.
  - Five basic steps for managing time:
    - Learn how to set priorities.
    - Be flexible and patient.
    - Cluster care.
    - Create the mental space to implement your time management skills by arriving early.
    - Take a break when you need it.

CRITICAL THINKING EXERCISES

1. An LPN is a team leader on a skilled care unit. When they return from dinner break, the UAP reports the following:
- One client vomited after receiving their 6 P.M. medications.
- A family member is upset that their mother pulled out her feeding tube and that it has not been replaced.
- A client's catheter seems to be leaking.
- A primary provider wants to order medications for the new client who had hip replacement surgery 2 weeks ago.

Prioritize these tasks—indicate what the LPN should attend to and what they can delegate.

2. An LVN is planning to change jobs from an acute care setting to a long-term care facility. They are concerned about their role in the new job as a team leader. They know that they will be working with UAPs. What should they know about their role in delegating tasks to UAPs if they take this new job?

3. An experienced LPN works nights at a rehabilitation hospital. As a charge nurse, the LPN is reluctant to delegate to the two UAPs because they are afraid the work will not be done right. As a result, this LPN is frequently stressed and feeling like they cannot keep up. What strategies could they employ to better utilize the UAPs and feel better about delegation of tasks?

4. The LVN provides appropriate direction as they delegate a task to the UAP. However, the UAP makes an error that causes injury to the client. Who is responsible?

NCLEX-STYLE REVIEW QUESTIONS PrepU

1. An LPN/LVN student is reviewing the different leadership styles. Which of the following examples best describes an authoritarian manager?
1. The manager allows the staff to determine client assignments.
2. The manager seeks consensus from the staff in a new policy.
3. The manager sends frequent directives to staff via e-mail.
4. The manager supports and encourages the staff in all situations.

2. The RN delegates a wound irrigation and dressing change to the LPN/LVN. The LPN/LVN has never done this particular type of wound irrigation but is hesitant to seek help. Which right of delegation did the RN neglect?
1. Right task
2. Right circumstances
3. Right person
4. Right communication

3. The LPN/LVN on the day shift is assigned a UAP to care for 12 clients on a skilled care unit. Which of the following tasks is most appropriate for the LPN/LVN to delegate to the UAP?
1. Assess the incision on a new client with a knee replacement.
2. Assist a newly admitted client to the bathroom.
3. Check the glucose level on a client who is difficult to arouse.
4. Take vital signs on all of the assigned clients.

4. An LPN/LVN expresses interest in leadership opportunities at the long-term care facility where they work. In recognition of the LPN/LVN's role, which of the following steps are appropriate? Select all that apply.
1. Apply for staff development position.
2. Chair staff education committee for unlicensed personnel.
3. Serve as night shift team leader.
4. Volunteer to organize staff holiday gatherings.
5. Write formal evaluations of co-assigned UAPs.

5. The RN asks the LPN/LVN to administer an oral pain medication to a client. Which statement by the LPN/LVN is correct?
1. "As an LPN/LVN, I am responsible for my own actions."
2. "Giving medications to another person's client is not appropriate."
3. "The RN is responsible for any delegated care."
4. "This task is not one that the RN should delegate."

WANT TO KNOW MORE? There are a wide variety of online resources available on thePoint to enhance learning and understanding of this chapter.

Go to **thePoint.lww.com/activate** and use the activation code found in the front of this text to unlock these online resources.

UNIT 2
Client Care Concerns

7 Nurse–Client Relationships

Words To Know

ad hoc interpreters
affective learner
affective touch
andragogy
caregiver
certified interpreter
cognitive learner
collaborator
comfort zone
communication board
deaf
delegator
educator
electrolarynx
empathy
expressive aphasia
finger spelling
formal teaching
geragogy
hard of hearing
hearing
informal teaching
intimate space
introductory phase
kinesics
learning capacity
learning needs
learning readiness
learning style
limited English proficiency
listening
motivation
nonverbal communication
nurse–client relationship
paralanguage
pedagogy
personal space

Learning Objectives

On completion of this chapter, you will be able to:

1. List four roles that nurses perform within the nurse–client relationship.
2. Describe four phases in a nurse–client relationship.
3. Differentiate between verbal, nonverbal, and therapeutic communication.
4. Give examples of therapeutic and nontherapeutic communication techniques.
5. List and explain five components of nonverbal communication.
6. Name and explain the four proxemic zones.
7. Explain what is meant by a client's "comfort zone."
8. Differentiate between task-oriented and affective touch.
9. Name three groups of clients for whom alternative communication modalities are required.
10. List six factors to consider before teaching clients.
11. Explain the learning styles of cognitive, affective, and psychomotor learners.
12. Compare informal with formal learning.
13. Discuss three techniques for evaluating learning comprehension.

The word *relationship* refers to an association between two or more people that develops over time. "The nurse-client relationship is conducted within boundaries that separate professional and therapeutic behavior from non-professional and non-therapeutic behavior. A client's dignity, autonomy and privacy are kept safe within the nurse-client relationship" (Nurse Client Relationship, n.d.). This chapter explores the scope of the nurse–client relationship, provides guidelines for effective interpersonal communication, and identifies principles for client teaching.

Words To Know (*continued*)

preinteraction phase
proxemics
psychomotor learner
public space
social space
task-oriented touch
teaching plan
telephonic interpreting
terminating phase
therapeutic communication
verbal communication
video interpreting
webcam
working phase

Gerontologic Considerations

- Preliminary information of the client's age may lead to assumptions regarding cognitive, physical, or interactive abilities (ageism). The nurse must be aware of the wide variation in function and abilities and carefully assess for strengths and needs of individual older adults.
- An appreciation of the older adult as an individual with unique needs and concerns is the foundation of a positive nurse–client relationship. Avoid using "older adult speak" that includes terms of endearment (e.g., honey, sweetie) and plural identity (e.g., "Let's take our medicine"), which can be perceived as patronizing or disrespectful.
- Take time to listen actively to the older adult and allow ample time for responses to questions; remember that the health history of an older adult may span more than 80 years. Involving support persons such as family or friends may be particularly important when establishing a relationship with the older client, especially if their memory is impaired. However, older adults may have preferences whether or not to include a particular support person in discussions or may be able to state a preference for which person is preferred to be included, even if some cognitive deficits exist.
- Potential sensory changes in older clients can pose a barrier to verbal communication. Older adults tend to lose the ability to hear high-pitched ranges, so it is best to lower the voice pitch when speaking, use a normal volume, and clearly enunciate consonants, especially at the beginning and ending of words.
- Communicate with hearing-impaired adults by using the client's preferred method of enhancing communication, such as writing, pictures, or sign language.
- When an older adult repeatedly tells the same story or asks the same question, make an effort to determine whether there is a hidden or unspoken fear or concern that the older adult is too apprehensive to discuss. For example, a client may repeatedly ask if you have gotten groceries for the week. A life review may reveal that the client had life segments of poverty during which obtaining food was unpredictable.
- In working with older adults who have English as a second language (ESL) or strong regional accents, hearing impairment may be assumed when what is more helpful is clarifying meaning of words by using synonyms or acting out motions to clarify meaning.
- This chapter discusses the use of touch in the nurse–client relationship. However, there is scant evidence to support the use of touch with an older adult. Therefore, touch should be used purposefully to reinforce verbal messages or in a manner that is culturally appropriate to convey concern or support. However, older adults may perceive touch as culturally inappropriate, offensive, or threatening. Frailty or vulnerability may also have an impact on the client's perception of touch; therefore, nursing judgment must be used in each situation.
- When communicating with older clients, assume a seated position if needed to establish horizontal eye level rather than standing above or over a client, which places the client in a position of vulnerability.
- Encourage the older client to reminisce. Ask about past events and relationships associated with positive experiences and feelings. Giving older adults an opportunity to talk about earlier times in their lives reinforces their value and unique identity. An older adult may desire to discuss past life events and lessons learned in an effort to leave a legacy or make a difference in the life of significant others, including health care providers. Be aware of the possibility that reminiscing may evoke painful memories or unresolved developmental tasks, which may lead to a need for referral for more in-depth counseling.

SCOPE OF THE NURSE–CLIENT RELATIONSHIP

The term *professional relationship* in this chapter refers to the association between nurses who bring knowledge and unique clinical skills that "protect, promote, and optimize health and abilities, prevent illness and injury, alleviate suffering, and advocate in the care of individuals, families, communities, and populations" (American Nurse Association [ANA], 2010b, p. 3). The **nurse–client relationship** exists during the period when the nurse interacts with clients, sick or well, to promote or restore their health, help them to cope with their illness, or assist them to die with dignity.

Communicating therapeutically, listening empathetically, sharing information, and providing client education are among the most basic processes that occur in the context of the nurse–client relationship. As in any effective relationship, each party has unique responsibilities to the other (Box 7-1).

Nursing Roles Within the Nurse–Client Relationship

The nurse–client relationship requires the nurse to respond to the client's needs. The National Council of State Boards of Nursing, which develops the National Council Licensure Examination for Practical Nurses (NCLEX-PN), identifies four categories of client needs as the structure for its test plan: (1) safe and effective care environment, (2) health promotion and maintenance, (3) psychosocial integrity, and (4) physiologic integrity. These content areas are consistently applied within nursing practice regardless of the stage in the client's life span or the setting for health care delivery.

To meet client needs, nurses perform four basic roles: caregiver, educator, collaborator, and delegator. Table 7-1 illustrates how these basic nursing roles correspond to examples of the client needs categories within the NCLEX-PN test plan.

BOX 7-1 Nurse–Client Responsibilities

Nursing Responsibilities

Possess current knowledge
Be aware of unique age-related differences
Perform technical skills safely
Be committed to the client's care
Be available and courteous
Allow client to participate in decisions
Remain nonjudgmental
Advocate on the client's behalf
Provide explanations in language that is easily understood
Promote independence

Client Responsibilities

Identify current problem
Describe desired outcomes
Answer questions honestly
Provide accurate historical and subjective data
Participate to the fullest extent possible
Be open and flexible to alternatives
Comply with the therapeutic regimen
Keep follow-up appointments

The Nurse as Caregiver

A **caregiver** is one who performs health-related activities that a person with sickness cannot perform independently (Fig. 7-1). The nurse's caregiving skills help to restore wellness, especially during an acute illness, or to maintain as

TABLE 7-1 Integration of NCLEX-PN Test Categories With Nursing Roles

CATEGORY	SUBCATEGORIES	NURSING ROLE
Safe and effective care environment	Coordinated care *Example:* Assigning assistive personnel to provide client care	• Collaborator • Delegator
	Safety and infection control *Example:* Ensuring availability and safe functioning of client care equipment	• Caregiver • Collaborator • Educator
Health promotion and maintenance	*Example:* Assisting clients with life transitions such as assisted living	• Caregiver • Collaborator • Educator
	Example: Identifying and educating clients in need of immunizations	• Caregiver • Educator • Collaborator
Psychosocial integrity	*Example:* Using therapeutic communication techniques *Example:* Providing care or support for client and family at the end of life	• Caregiver • Collaborator
Physiologic integrity	Basic care and comfort *Example:* Providing nonpharmacologic measures for pain relief	• Caregiver • Collaborator • Delegator
	Pharmacologic therapies *Example:* Reinforcing client teaching on possible effects of medications	• Educator
	Reduction of risk potential *Example:* Collecting specimens for diagnostic testing	• Caregiver • Delegator • Collaborator
	Physiologic adaptation *Example:* Responding to a client's life-threatening situation	• Caregiver • Delegator • Collaborator

NCLEX-PN, National Council Licensure Examination for Practical Nurses.
Adapted from National Council of State Boards of Nursing. (2020). *2020 NCLEX-PN detailed test plan.* National Council of State Boards of Nursing. Reprinted with permission from National Council of State Boards of Nursing.

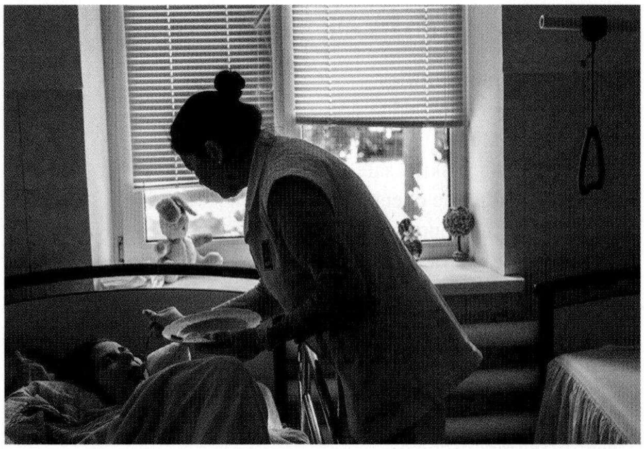

Figure 7-1 Nurses in the role of caregiver. (Source: shutterstock.com/Liukov)

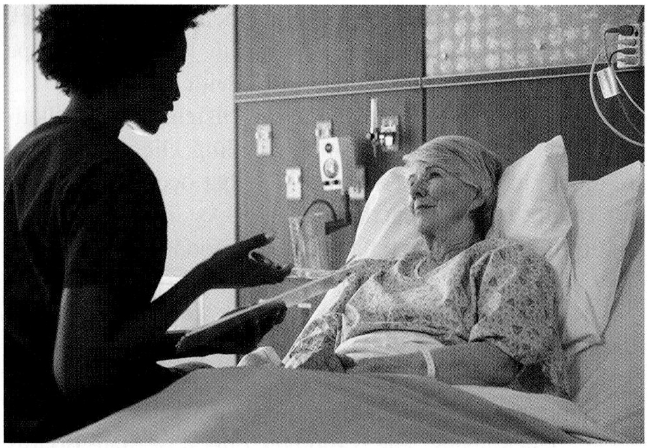

Figure 7-3 A nurse in the role of educator provides information to a client. (Source: shutterstock.com\MonkeyBusinessImages)

much function and independence as possible for a client with chronic physical or mental health problems.

Traditionally, nurses have been providers of physical care; however, caring also involves a close emotional relationship. Contemporary nurses understand that illness and injuries cause feelings of insecurity that may threaten a person's ability to cope. Consequently, the nurse becomes the client's guide, companion, and interpreter. The supportive relationship that develops establishes trust and reduces fear and worry.

Nurses use **empathy**, an intuitive awareness of what the client is experiencing, to perceive the client's emotional state and need for support (Fig. 7-2). Empathy helps the nurse become effective in providing for the client's needs while remaining compassionately detached.

>>> *Stop, Think, and Respond 7-1*

When you are assigned to one or more clients during clinical experience, what kinds of caregiving skills do you perform?

The Nurse as Educator

An **educator** is one who provides information. Nurses offer health teaching that is pertinent to each client's needs and knowledge base. Some examples include explanations about diagnostic test procedures, self-administration of medications, techniques for managing wound care, and restorative exercises such as those performed after a mastectomy (Fig. 7-3).

When it comes to treatment decisions, the nurse avoids giving advice, reserving the right of each person to make their own choices on matters affecting personal health and illness care. Instead, the nurse shares information on potential alternatives, allows the client the freedom to choose, and supports the client's ultimate decision.

Because nursing is considered a practice "without walls" (i.e., extending beyond the original treatment facility), nurses are resources for information about health services available in the community. This type of information empowers clients to become involved with self-help groups or those that offer rehabilitation, financial assistance, or emotional support.

The Nurse as Collaborator

A **collaborator** is one who works with others to achieve a common goal. Usually, many people are involved in a client's care (Fig. 7-4). The most obvious example of collaboration

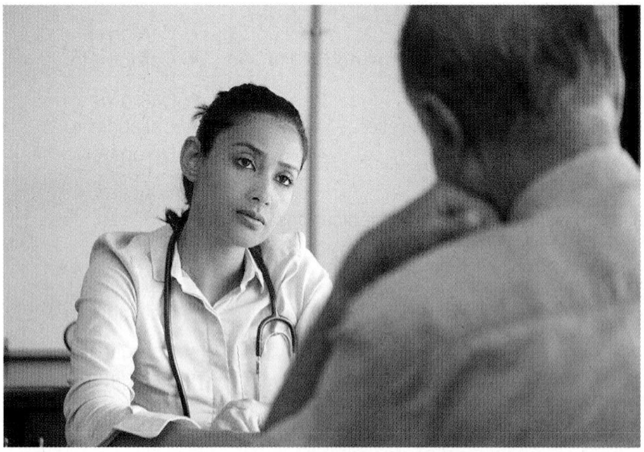

Figure 7-2 A nurse uses empathy during an interaction. (Source: shutterstock.com\AandNPhotography)

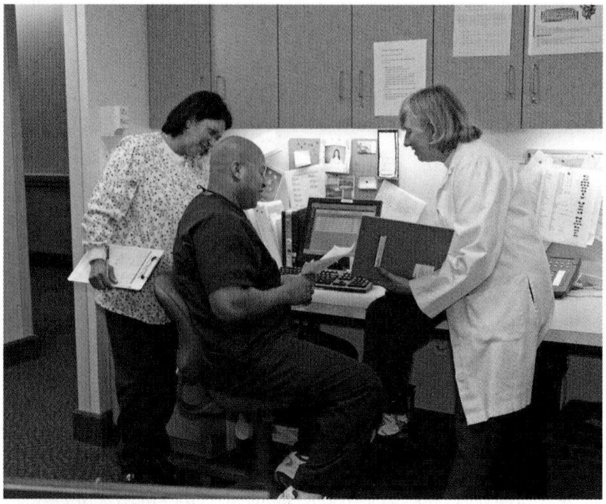

Figure 7-4 A nurse in the role of collaborator involves other members of the health care team.

occurs between the nurse who is responsible for managing care and those to whom the care is delegated. Collaboration also takes place when the nurse and primary provider share information and when they exchange information with other health care providers, such as the dietitian, physical therapist, respiratory therapist, and discharge planner.

>>> ***Stop, Think, and Respond 7-2***

What health care providers might be involved in managing the care of a client with a stroke?

The Nurse as Delegator

A **delegator** is one who assigns a task to someone (Fig. 7-5). Before assuming the role of delegator, the nurse must consider five basic aspects of delegation. The nurse must know what tasks are appropriate for particular health care providers. It is unsafe to delegate a task to someone who does not have the knowledge or expertise to perform it correctly. Once a task has been assigned, it is still the delegator's responsibility to check that the task has been performed and to determine the resulting outcome. For example, if a nurse asks a nursing assistant to change a client's position, the nurse must verify that the assistant has completed the job and obtain other pertinent information such as the condition of the client's skin. If the delegated task is not performed or is performed incorrectly, the nurse is held accountable for the inadequate client care.

>>> ***Stop, Think, and Respond 7-3***

What tasks might a staff nurse delegate to a student nurse?

Phases of the Nurse–Client Relationship

A nurse–client relationship is the culmination of interactions over a period of time. Its primary focus is to help clients achieve self-care and independence using knowledge and skills that are grounded in evidence-based nursing practice.

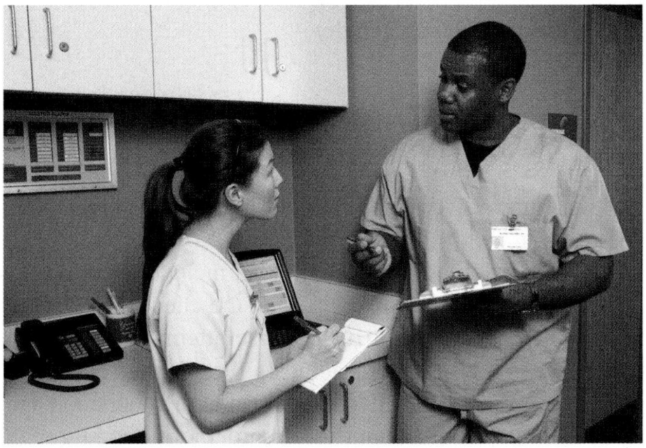

Figure 7-5 A nurse delegates tasks to a coworker.

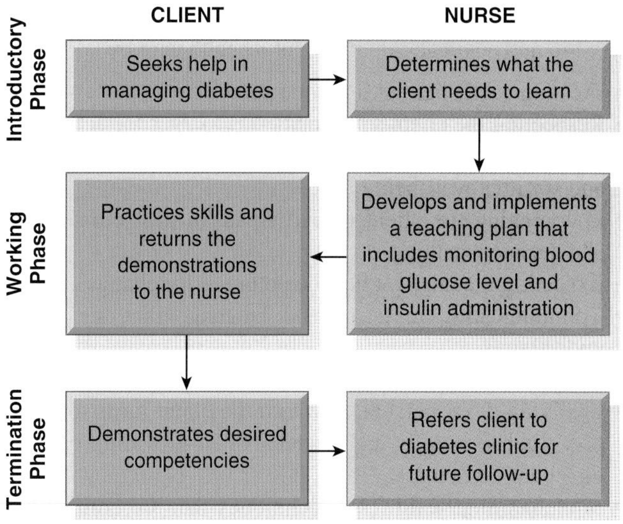

Figure 7-6 Examples of activities related to phases of the nurse–client relationship.

The nurse–client relationship progresses through several phases. The relationship initially begins in what has been called the **preinteraction phase** because it occurs before the nurse's first contact with the client. Once an interaction with clients takes place, the relationship progresses through three additional phases: the introductory phase, the working phase, and the terminating phase. Figure 7-6 gives an example of the activities that occur in each of the three interactive phases.

Preinteraction Phase

Prior to meeting with the client, the nurse prepares for the interaction. The first nursing action is to gather preliminary information about the client such as the initial diagnosis and age of the client. Previous medical records are potential sources of additional information. Other health care providers who have cared for the client may contribute more data as well.

Once the admitting diagnosis is identified, the nurse begins to formulate expectations of various problems the client may be experiencing. To validate the nurse's hypothetical predictions, the nurse selects a location that is appropriate for interviewing the client and allots sufficient time to accomplish a predetermined goal.

Introductory Phase

The **introductory phase** starts when the nurse and the client get acquainted and the client identifies one or more health problems for which they are seeking care. Both the nurse and the client bring preconceived ideas about the other to the initial interaction, and these assumptions eventually are confirmed or dismissed. Initial contact may begin with an exchange of names and a handshake if appropriate. Before calling a person by their first name, the nurse should obtain permission or wait to be invited to use a more familiar form of address, which some cultures reserve for family and close friends. The nurse demonstrates courtesy, active listening, empathy, competence, and appropriate communication skills to convey that they value the client. Nurses demonstrate partnership and advocacy in the client's health care by

- Treating each client as a unique person
- Respecting the client's feelings
- Striving to promote the client's physical, emotional, social, and spiritual well-being
- Encouraging the client to participate in problem-solving and decision-making
- Expecting that a client has the potential for change
- Communicating in terms and language that the client understands
- Using the nursing process to individualize the client's care
- Involving those persons to whom the client turns for support, such as family and friends, when providing care, if the client consents
- Implementing health care techniques that are compatible with the client's value system and cultural heritage

Working Phase

The **working phase** involves mutually planning the client's care and putting the plan into action. Both the nurse and the client participate. Each shares in performing those tasks that will lead to the desired outcomes identified by the client. During the working phase, attending to a client's personal dietary preferences demonstrates a respect for the unique characteristics of each person, which enhances the nurse–client relationship. The nurse supports the client's independence by allowing the client to pace their own care, even when this requires more time. Doing too much for the client is as harmful as doing too little. Allowing independence in self-care and decision-making promotes self-esteem and dignity.

Terminating Phase

The **terminating phase** occurs when the nurse and client mutually agree that the client's immediate health problems have improved and that the nurse's services are no longer necessary. Regression, evidenced by increased reliance on nursing assistance or the reemergence of physical symptoms, may indicate an underlying fear of having to assume independent responsibility for self-care. Initially, the nurse must ensure that the client is not developing health-related complications. Thereafter, a compassionate and caring attitude helps facilitate the client's transition to independent living or transfer to other health care services.

COMMUNICATION

Communication is an exchange of information. It involves both sending and receiving messages between two or more individuals. It is followed by feedback, indicating that the information is understood or needs further clarification (Fig. 7-7). The NCLEX includes questions and examples that relate to the use of therapeutic communication with clients.

In addition, The Joint Commission, the largest and most prestigious organization that accredits health care agencies in the United States, sets standards that promote high-quality, safe, and effective care across all health care settings. Several current standards and goals are specific to communication. Examples include the following:

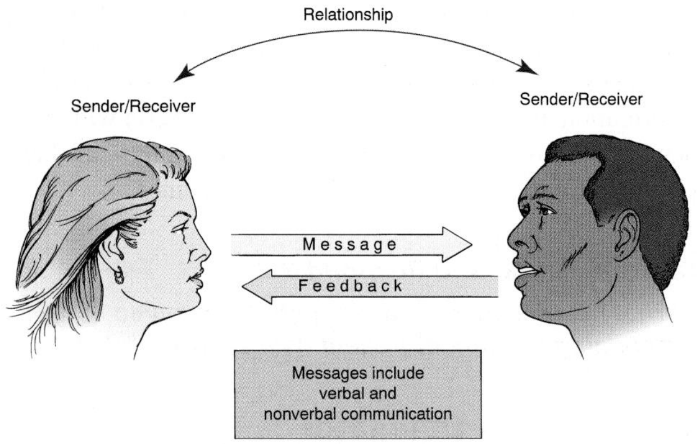

Figure 7-7 Communication is a two-way process.

- Demonstrate leadership commitment to effective communication, cultural competence, and client-/family-centered care.
- Improve the effectiveness of communication among caregivers.
- Encourage active involvement of clients in their own care as a client safety strategy.

Therefore, understanding principles of communication is essential for developing an effective nurse–client relationship, successfully passing the nurse licensure examination, and promoting sustained accreditation among health care organizations that employ nurses.

Verbal Communication

Verbal communication is communication that uses words. It includes speaking, reading, and writing. The following variables affect verbal communication between clients and nurses and other health care providers:

- Attention and concentration
- Language compatibility
- Verbal skills
- Hearing and visual acuity
- Motor functions involving the throat, tongue, and teeth
- Noise and distracting activity
- Interpersonal attitudes
- Literacy
- Cultural similarities
- Listening

Listening is as important during communication as speaking. In contrast with **hearing**, which refers to perceiving sounds, **listening** is an activity that includes attending to and becoming fully involved in what the client says. Empathetic listening implies that the nurse attempts to perceive the client's emotions and meanings. When the nurse conveys empathy to clients, it helps them to feel both understood and valued. Empathetic listening is often demonstrated through nonverbal means.

When communicating with most American clients, it is best to position oneself at the client's level and make frequent eye contact (see section "Culturally Influenced Characteristics" in Chapter 8). Nodding and encouraging the client to continue with comments, such as "Yes, I see," conveys interest in what the client is saying. The nurse guards against sending messages that indicate boredom, such as looking out a window or interrupting a comment.

Nonverbal Communication

Nonverbal communication is the exchange of information without using words. It is what is not said. Nonverbal communication consists of components such as kinesics, paralanguage, proxemics, touch, and silence. Table 7-2 lists examples of nonverbal behaviors and their meanings.

>>> ***Stop, Think, and Respond 7-4***

What nonverbal message is communicated when a person wears a white lab coat, a ring on the third finger of the left hand, or a badge and gun?

Kinesics

Kinesics refers to body language, or those collective nonverbal techniques that include facial expressions, postures, gestures, and body movements. Even clothing style and accessories (e.g., jewelry) can affect the context of communication.

Knowledge of kinesics is important for the nurse who is being evaluated by their clients and vice versa. The following are suggestions to create a positive impression during a nurse–client interaction:

- Stand tall.
- Relax arms, legs, and feet; do not cross any body part.
- Maintain eye contact approximately 60% to 70% of the time or as much as is appropriate for the culture (see Chapter 8); in a group, focus on the last person who spoke.
- Keep your head level both horizontally and vertically.
- Lean forward slightly to demonstrate interest and attention.
- Keep the arms where they can be seen.
- Strike a balance in arm movements, being neither too demonstrative nor too restrained.
- Keep the legs as still as possible.

TABLE 7-2 Examples of Body Language and Interpretations

BODY LANGUAGE	INTERPRETATION(S)
Positive	
Tilt of head	Interested
Open hands	Sincere
Brisk, erect walk	Confident
Hand to cheek	Contemplative
Rubbing hands	Anticipatory
Steepled fingers	Authoritative
Nod	Agreement
Negative	
Arms crossed	Blocking; oppositional
Clenched jaw	Angry; antagonistic
Downcast eyes	Remorseful; bored
Rubbing nose	Doubtful; deceitful
Drumming fingers	Impatient
Fondling hair	Insecure
Frown	Disagreement
Stroking chin	Stalling for time
Shifting from foot to foot	Desire to get away
Looking at watch	Bored

Paralanguage

Paralanguage refers to vocal sounds (not actually words) that communicate a message. Some examples include drawing in a deep breath to indicate surprise, clucking the tongue to show disappointment, and whistling to get someone's attention. Crying, laughing, and moaning are additional forms of paralanguage. Vocal inflections, volume, pitch, and rate of speech add yet another dimension to communication.

Concept Mastery Alert

Nonverbal Communication

Gestures and touch, such as smiling or rubbing a client's shoulder, are examples of how a nurse can practice therapeutic nonverbal communication when caring for a client and family who are awaiting the results of a diagnostic test. Listening to a client's frustration is also important but is considered verbal, not nonverbal, communication.

Proxemics

Proxemics refers to the use of space when communicating. In general, four proxemic zones are common when Americans communicate. The zones include **intimate space**, **personal space**, **social space**, and **public space** (Table 7-3).

Most Americans feel comfortable when strangers are 2 to 3 feet away, a distance that is often compromised within a nurse–client relationship. Determining the circumference of a person's **comfort zone**, the area that when intruded upon does not create anxiety, is important because physical closeness is common during nursing care. Approaches that relieve a client's anxiety about being close include explaining beforehand how a nursing procedure will be performed and ensuring that the client is properly draped.

Touch

Touch is a tactile stimulus produced by personal contact with another person or object. In the context of nursing, touch is task oriented or affective or both (Fig. 7-8). **Task-oriented**

TABLE 7-3 Proxemic Zones

ZONE	DISTANCE	PURPOSE
Intimate space	Within 6 inches	Lovemaking Confiding secrets Sharing confidential information
Personal space	6 inches to 4 feet	Interviewing Physical assessment Therapeutic interventions involving touch Private conversations
Social space	4–12 feet	Teaching one-on-one Group interactions Lecturing Conversations that are not intended to be private
Public space	12 feet or more	Giving speeches Gatherings of strangers

touch involves the personal contact that is required when performing nursing procedures. **Affective touch** is used to demonstrate concern or affection. Its intention is to communicate care and support. Most people respond positively to being touched; however, a nurse should use affective touching cautiously because there is a great deal of variation in responses among individuals. In general, nurses use affective touch therapeutically when a client is lonesome; uncomfortable; near death; anxious, insecure, or frightened; disoriented; disfigured; semiconscious or comatose; visually impaired; or sensory deprived.

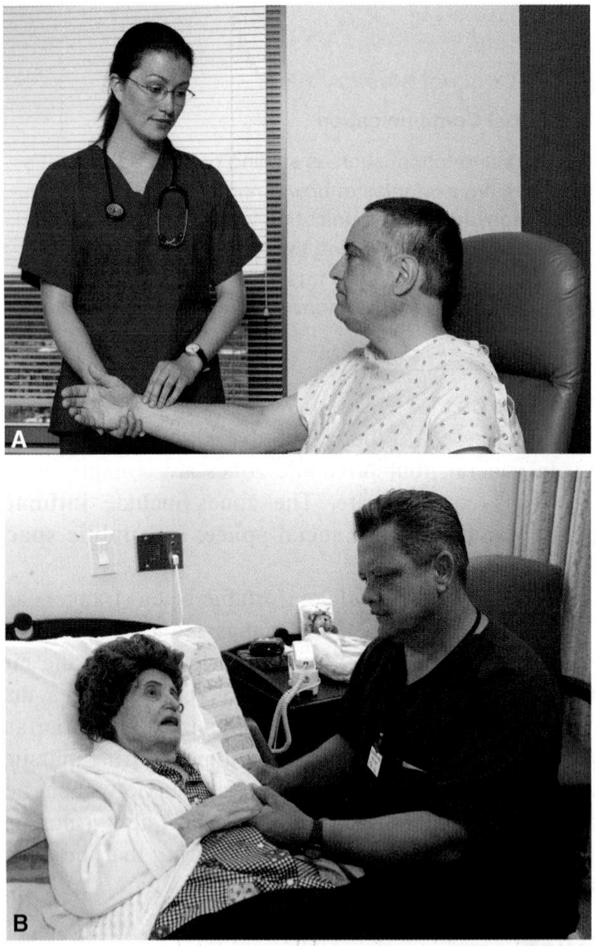

Figure 7-8 Types of touch: **(A)** Task-oriented touch. **(B)** Affective touch. (Reprinted with permission from Carter, P. J. (2012). *Lippincott's textbook for nursing assistants: A humanistic approach to caregiving* (3rd ed.). Wolters Kluwer Health/ Lippincott Williams & Wilkins.)

Silence

Silence is the art of remaining quiet. One of its therapeutic uses is to encourage a client's verbal communication. Other therapeutic uses include providing a personal presence and a brief period during which clients can process information or respond to a question.

Therapeutic Communication

Communication occurs on a social or a therapeutic level. **Therapeutic communication** refers to using verbal and nonverbal communication to promote a person's physical and emotional well-being. Techniques that are helpful are identified in Table 7-4.

››› *Stop, Think, and Respond 7-5*

Give an example of a therapeutic response to the following statement made by a client: "My family didn't visit me last evening."

When the client is quiet and uncommunicative, the nurse must avoid assuming that the client has no problems or understands everything. On the other hand, it is never appropriate to probe or press an unwilling client to communicate. It is best to wait for a response; reserved clients may share their feelings and concerns after they feel that the nurse is sincere and trustworthy.

The nurse must also respond delicately to a vocal and emotional client. For instance, when clients are angry or cry, the best nursing approach is to allow them to express their emotions without fear of retaliation or censure.

Although nurses have the best intentions of interacting therapeutically with clients, some fall into traps that block or hinder therapeutic communication. Table 7-5 lists common examples of nontherapeutic communication.

Communicating With Special Populations

Some clients, such as those who are verbally impaired or deaf, or those who have limited knowledge of English or none at all, have special communication needs that must be met to ensure client safety. According to The Joint Commission (2010), caregivers must

- Identify if the client has a sensory or communication need.
- Identify and address communication needs during assessment, treatment, discharge and transfer, and end-of-life care.
- Monitor changes in the client's communication status.
- Anticipate the communication needs of clients who are expected to develop communication impairments from scheduled treatments or procedures.

TABLE 7-4 Therapeutic Communication Techniques

TECHNIQUE	USE	EXAMPLE
Broad opening	Relieves tension before getting to the real purpose of the interaction	"Wonderful weather we're having."
Giving information	Provides facts	"Your surgery is scheduled at noon."
Direct questioning	Acquires specific information	"Do you have any allergies?"
Open-ended questioning	Encourages the client to elaborate	"How are you feeling?"
Reflecting	Confirms that the nurse is following the conversation	*Client:* "I haven't been sleeping well." *Nurse:* "You haven't been sleeping well."
Paraphrasing	Restates what the client has said to demonstrate listening	*Client:* "After every meal, I feel like I will throw up." *Nurse:* "Eating makes you nauseous, but you don't actually vomit."
Verbalizing what has been implied	Shares how the nurse has interpreted a statement	*Client:* "All the nurses are so busy." *Nurse:* "You're feeling that you shouldn't ask for help."
Structuring	Defines a purpose and sets limits	"I have 15 minutes. If your pain is relieved, I could go over how your test will be done."
Giving general leads	Encourages the client to continue	"Uh, huh" or "Go on."
Sharing perceptions	Shows empathy for how the client is feeling	"You seem depressed."
Clarifying	Avoids misinterpretation	"I'm afraid I don't quite understand what you're asking."
Confronting	Calls attention to manipulation, inconsistencies, or lack of responsibility	"You're concerned about your weight loss, but you didn't eat any breakfast."
Summarizing	Reviews information that has been discussed	"You've asked me to check on increasing your pain medication and getting your diet changed."
Silence	Allows time for considering how to proceed or arouse the client's anxiety to the point that it stimulates more verbalization	

TABLE 7-5 Nontherapeutic Communication Techniques

TECHNIQUE AND CONSEQUENCE	EXAMPLE	IMPROVEMENT
Giving False Reassurance		
Trivializes the client's unique feelings and discourages further discussion	"You've got nothing to worry about. Everything will work out just fine."	"Tell me about your specific concerns."
Using Clichés		
Provides worthless advice and curtails exploring alternatives	"Keep a stiff upper lip."	"It must be difficult for you right now."
Giving Approval or Disapproval		
Holds the client to a rigid standard; implies that future deviation may lead to subsequent rejection or disfavor	"I'm glad you're exercising so regularly."	"Are you having any difficulty fitting regular exercise into your schedule?"
	"You should be testing your blood sugar each morning."	"Let's explore some ways that will help you test your blood sugar each morning."
Agreeing		
Does not allow the client flexibility to change their mind	"You're right about needing surgery immediately."	"Having surgery immediately is one possibility. What others have you considered?"
Disagreeing		
Intimidates the client; makes the person feel foolish or inadequate	"That's not true! Where did you get an idea like that?"	"Maybe I can help clarify that for you."
Demanding an Explanation		
Puts the client on the defensive; the client may be tempted to make up an excuse rather than risk disapproval for an honest answer	"Why didn't you keep your appointment last week?"	"I see you couldn't keep your appointment last week."
Giving Advice		
Discourages independent problem-solving and decision-making; provides a biased view that may prejudice the client's choice	"If I were you, I'd try drug therapy before having surgery."	"Share with me the advantages and disadvantages of your options as you see them."

(*continued*)

TABLE 7-5 Nontherapeutic Communication Techniques *(continued)*

TECHNIQUE AND CONSEQUENCE	EXAMPLE	IMPROVEMENT
Defending		
Indicates such a strong allegiance that any disagreement to the contrary is not acceptable	"Ms. Johnson is my best nursing assistant. She wouldn't have let your light go unanswered that long."	"I'm sorry you had to wait so long."
Belittling		
Disregards how the client is responding as an individual	"Lots of people learn to give themselves insulin."	"You're finding it especially difficult to stick yourself with a needle."
Patronizing		
Treats the client condescendingly as less than capable of making an independent decision	"Are we ready for our bath yet?"	"Would you like your bath now, or should I check with you later?"
Changing the Subject		
Alters the direction of the discussion to a topic that is safer or more comfortable	*Client:* "I'm so scared that a mammogram will show I have cancer." *Nurse:* "Tell me more about your family."	"It is a serious disease. What concerns you the most?"

Consequently, nurses and other health care providers must find ways to help these clients effectively communicate their health problems and needs, give informed consent, or understand teaching about health practices that will have an impact on their recovery or health maintenance. Regardless of the barrier, The Joint Commission is adamant that health care providers facilitate communication with all clients by requiring that agencies develop a system to (1) provide auxiliary aids and services to address the communication needs of clients with hearing, visual, or speech impairments or literacy needs and (2) provide language interpreting and translation services for clients who do not speak English or who have limited English proficiency (LEP) (The Joint Commission, 2011).

Communicating With Verbally Impaired Clients

There are instances when nurses and clients cannot communicate verbally despite the fact that each is proficient in English. For example, clients who have had a stroke sometimes experience **expressive aphasia**, an inability to utilize verbal language skills. Clients who have artificial airways, such as an endotracheal or tracheostomy tube, or who have their jaws wired following facial trauma cannot speak. Other examples include clients with traumatic brain injury, cerebral palsy, and multiple sclerosis. Nevertheless, communication is still a nursing priority as mandated by The Joint Commission. The nurse may provide the verbally impaired client with a tablet and pencil or "magic slate," although this approach is time-consuming. In some cases, the client may not have the use of the hands or fine motor skills to use a writing device.

Other various communication tools are available to facilitate meeting the communication needs of verbally impaired clients. For example, the client may prefer to point to common phrases, spell with the alphabet, and identify numbers on a communication board (Fig. 7-9). A speaking valve may be used for clients who have a tracheostomy, and clients who have had a laryngectomy (removal of the larynx) may be assisted with an **electrolarynx**, a handheld device that when placed on the neck surface vibrates and mechanically resonates when words or sounds are mouthed.

Some assistive aids may meet temporary needs of verbally impaired clients, but for those who are affected long term, computerized technology has now made electronic "touch-to-speak" also known as "touch talk" alternative communication devices available (Fig. 7-10).

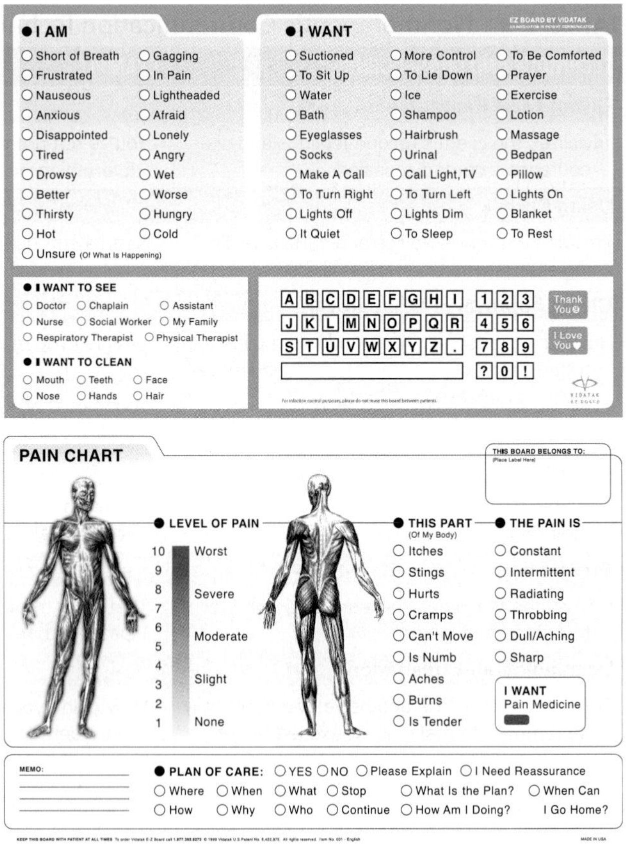

Figure 7-9 A client who is verbally impaired due to a stroke or intubation can communicate their needs to the nurse using a communication board. (Courtesy of Vidatak, LLC, Los Angeles, CA.)

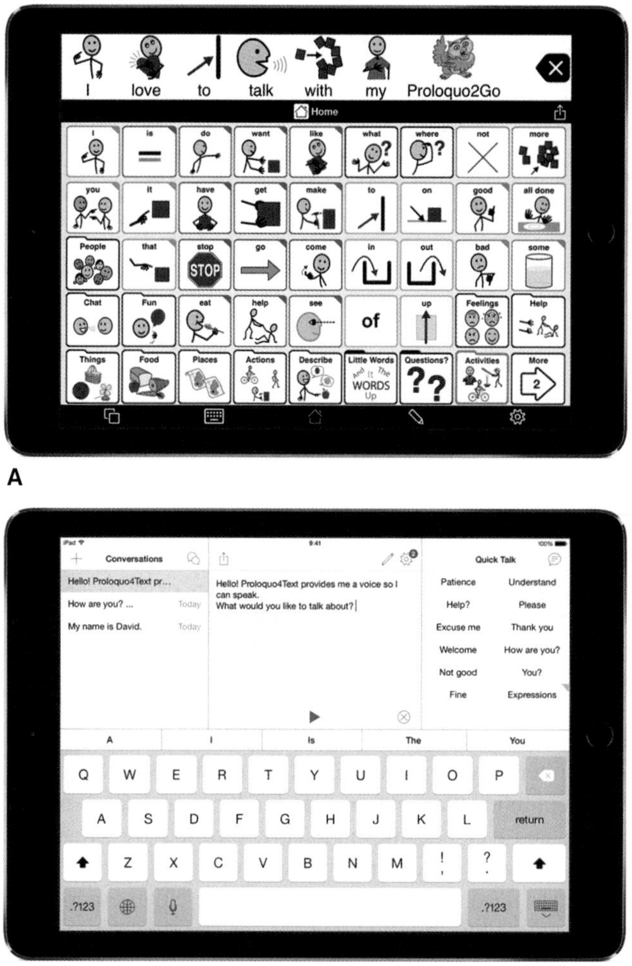

Figure 7-10 Computerized devices allow clients who are inarticulate to speak by placing a finger on a touch-sensitive screen to produce a computer-synthesized voice: **(A)** colorful images and **(B)** text only. (Proloquo2Go® **(A)** and Proloquo4Text™ **(B)** are AssistiveWare® products. Images used with permission.)

Communicating With Deaf Clients

A person who is **deaf** is unable to hear well enough to use hearing as a means of processing information, whereas a person who is **hard of hearing** has some hearing and is able to use it for communication purposes. If the deaf client can read and write, writing can facilitate communication. However, written communication may not be useful for all clients.

Many deaf clients, especially those who were born deaf or lost their hearing at a very early age, have learned to use American Sign Language (ASL). ASL uses signs made by hand movements and **finger spelling**, an alphabetical substitute for words that have no sign (Fig. 7-11). However, the health care agency may not have anyone available who is proficient in ASL. To overcome this barrier, some hospitals use a **webcam**, a video camera that allows viewing via the internet. The webcam allows **video interpreting** in which an ASL interpreter communicates with the deaf client through an internet video connection. Hospitals may also make a text telephone (TTY) or a telecommunication device for the deaf (TDD) available as an auxiliary aid so that deaf, hard of hearing, or speech-impaired clients can type messages rather than talking and listening. If these devices are not available, communication can be facilitated by using a free, telecommunications relay service (TRS), which is much like closed-captioned television. The service, which is available 24/7, connects the TTY caller with an operator who reads the typed words aloud to the contacted person and types back the response to the caller (see http://www.ultratec.com).

Communicating With Limited English Proficiency Clients

Individuals who report that they do not speak English well, or do not speak English at all, can be categorized as persons with **LEP**. An LEP client, by definition, is one who cannot understand English at a level that permits interacting

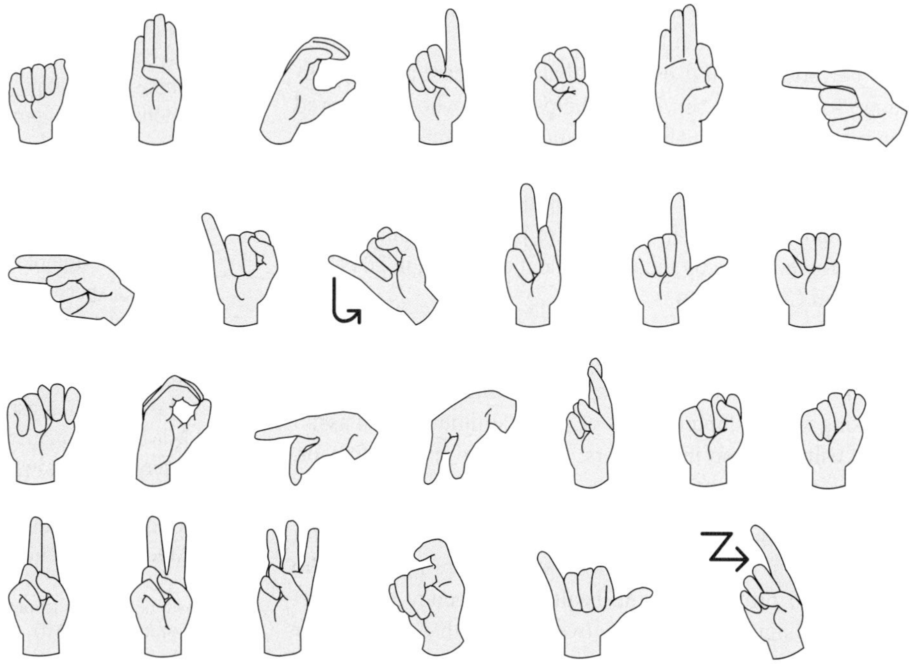

Figure 7-11 The alphabet in American Sign Language.

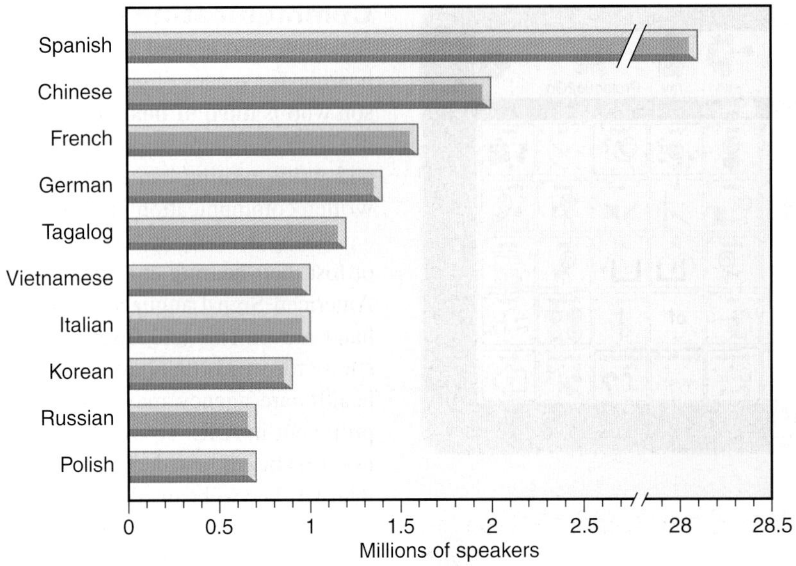

Figure 7-12 The top 10 languages other than English spoken in homes in the United States in 2014. (From Institute of Medicine. (2014). *Race, ethnicity, and language data: Standardization for healthcare quality improvement.* http://www.ahrq.gov/research/findings/final-reports/iomracereport/index.html

effectively with staff in health care settings, social service agencies, or public services without an interpreter (The Joint Commission, 2010).

The Center for Immigration Studies (2014) reports that there are 61.8 million people, or one in five people, who speak a language other than English at home. Of those, 41% indicate that they speak English less than very well (Zeigler & Camarota, 2014; Fig. 7-12).

The proportion of people who speak a particular language other than English varies geographically. For example, Spanish, the most common language other than English, is spoken in the southwest, whereas it is spoken by far fewer people in the northeast sections of the United States. Another weakness in the statistics is that U.S. Census questionnaires do not include those who communicate with ASL or use Braille as a written language.

Nevertheless, it is essential that health care agencies arrange for language services to help clients whose preferred language is not English. Furthermore, it is legally required under the Civil Rights Act of 1964 to avoid discrimination on the basis of race or national origin. The obligation to ensure linguistic access in health care programs continued to be reinforced again by the Department of Justice in 2011 and The Joint Commission.

Communication Methodologies

Health care agencies can comply with linguistic legislation by using certified interpreters or other communication assistance using ad hoc interpreters, telephonic interpreting, or, lastly, a communication board.

Certified Interpreters. The best form of communication with an LEP client is with a **certified interpreter**, a person who is paid and provided by the health care agency to convert spoken or signed language between a health care provider and non–English-speaking client into English. The certified interpreter may be present on-site or available by webcam. Once individuals meet age and education requirements, candidates can become nationally certified by satisfactorily passing a written and oral examination (Box 7-2). Interpreters must recertify every 5 years by either completing continuing education requirements or retaking the medical certification examination (National Board of Certification for Medical Interpreters, 2020). It is the responsibility of

BOX 7-2 Requirements for Interpreter Certification

To qualify for certification, candidates must meet the following requirements:

- Must be at least 18 years of age
- Demonstrate oral proficiency in English
- Demonstrate oral proficiency in the targeted language
- Pass a written examination that includes items on topics such as:
  - Roles of a medical interpreter
  - Medical interpreter ethics
  - Cultural competence
  - Medical terminology in working languages
  - Medical specialties in working languages
  - Interpreter standards of practice
  - Legislation and regulations
- Pass an oral examination that includes the following:
  - Mastery of linguistic knowledge of English
  - Mastery of linguistic knowledge of the other language
  - Interpreting knowledge and skills
  - Cultural competence
  - Medical terminology in working language
  - Medical specialties in working languages

Used with permission from the National Board of Certification for Medical Interpreters (NBCMI).

the health care agency to obtain qualified interpreters. The goal is to engage the services of individuals who are competent in the client's language of preference and who will convey information accurately and impartially and maintain confidentiality.

Ad Hoc Interpreters. When a certified interpreter is not available in person or by webcam, there are a variety of other options (see Chapter 8). In descending order of preference, the following may be utilized: untrained agency-employed, bilingual staff; self-declared bilingual volunteers; and family or friends, all of whom are referred to as **ad hoc interpreters**. The disadvantage in using ad hoc interpreters is that errors such as omissions, substitutions, editorializing, and additions often occur. The Joint Commission has not yet specified the type of training and competencies of individuals who are used as interpreters, but standards may be forthcoming.

Telephonic Interpreting. In the absence of a certified or ad hoc interpreter who provides a physical presence, **telephonic interpreting**—over-the-phone translation—is an alternative. AT&T USADirect In-Language Service provides translators in 170 languages whenever and wherever they are needed.

Communication Board. Although it does not meet all the needs of an LEP client, a **communication board** showing illustrations or translated words and phrases may be useful for immediate bedside interactions between the client and nursing staff.

CLIENT TEACHING

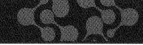

Sharing information and teaching are essential nursing activities. These activities promote the client's ability to understand the current health care environment and independently meet their own future health needs. Because hospitalization time is limited, nurses must begin teaching clients as soon as possible after admission. Teaching continues while nurses care for clients in their homes or refer them to educational programs in community settings. The most efficient teaching occurs when the nurse presents information compatible with the client's learning style. Teaching may be informal or formal. Box 7-3 lists suggestions for teaching adult client, and Evidence-Based Practice 7-1 discusses current ESL research related to special populations.

Learner Assessment

The nurse performs a learner assessment to determine various components of the client's learning status. Besides determining the style of learning a client prefers, the nurse assesses the client's learning style, age and developmental level, learning needs, learning capacity, motivation for learning, and learning readiness.

Learning Styles

A **learning style** is the manner in which a person best comprehends new information. Usually, people fall into one of three categories: cognitive, affective, or psychomotor learner (Box 7-4). The **cognitive learner** processes information

BOX 7-3 Teaching Adult Clients

- Identify the value or purpose for learning new information.
- Determine whether the client is comfortable at the moment.
- Make sure the client is wearing glasses or using a hearing aid if needed.
- Reduce noise and distractions in the environment.
- Sit at eye level (unless doing group teaching) and face the client(s).
- Use short sentences of 10 words or fewer.
- Avoid speaking rapidly.
- Minimize technical terms and medical jargon; define words whenever necessary.
- Use words that a seventh to ninth grader would understand.
- Present at least one but no more than three new ideas at each teaching session.
- Review frequently.
- Use the active form of the verb rather than passive (e.g., "Wipe straight down the center of the incision" rather than "The incision is wiped down the center").
- Use examples with which the learner can identify.
- Relate new information to prior learning.
- Build in a learner performance evaluation, such as asking the client to repeat or paraphrase prior information, demonstrate a skill, or apply the information to a hypothetical situation such as "What would you do if . . . ?"
- End teaching if the client cannot remain attentive.

Evidence-Based Practice 7-1

Client Teaching

Clinical Question

How can nurses improve communication with clients when English is not the first language?

Evidence

The Department of Health and Human Services (DHHS, 2018) states that "In the United States, approximately 20% of the adult population speaks a language other than English at home; of this group, almost half report speaking English less than very well and are considered to have limited English proficiency." The DHHS Patient Safety Network (PSNET) supports education for health care providers and provides numerous resources on communication. The resources can help guide language and cultural needs involved with communication.

Nursing Implications

Nurses learn therapeutic communication and diversity in training for practice. As our culture becomes more diverse, nurses need to have resources to communicate with non–English-speaking clients for care and education. Nurses must continue to be advocates for their clients in all areas of practice and be able to obtain resources if needed to guide and support the patients. Effective communication can influence client safety and the quality of care the client receives.

Reference

US Department of Health & Human Services. (2018). *When patients and providers speak different languages*. https://psnet.ahrq.gov/web-mm/when-patients-and-providers-speak-different-languages

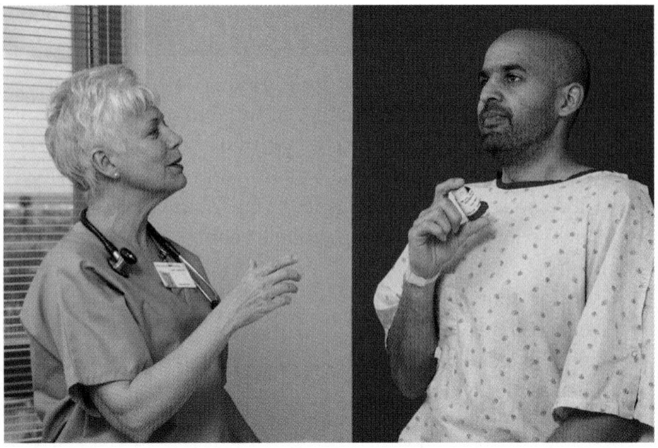

Figure 7-13 A psychomotor learner learns best by doing.

best by listening to or reading facts and descriptions. The **affective learner** learns best when presented with information that appeals to their feelings, beliefs, and values. The **psychomotor learner** prefers to learn by doing (Fig. 7-13).

One way to determine a client's learning style is to ask, "When you learned to add fractions, what helped you most: listening to the teacher's explanation, recognizing the value of fractions in cooking or carpentry, or working on sample problems?" Although most people favor one style of learning, presenting information through a combination of the three styles tends to optimize learning.

Age and Developmental Level

Nurses and all those who provide instruction must be aware of the basic learning characteristics of children, adults, older adult learners, and those learners who are developmentally compromised. Currently, there are three major categories:

- **Pedagogy** is the science of teaching children or those with cognitive ability comparable to children (although it often refers to the teaching of all individuals).
- **Andragogy** is the science of teaching adult learners.
- **Geragogy** is the science of teaching older adults.

Many clients with health problems are in their later years. Box 7-5 offers tips for tailoring client teaching to older adults. Nurse educators are also advised to prepare themselves to teach young adults who belong to "Generation X" and "Generation Y," also known as the Net Generation. **Generation X** refers to those born between 1961 and 1981, "millennials" (sometimes referred to as the Net Generation or cyberkids) were born after 1981, and Generation Z range from the mid-1990s through the second decade of this century. Technology and imposed independence as a consequence of growing up in single-parent households or homes in which both parents work have greatly affected the learning characteristics of these groups. In general, millennials may share some of the following learning characteristics:

- They are technologically literate, having grown up with computers (and are sometimes referred to as "digital natives" for that reason).
- They crave stimulation and quick responses.
- They expect immediate answers and feedback.
- They become bored with memorizing information and doing repetitious tasks.
- They like a variety of instructional methods from which they can choose.
- They respond best when they find the information to be relevant.
- They prefer visualizations, simulations, and other methods of participatory learning.

BOX 7-4 Activities That Promote Learning According to Styles

Cognitive Learners

Listing	Describing
Identifying	Summarizing
Naming	Selecting

Affective Learners

Advocating	Promoting
Supporting	Internalizing
Accepting	Valuing

Psychomotor Learners

Assembling	Filling
Changing	Adding
Emptying	Removing

BOX 7-5 Considerations for Teaching Older Adults

- Older adults have a lifetime of past experiences that can be used as a foundation for new learning.
- Before beginning a teaching session, ask the older adult about the need for glasses or a hearing aid or both. Make sure that the glasses are clean and/or the hearing aid is in good working order and turned on.
- Choose printed materials that positively portray persons of similar age.
- Avoid using printed materials that are cluttered with extensive information.
- Be sure that printed materials are of sufficient size for easy reading. Such materials usually should be in at least 14-point type for older adults.
- Booklets, pamphlets, and brochures that are printed in black on white or cream matte paper improve visual clarity.
- Healthy older adults maintain cognitive abilities and can learn new information. They do, however, learn more effectively when they are allowed to progress at their own pace, when information is hooked into prior knowledge, and when content is presented in chunks of information to promote recall.
- Learning motor skills may be more difficult for older adults because of physiologic changes. They may need more time to learn new activities or modifications in the equipment required for the skill.
- Asking the older adult to explain practices used to maintain health can provide insight into various cultural practices to be integrated in a health teaching plan (see Chapter 9).

Learning Needs

Client education begins with an assessment of learning needs. **Learning needs** are the skills and concepts that the client and family must acquire to restore, maintain, or promote health. For example, the client with diabetes needs to learn to self-administer insulin (a skill) and how diabetes affects circulation (a concept). Identifying the important skills and concepts that a client must learn and then assessing what the client already knows help in establishing goals, tailoring the teaching plan to the individual, and evaluating outcomes.

Learning Capacity

Learning capacity refers to a person's intellectual ability to understand, remember, and apply new information. Illiteracy, sensory deficits, and a shortened attention span require special adaptations when implementing client teaching. LEP clients may require translation of written information in order to understand and process information and instructions that enable them to make appropriate health decisions.

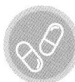

Pharmacologic Considerations

- Opioids and antianxiety drugs are frequently used, especially in conscious sedation for procedures. Amnesia results, even when the client appears to be coherent. Be sure to include written instructions or include another adult when teaching clients who have been medicated.

Motivation

Motivation is the desire to acquire new information. Learning occurs at an accelerated rate when a person has a purpose or reason for mastering it. Some motivating forces include restoring independence, preventing complications, facilitating discharge, and returning to or remaining in the comfort of home.

Learning Readiness

Learning readiness pertains to the optimal time for learning. Ideally, it occurs when a client is in a state of physical and psychological well-being. For example, a client who is in pain, uncomfortably warm or cold, anxious, or depressed is not in the best condition for learning. In these situations, it is best to restore comfort first and then attend to teaching.

Informal and Formal Teaching

Informal teaching is unplanned. It occurs spontaneously, usually at the client's bedside or while caring for the client at home. **Formal teaching** requires a plan to avoid being haphazard. A **teaching plan** is the organized arrangement of content in a specific time frame. It facilitates reaching goals, provides essential information, and ensures the client's comprehension before they assume responsibility for self-care. Developing a plan and implementing it gradually and sequentially avoid overwhelming the client with new information or learning skills that are difficult to perform.

Learning Comprehension

Effective teaching can be evaluated by assessing the learner's comprehension. To determine whether the information was understood correctly, caregivers can use one or combinations of the following techniques: (1) repeat back, (2) teach back, and/or (3) show back (The Joint Commission, 2007). *Repeat back* involves having the client restate or paraphrase the points that were taught. *Teach back* encourages the client to explain the essential information to validate comprehension of the instruction. *Show back* incorporates satisfactorily demonstrating a skill to a person who either taught the client or has similar expertise in the skill.

KEY POINTS

- The roles of the nurse in a nurse–client relationship:
  - Caregiver
  - Educator
  - Collaborator
  - Delegator
- Three phases in a nurse–client relationship:
  - Preinteraction phase: gather preliminary information about the client
  - Introductory phase: the nurse and the client get acquainted and the client identifies one or more health problems
  - Working phase: involves mutually planning the client's care and putting the plan into action
  - Terminating phase: the nurse and client mutually agree that the client's immediate health problems have improved and that the nurse's services are no longer necessary
- Communication:
  - Verbal: using words, hearing, and listening
  - Nonverbal: kinesics, paralanguage, proxemics, touch, and silence
  - Therapeutic: using verbal and nonverbal communication to promote a person's physical and emotional well-being
- Proxemics: the use of space when communicating
  - Intimate space: within 6 inches
  - Personal space: 6 inches to 4 feet
  - Social space: 4 to 12 feet
  - Public space: greater than 12 feet
- Task-oriented touch: involves the personal contact that is required when performing nursing procedures
- Affective touch: is used to demonstrate concern or affection
- Client teaching: sharing information and teaching are essential nursing activities. These activities promote the client's ability to understand the current health care environment and independently meet their own future health needs
- Learning styles:
  - Cognitive processes information best by listening to or reading facts and descriptions:

- Affective: learns best when presented with information that appeals to their feelings, beliefs, and values
- Psychomotor: prefers to learn by doing

- Techniques for evaluating learning comprehension:
  - Repeat back: involves having the client restate or paraphrase the points that were taught
  - Teach back: encourages the client to explain the essential information to validate comprehension of the instruction
  - Show back: incorporates satisfactorily demonstrating a skill to a person who either taught the client or has similar expertise in the skill

CRITICAL THINKING EXERCISES

1. Change the nontherapeutic interaction in the following example to one that is therapeutic:
Client: "I'm having second thoughts about having this breast reduction surgery."
Nurse: "You'll be happy with the results when it's over."

2. Studies have shown that older adults are not touched with the same frequency as clients in other age groups. Discuss reasons for this.

3. A client with a health problem does not speak English very well. How might you meet this client's communication needs?

4. What approaches should the nurse take when teaching an older adult with diabetes about their disease and its management?

NCLEX-STYLE REVIEW QUESTIONS PrepU

1. The nurse has been employed in an extended care facility. What outcome is the best evidence that the nurse's caregiving skills have been effective?
1. Clients make their own choices about health care.
2. Clients receive information about potential alternatives.
3. Clients become empowered and involved with self-help groups.
4. Clients with chronic physical problems maintain independence.

2. The nurse is notified that a new client will be admitted. What characteristic correlates with the introductory phase of a nurse–client relationship?
1. Developing goals with the client
2. Gathering health-related data
3. Performing nursing procedures
4. Teaching the client about self-care

3. The nurse is caring for a client who seems depressed. What statement is the best example of therapeutic communication at this time?
1. "You seem depressed."
2. "Why are you depressed?"
3. "Did your team lose last night?"
4. "You should count your blessings."

4. The nurse is caring for a client with LEP. What is the least desirable approach for communicating with an LEP client?
1. Utilizing a certified interpreter
2. Asking a family member to translate
3. Requesting the services of a bilingual employee
4. Contacting a telephonic interpreter

5. The nurse teaches a client how to perform breathing exercises. What is the best method for the nurse to evaluate the effectiveness of the teaching?
1. Requesting that the client explain the importance of breathing exercises
2. Asking the client to perform the breathing exercises as they were taught
3. Asking the client if they are performing the breathing exercises as required
4. Monitoring the client's respiratory rate several times a day

WANT TO KNOW MORE? There are a wide variety of online resources available on thePoint to enhance learning and understanding of this chapter.

Go to thePoint.lww.com/activate and use the activation code found in the front of this text to unlock these online resources.

8

Cultural Care Considerations

Words To Know

ageism
biocultural ecology
culture
cultural competence
ethnicity
ethnocentrism
generalization
health beliefs
health practices
race
stereotyping
subculture
transcultural nursing
underrepresented group

Learning Objectives

On completion of this chapter, you will be able to:

1. Define terms related to culture.
2. List the five population groups delineated in the United States.
3. Differentiate race from ethnicity and culture.
4. Contrast stereotyping and generalization.
5. Describe how cultural background and practices influence actions and behaviors.
6. Name three views that societies use to explain illness or disease.
7. Discuss biocultural assessment.
8. Describe cultural assessment.
9. Explain the meaning and characteristics of transcultural nursing.
10. List at least five ways to demonstrate culturally competent nursing care.

Health care providers are increasingly aware that high-quality care involves greater knowledge and appreciation of different linguistic and cultural backgrounds. Health care facilities in most large cities and many rural and suburban areas serve diverse populations. In every health care setting, clients and those providing health care have their own cultural values and beliefs about health care Thus, nurses must develop **cultural competence**, the ability to understand the client's worldview as well as their own and how these worldviews affect nursing care. This chapter provides information about cultural concepts, clinical variations among different ethnic and racial groups, and communication issues for various cultures. Knowledge of cultural differences and the ability to adapt to each client's cultural needs are crucial to providing quality care.

CULTURAL CONCEPTS

To deliver culturally competent care, nurses must understand terms related to culture. They must also view each person as a unique human being who may have a frame of reference that is similar to or different from that of the nurse.

Culture

Sir Edward Tyler, a British anthropologist, first used the term *culture* in 1871. He stated that culture includes knowledge, beliefs, art, morals, laws, customs, and other capabilities and habits. The term **culture** provides a means for understanding people's values and beliefs, including those that relate to health practices. Five basic concepts characterize

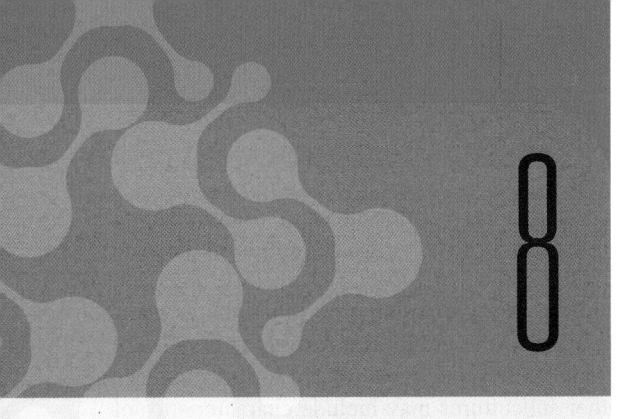

Gerontological Considerations

- Age may also be considered a cultural subgroup because older adults have shared experiences and resultant values and beliefs. **Ageism** is the stereotyping of older adult behavior or vulnerability based on an individual's prior experiences or anticipation of behaviors. Ageism may lead to discrimination against older persons or impact nurse beliefs regarding the delivery of care resources.
- Sensitivity and awareness when communicating with older adults in all cultures is critical for planning person-centered care.
- Older adults have had lifelong experiences with their own or family member health and illness, which may influence their foundational attitudes, desires, and expectations about health and health practices. These beliefs may conflict with those of their caregivers or health care providers.
- The nurse must be aware of possible events experienced by older adults at a younger age (e.g., possible trauma from war, refugee migration, natural disasters) that could influence health or health care decisions.
- Access to health care may be more difficult for older adults because of transportation issues or limited resources, thereby increasing the possibility of reverting to past health behavior practices, seeking nonprofessionals for health advice, or using alternative therapies.
- Although reimbursement issues have an impact on health behaviors, only about one-third of adults aged 50 to 64 years and less than half of those aged 65 and older are up to date on selected preventative screenings and immunizations (Healthy Aging, 2016).
- Health practices and beliefs may be affected by challenges inherent related to health literacy, navigating the health care delivery system, requirements for filing for reimbursement, transitions across settings of care, or the use of specialty providers for various comorbidities.
- Resources are available to assist with design of health care information and specific suggestions for cross-cultural communication effectiveness from the Centers for Disease Control and Prevention (CDC).
- An older adult's orientation to time, family, and self may create the potential for conflict with the health care system.
- In many African American families, a grandmother or an older aunt is considered the matriarch (woman leader). It may be appropriate to include this person in teaching sessions or ask if the client would like this person to be present.
- Aging people of Asian descent tend to be cared for by and live with one of their children. Suggesting the placement of an aging parent in a nursing home may be considered rude.
- Illnesses, especially those that cause obvious physical changes or dependence on a woman for care, may threaten an aging Latino man's self-image and security.

culture (Characteristics of Culture, n.d.). Culture is (1) learned from birth through language and socialization; (2) shared by members of the same cultural group and encompasses an internal and external perception of being distinct; (3) based on symbols, agreed upon by a specific culture; (4) influenced by specific conditions related to environment, technology, and availability of resources; and (5) dynamic and ever-changing.

Subculture

The United States is often referred to as a *melting pot*, implying that culturally diverse groups are assimilated in one society. Subcultures, however, are readily apparent. **Subculture** refers to a particular group that shares characteristics identifying the group as a distinct entity. These groups may have more subcultures related to specific place of origin. Other subcultures may include characteristics of region, religion, age, sex, social class, political party, ethnicity, racial or cultural identity, and occupation.

Underrepresented Groups

The phrase **underrepresented group** describes a population subgroup where cultural characteristics or physical characteristics or both differ from the majority of the population. People from the underrepresented group are perceived as "different," and the majority group may treat them unfairly. The U.S. Census formally defines five racial population groups: Native American or Alaska Native, Asian, Black or African American, Native Hawaiian or Other Pacific Islander, and White people. In addition, there are two additional categories: another race that is not listed and two or more races combined. People who are White are considered the majority race; the other groups are referred to as *ethnic underrepresented groups*. Groups such as people who are Hispanic or Latinx do not identify as a race, but as an ethnic underrepresented group. Other underrepresented groups can be based on sex or religion. The defining characteristics for an underrepresented group are not always on numbers, but rather on economic exploitation or marginalization. For example, women in the United States outnumber men, but women remain in lower paying jobs and less powerful positions and are considered an underrepresented group in many aspects. People in the LGBTQ community (lesbian, gay, bisexual, transgender, etc.) are a population underrepresented that refers to a coalition of groups. Society is more openly accepting of these groups, and more recognition will lead to exploration of differences in the people of the diverse groups that make up the LGBTQ community while also investigating the impact of their common experiences.

The influence of underrepresented groups is increasing in the United States related to increasing numbers and status. According to the latest U.S. Census Bureau statistics in 2020, it is predicted that by 2060, Whites will comprise 44% of the population. The fastest-growing racial or ethnic group in the United States are people who are two or more races and they are projected to grow some 200 percent by 2060 (US Census Bureau, 2020).

Ethnicity

Ethnicity is the bond or kinship that people feel with their country of birth or place of ancestral origin. It provides a sense of identity. People demonstrate pride in their ethnic heritage by valuing certain physical characteristics, giving children ethnic names, wearing unique items of clothing, and appreciating distinctive music, dance, food, customs, and/or holidays.

Race

The term **race** is often confused with ethnicity and culture. **Race** refers to genetically transmitted traits, such as skin color, bone structure, and eye shape. "All human beings are 99.9% identical in their genetic make-up. Differences in the remaining 0.1% hold important clues about the causes of diseases" (National Human Genome Research Institute, 2014). Many people associate physical differences, particularly skin color, with culture. Although ethnic and racial groups overlap, nurses must not equate skin color and other physical features with culture. Doing so may lead to erroneous assumptions that all people with certain physical attributes share essentially the same culture and ethnicity. This attitude leads to stereotyping.

Stereotyping

Stereotyping means assuming that all people in a particular cultural, racial, or ethnic group share the same values and beliefs, behave similarly, and are basically alike. For example, a nurse who thinks stereotypically may assign a client to a staff member who is of the same culture as the client simply because the nurse assumes that all people of that culture are alike. This same nurse may also believe that clients with the same skin color have similar social situations. Stereotypes are preconceived ideas unsupported by facts, so they are not real or accurate. In fact, they can be dangerous because they are dehumanizing and interfere with accepting others as unique individuals.

Generalization

Distinguishing between stereotyping and generalizing is important. Stereotyping has an end point; the assumption prevents one from seeing another person as unique. **Generalization**, however, acknowledges common trends in a group while recognizing that more information is needed. Cultural generalizations do not describe each client but provide a broad pattern of beliefs and behaviors for clients from a particular cultural group. This knowledge may assist health care providers to provide appropriate care. Nevertheless, generalization can lead to oversimplification and stereotyping, of which nurses must remain cognizant (Purnell, 2013). Increased awareness will assist them to see each client as a unique person.

››› *Stop, Think, and Respond 8-1*

You overhear a nurse talking about a client admitted with diabetes and a leg ulcer. The nurse says, "It figures they don't do what the doctors say—they have been in this country for 10 years and still can't speak English well. Those people are just stupid!" How would you respond?

Ethnocentrism

Ethnocentrism is the belief that one's own ethnic heritage is the "correct" one and superior to others. Nurses are human and certainly enter the nursing profession with their own ethnocentrism. They must be aware that their way is not the only or best way. Clients will sense that a nurse feels superior if they approach with a patronizing or condescending attitude. Clients bring their own values and practices, and having different beliefs does not mean clients are ignorant. Nurses must appreciate that their values and beliefs are not better than those of their clients—they simply are different.

Other Culture-Related Terms

Acculturation involves the process of adapting to or taking on the behaviors of another group. *Cultural blindness* is an inability to recognize the values, beliefs, and practices of others because of strong ethnocentric preferences. *Cultural imposition* is an inclination to impose one's cultural beliefs, values, and patterns of behavior on persons from a different culture. *Cultural taboos* are activities governed by rules of behavior that a particular cultural group avoids, forbids, or prohibits (Types of Taboos, 2018).

CULTURALLY INFLUENCED CHARACTERISTICS

Cultural upbringing influences a person's actions and behaviors. Socially acceptable conduct for one person may be unacceptable for another. Cultural background affects a person's actions and reactions to their environment. When considering cultural background, there is the danger of stereotyping. Issues such as personal space, touch, time, diet, verbal behaviors, and beliefs about the cause of illness are unique for each individual but may be culturally influenced.

Eye Contact

Nurses are taught to maintain eye contact with clients when they are speaking with them, but respecting and understanding behavior and providing a comfortable climate for clients are important considerations. The physical act of making eye contact may be culturally influenced. Americans of non-Hispanic White or Eurpoean origin typically value direct eye contact or "looking a person straight in the eye" while speaking. Such eye contact, however, may offend people of Asian origin, people who are Native Americans, and other cultural groups who view lingering eye contact as an invasion of privacy. Others, such as clients of Hispanic or Latinx ethnicity, may avoid eye contact with authority figures as a sign of respect.

Space and Distance

People are not always aware personal space needs until such needs are threatened. Health care situations, such as providing personal care or performing intricate procedures, reduce the accepted personal space along with causing personal discomfort. Furthermore, nurses often provide comfort and support through close physical proximity, but such closeness may threaten some clients. Nurses must observe how clients position themselves and respect their desire for space as much as possible. Simple explanations of the need for physical proximity during clinical procedures and personal care alleviate the discomfort that some clients may experience.

Space and distance are also factors affecting interactions between nurses and clients. For example, people of Hispanic or Latinx ethnicity are characteristically more comfortable sitting close to interviewers and letting interactions slowly unfold. People of Asian origin may feel comfortable positioned more than an arm's length from the interviewer.

Touch

There are great cultural differences in the use of touch. For example, some Native American people may interpret a White American person's custom of a strong handshake as offensive. They may be more comfortable with just a light passing of the hands. Arab culture prohibits male health care providers from physically examining women. In some Asian American cultures, touching the head is impolite because the spirit rests there. Orthodox Jewish women highly value their modesty and must keep their heads and limbs covered (Jewish Patient, n.d.). Nurses need to respect and adapt care to honor these and other differences related to touch.

Time

Throughout the world, people view clock time and social time. *Clock time* implies the orderly division of time into years, months, weeks, days, hours, minutes, and seconds. Calendars, clocks, sunrises, tides, and moons define clock time. *Social time* is based more on cultural habits, meals, celebrations, and other events and is related to punctuality and waiting. Aspects of social time vary among cultures. For example, some cultures highly value punctuality. A client from such a culture may be on time for an appointment and then have to wait, increasing their frustration with the health care system. Clients from other cultures may place priority more on activities, such as family needs, and less on punctuality for appointments. Recognizing that clients have different perceptions of time assists the nurse to provide more sensitive care.

Diet

The relationship between food-related behaviors and culture is complex (Box 8-1). Basically, food is a means of survival—it relieves hunger, promotes health, and prevents disease. Its social meanings encompass love, togetherness, and celebration. Food also has other connotations in terms of its use to reward or punish, relieve stress, and delineate social classes. Culture often dictates the types of food and how frequently a person eats, the types of utensils they use, and the status assigned to particular individuals (e.g., who eats first, who gets the most to eat). Religious practices also impose certain rules and restrictions, such as fasting, eliminating certain foods or following a vegetarian diet, and observing rituals (e.g., Passover Seder; Box 8-2). There are implications for health care when a client is diagnosed with

BOX 8-1 Selected Examples of Cultural Meanings of Food

- Critical life force for survival
- Relief of hunger
- Peaceful coexistence
- Promotion of health and healing
- Prevention of disease or illness
- Expression of caring for another
- Interpersonal closeness or distance
- Promotion of kinship and familial alliances
- Solidification of social ties
- Celebration of life events (e.g., birthday, marriage)
- Expression of gratitude or appreciation
- Recognition of achievement or accomplishment
- Business negotiations
- Information exchange
- Validation of social, cultural, or religious ceremonial functions
- Way to generate income
- Expression of affluence, wealth, or social status

BOX 8-2 Prohibited Foods and Beverages for Selected Religious Groups

Hindu
All meats
Animal shortenings

Islam
Alcoholic products and beverages (including extracts, such as vanilla and lemon)
Animal shortenings
Gelatin made with pork, marshmallow, and other confections made with gelatin
Pork

Judaism (Note: practiced primarily by Orthodox Jewish people, not by all Jewish groups)
Blood by ingestion (e.g., blood sausage, raw meat) (*Note:* blood by transfusion is acceptable.)
Mixing dairy products and meat dishes at same meal
Pork
Predatory fowl
Shellfish and scavenger fish (e.g., shrimp, crab, lobster, escargot, catfish) (*Note:* fish with fins and scales are permissible.)
Note: Packaged foods contain labels identifying kosher ("properly preserved" or "fitting") and pareve (made without meat or milk) items. Foods noted as pareve are neutral and can be consumed with milk or meat.

Members of the Church of Jesus Christ of Latter-Day Saints
Alcohol
Beverages containing caffeine stimulants (coffee, tea, colas, and selected carbonated soft drinks)
Tobacco

Seventh-Day Adventists
Certain seafood, including shellfish
Fermented beverages
Pork
Note: Optional vegetarianism is encouraged.

Rastafarianism
Pork
Scavengers
Shellfish
Salt, alcohol, milk, and coffee are restricted
Note: Most holy meals will be strictly vegetarian or vegan

Adapted from Stuckrath, T. (2018, January 24). *Religious dietary restrictions: Your essential quick reference guide*. https://thrivemeetings.com/2018/01/religious-dietary-restrictions-guide/

diabetes, hypertension, or other disorders that require dietary adjustments. Nurses must consider cultural and religious food preferences/requirements when instructing clients about the dietary restrictions related to a specific condition (Dietary Restrictions, 2018).

Nutrition Notes

The Culturally Diverse Client

- Culture defines what food is; how it is obtained, stored, prepared, and served; when it is eaten; differences in food habits based on age, sex, and status; and food's meaning. In any cultural or ethnic group, food habits can vary greatly. Generalizations are intended only as a guide.
- African American people are at increased risk for hypertension, stroke, diabetes, and obesity. Limiting fat, sodium, and excess calories may help prevent or treat these disorders. Because lactose intolerance is common, calcium intake may be inadequate. In the Southern United States, "soul food" refers to both cooking style (barbecued or fried) and particular foods consumed (e.g., pork, greens).
- Food practices are affected by availability, religion, climate, and tradition in different cultures around the world. Obesity, diabetes, and hypertriglyceridemia are common among people of Hispanic or Latinx ethnicity people. Calcium intake may be inadequate in people of Eastern European descent, people of Hispanic or Latinx ethnicity, people who are Native Americans, and people of Chinese origin due to high prevalence of lactose intolerance.
- The traditional Asian diet is plant based; common foods include rice, noodles, flat bread, potatoes, vegetables, nuts, seeds, beans, and soy foods. It is low in fat, saturated fat, and cholesterol and rich in fiber and nutrients. Meat traditionally serves more as a condiment than as a main entree. Preparing food usually takes longer than cooking it. Moderation is valued, and obesity is rare. Lactose intolerance is common. Because of the extensive use of soy sauce, limiting sodium intake is difficult.
- Native American and Alaskan Native people represent a heterogeneous group of more than 500 tribes and villages. Eating patterns and habits are widely diverse and influenced by cultural and religious beliefs, geography, and food availability. Although staples vary among tribes, corn, squash, and beans are used extensively. Many plant foods are also used in traditional medicinal practices. Obesity, diabetes, and lactose intolerance are common among Native American people.

Verbal Communication Patterns

General communication patterns are found among the major U.S. subcultures. The nurse must carefully observe or tactfully question clients about communication preferences and tailor the interview accordingly.

White Americans of non-Hispanic White or European origin are usually open to providing personal health information and expressing positive and negative feelings. Asian Americans tend to control their emotion and not reveal that they are physically uncomfortable (Asian American Patients, 2020), especially when among people with whom they are unfamiliar. Similarly, men who are of Hispanic or Latinx ethnicity may not show feelings or readily discuss symptoms because they may interpret doing so as less than manly (Hispanic Patients, 2020). Behavior for some men who are of Hispanic or Latinx ethnicity can be attributed to *machismo*, the belief that virile men are physically strong and must deal with emotions privately. They expect to be consulted in decision-making when a family member is the primary client.

Many Native American people are rather private and may hesitate to share much personal information with strangers. They may also be wary encounters with non–Native American health care providers because of the long history of the careless treatment of Native American people. Nurses should be client and listen carefully. In Native American cultures, listening is a valued skill, whereas impatience is seen as disrespectful (Native American Patients, 2020). Navajo people, currently the largest tribe of Native American people, feel that no person has the right to speak for another; they may refuse to comment on a family member's health problems. It might be necessary to write down notes after the client's visit or to explain how the notes will be used in the future to keep other members of the health care team informed.

Some clients may distrust health care providers because of negative past individual or group experiences. They may not trust health care providers to do the right thing. In order to establish rapport and trust, nurses can introduce themselves and respectfully address clients by their last names, preceded by Mr., Mrs., or Ms. Following up thoroughly with requests is essential, as are respecting privacy and asking open-ended rather than direct questions until trust is established.

Other cultures may view health care providers as authority figures. Clients from these backgrounds may feel uncomfortable asking questions. For example, Asian cultures consider it disrespectful to disagree with a person of authority or one who is more educated. They may consider it rude to imply that the person in authority did not teach properly or explain in enough detail. Asian Americans may not openly disagree with primary providers and nurses because of their respect for harmony. Their reticence can conceal a potential for nonadherence when a particular therapeutic regimen is unacceptable from their perspective.

Language

Communication with someone who speaks a different language presents unique challenges. With many different cultural groups living in the United States, many do not speak English or have learned it as their second language and do not speak it well. Others may communicate fairly well in English but are unfamiliar with English medical terminology. In addition, most people prefer to speak in their native tongue, especially when under stress. Because more than 350 languages (Language Maps, 2015) are spoken in the United States, it is unlikely that nurses can converse easily with most non–English-speaking clients.

When the client speaks a different language, nurses should use a translator, preferably one of the same sex identity as the client. Caution is needed when asking family members to interpret; embarrassment and lack of medical knowledge can result in miscommunication. Even when a nurse from one culture and a client from another speak the same language, the way they do so may cause miscommunication. An accepted pattern during verbal interactions for one may be unusual, rude, or offensive to the other. Understanding that unique cultural characteristics are related to verbal and nonverbal communication can facilitate the transition to culturally sensitive care. An interpreter is invaluable, but the nurse's actions, cultural respect, and nonverbal communication techniques will promote acceptance and cooperation. Box 8-3 outlines additional communication techniques.

BOX 8-3 Communicating With Clients Who Do Not Speak English

When clients do not speak English:

- Learn a second language, especially one spoken by a large ethnic population serviced by the health agency.
- Speak words or phrases in the client's language, even if it is not possible to carry on a conversation.
- Refer to an English/foreign language dictionary for bilingual vocabulary words.
- Construct a loose-leaf folder or file cards with words in one or more languages spoken by clients in the community.
- Develop a list of employees or individuals to contact in the community who speak a second language and are willing to act as translators; they should receive training to become competent interpreters for medical procedures and information. In an extreme emergency, international telephone operators may be able to provide assistance.
- Select a translator who is the same sex as the client and approximately the same age, if possible.
- Look at the client, not the translator, when asking questions and listening to the client's response.

When clients speak English, but they are still learning:

- Determine whether the client speaks or reads English, or both.
- Speak slowly, not loudly, using simple words and short sentences.
- Avoid using technical terms, slang, or phrases with a double or colloquial meaning, such as "Do you have to use the John?"
- Ask questions that can be answered by "yes" or "no."
- Repeat the question without changing the words if the client appears confused.
- Give the client sufficient time to process the question from English to the Native language and respond back in English.
- Rely heavily on nonverbal communication and pantomime if necessary.
- Avoid displaying impatience.
- Ask the client to "read this line" to determine the client's ability to follow written instructions, which are provided in English.

Health Beliefs and Health Practices

A person's beliefs about health and illness and how illness is treated are strongly influenced by culture. **Health beliefs** are a person's ideas about the role of the person who is ill, what causes the illness, how to restore health, and how one stays healthy. **Health practices** are the actions a person takes to maintain or restore health based on their health beliefs.

In general, societies use three views to explain illness or disease (Hinkle & Cheever, 2017):

- *Biomedical or scientific perspective:* This view, shared by many health care providers, embraces a cause-and-effect philosophy of human body functions. An example is the belief that bacterial or viral organisms cause meningitis.
- *Naturalistic or holistic perspective:* This view espouses that human beings are only one part of nature. Natural balance or harmony is essential for health. Native American people are one group who share this view. Many Chinese groups embrace *yin-yang theory*, which promotes the idea that energy forces exist between organisms and objects in the universe. The balance between these forces is health. Another example is the *hot/cold theory*, which says that diseases should be treated by adding or subtracting heat or cold or dryness or moisture to restore balance. Many people of Hispanic, African, and/or Arabian descent embrace beliefs based on the hot/cold theory.
- *Magico-religious perspective:* Supernatural forces dominate. Examples include faith healing in some Christian faiths and voodoo healing in some Caribbean cultures.

Nurses may disagree with a client's health/illness beliefs; however, they must appreciate and respect these beliefs to assist the client to achieve health care goals.

››› *Stop, Think, and Respond 8-2*

Hot/cold theory proposes that illnesses caused by heat or cold must be treated with substances having the opposite property. A Puerto Rican client believes they have arthritis because they rinsed their hands in cold water after washing dishes in hot water. They believe that if they eat "hot" foods (e.g., chili peppers), the symptoms will subside. How would you respond?

ASSESSMENT CONSIDERATIONS

Biocultural Assessment

When assessing any client, the nurse must consider general appearance and obvious physical characteristics—components that make up biocultural assessment. Andrews and Boyle (2016) delineate four areas for consideration:

- *Physical appearance:* age, sex, level of consciousness, facial features, and skin color, including evenness of tone, pigmentation, intactness, and lesions or other abnormalities
- *Body structure:* stature, nutrition, symmetry, posture, position, and overall body build or contour
- *Mobility:* gait and range of motion
- *Behavior:* facial expression, mood and affect, fluency of speech, ability to communicate, appropriateness of word choice, grooming, and attire or dress

Biocultural ecology is an area of study that examines biologic cultural differences, with a particular emphasis on adaptation and homeostasis (Giger & Davidhizar, 2013). This research has a focus on "a direct relationship between race and body structure, skin color, other visible physical characteristics, enzymatic and genetic variations, electrocardiographic patterns, susceptibility to disease, nutritional preferences and deficiencies, and psychological characteristics" (Giger & Davidhizar, 2013, p. 122). Safe and competent nursing care relies on research that determines such things as different reactions to drugs because of racial variations in drug metabolism and susceptibility to disease due to genetic distinctions. Table 8-1 provides a brief overview of some biocultural variations to consider in nursing assessment. Although gathering assessment data is the same for most individuals, the findings can vary depending on ethnic

TABLE 8-1 Biocultural Variations

	ASSESSMENT	VARIATIONS
Skin	Normal colors vary widely; melanin accounts for the shades and tones. Establish baseline tone to note future differences.	*Slate gray nevi* are irregular areas of deep blue pigmentation usually found in the sacral and gluteal areas of children of African, Asian, or Latin descent. They are not to be confused with bruising. *Vitiligo* is unpigmented skin patches. *Cyanosis* is difficult to assess in dark-skinned persons. Assess other factors such as respiratory rate, use of accessory muscles, and nasal flaring. People of Mediterranean descent normally have a dark blue tone around the mouth.
Jaundice	Jaundice is best observed in the sclera; establish normal scleral pigmentation.	African American people, Filipino American people, and other groups have heavy deposits of conjunctival fat, which contains carotene and may resemble jaundice.
Pallor	Generalized pallor is best observed in mucous membranes, lips, and nail beds; nail beds and conjunctiva are better to assess the pallor of anemia.	Dark-skinned clients may not have underlying red tones and exhibit pallor more as yellowish-brown or ashen-gray skin tones.
Erythema	Localized inflammation is characterized by reddened skin, which may not show in dark-skinned clients; also assess for increased warmth, tautness, or edema.	Conditions such as carbon monoxide poisoning, in which flushing is present, may be observed in the lips of dark-skinned clients.
Skin changes/normal aging	Light skin tends to show the effects of aging/sun exposure earlier; some people with darker skin tones may wrinkle.	Health care providers frequently assess age inaccurately based on their own cultural assumptions.
Secretions	Apocrine and eccrine sweat glands are important in fluid balance and thermoregulation. When skin flora contaminates sweat, odor results.	Alaskan Native people sweat less on their trunks and extremities but more on their faces.
Eyes	Biocultural differences are common in eye color and structure. Asian people have characteristic epicanthal eye folds.	Dark irises are associated with darker retinas and poorer night vision.
Skeletal system	The long bones of African American people are longer and more dense; hence, this population has a low incidence of osteoporosis. People who are of Asian origin or people who are Alasaka Natives have a lower bone density.	Many variations occur among all groups.
Laboratory tests	Biocultural variations occur in some laboratory results, such as hemoglobin/hematocrit, cholesterol, and blood glucose levels.	Be familiar with variations and their clinical significance.
Drug responses	Genetic or environmental factors may influence differences in pharmacokinetics.	Clients may respond differently to the same drug. For example, mydriatic drugs (drugs that cause eye dilation) produce less dilation in dark-colored eyes than in light-colored eyes.

differences. When caring for clients from diverse backgrounds, nurses need to review sources that provide more information about disease vulnerability and responses to medications for clients from culturally diverse backgrounds.

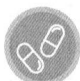

Pharmacologic Considerations

■ Genetic variations in racial groups can influence medication outcomes, "approximately 20% of the new drugs approved in the past several years have known racial/ethnic differences in disposition." For example, certain drug classes used for psychological illnesses (e.g., depression or schizophrenia) reduce symptoms better for African American and Asian clients than other classes of drugs do (Streetman, 2017).

Cultural Assessment

A cultural nursing assessment is a "systematic appraisal or examination of individuals, families, groups, and communities in terms of their cultural beliefs, values, and practices" (Streetman, 2017). The nurse should include cultural beliefs and health practices in any initial assessment (Box 8-4).

Assessing Cultural Heritage

Cultural ignorance can profoundly affect access to quality health care. It can provide the motivation for expanding one's knowledge base about different cultures. Recognizing all the areas in which cultural differences subtly manifest themselves is important. Examples include communication patterns; hygiene practices, including feelings about modesty and accepting help from others; use of special clothing or amulets; food preferences; management of symptoms such as pain, constipation, and depression; rituals surrounding birth and death; spiritual or religious orientation, especially as related to health care; family relationships, including expectations of older adults and children; and patterns of interacting with health care providers.

Assessing Health Beliefs and Practices

As described earlier, both health beliefs and practices are perpetuated and influenced by strong cultural affiliations. To discover a client's health beliefs and practices, the nurse will find it useful to ask specific questions (see Box 8-4). Assessment of these factors helps identify the client's beliefs about their values related to health or illness; recognize health-seeking behaviors on which to capitalize to promote health; view the situation from the client's perspective, recognizing there may be cultural sanctions and restrictions; distinguish beliefs and practices that may not contribute to health restoration, maintenance, or promotion; identify issues that can compromise the treatment plan; and establish a mutually agreed-on plan of care. Figure 8.1 delineates elements that should be included for a cultural nursing assessment.

BOX 8-4 Assessing Client Cultural Beliefs and Health Practices

- What is the client's country of origin? How long has the client lived in this country?
- What is the client's primary language and literacy level?
- What is the client's ethnic background? Does the client identify strongly with others from the same cultural background? Does the client live in a neighborhood with others of the same ethnic or cultural background?
- What is the client's religion, and is it important in their daily life? Are there religious rituals related to sickness, death, or health that the client observes?
- Does the client participate in cultural activities such as dressing in traditional clothing and observing traditional holidays and festivals?
- What are the client's food preferences or restrictions?
- What are the client's communication styles? Is eye contact avoided? How much physical distance is maintained? Is the client open and verbal about symptoms?
- To whom does the client turn for support? Who is the head of the family? Are they involved in decision-making about the client?
- What does the client do to maintain their health?
- What does the client call their health problem? What does the client think caused this problem?
- Has the client sought the advice of traditional healers? Have complementary and alternative therapies been used?
- What kind of treatment does the client think will help? What are the most important results the client hopes to get from this treatment?

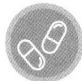

Pharmacologic Considerations

■ Eighty percent of the world's population relies on herbal preparations as part of their health care (Integrative Medicine, 2020). These preparations may have pharmacologic actions that interact with conventional medicines. It is important to assess for use before a problem arises.

TRANSCULTURAL NURSING

Transcultural nursing, founded by Leininger (1977), is considered a specialty in nursing. It refers to nursing care that is provided within the context of another's culture. Its characteristics are (1) accepting each client as an individual, (2) possessing knowledge of health problems that affect particular cultural groups, (3) assessing cultural background and health beliefs and practices, and (4) planning care compatible with the client's health belief system.

Leininger (1991) theorizes that *culturally congruent care* (care that fits a person's cultural values) assists a client to achieve better health outcomes. If a nurse respects a client's cultural values and beliefs, they can better teach diet modifications or lifestyle changes that promote healthier outcomes without insulting or patronizing the client. For

Cultural Nursing Assessment

Affiliations
- With what culture does the client self-identify?
- To what degree does the client identify with the cited cultural group?
- What is the client's place of birth?
- Where has the client lived? When? (If the patient is a recent U.S. immigrant, ask about or research prevalent diseases in the country of origin.)
- What is the client's current residence?
- What is the client's occupation?

Values
- How does the patient view birth and death?
- What is the client's view of health versus illness?
- How does the client regard health care providers?
- How does culture affect the client's body image and any changes resulting from illness or treatment? For example, what emphasis does the patient's culture place on appearance, beauty, and strength?
- Is cultural stigma associated with any of the client's illnesses or conditions?
- How does the client view work?
- What is the client's perspective on leisure?
- What are the client's views on education?
- How does the client feel about/perceive change?
- What effects on lifestyle do health, illness, treatments, and surgery pose for the client?
- What is the client's perspective on privacy? Courtesy? Touch? Age? Class? Gender?
- What perspective does the patient have regarding biomedical/scientific health care?
- How does the patient relate to those not from their culture?

Cultural Sanctions/Restrictions
- How do members of the client's culture typically express emotion and feelings?
- How do they view dying, death, and grieving?
- How do men and women show modesty? Does the culture place expectations on male–female relationships? The nurse–client relationship?
- Does the client have restrictions related to sexuality, body exposure, or type of surgery?
- Are there restrictions about discussing the dead or fears related to the unknown?

Communication
- What is the client's primary language? What other languages does the client speak or read? In what language would the client prefer to communicate with the nurse?
- What is the client's level of fluency in English (written and spoken)?
- Does the client need an interpreter?
- How does the client prefer to be addressed?
- How does the client's culture influence expectations about tempo of conversation, eye contact, topical taboos, confidentiality, and explanations?
- How does the client's nonverbal communication compare with those from other cultural backgrounds? How does it affect the health care relationship?
- How does the client view health care providers from different cultural backgrounds?
- Does the client prefer to receive care from a nurse of the same cultural background, gender, or age group?
- What are overall cultural characteristics of the client's language and communication?

Health-Related Beliefs/Practices
- To what cause(s) does the client attribute illness and disease (e.g., punishment from God, imbalance in hot/cold or yin-yang)?
- What are the client's beliefs about ideal body size and shape?
- What name does the client give to their health-related conditions?
- What does the client believe promotes health (e.g., certain foods, amulets)?
- What is client's religious background (if any)?
- Does the client rely on cultural healers (e.g., curandero, shaman, spiritualist, priest)?
- Who influences the client's choice/type of healer and treatment?
- In what types of cultural healing practices does the client engage (e.g., herbal remedies, potions, massage, talismans, healing rituals, incantations, prayers)?
- How does the client perceive biomedical/scientific health care providers? Nurses? Nursing care?
- What comprises appropriate "sick " behavior? Who determines what constitutes symptoms? Who decides when the client is no longer sick? Who cares for the patient?
- How does the client's culture view mental disorders? Are there differences in acceptable behaviors for physical versus psychological illnesses?

Nutrition
- How does the culture influence the client's nutritional factors?
- What is the meaning of food and eating for the client?

Figure 8-1 Sample of a comprehensive cultural nursing assessment inventory. (Adapted from Jensen, S. (2019). *Nursing Health Assessment* (3rd ed.). Wolters Kluwer; Andrews, M. M., Boyle, J. S., & Collins, J. (2020). *Transcultural concepts in nursing care* (8th ed.). Wolters Kluwer.)

example, clients from Middle Eastern cultures do not normally drink milk beyond childhood. They do, however, eat yogurt and also a goat or sheep cheese called *feta*. For such clients who need to increase calcium intake, nurses can inform them that these foods provide the needed calcium.

Developing Transcultural Sensitivity

Increasing one's awareness that the United States is a multicultural nation is a first step toward transcultural nursing. Examining personal beliefs, communication habits, and health care practices is another. The following recommendations will help to develop a growing expertise in culturally sensitive nursing care:

- Learn to speak a second language.
- Use techniques for facilitating interactions: sit within the client's comfort zone and make appropriate eye contact.
- Become familiar with physical differences among ethnic groups.
- Be aware of biocultural aspects of disease.
- Perform physical assessments using appropriate techniques that will provide accurate data.
- Perform cultural and health beliefs assessment and plan care accordingly.
- Consult the client about ways to solve health problems.
- Never ridicule a cultural belief or practice, verbally or nonverbally.
- Integrate cultural practices that are helpful or harmless into the plan of care.
- Modify or gradually change unsafe practices.
- Avoid removing religious medals or clothing that hold symbolic meaning for the client; if this must be done, keep them safe and replace them as soon as possible.
- Provide food that is customarily eaten.
- Advocate routine screening for diseases to which clients may be genetically or culturally prone.
- Facilitate rituals by whomever the client identifies as a healer within their belief system.
- Apologize if cultural traditions or beliefs are violated.

Being Culturally Competent

Providing culturally competent care is a process by which the nurse consistently endeavors to work within the cultural context of the client and their family and community. In doing so, the nurse must avoid stereotyping clients based on race or culture. The nurse must also listen to clients, acknowledge and respect their beliefs about health and illness, recognize culturally influenced health behaviors, communicate in a culturally sensitive manner, and adapt care to reflect cultural needs (see Evidence-Based Practice 8-1).

All individuals grow up with an ethnocentric perspective. The ethnocentrism reflects lack of knowledge and experience. Nurses must personally evolve from an ethnocentric viewpoint and develop a multicultural perspective that includes knowledge of their own as well as other cultures. They must also acknowledge any personal biases to develop a nonjudgmental attitude toward all clients.

The culturally competent nurse accepts each client as a unique individual. The first ethical principle in the American Nurses Association (ANA) Code of Ethics for Nurses states that "the nurse practices with compassion and respect for the inherent dignity, worth, and personal attributes of every person, without prejudice" (ANA, 2015, p. 1). This principle extends to providing culturally competent care to all individuals.

Evidence-Based Practice 8-1

Cultural Competence

Clinical Question

Why is it important for nurses to maintain cultural competence in practice?

Evidence

When nurses are practicing, they are taught to make eye contact when speaking to a client. This becomes challenging when they interact with different cultures. The health care world is more diverse with different cultures, and nurses must be prepared to communicate in all aspects of care. For example, the Latinx population makes up approximately 60% of the U.S. population in 2019 (24/7 Wall St, 2019). Caring for a different population or culture may lead to barriers in health care and also the quality of care received. The National Standards for Culturally and Linguistically Appropriate Services in Health and Health Care (the National CLAS Standards) have developed standards to improve and eliminate these barriers. The principal standard one "Provide effective, equitable, understandable, and respectful quality care and services that are responsive to diverse cultural health beliefs and practices, preferred languages, health literacy, and other communication needs" should be a guide in health care practice (US Department of Health and Human Services Office of Minority Health, n.d.).

Nursing Implications

Being a culturally competent nurse in this diverse era of health care will aid in misunderstandings and promote client safety and the quality of care received. Cultural competence is a continual learning process. Nurses should include in the assessment cultural beliefs and practices so that the client's trust and value are maintained.

References

24/7 Wall St. (2019). *Hispanic population in US hits new high.* https://247wallst.com/economy/2019/07/09/hispanic-population-in-us-hits-new-high/

U.S. Department of Health and Human Services Office of Minority Health. (n.d.). Culturally and Linguistically Appropriate Services (CLAS). https://thinkculturalhealth.hhs.gov/clas/what-is-clas

KEY POINTS

- Terms related to culture:
  - Cultural competence: the ability to understand the client's worldview as well as their own and how these worldviews affect nursing care
  - Subculture: refers to a particular group that shares characteristics identifying the group as a distinct entity
  - Underrepresented group: describes a group of people who differ from the majority in a society in terms of cultural characteristics or physical characteristics or both

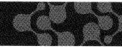

- Ethnicity: the bond or kinship that people feel with their country of birth or place of ancestral origin
- Race: refers to genetically transmitted traits, such as skin color, bone structure, and eye shape
- Stereotyping: assuming that all people in a particular cultural, racial, or ethnic group share the same values and beliefs, behave similarly, and are basically alike
- Cultural generalizations: provide a broad pattern of beliefs and behaviors for clients from a particular cultural group
- Ageism: the stereotyping of older adults' behavior or vulnerability based on an individual's prior experiences or anticipation of behaviors
- Ethnocentrism: the belief that one's own ethnic heritage is the "correct" one and superior to others
- Acculturation: involves the process of adapting to or taking on the behaviors of another group
- Cultural blindness: an inability to recognize the values, beliefs, and practices of others because of strong ethnocentric preferences
- Cultural imposition: an inclination to impose one's cultural beliefs, values, and patterns of behavior on persons from a different culture
- Cultural taboos: activities governed by rules of behavior that a particular cultural group avoids, forbids, or prohibits

- Health beliefs are a person's ideas about the role of the person who is ill, what causes the illness, how to restore health, and how one stays healthy
- Health practices: the actions a person takes to maintain or restore health based on their health beliefs
- Biocultural assessment: general appearance and obvious physical characteristics—components that make up biocultural assessment—physical appearance, body structure, mobility, and behavior
- Cultural assessment: is a systematic appraisal or examination of individuals, families, groups, and communities in terms of their cultural beliefs, values, and practices
- Transcultural nursing:
  - Accepting each client as an individual
  - Possessing knowledge of health problems that affect particular cultural groups
  - Assessing cultural background and health beliefs and practices
  - Planning care compatible with the client's health belief system
- Culturally competent nursing care: a process by which the nurse consistently endeavors to work within the cultural context of the client and their family and community. The nurse must avoid stereotyping clients based on race or culture. The nurse must also listen to clients, acknowledge and respect their beliefs about health and illness, recognize culturally influenced health behaviors, communicate in a culturally sensitive manner, and adapt care to reflect cultural needs.

CRITICAL THINKING EXERCISES

1. How could a culturally sensitive nurse prepare for the home care of a non–English-speaking client from Pakistan (or some other foreign country)?
2. How could a culturally sensitive nurse respond to a pregnant woman who wears a chicken bone around her neck to protect her unborn child from birth defects?
3. You are assigned with a nursing assistant to care for a client who is Jewish. Their care plan states that they practice religious dietary restrictions. The nursing assistant will be helping the client with meals. What factor is most important to tell the nursing assistant before they feed this client?
4. You are working in a health clinic. A recent immigrant to the United States is often late for appointments. What could you suggest to this client that may assist them to be on time for future appointments?

NCLEX-STYLE REVIEW QUESTIONS PrepU

1. A nurse is explaining why it is important that the client follow the diet prescribed by the primary provider, even though the diet includes meat, something this client does not eat based on religious observance.
   1. Advocacy
   2. Ethnocentrism
   3. Generalization
   4. Stereotyping
2. A nurse of the opposite sex identity needs to administer medications to a client of different heritage and check this client's blood pressure (BP). The client looks alarmed and covers up with the blankets. What is the nurse's best action?
   1. Ask a family member to stay while administering care.
   2. Explain to the client what the nurse plans to do.
   3. Ignore the client and carry out the procedures.
   4. Request that a nurse of the same sex give the meds and check the BP.
3. The licensed vocational nurse (LVN) needs to complete the admission data sheet for an Asian American client. This client may be offended by which of the following actions by the nurse?
   1. The nurse asks the client to speak more loudly.
   2. The nurse maintains minimal direct eye contact.
   3. The nurse sits to the side of the client while asking questions.
   4. The nurse touches the client's head as a gesture of empathy.

4. The nurse needs to reinforce principles of good body mechanics in the discharge teaching for a client who has had spinal surgery. The client speaks very little English. Which strategy will provide the best information regarding body mechanics for the non–English-speaking client?
1. Have the client watch a video.
2. Speak slowly while looking at the client.
3. Use colorful pictures or diagrams.
4. Write the instructions on paper.

5. A client from Japan who does not speak English arrives at a clinic. The client is accompanied by a family member of the opposite sex who speaks English and offers to serve as an interpreter. The licensed practical nurse (LPN) states that the clinic prefers that an interpreter assists with translation for which of the following reasons? Select all that apply.
1. The client may not want to discuss problems with a relative of the opposite sex present.
2. The nurse will be reluctant to ask questions of a sexual nature.
3. The family member may be embarrassed to answer some questions.
4. The relative may not understand the questions asked.

6. A client who is an African American person tells the nurse that the miseries continue following a surgical procedure. What is the nurse's best response?
1. "Can you explain or describe the miseries for me?"
2. "I am sorry you are miserable. What would help you?"
3. "Is there someone with you who can interpret for you?"
4. "Please use words that provide me with a better understanding."

WANT TO KNOW MORE? There are a wide variety of online resources available on thePoint to enhance learning and understanding of this chapter.

Go to **thePoint.lww.com/activate** and use the activation code found in the front of this text to unlock these online resources.

9 Integrative Medicine and Alternative Therapies

Words To Know

acupuncture
adequate intake
alternative medical systems
alternative therapies
apitherapy
aromatherapy
Ayurvedic medicine
biofeedback
bioidentical hormones
cannabinoids
Chinese medicine
chiropractic
compounding pharmacies
conventional medicine
dietary supplement
electromagnetic therapy
estimated average requirement
ethnobotanicals
herbal therapy
humor
hypnosis
imagery
integrative medicine
massage therapy
medical marijuana
mind–body medicine
Native American medicine
natural products
prebiotic
probiotic
recommended dietary allowances
reflexology
reiki
shiatsu
spirituality
tai chi
tolerable upper intake level
yoga

Learning Objectives

On completion of this chapter, you will be able to:

1. Explain the differences between Western medicine and alternative medical systems.
2. Describe the basic beliefs of Ayurvedic medicine, Chinese medicine, and Native American medicine.
3. Describe trends in Western medicine.
4. Define alternative therapy and its role in integrative medicine.
5. Name the federal agency that conducts research on alternative therapies.
6. Name two types of alternative modalities that are being researched.
7. Give examples of mind–body modalities and natural products that are being integrated into Western medicine.
8. Discuss the role nurses can play in relation to complementary and alternative therapies.

Most people in the United States and European countries turn to practitioners who represent traditional Western medicine for treatment of diseases and episodic care when symptoms arise. **Western medicine,** which is sometimes referred to as **conventional medicine**, utilizes drugs and surgery to care for clients who are not well. That is not necessarily the case in other areas of the world. There are older medical systems that have had their origins in ancient cultures in Asia, such as India and China, and even in North America prior to its settlement by Europeans. Each of these world areas has developed medical systems that are quite different from Western medicine.

Gerontologic Considerations

■ The National Institute of Health (NIH) found that older adults report frequent use of complementary therapies for health promotion or to help with specific health concerns, including exercise, home remedies, nutrition, supplements, herbs, over-the-counter medications, and prayer. Health information seeking was found to be associated with the use of complementary therapies for health self-management.

ALTERNATIVE MEDICAL SYSTEMS

From a conventional American standpoint, **alternative medical systems** are those whose theories of healing and practice evolved from other cultures. What most American people categorize as *alternative*

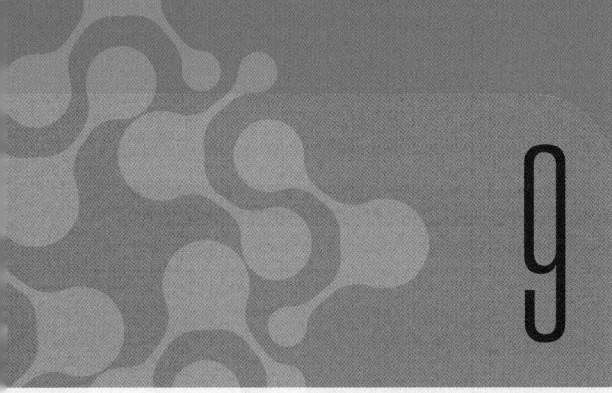

TABLE 9-1 Differences Between Alternative and Conventional Medical Systems

ALTERNATIVE MEDICAL SYSTEMS	CONVENTIONAL MEDICAL SYSTEMS
Originated in approximately 1500 BC or earlier	Originated with Hippocrates in approximately 5 BC
Believe that health results from harmony among the person, their environment (nature, universe), and energy force	Believe that health results from normal physiologic function
Focus on maintaining a healthy state	Focus on treating illness or injury
Do not correlate symptoms of disease with any specific organ or anatomic location	Correlate symptoms with the organ or location of the person's disorder
Identify with and are sensitive to cultural traditions	Recognize cultural differences but may not incorporate the client's beliefs into the treatment regimen
Incorporate religious principles	Do not reject spirituality, but do not apply any religious significance to a person's illness or recovery
Rely heavily on medicinal plants	Rely on manufactured pharmaceuticals
Accept the efficacy of treatment approaches based on traditional use rather than on specific scientific explanations	Demand scientific evidence for the mechanisms of treatment and replication of results through unbiased research
Do not have established educational standards for practitioners	Require practitioners to have formal education beyond college
Do not regulate practice	Require formal licensure for practice

medical systems, however, are considered *traditional* or *conventional* by the indigenous culture of origin, meaning that their system of healing existed before the beginning of Western medicine. Table 9-1 compares differences between alternative medical systems and conventional medical systems. The common thread among alternative medical systems is (1) the belief that one's body has the power to heal itself, and (2) that healing involves the mind, body, and spirit (Alternative Medicine, 2020). Some examples of alternative medical systems include Ayurvedic medicine practiced in India, traditional Chinese medicine, and Native American medicine in the United States.

Ayurvedic Medicine

Ayurvedic medicine has its roots in India and is the oldest system of medicine in the world. It is based on spiritual practices that developed among Tibetan monks. The object of Ayurvedic medicine is to help persons become unified with nature to develop a strong body, clear mind, and tranquil spirit. One belief is that the *prana*, or the life force, moves through various centers in the body called *chakras* (Fig. 9-1). The Ayurvedic practitioner prescribes modalities such as yoga, herbal medicine, fasting and eating cleansing foods, meditation, and massage to maintain or restore the dynamic flow of the *prana*.

Chinese Medicine

Although the term Chinese medicine is used, this medicine system also includes contributions from Japan, Korea, Vietnam, and other Southeast Asian countries. **Chinese medicine** proposes that health is the outcome of balancing *yin* and *yang*, opposite forces that must remain equalized to maintain *qi* (or *chi*), life's energy force (similar to the *prana* in Ayurvedic medicine). Forces that alter *qi*—either by depleting or obstructing it—cause illness. Correcting an imbalance between two attributes such as motion and stillness or hot and cold restores harmony and health. Treatment measures such as acupuncture, herbal remedies, diet, exercise, and massage are used to restore *qi* (Fig. 9-2).

Native American Medicine

Native American medicine practitioners view disease as resulting from disharmony with Mother Earth, possession by an evil spirit, or violation of a taboo. Followers rely on a *shaman*, a person in the tribal community who is both a medicine man (or woman) and a spiritual figure with the extraordinary ability to heal. The shaman has the power to achieve an altered state of consciousness to journey to the spirit world or assume the persona of another life form, such as an eagle or a mountain lion.

Native American medicine practitioners also believe that the shaman obtains knowledge from a higher power

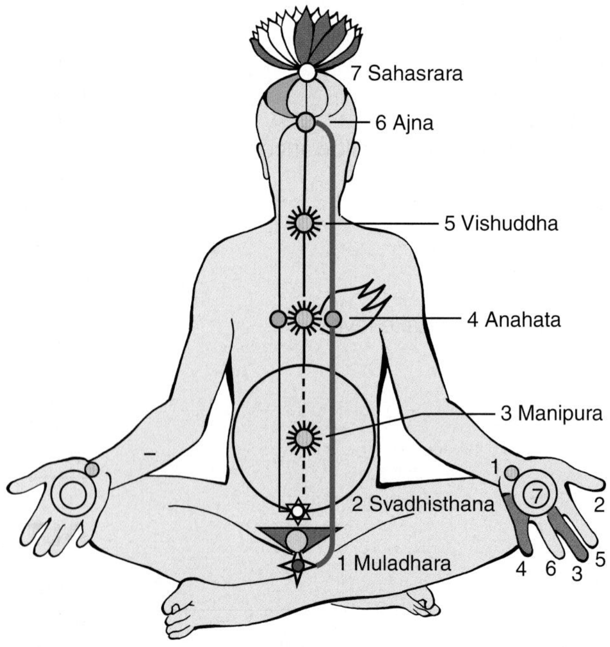

Figure 9-1 The chakras and channels of energy.

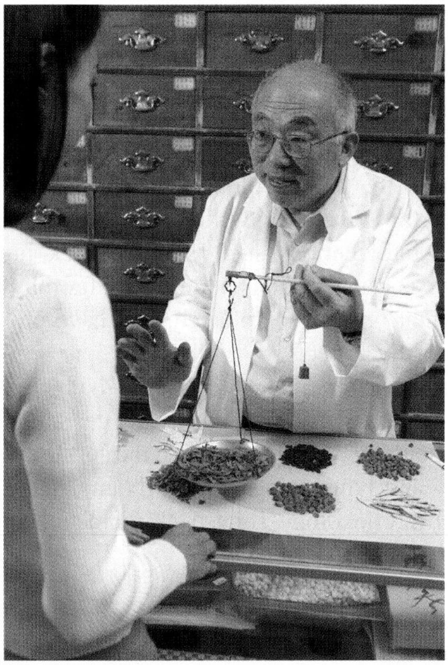

Figure 9-2 In Chinese medicine, one method for balancing the body's yin and yang energy is with herbs. (Reprinted with permission from Jensen, S. (2019). *Nursing health assessment: A best practice approach* (3rd ed.). Wolters Kluwer.)

during a trance-like state, that is induced through ritual. The knowledge allows the shaman to determine the cause and remedies for the person who is sick. Remedies may include herbs, meditation, fasting, and sweating. The shaman may fashion a talisman, a symbolic figure, that the person who is sick wears around the neck or another body location to ward off evil spirits or exorcise bad spirits.

CHANGES IN WESTERN MEDICINE

Many Americans are becoming dissatisfied with conventional Western medicine for a variety of reasons. Consequently, they are investigating alternative therapies and integrative medicine.

Alternative Therapies

A minority of Americans are turning to **alternative therapies**, nonorthodox methods with no current proven basis for their effectiveness at promoting health (Box 9-1). They are using alternative therapies in place of conventional medical treatment. Despite the number of people who exclusively use alternative therapies, the majority do not share that information with their primary provider or other health care providers. According to Johns Hopkins University, "more than 40 percent of Americans report using alternative medicine therapies for pain control when prescribed medications prove to be ineffective." Alternative medicine offers a combined approach to healing and may include interventions such as herbal remedies, reflexology, chiropractic, nutritional supplements, massage therapy, and acupuncture. More medical professionals are beginning to suggest the use of alternative therapies in combination with conventional medical treatments (Keffer, 2020).

BOX 9-1 Reasons for Adopting Alternative Therapies

- Reports from others that an alternative therapy has been personally beneficial
- Desire to become more active in decision-making and self-care
- Desire for comfort and control over chronic, incurable conditions
- Accumulating evidence of the benefits and safety of some alternative therapies
- Difficulty paying the rising costs of conventional health care
- Increased access to consumer health information via the Internet
- Growth of culturally diverse groups who do not share traditional American health beliefs and practices

Integrative Medicine

Currently, more and more clients and practitioners are turning to what is now called integrative medicine. **Integrative medicine** is a combination of conventional medical practice with nontraditional physical and nonphysical approaches for which there is some scientific evidence of safety and effectiveness (Weil, 2012). The latter is sometimes referred to as **complementary medicine**, or **complementary and alternative medicine (CAM)**. In other words, integrative medicine is not exclusively conventional medical practices or alternative therapies. It embraces selective treatments from both categories and draws upon the expertise of other disciplines like nutritionists, herbalists, massage therapists, yoga instructors, and the like. The goal is to safely help clients achieve better health and well-being. Box 9-2 identifies

BOX 9-2 Defining Principles of Integrative Medicine

1. Client and practitioner are partners in the healing process.
2. All factors that influence health, wellness, and disease are taken into consideration, including mind, spirit, and community, as well as the body.
3. Appropriate use of both conventional and alternative methods facilitates the body's innate healing response.
4. Effective interventions that are natural and less invasive should be used whenever possible.
5. Integrative medicine neither rejects conventional medicine nor accepts alternative therapies uncritically.
6. Good medicine is based on good science. It is inquiry-driven and open to new paradigms.
7. Alongside the concept of treatment, the broader concepts of health promotion and the prevention of illness are paramount.
8. Practitioners of integrative medicine should exemplify its principles and commit themselves to self-exploration and self-development.

From Andrew Weil Center for Integrative Medicine. (n.d.). *The defining principles of integrative medicine*. https://integrativemedicine.arizona.edu/about/definition.html

characteristics of integrative medicine. "CAM was most frequently used for pain control, and nearly 50% reported using CAM because their prescribed medications were ineffective" (CAM, n.d.).

Because integrative medicine provides a more comprehensive and holistic approach to health care, there is a growing consensus that alternative therapies and practices some of which are rooted in alternative medical systems deserve further research. This chapter provides an overview of various therapies that are undergoing scientific investigation, some of which are being used with and without definitive biomedical explanations.

RESEARCH AND DEVELOPMENT OF INTEGRATIVE MEDICINE

The National Center for Complementary and Integrative Health (NCCIH), a division of the Department of Health and Human Services, and the National Institute of Health, outline a research plan to assess the opportunities, to accomplish its mission; the NCCIH (2016a) has identified five strategic plans:

1. To advance research on mind and body interventions, practices, and disciplines.
2. To advance research on natural products (formerly referred to as biologically based practices) such as herbal medicines, botanicals, and probiotics.
3. To address the gaps in scientific evidence and public information on the effectiveness of alternative therapies and their outcomes on safety.
4. To bring together qualified experts from various alternative therapies and the biomedical sciences to carry out research.
5. To develop and disseminate objective, evidence-based information on alternative therapies.

Despite the absence of empirical evidence for the efficacy of some alternative therapies, the principle of "First, do no harm" prevails. That is, if the alternative therapy is not dangerous or unhealthy, it should be tolerated or even supported if it provides something perceived by the individual as being beneficial.

Modalities Under Study

The NCCIH subdivides its research into two general categories:

- **Mind–body medicine**—techniques that are administered or taught by a trained practitioner such as acupuncture, massage therapy, meditation, relaxation, spinal manipulation, and yoga.
- **Natural products**—diverse products derived from plants, bacteria, fungi, animal species, and marine organisms that include vitamins, minerals, and probiotics.

Practices among alternative medical systems, once considered an additional category in this list, are incorporated within the two categories of research. Many practices that were once categorized as belonging to alternative medical systems are now becoming accepted as conventional or integrative medical treatments.

Mind–Body Medicine

Mind–body medicine uses various techniques that rely on the power of the brain, emotions, social interactions, and spiritual factors to alter body functions or symptoms. Most mind–body interventions, such as biofeedback, imagery, humor, hypnosis, and spiritual healing, have few physical risks, can be taught or easily explained, and have provided evidence of positive effects.

Another category relegated to mind–body medicine pertains to techniques that focus on structures and systems of the body including bones and joints, the soft tissues, and the circulatory and lymphatic systems. Examples include massage therapy, reflexology, shiatsu, chiropractic, yoga, tai chi, reiki, and acupuncture.

Biofeedback

Biofeedback is a mind–body technique in which an individual voluntarily controls one or more physiologic functions, such as body temperature, heart rate, blood pressure (BP), and brain waves. Initially, clients are attached to a machine that transforms a physiologic activity, such as heart rate, into a pulsating waveform, digital numbers, or audible sound (Fig. 9-3). While receiving feedback from the machine, clients try to alter a particular function (e.g., decrease heart rate). If the machine's signal changes, it helps them determine if they are successful. Eventually, clients do not need to rely on the response from the device; they can alter their physiology at will. Biofeedback is currently being used in the United States to reduce hypertension and rapid heart rates, manage pain, abort seizures, relieve migraine

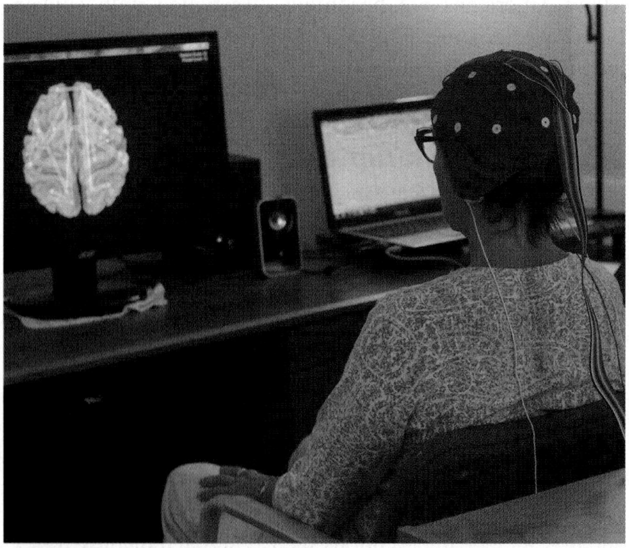

Figure 9-3 The client is participating in a 19-channel LORETA neurofeedback session. Her EEG and her brain's performance are monitored on one screen, and the client receives feedback about her brain's performance on the other screen. (Used with permission of Neurofeedback Associates Inc Greensboro, NC.)

headaches, and produce dilation of peripheral blood vessels in individuals with vascular disorders. The American Academy of Pediatrics (2013) endorsed biofeedback as a method for helping those with attention deficit hyperactivity disorder (ADHD) alter typical EEG patterns to a more focused, attentive state.

Imagery

Imagery is a psychobiologic technique that uses the mind to visualize a positive physiologic effect. When using imagery, clients conjure up mental images of their body waging and winning a battle with the disease process. For example, clients might visualize their body producing white blood cells in large numbers. They then imagine the white blood cells destroying cancer cells. Laboratory values of white blood cell counts taken before and after such imagery sessions often show that the numbers of white blood cells dramatically increase (Naparstek, 2011; Evidence-Based Practice 9-1).

Humor

Humor can be used therapeutically. Laughter stimulates the immune system by increasing the number of white blood cells and lowering cortisol, which suppresses immune function. Laughter can cause the release of neuropeptides (endorphins and enkephalins). Cousins (1981) shared his own pain-relieving and healing experiences using humor in his book, *Anatomy of an Illness*.

Hypnosis

Hypnosis is a therapeutic intervention that facilitates a physiologic change through the power of suggestion. Hypnotism has been used to help overcome habits such as smoking, relieve chronic pain, extinguish irrational fears, and end overeating to promote weight loss. Research is needed to find out how hypnotism works and why everyone cannot be hypnotized.

>>> ***Stop, Think, and Respond 9-1***

Which alternative medical system is associated with the following examples: (a) yoga, (b) acupuncture, and (c) wearing a talisman?

Spirituality

Of all the mind–body techniques, spirituality is one that the medical community has not yet entirely accepted as legitimately therapeutic. The premise of **spirituality**, not necessarily organized religion, is that it restores health through a higher power (God or some other metaphysical force). An intermediary person may channel the healing force, acting strictly as a facilitator. Sometimes, healing occurs through the prayers of the person who is sick or those said by others on their behalf. In "hopeless" cases, some would call the healing a miracle; however, spiritual healing is not limited to miracles. In his many books, such as *Prayer is Good Medicine* (Dossey, 1996) and *Healing Words: The Power of Prayer and the Practice of Medicine* (Dossey, 1993), the primary provider Larry Dossey notes that prayer-like thoughts offered from a distance have increased the healing rate of surgical wounds and sped the recovery of clients who have had surgery.

Evidence-Based Practice 9-1

Clinical Question

Can imagery encourage relaxation and support for clients in integrative medicine?

Evidence

Guided imagery (GI) is a technique that uses the mind and body as interventions in place of medication treatment. A study by Case et al. (2018) used GI to help with mood, fatigue, and quality of life in clients with multiple sclerosis. They looked at two groups: One group who were treated with GI, and the other group who journaled. The study concluded that the clients who had GI reported improved self-reported physical and mental well-being and additional benefits of changes in depressed mood and fatigue as well as improvements in the client's physical and mental quality of life. They concluded that the GI had a positive effect on the group.

Nursing Implications

In nursing practice, imagery is noninvasive and poses minimal risk to clients (Kubes, 2015). The technique can be integrated into nursing interventions and the outcomes evaluated. Many research studies have shown imagery to be positive and to reduce numerous symptoms. There are training sessions available at many schools that can help the nurse develop their technique.

References

Case, L. K., Jackson, P., Kinkel, R., & Mills, P. J. (2018). Guided imagery improves mood, fatigue, and quality of life in individuals with multiple sclerosis: An exploratory efficacy trial of healing light guided imagery. *Journal of Evidence-Based Integrative Medicine*. https://doi.org/10.1177/2515690X17748744

Kubes, L. F. (2015). Imagery for self-healing and integrative nursing practice. *American Journal of Nursing, 115*(11), 36–43. https://doi.org/10.1097/01.naj.0000473313.17572.60

Massage Therapy, Reflexology, and Shiatsu

Massage therapy involves applying pressure and movement to stretch and knead soft body tissues (Fig. 9-4). Massage

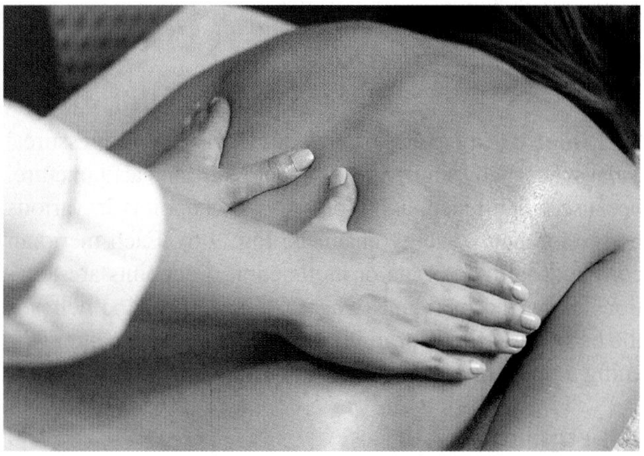

Figure 9-4 An example of a client receiving massage therapy. (Source: shutterstock.com/aerogondo2)

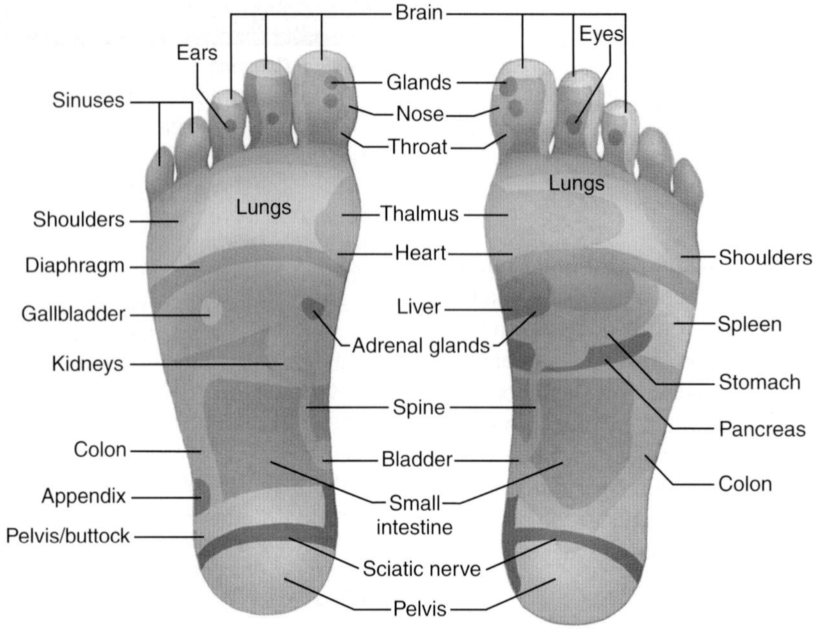

Figure 9-5 Reflex areas in the foot.

therapists use the warmth of their hands, elbows, and forearms and lubricating oils to stimulate circulation and relieve physical and psychological tension. The benefits of massage include relief from discomfort and improved mobility or functional use of affected parts of the body.

Reflexology is a complementary health practice in which manual pressure is applied to the feet and hands. The International Academy of Advanced Reflexology and those who practice reflexology claim that locations in the extremities contain reflex centers composed of more than 7,000 nerve endings linked to body organs and tissues (Spriggs, 2016). When pressure is applied to a reflex area, for instance in the foot (Fig. 9-5), the impulse travels from peripheral nerves to the spinal cord and brain. As a result, reflexologists believe that reconditioning or reprogramming the neural reflex improves the body's ability to facilitate natural healing.

››› *Stop, Think, and Respond 9-2*

Discuss physiologic and emotional responses that you have experienced during and after receiving a backrub or a similar type of massage.

Shiatsu is a Japanese word that means "finger pressure." Shiatsu has many similarities to acupressure and acupuncture, because practitioners apply pressure to acupoints in various body meridians (energy channels; Fig. 9-6). Each meridian correlates with an organ or its function. Acupoints are locations along the meridians where Chinese medicine believes the body's life force, or *qi*, moves. Unblocking and strengthening *qi* rebalances the body's energy and restores health.

Chiropractic

Chiropractic theory proposes that subluxation (malalignment) of the spinal vertebrae alters nerve activities that regulate body functions in distant organs. To treat various disorders, chiropractors, who are the single largest group of alternative–complementary therapy practitioners in the United States, perform spinal manipulation as a generic method for curing neuromuscular disorders and a host of other diseases (Fig. 9-7). Sciencebasedmedicine.org describes its mission as "exploring issues and controversies in the relationship between science and medicine," and offers the following critique of chiropractic theory: although subluxation, a partial dislocation or displacement of vertebrae, is the basis for most chiropractic practices, "there is no supportive evidence . . . for subluxation being associated with any disease process or suboptimal health conditions requiring intervention."

Despite the criticisms and controversies from many members of the scientific community, millions of people continue to seek chiropractic treatment with some improvement in their symptoms. Chiropractic treatment is further

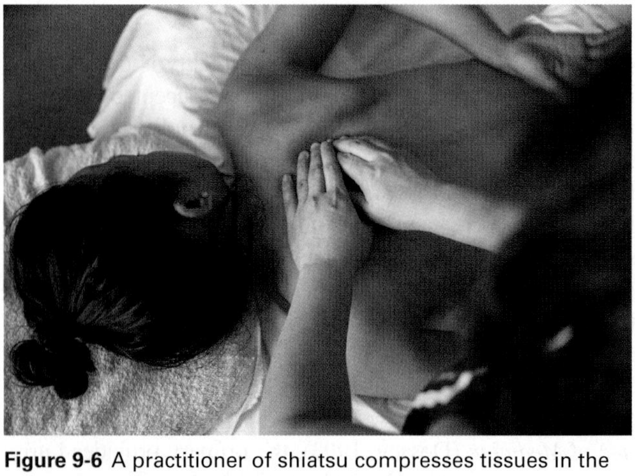

Figure 9-6 A practitioner of shiatsu compresses tissues in the client's back. (Source: Nicole De Khors/Burst)

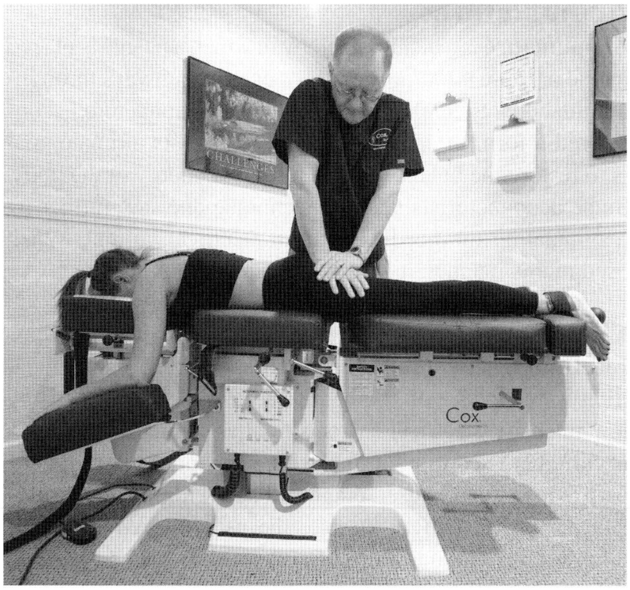

Figure 9-7 A chiropractor adjusts the client's spine. (Reprinted with permission from Cox, J. M. (2012). *Low back pain* (7th ed.). Wolters Kluwer Health/Lippincott Williams & Wilkins.)

legitimized because (1) many health insurance policies cover it, (2) the federal government provides Medicare and Medicaid reimbursement for it, and (3) the costs are an approved medical income tax deduction.

Some feel that chiropractic is a form of pseudomedicine that has attracted clients who are disgruntled with the outcomes of conventional medical care. Critics continue to suggest that there is no reason to justify practitioners who use "one cure" for all ailments. In fact, some hold that this type of philosophy can delay appropriate medical treatment. Many believe that spinal manipulation should be limited to medically trained specialists such as osteopaths, orthopedists, and physiatrists, primary providers who specialize in rehabilitation. But until the NCCIH conducts further scientific research, emotions and conjecture rather than facts will continue to fuel the controversy.

Yoga, Tai Chi, Qi Gong

Yoga was developed in India, and **tai chi** has its origins in China. Both incorporate techniques that combine mental and physical exercises for the purpose of integrating body and mind. There are several branches of yoga; hatha yoga is the most commonly practiced in the United States (Fig. 9-8). Advocates of hatha yoga attribute the following benefits to its practice:

- Relaxation and centeredness
- Relief of headaches, insomnia, anxiety, and pain
- Increased musculoskeletal flexibility
- Improved breathing
- Overall contentment

Chinese people believe that tai chi exercises restore *qi* or *chi*. The exercises require standing and shifting body weight from one foot to another while performing a series

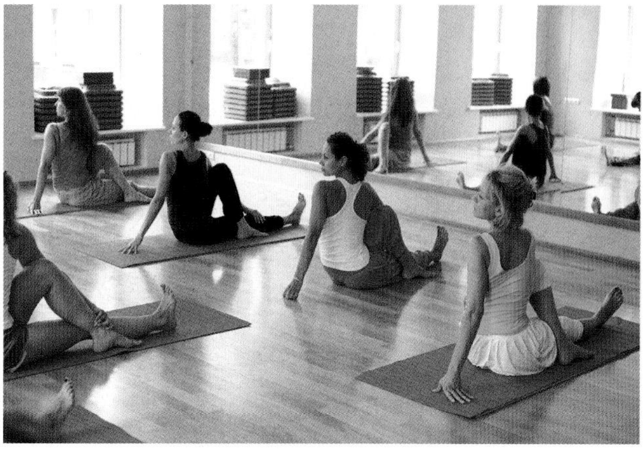

Figure 9-8 Participants learn to implement yoga positions and principles. (Reprinted with permission from DeLaet, R. (2011). *Introduction to health care & careers*. Wolters Kluwer Health/Lippincott Williams & Wilkins.)

of slow, choreographed arm movements (Fig. 9-9). To obtain full advantage of the physical exercise, it should be accompanied by slow, controlled breathing and visualization of energy circulating throughout the body.

Proponents believe that tai chi exercises tone the whole body without the exertion and cardiac risks associated with other aerobic forms of physical exercise, restore health, and prevent disease. In China, where a slightly different form of tai chi called *qi gong* is practiced, there are reports that people develop psychokinetic powers, the ability to move objects and people without touching them.

Reiki

Reiki (pronounced "ray-key") shares many features with what Westerners may call "therapeutic touch" and spiritual healing. **Reiki** is a Japanese method of healing that was introduced to the Western world in the 1800s. *Rei* means "spirit" and *ki* is translated like *qi* or *chi*. Those who use reiki believe that *ki* promotes health and healing. They further believe that when *ki* is blocked and a person is ill, a reiki practitioner can channel energy—not from their own body

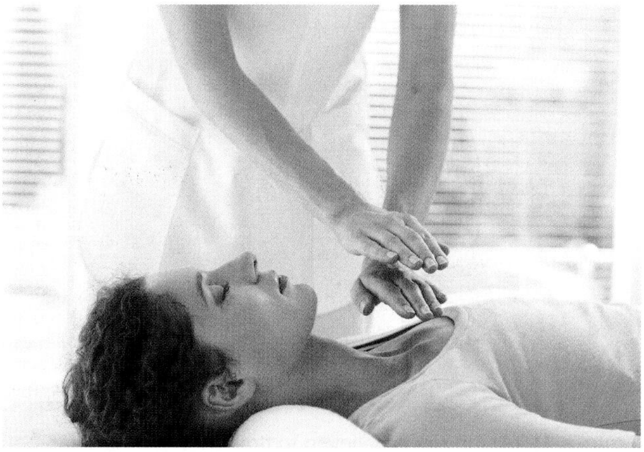

Figure 9-9 Tai chi, which mimics martial arts movements, is used to relieve stress and promote a sense of well-being. (Source: shutterstock.com/vanhurck)

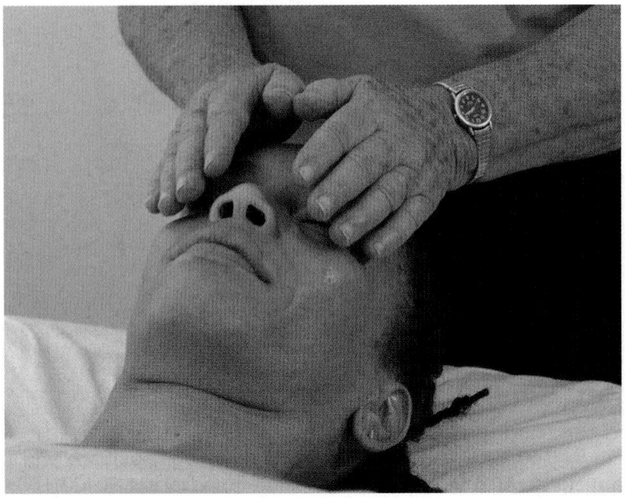

Figure 9-10 A client undergoes reiki to restore healing. (Source: shutterstock.com/wavebreakmedia)

but from the universe—to the body of the person who is sick. Once *ki* is restored, healing occurs.

The practitioner transfers the energy in the universe by laying on of hands (Fig. 9-10). Direct contact between the practitioner and client is the usual method of healing; however, healing can also occur from a distance, because Japanese people believe that the spirit is not confined by time or space. In other words, the practitioner and person who is ill can be geographically separate. The practitioner then moves their hands on an object that symbolically represents the person who is sick while visualizing the transmission of energy. The belief is that the recipient draws in the energy, which goes where it is needed.

Acupuncture

Acupuncture is a healing therapy in which a needle is placed in one or more *meridians*, pairs of energy pathways throughout the body, to unblock *qi* (Fig. 9-11). Acupuncture is considered a form of energy therapy, because its ultimate goal is to restore the balance and free flow of energy in the body. Some acupuncturists take the technique one step further by manipulating the needles with an electrical current. When used in this manner, it is referred to as *electroacupuncture*.

Electromagnetic Therapy

Electromagnetic therapy promotes healing using electricity, magnets, or both. Microcurrent therapy, using low-intensity electrical currents to alter cellular physiology, is currently used to treat nonhealing fractures and to relieve pain. Magnetism is used diagnostically with magnetic resonance imaging (MRI). Despite the use of electromagnetic therapies, several questions are yet unanswered: (1) How do these two forces produce healing? (2) What is the explanation for the anecdotal reports of symptom relief among people who wear magnets? and (3) if electromagnetic healing is validated, for what disorders is it best used?

The theory of electromagnetism is based on the physiologic principle that cellular membranes emit electrical currents. This electrical energy can be recorded using electrocardiograms, electroencephalograms (EEGs), and electromyelograms. Science also has confirmed that nerve stimulation causes the resting membrane potentials of cells to change to action potentials. Furthermore, a magnet can change the direction of an electrical current by separating charged ions. Consequently, speculation is that electromagnetic therapy (1) affects the cell membrane by changing the

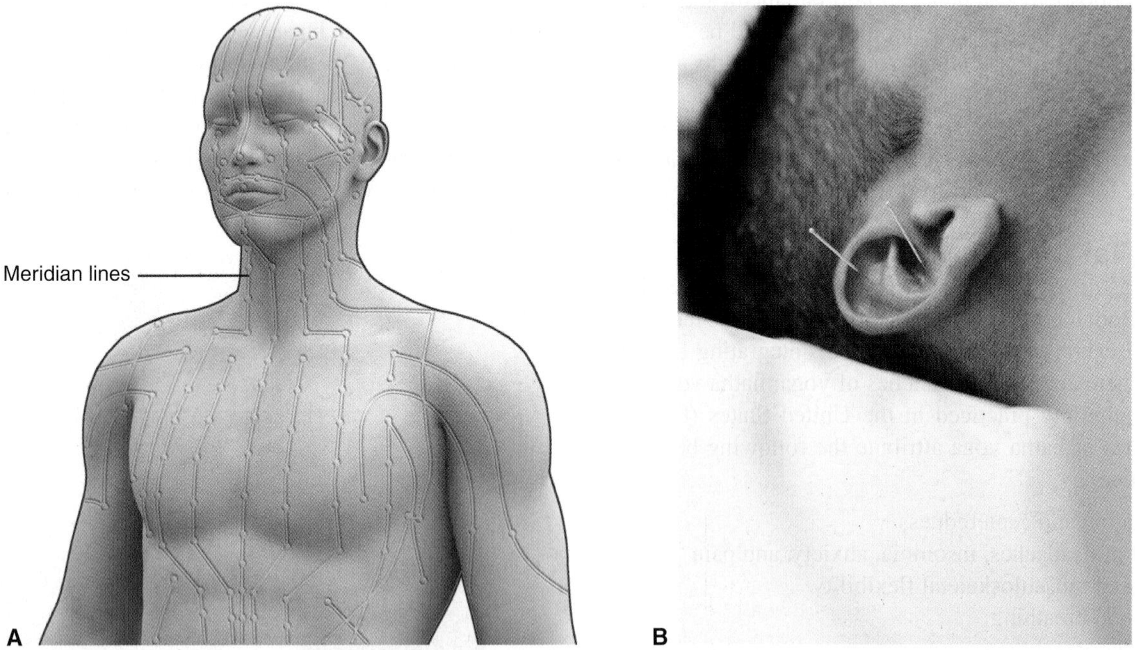

Figure 9-11 (**A**) Energy is believed to flow through meridian pathways. (**B**) Needles are placed in meridians to relieve disorders by unblocking pathways of energy. (A, reprinted with permission from Hoppenfeld, J. D. (2014). *Fundamentals of pain medicine: How to diagnose and treat your patients.* Wolters Kluwer; B, reprinted with permission from Mohr, W. (2013). *Psychiatric mental health nursing: Evidence-based concepts, skills, and practices* (8th ed.). Wolters Kluwer Health/Lippincott Williams & Wilkins.)

ion exchange of electrolytes such as calcium, sodium, and potassium; (2) stimulates the release of endorphins, naturally produced morphine-like chemicals, or other neurotransmitters through the cell's membrane; or (3) rebalances the electromagnetic field in the body.

Although questions about the what, why, and how of electromagnetic therapy remain largely unanswered, its use has been unscientifically expanded to include static magnet therapy and pulsed magnetic field therapy. Static magnet therapy refers to wearing stationary magnets, which are stronger than everyday refrigerator-type magnets, directly on the body. The static magnets are incorporated in bracelets, necklaces, belts, wraps, and even mattress pads. Pulsed magnetic field therapy uses devices that apply very-low-frequency electricity (50 Hz) to body areas at intervals of 25 pulses per second for 600 seconds (10 minutes) followed by an interval of rest. Supposedly, the pulsing effect produces rising and falling levels in the body's magnetic field.

Electromagnetic therapeutic devices continue to be used for a host of unrelated conditions such as fibromyalgia, postpolio syndrome, peripheral neuropathy, multiple sclerosis, depression, epilepsy, and urinary incontinence. Research must continue to determine if there is a legitimate scientific basis to its efficacy.

Natural Products

Natural products incorporate biologic-based practices such as using synthesized plant sources to make bioidentical hormones; plant or plant extracts (e.g., marijuana, to treat disease or symptoms); dietary supplements; aromatherapy products; and animal-derived extracts such as bee venom.

Bioidentical Hormones

Bioidentical hormones are those that are synthesized from plant chemicals. They are created in **compounding pharmacies** that combine, mix, or alter ingredients according to a primary provider's prescription to meet the specific needs of an individual. Most are designed to relieve menopausal symptoms. Although many are led to believe that compounded hormones are safer and more effective, scientific evidence does not support the claim. Bioidentical hormones have the same risks and benefits as nonbioidentical hormones made by pharmaceutical manufacturers (Harvard Medical School, 2015).

Concept Mastery Alert

Biologic-Based Practices

Biologic-based practices are integrative therapies that rely on natural substances such as herbs, healthy foods, and nutritional supplements. This is distinct from mind–body medicine, which utilizes the brain, emotions, social interactions, and spiritual factors.

Medical Marijuana

Medical marijuana refers to using the leaves, flowers, stems, and seeds of the marijuana plant for medicinal purposes. When inhaled or eaten, the plant contains *tetrahydrocannabinol* (THC) and *cannabidiol* (CBD), two of more than 100 other chemicals collectively called **cannabinoids.**

THC increases appetite and reduces nausea and is used by some with advanced cancer, those receiving chemotherapy, those with AIDS, and glaucoma to relieve their respective symptoms. Whereas, CBD is useful in reducing pain, inflammation, controlling epileptic seizures, and controlling muscle problems experienced by those with multiple sclerosis.

The possession and sale of marijuana is illegal in several states. As of May 2016, 25 states legalized some aspects of personal marijuana use. Four states and the District of Columbia have legalized marijuana for medical as well as recreational use (Governing Data, 2016). There is concern that abuse of natural marijuana may have serious health effects, such as pulmonary problems from inhaling smoke, impaired memory and learning, decreased motivation, distorted thinking manifested by paranoia and hallucinations, and possible harm to fetal brains among pregnant users. The U.S. Food and Drug Administration (FDA) has approved dronabinol (Marinol) and nabilone (Cesamet) synthetic THC. Taken orally, use of prescription synthetic cannabinoids is subject to abuse and the same side effects as those of the natural plant.

Dietary Supplements

The health food industry lobbied federal legislators in the early 1990s to "preserve the consumer's right to choose dietary supplements" (Barrett, 2015, p. 1). As a result, the Dietary Supplement Health and Education Act of 1994 (DSHEA) was passed. DSHEA defines a "**dietary supplement**" as something that supplies one or more dietary ingredients, including vitamins, minerals, amino acids, herbs, and other substances. See Nutrition Notes.

Nutrition Notes

The Client Taking Dietary Supplements

- The Office of Dietary Supplements publishes online fact sheets for individual dietary supplements that include what the supplement is used for, results of scientific research, potential side effects, cautions, and references. They are available at https://ods.od.nih.gov/.
- After a dietary supplement is marketed, it is up to the FDA to prove danger rather than being up to the manufacturer to prove safety. Check the FDA website at www.cfsan.fda.fda.gov/~dms for consumer advisories on supplements to be avoided.
- Generally, dietary supplements up to 10 times the RDA will not induce toxicity, but doses of no more than 100% of the RDA are recommended if supplements are used.

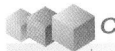

Vitamin and Mineral Supplements

Vitamin and mineral supplements are considered more legitimate for health than other biologically based practices. Scientists who advise the Food and Nutrition Board, a committee within the National Academy of Sciences, establish Dietary Reference Intakes, a set of four separate reference values used to plan and evaluate diets. The **estimated average requirement** is the intake that meets the estimated need of 50% of individuals in a specific group. The **recommended dietary allowances** (RDAs) represent the levels of essential nutrients necessary to meet the needs of most healthy persons. Special populations such as pregnant women, older adults, and people with medical disorders may have different RDA requirements. When there are insufficient data to determine the RDA, an **adequate intake** (AI) is set; it is the amount of a nutrient thought to meet or exceed requirements. The **tolerable upper intake level** (UL) is the highest level of daily nutrient intake that is likely to pose no risk of adverse health effects. The nutrient with the greatest risk for toxicity is vitamin A, especially for children and pregnant women.

Probiotics, Prebiotics, and Synbiotics

Additional types of supplements include probiotics and prebiotics. **Probiotics** are microorganisms that exert beneficial health effects, such as *Lactobacillus acidophilus* and *Bifidobacterium infantis*, which can lower the frequency or duration of diarrhea. **Prebiotics** include nondigestible food ingredients such as dietary fiber that enhance or maintain the growth of probiotic intestinal bacteria. When these two are combined, they are referred to as **synbiotics**, because they simultaneously provide a food source that supports the proliferation of probiotic bacteria (Sproule-Willoughby, 2015).

Herbal Supplements

The use of herbal supplements is based on **herbal therapy**, a technique of using plants to treat diseases and disorders (Fig. 9-12). Herbal therapy techniques have mostly been handed down orally from generation to generation. For centuries, humans have used **ethnobotanicals**, plants that grow in a region where specific groups of people live, for food, clothing, shelter, and medicine. The particular plants that are used by people from China, India, and people who are Native American, and other groups are different in various world locales, but their general purposes are largely the same. The use of plants and herbs is commonly referred to as *folk medicine* because the benefits are largely anecdotal rather than based on scientific investigation. However, the use of plants in medicine is not unique. In conventional medicine, approximately 25% of prescription drugs are derived from plants. Drugs manufactured from plant sources usually contain one or more extracts from the plant or a synthesized, molecularly similar structure.

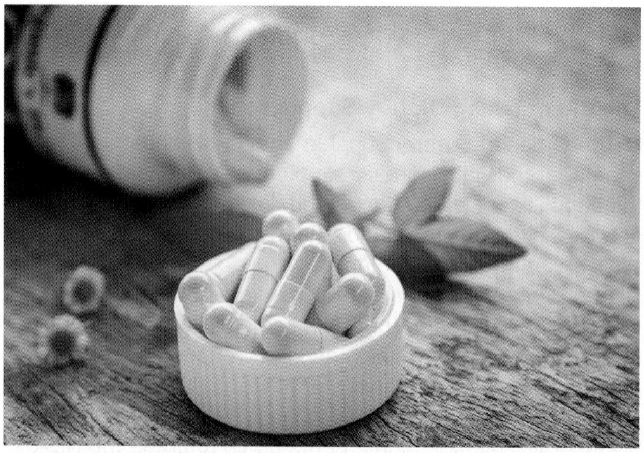

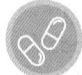

Figure 9-12 Various plants may be used to treat disorders or form the basis for developing new drugs. (Source: shutterstock.com/Fecundap stock)

Herbalists argue that using only parts of a plant changes the effects that are achieved from using the whole plant. Consequently, interest in self-treatment using herbs has been renewed (Table 9-2). Clients can use herbs in a variety of forms: liquified juice, mashed paste, steeped teas, compressed powders, fermented liquid, sweetened syrups, tinctures, liniments, and salves.

Herbal therapy is not regulated like pharmaceutical drugs are in the United States. Because herbs are classified as dietary supplements, they are not held to the same standards of unified dosages, safety, and efficacy as drugs. Manufacturers of herbal preparations, however, cannot claim that the herbal product prevents or treats a disease because that automatically places the substance in the category of a drug, which is highly regulated. To avoid federal regulation, labels on herbal products can make structural or functional claims, such as "boosts stamina," as long as they also contain a disclaimer that the FDA has not evaluated the product.

Herbal therapy is one of the greatest risk factors for adverse effects when combined with other conventional treatments, such as drugs. As the NCCIH studies herbs more scientifically, more than anecdotal information will become available. Until then, Dr. Roberta Lee, former vice chair of the Department of Integrative Medicine at the Continuum Center for Health and Healing at Beth Israel Medical Center in New York, advises consumers of herbs to (1) find out what they are using, (2) not to use a product if information is unavailable, (3) use the lowest dose initially, (4) increase the dose gradually, and (5) never exceed the maximum dose. Even herbs have possibly lethal side effects. Consulting with a primary provider before using herbs and disclosing that information before any medication is prescribed are best. Use of herbs also is not recommended for pregnant or lactating women, infants, and children younger than 6 years of age without the knowledge and approval of a primary provider.

Pharmacologic Considerations

- Certain herbs when taken can potentiate or eliminate the effectiveness of drugs. See Table 9-2 for examples.

TABLE 9-2 Popular Herbs Used in the United States

HERB/BOTANICAL NAME	CLAIM FOR USE	PRECAUTIONS	DRUG INTERACTIONS
Aloe vera *Aloe vera*	To inhibit infection and promote healing of minor burns and wounds; as a laxative	May cause burning sensation in wound. If taken internally as a laxative, do not take longer than 1–3 weeks without consulting primary health care provider.	(Internal use) Decrease blood sugar and triglycerides potential—glyburide Decreased potassium—digoxin, diuretics
Black cohosh *Actaea racemosa*	Management of menopausal symptoms, alternative to hormone replacement therapy; may be beneficial for hypercholesterolemia or peripheral vascular disease	Should not be used during pregnancy	Liver toxicity—when taken with other hepatotoxic drugs
Capsicum *Capsicum frutescens*	For neuralgic pain relief, bladder pain and hyperreflexia; as an antipruritic for psoriasis	Burning sensation upon application, apply with gloves—wash hands thoroughly before touching face or eyes.	
Chamomile *Chamomilla recutita*	Relieves digestive disorders	Avoid if allergic to ragweed, asters, chrysanthemums, or members of the daisy family.	Increases bleeding potential—anticoagulants, aspirin, NSAIDs Increases drowsiness—sedatives and hypnotics
Echinacea *Echinacea angustifolia*	Boosts immune function and speeds healing	Avoid if allergic to plants in the daisy family; prolonged use may reduce effects.	
Garlic *Allium sativum*	Lowers blood pressure, thins the blood	Possible side effects include intestinal gas; combining garlic with aspirin or other anticoagulants can prolong bleeding.	Increases bleeding potential—anticoagulants, aspirin, NSAIDs Reduced effectiveness of protease inhibitors (HIV Rx)
Ginkgo *Ginkgo biloba*	Improves memory	Possible side effects include gastrointestinal distress, headaches, and allergic reactions; use with caution if taking aspirin or other blood-thinning drugs.	Increases bleeding potential—anticoagulants, aspirin, NSAIDs Reduced effectiveness of monoamine oxidase inhibitor (MAOI) antidepressants
Kava *Piper methysticum*	Reduces stress and anxiety	Large doses can produce an intoxicating effect; long-term use can lead to dry, scaly skin.	
Ginseng *Panax gensema*	Increases energy and helps in dealing with stress	Use may raise blood pressure and serum glucose level and can increase the growth of estrogen-dependent cancer.	Risk of serotonin syndrome if used with selective serotonin reuptake inhibitor (SSRI) antidepressants
Marijuana, controlled substance not available in all states *Cannabis*	For pain, muscle spasms, and other conditions not relieved by standard treatment or medications.	Smoking may produce an effect in 10 minutes, whereas ingestion requires at least 30–60 minutes. Due to lag time for edible products, people may feel they have not taken enough for effect and may ingest more resulting in a dangerous overdose.	Increases drowsiness—sedatives, hypnotics, and opiates
Melatonin *Melatonin*	For insomnia; topically to protect against ultraviolet light	Do not take for prolonged periods, because effects of prolonged use are not known.	Reduced effectiveness of oral contraceptives
Red yeast *Monascus purpureus*	Reduces cholesterol levels in healthy people and can stimulate bone growth and prevent inflammation	Same reactions as statin drugs; headache, dizziness, nausea, constipation	Should not be taken with other antihyperlipidemia drugs.
St. John's wort *Hypericum perforatum*	Treats mild depression	Use may cause sensitivity to light.	Increases bleeding potential—anticoagulants, aspirin, nonsteroidal antiinflammatory drugs (NSAIDs) Reduced effectiveness of oral contraceptives, antiretrovirals Risk of serotonin syndrome if used with SSRI antidepressants

(continued)

TABLE 9-2 Popular Herbs Used in the United States (*continued*)

HERB/BOTANICAL NAME	CLAIM FOR USE	PRECAUTIONS	DRUG INTERACTIONS
Saw palmetto *Serenoa repens*	Relieves enlargement of the prostate gland	Avoid tea versions, because the herb dissolves poorly; nausea and gastrointestinal distress are possible.	Increases bleeding potential—anticoagulants, aspirin, NSAIDs
Valerian *Valeriana officinalis*	Relieves anxiety and insomnia	Possible side effects include blurred vision, excitability, and changes in heartbeat if taken in large doses or for more than 2 weeks.	Increases sedation—benzodiazepines, opioids, alcohol

Note. A more comprehensive listing can be found at https://www.urmc.rochester.edu/encyclopedia/content.aspx?contenttypeid=1&contentid=1169

Aromatherapy

Most people agree that they positively or negatively associate odors of certain substances with various people, places, or feelings. **Aromatherapy** is the use of scents to alter emotions and biologic processes. For therapeutic uses, scents from botanical oils of lavender, peppermint, and the like are released by adding them to bath water, permeating the air where they are inhaled, or rubbing them on the skin (Fig. 9-13). The olfactory nerves carry the scented molecules to the limbic system. The limbic system is the brain area used for learning, memory, and emotions. Once the limbic system is stimulated, it can trigger physiologic and psychological responses through neurotransmitters such as serotonin, endorphins, or norepinephrine released by the hypothalamus. The neurotransmitters can, in turn, affect nervous, endocrine, and immune system functions. Some believe that aromatherapy can help control BP and hormone secretions; relieve pain, depression, and anxiety; or promote higher states of alertness. More research is needed to validate the physiologic actions of various scents, evaluate how best to use them, and determine why one type of aroma affects people differently.

››› *Stop, Think, and Respond 9-3*

Discuss particular scents and the images or feelings they create for you. For example, the smell of the ocean may make you happy because of the pleasant memories that you associate with a holiday or former residence. On the other hand, odors such as the antiseptic smell of the dentist's office may create feelings of anxiety or fear because of its negative associations. Give other examples of scents or odors that personally evoke positive or negative effects.

Apitherapy

Apitherapy is the medicinal use of bee venom. To date, apitherapy has been used as an alternative for treating various inflammatory conditions of the joints such as rheumatoid arthritis and osteoarthritis. It is also used to treat multiple sclerosis, a neurologic condition. Although reports of the use of bee venom have dated from the mid-1800s, interest in apitherapy gained momentum around 1920. Bee venom does contain various enzymes that may stimulate the adrenal glands and induce the release of cortisol, an antiinflammatory and immunosuppressant hormone. Researchers at Washington University School of Medicine recently found that a toxin in bee venom can destroy human immunodeficiency virus (HIV) without harming surrounding cells (Strait, 2013). Primary providers currently consider apitherapy an unconventional treatment, however, and do not recommend its use or support a client's request for it. Nevertheless, clinical trials and researchers have demonstrated relief of symptoms among research volunteers. Under the supervision of the NCCIH, further study may validate (1) if bee venom therapy is effective; (2) if so, which types of disorders respond best when apitherapy is used; (3) which yields better results: the actual sting of the bee or chemically prepared apitoxin (bee venom); (4) how many stings or what apitoxin concentrations are necessary to achieve positive results; and (5) if there are any other side effects to consider besides discomfort and potential allergic reactions.

Hirudotherapy: Medical Leeches

Hirudotherapy or the use of medical leeches works "as a sort of reverse transfusion in cases of imbalanced blood circulation, the contemporary use of leeches is mostly limited to microsurgeons who reattach body parts like fingers, toes, thumbs, ears, lips, noses, or even bits of scalp" (Renault, 2019).

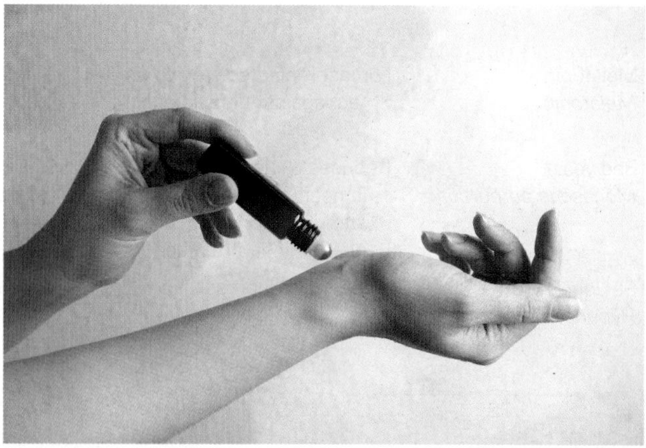

Figure 9-13 Essential oils are used in a variety of ways. (Source: shutterstock.com/New Africa)

NURSING ROLE IN INTEGRATIVE MEDICINE AND ALTERNATIVE THERAPIES

Because nursing is a holistic practice, it is essential to integrate both conventional medical therapies and alternative techniques that have demonstrated beneficial evidence-based outcomes. For those techniques that are still investigational, the nurse should teach the client regarding potential risk(s); however, it is important to respect and advocate for a client's choice of nontraditional medicine in combination with conventional medical treatment as long as there is no potential for harm.

Nursing can play a pivotal role in assisting clients to make knowledgeable choices about their health care by:

- Learning about alternative therapies.
- Assisting the client to obtain full disclosure about potential treatment options.
- Examining research findings to determine benefits and risks of alternative therapies.
- Empowering clients to assume autonomy for health care decisions.
- Supporting clients' choices as long as they are not potentially harmful.
- Preparing for possible untoward effects that may occur with nontraditional techniques.
- Avoiding the implementation of interventions that violate the legal scope of nursing practice.

KEY POINTS

- Western medicine: or conventional medicine, utilizes drugs and surgery to care for clients who are not well
  - Alternative medical systems: are those whose theories of healing and practice evolved from other cultures
- The basic beliefs of:
  - Ayurvedic medicine: developed by Tibetan monks, to help persons become unified with nature to develop a strong body, clear mind, and tranquil spirit
  - Chinese medicine: proposes that health is the outcome of balancing *yin* and *yang*, opposite forces that must remain equalized to maintain *qi* (or *chi*), life's energy force
  - Native American medicine: views disease as resulting from disharmony with Mother Earth, possession by an evil spirit, or violation of a taboo
- Changing trends in Western medicine:
  - Alternative medicine: offers a combined approach to healing and may include interventions such as herbal remedies, reflexology, chiropractic, nutritional supplements, massage therapy, and acupuncture
  - Integrative medicine: a combination of conventional medical practice with nontraditional physical and nonphysical approaches for which there is some scientific evidence of safety and effectiveness
- Biofeedback is a mind–body technique in which an individual voluntarily controls one or more physiologic functions, such as body temperature, heart rate, BP, and brain waves.
  - Imagery: a psychobiologic technique that uses the mind to visualize a positive physiologic effect
  - Humor: laughter stimulates the immune system by increasing the number of white blood cells and lowering cortisol, which suppresses immune function.
  - Hypnosis: a therapeutic intervention that facilitates a physiologic change through the power of suggestion
  - Spirituality: it works to restore health through a higher power (God or some other metaphysical force)
- Massage therapy: involves applying pressure and movement to stretch and knead soft body tissues
- Reflexology: believes that reconditioning or reprogramming the neural reflex improves the body's ability to facilitate natural healing
- Shiatsu: applies pressure to acupoints in various body meridians, to unblock and strengthen *qi* (body's life force), rebalances the body's energy, and restores health
- Chiropractic: proposes that subluxation (malalignment) of the spinal vertebrae alters nerve activities that regulate body functions in distant organs
- Yoga & Tai Chi: incorporate techniques that combine mental and physical exercises for the purpose of integrating body and mind
- Reiki: a Japanese method of healing; those who use Reiki believe that *ki* promotes health and healing and they believe that when *ki* (body's life force) is blocked, a person is ill.
- Acupuncture: a healing therapy in which a needle is placed in one or more *meridians*, pairs of energy pathways throughout the body, to unblock *qi*. It is considered a form of energy therapy, because its ultimate goal is to restore the balance and free flow of energy in the body.
- Electromagnetic therapy: promotes healing using electricity, magnets, or both. Microcurrent therapy, using low-intensity electrical currents to alter cellular physiology, is currently used to treat nonhealing fractures and to relieve pain.
- Natural products:
  - Bioidentical hormones are those that are synthesized from plant chemicals. They are created in compounding pharmacies that combine, mix, or alter ingredients according to a primary provider's prescription to meet the specific needs of an individual.
- Medical marijuana:
  - THC increases appetite and reduces nausea and is used by some with advanced cancer, those receiving chemotherapy, those with AIDS, and glaucoma to relieve their respective symptoms.

- CBD is useful in reducing pain, inflammation, controlling epileptic seizures, and controlling muscle problems experienced by those with multiple sclerosis.

- Dietary supplement, vitamins and mineral, probiotics, prebiotics, synbiotics, herbal supplements: supplies one or more dietary ingredients, including vitamins, minerals, amino acids, herbs, and other substances
- Aromatherapy: the use of scents to alter emotions and biologic processes
- Apitherapy: is the medicinal use of bee venom; it has been used as an alternative for treating various inflammatory conditions of the joints.
- Hirudotherapy/medical leeches: work as a sort of reverse transfusion in cases of imbalanced blood circulation; the of leeches is mostly limited to microsurgeons who reattach body parts like fingers, toes, thumbs, ears, lips, noses, or even bits of scalp

CRITICAL THINKING EXERCISES

1. What information is appropriate to offer a person who is interested in using herbs and botanicals for health-related benefits?
2. A woman who is experiencing menopausal symptoms has been advised by her primary provider to avoid hormone replacement treatment. Why might this woman and others in a similar situation turn to alternative therapies?
3. Discuss how prayer could be considered a complementary or alternative therapy.
4. Individuals such as Dr. Thomas Dooley (1927–1961), a humanitarian American primary provider in Laos, and Mother Teresa (1910–1997), an Albanian nun who worked among the sick and dying in India, integrated conventional medicine with traditional cultural practices. Discuss possible reasons why they were able to gain the trust of their "clients" even though the Laotians and Indians were unfamiliar with conventional medicine.

NCLEX-STYLE REVIEW QUESTIONS PrepU

1. The nurse is learning about health care in the United States. What are valid conclusions about conventional medicine, integrative medicine, and alternative therapies? Select all that apply.
   1. Alternative therapies are insensitive to cultural traditions.
   2. Alternative therapies are often based on word-of-mouth.
   3. Integrative medicine includes primary providers and many other types of practitioners.
   4. Conventional medicine focuses on treating diseases when they occur.
   5. Integrative medicine works in partnership with each client.
   6. Conventional medicine implements treatments based on biomedical science.
2. The nurse is caring for a client recently diagnosed with lung cancer. The client asks the nurse to provide an explanation of how imagery is used to fight the disease. What nursing response is most correct?
   1. "The mind uses mental pictures to promote a positive physical outcome."
   2. "The power of suggestion will help you to make physical changes."
   3. "This process provides you with feedback when you try to alter oxygen levels."
   4. "This technique helps to stimulate the immune system."
3. The nurse is caring for a client with irritable bowel syndrome characterized by bouts of cramping, bloating, intestinal gas, diarrhea, and constipation. The client asks the nurse to recommend a dietary change that will help relieve symptoms. What is best for the nurse to recommend?
   1. Wheat bran
   2. Granola
   3. Whole milk
   4. Cultured yogurt
4. The nurse responds to a friend who wants to add herbal therapy to current medical treatment. What should the nurse tell this person? Select all that apply.
   1. Herbs are nutritional supplements, so they are considered safe.
   2. Restrict daily usage to the FDA-recommended amount.
   3. Some herbs may adversely interact with prescribed medications.
   4. Consult your primary provider before purchasing a product.
   5. Use the Internet to learn which herbs are safe to use.
   6. Take the herb every other day initially to determine its effect on you.
5. The nurse is caring for a hospitalized client who asks the nurse to contact a reflexologist for the purpose of applying manual foot pressure. What nursing actions are appropriate? Select all that apply.
   1. Check that the reflexologist is certified.
   2. Contact a podiatrist who specializes in foot care.
   3. Determine the reason the client feels a need for reflexology.
   4. Recommend conventional medical treatment.
   5. Facilitate the services of the reflexologist.
   6. Communicate the request to the client's primary provider.

WANT TO KNOW MORE? There are a wide variety of online resources available on thePoint to enhance learning and understanding of this chapter.

Go to **thePoint.lww.com/activate** and use the activation code found in the front of this text to unlock these online resources.

10 End-of-Life Care

Words To Know
acceptance
advance directive
anger
bargaining
denial
depression
durable power of attorney (DPOA) for health care
Five Wishes document
grieving
hospice
living will
near-death experiences
nearing death awareness
palliative care
passive euthanasia
physician-assisted suicide
physician orders for scope of treatment (POST)
respite care
waiting for permission phenomenon

Learning Objectives

On completion of this chapter, you will be able to:

1. Define attitudes of society and health care providers toward death.
2. Discuss outcomes of informing a client about a terminal illness.
3. Explain how clients and families can maintain hopefulness during a terminal illness.
4. Name emotional reactions the dying client experiences.
5. Identify how the dying client can ensure that others carry out their wishes for terminal care.
6. Discuss the dilemma of physician-assisted suicide.
7. Describe physical phenomena that occur during the dying process.
8. Summarize psychological events that dying clients have reported.
9. Describe nursing management of the dying client and the family.

Although all of us will die, many Americans alive today ignore their potential for death because unlike previous generations, few are exposed to others who are dying or who have died. In the early 20th century, many people died in their homes, surrounded by family and loved ones. Later, it became more common to die in a hospital or nursing home. In the 1970s, the hospice movement began to promote care of dying clients at home or in hospice settings, providing a more dignified and supportive climate.

Increased technology and aggressive treatment have, in some ways, distorted the reality of dying and death even for health care providers. For some, death signifies a failure to save lives and act as healers. Death, however, is a natural and universal experience, a part of life, and a component of health care. Health care providers must acknowledge death as the final stage of growth and development (Kübler-Ross, 1975). They also must explore their own mortality and feelings about dying and death. This is the only way that they can then provide care and comfort to dying clients and their families.

Education about death helps health care providers become better informed about dying and death and to incorporate this knowledge into the care they give clients. Nurses who care for dying clients share emotional pain with them and their families. Denying death creates a barrier to becoming involved with clients and families and interferes with personal growth.

Death can occur in any health care setting; therefore, facing the death of clients is necessary for nurses. It is not partial to a particular age group or population. Death can be slow and tortuous or very sudden and unexpected. Preparing clients and their families for an expected death is usually very different from caring for grieving family members after an unexpected death. An essential component of quality care is recognizing that nursing care requires sensitivity and compassion for clients, families, and significant others.

Gerontologic Considerations

- Although older adults require as much emotional support as do young or middle-aged dying clients, ageism may involve the myth that all older adults are ready to die because future life has no meaning or personal value has diminished.
- Individual perspectives related to death vary according to social circumstances and prior life experiences throughout the age continuum; many older adults have unfulfilled life goals and expectations and are not ready to die.
- Older adults of 85+ years is expected to grow to over 19 million persons by 2050 (older population, 2020), which will increase the need for end-of-life care, including hospice care.
- Failure to refer clients to hospice or a delay in referral can leave people dying alone, in pain, and unwantedly attached to life support machines.
- A Physician Orders for Life-Sustaining Treatment (POLST) form may be part of a dying person's medical record. Depending on the laws of the state, this form is used to express the individual's wishes for levels of treatment, stating whether full treatment, including resuscitation attempts, is desired (see www.polst.org).
- Depending on state laws, an "allow natural death" (AND) order may be an alternative term for do-not-resuscitate (DNR) (see https://www.hospicealliance.org/services/advance-care-planning-tool-kit/).
- In institutional settings, nurses and unlicensed assistive personnel provide personal care for individuals who are dying and provide support for their families and significant others. Thus, it is imperative to include all staff in education regarding the needs of the dying and appropriate communication techniques.
  - The older adult may view dying as a natural part of life and therefore be more accepting of death than younger persons. Some older adults may fear prolonged illness, dependency, abandonment, loss of cognitive ability, or the unknown more than death itself.
  - Physical manifestations of grieving in older adults can include confusion, which may be falsely diagnosed as dementia.
- Older adults who have outlived most of their family may die alone, without support from family members, relatives, or close friends. The nurse may be the only person to give close emotional support during the final hours of life. Including older adults in as many aspects of care as possible helps maintain self-esteem and personal dignity.
- Depression or a sense of isolation in older adults can begin after the loss of a loved one. The nurse can help by listening and encouraging the bereaved older adult to talk about the loss and to describe the role that the deceased person held in their life. It may also be helpful for the bereaved person to understand that feelings of anger and guilt are normal.

SUPPORTING THE DYING CLIENT

Although most people recognize that death is inevitable, they do not spend time getting ready until actually faced with the prospect. Factors the nurse needs to consider when caring for dying clients include supporting informed clients, sustaining hope, assisting clients and families with emotional reactions, and recognizing client rights to make final decisions.

Supporting the Informed Dying Client

Nurses honor dying client rights to know the seriousness of their condition. The primary provider usually is responsible for informing clients of the nature and gravity of their illness. Even though some informed clients react negatively at first, outcomes of being truthful include the following:

- The nurse–client relationship is based on honesty rather than on the false pretense that recovery will occur.
- Client autonomy and right to determine how to spend the rest of their life are upheld.
- Clients can complete unfinished business—prepare for and arrange legal and personal affairs and complete any remaining tasks or goals.
- Clients can use inner resources and determination to survive and prolong life, often referred to as the *will to live*.
- Meaningful communication between clients and family members is promoted.

All members of the health care team must know what the client has been told regarding their prognosis. Lack of this knowledge greatly interferes with the nurse–client relationship. For example, the nurse may avoid all but the most superficial topics of conversation out of uncertainty about how to respond if asked, "Am I going to die?" Some nurses feel that, regardless of how others might try to conceal the truth, most clients gradually recognize clues that their illness is terminal. Avoidance alone tends to confirm their suspicions that they are dying. When uninformed clients are given the opportunity, they may give hints of their awareness of approaching death. Some may even indicate they are ready to discuss dying. If nurses reply to comments by saying, "Don't talk like that," they convey a message that the subject of dying is uncomfortable for the nurse. Often, clients will then avoid the subject in all future interactions (Evidence-Based Practice 10-1).

Sustaining Hope

Nurses must recognize the value of communicating a spirit of hopefulness. Hopefulness means that dying clients have a right to believe that the health care team will make their remaining days meaningful, use whatever treatment and comfort measures are appropriate, and dignify their approaching death. Both nurses and clients, however, should not confuse hope with unrealistic optimism. When clients learn that their condition is terminal, they must also understand that the health care team remains dedicated to providing palliative care, which reduces physical discomfort but does not alter a disease's progression (Box 10-1).

Evidence-Based Practice 10-1

End-of-Life Care

Clinical Question

What challenges do nurses experience when providing end-of-life care?

Evidence

A literature review on intensive care unit (ICU) critical care nurses by Isabell Fridh reviews the challenges for nurses in caring for dying clients in the ICU (Fridh, 2014). The review did not find many new concerns, but that nurses voice the same concerns such as: insufficient education in this area for nurses, the stressful ICU environment, being short-staffed in the ICU, unrealistic family wishes, disagreements among members of the care team, and clients and families that have little preplanning for these situations. The review found that all of the challenges also can cause moral stress for the nurse. In conclusion, although nurses can be educated better and work closely with the care team, there may also be a breakdown in the nursing process regarding communication with families and clients. The review includes a Norwegian study that found that nurses may avoid conversations that are stressful or difficult and can lead to a breakdown in communication and client and family satisfaction.

Nursing Implications

Employers will work within their health care facilities to improve in all categories through education and training. Nurses, however, should strive for a solid nursing process without a breakdown in communication. Nurses should seek the support of staff, the care team, unit, and mentors to help them through difficult conversations. The relationship between the nurse, client, and family is that of trust. Despite challenges and stress, client satisfaction with compassion is a goal for which to strive.

Reference

Fridh, I. (2014). Caring for the dying patient in the ICU: The past, the present and the future. *Intensive and Critical Care Nursing, 30*(6), 306–311. http://dx.doi.org/10.1016/j.iccn.2014.07.004

Assisting With Emotional Reactions

Although each dying client responds to terminal illness in unique ways, studies show a common emotional pattern. Elisabeth Kübler-Ross, a primary provider who studied death and dying extensively, describes a series of five reactions—(1) denial, (2) anger, (3) bargaining, (4) depression, and (5) acceptance—that dying clients often demonstrate. Clients do not always follow these stages in order. Some regress and then move forward again. Others may be in several stages at once (e.g., a client who is angry as well as depressed).

The first stage, **denial**, is a psychological coping mechanism (see Chapter 67) in which a person refuses to believe certain information. Dying clients usually first deny that the diagnosis is accurate. A common response is "No, not me—there must be some mistake." They may imagine that test results are erroneous or reports have been confused. Denial of the diagnosis may be followed by a refusal to accept that the condition is terminal.

During the second stage, **anger**, clients ask, "Why me?" Clients may say, "I'm still young. My children still need me. Why did I get this disease?" They may displace this anger onto others, such as the primary provider, nurses, family, or even God. They may express such anger in less obvious ways, such as complaining about their care or blaming anyone and everyone for the slightest aggravation.

The third stage, **bargaining**, is an attempt to postpone death. Usually, the client makes a secret bargain with God or some higher power. Clients attempt to negotiate a delay in dying until after a particularly significant event. They may say, "If I can just live until my daughter graduates from high school, I will accept death when it eventually comes."

The fourth stage is marked by depression. As clients realize the reality of their situation, they may mourn their potential losses, such as separation from their loved ones, the inability to fulfill their future goals, or loss of control.

In the fifth stage, **acceptance**, dying clients accept their fate and make peace spiritually and with those to whom they are close. Clients may begin to detach themselves from activities and acquaintances and seek to be with only a small circle of relatives or friends.

BOX 10-1 Principles of Palliative Care

Palliative care

- Affirms life and regards dying as a normal process
- Neither hastens nor postpones death
- Provides relief from pain and other distressing symptoms
- Integrates the psychological and spiritual aspects of care
- Offers a support system to help clients live as actively as possible until death
- Offers a support system to help client families cope during the client's illness and in their own bereavement

From HelloCare. (n.d.). *What is palliative care? The principles you need to know*. https://hellocaremail.com.au/principles-palliative-care-need-know/

>>> *Stop, Think, and Respond 10-1*

A client has learned that they have a terminal illness. They plead with God to allow them to live long enough to see the birth of their first grandchild. What is this stage called? What may have preceded this stage?

Supporting Final Decisions

During emotional turmoil, dying clients often must make some difficult decisions. The nurse presents options of where and how terminal care may be provided, respects client and family choices, and facilitates their preferences. As long as dying clients remain competent (retain the ability to understand the consequences of their choices), they have the right to request or refuse a variety of options and change their minds later. Problems arise when clients become incompetent before indicating their wishes about terminal care; at such times, they may become victims of decisions they would otherwise oppose.

Advance Directives

Dying clients or their families can control their destiny. Under a federal law called the Patient Self-Determination Act, which became effective in 1991, all health care facilities in the United States funded by Medicare must inform clients on admission of their right to refuse medical treatment and their right to prepare advance directives. An **advance directive** provides the client with the opportunity to identify their wishes concerning health care and treatment if too mentally or physically incapacitated to do so independently.

There are four types of advance directive formats: a living will, durable power of attorney (DPOA) for health care, the use of a document titled *Five Wishes*, and physician orders for scope of treatment (POST). Most agencies supply at least one of the necessary forms.

Living Will

A **living will** is a written or printed statement describing a person's wishes concerning medical care and life-sustaining treatments that are *wanted* or *unwanted* in the event that a person is unable to personally make those decisions (see Fig. 5-4, p. 54). Usually, a living will describes a desire to avoid being kept alive by artificial means or the use of heroic measures. It is considered a legal document when signed, dated, and witnessed by unrelated witnesses, none of whom are potential heirs or a personal health care provider. A living will helps others avoid indecision about whether to implement or continue life-sustaining treatment. Many primary providers try to abide by client wishes if they are known or stated in writing.

Durable Power of Attorney for Health Care

A **durable power of attorney (DPOA) for health care** (sometimes called medical power of attorney) or health care proxy is the person the client designates to make medical decisions when the client no longer can do so. It allows competent clients to identify exactly what life-sustaining measures they want implemented, avoided, or withdrawn and offers reassurance that others will carry out their wishes. Appointing a DPOA is more advantageous than a living will because a living will does not describe every possible life-threatening scenario, thus allowing the proxy to interpret the client's wishes in unique circumstances (Mayo Clinic, 2014). The appointee cannot exercise this authority at any other time or in any other matters. For obvious ethical reasons, the client's primary provider or other health care providers may not be designated as DPOA for health care. When a DPOA for health care document exists, the client brings it to the institution at admission, and a photocopy is attached to the chart.

Five Wishes Document

A third form of advance directive is the completion of a document titled *Five Wishes*, which meets the legal requirements for an advance directive in 44 states and the District of Columbia (Box 10-2). The remaining states allow clients to attach the *Five Wishes* **document** to their state's required form. The *Five Wishes* document, created by the Aging with Dignity Organization (2016), combines components of a living will with DPOA in order for clients to plan for their care before actually faced with a health care crisis. The *Five Wishes* are one or more statements that include (1) who can make proxy health care decisions, (2) the types of medical treatment desired and undesired, (3) actions that will promote personal comfort as death nears, (4) ways in which the person wants to be treated, and (5) information the person wants loved ones to know. It has been described nationwide as an innovative, comprehensive document that goes beyond medical issues because it deals with personal, emotional, and spiritual concerns of a person in the terminal stage before death.

Physician Orders for Scope of Treatment

Another form of an advance directive is called **physician orders for scope of treatment (POST)** (sometimes called POLST or medical orders for scope of treatment [MOST]). It is an advance care planning tool to safeguard a client's wishes for care during a serious illness and/or end-of-life care. The client provides specific information about resuscitation and medical interventions such as antibiotics, artificial feedings, comfort care, hospitalization, intubation, and mechanical ventilation. The client's preferences are documented as physician orders. In order to be activated, a primary provider must review the document and then sign off the orders. This form can be available and honored in all health care settings.

BOX 10-2 States That Have Legalized the Five Wishes Document

Alaska	Alabama	Arizona	Arkansas	California
Colorado	Connecticut	Delaware	Florida	Georgia
Hawaii	Idaho	Illinois	Iowa	Kentucky
Louisiana	Maine	Maryland	Massachusetts	Michigan
Minnesota	Mississippi	Missouri	Montana	Nebraska
Nevada	New Jersey	New Mexico	New York	North Carolina
North Dakota	Oklahoma	Pennsylvania	Rhode Island	South Carolina
South Dakota	Tennessee	Utah	Vermont	Virginia
Washington	West Virginia	Wisconsin	Wyoming	

The District of Columbia has also legalized the *Five Wishes* document. Fivewishes.org also states, "In the remaining 6 states, (Indiana, Kansas, New Hampshire, Ohio, Oregon, Texas) a statutory form is required, and one must attach the state document if one wishes to use the *Five Wishes* document as a guide."
Five Wishes. (n.d.). https://fivewishes.org/

INDIANA PHYSICIAN ORDERS FOR SCOPE OF TREATMENT (POST)

State form 55317 (6-13)
Indiana State Department of Health – IC 16-36-6

INSTRUCTIONS: Follow these orders first. Contact treating physician, advanced practice nurse, or physician assistant for further orders if indicated. Emergency Medical Services (EMS) should contact Medical Control per protocol. These medical orders are based on the patient's current medical condition and preferences. Any section not completed does not invalidate the form and implies full treatment for that section. HIPAA permits disclosure to health care professionals as necessary for treatment. Original form is personal property of the patient.

Patient Last Name	Patient First Name	Middle Initial
Birth date *(mm/dd/yyyy)*	Medical Record Number	Date prepared *(mm/dd/yyyy)*

A *Check One*

CARDIOPULMONARY RESUSCITATION (CPR): *Patient has no pulse AND is not breathing.*

☐ Attempt Resuscitation/CPR ☐ Do Not Attempt Resuscitation (DNR)

When not in cardiopulmonary arrest, follow orders in **B, C** and **D**.

B *Check One*

MEDICAL INTERVENTIONS: *If patient has pulse AND is breathing OR has pulse and is NOT breathing.*

☐ *Comfort Measures (Allow Natural Death):* Treatment Goal: Maximize comfort through symptom management. Relieve pain and suffering through the use of any medication by any route, positioning, wound care and other measures. Use oxygen, suction and manual treatment of airway obstruction as needed for comfort. Patient prefers no transfer to hospital for life-sustaining treatments. Transfer to hospital only if comfort needs cannot be met in current location.

☐ *Limited Additional Interventions:* Treatment Goal: Stabilization of medical condition. In addition to care described in Comfort Measures above, use medical treatment for stabilization, IV fluids (hydration) and cardiac monitor as indicated to stabilize medical condition. May use basic airway management techniques and non-invasive positive-airway pressure. Do not intubate. Transfer to hospital if indicated to manage medical needs or comfort. Avoid intensive care if possible.

☐ *Full Intervention:* Treatment Goal: Full interventions including life support measures in the intensive care unit. In addition to care described in Comfort Measures and Limited Additional Interventions above, use intubation, advanced airway interventions, and mechanical ventilation as indicated. Transfer to hospital and/or intensive care unit if indicated to meet medical needs.

C *Check One*

ANTIBIOTICS:

☐ Use antibiotics for infection only if comfort cannot be achieved fully through other means.

☐ Use antibiotics consistent with treatment goals.

D *Check One*

ARTIFICIALLY ADMINISTERED NUTRITION: Always offer food and fluid by mouth if feasible.

☐ No artificial nutrition.

☐ Defined trial period of artificial nutrition by tube. (Length of trial: ________ Goal: ______________________)

☐ Long-term artificial nutrition.

E

DOCUMENTATION OF DISCUSSION: ***Orders discussed with (check one):***

☐ Patient (patient has capacity) ☐ Health Care Representative

☐ Legal Guardian / Parent of Minor ☐ Health Care Power of Attorney

SIGNATURE OF PATIENT OR LEGALLY APPOINTED REPRESENTATIVE

My signature below indicates that my physician discussed with me the above orders and the selected orders correctly represent my wishes. If signature is other than patient's, add contact information for representative on reverse side.

Signature ***(required by statute)***	Print Name ***(required by statute)***	Date ***(required by statute)*** *(mm/dd/yyyy)*

F

SIGNATURE OF PHYSICIAN

Print Signing Physician Name ***(required by statute)***	Physician Office Telephone Number ***(required by statute)*** ( ) ______ – _______	License Number ***(required by statute)***
Physician Signature ***(required by statute)***	Date ***(required by statute)*** *(mm/dd/yyyy)*	Office Use Only

Figure 10-1 Indiana Physician Orders for Scope of Treatment (Post). (From Indiana State Department of Health-Ic 16-36-6.)

At least 26 states recognize this form of an advance directive. Figure 10-1 provides an example of a POST document.

CARE OPTIONS FOR THE DYING CLIENT

Some terminally ill clients spend their last days in an acute care setting using the best technology and resources available. Others prefer to be at home, with or without assistance from hospice home care. Others choose a hospice or extended care facility. Culture and family tradition may influence these choices (Tables 10-1 and 10-2). Regardless of the setting, clients need to know that their symptoms, particularly pain, will be controlled and that they will be a part of the planning process for their care.

Home Care

In the early stages of a terminal illness, clients usually remain at home. Nurses often coordinate community services and secure needed home equipment. Many clients experience greater emotional and physical comfort in their own home. They have greater security and personal integrity in a familiar environment. Family members also may experience fewer feelings of guilt when they are involved in caring for the client. In addition, children can interact more frequently and may be helped to understand death with less fear.

A negative factor of home care is the burden it places on the primary caregiver. If prolonged, the role of primary caregiver can be very isolating and physically exhausting because the responsibility for providing care continues 24 hours a day, day after day. Current financial restrictions related to reimbursement regulations may burden the caregiver even more. Home care nurses periodically need to assess the toll on the caregiver's physical and emotional health. If available, they may arrange **respite care** or care for the caregiver, to provide periodic relief.

Hospice Care

In 1967, Dr. Cicely Saunders founded St. Christopher's Hospice in Sydenham, England. This hospice has served as a model for hospice care in the United States. A **hospice** is a facility for the care of terminally ill clients who can live out their final days with comfort, dignity, and meaningfulness. Hospice care emphasizes helping clients live however they wish until they die. Clients receive services that relieve their physical symptoms and emotional distress and promote spiritual support. Pain is liberally controlled.

In the United States, facilities have implemented the hospice philosophy in various ways. In general, most hospice clients who usually have 6 months or less to live receive care in their own homes. A multidisciplinary team of hospice professionals and volunteers provides support to the dying client and caregivers. Services include personal care, homemaking services, companionship, and support programs for family members and significant others, including individual counseling during and after the death of the client (grief counseling). Box 10-3 outlines eligibility criteria for hospice care, and Box 10-4 lists home hospice care services covered by Medicare/Medicaid.

TABLE 10-1 Cultural Diversity and Death

ETHNIC GROUP	ROLE OF FAMILY	ENVIRONMENT	PREPARATION OF THE BODY
African American	Family members may expect health care providers to communicate with oldest family member. Public displays of emotion are acceptable.	Family members frequently care for dying older adults at home. They may believe that a death in the home will bring the family bad luck.	Family members often expect the health care team to clean and prepare a loved one's body. They may consider organ donation a taboo but may agree to an autopsy.
Chinese American	Family members may prefer that the client not be told of terminal illness or imminent death and may prefer to tell the client themselves.	Some believe that dying in the home brings the family bad luck. Others believe that the client's spirit may get lost if the client dies in the hospital. Family members may make use of special amulets or cloths.	Some family members prefer to wash the client themselves. They may believe that the body should be kept intact; organ donation and autopsy are uncommon.
Filipino American	Family members may want health care providers to communicate with the head of the family, out of the family's presence. Public displays of emotion are acceptable.	Terminally ill clients may prefer to die at home. If the family is Catholic, they may ask that a priest perform the "Sacrament of the Sick" and may use religious objects such as rosary beads and prayer.	Family members may want to wash the body and are likely to want time for all family members to say goodbye. They may not permit organ donation or autopsy.
Hispanic or Latinx American	Family members may expect extended family members to care for terminally ill loved ones, sharing information and decision-making. They may consider wailing as a sign of respect.	Dying in a hospital may not be desirable. Some believe that the client's spirit will get lost there. Special amulets, religious objects such as rosary beads, and prayer are used.	Relatives may help with care of the body and are likely to want time to say goodbye. Organ donation and autopsy are uncommon.

Adapted from Mazanec, P., & Tyler, M. K. (2003). Cultural considerations in end-of-life care. *American Journal of Nursing, 103*(3), 53. https://doi.org/10.1097/00000446-200303000-00019; Saccomano, S. J., & Abbatiello, G. A. (2014). Cultural considerations at the end of life. *The Nurse Practitioner, 39*(2), 24–31. https://doi.org/10.1097/01.NPR.0000441908.16901.2e

TABLE 10-2 Cultural and Ethnic Group Attitudes Toward Death

CULTURAL AND ETHNIC GROUP	ATTITUDES TOWARD DEATH
African American culture	Tend to display grief openly. Family and relatives usually present.
Amish culture	Death carries a lot of spiritual meaning.
Arab culture	May avoid discussions of impending death.
Cuban culture	Everything possible should be done.
East Asian culture	Reluctant to talk about death.
East Indian culture	Death should be discussed with family first, who may not inform the clients.
Filipino culture	A loud grieving process is typical. May avoid discussing.
Egyptian culture	Avoid discussions of death.
Iranian culture	Avoid discussions with the client.
Jamaican culture	Maybe very emotional with crying and mourning typically.
Japanese culture	May avoid discussion.
Ghanaian culture	Telling a client they are going to die is unacceptable. More culturally acceptable to say, "It is time to put your home in order."
Gypsy Roma culture	May involve wailing and calling out to God.
Haitian culture	Maybe very vocal regarding pain.
Hispanic culture	A large number of family members may be present. The family may not want to inform the client of the end stage of a terminal illness.
Indonesian culture	Greif may be filled with emotion.
Kenyan culture	Generally, desire life to be preserved at all costs.
Korean culture	Mourning and crying.
Libyan culture	Tend to be very emotional.
Native American culture	May avoid contact with dying. Verbal grieving may include wailing.
Native Hawaiian culture	Tend to celebrate life rather than death.
South African culture	Avoid the discussion as they believe talking about it will make it happen.
Vietnamese	Will have a tough time discussing death and do-not-resuscitate (DNR). These subjects stir deep emotions.

From Givler, A., Bhatt, H., & Maani-Fogelman, P. A. *The importance of cultural competence in pain and palliative care.* https://www.ncbi.nlm.nih.gov/books/NBK493154/

Institutionally Based Palliative Care

Some institutions provide **palliative care** to terminally ill clients who cannot maintain independent living. This care also may be referred to as *hospice care*. These units may be located in hospitals, long-term care facilities, or other, separate facilities. Nurses and other health care personnel provide 24-hour care. Factors that influence the decision to use institutionally based palliative care include the following:

- The client's weakness or immobility creates the need for more assistance than can be provided at home.
- The client cannot manage elimination needs.
- The client has uncontrolled or inadequately controlled pain or nausea.

BOX 10-3 Eligibility Criteria for Hospice Care

General
- Serious, progressive illness
- Limited life expectancy
- Informed choice of palliative care over cure-focused treatment

Hospice-Specific
- Presence of a family member or other caregiver continuously in the home when the client is no longer able to safely care for themselves (some hospices have created special services within their programs for clients who live alone, but this varies widely)

Medicare and Medicaid Hospice Benefits
- Your hospice doctor and your regular doctor (if you have one) certify that you're terminally ill (you're expected to live 6 months or less).
- You accept palliative care (for comfort) instead of care to cure your illness.
- You sign a statement choosing hospice care instead of other Medicare-covered treatments for your terminal illness and related conditions.

From Centers for Medicare & Medicaid Services. (n.d.). *Medicare hospice benefits*. https://www.medicare.gov/Pubs/pdf/02154-medicare-hospice-benefits.pdf

BOX 10-4 Services Covered Under Medicare in an Approved Hospice Program

Hospice and personal primary provider or nurse practitioner:
- Nursing care, available 24 hours a day
- Medical equipment, such as wheelchairs or walkers
- Medical supplies, such as bandages and catheters
- Prescription drugs for symptom control or pain relief
- Hospice aide and homemaker services
- Dietary counseling
- Physical and occupational therapy
- Speech-language pathology services
- Social worker services
- Dietary counseling
- Grief and loss counseling for client and family
- Short-term inpatient care (for pain and symptom management)
- Short-term respite care
- Any other Medicare-covered services needed to manage pain and other symptoms related to the terminal illness and related conditions, as recommended by the hospice team

From Centers for Medicare & Medicaid Services. (n.d.). *Medicare hospice benefits*. https://www.medicare.gov/Pubs/pdf/02154-medicare-hospice-benefits.pdf

- The family cannot provide adequate care.
- The client requires care that is too complex and demanding.
- The caregiver is too exhausted to provide care.

Many of the rules that govern traditional hospital and long-term care are relaxed for palliative care units. Visiting hours and ages of visitors are not restricted. In addition, the family is encouraged to bring in personal items for the client to enjoy and value.

Acute Care

Hospitals offer acute care with a 24-hour staff of nurses and other medical personnel, readily available resuscitative equipment, and access to a greater variety of medications than those in long-term care. This form of terminal care, however, is probably the most expensive. In this setting, the time and attention afforded to the supportive care of dying clients may be limited.

Physician-Assisted Suicide

Palliative care at the end of life is the ethical standard for most clients and health care providers in the United States. However, since 1997, five states—California (effective sometime in 2016), Montana, Oregon, Vermont, and Washington—have enacted legislation that decriminalizes **physician-assisted suicide**, the practice of providing a means by which a client can end their own life. Most believe that the act of helping someone die is counterintuitive to the Hippocratic Oath taken by primary providers, a position supported by most nurses. Some argue that failure to intervene when a terminally ill client voluntarily stops eating or drinking or when prescribing analgesics at a level that renders unconsciousness is akin to participating in a client's suicide, practices referred to as **passive euthanasia** because they facilitate death by letting nature take its course. Nurse practice acts prohibit nurses from assisting clients to die; however, nurses have a unique understanding of client wishes and suffering. Some nurses may face ethical dilemmas in advocating for their clients.

SIGNS OF APPROACHING DEATH

Although death is unique for each individual, common physical and psychological events occur when death is approaching.

Physical Events

Death usually occurs gradually over hours or days. Cells deteriorate from an underlying lack of sufficient oxygen, which leads to multisystem failure. The following are signs of impending death that alert the nurse that the client will die shortly:

- *Cardiac dysfunction*: Failing cardiac function is one of the first signs that a client's condition is worsening. At first, heart rate increases in a futile attempt to deliver oxygen to cells. The apical pulse rate may reach 100 or more beats/min. Cardiac output, the amount of blood the heart pumps per minute, may decrease, because a fast heart rate impairs the heart's ability to fill with blood. This may diminish the heart's own oxygen supply, which causes the heart rate to decrease and blood pressure to fall.
- *Peripheral circulation changes*: Reduced cardiac output compromises peripheral circulation, and impaired cellular metabolism produces less heat. The skin becomes pale or mottled, nail beds and lips may appear blue, and the client may feel cold.
- *Pulmonary function impairment*: Failure of the heart's pumping function causes fluid to collect in the pulmonary circulation. Breath sounds become moist. Oxygen does not diffuse very well, and the client cannot exhale carbon dioxide adequately, compounding the state of generalized hypoxia (low oxygenation).
- *Central nervous system alterations*: With hypoxia, the brain is less sensitive to accumulating levels of carbon dioxide; therefore, the client may experience periods of apnea (no breathing). Pain perception may be diminished, the client may stare blankly through partially open eyes, and the senses may become impaired, although hearing tends to remain intact. Eventually, the client becomes insensitive to all but extreme pressure.
- *Renal impairment*: Low cardiac output causes urine volume to diminish and toxic waste products to accumulate.
- *Gastrointestinal disturbances*: Peristalsis slows, causing gas and intestinal contents to accumulate. This buildup may stimulate the vomiting center, resulting in nausea and vomiting.
- *Musculoskeletal changes:* Reflexes become hypoactive. The client loses urinary and rectal sphincter muscle control, causing incontinence of urine and stool. The jaw and facial muscles also relax. As the tongue falls to the back of the throat, respirations become noisy. The accumulation of secretions in the respiratory tract coupled with noisy respirations is referred to as the *death rattle*. A brief period of restlessness may occur just before death.

Psychological Events

If they have reached the stage of acceptance, some terminally ill clients look forward to dying because it will end their suffering. Some clients, however, seem to forestall dying when they feel that their loved ones are not yet prepared to deal with their death. This has been described as the **waiting for permission phenomenon**, because death often occurs shortly after a significant family member communicates that they are strong enough and ready to "let go." Nurses must support family members at this time because family members may feel as though they have abandoned their loved one.

Near-death experiences (NDE), in which a person almost dies but is resuscitated, have been reported for some time. People who experience near death report similar events, such as

- Floating above their bodies
- Moving rapidly toward a bright light
- Seeing familiar people who have already died
- Feeling warm and peaceful
- Being told that it is not time yet for them to die
- Regretting having to return to their resuscitated body

Nearing death awareness is a phenomenon characterized by a dying client's premonition of the approximate time or date of death, or in general that death is near. In addition, as death approaches, clients may reach out, point, or open their arms as if to embrace someone or call them by name. These phenomena may be explained as "delirium or terminal restlessness," but according to Callanan and Kelley (2012), these phenomena are signs that clients are aware that something is happening to them. Acknowledging what the client is seeing or feeling provides an opportunity for the nurse to support the client in a more meaningful way. There can be greater comfort for the client and their loved ones by listening to and observing the client.

NURSING MANAGEMENT FOR END-OF-LIFE CARE

Nursing care of dying clients focuses on providing palliative care to the client and supporting family members and significant others. Client comfort is the primary goal, with the major long-term goal being that the client will die with dignity. Other client goals include control of pain, maintenance of basic physiologic functions, relief of fears and anxieties, completion of unfinished business, and acceptance of death. Having the client's family remain cohesive and supportive is another goal, as is providing a safe and secure environment.

Assessing Needs

Initially, nurses focus assessment on the client's basic physical needs, such as pain, breathing, nutrition, hydration, and elimination. They then include the psychosocial and spiritual needs of the client and family. Nurses must try not to repeat unnecessary assessments so as to allow the client to rest. They can make frequent checks without being physically intrusive. This frequency provides security so that the client does not feel abandoned.

Controlling Pain

The primary objective of pain control for dying clients is to block pain without suppressing level of consciousness or breathing. The nurse usually gives pain medications on a routine schedule around the clock to avoid causing intense discomfort followed by a period of heavy sedation. Regular dosing sustains a plateau of continuous pain relief and prevents exhausting the client who must use additional energy to cope with severe pain (see Chapter 11). The nurse also reassures the client that frequent use of opioid analgesia will not cause addiction when administered in a life-limiting illness. The primary provider may prescribe other medications such as mild antianxiety medications or antidepressants to reduce fear and anxiety. This is important because fear and anxiety can exacerbate pain. Other techniques such as imagery, humor, and progressive relaxation are useful in potentiating the effects of pain medication.

Facilitating Breathing

Placing the client in a Fowler's position may help ease difficulty with breathing. If the client cannot cough and raise secretions, the nurse gently suctions the client. Suctioning will not clear the lungs or ease breathing if the client has pulmonary edema (fluid in the lungs from heart failure). In this case, the primary provider may prescribe a sedative to relieve the anxiety created by the feeling of suffocation or a diuretic to reduce pulmonary congestion. Oxygen eventually may be used.

Pharmacologic Considerations

- Opiates, such as morphine, are found to reduce breathlessness in those with dyspnea. Fear of respiratory depression causes provider reluctance to prescribe and often time prevents the use of this drug.

Administering Food and Fluids

If the client can take oral fluids and food, the nurse offers nourishment frequently in small amounts and serves it at the appropriate temperature. They encourage the family to bring in foods that the client likes or have been a tradition in the family's diet (Nutrition Notes). Difficulty in swallowing, gastric and intestinal distention, and vomiting create a potential for aspiration of fluids as well as a decrease in food intake. The nurse administers medications for controlling nausea and vomiting 1 hour or so before meals. The nurse and family should not insist that the client eat or drink if these symptoms cannot be controlled. The nurse reports weight loss and inadequate intake so the team can consider alternative nutritional and fluid administration routes. If drooling occurs, the nurse may elevate and turn the client's head to the side or suction the oral cavity.

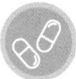

Pharmacologic Considerations

- The underlying cause of emesis should always be dealt with first, that is, new or rapid dosing of an opiate causing nausea and vomiting. Low-dose haloperidol is effective for reducing nausea as well as delirium (Haloperidol, 2021.).

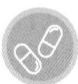

Pharmacologic Considerations

- Medications that have potential for more risks than benefits because of older adult altered absorption, metabolism, or excretion are listed in the Beers criteria for potentially inappropriate medication use in older adults (American Geriatrics Society, 2015). They are also addressed in the Screening Tool of Older People's potentially inappropriate Prescriptions (STOPP) and Screening Tool to Alert doctors to the Right Treatment (START; Gallagher et al., 2008).

Regulating Temperature

Skin temperature drops as death nears; the client may describe feeling cold. The nurse can give the client cotton socks, light blankets, and other light clothing if the client feels chilled. Gentle massaging of the arms and legs also may help because it transfers body heat from the hands to the skin surface and improves circulation. Touch also provides support and communicates personal concern.

Nutrition Notes

The Client at the End of Life

- Good nutrition becomes a quality-of-life issue for dying clients.
- Eating favorite foods with a mealtime companion may stimulate appetite and promote a sense of comfort. Loss of appetite and weight, however, may be inevitable.
- Offering small portions may result in a greater intake; normal and large amounts of food can diminish or suppress the appetite.
- Force feeding a dying client orally or through a tube may cause nausea and serves no useful purpose.
- If nausea is a problem, cool or cold foods may be better tolerated. The aromas of hot foods can increase the nausea.
- Assure family members that decreased appetite and altered gastrointestinal function are normal parts of the dying process.

Maintaining Skin and Tissue Integrity

A drop in blood pressure and rapid heart failure lead to poor tissue and organ perfusion. The nurse protects the client's skin from breakdown by changing the client's position at least every 2 hours. Poor tissue perfusion may cause inadequate drug absorption and decrease the effectiveness of drugs administered intramuscularly; in such cases, the nurse must consult with the primary provider. Drugs for raising blood pressure, improving tissue and organ perfusion, and correcting cardiac or circulatory problems may also be ordered.

Assisting With Self-Care and Activity

Dying clients may not tolerate physical activity well. The nurse may need to assist with personal hygiene. The client needs to be clean, well groomed, and free of unpleasant odors to promote dignity and self-esteem. The nurse gives oral care and ice chips, because mouth breathing makes the oral mucous membranes and lips dry. Petroleum jelly helps keep the lips lubricated. The nurse avoids glycerin applications because they tend to pull fluid from the tissue and eventually accentuate the drying problem.

Promoting Sleep

A disturbance in sleep pattern may occur because of anxiety, fear, pain, or other environmental stimuli, such as bright lights and disturbing noise. For this reason, nurses must cluster necessary activities to avoid awakening the client and to protect the client from a steady stream of health care workers or visitors. When possible, it is helpful to turn off or dim the lights at night and keep noise to a minimum. The radio, television, or recordings of the client's favorite music may mask the continuous hum of equipment and monitors.

Facilitating Elimination

The nurse can promote normal elimination by offering a bedpan or assisting the client to the bathroom or bedside commode. Incontinence of the bowel or bladder may occur because of the client's disease process or because the client is near death. The client needs absorbent pads when they have lost bowel or bladder control. The nurse assists with thorough cleaning. Occasionally, an indwelling or external catheter may be placed, particularly if skin breakdown is a potential problem.

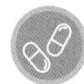

Pharmacologic Considerations

- Methylnaltrexone is the first drug of its kind which blocks the opioid binding specifically on gastrointestinal (GI) tract receptors, the cause of opiate-induced constipation. Clients need to be monitored for opioid withdrawal symptoms when taking this drug.

Addressing Fear, Social Isolation, Hopelessness, and Powerlessness

Because the dying client tends to become isolated from others, the nurse must spend time with them apart from the time necessary to provide physical care. It is important for nurses to be flexible and to interrupt physical care if and when the client indicates a need for companionship, support, and communication. During unplanned, spontaneous moments, clients often discuss fears or concerns that nurses should not ignore or rush. The nurse can communicate interest and a willingness to listen by sitting down, leaning forward in the client's direction, and making direct eye contact. Nodding, responsive comments such as "Yes," or brief periods of silence encourage the client to continue verbalizing.

Facilitating Grieving

Grieving is a painful yet normal reaction that helps clients cope with loss and leads to emotional healing. Grieving, the process that includes emotional, physical, spiritual, social, and intellectual responses and behaviors by which individuals, families, and communities incorporate an actual, anticipated, or perceived loss in their daily lives (Herdman & Kamitsuru, 2014), may begin before death for the client and family members. People express grief in a variety of ways: some become depressed and cry, some are angry and hostile, and some develop physical symptoms such as anorexia and insomnia. Family members may withdraw emotionally from the dying client because they find the experience too painful, whereas others draw closer, realizing they have only a short time to be with their loved one. The nurse is responsible for facilitating the grieving process and helping the client and family deal with their emotions. To do this, nurses may empathetically share perceptions of what the client and family is experiencing by saying something like, "It must be a very helpless feeling." Once the client and family sense they can speak freely, the nurse needs to listen in a nonjudgmental manner and avoid criticism or giving advice.

Addressing Spiritual Distress

Religious beliefs and cultural customs influence attitudes about death. Clients may find great comfort and support from their religious faith and may want someone associated with their religion to visit. If clients indicate such a desire, the nurse notifies appropriate clergy. If asked, the nurse may pray with clients or assist as indicated. When clients are too ill to express their wishes, the nurse must ask the family about spiritual care.

Promoting Family Coping

People often find it difficult to communicate frankly with a dying person. Failure to verbalize feelings, express emotions, and show tenderness for the dying person is often a source of regret for grieving relatives. Therefore, families must feel that they can express their feelings with nurses who are compassionate listeners. If nurses encourage family members and listen to them in their frank communication, family members may feel more prepared to carry on a similarly honest dialogue with the dying client. Once they mutually express feelings and break communication barriers, both relatives and the client often experience comfort in their meaningful relationship.

If possible, the family should have a **room** where they can talk with other relatives, cry, and rest. For emotional support, the nurse may sit with the family for a short time, express concern for their welfare, and listen to their concerns. The nurse explains measures taken to provide comfort and pain relief for the dying client. Families may find it helpful for the nurse to explain that as death draws near, the dying client may appear to become detached and unaware of those nearby and may slip into unconsciousness before death. The nurse is likely to be with the dying client and family at the moment of death. Some families may want to remain for a time with the body of the deceased. Therefore, the nurse allows a period of privacy before giving postmortem care. If family members or relatives seem unusually distraught, the nurse remains with them until a clergy member or other family member or friend arrives to be with them.

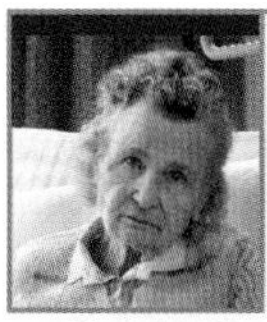

Clinical Scenario An 84-year-old woman who is terminally ill with advanced cancer is transferred from an acute care facility to a nursing home. The client's partner of 58 years is at the client's bedside along with two of their children. The client, who expects that she will die soon, fears she will not receive the same level of care in the nursing home. The family seems overwhelmed by their own grief. **What problems does the nurse encounter in this client's care and how can they be managed? See Nursing Care Plan 10-1.**

NURSING CARE PLAN 10-1 Care of the Dying Client

Assessment

In addition to performing physical assessments of the dying client:

- Assess feelings of the client and family about losses, isolation, grief, hopelessness, and distress.
- Assess family and client communication and coping patterns, strengths, and supports.
- Assess spiritual and cultural beliefs and practices.
- Assess family's ability to provide care at home.

Nursing Analysis. Grief related to functional losses and impending death

Expected Outcome. Client will verbalize grief and identify support systems.

Interventions	Rationales
Provide opportunities for client and family to share feelings.	*These opportunities allow client and family to discuss anticipated losses.*
Assist dying client to focus on the moment, review assets, and maintain relationships.	*Doing so helps client to remain connected to their world.*
If appropriate, encourage client to take care of any unfinished business.	*Doing so assists client to heal spiritually and move on.*
Identify support systems. Refer client and family to support groups and other resources.	*Contact with such groups and resources promotes positive bereavement experiences.*

Evaluation of Expected Outcome

Client and family grieve and become reconciled to impending death.

Nursing Analysis. Coping impairment related to client's inability to provide support to family and loved ones

Expected Outcome. Client and family verbalize resources to help deal with the situation.

(Continued)

NURSING CARE PLAN 10-1 Care of the Dying Client (*continued*)

Interventions	Rationales
Assist family to use coping skills that have been effective in other situations.	*Coping skills decrease stress and strengthen use of resources.*
Encourage family members to identify strengths and express feelings.	*These measures help family members to draw on one another's strengths and share feelings, which increases coping.*
Involve client and family in planning care.	*Such involvement encourages feelings of control.*
Refer family to appropriate resources.	*They can help the client deal with stressors such as child care, financial needs, and other needs.*

Evaluation of Expected Outcome

Client and family demonstrate use of other resources to increase coping with impending loss.

Nursing Analysis. Fear related to physical pain and concern that needs will not be met

Expected Outcome. Client will express trust that needs will be met.

Interventions	Rationales
Discuss client's fears with client and family.	*Such discussion provides an opportunity to empathize with and provide accurate information for the client.*
Encourage client to make decisions about care.	*Doing so gives client some control and decreases fear that needs will not be met.*
Plan care with client and family that addresses fears.	*Addressing fears enhances feelings of control.*
Discuss pain management program, including adjuncts to medication that promote comfort (see Chapter 11).	*Information about pain management decreases fear of physical pain.*

Evaluation of Expected Outcome

Client participates in decisions about care and expresses confidence that needs will be met.

Nursing Analysis. Psychosocial-spiritual needs related to desire to achieve harmony of mind, body, and spirit

Expected Outcome. Client will express feelings of hope.

Interventions	Rationales
Provide client time to meditate, pray, and contemplate changes in health status.	*Clients need time to be alone when health needs are changing.*
Help client develop and accomplish short-term goals and tasks.	*Such accomplishment increases self-esteem and self-worth.*
Help client to find reasons to live and look forward.	*Doing so promotes positive attitudes and ability to live for the moment.*
Provide requested religious materials, books, or music.	*They assist client to incorporate reading, music, imagery, or meditation into daily routine and spiritual life.*
Provide privacy for client to pray with others or for members of their faith to visit.	*Doing so demonstrates respect for and sensitivity to the client.*

Evaluation of Expected Outcome

Client demonstrates spiritual well-being as evidenced by statements of hope, purpose, and trust in their faith.

KEY POINTS

- Emotional reactions the dying client experiences according to EK-R a client who is dying will experience these emotional reactions:
  - The first stage, **denial**, is a psychological coping mechanism in which a person refuses to believe certain information.
  - In the second stage, **anger**, clients ask, "Why me?"
  - The third stage, **bargaining**, is an attempt to postpone death.
  - The fourth stage is **depression**. As clients realize the reality of their situation, they may mourn their potential losses.

- The fifth stage is **acceptance**, the dying clients accept their fate and make peace spiritually and with those to whom they are close.

- Advance Directives:
  - Living will: a written or printed statement describing a person's wishes concerning medical care and life-sustaining treatments that are *wanted* or *unwanted* in the event that a person is unable to personally make those decisions
  - DPOA: for health care (sometimes called medical power of attorney) or health care proxy is the person the client designates to make medical decisions when the client no longer can do so
  - *Five Wishes* document: meets the requirements of advanced directives in 44 states and the District of Columbia
  - The *Five Wishes* are one or more statements that include
    - who can make proxy health care decisions
    - the types of medical treatment desired and undesired
    - actions that will promote personal comfort as death nears
    - ways in which the person wants to be treated
    - information the person wants loved ones to know

- POST are medical orders for scope of treatment. It is an advance care planning tool to safeguard a client's wishes for care during a serious illness and/or end-of-life care.
- Palliative care: "Palliative care is an approach that improves the quality of life of patients and their families facing the problem associated with life-threatening illness, through the prevention and relief of suffering by means of early identification and impeccable assessment and treatment of pain and other problems, physical, psychosocial and spiritual" (WHO, 2020).
- Hospice care: the care of terminally ill clients who can live out their final days with comfort, dignity, and meaningfulness. Hospice clients who usually have 6 months or less to live receive care in their own homes. A multidisciplinary team of hospice professionals and volunteers provides support to the dying client and caregivers.
- Physician-assisted suicide: the practice of providing a means by which a client can end their own life; since 1997, five states—California (effective sometime in 2016), Montana, Oregon, Vermont, and Washington—have enacted legislation that decriminalizes physician-assisted suicide.

CRITICAL THINKING EXERCISES

1. Describe how nursing care of a young adult dying from AIDS might differ from the nursing care of an older adult dying from pneumonia.

2. A client with treatable cancer expresses a desire to go to Mexico where they offer coffee enemas and injections with sheep urine as a cure. How would you respond? Would your response change if the client's cancer were untreatable? Why?

3. If a client wanted to die at home, how would you help the family prepare for terminal home care?

4. A client you are caring for is transferring to a palliative care unit in a long-term care facility. They are concerned that the nurses there will not adequately treat their pain. What could you say to reassure them?

NCLEX-STYLE REVIEW QUESTIONS PrepU

1. When a client with cancer does not respond to medical treatment any longer and a restorative cure is unrealistic, which nursing action is most helpful initially to a client dealing with a terminal condition?
   1. Allow the client privacy to think alone.
   2. Let the client talk about how they are feeling.
   3. Provide the client with literature on death and dying.
   4. Suggest that the client get a second medical opinion.

2. Arrange the following reactions to terminal illness in the sequence they are most likely to occur. Use all the options.
   1. Bargaining
   2. Depression
   3. Anger
   4. Acceptance
   5. Denial

3. The family of a terminal client who has chosen to die at home with hospice care asks the nurse how they will know when death is near. Which of the following is correct information? Select all that apply.
   1. The client's pain will increase.
   2. The client's muscles will become tight and tense.
   3. The client's breathing will be irregular or stop temporarily.
   4. The client's extremities will feel warm.
   5. The client's respirations may sound noisy.
   6. The client's skin may appear mottled.

4. Which of the following interventions is best for the nurse to perform when drooling occurs in a dying client?
   1. Elevate and turn the client's head to the side.
   2. Help the client sit upright in a chair.
   3. Place the client in a Fowler's position.
   4. Move the client from sitting to supine.

5. The primary provider orders promethazine 25 mg IM q4h prn for nausea or vomiting. The label on a vial of promethazine indicates it contains 50 mg/mL. Fill in the blank with the volume the nurse should administer.

____

6. A hospice nurse is implementing the plan of care for a client with terminal cancer. Which interventions are most important to implement? Select all that apply.
   1. Ask the client if they have accepted their impending death.
   2. Assess the client's vital signs frequently.
   3. Control the client's pain with prescribed medications.
   4. Discuss the client's financial concerns.
   5. Encourage the client to express any fears.
   6. Insist that the client try to eat all of each meal.

UNIT 3

Foundations of Medical–Surgical Nursing

11

Pain Management

Words To Know

acute pain
addiction
adjuvant drugs
allodynia
breakthrough pain
chronic pain
cognitive behavioral therapy
cordotomy
endogenous opiates
equianalgesic dose
fifth vital sign
hyperalgesia
intractable pain
modulation
neuropathic pain
neuropeptides
nociceptive pain
nociceptors
opioid analgesics
pain
pain management
pain threshold
pain tolerance
palliative sedation
perception
percutaneous electrical nerve stimulation (PENS)
percutaneous neuromodulation therapy (PNT)
physical dependence
placebo
referred pain
rhizotomy
somatic pain
spinal cord stimulator
tolerance
transcutaneous electrical nerve stimulation (TENS)
transduction
transmission
visceral pain
withdrawal symptoms

Learning Objectives

On completion of this chapter, you will be able to:

1. Define the term *pain*.
2. Compare nociceptive pain with neuropathic pain.
3. Give characteristics distinguishing acute from chronic pain.
4. Describe four phases of pain transmission.
5. Differentiate between pain perception, pain threshold, and pain tolerance.
6. List at least three pain theories.
7. Describe essential components of pain assessment.
8. Explain why assessing pain is difficult.
9. Give examples of tools for assessing the intensity of pain.
10. Discuss The Joint Commission's standards on pain assessment and pain management.
11. Explain pain management and list examples of techniques commonly used.
12. Name categories of drugs used to manage pain.
13. Describe methods of administering analgesic drugs.
14. Discuss the issues of addiction, tolerance, and physical dependence associated with pain medication.
15. List examples of noninvasive techniques used to manage pain.
16. Identify three surgical procedures performed on clients with intractable pain.
17. List at least three nursing diagnoses besides acute pain and chronic pain that are common among clients with pain.
18. Discuss the nursing management of clients with pain.
19. Describe information pertinent to teach clients and family about pain management.

Pain is a privately experienced, unpleasant sensation usually associated with disease or injury. Pain also has an emotional component referred to as *suffering*. Extensive research is being conducted to discover more about various types of pain, pain transmission, and treatment. This chapter provides information about pain and the role of nursing and other disciplines in pain management. The American

Nurses Association states in their position statement that "Nurses have an ethical responsibility to relieve pain and the suffering it causes" (ANA, 2018).

Gerontologic Considerations

- Approximately 60% to 75% of people over the age of 65 years report having persistent pain. The percentage is believed to be considerably higher for people who are in assisted living or nursing homes (Larsson et al., 2017). About 20% take pain medications several times per week for joint- or muscle-related pain, lingering pain from previous injuries, cancer pain, and other types of chronic pain.
- Lack of an adequate pain assessment can contribute to undertreatment of pain in institutionalized older adults, especially those from cultural backgrounds that differ from those of care providers.
- Older adults may hesitate to relate pain, considering it a part of aging or from fear of being labeled as "difficult." Pain assessment must include attention to nonverbal and body positioning cues that conflict with verbal messages.
- Older adults frequently experience constipation from decreased fluid, decreased mobility secondary to pain with movement, or as an adverse reaction to pain medication. Providing fluid, fiber, or a stool softener along with pain medication can prevent discomfort from a prolonged lack of bowel movement or impaction.
- An older adult who receives pain medication around the clock (ATC) must have careful urine and bowel elimination assessment and documentation. Medication levels can increase to dangerous levels from prolonged absorption, metabolism, or elimination times. A change in level of consciousness may be an initial indicator of increasing medication levels.
- Some people assume that pain sensitivity and perception decrease with aging. Such an assumption can cause inaccurate assessment and undertreatment, leading to unnecessary suffering in older adults. All older clients should be asked about pain. Multiple factors may contribute to pain in older adults, causing difficulty determining individual causes (Larrson et al., 2017).
- Some older adults may be reluctant to report pain; they may prefer to describe pain as discomfort, burning, or aching.
- Cognitively impaired older adults may be unable to report pain; comparison of current behavior with previous behavior patterns and reports from caregivers can help in assessing pain in these clients.
- Pain may manifest as agitation; aggression; withdrawal; or changes in behavior, positioning, or sleep patterns.
- The client's use of distraction techniques such as television viewing or reading does not indicate they are not experiencing pain.
- Pain is the number one complaint of older Americans who take analgesics regularly. Some older adults skip doses or split their doses of prescribed medications to reduce their expense.
- A reduced dose of analgesics, especially opioid analgesics, may be prescribed for the older adult initially; the initial dose may be one-half to two-thirds the usual adult dose. Older adults experience a higher peak effect and longer duration of pain relief from an opioid. The risk of increased accumulation of narcotics, benzodiazepines, and/or antidepressants also increases the potential for falls from sedation and changes in cognitive functioning.
- Because constipation is a common side effect of opioid use, a bowel regimen to prevent constipation should be started when any older adult is treated with opioids. Older adults taking medications for multiple chronic and/or acute conditions have an increased susceptibility to drug reactions and interactions. Older adults taking nonsteroidal antiinflammatory drugs (NSAIDs) are at increased risk for renal toxicity and gastric ulceration.
- Analgesics given intramuscularly to older adults are less effective because of their diminished muscle mass.
- Older adults may avoid taking medication, especially opioids, out of fear of addiction or drug side effects. Nurses can educate older clients about opioids, facts about addiction, and effective treatment options for any breakthrough pain or side effects such as constipation.
- In older adults who experience diminished sensation, risk for burns can be minimized by careful monitoring of applications using heat. Monitoring is similarly required for cold pack applications to prevent hypothermia.

TYPES OF PAIN

Pain can be classified into categories according to (1) its source or (2) its onset, intensity, and duration. When classified according to its source, pain can be categorized as either nociceptive or neuropathic. When classified according to its onset, intensity, and duration, pain can be categorized as either acute or chronic.

Nociceptive Pain

Nociceptive pain is the noxious stimuli that are transmitted from the point of cellular injury over peripheral sensory nerves to pathways between the spinal cord and thalamus and eventually from the thalamus to the cerebral cortex of the brain (Fig. 11-1). Nociceptive pain is subdivided into somatic and visceral pain.

Somatic Pain

Somatic pain is caused by mechanical, chemical, thermal, or electrical injuries or disorders affecting bones, joints, muscles, skin, or other structures composed of connective tissue. *Superficial somatic pain*, also known as *cutaneous pain* (such as that from an insect bite or a paper cut), is perceived as sharp or burning discomfort. *Deeper somatic pain* such as that caused by trauma (e.g., a fracture) produces localized sensations that are sharp, throbbing, and intense. Dull, aching, diffuse discomfort is more common with long-term disorders such as arthritis.

Visceral Pain

Visceral pain arises from internal organs such as the heart, kidneys, and intestine that are diseased or injured. Causes for visceral pain are varied and include ischemia (reduced arterial blood flow to an organ), compression of an organ (as may be the case from a tumor), intestinal distention with gas, or contraction (spasm) as occurs with gallbladder or kidney stones. Visceral pain usually is diffuse, poorly localized, and accompanied by autonomic nervous system symptoms

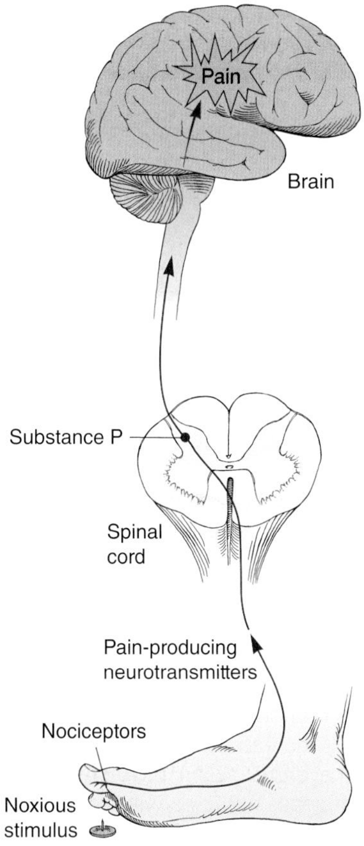

Figure 11-1 Nociceptive pain transmission pathway.

such as nausea, vomiting, pallor, hypotension, and sweating. **Referred pain** is a term used to describe discomfort that is perceived in a general area of the body but not in the exact site where an organ is anatomically located (Fig. 11-2).

Neuropathic Pain

Neuropathic pain is pain that occurs from a direct consequence of a disease or lesion that affects the peripheral nerves or pain-processing centers in the brain (Murnion, 2018). One theory is that the neurotransmitter glutamate, when released from a presynaptic neuron, activates postsynaptic neuron receptors for *N*-methyl-D-aspartate (NMDA), which sensitizes pain circuits in the spinal cord and brain. The outcome is a heightened level of pain.

An example of neuropathic pain is *phantom limb pain* or *phantom limb sensation*, in which individuals with an amputated arm or leg perceive that the limb still exists and that sensations such as burning, itching, and deep pain are located in tissues that have been surgically removed. Other examples include pain that is experienced by people with spinal cord injuries, strokes, diabetes, and herpes zoster (shingles).

Cancer pain may be either nociceptive or neuropathic. Nociceptive pain occurs when a tumor creates pressure in the organ or on adjacent tissue from its increased size. Neuropathic pain occurs when drugs or radiation used to treat the cancerous tumor causes nerve damage.

Acute Pain

Acute pain is discomfort that has a short duration (from a few seconds to less than 6 months). It is associated with tissue trauma, including surgery, or some other recent identifiable etiology. Although severe initially, acute pain eases with healing and eventually disappears. The gradual reduction in pain promotes coping with the discomfort because there is a reinforcing belief that the pain will resolve in time.

Acute and chronic pain both result in physical and emotional distress. Both also may be interrupted by pain-free periods, but that is where the similarities end.

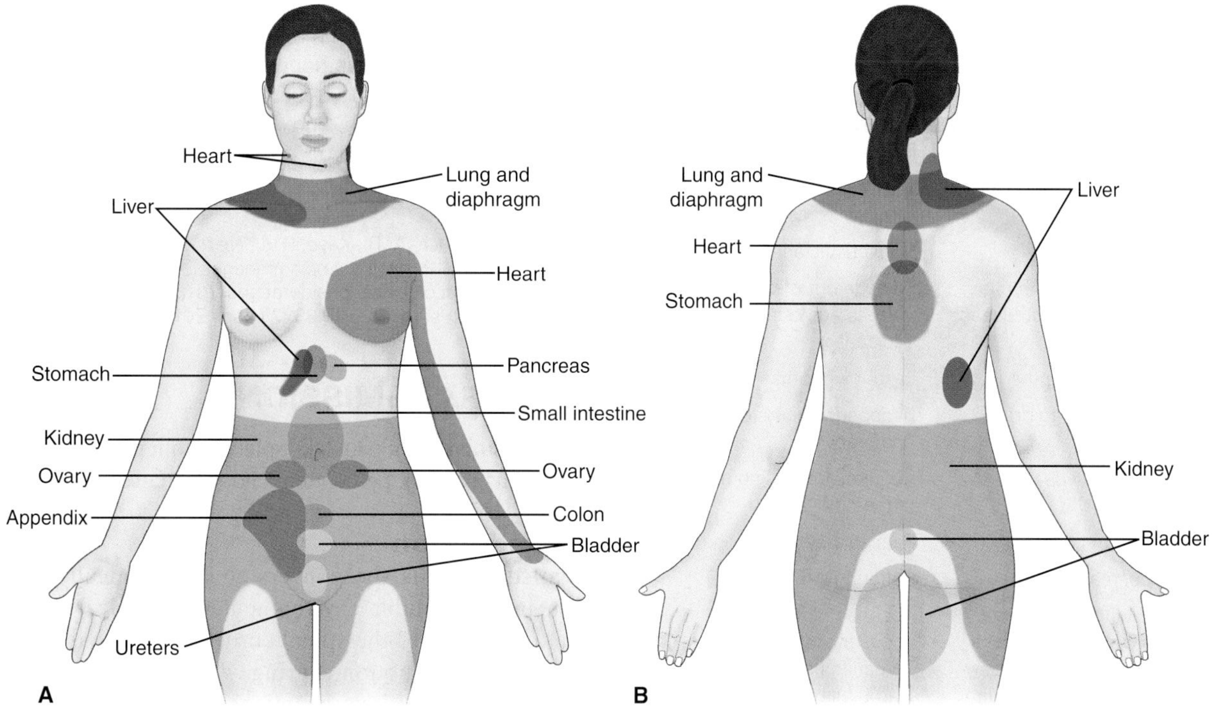

Figure 11-2 Common areas of referred pain. **(A)** Anterior view. **(B)** Posterior view.

Concept Mastery Alert

Acute pain is discomfort that has a short duration (from a few seconds to less than 6 months). It is associated with tissue trauma, including surgery, or some other recent identifiable etiology. Although severe initially, acute pain eases with healing and eventually disappears.

Chronic Pain

The characteristics of **chronic pain**, discomfort that lasts longer than 6 months, are almost totally opposite from those of acute pain (Table 11-1). Chronic pain sufferers may have periods of acute pain, which is referred to as **breakthrough pain**. The longer the pain exists, the more far-reaching its effects on the sufferer (Box 11-1). Others begin to show negative reactions to the chronic pain sufferer such as

- Anger for thinking the person with pain is not trying hard enough
- Anger with the medical system for not having answers
- Anger at insurance companies for denying or delaying approvals for procedures
- Guilt for being angry
- Guilt for wanting out of the relationship
- Feelings of being trapped
- Loneliness from social isolation
- Resentment for having to assume extra burdens
- Questioning if the person with pain is exaggerating to shirk responsibilities
- Becoming less attentive and withdrawing from intimacy (Black, 2015)

See Evidence-Based Practice 11-1 for research on assessing pain in older adults.

TABLE 11-1 Characteristics of Acute and Chronic Pain

ACUTE PAIN	CHRONIC PAIN
Recent onset	Remote onset
Symptomatic of primary injury or disease	Uncharacteristic of primary injury or disease
Specific and localized	Nonspecific and generalized
Severity associated with the acuity of the injury or disease process	Severity out of proportion to the stage of the injury or disease
Lasts less than 6 months	Lasts longer than 6 months
Responds favorably to drug therapy	Responds poorly to drug therapy
Requires gradually decreased drug therapy	Requires increasing drug therapy
Diminishes with healing	Persists beyond healing stage
Suffering decreases	Suffering intensifies
Associated with sympathetic nervous system responses such as hypertension, tachycardia, restlessness, anxiety	Absence of autonomic nervous system responses; manifests depression and irritability

BOX 11-1 Quality-of-Life Activities Affected by Chronic Pain

- Exercising
- Working around the house
- Sleeping
- Enjoying hobbies and leisure time
- Socializing
- Walking
- Concentrating
- Having sex
- Maintaining relationships with family and friends
- Working a full day at employment
- Caring for children

Evidence-Based Practice 11-1

Pain Assessment in Older Adults

Clinical Question

What challenges do nurses experience when assessing pain in older adults?

Evidence

"By 2040, the number of people aged 65 years and older worldwide will increase to 1.3 billion from the current 506 million" (Kaye et al., 2014, p. 15). As the population of older adults increases, nurses will likely care for an older client in their care settings. Barriers can exist that challenge the nurse in performing a pain assessment such as a client who underreports pain; confusion; poor memory; cost of medication; anxiety, sometimes depression; and multiple health issues. The barriers can lead to poor treatment and management of acute and chronic pain. As this population increases, the ability for nurses to assess clients and report findings to the health care team is crucial.

Nursing Implications

Nurses must understand how to do a thorough pain assessment in older adults and understand the barriers to an assessment for this population. Pain management for this population can be ensured with a thorough assessment, communication, and working with the health care team.

Reference

Kaye, A. D., Baluch, A. R., Kaye, R. J., Niaz, R. S., Kaye, A. J., Liu, H., & Fox, C. J. (2014). Geriatric pain management, pharmacological and nonpharmacological considerations. *Psychology & Neuroscience, 7*(1), 15–26. https://doi.org/10.3922/j.psns.2014.1.04

PAIN TRANSMISSION

The transmission of pain takes place in four phases: transduction, transmission, perception, and modulation (Fig. 11-3).

Transduction

Transduction is the conversion of chemical information in the cellular environment to electrical impulses that move toward the spinal cord. This phase is initiated by cellular disruption, during which affected cells release various noxious chemical mediators, collectively

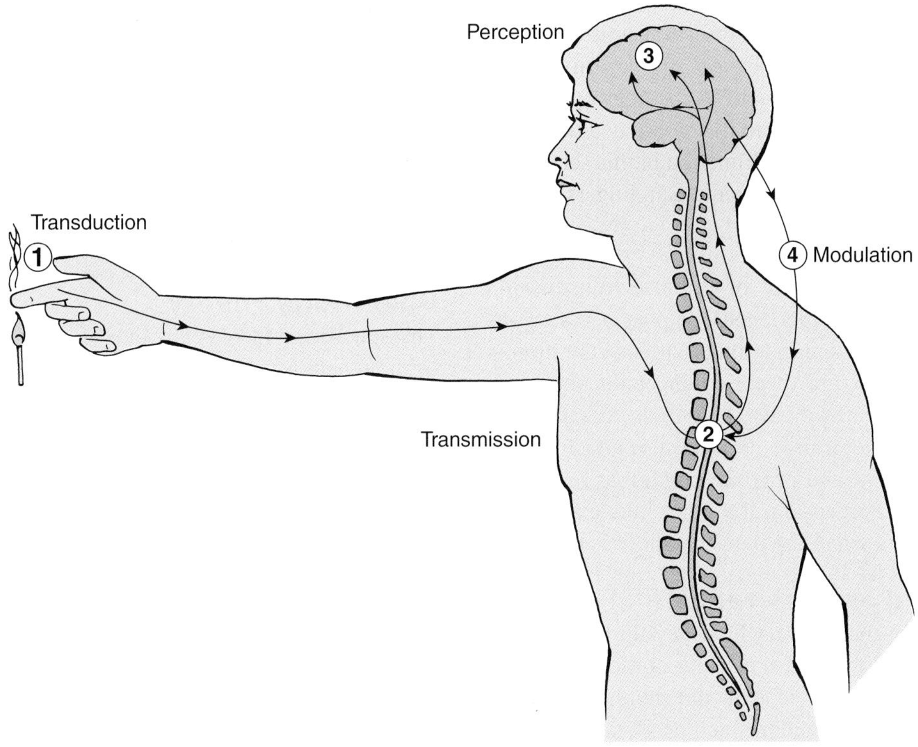

Figure 11-3 The phases of pain transmission.

referred to as **neuropeptides**, for example, prostaglandins, bradykinin, serotonin, histamine, substance P, and others. The neuropeptides stimulate **nociceptors**, specialized pain receptors located in the free nerve endings of peripheral sensory nerves (Dafny, n.d.) (Fig. 11-4). Nociceptors are located in the skin, bones, joints, muscles, and internal organs.

Nociceptors carry pain impulses by fast and slow nerve fibers. *A-delta fibers*, which are large and myelinated, carry impulses rapidly at a rate of approximately 5 to 30 m/s (Grossman & Porth, 2013). Impulses transmitted by the fast pain pathway result in sharp, acute initial sensations such as those that are felt when touching a hot iron. The result is that the person withdraws from the pain-provoking stimulus. After the fast transmission, impulses from small unmyelinated fibers known as *C-fibers* carry impulses at a slower rate of 0.5 to 2.0 m/s. They are responsible for the throbbing, aching, or burning sensation that persists after the immediate discomfort.

Transmission

Transmission is the phase during which peripheral nerve fibers form synapses with neurons in the spinal cord. With the help of substance P, pain impulses move to sequentially higher levels in the brain, such as the reticular activating system, thalamus, cerebral cortex, and limbic system. Prostaglandin, a chemical released from injured cells, speeds up the transmission. As the pain impulses are transmitted, pain receptors become increasingly sensitized, making established pain more difficult to suppress.

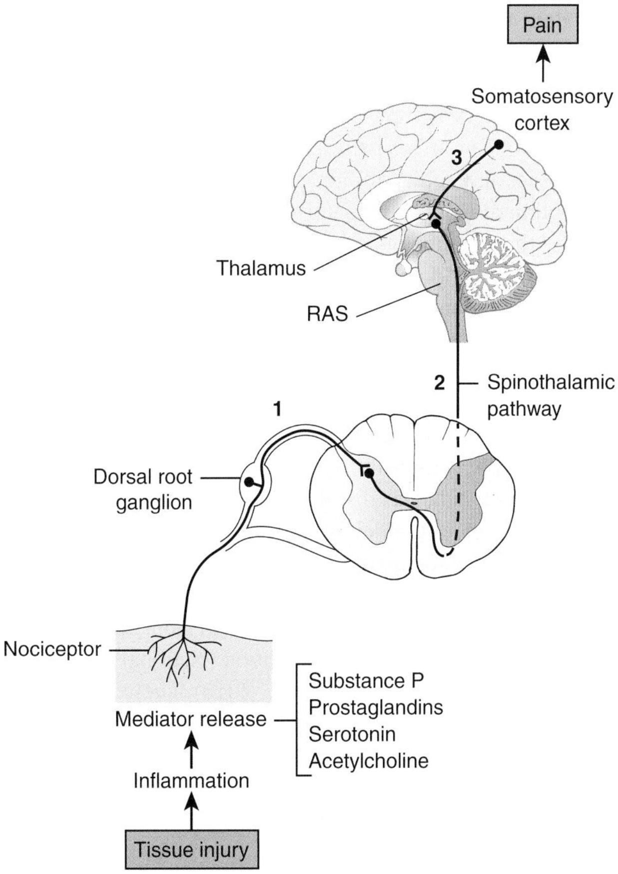

Figure 11-4 Mechanisms of acute pain. RAS, renin–angiotensin system. (Reprinted with permission from Norris, T. L. (2020). *Porth's Essentials of pathophysiology* (5th ed.). Wolters Kluwer.)

When pain impulses reach the thalamus within the brain, two responses occur. First, the thalamus transmits the message to the cortex, where the location and severity of the injury are identified. Second, it notifies the nociceptors that the message has been received and that continued transmission is no longer necessary. A malfunction in this secondary process may be one reason why chronic pain lingers.

Perception

Perception refers to the phase of impulse transmission during which the brain experiences pain at a conscious level, but many concomitant neural activities occur almost simultaneously. In addition to perceiving pain, the brain structures in the pain pathway also help to discriminate the location of the pain, determine its intensity, attach meaningfulness to the event, and provoke emotional responses (Peng et al., 2019). Perception, the conscious experience of discomfort, occurs when the pain threshold is reached.

Pain Threshold and Tolerance

The **pain threshold** is the point at which the pain-transmitting neurochemicals reach the brain, causing conscious awareness. **Hyperalgesia**, a lowered pain threshold, may occur when excitatory neurotransmitters such as glutamate sensitize the spinal cord to nociceptive input. In other words, the pain signals become amplified (French, n.d.; 2011). People tolerate or bear the sensation of pain differently.

Pain tolerance is the amount of pain a person endures once the threshold has been reached. The ability to endure a great deal of pain indicates a high pain tolerance; a low pain tolerance refers to very little ability to endure pain. Various factors can affect pain tolerance. For example, fatigue diminishes the ability to cope with pain and heightens the perception of pain. Anticipatory fear, the expectation of pain such as that accompanying an injection or root canal procedure, can lower pain tolerance. Concurrently dealing with multiple or accumulating stressors and depression decreases a person's ability to tolerate pain. Pain intolerance also is associated with social isolation or feeling socially abandoned. Cultural beliefs and values affect how a person deals with pain; some may be stoic, whereas others may be verbally and physically demonstrative in response to pain.

Research indicates that there are also gender differences in pain tolerance (Goldey et al., 2019; Keogh, 2014). Men tend to report lower pain intensity and demonstrate higher pain tolerance; women tend to rate their pain at higher levels and report pain in more body regions than men. Some believe that estrogen increases pain perception (National Institute of Neurological Disorders and Stroke, 2016). These gender differences must be viewed with caution because they may be examples of learned responses such as those associated with gender roles rather than physiologic differences.

Modulation

Modulation is the last phase of pain impulse transmission during which the brain transmits a response down the spinal nerves to the point where the pain transmission originated to alter the pain experience. At this point, the painful sensation is reduced with the release of pain-inhibiting neurochemicals such as endogenous opioids, which are discussed later in this chapter, and gamma-aminobutyric acid (GABA).

Theories of Pain

Several theories attempt to explain how pain is transmitted and reduced. No one theory is all-encompassing.

Specificity Theory

The specificity theory was one of the earliest explanations for how pain is transmitted. Its hypothesis, which originated in the 1800s, proposed that one type of sensory nerves were continuous from the periphery to the brain and functioned specifically to transmit pain signals. This theory has been discounted because the transmission and perception of pain and other sensations involves sensory nerves in the periphery and structures in the spinal cord before eventually reaching the brain.

Pattern Theory

The pattern theory proposed that sensory stimuli such as touch, heat, cold, and pain produce various patterns. Once a pattern develops, it is transmitted to the brain where the pattern is perceived as being either damaging or nondamaging.

Gate Control Theory

In the mid-1960s, Ronald Melzak, a Canadian psychologist, and his physiologist colleague, Patrick Wall, revolutionized the thinking of the scientific community with their gate control theory. Together they proposed that sensory information travels over slow small fibers as well as fast large fibers. Slow fibers, through which pain stimuli travel, open gates within the spinal cord allowing its transmission toward the brain. Fast fibers that are responsible for transmitting other types of sensory information can close the gates through which pain stimuli travel (Fig. 11-5). The gating mechanism helps to explain why competing sensory stimuli, such as heat, cold, massage, acupressure, and so on, can decrease the perception of pain or its intensity (Upendarrao, 2014).

Neuromatrix Theory

In 1999, Melzak offered another dimension to the pain experience when he introduced the neuromatrix theory. The neuromatrix theory expanded the original treatise on pain by incorporating biopsychosocial variables. Melzak indicated that the perception and modulation of the pain experience are affected by each person's unique psychological and cognitive thought processes. For example, past memories, current stressors, anxiety, and so on can either enhance or inhibit the experience of pain.

Endogenous Opioid Theory

The endogenous opioid theory is based on the fact that nociceptors contain receptors that can bind with morphine-like neurotransmitters called **endogenous opioids**—endorphins, dynorphins, and enkephalins that modulate pain. When endogenous opioids are released, they are thought to attach to sites on the nerve cell's membrane, blocking the

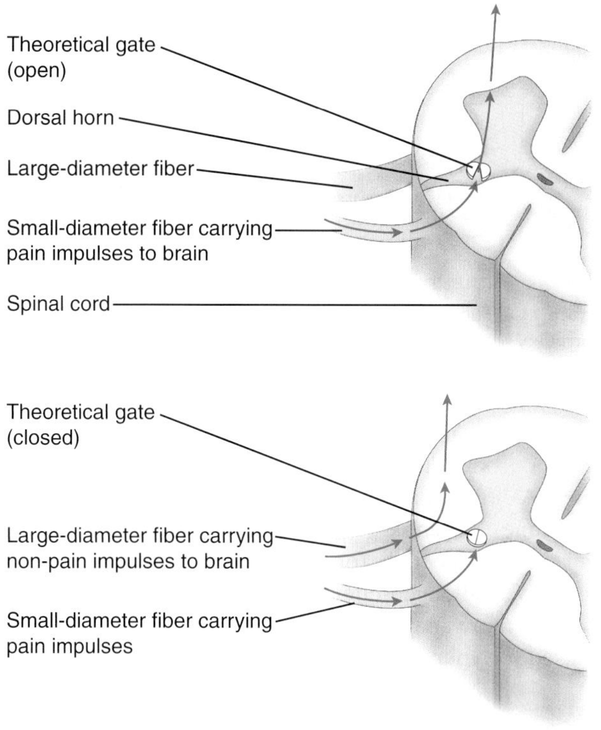

Figure 11-5 Pain impulse transmission and blocking according to the gate control theory. (Reprinted with permission from Taylor, C. R., Lynn, P. & Bartlett, J. L. (2019). *Fundamentals of nursing: The art and science of person-centered care* (9th ed.). Wolters Kluwer.)

transmission of pain-conducting chemicals such as substance P and prostaglandin (Fig. 11-6). If endogenous opioid production or storage is suppressed, pain of varying degrees will be experienced.

PAIN ASSESSMENT

There is no perfect way to determine if pain exists and how severe it is. In 1968, McCaffery, a nursing expert on pain, stated that pain is whatever the person says it is and exists whenever the person says it does. Individuals in pain may demonstrate a variety of nonverbal behaviors such as

- Positioning to avoid pain or being resistant to repositioning
- Rocking, fidgeting, or squirming

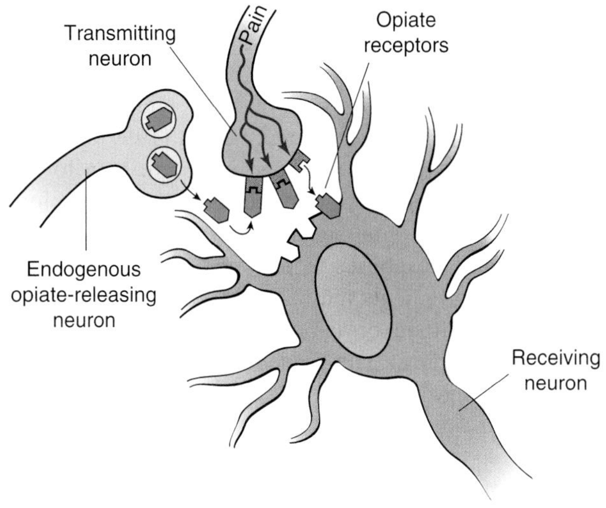

Figure 11-6 Opioid pain interference. (Reprinted with permission from Moreno, L. (2020). *Timby's fundamental nursing skills and concepts* (12th ed.). Wolters Kluwer.)

- Protective or guarding gestures
- Clenched jaw
- Frowning
- Sleep disturbances: increased sleep due to exhaustion or decreased sleep due to repeated awakening
- **Allodynia**, an exaggerated pain response due to increased sensitivity to stimuli such as air currents, pressure of clothing, or vibration
- Loss of interest in eating
- Moaning, crying, or sighing
- Emotional irritability
- Impaired thinking, confusion, or combativeness
- Reduced social interactions

A pain assessment includes the client's description of its onset, quality, intensity, location, and duration (Table 11-2). In addition, nurses assess for accompanying symptoms, such as nausea or dizziness, and what makes the pain better or worse. The American Pain Society has proposed that pain assessment should be considered the **fifth vital sign**. In other words, the nurse should check and document the client's pain every time they assess the client's temperature, pulse, respirations, and blood pressure.

TABLE 11-2 Basic Components of Pain Assessment

CHARACTERISTIC	DESCRIPTION	EXAMPLES
Onset	Time or circumstances under which the pain appeared	After eating, while shoveling snow, during the night
Quality	Sensory experiences and degree of suffering	Throbbing, crushing, agonizing, annoying
Intensity	Magnitude of the pain, such as moderate or severe; or a quantifying scale, such as from 0 to 10	None, slight, mild; a level of "7"
Location	Anatomic site	Chest, abdomen, jaw
Duration	Time span of the pain	Continuous, intermittent, hours, weeks, months

Assessment Biases

Despite the fact that the client is the only reliable source for quantifying pain, nurses do not respond consistently to the client's description of pain intensity with pain-relieving interventions. McCaffery and Ferrell (1999) observed that most nurses expect someone in severe pain to *look* as if they are suffering. Neither behavior nor other physiologic data such as vital signs, however, are reliable indicators of pain. Responses to pain and coping techniques are learned, and clients may express them in a variety of ways. If a client's expressions of pain do not match the nurse's expectations, pain management may not be readily forthcoming. Consequently, the client's pain may be undertreated.

Assessment Tools

Because there are no reliable objective indicators for pain, assessment tools are necessary. Common assessment tools for quantifying pain intensity include a numeric scale, a word scale, and a linear scale (Fig. 11-7). Clients identify how their pain compares with the choices on the assessment tool. One tool is not better than another. A numeric scale is commonly used when assessing adults. When using the numeric rating scale, the clients are asked to identify how much pain they are having by choosing a number from 0 (*no pain*) to 10 (*the worst pain imaginable*). A horizontal pain assessment tool can be used to determine a client's pain when a visual chart is needed (Fig. 11-8), especially for pediatric, culturally diverse, and mentally challenged clients. The use of pictures of faces showing more and more pain allows the assessment tool to be used for young children.

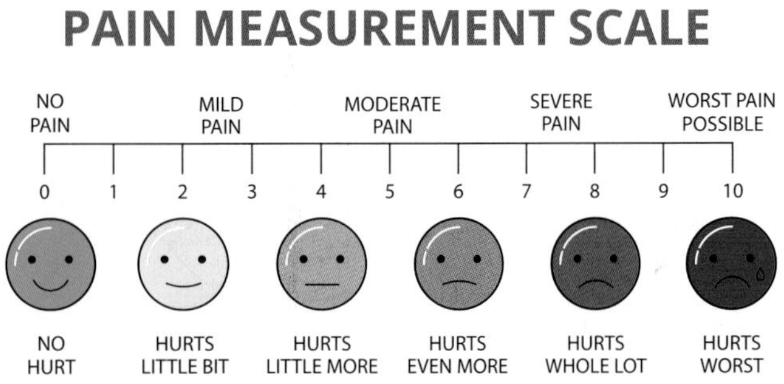

Figure 11-8 Faces Pain Scale, Revised. (Source: shutterstock.com/Oxy_gen)

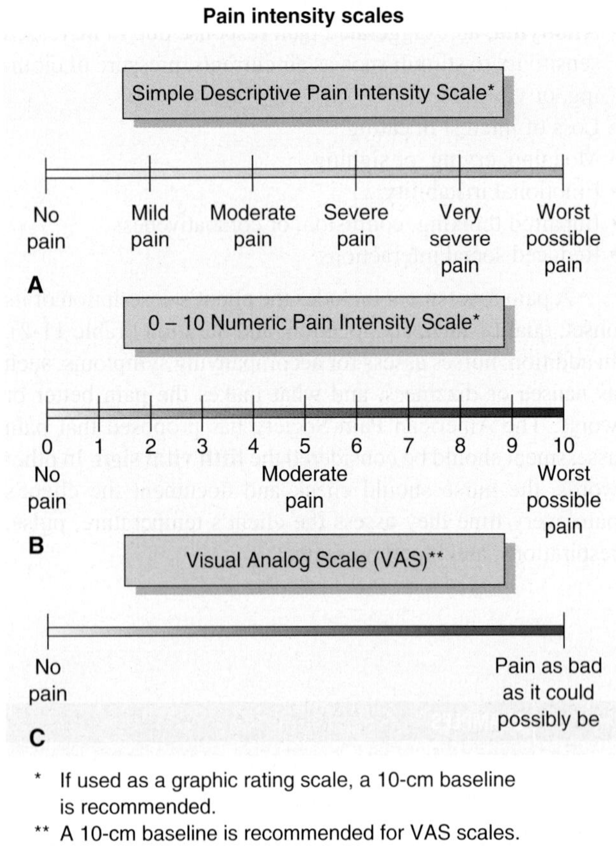

Figure 11-7 Pain assessment tools: **(A)** word scale, **(B)** numeric scale, and **(C)** linear scale.

>>> ***Stop, Think, and Respond 11-1***

When assessing the pain of two postoperative clients, the nurse is told by each client that incisional pain is a "10" using the numeric scale, in which "0" equals no pain and "10" is the most pain the person has ever felt. One of the clients is lying quietly in bed watching television. The other is restless and has placed both hands over the incisional area. Both have medical orders for 50 to 75 mg of meperidine intramuscularly (IM) every 3 to 4 hours as needed for pain. Both clients received 75 mg of meperidine IM 3 hours ago. What is the best nursing action at this time?

Assessment Standards

Since well over the previous decade, The Joint Commission (2020) has continued to address standards for pain assessment and management. All accredited health care organizations must comply with these standards. Table 11-3 lists components of an initial comprehensive pain assessment. Other aspects that are incorporated in the standards include the following:

- Everyone cared for in an accredited hospital, long-term care facility, home health care agency, outpatient clinic, or managed care organization has the right to assessment and management of pain.
- Pain is assessed using a tool that is appropriate for the person's age, developmental level, health condition, and cultural identity.
- Pain is regularly reassessed throughout health care delivery.
- Pain is treated in the health care agency or the client is referred elsewhere; both pharmacologic and

TABLE 11-3 The Joint Commission's Components of a Comprehensive Pain Assessment

COMPONENT	FOCUS OF ASSESSMENT
Intensity	Rating for present pain, worst pain, and least pain using a consistent scale
Location	Site of pain or identifying mark on a diagram
Quality	Description in client's own words
Onset	Time the pain began
Duration	Period that pain has existed
Variations	Pain characteristics that change
Patterns	Repetitiveness or lack thereof
Alleviating factors	Techniques or circumstances that reduce or relieve the pain
Aggravating factors	Techniques or circumstances that cause the pain to return or escalate in intensity
Present pain management regimen	Approaches used to control the pain and results and effectiveness
Pain management history	Past medications or interventions and responses; manner of expressing pain; personal, cultural, spiritual, or ethnic beliefs that affect pain management
Effects of pain	Alterations in self-care, sleep, dietary intake, thought processes, lifestyle, and relationships
Person's goal for pain control	Expectations for level of pain relief, tolerance, or restoration of functional abilities
Physical examination of pain	Assessment of structures that relate to the site of pain

Note. If clients have pain in more than one area, assessment data are collected for each.

nonpharmacologic strategies may be used. When pharmacologic strategies are proposed, both the benefits to the client as well as the risks of dependency, addiction, and abuse of opioids are considered.
- Health care providers are educated regarding pain assessment and management.
- Clients and their families are educated about effective pain management as an important part of care.
- The client's choices regarding pain management are respected.

PAIN MANAGEMENT

Pain management refers to the techniques used to prevent, reduce, or relieve pain. Achieving an optimum outcome often involves a multidisciplinary approach using drug and nondrug interventions (Fig. 11-9). The following are five general techniques for achieving pain management:

1. Blocking brain perception
2. Interrupting pain-transmitting chemicals at the site of injury
3. Combining analgesics with adjuvant drugs
4. Substituting sensory stimuli over shared pain neuropathways
5. Altering pain transmission at the level of the spinal cord

Any one or a combination of these techniques may be used.

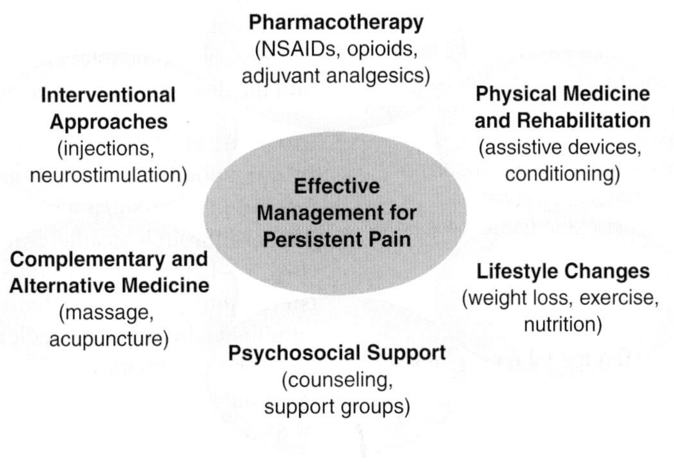

Figure 11-9 Multidisciplinary interventions for achieving pain management. NSAIDs, nonsteroidal antiinflammatory drugs. (From the American Pain Foundation. (2008). *A reporter's guide: Covering pain and its management.* https://assets.documentcloud.org/documents/277606/apf-reporters-guide.pdf)

Drug Therapy

Drug therapy is the cornerstone for managing pain. The World Health Organization (WHO) recommends following a three-tiered approach, according to the client's pain intensity and response to selected drug therapy (Fig. 11-10). A fourth step being considered for terminally ill clients with **intractable pain** (pain that is unresponsive to conventional treatment options) may include nerve blocks, analgesics administered *intrathecally* (in the subarachnoid or epidural spaces of the spine), electrical stimulation in the spinal cord, neurosurgical analgesic techniques, and palliative sedation. Examples of palliative sedation and neurosurgical analgesic techniques are discussed later in this chapter.

Opioid and opiate analgesics such as morphine and fentanyl are controlled substances often referred to as narcotics. Although the terms *opioid* and *narcotic* were once interchangeable, law enforcement agencies have generalized the term *narcotic* to mean a drug that is addictive and abused or used illegally. Health care providers use the term **opioid analgesics** to describe drugs used in pain relief. Opioids interfere with pain perception centrally (at the brain). Nonopioid analgesics relieve pain by altering neurotransmission at the peripheral level (site of injury) (Drug Therapy Table 11-1).

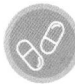

Pharmacologic Considerations

- Nonopioids are serious drugs. Instruct clients to consult their health care providers when using pain relievers for more than a few doses.
- Acetaminophen's effect on the liver makes drug overdose the primary cause of acute liver failure in children. To prevent hepatic damage, no more than 3250 to 4000 mg of acetaminophen should be taken per day. Individuals often are not aware they have exceeded the daily recommended dose when fever and pain relief drugs are coupled with over-the-counter cough and cold remedies that also contain acetaminophen.
- Likewise, some adults do not realize the anticoagulant (bleeding) effect of salicylate-based pain medications. Instruct clients taking the following drugs to tell all health care providers, when procedures are expected:
- Aspirin, including low-dose self-therapy (anticoagulant)
- Cold and cough product use (contains salicylates)
- NSAIDs such as ibuprofen and naproxen (increase gastrointestinal [GI] bleeding risk)

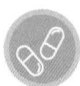

Pharmacologic Considerations

- The drug meperidine is less frequently used in a patient-controlled analgesia (PCA) machine. Some primary providers are less apt to prescribe the drug because it can potentially cause convulsions. Meperidine is metabolized into normeperidine by the body. When this metabolite is not excreted quickly, it builds up and can cause seizures.

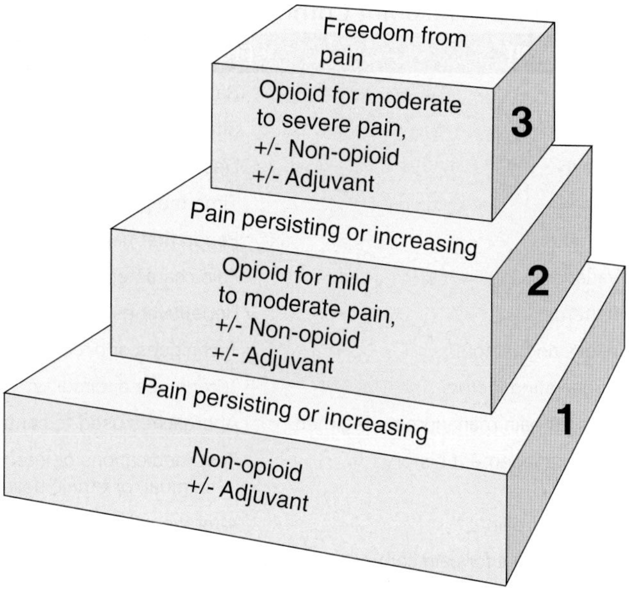

Figure 11-10 World Health Organization (WHO) analgesic ladder. (World Health Organization. (2012). *WHO's pain ladder.* https://www.who.int/images/default-source/infographics/cancer/guidelines-for-the-management-of-cancer-pain.jpg?sfvrsn=c9f27a68_6. Redrawn with permission.)

Methods of Administration

Analgesic drugs are administered by oral, rectal, transdermal, or parenteral (injected) routes, including a continuous infusion that may be instilled into the spinal canal or self-administered intravenously by clients. When changing from a parenteral to an oral route, it is best to administer an **equianalgesic dose**, an oral dose that provides the same level of pain relief as when the drug is given by a parenteral route (Table 11-4).

Patient-Controlled Analgesia

PCA allows clients to self-administer their own narcotic analgesic by means of an intravenous pump system (Fig. 11-11). The client infuses the drug by pressing a hand-held button. The dose and time intervals between doses are programmed into the device to prevent accidental overdose.

Intraspinal Analgesia

In intraspinal analgesia, a narcotic or local anesthetic is infused into the subarachnoid or epidural space of the spinal cord through a catheter inserted by a primary provider (Fig. 11-12). Depending on state nurse practice acts, registered nurses who are qualified as being competent may administer intraspinal medications through a catheter inserted by a primary provider or nurse anesthetist. The intraspinal analgesic is administered several times per day or as a continuous low-dose infusion. This method of analgesia relieves pain with minimal systemic drug effects. When used for clients who require long-term analgesia, there is less chance of affecting the subcutaneous tissues with repeated injections that may eventually lessen drug absorption.

DRUG THERAPY TABLE 11-1 Analgesic Drug Therapy

Category and Common Generic (Brand) Drugs	Intended Use	Common Side Effects	Safety Warnings for Nurses
Analgesics **Opioids**			
Opium derivatives Codeine Morphine (MS Contin) *Synthetics* Fentanyl (Sublimaze, Duragesic) Hydrocodone (Hysingla ER) Hydromorphone (Dilaudid) Meperidine (Demerol) Oxycodone (OxyContin) Tapentadol (Nucynta) Tramadol (Ultram)	Moderate-to-severe pain Acute pain only Neuropathic pain	Sedation, hypotension, vertigo, euphoria, nausea, vomiting, urinary retention, constipation (tolerance is not developed)	Watch for respiratory depression in opiate-naïve clients Treat constipation early with laxatives and fiber Use transdermal patches only when pain is not reduced by other routes, fold patches before disposal
Nonopioids			
Salicylate Aspirin or acetylsalicylic acid (Ascriptin, Bufferin)	Mild pain, antipyretic, antiinflammatory, stroke prevention in men (and women older than 65 years only)	Nausea, vomiting, epigastric distress	Anticoagulant, watch for bleeding and bruising Do not use in children under 12 years of age, risk of Rey syndrome Tinnitus (ringing in ears) can indicate overmedication use
Non-salicylate Acetaminophen (Tylenol)	Mild pain, antipyretic	Rare to see SE, itching	Liver toxicity with doses over 3500–4000 mg/day Used in cough/cold remedies, easy to go over daily max if taking with pain reliever
Nonsteroidal antiinflammatory drugs (NSAIDs) Celecoxib (Celebrex) ibuprofen (Motrin) indomethacin (Indocin) naproxen (Naprosyn)	Mild-to-moderate pain, antipyretic, antiinflammatory, rheumatoid disorders, dysmenorrhea	Nausea, dyspepsia, constipation	Risk of cardiovascular thrombosis, MI, and stroke Should not be used for postoperative cardiac surgery
Serotonin 5-HT Receptor Agonists			
Sumatriptan (Imitrex) Zolmitriptan (Zomig)	Acute migraine headache	Dizziness, fatigue, nausea, dry mouth, flushing	If taking with SSRI/SNRI antidepressant, monitor for serotonin syndrome Do not use injectable form if cloudy or yellow
Topical Analgesics			
Capsaicin cream (Zostrix) Lidocaine 5% patch (Lidoderm)	Minor aches, joint pain, nerve pain	Skin redness, irritation, or swelling	Avoid direct heat, e.g., heating pad, hot tub increases skin absorption Fold patches before disposal
Analgesic Adjuvants **Anticonvulsants**			
Carbamazepine (Tegretol) Levetiracetam (Keppra) Topiramate (Topamax) Valproic acid (Depakote) *Calcium Channel Binders* Gabapentin (Neurontin) Pregabalin (Lyrica)	Migraine headache Fibromyalgia, neuropathic pain syndromes, phantom limb pain	Dizziness, somnolence, nausea Weight gain	Increased fall risk due to sedative side effects Dose must be titrated down when stopping drug

(continued)

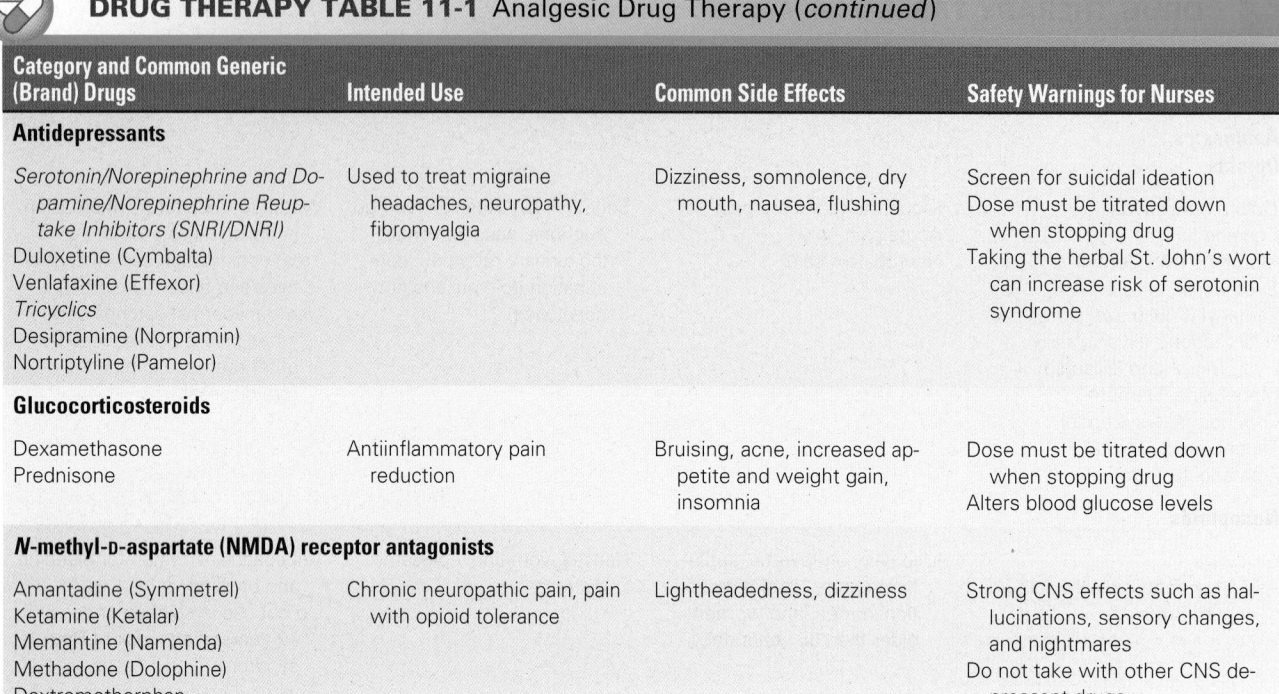

DRUG THERAPY TABLE 11-1 Analgesic Drug Therapy (*continued*)

Category and Common Generic (Brand) Drugs	Intended Use	Common Side Effects	Safety Warnings for Nurses
Antidepressants			
Serotonin/Norepinephrine and Dopamine/Norepinephrine Reuptake Inhibitors (SNRI/DNRI) Duloxetine (Cymbalta) Venlafaxine (Effexor) *Tricyclics* Desipramine (Norpramin) Nortriptyline (Pamelor)	Used to treat migraine headaches, neuropathy, fibromyalgia	Dizziness, somnolence, dry mouth, nausea, flushing	Screen for suicidal ideation Dose must be titrated down when stopping drug Taking the herbal St. John's wort can increase risk of serotonin syndrome
Glucocorticosteroids			
Dexamethasone Prednisone	Antiinflammatory pain reduction	Bruising, acne, increased appetite and weight gain, insomnia	Dose must be titrated down when stopping drug Alters blood glucose levels
***N*-methyl-D-aspartate (NMDA) receptor antagonists**			
Amantadine (Symmetrel) Ketamine (Ketalar) Memantine (Namenda) Methadone (Dolophine) Dextromethorphan	Chronic neuropathic pain, pain with opioid tolerance	Lightheadedness, dizziness	Strong CNS effects such as hallucinations, sensory changes, and nightmares Do not take with other CNS depressant drugs

5-HT, 5-hydroxytryptamine; CNS, central nervous system; MI, myocardial infarction; SE, side effects; SSRI, selective serotonin reuptake inhibitor.
The drugs in column 1 indicate the drug that matches up with explanations in columns 2 through 4.

Palliative Sedation

Palliative sedation is the controlled administration of sedative medication to eliminate an imminently dying client's intractable pain and suffering (American Academy of Hospice and Palliative Medicine, 2014; Kirk & Mahon, 2010). The aim of this approach is not to shorten survival or be completely irreversible, in other words, "to kill the pain—not the patient" (Doerflinger & Gomez, 2016).

Palliative sedation is used only when there is no other means available to alleviate suffering without speeding up or slowing down the dying process. In some cases, it may be used for only a predetermined period of time. Once awakened, the client's capacity to endure suffering is reassessed. Sedation may then be withheld for the time being or reestablished. In two cases reviewed by the U.S. Supreme Court in 1997, decisions were rendered establishing that palliative sedation is a safe, legal, and reasonable alternative to assisted suicide (Stanford School of Medicine, 2016). Caveats include that (1) the client and family are included in the decision-making process; (2) there is a 24-hour or longer waiting period before proceeding with palliative sedation; (3) one or two nurses are available at the client's bedside at all times, during which the client is continually assessed and basic needs for elimination, skin and mouth care, turning, and positioning are implemented; and (4) a primary provider must be accessible throughout its administration. Drugs that are commonly administered for palliative sedation include benzodiazepines, such as midazolam (Versed); neuroleptics,

TABLE 11-4 Examples of Adult Equianalgesic Doses

OPIOID AGONIST	PARENTERAL DOSE (mg)	ORAL DOSE (mg)	DURATION OF ACTION (h)
Morphine	10	30	3–4
Hydromorphone (Dilaudid)	1.5	7.5	2–3
Oxymorphone (Opana)	1	10	3–6

Adapted from Kishner, S. (2016). Opioid equivalents and conversions. *Medscape.* http://emedicine.medscape.com/article/2138678-overview

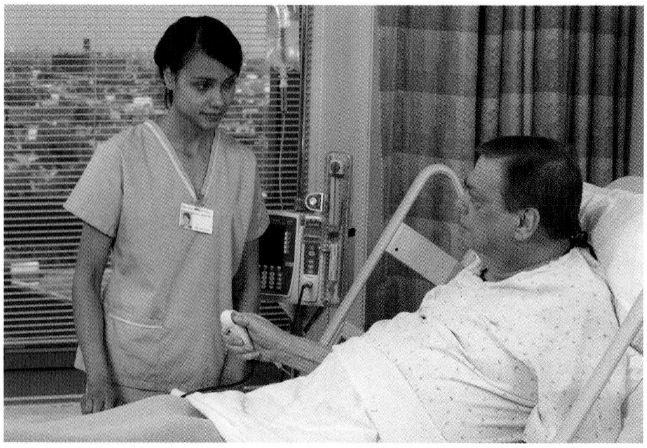

Figure 11-11 Patient-controlled analgesia allows the client to self-administer medication to control pain.

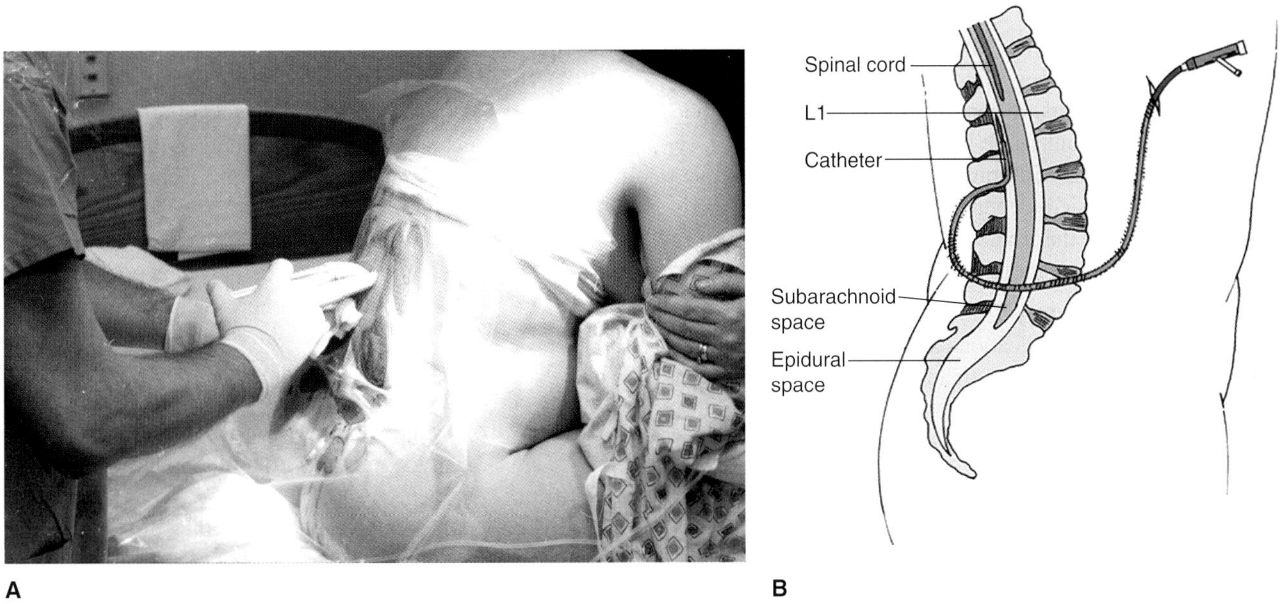

Figure 11-12 Intraspinal anesthesia. **(A)** Epidural catheter insertion. **(B)** Epidural catheter placement. (A, reprinted with permission from Ricci, S. S. (2017). *Essentials of maternity, newborn, and women's health nursing* (4th ed.). Wolters Kluwer. B, reprinted with permission from Lynn, P. B., & *Taylor, C. (2008). Taylor's clinical nursing skills: A nursing process approach* (2nd ed., p. 585). Wolters Kluwer Health/Lippincott Williams & Wilkins.)

such as haloperidol (Haldol); general anesthetics, such as propofol (Diprivan); and barbiturates, such as pentobarbital (Nembutal).

Addiction, Tolerance, and Physical Dependence

One of the leading factors interfering with adequate pain management is the fear of addiction. The American Society for Pain Management Nursing describes **addiction** as a chronic, relapsing, treatable disease—characterized by:

- Craving
- Dysfunctional behaviors
- Inability to control impulses regarding consumption of a substance
- Compulsive use despite harmful consequences (Oliver et al., 2012)

Addiction is a worldwide problem. The treatment and prescribing of opioid medications has been reduced due to the addictive properties of the drugs. In 2018, the National Institute on Drug Abuse (NIDA) reported that 128 Americans died daily from opioid overdose (2020). Unfortunately, the fear of addiction causes many clients to refuse or self-limit prescribed drug therapy. Nurses often assume that a client's desire to experience a drug's pleasant effects motivates their desire for frequent doses of narcotics. What may be happening is that the prescribed dose or frequency of administration is not controlling the pain. Clients with severe, unrelieved pain may be falsely labeled as being addicted because they are focused on receiving analgesics, when in reality they are only seeking relief from unrelenting discomfort. Consequently, nurses may administer subtherapeutic doses or may convince the primary provider to prescribe a **placebo**, an inactive substance intended to produce a beneficial effect without any physiologic alteration.

Although addiction rarely develops, tolerance is common. **Tolerance** is a condition in which a client needs increasingly larger doses of a drug to achieve the same effect as when the drug was first administered. Activation of NMDA receptors is believed to decrease the effect of opioids and the need to administer higher doses to achieve a therapeutic effect.

Although responses to drug therapy differ among individuals, tolerance may not develop until a client has taken an opioid drug regularly for 4 weeks or more (McCaffery & Ferrell, 1999). The development of tolerance is not an indication of addiction. The most appropriate nursing action is to consult with the primary provider regarding the need for an increased dose of the drug and not to reduce its dosage or frequency of administration. As a rule of thumb, an ineffective dose should be increased by 25% to 50% (McCaffery & Ferrell, 1999).

Because opioids depress the respiratory center in the brain, some nurses fear giving larger and larger doses of narcotic analgesics. In reality, respiratory depression is rare in those receiving opioids for prolonged periods of time. However, even if large doses of opioid analgesics coincidentally hasten death, the primary intention for their administration is controlling pain. The Hospice and Palliative Nurses Association (2020) and other professional organizations, therefore, acknowledge that it is an ethically acceptable intervention.

››› *Stop, Think, and Respond 11-2*

A medical order states meperidine hydrochloride 50 to 100 mg IM q3h prn for pain. If a client does not experience adequate pain relief after receiving 50 mg, what dose should the nurse administer?

Just as tolerance is not a characteristic of addiction, neither is physical dependence. **Physical dependence** means that a person experiences physical discomfort, known as **withdrawal symptoms**, when a drug that a person has taken routinely for some time is abruptly discontinued (see Chapter 71). To avoid withdrawal symptoms, drugs that are known to cause physical dependence are discontinued gradually. The dosage or the frequency of their administration is lowered over 1 week or longer.

Adjuvant Drug Therapy

Adjuvant drugs are medications that are ordinarily administered for reasons other than treating pain. When adjuvant drugs are combined with opioid and nonopioid analgesics, they may achieve any or all of the following: (1) improvement of analgesic effect without an increased analgesic dosage; (2) control of concurrent symptoms, such as inflammation, that worsen the pain; and (3) moderation of side effects of analgesics, such as nausea or sedation. Examples of adjuvant drugs used to manage pain include tricyclic antidepressants, corticosteroids, anticonvulsants, psychostimulants, and NMDA receptor antagonists (see Drug Therapy Table 11-1).

Nondrug Interventions

The pain management standards established by The Joint Commission include using nonpharmacologic methods for managing pain (see Chapter 9). Some are independent nursing measures; others may require collaboration with the client's primary provider and services provided within integrative medicine by individuals who have specialized training and expertise. Examples include applications of heat and cold, transcutaneous and percutaneous electrical nerve stimulation (TENS and PENS, respectively), acupuncture, and acupressure. The latter interventions are more likely to be used for clients with chronic pain or those for whom acute pain management techniques have been unsuccessful or are contraindicated.

Research is ongoing to determine how nondrug interventions relieve pain. Some question whether their effectiveness is the result of the placebo effect (see Chapter 67) or something more physiologic. Pasero and McCaffery (1999, p. 22) report that "the brain can accommodate a limited number of sensory signals. When individuals use techniques such as distraction, relaxation, and imagery to control pain, they direct their attention away from the pain sensation." Some believe that these techniques stimulate the visual portion of the brain's cortex in the right hemisphere, where abstract concepts and creative activities take place. In response, the body releases neurotransmitters such as GABA and serotonin that calm the body and promote emotional well-being. This may explain how some adjuvant drugs for pain relief such as anticonvulsants and antidepressants effect their actions.

Techniques such as electrical nerve stimulation, acupuncture, and acupressure may support the gate control and neuromatrix theories. They achieve benefits by stimulating sensory nerve fibers that conduct tactile or vibratory sensations over pathways shared for transmitting pain. The result is inhibition of pain transmission. Others speculate that these and other nondrug methods such as massage relieve pain by releasing **endogenous opiates** such as endorphins and enkephalins. Endogenous opiates are natural morphine-like substances in the body that modulate pain transmission by blocking receptors for substance P (see Fig. 11-6).

Heat and Cold

Applications of heat and cold (thermal therapy) are well-established techniques for relieving pain (Fig. 11-13). Pain associated with injury is best treated initially with cold applications such as an ice bag or chemical pack. A first aid measure following a soft tissue injury and for 24 to 48 hours thereafter is to follow the mnemonic **RICE: R**est, **I**ce, **C**ompression, **E**levation. The cold decreases vasodilation that reduces localized swelling, which may be useful for minor

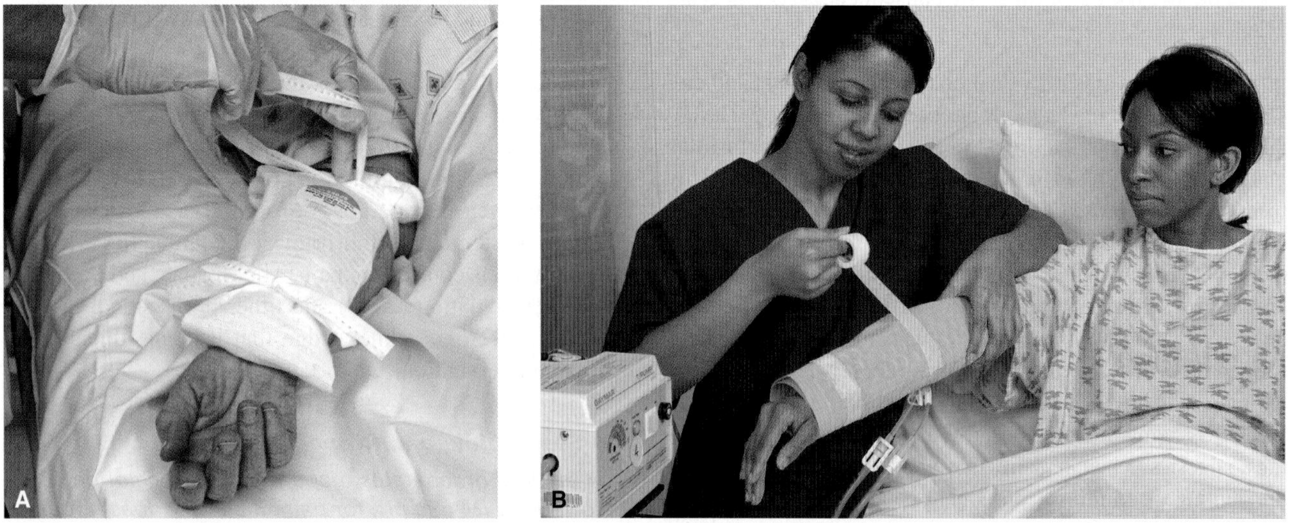

Figure 11-13 Examples of hot and cold applications. **(A)** Ice bag. **(B)** Warm compress covered by aquathermia pad. (A and B reprinted with permission from Springhouse. (2009). *Lippincott's visual encyclopedia of clinical skills.* Wolters Kluwer Health/ Lippincott Williams & Wilkins.)

or moderate pain. Cold applications using ice bags or compresses are repeatedly applied for 10 to 20 minutes, removed, and reapplied later. Regardless of whether hot or cold applications are used, they are never applied directly to the skin.

Applications of dry or moist heat, such as a heating pad, hot water bottle, warm baths, and hot tubs or whirlpools with water jets, are beneficial for chronic pain or several days following an injury. The heat reduces muscle tension and promotes relaxation; it increases blood flow, which brings healing blood cells to injured tissue.

Transcutaneous Electrical Stimulation

TENS is a pain management technique that delivers bursts of electricity to the skin and underlying nerves. It is safe for managing acute and chronic pain and does not produce systemic side effects or addiction. The electricity is delivered from a battery-operated TENS unit through electrode patches that are placed at appropriate sites, such as directly over the affected area, at areas along a nerve pathway, or at points distal to the painful area (Fig. 11-14). The client perceives the electrical stimulus as a pleasant tapping, tingling, vibrating, or buzzing sensation. Placement sites, intensity of electrical current, rate of electrical bursts, and duration can be changed according to the client's response.

Acupuncture and Acupressure

Acupuncture is a pain management technique in which long, thin needles are inserted into the skin. Acupressure uses tissue compression, rather than needles, to reduce pain. The location for needle placement and pressure is based on 2000-year-old traditions practiced in Chinese medicine (see Chapter 9). Relief of pain, especially in chronic transmission pathways, is not permanent, and repeated treatments are almost always necessary.

Although both techniques have been demonstrated to prevent or relieve pain, their exact mechanism is not completely understood. Some speculate that the twisting, vibration, and pressure are forms of cutaneous stimuli that close the gates to pain-transmitting neurochemicals. Another theory is that acupuncture and acupressure stimulate the body to release endorphins and enkephalins.

Percutaneous Electrical Nerve Stimulation

Two of the newest innovations in acute and chronic pain management are **PENS**, a form of electroacupuncture (see Chapter 9), and **percutaneous neuromodulation therapy (PNT)**, a variant of PENS. They combine the use of acupuncture needles with TENS. The practitioner inserts the needles in soft tissue near the area of the spine that is causing pain, and an electrical stimulus is conducted through the needles. PENS is considered superior to TENS in providing pain relief because the needles are located closer to nerve endings. The general treatment regimen for PENS and PNT therapy is 30 minutes once or twice a week for 8 to 10 sessions; some clients receive PENS or PNT for up to 8 weeks (National Medical Policy, 2016). The technique has been successful in research trials on clients with low back pain, pain caused by the spread of cancer to bones, shingles (acute herpes zoster viral infection), neuropathic pain among clients with diabetes or hemiplegia, and migraine headaches.

Other Noninvasive Techniques

Various other techniques are used alone or in addition to more traditional pain management techniques. Some include imagery, biofeedback, massage therapy, reflexology, chiropractic, and others (see Chapter 9). In addition, in some situations (e.g., clients with severe burns), hypnosis is used. Hypnosis is a technique in which a person assumes a trance-like state during which perceptions are altered. During hypnosis, a suggestion is made that a person's pain will be eliminated or that the client will experience the sensation in a more pleasant way.

Cotherapies also may include physical or occupational therapy and cognitive behavioral therapy. Physical therapy can help to strengthen muscles weakened by disuse. Occupational therapy may help inactive clients relearn to perform physical tasks without aggravating their preexisting condition. **Cognitive behavioral therapy** is a form of

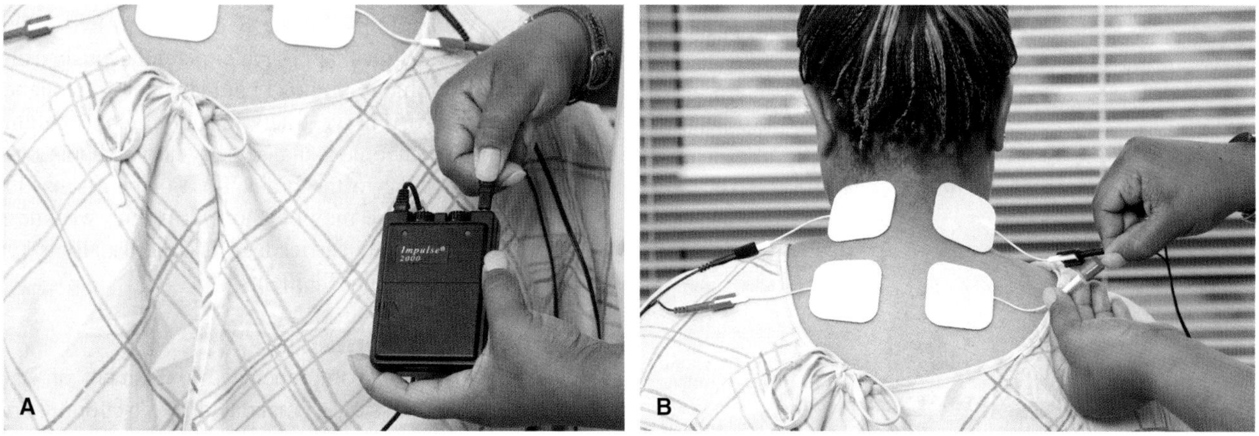

Figure 11-14 To activate various sensory nerves, a transcutaneous electrical nerve stimulation (TENS) unit **(A)** may be placed close to the pain source. The TENS unit floods the gates in the spinal cord, blocking pain perception. Site of placement **(B)** depends on the pain's location.

psychotherapy used to help clients change their unhealthy beliefs and behaviors.

Spinal Surgery Techniques

Intractable pain, pain that does not respond to analgesic medications, noninvasive nonpharmaceutical measures, or nursing management requires more drastic measures. Neurosurgical procedures that provide pain relief include implanting a spinal cord stimulator, rhizotomy, and cordotomy.

Spinal Cord Stimulation

A **spinal cord stimulator** is a pulse generator that is placed surgically under the client's skin and connects to a wire that leads to nerve fibers in the spinal cord (Fig. 11-15). The pulse generator transmits an electrical current that causes a tingling sensation, but ultimately interrupts pain transmission. Candidates for this device are clients for whom conservative pain management techniques have failed. Generally, most clients experience a 50% to 75% relief from pain. The battery for the pulse generator must be replaced every 2 to 5 years; however, some batteries are rechargeable and may be left in place for up to 10 years.

Rhizotomy

A **rhizotomy** is a procedure that destroys the medial branch sensory nerve that protrudes between spinal joints (Fig. 11-16). Destroying the spinal nerve prevents sensory impulses from entering the spinal cord and going to the brain. The result is relief of low back or cervical pain due to a loss of sensation in the area supplied by the affected nerve. More than one nerve may need to be sectioned to produce the desired results. Chemical rhizotomy (using chemicals such as alcohol or phenol to destroy the nerve) and percutaneous rhizotomy (using radiofrequency waves to destroy pain fibers) are alternatives to surgery that may provide the same result.

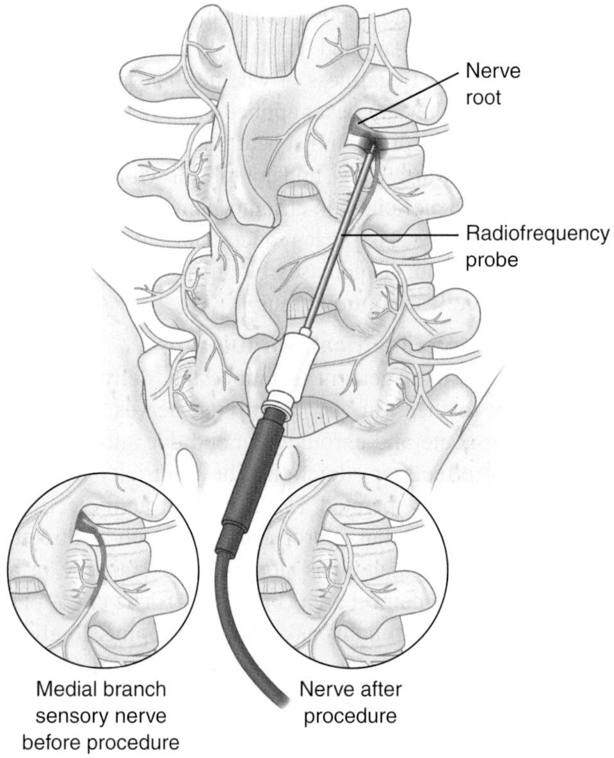

Figure 11-16 A sensory nerve root is destroyed to relieve pain when a rhizotomy is performed.

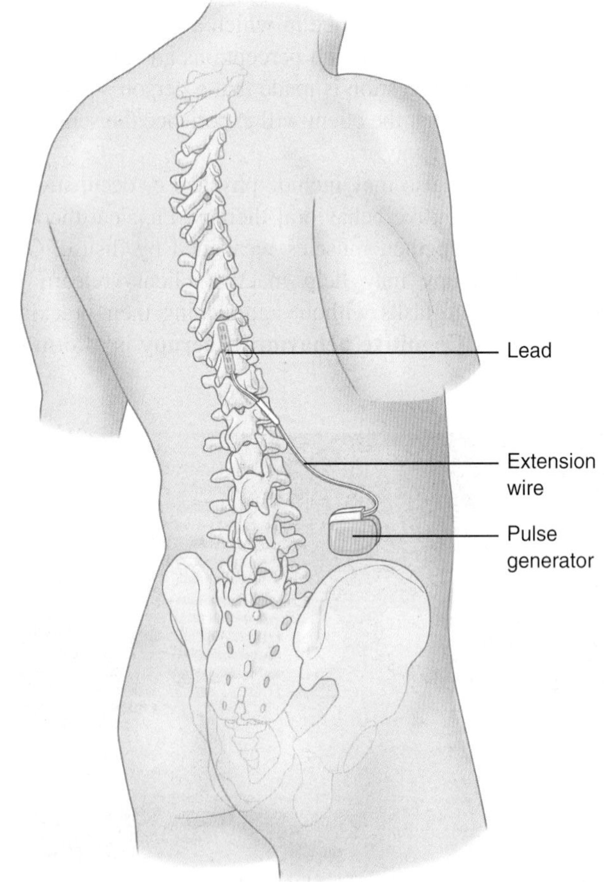

Figure 11-15 Spinal cord neurostimulator with percutaneous pulse generator.

Cordotomy

A **cordotomy** is an interruption of pain pathways in the spinal cord. The procedure is primarily indicated for those with a terminal illness with a life expectancy of less than 12 months. A cordotomy can be performed in two different ways: an open surgical approach or percutaneously using X-ray computed tomography (CT) guidance radiofrequency that destroys sensory nerve tracts in the vertebral column (Fig. 11-17). The outcome is that sensory nerve impulses are prevented from going to the brain. Loss of pain sensation is permanent, and there may be short-term limb weakness. Percutaneous cordotomy carries less risk and usually is better tolerated by terminally ill clients.

Nursing Management

The nurse performs a comprehensive assessment of each client's pain on admission as mandated by The Joint Commission (see Table 11-3). Regularly thereafter, the nurse determines the onset, quality, intensity, location, and duration of the client's pain. They explain the tool for assessing a

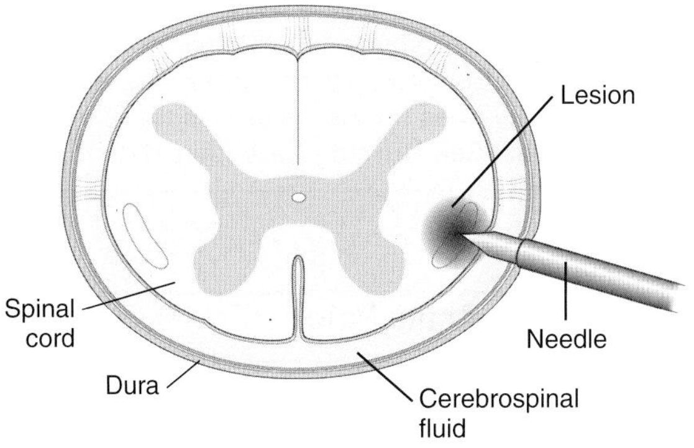

Figure 11-17 A percutaneous cordotomy creates a lesion within the spinal cord to eliminate the client's perception of pain.

client's pain so the client understands how to self-report their level of pain when the assessment tool is used again. Giving assurance that pain management is a nursing and agency priority is essential throughout the client's care. The nurse informs the client of available pain management techniques and incorporates any preferences or objections to interventions for pain management that the client may have when establishing a plan of care.

The nurse collaborates with each client about their goal for a level of pain relief and implements interventions for achieving the goal. The nurse never doubts or minimizes the client's description of pain or need for pain relief. If a client's goal for pain relief is not reached, the nurse collaborates with members of the health care team for other approaches that may do so. Scheduling the administration of analgesics every 3 hours rather than on an as-needed (prn) basis often affords a uniform level of pain relief. Providing a client with equipment to self-administer analgesics, as with a PCA pump, also promotes a more consistent level of pain relief.

When medications are administered, the nurse monitors for and implements measures for managing side effects (see Drug Therapy Table 11-1). Problems that may develop with opioid and opiate therapy include Impaired Gas Exchange related to respiratory depression, Constipation related to slowed peristalsis, Injury Risk related to drowsiness and unsteady gait, Malnutrition Risk related to anorexia and nausea, Dehydration related to reduced oral intake, and Sleep Deprivation (interrupted sleep) related to depression of the central nervous system. Some general nutrition considerations are listed in Nutrition Notes.

The nurse may administer adjuvant drugs or implement nondrug alternatives for pain management to enhance the effect of opioid and nonopioid analgesics or as a substitute when drug side effects jeopardize the client's safety. When planning the client's discharge from the health care agency, the nurse includes interventions for pain relief to facilitate a comfortable transition to the next level of care. Box 11-2 summarizes nursing responsibilities for managing pain.

An important component of pain management is client and family teaching (Client and Family Teaching 11-1).

Nutrition Notes

The Client Receiving Drug Therapy for Pain

- Administering pain medications 30 to 45 minutes before meals may relieve pain, enabling the client to consume an adequate nutritional intake.
- Small, frequent meals may help maximize intake in clients with drug-related or pain-related anorexia. Solicit food preferences.
- A high-fiber diet (i.e., a diet rich in whole-grain breads and cereals, fresh fruits, and vegetables) along with increased fluids may help ease constipation, a possible side effect of opioids.

BOX 11-2 Nursing Responsibilities for Managing Pain

- Assess for pain on a frequent and regular basis.
- Respond quickly to a client's or family's report of pain.
- Acknowledge the client's pain.
- Explain available options for managing pain.
- Encourage the client's participation in pain management decisions.
- Respect the client's choice for managing the pain.
- Implement measures to relieve pain in a timely manner.
- Evaluate the effectiveness of an intervention.
- Advocate on the client's behalf if pain is unrelieved or insufficiently relieved.
- Provide pain-relieving alternatives.
- Communicate with health care members concerning approaches and outcomes of a client's pain management.

Client and Family Teaching 11-1 Pain

The nurse encourages the client and family to

- discuss with the primary provider what to expect from the disorder, injury, or its treatment.
- talk with the primary provider about any concerns that relate to drug therapy.
- share information about what drugs or pain-relieving techniques have and have not been helpful during previous episodes.
- identify drug allergies to avoid adverse effects.
- inform the primary provider about other medications being taken to avoid drug–drug interactions.
- take prescribed drugs exactly as directed and report untoward effects.
- avoid taking over-the-counter drugs unless the primary provider has been consulted; follow label directions for administration.
- avoid alcohol and sedative drugs if the analgesic causes sedation.
- keep analgesic drugs out of the reach of children; request childproof caps.
- never share medications with others or take someone else's medications for pain.

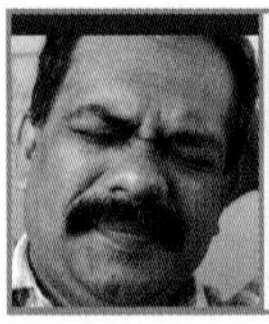

Clinical Scenario A client arrives at the emergency department of a hospital at 4 p.m. He reports that he has a "throbbing" pain in his left side that started this morning and hasn't stopped. He states that he has never felt this intense pain before today. "Please make it stop!" **How does the nurse assess this client and plan for his care? What data are needed for this assessment? See Nursing Care Plan 11-1.**

NURSING CARE PLAN 11-1 The Client With Acute Pain

Assessment

- Determine the following:
  - Source of client's pain; when it began; its intensity, location, characteristics, and related factors such as what makes the pain better or worse
  - How client's pain interferes with life, such as diminishing the ability to meet their own needs for hygiene, eating, sleep, activity, social interactions, emotional stability, concentration, and so forth
  - At what level client can tolerate pain
  - Pain-related behaviors such as grimacing, crying, moaning, and assuming a guarded position
- Measure vital signs.
- Perform a physical assessment, taking care to gently support and assist client to turn as you examine various structures. Use light palpation in areas that are tender. Show concern when assessment techniques increase client's pain.
- Postpone nonpriority assessments until client's pain has been reduced.

Nursing Diagnosis. Acute pain related to cellular injury or disease as manifested by stating, "I'm in severe pain"; rating pain at 10 using a numeric scale; pointing to the lower left abdominal quadrant; describing the pain as "continuous, throbbing, and starting this morning" without any known cause.

Expected Outcome. Client will rate the pain intensity at their tolerable level of "5" within 30 minutes of implementing a pain management technique.

Interventions	Rationales
Assess client's pain and its characteristics at least every 2 hours while awake and 30 minutes after implementing a pain management technique.	*Quick interventions prevent or minimize pain.*
Modify or eliminate factors that contribute to pain such as a full bladder, uncomfortable position, pain-aggravating activity, excessively warm or cool environment, noise, and social isolation.	*Multiple stressors decrease pain tolerance.*
Determine client's choice for pain relief techniques from among those available.	*Encourage and respect client's participation in decision-making.*
Administer prescribed analgesics or alternative pain management techniques promptly.	*Suffering contributes to the pain experience and can be reduced by eliminating delays in nursing response.*
Advocate on client's behalf for higher doses of prescribed analgesics or addition of adjuvant drug therapy if pain is not satisfactorily relieved.	*The Joint Commission standards mandate that nurses and other health care providers facilitate pain relief for clients.*
Administer a prescribed analgesic before a procedure or activity that is likely to result in or intensify pain.	*Prophylactic interventions facilitate keeping pain at a manageable level.*
Plan for periods of rest between activities.	*Fatigue and exhaustion interfere with pain tolerance.*
Reassure client that there are many ways to modify the pain experience.	*Suggesting that there are additional untried options helps alleviate frustration or despair that there is no hope for pain relief.*

Interventions	Rationales
Assist client to visualize a pleasant experience.	*Imaging interrupts pain perception.*
Help client focus on deep breathing, relaxing muscles, watching television, putting together a puzzle, or talking to someone on the phone.	*Diverting attention to something other than pain reduces pain perception.*
Apply warm or cool compresses to a painful sensory site.	*Flooding the brain with alternative stimuli closes the spinal gates that transmit pain.*
Gently massage a painful area or the same area on the opposite side of the body (contralateral massage).	*Massage promotes the release of endorphins and enkephalins that moderate the sensation.*

NURSING CARE PLAN 11-1 The Client With Acute Pain (*continued*)

Promote laughter by suggesting that client relate a humorous story or watch a video or comedy of their choice.	*Laughter releases endorphins and enkephalins that promote a feeling of well-being.*

Evaluation of Expected Outcomes

- Client reports that pain is gone or is at a tolerable level of "5" within 30 minutes.
- Client perceives the pain experience realistically and copes effectively.
- Client participates in self-care activities without undue pain.

KEY POINTS

- Pain Management
  - Types of pain
    - Nociceptive pain—noxious stimuli transmitted from point of cellular injury to the brain
      - Somatic pain—caused by mechanical, chemical, thermal, or electrical injuries or disorders
      - Visceral pain—arises from internal organs
    - Neuropathic pain—pain that is processed abnormally by the nervous system
    - Acute pain—discomfort for a short duration—seconds to less than 6 months
    - Chronic pain—pain that lasts longer than 6 months
  - Pain transmission
    - Transduction—conversion of chemical information in the cellular environment to electrical impulses that move toward the spinal cord
    - Transmission—phase where peripheral nerve fibers form synapse with neurons in the brain
    - Perception—the phase of impulse transmission, where one feels the pain
    - Pain threshold—the point at which the pain is felt
    - Pain tolerance—amount of pain a person endures
    - Modulation—last phase of pain impulse transmission
  - Theories of pain
    - Specific theory
    - Pattern theory
    - Gate control theory
    - Neuromatrix theory
    - Endogenous opioid theory
  - Pain Assessment—includes the client's description of the pain onset, quality, intensity, location, and duration, accompanying symptoms, what makes the pain better, what makes the pain worse
    - Assessment Biases
    - Assessment Tools
    - Assessment Standards
  - Pain Management—techniques used to prevent, reduce, or relieve pain
    - Drug Therapy
      - Methods of Administration
      - Palliative Sedation
      - Addiction, Tolerance, and Physical Dependence
      - Adjuvant Drug Therapy
    - Nondrug Interventions
      - Heat and Cold
      - Transcutaneous Electrical Nerve Stimulation
      - Acupuncture and Acupressure
      - Percutaneous Electrical Nerve Stimulation
    - Spinal Surgical Techniques
      - Spinal Cord Stimulation
      - Rhizotomy
      - Cordotomy
  - Nursing Management—The nurse performs a comprehensive assessment of pain upon admission, provides appropriate treatment, and reassesses routinely throughout the care of the client.

CRITICAL THINKING EXERCISES

1. What questions should the nurse ask when a client states that they have pain?
2. Discuss how acute pain after surgery is different from pain experienced by a client with chronic back pain.
3. Discuss nursing interventions that are appropriate if a client does not experience adequate pain relief from a prescribed analgesic.
4. What actions should a nurse take if a client who they assume to be in pain cannot verbalize discomfort?
5. If a client has an order for morphine sulfate 5 mg IM q3 to 4h prn and ibuprofen (Motrin) 800 mg po tid prn and has not experienced pain relief 2 hours after receiving the morphine, what could the nurse do?

NCLEX-STYLE REVIEW QUESTIONS PrepU

1. A nurse observes that the client who is experiencing abdominal pain is curled in a fetal position and rocking back and forth. What nursing action is best at the present time?
   1. Ask the client to rate the pain on a scale from 0 to 10.
   2. Determine if the client can stop moving about.
   3. Give the client a prescribed pain-relieving drug.
   4. Observe if the client is breathing heavily.

2. A postoperative client requests pain medication. Following the administration of morphine sulfate, what information is most important for the nurse to collect?
  1. Color and temperature of the skin
  2. Presence and activity of bowel sounds
  3. Rate and depth of respirations
  4. Rhythm and force of the heart rate

3. A primary provider orders ketamine 1 mg/kg IM now. The client weighs 220 lb. The vial of ketamine has been diluted to contain 50 mg/mL. Fill in the blank with the volume the nurse should administer. Record your answer in a whole number.

_________mL

4. A client has developed physical dependence on an opioid drug for pain relief. Which of the following interventions is appropriate first?
  1. Immediately discontinue all drug therapy.
  2. Replace the opioid with a nonopioid drug.
  3. Gradually decrease the dosage and frequency of the opioid.
  4. Increase the dosage but decrease the frequency of the opioid.

5. The nurse cares for a client with metastatic cancer, who is receiving hospice care and who has an advance directive that requests no aggressive treatment. If there is a primary provider's order for pain medication every 3 to 4 hours as necessary, which action by the hospice nurse is most appropriate in order to provide the client with maximum comfort at this time?
  1. Administer the medication every 3 hours.
  2. Ask the primary provider to prescribe a high dose.
  3. Give the medication immediately upon request.
  4. Give the medication when the pain is severe.

WANT TO KNOW MORE? There are a wide variety of online resources available on thePoint to enhance learning and understanding of this chapter.

Go to **thePoint.lww.com/activate** and use the activation code found in the front of this text to unlock these online resources.

12 Infection

Words To Know

bacteremia
carrier
chain of infection
colonization
communicable diseases
community-acquired infections
contagious diseases
culture
emerging infectious diseases
epidemics
fomites
health care–associated infections
host
immunizations
infection
leukocytosis
method of transmission
microorganisms
multidrug resistance
nonpathogens
opportunistic infections
pandemic
pathogens
phagocytosis
portal of entry
portal of exit
prion
reemerging infectious diseases
reservoir
sensitivity
sepsis
septicemia
severe sepsis
standard precautions
superinfections
susceptibility
transmission-based precautions
virulence
zoonotic pathogens

Learning Objectives

On completion of this chapter, you will be able to:

1. Describe types of infectious agents and list examples.
2. Differentiate between nonpathogens and pathogens.
3. Describe the six components of the chain of infection.
4. List factors that increase susceptibility to infection.
5. Explain the difference between mechanical and chemical defense mechanisms.
6. Describe events during the inflammatory process.
7. Differentiate localized from generalized infections.
8. List reasons why clients in health care agencies are at increased risk for infection.
9. Explain nursing actions to prevent or control transmission of infection in the hospital and in the community.
10. Describe measures to take if a needlestick injury occurs.
11. Name diagnostic tests ordered for clients suspected of having an infectious disorder.
12. Discuss the medical management of clients with infectious disorders.
13. Describe nursing care for the client with a potential or actual infection.

Infections have plagued humans since the beginning of time. Despite available vaccines, aggressive public health measures, and advances in drug therapy, respiratory infections rank eighth among the top 10 causes of death in the United States (Centers for Disease Control and Prevention [CDC], 2019), and about 1 in 31 develops at least one health care–associated infection (HAI) from which 75,000 die annually (CDC, 2019).

Although these statistics are significant in and of themselves, they do not take into account viral infections such as human immunodeficiency virus (HIV), human papillomavirus (HPV), and herpes simplex virus type 2, which, besides causing infections, play an etiologic role in various types of cancers (see Chapters 35 and 53), nor do they reflect infections caused by new and mutant microorganisms, nor the recent worldwide deaths from Ebola and COVID-19. When considered altogether, a logical conclusion is that infections continue to represent a global threat.

This chapter discusses the causes of infections, their transmission, methods for preventing and controlling infections, and techniques for managing the care of clients with infections.

Gerontologic Considerations

- Residents in nursing facilities tend to acquire infections through the urinary tract, skin, and respiratory tract portals of entry.
- Infections are often transmitted to vulnerable older adults through hospital equipment reservoirs such as indwelling urinary catheters, humidifiers, and oxygen equipment or through incisional sites such as those for IV tubing, parenteral nutrition, or tube feedings. Hand washing, standard precautions, and use of proper aseptic technique are essential preventive measures. Daily assessment for any signs of infection is imperative. Health care providers who are ill should take sick leave rather than expose susceptible older clients to infectious organisms.
- Pneumonia and influenza combined remain the eighth leading cause of death in adults over the age of 65 years (CDC, 2019). Immunizing older adults for pneumococcal pneumonia and influenza, combined with other health-promoting measures, can reduce morbidity and mortality.
- Symptoms of infections may be subtle or atypical among older adults. Older adults tend to have lower normal or baseline temperature, so a temperature that would typically be considered in the normal range may actually be elevated for the older adult. Common manifestations of infections in older adults include changes in behavior and mental status. Once established, infections are more likely to have a rapid course and life-threatening consequences.
- Older adults who had tuberculosis (TB) as children can experience reactivation of the disease if they become debilitated or experience a serious illness.
- The varicella zoster virus (the virus that causes chickenpox) can reactivate as shingles (herpes zoster), a painful, blistering rash that is more common in those older than age 60 years. Thus, education regarding the availability of a vaccination that may limit severe peripheral neuropathic pain should be included for all older adults.

INFECTIOUS AGENTS AND INFECTIOUS DISORDERS

Infection is the invasion of the body with pathogens or their toxins that have the potential to cause disease among susceptible individuals. Infection differs from **colonization**, a condition in which microorganisms are present, but the host does not manifest signs or symptoms of infection.

Infectious disorders can be classified in a variety of ways. **Communicable diseases** refer to those that are transmitted from one source to another. **Contagious diseases** are communicable diseases that can spread rapidly among individuals in close proximity to each other. **Community-acquired infections** are those that are not present or incubating prior to care; they may be labeled **health care–associated infections** (HAIs) when they are acquired in a health care facility.

Types of Infectious Agents

Types of infectious agents include microorganisms and prions. **Microorganisms**, commonly called *germs*, are so small they can be seen only with a microscope. Infectious microorganisms include bacteria, viruses, fungi, rickettsiae, protozoans, mycoplasmas, helminths, and prions.

Bacteria

Bacteria are single-celled microorganisms. They appear in various shapes (Fig. 12-1). Round bacteria are called *cocci* and are further classified by how they grow. Staphylococci are round bacteria that grow in clusters, streptococci are round bacteria that grow in chains, and diplococci are round bacteria that grow in pairs. Rod-shaped bacteria are called *bacilli*. Spiral-shaped bacteria are called *spirochetes*.

Bacteria may be aerobic or anaerobic. *Aerobic bacteria* require oxygen to grow and multiply, whereas *anaerobic bacteria* grow and multiply in an atmosphere that lacks oxygen.

Some bacteria, such as *Staphylococcus aureus*, *Streptococcus pneumoniae*, and *Escherichia coli*, are developing **multidrug resistance**, the ability to remain unaffected by antimicrobial drugs such as antibiotics.

Causes of antibiotic resistance, a consequence of bacterial mutations that interfere with the mechanism of antibiotic action, are related to the following:

1. Repeated and improper use of antibiotics
   - Taking antibiotics for minor or self-limiting infections
   - Taking antibacterials for viral infections
   - Not taking an entire course of prescribed antibiotics
   - Taking someone else's prescription of antibiotics
2. Lack of proper hand hygiene, causing the spread of pathogens in compromised individuals
3. Chemical pollution of the environment or provider
   - Improper disposal of antibiotics into toilets and nonhazardous trash
   - Reluctance to use personal protective equipment (PPE) during administration
4. Bacterial resistance in food animals from antibiotic overuse

Infections with multidrug-resistant microorganisms are very difficult to destroy with current pharmacologic agents, increasing the need to be vigilant about performing hand hygiene measures. The potential for death from drug-resistant infections is a major health problem.

Viruses

Viruses are so small that they can be seen only with a high-powered electron microscope. They are also filterable, meaning they pass through very small barriers. Viruses are divided into two types: (1) those whose nucleic acid is composed of DNA and (2) those whose nucleic acid is composed of RNA. Viruses use the metabolic and reproductive materials of living cells or tissues to grow and reproduce. Viruses may survive, albeit not very long, outside a living organism or host, but they cannot reproduce outside the host because they lack their own genetic components for this.

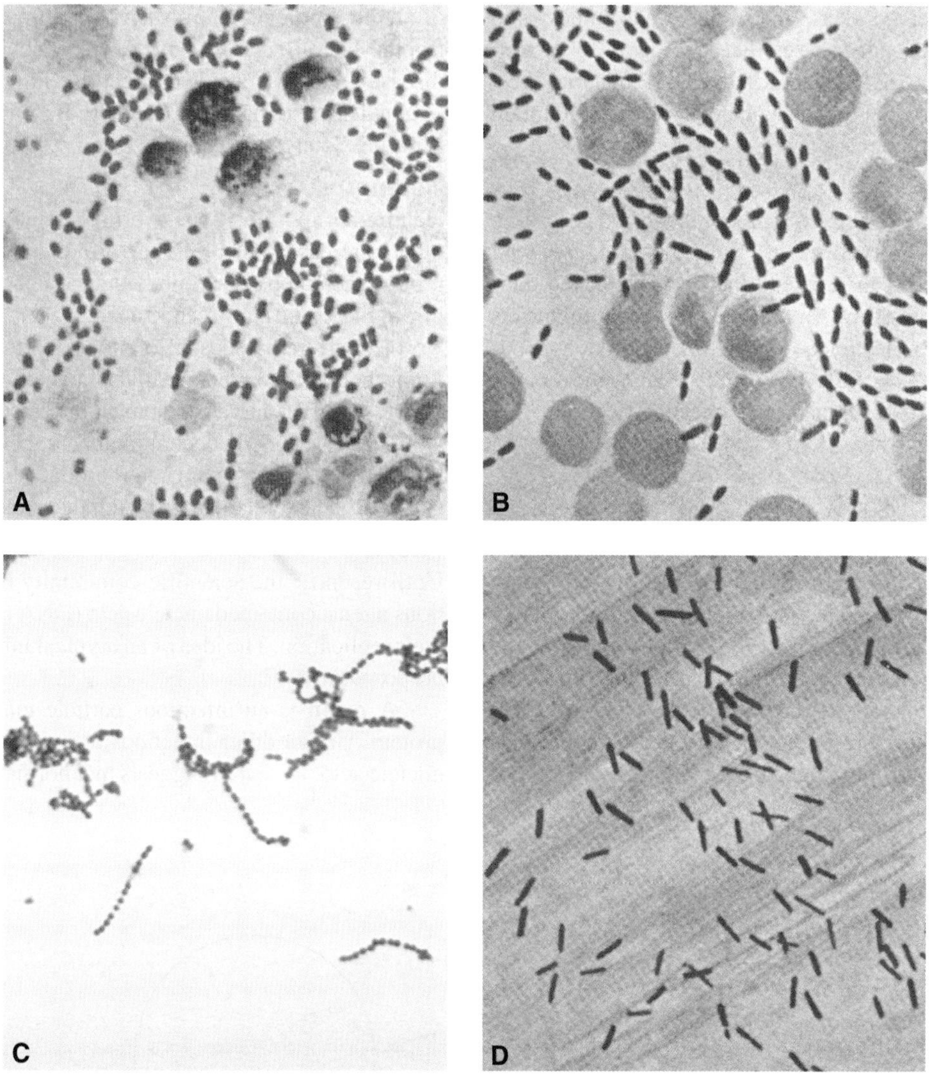

Figure 12-1 A sampling of microscopic bacteria demonstrating a variety of shapes and sizes: **(A)** bacilli known as *Yersinia pestis*, **(B)** diplococci known as *Streptococci pneumoniae*, **(C)** diplococci identified with Gram stain, **(D)** bacilli known as *Escherichia coli*. (From Public Images Library, Centers for Disease Control and Prevention. (2020). http://phil.cdc.gov.phil/home/asp)

Some viral infections, such as the common cold, are minor and *self-limiting*, that is, they terminate with or without medical treatment. Others, such as those that cause human immunodeficiency syndrome, rabies, and viral hepatitis, are more serious and may be fatal. Occasionally, viruses are dormant in a living host, reactivate periodically, and cause the infection to recur. Two examples are the herpes simplex virus, which causes periodic outbreaks of cold sores (fever blisters) long after the initial infection (see Chapter 56), and shingles in a person who has had chickenpox (see Chapter 65). The births of microcephalic infants has been linked with prenatal maternal infections from the Zika virus, which is spread by the bites from mosquitoes. Three coronaviruses, such as COVID-19, have caused worldwide spread of respiratory-based infections. This virus has caused many deaths for people with underlying medical conditions (CDC, 2020).

Fungi

Fungi are divided into two basic groups: yeasts and molds. Only a small number of fungi appear to produce diseases in humans. There are three types of fungal (mycotic) infections:

- *Superficial* (dermatophytoses), which affect the skin, hair, and nails; examples include *tinea corporis*, or ringworm, and *tinea pedis*, also known as athlete's foot (see Chapter 65)
- *Intermediate*, which chiefly affect subcutaneous tissues; an example is *candidiasis*, which affects the mucous membrane in the mouth, pharynx, or vagina (see Chapter 56)
- *Deep* (systemic), which affect internal tissues and organs; examples include pneumocystis pneumonia and histoplasmosis, both of which affect the lungs (see Chapter 35)

Rickettsiae

Rickettsiae resemble but are different from bacteria. Like viruses, they invade living cells and cannot survive outside a living organism or host. Arthropods (invertebrate animals with a segmented body; an external skeleton; and jointed, paired appendages) transmit rickettsial diseases. Examples of arthropods include fleas, ticks, lice, mosquitoes, and mites. Some rickettsial diseases that are spread by arthropods include Lyme disease (see Chapter 63), malaria, West Nile virus, eastern equine encephalitis, Rocky Mountain spotted fever, and bubonic plague.

Protozoans

Protozoans are single-celled organisms classified according to their motility (ability to move). Some possess *amoeboid motion*, meaning that they extend their cell walls and their intracellular contents flow forward. Others move by means of *cilia*, hairlike projections, or *flagella*, whiplike appendages. Still others have little or no independent movement. *Giardia* is a protozoan-transmitted intestinal disorder that results in severe diarrhea.

Mycoplasmas

Mycoplasmas are single-celled fungilike microorganisms that lack a cell wall and, therefore, are pleomorphic (assume many shapes), making them difficult to identify even with an electron microscope. They are similar to but not related to bacteria. They primarily infect the surface linings of the respiratory, genitourinary (GU), and gastrointestinal (GI) tracts. Infections can range from pneumonia to urethritis (inflammation of the urethra). Some believe that mycoplasmas are a cofactor in various other diseases, particularly those of an autoimmune nature such as multiple sclerosis, amyotrophic lateral sclerosis (ALS; also known as Lou Gehrig disease), Gulf War syndrome, chronic fatigue syndrome, and Crohn disease (Chapters 34 and 46; Baseman & Tully, 1997; Multiple Sclerosis Resource Center, 2009; Taylor, 2001).

Helminths

Helminths are infectious worms. Some are microscopic; others are easily visible. They are divided into three major groups: nematodes or roundworms, such as pinworms that infect the colon and rectum (Fig. 12-2); cestodes or tapeworms; and trematodes, also known as flukes or flatworms. Some helminths enter the body in the egg stage, whereas others spend the larval stage in an intermediate host, such as a dog, cat, or pork or beef animal, and then enter the human host. The organisms mate and reproduce in the infected host and are then excreted, after which the cycle begins again.

Prions

Until recently, the scientific community believed all infectious agents contained nucleic acid (DNA or RNA), enabling their replication. The idea of an atypical infectious agent was proposed in 1967.

A **prion** is an infectious particle made up entirely of protein. Unlike other infectious agents, it does not contain nucleic acid. Research suggests that normal prions present in

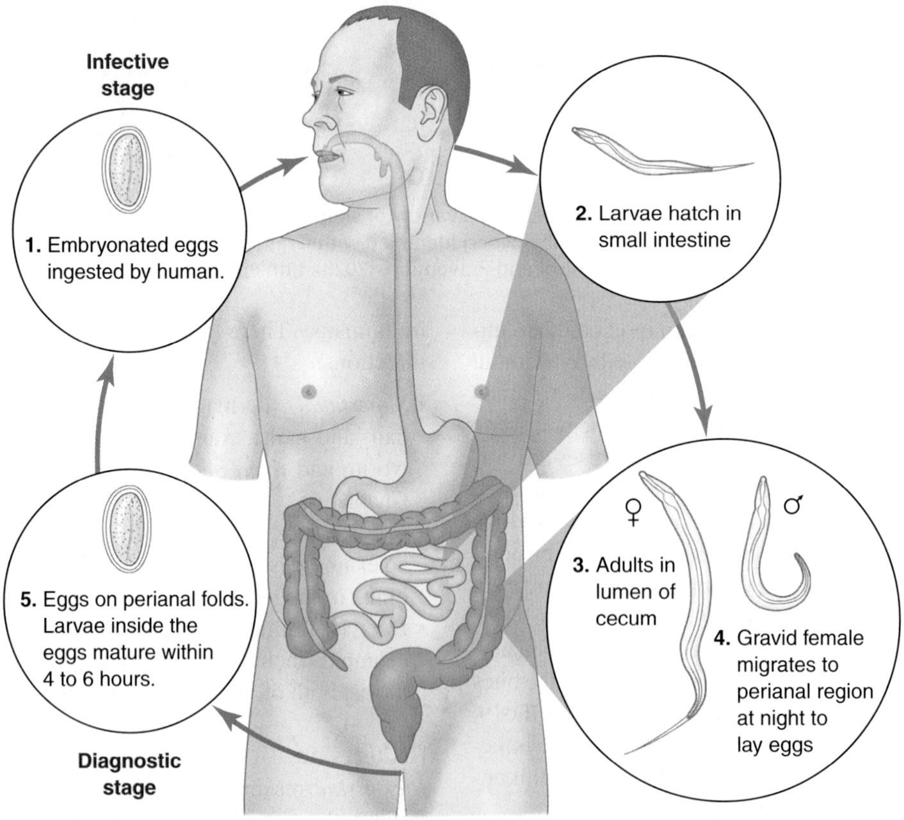

Figure 12-2 The life cycle of a pinworm infection begins (1) with hand-to-mouth transfer of pinworm eggs from a fecally contaminated environment; (2) once ingested, the eggs hatch in the small intestine of a human; (3) the eggs mature in the large intestine; (4) the mature female pinworms lay eggs in the perianal area and are shed by fecal elimination into the environment.

brain cells protect against dementia (see Chapter 72). When a prion mutates, however, it is capable of becoming an infectious agent and changing other normal prion proteins into similar mutant copies. The mutant prions, which can either be formed by genetic predisposition or acquired by transmission between the same or similar infected animal species, cause transmissible spongiform encephalopathies (TSEs). TSEs are so named because the brain becomes spongy (full of holes), the brain tissue withers, and uncoordinated movements develop in the affected person or animal. Examples of TSEs include bovine spongiform encephalopathy (BSE) or mad cow disease, scrapie in sheep, and Creutzfeldt–Jakob disease (CJD). Research conducted by the National Institute of Allergy and Infectious Diseases (2019) is ongoing to determine if mutant prions contribute to Alzheimer disease (see Chapter 72), Parkinson disease, and Huntington disease (see Chapter 37), or if clients with these disorders lack sufficient or have ineffective prions.

Mutant prions have been transmitted from sheep to cattle when cattle are fed waste parts of slaughtered infected sheep. Although one form of CJD is known to be inherited, a new variant form has developed in humans who have consumed beef infected with BSE in Europe. To prevent transmission of the new variant CJD, infected animals are destroyed, and potentially infected animal tissues are banned from human consumption. The CDC (2018) advises Americans traveling to Europe to avoid eating beef or beef products or to eat solid pieces of muscle meat from beef rather than ground meat products, which may contain tissues with infectious prions. Additionally, the American Red Cross adopted a policy placing restrictions on blood donations to prevent the potential for collecting prion-contaminated blood. The policy bans blood collection from anyone who has lived in the United Kingdom for a total of 6 months or longer between 1980 and 1996, lived in various countries in Europe including while serving in the military since 1980, received a blood transfusion in the United Kingdom, or lived 5 or more years in various European countries from 1980 to the present (Miller & Grima, 2016; Vacca, 2016).

Characteristics of Infectious Agents

Not all microorganisms and prions are dangerous. Some are **nonpathogens** because they generally are harmless to healthy humans. For example, nonpathogens in the intestine help synthesize vitamin B_{12}, biotin, vitamin K, and folic acid. **Pathogens**, on the other hand, have a high potential to cause infectious diseases. Given the right circumstances, however, both pathogens and nonpathogens can cause infections.

Once infectious agents invade the body, one of three events occurs: (1) the body's immune defense mechanisms eliminate them (see Chapter 33), (2) they reside in the body without causing disease, or (3) they cause an infection or infectious disease. Factors that influence whether a microorganism becomes a pathogen and whether an infection develops are the type of microorganism, its characteristics, and the components of the chain of infection.

TRANSMISSION OF INFECTION

The six components involved in the transmission of microorganisms are described as the **chain of infection**. All components in the chain of infection must be present to transmit an infectious disease from one human or animal to a susceptible host (Fig. 12-3): (1) infectious pathogen, (2) appropriate reservoir, (3) exit route, (4) method of transmission, (5) portal of entry, and (6) susceptible host.

Infectious Pathogen

Characteristics of the infectious pathogen that must be present include the ability to move or be moved from one place to another, **virulence** (power to produce disease), an adequate number, and the ability to invade a host.

Reservoir

A **reservoir** is the environment in which the infectious agent can survive and reproduce. It may be human, animal, or nonliving, such as contaminated food and water. A human or animal that harbors (or is the reservoir of) an infectious microorganism but does not show active evidence of infectious disease is a **carrier**. Nonliving reservoirs are **fomites**.

Portal of Exit

The **portal of exit** is the route by which the infectious agent escapes from the reservoir. Examples include the respiratory, GI, or GU tract; the skin and mucous membranes; stool; and blood and other body fluids.

Method of Transmission

A microorganism's **method of transmission** refers to how it is transferred or moved from its reservoir to the susceptible host. The five potential means of transmission are contact, droplet, airborne, vehicle, and vector (Table 12-1).

Portal of Entry

An infectious agent gains access to a susceptible host through a **portal of entry**. Some infectious agents may have only one portal of entry; others may use several. Staphylococci, for example, can cause disease by entering the respiratory tract (pneumonia), skin (boils), blood (internal abscesses), or the GI tract (food poisoning).

Susceptible Host

A **host** is the person on or in whom the infectious pathogen resides. Whether the host becomes infected depends on the host's duration of exposure to the infectious agent and the host's **susceptibility**, or ability to be compromised by or infected with disease. Unless and until a supporting host becomes weakened, microorganisms remain in check. Usually, available immunizations and natural body defenses (discussed later) protect most humans from infection.

Certain individuals are at increased risk for infection because their defenses are compromised in one or more ways. For example, older adults; premature infants; malnourished

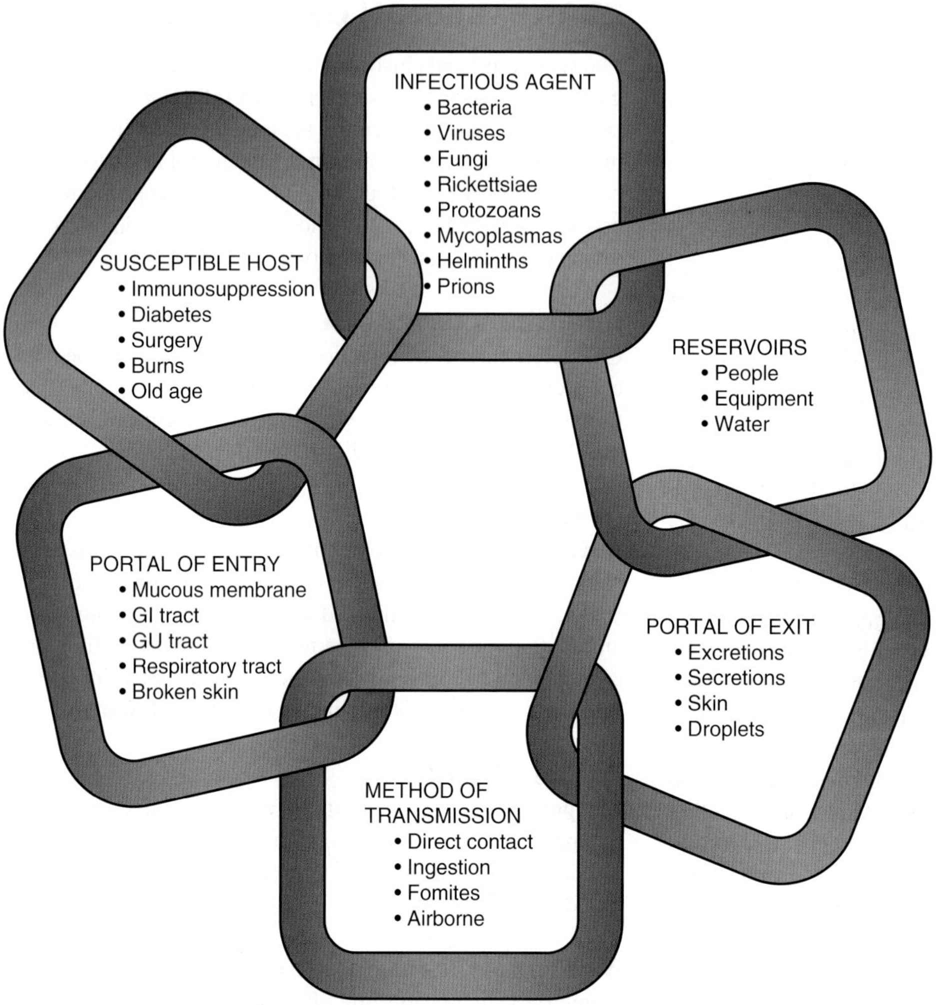

Figure 12-3 The chain of infection. GI, gastrointestinal; GU, genitourinary.

TABLE 12-1 Common Means of Transmission

ROUTE OF TRANSMISSION	DESCRIPTION	EXAMPLE
Contact		
Direct	Infected person to susceptible person	Sexual intercourse
Indirect	Contaminated substance to susceptible person	Handling a contaminated paper tissue
Droplet	Spray of moist particles within a 3-foot radius of infected person	Sneezing, coughing, talking
Airborne	Suspension and transport on air currents beyond 3 feet	Inhalation of microorganisms attached to dust particles
Vehicle	On or in contaminated food, water, objects, or equipment	Eating or drinking tainted products
Vector	Infected animal or insect to susceptible person	Transfer from bites of mosquitoes, bats, or ticks

and debilitated clients; clients receiving immunosuppressive agents such as corticosteroids and cancer chemotherapy drugs; and clients with impaired skin, bone marrow suppression, or disorders of the immune system are especially susceptible to virulent and nonvirulent strains of microorganisms.

>>> *Stop, Think, and Respond 12-1*

Identify the link in the chain of infection that each example represents:

1. *A client with cancer cannot produce sufficient blood cells after taking anticancer drugs.*
2. *A microorganism becomes especially virulent after developing resistance to multiple antibiotics.*
3. *A chef uses an unwashed counter to cut both raw chicken that contains infectious microorganisms and raw vegetables that they will incorporate into a salad.*
4. *A person with a common cold sneezes in a crowded elevator.*
5. *After a flood, raw sewage contaminates an aquifer for drinking water.*
6. *A health care provider receives a puncture from a needle used to give an injection to an HIV-positive client.*

DEFENSES AGAINST INFECTION

Humans and other animal species have both mechanical and chemical defense mechanisms to prevent infection with microorganisms. *Mechanical defense mechanisms* are physical barriers that prevent microorganisms from gaining entry or expel microorganisms before they multiply. Examples are the skin and mucous membranes, physiologic reflexes (e.g., sneezing, coughing, vomiting), and macrophages. *Chemical defense mechanisms* destroy or incapacitate microorganisms with naturally produced biologic substances. Examples include enzymes, antibodies, and secretions.

Mechanical Defenses

Skin and Mucous Membranes

The first line of defense against invading microorganisms is unbroken skin and mucous membranes, which separate underlying body tissues from environmental microorganisms. The normal flora (e.g., microorganisms) found on the skin compete with pathogens for nutrients, slowing pathogenic growth in these areas. In addition, the skin, which is acidic (because of the acetic acid in perspiration), creates an undesirable medium for pathogenic multiplication.

Mucus, a sticky substance secreted from mucous membranes, traps microorganisms and debris on its surface. For example, vaginal mucous membrane secretions favor the growth of nonpathogenic acid-producing bacteria, known as *Döderlein bacilli*. The acid environment is unfavorable for the multiplication of pathogenic bacteria and fungi. A change in vaginal pH or destruction of the normal flora, however, can promote the development of a vaginal infection (see Chapter 53).

Physiologic Reflexes

If microorganisms gain entry, sneezing, coughing, and vomiting can forcefully expel them. Coughing is promoted by cilia in the upper respiratory tract that beat upward.

Macrophages

Macrophages are specialized cells that make up the *mononuclear phagocyte* system, formerly known as the *reticuloendothelial system* (see Chapter 33). They are located throughout body tissues and in the liver (*Kupffer cells*), spleen, and lymphoid tissue (e.g., tonsils). *Polymorphonuclear leukocytes* are white blood cells (WBCs) capable of ameboid movement. Their primary function is **phagocytosis**, the ingestion of cells and foreign material, including microorganisms (Fig. 12-4).

Chemical Defenses

Enzymes

Lysozyme (e.g., muramidase), an enzyme capable of splitting (lysing) the cell wall of some Gram-positive bacteria, is present in tears, saliva, mucus, skin secretions, and some internal body fluids (e.g., gastric juices). Lysozyme is *bactericidal* (destroys bacteria) and thus defends against some pathogenic bacteria.

Antibodies

Antibodies, complex proteins also referred to as *immunoglobulins*, form when macrophages consume microorganisms and display the microorganisms' distinct cellular markers from their surfaces. Antibodies work with other WBCs by rendering microorganisms more easily ingested (phagocytized) in one of several ways: by *lysing* (dissolving or reducing size) them, *neutralizing* their *toxins* (poisons that some microorganisms release), *opsonizing* (coating) them, *agglutinating* (clumping) them, or *precipitating* (solidifying) them.

Secretions

The WBCs and other cells produce *interferon*, another chemical protein, in response to viral infections and other factors. Interferon appears to trigger infected cells to manufacture an antiviral protein. Because it also appears to inhibit cell reproduction, interferon is being used in the adjunctive

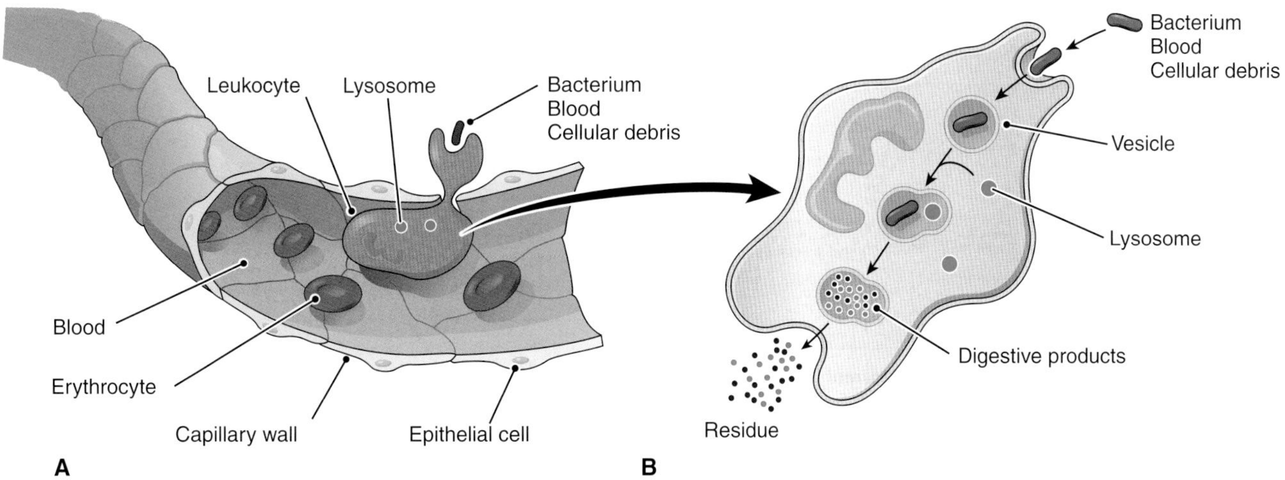

Figure 12-4 An example of the process of phagocytosis. **(A)** A phagocytic leukocyte exits through a capillary wall. **(B)** The debris is enclosed within a vesicle and digested by a lysosome. (Reprinted with permission from Donnelly-Moreno, L. A. (2020). *Timby's fundamental nursing skills and concepts* (12th ed.). Wolters Kluwer.)

treatment of some cancers and viral disorders with positive results.

PATHOPHYSIOLOGY OF INFECTION

Despite the various defense mechanisms, humans continue to succumb to infections. Regardless of the specific process, all infections share some common pathophysiologic characteristics. Most infections remain localized. Some lead to sepsis and complications such as septic shock.

Localized Infection

The initial localized reaction to an invading microorganism activates the inflammatory process (Fig. 12-5). The cellular response results in leakage of fluid, colloids, and ions from the capillaries into the tissues between the cells, producing swelling (Fig. 12-6). An ensuing vascular response produces redness and heat, whereas a chemical response causes pain. WBCs—neutrophils, macrophages, monocytes, and lymphocytes—move to the injury site to destroy the toxins produced by the pathogens and to remove debris from the area. The body manufactures more WBCs as needed, a process referred to as **leukocytosis**.

To prevent the spread of pathogens to adjacent tissues, a fibrin barrier forms around the injured area. Inside the barrier, a thick, white exudate (pus) accumulates. This collection of pus is called an *abscess*, which may break through the skin and drain or continue to enlarge internally (Fig. 12-7).

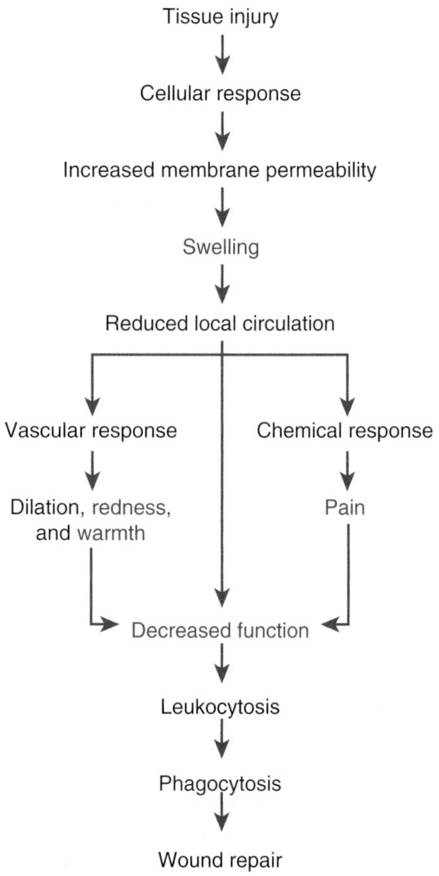

Figure 12-5 The inflammatory process.

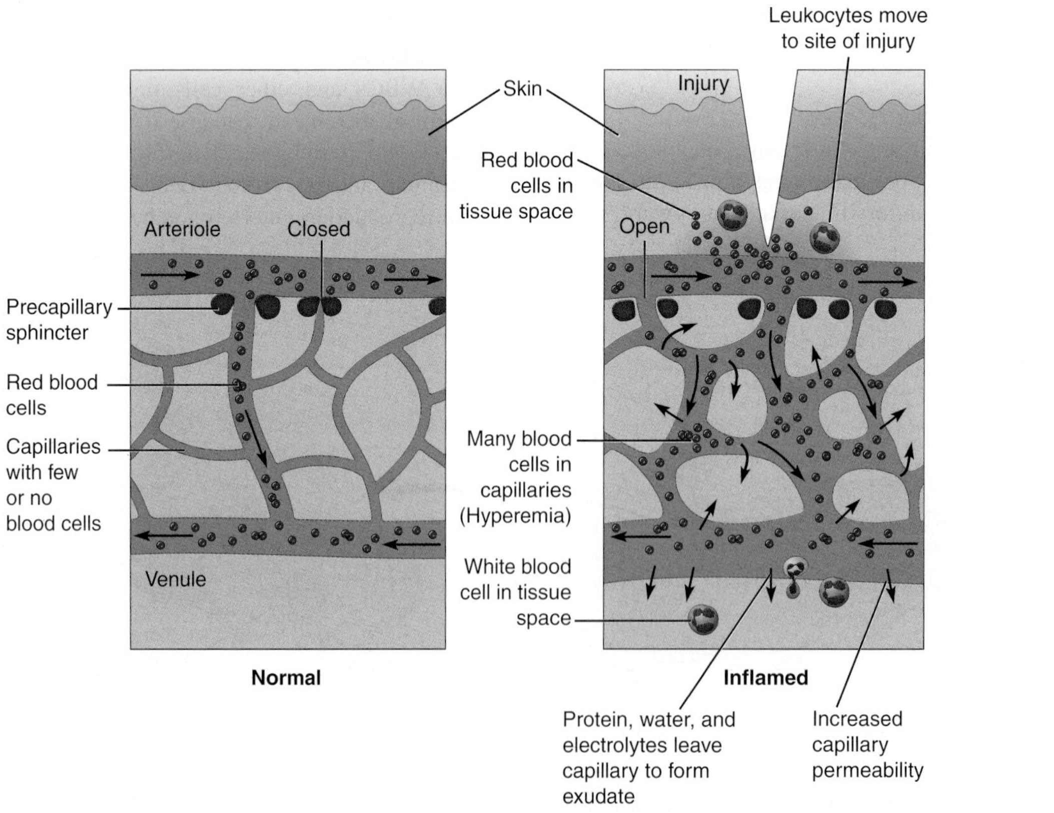

Figure 12-6 Vascular changes in acute inflammation. (Reprinted with permission from Premkumar, K. (2004). *The massage connection: Anatomy and physiology* (2nd ed.). Lippincott Williams & Wilkins.)

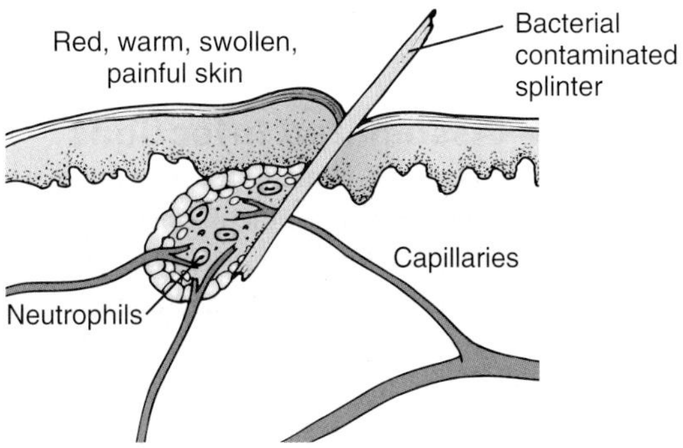

A Inflammation
Capillary dilation, fluid exudation, neutrophil migration

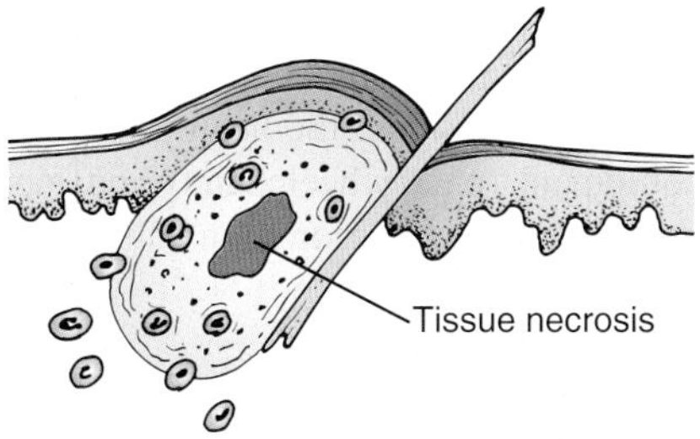

B Suppuration
Development of suppurative or purulent exudate containing degraded neutrophils and tissue debris

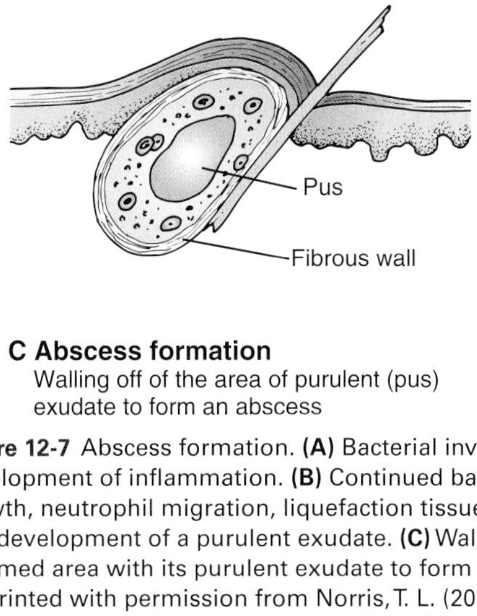

C Abscess formation
Walling off of the area of purulent (pus) exudate to form an abscess

Figure 12-7 Abscess formation. **(A)** Bacterial invasion and development of inflammation. **(B)** Continued bacterial growth, neutrophil migration, liquefaction tissue necrosis, and development of a purulent exudate. **(C)** Walling off of the inflamed area with its purulent exudate to form an abscess. (Reprinted with permission from Norris, T. L. (2019). *Porth's Pathophysiology: Concepts of altered health states* (10th ed.). Wolters Kluwer.)

Generalized Infection

If the infection becomes widespread or systemic, it is a generalized infection. Fever, which is the body's attempt to destroy the pathogen with heat, occurs in most people as an infection worsens. Exceptions may include older adults and clients who are immunocompromised; debilitated by malnutrition, chronic alcohol, or drug abuse; have kidney or liver failure; or are receiving corticosteroids or immunotherapy. These clients may have normal or low body temperature. The person with an elevated temperature feels chilled despite the fever because surface blood vessels constrict to prevent loss of body heat. Muscles may contract to produce additional heat, causing uncontrollable shivering. Sweating stops as circulation is diverted to blood vessels deep within the body. The pulse and respiratory rates rise in proportion to the fever.

When the lymph nodes become involved, they become enlarged and tender, an inflammatory condition referred to as *lymphadenitis*. If this defense mechanism cannot contain the infection, the microorganisms begin to travel from node to node (see Chapter 32). Because the lymphatic system drains into the venous system, the microorganisms may eventually reach the bloodstream, causing a condition called **bacteremia** or **septicemia**.

SEPSIS

Septicemia may lead to **sepsis**, a systemic inflammatory response syndrome resulting from infection. The pathophysiology of sepsis varies, depending on the virulence of the pathogen and condition of the host. Two or more of the following characterize sepsis:

- Temperature greater than 100.4°F (38°C) or less than 96.8°F (36°C)
- Heart rate greater than 90 beats/min
- Respiratory rate greater than 20 breaths/min or $PaCO_2$ less than 32 mm Hg (respiratory alkalosis secondary to hyperventilation)
- WBC count greater than 12,000 cells/mm^3 or 10% immature (band) forms

The body uses an inflammatory response to suppress the infectious process. Once the proinflammatory mechanisms achieve a beneficial effect, the body releases antiinflammatory mediators to restore homeostasis.

Severe Sepsis

The CDC (2020) indicates that there are over 1.5 million Americans who develop severe sepsis each year and estimates that one of three clients who die in hospitals has sepsis. Approximately 270,000 die due to sepsis each year. **Severe sepsis** is associated with organ dysfunction, hypotension, and hypoperfusion manifested by lactic acidosis, oliguria, and acute alteration in mental status. Basically, the system of proinflammatory mechanisms remains unchecked in severe sepsis. The proinflammatory response promotes coagulation of blood (microvascular clots) and suppression of fibrinolysis, the process by which clots are dissolved. Systemic microvascular clotting leads to multiple organ failure because it interferes with delivery of oxygen to cells.

Several biomarkers have been identified with determining if a client has sepsis. These biomarkers include C-reactive protein, neutrophil–lymphocyte count ratio (NLCR), and procalcitonin. The NLCR has been shown to correlate with the severity of the disease. At this time, there is not a specific individual test to determine and diagnose bacterial sepsis (Ljungström et al., 2017).

Severe sepsis remains quite lethal. Many with severe sepsis develop septic shock (see Chapter 17) and die. The main focus of treatment is to maintain and increase blood pressure with IV fluid therapy and vasopressors and administer one or more antibiotics within 3 hours after obtaining a blood culture (Rhee et al., 2020).

TYPES OF INFECTIONS

Infections can be described in terms of site (localized or generalized), source (communicable), and duration (acute or chronic/subacute). They may be further described by circumstances of infection (secondary or opportunistic). Table 12-2 explains these terms used to describe infections. The following sections discuss some of these types as well as the concern regarding emerging and reemerging infectious diseases.

Communicable Infections

Communicable infections, which are acquired in the community setting, are infectious contagious diseases, meaning that they are transmitted from one infected person or reservoir to another. Besides general systemic signs of infection (see Table 12-2), communicable diseases produce clusters of signs and symptoms that reflect dysfunction of the organs or tissues that the microorganisms have invaded. For example, a person with TB (see Chapter 21) develops a cough, lung congestion, and compromised gas exchange. A person with meningitis (see Chapter 37) develops a stiff neck, headache, arching of the back, and possibly seizures.

Health Care–Associated Infections

HAIs are infections acquired while receiving care in a health care agency that were not active, incubatory, or chronic at admission. They occur for many reasons. Hospitalized clients are more susceptible to infections than well people because they are exposed to pathogens in the health care environment, may have incisions or invasive equipment (e.g., IV lines) that compromise skin integrity, or may be immunosuppressed from poor nutrition, their disease process, or its treatment. Also, because health care providers are in frequent and direct contact with many clients who harbor various microorganisms, the risk for transmitting pathogenic microorganisms between and among clients is high. Visitors also may introduce pathogens into the health care environment, as may equipment (e.g., wheelchairs) and facilities shared among several people (e.g., common bathrooms).

Opportunistic Infections

In **opportunistic infections**, also called **superinfections**, nonpathogenic or remotely pathogenic microorganisms take advantage of favorable situations and overwhelm the host. For example, a prescribed antibiotic sometimes can upset biologic checks and balances. Although the antibiotic destroys

TABLE 12-2 Types of Infections

TYPE	DESCRIPTION	COMMON SIGNS AND SYMPTOMS	EXAMPLES
Localized	Confined to a small area	Pain, redness, warmth, swelling, collection of fluid that may be purulent, swollen lymph nodes, and leukocytosis	Furuncle (boil)
Generalized	Systemic or widespread in one or more organs	Fever, chills, shivering, rapid pulse and respirations, hypotension (see discussion of septic shock in Chapter 17), headache, fatigue, anorexia, and marked leukocytosis	Urosepsis
Communicable	Transmitted from one infected species to another	Same as generalized plus organ-specific or disease-specific manifestations (e.g., rash with chickenpox, diarrhea with dysentery)	Influenza, chickenpox, tuberculosis
Health care–associated	Acquired in a health care agency and not present before admission	Same as localized and generalized plus additional manifestations depending on the infected tissue	Methicillin-resistant *Staphylococcus aureus* (MRSA) infection
Acute	Sudden onset with serious and sometimes life-threatening manifestations	Symptoms appear suddenly	Appendicitis, an inflammation of the appendix secondary to a localized infection (see Chapter 46)
Chronic or subacute	An extended infection that resists treatment		Bacterial endocarditis, an inflammation of the inner muscle layer of the heart (see Chapter 24)
Secondary	A complication of some other disease process that occurred first		Infection in a person who has experienced severe burns
Opportunistic or super infections	Occur among immunocompromised hosts		Yeast infections in the mouth, bladder infections, gastroenteritis, and *Pneumocystis carinii* pneumonia (see Chapter 35)

one pathogen, other pathogens that the antibiotic does not affect grow and proliferate. Usually, however, common pathogens cause infections. Opportunistic infections commonly occur among immunocompromised clients.

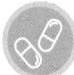

Pharmacologic Considerations

- The most common superinfections during antibiotic treatment are fungal and bacterial.
- Candidiasis is a common type of fungal superinfection that commonly occurs throughout the GI and reproductive systems. Symptoms include lesions of the mouth or tongue, vaginal discharge, and anal or vaginal itching.
- Overgrowth of the bacterium *Clostridium difficile (C. diff)* in the bowel can lead to a serious inflammation called *pseudomembranous colitis* (Fig. 12-8). Signs and symptoms include severe diarrhea with visible blood and mucus, fever, and abdominal cramps. These symptoms usually require immediate discontinuation of the antibiotic.

Emerging and Reemerging Infectious Diseases

Currently, there is concern about emerging and reemerging infectious diseases. **Emerging infectious diseases** are disorders caused by microorganisms that are new or by the evolution of existing organisms. Some examples include West Nile viral encephalopathy, avian influenza (bird flu), Lyme disease, Ebola hemorrhagic fever, and hantavirus pulmonary syndrome, severe acute respiratory syndrome (SARS), all of which are transmitted by **zoonotic pathogens** that are spread from microorganisms to animals and then to humans. **Reemerging infectious diseases** are caused by previously known pathogens that have developed genetic variations, recombinations, and adaptations forming new strains of older microorganisms. Examples of recent reemergent diseases include TB, malaria, and influenza. Infectious diseases for which there has been nonadherence to routine immunizations through vaccinations for measles, pertussis (whooping cough), and polio are also categorized as reemergent infections.

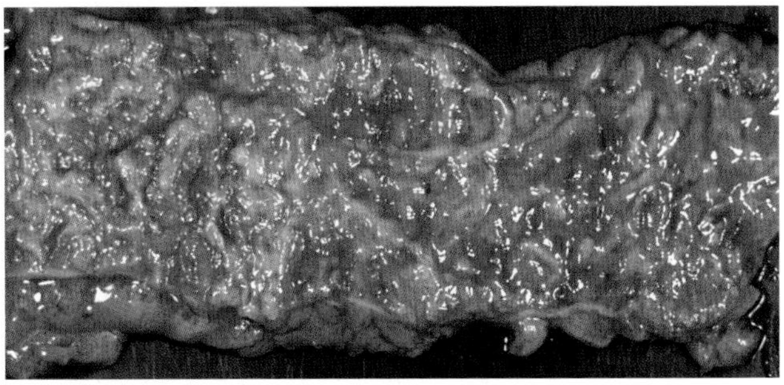

Figure 12-8 When pseudomembranous colitis develops, the colon becomes acutely inflamed with a surface covering of plaques containing necrotic tissue debris and exudates. (Reprinted with permission from Rubin, E., & Reisner, H. M. (2014). *Essentials of Rubin's pathology* (6th ed.). Wolters Kluwer Health/Lippincott Williams & Wilkins.)

Collectively, emerging and reemerging infectious diseases are spreading because of (1) mutations among existing organisms, (2) increased world travel, (3) ecologic changes in human and animal habitats, (4) antimicrobial resistance, (5) worldwide transport of animals and food products for human use, and (6) disregard for available vaccinations. If unchecked, emerging and reemerging infectious diseases may cause **epidemics**, widespread infections in a confined geographic area, or a **pandemic**, an infectious disorder that spreads to many different parts of the world in a relatively short period of time.

INFECTION CONTROL AND PREVENTION

Precautions and Asepsis

Nurses and other health care providers must take precautions to control infections when caring for all clients, regardless of diagnosis or infection status. These precautions are called **standard precautions**, measures for reducing the risk of transmitting pathogens from both recognized and unrecognized sources of infection (Box 12-1). Health care providers also must apply principles of medical asepsis, such as hand hygiene using an alcohol-based sanitizer or hand washing with soap and water (Nursing Guidelines 12-1). Hand hygiene is performed:

- When arriving at and leaving work
- Before and after contact with each client
- Before and after handling equipment
- Before and after gloving
- Before and after collecting specimens
- Before preparing medications
- After administering medications

For clients known to be or suspected of being infected with highly transmissible pathogens, nurses and other health care providers must also follow **transmission-based precautions** (Table 12-3, also Evidence-Based Practice 12-1). Because these precautions may isolate a client, it is important to consider the client's decreased social contact and lack of environmental stimulation. This isolation may increase confusion in older adults.

Prevention and Control of Health Care–Associated and Community-Acquired Infections

In addition to standard and transmission-based precautions and principles of medical asepsis, recommendations from the health care agency's infection control committee provide further guidance to prevent and control HAIs. Such committees usually consist of representatives from various areas and departments, such as medical staff, nursing service, clinical laboratories, pathology, operating room, housekeeping, and dietary service. Their responsibilities include conducting *surveillance;* the process of detecting, reporting, and recording HAIs; educating health care providers about methods to reduce HAIs; providing guidelines for prevention of infectious diseases; and investigating outbreaks of HAIs. Infection

BOX 12-1 Standard Precautions

- Wear clean gloves when touching:
  - Blood, body fluids, secretions, excretions, and items containing these body substances
  - Mucous membranes
  - Nonintact skin
- Perform hand washing immediately:
  - When there is direct contact with blood, body fluids, secretions, excretions, and contaminated items
  - After removing gloves
  - Between client contacts
- Wear a mask, eye protection, and face shield during procedures and client care activities that are likely to generate splashes or sprays of blood, body fluids, secretions, and excretions.
- Wear a cover gown during procedures and client care activities that are likely to generate splashes or sprays of blood, body fluids, secretions, or excretions or cause soiling of clothing.
- Remove soiled protective items promptly when the potential for contact with reservoirs of pathogens is no longer present.
- Clean and reprocess all equipment before reuse by another client.
- Discard all single-use items promptly in appropriate containers that prevent contact with blood, body fluids, secretions, and excretions; contamination of clothing; and transfer of microorganisms to other clients, health care workers, and the environment.
- Handle, transport, and process linens soiled with blood, body fluids, secretions, and excretions in such a way as to prevent skin and mucous membrane exposures; contamination of clothing; or transfer to other clients, health care workers, and the environment.
- Prevent injuries with used needles, scalpels, and other sharp devices by:
  - Never removing, recapping, bending, or breaking used needles
  - Never pointing the needle toward a body part
  - Using a one-handed "scoop" method, special syringes with a retractable protective guard or shield for enclosing a needle, or blunt-point needles
  - Depositing disposable and reusable syringes and needles in puncture-resistant containers
- Use a private room or consult with an infection control professional for the care of clients who contaminate the environment, or who cannot or do not assist with appropriate hygiene or environmental cleanliness measures.
- Use respiratory hygiene and cough etiquette.
  - Cover the mouth/nose with a tissue or use an upper sleeve or elbow when coughing or sneezing; dispose of used tissues promptly, followed by hand hygiene.
  - Have a client who is coughing use a surgical mask at the first point of encounter.
  - Distance persons with respiratory symptoms at least 3 feet from others in common waiting areas.
- Follow safe injection practices to prevent hepatitis B virus (HBV) and hepatitis C virus (HCV).
  - Use a sterile, single-use, disposable syringe for each injection.
  - Use single-dose vials rather than multidose vials of medication when administering to multiple clients.
- Special lumbar puncture procedure:
  - Provide a mask for the person performing the procedure to prevent respiratory transmission of the microorganism causing bacterial meningitis as well as other protective apparel.

NURSING GUIDELINES 12-1

Performing Hand Antisepsis and Hand Washing

- Use an alcohol-based hand-rubbing sanitizer containing 60% to 95% ethanol or isopropanol for hand antisepsis unless the hands are grossly contaminated. Alcohol-based hand rubs are the most efficacious agents for reducing the number of bacteria on the hands (CDC, 2020).
- Apply a dime-size amount of hand sanitizer onto the palm of one hand.
- Rub the hands together covering all surfaces of hands and fingers until dry (usually 15 seconds or less).
- For hand washing, lather the palms, back of hands, between fingers, and under nails with soap and water.
- Scrub for at least 20 seconds—the time it takes to hum "Happy Birthday" from beginning to end twice.
- Rinse soap from the wrists toward the fingers using running water. Directing the flow of rinse water toward the fingers avoids transferring microorganisms to cleaner skin areas.
- Use a paper towel to turn off a hand-operated faucet to avoid recontamination of the hands.

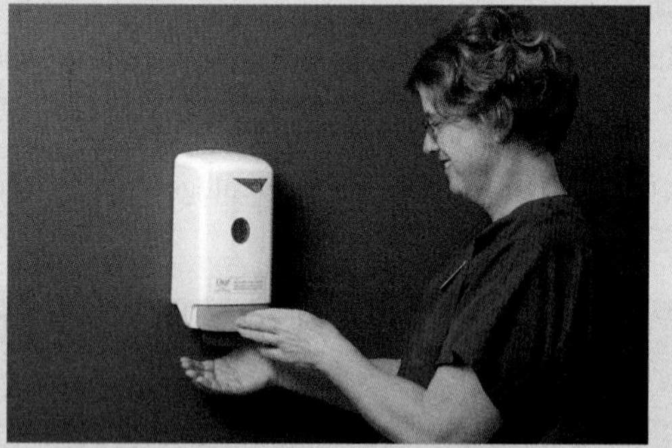

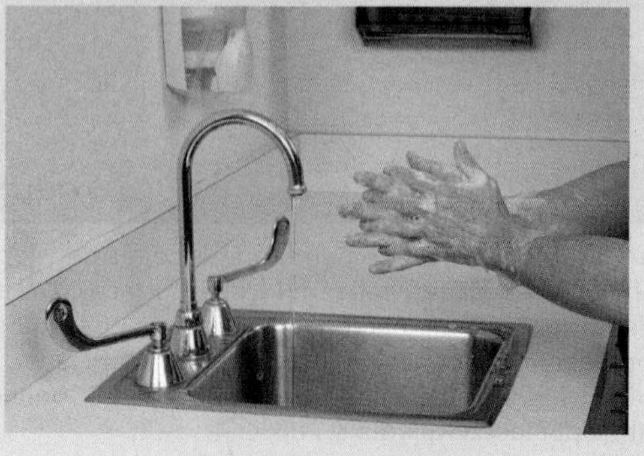

From Centers for Disease Control and Prevention. (2020). *Healthcare providers: Clean hands count for healthcare providers*. https://www.cdc.gov/handhygiene/providers/index.html

TABLE 12-3 Transmission-Based Precautions

TYPE OF PRECAUTION	LOCATION	PROTECTION	EXAMPLES OF DISEASES
Airborne	Private room Negative air pressure[a] Room air is discharged to environment or filtered before being circulated	Follow standard precautions. Wear a mask for airborne pathogens or particulate air filter respirator in the case of TB. Place a mask on the client if transport is required.	TB Measles Chickenpox
Droplet	Private room, or in a room with similarly infected client(s) or one with at least 3 feet between the client and other client(s) or visitors	Follow standard precautions. Wear a mask when entering the room, especially when within 3 feet of the infected client. Place a mask on the client if transport is required.	Influenza Rubella Streptococcal pneumonia Meningococcal meningitis SARS-associated coronavirus (SARS-CoV) Coronavirus (COVID-19)
Contact	Private room or in a room with similarly infected client(s), or consult with an infection control professional if the above options are not available	Follow standard precautions. Put on gloves before entering the room. Remove gloves before leaving the room. Change gloves after contact with infective material. Perform hand washing with an antimicrobial agent immediately after removing gloves. Wear a gown when entering the room if your clothing could touch the client or items in the room, or if the client is incontinent, has diarrhea, an ileostomy, or a colostomy, or wound drainage not contained by a dressing. Clean bedside equipment and client care items daily. Avoid transporting the client, but, if required, use precautions that minimize transmission. Clean bedside equipment and client care items daily. Use items such as a stethoscope, sphygmomanometer, and other assessment tools exclusively for the infected client and terminally disinfect them when precautions are no longer necessary.	Drug-resistant GI, respiratory, skin, or wound infections Acute diarrhea Draining abscess

GI, gastrointestinal; TB, tuberculosis.
[a]Negative air pressure pulls air from the hall into the room when the door is opened, as opposed to positive air pressure, which pulls room air into the hall.
From Centers for Disease Control and Prevention. (2019). *2007 Guideline for isolation precautions: Preventing transmission of infectious agents in healthcare settings.* https://www.cdc.gov/infectioncontrol/guidelines/isolation/index.html

Evidence-Based Practice 12-1

Health Care–Associated Infections

Clinical Question

Do nurses contribute to health care–associated infections?

Evidence

Infections that clients acquire while being treated in a health care facility are considered health care–associated infections (HAIs). The Centers for Disease Control and Prevention (CDC) estimate that each day approximately 1 in 31 clients acquires an HAI. The CDC concludes that when all members of a health care team in a facility are aware of the statistics and aid in prevention, the infection rate of HAIs can be reduced up to approximately 70% (CDC, 2019). One of the proposed goals of *Healthy People 2030* is to "Reduce hospital-onset Clostridioides difficile infections and Reduce hospital-onset MRSA bacteremia" in HAIs (*HealthyPeople.Gov,* 2020). *Healthy People 2030* continues with research to show that education and prevention are key to reduction in infections and that prevention is also best practice.

Nursing Implications

Nurses are part of the health care team both in acute care and the community setting. HAIs can occur in either setting and client safety is at risk. Nurses should update and maintain education and practice in infection control to align themselves with best practice and national guidelines.

References

Centers for Disease Control and Prevention. (2019). *HAI data and statistics.* https://www.cdc.gov/hai/data/portal/progress-report.html
HealthyPeople.Gov. (2020). *Health care associated infections.* https://www.healthypeople.gov/2020/About-Healthy-People/Development-Healthy-People-2030

control guidelines usually establish policies for preemployment and postemployment health examinations, sterilization procedures and methods, disposal of garbage and biologic wastes, and housekeeping techniques; designate precautions to follow for specific infections; and define procedures for managing contaminated materials such as linens, equipment, and supplies used in the care of infectious clients.

Many communicable infections have been contained or eliminated because of advances in the prevention and treatment of infectious diseases. These advances include the discovery and use of antibiotics, the development of immunizing agents, guidelines for the proper disposal of human wastes, legislation controlling the preparation and sale of foods, immunization programs, and public education. Local, state, and federal public health agencies and the World Health Organization (WHO) cooperate in the detection and control of communicable diseases. Their combined efforts have reduced the incidence of many infectious diseases and virtually eliminated others (e.g., smallpox). To help prevent and control community-acquired infections, nurses encourage childhood and adult **immunizations**, vaccines that stimulate the body to produce antibodies against a specific disease organism. (Recommended immunization schedules are available on the CDC website at www.cdc.gov/vaccines/) Apathy, religious beliefs, unfounded fear that certain immunizations will cause illness or disorders such as autism, or inability to afford health care, however, can pose potential barriers to obtaining immunizations. Immunizations protect all people—children as well as adults who may not have developed sufficient immunity.

Additional nursing measures to prevent infection transmission include the following:

- Wear a clean uniform, preferably donned in the place of employment. The United Kingdom nationwide and many facilities in the United States have policies in place that have nurses put on a clean uniform upon arriving at work and change before going home. In keeping with a "bare below the elbows" policy, uniforms with short sleeves are also advised to be worn to reduce nosocomial infections because they facilitate adequate hand hygiene (Bearman et al., 2018)
- Do not wear hand or arm jewelry.
- Avoid artificial nails and keep natural nails short and free of chipped nail polish.
- Remain home when ill.
- Advise sick visitors to refrain from contact with the client.
- Protect immunosuppressed clients from pathogens.
- Educate clients and families about ways to prevent infections at home (Client and Family Teaching 12-1).

>>> *Stop, Think, and Respond 12-2*

Nearly 2 million clients in U.S. hospitals develop HAIs because health care providers of all disciplines consistently fail to adhere to adequate hand hygiene practices. What are some reasons that health care providers are lax in this basic method of preventing infection?

Client and Family Teaching 12-1
Reducing Infections

To reduce potential infections, the nurse teaches the following measures:

- Perform frequent hand washing, especially before eating, after using the toilet, and after contact with nasal secretions.
- Bathe and perform other personal hygiene (e.g., oral care) daily.
- Keep the home environment clean; household bleach diluted 1:10 or 1:100 is an excellent disinfectant.
- Keep immunizations current. Tetanus vaccine is recommended every 10 years, influenza vaccine is repeated yearly, and one dose of pneumococcal pneumonia vaccine lasts a lifetime. The Advisory Committee on Immunization Practices (ACIP) recommends a two-dose subcutaneous injection of zoster (shingles) vaccine for adults aged 50 years or older (CDC, 2020).
- Investigate the need for vaccinations, water purification techniques, and foods to avoid when traveling outside the United States.
- Eat the recommended proportions of fruit, vegetable, grains, protein, and dairy from MyPlate, and use safe food-handling practices.
- Use and immediately discard disposable paper tissues rather than reuse cloth handkerchiefs.
- Avoid sharing washcloths, drinking cups, and other personal care items.
- Follow safe sex practices.
- Stay home from work or school when ill rather than expose others to infectious pathogens.
- Avoid crowds and public places during local outbreaks of influenza.
- Follow posted infection control instructions when visiting hospitalized family members and friends.
- Understand that antibiotic therapy is not appropriate for every infectious disease, but when it is, take the full dose for the prescribed period.

Prevention of Infection from Needlestick Injuries

One of the greatest threats to health care providers is the potential for acquiring blood-borne infectious diseases such as hepatitis B virus (HBV) infection and AIDS. Following standard precautions reduces but does not eliminate this risk because gloves are not impervious to penetration by sharp objects (e.g., needles) that may contain blood. Despite following policies and precautions for avoiding blood-borne pathogens and using new needleless access devices on IV lines, needlestick injuries continue to occur.

Should a needlestick injury or other exposure to a potential blood-borne pathogen occur, health care providers are advised to follow postexposure recommendations:

- Report the injury or exposure to one's supervisor immediately.

- Document the injury in writing.
- Identify the person or source of blood, if possible.
- Obtain the HIV and HBV statuses of the source of blood if it is legal to do so. Unless the client gives permission, testing and revealing HIV status are prohibited.
- Obtain counseling on the potential for infection.
- Receive the most appropriate postexposure prophylaxis.
- Be tested for disease antibodies at appropriate intervals.
- Receive instructions on monitoring potential symptoms and medical follow-up.

CARE OF THE CLIENT WITH INFECTION

Signs and Symptoms

Signs and symptoms vary depending on whether the infection remains localized, becomes generalized, or develops into sepsis (see Table 12-2). Manifestations for specific infections are discussed in relevant chapters in this text. Regardless of the type of infection, however, the infection process follows a similar course (Table 12-4).

Diagnostic Tests

A thorough history and physical examination are essential for the diagnosis of an infectious disease. Diagnosis of some infectious diseases, however, requires additional tests and laboratory examinations to identify the microorganism.

White Blood Cell Count and Differential

Elevation in the number and type of WBCs, especially polymorphonuclear (PMN) leukocytes such as neutrophils, whose main function is phagocytosis, indicates an inflammatory and possibly infectious process. Although a total WBC count provides important information, a differential—one that indicates the percentage of WBC subtypes—is even more valuable. Elevated neutrophils, the largest subtype of WBCs, indicate that the body is in the early stages of responding to an invading pathogen. As the number of neutrophils becomes depleted, bone marrow produces additional cells called *band cells* (bands) that eventually mature and replace them. Elevated monocytes, the largest-sized subtype of WBCs, are the body's second line of defense.

Culture and Sensitivity Test

A **culture** identifies bacteria in a specimen taken from a person with symptoms of an infection. The source of the specimen may be body fluids or wastes, such as blood, sputum, urine, or feces, or the *purulent exudate*, collection of pus, from an open wound. The specimen is cultured, which involves placing a small amount of it in or on a special growth medium (Fig. 12-9). The specimen is incubated for a specific period (usually 48–72 hours) and then examined microscopically. To facilitate examination, it is stained or dyed (colored). One stain is the Gram stain. Those bacteria that absorb the color of the stain are classified as *Gram positive*; those that do not are classified as *Gram negative*. A coagulase test also may be used to test the microorganisms for pathogenicity or virulence. When a culture is reported as *coagulase positive*, it is more virulent than a culture of the same microorganism that produces a negative (*coagulase negative*) response.

Sensitivity studies are done to determine which antibiotic(s) inhibits the growth of a nonviral microorganism and will be most effective in treating the infection.

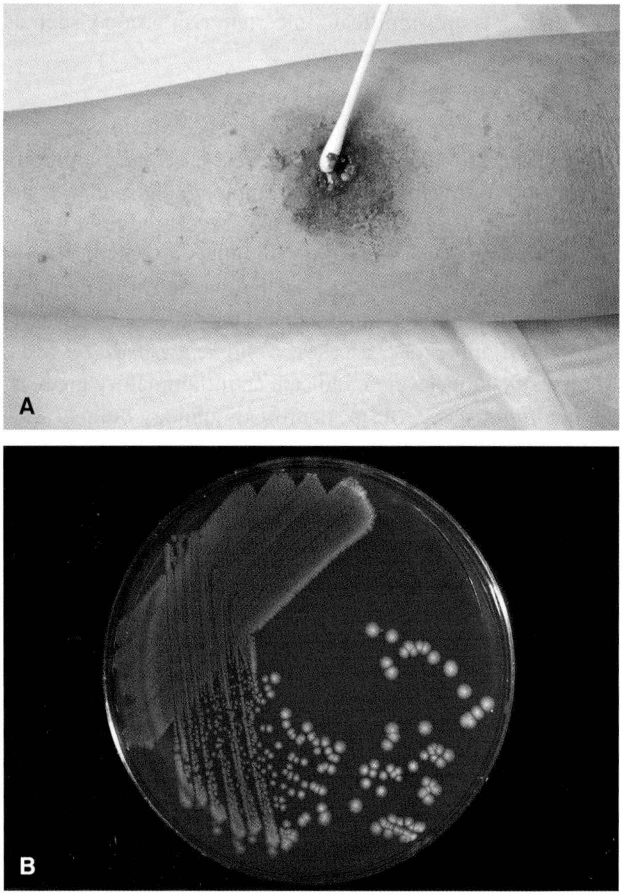

Figure 12-9 Bacterial culture. **(A)** A sterile culture swab is inserted in a wound to obtain a sample of exudates. **(B)** Variability of the macroscopic appearance of bacteria cultured on solid, agar-containing medium. (Part B, reprinted with permission from Porth, C. M. (2007). *Essentials of pathophysiology: Concepts of altered health states* (2nd ed.). Wolters Kluwer Health/Lippincott Williams & Wilkins.)

TABLE 12-4 The Course of an Infectious Disease

STAGE	CHARACTERISTIC
Incubation period	The infectious agent reproduces. The host displays no recognizable symptoms; however, the infectious agent may exit the host at this time and infect others.
Prodromal stage	Initial symptoms appear; they may be vague and nonspecific. Possible symptoms include mild fever, headache, and loss of usual energy.
Acute stage	Symptoms become severe and specific to the affected tissue or organ. For example, tuberculosis is manifested by respiratory symptoms.
Convalescent stage	Symptoms subside as the host overcomes the infectious agent.
Resolution	The pathogen is destroyed. Health improves or is restored.

Examination for Ova and Parasites

Most ova (eggs) and parasites (those that live at the expense of the host) are intestinal worms. Therefore, the client's stool is examined for evidence of any forms in the infecting microorganism's life cycle. Usually, three separate random samples of stool are collected from a bedpan, not the toilet. Urine and toilet paper may alter the specimen and therefore must be disposed of separately. Clients suspected of having intestinal ova and parasites should perform scrupulous hand washing to avoid reinfecting themselves and others.

Skin Tests

Skin testing determines the presence of a specific active or inactive infection. Diseases for which skin testing may be done include histoplasmosis, mumps, TB, diphtheria, and coccidioidomycosis. The material for skin testing is injected intradermally. The reaction is read after a specified period (usually 48–72 hours). The size of the *induration* (hard, elevated tissue), not including the surrounding area of *erythema* (redness), is measured in millimeters. The measurement determines whether the reaction is significant. For example, a tuberculin skin test is considered positive if the induration (hardened area) is 10 mm or greater in persons with no known risk factors for TB (see Chapter 21); smaller measurements are significant in certain risk groups, such as immunocompromised clients.

Immunologic Tests

Immunologic tests determine the presence of *antigen* (substances that stimulate an immune response) and antibody reactions (see Chapter 33). For example, *agglutination* tests, such as the cold agglutinins test, may reveal the presence of high antibody titers confirming immunity to rubella (measles). *Precipitation tests*, such as the C-reactive protein test and erythrocyte sedimentation rate, produce elevated rates in some inflammatory diseases. *Complement fixation* tests, when results are elevated, indicate an inflammatory process. *Immunofluorescence* tests identify immunoglobulins, antibodies formed by the immune system.

Other Tests

Depending on the disease, other diagnostic tests may be used. Radiography (plain films or contrast studies), computed tomography (CT) scanning, and magnetic resonance imaging (MRI) may be used to locate abscesses, identify displacement of organs or structures that may indicate abscess formation, and detect changes in tissues in areas such as the bones or lungs.

Medical Management

In some cases, supportive therapy such as rest, fluids, adequate nutrition, and antipyretics (e.g., aspirin or acetaminophen [Tylenol]) for a significantly elevated fever may be advised while the infectious disease runs its course. If the etiology is responsive to drug therapy, antimicrobials (e.g., antibiotics, sulfonamides, antiviral drugs) are prescribed.

Infected wounds may be *debrided*, a process of removing dead and damaged tissue. Wound irrigations, hydrotherapy (whirlpool), and application of wet-to-dry dressings may accomplish the same objective.

Treatment of a primary condition may relieve the infectious process. Bone marrow transplantation or administration of drugs that boost WBC production, such as filgrastim (Neupogen), may help immunosuppressed clients.

Pharmacologic Considerations

- Nausea, vomiting, anorexia, and diarrhea are common adverse effects of antibiotic treatment as well as symptoms of infection. Accurate assessment and thorough client teaching will help distinguish between symptoms related to the infectious disease and those possibly caused by antibiotic therapy. Be sure outpatient instructions include taking antibiotics as directed and for the full course of the prescription.

Nursing Management

Nursing management for the client with a potential or actual infection focuses on preventing or controlling the transmission of infection among clients, visitors, and health care workers and preventing complications. Some nursing actions include the following:

- Maintaining the client's skin integrity
- Monitoring vital signs, especially temperature and pulse rate
- Promoting adequate nutrition and hydration
- Regulating blood sugar within normal limits; sugar supports the growth of microorganisms
- Inspecting the client's body for signs of redness, swelling, and purulent drainage
- Reviewing WBC counts from laboratory test results and reporting elevations above normal
- Obtaining cultures and transmitting them immediately to the laboratory
- Keeping fresh wounds intact and covered for 24 to 48 hours
- Following aseptic principles when changing dressings
- Disposal of soiled substances in a waterproof container
- Administering antimicrobial drugs as prescribed
- Promoting urination to avoid catheterization
- Encouraging coughing and deep breathing to clear secretions from the airways
- Following transmission-based precautions

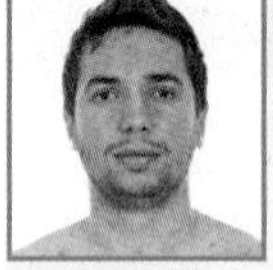

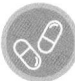

Clinical Scenario A client is being seen in the health clinic for a rash that appears as itchy blisters covering the abdomen, face, and scalp. Some lesions have formed crusts. He also reports feeling tired and has not had any appetite. The client recalls having had contact with a friend who recently developed shingles. The client does not remember ever having had chickenpox as a child. The tentative diagnosis is that the client's rash is an adult form of chickenpox as a result of acquiring the herpes zoster virus. The client will remain at home until all lesions have formed crusts and there are no new outbreaks of lesions. **What nursing actions are needed in caring for this client? See the following Nursing Process section.**

NURSING PROCESS FOR THE CLIENT WITH A POTENTIAL OR ACTUAL INFECTION

Assessment

Obtain the client's history, paying particular attention to information that might suggest exposure to someone with an infectious illness or other reservoirs of infection, immunization status, recent travel to a foreign country, treatment with antimicrobial or immunosuppressive drugs, and current medical disorders. Weigh the client to gain information about nutritional status and measure vital signs to detect temperature, heart and respiratory rates, and blood pressure. A head-to-toe physical assessment helps detect manifestations of an inflammatory response, impaired skin, and evidence of unusual drainage. Questioning about feelings of lassitude (tiredness) and anorexia is important. After preparing the client for diagnostic tests and collecting specimens, monitor the results of the laboratory findings and observe the response to skin tests.

Analysis, Planning, and Interventions

Implement measures to prevent or interrupt components of the chain of infection. Examples include supporting nutrition and hydration, maintaining intact skin and mucous membranes, and following aseptic principles. Administer prescribed drug therapy and observe for evidence of improvement. Also, implement measures that promote comfort (e.g., reducing fever).

Analysis, expected outcomes, and interventions for the client described previously include the following:

Impaired Comfort: Related to itching
Expected Outcome: The client will experience relief from distressful itching.

- Recommend applying cool compresses, an ice pack, or a cold gel pack to lesions. *Cooling the surface of the skin reduces blood flow to cutaneous peripheral nerves, inhibiting the sensory transmission of itching.*
- Suggest soaking in a cool water bath with baking soda or colloidal oatmeal for 20 minutes every 3 to 4 hours as needed. *Baking soda is an alkaline substance that soothes the discomfort of itching; colloidal oatmeal is an emollient that moisturizes skin and reduces dryness that contributes to itching.*
- Remind the client to pat rather than rub the skin dry. *Patting preserves skin integrity. Rubbing stimulates the cutaneous nerves, which may perpetuate itching.*
- Advise the client to trim fingernails short. *Scratching contributes to the itch–scratch–itch cycle; trimming the fingernails reduces the potential for trauma to the skin.*
- Explain that following label directions for an over-the-counter topical antihistamine such as Caladryl, a combination of calamine and diphenhydramine (Benadryl), or an oral antihistamine such as diphenhydramine (Benadryl), loratadine (Claritin), or cetirizine (Zyrtec) is a treatment option. *Antihistamines compete with histamine receptors to relieve itching.*

Infection Risk: Related to exposure to susceptible contacts
Expected Outcome: The client's infection will be limited to this solitary case.

- Restrict direct contact with anyone who has not been immunized for chickenpox or had chickenpox as a child. *A pathogen that remains infectious over a long distance when suspended in the air has the potential for being transmitted to susceptible persons via direct contact to an uncrusted lesion or via inhalation.*
- Explain that it is necessary to remain homebound until all lesions have dried and formed crusts. *Chickenpox is contagious from 1 to 2 days before the rash appears and until all blisters have formed scabs.*
- Inform the client that should it become necessary to see the primary provider, they should call ahead and understand that the primary provider will need to take certain precautions, such as isolation in a separate area with the door closed and the use of a mask. *Chickenpox is transmitted by direct contact and by inhalation of airborne secretions.*
- Follow hand antisepsis and hand hygiene guidelines (see Nursing Guidelines 12-1). *Hand hygiene remains the single most important measure to prevent the spread of infection. It reduces the number of transient and resident microorganisms.*
- Advise the client to avoid touching any areas of impaired skin. Hands contain microorganisms that clients can transfer to tissue and blood vessels beneath impaired skin.
- Recommend nutritious supplements if appetite is suppressed (Nutrition Notes). *Sufficient intake helps restore biologic defense mechanisms (e.g., adequate WBCs, wound healing).*
- Follow label directions for self-application of a prescribed topical antimicrobial. *Antimicrobials reduce microorganisms at the site of impaired skin.*
- Monitor for signs of superinfection: diarrhea, vaginal discharge, and inflammation of oral mucous membranes. *Drug therapy or a debilitated state may cause microorganisms to overgrow elsewhere in the body.*

Altered Skin Integrity Risk

Expected Outcomes: The nurse will monitor for, manage, and minimize complications of chickenpox.

- Inform the client and family member to report a fever over 101°F, purulent drainage from one or more lesions, change in mental status, decreased urination, rapid or labored breathing. *Secondary bacterial infections can be sequelae of chickenpox.*
- Follow transmission-based precautions (see Table 12-3) if symptoms of complications develop. *They interfere with the ways a particular pathogen is spread.*
- Administer antimicrobials as prescribed. *Systemic antimicrobial therapy may be necessary to prevent, control, and eliminate an infection.*
- Report worsening of client's condition and signs of organ dysfunction to the primary provider. *Severe sepsis may lead to septic shock and death.*

(*continued*)

NURSING PROCESS FOR THE CLIENT WITH A POTENTIAL OR ACTUAL INFECTION (continued)

Evaluation of Expected Outcomes

Expected outcomes include a WBC count below 10,000 cells/mm^3, body temperature less than 99°F, no purulent drainage from impaired skin, wound culture free of virulent pathogens, and no signs of superinfection. Changes in vital signs, mental status, and leukocyte count are detected early. The infection resolves and no complications occur.

Nutrition Notes

The Client With Infection

- Malnutrition is the main cause of a suppressed immune system; ensuring that older adults are well nourished and that they maintain their body weight is one of the best ways to protect their aging immune systems.
- Fever is a major determinant of caloric needs during infection. Basal metabolic rate (BMR) increases 7% for each degree Fahrenheit that the temperature is above normal. For instance, the BMR for a person with a temperature of 103.6°F is increased 35% (5°F above normal × 7% = 35% increase). This translates into an extra 350 to 700 calories needed per day based on an average BMR of 1000 to 2000 calories/day.
- Protein needs can increase to 1.5 to 2.0 g/kg of body weight for severe infections (normal protein requirement is 0.8 g/kg). Milk, milk drinks, and commercial supplements may be used to add significant proteins and calories.
- Fluid needs depend on the severity of fever and any complicating factors (e.g., diarrhea, vomiting, excessive sweating). Encourage the intake of ice water, broth, fruit juices, milk, popsicles, and gelatin. Clients should avoid tea, coffee, and carbonated beverages containing caffeine, which promote diuresis.
- Acutely ill clients may accept and tolerate a full liquid diet with in-between–meal supplements better than solid food. Advance the diet as tolerated to maximize intake.
- For clients who require transmission-based precautions, meals are served on disposable dinnerware. The tray is made as attractive as possible to encourage eating. Uneaten food is disposed of in the toilet, and plastic containers are deposited in sealed bags before removal.

From Sandrock, C. E., & Albertson, T. E. (2010). *Controversies in the treatment of sepsis. Seminars in Respiratory and Critical Care Medicine, 31(1): 66–78.* https://doi.org/10.1055/s-0029-1246290

KEY POINTS

- Infectious diseases: Spread by pathogens or toxins among susceptible individuals
- Communicable diseases: Transmitted from one source to another by infectious bacteria or viral organisms
- Contagious diseases: Communicable diseases that can spread rapidly among individuals in close proximity to each other.
- Community-acquired infections: Those that are not present or incubating prior to care provided by health care providers.
- HCAIs: Acquired within health care facilities
- Types of infectious agents: All can cause illness but must be treated based on type:
  - Bacteria
  - Viruses
  - Fungi
  - Rickettsiae
  - Protozoan
  - Mycoplasmas
  - Helminths
  - Prions
- Transmission of infection: The sequence that enables the spread of disease-producing microorganisms that must be in place if pathogens are to be transmitted from one location or person to another.
  - An infectious agent
  - A reservoir for growth and reproduction
  - An exit route from the reservoir
  - A means of transmission
  - A portal of entry
  - A susceptible host
- Defenses against infection: Humans have these defenses to help prevent infection.
  - Mechanical defenses: physical barriers that prevent microorganisms from gaining entry or expel them before they multiply
    - Skin and mucus membranes
    - Physiologic reflexes
    - Macrophages
  - Chemical defenses: destroy or incapacitate microorganisms with naturally produced biologic substances
    - Enzymes
    - Antibodies
    - Secretions
- Infections can be localized or generalized; severe infections can lead to sepsis.
  - Types of infections:
    - Communicable
    - Health care–associated
    - Opportunistic
    - Emerging and reemerging infectious diseases
- Infection control and prevention: ways to reduce or prevent infections
  - Precautions and asepsis
  - Prevention and control of health care–associated and community-acquired infections
  - Prevention of infection from needlestick injuries

- Care of the client with infection:
  - Determine the signs of symptoms being presented
  - Understand which diagnostic tests should be performed
  - Understand the needed medical management for specific cases
  - Provide appropriate nursing management

CRITICAL THINKING EXERCISES

1. Use the chain of infection illustrated in Figure 12-3 to trace the viral transmission of a common cold from one person to another.
2. Give a specific example of how pathogens are spread among clients and health care workers and then identify techniques for preventing their transmission.
3. Select any community-acquired infection and identify the type of microorganism that causes it and its usual reservoir, portal of exit, means of transmission, and portal of entry.
4. Develop a list of suggestions for improving hand hygiene practices in health care agencies.

NCLEX-STYLE REVIEW QUESTIONS PrepU

1. When monitoring a client with an infection, what signs correlate with the development of sepsis? Select all that apply.
   1. Blood pressure of 90/60 mm Hg
   2. Tympanic temperature of 102°F (38.9°C)
   3. Apical heart rate of 110 beats/min
   4. Respiratory rate of 28 breaths/min
   5. Vesicular breath sounds in lung periphery
   6. WBC count of 22,000 cells/mm^3
2. The client tells the nurse that the doctor identified a HAI affecting the bladder and kidneys. Which of the following statements provides the best explanation of a HAI for the client?
   1. "Your infection is affecting more than one organ and may become widespread."
   2. "Your infection is related to the wound infection you came in with."
   3. "This infection is confined to your urinary system."
   4. "This infection was acquired while you were hospitalized."
3. A client with TB is in a private room on a medical unit. A diagnosis of TB requires the use of airborne precautions. What personal protection equipment must the nurse wear when caring for this client?
   1. Face mask
   2. Isolation gown
   3. Particulate air filter respirator
   4. Nonsterile gloves
4. What health care measure is best for preventing all types of infections?
   1. Cover the mouth and nose when coughing or sneezing.
   2. Keep immunizations updated throughout life.
   3. Perform hand hygiene before and after contact with clients.
   4. Implement infection control policies for contagious diseases.
5. When changing a sterile dressing, what nursing action violates the principles of surgical asepsis?
   1. The nurse cleans the wound from the outer edge toward the center.
   2. The nurse puts on clean gloves to remove the soiled dressing.
   3. The nurse performs hand washing before putting on sterile gloves.
   4. The nurse places the soiled dressing in a moisture-resistant bag.

WANT TO KNOW MORE? There are a wide variety of online resources available on thePoint to enhance learning and understanding of this chapter.

Go to **thePoint.lww.com/activate** and use the activation code found in the front of this text to unlock these online resources.

13 Intravenous Therapy

Words To Know

ABO system
albumin
blood products
blood substitute
central venous sites
coagulopathies
colloid solutions
cryoprecipitate
crystalloid solutions
drop factors
drop size
electronic infusion device
emulsion
hypertonic solution
hypotonic solution
infusion pump
in-line filter
intravenous (IV) therapy
isotonic solution
macrodrip tubing
medication lock
microdrip tubing
midline catheter
oxygen therapeutics
packed cells
peripheral venous sites
phlebitis
plasma
plasma expanders
platelets
pressure infusion sleeve
primary tubing
Rh factor
salvaged blood
secondary tubing
thrombus formation
total parenteral nutrition (TPN)
universal donors
universal recipients
unvented tubing
venipuncture
vented tubing
volumetric controller
whole blood
Y-administration tubing

Learning Objectives

On completion of this chapter, you will be able to:

1. Explain common indications for intravenous (IV) therapy.
2. Differentiate between crystalloid and colloid solutions and give examples of each.
3. Describe the difference between isotonic, hypotonic, and hypertonic solutions.
4. Explain the difference between whole blood, packed cells, blood products, and plasma expanders.
5. Describe nursing responsibilities for preparing IV solutions, selecting tubing, and selecting an infusion technique.
6. Identify nursing responsibilities when preparing the client for IV therapy.
7. Describe nursing actions involved in performing a venipuncture, including sites and devices commonly used.
8. Explain the equipment that must be replaced during IV therapy.
9. List complications of IV therapy and signs and symptoms for which the nurse monitors.
10. Explain how the nurse discontinues IV therapy.
11. Discuss the purpose of a medication lock.
12. Describe the nursing process for the client requiring IV therapy.
13. Discuss the purpose of total parenteral nutrition, and name one solution often administered concurrently.
14. Explain special considerations for blood transfusion therapy, including the equipment used, blood compatibility, and complications.

Intravenous (IV) therapy is the parenteral administration of fluids and additives into a vein. State nurse practice acts specify the qualifications for licensed practical/vocational nurses who can administer or participate in IV therapy; only nurses who meet these qualifications and receive appropriate training can administer this particular therapy. All registered nurses can administer IV therapy. IV administration demands skillful administration techniques, close observation of the client, and nursing considerations, all of which are discussed in this chapter.

INDICATIONS FOR INTRAVENOUS THERAPY

IV therapy is used to maintain or restore fluid balance when oral replacement is inadequate or impossible, to maintain or replace electrolytes, to administer water-soluble vitamins, to administer drugs, to provide a source of calories and nutrients, and to replace blood and blood products.

Gerontological Considerations

- Rigidity of veins and poor skin turgor may make venipuncture in the older client more difficult. To avoid skin trauma, place a soft cloth or material between the skin and tourniquet. Use of a tourniquet may not be necessary prior to venipuncture because the veins may already be sufficiently distended and easily visualized. Use of a tourniquet may further increase venous distention and venous pressure to a point that the vein ruptures when pierced, causing a hematoma, blood within the skin, or gross bleeding from the puncture site.
- Monitor responses to IV infusions closely since the older adult may be unable to tolerate the same volumes or rates of infusion as younger adults, especially if respiratory, cardiac, or renal disorders are present.
- Older adults, especially those with chronic conditions, are at risk for fluid overload and electrolyte imbalances; observe for signs and symptoms such as alteration in cognitive function or heart rhythm, weight gain, and shortness of breath.
- Observe confused or disoriented clients frequently, as excessive movement or pulling on the IV tubing may dislodge the venipuncture device.
- Transfusion is common in older adults and may be anticipated in those who smoke; have low body mass index; and a history of anemia, cancer, diabetes mellitus, end-stage renal disease, or heart disease (Burney, Ahmad, & Masroor, 2016).

IV therapy may be used to administer medications, because drugs given by the IV route have a more rapid effect than other routes of administration. Only drugs labeled for IV use are given by this route. Administering a drug IV may be indicated in the following circumstances:

- A rapid drug effect is required.
- Oral intake is restricted.
- A client cannot swallow.
- Gastrointestinal absorption is impaired.
- A continuous therapeutic blood level is desired.

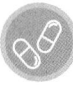

Pharmacologic Considerations

- Most drugs added to an IV solution are done so by clinical pharmacists. If a medication is added on the unit by a nurse, the solution container should be labeled with the name and dose of the drug, the date and time, and the name of the nurse who added the drug.

IV therapy designed to meet nearly all the caloric and nutritional needs of a client is called **total parenteral nutrition (TPN)**. Clients who are severely malnourished or cannot consume food or liquids for a long time may require TPN. Special considerations for administering IV therapy for TPN and blood transfusions are discussed later in this chapter.

TYPES OF INTRAVENOUS SOLUTIONS

The two types of IV solutions are crystalloid and colloid solutions. **Crystalloid solutions** consist of water and uniformly dissolved crystals such as salt (sodium chloride) or sugar (glucose, dextrose; Fig. 13-1). **Colloid solutions** consist of water and molecules of suspended (undissolved) substances such as blood cells and blood products.

Crystalloid Solutions

Crystalloid solutions are divided into isotonic, hypotonic, and hypertonic solutions (Table 13-1). These terms refer to the concentration of dissolved substances in relation to the plasma into which they are instilled. When crystalloid solutions are administered to clients, the concentration influences the osmotic distribution of body fluid (Fig. 13-2).

Isotonic Solutions

An **isotonic solution** contains the same concentration of dissolved substances as is normally found in plasma. Isotonic solutions are administered to maintain fluid balance when clients temporarily cannot eat or drink. Because of its equal concentration to plasma, an isotonic solution causes no appreciable redistribution of body fluid on administration.

Hypotonic Solutions

A **hypotonic solution** contains fewer dissolved substances compared with plasma. Hypotonic solutions effectively rehydrate clients experiencing fluid deficits; therefore, they are administered to clients experiencing fluid losses in excess of fluid intake, such as those who have diarrhea or are vomiting. Because a hypotonic solution is dilute, the water in the solution passes through the semipermeable membrane of blood cells, causing them to swell. This swelling can temporarily increase blood pressure (BP) because it expands the circulating volume. The water also may pass through capillary walls and become distributed in other body cells and interstitial spaces.

Hypertonic Solutions

A **hypertonic solution** is more concentrated (contains more dissolved substances) than body fluid. Consequently, it draws fluid into the intravascular compartment from the

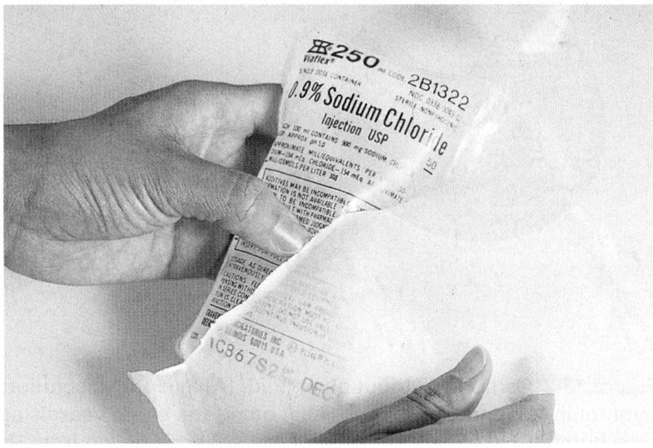

Figure 13-1 Crystalloid solution. (Photo by B. Proud.)

TABLE 13-1 Types of Crystalloid Solutions

SOLUTION	COMPONENTS	SPECIAL COMMENTS
Isotonic Solutions		
0.9% saline, also called normal saline (NS)	0.9 g sodium chloride/100 mL water	Contains sodium and chloride in amounts physiologically equal to those in plasma
5% dextrose in water, also called D_5W	5 g dextrose (glucose/sugar)/100 mL water	Isotonic when infused, but the glucose is metabolized quickly, leaving a solution of dilute water
Ringer's solution or lactated Ringer's	Water and a mixture of sodium, chloride, calcium, potassium, bicarbonate, and, in some cases, lactate	Replaces electrolytes in amounts similarly found in plasma; lactate, when present, helps maintain acid–base balance
Hypotonic Solutions		
0.45% sodium chloride, also called half-strength saline	0.45 g sodium chloride/100 mL water	Contains a smaller proportion of sodium and chloride than found in plasma, causing it to be less concentrated in comparison
5% dextrose in 0.45% saline	5 g dextrose and 0.45 g sodium chloride/100 mL water	The sugar provides a quick source of energy, leaving a hypotonic salt solution
Hypertonic Solutions		
10% dextrose in water, also called $D_{10}W$	10 g dextrose/100 mL water	Contains twice the concentration of glucose found in plasma
3% saline	3 g sodium chloride/100 mL water	The high concentration of salt in the plasma dehydrates cells and tissue
20% dextrose in water	20 g dextrose/100 mL water	Rapidly increases the concentration of sugar in the blood, causing a fluid shift to the intravascular compartment

more dilute areas in the cells and interstitial spaces. Hypertonic solutions are used infrequently, except when it is necessary to reduce cerebral (brain) edema, expand circulatory volume rapidly, administer nutrition parenterally, or treat severe hyponatremia (low serum sodium).

Colloid Solutions

Colloid solutions are used to replace circulating blood volume because the suspended molecules in the solutions pull fluid from other fluid compartments in the body. Examples include blood (whole blood and packed cells), blood products such as albumin, and solutions known as plasma expanders.

Blood

Whole blood and packed cells probably are the most commonly administered colloid solutions. One unit of **whole blood** (Fig. 13-3) contains approximately 475 mL of blood cells and plasma, with 60 to 70 mL of preservative and anticoagulant added. Whole blood is administered when clients need fluid restoration as well as blood cells. **Packed cells** have most of the plasma (fluid) removed, resulting in an average volume of 285 to 300 mL. Packed cells are preferred for clients who need cellular replacements but do not need and may be harmed by the administration of additional fluid. Such clients include those who have an adequate oral intake of fluid and clients at risk for heart failure (see Chapter 28).

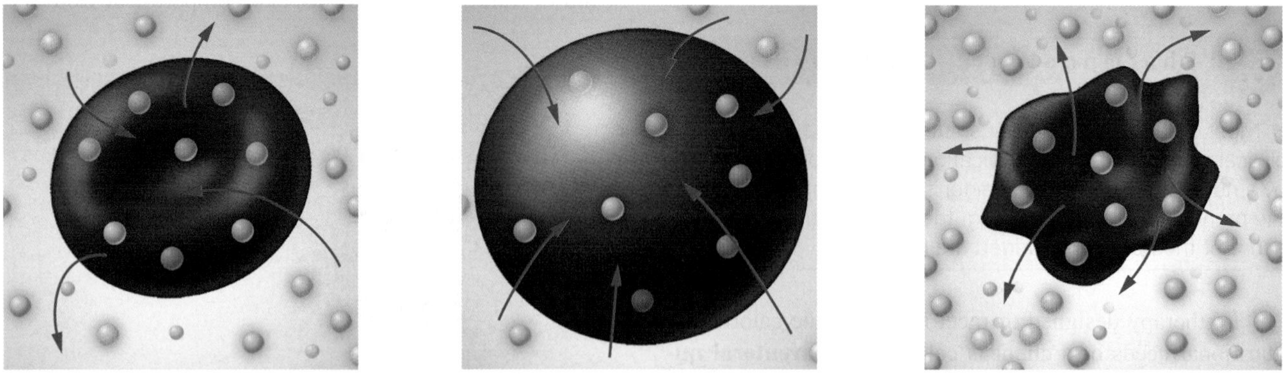

A B C

Figure 13-2 Osmotic distribution of fluid. **(A)** In isotonic solutions, cells maintain normal size because of fluid balance. **(B)** In hypotonic solutions, body fluids shift out of the blood vessels and into the cells and the interstitial space. The cells fill with fluid and may burst. **(C)** In hypertonic solutions, the fluid is pulled from the cells and the interstitial tissues into the vascular space. (Adapted from McConnell, T. H., & Hull, K. L. (2011). *Human form, human function.* Lippincott Williams & Wilkins.)

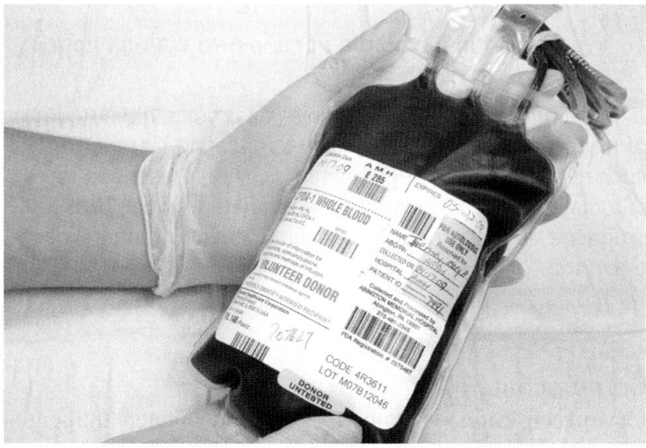

Figure 13-3 Unit of whole blood.

Blood transfusion, equipment, blood compatibility, and complications are discussed later in this chapter.

Blood Products

Several types of solutions contain **blood products**, components extracted from blood, such as fresh-frozen plasma (FFP), albumin, platelets, granulocytes, and cryoprecipitate (Table 13-2). Blood products are administered to clients who need specific blood substances but not all the fluid and cellular components in whole blood.

Fresh-Frozen Plasma

Plasma is the liquid noncellular component of blood. It contains nutrients; hormones; enzymes; plasma proteins such as albumin, globulin, and fibrinogen; and especially, all known coagulation factors. Plasma is separated from blood cells within 8 hours after collection and subsequently frozen. Frozen plasma is used primarily to manage **coagulopathies**, clotting disorders of various types, and control or eliminate hemorrhage caused by an overdose of anticoagulants. However, when the specific clotting factor is known or an antidote for the anticoagulant is available and the client is not in immediate danger, it is more efficacious to administer more definitive treatment rather than use a generalized approach. Although reactions are rare, FFP should be typed and crossmatched for compatibility (see "Blood Compatibility" discussed later in this chapter).

Pharmacologic Considerations

- Protamine should only be used as a heparin neutralization or reversal (Boer et al., 2018). Instead, Octaplas—a pooled plasma product—is being used in liver disease or transplant and cardiac surgery where coagulation problems arise.

Albumin

Albumin is a large plasma protein that does not normally move across semipermeable membranes like those in capillaries. Consequently, it plays a major role in maintaining blood volume. In other words, its presence attracts fluid to the intravascular space, a function described as providing *colloidal osmotic pressure*. When a person experiences hypoalbuminemia, colloidal osmotic pressure decreases, which results in movement of intravascular fluid into extravascular areas, evidenced by peripheral edema in the limbs, organ edema, or cavity effusion such as ascites (see Chapter 47).

Human albumin is isolated from pooled human plasma and administered to restore fluid balance in intracellular and extracellular compartments. It is supplied in strengths of 5% or 25% in 50- or 100-mL glass containers with special tubing for administration. A container of albumin must be hung at least 3 feet higher than the client's heart and infused through a large-lumen needle or catheter to achieve an infusion within 30 to 60 minutes. The client must be monitored during and after the infusion to detect hypervolemia as extravascular fluid is pulled into the intervascular space. Sometimes, the primary provider may order a diuretic by the IV route to avoid fluid volume overload.

Platelets

Platelets, also known as thrombocytes, are cell-like structures within blood that aggregate (clump together) and release chemicals that produce fibrin at the site of an injury (Fig. 13-4). Together with clotting factors, platelets play a role in hemostasis (clotting).

Platelets intended for transfusion are derived from the whole blood of pooled or single donors from which platelets have been isolated. Collected platelets are stored at

TABLE 13-2 Types of Blood Products

BLOOD PRODUCT	DESCRIPTION	PURPOSE FOR ADMINISTRATION
Platelets	Disk-shaped cellular fragments that promote coagulation of blood	Restores or improves the ability to control bleeding
Granulocytes	Types of WBCs	Improves the ability to overcome infection
Plasma	Serum without blood cells	Replaces clotting factors or increases intravascular fluid volume by increasing colloidal osmotic pressure
Albumin	Plasma protein	Pulls third-spaced fluid by increasing colloidal osmotic pressure
Cryoprecipitate	Mixture of clotting factors	Treats blood-clotting disorders such as hemophilia

WBC, white blood cell.

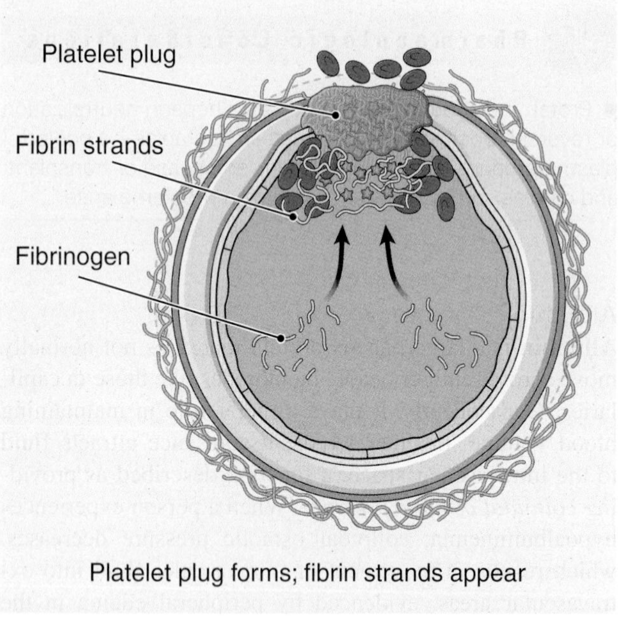

Figure 13-4 Platelets and strands of fibrin accumulate at the site of an injury to form a temporary plug to control bleeding. (Reprinted with permission from McConnell, T. H. (2014). *The nature of disease: Pathology for the health professions* (2nd ed.). Wolters Kluwer Health/Lippincott Williams & Wilkins.)

room temperature for no more than 5 days. Candidates for platelet transfusion are those whose platelet count, which normally is 150,000 to 450,000/mm^3, falls below 10,000 to 20,000/mm^3. One unit of 100 mL is infused IV over 15 to 30 minutes through a Y-set containing a filter that is primed with normal saline. As many as 6 units may be combined in one container. Each unit is expected to raise the platelet count by 10,000/mm^3 within an hour after administration. Preferably, platelet donors and recipients should be of compatible blood cell and Rh types to avoid potential reactions and *platelet refractoriness*, a less than effective response. Clients are monitored for minor febrile or possibly severe allergic reactions that may occur during or up to an hour after an infusion.

Granulocytes

Granulocytes are white blood cells (WBCs), also known as polymorphonuclear leukocytes, specifically neutrophils, eosinophils, and basophils. Neutrophils are the major type of blood cells that defend against infection. Consequently, a person with a low granulocyte or neutrophil count is highly susceptible to succumbing to a life-threatening infection.

Granulocytes are separated from whole blood and must be transfused within 48 hours of collection. Clients such as those who are undergoing stem cell transplantation or those for whom aggressive drug therapy to treat infection and neutropenia (low neutrophil count) are unsuccessful may be given one 400-mL unit of granulocytes per day through standard Y-set tubing with normal saline until an acceptable granulocyte count is achieved. Vital signs are assessed every 15 minutes during the infusion.

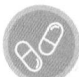

Pharmacologic Considerations

- In situations when neutropenia is a predictable outcome of treatment, granulocyte colony-stimulating factors (G-CSF) such as filgrastim or pegfilgrastim may be prescribed to stimulate bone marrow production of neutrophils. These drugs are used to support recovery from neutropenia, not prevent it.

Cryoprecipitate

Cryoprecipitate, also known as cryoprecipitated antihemophilic factor, is an acellular blood component that contains fibrinogen and multiple clotting factors. Its name is derived from the fact that it is prepared by thawing FFP and recovering the cold, insoluble precipitate. The precipitate is then refrozen within 1 hour.

Cryoprecipitate is given for actual or potential bleeding disorders (1) when the specific clotting factor, for example, factor VIII, is unavailable; (2) following cardiac surgery to clients experiencing hemodilution, hypothermia, or acidosis; or (3) to clients who require massive blood transfusions.

After thawing, the cryoprecipitate is diluted with normal saline and transfused as soon as possible or at least within 4 to 6 hours. Preferably, the donor and recipient should have compatible blood types. Each unit of cryoprecipitate contains 15 mL; the usual dose is 1 unit per 7 to 10 kg of body weight. Up to 10 units may be required and administered at a rate of 10 mL/minute (American Red Cross, 2016).

Blood Substitutes

A **blood substitute** is an experimental fluid **emulsion**, a mixture of two liquids, one of which is insoluble but remains dispersed in the other. When transfused, a blood substitute carries and distributes oxygen to cells, tissues, and organs. Many practitioners feel that blood substitutes should be more accurately called **oxygen therapeutics** because they do not replace all the functions of human blood.

Currently, oxygen therapeutics fall into two categories: *perfluorocarbons* (PFCs) and *hemoglobin-based oxygen carriers* (HBOCs). PFCs are solutions containing fluorine and carbon that have the potential to carry 50 times more oxygen than plasma. HBOCs are derived from three sources: (1) hemoglobin harvested from outdated human blood, (2) hemoglobin from bovine (cattle) blood, and (3) cultured bacteria in which the gene for human hemoglobin is inserted (recombinant technology), much like the production of human insulin.

PFCs are now in the second generation of development; first-generation PFCs have been placed on hold or abandoned because of safety issues. Hemopure is an HBOC that has been approved by the Food and Drug Administration (FDA) to use as a blood alternative.

Many believe that once blood substitutes are safer and approved for use, their value will lie in reducing exclusive reliance on stored human blood that has a limited shelf life and as an option in managing life-threatening situations when blood is needed but nothing else is available. Although clinical trials continue, there are current concerns about the safety of artificial blood substitutes that continue to delay their approval.

Plasma Expanders

Plasma expanders are nonblood, polysaccharide colloid solutions derived from beet sugar or corn starch. Examples include dextran 70, 6% (Macrodex); dextran 40, 10% (Rheomacrodex); and hetastarch 6% (Hespan). Plasma expanders pull fluid into the vascular space more effectively than hypertonic crystalloid solutions. They are used as an economical and virus-free substitute for blood and blood products when treating clients with hypovolemic shock. However, they can affect coagulation and cause renal toxicity, intravascular fluid overload, and allergic reactions.

ADMINISTERING INTRAVENOUS THERAPY

CONCEPTS IN ACTION

Selecting and Preparing Equipment

Equipment commonly used when administering IV therapy includes the solution, IV tubing, and an IV pole or infusion device. A fluid warmer may be used to raise the temperature of parenteral solutions when it is beneficial to ensure stable body temperature. The nurse selects and prepares the fluid that will be administered, chooses appropriate tubing, and decides on an infusion technique.

Preparing Intravenous Solutions

Crystalloid solutions are stored in plastic bags containing volumes of 1000, 500, 250, 100, and 50 mL. Only a few solutions are in glass containers. The primary provider specifies the type of solution, additional additives, and the volume to infuse over a specific period. To reduce the potential for infection, standard practice is to replace IV solutions every 24 hours even if the total volume in a container has not been infused. Before preparing the solution, the nurse inspects the container and determines that the type of solution is the one prescribed, the solution is clear and transparent, the expiration date has not elapsed, no leaks are apparent, and a separate label is attached identifying the type and amount of drugs added to the original solution.

Selecting Intravenous Tubing

IV tubing consists of a spike for piercing the container of solution, a drip chamber for holding a small amount of fluid, a length of plastic tubing with one or more ports for instilling IV medications or additional solutions, and a roller or slide clamp for regulating the rate of the infusion (Fig. 13-5). Despite the common components, the nurse selects from various options in tubing design:

- Primary, secondary, or Y-administration tubing
- Vented or unvented tubing
- Drop size options (macrodrip or microdrip tubing)
- Filtered or unfiltered tubing

Primary, Secondary, or Y-Administration Tubing

Primary tubing is used to administer a large volume of IV solution over a long period or a small volume through a medication lock (discussed later). Primary tubing is usually quite long to span the distance from the solution, which hangs several feet above the infusion site, to the site itself. **Secondary tubing**, which is shorter, is used to administer smaller volumes of solution through a port in the primary tubing in a relatively short time. **Y-administration tubing**, used to administer whole blood, packed cells, and various blood products, is discussed later.

Vented Versus Unvented Tubing

IV tubing may be vented or unvented (Fig. 13-6). **Vented tubing** draws air into the container of solution and is used for administering solutions packaged in glass containers to facilitate their flow. **Unvented tubing** does not draw air into the container of solution and is used for solutions packaged in plastic bags.

Drop Size

The opening through which fluid passes from the solution container into the drip chamber determines the **drop size**. Tubing manufacturers design the drop size to deliver large-sized drops (**macrodrip tubing**) or small-sized drops (**microdrip tubing**).

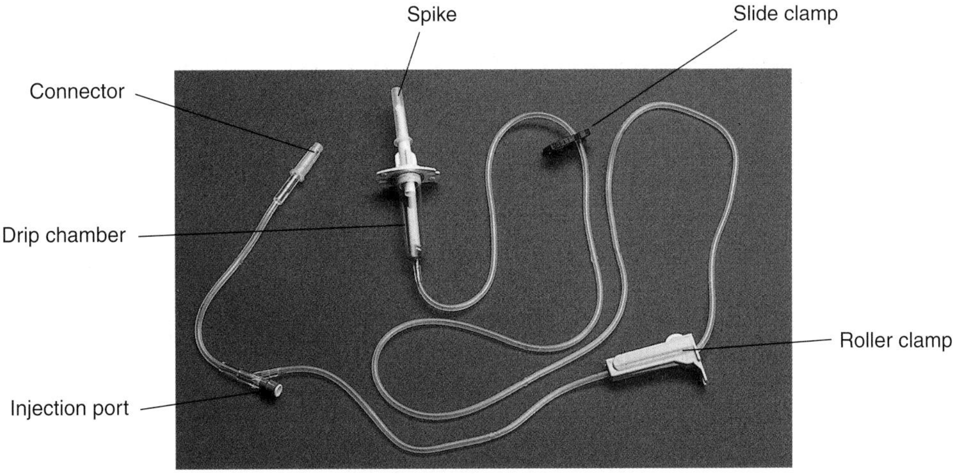

Figure 13-5 Basic components of intravenous tubing. (Courtesy of Abbott Laboratories, North Chicago, IL.)

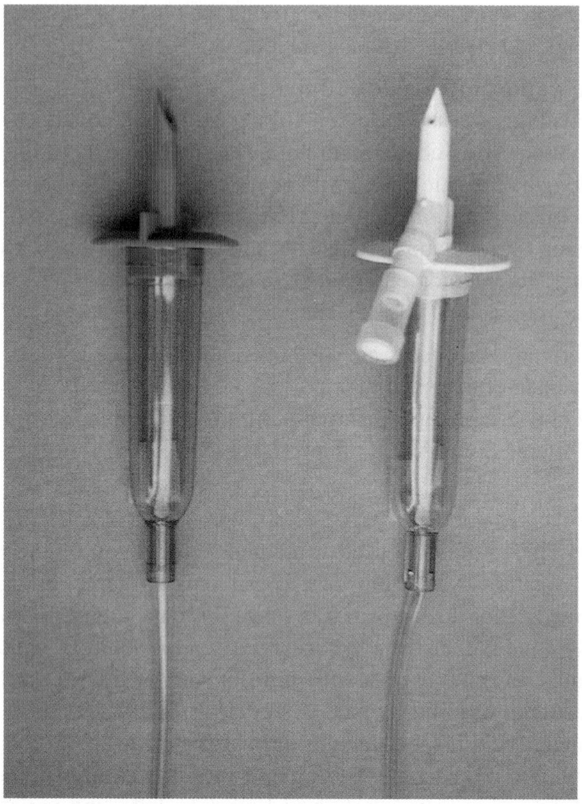

Figure 13-6 (Left) Unvented tubing and **(Right)** vented tubing. (Photo by Ken Timby.)

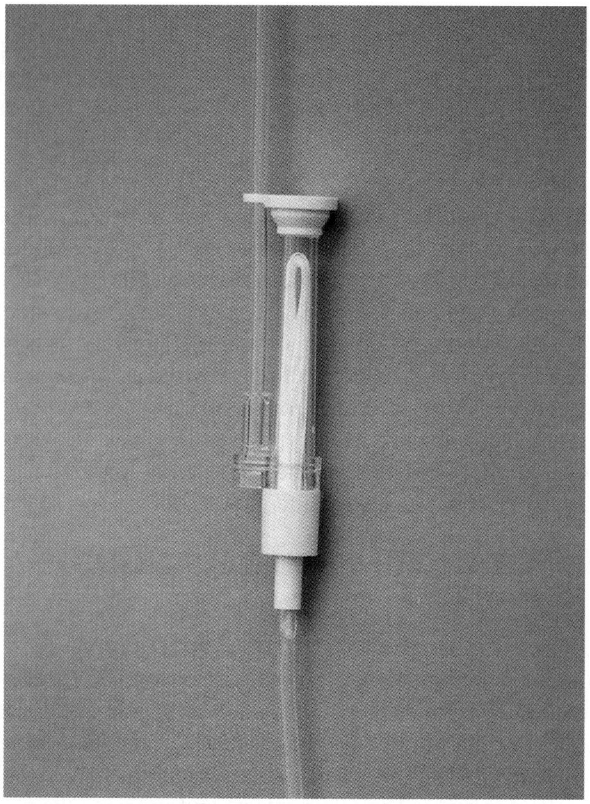

Figure 13-7 An in-line filter. (Photo by Ken Timby.)

The nurse determines the one to be used. When a solution infuses by gravity at a fast rate such as over 100 mL/hour, it is usually easier to count fewer larger drops than to count many smaller ones. When the rate must be infused very precisely or at a slow rate, smaller drops are preferred.

Microdrip tubing, regardless of the manufacturer, delivers a standard volume of 60 drops (gtt)/mL. Macrodrip tubing, however, varies in the drop size among manufacturers. Common macrodrip **drop factors**, the ratio of drops per milliliter, are 10, 15, and 20 gtt/mL. The nurse determines the drop factor, which is important in calculating the gravity infusion rate, by reading the package label.

Most IV solutions are infused using an electronic infusion device (discussed later). The drop size is of no consequence with infusion devices because the rates are programmed electronically in milliliters per hour (mL/hour).

Filters

An **in-line filter** (Fig. 13-7) is a device that removes air bubbles as well as undissolved drugs, bacteria, and large molecules from the infusing solution. Filtered tubing is used when administering TPN, blood and packed cells, and solutions to immunosuppressed or pediatric clients.

Another factor that may affect the type of tubing selected is the technique that will be used to administer the IV solution.

Selecting an Infusion Technique

IV solutions are instilled by gravity or with an **electronic infusion device**, a machine that regulates and monitors the administration of IV solutions. In some cases, the use of an electronic infusion device affects the type of tubing used.

The method for calculating the rate of infusion varies depending on the infusion technique (Box 13-1). If the solution is infused by gravity, the rate is calculated in drops per minute (gtt/minute). When an electronic infusion device is used, the rate is calculated in milliliters per hour.

Gravity Infusion

When IV solutions are infused by gravity, the height of the IV solution in relation to the infusion site influences the rate of flow. To overcome the pressure in the client's vein, which

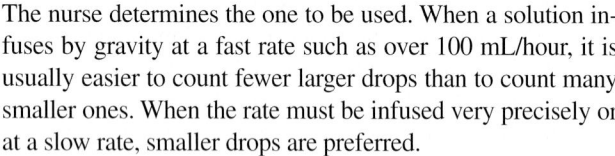

BOX 13-1 Calculating Infusion Rates

When using an electronic infusion device:

$$\frac{\text{Total volume in mL}}{\text{Total}} = \text{mL/hour}$$

Example:

$$\frac{1000\text{ mL}}{8\text{ hours}} = 125\text{ mL/hour}$$

When infusing by gravity:

$$\frac{\text{Total volume in mL}}{\text{Total time in minutes}} \times \text{drop factor*} = \text{gtt/minute}$$

Example:

$$\frac{1000\text{ mL}}{480\text{ minutes}} \times 20 = 42\text{ gtt/minute}$$

*The macrodrip drop factor varies among manufacturers.

is higher than atmospheric pressure, the nurse must elevate the solution at least 18 to 24 inches (45 to 60 cm) above the infusion site. The higher the solution, the faster it infuses, and vice versa. The nurse uses the roller clamp to adjust the rate of flow. In some cases, they may apply a **pressure infusion sleeve** around the bag of solution. The sleeve exerts a squeezing action around the solution bag to facilitate rapid infusion.

Electronic Infusion Devices

Electronic infusion devices, such as infusion pumps and volumetric controllers, are machines programmed to deliver a preset volume per hour and sound audible and visual alarms if the infusion is not progressing at the preprogrammed rate (Fig. 13-8). They also produce an audible sound when the infusion container is nearly empty, air is inside the tubing, or an obstruction or resistance to delivering the fluid occurs.

Infusion Pumps. An **infusion pump** is a device that exerts positive pressure to infuse solutions. Infusion pumps usually require special tubing that contains a cassette for creating sufficient pressure to push fluid into the vein. The machine adjusts the pressure according to the resistance it meets. This feature accounts for one of its major disadvantages: If the catheter or needle within the vein becomes displaced, the pump may continue to infuse fluid into the tissue until a default pressure is reached.

Volumetric Controllers. A **volumetric controller** is a device that infuses IV solutions by gravity by compressing the tubing at a certain frequency to infuse the solution at a precise preset rate. Volumetric controllers may or may not require special tubing. Some models allow the nurse to program the infusion of more than one solution. In some cases, when one container of fluid finishes infusing, the controller automatically shifts to infuse another. Volumetric controllers are minimally used in many facilities, as the use of an infusion pump has become more popular and safer for pediatric and geriatric clients.

>>> *Stop, Think, and Respond 13-1*

The primary provider orders an IV infusion of 1000 mL of 5% dextrose in water (D_5W) that will infuse over 8 hours. The nurse asks you to collect the fluid infusion supplies. What will you assemble?

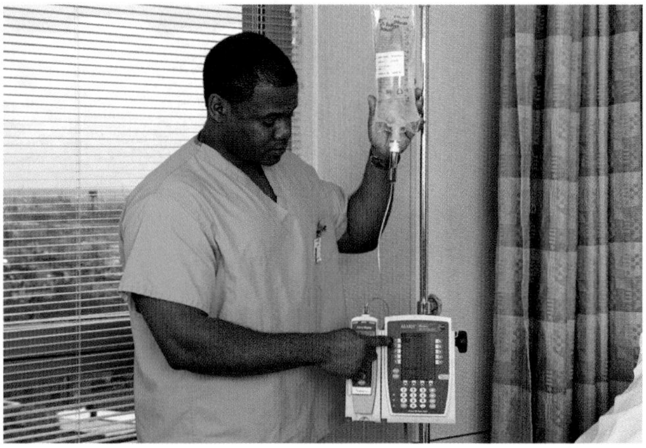

Figure 13-8 Electronic infusion devices are programmed to deliver a preset volume of intravenous solution per hour.

Preparing the Client

The identity of the client must be verified by checking the wrist band or scanning the band's bar code and asking additional questions such as the client's name and birth date. The nurse explains the purpose of the IV therapy to clients at their level of understanding. It is best to do so before bringing the equipment to the client's room. The nurse tries to make the explanation as clear, concise, and informative as possible without causing the client undue anxiety. They also allow time to answer the client's questions. The nurse may address the following points: the reason that the client needs IV therapy, approximately how long the procedure will take, the site to be used, the amount of discomfort that normally accompanies insertion of the needle or catheter, and any instructions regarding limitation of activities.

Performing a Venipuncture

Venipuncture is the method for gaining access to the venous system by piercing a vein with one of a variety of devices. Venipunctures are performed by trained nurses. The nurse assesses the client to detect alterations in fluid volume and implements the primary provider's orders for IV fluid therapy. While the client undergoes fluid therapy, the nurse monitors to detect an increase, decrease, or rapid shift from one fluid compartment to another. The nurse follows the agency's infection control policies as they relate to IV fluid therapy, uses aseptic techniques when caring for the venipuncture site or changing equipment, and gathers data as they relate to the presence of an infection.

For all venipunctures, the following items are necessary: venipuncture device, gloves, tourniquet, antiseptic swabs to clean the skin, a transparent dressing, tape for securing the catheter or needle, tubing, and solution. An armboard or splint may be needed to prevent dislodging of the venipuncture device.

Venipuncture Sites

IV therapy is administered through peripheral venous sites or central veins. Short-term **peripheral venous sites** are superficial veins of the arm and hand (antecubital fossa, or inner elbow; dorsum, or back, of the hand; and forearm veins; Fig. 13-9). They are the most common sites for infusing IV fluids. Scalp veins may be used in infants. Veins in the foot are avoided because infusions in the lower extremities restrict mobility and increase the risk for forming blood clots. **Central venous sites** are those that deliver solutions into a large central vein, such as the superior vena cava.

Selection of a vein depends on several factors, such as the client's age, condition of the veins, duration of IV therapy, IV solution ordered, size of venipuncture device, and client cooperation.

Venipuncture Devices

Peripheral Venous Access Devices

Several devices are used for accessing a vein: a butterfly needle, an over-the-needle catheter (most commonly used; Fig. 13-10), or a through-the-needle catheter. All of these types of venipuncture devices come in various diameters or

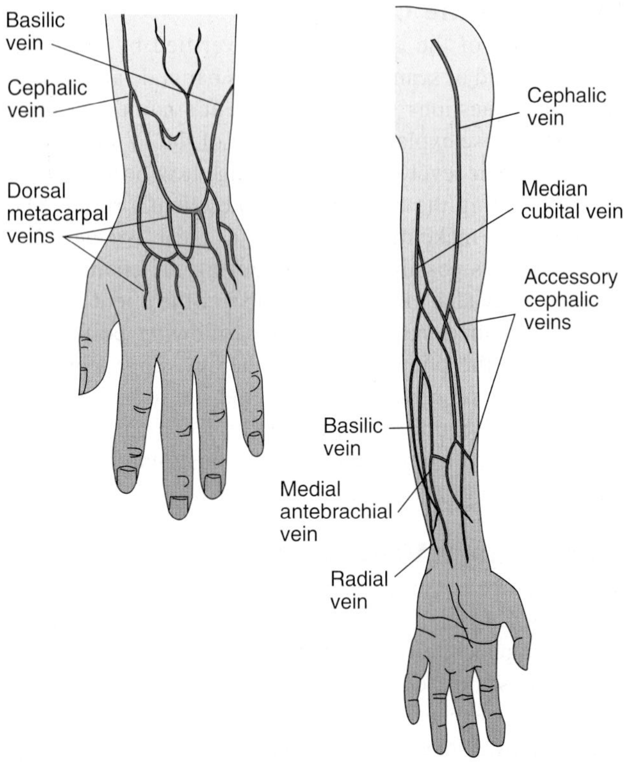

Figure 13-9 Venipuncture sites.

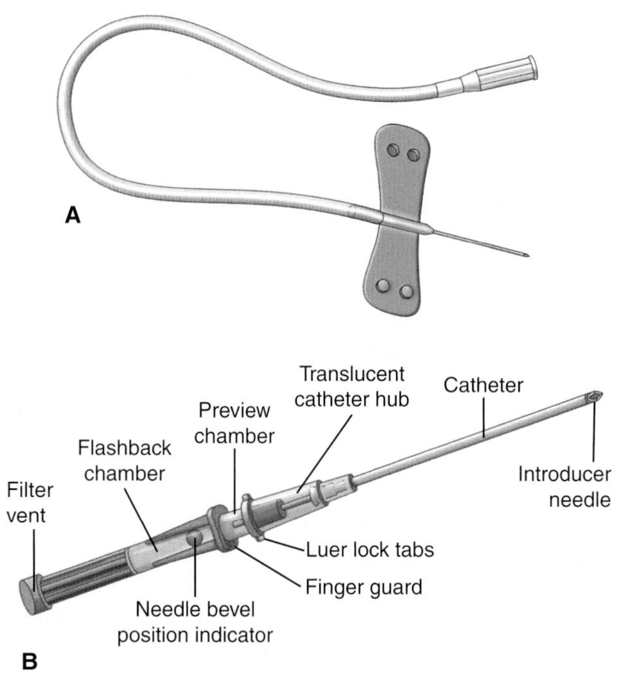

Figure 13-10 Examples of venipuncture devices. **(A)** Butterfly needle. **(B)** Over-the-needle catheter.

gauges; the larger the gauge number, the smaller the diameter. The diameter of the venipuncture device always should be smaller than the vein into which it will be inserted to reduce the potential for occluding blood flow. The 18-, 20-, or 22-gauge venipuncture devices are the sizes most used for adults.

Registered nurses who are certified may insert tunneled venous access devices such as a **peripherally inserted central catheter (PICC)** or midline catheter. Depending on the manufacturer, a PICC may measure 11 to 27 inches to reach from the median basilic vein to the superior vena cava depending on the size of the client. A **midline catheter** is 7 to 8 inches long, but only 3 to 6 inches of the catheter are inserted from just above or below the antecubital area until the tip rests in the upper arm just short of the axilla (Fig. 13-11). Peripherally inserted tunneled catheters are best suited for clients who have limited peripheral veins or who require several weeks of IV therapy before they need replacement.

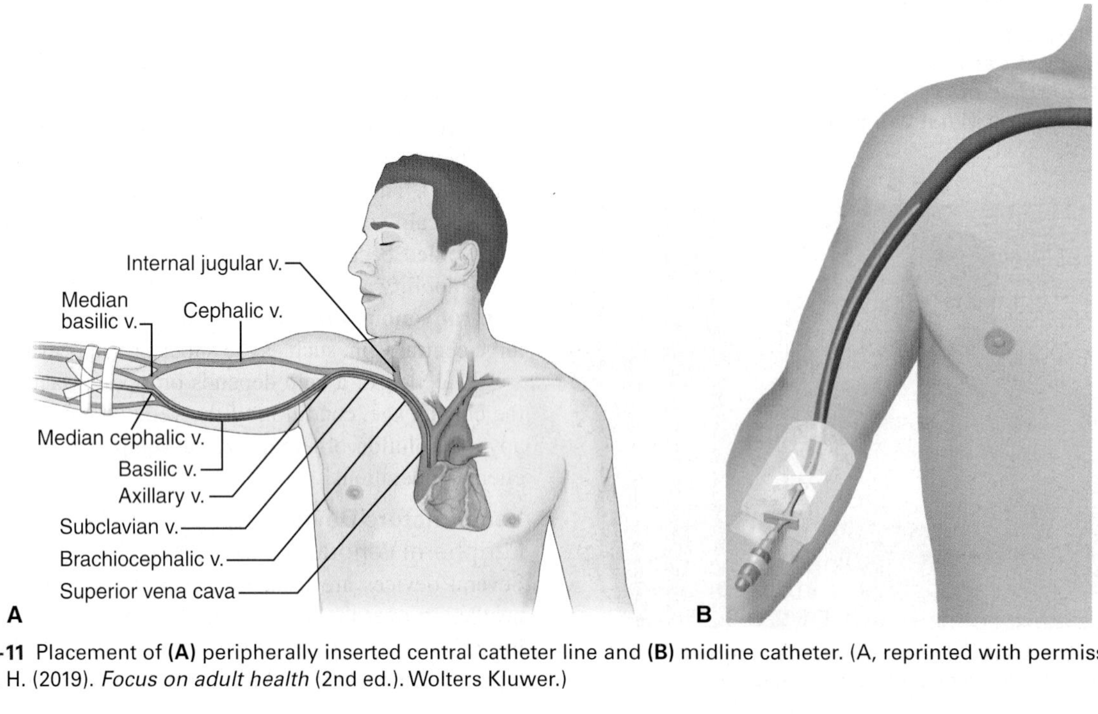

Figure 13-11 Placement of **(A)** peripherally inserted central catheter line and **(B)** midline catheter. (A, reprinted with permission from Pellico, L. H. (2019). *Focus on adult health* (2nd ed.). Wolters Kluwer.)

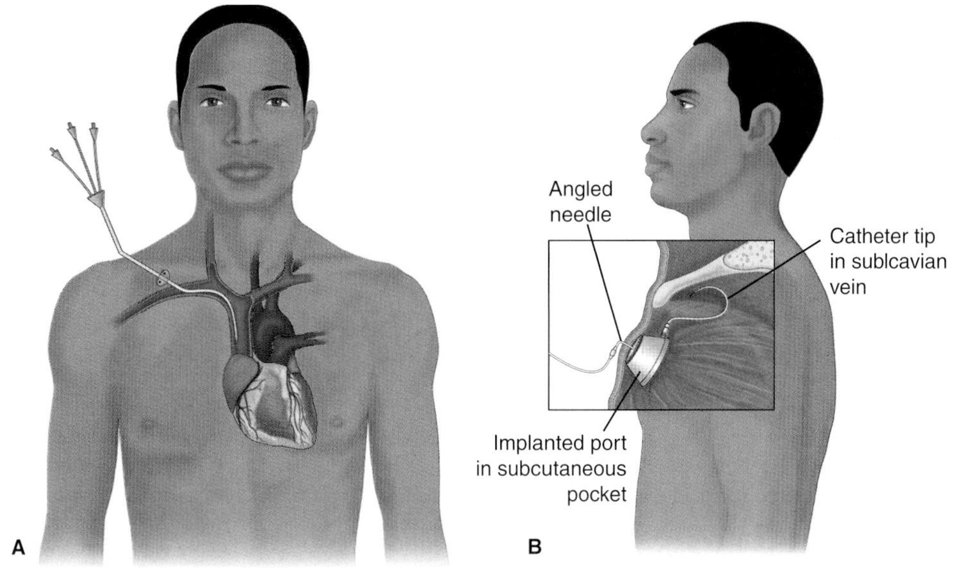

Figure 13-12 **(A)** Placement of triple-lumen nontunneled percutaneous central venous catheter. **(B)** Placement of an implanted port with the tip in the subclavian vein. Angled needle is inserted through skin and rubber septum into port.

Central Venous Access Devices

A primary provider inserts a central venous catheter into the jugular or subclavian vein until the tip is located just above the heart (Fig. 13-12). Central venous catheters are inserted when providing TPN, monitoring central venous pressure, or administering concentrated or irritating IV solutions; when peripheral veins have collapsed; or when long-term IV therapy or thrombophlebitis (inflammation of a vein) and infiltration have reduced the availability of peripheral veins. After insertion of the catheter, a chest radiograph is taken to confirm catheter placement and to rule out an accidental puncture of the pleural membrane, which can cause a pneumothorax (see Chapter 21).

››› *Stop, Think, and Respond 13-2*

A client with cancer has a central venous catheter through which they receive antineoplastic drugs. Why is the medication infused through a central venous catheter and filtered tubing?

Replacing Equipment

Replacing equipment is important to reduce the potential for infection. Solutions are replaced when they finish infusing or every 24 hours, whichever comes first. Most IV tubing is changed every 72 hours, but the exact parameters depend on agency policy. Some exceptions include tubing used to administer TPN and intermittent secondary infusions. Y-administration tubing used to administer blood can be reused one time for a second unit that immediately follows the first. Medication locks (discussed later) can remain in place for 72 hours, and venipuncture devices are replaced every 72 to 96 hours or immediately if evidence of complications develops. Central catheters remain in the same site indefinitely.

Monitoring for Complications

The nurse is responsible for monitoring the IV site at least once per shift and anytime the client is symptomatic or reports localized discomfort (Fig. 13-13). Several complications are associated with the infusion of IV solutions. When the integrity of the skin is compromised with a venous access device such as a catheter or needle, the client is at risk for infection. Because the venous access device traumatizes the vein wall and disturbs the flow of blood cells in the vein,

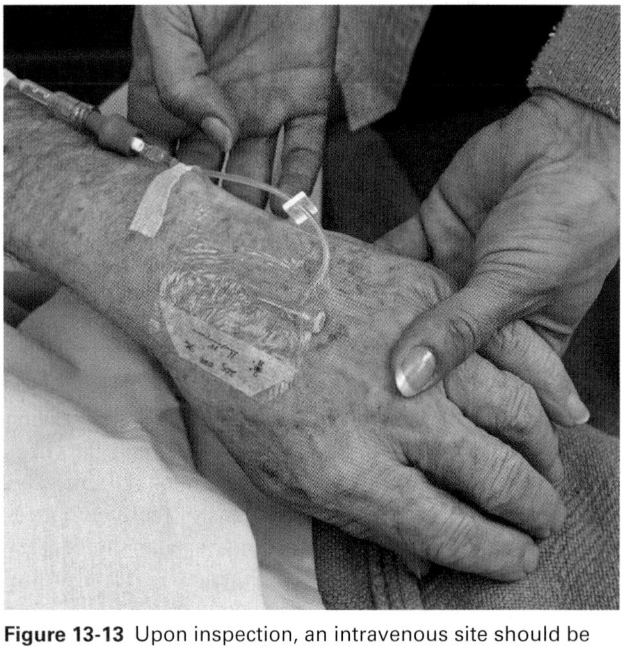

Figure 13-13 Upon inspection, an intravenous site should be free of redness, swelling, and discomfort. The surrounding tissue should be of similar temperature. (Reprinted with permission from Taylor, C. R., Lillis, C., & Lynn, P. (2015). *Fundamentals of nursing: The art and science of nursing care* (8th ed). Wolters Kluwer.)

TABLE 13-3 Complications of IV Therapy

COMPLICATION	SIGNS AND SYMPTOMS	CAUSE(S)	ACTION
Infection	Swelling, discomfort, redness at site, drainage from site	Growth of microorganisms	Change site Apply antiseptic and dressing to previous site Report findings
Circulatory overload	Elevated BP, shortness of breath, bounding pulse, anxiety	Rapid infusion Reduced kidney function Impaired heart contraction	Slow the IV infusion rate Contact the primary provider Elevate the client's head Give oxygen
Infiltration (extravasation)	Swelling at the site, discomfort, decrease in infusion rate, cool skin temperature at the site	Displacement of the venipuncture device	Restart the IV Elevate the arm
Phlebitis	Redness, warmth, and discomfort along the vein	Administration of irritating fluid Prolonged use of the same vein	Restart the IV Report the findings Apply warm compresses
Thrombus formation	Swelling, discomfort at site, slowed infusion	Stasis of blood at the catheter, needle tip, or vein	Restart the IV Report the findings Apply warm compresses
Pulmonary embolus	Sudden chest pain, shortness of breath, anxiety, rapid heart rate, drop in BP	Movement of previously stationary blood clot	Stay with the client Call for help Administer oxygen
Air embolism	Same as pulmonary embolus	Failure to purge air from the tubing Disconnected tubing from central venous catheter	Same as for pulmonary embolus but also place the client's head lower than the feet Position the client on left side

BP, blood pressure; IV, intravenous.

there is a potential for **phlebitis**, inflammation of the vein, and **thrombus formation** (development of a clot). If the clot breaks free, it may travel to the lungs and cause a pulmonary embolism, which can be fatal. A bolus of air traveling through the venous system to the lungs is just as serious. If the venous access device fails to remain in the vein, fluid infiltrates the tissue, causing localized edema. Lastly, circulatory overload can develop if the volume of infusing solution exceeds the heart's ability to circulate it effectively.

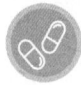

Pharmacologic Considerations

- Some IV medications have vesicant properties, meaning they can cause tissue necrosis if they infiltrate or leak into soft tissue. Extravasation kits should be kept close when vesicants are infused, and emergency treatment protocols included when these drugs are prescribed.

Inspecting the venipuncture site routinely and observing for signs of infection, infiltration, phlebitis, and thrombus formation are important nursing interventions. Table 13-3 identifies the causes and manifestations of these complications and appropriate nursing actions to take should they occur. Also see Evidence-Based Practice 13-1, regarding multiple IV infusions and client safety.

The nurse documents site appearance daily in the client's medical record. A common practice is to change the dressing over the venipuncture site every 24 to 72 hours according to the agency's infection control policy or immediately if complications develop.

Evidence-Based Practice 13-1

Client Safety and Multiple IV Infusions

Clinical Question

Is client safety at risk if multiple IV infusions are given to a single client?

Evidence

A research study in Ontario collected data from two national incident reporting databases and concluded that clients with multiple IV therapy infusions were at risk for harm. (Cassano-Piché et al., 2012). The study occurred in phases. The first phase looked at a group of 12 hospitals and collected data on safety concerns with multiple infusions and how nurses were educated on the risks of harm. The data indicated a need for continuing education on multiple infusions, IV therapy technology, and best practice guidelines for nurses to reduce the potential risk of harm to clients. Within this research study, other research was reviewed showing common safety risks as programmer error, error in secondary infusion setup, and multiple medications causing an adverse drug reaction. These common errors may all lead to client safety risks.

Nursing Implications

Nurses are responsible to know how to use infusion equipment properly and know the facility policies and guidelines. Standard practice should include verifying orders, checking IV setup, and limiting distractions when administering multiple infusions to decrease the common errors in IV therapy and reduce potential harm to clients.

Reference

Cassano-Piché, A., Fan, M., Sabovitch, S., Masino, C., Easty, A. C., Health Technology Safety Research Team, & Institute for Safe Medication Practices Canada. (2012). Multiple intravenous infusions phase 1b: Practice and training scan. *Ontario Health Technology Assessment Series, 12*(16), 1–132.

NURSING GUIDELINES 13-1

Discontinuing an Intravenous Infusion

- Wash your hands.
- Put on clean gloves.
- Clamp the tubing and remove the dressing holding the venipuncture device in place.
- Gently press a dry, sterile gauze square over the site (use of an alcohol swab interferes with blood clotting).
- Remove the venipuncture device by pulling it out without hesitation, following the course of the vein.
- Continue to apply pressure to the site for 30 to 45 seconds while elevating the forearm to control bleeding.
- Cover the site with a dressing or bandage.
- Remove the gloves and wash your hands.
- Record the time the IV infusion was discontinued, the amount of fluid infused, and the appearance of the venipuncture site.

Discontinuing Intravenous Therapy

IV infusions are discontinued when the solution has infused and no more is scheduled to follow (Nursing Guidelines 13-1). Alternatively, the venipuncture device may be temporarily capped and kept patent with the use of a **medication lock**, many times called a saline lock, which is a sealed chamber that allows intermittent access to a vein. The nurse inserts the lock into the venipuncture device (Fig. 13-14). Flushing the lock with saline or heparinized saline keeps the vein patent. Medication locks are used when the client no longer needs continuous infusions, needs intermittent IV medication administration, or may need emergency IV fluids or medications.

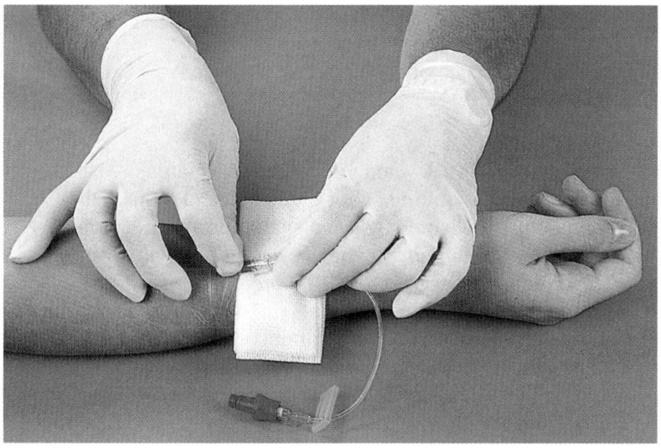

Figure 13-14 Attaching a lock device with extension tubing to the intravenous catheter hub. (Photo by B. Proud.)

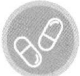

Pharmacologic Considerations

- Be aware of drug name and strength when preparing flush solutions. Mistakes can occur because vials of heparin come in various dosages—for example, 20,000, 10,000, 5000, or 1000 units/mL. Carefully examine orders and vials supplied when administering the drug.

Nutrition Notes

The Client Receiving Intravenous Fluid Therapy

- When administered parenterally, dextrose provides 3.4 cal/g, not 4 cal/g as with carbohydrates consumed orally. Therefore, 1 L of 5% D_5W, which contains 50 g dextrose, provides a total of 170 calories; 3 L of D_5W infused over 24 hours provides only 510 calories.
- Because simple IV solutions (i.e., D_5W) are nutritionally and calorically inadequate, it is best to avoid maintaining clients on them longer than 1 to 2 days.

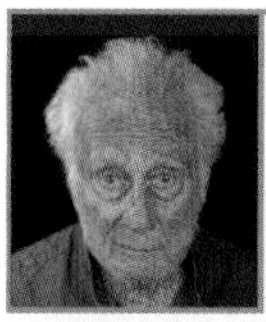

Clinical Scenario The client, an 81-year-old man, was observed by his neighbor to be confused. The neighbor called an ambulance but could not provide the emergency medical team with any information about whether or not the client had eaten or consumed any beverages. When examined by the nurse at the emergency department, the client appeared to be dehydrated. An indwelling catheter revealed very little urine. The plan for care includes rehydrating the client with IV therapy and evaluating his ability to resume oral nutrition. **What are the client's current problems related to the IV rehydration? See the following Nursing Process section.**

NURSING PROCESS FOR THE CLIENT REQUIRING INTRAVENOUS THERAPY

Assessment

Before initiating fluid therapy, gather clinical data related to fluid status (see Chapter 16). Examples include vital signs; body weight; color, volume, and specific gravity of urine; skin turgor; characteristics of oral mucous membranes; respiratory effort; and level of consciousness. Also review laboratory test results such as blood cell count and hematocrit and serum electrolyte levels. Identify the purpose(s) for administering IV fluid therapy.

Before performing the venipuncture, use at least two identifiers to validate that the client is the correct person for the intended procedure (Evidence-Based Practice 13-1). Ask the client to indicate their nondominant hand. The nondominant hand or forearm is preferred unless there are contraindications to its use, such as having had a breast and lymph nodes removed on that side or having had vascular surgery for kidney dialysis. If the client cannot respond, assume that the client is right-handed because that is more common. To determine which vein is most appropriate, first assess the size and condition of the veins in the hand or wrist area. If they are exceptionally small, tortuous, or traumatized by previous venipunctures, inspect veins in more proximal areas, trying to avoid the veins in the antecubital fossa, where the elbow bends, if at all possible. Read the label on the IV fluid at least three times to confirm

(continued)

NURSING PROCESS FOR THE CLIENT REQUIRING INTRAVENOUS THERAPY (continued)

that it is the volume and type of solution the primary provider has ordered for the client.

After performing the venipuncture, monitor the IV site for swelling, warmth, pain, and induration (hardening). Assess at least hourly the rate at which fluid is infusing and the client's condition. Examine the electronic infusion device, if one is used, to ensure that it is correctly programmed and functioning properly. Throughout fluid therapy, measure intake and output volumes to determine trends in fluid balance. Auscultate lung sounds and heart sounds each shift or more often to evaluate the client's capacity to circulate the infusing fluid without complications. Inspect the venipuncture site at least once a day for signs of inflammation or infection, and observe the condition of the dressing, which should be dry and intact.

Analysis, Planning, and Interventions

Fluid Overload/Fluid Overload Risk: Related to rate of infusion that exceeds circulatory capacity or a shift in a fluid compartment
Expected Outcomes: (1) Fluid volume will be maintained or restored. (2) Client will not experience cardiopulmonary complications secondary to the IV infusion of fluid.

- Calculate the rate of fluid infusion accurately, and correctly regulate the drip rate or program the electronic infusion device with the prescribed hourly infusion volume. *Errors in calculating or regulating the prescribed rate of fluid infusion can compromise the heart's ability to circulate the fluid or delay restoration of fluid balance.*
- Monitor the time strip on the container of IV solution hourly. *Reading the time strip is a quick method for determining whether fluid is infusing at the predetermined hourly rate.*
- Respond when an electronic infusion device sounds an alarm. *Audible alarms call attention to a problem associated with the infusion of IV fluid.*
- Inspect the site where the fluid is infusing for signs of localized edema. *Parenteral fluid should be instilled in the vein; local edema suggests that the fluid is entering interstitial spaces, where it is more slowly absorbed.*
- Maintain an accurate intake and output record. *Fluid intake should approximate fluid output.*
- Note the amount of fluid the client takes orally and report when the combined volume of oral and parenteral fluid exceeds 3000 mL in 24 hours. *Normal adult fluid intake generally is 1500 to 3000 mL/24 hours. Volumes that exceed 3000 mL/day may be excessive unless the client is dehydrated or losing large volumes of fluid simultaneously.*
- Reassess fluid status at regular intervals according to the client's acuity level. *Changes in weight (e.g., 2 lb in 24 hours), elevated BP, dyspnea or adventitious lung sounds, abnormal heart sounds, peripheral edema, intake that significantly exceeds output, distended neck veins, anxiety, or diminished level of consciousness suggest excessive fluid volume.*

Infection Risk: Related to disrupted skin integrity secondary to venipuncture and presence of a venous access device
Expected Outcome: Client will remain free of localized or generalized infection.

- Follow agency protocol for changing IV sites and venipuncture devices. *To avoid infection, the standard of care is to change IV sites every 48 to 72 hours. Clients with a suppressed immune system may require the use of tubing with a bacterial filter and more frequent site changes.*
- Check the initial date of use on the IV fluid container and tubing, and change equipment according to the agency's infection control policies. *Infection control policies usually advise changing IV solution containers every 24 hours; IV tubing can be used for up to 72 hours, provided solution is continuously infusing through it. Nurses change tubing for intermittent infusions more frequently.*
- Use aseptic technique when changing IV site dressings, tubings, and solution containers. *Preventing or reducing the entrance of bacteria in the venipuncture site or vascular system decreases the potential for infection.*
- Assess for signs and symptoms of infection such as redness, warmth, tenderness, and purulent drainage at the venipuncture site; elevated temperature; and an increased WBC count. Discontinue the IV infusion and remove the venipuncture device if signs and symptoms of infection exist. *Removing the venipuncture device enables the impaired skin to heal and restores the barrier to microorganisms.*
- Document and report assessments that relate to an infection; follow agency protocols for obtaining a culture of the wound and its drainage. *Local antimicrobial therapy or systemic antibiotic therapy may be indicated in some cases of infection.*
- Elevate the extremity and apply warm compresses if an infection is suspected. *Elevation promotes venous circulation and reduces swelling. Warmth dilates blood vessels, relieves discomfort, and facilitates a reduction in local edema.*
- Restart the IV infusion in another site, preferably in the opposite upper extremity. *Fluid therapy should not be interrupted if it is still necessary.*

Malnutrition Risk: Related to an inadequate nutritional intake from crystalloid solutions without oral nutrition
Expected Outcome: The client will have adequate nutrition to meet the needs for growth and repair of tissue.

- Weigh the client daily. *Although short-term weight changes usually relate to fluids, long-term weight loss may indicate inadequate caloric intake* (Nutrition Notes).
- Monitor laboratory test results such as blood cell count and hemoglobin, albumin, and transferrin levels. *A drop in specific laboratory findings indicates insufficient protein to ensure their normal production or replacement.*
- Implement the primary provider's orders to provide TPN if it becomes necessary. *TPN provides the client with protein, vitamins, and minerals as well as glucose and water. Intermittent fat emulsions complete the requirements for adequate nutrition.*

NURSING PROCESS FOR THE CLIENT REQUIRING INTRAVENOUS THERAPY (continued)

Evaluation of Expected Outcomes

Expected outcomes are that the client's fluid status is improved or maintained within normal range, with approximately equal intake and output volumes and normal vital signs. Breathing remains quiet and effortless, with no signs of localized or generalized edema. The IV site is not red, tender, or warm and shows no drainage. The client's body temperature remains within normal range. The client uses the extremity with minimal inconvenience from the IV infusion. They maintain preillness weight. Blood cell count and hemoglobin, albumin, and transferrin levels are within normal limits.

>>> ***Stop, Think, and Respond 13-3***

A client had surgery 2 days ago, at which time they lost approximately 500 mL of blood. After surgery, they are not allowed to have anything orally because they have a nasogastric tube connected to suction. In the meantime, they have also developed diarrhea, a side effect that the primary provider attributes to the parenteral antibiotic they are receiving. When you assess this client, their BP is 104/62 mm Hg, much lower than their admission BP of 132/86 mm Hg. Their skin is dry and tents when you assess turgor; urine output has been 350 mL over the past 8 hours, and the urine appears dark yellow.

1. *What additional information would you gather to assess the client's fluid status?*
2. *If IV fluids are administered, which type of solution is most appropriate to use and why?*

SPECIAL CONSIDERATIONS FOR INTRAVENOUS THERAPY

WATCH & LEARN

Total Parenteral Nutrition

The primary provider may order TPN for a client who is severely malnourished or cannot consume food or liquids for a long time (Box 13-2). TPN uses a solution of nutrients to meet the client's caloric and nutritional needs. The composition of a TPN solution is individualized according to the client's nutritional requirements and medical condition. Because concentrations of protein, carbohydrate, and fat are standard in standard volumes, however, individualization is somewhat limited.

BOX 13-2 Candidates for Total Parenteral Nutrition

Candidates for TPN include clients:

- Who have not eaten for 5 days and are not likely to eat during the next week
- Who have had a 10% or more loss of body weight
- Exhibiting self-imposed starvation (anorexia nervosa)
- With cancer of the esophagus or stomach
- With postoperative gastrointestinal complications
- With acute inflammatory bowel disease
- With major trauma or burns
- With liver and renal failure

TPN solutions, which are extremely concentrated (hypertonic), are instilled into the central circulation, where they are diluted in a fairly large volume of blood. Because of their immediate dilution, TPN solutions do not dehydrate cells.

A lipid emulsion is sometimes administered intermittently with TPN (Fig. 13-15). Lipid emulsions contain fat from soybean and safflower oils, phospholipids from egg yolks that act as emulsifying agents, and glycerol to make the solution isotonic. Lipid emulsions provide essential fatty acids and are often used to meet 20% to 30% of the client's total calorie needs. However, lipid emulsions may be contraindicated in clients with elevated triglyceride levels.

Before TPN is initiated, the primary provider gains access to the central circulation using a central venous catheter. Trained nurses administer TPN using filtered tubing and an electronic infusion device (Nursing Guidelines 13-2).

For clients receiving TPN at home or as a supplement to an inadequate oral diet, cyclical TPN is most often used. Cyclical TPN is infused in cycles over 10 to 16 hours, followed by 8 to 14 hours of rest. Cyclical TPN offers the client more mobility, especially if infused during the night, and has the advantage of allowing enzyme and hormone levels to drop to normal during the rest periods. To give the body time to adjust to the decreasing glucose load (and prevent rebound hypoglycemia), the infusion should be tapered near the end of each cycle. The nurse should monitor the client's blood glucose level because the glucose levels in TPN can cause hyperglycemia.

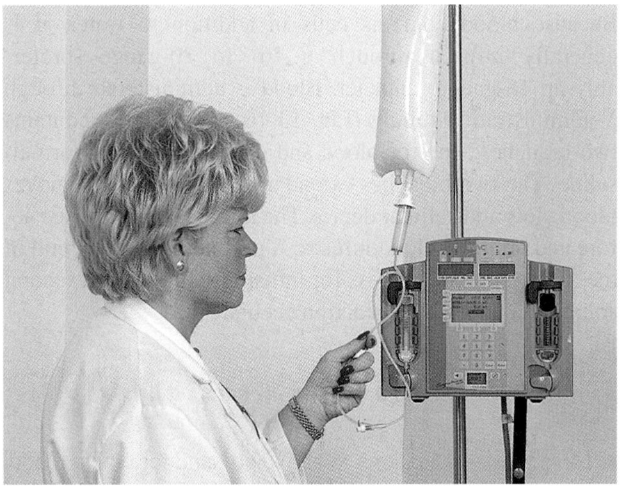

Figure 13-15 A lipid emulsion appears milky white. It is infused through standard intravenous tubing by gravity or with an electronic infusion device. (Photo by B. Proud.)

NURSING GUIDELINES 13-2

Administering Total Parenteral Nutrition

- Weigh client daily.
- Use tubing that contains a filter; however, bypass the filter when administering lipid emulsions to prevent large fat molecules from obstructing the filter.
- Label the tubing used for TPN to ensure that it is used exclusively for TPN and not IV medications or blood products.
- Change TPN tubings daily.
- Tape all connections in the tubing to prevent accidental separation and the potential for an air embolism.
- Clamp the central catheter whenever separating the tubing from its catheter connection.
- Use an electronic infusion device to administer TPN.
- Infuse initial TPN solutions gradually (e.g., 25 to 50 mL/hour); increase rate according to the agency's standard of care or the primary provider's medical orders.
- Monitor blood glucose levels regularly to assess the client's ability to metabolize the concentrated glucose.
- Administer insulin on a sliding scale according to blood glucose levels.
- Wean client from TPN gradually to avoid a sudden drop in blood glucose level.
- Infuse IV lipids three times a week.
- Monitor the following laboratory test results to evaluate the nutritional status of the client receiving TPN and lipids: serum transferrin, serum osmolality, cholesterol, triglycerides, electrolytes, blood urea nitrogen (BUN), and urine creatinine.
- Initiate nutrition consult as per institutional protocol.

Blood Transfusion

Blood that is administered usually comes from nonautologous donors, meaning that it comes from a person other than the person who will receive the blood. Blood contains cells and additives and preservatives that enable it to be stored in a refrigerated state for approximately 6 weeks without clotting. For these reasons, administering blood IV requires special considerations.

Blood Transfusion Equipment

Because blood contains cells in addition to water, it is generally infused through a 16- to 20-gauge (preferably an 18-gauge) catheter. Blood is administered through Y-administration tubing (Fig. 13-16). This tubing contains two branches: one for blood and one for isotonic (normal) saline. The two branches extend above a filter that removes blood clots and cellular debris. The normal saline infuses before and after the blood infuses. A port near the distal end of the tubing provides access for infusing saline from a second source if a transfusion reaction occurs.

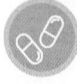

Pharmacologic Considerations

- Never add medications to an IV line used for whole blood or blood products. Interaction can result in hemolysis of the blood cells.

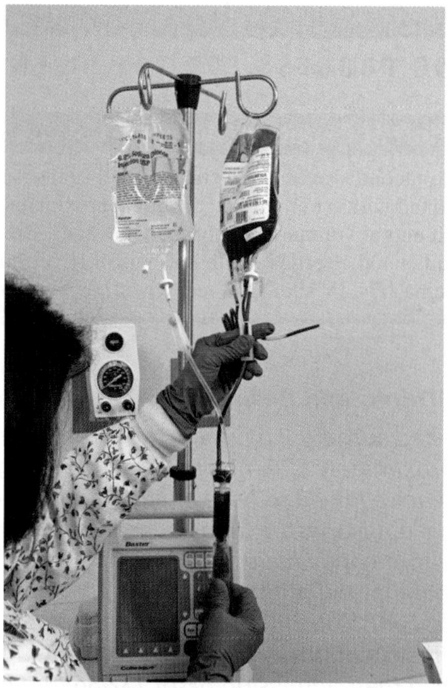

Figure 13-16 Blood administration set using Y-administration tubing. (Reprinted with permission from Taylor, C. R., Lillis, C., & Lynn, P. (2015). *Fundamentals of nursing: The art and science of nursing care* (8th ed). Wolters Kluwer.)

Blood Compatibility

There are several hundred differences among the proteins in the blood of a donor and recipient. These differences can cause minor or major transfusion reactions. One of the most dangerous differences involves the antigens, or proteins on the membranes of red blood cells (RBCs). Antigens determine the characteristic blood groups A, B, AB, and O, referred to as the **ABO system**.

Before blood is administered, it must be examined to make sure the donor and recipient blood types are compatible. Blood is typed according to the ABO system. Everyone has one of four blood types: A, B, AB, or O. RBCs of types A, B, and AB blood have a protein on their surface called an antigen. Type A blood has antigen A, type B has antigen B, and type AB has both antigen A and antigen B. Type O has neither A nor B antigen.

The blood type is important when transfusing blood because antibodies in the blood plasma will react against transfused blood cells that have a different antigen on their surface. For example, if a person who has type A blood receives type B blood, anti–B antibodies will destroy the transfused blood cells carrying antigen B, with life-threatening consequences. Because type O blood has neither A nor B antigen on its surface, type O can be given to a person with any type of blood. For this reason, people with type O blood are referred to as **universal donors**. However, a person with type O blood cannot receive a type other than type O because anti–A and anti–B antibodies will attack the cells in the donated blood. Persons with type AB blood can receive AB, A, B, or O blood because they do not have anti–A or anti–B antibodies. Consequently, persons with type AB blood are called **universal recipients**.

TABLE 13-4 Blood Groups and Compatible Types

BLOOD GROUPS	PERCENTAGE OF POPULATION	COMPATIBLE BLOOD TYPES
A	41%	A and O
B	9%	B and O
O	47%	O
AB	3%	AB, A, B, and O
Rh-positive	85% Whites 95% African Americans	Rh-positive and Rh-negative
Rh-negative	15% Whites 5% African Americans	Rh-negative only

Some blood cells have an additional protein surface marker known as the **Rh factor**. It acquired its name because the protein was first discovered in rhesus monkeys. Approximately 85% of humans have this additional protein on their blood cells, which makes them Rh-positive (+). Those who lack the protein are Rh-negative (−). The Rh factor acts as an antigen that will cause a fatal reaction if given to a person with Rh-negative blood. On the other hand, a person with Rh-positive blood will not be affected by type compatible blood that is Rh-negative because it does not have the antigenic protein on the cells' surface.

Whole blood and packed cells are typed and cross-matched in the laboratory before administration to ensure that the donor's and recipient's blood types and Rh factor are compatible (Table 13-4).

>>> ***Stop, Think, and Respond 13-4***

What blood type(s) are compatible for a client with an AB Rh-positive blood type, a client with an O Rh-negative blood type, and a client with a B Rh-positive blood type?

Each client who needs a blood transfusion has an additional identification bracelet that is attached when the laboratory draws a sample of blood for typing and cross-matching. Before a blood transfusion is initiated, two nurses must check the identifying numbers on the bracelet to confirm that they match the numbers on the unit of blood from the blood bank (Fig. 13-17).

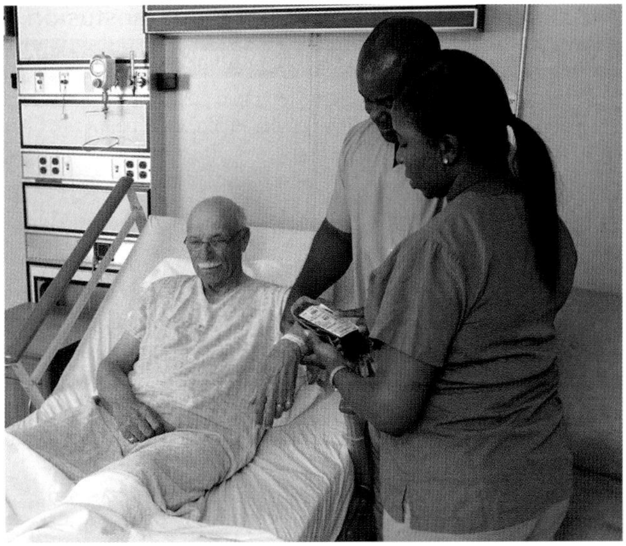

Figure 13-17 When blood is administered, two nurses are required to compare the numbers on the blood and the numbers on the client's wrist band. (Reprinted with permission from Craven, R. F., Hirnle, C. J., & Henshaw, C. M. (2017). *Fundamentals of nursing: Human health and function* (8th ed.). Wolters Kluwer.)

Complications of Blood Transfusion

Clients who receive blood are at risk for the same complications as those receiving crystalloid fluids. They also face additional risks, however. A **transfusion reaction** is an untoward event at the time that blood is being administered. One of the most life-threatening transfusion reactions is an incompatibility reaction that occurs when the donor and recipient blood types are incorrectly matched. In this instance, the recipient's antibodies destroy the donor cells. Although an incompatibility reaction occurs infrequently, when acute hemolytic reactions do occur, they are accompanied by a high rate of fatality. An acute hemolytic reaction occurs within minutes of infusing the donor blood. Milder allergic reactions such as hives and itching or a febrile response may occur if the recipient is sensitive to noncellular substances in the donor blood. Delayed reactions, which are milder than incompatibility reactions, can occur weeks to months after a transfusion. Delayed reactions are more likely the result of an immune response against the antigens of the Rh component of blood cells.

Because serious transfusion reactions generally occur within the first 5 to 15 minutes of the infusion, many health care agencies require that a nurse remains with and monitors the client during this critical time. Because a transfusion reaction can occur at any time, however, nurses monitor clients frequently throughout a transfusion for signs of a reaction or other complications associated with receiving blood (Table 13-5). Clients are instructed to call for assistance if they feel unusual while receiving the infusion of blood. In cases of a suspected transfusion reaction, it is appropriate to stop the infusion of blood and infuse a solution of normal saline while continuing to assess the client.

Nonimmune complications are also possible after blood transfusion. Clients may become septic if pathogens have grown and multiplied in the stored blood or during the interim when blood is being infused. A universal standard is to keep the blood refrigerated until just before use and to infuse the blood in 4 hours or less to prevent a septic reaction from bacterial contamination. Some clients have shaking chills and a fever during a septic or febrile reaction. Monitoring the client's temperature before, during, and after a blood transfusion is necessary to determine whether chilling is the result of an emerging complication or of infusing cold blood.

Reduced levels of serum calcium can produce symptoms in clients who receive massive transfusions of blood over a very short time. Citrate, which is added to the donor blood to prevent clotting while in storage, binds with calcium in the recipient's blood, causing hypocalcemia.

TABLE 13-5 Complications of Blood Transfusion

COMPLICATION	SIGNS AND SYMPTOMS	CAUSE(S)	ACTIONS
Incompatibility reaction	Hypotension, rapid pulse rate, difficulty breathing, back pain, flushing	Mismatch between donor and recipient blood groups	Stop the infusion of blood Infuse saline at a rapid rate Call for assistance Administer oxygen Raise the feet higher than the head Be prepared to administer emergency drugs Send first urine specimen to laboratory Save the blood and tubing
Febrile reaction	Fever, shaking chills, headache, rapid pulse, muscle aches	Allergy to foreign proteins in the donated blood	Stop the blood infusion Start infusing saline Check vital signs Report findings
Septic reaction	Fever, chills, hypotension	Infusion of blood that contains microorganisms	Stop the infusion of blood Start infusing saline Report findings Save the blood and tubing
Allergic reaction	Rash, itching, flushing, stable vital signs	Minor sensitivity to substances in the donor blood	Slow the rate of infusion Assess the client Report findings Be prepared to give an antihistamine
Moderate chilling	No fever or other symptoms	Infusion of cold blood	Continue the infusion Cover and make the client comfortable
Circulatory overload	Hypertension, difficulty breathing, moist breath sounds, bounding pulse	Large volume or rapid rate of infusion; inadequate cardiac or kidney function	Reduce the rate of infusion Elevate the head Give oxygen Report findings Be prepared to give a diuretic
Hypocalcemia (low calcium)	Tingling of fingers, hypotension, muscle cramps, convulsions	Multiple blood transfusions containing anticalcium agents	Stop the blood infusion Start infusing saline Report findings Be prepared to give antidote—calcium chloride
HIV and hepatitis B virus transmission	Opportunistic infections; elevated antibody titers, abnormal blood cell counts or liver enzyme levels	Blood collected from infected donors that passed screening examinations	Encourage autologous (self) blood collection if possible

Blood-borne infections such as hepatitis A, B, and C and HIV infection also can be transmitted through blood from infected donors. Donors are asked questions about their infection history, foreign travel, and risk behaviors when being screened before donating blood. Donated blood is also tested for hepatitis virus and HIV antibody levels. Although it is impossible to guarantee that all donated blood is free of blood-borne pathogens, the incidence of transmission is much smaller than it was at one time. Table 13-5 provides an overview of potential complications from blood transfusion and specific nursing actions.

To avoid the use of publicly donated blood, some surgeons administer salvaged blood. **Salvaged blood** is blood collected from a client during a surgical procedure and reinfused while surgery is being performed or shortly thereafter. Salvaging blood involves using a device known as a cell saver system. In this system, blood drains from the surgical site into a collection device; a reservoir sends debris into a separate waste container, and salvaged blood is reinfused IV to the client. Salvaged blood is commonly reclaimed during cardiothoracic and orthopedic joint replacement surgery. Using salvaged blood eliminates the potential for transmission of blood-borne diseases, provides type-specific blood, and frees stored blood in the blood bank so that it is available to other clients who may require a blood transfusion.

KEY POINTS

- Indications for IV therapy:
  - A rapid drug effect is required.
  - Oral intake is restricted.
  - Client cannot swallow.
  - Gastrointestinal absorption is impaired.
  - A continuous therapeutic blood level is desired.
- Types of IV solutions:
  - Crystalloids: made of water and other uniformly dissolved crystals such as salt and sugar
    - Isotonic: sodium and chloride equal to those found in plasma
    - Hypotonic: sodium and chloride less than found in plasma, less concentrated

        - Hypertonic: twice the concentration of glucose than found in plasma
    - Colloids: made of water and molecules of suspended substances such as blood cells and blood products
        - Blood
        - Blood products
            - FFP
            - Albumin
            - Platelets
            - Granulocytes
            - Cryoprecipitate
        - Blood substitutes
        - Plasma expanders
- Administering IV therapy
    - Selecting and preparing equipment
        - Preparing IV solutions
        - Selecting IV tubing
        - Primary (long), secondary (short), or Y-Administration tubing
        - Vented or unvented tubing
        - Drop size
            - Microdrip (small drops)
            - Macrodrip (large drops)
        - Unfiltered or filtered tubing
    - Selecting infusion technique
        - Gravity infusion
        - Electronic infusion device
            - Infusion pump
            - Volumetric controllers
    - Preparing the client
    - Performing venipuncture
        - Venipuncture sites
    - Venipuncture devices
        - Peripheral venous access devices
        - Central venous access devices
    - Monitoring for complications
        - Phlebitis
        - Thrombus
    - Discontinuing IV therapy
        - Medication lock (saline lock)
- Special considerations for IV therapy
    - TPN
    - Blood transfusion
        - Equipment
        - Compatibility
        - Complications

CRITICAL THINKING EXERCISES

1. Determine the rate of infusion for 1000 mL of solution ordered to infuse by gravity over 10 hours. You have tubing with a drop factor of 15 gtt/mL. Explain how you determine if the solution is infusing according to the calculated rate.
2. How is the administration of IV fluid different for an older adult compared with an individual who is middle age or younger?
3. If a unit of type A Rh-negative blood is obtained from the blood bank for administration to a client who is type A Rh-positive, what action is appropriate?
4. What action is appropriate if the site where an IV fluid is infusing appears swollen and feels cool and tender when palpated?
5. Explain whether it would be better to infuse 1000 mL of IV solution in 8 hours using a gravity infusion method or an electronic infusion device for a client who is confused and restless.

NCLEX-STYLE REVIEW QUESTIONS PrepU

1. What nursing intervention is most appropriate for relieving the anxiety of a client who is startled and worried about an alarm that sounded from an electronic IV infusion pump?
    1. Explain why the alarm sounded.
    2. Give a prescribed tranquilizer.
    3. Infuse the solution by gravity.
    4. Assure the client nothing is wrong.
2. Calculate the hourly infusion rate for a 1-L solution of dextrose 5% and normal saline (D_5NS) that should infuse in 8 hours using a volumetric controller. Record the answer in the nearest whole number.

    _________ mL/hour
3. When inspecting a current site used for IV therapy, what signs suggest that the IV fluid has infiltrated? Select all that apply.
    1. Redness at the venipuncture site
    2. Warmth along the vein
    3. Swelling at the site
    4. Decreased rate of infusion
    5. Elevated BP
    6. Drainage from the site
4. When discontinuing the administration of IV fluid, what nursing action is essential?
    1. Putting on clean gloves
    2. Weighing the client
    3. Pulling the privacy curtain
    4. Taking vital signs
5. What nursing assessment is essential for evaluating a client's response to the administration of TPN?
    1. Measuring the arterial pulse pressure
    2. Monitoring the capillary blood glucose
    3. Obtaining an apical–radial pulse rate
    4. Testing the urine's specific gravity

WANT TO KNOW MORE? There are a wide variety of online resources available on thePoint to enhance learning and understanding of this chapter.

Go to **thePoint.lww.com/activate** and use the activation code found in the front of this text to unlock these online resources.

14 Perioperative Care

Words To Know

ambulatory surgery
anesthesia
anesthesiologist
anesthetist
dehiscence
embolus
evisceration
intraoperative
malignant hyperthermia
paralytic ileus
perioperative
phlebothrombosis
postoperative
preoperative
procedural sedation
surgical asepsis
thrombophlebitis

Learning Objectives

On completion of this chapter, you will be able to:

1. Describe why surgical procedures may be performed.
2. Differentiate the phases of perioperative care.
3. Outline preoperative assessments needed to identify surgical risk factors.
4. List components of a preoperative teaching plan.
5. Describe physical preparation of the client for surgery.
6. List preoperative medications that may be ordered.
7. Discuss psychosocial preparation of the client for surgery, including strategies for alleviating clients' preoperative anxiety.
8. Compare types of anesthesia.
9. Describe the roles and functions of the surgical team members.
10. Describe nursing management of the intraoperative client.
11. Discuss assessments needed to prevent postoperative complications.
12. Describe standards of care, nursing analyses, and common interventions for general surgical clients in the later postoperative period.

Clients undergo surgery for a variety of reasons (Table 14-1). No matter how minor, surgery causes stress and poses risks for complications for the client. Many variables, such as the procedure performed, age of the client, and coexisting medical conditions, determine the care clients need before, during, and after surgery. However, administering anesthesia and disrupting physiologic processes (i.e., through creation of the surgical wound and the operation itself) subject all clients undergoing surgery to a common set of problems. These problems require standardized, in addition to individualized, assessments and interventions. As much as possible, clients require comprehensive education before and after surgery. Table 14-2 categorizes surgery in terms of urgency.

Gerontologic Considerations

- Diminished abilities to hear, see, and understand may interfere with preoperative and postoperative teaching. Removal of assistive devices such as eyeglasses or hearing aids before surgical procedures may cause sensory deprivation or contribute to confusion.
- Nurses may need to repeat explanations and demonstrations and include family members or significant others, always being aware of potential for cognitive changes

Gerontologic Considerations (*continued*)

due to physical condition, pain, effects of medications, or change in environment.

- Techniques of motivational interviewing include encouraging the person's belief that change is needed and is possible (see https://motivationalinterviewing.org/understanding-motivational-interviewing). For example, when discussing deep breathing and coughing, include the intended outcome of clearing mucus from the lungs and express confidence and encouragement that the person will be able to do so.
- Asking the client or family member to teach back important components of any instructions helps the nurse to ascertain understanding and areas that may need to be clarified.
- During the preoperative phase, discussion among all health care providers can improve assessment in nine categories (cognitive/behavioral disorders, cardiac, pulmonary, function/performance, nutrition, frailty, client counseling, preoperative testing, and management of essential and nonessential medications).
- Medications such as anesthesia, narcotics, and barbiturates may cause confusion, disorientation, and other physiologic alterations. Opioid-sparing techniques can be used in the preoperative, intraoperative, and postoperative periods.
- An age-related loss of elasticity of blood vessels may place the older client at higher risk for injury related to prolonged surgical positioning. Therefore, pressure relief is needed every 1.5 to 2 hours based on the skin assessment of blanching. Presence of chronic conditions such as arthritis may necessitate special positioning. Chronic health conditions and age-related physical changes (e.g., cardiac, renal, respiratory, immunologic conditions) may also increase the risks associated with surgical procedures. Specific assessment tools for older adults can help identify potential intraoperative complications.
- A major adverse reaction to anesthesia in older adults is decreased mental functioning, which can manifest with symptoms similar to delirium or dementia.
- Medications such as narcotics and barbiturates may cause confusion and disorientation in older adults, even when given in standard doses. The respiratory depressive effects of narcotics may also be increased in older adults.
- A thinning of the skin and loss of subcutaneous tissue accompany the aging process. This may lead to poor wound healing, tissue breakdown caused by excessive pressure on a part, or inadequate development of granulation tissue in healing wounds. Additionally, older adults may have a diminished immunologic response, leading to a higher risk for infection.
- Older adults are more prone to postoperative complications such as shock, atelectasis, pneumonia, paralytic ileus, gastric dilatation, and venous stasis. The increased risk is due to age-related changes in metabolism of anesthetics and vulnerability of organ systems as well as chronic illness. Cognitive changes may be an indication of urinary tract infection.
- If an older adult lives alone or with a spouse who is experiencing functional decline, additional considerations must be given to discharge planning. This client may require the services of relatives or friends, a public health nurse, a visiting nurse, or home health care personnel during the recovery period. In some instances, admitting the client to a skilled nursing facility for rehabilitation is necessary.

TABLE 14-1 Reasons for Surgery

TYPE OF SURGERY	PURPOSE	EXAMPLES
Diagnostic	Removal and study of tissue to make a diagnosis	Breast biopsy Biopsy of skin lesion
Exploratory	More extensive means to diagnose a problem; usually involves exploration of a body cavity or use of scopes inserted through small incisions	Exploration of abdomen for unexplained pain Exploratory laparoscopy
Curative or reparative	Removal of a tumor or diseased organ, replacement of defective tissue to restore function, or repair of multiple wounds	Cholecystectomy Total hip replacement
Palliative	Relief of symptoms or enhancement of function without cure	Resection of a tumor to relieve pressure and pain
Cosmetic	Reshape normal body structures or improve appearance or change a physical feature	Rhinoplasty Cleft lip repair Mammoplasty
Preventive or prophylactic	Removal of tissue that does not yet contain cancer cells, but has a high probability of becoming cancerous in the future	Prophylactic bilateral oophorectomy (removal of both ovaries)
Reconstructive	Repair or reconstruct physical deformities and abnormalities caused by traumatic injuries, birth defects, developmental abnormalities, or disease	Breast reconstruction following mastectomy Cleft lip repair

TABLE 14-2 Categories of Surgery Based on Urgency

CLASSIFICATION	CONDITIONS	EXAMPLES
Emergency	Immediate; condition is life threatening, requiring surgery at once	Gunshot wound Severe bleeding Small bowel obstruction
Urgent	Within 24–30 hours; client requires prompt attention	Kidney stones Acute gallbladder infection Fractured hip
Required	Planned for a few weeks or months after decision; client requires surgery at some point	Benign prostatic hypertrophy Cataracts Hernia without strangulation
Elective	Client will not be harmed if surgery is not performed but will benefit if it is performed	Revision of scars Vaginal repairs
Optional	Personal preference	Cosmetic surgery

Adapted from Hinkle, J. L., & Cheever, K. H. (2018). *Brunner & Suddarth's textbook of medical-surgical nursing* (14th ed.). Wolters Kluwer.

Traditionally, any surgical procedure required admitting the client to the hospital. However, many diagnostic or short therapeutic surgical procedures—such as bone marrow biopsy, endoscopy, or cardiac catheterization—are now performed in outpatient settings and ambulatory surgical centers. **Ambulatory surgery**, sometimes referred to as *same-day* or *outpatient surgery*, is defined as surgery that requires fewer than 24 hours of hospitalization. These short-term admissions may be as brief as 1 to 2 hours or extend to overnight. Ambulatory surgical units are located either in a hospital or in a separate building that the hospital owns. Others are freestanding, privately owned facilities not affiliated with a hospital.

The increase in the number of ambulatory surgical procedures is related to advances in surgical techniques and methods of anesthesia, prospective reimbursement, managed care, and changes in Medicare and Medicaid provisions. A client admitted for ambulatory surgery must meet the following criteria:

- The client is not critically ill.
- The surgical procedure is not extensive and does not require many hours of general anesthesia.
- The client has few, if any, coexisting and disabling illnesses.
- Recovery is expected to be quick, with minimal specialized care after surgery.
- The client or family can provide adequate postoperative care.

Regardless of the setting, nursing goals when caring for surgical clients are to minimize clients' anxiety, prepare them for surgery, monitor for complications during surgery, and assist in a speedy, uncomplicated recovery. **Perioperative** is a term used to describe the entire span of surgery, including before and after the actual operation. The three phases of perioperative care are as follows:

1. **Preoperative:** begins with the decision to perform surgery and continues until the client reaches the operating area
2. **Intraoperative:** includes the entire surgical procedure until transfer of the client to the recovery area
3. **Postoperative:** begins with admission to the recovery area and continues until the client receives a follow-up evaluation at home or is discharged to a rehabilitation unit

Each phase requires specific assessments and nursing interventions.

BOX 14-1 Preoperative Assessment

Review Preoperative Laboratory and Diagnostic Studies
- Complete blood count
- Blood type and crossmatch
- Serum electrolytes
- Urinalysis
- Chest X-ray
- Electrocardiogram
- Other tests related to procedure or client's medical condition (e.g., prothrombin time, partial thromboplastin time, blood urea nitrogen, creatinine, other radiographic studies)

Review Client's Health History and Preparation for Surgery
- History of present illness and reason for surgery
- Past medical history
  - Medical conditions—acute and chronic
  - Previous hospitalizations and surgeries
  - Any past problems with anesthesia
  - Allergies
  - Present medications
- Substance use: alcohol, tobacco, street drugs
- Review of systems

Assess Physical Needs
- Ability to communicate
- Vital signs
- Level of consciousness
  - Confusion
  - Drowsiness
  - Unresponsiveness
- Weight and height
- Skin integrity
- Ability to move/ambulate
- Level of exercise
- Prostheses
- Circulatory status

Assess Psychological Needs
- Emotional state
- Level of understanding of surgical procedure and preoperative and postoperative instructions
- Coping strategies
- Support system
- Roles and responsibilities

Assess Cultural Needs
- Language—need for an interpreter
- Particular customs related to surgery, privacy, disposal of body parts, and blood transfusions

PREOPERATIVE CARE

Time for preoperative assessment, nursing analyses, and evaluation of nursing management may be limited when a client is admitted for ambulatory surgery or shortly before surgery. Recognition of the client's immediate preoperative needs is important, however, and preparation for surgery still requires the nursing process.

Assessment

Preoperative care requires a complete assessment of the client (Box 14-1). The assessment varies depending on the urgency of the surgery and whether the client is admitted the same day of surgery or earlier. For any preoperative client, however, the nurse must make every effort to gather as much data as possible.

On admission, the nurse reviews preoperative instructions, such as diet restrictions and skin preparations, to ensure the client has followed them. If the client has not carried out a specific portion of the instructions, such as withholding foods and fluids, the nurse immediately notifies the surgeon. They identify the client's needs to determine if the client is at risk for complications during or after the surgery. General risk factors are related to age; nutritional status; use of alcohol, tobacco, and other substances; and physical condition (Table 14-3).

When surgery is not an emergency, the nurse performs a thorough history and physical examination. They assess the client's understanding of the surgical procedure, postoperative expectations, and ability to participate in recovery. The nurse also considers the client's cultural needs, specifically as they relate to beliefs about surgery, personal privacy, disposal of body parts, blood transfusions, and presence of family members during the preoperative and postoperative phases (see Chapter 8).

If the surgical procedure is an emergency, the nurse may have to omit some tasks because of the client's condition or need for rapid preparation. There may not be time to perform a thorough assessment or write a complete care plan. Assessment of the surgical client is essential, but the situation dictates the extent of this process.

»> *Stop, Think, and Respond 14-1*

A client who is admitted for knee replacement surgery is 100 lb overweight. What are the potential postoperative concerns?

Surgical Consent

Before surgery, the client must sign a surgical consent form or operative permit. When signed, this form indicates that the client consents to the procedure and understands its risks and benefits as explained by the surgeon. Box 14-2 describes the criteria needed for valid informed consent. If the client has not understood the explanations, the nurse notifies the surgeon before the client signs the consent form. Clients must sign a consent form for any invasive procedure that requires anesthesia and has risks of complications. (See also Evidence-Based Practice 14-1.)

If an adult client is confused, unconscious, or not mentally competent, a family member or guardian must sign the consent form. If the client is younger than 18 years of age, a parent or legal guardian must sign the consent form. Persons younger than 18 years of age living away from home and supporting themselves are regarded as emancipated minors and sign their own consent forms. In an emergency, the surgeon may have to operate without consent. Health care providers, however, make every effort to obtain consent by telephone and e-mail. Each nurse must be familiar with agency policies and state laws regarding surgical consent forms.

TABLE 14-3 Surgical Risk Factors and Potential Complications

VARIABLE	POTENTIAL COMPLICATION
Age	
Very young—immaturity of organ systems and regulatory mechanisms	Respiratory obstruction, fluid overload, dehydration, hypothermia, and infection
Older adults—multiple organ degeneration and slowed regulatory mechanisms	Decreased metabolism and excretion of anesthetics and pain medications, fluid overload, renal failure, formation of blood clots, delayed wound healing, infection, confusion, and respiratory complications
Nutritional Status	
Malnourished—low weight and nutrient deficiencies	Fluid and electrolyte imbalances, cardiac dysrhythmias, delayed wound healing, wound infections
Obese—stressed cardiovascular system, decreased circulation, decreased pulmonary function	Atelectasis, pneumonia, blood clots, delayed wound healing, wound infection, delayed metabolism and excretion of anesthetics and pain medication
Substance Abuse	
Altered respiratory function, nutritional status, or liver function	Atelectasis, pneumonia, altered effectiveness of anesthetics and pain medications, drug interactions, drug withdrawal
Medical Problems	
Immune—allergies and immunosuppression secondary to corticosteroid therapy, transplants, chemotherapy, or diseases such as AIDS	Adverse reactions to medications, blood transfusions, or latex; infection
Respiratory—acute and chronic respiratory problems and history of tobacco use	Atelectasis, bronchopneumonia, respiratory failure
Cardiovascular—hypertension, coronary artery disease, peripheral vascular disease	Hypotension, hypertension, fluid overload, congestive heart failure, shock, dysrhythmias, myocardial infarction, stroke, blood clots
Hepatic—liver dysfunction	Delayed drug metabolism leading to drug toxicity, disrupted clotting mechanisms leading to excessive bleeding or hemorrhage, confusion, increased risk of infection
Renal—kidney disease, chronic renal insufficiency, renal failure	Fluid and electrolyte imbalances, congestive heart failure, dysrhythmias, delayed excretion of drugs leading to drug toxicity
Endocrine—diabetes	Hypoglycemia, hyperglycemia, hypokalemia, infection, delayed wound healing

BOX 14-2 Criteria for Valid Informed Consent

Voluntary Consent
Valid consent must be freely given, without coercion. Client must be at least 18 years of age (unless an emancipated minor), a primary provider must obtain consent, and a professional staff member must witness the client's signature.

Incompetent Client
Legal definition: individual who is *not* autonomous and cannot give or withhold consent (e.g., individuals who are cognitively impaired, mentally ill, or neurologically incapacitated).

Informed Subject
Informed consent should be in writing. It should contain the following:

- Explanation of procedure and its risks
- Descriptions of benefits and alternatives
- An offer to answer questions about procedure
- Instructions that the client may withdraw consent
- A statement informing the client if the protocol differs from customary procedure

Client Able to Comprehend
If the client is non-English speaking, it is necessary to provide consent (written and verbal) in a language that is understandable to the client. A trained medical interpreter may be consulted. Alternative formats of communication (e.g., Braille, large print, sign interpreter) may be needed if the client has a disability that affects vision or hearing. Questions must be answered to facilitate comprehension if material is confusing.

Clients must sign the consent form before receiving any preoperative sedatives. When the client or designated person has signed the permit, a professional staff member serves as a witness and signs the permit to indicate that the client or designee signed voluntarily. The nurse is responsible for ensuring that all necessary parties have signed the consent form and that it is in the client's chart before the client goes to the operating room (OR).

Preoperative Teaching

Teaching clients about their surgical procedure and expectations before and after surgery is best done during the preoperative period. Clients are more alert and free of pain at this time. Clients and family members can better participate in recovery if they know what to expect. The nurse adapts instructions and explanations to the client's ability to understand. When clients understand what they can do to help themselves recover, they are more likely to follow the preoperative instructions and work with health care team members.

Information to include in a preoperative teaching plan varies with the type of surgery and the length of the hospitalization. The following are examples of information to include in preoperative teaching:

- Preoperative medications—when they are given and their effects
- Postoperative pain control
- Explanation and description of the postanesthesia recovery room or postsurgical area
- Discussion of the frequency of assessing vital signs and use of monitoring equipment

The nurse also explains and demonstrates deep-breathing and coughing exercises, use of incentive spirometry, how to splint the incision for breathing exercises and moving, position changes, and feet and leg exercises. In addition, the nurse must inform the client about intravenous (IV) fluids

Evidence-Based Practice 14-1

The Nurse's Role in Informed Consent

Clinical Question

What is the nurse's role in informed consent of a client?

Evidence

A research study was completed in Southeast Asia with primary providers and nurses to compare views on both of their roles in informed consent. Three factors were surveyed: the views of roles, barriers, and adequacy of information were included in a survey between two hospitals that included 129 primary providers and 616 nurses (Susilo et al., 2014). The study found that there was a gap in what the primary providers and nurses viewed as their roles. The informed consent policies also differed between facilities. The study felt that legal and ethical knowledge in informed consent and interpersonal communication would be supportive to the views of these roles and what each practitioner is responsible for. In conclusion, the study identified gaps in the above three factors and recommended that an interdisciplinary approach to educating staff be implemented. It was also suggested that individual facilities provide a survey type assessment first of their nurses and primary providers to see where the gaps are in informed consent roles and then formulate their education processes.

Nursing Implications

Interdisciplinary communication takes place in nursing with different staff and practitioners. Nurses have a role responsibility in informed consent of a client. The above study identified gaps between practitioners in the health care facility. Nurses should be current in their state law on ethics and standards of practice in informed consent. In the nursing role, it is also important to know the primary provider's role responsibilities to make sure that the client is informed correctly before any type of care or treatment occurs. Increasing nurse communication in an interdisciplinary approach may decrease gaps, barriers, and ultimately the client's experience.

Reference

Susilo, A. P., Dalen, J. V., Chenault, M. N., & Scherpbier, A. (2014). Informed consent and nurses' roles: A survey of Indonesian practitioners. *Nursing Ethics, 21*(6), 684–694. https://doi.org/10.1177/0969733014531524

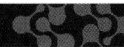

and other lines and tubes. Sometimes, IV fluids are initiated before surgery, along with indwelling catheters or nasogastric tubes. When clients receive demonstrations, it is important that they practice these skills and provide an opportunity for the nurse to assess whether they understood the instructions. Preoperative teaching time also gives clients the chance to express any anxieties and fears and for the nurse to provide explanations that will help alleviate those fears.

When clients are admitted for emergency surgery, time for detailed explanations of preoperative preparations and the postoperative period is usually unavailable. If the client is alert, however, the nurse provides brief explanations as much as possible. During the postoperative period, explanations will be more complete. Family members require as many preoperative explanations as possible.

The purpose of adequate preoperative teaching/learning is for the client to have an uncomplicated and shorter recovery period. They will be more likely to deep breathe and cough, move as directed, and require less pain medication. The client and family members will demonstrate sufficient knowledge of the surgical procedure, preoperative preparations, and postoperative procedures and can participate fully in the client's care.

Physical Preparation

Preparing a client for surgery is an essential element of preoperative care. Depending on the time of admission to the hospital or surgical facility, the nurse may perform some of the physical preparation, which includes the following:

- *Skin preparation:* Skin preparation depends on the surgical procedure and the policies of the surgeon or institution. The goal is to decrease bacteria without compromising skin integrity. For planned surgery, the client may be asked to cleanse the particular area with detergent germicide soap for several days before surgery. Hair usually is not removed before surgery unless it is likely to interfere with the incision. In that case, the hair is removed with electric clippers at the time of surgery.
- *Elimination:* The nurse may need to insert an indwelling urinary catheter preoperatively for some surgeries, particularly of the lower abdomen. A distended bladder increases the risk of bladder trauma and difficulty in performing the procedure. The catheter keeps the bladder empty during surgery. If a catheter is not inserted, the nurse instructs the client to void immediately before receiving preoperative medication. Enemas or laxatives may be ordered to clean out the lower bowel if the client is having abdominal or pelvic surgery. A clean bowel allows for accurate visualization of the surgical site and prevents trauma to the intestine or accidental contamination by feces to the peritoneum. A cleansing enema or laxative is prescribed the evening before surgery and may be repeated the morning of surgery.
- *Food and fluids:* The primary provider gives specific instructions about how long before surgery food and fluids are to be withheld, often at least 8 to 10 hours before surgery. After midnight the night before surgery, the client may not be allowed to have anything by mouth (NPO). According to new recommendations, healthy clients having elective surgery may be told they can have clear liquids up to 2 hours before surgery. Many ambulatory surgical centers allow clear fluids up to 3 or 4 hours before surgery. Before these times, the nurse encourages the client to maintain good nutrition to help meet the body's increased need for nutrients during the healing process. Adequate intake of protein and ascorbic acid (vitamin C) is especially important in wound healing.
- *Care of valuables:* The nurse encourages the client to give valuables to a family member to take home. If this is not possible, however, the nurse itemizes the valuables, places them in an envelope, and locks them in a designated area. The client signs a receipt, and the nurse notes their deposition on the client's chart. If the client is reluctant to remove a wedding band, some facilities allow the nurse to slip gauze under the ring, then loop the gauze around the finger and wrist or apply adhesive tape over a plain wedding band. The client also removes eyeglasses and contact lenses, which the nurse places in a safe location or gives to a family member.
- *Attire/grooming:* Usually, clients wear a hospital gown and a surgical cap in the OR. Hair ornaments and all makeup and nail polish must be removed. If the client is having minor surgery performed under local anesthesia in a room separate from the general surgical suites, the nurse instructs the client on what clothing and cosmetics to remove and provides appropriate hospital attire. The primary provider may order thigh-high or knee-high antiembolism stockings or order the client's legs to be wrapped in elastic bandages before surgery to help prevent venous stasis during and after the surgery. Removal of cosmetics assists the surgical team to observe the client's lips, face, and nail beds for cyanosis, pallor, or other signs of decreased oxygenation. If a client has acrylic nails, one usually is removed to attach a pulse oximeter, which measures oxygen saturation (see Chapter 19).
- *Prostheses:* Depending on agency policy and primary provider preference, the client removes full or partial dentures. Doing so prevents the dentures from becoming dislodged or causing airway obstruction during administration of a general anesthetic. Some anesthesiologists prefer that well-fitting dentures be left in place to preserve facial contours. If dentures are removed, the nurse usually places them in a denture container and leaves them at the client's bedside or places them with the client's belongings. Other prostheses, such as artificial limbs, also are removed, unless otherwise ordered.

Preoperative Medications

The anesthesiologist frequently orders preoperative medications, although these may be used more infrequently in an ambulatory surgery setting. Common preoperative medications include one or more of the following:

- *Antianxiety drugs*, such as lorazepam, reduce preoperative anxiety, cause slight sedation, slow motor activity, and promote the induction of anesthesia.
- *Histamine-2 receptor antagonists*, such as cimetidine, decrease gastric acidity and volume.

- *Anticholinergics*, such as glycopyrrolate, decrease respiratory secretions, dry mucous membranes, and prevent vagal nerve stimulation during endotracheal intubation.
- *Neuromuscular blocking agents*, such as succinylcholine, promote skeletal muscle relaxation during procedure, allowing for rapid intubation.
- *Opioids*, such as fentanyl, sedate and decrease the amount of anesthesia.
- *Sedatives*, such as midazolam, promote sleep or amnesia and decrease anxiety.
- *Antibiotics,* such as kanamycin, destroy enteric microorganisms.

Drug Therapy Table 14-1 provides more information about dosages and the desired and adverse effects of preoperative medications.

Before administering preoperative medications, the nurse checks the client's identification bracelet, asks about drug allergies, obtains blood pressure (BP) and pulse and respiratory rates, asks the client to void, and makes sure the surgical consent form has been signed. The nurse also reviews with the client what to expect after receiving the medications. Immediately after giving the medications, the nurse instructs the client to remain in bed; they place side rails in the up position and ensure that the call button is within easy reach.

Pharmacologic Considerations

- Clients are frequently instructed to take preoperative or routine medications at home before procedures; this is especially important for those who take heart, hypertension, or diabetes medications. It is critical for the primary provider to know when and what dose was taken for appropriate monitoring during procedures.

DRUG THERAPY TABLE 14-1 Preoperative Medications

Category and Common Generic (Brand) Drugs	Intended Use	Common Side Effects	Safety Warnings for Nurses
Antianxiety/Sedative			
Benzodiazepines Diazepam (Valium) Lorazepam (Ativan) Midazolam *Non-benzodiazepines* Hydroxyzine (Vistaril) Propofol (Diprivan)	Reduce preoperative anxiety and promote induction of anesthesia. Hydroxyzine also works as an antiemetic.	Dry mouth, drowsiness	Depressed breathing, monitor if given with opiate Increased fall risk due to sedative side effects
Gastric Acid Reducers			
H2 receptor antagonists Cimetidine (Tagamet), ranitidine (Zantac), famotidine (Pepcid) *Protein pump inhibitors* Omeprazole (Prilosec) Lansoprazole (Prevacid)	Reduce GI acidity and gastric volume.	Headache, dizziness, drowsiness, nausea, gas	Cimetidine can cause mental confusion in the older adult.
Anticholinergics			
Atropine Glycopyrrolate (Robinul) Scopolamine	Decrease oral, respiratory, and gastric secretions; prevent laryngospasm and reflex bradycardia.	Dry mouth, tachycardia, urinary retention	Increased fall risk due to sedative side effects
Neuromuscular Blocking Agents			
Succinylcholine (Anectine)	Promote skeletal muscle relaxation during procedure; allow for rapid intubation.	Respiratory depression	Monitor for hyperkalemia.
Analgesics			
Opioid Fentanyl (Sublimaze) NSAID Ketorolac (Toradol)	Sedate and decrease the amount of anesthesia needed, control post-op shivers.	Sedation, hypotension, vertigo, euphoria, nausea, vomiting, urinary retention, constipation	Watch for respiratory depression in opiate-naïve clients. Treat constipation early with laxatives and fiber.
Antiemetics			
Ondansetron (Zofran) Promethazine (Phenergan)	Reduce nausea, prevent emesis, and enhance preoperative sedation. Ondansetron is given end of procedure to reduce post-op nausea.	Lightheadedness, dry mouth; urinary retention; hypotension	Ondansetron may cause abnormal cardiac electrical activity. Promethazine has extravasation potential if it leaks into soft tissue.

GI, gastrointestinal; NSAID, nonsteroidal antiinflammatory drug.

Psychosocial Preparation

Preparing the client emotionally and spiritually is as important as doing so physically. Psychosocial preparation should begin as soon as the client is aware that surgery is necessary. Anxiety and fear, if extreme, can affect a client's condition during and after surgery. Anxious clients have a poor response to surgery and are prone to complications. Many clients are fearful because they know little or nothing about what will happen before, during, and after surgery. Careful preoperative teaching and listening by the nurse about what will happen and what to expect can help allay some of these fears and anxieties. The nurse also must assess methods the client uses for coping. Religious faith is a source of strength for many clients; therefore, nurses facilitate contact with a client's clergyperson or the hospital chaplain if requested.

Preoperative Checklist

Most clients are transported to the OR on a stretcher. To provide privacy, safety, and warmth, the nurse covers the client with a blanket and fastens restraint straps around the client. Before the client leaves the room, the nurse records all necessary information on the client's chart: vital signs, weight, preoperative medications administered, procedures performed, whether the client has voided, disposition of valuables and dentures, and pertinent observations.

Most hospitals or surgical facilities use a preoperative checklist to ensure that all assessments and procedures for the client are complete before surgery. A checklist (Fig. 14-1) usually includes the following:

- *Assessment:* includes the identification and allergy bracelet; identification of allergies; list of current medications; last time the client ate or drank; disposition of valuables,

1. Client's name: ________ Date: ________ Height: ________ Weight: ________
   Identification band present: ________
2. Informed consent signed: ________ Special permits signed: ________
3. Surgical site: ________ (Ex: Sterilization)
4. History & physical examination report present: ________ Date: ________
5. Laboratory records present: ________
   CBC: ________ Hgb: ________ Urinalysis: ________ Hct: ________

6.

Item	Present	Removed
a. Natural teeth	________	________
Dentures: upper, lower, partial	________	________
Bridge: fixed, crown	________	________
b. Contact lenses	________	________
c. Other prostheses—type: ________	________	________
d. Jewelry:		
Wedding band (taped/tied)	________	________
Rings	________	________
Earrings: pierced, clip-on	________	________
Neck chains	________	________
Any other body piercings	________	________
e. Make-up	________	________
Nail polish	________	________

7. Clothing

a. Clean client gown	________	________
b. Cap	________	________
c. Sanitary pad, etc.	________	________

8. Family instructed where to wait? ________
9. Valuables secured? ________
10. Blood available? ________ Ordered? ________ Where? ________
11. Preanesthetic medication given: ________
    Type: ________ Time: ________
12. Voided: ________ Amount: ________ Time: ________ Catheter: ________
    Mouth care given: ________
13. Vital signs: Temperature: ________ Pulse: ________ Resp: ________ Blood pressure: ________
14. Special problems/precautions (Allergies, deafness, etc.): ________
15. Area of skin preparation: ________
16. ________ Date: ________ Time: ________
    Signature: Nurse releasing client

Figure 14-1 Example of a preoperative checklist.

dentures, or prostheses; removal of makeup and nail polish; and wearing of hospital attire

- *Preoperative medications:* includes route and time administered
- *IV:* includes location, type of solution, and rate
- *Preoperative preparations:* includes, as appropriate, skin preparation, indwelling urinary catheter or nasogastric tube insertion, times and results of enemas or douches, application of antiembolism stockings or wraps, and time and amount of last voiding
- *Medical record:* includes signed surgical consent, history and physical completed by primary provider, old records, and ordered test results (e.g., electrocardiogram, complete blood count, urinalysis, type and screen or type and crossmatch for blood transfusions)
- *Other information:* as required by agency policy
- *Signature(s):* of nurse and other personnel involved with preparing the client for surgery and transporting the client to the OR

When the preoperative checklist is complete, the client is ready to go to the operating suite. Personnel from the OR assist in the transfer of the client to the stretcher and then to the OR or surgical holding area.

There is an increased emphasis on making sure that the right client has the right procedure at the right site. To prevent "wrong site, wrong procedure, wrong person surgery," The Joint Commission (2020) established a universal protocol to achieve this goal (Box 14-3).

BOX 14-3 Universal Protocol for Preventing Wrong Site, Wrong Procedure, Wrong Person Surgery

Conduct a Preprocedure Verification Process

Address missing information or discrepancies before starting the procedure.

- Verify the correct procedure, for the correct client, at the correct site.
- When possible, involve the client in the verification process.
- Identify the items that must be available for the procedure.
- Use a standardized list to verify the availability of items for the procedure (it is not necessary to document that the list was used for each client). At a minimum, these items include:
  - Relevant documentation. *Examples:* history and physical, signed consent form, preanesthesia assessment
  - Labeled diagnostic and radiology test results that are properly displayed
  - Any required blood products, implants, devices, special equipment
- Match the items that are to be available in the procedure area to the client.

Mark the Procedure Site

At a minimum, mark the site when there is more than one possible location for the procedure and when performing the procedure in a different location could harm the client.

- For spinal procedures, mark the general spinal region on the skin. Special intraoperative imaging techniques may be used to locate and mark the exact vertebral level.
- Mark the site before the procedure is performed.
- If possible, involve the client in the site-marking process. The site is marked by a licensed independent practitioner who is ultimately accountable for the procedure and will be present when the procedure is performed.
- In limited circumstances, site marking may be delegated to some medical residents, physician assistants (PA), or advanced practice registered nurses (APRN).
- Ultimately, the licensed independent practitioner is accountable for the procedure, even when delegating site marking.
- The mark is unambiguous and is used consistently throughout the organization.
- The mark is made at or near the procedure site.
- The mark is sufficiently permanent to be visible after skin preparation and draping.
- Adhesive markers are not the sole means of marking the site.
- For clients who refuse site marking or when it is technically or anatomically impossible or impractical to mark the site (see examples below): Use your organization's written, alternative process to ensure that the correct site is operated on. Examples of situations that involve alternative processes:
  - mucosal surfaces or perineum
  - minimal access procedures treating a lateralized internal organ, whether percutaneous or through a natural orifice
  - teeth
  - premature infants, for whom the mark may cause a permanent tattoo

Perform a "Time-Out"

The procedure is not started until all questions or concerns are resolved:

- Conduct a time-out immediately before starting the invasive procedure or making the incision.
- A designated member of the team starts the time-out.
- The time-out is standardized.
- The time-out involves the immediate members of the procedure team: the individual performing the procedure, anesthesia providers, circulating nurse, operating room technician, and other active participants who will be participating in the procedure from the beginning.
- All relevant members of the procedure team actively communicate during the time-out.
- During the time-out, the team members agree, at a minimum, on the following:
  - Correct client identity
  - Correct site
  - Procedure to be done
- When the same client has two or more procedures: If the person performing the procedure changes, another time-out needs to be performed before starting each procedure.
- Document the completion of the time-out. The organization determines the amount and type of documentation.

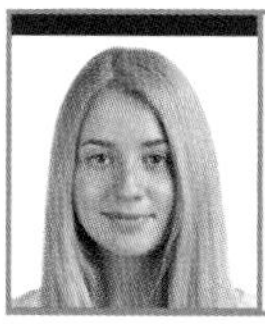

Clinical Scenario A 25-year-old client is scheduled for an appendectomy in a short-stay facility (less than 24 hours). The client has never been hospitalized nor had any type of surgical procedure before. **What is important for the nurse to include in the plan of care? What questions should the nurse ask when assisting the client preoperatively? See the following Nursing Process section.**

NURSING PROCESS FOR PREOPERATIVE CARE

Assessment

Assess the client's physical and psychological status, as described earlier in this section. Include questions about the client's fears and concerns, knowledge about surgery in general, and about appendectomies in particular. Ask the client about what information the surgeon has provided.

Analysis, Planning, and Interventions

Acute Anxiety: Related to impending surgery, results of surgery, and postoperative pain
Expected Outcome: Client will verbalize feelings of anxiety.

- Ask what concerns the client has about the upcoming surgery. *Such discussion provides specific information about the client's fears.*
- Provide appropriate explanations for preoperative procedures and postoperative expectations. *Clients experience less anxiety if they know what to expect.*
- Maintain as much contact as possible with the client. *Being present and approachable encourages communication.*

Knowledge Deficiency: Related to preoperative procedures and postoperative expectations
Expected Outcome: Client will verbalize understanding of preoperative and postoperative procedures.

- Assess client's level of knowledge about the perioperative plans. *Building on a client's knowledge assists in reinforcing instructions and helps to correct false information.*
- Use audiovisual aids to present information. *Verbal reinforcement of other forms of instruction promotes learning.*
- Include family members or significant others in preoperative instructions. *These people help in reinforcing instructions and providing support to the client.*

Evaluation of Expected Outcomes

The client reports minimal anxiety, demonstrates knowledge of the preoperative instructions, and verbalizes understanding of what they can expect postoperatively.

INTRAOPERATIVE CARE

The intraoperative period begins when the client is transferred to the operating table. The surgical team is responsible for the client's care during this time.

Anesthesia

Anesthesia is the partial or complete loss of the sensation of pain with or without loss of consciousness. Surgical procedures are performed with general, regional, or local anesthesia. Procedural sedation may also be used for ambulatory surgery. Clients need to be informed about the types of anesthesia and any associated risks. The Joint Commission has a Speak Up document related to anesthesia and sedation that provides important information for clients to review.

General Anesthesia

General **anesthesia** acts on the central nervous system to produce loss of sensation, reflexes, and consciousness. Anesthesia is used to induce a state of *narcosis*, in which medications are used to induce deep central nervous system depression, *analgesia* (absence of pain sensation), relaxation, and loss of reflexes. Vital functions such as breathing, circulation, and temperature control are not regulated physiologically when general anesthetics are used. General anesthetics are administered as IV, intramuscular (IM), inhaled (Fig. 14-2), or rectal medications. Four stages are used to describe the induction of general anesthesia.

- *Stage 1, Induction:* This short period is crucial for producing unconsciousness. The client experiences dizziness, detachment, a temporary heightened sense of awareness to noises and movements, and a sensation of "heavy" extremities and being unable to move them. Inhaled or IV anesthetics are used to produce this phase. When the client becomes unconscious, their airway is secured with an endotracheal tube.
- *Stage 2, Excitement:* During this stage, the client may struggle, shout, talk, sing, laugh, or cry. They may make

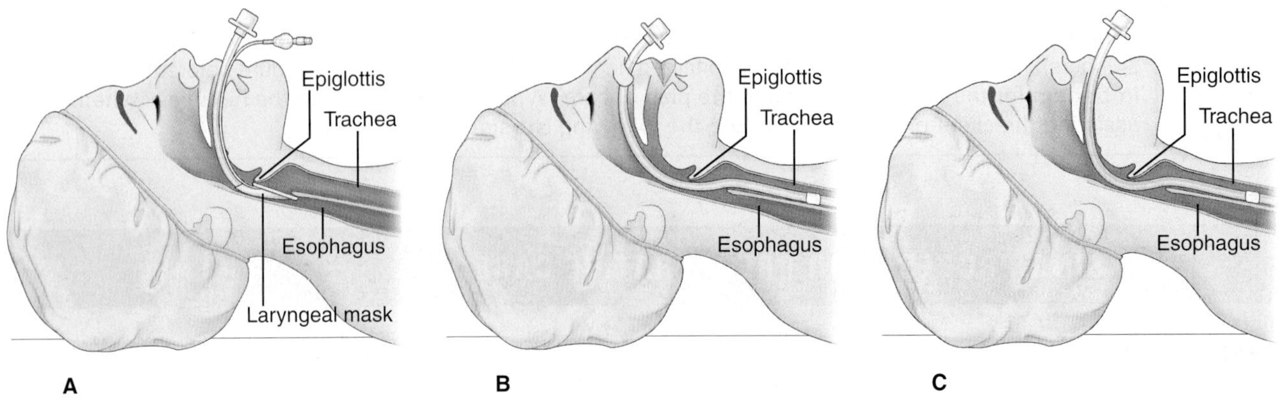

Figure 14-2 Inhaled anesthetic delivery methods: **(A)** laryngeal mask, **(B)** nasal endotracheal catheter (in position), and **(C)** oral endotracheal intubation (tube in position with cuff inflated).

uncontrolled movements, so team members must protect the client from falling or other injury. Quick and smooth administration of anesthesia can prevent this phase.

- *Stage 3, Surgical anesthesia:* In this stage, the client remains unconscious through continuous administration of the anesthetic agent. The muscles are relaxed and breathing is depressed. This level of anesthesia may be maintained for hours with a range of light to deep anesthesia.
- *Stage 4, Medullary depression:* This stage occurs when the client receives too much anesthesia. The client will have shallow respirations, weak pulse, and widely dilated pupils unresponsive to light. Without prompt intervention, death can occur.

Usually, with even, careful administration of general anesthesia, there is no major division between the first three stages, and the fourth stage does not occur. Throughout the duration of and recovery from anesthesia, team members closely monitor the client for effective breathing and oxygenation, effective circulatory status including BP and pulse within normal ranges, effective regulation of temperature, and adequate fluid balance. When anesthetics are carefully withdrawn at the end of a surgical procedure, the client will wake enough to follow commands and breathe independently. The endotracheal tube used for inhaled anesthetics may be removed before the client leaves the OR. The recovery period can be brief or long. Many effects of general anesthesia take some time for the client to eliminate completely. Usually, clients do not remember much about the initial recovery period.

Regional Anesthesia

Regional anesthesia uses local anesthetics to block the conduction of nerve impulses in a specific region (Drug Therapy Table 14-2). The client experiences loss of sensation and decreased mobility to the specific anesthetized area. They do not lose consciousness. Depending on the surgery, the client may be given a sedative before the local anesthetic to promote relaxation and comfort during the procedure. Types of regional anesthesia include local anesthetics, spinal anesthesia, and conduction blocks (Fig. 14-3).

Concept Mastery Alert

Regional anesthesia involves injecting an anesthetic agent around the nerves so that the area supplied by these nerves is anesthetized. Local anesthesia is one of several types of regional anesthesia that can be given by injection or topically.

DRUG THERAPY TABLE 14-2 Types of Regional Anesthesia

Type of Anesthesia	Administration and Intended Use	Drug Examples
Local anesthesia	Administered topically or by local infiltration. Palliative pain management may be delivered by pump into subcutaneous tissue. Provides local loss of sensation. Used with epinephrine to keep in local tissue and reduce bleeding. Used primarily for dental, eye, and minor surgeries.	Lidocaine (Xylocaine), procaine (Novocaine), tetracaine
Spinal anesthesia	Local anesthetic injected into the subarachnoid space of the lumbar area. Used for surgery involving the abdomen, perineum, and lower extremities.	Bupivacaine (Marcaine), lidocaine (Xylocaine), tetracaine
Conduction nerve block	Local anesthetic injected into or near a specific nerve trunk Uses vary widely—Epidural for obstetrics or brachial plexus block for arm/hand surgeries, trigeminal facial pain.	Bupivacaine (Marcaine), lidocaine (Xylocaine)

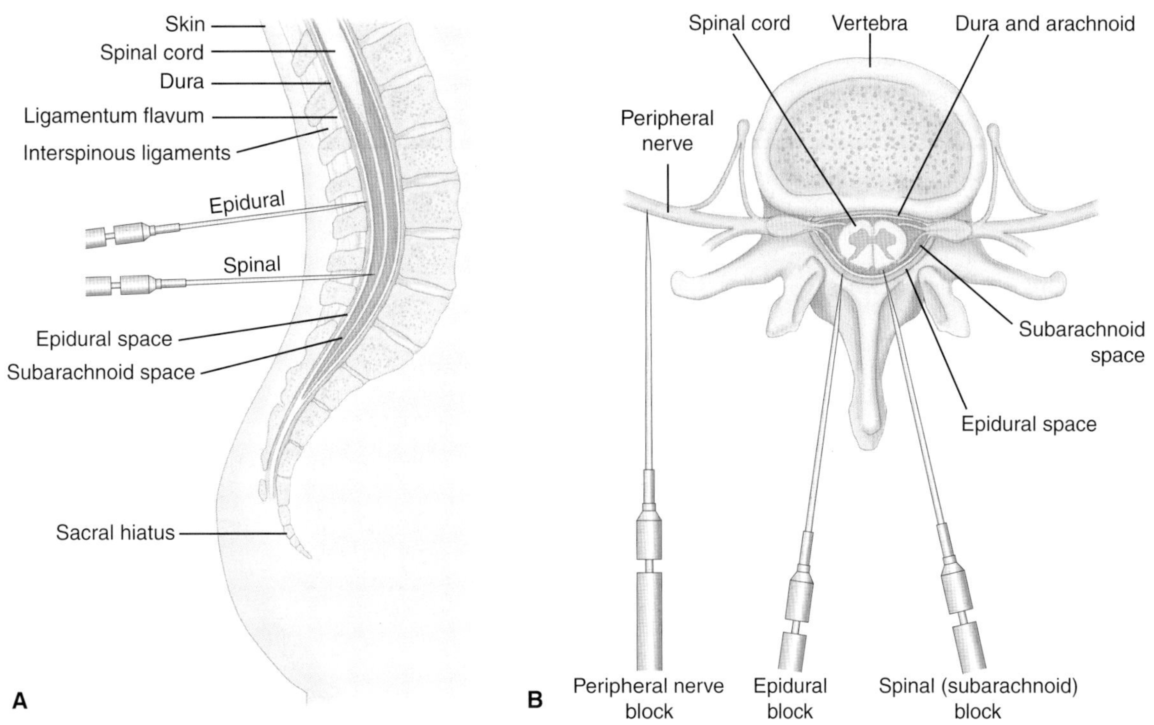

Figure 14-3 **(A)** Injection sites for spinal and epidural anesthesia. **(B)** Cross-section of injection sites for peripheral nerve, epidural, and spinal blocks. (Reprinted with permission from Hinkle, J. L., & Cheever, K. H. (2018). *Brunner & Suddarth's textbook of medical-surgical nursing* (14th ed.). Wolters Kluwer.)

Procedural Sedation

For many ambulatory surgery procedures, clients are sedated but not unconscious. *Sedation* refers to a pharmacologically induced state of relaxation and emotional comfort. *Analgesia* is the absence or relief of pain. **Procedural sedation** (also known as *moderate sedation* or *conscious sedation*) describes a state in which the client is free of pain, fear, and anxiety and can tolerate unpleasant procedures; the client maintains independent cardiorespiratory function and the ability to respond to verbal commands and tactile stimulation. IV anesthesia usually is used to induce procedural sedation. If other routes are used, the client must have venous access for treatment of possible adverse effects, such as anaphylaxis.

The presedation evaluation determines which clients are suitable for administration of sedative medications. It is similar to the preoperative evaluation. The nurse considers past adverse reactions to sedative medication. The client's age and weight help determine the amount of medication they will need.

The three phases of the sedation process are as follows:

1. Titration of sedative medications, which is the administration of multiple small doses of medication until the desired drug effect is achieved
2. Performance of the diagnostic or therapeutic procedure
3. Recovery phase

In each phase, the client requires careful monitoring for complications. Levels of sedation range from slight drowsiness to anesthesia. Unpredictable absorption, metabolism, and excretion of medications make the client vulnerable to complications of undersedation or oversedation. Increased vigilance is necessary during titration of medications and recovery phases. At these times, the client has the greatest potential to become more deeply sedated because there is no painful stimulus. Even when the client does not seem to be sedated at the end of the procedure, late sedation may develop from continued drug uptake, delayed excretion, pharmacodynamics, or lack of stimulation.

Nurses who care for clients receiving sedation must be aware of the effects, side effects, and desired doses of sedative. Benzodiazepines, opioids, sedative-hypnotics, and barbiturates are the drug classes used in procedural sedation (Drug Therapy Table 14-3). These drugs can cause nausea, dizziness, euphoria or depression, flushed skin, coughing, jerking movements, and unusual eye and tongue movements. Although harmless, such side effects can frighten clients. Because virtually all sedative medications carry a risk of respiratory depression, the nurse also must be prepared for respiratory or cardiopulmonary arrest.

Antagonists, also called *reversal drugs*, reverse the effects of opioids or benzodiazepines. Drugs from this class should be readily available whenever narcotics or benzodiazepines are used. If reversal drugs are required, the nurse *must* observe the client for an extended period because the reversal effects nearly always are shorter than the effects of the drugs being reversed. This may result in resedation. Naloxone (Narcan) reverses opioids; flumazenil (Romazicon) reverses benzodiazepines.

DRUG THERAPY TABLE 14-3 Agents Used to Sedate Clients for Diagnostic and Therapeutic Procedures

Category and Common Generic (Brand) Drugs	Intended Use	Common Side Effects	Safety Warnings for Nurses
Antianxiety			
Benzodiazepines Lorazepam (Ativan) Midazolam	Reduce preprocedure anxiety. Midazolam has rapid onset.	Dry mouth, drowsiness	Depressed breathing; monitor if given with opiate. Increased fall risk due to sedative side effects
Amnesics			
Dexmedetomidine (Precedex) Etomidate (Amidate) Ketamine (Ketalar) Propofol (Diprivan)	Alters consciousness with ability to follow directions, and reduces memory of procedure	Increased oropharyngeal secretions, with propofol; there is pain upon injection.	Depressed breathing, when rapidly administered Ketamine causes delirium when emerging from sedation.
Analgesics			
Opioid Fentanyl (Sublimaze) *NSAIDs* Ketorolac (Toradol)	Sedate and provide pain relief during procedures. Ketorolac is an antiinflammatory.	Sedation, hypotension, vertigo, euphoria, nausea, vomiting, urinary retention, constipation	Watch for respiratory depression in opiate-naïve clients, those with underlying respiratory conditions. Treat constipation early with laxatives and fiber.
Antidotes			
Flumazenil Naloxone (Narcan)	Reverses opiates Reverses benzodiazepines		Attaches to all receptors, gets immediate response

NSAID, nonsteroidal antiinflammatory drug.
Drugs in column 1 indicate the drug that matches up with explanations in the other three columns.
From Juels, A. (2019). Procedural sedation. *Medscape.* https://emedicine.medscape.com/article/109695-overview#a3

Surgical Team

The surgical team consists of an anesthesiologist or anesthetist, surgeon and their assistants, and intraoperative nurses.

The **anesthesiologist** is a primary provider who has completed 2 years of residency in anesthesia. This person is responsible for administering anesthesia to the client and for monitoring the client during and after the surgical procedure. The anesthesiologist assesses the client before surgery, writes preoperative medication orders, informs the client of the options for anesthesia, and explains the risks involved.

The **anesthetist** may be a medical doctor who administers anesthesia but has not completed a residency in anesthesia, a dentist who administers limited types of anesthesia, or a registered nurse (RN) (master's-prepared) who has completed an accredited nurse anesthesia program and passed the certification examination (Certified Registered Nurse Anesthetist [CRNA]). The anesthesiologist oversees the work of the anesthetist, who may assess the client before surgery, discuss options for anesthesia, write preoperative medication orders, administer anesthesia, and monitor the client during and after surgery. The anesthesiologist and anesthetist are not sterile members of the surgical team, meaning that they wear OR attire but they do not wear sterile gowns or work within the sterile field.

Anesthesiologists or anesthetists classify clients according to their general physical status and assign a risk potential. They use the American Society of Anesthesiologists (ASA) Physical Status Classification System (Table 14-4).

The *surgeon* heads the surgical team. They are a primary provider, oral surgeon, or podiatrist with specific training and qualifications. The surgeon is responsible for determining the surgical procedure required, obtaining the client's consent, performing the procedure, and following the client after surgery.

Surgical assistants are classified as either first, second, or third assistants. The *first assistant* assists in the surgical procedure and may be involved with the client's preoperative and postoperative care. They might be another primary provider, a surgical resident, or an RN who has appropriate approval and endorsement from the American Operating Room Nurses (AORN) and the American College of Surgeons. The Registered Nurse First Assistant (RNFA) is a designation that denotes a perioperative RN working in an expanded role. This nurse will be involved with managing tissue specimens, exposing the operative field, suturing, and controlling *hemostasis* (stopping bleeding). Second or third assistants are RNs, licensed practical or vocational nurses (LPNs/LVNs), or surgical technologists who assist the surgeon and first assistant. All assistants are sterile members of the surgical team—they wear sterile gloves and gowns over OR attire and work within the sterile field.

Intraoperative nurses include the *scrub nurse* and *circulating nurse*. The scrub nurse (may be an RN, LPN/LVN, or surgical technologist) wears a sterile gown and gloves and assists the surgical team by handing instruments to the surgeon and assistants, preparing sutures, receiving specimens for laboratory examination, and counting sponges and needles.

TABLE 14-4 American Society of Anesthesiologists (ASA) Physical Status (PS) Classification System

Anesthetists and anesthesiologists use the ASA PS Classification System to describe the client's general status and identify potential risks during surgery. There are six classes of PS:

ASA PS CLASSIFICATION	DEFINITION	EXAMPLES, INCLUDING, BUT NOT LIMITED TO
ASA I	A normal healthy client	Healthy, nonsmoking, no or minimal alcohol use
ASA II	A client with mild systemic disease	Mild diseases only without substantive functional limitations. Examples include (but are not limited to): current smoker, social alcohol drinker, pregnancy, obesity (30 < BMI < 40), well-controlled DM/HTN, mild lung disease.
ASA III	A client with severe systemic disease	Substantive functional limitations; one or more moderate-to-severe diseases. Examples include (but are not limited to): poorly controlled DM or HTN, COPD, morbid obesity (BMI ≥ 40), active hepatitis, alcohol dependence or abuse, implanted pacemaker, moderate reduction of ejection fraction, ESRD undergoing regularly scheduled dialysis, premature infant PCA < 60 weeks, history (>3 months) of MI, CVA, TIA, or CAD/stents.
ASA IV	A client with severe systemic disease that is a constant threat to life	Examples include (but are not limited to): recent (<3 months) MI, CVA, TIA, or CAD/stents, ongoing cardiac ischemia or severe valve dysfunction, severe reduction of ejection fraction, sepsis, DIC, ARD, or ESRD not undergoing regularly scheduled dialysis.
ASA V	A moribund client who is not expected to survive without the operation	Examples include (but are not limited to): ruptured abdominal/thoracic aneurysm, massive trauma, intracranial bleed with mass effect, ischemic bowel in the face of significant cardiac pathology or multiple organ/system dysfunction.
ASA VI	A declared brain-dead client whose organs are being removed for donor purposes	

ARD, acute respiratory distress; BMI, body mass index; CAD, coronary artery disease; COPD, chronic obstructive pulmonary disease; CVA, cerebrovascular accident; DIC, disseminated intravascular coagulation; DM, diabetes mellitus; ESRD, end-stage renal disease; HTN, hypertension; MI, myocardial infarction; PCA, patient-controlled anesthesia; TIA, transient ischemic attack.

Note: The addition of "E," such as ASA IV-E, denotes emergency surgery (an emergency is defined as existing when delay in treatment of the client would lead to a significant increase in the threat to life or body part).

Excerpted from ASA Physical Status Classification System, 2020 of the American Society of Anesthesiologists. A copy of the full text can be obtained from ASA, 1061 American Lane Schaumburg, IL 60173-4973 or online at www.asahq.org.

The circulating nurse (RN) wears OR attire but not a sterile gown and is responsible for overseeing the health and safety of the client by monitoring all activities of the surgical team. Responsibilities include assessment of the client for signs of injury, intervening as needed, and maintaining the safety checks required to protect the client from injury. This RN also is involved with obtaining and opening wrapped sterile equipment and supplies before and during surgery, keeping records, adjusting lights, receiving specimens for laboratory examination, and coordinating activities of other personnel, such as the pathologist and radiology technician.

The Operating Room Environment

The OR or surgical suite environment is physically isolated from other areas of the hospital or surgical clinic. This restricts access to the area to only authorized OR personnel and surgical clients. In the surgical suite, air is filtered and positive pressure is maintained to reduce the number of possible microbes that can cause infection. Three designated zones help to separate clean and contaminated areas and decrease the presence of microbes:

- *Unrestricted zone*—includes a central point to monitor the arrival of clients, personnel, and supplies. Street clothes are allowed in this area.
- *Semi-restricted zone*—includes the peripheral support areas of the surgical suite, with storage area for sterile and clean supplies, work areas for processing and storage of instruments, and corridors leading to the restricted area of the OR. Personnel are required to wear surgical attire, including two-piece pantsuits, cover jackets, and caps. Masks are not required in this area.
- *Restricted zone*—includes the OR and procedure room, the clean core, and scrub sink areas. Personnel are required to wear full surgical attire and cover all head and facial hair, including sideburns, beard, and necklines. Full surgical attire includes two-piece pantsuits, cover jackets, head coverings, shoes/shoe covers, masks, protective eyewear, and other protective barriers as indicated.

Surgical suites are designed to be efficient, in that the needed equipment and supplies are immediately available for use. Usually, the furniture is made of stainless steel for easy cleaning and disinfecting. The temperature in the OR is kept below 70°F to provide a cooler environment that does not promote bacterial growth, to offer more comfort for OR personnel working in bright lights and wearing surgical attire, and to maintain a temperature that enhances client comfort and safety.

OR personnel wear specific attire that decreases the opportunity for microbial growth. They strictly adhere to rules about where to change clothes and what to wear in the OR, including protective attire (Box 14-4). In addition, OR personnel must report any symptoms of infection they are

BOX 14-4 Surgical Attire

- *Scrub attire* includes tops, pants with cuffs, and jackets with cuffs. Changing rooms are located near the operating room (OR); personnel change into OR attire before entering the OR and take OR attire off when they leave.
- *Masks* are worn at all times in the OR; personnel change masks between surgical procedures or if masks become wet.
- *Headgear* is worn to cover the hair and hairline. Beards and sideburns must also be covered.
- *Shoes* should be comfortable. Agencies vary in specific requirements. Shoe covers also are worn over the shoes. The conductive covers provide an electrical ground.
- *Personal protective equipment* includes intact gloves, gowns, masks, and eye protection (face shields, goggles, and glasses with side shields).

experiencing because colds, sore throats, and skin infections are potential sources of infection to the client.

Nursing Management

Nursing management during the intraoperative period depends on routine tasks performed during surgery as well as on variables such as type of surgery performed, type of anesthesia used, client's age and condition, and any complications. Asepsis in the OR is the responsibility of all OR personnel. **Surgical asepsis** prevents contamination of surgical wounds. The risk of infection is high because of the break in skin integrity from the surgical incision. The client's own pathogens, plus those found in the OR, create an unsafe environment if personnel neglect to uphold strict aseptic technique. Thus, they strictly follow asepsis protocols to protect the client as much as possible. The client's safety and protection during surgery are essential.

Intraoperative Assessment

Assessment of the client in the OR is based largely on the type or extent of surgery, the client's age, and any preexisting conditions. Depending on circumstances, assessment before the administration of the anesthetic may include the following:

- BP and pulse and respiratory rates
- Level of consciousness
- General physical condition
- Presence of catheters and tubes
- Review of client's medical record, including a signed consent form, administration of preoperative medications (time, dose, client response), voiding, skin preparation, carrying out other preoperative orders, and laboratory and diagnostic tests

››› *Stop, Think, and Respond 14-2*

A client was told not to take their morning medications on the day of surgery. When they arrive at the OR, they inform the RN that they took their morning diuretic by mistake a few hours ago. What implications does this have for their care during surgery?

Prevention of Intraoperative Complications

Nurses who work in the OR assess the client continuously and protect the client from potential complications, including the following:

- ***Infection:*** Strict aseptic technique is absolutely necessary before and during surgery. If a nurse notes a break in technique, they immediately notify the surgeon and OR personnel. Clients are also at risk for the retention of foreign objects in the wound. The scrub nurse and circulating nurse count surgical instruments, gauze sponges, and sharps to prevent this problem. The circulating nurse records the counts on the intraoperative record.
- ***Fluid volume excess or deficit:*** The anesthesiologist usually adds fluids to the IV lines, but the circulating nurse also may perform this function. The circulating nurse is responsible for recording and keeping a running total of IV fluids administered. If the client has an indwelling catheter, the nurse measures urine output during surgery.
- ***Injury related to positioning:*** The OR staff positions the client on the OR table according to the type of surgery. Careful positioning and monitoring help to prevent interruption of blood supply secondary to prolonged pressure, nerve injury related to prolonged pressure, postoperative hypotension, dependent edema, and joint injury related to poor body alignment.
- ***Hypothermia:*** During the procedure, the client may be at risk for hypothermia related to the low temperature in the OR, administration of cold IV fluids, inhalation of cool gases, exposure of body surfaces for the surgical procedure, opened incisions/wounds, and prolonged inactivity. For some surgeries, the body temperature is deliberately lowered. This is referred to as therapeutic hypothermia. There is ongoing research to determine the benefits for clients undergoing cardiac surgery, organ transplant, spinal cord trauma surgery, or other procedures. Careful monitoring of the client is essential if the temperature is deliberately lowered.
- ***Malignant hyperthermia:*** **Malignant hyperthermia** (MH) is an inherited disorder that occurs when body temperature, muscle metabolism, and heat production increase rapidly, progressively, and uncontrollably in response to stress and some anesthetic agents. There are two tests that indicate if a client is susceptible to MH: skeletal muscle biopsy, which determines muscle contractile qualities, and a blood test for a genetic mutation linked to MH. Certain anesthetic agents trigger uncontrolled calcium release within skeletal muscle cells, which leads to muscle rigidity and a hypermetabolic state (Yang et al., 2020). Signs and symptoms include jaw muscle rigidity, rapidly rising temperature, elevated $PaCO_2$ and serum potassium levels, metabolic acidosis, tachycardia, tachypnea, diaphoresis, mottled skin, hypotension, irregular heart rate, decreased urine output, eventual kidney failure, and, if untreated, cardiac arrest. Prevention of MH is essential because the mortality rate is high. Clients at risk include those with strong, bulky muscles, those who

experience muscle cramps or muscle weakness and temperature elevation for no apparent reason, and those who have a relative who had an acute febrile episode and died suddenly without explanation (Gray & Thomas, 2017). The circulating nurse closely monitors the client for signs of hyperthermia. If the client's temperature begins to rise rapidly, anesthesia is discontinued and the OR team implements measures to correct physiologic problems, such as fever or arrhythmias.

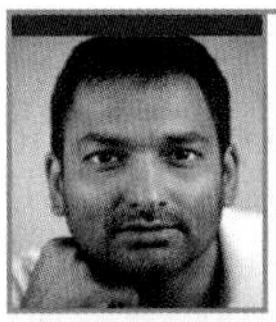

Clinical Scenario A client is scheduled for an exploratory laparoscopy. It is expected that the procedure will not be any longer than 2 hours. The client will be able to go home after recovering from the anesthesia. What information does the nurse need to collect? What are important considerations for the nurse to monitor while the client is sedated? See the following Nursing Process section.

NURSING PROCESS FOR THE CLIENT UNDERGOING PROCEDURAL SEDATION

The client undergoing procedural sedation requires special considerations for intraoperative nursing management.

Assessment

Before sedation, the nurse gathers important client data, records baseline vital signs and oximeter readings, and provides education to clients and their families. Education includes instructions specific to the procedure, preparations for the procedure, likely sensations (pain, discomfort, cramping, gagging, nausea), and common side effects of medications.

During sedation, the nurse continuously evaluates the client. Monitoring during all phases includes assessment of heart rate, respiratory rate, BP, oxygen saturation, and level of consciousness. The nurse monitors cardiac rhythm in clients who are at risk for arrhythmias or cardiovascular compromise. If vital signs deviate significantly during sedation, the nurse collects additional information to help determine if those deviations are secondary to an adverse reaction to the sedation or to the procedure itself. When the client shows signs of distress (i.e., deviation in vital signs, respiratory compromise), the nurse immediately reports these signs to the primary provider and provides interventions such as suctioning, gentle tactile stimulation, or administration of oxygen. They continue to monitor the client's response until the level of consciousness and vital signs are at baseline. The nurse documents these observations at intervals specified by the institution.

Analysis, Planning, and Interventions

Altered Breathing Pattern: Related to effect of sedative medications
Expected Outcome: Client will maintain an effective breathing pattern without signs of cyanosis, hypoxia, and with arterial blood gases in normal range.

- Position client in an upright or semi-Fowler's position. *These positions facilitate lung expansion and oxygenation.*
- Observe for signs and symptoms of distress related to inappropriate head position (stridor, increased respiratory effort); reposition head as indicated. *Early intervention prevents further complications.*
- Encourage client to take deep breaths and cough at least every hour. *Deep breathing and coughing improve oxygenation and assist in clearing the effects of anesthesia.*

Perioperative Injury Risk: Related to sensory/perceptual disturbances due to anesthesia
Expected Outcome: Client will remain safe and free of injury while recovering from the effects of anesthesia.

- Provide safety by preventing client from falling out of bed, stretcher, or recliner; assisting with ambulation; and carefully monitoring all activities. *Clients recovering from sedation may have impaired judgment and reflexes; the nurse must protect them from injury.*
- Monitor client for return to presedation level of consciousness. *Until client is fully responsive, they continue to be at risk for a perioperative injury.*
- Discharge client to the care of a person who has received instructions regarding client safety. *Sedative effects may last for several more hours; the client requires continued care after discharge.*

Evaluation of Expected Outcomes

The client has a patent airway and effective breathing patterns. They are alert and oriented and able to follow instructions related to deep breathing and coughing and maintaining safety. The client has not experienced any perioperative injury. The client's caregiver verbalizes the need to keep the client safe while recovering from the effects of anesthesia.

POSTOPERATIVE CARE

The postoperative period designates the time that the client spends recovering from the effects of anesthesia. Factors such as the client's age and nutritional status, preexisting diseases, type of surgery, and length of anesthesia may affect the duration, type, and extent of nursing management.

Transport of the Client

Immediately after the surgical procedure is complete, the client is transported to the postanesthesia care unit (PACU), also known as the *postanesthesia recovery room*, located near the OR. The nursing staff there is specifically knowledgeable in the care of clients recovering from anesthesia. Specialized equipment is available to monitor and treat the client. Surgical and anesthesia personnel are immediately available for any emergencies.

Nursing Management

Immediate Postoperative Period

When clients are transferred from the OR to the PACU, the anesthesiologist or anesthetist is responsible for the client's safety. Critical considerations include maintaining an intact surgical site (incision), observing for potential vascular changes, and keeping the client warm. Position of the client is also important so that the incision is not compromised, drains do not obstruct, and the client does not experience *orthostatic hypotension*. The nurse receiving the client from the OR needs the following information:

- Client's name, gender, age
- Allergies
- Surgical procedure
- Length of time in the OR
- Anesthetic agents and reversal agents used
- Estimated blood/fluid loss
- Fluid/blood replacement
- Last set of vital signs and any problems during the procedure
- Complications encountered (anesthetic or surgical)
- Medical comorbidities (e.g., diabetes, hypertension)
- Considerations for immediate postoperative period (pain management, reversals, ventilator settings)
- Language barrier
- Location of client's family

The anesthesia provider should stay with the client until the nurse confirms that the client's airway has effective function and the client overall is in stable condition. The most important aspect of nursing management is close observation and monitoring of the client during emergence from anesthesia.

Initial Postoperative Assessment

Initial postoperative assessments include airway patency; effectiveness of respirations; presence of artificial airways, mechanical ventilation, or supplemental oxygen; circulatory status; vital signs; wound condition, including dressings and drains; fluid balance, including IV fluids, output from catheters and drains, and ability to void; level of consciousness; and pain. The nurse's major responsibilities during the client's PACU stay are to ensure a patent airway; help maintain adequate circulation; prevent or assist with the treatment of shock; maintain proper position and function of drains, tubes, and IV infusions; and monitor for potential complications.

An important assessment is determining how the client is recovering from anesthesia. A useful assessment tool is the Aldrete scale, which rates the client's mobility, respiratory status, circulation, consciousness, and pulse oximetry (Table 14-5). A score of 9 or greater indicates that the client has recovered from anesthesia.

Prevention of Postoperative Complications

Hemorrhage. Hemorrhage can be internal or external. If the client loses a lot of blood, they will exhibit signs and symptoms of shock (see Chapter 17). Table 14-6 provides classifications of hemorrhage. The nurse inspects dressings frequently for signs of bleeding and checks the bedding

TABLE 14-5 Modified Aldrete Scale for Assessing Recovery From Anesthesia

	SCORE[a]		
	0	**1**	**2**
Activity	Unable to move extremities voluntarily or on command	Able to move two extremities voluntarily or on command	Able to move all extremities voluntarily or on command
Respiration	Apneic	Dyspnea, shallow, or limited breathing	Able to breathe deeply and cough freely
Circulation	BP $\pm$ 50 mm Hg of preanesthesia level	BP $\pm$ 20–50 mm Hg of preanesthesia level	BP $\pm$ 20 mm Hg of preanesthesia level
Consciousness	Unresponsive	Arousable with verbal stimuli	Fully awake
SpO_2	$<$90% with supplemental oxygen	Needs supplemental oxygen to maintain $>$90%	$>$92% on room air

BP, blood pressure; SpO_2, oxygen saturation.
[a]Add the scores for all criteria for a total score; a score of 9 or greater on this modified Aldrete scale means that the client has recovered from anesthesia.
Pusey-Reid, E. (2018). Patient readiness for PACU discharge. *Nursing Critical Care, 13*(5), 31–34. https://doi.org/10.1097/01.CCN.0000544399.76592.be

TABLE 14-6 Classifications of Hemorrhage

CLASSIFICATION	DEFINING CHARACTERISTIC
Time Frame Categories	
Primary	Intraoperative hemorrhage—occurs during surgery
Intermediary or reactive	Hemorrhage occurs 24 hours of surgery when the rise of blood pressure to its normal level dislodges insecure clots from untied vessels.
Secondary	Hemorrhage may occur 7–10 days following surgery if a suture slips because a blood vessel was not securely tied, became infected, or was eroded by a drainage tube.
Type of Vessel	
Capillary	Hemorrhage is characterized by a slow, general ooze.
Venous	Darkly colored blood bubbles out quickly.
Arterial	Blood is bright red and appears in spurts with each heartbeat.
Visibility	
Evident	Hemorrhage is on the surface and can be seen.
Concealed	Hemorrhage is in a body cavity and cannot be seen.

Adapted from Hinkle, J. L., & Cheever, K. H. (2018). *Brunner & Suddarth's textbook of medical-surgical nursing* (14th ed.). Wolters Kluwer.

under the client because blood may pool under the body and be evident on the bedding. If bleeding is internal, the client may need to return to surgery for ligation of the bleeding vessels. Blood transfusions may be necessary to replace lost blood. When bleeding occurs, the nurse notes the amount and color on the chart. Bright red blood signifies fresh bleeding; dark, brownish blood indicates older blood. The nurse may need to reinforce soiled or saturated dressings. A written order is needed to change dressings. The nurse also must be aware of any wound drains and the type and amount of drainage expected. If such drainage is expected, the nurse explains to the client that the drainage is normal and does not indicate a complication. They place incontinence pads under the client if drainage occurs.

Shock. Fluid and electrolyte loss, trauma (both physical and psychological), anesthetics, and preoperative medications all may contribute to shock. Signs and symptoms include pallor, fall in BP, weak and rapid pulse rate, restlessness, and cool, moist skin (see Chapter 17). Shock must be detected early and treated promptly because it can irreversibly damage vital organs such as the brain, kidneys, and heart.

Narcotics are not administered to a client in shock until a primary provider evaluates the client, who should remain supine. Some primary providers advocate elevating the legs to enhance the flow of venous blood to the heart. Treatment of shock varies and depends on the cause, if known. Blood, plasma expanders, parenteral fluids, oxygen, and medications such as adrenergic agonists may be used (see Chapter 17).

Hypoxia. Factors such as residual drug effects or overdose, pain, poor positioning, pooling of secretions in the lungs, or obstructed airway predispose the client to hypoxia (decreased oxygen). Oxygen and suction equipment must be available for immediate use. The nurse observes the client closely for signs of cyanosis and dyspnea. Breathing may be obstructed if the tongue falls back and blocks the nasopharynx. If this occurs, the nurse pulls the lower jaw and inserts an oropharyngeal airway (Fig. 14-4). Positioning the client on their side also may relieve nasopharyngeal obstruction. Restlessness, crowing or grunting respirations, diaphoresis, bounding pulse, and rising BP may indicate respiratory obstruction. If a client cannot breathe effectively, mechanical ventilation is used.

Aspiration. Danger of aspiration from saliva, mucus, vomitus, or blood exists until the client is fully awake and can swallow without difficulty. Suction equipment must be kept at the client's bedside until the danger of aspiration no longer exists. The nurse closely observes the client for difficulty swallowing or handling of oral secretions. Unless contraindicated, the nurse places the client in a side-lying position until the client can swallow oral secretions.

Later Postoperative Period

The later postoperative period begins when the client arrives in the hospital room or postsurgical care unit. Because the nurse can anticipate, prevent, or minimize many postoperative problems, they must approach the care of the client systematically.

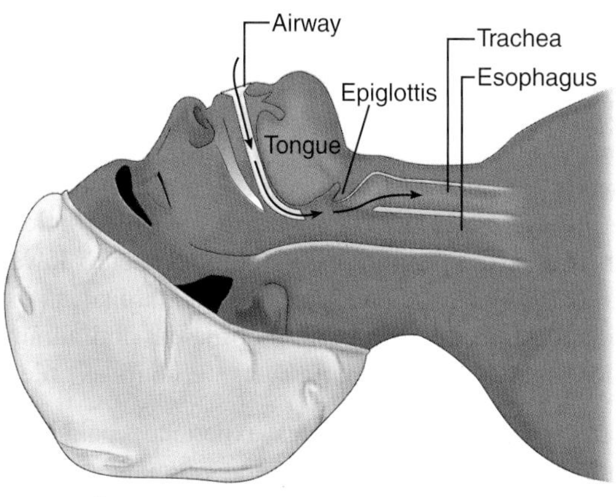

Figure 14-4 Oropharyngeal airway in place.

Ongoing Assessments

Assessment during this period includes respiratory function; general condition; vital signs; cardiovascular function and fluid status; pain level; bowel and urinary elimination; and dressings, tubes, drains, and IV lines.

Respiration. The nurse focuses on promoting gas exchange and preventing atelectasis. Hypoventilation related to anesthesia, postoperative positioning, and pain is a common problem. Preoperative and postoperative instructions include teaching the client to deep breathe and cough and how to splint the incision to minimize pain. Clients who have abdominal or thoracic surgery have greater difficulty taking deep breaths and coughing. Some clients require supplemental oxygen. Nursing management to prevent postoperative respiratory problems includes early mobility, frequent position changes, deep-breathing and coughing exercises, and use of incentive spirometer.

Hiccups (singultus) also may interfere with breathing. They result from intermittent spasms of the diaphragm and may occur after surgery, especially abdominal surgery. They may be mild and last for only a few minutes. Prolonged hiccups not only are unpleasant but also may cause pain or discomfort. They may result in wound dehiscence or evisceration; inability to eat; nausea and vomiting; exhaustion; and fluid, electrolyte, and acid–base imbalances. If hiccups persist, the nurse needs to notify the primary provider.

Circulation. The nurse must assess the client's BP and circulatory status frequently. Although problems with postoperative bleeding decrease as the recovery time advances, the client is still at risk for bleeding. Some clients experience syncope when moving to an upright position. To prevent this (and the danger of falling), the nurse helps the client to move slowly to an upright or standing position.

The client also is at risk for impaired venous circulation related to immobility. When clients lie still for long periods without moving their legs, blood may flow sluggishly through the veins (venous stasis). Venous stasis predisposes the client to venous inflammation and clot formation in the veins (**thrombophlebitis**), or clot formation with minimal or absent inflammation (**phlebothrombosis**). These two conditions are most common in the lower extremities. A clot (**embolus**) traveling in the bloodstream may obstruct circulation to a vital organ, such as the lungs, and cause severe symptoms and possibly death.

To prevent venous stasis and other circulatory complications, the nurse encourages the client to move their legs frequently and do leg exercises. The nurse also does not place pillows under the client's knees or calves unless ordered. They avoid placing pressure on the client's lower extremities, apply elastic bandages or antiembolism stockings as ordered, ambulate the client as ordered, and administer low-dose subcutaneous heparin every 12 hours as ordered.

Pain Management. Most clients experience pain after an operation, and a range of postoperative analgesics usually are ordered. Postoperative pain reaches its peak between 12 and 36 hours after surgery and diminishes significantly after 48 hours. Pain creates varying degrees of anxiety and emotions. If accompanied by great fear, the degree of pain can increase. Clients must receive pain and discomfort relief. When patient-controlled analgesia (PCA) is used, clients administer their own analgesic (see Chapter 11).

The nurse assesses for adverse effects of analgesics, timing of the medication in relation to other activities, effects of other comfort measures, contraindications, and source of the pain. The need for pain medications depends on the type and extent of the surgery and the client. Pain unrelieved by medication may signal a developing complication, which underscores the need for a thorough assessment of the cause and type of pain (see Chapter 11).

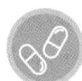

Pharmacologic Considerations

- Opioid-naïve (infrequent user of opiates) clients are at greatest risk for respiratory depression. Promethazine can also increase the sedation and respiratory depression when used with an opiate.

Fluids and Nutrition. IV fluids usually are administered after surgery. Length of administration depends on the type of surgery and the client's ability to take oral fluids. The nurse monitors the IV fluid flow rate and adjusts it as needed. They also assess for signs of fluid excess or deficit (see Chapter 16) and notify the primary provider of any such signs. Dietary progression depends on the type of surgery, the client's progress, and primary provider preference. The following items must be considered:

- Each client is different, as is their surgery. Any postoperative client may get abdominal distention from gas in the intestinal tract, swallowed air during surgery, and the continued production and accumulation of gastrointestinal (GI) tract secretions.
- Taking oral fluids stimulates normal functions of the GI system, so clients should be offered fluids as soon as possible after surgery, depending on their recovery.
- Resumption of stomach activity may not occur for 24 to 48 hours.
- Manipulation of GI organs can delay peristalsis for 24 to 48 hours.
- Nausea and vomiting may occur postoperatively and need to be managed before the client can resume oral intake.

If vomiting and/or abdominal distention is a risk because of the nature of the surgery, a nasogastric tube may be placed before, during, or after surgery. Assessment of the client is crucial while making decisions about resumption of fluids and nutrition. The nurse will ensure that the client progresses at their own pace in order to avoid or minimize any GI discomfort or complications. Nursing Guidelines 14-1 includes factors to consider before resuming oral fluids. IV fluids

NURSING GUIDELINES 14-1

Resuming Oral Fluids After Surgery

- Most clients can begin to take fluids within 4 to 24 hours after surgery (except when surgery involves the GI tract). Check primary provider's orders to ensure that fluids can be given.
- If not allowed oral fluids, provide the client with mouth rinses and a cool, wet cloth or ice chips against the lips to relieve dryness.
- Before giving fluids, assess that the client has recovered sufficiently from anesthesia to swallow. Ask the client to try swallowing without drinking anything. If the client can do so, offer a small sip of water or a few ice chips.
- Give only a few sips of water or ice chips at a time. Introduce fluids slowly and give them in small amounts to prevent vomiting. The client can take fluids through a straw so they do not have to sit up. Once the client can sit up, however, straws are discouraged because clients tend to swallow air as well, which can lead to abdominal distention and gastric discomfort.
- If the client vomits, reassure them that it should cease shortly. Offer mouthwash to remove the taste of anesthetics and vomitus. Administer antiemetics as indicated.

usually are discontinued when the client can take oral fluids and food and nutritional needs are met (Nutrition Notes).

››› *Stop, Think, and Respond 14-3*

Postoperatively, the client complains of nausea. What is an important nursing action?

If the client is malnourished, hypermetabolic, or not expected to resume an oral intake within a few days, a needle catheter jejunostomy tube may be inserted during surgery so that enteral feedings can be given.

Skin Integrity/Wound Healing. A surgical incision is a wound or injury to skin integrity. Initially, the client may have a wound or incisional drain, which is a tube that exits from the peri-incisional area into either a dressing or portable wound suction device. Figure 14-5 depicts three types of wound devices: Penrose, Jackson–Pratt, and Hemovac drains.

When assessing the wound, the nurse inspects for approximation of the wound edges, intactness of staples or sutures, redness, warmth, swelling, tenderness, discoloration, or drainage. They also note any reactions to the tape or dressings. The first phase of wound healing is the *inflammatory stage*, which is when a blood clot forms, swelling occurs, and phagocytes ingest the debris from damaged tissue and the blood clot. This phase lasts 1 to 4 days. The second phase is the *proliferative phase*, in which collagen is produced and granulation tissue forms. It occurs over 5 to 20 days. The last phase is referred to as the *maturation* or *remodeling phase* and lasts from 21 days to several months and even 1 to 2 years. During this phase, the tensile strength of the wound increases through synthesis of collagen by fibroblasts and lysis by collagenase enzymes.

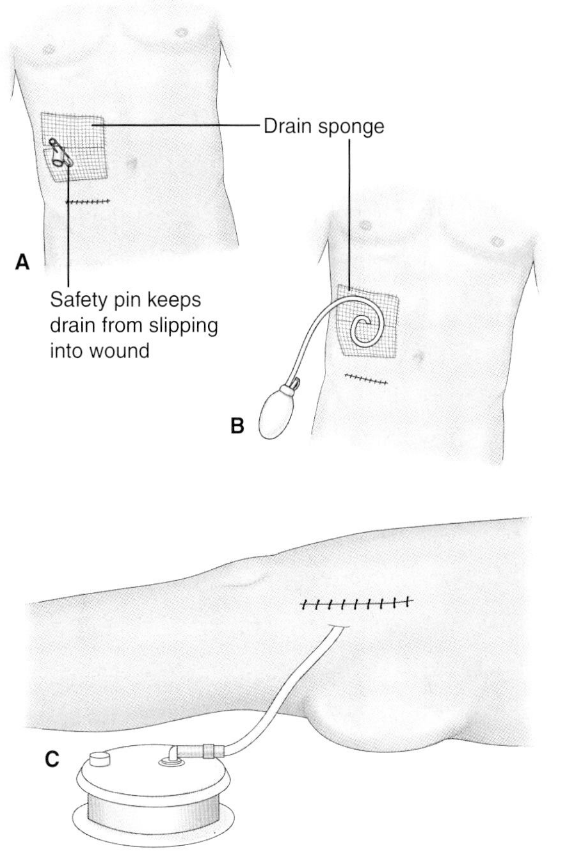

Figure 14-5 Types of surgical drains: **(A)** Penrose, **(B)** Jackson–Pratt, and **(C)** Hemovac.

Nutrition Notes

The Postoperative Client

- Progress the diet as soon as possible after surgery to promote an adequate oral intake.
- Encourage clients who are anorexic or nauseated to consume small, frequent feedings. They may tolerate high-protein, low-fat liquids better than traditional meals.
- If possible, schedule pain medications enough in advance to allow the client a pain-free mealtime.
- Normal weight loss during the early postoperative period is about half a pound daily. Weight gain during this period signifies fluid accumulation.
- Protein, calories, vitamins A and C, and zinc are important for wound healing and immune system functioning; actual requirements depend on the client's nutritional status, extent of surgery, and development of complications.
- Unlike the stomach, which does not regain motility for 24 to 48 hours after surgery, the small intestine resumes peristalsis and the ability to absorb nutrients within several hours after surgery.

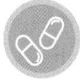

Pharmacologic Considerations

- Antibiotics to prevent or fight infection may be ordered before as well as after surgery. The drugs must be given at specified intervals to maintain consistent therapeutic blood levels.

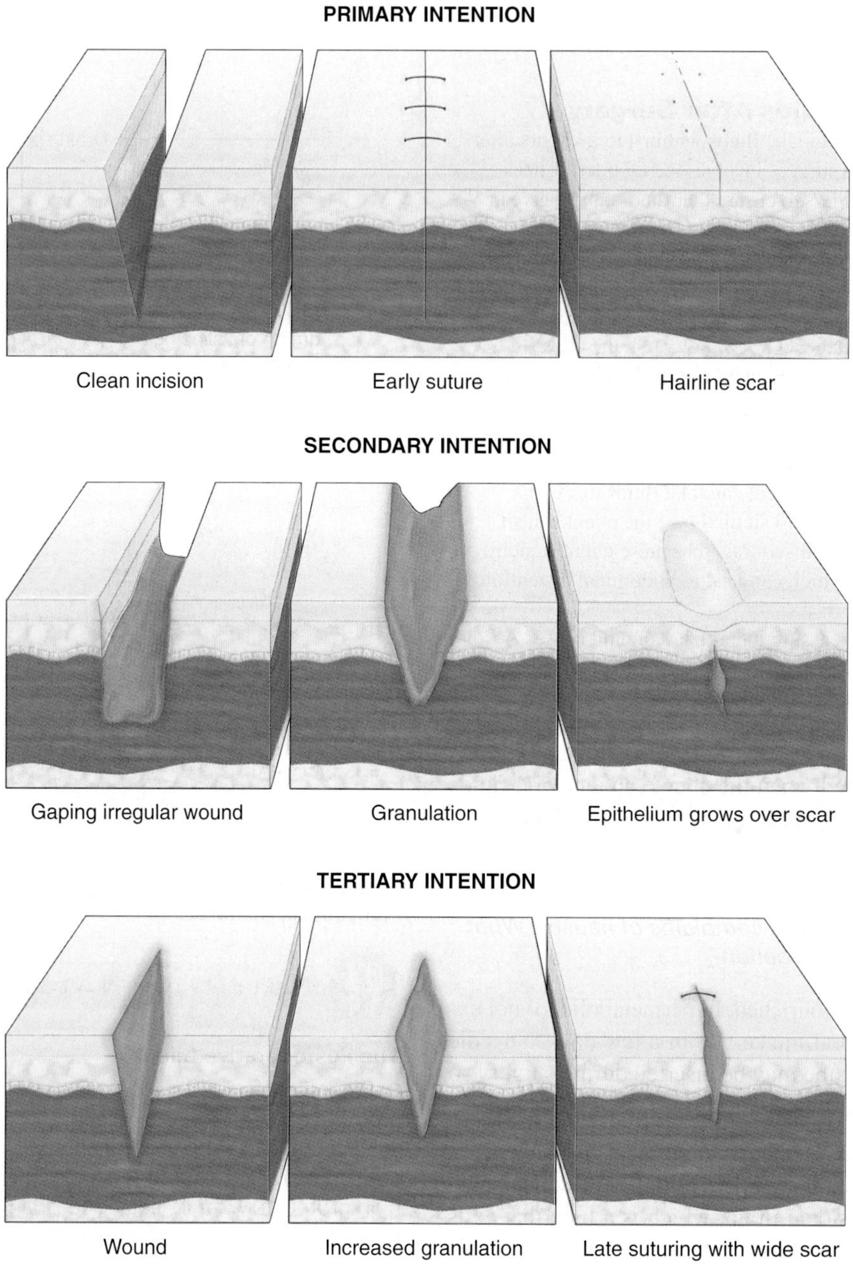

Figure 14-6 Types of wound healing.

In addition, surgical wounds are formed aseptically depending on the nature of the incision and the underlying condition. There are three modes of wound healing (Fig. 14-6):

- *Primary intention:* The wound layers are sutured together so that wound edges are well approximated. This type of incision usually heals in 8 to 10 days with minimal scarring.
- *Secondary intention:* Granulating tissue fills in the wound for the healing process. The skin edges are not approximated. This method is used for ulcers and infected wounds. This type of wound healing is slow, although new products, such as antimicrobial underdressings or calcium alginate dressings, promote healing.
- *Tertiary intention:* The approximation of wound edges is delayed secondary to infection. When the wound is drained and cleaned of infection, the wound edges are sutured together. The resulting scar is wider than that with primary intention.

The key to healing is adequate blood flow. Poor blood supply to the wound delays healing, as can excessive tension or pulling on wound edges. The nurse must be alert for signs and symptoms of impaired circulation, such as swelling, coldness, absence of pulse, pallor, or mottling, and report them immediately. Other factors that interfere with healing include malnutrition, impaired inflammatory and immune responses, infection, foreign bodies, and age. Obesity may also contribute to poor wound healing, secondary to impaired oxygenation, hyperglycemia, immobility, and nutritional deficits. Studies show that obese clients are more likely to have wound infections as well as dehiscence, pressure ulcers, and deep tissue injury. Excess fat prolongs the length of surgery and necessitates the use of more forceful retraction (holding surgical openings open with instruments), which contributes to tissue damage. It also adds to pressure on wound edges, decreasing blood flow and increasing the danger of dehiscence.

The nurse must be careful when changing dressings to avoid damaging new tissue as well as causing the client unnecessary discomfort. Using normal saline to soak packings and dressings that adhere to the wound bed may ease removal.

The nurse closely monitors the client for signs and symptoms of wound infection, such as increased incisional pain; redness, swelling, and heat around the incision; purulent drainage; fever and chills; headache; and anorexia. Treatment of wound infections includes antibiotics, wound care, and measures to promote healing such as adequate nutrition and rest. Surgical site infections (SSIs) from any inpatient surgery accounted for almost 22% of health care–associated infections, with no change being reported from 2015 to 2018. The Joint Commission formed a national partnership of health care organizations called the Surgical Care Improvement Project (SCIP). With this project, there is a target of a 30% reduction in SSIs during the measurement time of 2015 to 2020, with reports remaining pending. Their goal is to prevent and reduce SSIs through the appropriate use of perioperative prophylactic antibiotics, control of glucose levels in cardiac surgical clients, use of appropriate methods for hair removal, removal of urinary catheters postoperatively, management of temperatures during the perioperative period, management of clients on beta-blockers, and management of clients with appropriate venous thromboembolism prophylaxis.

Other complications of wound healing are dehiscence and evisceration. Wound **dehiscence** (Fig. 14-7A) is the separation of wound edges without the protrusion of organs. **Evisceration** (Fig. 14-7B) occurs when the wound completely separates and organs protrude. These complications are most likely to occur within 7 to 10 days after surgery. Risk factors for wound disruption are identified in Box 14-5.

The client may complain of something "giving way." Pinkish drainage may appear suddenly on the dressing. If wound disruption is suspected, the nurse places the client in a position that puts the least strain on the operative area. If evisceration occurs, the nurse places sterile dressings moistened with normal saline over the protruding organs and tissues. For any wound disruption, the nurse notifies the primary provider immediately.

Postoperative wound care also must include teaching the client and family members about wound care while in the hospital and when discharged (Client and Family Teaching 14-1).

Activity. When possible, the client begins ambulatory activities shortly after surgery. Factors such as pain tolerance, response to analgesics, general physical condition, and desire

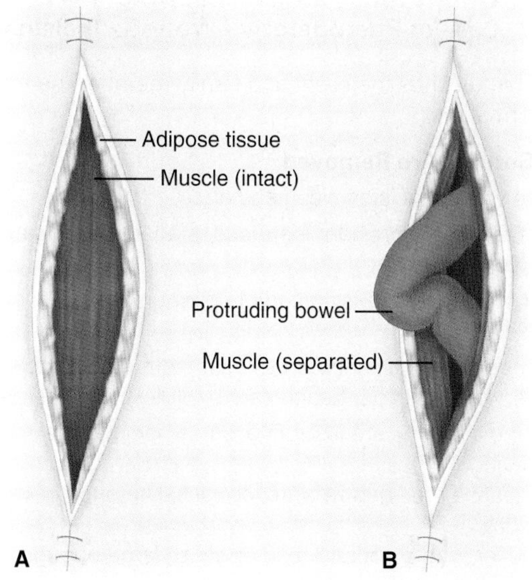

Figure 14-7 **(A)** Wound dehiscence. **(B)** Wound evisceration.

to participate affect the client's ability to be active. Some clients need encouragement. The nurse must emphasize the importance of increasing activities. They assist the client to a sitting position at the side of the bed. If the client becomes dizzy longer than momentarily, the nurse returns the client to a supine position. When the client can stand, the nurse assists and supports the client. The nurse continues to assist with ambulation until the client can walk without help. Some clients experience moderate-to-severe fatigue after surgery. For these clients, the nurse spaces activities such as ambulation and personal care throughout the day.

If the client has received regional anesthesia, activity may initially be restricted. At first, the client experiences numbness and a feeling of heaviness in the anesthetized

BOX 14-5 Risk Factors for Wound Dehiscence

- Advanced age—older than 65 years
- Chronic disease such as diabetes, hypertension, or obesity
- History of radiation or chemotherapy
- Malnutrition, particularly insufficient protein and vitamin C
- Hypoalbuminemia
- Increased intra-abdominal pressure or tension related to distended bowel, coughing, hiccupping, or vomiting
- Obesity or enlarged abdomen
- Tobacco use
- Use of some medications, such as anticoagulants, aspirin, corticosteroids, or chemotherapeutic agents
- Wound complication, such as infection, hematoma, or inadequate closure
- Abdominal wall weakened by previous surgeries

Adapted from Walming, S., Angenete, E., Block, M., Bock, D., Gessler, B., & Haglind, E. (2017). Retrospective review of risk factors for surgical wound dehiscence and incisional hernia. *BMC surgery, 17*(1), 19. https://doi.org/10.1186/s12893-017-0207-0. https://creativecommons.org/licenses/by/4.0/.

Client and Family Teaching 14-1
Care of Postoperative Wounds/Incisions

The nurse teaches the client and family member the following information:

Until Sutures Are Removed

- Keep wound/incision clean and dry.
- Follow primary provider instructions about bathing and showering.
- Do not remove dressing and/or splint unless it is wet or soiled.
- If wet or soiled, change dressing if instructed to do so. Otherwise, call your health care provider for guidance.
- Wound/incision care instructions may include the following:
  - Cleanse area gently with normal saline once or twice a day.
  - Cover with a nonstick pad or gauze large enough to cover the wound/incision.
  - Tape with hypoallergenic tape (adhesive is difficult to remove without injury).
- Immediately report any signs of infection:
  - Redness and/or marked swelling exceeding 1/2 inch surrounding the wound/incision
  - Increased tenderness or warmth around the wound/incision
  - Red streaks in skin near wound/incision
  - Pus, discharge, foul odor
  - Chills or temperature above 37.5°C (100°F)
- If there is soreness or pain at the site of the wound/incision, apply an ice pack or cold water pack. Do not use a wet pack. Take pain medications according to directions.
- Swelling after surgery is common. To help reduce swelling, elevate the affected part to the level of the heart.

After Sutures Are Removed

- Follow directions regarding the level of activity allowed.
- Keep suture line clean and dry.
- Wash, dry, and apply dressing as directed.
- Wound edges may look slightly raised and red—this is normal.
- If the wound/incision site looks red and thick and is painful to touch 8 weeks after sutures are removed, contact the primary provider (excessive collagen may have formed).

Adapted from Hinkle, J. L., & Cheever, K. H. (2018). *Brunner & Suddarth's textbook of medical-surgical nursing* (14th ed.). Wolters Kluwer.

area. Reassuring the client that numbness is typical and will subside shortly may be necessary. Unless ordered otherwise, the client who has received spinal anesthesia remains flat for 6 to 12 hours. If permitted, the nurse turns the client from side to side at least every 2 hours. As the anesthesia wears off, the client begins to have a "pins-and-needles" sensation in the anesthetized parts and to feel pain in the operative area. Clients who develop a headache after spinal anesthesia may have to remain lying flat for a longer period.

Bowel Elimination. Constipation may develop after the client begins to take solid food. Causes of this constipation include inactivity, diet, and narcotic analgesics. Some clients may experience diarrhea as a result of diet, medications such as antibiotics, or the surgical procedure. The nurse maintains a record of bowel movements and notifies the primary provider of either problem.

Abdominal distention results from the accumulation of gas (flatus) in the intestines because of failure of the intestines to propel gas through the intestinal tract by peristalsis. Contributing factors include manipulation of the intestines during abdominal surgery, inactivity after surgery, interruption of normal food and fluid intake, swallowing of large quantities of air, and anesthetics and medications given during or after surgery. If the symptoms are mild, they can be treated with nursing measures. The nurse encourages and assists clients who are permitted out of bed to ambulate. Sometimes walking, plus privacy in the bathroom, enables the client to expel the gas. The nurse encourages clients to change position frequently and to eat as normally as possible within the allowed dietary limits. If discomfort is severe or not relieved promptly by nursing measures, the nurse must contact the primary provider.

Sometimes a serious condition called **paralytic ileus** occurs in which the intestines are paralyzed and, thus, peristalsis is absent. Fluids, solids, and gas do not move through the intestinal tract. Bowel sounds are absent, the abdomen is distended, and abdominal pain often is severe. Vomiting also may occur. If the client complains of severe abdominal pain, assessment includes inspecting the abdomen for distention, palpating for rigidity, and auscultating for bowel sounds. If bowel sounds are absent or abnormal or the abdomen is distended or rigid, the nurse notifies the primary provider immediately. A nasogastric tube usually is inserted and food and fluids withheld until bowel sounds return.

Acute gastric dilatation, a condition in which the stomach becomes distended with fluids, is a complication similar to paralytic ileus. The client may regurgitate small amounts of liquid; the abdomen appears distended; and as the condition progresses, symptoms of shock may develop. Treatment includes inserting a nasogastric tube, applying suction, and removing the gas and fluid. Some surgeons routinely use suction of the GI tract to prevent paralytic ileus and acute gastric dilatation.

Urinary Elimination. Some clients experience difficulty voiding after surgery, particularly lower abdominal and pelvic surgery. Operative trauma in the region near the bladder may temporarily decrease the voiding sensation. Fear of pain also causes tenseness and difficulty voiding. Signs and symptoms of bladder distention include restlessness, lower abdominal pain, discomfort or distention, and fluid intake without urinary output. If the client does not have a catheter, the nurse assesses the client's ability to void and measures urine output. If the client cannot void within 8 hours following surgery, the nurse uses methods to encourage voiding, such as running water or having the client stand or use a bedside commode or toilet if permitted. If this does not work, the nurse notifies the primary provider, unless catheterization orders are in place.

Psychosocial Status. Many clients experience anxiety and fear after surgery as well as an inability to cope with changes in body image, lifestyle, and other factors. The nurse assesses what the client is experiencing and how the client is dealing with those issues. Many clients need referrals for counseling, support groups, and social services. The nurse acts as an effective listener, identifies areas of concern, and works with other health care professionals to assist the client and family to work through the problems. Box 14-6 lists the potential complications that clients may experience postoperatively.

Client and Family Teaching and Discharge

Before discharge, the client needs to receive instructions on how to carry out treatments at home. The nurse conveys the discharge instructions verbally and in writing. The nurse evaluates clients to determine their ability to carry out their care and to determine their specific needs, such as the need for the following:

- Supervised home care (e.g., visiting nurse, other health care agencies and providers)
- Supplies (e.g., dressings, tape, ostomy supplies, crutches)

BOX 14-6 Potential Postoperative Complications

Respiratory	**Gastrointestinal**
Atelectasis	Constipation
Pneumonia	Paralytic ileus
Pulmonary embolism	Bowel obstruction
Aspiration	**Functional**
Cardiovascular	Weakness
Shock	Fatigue
Thrombophlebitis	Functional decline
Urinary	**Wound**
Acute urine retention	Infection
Urinary tract infection	Dehiscence
Neurologic	Evisceration
Delirium	Delayed healing
Stroke	Hemorrhage
	Hematoma

Client and Family Teaching 14-2
Postoperative Instructions

The nurse develops a teaching plan to meet the client's needs. Points may include the following:

- Follow primary provider's instructions about cleaning the incision, applying the dressing, bathing, diet, and physical activity.
- Notify primary provider of any of the following: chills or fever; drainage from the incision (some drainage may be expected in certain cases); foul odor or pus from the incision; redness, streaking, pain, or tenderness around the incision; other symptoms not present at discharge (e.g., vomiting, diarrhea, cough, or chest or leg pain).
- Take medications as prescribed, including pain medications. Do not omit or change the dose unless the primary provider advises to do so.
- Do not take nonprescription medications unless approved by the primary provider.
- Follow dietary advice and drink fluids liberally, unless directed otherwise.
- Do not drive or operate machinery until cleared by the primary provider.
- Keep all postoperative appointments.
- Tell the primary provider about any problems during recovery.

- Special dietary needs
- Adjustments to the living environment (e.g., special bed, portable commode, wheelchair access)

Because sedative medications affect memory for events surrounding their administration, the nurse must review discharge instructions with an adult who will be responsible for the client after discharge. They instruct the client not to drink alcoholic beverages for a specified period after the procedure and to resume prescription and nonprescription medications when appropriate. The nurse must instruct the client about when it is appropriate to begin taking pain medications because they may have an additive effect with the sedative medications that were administered. Client and Family Teaching 14-2 outlines key information to teach postoperatively.

For clients who have undergone ambulatory surgery, surgical units use outcome criteria to determine if the client's condition is stable and if they can safely leave the hospital or outpatient setting. These criteria include that the client

- has stable cardiovascular function and a patent airway;
- is easily aroused;
- has intact protective reflexes;
- can talk;
- can sit up unaided;
- is adequately hydrated.

NURSING PROCESS FOR POSTOPERATIVE CARE

Nurses must follow current practice standards of care for postoperative clients. The following material provides commonly used nursing analyses and interventions in postoperative care. It does not provide a complete list but contains minimum standards for the general surgical client.

Overall Goal: Respiratory Function Is Maintained

Ineffective Airway Clearance Risk: Risk for ineffective airway clearance related to immobility, effects of anesthesia and analgesics, and pain
Expected Outcome: Client will have clear lungs and full and unlabored respirations.

- Monitor respiratory rate and characteristics.
- Auscultate lung sounds once per shift or more often if indicated.
- Help client turn and deep breathe every 1 to 2 hours.
- Reinforce use of incentive spirometer.
- Show client how to splint incision before coughing.
- Assess client's ability to mobilize secretions; suction if necessary.
- Administer oxygen as ordered.
- Refrain from administering narcotic analgesics if respiratory rate is less than 12 breaths/min.
- Encourage early ambulation.

Overall Goal: Circulatory Function Is Maintained

Electrolyte Imbalance Risk

Expected Outcome: The nurse will manage imbalances in fluid and electrolytes.

- Assess vital signs and monitor laboratory values.
- Ensure that IV fluids are infusing at the prescribed rate and that the IV site is patent.
- Monitor postoperative intake and output for at least 48 hours or until all drains and tubes have been removed, client is tolerating oral intake, and urine output is normal.
- Report discrepancies in intake and output, hypotension, dizziness, palpitations, or abnormal laboratory values (see Chapter 16 for additional information on management of fluid and electrolyte imbalance).

Bleeding Risk/Hypovolemia: Potential for Bleeding and Shock

Expected Outcome: The nurse will manage and minimize hemorrhage and shock.

- Monitor for signs or symptoms of shock: tachycardia; hypotension; decreased urine output; cold, clammy skin; and restlessness.
- Keep head of bed flat unless contraindicated.
- Maintain patent IV line.
- Assess surgical site for excessive external bleeding.
- Reinforce dressing or apply pressure if bleeding is frank (obvious or clinically evident).
- Monitor for internal bleeding: peri-incisional hematoma and swelling, abdominal distention if abdominal surgery was performed, excessive bloody output in wound drainage collection devices, falling hemoglobin and hematocrit levels, orthostatic hypotension, and signs of impending shock (see Chapter 17 for additional information on management of shock).
- Report findings immediately.

Overall Goal: Pain and Nausea Are Recognized and Effectively Treated

Acute Pain: Related to surgical incision and manipulation of body structures
Expected Outcome: Client will experience relief of pain.

- Assess pain level using an established scale (visual or numerical).
- Determine source of pain (e.g., incision, body position, flatus, IV lines or drainage tubes, distended bladder).
- Provide pain medication and evaluate effectiveness 30 minutes after administration.
- Reposition client to improve comfort.
- Teach client nonpharmacologic methods of pain relief: breathing exercises, relaxation techniques, and distraction (see Chapter 11).

Nausea: Related to effects of anesthesia or side effects of narcotics
Expected Outcome: Client will report relief of nausea and vomiting.

- Encourage client to breathe deeply to help eliminate inhaled anesthetics.
- Help client sit up and turn head to one side while vomiting to avoid aspiration.
- Record intake and output.
- Offer small sips of flat ginger ale or cola or ice chips if permitted.
- Administer antiemetics as ordered.
- Provide mouth care and fresh linens after vomiting.
- Monitor intake and output and assess for signs or symptoms of dehydration or electrolyte imbalance (see Chapter 16).

NURSING PROCESS FOR POSTOPERATIVE CARE (continued)

Sleep Deprivation: Related to difficulty in assuming comfortable position secondary to surgery, unusual environment, noise, and interruptions
Expected Outcome: Client will report enhanced sleep pattern.

- Identify factors contributing to poor sleep (noise, room temperature, position, daytime sleeping, hospital routines).
- Reduce environmental distractions—use night lights, close door.
- Schedule nursing activities to coincide with client's schedule.
- Teach client progressive relaxation techniques and deep-breathing exercises to facilitate sleep.
- Provide back rub.
- Assist with hygiene; provide clean gown and linens.
- Limit daytime sleeping; encourage increased daytime activity.
- Collaborate with primary provider about sleeping medication if other methods fail.

Overall Goal: Client Safety Is Maintained

Injury Risk: Related to decreased alertness secondary to effects of anesthesia and pain medication
Expected Outcome: Client will remain free of injury.

- Place bed in low position and elevate side rails.
- Place call bell within reach.
- Ensure that tubings are long enough or properly secured to allow for movement. Inspect drainage tubes for kinks.
- Ensure that all equipment is functioning properly.
- Provide emesis basin, tissues, ice chips (if allowed), bedpan, and urinal within easy reach.
- Instruct clients to call for assistance with any activity.

Overall Goal: Wound Healing Is Promoted and Wound Management Is Provided

Infection Risk: Related to break in skin integrity (surgical incision, wound drainage devices)
Expected Outcome: Client will have uncomplicated wound healing free of infection.

- Inspect surgical site and peri-incisional drain sites for signs or symptoms of infection (redness, warmth, tenderness, separation of wound edges, purulent drainage).
- Wash hands before and after dressing changes; follow aseptic or sterile technique.
- Change wet dressings frequently (surgeon usually does first dressing change).
- Use skin barrier to protect skin and wound from irritating drainage.
- Avoid using excessive tape.
- Keep drainage tube exit sites clean.
- Prevent excess tension on drainage tubes by securing tubes to dressing.
- Empty collection devices frequently to promote drainage; note characteristics of drainage.
- Teach client to splint wound when coughing or changing position.

Overall Goal: Complication Potential Is Continuously Assessed and Any Complications Are Immediately and Effectively Treated

Venous Thomboembolism Risk: Deep Vein Thrombosis

Expected Outcome: The nurse will manage and minimize risk of phlebitis/thrombosis.

- Reinforce need to perform leg exercises every hour while awake.
- Instruct client not to cross legs or prop pillow under knees.
- Apply compression and antiembolic stockings as ordered.
- Monitor for signs and symptoms of thrombophlebitis: calf pain, tenderness, warmth, or redness; swelling of the extremity; low-grade fever. Notify primary provider of any such signs or symptoms, and maintain bed rest until client can be further evaluated.
- Ambulate or encourage client to ambulate for a few minutes each hour while awake.
- Help client avoid prolonged sitting and poorly fitting, constrictive antiembolic hose.
- Do not massage calves or thighs.
- Administer anticoagulant medication as ordered; monitor laboratory values for therapeutic levels.

Urinary Retention: Inability to Empty Bladder Fully

Expected Outcome: The nurse will manage and minimize risk of urinary retention.

- Assess for bladder distention, discomfort, and urge to void.
- Encourage client to try to void within the first 4 hours after surgery.
- Assess volume of first voided urine to determine adequacy of output (voiding frequent, small amounts indicates retention of urine with elimination of overflow only).
- If client has difficulty voiding in the bedpan or using the urinal in bed, stand male clients (if allowed) and ambulate female clients to bathroom (if allowed).
- If client cannot void within 8 hours of surgery, consult with primary provider regarding instituting intermittent catheterization until voluntary voiding returns.

(continued)

NURSING PROCESS FOR POSTOPERATIVE CARE (continued)

Risk for Complications: Paralytic ileus
Expected Outcome: The nurse will manage and minimize risk for developing postoperative paralytic ileus.

- Assess bowel sounds every shift or more often if indicated.
- Assess returning bowel function as evidenced by passage of flatus or stool.
- Maintain NPO status until bowel sounds return.
- Report large amounts of emesis (more than 300 mL).
- Provide client with moistened gauze to wet lips and tongue until oral intake is allowed.
- Assist with passage of nasogastric tube, if ordered.

Overall Goal: Gastrointestinal Function Is Maintained

Constipation Risk: Related to effects of anesthesia, surgery (manipulation of abdominal organs), side effects of narcotics, and decreased intake of fluids and fiber
Expected Outcome: Client will have regular bowel movements.

- Once bowel sounds have returned and client resumes oral intake, encourage intake of sufficient fluids and fiber.
- Encourage ambulation to promote peristalsis.
- Encourage use of bathroom if possible. Provide privacy if client must use bedside commode or bedpan.
- Administer bulk-forming laxatives or stool softeners prophylactically if ordered.
- Notify primary provider if client has had no bowel movement within 2 to 3 days after surgery.

Overall Goal: Self-Care and Mobility Are Encouraged as Appropriate

Activity Intolerance: Related to decreased mobility and weakness secondary to anesthesia and surgery
Expected Outcome: Client will regain strength and activity tolerance.

- Encourage progressive activity.
- Help client dangle legs over bedside the evening of surgery or the next morning, if allowed, followed by sitting out of bed for 15 minutes (or more if tolerated).
- Progress to ambulation in room and hallway.
- Collaborate with client in establishing goals to increase ambulation.
- Help client with hygiene the evening of surgery; encourage increased self-care as appropriate.
- Schedule regular rest periods.

Overall Goal: Psychosocial Needs Are Recognized and Effectively Managed

Acute Anxiety: Related to unfamiliar environment, loss of privacy, threat to biologic integrity, and fear secondary to illness and surgery
Expected Outcome: Client will share anxieties and report increased psychological comfort.

- Ask client to rate anxiety level on a scale of 0 (*none*) to 10 (*unbearable*).
- Explore reasons for anxiety (concerns about health, financial status, family coping, effects on independence). Provide information and reassurance.
- Provide referrals if appropriate.
- Encourage client to use anxiety-reduction techniques (see Chapter 68).
- Determine how to modify the environment to improve relaxation (e.g., close or open curtains, reduce noise, move client closer to nurses' station).
- Assess anxiety level after interventions.

Overall Goal: Discharge Instructions Including Follow-Up Care and Home Health Services Are Provided

Knowledge Deficiency: Related to incomplete knowledge of wound care, activity and diet restrictions, medications, reportable signs and symptoms, and follow-up care
Expected Outcome: Client and/or family will demonstrate ability to provide wound care, restate specific instructions regarding diet and activity, and identify signs and symptoms of complications and needed follow-up care.

- Explain, demonstrate, and provide written instructions about care of surgical wound.
- Observe the client or family performing care.
- Discuss signs and symptoms of wound infection and instruct client and family to contact health care provider if they develop.
- Describe and provide written instructions about activity restrictions and when to resume normal activity.
- Include information on walking, bending, lifting, climbing stairs, bathing, showering, driving, and engaging in sexual activity.
- Explain need for adequate nutrition and fluids and how to manage constipation, which can result from decreased fluid intake, decreased activity, and narcotic pain relievers.
- Review all medications, including dose, route of administration, intended effect, side effects, and duration of prescription.
- Review signs and symptoms of complications such as shortness of breath, fever, productive cough, weakness, new or unusual pain, pain unrelieved by medication, calf tenderness and swelling, and wound drainage.
- Evaluate client's and family's understanding of discharge instructions.

KEY POINTS

- Perioperative care has three sections:
  - Preoperative: begins with decision to perform surgery and continues until operating area
  - Intraoperative: includes the entire surgical procedure until transfer to the recovery area
  - Postoperative: begins with admission to recovery area until discharge home or to a unit
- Preoperative care: preparing the client for surgery
  - Assessment
  - Surgical consent
  - Preoperative teaching
  - Physical preparation
  - Preoperative medications
  - Psychosocial preparation
  - Preoperative checklist
- Intraoperative care: begins when the client is transferred to the operating table
  - Anesthesia
    - General
    - Regional anesthesia
    - Procedural sedation
  - Surgical team
    - Anesthesiologist
    - Anesthetist
    - Surgeon
    - Surgical assistants
    - Intraoperative nurses
      - Scrub nurse
      - Circulating nurse
  - OR environment
    - Unrestricted zone: street clothes allowed
    - Semi-restricted zone: surgical attire required but not masks
    - Restricted zone: full surgical attire required
  - Nursing management
    - Intraoperative assessment
    - Prevention of intraoperative complications
- Postoperative care: designates the time spent recovering from the effects of anesthesia
  - Transport of the client
  - Nursing management
    - Immediate postoperative period
      - Initial postoperative assessment
      - Prevention of postoperative complications
        - Hemorrhage
        - Shock
        - Hypoxia
        - Aspiration
    - Later postoperative period
      - Ongoing assessments
        - Respiration
        - Circulation
        - Pain management
        - Skin integrity/wound healing
        - Bowel elimination
        - Urinary elimination
        - Psychosocial status
      - Client and family teaching and discharge

CRITICAL THINKING EXERCISES

1. The nurse is checking to ensure that a client's surgical consent form is signed and on the medical record the evening before surgery. When the nurse assesses this client, the client reports that they are uncertain about having the surgery and does not understand what is expected or its long-term consequences. What steps should the nurse take? What must the nurse document?
2. A client reports to the nurse that their family has lost several family members unexpectedly during surgery. The client is very scared about their upcoming surgery. What actions should the nurse take? What should the nurse document?
3. It is the fifth day of a client's postoperative period (5 days post-op). They complain of incisional pain, feeling warm, and nausea. What assessments should the nurse make? What should they document?
4. What concerns should nurses have when caring for postoperative clients with a history of smoking at least one pack of cigarettes per day for many years?

NCLEX-STYLE REVIEW QUESTIONS PrepU

1. A nurse is reviewing the list of clients scheduled for outpatient surgery the following day. What clients would be of most concern to the nurse?
   1. A client having a breast biopsy to rule out malignancy (cancer).
   2. A client scheduled for cataract removal at an eye surgical center.
   3. A client who reports a blood clotting problem having abdominal hernia repair.
   4. A client with chronic knee pain having an arthroplastic procedure.
2. The nurse is caring for a 16-year-old client who requires surgery to realign the bones in a fractured tibia sustained while backpacking with a youth group. In this case, from whom is it most appropriate to obtain consent to perform the surgical procedure?
   1. The client
   2. The client's parents
   3. The client's primary provider
   4. The client's youth leader

3. The nurse recognizes that more preoperative teaching is needed when hearing the client state which of the following statements?
1. "I can have a small breakfast of juice and coffee the morning of surgery."
2. "I do not need to bring my jewelry to the hospital the day of surgery."
3. "I will bathe with the special soap I was given the night before the surgery."
4. "I will need to empty my bladder before I receive my preoperative medications."

4. A nurse is caring for a client scheduled for right rotator cuff repair (right shoulder). The client expresses concern about having the wrong shoulder operated on. What responses by the nurse should help to relieve the client's fears? Select all that apply.
1. "A zero with a line through it is marked on the left shoulder to avoid surgery on that one."
2. "The nurses always make sure nothing like that ever happens at this hospital."
3. "The OR nurse will ask you to identify which shoulder is being operated on."
4. "You are asked to mark your right shoulder with an 'X' to ensure the surgery is on the correct side."
5. "Your surgeon will have to verify that the right shoulder is correct, placing their initials on the right shoulder."

5. A nurse needs to explain to a postoperative client the importance for performing leg exercises after surgery. What is the nurse's best explanation?
1. "Contracting and relaxing leg muscles prevent the development of varicose veins."
2. "Contracting and relaxing leg muscles prevent the formation of blood clots."
3. "Contracting and relaxing leg muscles prevent the loss of muscle strength."
4. "Contracting and relaxing leg muscles prevent the swelling of the extremities."

6. The nurse observes that a surgical client is experiencing abdominal incisional discomfort when coughing postoperatively. Which nursing intervention is most appropriate for reducing the client's discomfort?
1. Administer an analgesic soon after coughing.
2. Apply light pressure to the incision with a pillow.
3. Have the client lie supine before trying to cough.
4. Tell the client to flex both knees while coughing.

7. The nurse notes that a postoperative client is on a clear liquid diet. Which food item is most appropriate to provide?
1. A bowl of ice cream
2. A cup of creamed soup
3. A dish of gelatin
4. A glass of milk

8. The nurse explains the purpose of the Penrose drain positioned in the postoperative client's abdomen. What is the nurse's best explanation?
1. "An open wound drain decreases the formation of scar tissue."
2. "An open wound drain provides a means for irrigating the wound."
3. "An open wound drain releases accumulating intestinal gas."
4. "An open wound drain removes fluid from the surgical area."

9. The nurse notes that a postoperative abdominal surgical client who is NPO is complaining of a dry mouth. What is the best action for the nurse to take?
1. Allow the client to have a few ice chips.
2. Apply petrolatum to the inside of the client's mouth.
3. Assist the client to perform frequent oral hygiene.
4. Increase the rate of the IV fluids.

WANT TO KNOW MORE? There are a wide variety of online resources available on thePoint to enhance learning and understanding of this chapter.

Go to **thePoint.lww.com/activate** and use the activation code found in the front of this text to unlock these online resources.

15 Disaster Situations

Words To Know

anthrax
biologic disaster
blistering agents
bombs
botulism
chemical disasters
chlorine
cyanide
dirty bomb
disaster
earthquakes
external radiologic contamination
fallout
fault lines
flooding
human disasters
hurricanes
improvised explosive devices
internal radiologic contamination
natural disasters
nerve agents
nuclear blast
phosgene
potassium iodide
respiratory toxins
sarin
smallpox
tectonic plates
terrorists
tornadoes
toxins
triage system
tsunami
vesicants
wildfires
worried well

Learning Objectives

On completion of this chapter, you will be able to:

1. Define disaster.
2. List characteristics of a disaster.
3. Differentiate between natural and human disasters and give examples.
4. Identify three categories of human disasters that may result from acts of terrorism.
5. Explain the difference between external and internal radiation contamination.
6. List possible indications of a bioterrorism attempt.
7. Name three biologic agents likely to be used as terrorist weapons.
8. List possible indications of a chemical terrorism attempt.
9. Name four types of chemical agents that may be used to create a human disaster.
10. Name and describe phases involved in disaster management.
11. Discuss the role of nursing during a disaster.
12. List four triage categories used to prioritize victims' need for treatment.
13. Provide examples of collaborative problems and nursing analyses that the nurse may be required to manage in a disaster.

The American College of Emergency Physicians (2020) defines a **disaster** as one in which "an event that requires resources beyond the capability of a community and requires a multiple agency response." The magnitude of the disaster is related to the causal event. Disasters challenge emergency and health care services when victims overwhelm the health care system and health care providers who respond to their care and treatment. This chapter describes various types of disasters and the role of nurses and others who help manage the needs of victims.

Gerontologic Considerations

■ In a disaster situation, older adults may have increased vulnerability due to individual physical or mental needs, need for assistive devices and medications, lack of family or access to transportation, or need for special placement within a shelter. Various assessment instruments have been developed for rapid determination of priority needs (Baylor College of Medicine & The American Medical Association, n.d.).

(continued)

Gerontologic Considerations (*continued*)

- However, allocation of scarce medical and health care supplies can pose ethical challenges to nurses and other health care providers. Predisaster planning for evacuation and for triage principles involving various levels of health care providers and settings is crucial for effective response (U.S. Department of Health and Human Services, 2020).
- Changes related to aging involve temperature-regulating mechanisms, thus placing older adults at higher risk for hypothermia or hyperthermia if electricity is unavailable. Planning for methods to maintain temperature should be part of disaster planning in community or health care systems. Resources such as generators will be needed to maintain oxygen and other supportive equipment.

CHARACTERISTICS OF DISASTERS

Disasters are a type of extreme emergency. They tend to exceed the capacity of the community to function normally. They create demands that cannot be adequately met by the community (or country) without help from others. Some common characteristics of disasters include the following:

- Sudden
- Unpredicted
- Large-scale destruction
- Unfamiliarity with event
- Communication failure
- Disruption of resources
- Vulnerable victims
- Fear and helplessness

An emergency department (ED) is the usual location for managing extraordinary events that require a rapid response. However, a disaster exponentially increases an ED's stress and chaos. It requires multiple community resources and responders.

TYPES OF DISASTERS

There are basically two types of disasters: natural and human (man-made). Examples of **natural disasters** are generally weather related. Examples of **human disasters** are those that are the result of *unintentional* and *intentional* causes. An example of an unintentional human disaster is an explosion that occurs within a mine, at a fertilizer plant, industrial accident, or during the transport of incendiary materials. An intentional human disaster is often the result of acts of terrorism by people whose objective is to manipulate the politics and policies of a country by frightening and maiming the civilian population. Intentional disasters generally involve types of bombs, biologics, or chemicals. Both natural and human disasters may result in mass trauma and disruption of services.

Natural Disasters

Four types of natural disasters result in high **morbidity**, the incidence of health-related effects, and **mortality**, deaths within a population. Examples of natural disasters include earthquakes, floods, wild fires, and those caused by storms such as hurricanes, tornadoes, and blizzards.

Earthquakes

Earthquakes occur when two **tectonic plates**, sublayers of the earth's crust, cause the ground to shift. Locations where earthquakes occur are usually along **fault lines**, cracks between subterranean layers of rocks. Most are familiar with the San Andreas fault line in California where many predict a major earthquake will occur. However, a second potentially more deadly fault line is in the Pacific Northwest that follows the Cascadia mountain range. It runs from Vancouver, Canada, in the north, through Washington state, Oregon, and California. Alaska also has experienced earthquakes and may do so again. There is even a vulnerable fault line in New York.

In 2011, an earthquake in Japan caused devastating human casualties, floods, and damage to infrastructures. It damaged the Fukushima nuclear plant and set off a massive **tsunami** (tidal wave) containing potentially radioactive materials, cars, boats, and other debris that reached the shores of north coastal regions of the United States. Other recent earthquake locations have occurred in Nepal, India, Haiti, and New Guinea.

More people have been killed by earthquakes than any other natural disaster. For example, 220,000 people died in the earthquake that struck Haiti in 2010 and 300,000 were injured (Mesidor & Sly, 2019). Most earthquakes have devastating effects when they occur in developing countries. Besides the loss of human life, earthquakes are generally accompanied by landslides, fires, flooding, dam breaches, downed power lines, and spills of hazardous materials. Life-sustaining commodities like food and water may be temporarily unavailable.

Floods

Flooding, the overflow of water beyond its normal confines, occurs in a variety of situations: excessive rain, dam or levee failure, rapid snow melt, and tsunamis. When flooding occurs in a few hours of time, it can have disastrous effects. Floods account for 40% of all the world's disasters and do the greatest amount of damage. Many deaths are the result of driving into deep water or becoming trapped in fast-flowing water. Secondary health-related deaths can result when the high water disrupts sewage disposal systems and toxic waste sites, or chemicals stored above ground. Morbidity and mortality can be reduced by identifying flood-prone areas, inspecting and repairing dams and levees, and issuing early warnings of floods.

Storms

The terms **hurricanes** and **tornadoes** refer to storms that occur with rotating wind systems in which spinning air creates explosive forces. Tornadoes can reach wind speeds as high as 300 miles/hour. Most victims of hurricanes are coastal residents, those involved in boating and shipping, and those involved in emergency evacuations. Residents in lightweight mobile homes or driving small automobiles are often casualties of tornadoes. The National Weather Service in the United States identifies conditions that are conducive to the formation of tornadoes, but some civilians have no place to take shelter. Blizzards, which are accompanied by snow, high winds, and freezing rain, can also be considered a form of a natural disaster.

Wildfires

A **wildfire** is the large combustion of vegetation that spreads quickly and is difficult to extinguish. Wildfires can be ignited by careless smokers, campers, and lightning. Large acres of property are destroyed. Domestic and wild animals perish. The human death toll occurs largely among firefighters who die from heat stroke and carbon monoxide inhalation, and those who resist leaving their homes.

HUMAN DISASTERS

There are three categories of intentional human disasters discussed in this chapter. They are (1) bombings, an explosion that may or may not result in radiation exposure; (2) biologic disasters; and (3) chemical disasters. The actual or potential threat from these three forms of human disasters recently has been attributed to **terrorists**, people who use violence directed against civilian targets in pursuit of political, religious, or ideologic goals. Terrorist attacks accounted for nearly 92% of worldwide incidents, with approximately 8% occurring in the United States within the previous 50 years (The Heritage Foundation, 2011). Despite the lower percentage, those in the United States were quite deadly as a consequence of the casualties from the World Trade Center, Pentagon, and Shanksville, Pennsylvania, attacks on September 11, 2001, and those at the Boston Marathon bombing in 2013 (The Heritage Foundation, 2011).

Bombs

Bombs are devices designed to explode on impact or when detonated to kill people, damage or destroy property.

Improvised Explosive Devices

Currently, the types of bombs favored by terrorists are **improvised explosive devices** (IEDs) made from triacetone triperoxide (TATP), nicknamed *Mother of Satan*. Unfortunately, the ingredients for TATP can be obtained easily from home and garden stores, retail stores, and drug stores. Once made, the substance is highly unstable, making bombs of this kind easy to detonate. Terrorists have been adding **shrapnel**, pieces of metal ejected during the explosion, which cause penetrating wounds that can be as lethal as the pressure changes caused by the explosion. The attacks in Paris and Brussels in 2015 and 2016, respectively, involved TATP. In the United States, the bombs used in the Boston Marathon in 2013; the foiled bomb threats of Richard Reid, the shoe bomber; the Christmas day underwear bombing attempt in 2009; and the bombs found secreted in printer cartridges on air cargo planes originating from Yemen in 2010 indicate that this type of disaster continues to be a major threat.

Dirty Bombs

A **dirty bomb** combines radioactive material with conventional explosives. When detonated, it scatters radiation. Although it generally does not cause mass casualties, it can cause a fire, radiation poisoning, fear among those who were exposed, and costly decontamination of locations in the immediate environment. When a dirty bomb is released, responders focus attention on caring for injured victims and those referred to as the **worried well**, unaffected people who believe they are at risk for physical consequences.

Nuclear Power Plant Disasters

Nuclear power plants use radioactive materials as a source of fuel to create electrical energy for consumers. The devices that initiate, control, and sustain the nuclear reactions as well as spent fuel are potential concerns for the escape of radiation. Accidents involving nuclear power plants occurred at Three Mile Island, Pennsylvania, in 1979; Chernobyl in the Ukraine in 1986; and the earthquake-damaged Fukushima plant in Japan in 2011.

The U.S. Nuclear Regulatory Commission (USNRC) oversees civilian use of nuclear materials to ensure adequate protection of public health and safety. The chairman of the NRC has indicated that nuclear power plants can resist damage from hurricanes, tornadoes, earthquakes, and the impact of a small plane. However, nuclear power plants have not been built to withstand a crash from a large airliner like those used in the September 11, 2001, terrorist attack. Although the risk of radiologic sabotage is lower in the United States than in other countries with less rigorous regulations, the Government Accounting Office has continued to recommend that the NRC evaluate and implement measures to strengthen the defense of nuclear power plants against terrorists seeking to cause the release of radioactive materials (USNRC, 2020). The NRC currently requires states with a population within 10 miles of a commercial nuclear plant to have immediate access to a supply of **potassium iodide** (KI) tablets, prophylaxis for protecting the thyroid gland from absorption of radiation, and to provide a place for shelter during a power plant accident.

Nuclear Blast

A **nuclear blast** such as that used in Hiroshima and Nagasaki, Japan, in 1945 is an explosion that produces an intense wave of heat, light, air pressure, and radiation. The explosion creates a fireball and mushroom cloud that contains radioactive material and vaporized particles. When the vapor cools, it condenses and drops back to earth, whereupon it is known as **fallout**. Wind currents can carry the fallout long distances (CDC, 2018).

The consequences for survivors of a nuclear blast include severe burns, trauma from debris, blindness, radiation sickness, and cancer, all of which result from external and internal radiologic contamination. **External radiologic contamination** occurs from exposure to fallout that lands on the skin, hair, and clothing. **Internal radiologic contamination** occurs when fallout enters an open wound, is inhaled via contaminated air, or is consumed through contaminated food and water.

To avoid the potential for nuclear destruction, representatives of 191 countries including the United States, Russia, the United Kingdom, France, and China, all of whom possess nuclear weapons, signed the Treaty on the Non-Proliferation of Nuclear Weapons in 1968. The treaty in essence is an agreement to prevent the spread of nuclear weapons, to promote peaceful uses of nuclear energy, and to work toward nuclear disarmament (Nuclear Threat Initiative, 2020). Nonproliferation and Disarmament Initiative (NPDI) was established in 2010 and continues working to reduce the global threats from nuclear, biologic, and chemical weapons.

See Evidence-Based Practice 15-1 for research on disaster preparedness for nurses.

Evidence-Based Practice 15-1

Disaster Preparedness Training for Nurses

Clinical Question

Is disaster preparedness training beneficial for nurses?

Evidence

A research study was completed in Ohio with public health nurses to see if a blended training method was effective when put through disaster competencies. The study did a pre- and postsurvey among nurses to collect data on confidence in training and if there is further training needed to prepare for disasters (Chiu et al., 2012). The need for nurses who are trained in population health may increase as there are more global threats, terrorism, and natural disasters. Public health nurses fall into this category as they are working in communities and are connected with resources and community needs. The education that the study examined was a blend of in-class training and self-learning modules. Presurveys were sent out to 182 Ohio public health nurses who had worked at six designated hospitals. Fifty-four postsurveys were returned. The survey results showed that in all three areas of disaster preparedness, the nurses felt that their confidence increased. The survey also showed that the nurses felt the need for further training was decreased. The survey looked at responses of nurses with <5 years' experience and nurses with >5 years' experience and showed no significant gap.

Nursing Implications

Although the study focused on public health nurses, all nurses may be in contact with a disaster at some point in their practice as our global world and environment change. Nurses should take advantage of educational offerings and be aware of their role in a disaster. Blended education offerings may reach many nurses who learn at different levels and increase confidence in their role in these situations.

Reference

Chiu, M., Polivka, B. J., & Stanley, S. R. (2012). Evaluation of a disaster-surge training for public health nurses. *Public Health Nursing, 29*(2), 136–142. http://doi.org/10.1111/j.1525-1446.2011.00984.x

BIOLOGIC DISASTERS

A **biologic disaster** is one in which pathogens or their **toxins**, pathologic substances produced by microorganisms, cause harm to many humans and other living species. Examples of biologic disasters include the outbreak of bubonic plague in Eurasia in the 12th century and the influenza epidemic in the United States during the early 20th century. Although these disasters occurred naturally, the current concern is the deliberate use of biologic agents as weapons of mass destruction. Box 15-1 lists possible indications of the use of a bioterrorist agent.

Biologic agents are classified into three categories: A, B, and C according to their risk to national security and public health preparedness (Box 15-2). Three high-priority agents likely to be used in bioterrorist warfare include anthrax, botulism, and smallpox. These agents pose a high threat because they are (1) stable and simple to mass produce, (2) easy to deliver to a large population, (3) associated with high mortality, and (4) likely to cause public fear (CDC, 2018).

BOX 15-1 Indications of Bioterrorism

- High outbreak of similar symptoms among previously healthy people
- Increased numbers of people who are sick seeking health care
- Atypical incidence of illness for the time of year and geographic location
- Clusters of people who are sick from a shared locale
- Unusual mortality rates among people following a brief illness
- Unexplained deaths or illness among domestic and wild animals

Adapted from San Francisco Department of Public Health (2020). *Recognizing bioterrorism*. https://www.sfcdcp.org/health-alerts-emergencies/recognize-an-illness-associated-with-bioterrorism/

BOX 15-2 Examples of Biologic Agents Listed by Potential Morbidity and Mortality

Category A (Highest Mortality)
- *Bacillus anthracis* (anthrax)
- *Clostridium botulinum* (botulism)
- *Variola major* (smallpox)
- Viral hemorrhagic fevers (Dengue, Ebola, and Marburg viruses)

Category B (Moderate Morbidity; Low Mortality)
- *Salmonella* species
- *Escherichia coli*
- *Brucella* species (brucellosis)

Category C (Not Presently Likely to Be Used for Bioterrorism)
- Hantaviruses (pulmonary syndrome)
- Flavivirus (yellow fever)
- Mycobacterium tuberculosis (multidrug-resistant tuberculosis)

From National Institute of Allergy and Infectious Diseases. (2018). *NIAID emerging infectious diseases/pathogens*. http://www.niaid.nih.gov/topics/biodefenserelated/biodefense/pages/cata.aspx

Anthrax

Anthrax is a spore-forming bacterium known as *Bacillus anthracis*. Anthrax is fairly easy to promulgate because in its spore form, it is inactive and causes disease only when inhaled, ingested, or introduced into nonintact skin. Skin infection is the least deadly form and the only one that may be transmitted by direct contact. It is characterized by painless lesions usually on the head, hands, and arms that develop into black-centered blisters that eventually ulcerate (Fig. 15-1). Once inside the body, the spores multiply and produce toxins. Anthrax sent in powdered form within letters delivered by the U.S. Postal Service caused 22 infections and 5 deaths among Americans in 2001 (CDC, 2016). Standard precautions, measures for reducing the risk of transmitting pathogens (see Chapter 12), are sufficient when caring for clients infected with anthrax.

Anthrax is treated fairly successfully with antibiotic therapy. The preferred antibiotic is ciprofloxacin (Cipro) or levofloxacin (Levaquin), both of which are fluoroquinolones; the treatment lasts 4 weeks or longer for an inhalant infection. A vaccine has been developed to prevent infection with anthrax, but currently only military personnel and at-risk civilians are being targeted as recipients.

Botulism

Botulism is a disease that develops from the neurotoxin produced by *Clostridium botulinum*, an anaerobic bacterium (see Chapter 12). The pathogen is generally food-borne, but it also can be acquired through inhalation. People infected with botulinum toxin are not a risk to others; there have been no reports of person-to-person transmission. If used as a weapon of mass destruction, the pathogen most likely would be spread via toxin-contaminated food or aerosolization.

The botulinum toxin blocks acetylcholine, a parasympathetic neurotransmitter. Acetylcholine is responsible for the transmission of neural impulses to muscles. Blockage of acetylcholine results in paralysis of motor and autonomic nerves (Fig. 15-2). The greatest potential for lethality occurs with paralysis of the respiratory muscles. Even when a person survives, respiratory difficulty and muscular weakness may continue for years. Botulinum antitoxin is the only immediate treatment after exposure to lessen the severity of botulism. An antitoxin is a form of antibody therapy designed to provide rapid but short-term protection against a toxin. Botulinum antitoxin is available from the state's public health department or the CDC.

Smallpox

Smallpox is a highly contagious disease caused by the variola virus. The disease acquired its name because of the raised bumps that appear on the face and body.

The World Health Organization proclaimed eradication of smallpox in 1980 following the success of aggressive vaccination programs. Believing that smallpox had been conquered, the United States stopped administering routine childhood vaccinations in 1972 (CDC, 2019). The status of immunity among adults vaccinated prior to that date is unknown. Consequently, estimates are that many susceptible people could die if the smallpox virus that has been stored in two laboratories—one in the United States and one in Russia—were released as a bioterrorist act.

Smallpox may be mistaken for chickenpox (*varicella*), although the outbreak and progression of the rash are opposite in these illnesses (Fig. 15-3). The rash associated with smallpox begins on the face and progresses to the extremities, including the palms and soles, with few lesions on the trunk. The rash of chickenpox begins heavily on the trunk and spreads lightly to the face and extremities but tends to be missing or sparse on the palms and soles. Smallpox lesions are generally all in the same stage of development, but successive crops of chickenpox macules and papules appear every few days. Smallpox has no specific treatment.

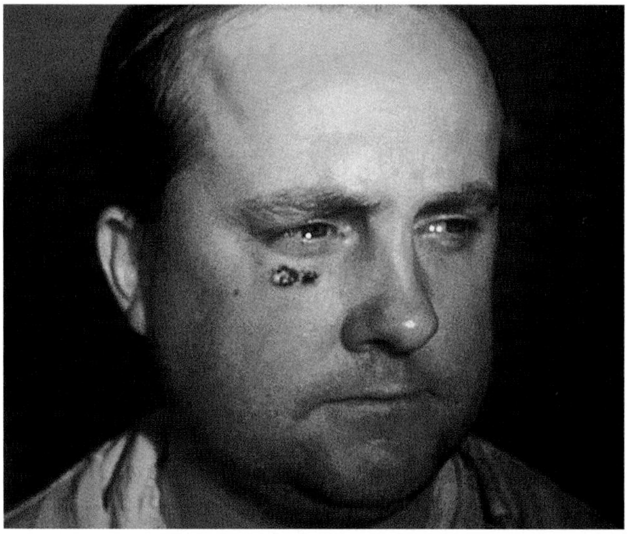

Figure 15-1 Appearance of anthrax skin lesion. (Courtesy of the Public Health Image Library, Centers for Disease Control and Prevention.)

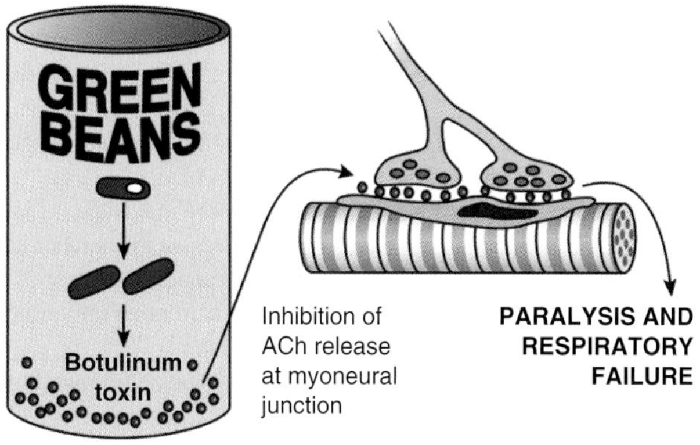

Figure 15-2 Botulinum toxin inhibits acetylcholine (ACh) at the myoneural junction, causing paralysis and respiratory failure. (Reprinted with permission from Strayer, D. S., Saffitz, J. E., & Rubin, E., (Eds.). (2019). *Rubin's pathology: Mechanisms of human disease* (8th ed.). Wolters Kluwer.)

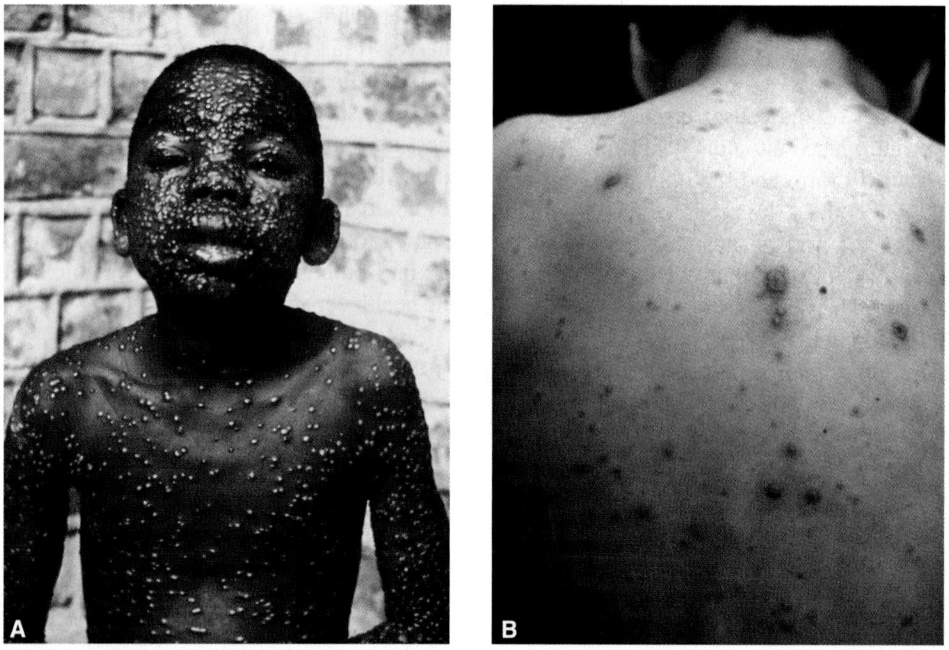

Figure 15-3 Smallpox may be mistaken for chickenpox. **(A)** Characteristic lesions of smallpox; the rash begins on the face and progresses to the extremities. **(B)** Characteristic lesions of chickenpox; the rash begins on the trunk and spreads lightly to the face and extremities. (Images courtesy of the Public Health Image Library, Centers for Disease Control and Prevention.)

Supportive measures such as fluid therapy, antipyretics, and antibiotics for secondary bacterial infections reduce symptoms and help prevent death.

The U.S. government has proactively stockpiled sufficient smallpox vaccine to administer to everyone in the country, if necessary. It may take up to 12 hours for the vaccine to arrive at any needed destination, however, which could be problematic in the event of a wide-scale attack. The smallpox vaccine is effective in preventing infection or rendering the illness less severe if administered within 3 days of exposure to the virus; however, in most cases, a person may be unaware of having been exposed. The vaccine is useless for a person who is already symptomatic. No one who has been exposed to smallpox will be vaccinated forcibly, but they may be placed in isolation for at least 18 days to monitor for symptoms.

Nurses would play a major role in vaccinating the public during a potential or actual outbreak of smallpox (Nursing Guidelines 15-1). They would also teach anyone vaccinated for smallpox how to care for the vaccination site (Client and Family Teaching 15-1).

NURSING GUIDELINES 15-1

Administering a Smallpox Vaccination

When administering a smallpox vaccination, the nurse will

- Use the deltoid site for vaccination.
- Avoid the use of alcohol as a skin disinfectant because alcohol inactivates the virus.
- Dip the bifurcated needle once into the multidose vial of vaccine to create a tiny drop at the tip.
- Hold the needle perpendicular to the site.
- Pierce the skin rapidly in a 5-mm area 15 times, or the number identified on the vial, to cause a trace of blood to appear (see figure).
- Dab the site with dry sterile gauze and discard in an infection control receptacle.
- Cover the site of the vaccination with loose gauze followed by adhesive tape.

Adapted from Centers for Disease Control and Prevention. (2018). *Smallpox vaccination method.* https://www.cdc.gov/smallpox/clinicians/vaccination-administration2.html

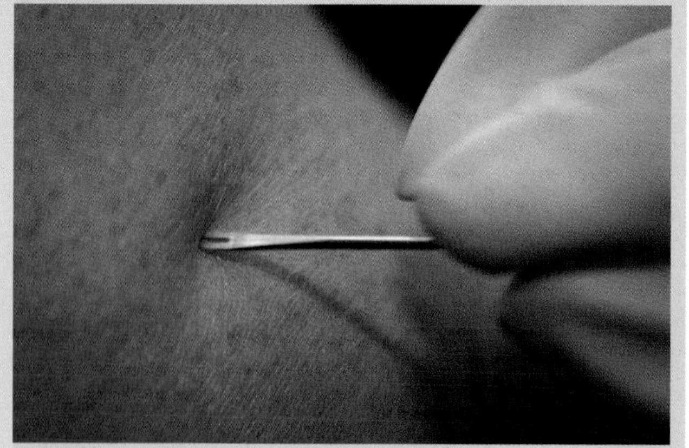

A bifurcated needle is used to administer a smallpox vaccination. (Courtesy of Public Health Image Library, Centers for Disease Control and Prevention. Photo Credit: James Gathany.)

Client and Family Teaching 15-1 Caring for a Smallpox Vaccination Site

The nurse teaches the client and family to do the following:

- Avoid scratching or rubbing the site of vaccination.
- Keep the site covered with a gauze dressing.
- Place a waterproof cover over the site when bathing.
- Change the gauze dressing every 1 to 2 days or if it becomes wet.
- Discard the soiled dressing, waterproof covering, and scab when it is shed in a sealable plastic bag.
- Wash hands thoroughly or use an alcohol-based handrub after touching the site or dressings, clothing, towels, or sheets in contact with the site.
- Separate and wash clothes, towels, and bed linens that come in contact with the vaccination site in hot water, detergent, or bleach.
- Call a health care provider if there are concerns about the vaccination site.
- Have the site checked 7 days following the vaccination.

Adapted from Centers for Disease Control and Prevention. (2017). *Smallpox vaccination method.* https://www.cdc.gov/smallpox/vaccine-basics/who-gets-vaccination.html#care-for

CHEMICAL DISASTERS

Chemical disasters result from the release of toxic man-made substances with a potential for causing mass casualties. Release of chemical agents among a population may occur either through an industrial accident or during transport. Terrorists also can use chemical agents as weapons. Examples of extremely toxic chemicals include nerve agents, cyanide, respiratory toxins, and blistering agents.

Detecting a chemical accident or attack is difficult because most chemical agents are liquids that vaporize quickly with either no odors or odors that may be attributed to other substances (e.g., garlic, onions). Box 15-3 lists some indications of a chemical release.

BOX 15-3 Indications of Chemical Terrorism

- Numerous dead animals such as birds, domestic pets, fish, or insects in a confined area
- Dead or dying vegetation
- Sick, dying, and dead humans, especially indoors or downwind
- Unexplained odor atypical for the location
- Fog-like or low-lying cloud in the atmosphere
- Abandoned devices that could be used for spraying chemicals

Adapted from U.S. Department of Health and Human Services. (2020). *Surveillance for possible chemical emergencies. https://chemm.nlm.nih.gov/surveillance.htm*

Nerve Agent Poisoning

Nerve agents, the most toxic of all chemical agents, are potent organophosphate compounds that cause fatal consequences by inhibiting acetylcholinesterase. Acetylcholinesterase is an enzyme that inactivates acetylcholine, a neurotransmitter of the parasympathetic (cholinergic) nervous system. Consequently, in cases of attacks with nerve agents, the functions of the parasympathetic nervous system will be active without any potential for disinhibition.

One example of a nerve agent is the commonly used insecticide Malathion. Malathion is highly toxic to insects but not to humans or the environment when applied following the labeled directions (U.S. Environmental Protection Agency, 2016). If released in large quantity or indiscriminately, however, it could be toxic to large numbers of people. Dangerous nerve agents such as **sarin**, which was released in a Tokyo subway in 1995, are 100 to 150 times more potent.

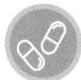

Pharmacologic Considerations

- Three drugs are given to manage the effects of nerve agent toxicity. They are atropine sulfate, which counteracts excess acetylcholine at muscarinic sites, pralidoxime chloride (2-PAM), which reactivates acetylcholinesterase, and diazepam (Valium) to control possible seizures.

Cyanide Poisoning

Cyanide is a solid salt or volatile liquid chemical that causes death in minutes. It is used currently in gas chambers to execute prisoners. The Nazis used cyanide known as Zyklon B to exterminate Jews in gas chambers of concentration camps during World War II. The mechanism of cyanide's action is the inhibition of an enzyme, cytochrome oxidase, needed for oxygen metabolism and cellular energy. The gas that forms with release of cyanide is colorless and may have a faint odor of "bitter almonds." Inhalation, especially in an enclosed space, is the most deadly type of poisoning. Cyanide also can be ingested by eating foods laced with it or in accidental poisoning when consuming various industrial chemicals that break down into a cyanide-containing by-product. An example is the compound used to remove artificial fingernails. Cyanide can also be absorbed through the skin.

Nurses and other health care providers must wear protective garments and respirator masks if the victim's clothing contains cyanide. Contaminated clothing is removed and placed in a sealed container while resuscitation proceeds.

Pharmacologic Considerations

- One or all of the following, which are contained in a cyanide antidote kit, are administered: (1) amyl nitrite, a temporary measure administered by inhalation until intravenous (IV) access is achieved; (2) sodium nitrite by the IV route; and (3) IV sodium thiosulfate. Amyl nitrite promotes the formation of methemoglobin, which combines with cyanide to form nontoxic cyanmethemoglobin.
- Nursing Guidelines 15-2 provides information on administering amyl nitrite. If a victim does not respond to amyl nitrite, additional treatment with sodium nitrite is necessary. Sodium nitrite, administered intravenously for at least 5 minutes, attracts cyanide from the heme group of cytochrome oxidase. Intravenous sodium thiosulfate is given following sodium nitrite. It produces thiocyanate, a nontoxic substance that detoxifies cyanide. Most clients can be revived in 1 to 2 hours.

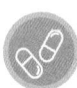

Pharmacologic Considerations

- Amyl nitrite causes rapid vasodilation, which may increase intraocular and intracranial pressure. It should be used with caution in people with glaucoma, recent head injury, or hemorrhagic stroke.
- Methemoglobin can cause cyanosis if it exceeds 15% to 20% in an adult. More severe symptoms such as headache, weakness, confusion, chest pain, and arrhythmias can occur when percentages rise above 25% to 70% (Densahw-Burke, 2016). If amyl nitrite is administered in the recommended doses, toxic levels of methemoglobin should not develop.
- It is not easy to control the fumes from broken amyl nitrite pearls and from the saturated cloth held over the victim's nose and mouth, resulting in overdosing or underdosing or causing adverse effects in the rescuer.

Respiratory Toxin Poisoning

Respiratory toxins are chemical agents that primarily cause pulmonary edema when inhaled. Two common examples are **chlorine** and **phosgene**, liquids that become gases when released in the atmosphere. When vaporized, the gas settles and remains close to ground level for some time.

Chlorine is used in households and commercially as a cleaning agent; it is effective in reducing the growth of microorganisms in water and pools. Phosgene has multiple industrial uses and helps produce polyurethane, insecticides, and solvents. Phosgene is a by-product when Freon, a gas used in refrigerators and air-conditioners, burns (CDC, 2019). Both chemicals are used widely and therefore available for legitimate or possible terrorist purposes.

Exposure to these respiratory toxins leads to tearing, coughing, bronchospasms, and laryngospasms with airway obstruction from localized swelling. Phosgene actually breaks down alveolar tissue. The consequences of exposure to chlorine or phosgene are related to the amount, route, and length of chemical exposure. Death occurs as fluid infiltrates the pulmonary air spaces and terminal bronchioles interfering with gas exchange. Following recovery from an acute event, victims may develop chronic bronchitis and emphysema.

NURSING GUIDELINES 15-2

Administering Amyl Nitrite

To give amyl nitrite to a victim of cyanide poisoning, the nurse proceeds as follows:

- Break an ampule (perle) of amyl nitrite into a piece of cloth or gauze square.
- Insert the cloth or gauze containing amyl nitrite under the lip of an oxygen mask.
- Place the oxygen mask with 100% concentration of oxygen and the cloth containing amyl nitrite over the victim's nose and mouth.
- Inhale for 30 seconds every minute.
- Use a fresh ampule of amyl nitrite every 3 minutes.
- If the client has not responded to oxygen and amyl nitrite treatment, infuse 10 mL of sodium nitrite intravenously in a 3% solution (300 mg), starting the infusion as soon as possible and infusing over no less than 5 minutes.
- Monitor blood pressure and stop administering sodium nitrite if hypotension develops.
- Next, infuse sodium thiosulfate intravenously, 50 mL of a 25% solution (12.5 g) infused over 10 to 20 minutes. Repeat one-half of the initial dose 30 minutes later if there is an inadequate clinical response.

From Agency for Toxic Substances & Disease Registry. (n.d.). *Hydrogen cyanide (HCN)*. https://www.atsdr.cdc.gov/MHMI/mmg8.pdf.

Blistering Agents

Blistering agents, also known as **vesicants**, are chemicals that damage exposed skin and mucous membranes on contact. If inhaled, blistering agents also can damage respiratory tissues. Two examples of vesicants that have been used in chemical warfare include sulfur mustard (referred to as *mustard gas* during World War I) and lewisite, which was developed during World War I but never used.

In addition to being a contactant, vesicants can penetrate fabric. When in contact with skin, these chemicals combine with perspiration to form a solution that penetrates the skin and becomes anchored to dermal cells, forming blisters via enzymatic protein digestion. The impaired skin creates the potential for infection. Inhalation of the vesicant is almost sure to cause death within 24 hours from airway obstruction with blisters within the respiratory passages. Some chemical enters the circulation and potentially can affect major internal organs. For example, vesicants damage the DNA of rapidly growing cells, which may explain why nitrogen mustard continues to be a chemotherapeutic agent for cancer.

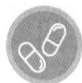

Care for the skin lesions is similar to burn wound management (see Chapter 66). Damaged skin may take several months to heal and longer if the wound becomes infected. Breathing is supported with mechanical ventilation. Blood transfusions or administration of colony-stimulating factors such as erythropoietin (Epogen, Procrit) and filgrastim (Neupogen) may be necessary if bone marrow function becomes suppressed.

››› *Stop, Think, and Respond 15-1*

For which agent are the following antidotes used: amyl nitrite, atropine sulfate, and dimercaprol?

Pharmacologic Considerations

■ Only one vesicant antidote is available, and it is effective only for lewisite. The antidote, known as dimercaprol, or British anti-lewisite (BAL), is most effective if given as soon as possible after exposure. It can also be used to treat heavy metal poisoning from arsenic, mercury, or gold.

››› *Stop, Think, and Respond 15-2*

Which of the three biologic agents discussed in this chapter is the most dangerous? Explain your answer.

DISASTER MANAGEMENT

Although natural and human disasters can develop under many circumstances, the key to limiting their effect requires four phases: mitigation, also called the prevention phase; preparedness; response; and recovery (Fig. 15-4; Table 15-1).

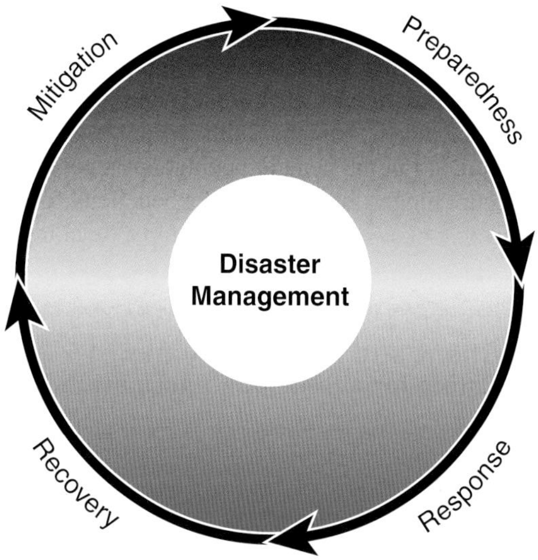

Figure 15-4 The disaster management continuum.

TABLE 15-1 Phases of Disaster Management

PHASE	DESCRIPTION	ACTIVITIES
Mitigation (takes place before and after disaster)	Prevent disaster Reduce future occurrence Limit damaging effects	Assess existing hazards Repair or reinforce dams, levees Enforce building codes Revise zoning and land use Provide public awareness
Preparedness (takes place before disaster occurs)	Plan for saving lives	Develop early warning system Determine evacuation routes Stockpile food, water, medications Designate location of shelters Conduct training and mock disaster response drills
Response (takes place during disaster)	Limit injuries and deaths Reduce property damage	Activate the disaster plan Conduct search, rescue, recover bodies Provide emergency care Communicate information to public Mobilize distribution of water and food Provide for sanitation needs Shut off damaged utilities such as water and leaking gas Control looting
Recovery (takes place immediately and after disaster occurs)	Return to normal Restore safety	Reunite victims with family Reconstruct infrastructure Integrate state and federal resources Provide services for emotional, social, economic, and physical well-being Revise original disaster plan

THE ROLE OF NURSES IN A DISASTER

Nurses are just one group of health care providers involved in a disaster. Others include police; firefighters; emergency medical technicians and paramedics; and local, state, and federal disaster workers under the direction of the American Red Cross, the Federal Emergency Management Agency (FEMA), and the U.S. Department of Health and Human Services. Many nurses are involved in triage activities in the field as well as caring for victims in shelters or EDs.

Although nurses have always played an integral role in disaster relief efforts, nursing skills are an essential component in preparing the general population in case an event should occur. Suggestions that may be beneficial for temporary survival are listed in Client and Family Teaching 15-2.

During an actual disaster, the first nursing action involves assessing as many victims as possible at the scene of the disaster to manage time efficiently and to avoid overwhelming valuable resources. Following a head-to-toe examination, nurses assign one of four categories in the standard **triage system** to prioritize victims' needs for treatment: *immediate*, *delayed*, *minimal*, and *expectant* (Table 15-2). Ideally, victims are tagged after assessing them to prevent duplication of assessments by another nurse or emergency worker (Fig. 15-5).

Although seemingly counterintuitive, nurses must adapt to the futility of trying to save casualties who are in imminent danger of dying. When supplies, equipment, and personnel are limited, nurses must be creative in implementing alternatives. They are often called upon to utilize and supervise volunteers.

Client and Family Teaching 15-2
Caring for a Smallpox Vaccination Site Preparing for a Disaster

The nurse teaches the following points for disaster preparedness:

- Keep a 7-day supply of medications and extra hearing aids or eyeglasses on hand at all times in case of a disaster.
- Store a supply kit with a flashlight, battery-operated radio, and extra batteries in case of loss of electricity.
- Keep a supply of canned or dried packaged food and bottled water on hand.
- In the event of biologic, chemical, or radiologic disaster, avoid consuming fresh food or water from the faucet because these items also might be contaminated with pathogens, chemicals, or fallout.
- Affix a tag to a pet's collar with a name, address, and phone number in case the pet is rescued and taken to an animal shelter.
- Create a network of persons who could provide support during and after a disaster, especially if older or disabled.

TABLE 15-2 Triage Categories

CATEGORY	COLOR COORDINATE	DESCRIPTION	EXAMPLES
Immediate	Red	Life-threatening but survivable if rapid medical attention is provided	Significant hemorrhage, pneumothorax, partial- or full-thickness burns of the face and neck
Delayed	Yellow	Serious but stable enough to survive if treatment is delayed 6–8 hours	Penetrating abdominal wound, fractures, partial- or full-thickness burns not involving the head
Minimal	Green	Minor injuries that can wait longer for treatment	Minor lacerations, superficial burns, contusions
Expectant	Black	Soon to die; lack of spontaneous respirations after opening the airway	Head injury with a Glasgow Coma score less than 8, multisystem trauma, partial- or full-thickness burns over 85% of body surface

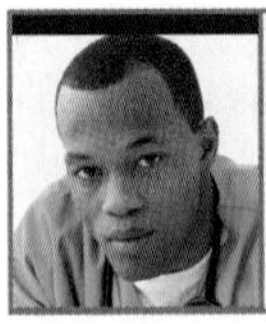

Clinical Scenario A student nurse is joining their classmates in a disaster drill. The disaster may involve a bomb or radiologic incident, biologic, or chemical agent. What actions should the nursing students take to identify victims, what problems might they encounter, and what interventions are appropriate? See the following Nursing Process section.

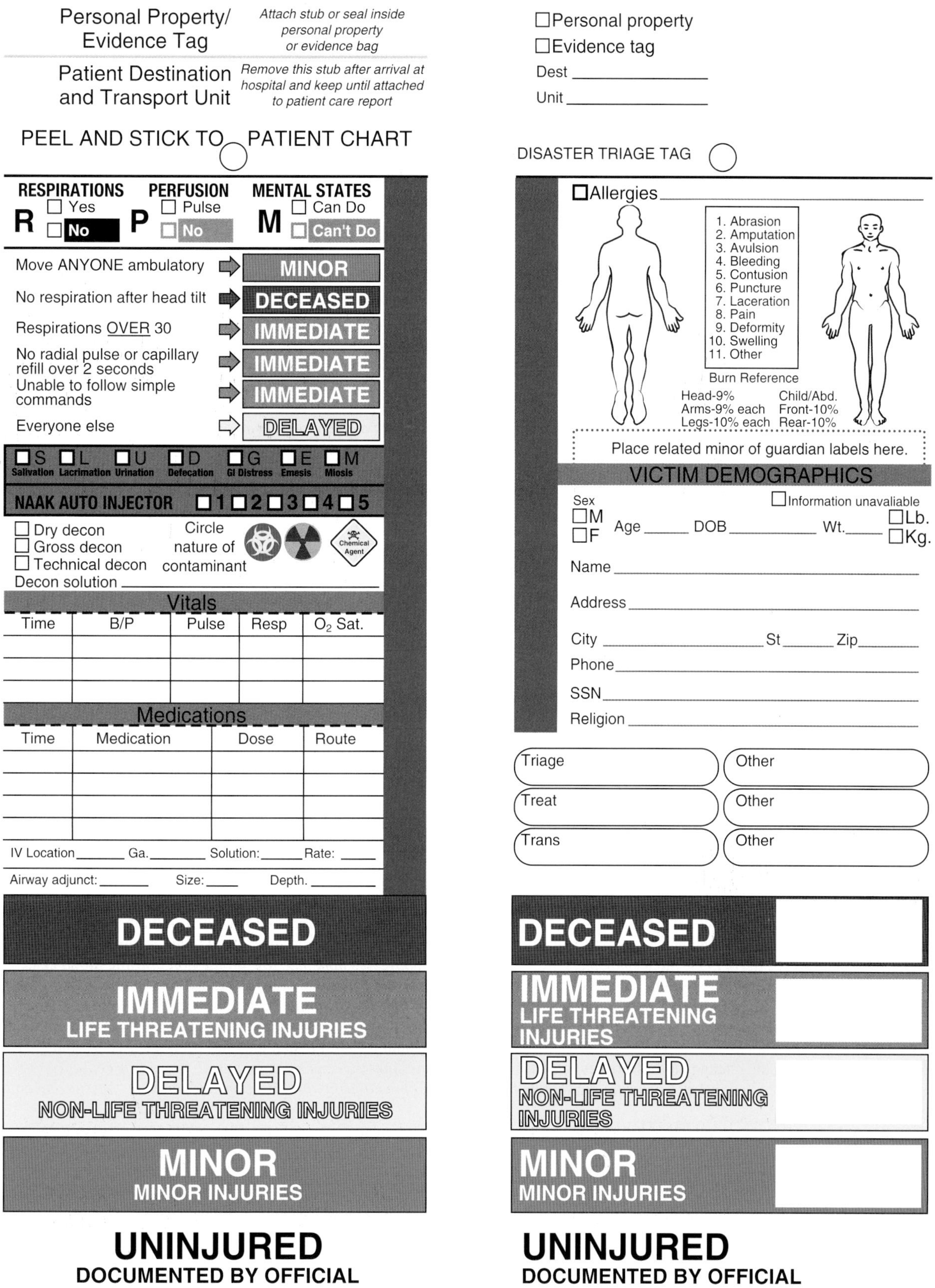

Personal Property/ Evidence Tag — *Attach stub or seal inside personal property or evidence bag*

Patient Destination and Transport Unit — *Remove this stub after arrival at hospital and keep until attached to patient care report*

PEEL AND STICK TO PATIENT CHART

RESPIRATIONS	PERFUSION	MENTAL STATES
R ☐ Yes ☐ No	P ☐ Pulse ☐ No	M ☐ Can Do ☐ Can't Do

Move ANYONE ambulatory	MINOR
No respiration after head tilt	DECEASED
Respirations OVER 30	IMMEDIATE
No radial pulse or capillary refill over 2 seconds	IMMEDIATE
Unable to follow simple commands	IMMEDIATE
Everyone else	DELAYED

☐S Salivation ☐L Lacrimation ☐U Urination ☐D Defecation ☐G GI Distress ☐E Emesis ☐M Miosis

NAAK AUTO INJECTOR ☐1 ☐2 ☐3 ☐4 ☐5

☐ Dry decon
☐ Gross decon
☐ Technical decon
Circle nature of contaminant — Chemical Agent
Decon solution ______

Vitals

Time	B/P	Pulse	Resp	O_2 Sat.

Medications

Time	Medication	Dose	Route

IV Location______ Ga.______ Solution:______ Rate: ______

Airway adjunct: ______ Size: ______ Depth. ______

DECEASED

IMMEDIATE
LIFE THREATENING INJURIES

DELAYED
NON-LIFE THREATENING INJURIES

MINOR
MINOR INJURIES

UNINJURED
DOCUMENTED BY OFFICIAL

☐Personal property
☐Evidence tag
Dest ______
Unit ______

DISASTER TRIAGE TAG

☐Allergies ______

1. Abrasion
2. Amputation
3. Avulsion
4. Bleeding
5. Contusion
6. Puncture
7. Laceration
8. Pain
9. Deformity
10. Swelling
11. Other

Burn Reference
Head-9% Child/Abd.
Arms-9% each Front-10%
Legs-10% each Rear-10%

Place related minor of guardian labels here.

VICTIM DEMOGRAPHICS

Sex ☐M ☐F ☐Information unavaliable
Age ______ DOB ______ Wt.______ ☐Lb. ☐Kg.
Name ______
Address ______
City ______ St______ Zip______
Phone ______
SSN ______
Religion ______

Triage | Other
Treat | Other
Trans | Other

DECEASED

IMMEDIATE
LIFE THREATENING INJURIES

DELAYED
NON-LIFE THREATENING INJURIES

MINOR
MINOR INJURIES

UNINJURED
DOCUMENTED BY OFFICIAL

Figure 15-5 An example of a triage tag that identifies a person's category by color code and includes additional identifying information.

NURSING PROCESS FOR THE CLIENT IN A DISASTER SITUATION

Assessment

Assess as many victims as possible at the scene of the disaster to manage time efficiently and to avoid overwhelming valuable resources. Wear protective garments and start with the closest victim, working outward from there. Begin by assessing a victim's airway, breathing, and circulation. Cut off clothing in a sequence from head to foot. Logroll the client to examine the body's posterior surface. Follow a head-to-toe examination.

Analysis, Planning, and Interventions

Bleeding Risk/Thermal Injury Risk

Expected Outcome: The nurse will monitor for, manage, and minimize life-threatening but survivable injuries.

- Provide comfort and emotional support to victims in an expectant triage category; reassess them again after managing those in the immediate triage category. Do not totally abandon victims in the expectant category; transport them for treatment when resources become available. *Victims who have injuries that are treatable are the priority for attention, but those who may soon die should not be neglected.*
- Administer first aid to victims in the immediate triage category by keeping the airway open, loosely covering an open chest wound, controlling bleeding, and splinting fractures; facilitate transport to a treatment facility. *Stabilizing a client in the immediate triage category helps facilitate a better outcome where more advanced medical services are available.*
- Direct victims with injuries that can withstand a delay in treatment for up to 10 hours to a separate waiting area. *Delaying treatment for stable victims helps to avoid overwhelming advanced treatment facilities needed for victims in critical condition.*
- Delegate the care of those with minimal health needs to volunteers with first aid skills. *Assistive personnel can manage victims with minor injuries with negligible consequences.*

Altered Skin Integrity: Related to prior or concurrent trauma or thermal or chemical burns as manifested by a disruption in epidermal and dermal tissue
Expected Outcome: The client's skin will become intact.

- Cleanse the wound using standard precautions. *Cleansing reduces pathogens; standard precautions protect the nurse from contact with pathogens.*
- Apply a semiocclusive dressing over the wound. *A moist wound increases the rate of epithelialization.*

Infection Risk: Related to possible exposure to a biologic agent or exposure to gamma radiation
Expected Outcome: Clients in the triage and treatment area will have their risk for infection reduced and their risk for internal radiologic contamination minimized.

- Restrict public access to clients who are nauseated, vomiting, or experiencing diarrhea. *Separating infected from uninfected people helps reduce spread of contamination.*
- When providing client care, wear personal protective equipment such as gloves, mask, gown, eye protection, or a self-contained respirator and vapor-protective suit, depending on the potential pathogen. *Personal protective equipment can prevent the transmission of an infectious agent to the nurse and others.*
- Double bag and dispose of all clothing and body waste in biohazard containers. *Confining sources of possible pathogens and radiologic contaminants reduces the potential for direct and indirect contact.*
- Have victims shower and change clothes; irrigate or wash open wounds with soap and water. *Cleansing the skin helps to reduce the transition from external to internal radiologic contamination.*
- Bandage any decontaminated wound with a sterile waterproof dressing. *A waterproof dressing acts as a barrier to the entrance of pathogens or external radiologic contaminants.*
- Administer a prescribed colony-stimulating agent such as filgrastim (Neupogen). *Exposure to high-dose gamma radiation suppresses bone marrow production of white blood cells. Filgrastim promotes white blood cell production, making victims of radiologic contamination less susceptible to infections.*
- Immunize against smallpox or administer vaccinia immune globulin (VIG) if smallpox has been released. *A smallpox vaccination given early enough will prevent susceptible people from acquiring this infection. VIG provides passive immunity.*

Coping Impairment: Related to lack of information and fear of personal danger
Expected Outcome: The client will cope effectively as evidenced by expressing emotions appropriately and cooperating with directives from disaster workers.

- Minimize panic by providing information on the type and extent of the disaster. *Coping effectively depends on acquiring accurate information to facilitate a realistic perception of the disaster.*
- Reassure the client that they will receive care and shelter. *Relieving insecurity facilitates a sense that the situation is under control.*
- Encourage the client to express feelings and concerns. *Verbalizing allows an opportunity for clarifying misperceptions, obtaining answers to questions, and putting fears in perspective.*
- Listen nonjudgmentally to the victim recount the horror that they have just experienced. *Convey that a victim is not atypical and feels similar to other people who have lived through a catastrophic event.*
- Reunite family members or provide information concerning their whereabouts and condition. *Family members are the strongest links to emotional support.*

NURSING PROCESS FOR THE CLIENT IN A DISASTER SITUATION (continued)

Evaluation of Expected Outcomes

The nurse assesses triaged victims accurately and gives them appropriate treatment. The client's impaired skin is clean and covered with a dressing. Risks for infection and contamination are prevented or reduced. The client copes effectively with the physical and emotional trauma of having survived a disaster.

KEY POINTS

- Characteristics of disasters: a disaster is a type of extreme emergency, exceeding the capacity of the community to function normally.
- Types of disasters
  - Natural disasters: generally weather related
    - Earthquakes: may cause tsunamis
    - Floods
    - Storms: hurricanes and tornadoes
    - Wildfires
  - Human disasters: result from unintentional and intentional causes
    - Bombs: devices that are designed to explode on impact or when detonated
      - IED
      - Dirty bombs
      - Nuclear power plant disasters
      - Nuclear blast
  - Biologic disasters: pathogens or their toxins cause harm—intentional or unintentional
    - Anthrax
    - Botulism
    - Smallpox
  - Chemical disasters: release of a toxic man-made substance to cause mass casualties
    - Nerve agent poisoning
    - Cyanide poisoning
    - Respiratory toxin poisoning
    - Blistering agent
- Disaster management—four phases: mitigation (prevention), preparedness, response, and recovery
  - Role of nurse: essential for triage, rapid assessment, care of multiple clients

CRITICAL THINKING EXERCISES

1. What types of transmission-based precautions should be used when caring for clients with a possible diagnosis of anthrax exposure, botulism poisoning, and smallpox?
2. What drug should be dispensed quickly following a nuclear bomb or power plant disaster to prevent or limit damage to the thyroid gland?
3. Discuss why triage does not mean "first come, first served."
4. Which triage category should the nurse assign to victims with the following assessment data?
   - Victim A is conscious, clothing is bloody, pulse is 110 beats/min and weak, and respirations are 40 breaths/min.
   - Victim B is alert and crying, an obvious deformity of the arm suggests a fracture, and pulse and respirations are rapid but within normal range.
   - Victim C is unresponsive, respirations are 4 breaths/min after opening the airway, and gurgling is heard with each respiration.
   - Victim D is conscious and hysterical, there is evidence of abrasions on exposed skin, and the person pleads to be transported in an emergency vehicle for further treatment.

NCLEX-STYLE REVIEW QUESTIONS PrepU

1. Homeland security has received information that there is a credible terrorist threat against the United States. What information can a nurse provide for preparing for a potential disaster? Select all that apply.
   1. Take shelter in an enclosed area of the home.
   2. Stock canned and packaged food.
   3. Obtain a supply of bottled water.
   4. Lock all windows and doors.
   5. Store a week's supply of medications.
   6. Stay indoors until danger has passed.
2. A nurse in the military vaccinates soldiers for smallpox. What actions are correct? Select all that apply.
   1. The nurse selects the deltoid site.
   2. The nurse disinfects the site with alcohol.
   3. The nurse inserts the needle into the muscle.
   4. The nurse massages the site of administration.
   5. The nurse covers the injection site with gauze.
   6. The nurse checks the site in 72 hours.
3. Which side effect is the nurse most likely to detect when administering pearls of amyl nitrite?
   1. Bradycardia
   2. Muscle weakness
   3. Hypotension
   4. Skin pallor

4. An ED receives a report of an overturned truck that was transporting liquid chlorine. What preparation should the nursing staff make first for potential admissions to the ED?
1. Contact the nursing supervisor for additional staff to care for multiple clients.
2. Notify respiratory therapy staff of possible need for ventilatory support for affected clients.
3. Call the physical therapist to initiate chest physical therapy for clients with breathing issues.
4. Contact the cardiac care primary provider on call to assess clients for heart damage.

5. When a nurse participates in a community-wide mock disaster drill, which one of the following victims should be triaged with a red tag indicating a need for immediate attention?
1. A victim with a compound fracture of the femur
2. A victim with 85% body surface full-thickness burns
3. A victim who has evidence of significant hemorrhage
4. A victim with a penetrating abdominal wound

WANT TO KNOW MORE? There are a wide variety of online resources available on thePoint to enhance learning and understanding of this chapter.

Go to **thePoint.lww.com/activate** and use the activation code found in the front of this text to unlock these online resources.

UNIT 4
Caring for Clients With Multisystem Disorders

16 Caring for Clients With Fluid, Electrolyte, and Acid–Base Imbalances

Words To Know

acidosis
acids
active transport
alkalosis
anion gap
anions
baroreceptors
bases
bicarbonate–carbonic acid
buffer system
cation
Chvostek sign
circulatory overload
compensation
dehydration
dependent edema
electrolytes
extracellular fluid
facilitated diffusion
filtration
generalized edema
hemoconcentration
hemodilution
hypervolemia
hypovolemia
interstitial fluid
intracellular fluid
intravascular fluid
ions
natriuretic peptides
osmoreceptors
osmosis
passive diffusion
pitting edema
renin–angiotensin–aldosterone system
serum osmolality
skin tenting
third-spacing
Trousseau sign

Learning Objectives

On completion of this chapter, you will be able to:

1. List three chemical substances that are components of body fluid.
2. Name the two main fluid locations in the human body and two subdivisions.
3. Give the average fluid intake per day for adults.
4. List four ways in which the body normally loses fluid.
5. Identify five processes by which water and dissolved chemicals are relocated in the body.
6. Name three mechanisms that help regulate fluid and electrolyte balance.
7. List two types of fluid imbalance.
8. Explain the difference between hypovolemia and dehydration.
9. Explain hemoconcentration and hemodilution.
10. Identify assessment findings of and nursing interventions for hypovolemia.
11. List and identify the differences in three types of edema.
12. Identify assessment findings of and nursing interventions for hypervolemia.
13. Explain third-spacing and medical techniques for relocating this fluid.
14. List factors that contribute to electrolyte loss and excess.
15. Name four electrolyte imbalances that pose a major threat to well-being.
16. Discuss the nursing management of clients with electrolyte imbalances.
17. Discuss the role of acids and bases in body fluid.
18. Explain pH and identify the normal range of plasma pH.
19. Identify two chemicals and two organs that play major roles in regulating acid–base balance.
20. Give the names of two major acid–base imbalances and subdivisions of each.
21. List three components of arterial blood gas findings used to determine acid–base imbalances.
22. Discuss the nursing management of clients with acid–base imbalances.

Body fluids consist of water and chemicals, including electrolytes, acids, and bases. **Electrolytes** are substances that carry an electrical charge when dissolved in fluid. **Acids** are substances that release hydrogen into fluid, and **bases** are substances that bind with hydrogen. The delicate balance of fluids, electrolytes, acids, and bases is ensured by an adequate intake of water and nutrients, physiologic mechanisms that regulate fluid volume, and chemical processes that buffer the blood to keep its pH nearly neutral. This chapter discusses fluid, electrolyte, and acid–base balance and the disorders that occur when there are imbalances.

Gerontologic Considerations

- The most common fluid imbalance in older adults is dehydration. Older adults frequently experience reduced thirst sensation, causing them to drink less water. Use of diuretic medications, laxatives, or enemas may also deplete fluid volume. Chronic fluid volume deficit can lead to other problems, such as electrolyte imbalances.
- Aging causes skin to lose elasticity. Thus, assessing skin turgor may be ineffective in detecting fluid volume deficit in older adults. If assessing skin turgor in older clients, use the skin of the forehead or sternum. Assessing daily weight is a more accurate measure of fluid volume changes in older adults.
- Several factors can lead to fluid and electrolyte imbalances in older adults. Thirst sensation may decrease, causing inadequate intake or intake of caffeinated beverages, which may increase diuresis. Decreased renal function can cause an inability to concentrate urine. Enema use can also potentially cause fluid and electrolyte imbalance. Additionally, laxatives draw fluid into the intestine and may lead to fluid depletion if not administered with water. A poor appetite, erratic meal patterns, inability to prepare nutritious meals, or financial circumstance may influence nutritional status, resulting in fluid and electrolyte imbalances.
- Older adults are at increased risk for hyponatremia related to the kidneys' inability to excrete water and the sluggish renin–angiotensin–aldosterone response.
- Hypernatremia is also common in older adults who may desire increased salt in food when taste sensation diminishes or from the increased sodium concentration that accompanies dehydration; it may be manifested as confusion, lethargy, irritability, or weakness.
- Older adults should be taught that prolonged laxative use can lead to hypernatremia and hypermagnesemia (discussed later).
- Older adults may use magnesium sulfate (e.g., Epsom salt) soaks, leading to absorption of magnesium through the skin.
- If magnesium sulfate is taken orally as a laxative self-treatment, large amounts of magnesium may be absorbed through the digestive tract.
- Older adults may avoid consulting a health care provider for the management of gastric hyperacidity; rather, they may be self-treating with household baking soda (sodium bicarbonate [$NaHCO_3$]) as an inexpensive substitute for a commercial antacid. Overuse of sodium bicarbonate may lead to metabolic alkalosis.
- Poor respiratory exchange as the result of decreased lung expansion from inactivity, remaining in the same position for prolonged periods, thoracic skeletal changes, or chronic lung disease may lead to chronic respiratory acidosis.

FLUID AND ELECTROLYTE BALANCE

Body Fluid Compartments

About 60% of the adult human body is water. Put another way, for every 100 lb of body weight, approximately 60 lb is water. Most body water is located within cells (**intracellular fluid**). The rest is outside cells (**extracellular fluid**). Extracellular fluid includes the water between cells (**interstitial fluid**) and in the plasma (serum) portion of blood (**intravascular fluid**; Fig. 16-1).

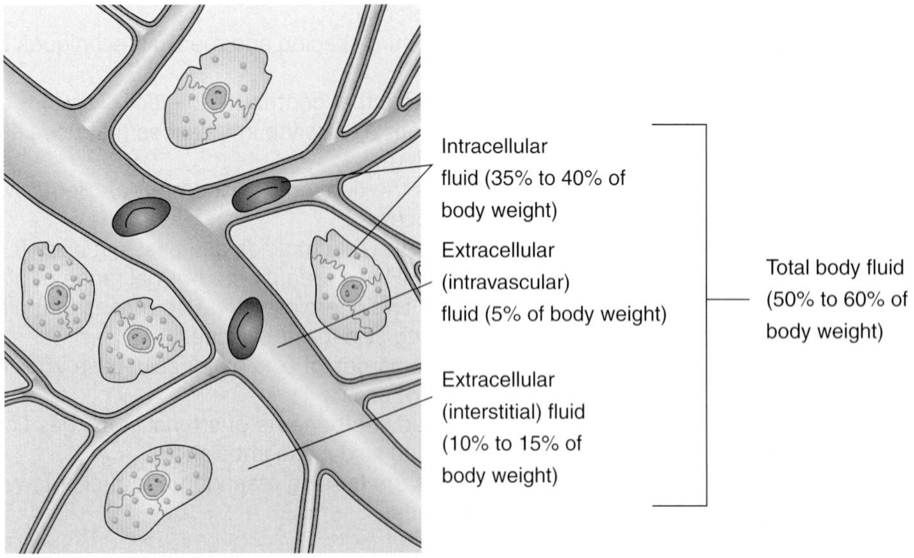

Figure 16-1 Distribution of body fluid at the cellular level. Total body fluid represents 50% to 60% of body weight in an average adult. Location of body fluid at the cellular level.

TABLE 16-1 Percentages of Body Fluid According to Age and Sex

FLUID COMPARTMENT	INFANTS (%)	MALE ADULTS (%)	FEMALE ADULTS (%)	OLDER ADULTS (%)
Intravascular	4	4	5	5
Interstitial	25	11	10	15
Intracellular	48	45	35	25
Total	77	60	50	45

The volume of fluid in each location varies with age and sex (Table 16-1).

Intake and Output

In healthy adults, oral fluid intake averages about 2500 mL/day; however, it can range between 1800 and 3000 mL/day, with a similar volume of fluid loss. A standard formula for calculating daily fluid intake is as follows:

- 100 mL/kg for the first 10 kg of weight, plus
- 50 mL/kg for the next 10 kg of weight, plus
- 15 mL/kg per remaining kilogram of weight

The primary sources of body fluid are food and liquids. As fluid volume increases, the body loses fluid, primarily through urination, in a proportionate volume to maintain or restore equilibrium. Other mechanisms of fluid loss include bowel elimination, perspiration, and breathing. Losses from sweat and the vapor in exhaled air are referred to as *insensible losses* because they are, for practical purposes, unnoticeable and unmeasurable (Fig. 16-2).

»» *Stop, Think, and Respond 16-1*

Using the formula for calculating fluid intake requirements according to weight, how much oral fluid per day is considered adequate for a client who weighs 176 lb?

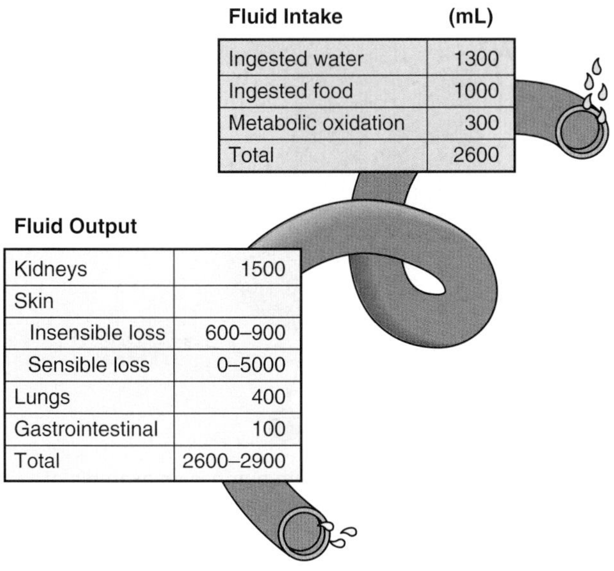
Fluid Intake (mL)
Ingested water 1300
Ingested food 1000
Metabolic oxidation 300
Total 2600
Fluid Output
Kidneys 1500
Skin
Insensible loss 600–900
Sensible loss 0–5000
Lungs 400
Gastrointestinal 100
Total 2600–2900

Figure 16-2 In a healthy person, fluid intake and output are about equal. The amounts indicated are average daily fluid sources and losses.

Distribution of Fluids and Electrolytes

Translocation (movement back and forth) of fluid and exchange of chemicals—including electrolytes, acids, and bases—is continuous in and among all areas where water is located. Physiologic processes govern the movement and relocation of fluids and chemicals at the cellular level. These processes include osmosis, filtration, passive and facilitated diffusion, and active transport.

Osmosis

Osmosis is the movement of water through a *semipermeable membrane*—one that allows some but not all substances in a solution to pass through from a diluted area to a more concentrated area. *Tonicity* refers, in this case, to the quantity (concentration) of substances dissolved in the water. The power to draw water toward an area of greater concentration is referred to as *osmotic pressure*. *Colloids*, large-sized substances such as serum proteins (e.g., albumin, globulin, fibrinogen) and blood cells, do not readily pass through cell and tissue membranes. They contribute to fluid concentration and act as a force for attracting water—a property referred to as *colloidal osmotic pressure*.

Fluid distribution through osmosis occurs in the following ways. If the solute concentration is higher in the cell, water is drawn through the membrane into the cell from the interstitial space. The process continues until the concentration is the same (*isotonic*) on both sides of the membrane. The reverse also is true: If the solute concentration is higher in the interstitial space, water is pulled into the interstitial space from the cell (Fig. 16-3).

Filtration

Filtration promotes the movement of fluid and some dissolved substances through a semipermeable membrane according to pressure differences. It relocates water and chemicals from an area of high pressure to an area of lower

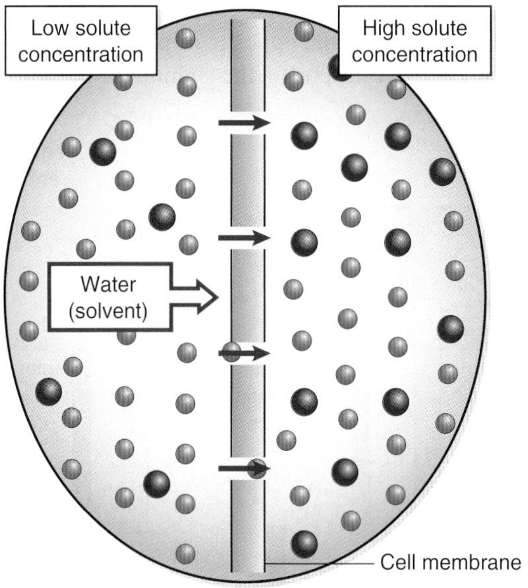
Low solute concentration
High solute concentration
Water (solvent)
Cell membrane

Figure 16-3 Osmosis. (Reprinted with permission from Taylor, C. R., Lynn, P., & Bartlett, J. L. (2019). *Fundamentals of nursing: The art and science of person-centered care* (9th ed.). Wolters Kluwer.)

pressure. For example, fluid is under higher pressure at the arterial end than at the venous end of capillaries. Filtration causes the fluid and some dissolved substances (e.g., oxygen) to move into the interstitial space. Most of the water is then reabsorbed at the venous end of the capillaries by colloidal osmotic pressure (Fig. 16-4). Filtration also affects how the kidneys excrete fluid and wastes and then selectively reabsorb water and other chemicals that need to be conserved. The kidneys filter about 180 L of fluid from the blood each day; all but 1 to 1.5 L is reabsorbed.

Diffusion

Passive diffusion is a physiologic process by which dissolved substances (e.g., electrolytes) move from an area of high concentration to an area of lower concentration through a semipermeable membrane. Passive diffusion, like osmosis, remains fairly static (unchanged) once equilibrium occurs.

Facilitated diffusion is the process in which certain dissolved substances require the assistance of a carrier molecule to pass from one side of a cellular membrane to the other (Fig. 16-5). Facilitated diffusion distributes substances from an area of higher concentration to one that is lower. Glucose is an example of a substance that requires facilitated diffusion because once in the blood stream, glucose cannot permeate cell walls. Glucose is made available to cells in combination with insulin and glucose transport (GLUT) proteins located within cellular membranes. Without insulin, glucose transport is very low; in the presence of insulin, glucose transport is rapidly stimulated. The GLUT proteins (1) bind with glucose in plasma on the outside of the cell membrane; then (2) the glucose transporters change shape so as to face the inner area of the cell; and (3) the glucose moves into the cell (Cooper & Hausmann, 2013).

Active Transport

Active transport requires an energy source, a substance called *adenosine triphosphate* (ATP), to drive dissolved chemicals from an area of low concentration to an area of higher concentration—the opposite of passive diffusion. An example of active transport is the sodium–potassium pump system. Its function is to move potassium from lower concentrations in the extracellular fluid into cells where potassium is highly concentrated. The pump also moves sodium, which is in lower amounts in the cells, to extracellular fluid where it is more abundant (Fig. 16-6). Metabolic disorders that diminish ATP, such as hypoxia, seriously affect normal cellular functions by impairing the distribution of chemicals in intracellular and extracellular fluid. Any significant change in fluid volume or its distribution can disrupt normal body functioning.

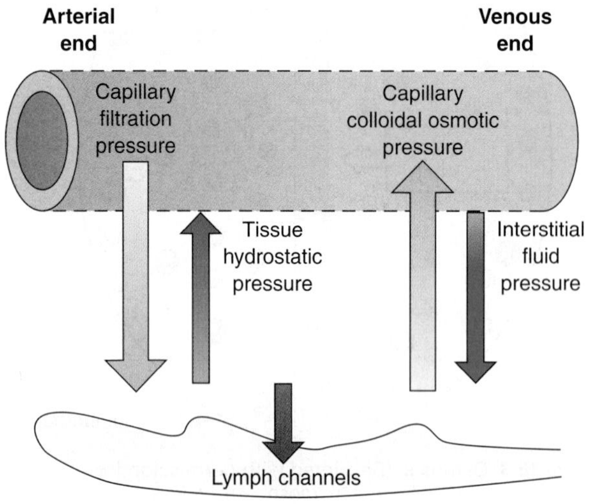

Figure 16-4 Fluid exchange at the capillary level.

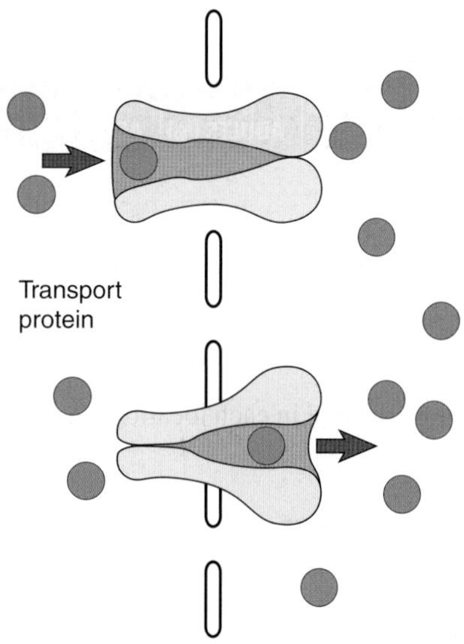

Figure 16-5 Glucose transport proteins facilitate diffusion of insulin into cells. (Reprinted with permission from Donnelly-Moreno, L. A. (2020). *Timby's fundamental nursing skills and concepts* (12th ed.). Wolters Kluwer.)

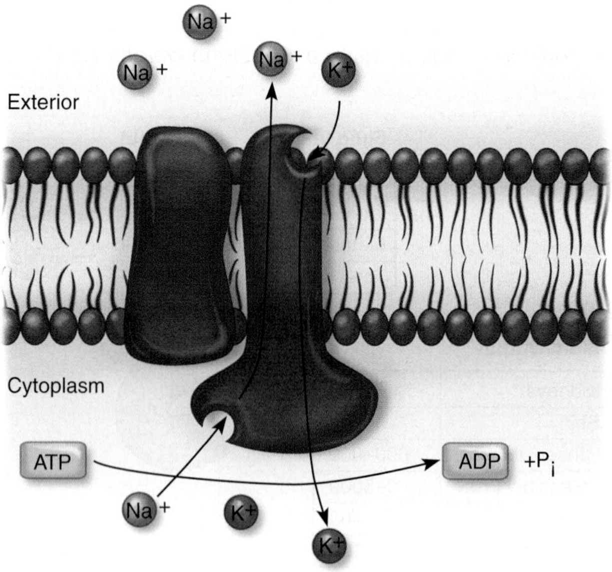

Figure 16-6 The sodium–potassium pump is an example of active transport. Energy provided by adenosine triphosphate (ATP) is used to actively pump sodium that diffuses into the cell through a pore in the cell membrane. Similarly, the pump actively replaces potassium that diffuses from the cell with adenosine diphosphate (ADP).

>>> *Stop, Think, and Respond 16-2*

If a client takes an oral potassium supplement or receives potassium in an intravenous (IV) solution, for example, 20 mEq in 1000 mL of solution, which physiologic process relocates the potassium within cells?

Mechanisms of Fluid and Electrolyte Regulation

Under normal conditions, several mechanisms maintain normal fluid volume and electrolyte concentrations. They include those promoted by osmoreceptors (i.e., the release or inhibition of antidiuretic hormone [ADH]), the renin–angiotensin–aldosterone system, and the secretion of natriuretic peptides.

Osmoreceptors

Fluid volume is regulated primarily by the excretion of water in the form of urine and the promotion of thirst. These processes are, in turn, regulated in the hypothalamus by **osmoreceptors**, specialized neurons that sense the **serum osmolality**, or concentration of substances, in blood. When the blood becomes overly concentrated, osmoreceptors stimulate the hypothalamus to synthesize ADH, released by the posterior lobe of the pituitary gland. Release of ADH inhibits urine formation by increasing reabsorption of water from the distal and collecting tubules in the nephrons of the kidneys. The reabsorbed water restores normal serum osmolality, increases circulating blood volume, improves cardiac output, and maintains blood pressure (BP).

Osmoreceptors also are sensitive to changes in blood volume and BP through information relayed by baroreceptors. **Baroreceptors** are stretch receptors in the aortic arch and carotid sinus that signal the brain to release ADH when blood volume decreases by 10%, systolic BP falls below 90 mm Hg, or the right atrium is underfilled (Miller & Arnold, 2018). They signal the brain to suppress ADH when blood volume increases, systolic BP rises, or the right atrium is overfilled.

Osmoreceptors also trigger thirst, a mechanism that promotes increased intake of oral fluid. A person senses thirst when extracellular volume decreases by approximately 700 mL, an amount that equals about 2% of body weight (Gizowski & Bourque, 2018).

Renin–Angiotensin–Aldosterone System

The **renin–angiotensin–aldosterone system** is a series of chemicals released to increase both BP and blood volume. It is triggered by the *juxtaglomerular apparatus*, a ring of pressure-sensing cells that surround the arterioles leading to each glomerulus in the kidneys. When the volume of arterial blood supplying the glomeruli is reduced, the juxtaglomerular cells release renin. Renin begins the transformation of angiotensinogen to angiotensin I to angiotensin II. Angiotensin II causes vasoconstriction and raises BP; it also stimulates release of aldosterone from the adrenal cortex. Aldosterone causes the kidneys to reabsorb sodium, which, in turn, increases blood volume and BP (Fig. 16-7).

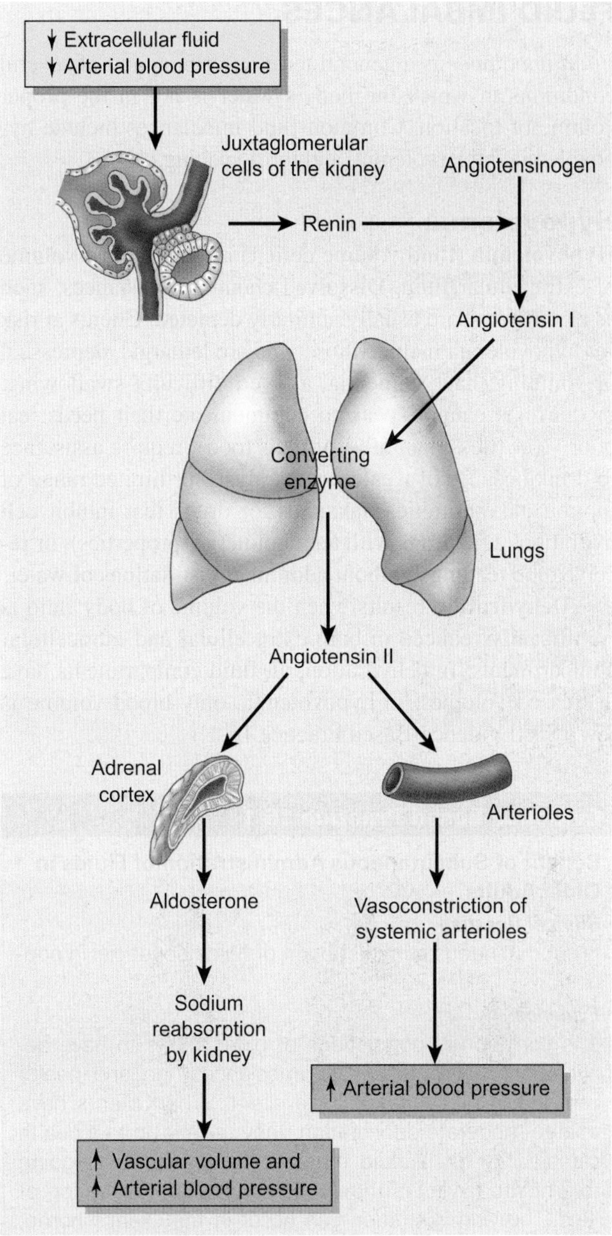

Figure 16-7 Control of blood pressure by the renin–angiotensin–aldosterone system.

Natriuretic Peptides

Natriuretic peptides are hormone-like substances that act in opposition to the renin–angiotensin–aldosterone system. Three main natriuretic peptides have been identified: (1) atrial natriuretic peptide (ANP), produced by the heart's atrial muscle; (2) brain natriuretic peptide (BNP), synthesized in the ventricles of the heart, despite originally being attributed to the brain; and (3) C-type natriuretic peptide (CNP), which is made in the brain. ANP and BNP are released in response to overstretching of the atrial and ventricular walls. They are vasodilators that reduce blood volume by promoting the excretion of sodium, inhibiting the release of renin which eventually limits the formation of angiotensin II and cause diuresis by inhibiting ADH (see Chapter 28).

FLUID IMBALANCES

Fluid imbalance is a general term describing any of several conditions in which the body's water is not in the proper volume or location. Common fluid imbalances include hypovolemia, hypervolemia, and third-spacing.

Hypovolemia

Hypovolemia (fluid volume deficit) refers to a low volume of extracellular fluid. Dissolved chemical substances, such as electrolytes, are usually similarly depleted. Clients at risk for hypovolemia include those who are lethargic, depressed, or vomiting; have dementia, a fever, difficulty swallowing, or diarrhea; cannot speak to communicate their needs; eat poorly (i.e., less than 50% of their food); require assistance to drink because of weakness, paralysis, or limited range of motion; take diuretics, laxatives, or drugs that inhibit cell hydration (e.g., drugs with anticholinergic properties); or receive tube feedings without additional instillations of water.

Dehydration results when the volume of body fluid is significantly reduced in both extracellular and intracellular compartments. In dehydration, all fluid compartments have decreased volumes; in hypovolemia, only blood volume is low. (See Evidence-Based Practice 16-1.)

Evidence-Based Practice 16-1

Benefit of Subcutaneous Administration of Fluids in Older Adults

Clinical Question

Is subcutaneous administration of fluids beneficial in populations of older adults?

Evidence

It is common in populations of older adults to have dehydration, which is a fluid imbalance. Age and health can affect the hydration of a client. When clients have mild-to-moderate dehydration, they usually go to a health care facility for IV fluid therapy. An alternative to going to a health facility is the subcutaneous administration of fluid. This administration can occur in the client's home, which helps the client with transportation, comfort, and decreased cost.

Subcutaneous fluid administration offers an alternative to being admitted to the hospital. The treatment may not be an option for every client; however, it is one choice to support the client either at home or in an agency's care.

Nursing Implications

Older adult clients may have a complex health history and care needs that require planning, resources, and education. The client assessment is important so that the best site for placement is determined and the device is secure during administration of fluids. The nurse working with an older dehydrated adult client will need to work with the client, family, and care team for the best options and resources for the client.

Reference

Gabriel, J. (2014). Subcutaneous fluid administration and the hydration of older people. *British Journal of Nursing, 23*(14), S10–S14. https://doi.org/10.12968/bjon.2014.23.Sup14.S10

Pathophysiology and Etiology

Factors that contribute to hypovolemia include inadequate fluid intake; fluid loss in excess of fluid intake such as with hemorrhage, prolonged vomiting or diarrhea, wound loss (as with burn injury), or profuse urination or perspiration; and translocation of fluid to compartments where it is trapped, such as the abdominal cavity or interstitial spaces (e.g., third-spacing). When circulatory volume is decreased, BP falls and the heart compensates by increasing the heart rate to maintain adequate cardiac output (see Chapter 22). BP falls with postural changes, or it may become severely lowered when blood is rapidly lost. **Hemoconcentration**, a high ratio of blood components in relation to watery plasma, increases the potential for blood clots and urinary stones and compromises the kidney's ability to excrete nitrogen wastes. Hypovolemia eventually depletes intracellular fluid, which can affect cellular functions. One example is the change in mentation that usually occurs.

Assessment Findings

One of the earliest symptoms of hypovolemia is thirst. Other signs and symptoms are listed in Table 16-2. Evidence of hemoconcentration is reflected in elevated hematocrit level and blood cell counts, a consequence of water deficiency. Urine specific gravity is high. Serum electrolyte levels tend to remain normal because they are depleted in proportion to

TABLE 16-2 Signs and Symptoms of Fluid Volume Deficit and Excess

ASSESSMENT	FLUID DEFICIT	FLUID EXCESS
Weight	Weight loss ≥2 lb/24 hours	Weight gain ≥2 lb/24 hours
Blood pressure	Low	High
Temperature	Elevated	Normal
Pulse	Rapid, weak, thready	Full, bounding
Respirations	Rapid, shallow	Moist, labored
Urine	Scant, dark yellow	Light yellow
Stool	Dry, small volume	Bulky
Skin	Warm, flushed, dry	Cool, pale, moist
Skin turgor	Poor, tents	Pitting and dependent edema
Mucous membranes	Dry, sticky	Moist
Eyes	Sunken	Swollen
Lungs	Clear	Crackles, gurgles
Breathing	Effortless	Dyspnea, orthopnea
Energy	Weak	Fatigues easily
Jugular neck veins	Flat	Distended
Cognition	Reduced	Reduced
Mental state	Sleepy	Anxious

the water loss (Gizowski & Bourque, 2018). Central venous pressure (CVP; see Chapter 29) is below 2 to 3 mm Hg.

Medical Management

Fluid deficit is restored by treating its etiology, increasing the volume of oral intake, administering IV fluids (see Chapter 13), and controlling fluid losses.

Nursing Management

The nurse gathers assessment data that provide evidence of fluid status (Nursing Care Plan 16-1). If they reflect a fluid deficit, they plan measures to restore fluid balance (Nursing Guidelines 16-1; Evidence-Based Practice 16-1) and evaluates the outcomes of interventions. In addition, the nurse teaches clients who have a potential for hypovolemia and their families to

- Respond to thirst because it is an early indication of reduced fluid volume.
- Consume at least 8 to 10 (8 oz) glasses of fluid each day and more during hot, humid weather.
- Drink water as an inexpensive means to meet fluid requirements.
- Avoid beverages with alcohol and caffeine because they increase urination and contribute to fluid deficits.
- Do not restrict salt or sodium intake.
- Rise slowly from a sitting or lying position to avoid dizziness and potential injury.

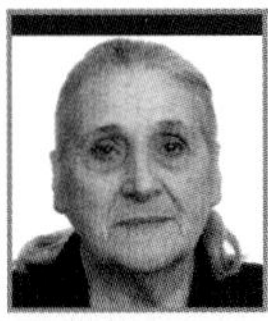

Clinical Scenario A 73-year-old woman has a food-borne case of gastroenteritis. She has been vomiting with accompanying diarrhea for 2 days. Because of her weakened condition and because she lives alone, the primary provider has admitted the client for supervised rehydration. **What measures can the nurse use to restore the client's fluid volume without contributing to a prolongation of her symptoms? See Nursing Care Plan 16-1.**

NURSING CARE PLAN 16-1 The Client With Hypovolemia

Assessment

- Look for gross sources of fluid loss: vomiting, diarrhea, bleeding, wound drainage, gastrointestinal (GI) suctioning, and diaphoresis.
- Weigh client daily at the same time, on the same scale, and dressed similarly. Report a loss of 2 lb (1 kg) or more in 24 hours (a 2-lb loss equals 1 L of body fluid).
- Note medications. Daily diuretic therapy or chronic laxative use may promote excess fluid losses.
- Record vital signs regularly; the frequency depends on client's acuity level. Check for postural hypotension (a drop in systolic pressure of 15 mm Hg after client rises from a sitting or recumbent position). Increased insensible losses may cause or result from elevated body temperature.
- Ask if client is thirsty.
- Examine skin for dryness. Assess turgor (elasticity) by lifting the skin over the sternum, inner thigh, or forehead each shift. **Skin tenting**, skin that remains elevated and is slow to return to underlying tissue, indicates dehydration.
- Observe the tongue for furrowing (linear lines) and look for dry oral mucous membranes.
- Determine cognition by performing a Mini-Mental Status Examination (see Chapter 67).
- Examine urine. Urine that is dark yellow, has a strong odor, or has a specific gravity of 1.020 or more indicates low fluid volume.
- Monitor blood test results for hemoconcentration (high hematocrit level and blood cell counts).
- Keep a daily record of fluid intake and output. Report output that is less than 500 mL/24 hours or less than 50 mL if measuring hourly volumes.
- Observe if client has the strength, ability to swallow, and mental capacity to drink fluid without assistance.

Nursing Diagnosis. Hypovolemia: Related to fluid loss greater than intake as manifested by vomiting and diarrhea secondary to gastroenteritis, oral intake of 500 mL, fluid loss of 1700 mL in previous 24 hours, concentrated urine, postural hypotension, tachycardia, and dry mucous membranes

Expected Outcome. Client will have a fluid intake of at least 1500 mL/24 hours and urine output within 500 mL of oral intake (i.e., at least 1000 mL/24 hours).

Interventions	Rationales
Withhold solid food for 8 hours.	*Solid food can irritate gastric mucosa.*
Provide diluted mouthwash or weak salt water as an oral rinse after vomiting.	*An oral rinse reduces the unpleasant aftertaste of emesis that may trigger additional vomiting.*
Empty the emesis basin and change linens soiled with vomitus.	*The sight and smell of emesis perpetuate the cycle of vomiting.*
Encourage slow, deep breaths when the client experiences waves of nausea.	*Breathing distracts the client from the nausea until the reversed peristaltic action passes.*
Avoid jarring the bed or activities that require movement on the client's part.	*The vestibular center in the ear is sensitive to movement of the head and can stimulate the vomiting center (as in motion sickness).*

(continued)

NURSING CARE PLAN 16-1 The Client With Hypovolemia (*continued*)

Administer prescribed antiemetics according to the primary provider's written orders.	*Antiemetics may inhibit the vomiting center directly or help control vomiting by other mechanisms (e.g., slowing GI peristalsis).*
Provide sips of liquids like weak tea, flat carbonated soft drinks, and water as often as the client can tolerate them.	*Small volumes of fluids that are not strongly flavored or highly carbonated are less likely to cause nausea or distend the stomach.*
Progress fluid selection to include gelatin, bouillon, Gatorade, or Pedialyte when the client can tolerate fluids identified earlier.	*These products provide glucose, sodium, chloride, and other electrolytes.*
Eliminate dairy products if the client is lactose intolerant.	*Clients who do not produce lactase, the enzyme that aids in milk digestion, develop cramps and diarrhea when they consume dairy products.*
Offer dry crackers or toast if the client is able to tolerate fluids.	*Solid foods in readily digestible carbohydrates are tolerated better than other types of food.*
Administer prescribed antidiarrheals as medically ordered.	*They reduce the frequency and consistency of watery stools by adsorbing excess liquid from and soothing the bowel and slowing bowel motility.*
Increase to a low-residue diet, starting with the BRAT (bananas, rice, applesauce, toast) diet when diarrhea is controlled.	*Low-residue foods reduce stool bulk and slow GI transit time; the BRAT diet contains foods that are high in pectin, which helps make stools firm.*

Evaluation of Expected Outcomes

Intake is 1500 mL and output is 1750 mL, 500 mL of which is emesis. Episodes of vomiting and diarrhea are reduced. BP is stable at 110/68 mm Hg in both lying and sitting positions. Urine is medium yellow. Client is tolerating clear fluids, saltines, and dry white toast.

NURSING GUIDELINES 16-1

Managing Deficient Fluid Volume

- Inform client that they must increase consumption of oral fluids. Set a target goal for intake per hour, shift, and 24-hour period; a goal of 3000 to 4000 mL is not excessive for dehydrated clients. Schedule the bulk of fluid intake at meals and when the client is awake (i.e., more intake during daytime than throughout the night).
- Offer at least 180 mL of fluid when administering oral medications.
- Implement a frequent fluids plan by which anyone entering the room offers the client at least 60 mL of fluid.
- Obtain a list of fluids the client prefers; include gelatin, popsicles, ice cream, and sherbet if they are allowed.
- Provide various liquids, replace with a fresh supply periodically, and ensure they are at an appropriate temperature.
- Modify fluid containers to accommodate for client's strength and physical skills (e.g., cups with handles, covered cups with an opening for the mouth or insertion of a straw).
- Offer small volumes frequently rather than expecting the client to consume a large volume at once.
- Thicken watery fluid with a commercial thickener if the client has difficulty swallowing.
- Relieve nausea, vomiting, mouth discomfort, and other problems that interfere with drinking.
- Ensure that clients prone to low fluid volume have fasting tests done expeditiously to reduce the time they remain without food or fluids.
- Evaluate goals by recollecting assessment data and analyzing trends, especially in intake and output totals. Report results to the primary provider, especially if collaborative efforts fall short.

Hypervolemia

Hypervolemia (fluid volume excess) means there is a high volume of water in the intravascular fluid compartment.

Pathophysiology and Etiology

Hypervolemia is caused by fluid intake that exceeds fluid loss, such as from excessive oral intake or rapid IV infusion of fluid. It also is a consequence of heart failure (see Chapter 28) when the heart cannot adequately distribute fluid to the kidneys for filtration. It also can result from inadequate fluid elimination, as may accompany kidney disease (see Chapter 58). Fluid retention (reduced fluid loss) also can occur secondary to excessive salt intake (sodium chloride), adrenal gland dysfunction (see Chapter 50), or administration of corticosteroid drugs such as prednisolone (Delta-Cortef).

Clients at risk for hypervolemia include those who:

- Have altered cardiac or kidney function;
- Have increased ADH production, which sometimes accompanies brain trauma;
- Are receiving corticosteroid therapy, large rapid volumes of IV fluid, or IV colloid solutions (e.g., albumin);
- Consume oral fluids to excess, such as clients with schizophrenia who can develop water intoxication;
- Ingest highly salted food or foods that contain large amounts of sodium.

Hypervolemia can lead to **circulatory overload**, a fluid volume that exceeds what is normal for the intravascular space and can potentially compromise cardiopulmonary function. The excess volume raises BP and causes the heart to increase its force of contraction.

Assessment Findings

Signs and Symptoms

Early signs of hypervolemia (see Table 16-2) are weight gain, elevated BP, and increased breathing effort. As the excess fluid volume is distributed to the interstitial space, **pitting edema**, indentations in the skin after compression, may be noted (Fig. 16-8). Pitting edema usually does not occur, however, until there is a 3 L excess in the intravascular volume. There may be evidence of **dependent edema** (edema in body areas most affected by gravity, such as the feet, ankles, sacrum, or buttocks) in clients confined to bed. Rings, shoes, and stockings may leave marks in the skin. The jugular neck veins may appear prominent when the client sits. Eventually, fluid congestion in the lungs leads to moist breath sounds.

Diagnostic Findings

The blood cell count and hematocrit level are low as the result of **hemodilution**, a reduced ratio of blood components to watery plasma. Urine specific gravity is also low, reflecting the larger proportion of water. CVP is elevated above its normal range of 2 to 6 mm Hg.

Medical Management

The condition causing the fluid excess is treated. Oral and parenteral fluid intake is restricted. Diuretics, drugs that promote urinary excretion, are prescribed. Salt and sodium intake is limited.

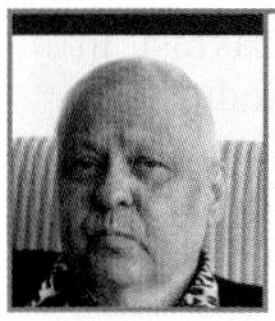

Clinical Scenario While making a home visit, a nurse finds that the 78-year-old client has gained 8 lb since the previous visit 1 week ago. The client's feet and lower legs are edematous to the point that the client can no longer wear their shoes. The nurse consults the primary provider who prescribes a diuretic. A plan of care is discussed among the nurse, the client, and the client's live-in daughter to help relieve the excess volume of fluid. The nurse will return in 3 days to evaluate the effectiveness of the planned interventions. **What data should the nurse gather at this time for a future comparison? What are the client's priority problems and how might they be managed? See the following Nursing Process section.**

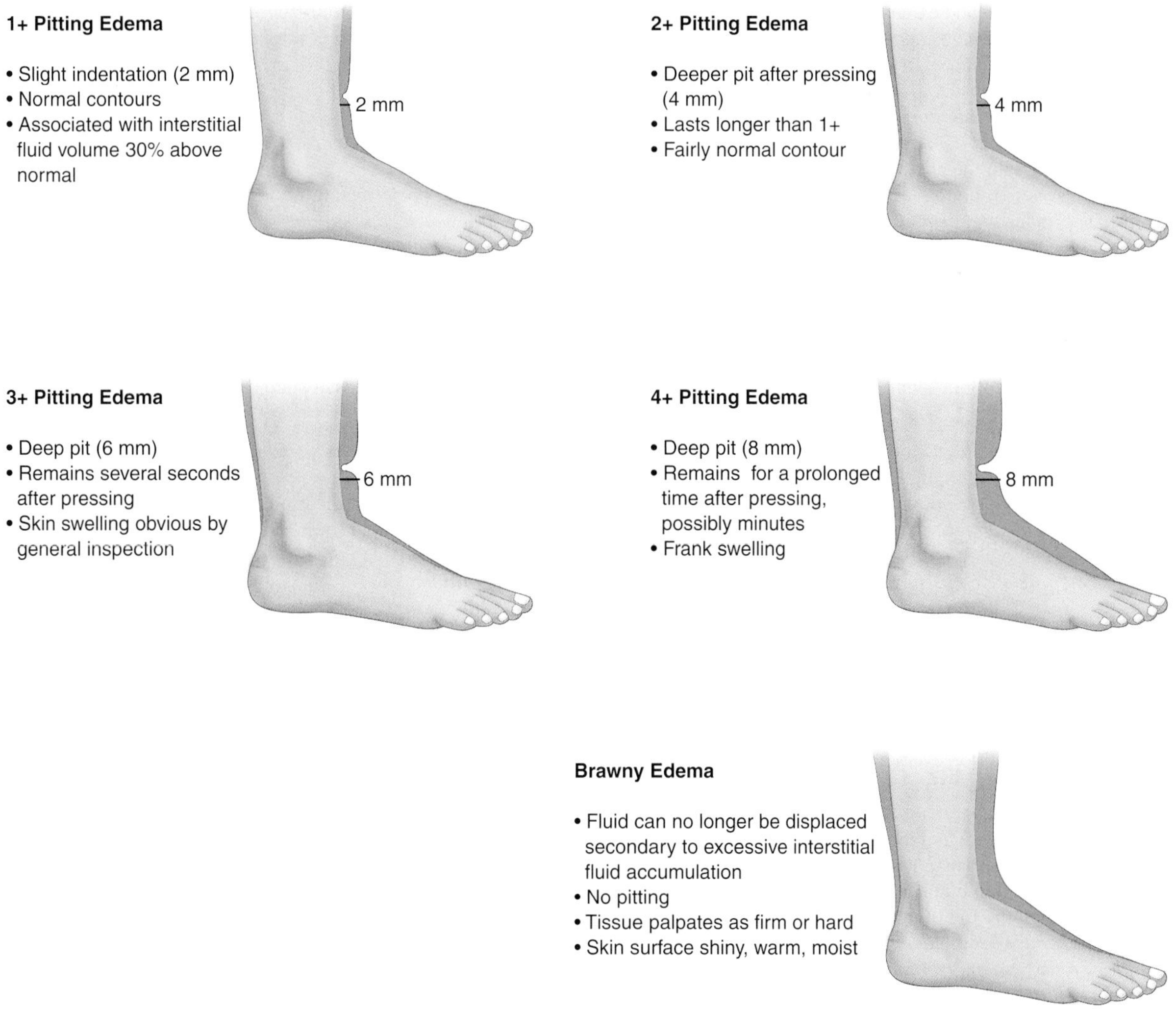

1+ Pitting Edema
• Slight indentation (2 mm)
• Normal contours
• Associated with interstitial fluid volume 30% above normal
2 mm
2+ Pitting Edema
• Deeper pit after pressing (4 mm)
• Lasts longer than 1+
• Fairly normal contour
4 mm
3+ Pitting Edema
• Deep pit (6 mm)
• Remains several seconds after pressing
• Skin swelling obvious by general inspection
6 mm
4+ Pitting Edema
• Deep pit (8 mm)
• Remains for a prolonged time after pressing, possibly minutes
• Frank swelling
8 mm
Brawny Edema
• Fluid can no longer be displaced secondary to excessive interstitial fluid accumulation
• No pitting
• Tissue palpates as firm or hard
• Skin surface shiny, warm, moist

Figure 16-8 Grading edema is somewhat subjective; assessment findings may vary depending on the clinician. These criteria are offered to assist in documentation.

NURSING PROCESS FOR THE CLIENT WITH HYPERVOLEMIA

Assessment

Obtain baseline weight and weigh the client daily thereafter on the same scale and at the same time before breakfast, in similar clothing. A 2-lb weight gain in 24 hours indicates that the client is retaining 1 L of fluid. Maintain accurate intake and output records, and report significant differences in the two measurements. Auscultate the lungs to detect abnormal breath sounds. Determine if an S_3 heart sound is present and inspect the neck veins to assess for distention (see Chapter 22). Measure BP, heart rate, and respiratory rate regularly. Note the client's activity tolerance. To detect pitting edema, gently press the skin over a bony area, such as the tibia or dorsum of the foot, for up to 5 seconds and observe the results (see Fig. 16-8). Inspect edematous skin for cracks and breakdown.

Diagnosis, Planning, and Interventions

Implement prescribed interventions such as limiting sodium and water intake and administering ordered medications that promote fluid elimination. Elevating the client's head can relieve labored breathing. Take measures to prevent skin breakdown in cases of peripheral edema. Reassessment is necessary to determine if planned interventions have restored fluid volume balance.

Also perform necessary teaching with the client and family. Show common containers and indicate the volume that each holds. Instruct clients to avoid foods that are high in salt or sodium (Box 16-1). Teach how to read food labels and look for the words *salt*, *sodium*, and other sources of sodium such as baking soda or baking powder. Provide information concerning diuretic drug therapy. List ways to determine if fluid excess is recurring or has resolved.

Fluid Overload: Related to intake that exceeds fluid loss (or reduced fluid loss in relation to intake)
Expected Outcome: Fluid status will return to normal as evidenced by weight loss, reduced edema, BP within normal limits, and urine output of at least 2000 mL/day.

- Assess vital signs, daily weight, intake and output, breath sounds, and location and extent of edema as often as necessary. *Focused assessments help determine if interventions are reducing or eliminating the problem.*
- Use guidelines established by the primary provider for restricting oral fluid. *Limiting fluid intake helps reduce the volume absorbed into the vascular system.*
- Develop a plan with the client for distributing the allotted oral volume over 24 hours. *Involving the client in care promotes compliance and demonstrates that health care professionals value and respect the client's preferences.*
- Ration fluid so that the client can consume approximately 20% to 25% at times other than meals. *The client should be able to consume some fluid whenever thirsty; restricting fluids to meals only is inappropriate.*
- Collaborate with the dietitian to modify the diet to meet salt/sodium restrictions and to avoid sweet or dry foods. *The higher the concentration of sodium (salt) in the blood, the greater the serum osmolality, with a proportionate increase in fluid volume. Sweet or dry food increases a client's desire to consume fluid.*
- Administer prescribed diuretics. *They promote sodium excretion and water elimination.*
- Prepare client and assist with medical interventions such as dialysis (see Chapter 58). *Dialysis uses principles of osmosis and filtration to promote fluid elimination from the blood.*

Impaired Comfort: Dry Mouth and Thirst: Related to restricted oral fluid
Expected Outcomes: (1) Client's mouth will be moist despite fluid restrictions. (2) Client will state that thirst is tolerable.

- Provide supplies for frequent oral hygiene. *Keeping the mouth clean and moist reduces discomfort.*
- Substitute ice chips for oral liquids. *The volume of melted ice is half that of solid ice. Holding ice chips in the mouth gives the psychological impression of consuming more fluid. Because melting ice chips stay in the mouth longer than water, they promote the sensation that larger volumes are being ingested.*
- Instruct client to wet the mouth with a measured volume of fluid in a squeezable squirt bottle or spray atomizer. *Squirting or spraying water in the oral cavity moisturizes the surface of the oral mucous membranes with a small volume of fluid and reduces dryness and thirst.*

Altered Skin Integrity Risk: Related to compromised circulation secondary to edema
Expected Outcome: The client's skin will remain intact.

- Change client's position every 2 hours. *Doing so relieves pressure on capillaries. If capillary pressure falls below 32 mm Hg for more than 2 hours, the skin and underlying tissue are deprived of oxygenated blood, predisposing the client to cell death and skin breakdown.*
- Evaluate client's skin blanching at area of contact with bed or chair by applying light finger pressure. *Light finger pressure should cause brief blanching followed by prompt skin capillary refill. Prolonged blanching may indicate lack of sufficient BP or circulatory volume; this finding may necessitate more frequent position changes than every 2 hours.*
- Keep client's legs elevated higher than the heart. *Doing so facilitates return of venous blood to the heart. Improved circulation reduces metabolic waste products and their toxic effects.*
- Encourage ambulation or isometric bed exercises within client's level of tolerance. *Activity increases respiratory and heart rates; muscle contraction promotes venous return to the heart. All these factors improve delivery of oxygenated blood to the skin and other body cells and removal of metabolic wastes.*
- Apply elastic stockings. *They support valves in the veins and prevent fluid from pooling in dependent areas like the feet and ankles.*

NURSING PROCESS FOR THE CLIENT WITH HYPERVOLEMIA (continued)

Evaluation of Expected Outcomes

Expected outcomes are a daily weight loss of approximately 1 lb, decreased edema from previous assessments, clear lungs, and unlabored respirations. Laboratory values for red blood cells, hematocrit, urine specific gravity, and electrolytes return to normal. Elevations in BP or heart rate resolve. Oral mucous membranes are moist, and the client reports that the distribution of oral fluids controls thirst within a tolerable level. The client shows no evidence of skin breakdown, with reduced or eliminated edema. The toes and feet are warm. Blood returns to the nail bed within 2 to 3 seconds after release of the compressed area.

Third-Spacing

Third-spacing describes the translocation of fluid from the intravascular or intercellular space to tissue compartments, where it becomes trapped and useless. It is associated with the loss of colloids, as may accompany *hypoalbuminemia* (low level of albumin in the blood) or burns, and severe allergic reactions that alter capillary and cellular membrane permeability. Fluid translocation follows the shift in osmotic pressure to other locations. If the translocation depletes fluid volume in the intravascular area, it can lead to hypotension, shock, and circulatory failure (see Chapter 17).

Assessment Findings

The client manifests signs and symptoms of hypovolemia with the exception of weight loss. Fluid volume remains relatively unchanged, but the percentages in various locations are altered. There may be signs of localized enlargement of organ cavities (such as the abdomen) if they fill with fluid, a condition referred to as *ascites* (see Chapter 47). There may be **generalized edema** in all the interstitial spaces, which sometimes is called *brawny edema* or *anasarca* (see Fig. 16-7). Results of laboratory blood tests and urine specific gravity are borderline normal or reveal evidence of hemoconcentration. CVP is below normal, as are other hemodynamic measurements (pressure as it relates to intravascular volume; see Chapter 29).

BOX 16-1 Foods High in Salt or Sodium

- Processed meats (hot dogs and cold cuts)
- Most fast-food choices
- Most frozen convenience meals
- Salted and smoked fish
- Cheeses, especially processed varieties
- Powdered cocoa and hot chocolate mixes
- Canned vegetables
- Foods preserved in brine (pickles, olives, sauerkraut)
- Tomato and tomato vegetable juices
- Canned soup and instant soups or bouillon
- Boxed casserole mixes
- Salted snack foods
- Seasonings: catsup, gravy mixes, soy sauce, monosodium glutamate (MSG), pickle relish, tartar sauce, mustard, horseradish, barbecue sauce, steak sauce

Medical Management

The medical priority is to restore circulatory volume in clients with hypotension and eliminate the trapped fluid. This is done by administering IV solutions—sometimes at rapid rates—and blood products, such as albumin, to restore colloidal osmotic pressure. Administration of albumin pulls the trapped fluid back into the intravascular space. When this occurs, clients who were previously hypovolemic can suddenly become hypervolemic. An IV diuretic may be ordered to reduce the potential for circulatory overload.

Nursing Management

Nursing care combines the assessment techniques for detecting both hypovolemia and hypervolemia. Policies and practices vary concerning how much responsibility licensed practical/vocational nurses (LPNs/LVNs) may assume with regard to IV fluid therapy and administration of IV medications (see Chapter 13).

ELECTROLYTE IMBALANCES

Electrolytes are in both intracellular and extracellular water. They include **ions**, positively and negatively charged particles, such as potassium, magnesium, sodium, phosphate, sulfate, calcium, chloride, HCO_3, protein, and organic acids. Sodium, calcium, and chloride ion concentrations are higher in extracellular fluid, whereas potassium, magnesium, and phosphate concentrations are higher in the cells. These differences are responsible for electrical potentials that develop across cell membranes and perhaps for the degree of cell membrane permeability.

Electrolyte imbalances occur when there is a deficit or an excess of electrolytes or when electrolytes are translocated to any one or more fluid compartments. A loss or gain in fluid usually is accompanied by a similar change in electrolytes. Electrolyte imbalances are identified primarily by measuring their levels in the serum (watery portion of blood).

Electrolyte deficits sometimes result from inadequate intake of food that provides their natural source. Other causes include administering IV solutions that contain no or only some needed electrolytes and conditions that deplete water and substances dissolved therein (e.g., vomiting, diarrhea). Administration of certain medications (e.g., diuretics) also depletes electrolytes.

Factors that contribute to excess electrolytes include an overabundance of orally consumed or parenterally administered electrolytes, kidney failure, and endocrine (glandular) dysfunction, especially of the pituitary gland or adrenal cortex. Electrolytes move from within cells into serum when cell membranes are damaged, such as in crushing injuries or burns. Sodium, potassium, calcium, and magnesium deficits or excesses are of particular concern.

Sodium Imbalances

Sodium (Na^+), the chief **cation** (positively charged electrolyte) in extracellular fluid, is essential for maintaining normal nerve and muscle activity, regulating osmotic pressure, and preserving acid–base balance. The principal role of sodium is to regulate and distribute fluid volume in the body. Normal concentration ranges from 135 to 145 mEq/L. Lower-than-normal serum sodium level is *hyponatremia*; higher than normal serum sodium level is *hypernatremia*.

Hyponatremia

Causes of hyponatremia include profuse diaphoresis, excessive ingestion of plain water or administration of nonelectrolyte IV fluids, profuse diuresis, loss of GI secretions (e.g., in prolonged vomiting, GI suctioning, draining fistulas), and Addison disease (see Chapter 50).

Manifestations include mental confusion, muscular weakness, anorexia, restlessness, elevated body temperature, tachycardia, nausea, vomiting, and personality changes. If the deficit is severe, symptoms are more intense, and convulsions or coma can occur. In such cases, the serum sodium level is below 135 mEq/L.

When possible, the underlying cause is corrected. Treatment of mild deficits includes oral administration of sodium (foods high in sodium, water to which salt has been added, and salt tablets). For severe deficits, administration of IV solutions containing sodium chloride (see Chapter 13) is prescribed.

Hypernatremia

Hypernatremia is excess sodium in the blood. Causes include profuse watery diarrhea, excessive salt intake without sufficient water intake, high fever, decreased water intake (e.g., in older adults; debilitated, unconscious, or developmentally delayed clients), excessive administration of solutions that contain sodium, excessive water loss without an accompanying loss of sodium, and severe burns.

Hypernatremia results in thirst; dry, sticky mucous membranes; decreased urine output; fever; a rough, dry tongue; and lethargy, which can progress to coma if the excess is severe. In such cases, the serum sodium level is above 145 mEq/L.

Treatment depends on the cause and includes oral administration of plain water or IV administration of a hypotonic solution, such as 0.45% sodium chloride or 5% dextrose.

Nursing Management for Sodium Imbalances

Nursing management includes early detection, especially in clients at risk for hyponatremia or hypernatremia. The nurse apportions oral fluids according to target volumes, maintains accurate intake and output measurements, assesses vital signs every 1 to 4 hours, and closely monitors the infusion of IV fluids. They implement prescribed dietary restrictions or supplements (Nutrition Notes). The nurse gathers data that indicate increased or decreased symptoms and notifies the primary provider if symptoms worsen or laboratory values show a significant change.

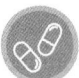

Pharmacologic Considerations

- Sodium can be hidden in routine drugs. When a client is on sodium restriction (especially those with edema, heart or renal failure), be aware of drugs that contain sodium such as some antacids, laxatives, and nonsteroidal antiinflammatory drugs (NSAIDs).

>>> Stop, Think, and Respond 16-3

Which sodium imbalance is likely in a client who manifests mental confusion, muscular weakness, anorexia, restlessness, elevated body temperature, tachycardia, nausea, vomiting, and personality changes?

Potassium Imbalances

The potassium (K^+) cation is the chief electrolyte found in intracellular fluid. Potassium has the same functions intracellularly as sodium has extracellularly. A deficit of potassium in the blood is called *hypokalemia*; an excess is called *hyperkalemia*.

Nutrition Notes

The Client With a Sodium Imbalance

- Under normal circumstances, the body maintains sodium balance over a wide range of intakes by regulating urinary sodium excretion.
- A rule of thumb guideline for determining if a food is high or low in sodium is to look at the % Daily Value (DV) on the Nutrition Facts label. If an item provides ≤5% of the DV for sodium, it is considered low in sodium. If it provides ≥20%, that food is high in sodium.
- Each teaspoon of salt added to food provides approximately 2000 mg of sodium.
- Because salt and sodium compounds are used extensively in food processing and manufacturing, processed and convenience foods are estimated to account for 75% of the sodium in the average American diet. Naturally occurring sources of sodium (e.g., in milk, meats, certain vegetables) provide 12%.
- Five percent comes from salt added during cooking and 6% at the table.

Hypokalemia

Potassium-wasting diuretics such as furosemide (Lasix), ethacrynic acid (Edecrin), and hydrochlorothiazide (HydroDIURIL) contribute to hypokalemia. Loss of fluid from the GI tract (as with severe vomiting or diarrhea, draining intestinal fistulae, or prolonged suctioning) also causes potassium deficit. Large doses of corticosteroids, IV administration of insulin and glucose, and prolonged administration of nonelectrolyte parenteral fluids can deplete potassium. Hypokalemia causes fatigue, weakness, anorexia, nausea, vomiting, cardiac arrhythmias (abnormal heart rate or rhythm, especially in people receiving cardiac glycosides such as digitalis preparations), leg cramps, muscle weakness, and paresthesias (abnormal sensations). Severe cases result in hypotension, flaccid paralysis, and even death from cardiac or respiratory arrest. Hypokalemia produces characteristic changes in the electrocardiogram (ECG) waveform (Fig. 16-9B). The serum potassium level is below 3.5 mEq/L. Symptoms may not develop, however, until the serum potassium level is below 3.0 mEq/L.

Pharmacologic Considerations

- Reconcile medications for digitalis preparations when a client is hypokalemic. Digitalis toxicity is more likely to occur with both potassium and magnesium deficiencies.

Treatment includes elimination of the cause (when possible). The primary provider may substitute a potassium-sparing diuretic such as spironolactone (Aldactone) for one that causes excretion of potassium. Mild hypokalemia is treated by increasing oral intake of potassium-rich foods or using a prescribed potassium oral replacement such as K-Dur, K-Lyte CL, or Klorvess. Severe hypokalemia is treated with IV administration of solutions containing a potassium salt, such as potassium chloride.

Hyperkalemia

Hyperkalemia can occur with severe renal failure in which the kidneys cannot excrete potassium; severe burns; administration of potassium-sparing diuretics; overuse of potassium supplements, salt substitutes or some diet sodas (which contain potassium instead of sodium), or potassium-rich foods; crushing injuries; Addison disease; and rapid administration of parenteral potassium salts.

Symptoms include diarrhea, nausea, muscle weakness, paresthesias, and cardiac arrhythmias. The serum potassium level is above 5.5 mEq/L. Hyperkalemia also causes unique changes in ECG waveforms (see Fig. 16-9C) that can forewarn of sudden cardiac death.

Treatment depends on the cause and severity. Mild hyperkalemia is treated by decreasing the intake of potassium-rich foods or discontinuing oral potassium replacement until

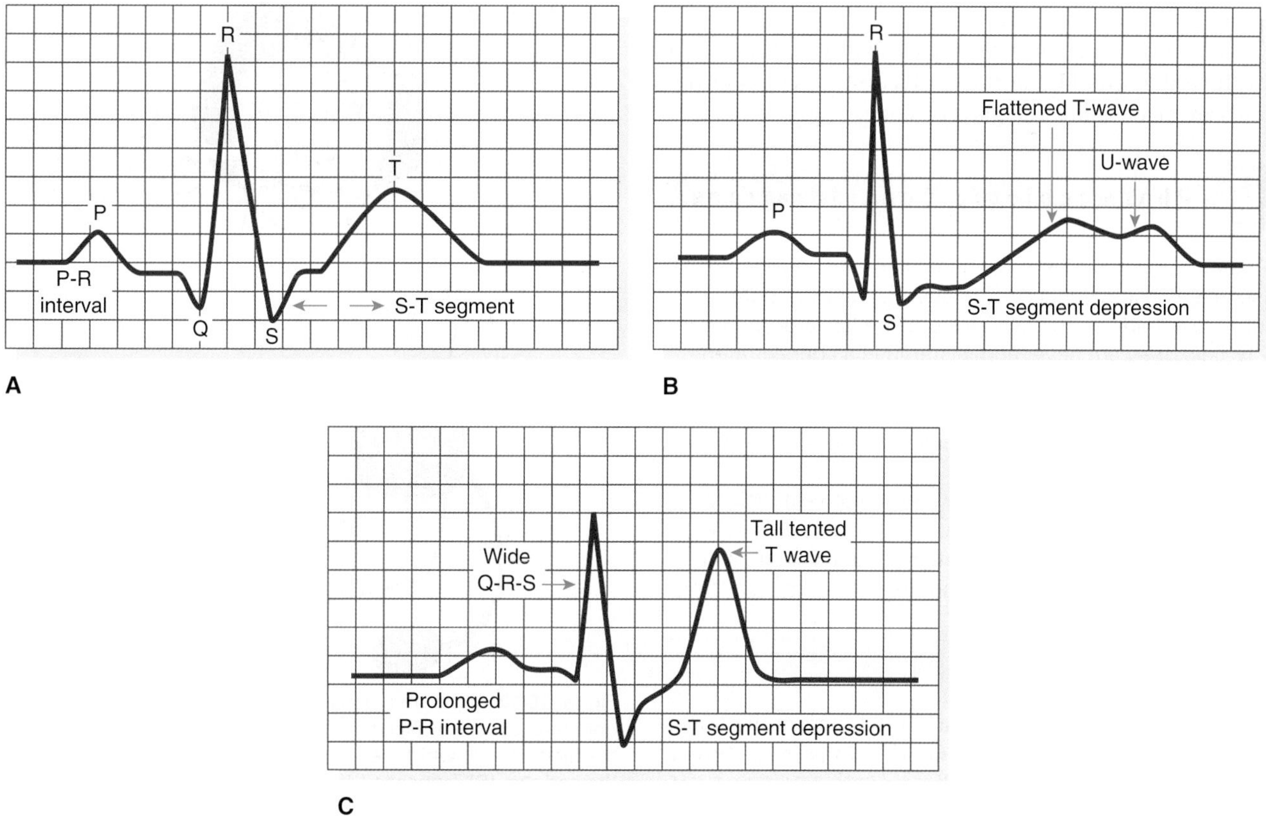

Figure 16-9 Effects of potassium on electrocardiogram (ECG). **(A)** Normal tracing. **(B)** Serum potassium level below normal (hypokalemia) results in ST-segment depression, flattened T wave, and a U wave. **(C)** High potassium level (hyperkalemia) produces prolonged PR interval; widened QRS; ST-segment depression; and a tall, peaked T wave. (From Porth, C. (2015). *Essentials of pathophysiology: Concepts of altered health states* (4th ed.). Wolters Kluwer.)

laboratory values are normal. Severe hyperkalemia is treated by intravenously administering a combination of regular insulin and glucose that temporarily shifts serum potassium into cells within 30 minutes of administration (Paparella, 2018). Peritoneal dialysis or hemodialysis, techniques for removing toxic substances from the blood, also may be used (see Chapter 58).

Nursing Management for Potassium Imbalances

The nurse assesses clients for conditions with the potential to cause potassium imbalances, identifies signs and symptoms associated with potassium imbalances, monitors laboratory findings measuring serum potassium, administers medications that restore potassium balance, and evaluates the client's response to medical therapy. The nurse consults with the primary provider when a client is receiving prolonged IV fluid therapy without added potassium. If IV potassium is ordered, it must be diluted in an IV solution and administered at a rate below 10 mEq/hour. The nurse observes the infusion frequently to verify it is being administered at the appropriate rate. They also inform clients at risk for potassium imbalances and their families about:

- Medications that cause urinary excretion of potassium, such as non–potassium-sparing diuretics;
- Food sources of potassium: vegetables, dried peas and beans, wheat bran, bananas, oranges, orange juice, melon, prune juice, potatoes, and milk;
- Taking oral potassium supplements shortly after meals or with food to avoid GI distress; effervescent tablets or liquids are taken with a full glass of water.

Pharmacologic Considerations

- Potassium should never be administered to a client with insufficient kidney function. Therapeutic doses of potassium are administered orally or are diluted in large volumes of IV fluid; they are never administered in a concentrated strength by IV.
- When given as an IV bolus, potassium depresses heart contraction, causing bradycardia (slow heart rate) and cardiac arrest.
- Clients may experience burning along the vein with IV infusion of potassium in proportion to the infusion's concentration. If the client can tolerate the fluid, consult with the primary provider about diluting the potassium in a larger volume of IV solution.

Calcium Imbalances

Most of the body's calcium (Ca^{++}) is found in the bones and teeth. A small percentage (about 1%) is in the blood. The parathyroid glands regulate the serum calcium level. Calcium is necessary for blood clotting; smooth, skeletal, and cardiac muscle function; and transmission of nerve impulses. Vitamin D is needed for calcium absorption in the intestines and uptake in the bones. *Hypocalcemia* occurs when the serum calcium level is lower than normal; *hypercalcemia* occurs when the level is higher than normal.

Hypocalcemia

Causes of hypocalcemia include vitamin D deficiency, hypoparathyroidism, severe burns, acute pancreatitis, certain drugs such as corticosteroids, rapid administration of multiple units of blood that contain an anticalcium additive, intestinal malabsorption disorders, and accidental surgical removal of the parathyroid glands.

Hypocalcemia is evidenced by tingling in the extremities and the area around the mouth (*circumoral paresthesia*), muscle and abdominal cramps, positive **Chvostek sign** (spasms of the facial muscles when the facial nerve is tapped; Fig. 16-10A), carpopedal spasms referred to as **Trousseau sign** (Fig. 16-10B), mental changes, laryngeal spasms with airway obstruction, *tetany* (muscle twitching), seizures, bleeding, and cardiac arrhythmias. The client has hypocalcemia if the total serum calcium level is below 8.8 mg/dL (normal range: 9 to 11 mg/dL) or the ionized calcium level is below 4.4 mg/dL (normal range: 4.4 to 5.4 mg/dL).

Treatment includes administration of oral calcium and vitamin D for mild deficits and IV administration of a calcium salt, such as calcium gluconate, for severe hypocalcemia.

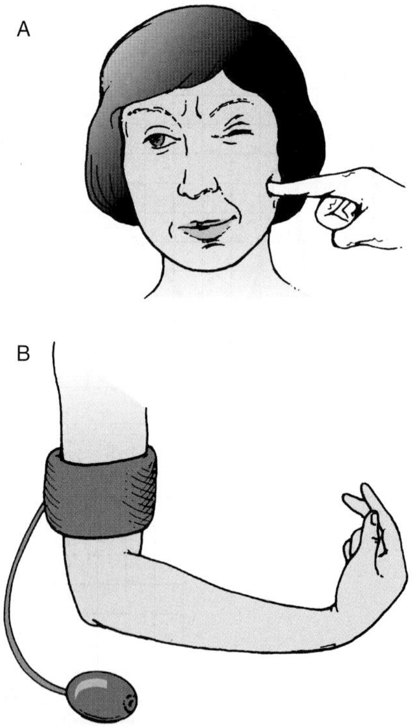

Figure 16-10 Signs of hypocalcemia. **(A)** Chvostek sign, unilateral spasm of facial muscles, is elicited by tapping over the facial nerve, which lies approximately 2 cm anterior to the earlobe. **(B)** Trousseau sign is evidenced by a spasm of the fingers, hand, and wrist when a blood pressure cuff is inflated to a level between the client's systolic and diastolic blood pressure for 3 minutes. (Reprinted with permission from Nettina, S. M. (2006). *Lippincott manual of nursing practice* (8th ed.). Lippincott Williams & Wilkins.)

Hypercalcemia

Hypercalcemia is associated with parathyroid gland tumors, multiple fractures, Paget disease, hyperparathyroidism, excessive doses of vitamin D, prolonged immobilization, some chemotherapeutic agents, and certain malignant diseases (multiple myeloma, acute leukemia, lymphomas).

Hypercalcemia causes deep bone pain, constipation, anorexia, nausea, vomiting, polyuria, thirst, pathologic fractures, and mental changes such as decreased memory and attention span. Chronic hypercalcemia can promote the formation of kidney stones. The total serum calcium level is above 10 mg/dL, and the ionized calcium level is above 5.4 mg/dL.

Treatment includes determining and correcting the cause when possible. Mild hypercalcemia is treated by increasing oral fluid intake and limiting calcium consumption until laboratory findings are normal. Acute hypercalcemia is treated by administering one or more of the following: IV sodium chloride solution (0.45% or 0.9%) and a diuretic such as furosemide (Lasix) to increase calcium excretion in the urine; oral phosphates; or calcitonin (Miacalcin), a synthetic hormone for regulating calcium levels. Hypercalcemia associated with cancer or chemotherapy is treated on an individual basis. A decrease in drug dosage or discontinuation of therapy may be necessary. Corticosteroids or plicamycin (Mithracin), an antineoplastic agent, also may be used to treat hypercalcemia of malignant diseases that do not respond to other forms of therapy.

Nursing Management for Calcium Imbalances

The nurse closely monitors the client with hypocalcemia for neurologic manifestations (tetany, seizures, spasms), cardiac arrhythmias, and airway obstruction because emergency interventions may be necessary. If the deficit is severe, seizure precautions are necessary. Clients with severe muscle cramping remain on bed rest for comfort and to avoid falls. Because a low calcium level interferes with clotting, the nurse routinely checks for signs of bruising or bleeding.

The nurse encourages the client with mild hypercalcemia to drink many oral fluids and collaborates with the dietitian to limit food sources of calcium when calcium is restricted from the diet. Encouraging ambulation as tolerated is important. The nurse provides assistance and instructs the client to wear shoes to avoid falls that may result in pathologic fractures.

A teaching plan for the client with hypocalcemia or hypercalcemia includes the following points:

- Follow the primary provider's recommendations regarding the addition or restriction of calcium to the diet. Milk, yogurt, and hard cheese are rich sources of dietary calcium. Nondairy sources are turnip and mustard greens, collards, kale, broccoli, canned fish with bones, and calcium-fortified orange juice.
- Lactose-free milk and nonprescription lactase enzymes are available for lactose-intolerant clients.
- Take prescribed or primary provider–recommended drugs as directed; do not exceed or omit a dose.

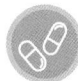

Pharmacologic Considerations

- Calcium replacement is given cautiously to clients with a history of kidney stones because high calcium levels in the kidney tubules may contribute to stone formation.

Magnesium Imbalances

Magnesium (Mg^{++}) is found in bone cells and specialized cells of the heart, liver, and skeletal muscles. Only a small percentage of the total magnesium in the body is found in extracellular fluid. Magnesium is involved in the transmission of nerve impulses and muscle excitability and activates several enzyme systems, including the functioning of B vitamins and use of potassium and calcium. A lower-than-normal serum level of magnesium is *hypomagnesemia*; higher than normal is *hypermagnesemia*.

Hypomagnesemia

Conditions that can result in hypomagnesemia include chronic alcoholism, diabetic ketoacidosis, severe renal disease, severe burns, severe malnutrition, pregnancy-induced hypertension, intestinal malabsorption syndromes, excessive diuresis (drug induced), hyperaldosteronism (see Chapter 50), and prolonged gastric suction. Physical stress or high intake of calcium, protein, or alcohol may increase the need for magnesium.

Signs and symptoms include tachycardia and other cardiac arrhythmias, neuromuscular irritability, paresthesias of the extremities, leg and foot cramps, hypertension, mental changes, positive Chvostek and Trousseau signs (see Fig. 16-9), dysphagia (difficulty swallowing), and seizures. The serum magnesium level is below 1.3 mEq/L (normal range: 1.3 to 2.1 mEq/L).

Treatment includes administration of oral or parenteral magnesium salts or the magnesium-rich foods to the diet. Magnesium is found in green leafy vegetables, whole grains (especially wheat germ and bran), nuts, cocoa, chocolate, nuts, soybeans, seafood, and dried peas and beans. A severe magnesium deficit is treated with IV administration of magnesium sulfate.

Hypermagnesemia

Hypermagnesemia can be a consequence of renal failure, Addison disease, excessive use of antacids or laxatives that contain magnesium, and hyperparathyroidism. Clients with hypermagnesemia experience flushing, warmth, hypotension, lethargy, drowsiness, *bradycardia*, muscle weakness, depressed respirations, and coma. The serum magnesium level is above 2.1 mEq/L.

Treatment includes decreasing oral magnesium intake or discontinuing administration of parenteral replacement. In severe hypermagnesemia, hemodialysis may be necessary. If respiratory failure occurs, mechanical ventilation is essential.

Nursing Management for Magnesium Imbalances

The nurse closely observes clients with hypomagnesemia for arrhythmias and early signs of neuromuscular irritability, which they report to the primary provider immediately. If administering IV magnesium sulfate, the nurse checks BP frequently because such administration can produce vasodilation and subsequent hypotension. Calcium gluconate is kept available as an antidote for an adverse reaction during administration of magnesium sulfate. If dysphagia occurs, the nurse consults with the primary provider and dietitian about alternatives or modifications to dietary management.

Vital signs of clients with actual or potential hypermagnesemia require close monitoring. The nurse notifies the primary provider immediately of significant changes, especially in respiratory rate, rhythm, or depth. Teaching points include the following:

- Check with the primary provider, pharmacist, or nurse concerning antacids or laxatives that contain magnesium.
- If use of an antacid or laxative is allowed, follow the primary provider's recommendations regarding the frequency of use.

Pharmacologic Considerations

■ When administering electrolytes to correct or prevent a deficiency, measure the dose carefully and give only as directed by the prescriber because these agents are potentially dangerous.

>>> *Stop, Think, and Respond 16-4*

Identify the electrolyte imbalance each client is most likely manifesting:

Client A is nauseous and weak. The ECG shows a U wave.

Client B has muscle twitching and tingling around the mouth.

Client C is thirsty, lethargic, and excreting only scant urine.

ACID–BASE BALANCE

In addition to water and electrolytes, body fluid also contains acids and bases. One of the chief acids is carbonic acid. An example of a base, sometimes referred to as an *alkaline substance*, that neutralizes acids is HCO_3. Acid and base content influence the pH of body fluid. The symbol *pH* refers to the amount of hydrogen ions in a solution; pH can range from 1, which is highly acidic, to 14, which is highly basic. A pH of 7 is neutral. The more hydrogen ions in a solution, the more acidic it is. Acidity is indicated by a pH below 7. The degree of alkalinity is identified by a pH above 7. Normal plasma pH is 7.35 to 7.45, or slightly alkaline. The body maintains the normal plasma pH by two mechanisms: chemical regulation and organ regulation.

Chemical Regulation

Chemical regulation occurs through one or more buffering systems by which hydrogen ions are either added or eliminated. Adding hydrogen ions increases acidity; removing them promotes alkalinity. The major chemical regulator of plasma pH is the **bicarbonate–carbonic acid buffer system**. A ratio of 20 parts HCO_3 to 1 part H_2CO_3 maintains normal plasma pH.

Organ Regulation

The lungs and kidneys facilitate the ratio of HCO_3 to H_2CO_3. Carbon dioxide (CO_2) is one of the components of carbonic acid:

$$CO_2 + H_2O \text{ (water)} = H_2CO_3$$

The lungs regulate H_2CO_3 levels by releasing or conserving CO_2 by increasing or decreasing the respiratory rate, volume, or both. The kidneys assist in acid–base balance by retaining or excreting bicarbonate ions. If an imbalance in acids or bases occurs, these regulatory processes are accelerated, which is referred to as **compensation**.

ACID–BASE IMBALANCES

An imbalance in acids or bases is life threatening. Death occurs quickly if plasma pH is outside the range of 6.8 to 7.8 (Sherwood, 2011). Arterial blood gas (ABG) results are the main tool for measuring blood pH, CO_2 content ($PaCO_2$), and HCO_3. An acid–base imbalance may accompany a fluid and electrolyte imbalance.

There are essentially two types of acid–base imbalances: acidosis and alkalosis (Fig. 16-11). **Acidosis** means excessive accumulation of acids or excessive loss of bicarbonate in body fluids. **Alkalosis** means excessive accumulation of bases or loss of acid in body fluids. Either can stem from metabolic or respiratory alterations. There are four subtypes: metabolic acidosis, metabolic alkalosis, respiratory acidosis, and respiratory alkalosis.

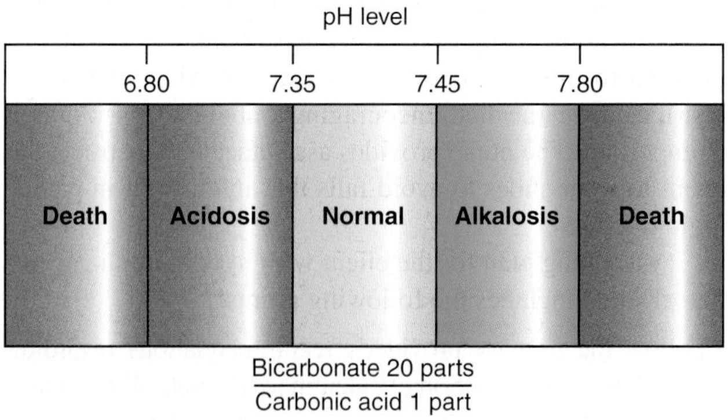

Figure 16-11 Acid–base balance and imbalances. Note that acidosis is used to describe the condition when pH is between 6.8 and 7.35. *Alkalosis* describes the condition when pH is between 7.45 and 7.80. When the pH exceeds these limits in either direction, death can occur. Dangerous cardiac arrhythmias can develop, and the force of cardiac contractions can be weakened. In severe stages, stupor and coma occur, and death may follow shortly.

Metabolic Acidosis

Metabolic acidosis is a condition that results in decreased plasma pH because of increased organic acids (acids other than H_2CO_3) or decreased bicarbonate. Organic acids increase during periods of anaerobic metabolism, when cells attempt to produce ATP without oxygen. Anaerobic metabolism is much less efficient than aerobic (with oxygen) metabolism and produces by-products such as lactic acid. It occurs during shock and cardiac arrest. Acids also increase in starvation and diabetic ketoacidosis (see Chapter 51), as fatty acids accumulate because the body cannot use glucose for energy. Accumulation of acids also may follow renal failure because the kidneys cannot reabsorb bicarbonate to buffer the blood. They also accumulate with aspirin (acetylsalicylic acid) overdosage or profuse diarrhea. Another cause of acid accumulation is loss of intestinal fluid through wound drainage in which bicarbonate can be lost in disproportionate amounts.

Assessment Findings

Signs and Symptoms

Metabolic acidosis is accompanied by deep and rapid breathing (*Kussmaul breathing*), a compensatory mechanism to rid the body of CO_2 and thus prevent carbonic acid from forming. The client may experience anorexia, nausea, vomiting, headache, confusion, flushing, lethargy, malaise, drowsiness, abdominal pain or discomfort, and weakness.

Diagnostic Findings

The ABG values usually show decreased pH and plasma HCO_3. Initially, $PaCO_2$ is normal, a condition referred to as an *uncompensated state*. As the rapid and deep breathing becomes effective, $PaCO_2$ decreases. Until pH returns to normal, it is referred to as a *partially compensated state*. When pH returns to normal, it is referred to as *a fully compensated state*, even though HCO_3 and $PaCO_2$ values are abnormal (Table 16-3). In a fully compensated state, regardless of the initial imbalance and current abnormal values, the client is out of danger.

TABLE 16-3 Arterial Blood Gas Trends in Acid–Base Imbalances

CONDITION	pH	HCO_3 (mEq/L)	$Paco_2$ (mm Hg)
Acid–base balance	7.35–7.45	22–26	35–45
Metabolic Acidosis			
Uncompensated	<7.35	<22	Normal
Partially compensated	<7.35	<22	<35
Fully compensated	7.35–7.45	<22	<35
Metabolic Alkalosis			
Uncompensated	>7.45	>26	Normal
Partially compensated	>7.45	>26	>45
Fully compensated	>7.45	>22	>45
Respiratory Acidosis			
Uncompensated	<7.35	Normal	>45
Partially compensated	<7.35	>26	>45
Fully compensated	7.35–7.45	>26	>45
Respiratory Alkalosis			
Uncompensated	7.45	Normal	<35
Partially compensated	7.45	<22	<35
Fully compensated	7.35–7.45	<22	<35

The anion gap also is used to identify metabolic acidosis. The **anion gap** is the difference between sodium and potassium cation (positive ion) concentrations and the sum of chloride and bicarbonate **anions** (negative ions) in the extracellular fluid. The measured cations usually exceed the measured anions; the gap reflects the remaining unmeasured anions, such as phosphates, sulfates, organic acids, and proteins. The normal anion gap is 12 ± 4 mEq/L. An anion gap that exceeds 16 mEq/L indicates, but is not absolutely diagnostic for, metabolic acidosis. Low or negative anion gaps are relatively rare, usually resulting from a laboratory error.

The measurement of all base buffers—sometimes referred to as the *base excess* or *deficit*—is used to identify acid–base imbalances. The base buffers include bicarbonate, phosphate, protein, and hemoglobin. To determine if the base is in excess or deficit, the laboratory determines the amount of a fixed acid or base that is necessary to reach a pH of 7.4 in a sample of the client's blood (Porth, 2014). The normal range is ±3.0 mEq/L. A base deficit indicates metabolic acidosis; a base excess indicates metabolic alkalosis.

Medical Management

Treatment includes eliminating the cause and replacing fluids and electrolytes that may have been lost. IV bicarbonate is administered for severe metabolic acidosis.

>>> *Stop, Think, and Respond 16-5*

Calculate the anion gap using the following measurements and indicate if they indicate metabolic acidosis or metabolic alkalosis.

Sodium (Na^+): 165 mEq/L
Potassium (K^+): 4.0 mEq/L
Chloride (Cl^-): 112 mEq/L
Bicarbonate (HCO_3): 32 mEq/L

Metabolic Alkalosis

Metabolic alkalosis results in increased plasma pH because of accumulated base bicarbonate or decreased hydrogen ion concentrations. Factors that increase base bicarbonate include excessive oral or parenteral use of bicarbonate-containing drugs or other alkaline salts, a rapid decrease in extracellular fluid volume (e.g., in diuretic therapy), and loss of hydrogen and chloride ions (e.g., in vomiting, prolonged gastric suctioning, hypokalemia, hyperaldosteronism). The result is retention of sodium bicarbonate and increased base bicarbonate.

Assessment Findings

Clients in metabolic alkalosis can manifest anorexia, nausea, vomiting, circumoral paresthesias, confusion, carpopedal spasm, hypertonic reflexes, and tetany. The respiratory rate and volume decrease in a compensatory effort to produce more carbonic acid to increase and restore the acidic level in the blood. Initially, ABGs show increased pH and HCO_3 and normal $PaCO_2$ levels (see Table 16-3). As compensatory respiratory mechanisms result in slower and shallower breathing, the $PaCO_2$ level is elevated; eventually, pH may return to normal.

Medical Management

Treatment involves eliminating the cause. The primary provider may prescribe potassium (as a potassium salt) if hypokalemia is present. In hypokalemia, hydrogen ions shift to the intracellular space to ensure the appropriate level of cations; the intracellular shift of hydrogen raises blood pH. Administering potassium allows hydrogen to return to the intravascular space and reestablishes a normal blood pH (Thomas, 2020).

Treatment may also involve prescribing sodium chloride. When sodium is reabsorbed in the kidney tubules, hydrogen ions are excreted, contributing to a state of alkalosis. Maintaining an adequate sodium level reduces the excretion of hydrogen ions and offsets the rising pH.

Respiratory Acidosis

Respiratory acidosis, which may be either acute or chronic, is caused by excess carbonic acid, which causes the blood pH to drop below 7.35. Conditions that predispose to respiratory acidosis include pneumothorax, hemothorax, pulmonary edema, acute bronchial asthma, atelectasis, hyaline membrane disease or other forms of respiratory distress in the newborn, pneumonia (see Chapter 21), some drug overdoses, and head injuries. Chronic respiratory acidosis is associated with disorders such as emphysema, bronchiectasis, bronchial asthma, and cystic fibrosis.

Assessment Findings

Acute respiratory acidosis is associated with extreme respiratory insufficiency. The client may make frantic efforts to breathe, breathe slowly or irregularly, or stop breathing. Expiratory volumes are decreased. Lung sounds may be moist or absent in some lobes. Tachycardia usually is present, and cardiac arrhythmias can develop. In later stages, *cyanosis*, a dusky appearance to the skin, may be evident. The accumulation of CO_2 leads to behavioral changes (mental cloudiness, confusion, disorientation, hallucinations), tremors, muscle twitching, flushed skin, headache, weakness, stupor, and coma. Responses to chronic respiratory acidosis are less prominent and can include an increased breathing effort, lack of energy, reduced activity, dull headache, and weakness.

ABG values show a decreased pH and an increased $PaCO_2$ above 45 mm Hg. As the kidney attempts to compensate, which may take 2 to 3 days, the HCO_3 rises, followed by a return to normal pH if full compensation occurs (see Table 16-3).

Medical Management

Treatment is individualized depending on the cause of the imbalance and whether the condition is acute or chronic. Mechanical ventilation may be necessary to support respiratory function. IV sodium bicarbonate is administered when ventilation efforts do not adequately restore a balanced pH. Heart rate and rhythm are monitored to detect sudden cardiac changes. In less acute situations, treatment may include the administration of pharmacologic agents, such as bronchodilators and antibiotics, to improve breathing. Airway suctioning may be necessary if the client is too weak to cough secretions.

Respiratory Alkalosis

Respiratory alkalosis results from a carbonic acid deficit that occurs when rapid breathing releases more CO_2 with expired air. *Tachypnea* (rapid breathing) may result from acute anxiety, high fever, thyrotoxicosis (overactive thyroid), early salicylate (aspirin) poisoning, *hypoxemia* (low oxygen in the blood), or mechanical ventilation.

Assessment Findings

The most obvious manifestation is an increased respiratory rate. Accompanying symptoms include lightheadedness, numbness and tingling of the fingers and toes, circumoral paresthesias, sweating, panic, dry mouth, and, in severe cases, convulsions. The ABG values indicate a pH above 7.45 and a $PaCO_2$ below 35 mm Hg. If the kidney compensates by excreting bicarbonate ions, the HCO_3 falls below 22 mEq to restore pH (see Table 16-3).

Medical Management

Treatment aims to correct the cause of the rapid breathing. Having the client breathe into a paper bag held over the nose and mouth and rebreathe expired air may be useful temporarily. Sedation may be necessary when extreme anxiety is the cause of tachypnea.

Concept Mastery Alert

Respiratory Alkalosis

Clients experiencing respiratory alkalosis (which can be brought on by a severe anxiety attack and associated hyperventilation) would have a pH greater than 7.45.

Nursing Management for Acid–Base Imbalances

The nurse carefully documents all presenting signs and symptoms to provide accurate baseline data. They monitor laboratory values, compare ABG findings with previous results (if any), and report current results to the primary provider as soon as they are obtained. The same applies to abnormal electrolyte levels. The nurse maintains accurate intake and output records to monitor fluid status. They implement prescribed medical therapy, such as administering fluid and electrolyte replacements, suctioning the airway, maintaining mechanical ventilation, and monitoring cardiac rate and rhythm (see Chapters 20 and 21). The nurse administers cardiopulmonary resuscitation whenever necessary.

KEY POINTS

- Fluid and electrolyte balance: maintained by:
  - Intake and output
  - Distribution of fluids and electrolytes
    - Osmosis: movement of water through a semipermeable membrane
    - Filtration: movement of fluid according to pressure differences
    - Diffusion: passive (high to lower concentration) and facilitated (assistance required)
    - Active transport: requires energy source
- Fluid imbalances:
  - Hypovolemia: fluid volume deficit
  - Hypervolemia: fluid volume excess
  - Third-spacing: fluid in tissue compartments
- Electrolyte imbalances: Hypo—low, Hyper—high
  - Sodium imbalances: essential for maintaining normal nerve and muscle activity, regulating osmotic pressure, and maintaining acid–base balance
  - Potassium imbalances: chief electrolyte in the cells, essential for maintaining cardiac function
  - Calcium imbalances: most of calcium found in bones, essential for blood clotting, muscle function, and transmission of nerve impulses
  - Magnesium imbalances: involved in transmission of nerve impulses and muscle excitability
- Acid–base balance: influences the pH of the body, maintained by chemical and organ regulation
- Acid–base imbalances
  - Metabolic acidosis: decreased plasma pH due to increased organic acids or decreased bicarbonate
  - Metabolic alkalosis: increased plasma pH due to accumulated base bicarbonate or decreased hydrogen ion concentrations
  - Respiratory acidosis: excess carbonic acid caused blood pH to drop below 7.35
  - Respiratory alkalosis: deficient carbonic acid that occurs from rapid breathing releasing increased amounts of CO_2.

CRITICAL THINKING EXERCISES

1. Describe the relationship of water to imbalances in electrolytes, acids, and bases.
2. Explain the action that occurs when an IV bolus of potassium is used to execute criminals by lethal injection.
3. Which respiratory acid–base imbalance do you think is more common? Support your answer.
4. What imbalances are likely to occur among athletes, and what steps are taken to help avoid serious consequences?

NCLEX-STYLE REVIEW QUESTIONS PrepU

1. A nurse calculates that the 24-hour total oral fluid intake for an afebrile 110 lb client has been 1725 mL. What conclusion is accurate?
   1. The client's oral fluid intake is adequate for the client's weight.
   2. The client's oral fluid intake is below the standard for this client.
   3. The client's oral fluid intake should be supplemented with IV fluid.
   4. The client's oral fluid intake should be increased by approximately 100 mL.
2. A hypertensive client will begin taking furosemide (Lasix), a potassium-wasting diuretic, every day. The nurse knows that teaching regarding the need for potassium-rich foods is successful when the client makes which of the following statements?
   1. "I can have a daily serving of gelatin."
   2. "I need to have more fruits like bananas and nectarines."
   3. "I will add more servings of broiled white fish."
   4. "I will eat more pasta and cheese."
3. Following a subtotal thyroidectomy, which client statement is most indicative that the client is experiencing hypocalcemia?
   1. "I don't have much of an appetite."
   2. "I feel so weak when I ambulate."
   3. "Light seems to bother my eyes."
   4. "My lips feel numb and tingly."
4. A client has been taking aluminum and magnesium hydroxide (Maalox), an antacid, for many days because of gastric discomfort. The nurse suspects that the client's magnesium level is elevated because of which symptoms? Select all that apply.
   1. Bradycardia
   2. Hyperventilation
   3. Hypotension
   4. Insomnia
   5. Shivering

5. The nurse observes this abnormal appearance on the cardiac monitor.

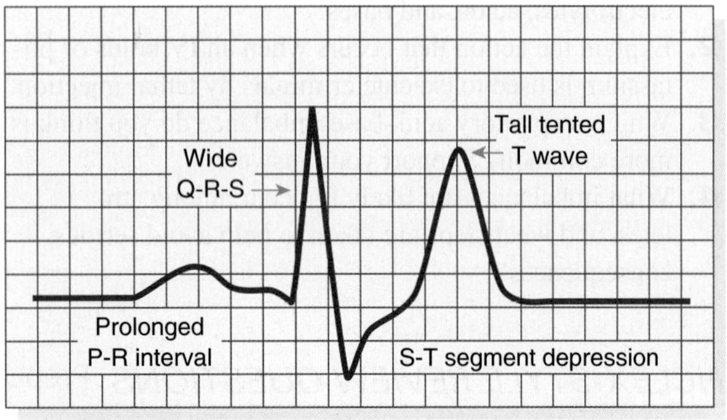

Which electrolyte imbalance should the nurse suspect?

1. Hypercalcemia
2. Hypocalcemia
3. Hyperkalemia
4. Hypokalemia

WANT TO KNOW MORE? There are a wide variety of online resources available on thePoint to enhance learning and understanding of this chapter.

Go to **thePoint.lww.com/activate** and use the activation code found in the front of this text to unlock these online resources.

17 Caring for Clients in Shock

Words To Know

adenosine triphosphate
adrenocorticotropic hormone
anaerobic metabolism
anaphylactic shock
antidiuretic hormone
cardiac output
cardiogenic shock
catecholamines
compensation stage
corticosteroid hormones
decompensation stage
distributive shock
endotoxins
hypovolemic shock
hypoxia
irreversible stage
ischemia
multiple organ dysfunction syndrome
neurogenic shock
obstructive shock
oliguria
positive inotropic agents
septic shock
shock
systemic inflammatory response syndrome
vasopressors

Learning Objectives

On completion of this chapter, you will be able to:

1. Define shock.
2. Name four general categories of shock.
3. Identify the subcategories of distributive shock.
4. List pathophysiologic consequences of shock.
5. Name the three stages of shock.
6. Identify three physiologic mechanisms that attempt to compensate for shock.
7. Discuss signs and symptoms manifested by clients in shock.
8. Name three diagnostic measurements used when monitoring clients in shock.
9. Give three medical approaches for treating shock.
10. List complications of shock.
11. Discuss the nursing management of clients with shock.

This chapter discusses shock and its various types, pathophysiologic consequences, and assessment findings, which may vary according to type. It also presents the medical and nursing management of clients in shock.

Gerontologic Considerations

- Older adults, particularly those with cardiac disease, are prone to cardiogenic shock.
- They also have a decreased percentage of body water and are more likely to develop hypovolemic shock.
- Owing to a decreased immune response, which hinders the body's ability to fight infection, older adults may be at higher risk for developing septic shock.

SHOCK

Shock is a life-threatening condition that occurs when arterial blood flow and oxygen delivery to tissues and cells are inadequate. Shock develops as a consequence of one of three events: (1) blood volume decreases, (2) the heart fails as an effective pump, or (3) peripheral blood vessels massively dilate. The body implements compensatory mechanisms to counteract the effects of shock. When compensatory mechanisms become ineffective, shock progresses until therapeutic measures are implemented. If physiologic and therapeutic measures are inadequate, organs are damaged and death may follow.

Types of Shock

The four main categories of shock are hypovolemic, distributive, obstructive, and cardiogenic, depending on the cause. Distributive shock is subdivided into neurogenic, septic (toxic), and anaphylactic shock (Silva et al., 2018; Table 17-1). More than one type of shock can develop simultaneously.

Hypovolemic Shock

In **hypovolemic (hemorrhagic) shock**, the most common type of shock, the volume of extracellular fluid is significantly diminished, primarily because of lost or reduced blood or plasma (serum; see Chapter 16). Because the intravascular, interstitial, and intracellular fluid volumes are interdependent, a loss from one location results in a similar depletion in the others. Thus, a deficit of intravascular volume (plasma) reduces the net circulating volume. Hypovolemic shock can develop when overall fluid volume is depleted from significant bleeding, such as during surgery, after trauma, or after delivery of an infant. It may also result from significant fluid

TABLE 17-1 Types of Shock

TYPE	CAUSE	ILLUSTRATION	EXAMPLES
Hypovolemic shock	Decreased blood volume with decreased filling of the circulatory system	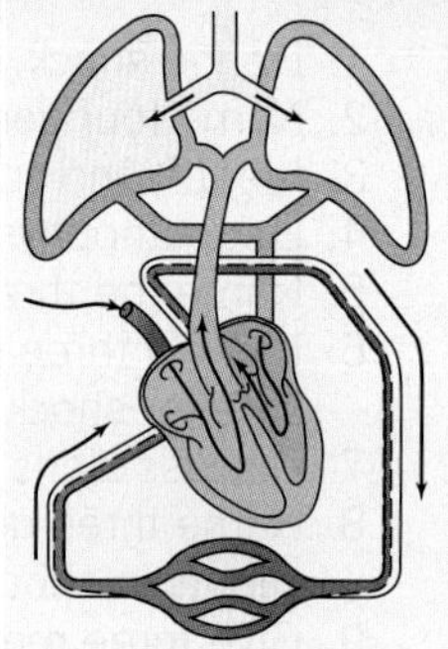	Hemorrhage (frank and internal) Extreme diuresis Severe diarrhea or vomiting Dehydration Third-spacing
Distributive shock (*Neurogenic, Septic, Anaphylactic*)	Enlargement of the vascular compartment and redistribution of intravascular fluid from arterial circulation to venous or capillary areas	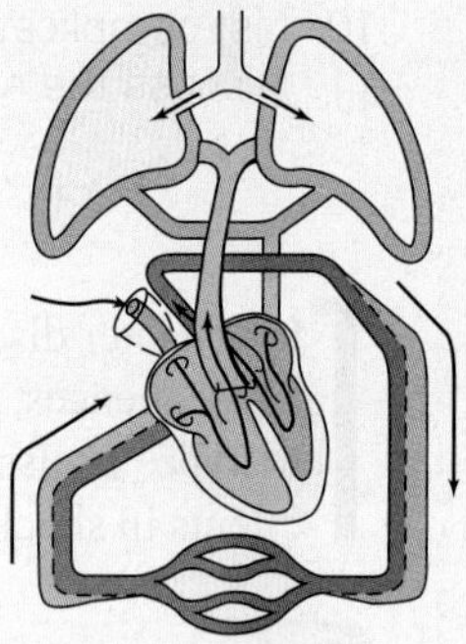	*Neurogenic*: Spinal cord injury *Septic*: Toxic reaction to gram-negative bacterial infection *Anaphylactic*: Severe allergic reaction
Obstructive shock	Impaired filling of heart with blood due to mechanical impediment	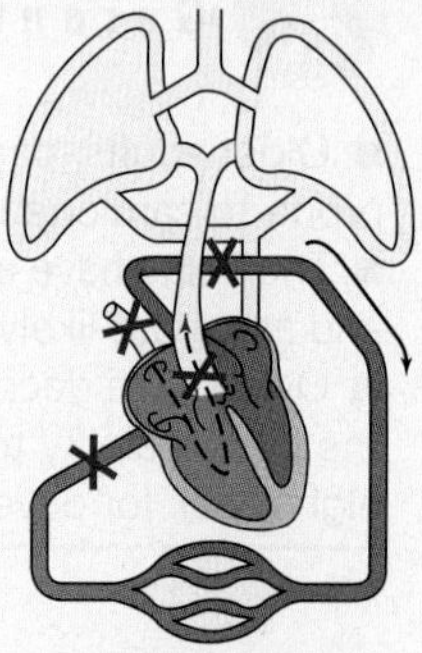	Cardiac tamponade (see Chapter 23) Dissecting aneurysm Tension pneumothorax (see Chapter 21)
Cardiogenic shock	Decreased force of ventricular contraction leading to inadequate intravascular volume and tissue hypoxia	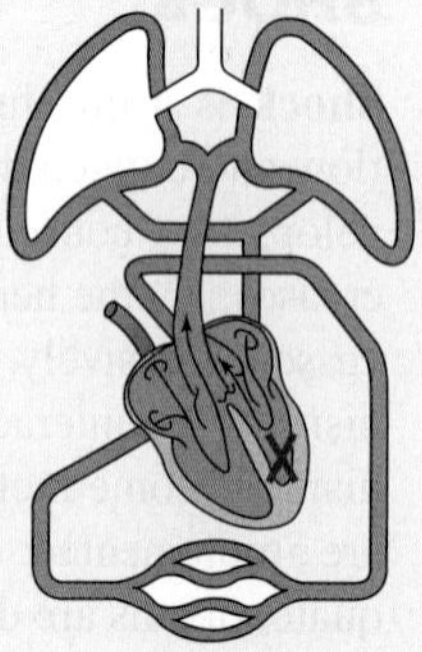	Myocardial infarction (see Chapter 25) Cardiac arrhythmia (see Chapter 26)

Reprinted with permission from Porth, C. M. (2015). *Essentials of pathophysiology: Concepts of altered health states* (4th ed.). Wolters Kluwer.

loss, as with burns, large draining wounds, reduced fluid intake, prolonged gastrointestinal (GI) suctioning, or disorders in which fluid losses exceed fluid intake, such as diabetes insipidus (see Chapter 50). Table 17-2 identifies how symptoms escalate, ranging from 15% (750 mL) or less loss of fluid volume to over 40% (in excess of 2000 mL). Most require blood and fluid replacement when there is a 30% to 40% loss of fluid. A fluid loss that exceeds 40% is life-threatening (Hill & Mitchell, 2020).

Distributive Shock

Distributive shock is sometimes called *normovolemic* shock because the amount of fluid in the circulatory system is not reduced, yet the fluid circulation does not permit effective tissue perfusion. Vasodilatation, a prominent characteristic of distributive shock, increases the space in the vascular bed. Central blood flow is reduced because peripheral vascular or interstitial areas exceed their usual capacity. Three types of distributive shock are neurogenic, septic, and anaphylactic shock.

Neurogenic Shock

Neurogenic shock, the rarest type of shock, results from injury that affects the vasomotor center in the medulla of the brain or to the peripheral nerves that extend from the spinal cord to the blood vessels. Injury to the spinal cord or head or overdoses of opioids, tranquilizers, or general anesthetics can cause neurogenic shock. The tone of the sympathetic nervous system is impaired, resulting in decreased arterial vascular resistance, vasodilatation, and hypotension. Because blood remains distributed in the periphery, the heart does not fill adequately, cardiac output is reduced, tissue perfusion is compromised, cells are deprived of oxygen and switch to anaerobic metabolism, and metabolic acidosis develops from an increase in lactic acid.

Septic Shock

Septic shock (toxic shock) has the highest mortality rate of the various types of shock. Client deaths occur in 40% to 60% of those who develop septic shock despite aggressive treatment (Cecconi et al, 2018). It is associated with overwhelming bacterial infections (see Chapter 12). Septic shock is preceded by a **systemic inflammatory response syndrome** (SIRS), an inflammatory state without a proven source of infection (Box 17-1). SIRS progresses to sepsis when symptoms of SIRS are present and an infection is proven. Severe sepsis is a preseptic shock condition that develops when sepsis is combined with organ hypoperfusion (see Chapter 12). Once septic shock, which is accompanied by hypotension, develops, the client may deteriorate to the point of **multiple organ dysfunction syndrome**, a complication of overwhelming inflammation that results in massive cellular, tissue, and organ injury.

Septic shock occurs most commonly in clients with gram-negative bacteremia (bacteria in the blood) caused by such pathogens as *Escherichia coli*, species of *Pseudomonas*, and gram-positive drug-resistant *Staphylococcus aureus* and streptococcal species. **Endotoxins**, harmful chemicals released by bacterial cells, are probably the major cause of septic shock. They trigger an immune response in which vasoactive chemicals, such as cytokines (see Chapter 33), dilate the blood vessels and increase capillary permeability, causing vascular fluid to shift to the interstitium. Unlike other forms of shock, clients with septic shock have an elevated leukocyte count and initially manifest a fever accompanied

TABLE 17-2 Classifications of Hypovolemic Shock

STAGE	FLUID VOLUME LOSS	SIGNS AND SYMPTOMS
Class I	0%–15% (≤750 mL)	Stable blood pressure Slight tachycardia Sudden anxiety
Class II	15%–30% (750–1000 mL)	Tachycardia Tachypnea Stable blood pressure Increased diastolic pressure Cool clammy skin Decreased urine output Delayed capillary refill
Class III	30%–40% (1500–2000 mL)	Marked tachycardia (>120 beats/min) Marked tachypnea (>30 breaths/min) Decreased systolic blood pressure (<100 mm Hg) Oliguria (<20 mL) Confusion or agitation Skin pale, cold, and sweating noted
Class IV	≥ 40% (>2000 mL)	Systolic blood pressure <70 mm Hg Weak pulse Marked oliguria Cold, pale skin Extreme sweating Unconscious

Adapted from Hill, B., & Mitchell, A. (2020). Hypovolaemic shock. *British Journal of Nursing, 29*(10), 557–560. https://doi.org/10.12968/bjon.2020.29.10.557.

BOX 17-1 Criteria for Systemic Inflammatory Response Syndrome

Systemic inflammatory response syndrome (SIRS) is diagnosed when two or more of the following are present and there is a strong suspicion of inflammation such as microbial infection, pancreatitis, and multiple trauma:

- Heart rate greater than 90 beats/min
- Body temperature less than 36°C (96.8°F) or greater than 38°C (100.8°F)
- Respiratory rate over 20 breaths/min or blood gas measurement of carbon dioxide ($PaCO_2$) of less than 32 mm Hg (normal is 35–45 mm Hg)
- White blood cell count less than 4000 cells/mm^3 or greater than 12,000 cells/mm^3 or the presence of more than 10% immature neutrophils

From Chakraborty, R. K., & Burns, B. (2020). Systemic inflammatory response syndrome. *StatPearls* [Internet]. StatPearls Publishing.

by warm, flushed skin and a rapid, bounding pulse. As septic shock progresses, however, affected clients eventually develop cold, pale, or mottled skin and hypotensive symptoms, findings common with other forms of shock.

Anaphylactic Shock

Anaphylactic shock is a severe allergic reaction that follows exposure to a substance to which a person is extremely sensitive (see Chapter 34). Common allergic substances include bee venom, latex, fish, nuts, and penicillin. The body's immune response to the allergic substance causes mast cells in the connective tissues, bronchi, and GI tract to release histamine and other chemicals. The results are vasodilatation, increased capillary permeability accompanied by swelling of the airway and subcutaneous tissues, hypotension, and hives or an itchy rash.

Obstructive Shock

Obstructive shock occurs when there is interference with the circulation of blood into and out of the heart, compromising the volume of blood that enters and leaves the heart en route to the lungs and tissues. Any condition that fills the thoracic cavity with fluid, air, or tissue can lead to obstructive shock. Examples include increased fluid or blood in the pericardial sac (cardiac tamponade; see Chapter 23); air that accumulates between the layers of pleura (tension pneumothorax; see Chapter 21); or abdominal tissue, fluid, or air that crowds the diaphragm, as in an enlarged liver and ascites (see Chapter 47), thus reducing the size of the thorax.

Cardiogenic Shock

In **cardiogenic shock**, heart contraction is ineffective, which reduces **cardiac output**, the volume of blood ejected from the left ventricle per minute. A myocardial infarction (MI) with subsequent heart failure (see Chapters 25 and 28) is a leading cause of cardiogenic shock.

››› *Stop, Think, and Respond 17-1*

Indicate the type of shock each client is most likely experiencing:

- *Client A has had an MI and cardiac arrest; paramedics resuscitated the client. They are now having difficulty breathing, a rapid heart rate, and chest pain. Urine output is 50 mL in the last 4 hours.*
- *Client B was involved in a motor vehicle collision. Paramedics note a substantial bruise on their right upper thigh, which is much larger than the left upper thigh. Based on assessment findings and a distorted alignment of the right leg, they suspect a fractured pelvis or femur. They also suspect a ruptured spleen because the client has abdominal tenderness. The client is hypotensive with pale and cool skin.*
- *Client C was pruning roses when a bee stung her. Within minutes, the client had difficulty breathing and lost consciousness. The neighbor called 911. Paramedics note that the client is hypotensive, tachycardic, and barely able to breathe.*

Stages and Pathophysiology

Regardless of the type, many complex events accompany shock, which usually progresses through three stages: (1) compensation, (2) decompensation, and (3) irreversible.

Compensation Stage

The **compensation stage** is the first stage of shock, during which several physiologic mechanisms attempt to stabilize the spiraling consequences. If these mechanisms are successful, homeostatic stability may be achieved. If natural or medical means can reverse shock, the chances of uncomplicated recovery are greatly improved. As shock progresses, positive outcomes are less predictable. Compensatory mechanisms include the release of catecholamines, activation of the renin–angiotensin–aldosterone system, and production of antidiuretic and **corticosteroid hormones** (Fig. 17-1).

Catecholamines

Catecholamines are neurotransmitters that stimulate responses via the sympathetic nervous system (Table 17-3). To compensate in shock, the sympathetic nervous system releases endogenous catecholamines, epinephrine and norepinephrine, into the circulation. The adrenal medulla secretes epinephrine, whereas the endings of sympathetic nerve fibers secrete norepinephrine. Epinephrine and norepinephrine increase heart rate and myocardial contractility, which may be counterproductive in cardiogenic shock because it increases a demand for oxygen by an already compromised heart. Venous return to the right atrium subsequently increases, as does blood sent to the lungs. Bronchial dilatation increases the amount of oxygenated air entering the lungs, followed by a more efficient exchange of oxygen and carbon dioxide (CO_2).

Renin–Angiotensin–Aldosterone System

The renin–angiotensin–aldosterone system is a mechanism that restores blood pressure (BP) when circulating volume is diminished (see Fig. 16-7, p. 223). In response to low renal (kidney) blood perfusion, the juxtaglomerular cells release renin, an enzymatic hormone in the nephrons of the kidneys. Release of renin causes a series of chemical reactions that eventually produce angiotensin II, a potent vasoconstrictor that raises BP. Angiotensin II also stimulates the hypothalamus to signal the adrenal cortex via the pituitary gland to release aldosterone, a mineralocorticoid that promotes reabsorption of sodium and water by the kidneys, which serves to increase blood volume.

Antidiuretic Hormone and Corticosteroid Hormones

Low blood volume also stimulates the pituitary to secrete **antidiuretic hormone** (ADH), also known as *vasopressin*, and **adrenocorticotropic hormone** (ACTH). ADH promotes reabsorption of water that the kidneys would

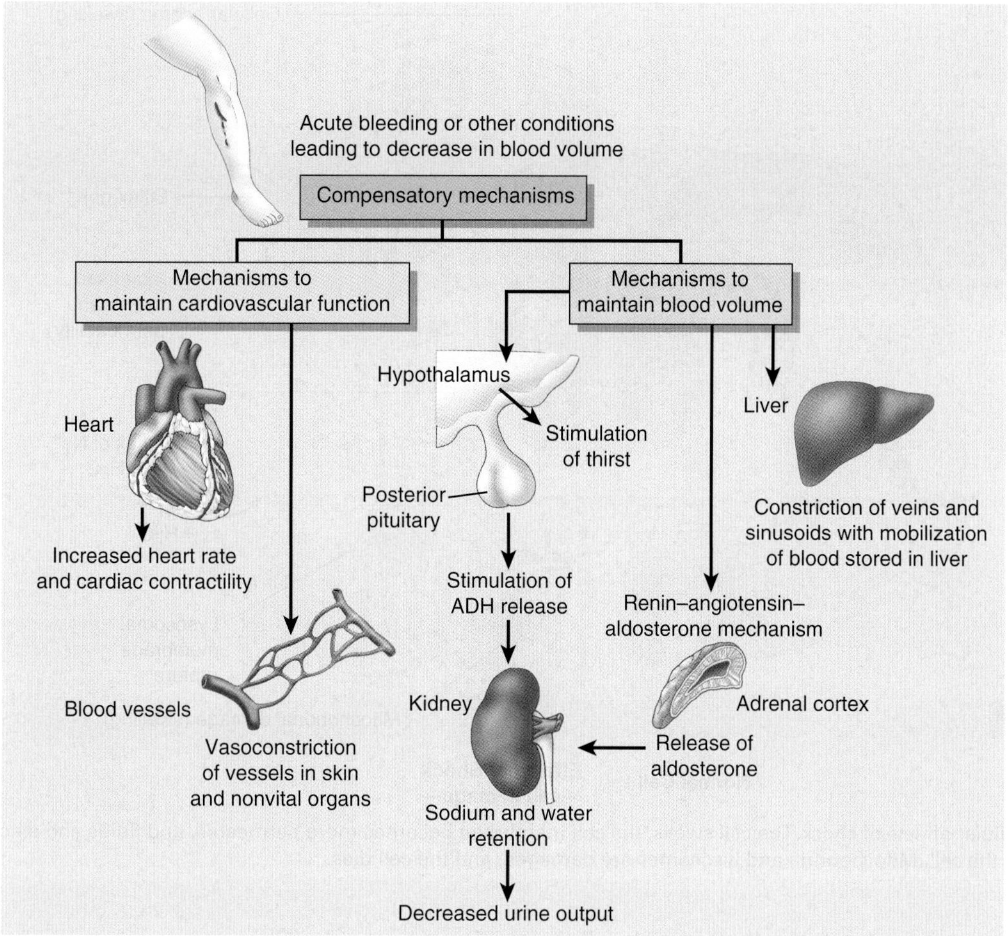

Figure 17-1 Compensatory mechanisms during shock. (Reprinted with permission from Grossman, S. C., & Porth, C. M. (2014). *Porth's pathophysiology: Concepts of altered health states* (9th ed.). Wolters Kluwer Health/Lippincott Williams & Wilkins.)

ordinarily excrete. ACTH stimulates the adrenal glands to secrete corticosteroid hormones, which include glucocorticoids and mineralocorticoids. *Glucocorticoids* help the body respond to stress. *Mineralocorticoids*, such as aldosterone, conserve sodium and promote potassium excretion. Thus, they play an active role in controlling sodium and water balance. Both ADH and corticosteroid hormones promote fluid reabsorption and retention.

Decompensation Stage

The **decompensation stage** occurs as compensatory mechanisms fail. The client's condition spirals into cellular hypoxia, coagulation defects, and cardiovascular changes.

Cellular Hypoxia

Hypoxia refers to decreased oxygen reaching the cells. Hypoxic cells are forced to switch from aerobic metabolism to **anaerobic metabolism**, a less efficient mechanism for

TABLE 17-3 Effects of Endogenous Catecholamines

EFFECT	CONSEQUENCES
Constriction of arterioles of skin, mucous membranes, subcutaneous tissues	Sends blood to larger blood vessels supplying vital organs
Dilatation of arterioles of skeletal muscles	Increases blood supply to skeletal muscles
Dilatation of coronary arteries	Increases oxygen to myocardium
Increased contractility of myocardium	Increases amount of blood leaving the left ventricle each time ventricle contracts (cardiac output)
Increased heart rate	Increases blood supply to body, especially vital organs
Bronchial dilatation	Increases amount of air entering the lungs on inspiration
Release of glycogen stored in the liver	Provides energy

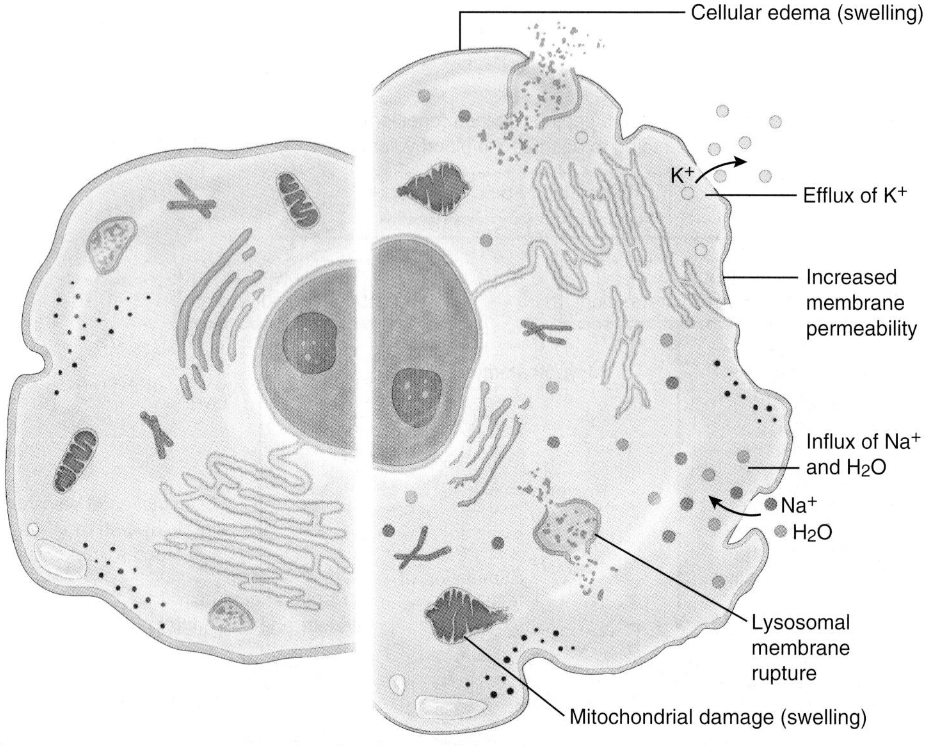

Figure 17-2 Cellular effects of shock. The cell swells, the cell membrane becomes more permeable, and fluids and electrolytes seep out of and into the cell. Mitochondria and lysosomes are damaged, and the cell dies.

meeting energy requirements. As the energy supply falls below the demand, pyruvic and lactic acids increase, causing metabolic acidosis. The structural integrity of cells is impaired because without sufficient **adenosine triphosphate** (ATP), the energy source for operating the sodium and potassium pumps, sodium and water enter the cell, and potassium exits into the extracellular fluid (Fig. 17-2). Eventually, the cells swell and rupture, disrupting their ability to carry out electrochemical processes. Lysosomes, the cellular structure for breaking down cellular waste, leak enzymatic fluid and contribute to further cellular destruction. Gradually, significant numbers of cells are damaged.

Coagulation Defects

As cells become damaged, an inflammatory response ensues. Platelets become sticky and accumulate in the blood vessels of the volume-depleted client, predisposing him or her to the formation of microemboli. Clots further compromise the ability of the red blood cells (RBCs) to deliver oxygen throughout the body. Cell and organ death are potentiated.

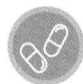

Pharmacologic Considerations

■ Heparin reduces 28-day mortality of clients in severe septic shock. Additionally, the administration of the anticoagulant does not appear to increase bleeding episodes (Wang, 2004).

Cardiovascular Changes

Impaired myocardial cells cannot maintain sufficient heart rate and force of contraction to circulate blood efficiently. Subsequently, brain cells in the medulla can no longer sustain the stimulus for vasoconstriction. The blood vessels dilate, blood pools in the periphery or leaks into the interstitium, cardiac output decreases, and BP falls. Clinical signs are more obvious and include bradycardia; hypotension; confusion; lethargy; decreased urine production; cold, pale skin; and reduced peristalsis. Aggressive interventions are necessary to prevent the irreversible stage of shock and ensure the client's survival.

Irreversible Stage

The **irreversible stage** occurs when significant cells and organs become damaged. The client's condition reaches a "point of no return" despite treatment efforts. The client no longer responds to medical interventions. Multiple systems begin to fail. When the kidneys, heart, lungs, liver, and brain cease to function, death is imminent (Fig. 17-3).

Assessment Findings

Signs and Symptoms

The nurse monitors the client for evidence that blood volume or circulation is becoming compromised. Although shock can develop quickly, early signs and symptoms are evident during the decompensation stage. Critical assessments include vital signs, changes in mentation, skin, and urine output.

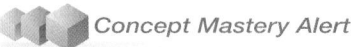

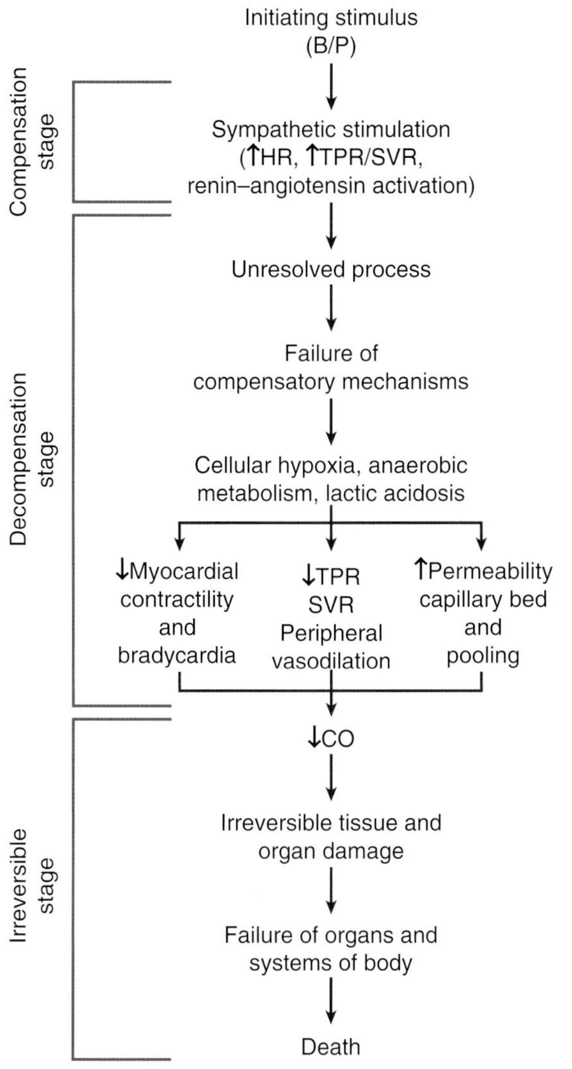

Figure 17-3 Stages of shock. BP, blood pressure; CO, cardiac output; HR, heart rate; SVR, systemic vascular resistance; TPR, total peripheral resistance.

Some health care providers use the APACHE scoring system, which stands for **A**cute **P**hysiology, **A**ge, and **C**hronic **H**ealth **E**valuation, to arrive at a number that reflects the severity of the client's status and predicts the potential length of stay in a critical care setting. The most recent version, APACHE IV, requires entering 27 variables that are unique to the client, such as diagnosis, age, vital signs, and laboratory values. The point value increases according to age and complexity of health problems. An increasing score correlates with a higher risk for hospital death.

Arterial Blood Pressure

In shock, both systolic and diastolic arterial BPs fall because cardiac output decreases or the vascular bed increases due to vasodilation. Hypotension may be rapid and sudden or slow and insidious. For the normotensive (normal BP) adult, the systolic BP is slightly less than 120 mm Hg. A systolic BP of 90 to 100 mm Hg indicates impending shock, whereas 80 m Hg or below indicates shock.

Concept Mastery Alert

Decompensation Stage of Shock

Early signs and symptoms of shock, particularly a dropping BP, are evident during the decompensation stage. During this first phase of shock, physiologic mechanisms attempt to stabilize the spiraling consequences.

To determine the presence of shock, the client's previous BP must be known. Regardless of the numeric figure, a significant and progressive fall in BP from baseline is serious. For example, a BP of 120/82 mm Hg is usually considered normal; however, if an individual with an original BP of 190/112 mm Hg has a BP of 120/82 mm Hg, shock is developing. The nurse must make the primary provider aware of any trends such as a significant fall below the client's usual systolic BP or any trend in progressively decreasing BP. Direct BP monitoring (intra-arterial) is more accurate than indirect monitoring—the usual, auscultatory method using a BP cuff (see Chapter 22)—but it is implemented primarily in critical care areas.

Pulse Pressure

Pulse pressure is the numeric difference between systolic and diastolic BP. If a client has a BP of 120/80 mm Hg, the pulse pressure is 40 mm Hg. A pulse pressure between 30 and 50 mm Hg is considered normal, with 40 mm Hg being a healthy average. In shock, the pulse pressure tends to narrow (decrease) as the falling systolic pressure nears the diastolic pressure.

Pulse Rate, Volume, and Rhythm

In shock, health care personnel use the pulse rate and other assessment data to identify the severity of shock and estimate the approximate reduction in blood volume. As cardiac output decreases, compensatory tachycardia initially develops to increase cardiac output. In neurogenic shock, bradycardia occurs because there is a loss of compensatory sympathetic nervous system response. Pulse volume becomes weak and thready as circulating volume diminishes. In the later stages, the pulse may be slow and imperceptible. Pulse rhythm may change from regular to irregular. Hypoxia, especially when it affects heart tissue, is a leading cause of dangerous cardiac arrhythmias such as ventricular fibrillation (see Chapter 26).

Respirations

In shock, tissues receive less oxygen. In response, the body tries to obtain more oxygen by breathing faster. Rapid respirations help move blood in the large veins toward the heart. Respirations are shallow, and the client may be heard grunting. In early stages, the client is hungry for air, but in profound shock, as death nears, the respiratory rate decreases.

Temperature

Heat-regulating mechanisms are depressed in shock, and added diaphoresis increases heat loss. With the possible exception of septic shock, subnormal body temperature is characteristic.

Mentation

Altered cerebral function is often the first sign of inadequate oxygen delivery to the tissues. Mild anxiety, increasing restlessness, agitation, and confusion can accompany shock. As the condition deteriorates, the client becomes listless and stuporous, ultimately losing consciousness.

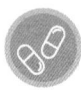

Pharmacologic Considerations

- Morphine may be administered to decrease anxiety and pain. It also decreases stress on the sympathetic branch of the peripheral nervous system, which helps reduce cardiac preload.

Skin

In all but the early stages of septic and neurogenic shock, the skin is cold and clammy. As peripheral blood vessels constrict to direct blood from the skin to more vital organs (heart, kidneys, brain), the skin becomes pale. Eventually, the skin may appear mottled (i.e., a mix of pale and cyanotic areas lacking any uniform color). Capillary filling longer than 3 seconds and cyanosis, especially of the nail beds, lips, and earlobes, indicate oxygen deficiency. In clients with highly pigmented skin (such as African Americans), cyanosis is more accurately detected by inspecting the conjunctiva and oral mucous membranes. Lack of cyanosis, however, does not prove the absence of hypoxia because cyanosis is one of the last signs to appear.

Urine Output

Reduced cardiac output decreases renal blood flow, which leads to decreased urine output. Vasoconstriction, the physiologic response to shock, also contributes to markedly reduced renal blood flow. In many instances, the rate of urine formation is an important indicator of the status of a client in shock (see Table 17-3). When shock is quickly reversed, urine output usually returns to normal. Continued **oliguria** (decreased urine formation) indicates renal damage caused by reduced blood flow to the kidneys.

>>> *Stop, Think, and Respond 17-2*

Which stage of shock is characterized by the following physiologic changes?

1. *Client is unconscious with a slow pulse, systolic BP of 85 mm Hg, and mottled skin color.*
2. *Client is alert and oriented with tachycardia but normal BP and skin color.*
3. *Client is somewhat disoriented with BP lower than earlier assessment and pale skin.*

Diagnostic Findings

Arterial blood gas (ABG), central venous pressure (CVP), and pulmonary artery pressure (PAP) measurements can support a diagnosis of shock. They also are used to monitor response to treatment.

Arterial Blood Gas Measurements

ABG specimens are drawn from a direct arterial puncture or an indwelling arterial catheter (see Chapter 29). In shock, the partial pressure of oxygen in arterial blood (PaO_2; normally 80 to 100 mm Hg) falls below 60 mm Hg. The partial pressure of CO_2 in arterial blood ($PaCO_2$) may be normal, decreased with hyperventilation, or increased with hypoventilation. A pulse oximeter, sometimes used to monitor oxygenation continuously, measures the amount of oxygen bound to hemoglobin, or the saturated oxygen (SpO_2) level, which is normally 95% to 100%. If the SpO_2 level is above 90%, it can be assumed that the PaO_2 is 60 mm Hg or above.

Central Venous Pressure

CVP is the pressure of the blood in the right atrium or venae cavae. It distinguishes relationships among hemodynamic variables in shock: venous return, quality of right ventricular function, and vascular tone. CVP measurements, especially trends in readings, are useful in the management of a client in shock (see Chapter 29). Normal CVP is 2 to 7 mm Hg or 4 to 10 cm H_2O, depending on how it is measured. In hypovolemic shock, the CVP is lower than normal owing to a low blood volume; in cardiogenic shock, it is usually above normal because there is venous congestion due to low cardiac output. The trend in CVP measurements is more helpful than isolated readings.

Pulmonary Artery Pressure

Although CVP measurements can indicate the status of right ventricular function, they do not provide information about left ventricular function. Because left ventricular function is more pertinent to circulation than right, knowing fluid pressures on the left side of the heart is more meaningful. To assess left ventricular function, a two-, three-, or four-lumen catheter is inserted into the vena cava and advanced through the right atrium and right ventricle into the pulmonary artery (Fig. 17-4). The catheter is connected to a monitor from which the PAP or *pulmonary capillary wedge pressure* (PCWP) is measured (see Chapter 29). Normal PAP ranges from 20 to 30 mm Hg systolic and from 8 to 12 mm Hg diastolic. Normal PCWP ranges from 4 to 12 mm Hg. In shock, PAP measurements are usually low because they reflect the low volume of blood in the arterial system.

Medical Management

Aggressive treatment of conditions that predispose to shock may prevent it. Once shock develops, treatment depends on its type and level and usually includes one or more of the following: intravenous (IV) fluid therapy, vasopressor drug therapy, and mechanical devices that restore blood circulation to cells.

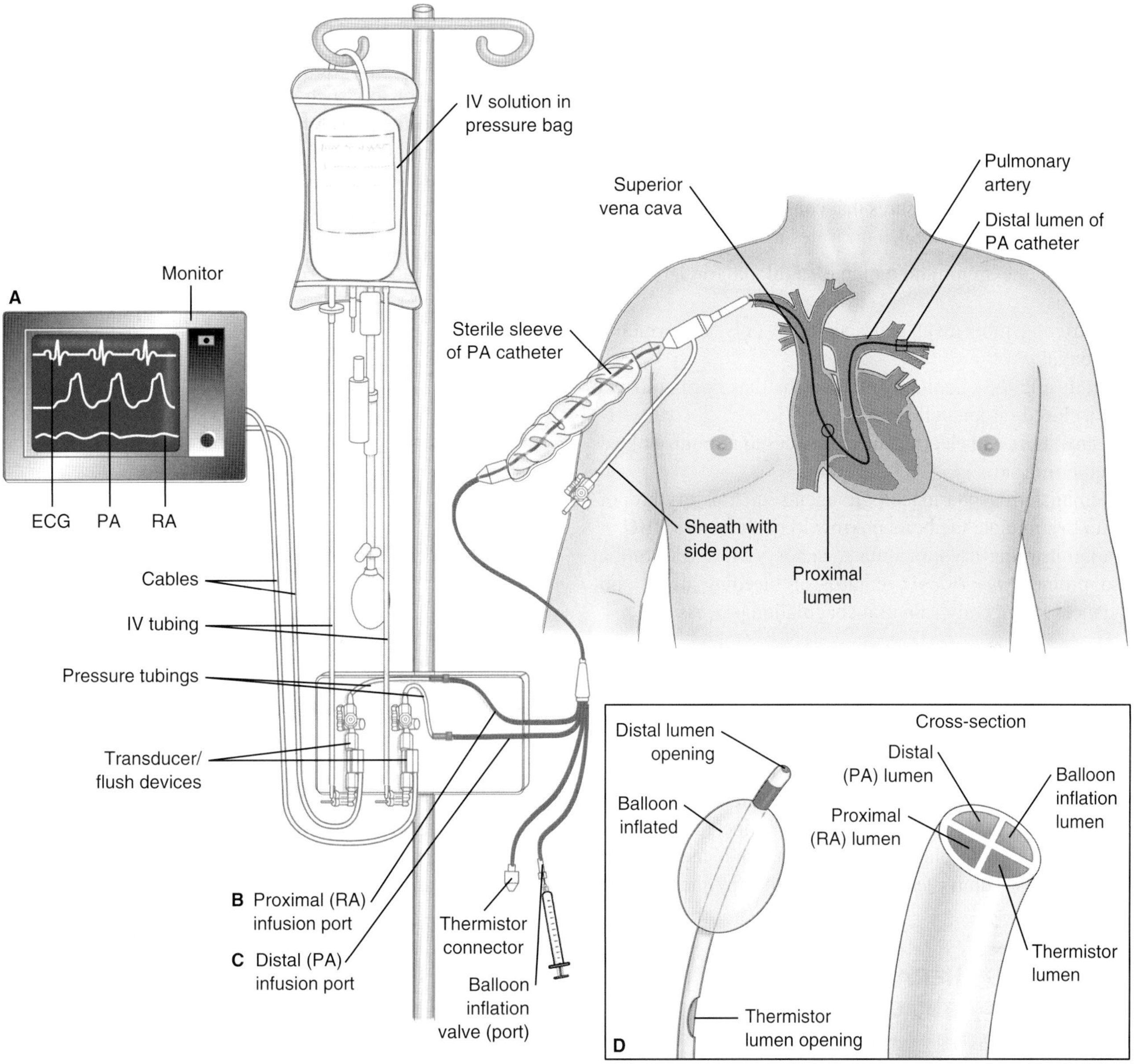

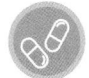

Figure 17-4 Example of a pulmonary artery (PA) catheter and pressure monitoring system. **(A)** Bedside cardiac monitoring. **(B)** Right atria (RA) or central venous pressure monitoring system connected to proximal infusion lumen hub. **(C)** PA monitoring system connected to distal infusion lumen hub. Each system is attached to pressurized IV fluid, a transducer with stopcock and flush device, and pressure tubing. A cable attaches each transducer to the bedside monitor. **(D)** Magnified view of distal end of PA catheter with cross-section of catheter lumen.

Intravenous Fluid Therapy

Intravenous fluids are prescribed to restore intravascular volume. The total volume, type of solution(s), and rate of administration vary according to the etiology of shock. Usually, a ratio of 3:1 is followed; that is, 3 L of fluid is administered for every 1 L of fluid lost. This amount stabilizes the client, replaces the deficit, and provides a reserve to prevent shock from recurring. Initially, as much as 250 to 500 mL may be infused in 1 hour. Solutions may include crystalloid solutions, those containing dissolved substances such as sodium, other electrolytes, or glucose in water; colloid solutions, those containing proteins (such as albumin) to increase osmotic pressure; and blood and blood products if blood loss has been major (see Chapter 13).

Pharmacologic Considerations

- Ringer lactate (RL) and 0.9% saline (isotonic solutions) work equally well with hypovolemic shock. RL is preferred in hemorrhagic shock because it minimizes acidosis. For shock involving acute brain injuries, 0.9% saline is used.

To ensure oxygenation of tissues, especially in cases of hemorrhage or if the hemoglobin level is 7 g/dL or less, administering whole blood or packed RBCs is best. One unit of RBCs can increase an adult's hemoglobin by 1 g/dL (Roubinian et al., 2019). Clients who are alert and capable of making informed decisions but refuse blood transfusions on the basis of religious beliefs (e.g., Jehovah's Witnesses) require bloodless alternatives and measures that conserve blood and its oxygen-carrying capacity. Such measures include the following:

- Drawing the minimum volume of blood for laboratory analysis
- Restricting movement and activity to only that which is essential
- Reinfusing the client's own blood that has been collected in a closed-circuit cell saver
- Using lasers and electrocautery devices to minimize bleeding during surgery
- Administering pharmacologic agents such as erythropoietin to stimulate the bone marrow to manufacture RBCs
- Administering cryoprecipitate, factor VIII, and thrombin to promote *hemostasis,* control of bleeding using substances in the body's natural coagulation process

Drug Therapy

Medical management of shock is extremely complex; drugs are carefully titrated and used alone or in combination to improve cardiovascular status (Drug Therapy Table 17-1). Adrenergic drugs are the main medications used to treat shock. **Vasopressors**, drugs with alpha-adrenergic activity, increase peripheral vascular resistance and raise BP. Examples include dopamine (Intropin), norepinephrine (Levophed), and metaraminol. They are best administered after fluid therapy increases the intravascular fluid volume; otherwise, the vasoconstrictive qualities further impair cellular circulation, which is already compromised by the effects of angiotensin. If infusions of first-line vasopressors such as dopamine and norepinephrine become ineffective, vasopressin may be used. Vasopressin, also known as ADH, causes contraction of arterial smooth muscles, raises BP, and diverts blood to vital organs.

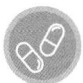

Pharmacologic Considerations

■ When treating shock, drugs are titrated to client responses. Because the dose can change frequently, vasopressor drugs, for example, dopamine, are premixed in an IV solution. The dosage of the drug is delivered by changing the infusion rate of the IV.

Drugs with beta-adrenergic activity that increase heart rate and improve the force of heart contraction are **positive inotropic agents** (*inotropic* means affecting the force of muscular contraction). Digoxin (Lanoxin), isoproterenol (Isuprel), dobutamine (Dobutrex), milrinone (Primacor), and amrinone (Inocor) are examples.

Many drugs have combined alpha- and beta-adrenergic effects. Epinephrine is an example and is the drug of choice in anaphylactic shock. Dopamine also has combined actions. Anaphylactic shock may also be treated with an antihistamine, ACTH, or adrenal corticosteroids to counter the allergen. Other drug categories, such as antiarrhythmics and drugs that reduce peripheral vascular resistance, such as calcium channel blockers, angiotensin-converting enzyme inhibitors, and vasodilators such as nitrates, are appropriate for cardiogenic shock.

DRUG THERAPY TABLE 17-1 Agents to Treat Shock

Drug Category and Common Examples	Intended Use	Common Side Effects	Safety Warnings for Nurses
Vasopressor Agents: Sympathomimetic (Alpha-Adrenergic Activity)			
Metaraminol Norepinephrine (Levophed) Phenylephrine (Neo-Synephrine)	Raise blood pressure by constricting peripheral blood vessels	Headaches, restlessness, palpitations, nausea, vomiting, anxiety, dizziness	Photophobia, Protect eyes from light Avoid abrupt withdrawal
Hormonal Vasoconstrictor			
Vasopressin	Contraction of smooth muscle, divert blood flow, raise blood pressure	Sweating, headaches, nausea, vomiting, anxiety, dizziness	Water intoxication may occur
Positive Inotropic Agents: Sympathomimetic (Beta-Adrenergic Activity)			
Dobutamine (Dobutrex) Isoproterenol (Isuprel) Milrinone (Primacor)	Strengthen cardiac contraction and increase cardiac output and heart rate, used in pediatrics	Headaches, restlessness, nausea, vomiting	If client has atrial fibrillation, watch ventricular response
Vasoconstrictor: Sympathomimetic (Combined Alpha- and Beta-Adrenergic Activity)			
Dopamine (Intropin) Epinephrine (Adrenalin)	Increases myocardial contractions, diverts blood flow to internal organs	Headaches, nausea, vomiting, dizziness	Rapid elevation of BP in older persons Do not add other drugs to dopamine infusion Can cause hyperglycemia

The drugs in column 1 indicate the drug that matches up with explanations in columns 2 through 4.

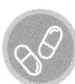

Pharmacologic Considerations

■ Evidence suggests that low-dose hydrocortisone reduces mortality in cases of severe septic shock. Corticosteroid use is not proven to be helpful in other forms of shock.

Mechanical Devices

Mechanical devices help improve cardiac output or redistribute blood. Those used in the treatment of cardiogenic shock include the intra-aortic balloon pump (IABP) and ventricular assist device (VAD; see Chapter 28). In the past, first responders (paramedics) used a pneumatic antishock garment (PASG), also called *military antishock trousers* (MAST), to redistribute blood from the lower extremities to the central circulation. The use of PASGs, however, is somewhat controversial because (1) incorrect application or removal is life-threatening, (2) poor outcomes have occurred when such garments have been used indiscriminately to manage types of shock other than hypovolemic, and (3) their application lengthens the time between the field treatment of the client and transport to a trauma center.

Because of the potential disadvantages regarding PASGs, a new type of nonpneumatic antishock garment (NASG), in contrast to PASGs, the DMAST is made of five segments of manually applied elastic neoprene that fasten with Velcro straps (Fig. 17-5). The garment, which can be applied in less than 60 seconds, encloses the body from the ankles to the diaphragm. As a result of the circumferential pressure, blood is shunted to the heart, lungs, and brain, helping to reverse hypovolemic shock and stabilize individuals until blood transfusions can be administered or surgery can be performed.

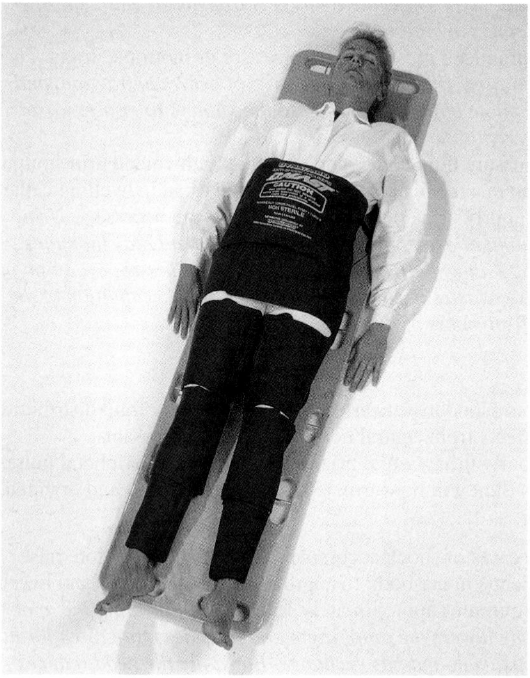

Figure 17-5 Dyna Med antishock trousers (DMAST).

Prognosis and Complications

When shock is treated adequately and promptly, the client usually recovers. Recovery may be tenuous, however, because of secondary complications, which almost always result directly from tissue hypoxia and organ **ischemia** due to reduced oxygenation. Life-threatening complications include kidney failure, neurologic deficits, bleeding disorders such as disseminated intravascular coagulation, acute respiratory distress syndrome (see Chapter 21), stress ulcers, and sepsis that can lead to multiple organ dysfunction (see Chapter 12). (See Evidence-Based Practice 17-1.)

Evidence-Based Practice 17-1

Nursing Teamwork in Medical Emergencies

Clinical Question

How do nurses and student nurses perform teamwork and leadership in simulated medical emergencies?

Evidence

A study was done to determine leadership and teamwork in deteriorating clients during simulated medical emergencies. The study looked at nurses and nursing students during three simulation scenarios (Endacott, Bogossian, Cooper, Forbes, Kain, Young, Porter, & First2Act Team, 2015). The participants in the study were from two universities and a hospital. The participants were put through simulations on chest pain, respiratory distress, and hypovolemic shock. The study evaluated if there were any differences between nurses and nursing students in caring for clients who were deteriorating in a simulation scenario; if nurses and nursing students displayed a different behavior during the care of the client in the simulation; and if there was any type of correlation in nontechnical and technical scores between the two groups. The study found that there was a correlation between technical and nontechnical skills for both the nurses and the nursing students. There was a difference in behaviors that occurred during the simulations. Nurses relied on experience, and it was evident when there was no experience. Neither group asked for more help or support. Students appeared unsure about the leadership role, whereas nurses were able to display this behavior. In conclusion, the study suggests that simulation is a safe way to encourage less experienced staff and students to embrace leadership roles and teamwork.

Nursing Implications

Simulation is a positive way for students and nurses to increase confidence in all areas of practice. Leadership is an important part of practice along with teamwork and task management. Nurses need to be able to act quickly and perform as a team in various medical emergencies.

Reference

Endacott, R., Bogossian, F. E., Cooper, S. J., Forbes, H., Kain, V. J., Young, S. C., Porter, J. E., & First2Act Team. (2015). Leadership and teamwork in medical emergencies: performance of nursing students and registered nurses in simulated patient scenarios. *Journal of Clinical Nursing, 24*(1/2), 90–100. https://doi.org/10.1111/jocn.12611

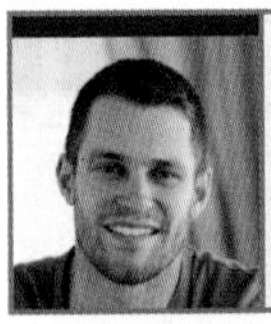

Clinical Scenario A client is exhibiting early stages of shock. What client assessments are critical? What problems are common among clients experiencing shock, and how are they managed by the nurse if they are manifested? See the following Nursing Process section.

NURSING PROCESS FOR THE CLIENT IN SHOCK

Regardless of the cause, prolonged shock is incompatible with life. In few instances is the careful attention to nursing practices and principles more important than in the management of a client in impending or actual shock (see Evidence-Based Practice 17-1).

Assessment

Assess for early signs of shock and report such findings to the primary provider immediately. Check vital signs on initial contact and frequently thereafter to closely monitor the client's condition. An automatic BP device may be substituted for manual assessments. Observe skin color and temperature and assess the rate and quality of radial and peripheral pulses. Monitor urine output and determine respiratory rate and effort to detect evidence of dyspnea or airway obstruction resulting from edema, which accompanies anaphylactic shock. Inspect for bleeding or other causes that may explain the developing symptoms of shock. Determine level of consciousness and orientation status regularly to detect changes. In cases of suspected cardiogenic shock, auscultate the chest for abnormal lung and heart sounds. Check laboratory test results for evidence of low RBCs and hemoglobin, findings that correlate with hypovolemic shock. An elevated WBC count supports septic shock. Analysis of ABG findings is essential for evidence of hypoxemia and metabolic acidosis. Elevated serum lactate levels suggest lactic acidosis precipitated by sepsis and septic shock. Apply a pulse oximeter to monitor Sp_2. Monitor the results of coagulation tests such as platelet counts, the international normalized ratio, prothrombin time, and partial thromboplastin time.

Diagnosis, Planning, and Interventions

Implement measures to control bleeding, other fluid losses, or fluid maldistribution and to promote blood circulation to the brain and vital organs. Support breathing to ensure adequate blood oxygenation. Use measures to maintain normal body temperature and implement medical therapy as directed. Other care includes, but is not limited to, the following:

Hypotension/Hypotension Risk: Related to (specify) blood loss, impaired fluid distribution, impaired circulation, massive vasodilatation

Expected Outcome: Cardiac output will be of adequate volume, as evidenced by heart rate between 60 and 100 beats/min, systolic BP near 119 mm Hg, urine output greater than 35 to 50 mL/hour, alert mental status, and warm, dry skin.

- Restrict activity to total rest. *Rest decreases cellular oxygen requirements, which are already compromised in shock. Inactivity reduces heart rate, allowing the heart to fill with more blood between contractions. The force of heart contraction, which promotes cardiac output, is related to myocardial stretch as the heart fills with blood.*
- Establish at least one and preferably two IV sites with large-gauge catheters. *Access to the intravascular fluid compartment ensures quick replacement of circulating fluid. Cardiac output depends on circulating volume and adequate contraction of heart muscle. Emergency medications are usually administered by the IV route. If the client is volume depleted, IV fluid therapy with or without whole blood or packed cells may be necessary.*
- Administer IV fluids or blood products at the prescribed rate, ensuring patency of the IV catheter(s). *IV fluids replace fluid lost or trapped in the interstitial space. Administration of whole blood or packed cells increases tissue and cellular oxygenation. IV fluids are delivered through a high-volume infusion device at 1 L in 10 to 15 minutes in severe hemorrhage; type O negative blood is transfused until type-specific blood is available.*
- Administer prescribed vasopressor or inotropic drugs. *They can raise BP, increase the force of heart contraction, and promote blood circulation to the kidneys to ensure waste excretion.*
- Measure fluid intake and compare with voided urine output; obtain a medical order for insertion of an indwelling catheter if hourly urine output measurements are necessary. *Urine output above 35 to 50 mL/hour or 500 mL/day indicates that kidney perfusion is sufficient to ensure the excretion of toxic wastes. Urinary volume aids in the evaluation of the effectiveness of therapeutic interventions.*

Altered Tissue Perfusion: Related to reduced cardiac output secondary to blood loss, heart failure, altered body fluid distribution, vasodilation, and bradycardia secondary to neurologic trauma or adverse effects from central nervous system depressants

Expected Outcomes: (1) Systolic BP will be at least 90 mm Hg, with hourly urine output 50 mL or greater. (2) Peripheral pulses will be strong. (3) Capillary refill time will be between 2 and 3 seconds. (4) Skin will be warm. (5) Client will be alert and oriented.

- Control frank bleeding by applying direct pressure to the site. *Pressure compresses the area and slows blood loss from the vascular system.*
- Maintain client in a supine position with legs elevated 12 inches (higher than the heart) unless there is head injury, heart failure, increased intracranial pressure, possible spinal cord injury, or dyspnea. *Elevating the legs promotes blood perfusion to heart, lungs, and brain.*
- In cases of shock accompanied by lung congestion, raise client's upper body to approximately 45 degrees and lower extremities approximately 15 degrees. *Elevating the upper body lowers the diaphragm and provides more room for lung expansion and gas exchange. Elevating the head reduces intracranial pressure. Elevating the legs promotes blood perfusion to heart, lungs, and brain.*

NURSING PROCESS FOR THE CLIENT IN SHOCK (continued)

- Administer oxygen by the medically prescribed method and percentage. *Administration at higher percentages than in room air increases the oxygen bound to hemoglobin and dissolved in blood so that cells can maintain aerobic metabolism.*
- Collaborate with the primary provider about alternative techniques to control internal bleeding such as esophageal gastric balloon tamponade with a Sengstaken–Blakemore tube (see Chapter 47) used to manage bleeding esophageal varices. *An internally inflated balloon is used to apply internal pressure to esophageal and gastric areas of venous bleeding that are impossible to reach manually.*
- Increase the rate of IV fluid infusion if BP falls during deflation of the PASG. *Increasing the circulating fluid volume maintains BP.*
- Implement measures to reduce the work of the heart in cardiogenic heart failure, such as administering diuretics, vasodilators, and antiarrhythmics. *A heart in failure is best supported by reducing the volume it must circulate, decreasing the arterial resistance that it must overcome to eject blood, and slowing the heart to reduce its oxygen requirements.*
- Prepare the client in cardiogenic shock for insertion of an IABP or VAD. *Mechanically supporting or enhancing natural heart contractions improves cardiac output and tissue perfusion* (see Chapter 29).
- Immobilize possible spinal injuries and splint fractures. *Reducing complications from trauma can minimize the potential for neurogenic and hypovolemic shock.*

Impaired Gas Exchange: Related to edema of the airway secondary to a severe allergic reaction leading to anaphylactic shock
Expected Outcomes: (1) SpO_2 level will be at least 90%, PaO_2 will be 80 to 100 mm Hg, and $PaCO_2$ will be 35 to 45 mm Hg. (2) Airway will be patent, respiratory rate will be no more than 24 breaths/min at rest, and breathing will be quiet and effortless.

- Assist with the insertion of an artificial airway and ventilatory support (see Chapter 21). *Intubation facilitates maintenance of a patent airway; artificial ventilation ensures that respiratory gases enter and leave the lungs.*
- Suction the airway when secretions compromise gas exchange. *Suctioning removes fluid that occupies space in the airways needed for the movement and exchange of gases.*
- Administer prescribed adrenergic, bronchodilating, antiinflammatory, and antihistamine medications. *Drug therapy helps to improve the potential for gas exchange.*

Hypothermia: Related to hemorrhage
Expected Outcome: Body temperature will be restored to normal range.

- Keep client dry and covered. *Measures that prevent evaporation and heat loss from radiation interfere with the loss of body heat.*
- Raise the room temperature to approximately 80°F. *Using the physics of convection, warming the environment can raise body temperature.*
- Place client on a warming blanket or direct warming lights to the client's body. *Conduction and radiation transfer heat.*
- Keep client's head covered with a turban made of stockinette or other material. *Body heat is lost in significant amounts from the head; covering the head reduces heat loss.*
- Warm IV solutions and blood products. *Warmed infusions raise the temperature of tissues where they are circulated.*
- Warm the humidified air that is mixed with oxygen during mechanical ventilation. *Inhalation of warmed air increases core body temperature.*

Hyperthermia: Related to altered temperature regulation secondary to sepsis
Expected Outcome: Body temperature will be reduced to normal range.

- Administer prescribed antipyretics. *They block the production of prostaglandins, which elevate the temperature set point within the hypothalamus.*
- Place client on a cooling mattress. *Contact with a cool surface lowers body temperature.*
- Control shivering. *Shivering increases body heat through the contraction of skeletal and pilomotor muscles in the skin.*
- Administer a tepid sponge bath. *Body temperature is lowered when the heat of the skin vaporizes water.*
- Administer prescribed antibiotics. *They reduce or destroy pathogens responsible for sepsis.*

Evaluation of Expected Outcomes

Vital signs are stable. Tissue perfusion is satisfactory, as evidenced by adequate urine output; strong, palpable peripheral pulses; warm, dry skin; and intact sensorium. Capillary refill is immediate. ABGs are within normal range. Blood pH is between 7.35 and 7.45. The client is normothermic.

KEY POINTS

- Shock: four main types
  - Hypovolemic (hemorrhagic): loss of blood or plasma
  - Distributive (normovolemic): no fluid loss, but fluid circulation does not permit effective tissue perfusion
    - Neurogenic: injury that affects vasomotor center or to the nerves that extend from the spinal cord to the blood vessels
    - Septic (toxic shock): large amounts of bacteria in the blood cause endotoxins
    - Anaphylactic: severe allergic reaction
  - Obstructive: interference with the circulation of blood into and out of the heart
  - Cardiogenic: heart contraction is ineffective, reducing cardiac output
- Stages of shock
  - Compensation stage: first stage, where the body tries to stabilize itself
  - Decompensation stage: second stage, occurs as compensatory mechanisms fail
  - Irreversible: last stage, significant cells and organs are damaged, multiple organ failure occurs
- Signs and symptoms worsen as each stage progresses
- Medical management: IV fluids, drug therapy closely titrated, possibly mechanical devices used
- Prognosis: client can recover if treated promptly, but recovery may be long and have many complications.

CRITICAL THINKING EXERCISES

1. Which types of shock are usually accompanied by warm skin rather than cool skin?
2. In which type of shock does the client manifest a slow rather than a rapid heart rate?
3. Although all forms of shock are serious, which type of shock do you feel would have the best outcome? Support your answer with rationales.
4. Explain reasons that make septic shock the type of shock with the highest mortality.

NCLEX-STYLE REVIEW QUESTIONS PrepU

1. If the primary provider ordered all of the following tests on a client with septic shock, which test result is most important for the nurse to review?
   1. Blood urea nitrogen (BUN)
   2. White blood cell (WBC) count
   3. Erythrocyte sedimentation rate (ESR)
   4. Aspartate aminotransferase (AST)
2. A primary provider orders 0.3 mg epinephrine subcutaneous stat for a client experiencing anaphylaxis. Calculate the amount the nurse should administer if the label indicates that the drug is supplied in a 1:1000 strength solution. Record your answer using one decimal place.

   __________mL
3. Place the pathophysiologic processes that accompany shock in the sequence in which they occur. Use all the options.
   1. Organ failures
   2. Decreased urine output
   3. Tachycardia
   4. Anaerobic metabolism
   5. Decreased blood pressure
   6. Cellular hypoxia
4. Which of the following are signs manifested by a client in most types of shock? Select all that apply.
   1. Flushed, warm skin
   2. Low urine output
   3. Bradycardia
   4. Tachypnea
   5. Hypotension
   6. Weak pulse
5. If an adequate urine output is 0.5 mL/kg/hour, calculate the expected hourly urine output for a client recovering from shock who weighs 185 lb? Record your answer in a whole number.

   ______________ mL/hour

WANT TO KNOW MORE? There are a wide variety of online resources available on thePoint to enhance learning and understanding of this chapter.

Go to **thePoint.lww.com/activate** and use the activation code found in the front of this text to unlock these online resources.

18

Caring for Clients With Cancer

Words To Know

alopecia
antineoplastic
benign
biologic response modifiers
brachytherapy
cancer
carcinogenesis
carcinogens
chemotherapy
engraftment
extravasation
gene therapy
leukopenia
malignant
metastasis
myelosuppression
neoplasms
neutropenia
oncology nursing
radiation therapy
stomatitis
targeted therapies
thrombocytopenia
tumor-specific antigens
vesicants
xerostomia

Learning Objectives

On completion of this chapter, you will be able to:

1. Discuss the pathophysiology and etiology of cancer.
2. Differentiate benign and malignant tumors.
3. Name factors that contribute to the development of cancer.
4. Identify the warning signs of cancer.
5. Describe ways to reduce risks of cancer.
6. Explain methods for diagnosing cancer.
7. Describe systems for staging and grading malignant tumors.
8. Differentiate various treatments and methods for managing cancer.
9. Discuss various adverse effects and complications that occur with cancer treatments and methods used to treat those effects.
10. Describe emotions associated with the diagnosis and treatment of cancer.
11. Clarify nursing care required for clients experiencing cancer and cancer treatments.

Cancer is characterized by abnormal, unrelated cell proliferation. Cancerous tumors invade healthy tissues and compete with normal cells for oxygen, nutrients, and space. The nursing specialty related to care of clients with cancer is **oncology nursing**. However, nurses in all settings care for clients of all ages with cancer—a complex and challenging endeavor. A diagnosis of cancer is frightening to most people, although reactions depend on the particular diagnosis, location, stage, treatment, effects on bodily functions, and prognosis.

Gerontologic Considerations

- Prolonged, cumulative exposure of older adults to sunlight over many years may contribute to an increased risk for skin cancers such as basal cell and squamous cell carcinomas.
- Normal changes of aging and/or chronic conditions may complicate cancer screening and treatment decisions in older adults. Evidence indicates that primary provider's recommendation most affected decisions of older adults to accept or decline treatment.
- In addition, the client's values and preferences should be included for an honest discussion of anticipated risks/benefits of cancer screening and treatments.
- The skin of older adults is often dry and/or extremely thin owing to changes in subcutaneous tissue. They may experience intense itching and dryness during and after radiation

(continued)

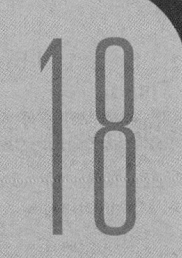

Gerontologic Considerations (continued)

therapy; therefore, additional treatment of skin problems may be necessary. Inspect the skin frequently for signs of breakdown, excessive scratching, and infection.

- The risk for infection with cancer may be increased in older clients because of age-related changes in the immune response.
- Older adults may have problems with nutrition and adequate fluid intake, possibly complicated by normal aging changes in taste sensation and appetite, especially if stomatitis occurs.
- Additional skin care problems and complications related to inactivity may be present. Assessment of functional abilities is crucial to determine increased fall risk.
- Also, because older adults are more prone to electrolyte imbalance, any vomiting or diarrhea during or after cancer treatments may result in a serious electrolyte disturbance.
- Older adults who have chronic conditions must weigh the risks and benefits of cancer treatment against prognosis. Included in this consideration is the potential interaction of medications or treatments for cancer with medications or treatments for other conditions, possibly increasing or limiting the effects, that could result in complicated outcomes from the preexisting conditions.

UNDERSTANDING CANCER

Pathophysiology

The cell is the basic structural unit in plants and animals. Differentiated cells work together to perform specific functions. Cell regeneration occurs through cell division and reproduction. Abnormal changes in cells develop for many reasons. These abnormal cells reproduce in the same way as normal cells, but they do not have the regulatory mechanisms to control growth. Thus, abnormal cell growth proliferates in an uncontrolled and unrestricted way.

New growths of abnormal tissue are called **neoplasms** or *tumors*. The first part of the tumor's name indicates the particular cell or tissue. The suffix *-oma* indicates it is a tumor. Four main cancerous tumor classifications according to tissue type are *carcinomas* (cancers originating from epithelial cells), *lymphomas* (cancers originating from organs that fight infection), *leukemias* (cancers originating from organs that form blood), *myelomas* (cancers originating from plasma cells, and *sarcomas* (cancers originating from connective tissue, such as bone or muscle). Table 18-1 depicts names of benign and malignant tumors based on the tissue type. Tumors are also classified according to their cell of origin and whether their growth is **benign**, not invasive or spreading, or **malignant**, invasive, and capable of spreading (Table 18-2).

Benign tumors remain at their site of development. They may grow large, but their growth rate is slower than that of malignant tumors. They usually do not cause death unless

TABLE 18-1 Selected Benign and Malignant Tumors by Tissue Type

TISSUE TYPE	BENIGN TUMORS	MALIGNANT TUMORS
Epithelial		
Surface	Papilloma	Squamous cell carcinoma
Glandular	Adenoma	Adenocarcinoma
Connective		
Fibrous	Fibroma	Fibrocarcinoma
Adipose	Lipoma	Liposarcoma
Cartilage	Chondroma	Chondrosarcoma
Bone	Osteoma	Osteosarcoma
Blood vessels	Hemangioma	Hemangiosarcoma
Lymph vessels	Lymphangioma	Lymphangiosarcoma
Lymph tissue		Lymphosarcoma
Muscle		
Smooth	Leiomyoma	Leiomyosarcoma
Striated	Rhabdomyoma	Rhabdomyosarcoma
Neural		
Nerve cell	Neuroma	Neuroblastoma
Glial tissue	Glioma	Glioblastoma
Meninges	Meningioma	Meningeal sarcoma
Hematologic		
Erythrocytic		Erythrocytic leukemia
Plasma cells		Multiple myeloma
Lymphocytic		Lymphocytic leukemia or lymphoma
Endothelial		
Blood vessels	Hemangioma	Hemangiosarcoma
Lymph vessels	Lymphangioma	Lymphangiosarcoma

Adapted from Norris, T. L. (2019). *Porth's pathophysiology: Concepts of altered health states* (10th ed.). Wolters Kluwer.

TABLE 18-2 Characteristics of Benign and Malignant Neoplasms

CHARACTERISTICS	BENIGN	MALIGNANT
Cell characteristics	Well-differentiated cells that resemble cells in the tissue of origin	Undifferentiated cells that often bear little resemblance to cells in the tissue of origin
Mode of growth	Grows by expansion without invading the surrounding tissues; usually encapsulated	Grows by invasion, sending out processes that infiltrate the surrounding tissues
Rate of growth	Usually progressive and slow; may stop or regress.	Variable and depends on level of differentiation; the more undifferentiated the cells, the more rapid the rate of growth.
Metastasis	Does not spread by metastasis	Gains access to the blood and lymph channels to metastasize to other areas of the body

Adapted from Norris, T. L. (2019). *Porth's pathophysiology: Concepts of altered health states* (10th ed.). Wolters Kluwer.

their location impairs the function of a vital organ, such as the brain. Malignant tumors have uncontrolled growth and, unless completely removed, are likely to undergo **metastasis** (spreading). Characteristics of malignant cells include alterations in the cell membrane that affect fluid movement in and out of the cell. There are also **tumor-specific antigens**, proteins located in the cell membrane, which develop as cells become less differentiated. These antigens categorize benign and malignant cells from the same tissue type. In addition, there are genetic differences that promote cellular mutation, proliferation, and growth. Tumors grow and spread through projections that invade surrounding tissues.

Cancers produce enzymes that break down proteins and promote infiltration, invasion, and penetration of surrounding tissues. Seeding of cancer cells occurs when tumors shed cells in body cavities. Metastasis is the development of a secondary tumor from the primary tumor at a distant location, which occurs through the lymph channels and blood vessels.

Metastasis is one of cancer's most discouraging characteristics because even one malignant cell can give rise to a metastatic lesion in a distant part of the body. Metastatic tumors are treated aggressively when possible to improve quality of life and lengthen survival time. Cancer is known to spread to the lymph nodes that drain the tumor area. The *sentinel node* is the first lymph node to which a primary tumor drains. When a malignant tumor is removed, lymph node dissection may also be done, along with a wide excision of the tumor, to ensure that the margins surrounding the tumor are cancer free.

Carcinogenesis is the process of malignant transformation. The initial *(initiation)* process involves **carcinogens** (factors that contribute to the development of cancer; see following discussion) that alter the genetic structure of DNA within the cells. Repeated exposure to carcinogens (*promotion*) transforms the genetic information so that cells begin to produce mutant cell populations. The final step involves malignant behavior (*progression*), in which malignant cells demonstrate an ability to invade adjacent tissues and metastasize.

Etiology

Cancer is the second leading cause of death in the United States, where one in two of all men and one in three of all women will develop cancer at some point during their lives (Siegel et al., 2020). Lung cancers account for more cancer-related deaths in both men and women than any other type of cancer. Common cancers in men include prostate, lung, and colorectal. Breast, lung, and colorectal cancers most commonly affect women.

Genetics

Damage to cellular DNA causes cancer cells to develop. In many cases, the body repairs such damage. In cancer cells, the DNA remains mutated or damaged. Inherited gene mutations occur when the damaged DNA is passed to the next generation. Acquired mutations may occur at some point in a person's life and are not inherited. It is known that genes play a major role in cancer prevention or development. *Defective genes* are responsible for diverse cancers. Some types of leukemia, retinoblastoma (an eye tumor in children), and skin cancer are associated with genetic factors. Breast, prostate, and colorectal cancers are also associated with defective genes. The following information describes the genetic components linked to the development of cancer:

- *Oncogenes*—These are mutated forms of specific normal genes known as *proto-oncogenes* that control cell growth and replication. When a proto-oncogene mutates, it activates out-of-control cell growth and causes cancer.
- *Tumor suppressor genes*—These are normal genes that slow cell growth, repair DNA mistakes, and promote normal cell death. When tumor suppressor genes mutate, the functions are inactivated, and cell growth becomes out of control and causes cancer.

Other factors contribute to carcinogenesis and include chemical agents, environmental factors, dietary substances, viruses, lifestyle factors, and medically prescribed interventions.

Chemical Agents in the Environment

Chemical agents in the environment are believed to account for 75% of all cancers. The effects of tobacco smoke and nicotine, as well as chewing tobacco and secondhand smoke, are related to cancers of the lung, mouth, throat, neck, esophagus, pancreas, cervix, and bladder. Prolonged exposure to chemicals such as asbestos and coal dust is associated with some cancers. Chemical substances in workplaces can cause cancer. Potential chemical substances include aromatic amines and aniline dyes; pesticides and formaldehydes; arsenic, soot, and tars; asbestos; benzene; betel nut and lime; cadmium; chromium compounds; nickel and zinc ores; wood dust; beryllium compounds; and polyvinyl chloride (American Cancer Society, 2019). Organs most affected are the lungs, liver, and kidneys because they are involved with biotransformation and excretion of chemicals.

Other Environmental Factors

Environmental factors include prolonged exposures to sunlight, radiation, and pollutants. Electromagnetic fields from microwaves, power lines, and cellular phones are other possible carcinogens, although study results related to such factors are conflicting. People who live in the vicinity of nuclear power plants appear to have a higher incidence of leukemia; multiple myeloma; and lung, bone, breast, or thyroid cancers.

Diet

Diet is an important variable. What a person fails to consume is as important as what they do consume (Box 18-1). Foods high in fat and those smoked or preserved with salt, alcohol, or nitrates are associated with an increased cancer risk. Foods believed to reduce cancer risk are high in fiber, cruciferous (e.g., cabbage, broccoli), and high in carotene (e.g., winter squash, carrots, and cantaloupe). Vitamins A, C, and E also seem to have anticancer value. There is evidence that

BOX 18-1 Dietary Recommendations for Cancer Prevention

- Maintain or achieve a healthy weight. Some cancers, such as colorectal cancer and pancreatic cancer, are associated with obesity and belly fat.
- Limit added sugars and solid fats such as sugar-sweetened beverages, desserts, and highly processed snacks. This measure helps with weight control and encourages intake of healthier foods.
- Increase intake of vegetables, fruits, whole grains, and legumes. An easy method is to have one half of a plate filled with fruits and vegetables, or measure 1½ cups. When selecting grains, make half of them whole grain. Beans and peas should be included and can be substituted for protein as well as vegetables. Limit the use of creamy sauces, dips, or dressings. All of these measures are beneficial for maintaining a healthy weight and lowering the risk of some cancers, such as colon, stomach, and esophageal cancers.
- Modify meat intake so that red meat and processed meat intake is greatly reduced (associated with an increased risk of colon cancer). Use smaller and leaner portions and select more poultry and fish. Frying and charbroiling meat should be very limited. Choose beans and other plant proteins as a substitute for meat.
- Limit alcohol intake. Increased alcohol intake increases the risk for liver, stomach, and other cancers. Recommended amounts are one drink per day for women (12 ounces of beer, 5 ounces of wine, or 1 ½ ounces of 80-proof hard liquor) and two drinks per day for men.
- Choose foods first that have natural nutrients, because these can offer a protective effect. Supplements do not appear to offer the same protection as can intake from whole foods and beverages.

Adapted from Eat Right. Academy of Nutrition and Dietetics (2020). *7 cancer prevention tips for your diet*. https://www.eatright.org/health/diseases-and-conditions/cancer/7-cancer-prevention-tips-for-your-diet

obesity is associated with endometrial and postmenopausal breast cancers as well as pancreatic, colon and rectum, gallbladder, thyroid, ovarian, and cervical cancers as well as placing clients at higher risk for multiple myeloma, Hodgkin lymphoma, and certain types of prostate cancer (American Cancer Society, 2019).

Viruses and Bacteria

Viruses and bacteria are implicated in many cancers. The cell changes that a virus incorporates into the genetic information may cause cancerous cells to form. An example of a viral connection to cancer is Kaposi sarcoma, which is associated with HIV and AIDS (see Chapter 35). *Helicobacter pylori* (see Chapter 45) is associated with gastric cancers.

Medically prescribed interventions such as immunosuppressive drugs, hormone replacements, and anticancer drugs have been associated with increased incidence of cancer in people or their offspring exposed in utero.

Role of the Immune System

The immune system is a major factor in the prevention or development of cancer. An intact immune system fights cancer in the following ways:

- Immune T cells or antibodies, known as tumor antigens, recognize most molecular makeups of tumor cells (Norris, 2019). These fall into two categories:
- Unique tumor-specific antigens, found only on tumor cells
- Tumor-associated antigens, found on tumor cells and normal cells; the qualitative and quantitative differences allow the tumor-associated antigens to distinguish normal from abnormal.
- Macrophages, T lymphocytes, B lymphocytes, antibodies, and natural killer (NK) cells work to eradicate malignant cells
- Interferon, generated in response to a viral invasion, has some ability to fight malignant cells.

If the immune system fails to recognize malignant cells or is not stimulated in any way to fight cancer cells, tumor growth is not inhibited. Malignant cells survive and proliferate.

Assessment Findings

Signs and Symptoms

Cancer presents differently because it is not one disease and does not have one cause. Depending on the type of cancer, one or more organ systems may be involved, and the presenting signs and symptoms may or may not be readily apparent. This factor underscores the importance of educating clients about prevention and self-examination so that cancer can be diagnosed as early as possible. The American Cancer Society (2014) states that general signs and symptoms of cancer include the following:

- *Unexplained weight loss*: a loss of 10 pounds or more without an apparent cause. This is particularly significant for cancers of the pancreas, stomach, esophagus, and lungs.
- *Fever*: fever is common with cancers but is particularly significant when a cancer has metastasized or as an early sign of leukemia or lymphoma.
- *Fatigue* that does not get better with rest. Fatigue worsens as cancer progresses, but it may also be an early sign of leukemia or cancers that are causing blood loss, such as colon cancer.
- *Pain*: this varies with the type of cancer:
  - Early symptom with bone cancers or testicular cancer.
  - A headache that does not get better may be likened to a brain tumor.
  - Back pain that has no other cause may be associated with colorectal or ovarian cancer.
  - Most pain related to cancer is a sign of metastasis.
- *Skin changes*: these include changes associated with skin cancers, but also the following:
  - Hyperpigmentation (darker looking skin)
  - Jaundice (yellowish skin and sclera)
  - Erythema (reddened skin)
  - Pruritus (itching)
  - Excessive hair growth

Other signs may include changes in bowel habits or bladder function, sores that do not heal, leukoplakia or white patches in the mouth or on the tongue, unusual bleeding or discharge, thickening or lump in breast or other tissue, indigestion or trouble swallowing, recent change in a mole or wart, or nagging cough or hoarseness. Box 18-2 describes possible warning signs of specific cancers.

Better education has improved awareness of both warning signals and factors that may influence cancer development. Public education focuses on periodic physical examinations and cancer screening programs. Health care providers must emphasize and teach self-examination of the breasts, testicles, and skin. Avoidance of factors that predispose people to cancer and early detection of cancer increase the chances of cure. Box 18-3 describes healthy habits that reduce cancer risk.

››› *Stop, Think, and Respond 18-1*

Review the general warning signs for cancer and the possible warning signs for specific cancers. If you were caring for a client who complained of chronic fatigue, abdominal bloating, and intermittent constipation, what further information is needed?

BOX 18-2 Possible Warning Signs of Specific Types of Cancers

- *Bladder and kidney:* blood in urine, pain and burning with urination, increased frequency of urination
- *Breast:* lump(s), thickening, and/or other physical changes in the breast; itching, redness, and/or soreness of the nipples not associated with breastfeeding or menstruation
- *Cervical and uterine:* bleeding between menstrual periods, unusual discharge, painful menstrual periods, heavy periods
- *Colon:* rectal bleeding, blood in stool, changes in bowel habits (persistent diarrhea and/or constipation)
- *Endometrial:* same signs as for cervical and uterine cancers
- *Laryngeal:* persistent cough, hoarse throat
- *Leukemia:* paleness, fatigue, weight loss, repeated infections, easy bruising, bone and joint pain, nosebleeds
- *Lung:* a persistent cough, sputum with blood, heavy chest, and/or chest pain
- *Lymphoma:* enlarged, rubbery lymph nodes; itchy; night sweats; unexplained fever and/or weight loss
- *Mouth and throat:* a chronic ulcer of the mouth, tongue, or throat that does not heal
- *Ovarian:* often no obvious symptoms until it is in later stages of development
- *Prostate:* weak and interrupted urine flow; continuous pain in lower back, pelvis, and/or upper thighs
- *Skin:* tumor or lump under the skin, resembling a wart or an ulceration that never heals; moles that change color or size; flat sores; lesions that look like moles
- *Stomach:* indigestion and pain after eating, weight loss, blood in vomit
- *Testicular:* lump(s), enlargement of a testicle, thickening of the scrotum, sudden collection of fluid in the scrotum, pain and discomfort in a testicle or in the scrotum, mild ache in the lower abdomen or groin, enlargement or tenderness of the breasts

BOX 18-3 Recommendations for Cancer Prevention

- Achieve and maintain a healthy body weight throughout life
- Be physically active for 150–300 minutes of moderate intensity activity every week. Limit sedentary behavior.
- Follow a healthy eating pattern at all ages. This includes foods that are high in nutrients and eating a variety of vegetables, legumes (beans), whole fruits, and whole grains.
- Limit consumption of red meats (beef, pork, lamb) and avoid processed meats. Limited sugar-sweetened beverages and highly processed foods.
- If consumed at all, limit alcoholic drinks to two for men and one for women a day.
- Do not use supplements to protect against cancer.
- After treatment, cancer survivors should follow the recommendations for cancer prevention.
- Abstain from smoking or using tobacco products.
- Avoid overexposure to the sun using sunscreen with a sun protection factor (SPF) of at least 15.

Adapted from Rock et al. (2020). American Cancer Society guideline for diet and physical activity for cancer prevention. *CA: A Cancer Journal for Clinicians, 70*, 245–271. https://doi.org/10.3322/caac.21591

Diagnostic Findings

A client's history, physical examination, and diagnostic studies contribute to the diagnosis of cancer. In some cases, physical examination findings are unremarkable, but the client's history is suspect. In addition, the client is evaluated for risk factors. Many diagnostic studies are used to establish a diagnosis of cancer. The primary provider, using information obtained during the history and physical examination, selects tests that help to establish a diagnosis.

Laboratory Tests

Specific cancers alter the chemical composition of blood and other body fluids. Specialized tests have been developed for *tumor markers*, specific proteins, antigens, hormones, genes, or enzymes that cancer cells release (Table 18-3). Normally, tumor markers are not present in or not found in large quantities in the blood.

Other laboratory tests may be useful in establishing a diagnosis. Although abnormal values do not directly indicate a malignant process, they may help to formulate a total clinical picture. For example, a complete blood count may indicate anemia in a client with possible colon cancer. Occult blood in the stool may indicate colorectal cancer.

Radiologic and Imaging Tests

X-ray Imaging. X-rays are quick and painless tests that produce images of body structures. These images are produced based on absorption of the X-rays. Bones absorb the most; soft tissues much less. Air absorbs very little, and thus lungs show up as black on the radiograph. For some tests, a *contrast medium*, such as iodine or barium, is used to highlight, outline, or provide more detail. A barium enema is an example of a study done with contrast medium.

TABLE 18-3 Selected Specific Tumor Markers

MARKER	SIGNIFICANCE
Alpha-fetoprotein (AFP)	Used to diagnose liver cancer; may also be elevated in acute and chronic hepatitis, but levels will not be as high as with liver cancer
Carcinoembryonic antigen (CEA)	Used to predict a client's prognosis with colorectal cancer after diagnosis is established by other methods
Prostate-specific antigen (PSA)	PSA levels can be elevated in the presence of prostate cancer but may also be elevated in other conditions, such as benign prostatic hyperplasia (BPH).
CA 15-3	Elevated in metastatic breast cancer; a smaller percentage is elevated in primary breast cancer, but the marker may be elevated in benign breast disease and gastrointestinal disease.
CA 19-9	Antibody developed against tumor-associated antigens from gastrointestinal and, more specifically, from pancreatic cancers
CA 125	Used to follow women diagnosed with ovarian cancer during and after treatment for ovarian cancer
CA 27.29	Used to follow women diagnosed with breast cancer during or after treatment
Human chorionic gonadotropin (hCG)	Elevated in some types of testicular and ovarian cancer; also used to follow these cancers after treatment; many different uses for this test.

CA, cancer antigen.

Computed Tomography. The computed tomography (CT) scan, using computer-controlled X-rays, provides three-dimensional cross-sectional views of tissues to determine tumor density, shape, size, volume, and location as well as highlighting blood vessels that feed the tumor. The views are made through a computer and can be enlarged for better viewing. Contrast medium may be used to better define boundaries between organs and/or tumors. CT is useful in diagnosing many types of cancer.

Magnetic Resonance Imaging. Producing detailed sectional images, magnetic resonance imaging (MRI) uses radio frequency signals in the presence of a magnetic field to differentiate diseased tissue from healthy tissue and to study blood flow. It helps to visualize tumors hidden by bone or other structures.

Nuclear Imaging. Clients ingest or receive intravenous (IV) radioisotopes (also known as tracers). After specific time intervals, images are taken of tissues that are affected by cancer or other diseases; the images distinguish tissues or portions of tissues that absorb more or less of the tracer. "Hot spots" show on an image of a tumor that has increased concentrations of the tracer, whereas "cold spots" can be the image of a tumor that has decreased concentration of the tracer. Examples of specific types of nuclear scans include the following:

- *Positron emission tomography (PET).* The PET scan uses computed cross-sectional images of increased concentrations of radioisotopes in malignant cells. It provides information about the biologic activity of the cells and assists in differentiating benign and malignant processes and responses to treatment. PET is principally used for brain, lung, colon, liver, and pancreatic cancers.
- *Single photon emission computed tomography (SPECT) scan.* A newer imaging machine called SPECT incorporates PET scanning with CT scanning and contrast, allowing for better details related to increased cellular activity and thus improving the ability to locate tumors.
- *Radioimmunoconjugates.* Monoclonal antibodies, labeled with radioisotopes and injected intravenously, accumulate at the tumor site. Scanners may then visualize the tumor. These studies are particularly useful for colorectal, breast, ovarian, head, and neck tumors. They may be also used for lymphomas and melanomas.

Ultrasound. Ultrasound uses high-frequency sound waves to detect abnormalities of a body organ or structure. The sound wave reflections (echoes) are projected on a screen and may be recorded on film. These studies help differentiate solid and cystic tumors of the abdomen, breasts, pelvis, and heart.

Fluoroscopy. Fluoroscopy is a type of imaging used to show continuous X-ray images on a monitor. The movement of a body structure can be viewed, or the examiner can view the movement of contrast agent or a specific instrument within a body structure. The views are transmitted to a monitor so that both the body part and its motion are examined in detail. An example of fluoroscopy is a barium study (to view the movement of barium through the gastrointestinal [GI] system) or visualization of a catheter as it is inserted into a specific organ (cardiac catheterization). Fluoroscopy can also be used to visualize blood flow to organs.

Vascular Imaging. Vascular imaging uses contrast agents that are injected directly into veins and arteries to assess the vasculature of a tumor. MRI, CT, or fluoroscopy is used to track the contrast agent. This type of imaging is particularly useful prior to surgical procedures for liver and brain cancers.

Other Studies

Biopsy. Tissue samples excised from the body are directly examined microscopically for malignant or premalignant processes. Tissue samples may be obtained during surgery, via insertion of a biopsy needle under local anesthesia, or by endoscopic procedures. A biopsy provides the most definitive method for diagnosing cancer. More information related to biopsies is provided in the surgery section.

Frozen Section. During some surgeries, when a tumor or node is removed, it is taken to the pathologist for immediate examination. The specimen is quickly frozen and then sliced into very thin pieces so that it may be examined under a microscope. Once the preliminary findings are known, the surgeon decides the type of surgery needed. Health care providers make the client aware of the possibilities before surgery.

Endoscopy. Fiber-optic instruments are flexible tubes that contain optical fibers, which enable light to travel in a straight line or at various angles and illuminate the area being examined. Specific body areas can be examined with gastroscopy, bronchoscopy, and colonoscopy. Tissue biopsies may be done if a malignancy is suspected.

Cytology. Microscopic examination of cells from various body areas may be used to diagnose malignant or premalignant disorders. Cells are obtained by needle aspiration, scraping, brushing, or sputum. An example of a cytologic test is the Papanicolaou (Pap) smear used to diagnose changes in the endometrium, cervix, and vagina (see Chapter 53).

Staging of Tumors

Tumors are staged and graded based on how they tend to grow and the cell type before a client is treated for cancer. The American Joint Committee on Cancer developed a staging system referred to as the *TNM classification*: *T* indicates the size of the tumor, *N* stands for the involvement of regional lymph nodes, and *M* refers to the presence of metastasis (Table 18-4). Once the TNM descriptions are established, they are grouped together in a simpler set of stages that include tumor size, evidence of metastasis, and lymph node involvement:

- *Stage 0:* The cancer is in situ (CIS), which means the malignant cells are confined to the layer of cells in which they began, with no signs of metastasis.
- *Stages I, II, and III:* Higher numbers indicate that the tumor is of greater size and/or the spread of cancer is to nearby lymph nodes and/or organs near the primary tumor.
- *Stage IV:* Cancer has invaded or metastasized to other organs of the body.

Grading of tumors involves the differentiation of the malignant cells. Basically, there are two classifications: differentiated and undifferentiated. Cancer cells are evaluated in comparison with normal cells. *Well-differentiated* cells are those that most closely resemble the tissue of origin. *Undifferentiated* cells bear little resemblance to the tissue of origin. Cell differentiation is graded from I to IV. The higher the number, the less differentiated the cell type. Tumors with poorly differentiated cells are graded IV; these tumors are very aggressive and unpredictable, and the prognosis is usually not good. Grade IV tumors do not respond well to cancer treatments.

TABLE 18-4 TNM Staging System and Classification

SYMBOL	MEANING
T	Tumor
TX	Primary tumor cannot be evaluated
T0	No evidence of primary tumor
Tis	Carcinoma in situ (CIS); abnormal cells present but have not spread to surrounding tissue
T1, T2, T3, T4	Progressive increase in tumor size and extension; the higher the number, the larger the tumor and the greater the extension
N	Regional lymph nodes
NX	Regional lymph nodes cannot be evaluated
N0	No regional lymph node involvement
N1, N2, N3	Increase in regional lymph node involvement; the higher the number, the greater the lymph node involvement
M	Distant metastasis
MX	Cannot be evaluated
M0	No distant metastasis
M1	Distant metastasis present
Example: T2, N1, M0	Indicates the primary tumor has grown and spread to regional lymph nodes but has not metastasized
GX	Grade cannot be evaluated
G1	Well differentiated (low grade; the cancer cells look very similar to normal cells)
G2	Moderately differentiated (intermediate grade)
G3	Poorly differentiated (high grade)
G4	Undifferentiated (high grade); G4 is linked to the worst outcome

TREATMENT OF CANCER

Four primary treatment options are used to treat cancer: (1) surgery, (2) radiation therapy, (3) chemotherapy, and (4) hematopoietic stem cell transplantation (HSCT). Immunotherapy, gene therapy, and other alternative therapies may also be used. Cancer is frequently treated with a combination of therapies using standardized protocols.

Surgery

Surgery continues to be a primary method for diagnosing, staging, and treating cancer. Newer and less invasive surgical techniques allow for removal of tumors while preserving as much normal tissue and function as possible. Surgery may range from tumor excision alone to extensive excision, including removal of the tumor and adjacent structures such as bone, muscle, and lymph nodes. The type and extent of surgery depend on the extent of the disease, actual pathology, client's age and physical condition, and anticipated results. When tumors are confined and have not invaded vital organs, the surgery is more likely to be curative and is referred to as the *primary treatment*. In some cases, the entire tumor cannot be removed, but as much of it as possible is removed, which is referred to as *debulking* or *cytoreductive surgery*.

BOX 18-4 Common Biopsy Procedures

Fine needle aspiration biopsy: A very thin needle attached to a syringe is used to extract a small amount of tissue from a tumor. Ultrasound or other imaging method may be used to guide the needle into the tumor.

Core needle biopsy: The procedure is similar to fine needle aspiration, but a slightly larger needle is used to remove some tissue. More tissue can be obtained, ensuring a more accurate diagnosis.

Excisional or incisional biopsy: An incision is made to remove the entire tumor (excisional biopsy) or a small part of the tumor (incisional biopsy). The procedures can often be done with local or regional anesthesia.

Two types of excisions are generally done. The first is *local excision*, in which the tumor is removed along with a small margin of healthy tissue. The other type is *wide* or *radical excision*, which removes the primary tumor, lymph nodes, any involved adjacent structures, and surrounding tissues that pose a risk for metastasis. *Diagnostic and staging procedures* are also done to obtain tissue samples used to determine cell type and the extent of the cancer. Box 18-4 describes common biopsy methods.

Prophylactic or *preventive surgery* may be done if the client is at considerable risk for cancer. Prophylactic surgery may be discussed when there is a family history or genetic predisposition; the ability to detect cancer is at an early stage; or the client is able to accept the postoperative outcome regardless of the findings. Examples of prophylactic surgery include mastectomy and hysterectomy. Clients who choose prophylactic surgery require careful preoperative counseling and teaching so that they are fully aware of the consequences of surgery (American Cancer Society, 2019).

Concept Mastery Alert

The surgery done after cancer returns is known as salvage surgery. Prophylactic surgery is done to prevent a malignancy.

Surgery that helps to relieve uncomfortable symptoms or prolong life is considered *palliative*. Some palliative surgeries are used to remove excess fluid and increase comfort, such as *paracentesis* (removal of fluid from the abdominal cavity) and *thoracentesis* (removal of fluid from the chest). Surgical procedures used to relieve pain include nerve blocks, placement of epidural catheters for administration of epidural analgesics, and placement of venous access devices for administration of parenteral analgesics. *Reconstructive* or *plastic surgery* may be done after extensive surgery to correct defects caused by the original surgery. Some surgeries are disfiguring or so profound that the client may have difficulty adjusting to body changes. In these cases, radiation therapy may be a better option.

Other surgical interventions include the following:

- *Cryosurgery*: uses liquid nitrogen spray or a very cold probe to freeze and kill abnormal cells
- *Electrosurgery*: uses a high-frequency electric current to destroy tumor cells
- *Laser (light amplification by stimulated emission of radiation) surgery*—uses photoablation and photocoagulation lasers to aim light and energy directly at an exact tissue location and depth to vaporize cancer cells, destroying tissue or sealing tissues or vessels
- *Radiofrequency ablation*: uses high-energy radio waves through a needle to heat and destroy cancer cells
- *Mohs surgery (formerly called chemosurgery)*: involves shaving off one thin layer of skin at a time. Each layer is examined microscopically. Surgery ends when all cells look normal. *Chemosurgery* involves the use of topical chemicals as layers are removed but is not part of Mohs surgery.
- *Laparoscopic surgery*: uses a long flexible scope through a small incision to inspect and remove pieces of tissue. This type of surgery is selectively used for some cancers.
- *Robotic surgery*: similar to laparoscopic surgery, the surgeon sits at a control table and guides precise robotic arms to pass a scope through a small incision to inspect and remove tissue.

Perioperative care is discussed in Chapter 14. Specific surgeries are addressed in separate chapters.

Radiation Therapy

Radiation therapy uses high-energy ionizing radiation, such as high-energy X-rays, gamma rays, and radioactive particles (alpha and beta particles, neutrons, and protons), to destroy cancer cells, shrink tumors, and relieve symptoms. Radiation destroys cells by breaking a strand of the DNA molecule in the cell, thereby preventing the cell from growing and dividing. Cell death can occur immediately or when the cell can no longer reproduce.

The goal of radiation therapy is to destroy malignant, rapidly dividing cells without permanently damaging surrounding healthy tissues. Although radiation therapy may also destroy some normal cells, rapidly reproducing malignant cells are more sensitive to radiation; it affects cells undergoing mitosis (cancer cells) more than cells in slower growth cycles (normal cells). Radiation therapy may be applied externally or internally, both with curative and palliative intent. About 60% of all clients with cancer receive some form of radiation therapy.

External Radiation Therapy

External beam radiation therapy (EBRT) uses high-energy electromagnetic radiation aimed at a specific body location. Higher energy levels are used to achieve deeper penetration into the body. A treatment plan is developed and customized for each client. Various types of EBRT may be used (Box 18-5).

EBRT enables treatment of targeted tumors and nearby lymph nodes. Clients usually have daily radiation treatments over several weeks on an outpatient basis. Their skin is marked with a marker or tattoo to identify the reference points for the treatment plan. Clients are instructed not to wash off these markings until the therapy is complete. Clients are not radioactive when receiving EBRT, because there is not a source of radiation in the body at any time.

Internal Radiation Therapy

Internal radiation therapy (**brachytherapy**) refers to the direct application of high doses of radiation therapy to a

BOX 18-5 Types of External Beam Radiation Therapy (EBRT) Procedures

Stereotactic Radiosurgery (SRS)/Stereotactic Radiation Therapy
A device called a *gamma knife* delivers large, precise radiation doses to a small tumor area with well-defined margins. Although there is no actual surgery, the gamma knife is referred to as "surgery" because of its accuracy. Another type of SRS uses heavily charged particle beams, such as protons, to deliver radiation to the tumor. Different angles can be used in order to deliver the radiation at precise depths, limiting damage to healthy tissue. Head frames or other devices are required to immobilize the client. Angiography, CT, or MRI locates the tumor. Treatment outside the brain is called stereotactic body radiation therapy (SBRT). SBRT may be used for certain lung, spine, and liver tumors.

Three-Dimensional Conformal Radiation Therapy (3D-CRT)
Special computers precisely map the cancer's location. A plastic mold or cast keeps the body part stabilized so that radiation beams can be more accurately aimed from several directions. It is hoped that radiation damage to normal tissues will decrease as the radiation dose to the cancer increases.

Image Guided Radiation Therapy (IGRT)
A form of 3D-CRT where imaging scans (like a CT scan) are done before each treatment. This allows the radiation oncologist to adjust the position of the client or refocus the radiation as needed to be sure that the radiation beams are focused on the tumor exactly and that exposure to normal tissues is limited.

Intensity-Modulated Radiation Therapy (IMRT)
Technology similar to 3D-CRT aims photon beams from several directions. The intensity can be adjusted, allowing for a higher dose to the tumor but less to the normal tissue. The person being treated must remain absolutely still; thin casts or molds are used.

Helical-Tomotherapy
This technology is a type of IMRT using a tomotherapy machine, which combines a CT imaging scanner with an EBRT machine. It allows for an image of the client's tumor immediately before treatment, promoting accurate targeting of the tumor and sparing healthy tissue. For this treatment, the radiation machine delivers many small beams of radiation at the tumor from different angles around the body. This may allow for radiation to be even more precisely focused.

Conformal Proton Beam Radiation Therapy
This type of radiation therapy is similar to 3D-CRT except that proton beams are used instead of X-rays. The advantage is that more radiation can be delivered to the tumor with less effect on normal tissues. A special piece of equipment called a cyclotron or synchrotron must be used, which increases the cost greatly and requires specially trained technicians.

Intraoperative Radiation Therapy (IORT)
Radiation therapy is delivered directly to the tumor during surgery. It is usually used on abdominal and pelvic cancers or those cancers that are most likely to recur. IORT reduces damage to normal tissues because they can be moved out of the way during surgery and protected from radiation. Higher doses of radiation can be delivered in this manner. Surgical departments generally have special operating rooms with radiation-shielding walls so that the client remains in the same room for surgery and radiation therapy.

Adapted from American Cancer Society. (2019). *Getting External Beam Radiation Therapy*. https://www.cancer.org/treatment/treatments-and-side-effects/treatment-types/radiation/external-beam-radiation-therapy.html

small or localized site in or near the tumor. The advantage of brachytherapy is that it applies less radiation to adjacent normal tissues. It may be used alone or combined with surgery, chemotherapy, and external radiation therapy. The most common methods of brachytherapy include interstitial implants, intracavitary implants, and systemic therapy.

Interstitial implants and intracavitary implants use *sealed radiation sources* in the forms of needles, seeds, pellets, wires, catheters, ribbons, balloons, or capsules. Brachytherapy may be implanted temporarily or permanently. In interstitial radiation therapy, the radioactive source is inserted directly into a tumor or into tissue near the tumor, such as a tumor in the head or neck. For intracavitary implants, the radioactive source is placed directly in the body cavity, and an applicator holds it in place. When temporary implants are removed, radioactivity is not left in the body (American Cancer Society, 2017).

Permanent implants cease to be radioactive when they decay over several weeks or months, depending on the radioactive element's *half-life* (the time for 50% of the isotope to lose its radioactivity). Clients usually go home if they have permanent implants. Clients must stay away from other people for a few days while the radiation is most active. Once the radiation is gone, the implants are not active.

A client is hospitalized when receiving temporary implantable radiation sources because they will emit radiation during therapy. Specific orders for treatment and precautions to be taken as well as the type and dosage of the radioactive substance, time and area of insertion, type of applicator used, and when to remove the material are noted in the client's chart. If any orders are unclear, the nurse should contact the radiation oncologist or radiation safety officer. Box 18-6 lists safety measures when a client is receiving sealed radiation therapy. Everyone involved in the client's care must recognize the necessity to limit radiation exposure. The degree of possible hazard depends on the type and amount of radioactive material used. Usually, no special precautions are required when a small amount of a radioactive substance is used for diagnostic studies. If necessary, the radiation oncologist specifies precautions, informs personnel, and posts a radiation sign (Fig. 18-1).

Systemic internal radiation therapy uses *unsealed radiation sources* (radiation in a suspension or solution or radiopharmaceutical therapy), such as iodine-131. These sources may be administered orally, intravenously, or into a body cavity. Various body parts take up these sources in doses sufficient to treat cancer or, if received in small amounts, to diagnose cancer. This type of radiation has systemic effects

BOX 18-6 Safety Measures for Protecting Health care Personnel and Visitors From Excessive Exposure to Radiation—Time, Distance, and Shielding

- Client is placed in private room; some rooms have walls that are lined with lead.
- Standardized sign (see Fig. 18-1) is placed on door to designate the room as a radiation room.
- Anyone entering the room must have knowledge of the precautions required, including what shielding equipment is required. Children younger than 18 years and pregnant women are generally not permitted in the room.
- Health care providers limit time spent in the room and limit distance from source of radiation by working as far from the source of radiation as possible.
- The primary provider and radiation safety personnel are notified if the sealed sources become dislodged.
- When the client has unsealed sources, gloves must be worn at all times. Policies regarding disposal of body fluids and contaminated articles such as dressings must be adhered to.

and is excreted primarily in urine but also through saliva, sweat, and feces. As an example, the half-life for iodine-131 is 8.02 days (U.S. Environmental Protection Agency, 2019). To reduce exposure, clients are asked to:

- Wash hands carefully after going to the bathroom.
- Flush toilet several times after each use.
- Use separate eating utensils and towels.
- Wash laundry separately.
- Drink plenty of fluids to help flush radioactive substances away.
- Avoid kissing and sexual contact.
- Maintain an arm's length distance between yourself and those who spend more than 2 hours within a 24-hour period with you. It is recommended that clients sleep alone for a week or so.
- Minimize contact with infants, children, women who are pregnant, and pets.

A more recently developed method of brachytherapy, known as selective internal radiation therapy (SIRT), delivers millions of microscopic radioactive beads or microspheres via a hepatic pump targeted directly to the malignant tissue to treat tumors from the inside out. The surrounding tissue is relatively unaffected. This type of therapy is effective for shrinking tumors of the liver and improving quality of life.

Expected side effects of radiation therapy may result from the destruction of normal cells in the area being irradiated and are specific to the anatomic site treated. They include the following:

- **Alopecia** (hair loss)
- Erythema (local redness and inflammation of the skin)

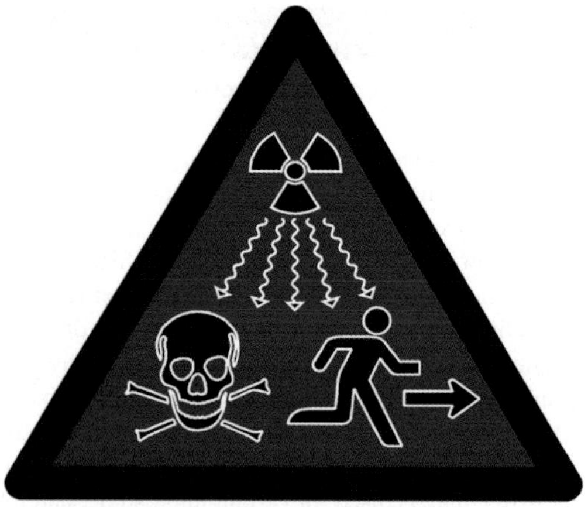

Figure 18-1 International radiation symbol. (©ISO. This material is reproduced from ISO 21482:2007, with permission of the American National Standards Institute (ANSI) on behalf of the International Organization for Standardization. All rights reserved.)

- Desquamation (shedding of epidermis, which can be dry or moist)
- Alterations in oral mucosa, including **stomatitis** (inflammation of the mouth), **xerostomia** (dryness of the mouth), change or loss in taste, and decreased salivation
- Anorexia (loss of appetite)
- Nausea and vomiting
- Diarrhea
- Cystitis (inflammation of the bladder)
- Pneumonitis (inflammation of the lungs)
- Fatigue
- **Myelosuppression** (depression of bone marrow function) if marrow-producing sites are irradiated, resulting in anemia (decreased red blood cells [RBCs], hemoglobin, or volume of packed RBCs); **leukopenia** (decreased white blood cell [WBC] count); and **thrombocytopenia** (decreased platelet count)

Effects of radiation are cumulative. Often, the client experiences chronic or long-term side effects after completing therapy. Many times, these effects result from decreased blood supply and normal tissue destruction. The changes are irreversible. Possible effects include fibrosis (abnormal formation of scar tissue) in the small intestine, lungs, and bladder; cataracts; disturbances in blood cell formation; sterility; and new cancers.

Radiation Safety

The National Council on Radiation Protection and Measurements publishes guides for radiation safety. The effects of long-term and short-term exposures must be considered. The latent period between the exposure and the accumulated biologic effect is often long, and great care is taken to protect occupationally exposed workers from radiation injury that can accumulate over years. Pregnant women should avoid exposure to radioactive substances. Nursing Guidelines 18-1 provide standard interventions for clients receiving radiation therapy. When nurses provide information, clients need to know the type and duration of treatment, what is required

NURSING GUIDELINES 18-1

Managing Clients Receiving Radiation Therapy

- Provide information regarding the safety of radiation: effects on others, effects on tumor, and side effects related to radiation.
- Teach client about the actual procedure of external or internal radiation therapy.
- Explain the need for optimal nutritional intake.
- Perform additional client and family teaching related to protecting the skin and mucous membranes (see Client and Family Teaching 18-1).
- Protect the skin from irritation.
- Assess skin and mucous membranes for changes, particularly the areas being treated. Effects of radiation on skin include redness, tanning, peeling, itching, hair loss, and decreased perspiration.
- Cleanse the client's skin with mild soap (be careful not to wash radiation marks) and tepid water.
- Moisturize with mild, water-based lubricant lotions.
- Maintain intact oral mucous membranes.
- Assess lesions—culture as necessary.
- Monitor client for signs of bone marrow suppression: decreased leukocyte, erythrocyte, and platelet counts.
- Assess for signs of bleeding; assess lesions and culture as necessary.
- Monitor for signs and symptoms related to area of irradiation: cerebral edema, malabsorption, pleural effusion, pneumonitis, esophagitis, cystitis, and urethritis.
- Encourage client to share fears and anxieties related to radiation therapy.
- Inform client that fatigue is a common effect of radiation therapy.

Pharmacologic Considerations

■ Medications are used for symptom management of radiation side effects. Ibuprofen or acetaminophen for pain or inflammation, antiemetics for GI distress, antidiarrheal agents, and various topical agents for skin irritation.

of the client, possible side effects, skin and mouth care, nutritional and dietary concerns, and precautions needed. Client and Family Teaching 18-1 provides additional teaching points.

When radioisotopes are used to treat cancer, three safety principles must always be kept in mind: time, distance, and shielding (where applicable).

Time

Time refers to the length of exposure. The less time spent in the vicinity of a radioactive substance, the less radiation is received. Health care personnel must plan carefully and work quickly and efficiently to spend minimal time at the bedside. Clients are placed in private rooms. Health care personnel who are involved in the care of the client wear dosimeter badges. Careful psychological preparation helps the client accept the limited amount of nursing time. Visitors are limited to 30 minutes/day.

Client and Family Teaching 18-1
Radiation Therapy

The nurse instructs clients who receive radiation therapy on an outpatient basis as follows:

- Be aware that effects of radiation on skin include redness, tanning, peeling, itching, hair loss, and decreased perspiration.
- Avoid using ointments or creams on the area receiving radiation therapy unless prescribed or instructed to by a primary provider or radiation therapist.
- Wear loose, cotton clothing to avoid irritating the irradiated areas of skin.
- Avoid extremes of heat or cold, including heating pads, heat lamps, ultraviolet light, diathermy, whirlpool, sauna, steam baths, or direct sunlight.
- Protect skin from sun exposure, chlorine, and wind.
- Report any blistering.
- If receiving radiation to the head or scalp, avoid shampooing with harsh shampoos (baby or mild shampoo is acceptable), tinting, permanent waving, hair dryers, curling irons, and any hair products or treatments unless approved by the primary provider or radiation therapist.
- Bathe carefully. Avoid using soap and friction over the irradiated area. Do not wash off skin markings, because they serve as guides for setting and adjusting the treatment machine over the area to be radiated.
- Shave with an electric razor.
- Report oral burning, pain, open lesions, or problems with swallowing; use nonalcoholic mouthwash.
- Brush with soft toothbrush and avoid electric toothbrushes.
- Floss gently; use Waterpik cautiously.
- Keep lips moist with lip balm.
- Avoid alcoholic beverages, very hot drinks and foods, highly seasoned foods, acidic foods, and tobacco products.

Distance

Distance refers to the length in feet between the person entering the room and the radioactive source (client). The inverse square law applies to radiation exposure. The rate of exposure varies inversely with the square of the distance from the source (client). For example, nurses standing 4 feet from the source of radiation receive 25% of the radiation they would receive if they stood 2 feet from the source. Visitors must maintain a distance of at least 6 feet from the client.

Shielding

Shielding is the use of any type of material to decrease the radiation that reaches an area. The material usually used is lead, such as lead-lined gloves and lead aprons. Other materials, such as concrete walls, are capable of shielding.

Chemotherapy

Chemotherapy uses **antineoplastic** agents that work by interfering with cellular function and reproduction. These agents may be used alone or combined with other therapies to cure cancer, prevent it from metastasizing, slow its growth, destroy tumor cells that have metastasized, or relieve symptoms.

Antineoplastic agents are classified according to their relationship to cell division and reproduction. Healthy and malignant cells follow a cell cycle pattern, which involves division of the cell and reproduction of two identical daughter cells. There are distinct phases within the cell cycle (Norris, 2019):

1. *Synthesis (S) and mitosis (M)*: These are the two major phases of the cell cycle. The S phase (10 to 12 hours) involves DNA synthesis and replication of chromosomes. The M phase (usually less than 1 hour) includes mitotic spindle formation and cell division with the formation of two daughter cells.
2. *Gaps 1 and 2 (G1 and G2)*: Gaps are part of the cell cycle because cells require time to grow and double their mass of proteins and organelles. G1 is the stage when protein synthesis and organelle and cytoskeletal elements increase to prepare for DNA replication and mitosis. G2 is the premitotic phase in which enzymes and other proteins needed for cell division are synthesized and moved to the appropriate sites.
3. *Gap 0 (G0)*: G0 is the stage after mitosis in which a cell can leave the cell cycle and remain inactive or reenter the cell cycle at another time. Examples include the following:
   - Labile cells such as blood cells do not enter G0 but continue recycling.
   - Stable cells such as hepatocytes enter G0 after mitosis but can reenter the cell cycle when stimulated by the loss of other cells.
   - Permanent cells such as neurons are differentiated after mitosis and leave the cell cycle and never return. As such, they are incapable of cell renewal.
4. *Checkpoints and cyclins*—Most cells have checkpoints in the cell cycle that can be arrested if previous events are not complete. For example:
   - The G1/S checkpoint monitors whether there is damage to the DNA in the chromosomes caused by radiation or chemicals.
   - The G2/M checkpoint prevents entry into mitosis if DNA replication is incomplete.

In addition, cyclins are proteins that control the entry and progression of cells through the cell cycle. The function occurs through activation of proteins called *cyclin-dependent kinases* (CDKs). Different combinations of cyclins and CDKs are involved with each stage in the cell cycle. CDK inhibitors regulate the cyclin–CDK complexes and are most important in regulating cell cycle checkpoints for repairs of mistakes in DNA replication.

Cell Cycle–Specific Drugs

Antineoplastic drugs are most effective during cell division. Cell cycle–specific drugs are used to treat rapidly growing tumors because they attack cancer cells when they enter a specific phase of cell reproduction. Most chemotherapeutic agents affect cells in the S phase by interfering with RNA and DNA synthesis. Others are more specific to the M phase. Chemotherapy is administered in multiple, repeated doses to produce a greater cell kill and to halt the growth of tumor cells. Examples of cell cycle–specific agents are topoisomerase I inhibitors, antimetabolites, mitotic spindle poisons, and some of the miscellaneous agents (Drug Therapy Table 18-1).

Cell Cycle–Nonspecific Drugs

Cell cycle–nonspecific drugs are effective during any phase of the cell cycle, whether reproducing or resting. They are used for large, slow-growing tumors. The amount of drug given is more important than the frequency. Cell cycle–nonspecific drugs have more prolonged effects on cells, which results in cell damage and destruction. They are often given in combination with cell cycle–specific drugs and may also be combined with or follow radiation therapy. Examples of cell cycle–nonspecific agents are alkylating agents, antitumor antibiotics, nitrosoureas, hormones, and some of the miscellaneous agents (see Drug Therapy Table 18-1).

Routes and Devices for Administration of Chemotherapy

Chemotherapeutic drugs are administered by several routes. The most common are the oral and IV routes, but they may also be given via intramuscular, subcutaneous, intraperitoneal, arterial, intrapleural, topical, or intrathecal routes or directly into a cavity. Dosage is based on the client's total body surface area, prior responses to chemotherapy and other therapies, function of the major organs, and the client's health status. IV administration is monitored closely to prevent the drug from leaking into surrounding tissues, referred to as **extravasation**. Inspecting the site daily for signs of thrombophlebitis, such as tenderness, pain, swelling, and induration, is also important. Most antineoplastic agents can be very irritating. Blistering and tissue necrosis are possible effects of extravasation. If a client complains of burning or pain during the chemotherapy infusion, the drug must be discontinued. **Vesicants** are particularly damaging antineoplastics, in that they cause tissue necrosis of underlying tendons, nerves, and blood vessels. Sloughing and ulceration of the skin may be so severe that the client needs skin grafts. If vesicants are being administered, there are protocols for treating the extravasation (Box 18-7). In addition, there are safety issues for the nurse who administers chemotherapy (Box 18-8).

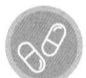

Pharmacologic Considerations

- Most antineoplastic agents are teratogenic to both handlers and clients. Nurses should not handle agents early in pregnancy or if attempting to conceive. Pregnant nurses have the right to opt out of chemotherapy treatment. Clients should use effective birth control during chemotherapeutic treatment.

DRUG THERAPY TABLE 18-1 Antineoplastic Agents

Drug Category and Common Examples	Intended Use	Therapy-Related Side Effects
Cell Cycle–Specific Agents		
Plant Alkaloids		
Vinca Alkaloids Vinblastine Vincristine Vinorelbine (Navelbine)	Leukemia/lymphomas: Hodgkin disease, other lymphomas Solid tumors: testicular, breast, non–small cell lung cancer (NSCLC), Kaposi sarcoma (KS) Nonmalignant: mycosis fungoides, idiopathic thrombocytopenic purpura	Immediate: extravasation potential During therapy cycles: alopecia, anemia, leukopenia, paresthesia, nausea, vomiting, constipation Long term: fertility problems
Taxanes Cabazitaxel (Jevtana) Docetaxel[a] (Taxotere) Paclitaxel (Abraxane)	Solid tumors: breast, NSCLC, prostate, ovary, KS	Immediate: hypersensitivity reaction, extravasation potential[a] During therapy cycles: nausea, fever, anemia, leukopenia, vomiting, diarrhea, constipation, stomatitis, hematuria Long term: fertility problems
Podophyllotoxins Etoposide Teniposide (Vumon)[a]	Leukemia/lymphomas: acute lymphocytic leukemia (ALL) Solid tumors: testicular, small cell lung cancer (SCLC)	Immediate: extravasation potential[a] During therapy cycles: anemia, leukopenia, thrombocytopenia, alopecia, nausea, vomiting
Camptothecin Analogs Irinotecan (Camptosar, Onivyde) Topotecan (Hycamtin)	Solid tumors: metastatic colon or rectal, ovarian, SCLC	Immediate: nausea, vomiting, diarrhea, inflammation potential (IV site) During therapy cycles: diarrhea, anemia, leukopenia, thrombocytopenia, asthenia, alopecia
Antimetabolites		
Azacitidine (Vidaza) Capecitabine (Xeloda)[a] Cladribine Clofarabine (Clolar)[b] Cytarabine (Cytosar-U) Decitabine (Dacogen) Fludarabine Fluorouracil (5-FU)[c] Gemcitabine (Gemzar) Mercaptopurine (Purixan)[b] Methotrexate (Trexall)[d] Nelarabine (Arranon)[e] Pemetrexed (Alimta) Pentostatin (Nipent) Pralatrexate (Folotyn) Thifluridine/tipiracil (Lonsurf) Thioguanine	Leukemia/lymphomas, Hodgkin lymphoma, myelodysplastic syndrome Solid tumors: breast, colon, head/neck, choriocarcinomas, osteosarcomas Palliative treatment for solid tumors: breast, stomach, pancreas, colon, rectum Nonmalignant: mycosis fungoides, severe psoriasis, rheumatoid arthritis	During therapy cycles: anemia, leukopenia, thrombocytopenia, nausea, vomiting, diarrhea, Hand and foot syndrome[a] Hyperuricemia[b] Alopecia[c] Renal damage[d] Neurologic toxicity[e] Long term: hepatotoxicity[d]
Miscellaneous Agents Ixabepilone (Ixempra)	Solid tumors: advanced breast	During therapy cycles: fatigue, peripheral neuropathy, neutropenia, alopecia, nausea, diarrhea
Cell Cycle–Nonspecific Agents		
Alkylating Drugs		
Nitrogen Mustard Derivatives Chlorambucil (Leukeran) cyclophosphamide[a] Ifosfamide (Ifex)[a–c] Mechlorethamine (Mustargen)[a,b,d] Melphalan (Alkeran)	Leukemia/lymphomas: chronic lymphocytic leukemia (CLL), lymphomas, Hodgkin disease, ALL, AML, CLL, advanced lymphomas Solid tumors: breast, ovary, neuroblastoma, retinoblastoma Nonmalignant: mycosis fungoides, nephrotic syndrome (children), rheumatoid arthritis, systemic lupus erythematosus, multiple sclerosis	Immediate[b]: nausea, vomiting, extravasation potential[d] During therapy cycles: anemia, leukopenia, thrombocytopenia, leukopenia, hemorrhagic cystitis,[a] alopecia,[c] somnolence, confusion, hyperuremia[d] Long term: fertility problems, secondary cancers[a]
Ethyleneimines Altretamine (Hexalen)[a] Bendamustine (Treanda) Thiotepa[b]	Leukemia/lymphomas: CLL, non-Hodgkin lymphoma Solid tumors: breast, ovary, bladder Palliative treatment for solid tumors: ovary	During therapy cycles: anemia, leukopenia, thrombocytopenia, nausea, vomiting, dizziness, peripheral neuropathy,[a] alopecia[b] Long term[b]: fertility problems
Alkyl Sulfonate Busulfan (Busulfex, Myleran)	Palliative treatment for CML	Immediate: induce seizures During therapy cycles: anemia, leukopenia, thrombocytopenia, hyperuremia, graft-versus-host disease Long term: fertility problems

(continued)

DRUG THERAPY TABLE 18-1 Antineoplastic Agents (*continued*)

Drug Category and Common Examples	Intended Use	Therapy-Related Side Effects
Hydrazines Dacarbazine (DTIC) Procarbazine (Matulane)[b,c] Temozolomide (Temodar)[a,c]	Leukemia/lymphomas: Hodgkin disease Solid tumors: melanoma, glioblastoma,[a] astrocytoma	Immediate: nausea, vomiting During therapy cycles: anemia, leukopenia, thrombocytopenia, alopecia,[c] peripheral neuropathy[b]
Nitrosoureas Carmustine (BiCNU, Gliadel) Lomustine (CCNU) Streptozocin (Zanosar)	Leukemia/lymphomas: secondary treatment for Hodgkin disease Solid tumors: pancreatic Palliative treatment for Hodgkin disease, multiple myeloma, various brain tumors	Immediate: nausea, vomiting During therapy cycles: leukopenia, thrombocytopenia Long term: pulmonary fibrosis
Platinum-Based Drugs Cisplatin[a] Oxaliplatin (Eloxatin)[b] Carboplatin	Solid tumors: ovarian, testicular, bladder	Immediate: nausea, vomiting, renal damage[a] During therapy cycles: anemia, leukopenia, thrombocytopenia tinnitus,[a] hyperuricemia,[a] peripheral neuropathy[b]
Antibiotics Bleomycin[a] Dactinomycin (Cosmegen)[b] Daunorubicin (Cerubidine)[b] Doxorubicin (Doxil)[b] Epirubicin (Ellence)[b] Idarubicin[b] Mitomycin[b] Mitoxantrone[b] Valrubicin (Valstar)	Leukemia/lymphomas; ALL, AML, and various lymphomas Solid tumors: various sarcomas, Wilms tumor, thyroid, breast, gestational neoplasia, testicular Palliative treatment for lymphomas, pleural effusion Solid tumors: testicular, various types	Immediate[b]: nausea, vomiting, extravasation potential During therapy cycles: anemia, leukopenia, thrombocytopenia, vomiting, alopecia, skin erythema, cutaneous changes Long term: pneumonitis,[a] pulmonary fibrosis
Hormonal Agents		
Adrenal Steroid Inhibitors Aminoglutethimide (Cytadren)	Metastatic breast, prostate cancers	Drowsiness, skin rash, nausea, vomiting
Gonadotropin-Releasing Hormone Analogs Degarelix (Firmagon) Goserelin (Zoladex) Histrelin (Vantas) Leuprolide (Eligard, Lupron) Triptorelin (Trelstar)	Prostate and breast cancer, endometriosis, endometrial thinning	Headache, emotional lability, depression, sweating, acne, breast atrophy, sexual dysfunction, vaginitis, hot flashes, pain, edema
Antiandrogens Abiraterone (Zytiga) Bicalutamide (Casodex) Flutamide (Eulexin) Nilutamide (Nilandron)	Prostate cancer	Hot flashes, nocturia, urinary frequency, peripheral edema, general pain, upper respiratory infection
Estrogen Estramustine (Emcyt)	Prostate cancer	Breast tenderness and enlargement, nausea, diarrhea, edema
Androgen Testolactone (Teslac)	Palliative treatment: breast cancer	Paresthesia, glossitis, anorexia, nausea, vomiting, maculopapular erythema, aches, alopecia, edema of the extremities, increase in blood pressure
Aromatase Inhibitors Anastrazole (Arimidex) Exemestane (Aromasin) Letrozole (Femara)	Breast cancer	Vasodilation, mood disturbances, nausea, hot flashes, pharyngitis, asthenia, pain
Progestins Medroxyprogesterone (Depo-Provera) Megestrol (Megace)	Breast, renal, or endometrial cancer	Fatigue, nervousness, rash, pruritus, acne, edema, weight gain
Antiestrogen Fulvestrant (Faslodex)	Breast cancer	Nausea, vomiting, asthenia, pain, pharyngitis, headache

Superscripts (e.g., [a]) on drugs in column 1 matches up the the specific therapy-related side effects in column 3

BOX 18-7 Treatment of Extravasation

General Measures
- Stop administration of drug.
- Leave needle in place.
- Gently aspirate residual drug and blood into tubing or needle.
- Inject neutralizing solution such as sodium thiosulfate, hyaluronidase, or sodium bicarbonate to reduce tissue damage. Selection of neutralizing agent depends on vesicant.

Vesicant-Specific Measures
- Doxorubicin
- Elevate and rest extremity.
- Apply topical cooling for 24 hours.
- Give hydrocortisone as ordered.
- Nitrogen mustard
- Apply cold compresses.
- Administer thiosulfate as ordered.
- Vinca alkaloids (vinblastine, vincristine, vindesine)
- Apply warm compresses.
- Do not apply ice—increases skin toxicity.
- Administer hyaluronidase as ordered.
- Mitomycin
- Apply ice.
- Administer dimethyl sulfoxide (DMSO) as ordered.

Various vascular devices are used to administer chemotherapy and are particularly beneficial for long-term chemotherapy. The client does not have to endure repeated venipunctures. In addition, they are beneficial when a client has poor veins. One method used is the insertion of venous access devices, which are special catheters inserted into a peripheral or central vein so that the catheter tip is located in the superior vena cava or right atrium. Examples include peripheral indwelling catheters (PIC lines), peripherally inserted central catheters (PICC lines), and external catheters (Hickman catheters, Broviac catheters). Another type is the implanted vascular access device (IVAD), also referred to as a *port*. A metal or plastic port encloses a self-sealing silicone rubber septum. The port is surgically implanted subcutaneously. A silicone catheter attached to the port is threaded subcutaneously to the right atrium. To access the port, a needle is inserted in the self-sealing septum of the port.

Chemotherapy infusion pumps are used for some cancers. They provide constant infusion of an antineoplastic drug directly into the cancerous organ. A small pump (similar in size to a hockey puck) is surgically implanted subcutaneously in the abdomen or attached externally.

BOX 18-8 Safety Measures When Administering Chemotherapy

- Prepare chemotherapy in designated biologic safety area.
- Use gloves when handling chemotherapy drugs and excretions from clients receiving chemotherapy.
- Wear disposable long-sleeved gowns when preparing and administering chemotherapy.
- Use Luer-Lok fittings on IV tubing used in delivering chemotherapy.
- Dispose of all equipment used in chemotherapy preparation and administration in designated containers.
- Dispose of all chemotherapy wastes as hazardous materials.

Adverse Effects of Chemotherapy

Some clients experience little discomfort or few adverse effects. Others have a wide range of symptoms. The tissues most susceptible to chemotherapy are those with rapidly growing cells, such as epithelial tissue, hair follicles, and bone marrow. Chemotherapy can potentially harm all body systems. Common adverse effects associated with chemotherapy are as follows:

- Nausea and vomiting are common during the first 24 hours after chemotherapy administration; use of concurrent antiemetics helps to reduce the incidence and severity.
- Stomatitis and mouth soreness or ulceration may result from destruction of the epithelial layer.
- Alopecia develops because chemotherapy affects rapidly growing cells of the hair follicles.
- Myelosuppression results from inhibition of the manufacture of RBCs and WBCs and platelets. Severe anemia, bleeding tendencies, leukopenia, **neutropenia** (decreased neutrophils), and thrombocytopenia are possible if bone marrow depression is profound. Blood transfusions as well as protection of the client from infections may be necessary.
- Fatigue results from the aforementioned effects, the chemotherapy itself, and the increased metabolic rate that accompanies cell destruction.

Antineoplastic drugs are potentially toxic. Nurses must be thoroughly familiar with their adverse effects and toxicity. The dose or length of treatment depends, in some cases, on the client's response to therapy.

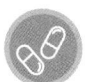

Pharmacologic Considerations

- Treating oral mucositis with a lidocaine product can numb the oral cavity. Teach the client to test for absence of gag reflex before eating or drinking when using lidocaine gel for oral pain.

Nursing Management

Nursing management of the client receiving chemotherapy varies depending on the drug, dose administered, and route used (Nursing Guidelines 18-2). Client teaching is an important nursing responsibility (Client and Family Teaching 18-2). In addition, there are recommended safety procedures that nurses must follow when caring for clients receiving chemotherapy (Box 18-9).

››› *Stop, Think, and Respond 18-2*

You are assigned to a client who was recently diagnosed with lung cancer. Surgery is planned, followed by chemotherapy. Your client says that he has heard that large doses of vitamin C would contribute to postoperative healing and would also enhance chemotherapy. He asks if he should begin megadoses of vitamin C. How should you respond?

NURSING GUIDELINES 18-2

Managing Clients Receiving Chemotherapy

- Monitor client for symptoms of anaphylactic reaction: urticaria (hives), pruritus (itching), sensation of lump in throat, shortness of breath, wheezing.
- Assess for electrolyte imbalances (see Chapter 16).
- Prevent extravasation of vesicant drugs. Implement measures to treat extravasation of vesicant medications if it occurs (see Box 18-7).
- Assess for signs of bone marrow depression: decreased white and red blood cell, granulocyte, and platelet counts.
- Assess for signs of bleeding and infection.
- Monitor for signs of renal insufficiency:
- Elevated urine specific gravity
- Abnormal electrolyte values
- Insufficient urine output (<30 mL/hour)
- Elevated blood pressure, blood urea nitrogen (BUN), and serum creatinine
- Inform client about the reasons for nausea and vomiting.
- Administer antiemetics before and during administration of chemotherapy or as indicated.
- Assess oral mucosa for dryness, redness, swelling, lesions, ulcerations, viscous (sticky) saliva, or white patches.

Client and Family Teaching 18-2 Chemotherapy

The nurse instructs clients receiving chemotherapy on an outpatient basis to

- Keep all appointments for chemotherapy treatments.
- If hair loss is anticipated, purchase a wig, cap, or scarf before therapy begins. Hair usually begins to grow again within 4 to 6 months after therapy; new growth may have a slightly different color and texture.
- Make the following dietary modifications:
  - Eat small, frequent meals.
  - Eat slowly.
  - Eat cool, bland foods and liquids.
  - Suck on hard candy during chemotherapy if taste alterations occur.
  - Avoid hot or very cold liquids, food with fat and fiber, spicy foods, and caffeine.
- Increase fluid intake to 2500 to 3000 mL/day (unless contraindicated or advised by primary provider).
- Report excessive fluid loss or gain, change in level of consciousness, increased weakness or ataxia (lack of muscle coordination), paresthesia (numbness, prickling, or tingling), seizures, persistent headache, muscle cramps or twitching, nausea and vomiting, or diarrhea.
- Have periodic evaluations and examinations as recommended.

BOX 18-9 Safety Precautions When Caring for Clients Receiving Chemotherapy

- Use protective equipment (gloves and gowns) when handling body fluids; wear a face shield if splashing is possible.
- Encourage clients to use toilets if possible. In addition, ask male clients to sit to void instead of standing to reduce splashing.
- Protect the skin of incontinent clients with moisture-barrier products to the perineal and perirectal area.
- Flush toilets twice with lids down to avoid aerolization of chemotherapeutic agents.
- Dispose of contaminated equipment and linens in appropriate leak-proof and puncture-proof containers.
- Dispose of all chemotherapy wastes as hazardous materials.
- Maintain chemotherapy precautions for 48 hours post administration of chemotherapy.

Adapted from American Cancer Society (2019). *Chemotherapy safety*. https://www.cancer.org/treatment/treatments-and-side-effects/treatment-types/chemotherapy/chemotherapy-safety.html

Stem Cell Transplantation

Cancers that are very sensitive to high doses of chemotherapy and radiation therapy may be treated with stem cell transplantation. *Stem cell transplantation* or HSCT is done to restore stem cells destroyed by disease or cancer treatments—chemotherapy and/or radiation therapy. Stem cells refer to young (immature) cells called *hematopoietic (blood-forming) stem cells*. They are responsible for the formation of RBCs and WBCs and platelets. They are mostly found in the bone marrow, but are also in the blood stream—referred to as peripheral stem cells—and in umbilical cord blood.

For some types of cancer, such as leukemia, the WBCs from the donor identify any remaining cancer cells and destroy them. In addition, the new stem cells develop into healthy blood cells, settling into bone marrow and producing new blood cells, a process referred to as **engraftment**. For adults, stem cells are generally obtained from bone marrow or peripheral blood. Umbilical cord blood is also a source for children but can be used for small adults as well. There are three types of stem cell transplants: autologous, allogeneic, and syngeneic.

Autologous Stem Cell Transplantation

Autologous stem cell transplants are obtained or harvested from the client, either from bone marrow or circulating blood. The stem cells are removed before other cancer treatments and frozen to be reinfused after cancer treatment is complete. Clients having autologous stem cell transplants do not require immunosuppressant drugs, but they can still be at risk for graft (transplant) failure. There are risks: there may be tumor cells present in the stem cells, and/or the client's immune system has not changed and still cannot fight off cancer cells. A process called "purging" may be used to remove the cancer cells with chemotherapy. Autologous stem cell transplants are used for some leukemias, lymphomas, and multiple myeloma. Research is ongoing to use this type of HSCT for other diseases, such as autoimmune disorders and other cancers.

Allogeneic Stem Cell Transplantation

Allogeneic stem cell transplantation uses stem cells from a donor whose tissue type matches the client's. Typically, blood relatives are tested for their potential to be the donor, but a donor may be found from a national registry. The donor can donate additional stem cells if required because they are obtained from peripheral blood. Donor stem cells produce immune cells that can destroy any remaining cancer cells—referred to as graft versus cancer effect. Engraftment may not occur with allogeneic transplantation. Recipients are also prone to infections carried by the donor, although donors are carefully screened. Another risk is graft-versus-host disease (GVHD), in which the donor cells produce new immune cells that attack the recipient's healthy cells. To prevent GVHD, clients receive immunosuppressant drugs. Allogeneic transplants are primarily used for cancers affecting blood, such as leukemia, and other bone marrow disorders.

A more recently developed type of allogeneic transplant is called a reduced-intensity transplant or a *nonmyeloablative transplant* or *minitransplant*. Clients having this type of transplant have reduced doses of chemotherapy and/or radiation therapy. The donor cells are then able to assist in the destruction of tumor cells and with time replace the recipient's own bone marrow cells. This method is most effective in clients whose disease is slower growing and less extensive.

Syngeneic Stem Cell Transplantation

Syngeneic stem cell transplantation is rarely done because it is possible only if the client has an identical sibling with identical tissue type. Syngeneic stem cell transplant does not cause GVHD—a distinct advantage. However, all cancer cells must be destroyed prior to transplantation because the donor stem cells cannot destroy any remaining cancer cells.

Nursing Management

Nursing management for the client receiving any form of stem cell transplantation is crucial. Before the procedure, the nurse thoroughly evaluates the client's physical condition, organ function, nutritional status, complete blood studies (including assessment for past antigen exposure such as HIV, hepatitis, or cytomegalovirus), and psychosocial status.

Prior to receiving stem cells, clients usually undergo intensive chemotherapy and possibly whole-body radiation, referred to as conditioning or bone marrow preparation or *myeloablation*. Because a large amount of tissue is treated, nausea, vomiting, diarrhea, and stomatitis are common. In addition, until transplanted stem cells begin to multiply and make new blood cells, usually within 2 to 6 weeks, these clients have no physiologic means to fight infection, making them very prone to infection. They are at high risk for dying from sepsis and bleeding before engraftment. Nurses must monitor clients closely and take measures to prevent infection. Clients are also at risk for bleeding, renal complications, and liver damage.

After stem cell transplantation, the recipient client is closely monitored for at least 3 months because complications related to the transplant are still possible. Getting blood counts back to normal may take 6 to 12 months. Infections are possible, as is GVHD. The client's immune system is deficient because of the chemotherapy, radiation therapy, and decreased blood counts. Throughout the entire process, the nurse assesses the client's psychological status. Clients experience many mood swings and need support and assistance throughout this process. Their families and significant others also require support. See Nursing Guidelines 18-3.

Targeted Therapies

Targeted therapies either use the client's own immune system to stimulate the body's natural immunity to restrict and destroy cancer cells or involve receiving immune system components to do the same. These drugs are developed as a result of the research done on genetic changes that occur in cancer cells. The purpose of targeted therapies is to manipulate the natural immune response by restoring, modifying, stimulating, or augmenting the natural defenses. Although a type of chemotherapy, targeted therapies work on cancer cells but do less damage to normal cells. *Carcinogenesis* is

NURSING GUIDELINES 18-3

Managing Clients Receiving Stem Cell Transplantation

- Assess client's nutritional status.
- Monitor for signs and symptoms of infection and renal insufficiency (see Nursing Guidelines 18-2).
- Assess for signs and symptoms of GVHD: irritability, pulmonary infiltration, hepatitis, enlarged spleen, enlarged lymph nodes, anemia, sepsis, diarrhea, maculopapular rash, and skin desquamation.
- Implement standard precautions and use protective isolation as needed.
- Assist with thorough hygiene.
- Review information related to prevention of infection, signs of rejection, importance of adherence to medical regimens and follow-up, medication instructions, and dietary needs.
- Encourage client to discuss anxieties and fears.
- Provide ongoing information about recovery phase and status of recuperation.

the process that occurs when a normal cell becomes malignant. Continued research is focused on developing drugs/therapies that interfere with carcinogenesis. The drugs are divided into three categories:

- *Enzyme inhibitors*: these targeted therapies block the ability for cancer cells to grow or spread. This in turn may assist other therapies to be more effective.
- *Apoptosis-inducing drugs*: these drugs target specific proteins within a cancer cell and cause the cell to die.
- *Angiogenesis inhibitors*: these drugs interfere with a tumor's ability to develop new blood vessels, thus cutting off the blood supply and halting its growth.

Types of targeted therapies are described in the next section.

Biologic Response Modifiers

Biologic response modifiers (BRMs) alter the interaction between the immune defenses and cancer cells. This interaction serves to destroy or halt the growth of malignant cells. BRMs can be naturally occurring or genetically engineered (recombinant).

Nonspecific Biologic Response Modifiers

Nonspecific BRMs use nonspecific agents such as bacillus Calmette-Guérin (BCG) or *Corynebacterium parvum* to act as antigens to stimulate an immune response. When these agents are injected into a client, the goal is for the stimulated immune system to destroy malignant growths. These agents are useful in treating localized melanoma and localized bladder cancer. Adjuvants are substances used in addition to the primary treatment to boost the immune system and enhance the main treatment.

Cytokines

Cytokines, another type of nonspecific BRMs, are substances that immune system cells produce to enhance the immune system. Common types of cytokines are interferons, interleukin-2, colony-stimulating factors, and tumor necrosis factor (Table 18-5). In general, they stimulate the immune system or assist in inhibiting tumor growth. Side effects include flu-like symptoms, GI disturbances, alopecia, and low blood counts.

Monoclonal Antibody Immunotherapy

Monoclonal antibody immunotherapy uses monoclonal antibodies (MoAbs or mAbs) to target antigen proteins on the tumor's surface not found in normal tissue. MoAbs are produced in the lab and are specific for various diseases, including some cancers. There are several uses for MoAbs:

- *Diagnostic*—radioactive substances are attached to the MoAbs to detect tumors (radioimmunodetection)
- *Treatment*—purge remaining tumor cells from blood or bone marrow for clients who are having a peripheral stem cell transplant
- *Cancer therapy*—destroys tumor cells directly

The goal is for the MoAbs to overwhelm and destroy the tumor cells. Some MoAbs are currently treating non-Hodgkin lymphoma, some types of metastatic breast cancer, and some forms of leukemia. More recently, some MoAbs have been approved for the treatment of colorectal cancer and lung cancers. More research is being done to treat other types of cancer.

Cancer Vaccines

The development of cancer vaccines is relatively new and mostly still in clinical trials. Vaccines may be used

TABLE 18-5 Cytokines or Immunomodulating Agents

CATEGORY AND COMMON EXAMPLES	INTENDED USE	THERAPY-RELATED SIDE EFFECTS
Interferons: Antiviral properties and regulate the immune response		
Alpha Interferon alfa (Roferon)	Treat various leukemia, lymphomas, and melanoma	Flu-like symptoms, fatigue, pancytopenia
Beta Interferon beta-1a (Rebif)	Treat flare-ups of multiple sclerosis	
Interleukins: direct immune cells to a site of inflammation		
Aldesleukin (IL-2) (Proleukin)	Renal cell cancer and metastatic melanoma	Flu-like symptoms, flush, skin rash, nausea, vomiting, fatigue, swelling, pancytopenia
Hematopoietic (colony-stimulating factors [CSF]): stimulate production of blood cells: neutrophils, platelets, erythrocytes		
Filgrastim (Neupogen)	Treat or prevent severe neutropenia	Bone pain, nausea, vomiting, diarrhea, alopecia
Oprelvekin (Neumega)	Treat or prevent severe thrombocytopenia associated with cancer chemotherapy	Edema, dyspnea, tachycardia, palpitations, syncope, fever
Darbepoetin alfa (Aranesp)	Anemia associated with chronic kidney disease (CKD) and nonmyeloid cancers	Hypertension, hypotension, headache, diarrhea, vomiting, nausea, myalgia, arthralgia
Tumor necrosis factor: regulates immune cells and inflammation		
Used with the chemotherapy agent melphalan	Advanced soft tissue sarcoma	Same as the chemo agent used

to treat cancer (therapeutic) or prevent cancer (prophylactic). A vaccine that is approved for use in the United States is the human papillomavirus (HPV), which is given to prevent women from getting cervical cancer. Vaccines not yet approved are being developed to boost the immune system's ability to attack a cancer that already exists.

Hyperthermia

Hyperthermia or thermal therapy uses temperatures greater than 106.7°F (41.5°C) to destroy tumor cells. There are three general types of hyperthermia:

- Local hyperthermia, in the form of high-energy waves or delivered through needles or probes directly into the tumor, is used to directly kill cancer cells and the surrounding blood vessels. Radiofrequency ablation is the most common type of local hyperthermia.
- Regional hyperthermia involves heating a larger area, such as an organ or body cavity in combination with other therapies such as chemotherapy to treat cancer. An example is regional or isolation perfusion, in which blood in a specific body part is pumped into a heating device and then pumped back to heat the body part. Chemotherapy may be infused at the same time.
- Whole-body hyperthermia raises a client's body temperature with heating blankets, immersion in warm water, or with the use of a thermal chamber. It is theorized that this briefly boosts a person's immunity and raises cell-killing elements in the blood.

Hyperthermia is combined with other therapies. When used with radiation therapy, the tumor cells are more sensitive to the radiation and cannot repair themselves at all. Hyperthermia alters cell membrane permeability so that uptake of chemotherapy is increased. It enhances the function of immunotherapeutic agents. Clients receiving hyperthermia may experience local burns and tissue damage, electrolyte imbalances, fatigue, GI disturbances, and neuropathies.

Photodynamic Therapy

Photodynamic therapy (PDT) or phototherapy uses a photoactive drug like porfimer (Photofrin), which, when administered intravenously, is stored in higher concentrations in malignant tissues. After a prescribed interval, laser light applied to the tumor activates the drug and destroys the malignant cells. Damage to healthy tissues is minimal (American Cancer Society, 2015c). This type of therapy requires a commitment from clients to protect their eyes and skin from sunlight and bright indoor light for at least 6 weeks after receiving the photoactive drug. Failure to adhere to this warning can result in a severe sunburn-like reaction that may require hospitalization for pain, dehydration, and local skin care. This therapy is currently used to treat esophageal and lung cancers, but not to a large extent. Research is ongoing.

Gene Therapy

Scientists theorize that many cancers result from gene alterations, which can include mutations, amplifications or deletions of specific elements of the gene, or relocation of specific elements. Strategies to confront this problem include **gene therapy**, which currently has three primary strategies: replacing altered or mutated genes with correct genes, inhibiting or "silencing" defective genes, and/or introducing substances that destroy genes or cancer cells (American Society of Gene and Cell Therapy, 2020). Scientists predict that gene therapy will play a significant role in the future prediction, diagnosis, and treatment of cancer. Gene therapy is currently being investigated in the treatment of brain tumors; melanoma; and renal, breast, ovarian, lung, and colon cancers.

Clinical Trials

Clinical trials provide methods to test new treatments for specific cancers. The trials may involve a new drug, a new combination of existing drugs, or new therapies. The process for new treatments to become accepted practice is lengthy. Before testing on humans, there is testing on laboratory animals to ascertain safety and effectiveness. After animal testing, there are four phases:

1. *Phase I:* Treatment is given to a small group of people to determine dosing, schedule for treatment, and toxicity. Participants are usually clients for whom standard treatment has been ineffective. Clients are fully aware of the trial's experimental nature.
2. *Phase II*: Treatment is given to a larger group of clients to further determine effectiveness with specific cancers and to get better information about dosing, side effects, and toxicity. Clients are similar to those selected for phase I.
3. *Phase III:* If the treatment appears effective in phase II, then a larger number of clients are selected and compared with clients receiving accepted treatments for a particular type of cancer. At this point, the new treatment has had significant testing and review.
4. *Phase IV*: During this phase, more studies are done after the drug is on the market to gain more knowledge of the drug's effect on various populations and side effects with long-term use.

Complementary and Alternative Therapies

Complementary and alternative therapies include treatments used in conjunction with prescribed medical treatments and may be such things as acupuncture relaxation techniques. Many are safe to use and provide pain relief and comfort to the client. It is important to instruct clients about safe alternative therapies and to limit treatments to those where evidence supports their use. Table 18-6 provides some information about various therapies that may be used for clients with cancer.

TABLE 18-6 Complementary and Alternative Methods of Cancer Treatment

METHOD	DESCRIPTION
Imagery, relaxation techniques, stress reduction exercises, yoga, biofeedback, massage, and music therapy	These methods are used to reduce pain, promote relaxation, and enhance conventional treatment methods based on beliefs that there is a link between the immune system and cancer and that these methods boost the immune system's ability to fight the cancer cells.
Medicinal agents	Many "cures" for cancer have been concocted from plants, herbs, flowers, and fluids of humans and animals. Although a few merit scientific investigation, many are considered quackery. The use of vitamins, minerals, proteins, and other ingredients is advocated for treatment of many cancers and prevention or treatment of side effects.
Special diets	Many diet regimens are advocated as treatment for certain cancers or as adjuncts to treatment. Examples include organic foods, macrobiotic diets, and particular foods that reportedly kill cancer cells. Clinical evidence indicates that a low-fat, high-fiber diet rich in antioxidants and beta-carotene is the most effective diet treatment.
Spiritual methods	These methods are derived from powers of faith that people believe will help them to overcome cancer. Examples include faith healing, laying on of hands, and prayer.

It is difficult for health care providers to condone unconventional therapies because many of the methods do not have a scientific foundation. There are also legal and ethical implications if health care providers participate in unaccepted treatments. Information that they provide to clients must be factual and understandable. Although some alternative methods have successfully augmented conventional treatments, many methods have no positive effects and, indeed, some are actually harmful.

NURSING MANAGEMENT OF THE CLIENT WITH CANCER

Managing the care of clients with cancer is challenging. The diagnosis itself implies multiple problems, and the treatments result in many secondary problems. This care requires a comprehensive plan designed to meet or assist the client and family's needs (Nursing Care Plan 18-1).

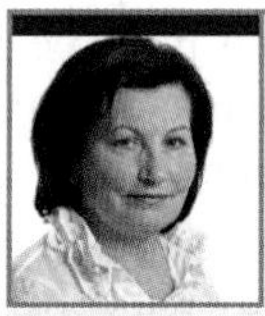

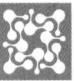

Clinical Scenario A client with a diagnosis of colon cancer had surgery to remove the tumor and will begin chemotherapy this week. **What are important nursing actions when caring for this client? See Nursing Care Plan 18-1.**

NURSING CARE PLAN 18-1 The Client With Cancer

Assessment

- Assess client's level of understanding about the diagnosis, treatment, and follow-up care.
- Determine the client's strengths, coping mechanisms, response to diagnosis, and emotional and physical support systems
- Evaluate the family's response to illness.
- Check client's overall physical condition, energy and pain levels, and nutritional and fluid status.

Nursing Diagnosis. **Fatigue** related to side effects of treatments, weakness from cancer, and physical and psychological stress

Expected Outcomes. (1) Client will participate in daily care as much as possible. (2) Client will identify measures to conserve and improve energy.

Interventions	Rationales
Identify energy level by asking client to evaluate it on a scale of 0 (*not tired*) to 10 (*totally exhausted*).	*Such identification establishes current level of fatigue.*
Plan care around energy level and include rest periods.	*Rest reduces physical stress and conserves energy.*
Promote reduced workload and increased assistance with daily chores.	*Reducing work levels conserves energy and decreases physical stress.*
Encourage adequate protein and calorie intake.	*Adequate protein and caloric intake increases activity tolerance.*
Encourage use of relaxation techniques and mental imagery.	*They promote relaxation and reduce psychological stress.*

Evaluation of Expected Outcomes

Client can participate in care without becoming exhausted.
Client can identify need for rest.
Diet consumed consists of recommended protein and calories.
Able to use relaxation techniques and imagery to enhance rest and alleviate stress and anxiety.

NURSING CARE PLAN 18-1 The Client With Cancer (*continued*)

Nursing Diagnosis. Grief related to potential loss and altered role status

Expected Outcomes. (1) Client will identify and verbalize feelings. (2) Client will continue to make future-oriented plans, even if one day at a time. (3) Client will verbalize understanding of the dying process. Refer to Chapter 10 for nursing interventions.

Evaluation of Expected Outcomes

(1) Client expresses feelings of guilt, anger, or sorrow. (2) Client plans for future one day at a time.

Nursing Diagnosis. Chronic Pain related to disease, metastasis, effects of surgery and treatments

Expected Outcomes. (1) Client will report pain relief. (2) Client will use relaxation methods and other alternatives to reduce pain and discomfort. Refer to Chapter 11 for nursing interventions.

Evaluation of Expected Outcomes

Client states that pain medications are effective.

Nursing Diagnosis. Altered Body Image Perception related to side effects of treatments, weight loss, and changes in appearance

Expected Outcomes. (1) Client will verbalize understanding of changes in appearance. (2) Client will demonstrate coping methods and adaptation to changes they are experiencing.

Interventions	Rationales
Explore strengths and resources with client.	*Emphasizing strengths promotes a positive self-image.*
Discuss possible changes in weight and hair loss. Suggest that the client select a wig before hair loss occurs.	*Planning for an event such as weight or hair loss decreases anxiety associated with a change in appearance.*
Acknowledge client's anger, sadness, or depression.	*Body image changes cause anxiety and other feelings; acknowledging such feelings assists the client to cope.*
Refer client to a support group or counseling.	*Support groups and counseling allow the client to share feelings and to recognize that they are not alone.*

Evaluation of Expected Outcomes

Client states acceptance of change or loss and demonstrates ability to adjust.

Nursing Diagnosis. Malnutrition Risk related to loss of appetite, difficulty swallowing, side effects of chemotherapy, or obstruction by tumor

Expected Outcomes. (1) Client will increase dietary intake. (2) Client will demonstrate understanding of the need for adequate intake of nutrients and fluids.

Interventions	Rationales
Monitor daily food intake.	*Such monitoring provides baseline data.*
Encourage intake of sufficient calories, nutrients, and fluids (see Nursing Guidelines 18-2); offer small, frequent meals and fluids.	*These measures reduce the sensation of fullness and decrease the stimulus to vomit.*
Administer antiemetics as ordered before meals.	*They are more effective when given before nausea.*
Monitor laboratory studies for signs of dehydration, biochemical imbalances, and malnutrition.	*Such monitoring reveals evidence of imbalances and assists in making needed interventions.*

Evaluation of Expected Outcomes

Client demonstrates minimal weight loss and verbalizes necessity to have adequate intake.

Nursing Diagnosis. Altered Skin Integrity related to immunologic deficits, effects of chemotherapy and radiation therapy, poor nutrition, immobility, and altered oral flora

Expected Outcome. Client will demonstrate measures to prevent complications from skin or tissue impairment or to promote tissue or skin healing. Refer to Chapter 12 for interventions.

Evaluation of Expected Outcomes

Client manages treatment for skin impairment and has minimal impairment of oral mucous membranes.

Pain is a major problem for clients with cancer (see Chapter 11). Sources of pain include bone metastasis; nerve compression; obstructed blood vessels, lymph systems, or organs; inflammation; ulceration; infection; or necrosis. Pain ranges from dull and aching to sharp, unrelenting, and throbbing.

Clients with cancer also experience fatigue, which is a frequent side effect of cancer treatments that rest fails to relieve. Fatigued clients are constantly weary, lack energy, and often feel too weak to carry out normal activities. The nurse must assess the client for other stressors that contribute to fatigue, such as pain, nausea, fear, and lack of adequate support. The nurse works with other health care team members to treat the client's fatigue.

Another major problem for clients with cancer is infection. Many factors predispose clients with cancer to infection: impaired skin and mucous membranes, chemotherapy, radiation and other therapies, the malignancy itself, malnutrition, medications, invasive catheters and IV lines, contaminated equipment, age, chronic illness, and prolonged hospitalization. Clients should avoid crowds and people with colds, flu, or other infectious diseases. Nurses must provide scrupulous care to clients with cancer and monitor for signs and symptoms of infection, including fever, elevated WBC levels, pain, redness, swelling, and drainage. (See Nutrition Notes for nutrition considerations.)

Other potential issues that clients with cancer face are as follows:

- Bleeding: may result from bone marrow suppression, medications that interfere with coagulation and platelet function, or both
- Impaired skin integrity: may result from chemotherapy, radiation therapy, surgery and other invasive procedures, nutritional deficits, and incontinence
- Hair loss
- Alterations in body image
- Changes in psychological and mental status
- Grieving: coping with a cancer diagnosis and treatments is frequently overwhelming.

Although cancer is not necessarily fatal, it does change a person's life in many ways. For those clients facing long and intense treatments and for those with few options for treatment, nurses must be supportive and guide them to resources.

Nutrition Notes

The Client With Cancer

- Improving the client's nutritional status not only improves quality of life but may also make cancer cells more susceptible to treatment. Good nutrition also promotes rehabilitation, may lessen the side effects of treatment, and may increase the chances of survival. Conversely, poor nutritional status may potentiate the toxicity of cancer treatments.
- Malnutrition is not an inevitable consequence of cancer; once established, however, it can be difficult to reverse. To prevent malnutrition, it is usually more effective to increase the nutrient density of foods consumed rather than to expect a client to eat more food. Fortifying casseroles, beverages, cereals, and other foods with skim milk powder, whole milk, cheese, cream cheese, peanut butter, eggs, butter, and honey increases nutrient density without increasing volume. Small, frequent feedings are also beneficial.
- Side effects of cancer and cancer therapies can devastate the client's ability to eat, which may change daily or as often as with each meal. Clients with nausea fare better with low-fat foods and "dry" meals (taking liquids between meals). Clients receiving chemotherapy should avoid eating or drinking for 1 to 2 hours after treatment to avoid nausea. Clients with anorexia should consume small, frequent meals. Encourage clients to view eating as part of therapy, not a voluntary activity.
- Clients with vomiting need to replenish fluids by taking water or noncarbonated, noncaffeinated beverages every 10 to 15 minutes.
- Clients who develop taste alterations from chemotherapy often complain that meat tastes "bad" or "rotten." Offer cold protein alternatives such as cheese, cottage cheese, protein beverages, and sandwiches. Assure the client that eating meat is not the only way to consume adequate protein. Sucking on hard candy during chemotherapy infusion may prevent a bitter or metallic taste.
- Clients with fatigue should rest before meals and avoid items that require a lot of chewing.
- Clients with difficulty swallowing should use gravies and sauces liberally. They may tolerate semisolid foods better than liquids. They should avoid extremely hot foods.
- If the client has difficulty due to lack of saliva, rinsing the mouth with water or using artificial saliva just prior to eating and frequent sips throughout meals may ease mealtimes.
- A high fluid intake is necessary to promote excretion of chemotherapeutic drugs. Water, milk, fruit juices, and high-protein beverages are all good choices; clients should avoid beverages containing caffeine and limit soft drinks, which are high in empty calories.
- Clients with a sore mouth should avoid highly seasoned foods, acidic juices, salty items, and coarse breads and cereals. They may tolerate cold food and beverages better than warm items. For clients receiving palliative care, do not force feedings, weigh clients, or use nutritional support.

Psychological Support

The diagnosis of cancer is frightening and frequently overwhelming. Psychological support is as important as medical treatments and physical care. Clients have many reactions, ranging from anxiety, fear, and depression to feelings of guilt related to viewing cancer as a punishment for past actions or failure to practice a healthy lifestyle. They may also express anger related to the diagnosis and their inability to be in control. Clients have the right to know their diagnosis, treatment plan, and prognosis so that they can make informed decisions. A client may never accept a cancer diagnosis. When provided with adequate information and supported psychologically, however, clients are more likely to face their diagnosis and be involved with their care and treatment. Families and significant others also require support.

Client and Family Teaching

Clients and their families or significant others require education to understand the diagnostic procedures, make treatment choices, participate in preventing complications, and recognize side effects and other adverse signs. Teaching focuses on:

- Medications, treatments, and procedures
- Adverse effects associated with treatment
- Possible changes in body image or function
- Resources for support
- Follow-up needed after discharge from the hospital

When developing a plan for client and family teaching, the nurse must consider facts such as the type of malignancy, treatment given, proposed treatments, client's condition, and effectiveness of the family support system (Evidence-Based Practice 18-1). These facts will determine the areas to discuss in more detail. The nurse should be aware of any explanations or information that other health care providers give to the client and family and must also allow time for clients to express their feelings or discuss home care. Doing so also helps identify issues the client or family does not understand.

Care of the Terminally Ill Client

Nursing management of the terminally ill client can be both physically and emotionally difficult. It must include both client and family. The nurse must carry out tasks gently to reduce the possibility of pain and discomfort and to keep the client as comfortable as possible. Nursing care is focused on controlling pain, providing adequate fluid and nutrition, keeping the client warm and dry, and controlling odors (when present). An important part of nursing care is to help the client maintain dignity despite an illness that often requires dependence on others for activities of daily living. (See Chapter 10 for more information on nursing and hospice care.)

Evidence-Based Practice 18-1

Shared Decision Making for Clients With Cancer

Clinical Question

Would Shared Decision Making (SDM) be an effective communication tool for clients with a cancer diagnosis?

Evidence

A study was initially conducted in 2007 and repeated in 2016 to look at who initiates a discussion with clients of poor prognosis and who is responsible for leading these discussions. The study was developed based on research and discussions of effective communication at the "end of life" for clients and the author Jane Price's nursing experience in providing dignity with care (Price, 2016). The author explored the benefits of SDM in two countries to see how the tool benefited clients and families with poor prognosis. She also explored whether using the SDM tool caused earlier discussions about "end-of-life decisions" and if an increase in therapeutic communication occurred. The author looked at data collected from the United States and the United Kingdom. The data revealed that in the United States a majority of people still die in the hospital, whereas in the United Kingdom, the wish of clients is to die at home. In conclusion of the study, it suggests that there is a patient care approach to "end-of-life care"; however, there remain inconsistency and gaps in regard to how this process occurs. The author feels that the SDM tool that brings earlier choice decisions and preplanning for the end of a poor diagnosis could greatly impact the therapeutic relationship and experience of the client and family.

Nursing Implications

Nurses are patient advocates. Assessing the patient's family, needs, and support system and encouraging resources are an important part of caring for cancer clients. The nurse must work well with the health care team and related the assessment findings so that an early team approach occurs. The nurse spends the most time with the client and family and plays a crucial role in relaying the information. Effective communication and building a trusting relationship will help support clients with a poor prognosis.

Reference

Price, J. (2016). Informed shared decision-making in planning for the end of life. *British Journal of Nursing, 25*(7), 378–383. https://doi.org/10.12968/bjon.2016.25.7.378

KEY POINTS

- Cancer is characterized by abnormal, unrelated cell proliferation that invades healthy tissues
- Pathophysiology: neoplasms can be benign or malignant
- Etiology can be from genetics, chemical agents in the environment, diet, viruses and bacteria, and from the role of the immune system
- Assessment findings include unexplained weight loss, fever, fatigue, pain, and skin changes
- Diagnostic findings are based on laboratory tests, radiologic and imaging tests, and from biopsies, endoscopies, frozen sections, and cytology examinations.
- Staging is done to determine the advancement of the cancer
- Treatment consists of:
  - Surgery: removal of cancer tumor
  - Radiation therapy: treatment with high-energy ionizing radiation
  - Chemotherapy: use of antineoplastic agents
  - Stem cell transplantation: restore stem cells destroyed by disease or cancer treatments
  - Targeted therapies: uses the client's own immune system to stimulate the body to destroy cancer cells
  - Hyperthermia: uses temperatures greater than 106.7°F to destroy tumor cells

- PDT: uses a photoactive drug that then allows laser lights to destroy malignant cells
- Gene therapy: gene alterations are done and are used to replace defective genes
- Clinical trials: experimental new therapies
- Complementary and alternative therapies: include treatments used in conjunction with medical treatments, such as acupuncture relaxation techniques
- Psychological support: needed for the client and their family members
- Client and family teaching: needed for treatments, medications, procedures, adverse effects, resources for support, follow-up appointments
- Care of the terminally ill client: done for the client and their family members, helping to maintain dignity of the client

CRITICAL THINKING EXERCISES

1. A client with endometrial cancer has been told that they will be treated with internal radiation therapy. Discuss what information to include in their teaching plan.
2. A client has been receiving chemotherapy while in the hospital. The registered nurse (RN) identified a nursing diagnosis of Risk for Infection related to altered immunologic response. As the licensed practical nurse (LPN) caring for this client, what steps should you take to minimize the client's risk of infection?
3. A client tells you that they are afraid of losing their hair related to treatment for cancer. What strategies may assist them with coping with alopecia?
4. Often, clients are most fearful of pain and pain control options when dealing with cancer. What would reassure this client?

NCLEX-STYLE REVIEW QUESTIONS PrepU

1. A nurse instructs a group of young adults at a community center about behaviors that can decrease the risk of cancer. Which information is most applicable for this age group?
   1. Avoid smoking and prolonged sun exposure.
   2. Eat a diet low in salt and fat.
   3. Perform self-examination techniques four times per year.
   4. Schedule yearly mammograms or prostate examinations.
2. The nurse's client is told that the malignant tumor is at stage T2, N0, M0. The client asks the nurse what this means. What is the nurse's best response?
   1. "The cancer is widespread beyond the tumor margins."
   2. "There is evidence of metastasis to another organ."
   3. "The tumor has spread to the surrounding lymph nodes."
   4. "This tumor can be measured but has not extended or metastasized."
3. A client newly diagnosed with cancer receives external radiation therapy. Which nursing instruction regarding bathing is most appropriate?
   1. Avoid getting the irradiated skin wet.
   2. Cover the reddened irradiated area with clear plastic.
   3. Use alcohol instead of soap on the irradiated skin.
   4. Use a soft washcloth to wash the irradiated skin.
4. A client is receiving chemotherapy for cancer. After several treatments, blood studies demonstrate that the client is experiencing bone marrow suppression. The LPN can expect that the client will exhibit which of the following signs and symptoms? Select all that apply.
   1. Bleeding from gums
   2. Bone pain
   3. Easy bruising
   4. Fatigue
   5. Headaches
5. The nurse is caring for a client who is experiencing a poor appetite while receiving chemotherapy. Which of the following strategies is most appropriate for the nurse to use to increase the patient's nutritional intake?
   1. Add instant breakfast or milk powder, cheese, or peanut butter to selected foods.
   2. Avoid liquid protein supplements to encourage eating at mealtime.
   3. Increase intake of liquids at mealtime to stimulate the appetite.
   4. Serve three large meals per day plus snacks between each meal.
6. A client diagnosed with cancer comes to the clinic after receiving a combination of radiation and chemotherapies. The client complains of nausea, vomiting, and diarrhea. Which of the following signs requires an initial focused assessment by the nurse?
   1. Anemia
   2. Dehydration
   3. Fatigue
   4. Infection
7. At a routine clinic visit, the nurse weighs a client who has cancer and finds that the client has lost 40 kg since beginning cancer treatment. What is the nurse's best suggestion for increasing the client's caloric intake?
   1. Advise the client to eat small, frequent meals.
   2. Inform the client to eat foods high in fat.
   3. Suggest that the client eat larger portions.
   4. Tell the client to increase red meat intake.

WANT TO KNOW MORE? There are a wide variety of online resources available on thePoint to enhance learning and understanding of this chapter.

Go to **thePoint.lww.com/activate** and use the activation code found in the front of this text to unlock these online resources.

UNIT 5
Caring for Clients With Respiratory Disorders

19 Introduction to the Respiratory System

Words To Know

adenoids
alveoli (singular alveolus)
bronchi (singular bronchus)
bronchioles
carina
cilia
diaphragm
diffusion
epiglottis
ethmoidal sinuses
frontal sinuses
glottis
hilus
interstitium
larynx
lungs
maxillary sinuses
mediastinum
nasal septum
nasopharynx
oropharynx
paranasal sinuses
parietal pleura
perfusion
pharynx
pleura
pleural space
respiration
sphenoidal sinuses
thoracentesis
tonsils
trachea
turbinates (conchae)
ventilation
visceral pleura
vocal cords

Learning Objectives

On completion of this chapter, you will be able to:

1. Describe the structures of the upper and lower airways.
2. Explain the normal physiology of the respiratory system.
3. Differentiate respiration, ventilation, diffusion, and perfusion.
4. Describe oxygen transport.
5. Define forces that interfere with breathing, including airway resistance and lung compliance.
6. Identify elements of a respiratory assessment.
7. List diagnostic tests that may be performed on the respiratory tract.
8. Discuss preparation and care of clients having respiratory diagnostic procedures.

The respiratory system provides oxygen for cellular metabolic needs and removes carbon dioxide (CO_2), a waste product of cellular metabolism. Respiratory disorders and diseases are common, ranging from mild to life threatening. Disorders that interfere with breathing or the ability to obtain sufficient oxygen greatly affect respiratory and overall health status.

Gerontologic Considerations

■ As adults age, the cartilage of the nasal septum increases in length and may harden, resulting in airflow changes such as septal deviations, increasing the risk for obstructive apnea. Although the number of alveoli remains stable with age, the alveolar walls become thinner and contain fewer capillaries, resulting in decreased gas exchange. The lungs also lose elasticity, diminishing lung expansion and increasing dead space. Muscle tone, the cough reflex, and the number of cilia decrease. These changes place older adults at increased risk for respiratory disease.

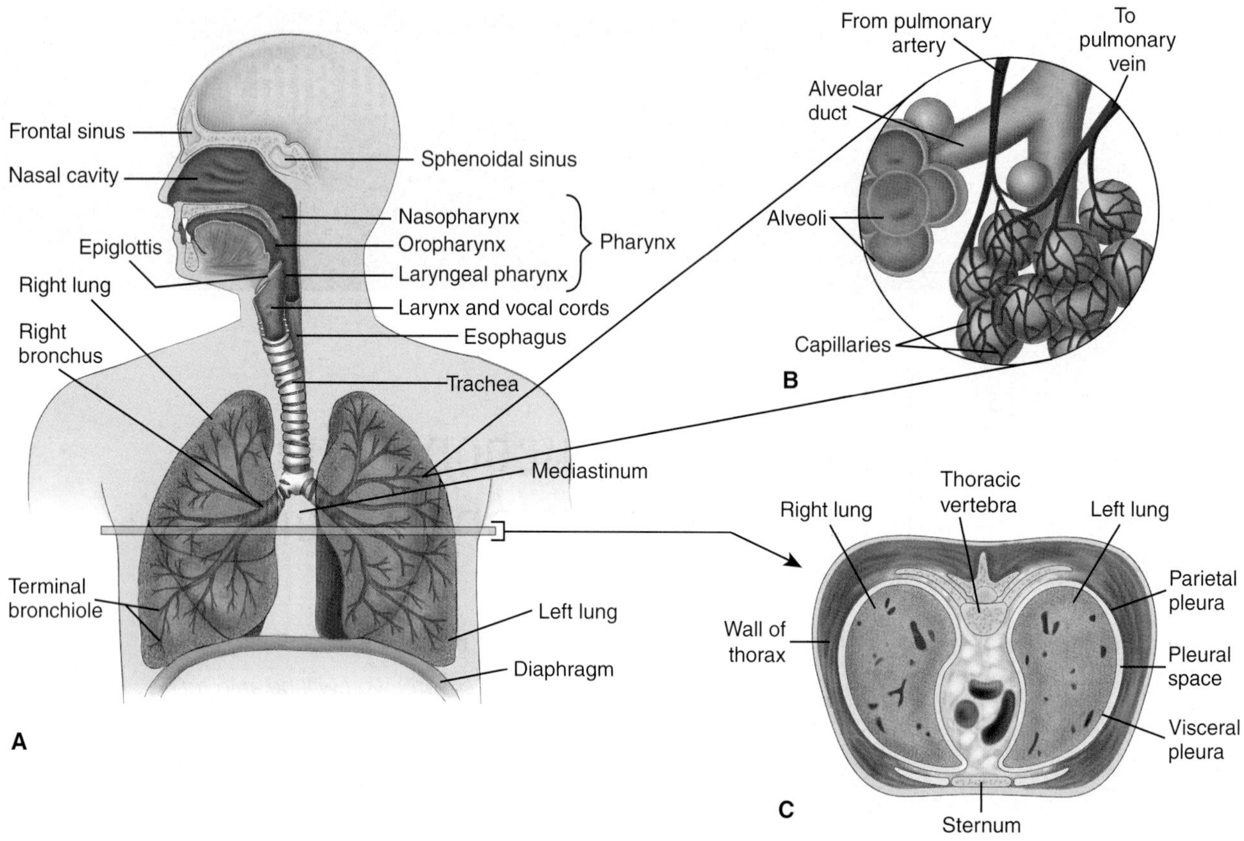

Figure 19-1 Major structures of the respiratory system. **(A)** Overview. **(B)** Alveoli (air sacs) of the lungs and the blood capillaries. **(C)** Transverse section through the lungs.

RESPIRATORY ANATOMY

The respiratory system (Fig. 19-1) is divided into the upper airway and lower airway.

Upper Airway

The upper airway consists of the nose, sinuses, turbinates, pharynx, and larynx.

Nose

Nasal bones and cartilage support the external nose. The nares are the external openings of the nose. The internal nose is divided into two cavities separated by the **nasal septum**. Each nasal cavity has three passages created by the projection of turbinates or conchae from the lateral walls. The vascular and ciliated mucous lining of the nasal cavities warms and humidifies inspired air. Mucus secreted from the nasal mucosa traps small particles (e.g., dust, pollen). **Cilia** (fine hairs) move the mucus to the back of the throat. This movement helps prevent irritation to and contamination of the lower airway. The nasal mucosa also contains olfactory sensory cells that are responsible for the sense of smell.

The olfactory area lies at the roof of the nose. The cribriform plate forms part of the roof of the nose and the floor of the anterior cranial fossa. Trauma or surgery in this area carries the risk of injuring or causing infection in the brain.

Paranasal Sinuses

The **paranasal sinuses** are extensions of the nasal cavity located in the surrounding facial bones (Fig. 19-2). They lighten the weight of the skull and give resonance to the voice. There are four pairs of these bony cavities. The two **frontal sinuses** lie in the frontal bone that extends above the orbital cavities. The ethmoid bone, located between the eyes, contains a honeycomb of small spaces called the **ethmoidal sinuses**. The **sphenoidal sinuses** lie behind the nasal cavity. The **maxillary sinuses** are found on either side of the nose in the maxillary bones. The maxillary sinuses are the largest sinuses and the most accessible to treatment.

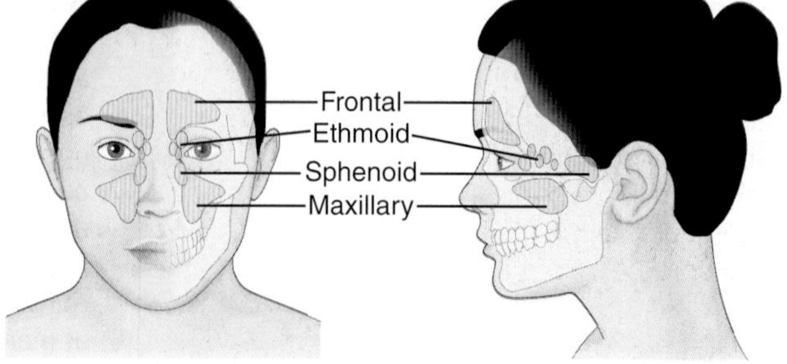

Figure 19-2 The paranasal sinuses.

The lining of the sinuses is continuous with the mucous membrane lining of the nasal cavity. Mucus traps particles that cilia sweep toward the pharynx. Immunoglobulin A (IgA) antibodies in the mucus protect the lower respiratory tract from infection.

Concept Mastery Alert

The paranasal sinuses provide the resonating chamber that serve in speech. This is why a person's voice sounds different when they have a cold.

Turbinate Bones (Conchae)

The **turbinates** (or **conchae**) are bones that change the flow of inspired air to moisturize and warm it better. As air is inhaled, the turbinates deflect it toward the roof of the nose. They have a large, moist, and warm mucous membrane surface that can trap almost all dust and microorganisms. They also contain sensitive nerves that detect odors or induce sneezing to remove irritating particles, such as dust or soot.

Pharynx

The **pharynx**, or throat, carries air from the nose to the larynx and food from the mouth to the esophagus. The pharynx is divided into three continuous areas: the **nasopharynx** (near the nose and above the soft palate), the **oropharynx** (near the mouth), and the *laryngeal pharynx* (near the larynx). The nasopharynx contains the adenoids and openings of the eustachian tubes. The eustachian tubes connect the pharynx to the middle ear and are the means by which upper respiratory infections spread to the middle ear. The oropharynx contains the tongue. The muscular nature of the pharynx allows for closure of the epiglottis during swallowing and relaxation of the epiglottis during respiration.

Tonsils and adenoids, which do not contribute to respiration but instead protect against infection, are found in the pharynx. Palatine **tonsils** consist of two pairs of elliptically shaped bodies of lymphoid tissue. They are located on both sides of the upper oropharynx. **Adenoids**, or pharyngeal tonsils, also composed of lymphoid tissue, are found in the nasopharynx. Chronic throat infections often lead to removal of the tonsils and adenoids. In adults, adenoids may shrink and become nonfunctional.

Larynx

The **larynx**, or voice box, is a cartilaginous framework between the pharynx and trachea. Its primary function is to produce sound. The larynx also protects the lower airway from foreign objects because it facilitates coughing.

Important structures in the larynx include the **epiglottis**, a cartilaginous valve flap that covers the opening to the larynx during swallowing; the **glottis**, an opening between the vocal cords; and the **vocal cords**, folds of tissue in the larynx that vibrate and produce sound as air passes through. The pharynx, palate, tongue, teeth, and lips mold the sounds made by the vocal cords into speech. Table 19-1 reviews laryngeal structures.

Lower Airway

The lower respiratory airway consists of the trachea, bronchi, bronchioles, lungs, and alveoli (see Fig. 19-1). Accessory structures include the diaphragm, rib cage, sternum, spine, muscles, and blood vessels.

Trachea

The **trachea** is a hollow tube composed of smooth muscle and supported by C-shaped cartilage. The cartilaginous rings are incomplete on the posterior surface. The trachea transports air from the laryngeal pharynx to the bronchi and lungs.

Bronchi and Bronchioles

The trachea bifurcates (divides) at the **carina** (lower end of the trachea) to form the left and right **bronchi**. Stimulating the carina results in coughing and *bronchospasm* (spasm of the bronchial smooth muscle, causing narrowing of the lumen). The right mainstem bronchus is shorter, more vertical, and larger than the left mainstem bronchus. Aspiration of foreign objects is more likely to occur in the right mainstem bronchus and right upper lung. Mucous membrane continues to line this portion of the respiratory tract. Cilia sweep mucus and particles toward the pharynx.

The right and left mainstem bronchi divide into three secondary right bronchi and two secondary left bronchi. Each secondary bronchus supplies air to the three right lobes and two left lobes of the lung. The entrance of the bronchi to the lungs is called the **hilus**. The bronchi branch enters each lobe and continues to branch to form smaller bronchi and, finally, terminal **bronchioles** (smaller subdivisions of bronchi).

Lungs and Alveoli

The **lungs** are paired elastic structures enclosed by the thoracic cage. They contain the **alveoli**, small, clustered sacs that begin where the bronchioles end. Adult lungs contain approximately 300 million alveoli, which form most of the pulmonary mass. Each alveolus consists of a single layer of squamous epithelial cells. Capillaries surround these thin-walled alveoli and are the site of exchange of oxygen and CO_2.

TABLE 19-1 Structures of the Larynx

STRUCTURE	DESCRIPTION
Epiglottis	Valve flap of cartilage that covers the opening of the larynx during swallowing
Glottis	Opening between the vocal cords in the larynx
Thyroid cartilage	Largest cartilage in the trachea; part of it forms the Adam's apple
Cricoid cartilage	Only complete cartilaginous ring in the larynx, located below the thyroid cartilage
Arytenoid cartilages	Used in vocal cord movement with the thyroid cartilage
Vocal cords	Ligaments controlled by muscular movement that produce vocal sounds

Adapted from Hinkle, J. L., & Cheever, K. H. (2014). *Brunner & Suddarth's textbook of medical-surgical nursing* (13th ed.). Wolters Kluwer Health/ Lippincott Williams & Wilkins.

The epithelium of the alveoli consists of the following types of cells:

- Type I alveolar cells: line 95% of alveolar surfaces
- Type II alveolar cells: line about 5% of alveolar surfaces and synthesize *surfactant*, a mixture of phospholipid, neutral lipids, and proteins that reduces the surface tension of alveoli, preventing their collapse during expiration and limiting their expansion during inspiration
- Alveolar macrophages: remove foreign material, such as particulate matter and bacteria

The **interstitium** lies between the alveoli and contains the pulmonary capillaries and elastic connective tissue. Elastic and collagen fibers allow the lungs to have *compliance*, the ability to expand. Lung expansion creates a negative or subatmospheric pressure, which keeps the lungs inflated. If air gets into the space between the lungs and the thoracic wall, the lungs will collapse.

Accessory Structures

The **diaphragm** separates the thoracic and abdominal cavities. On inspiration, the respiratory muscles contract. The diaphragm also contracts and moves downward, enlarging the thoracic space and creating a partial vacuum. On expiration, the respiratory muscles relax, and the diaphragm returns to its original position.

The **mediastinum** is a wall that divides the thoracic cavity into two halves. This wall has two layers of **pleura**, a saclike serous membrane. The **visceral pleura** covers the lung surface, whereas the **parietal pleura** covers the chest wall. Serous fluid within the **pleural space** separates and lubricates the visceral and parietal pleurae. The remaining thoracic structures are located between the two pleural layers.

RESPIRATORY PHYSIOLOGY

The main function of the respiratory system is to exchange oxygen and CO_2 between the atmospheric air and the blood and between the blood and the cells. This process is called **respiration**. Other terms related to respiration are defined in Table 19-2.

TABLE 19-2 Terms Related to Respiration

TERM	DEFINITION
Ventilation	Movement of air into and out of the lungs sufficient to maintain normal arterial oxygen and carbon dioxide tensions
Inspiration	Movement of oxygen into the lungs
Expiration	Removal of carbon dioxide from the lungs
Diffusion	Transfer of a substance from an area of higher concentration or pressure to an area of lower concentration or pressure; exchange of oxygen and carbon dioxide across the alveolar capillary membrane and at the cellular level
Perfusion	Flow of blood in the pulmonary circulation
Distribution	Delivery of atmospheric air to the separate gas exchange units in the lungs

Ventilation

Ventilation is the actual movement of air in and out of the respiratory tract. Air must reach the alveoli for gas to be exchanged. This process requires a patent airway and intact and functioning respiratory muscles. Pressure gradients between atmospheric air and the alveoli enable ventilation. Air flows from an area of higher pressure to an area of lower pressure.

Mechanics of Ventilation

During inspiration, the diaphragm contracts and flattens, which expands the thoracic cage and increases the thoracic cavity. The pressure in the thorax decreases to a level below atmospheric pressure. As a result, air moves into the lungs. When inspiration is complete, the diaphragm relaxes, and the lungs recoil to their original position. The size of the thoracic cavity decreases, increasing the pressure to levels greater than the atmospheric pressure. Air then flows out of the lungs into the atmosphere (Fig. 19-3).

Neurologic Control of Ventilation

Several mechanisms control ventilation. The respiratory centers in the medulla oblongata and pons control rate and depth. Central chemoreceptors in the medulla respond to changes in CO_2 levels and hydrogen ion (H^+) concentrations (pH) in the cerebrospinal fluid. They convey a message to the lungs to change the depth and rate of ventilation. Peripheral chemoreceptors in the aortic arch and carotid arteries respond to changes in the pH and levels of oxygen and CO_2 in the blood. Table 19-3 describes other neurologic controls of ventilation.

Diffusion

Diffusion is the exchange of oxygen and CO_2 through the alveolar capillary membrane. Concentration gradients determine the direction of diffusion. During inspiration, the concentration of oxygen is higher in the alveoli than in the capillaries. Therefore, oxygen diffuses from the alveoli to the capillaries and is carried to the arteries. The concentration of oxygen in the arteries is higher than that in the cells; thus, oxygen diffuses into the cells.

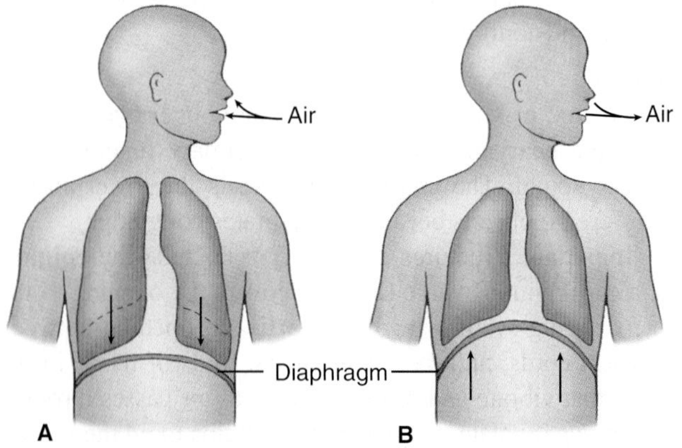

Figure 19-3 The mechanics of ventilation: **(A)** inspiration, **(B)** expiration.

TABLE 19-3 Neurologic Control of Respiration

CONTROL	DESCRIPTION
Hering–Breuer reflex	Stretch receptors located in the alveoli are activated during inspiration so that inspiration is inhibited and lungs are not overdistended.
Proprioceptors	Exercise stimulates breathing. Movement activates proprioceptors located in the muscles and joints and increases ventilation.
Baroreceptors	These receptors in the aortic and carotid bodies respond to changes in arterial blood pressure (BP). Elevated arterial BP causes a reflex hypoventilation; lowered BP causes a reflex hyperventilation.

As cellular CO_2 gradients increase, CO_2 diffuses from the cells into the capillaries and then into the venous circulatory system. As CO_2 travels to the pulmonary circulation, its concentration is higher there than in the alveoli. Therefore, CO_2 diffuses into the alveoli.

Alveolar Respiration

Alveolar respiration determines the amount of CO_2 in the body. Increased CO_2, which is present in body fluids primarily as carbonic acid, causes the pH to decrease below the normal 7.4. Decreased CO_2 causes the pH to increase above 7.4. The pH affects the rate of alveolar respiration by a direct action of H^+ on the respiratory center in the medulla oblongata.

The kidneys contribute to maintaining normal pH by excreting excess H^+, which in turn keeps serum bicarbonate (HCO_3) levels near normal. The lungs and kidneys combine to maintain the ratio of carbonic acid to HCO_3 at 1:20, fixing the pH at approximately 7.4.

In a client who is critically ill, various homeostatic mechanisms compensate for alterations. In an attempt to maintain normal pH, two mechanisms may occur:

- The lungs eliminate carbonic acid by blowing off more CO_2. They also conserve CO_2 by slowing respiratory volume and reabsorbing HCO_3.
- The kidneys excrete more HCO_3.

A client's condition remains compensated if the carbonic acid-to-HCO_3 ratio remains 1:20.

Disturbances in pH that involve the lungs are considered respiratory. Disturbances in pH involving other mechanisms are termed *metabolic*. At times, respiratory and metabolic disturbances coexist (see Chapter 16).

››› *Stop, Think, and Respond 19-1*

Explain the differences between ventilation and respiration.

Transport of Gases

Oxygen transport occurs in two ways: (1) a small amount is dissolved in water in the plasma, and (2) a greater portion combines with hemoglobin in red blood cells (RBCs; oxyhemoglobin). Dissolved oxygen is the only form that can diffuse across cellular membranes. As this oxygen crosses cellular membranes, oxygen from the hemoglobin rapidly replaces it. Large amounts of oxygen are transported in the blood as oxyhemoglobin. The formula for this process is $O_2 + Hgb \rightarrow HgbO_2$.

CO_2 diffuses from the tissue cells to the blood. Bicarbonate ions (HCO_3^-) are then transported to the lungs for excretion. Most of the CO_2 enters the RBCs, although some combines with hemoglobin to form carbaminohemoglobin. Much of the CO_2 combines with water in the cells and exits as HCO_3^-, which the plasma transports to the kidneys. A small portion remains in the plasma and is called *carbonic acid*. The formation of carbonic acid yields H^+. The amount of H^+ determines the pH, which also determines the amount of CO_2 for the lungs to excrete. Refer to Chapter 16 for a review of acid–base balance. Briefly, acid–base imbalances are compensated in the following ways:

- Respiratory acidosis: kidneys retain more HCO_3 to raise the pH
- Respiratory alkalosis: kidneys excrete more HCO_3 to lower pH
- Metabolic acidosis: lungs "blow off" CO_2 to raise pH
- Metabolic alkalosis: lungs retain CO_2 to lower pH

Pulmonary Perfusion

Perfusion refers to blood supply to the lungs through which the lungs receive nutrients and oxygen. The two methods of perfusion are the bronchial and pulmonary circulation.

Bronchial Circulation

The bronchial arteries, which supply blood to the trachea and bronchi, arise in the thoracic aorta and intercostal arteries. The bronchial arteries also supply the lungs' supporting tissues, nerves, and outer layers of the pulmonary arteries and veins. This circulation returns either to the left atrium through the pulmonary veins or to the superior vena cava through the bronchial and azygos veins. Bronchial circulation is not involved with gas exchange.

Pulmonary Circulation

The pulmonary artery transports venous blood from the right ventricle to the lungs. It divides into the right and left branches to supply the right and left lungs. The blood circulates through the pulmonary capillary bed where diffusion of oxygen and CO_2 occurs. The blood then returns to the left atrium through the pulmonary veins.

Pulmonary circulation is referred to as a low-pressure system. This means that gravity, alveolar pressure, and pulmonary artery pressure affect pulmonary perfusion. A person in an upright position has less perfusion to the upper lobes. If a person is in a side-lying position, perfusion is greater to the dependent side. In addition, increased alveolar pressure can cause pulmonary capillaries to narrow or collapse, affecting gas exchange. Decreased pulmonary artery pressure results in decreased perfusion to the lungs. Clients with lung and cardiovascular diseases may have decreased pulmonary perfusion.

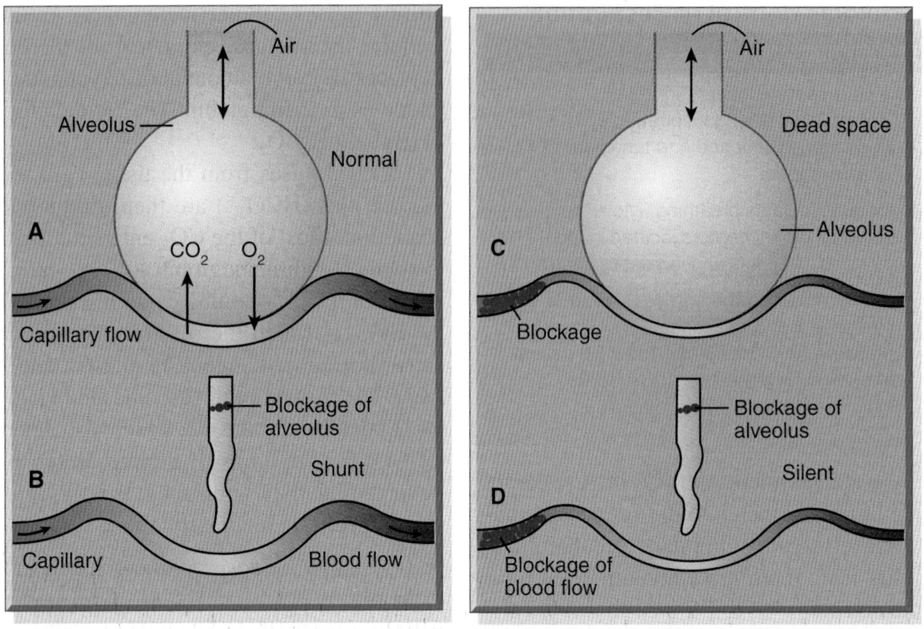

Figure 19-4 **(A)** Normal ratio. In the healthy lung, a given amount of blood passes an alveolus and is matched with an equal amount of gas. The ventilation/perfusion (V/Q) ratio is 1:1 (ventilation matches perfusion). **(B)** Low V/Q ratio: Shunts. Low V/Q states may be called shunt-producing disorders. When perfusion exceeds ventilation, a shunt exists. Blood bypasses the alveoli without gas exchange occurring. This is seen with obstruction of the distal airways, such as pneumonia, atelectasis, tumor, or a mucus plug. **(C)** High V/Q ratio: Dead space. When ventilation exceeds perfusion, dead space results. The alveoli do not have an adequate blood supply for gas exchange to occur. This is characteristic of a variety of disorders, including pulmonary emboli, pulmonary infarction, and cardiogenic shock. **(D)** Silent unit. In the absence of both ventilation and perfusion, or with limited ventilation and perfusion, a condition known as a silent unit occurs. This is seen with pneumothorax and severe acute respiratory distress syndrome.

Ventilation/Perfusion Ratio

A client's cardiopulmonary status involves several factors; in particular, the client's ventilation/perfusion ratio (V/Q ratio) indicates the effectiveness of airflow within the alveoli (ventilation) and the adequacy of gas exchange within the pulmonary capillaries (perfusion). Figure 19-4 depicts normal and abnormal V/Q ratios and their implications.

Problems in Respiratory Physiology

The respiratory system usually has sufficient reserves to maintain the normal partial pressures or tension of oxygen and CO_2 in the blood during times of stress. Respiratory insufficiency develops if there is too much interference with ventilation, diffusion, or perfusion. Abnormalities in these processes can lead to hypoxia, hypoxemia, hypercapnia, and hypocapnia (Table 19-4).

Several factors influence the work of breathing. Pressures needed to overcome the forces interfering with breathing determine the respiratory effort needed. Forces that interfere with breathing include airway resistance and lung compliance.

Airway resistance is related to airway diameter, rate of airflow, and speed of gas flow. As the rate of breathing increases, so does the resistance. A narrowed airway results from increased or thick mucus, bronchospasm, or edema. Conditions that may alter bronchial diameter and affect airway resistance include contraction of bronchial smooth muscle (e.g., asthma); thickening of bronchial mucosa (e.g., chronic bronchitis); airway obstruction by mucus, a tumor, or a foreign body; and loss of lung elasticity (e.g., emphysema). Decreased surfactant, fibrosis, edema, and atelectasis (alveolar collapse) affect lung compliance. Greater pressure gradients are needed when lungs are stiff.

TABLE 19-4 Conditions Related to Abnormalities in Ventilation, Perfusion, Diffusion, and Distribution

CONDITION	DESCRIPTION
Hypoxia	Decreased oxygen in inspired air
Hypoxemia	Decreased oxygen in the blood
Hypercapnia	Increased carbon dioxide in the blood
Hypocapnia	Decreased carbon dioxide in the blood

ASSESSMENT

Assessment of the respiratory system includes obtaining information about physical and functional issues related to breathing. It also means clarifying how these issues may affect the client's quality of life.

History

Often, a client seeks medical attention because of respiratory problems related to one or more of the following: dyspnea (labored or difficult breathing), pain on inspiration, increased or more frequent cough, increased sputum production or change in the color/consistency of the mucus, wheezing, or hemoptysis (blood in the sputum). The nurse obtains information about the client's general health history and family history and asks the client about the frequency of respiratory illnesses, allergies, smoking history, nature of any cough, sputum production, dyspnea (Box 19-1), and wheezing. Questioning the client about respiratory treatments or medications (prescription and over the counter) is essential. In addition, the nurse inquires about recent pulmonary tests (chest X-ray, tuberculosis test), including questions about occupation, exercise tolerance, pain, and level of fatigue.

Physical Examination

The physical examination begins with a general examination of overall health and condition. Clients with respiratory problems may show signs of shortness of breath when speaking, or they may have a certain posture or position to facilitate breathing. Other observations include skin color; level of consciousness; mental status; respiratory rate, depth, effort, and rhythm; use of accessory muscles; and shape of the chest and symmetry of chest movements. Extremities are assessed for finger clubbing, a condition in which the tips of the fingers or toes are enlarged because the soft tissue beneath the nail beds is increased. Although it is not always clear why this occurs, it may be related to levels of proteins that stimulate blood vessel growth or to genetic factors. Finger clubbing seems to occur with some lung diseases such as lung cancer but not with others such as asthma; it can also occur with congenital heart, liver, and thyroid diseases.

The nurse inspects the nose for signs of injury, inflammation, symmetry, and lesions and examines the posterior pharynx and tonsils with a tongue blade and light. Nursing notes document any evidence of swelling, inflammation, or exudate; changes in the color of the mucous membranes; and any difficulty with swallowing or hoarseness.

A health care provider inspects the larynx either directly with a laryngoscope or indirectly with a light and laryngeal mirror. Both procedures require a local anesthetic to suppress the gag reflex and reduce discomfort.

The nurse inspects and gently palpates the trachea to assess for placement and deviation from the midline, noting any lymph node enlargement. The nurse also examines the anterior, posterior, and lateral chest walls for lesions, symmetry, deformities, skin color, and evidence of muscle weakness or weight loss. Checking the contour of the chest walls is important. Normally, the anteroposterior diameter of the chest wall is half the transverse diameter; however, some pulmonary conditions (e.g., emphysema) change the chest dimensions.

An experienced nurse palpates the chest wall to detect tenderness, masses, swelling, or other abnormalities (Table 19-5). Tactile or vocal *fremitus* (vibrations from the client's voice transmitted to the examiner's fingers) depends on the capacity to feel sound through the fingers and palm placed on the chest wall. The palpable vibrations occur when the client speaks. The examiner uses the palmar surfaces of the fingers and hands to palpate and asks the client to repeat "99" as the examiner moves their hands. If the client is healthy and thin, the fremitus will be highly palpable. Conditions that affect fremitus include a thick or muscular chest wall (decreased fremitus); lung diseases such as emphysema and pneumonia (increased fremitus); and fluid, air, or masses in the pleural space (decreased fremitus).

The experienced nurse performs percussion of the chest wall to assess normal and abnormal sounds. With the client sitting, the examiner places their middle finger on the chest wall and taps that finger with the middle finger of the opposite hand. Table 19-6 describes the types of sounds heard with percussion.

The experienced nurse auscultates breath sounds from side to side, moving from the upper to the lower chest (Fig. 19-5). They listen anteriorly, laterally, and posteriorly. Normal breath sounds include the following:

- *Vesicular sounds*: Produced by air movement in bronchioles and alveoli, these sounds are heard over the lung fields; they are quiet and low pitched, with long inspiration and short expiration.
- *Bronchial sounds*: Produced by air movement through the trachea, these sounds are heard over the trachea and are loud with long expiration.
- *Bronchovesicular sounds*: These normal breath sounds are heard between the trachea and upper lungs; pitch is medium with equal inspiration and expiration.

BOX 19-1 Questions for the Client With Dyspnea

- What makes you short of breath?
- Do you cough when you are short of breath?
- Do you have other symptoms when you are short of breath?
- Do you get short of breath suddenly or gradually?
- When do you usually have difficulty breathing?
- Can you lie flat in bed?
- Do you get short of breath when you rest? With exercise? Running? Climbing stairs?
- How far can you walk before you get short of breath?
- How severe is the shortness of breath? On a scale of 1 to 10 (1 is not breathless at all and 10 is very breathless), how hard is it to breathe?

TABLE 19-5 Common Abnormalities of the Chest

CONTROL	DESCRIPTION
Kyphosis	Exaggerated curvature of the thoracic spine; congenital anomaly or associated with injuries and osteoporosis
Scoliosis	Lateral S-shaped curvature of the thoracic and lumbar spine
Barrel chest	Anteroposterior diameter increases to equal the transverse diameter; chest is rounded; ribs are horizontal; sternum is pulled forward; associated with emphysema and aging
Funnel chest	Also known as *pectus excavatum*; the sternum is depressed from the second intercostal space—more pronounced with inspiration; a congenital anomaly
Pigeon chest	Also known as *pectus carinatum*; the sternum abnormally protrudes; the ribs are sloped backward; a congenital anomaly

TABLE 19-6 Sounds Heard With Chest Wall Percussion

SOUND	DESCRIPTION	IMPLICATIONS
Flat	High pitch, little intensity, decreased duration	Heard during percussion of a solid area, such as a mass or pleural effusion
Dull	Medium pitch, medium intensity, medium duration	Heard when no air or fluid is in the lung (e.g., atelectasis, lobar pneumonia)
Tympanic	High pitch, loud intensity, long duration	Normal sounds heard over stomach and bowel; abnormal sounds heard over lungs, such as in a pneumothorax
Resonant	Low pitch, loud intensity, long duration	Normal lung sounds
Hyperresonant	Lower pitch, very loud, longer duration	Abnormal sounds that occur when free air exists in the thoracic cavity (e.g., emphysema, pneumothorax)

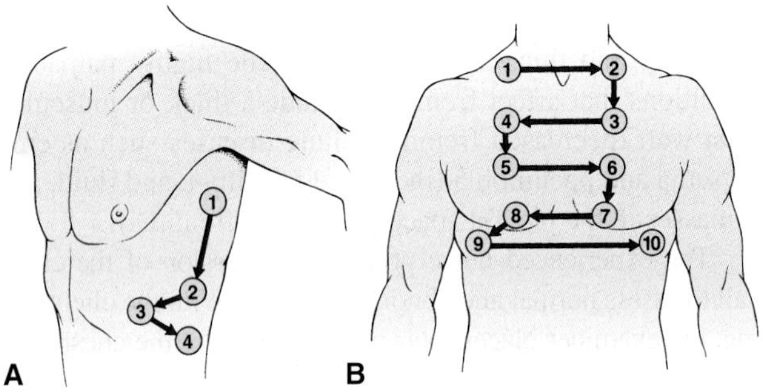

Figure 19-5 (A) Each side of the chest is auscultated and compared. **(B)** The anterior chest is systematically examined over each lung field.

Adventitious or abnormal breath sounds are categorized as crackles or wheezes. *Crackles* (formerly called *rales*) are discrete sounds that result from the delayed opening of deflated airways. They resemble static or the sound made by rubbing hair strands together near one's ear. Sometimes they clear with coughing. They may be present because of inflammation or congestion. Crackles that do not clear with coughing may indicate pulmonary edema or fluid in the alveoli. Wheezes may be sibilant (hissing or whistling) or sonorous (full and deep). Sibilant wheezes (formerly called wheezes) are continuous musical sounds that can be heard during inspiration and expiration. They result from air passing through narrowed or partially obstructed air passages and are heard in clients with increased secretions. Sonorous wheezes (formerly called rhonchi) are lower pitched and are heard in the trachea and bronchi. Friction rubs are heard as crackling or grating sounds on inspiration or expiration. They occur when the pleural surfaces are inflamed and do not change if the client coughs.

Diagnostic Tests

Arterial Blood Gases

Oxygenation of body tissues depends on the amount of oxygen in arterial blood. Arterial blood gases (ABGs) determine the blood's pH; oxygen-carrying capacity; and levels of oxygen, CO_2, and HCO_3^-. Blood gas samples are obtained through an arterial puncture at the radial, brachial, or femoral artery. A client also may have an indwelling arterial catheter from which arterial samples are obtained. If an arterial blood sample cannot be obtained, a mixed venous sample will be used, adjusting for normal values for mixed venous blood.

ABGs frequently are ordered when a client is acutely ill or has a history of respiratory disorders. If the partial pressure of oxygen in arterial blood (PaO_2) is decreased, body tissues do not receive sufficient oxygen. Table 19-7 presents the descriptions and measures of normal ABGs, both arterial and mixed venous.

Clients with respiratory disorders can neither get oxygen into the blood nor get CO_2 out of the blood. Some conditions that affect ABGs are as follows:

- Hyperventilation during collection of ABGs, causing elevated PaO_2
- Hypoventilation with neuromuscular disease, chronic obstructive pulmonary disease (COPD), or insufficient oxygen in the atmosphere, causing decreased PaO_2
- Elevated $PaCO_2$ in clients with COPD, inadequate ventilation with a mechanical ventilator, or decreased respiratory rates
- Decreased $PaCO_2$ in clients who are nervous or anxious or have a condition that causes hyperventilation or a rapid respiratory rate

TABLE 19-7 Normal Values for Arterial Blood Gases

PARAMETERS	NORMAL VALUES ARTERIAL BLOOD	NORMAL VALUES MIXED VENOUS BLOOD
pH, hydrogen ion concentration, acidity or alkalinity of the blood	7.35–7.45	7.32–7.42
PaO_2,[a] partial pressure of oxygen in arterial blood	80–100 mm Hg	38–52 mm Hg
$PaCO_2$, partial pressure of carbon dioxide in arterial blood	35–45 mm Hg	24–48 mm Hg
HCO_3^-, bicarbonate ion concentration in the blood	22–26 mEq/L	19–25 mEq/L
SaO_2%, arterial oxygen saturation or percentage of the oxygen-carrying capacity of the blood	>94%	65%–75%

[a]At altitudes of 1000 feet and higher, age dependent
Adapted from Fischbach, F., & Fischbach, M. (2019). *A manual of laboratory tests and diagnostic tests* (10th ed.). Wolters Kluwer.

NURSING GUIDELINES 19-1

Performing Pulse Oximetry

- Explain the procedure to the client.
- Assess potential sensor sites for quality of circulation, edema, tremor, restlessness, nail polish, or artificial nails.
- Review the medical history for data indicating vascular or other pathology (e.g., anemia, carbon monoxide poisoning).
- Check prescribed medications for vasoconstrictive effects.
- Assess the client's understanding of pulse oximetry.
- Position the sensor so that the light emission is directly opposite the detector.
- Observe the numeric display, audible sound, or waveform on the oximeter.
- Set the high and low alarms according to the manufacturer's directions.

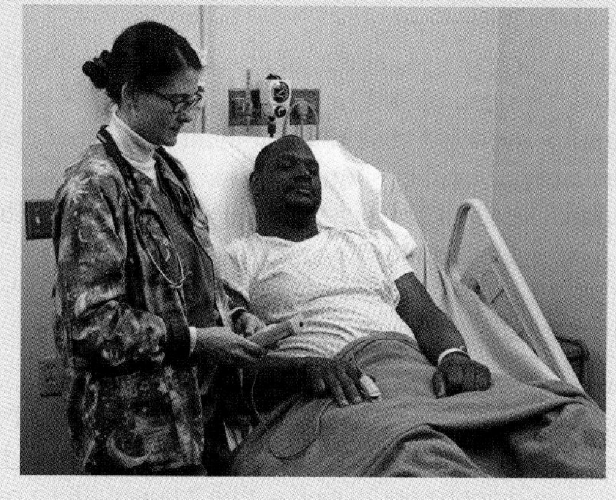

Portable pulse oximetry unit, used to measure oxygen saturation (SpO_2) of arterial blood.

Pulse oximetry is a noninvasive method that uses a light beam to measure the oxygen content of hemoglobin (arterial oxygen saturation [SaO_2]). The monitoring device attaches to the client's earlobe or fingertip and connects to the oximeter monitor. The monitor registers wavelengths of light passing through the earlobe or fingertip and uses them to calculate the SaO_2. Normal values are 94% or higher (Nursing Guidelines 19-1).

Pulmonary Function Studies

Pulmonary function studies measure the functional ability of the lungs. These studies are done to diagnose pulmonary conditions and to assess preoperative respiratory status (Evidence-Based Practice 19-1). They also may be used to determine the effectiveness of bronchodilators or to screen employees who work in environments that are hazardous to pulmonary health. Measurements of pulmonary function are obtained with a spirometer and include the following:

- Tidal volume: volume of air inhaled and exhaled with a normal breath
- Inspiratory reserve volume: maximum volume of air that normally can be inspired
- Expiratory reserve volume: maximum volume of air that normally can be exhaled by forced expiration

Evidence-Based Practice 19-1

Technology and Client Assessment

Clinical Question

Does technology interfere with a thorough client assessment in nursing?

Evidence

A small research study involving 10 nurses in New Zealand investigated the effects of technology and nursing assessments through interviews (Ansell, Meyer, & Thompson, 2015). The data resulted in three findings: impacts that technology has on assessments, how early warning signs (EWS) are affected with technology, and nurse autonomy. It was reported through interviews of nurses that technology for vital signs does not include the respiratory rate and must be done by hand. The nurses admitted that sometimes the respiratory rate is only recorded when the nurse deems it important and takes the time to manually take it. Others reported seeing documentation of respiratory rates, but noted that the nurse did not have a watch or clock to take the rate properly, and therefore documentation may be false. The study reported that some hospitals used EWS-type system trackers and score systems that would help nurses identify when clients started deteriorating quickly.

The data revealed that facilities using an EWS scoring system had improvements in recording respiratory rates; however, some nurses felt it did not help nurses understand the reason for actually taking the rate and recording it. Lastly, the data showed that while nurses included autonomy and accountability in their practice by recording the respiratory rate, they did not always understand the *why* part of the process. Understanding a practice is also part of accountability to practice. As the aging population increases with more complex health problems, technology and time-saving tools can help nurses with time management. However, nurses are still accountable for assessment and client safety.

Nursing Implications

Nurses are legally accountable to clients and their safety. Part of a registered nurse's practice includes assessment. As new nurses gain experience, good assessment skills are needed to prepare for clients in deteriorating situations. Embracing technology and innovation will help professionals grow; however, time for crucial assessments must still be addressed.

Reference

Ansell, H., Meyer, A., & Thompson, S. (2015). Technology and the issues facing nursing assessment. *British Journal of Nursing, 24*(17), 886–889. https://doi.org/10.12968/bjon.2015.24.17.886

- Residual volume: volume of air left in the lungs after maximal expiration
- Vital capacity: maximum amount of air that can be expired after maximal inspiration
- Forced vital capacity: amount of air exhaled forcefully and rapidly after maximal inspiration
- Inspiratory capacity: maximum amount of air that can be inhaled after normal expiration
- Functional residual capacity: amount of air left in the lungs after a normal expiration
- Total lung capacity: total volume of air in the lungs when maximally inflated

Pulmonary function results vary according to age, sex, weight, and height. The maximum lung capacities and volumes are best achieved when the client is sitting or standing. The test should not be performed within 2 hours after a meal. The nurse explains the procedure to the client and instructs them to wear loose-fitting clothing. A nose clip prevents air from escaping through the client's nose when blowing into the spirometer. Bronchodilators may be used after the initial spirometry to see if there is any improvement or response with the inhaled medication. Although the test is simple, the client may be tired afterward.

Sputum Studies

Sputum specimens are examined for pathogenic microorganisms and cancer cells. Culture and sensitivity tests are done to diagnose infections and prescribe antibiotics. Negative results on the examination of sputum smears do not always indicate the absence of disease, so collection of sputum for successive days may be necessary. Sputum is collected by having the client expectorate a specimen (Nursing Guidelines 19-2), by suctioning the client, or during a bronchoscopy (see later discussion).

Imaging Studies

Chest X-rays show the size, shape, and position of the lungs and other structures of the thorax. Their purpose is to screen for asymptomatic disease and diagnose tumors, foreign bodies, and other abnormal conditions. Fluoroscopy enables the primary provider to view the thoracic cavity with all its contents in motion. It more precisely diagnoses the location of a tumor or lesion. Computed tomography scanning or magnetic resonance imaging may be used to produce axial views of the lungs to detect tumors and other lung disorders during the early stages.

Pulmonary Angiography

Pulmonary angiography is a radioisotope study that allows the primary provider to assess the arterial circulation of the lungs, particularly to detect pulmonary emboli or any abnormalities. A catheter is introduced into an arm vein and threaded through the right atrium and ventricle into the pulmonary artery. Contrast medium is rapidly injected into the femoral artery, and X-rays are taken to see the distribution of the radiopaque material.

During pulmonary angiography, the nurse obtains data about the client's level of anxiety and knowledge of the procedure. The nurse provides explanations and reinforces the client's understanding. The client will experience a feeling of pressure on catheter insertion. When the contrast medium is infused, the client will sense a warm, flushed feeling and an urge to cough.

The nurse must determine if the client has any allergies, particularly to iodine, shellfish, or contrast dye. During the procedure, the nurse monitors for signs and symptoms of allergic reactions to the contrast medium, such as itching, hives, or difficulty breathing. Infusion of contrast dye is discontinued immediately if the client has an allergic reaction.

After the procedure, the nurse inspects the puncture site for swelling, discoloration, bleeding, or hematoma. The nurse assesses distal circulation and sensation to ensure that circulation is unimpaired. If bleeding occurs, pressure must be applied to the site. The nurse must notify the primary provider about diminished or absent distal pulses, cool skin temperature in the affected limb, poor capillary refill, client complaints of numbness or tingling, and bleeding or hematoma. The client remains on bed rest for 2 to 6 hours after the procedure. The pressure dressing, applied after the catheter is removed, remains in place for this period.

Lung Scans

Several types of lung scans may be done for diagnostic purposes: the ventilation-perfusion scan, referred to as a *V-Q scan*; the gallium scan; or the positron emission tomography (PET) scan. The V-Q scan requires the use of radioisotopes and a scanning machine to detect patterns of blood flow through the lungs and patterns of air movement and distribution in the lungs. V-Q scans are particularly useful in diagnosing pulmonary emboli. They are also used to diagnose lung cancer, COPD, and pulmonary edema.

A radioactive contrast medium is administered intravenously for the *perfusion scan* and by inhalation as a radioactive gas for the *ventilation scan*. Before the perfusion scan, nurses must assess the client for allergies to iodine. During the procedure, the radiologist asks the client to change positions. During inhalation, the client may need to hold their breath for short periods as scanning images are obtained. The client must receive adequate explanations before the procedure to reduce anxiety. The nurse must reassure the client that the amount of radiation from this procedure is less than that used during a chest X-ray.

NURSING GUIDELINES 19-2

Collecting a Sputum Specimen

- Explain the procedure to the client.
- Collect a sputum specimen early in the morning or after an aerosol treatment.
- Collect the specimen in a sterile specimen container.
- Instruct the client to rinse the mouth with tap water.
- Instruct the client to take several deep breaths, cough forcefully, and expectorate into the container.
- Collect at least 1 to 3 mL (½ teaspoon).
- Deliver the specimen to the laboratory as soon as possible. The container should be transported in a sealed plastic bag with the appropriate requisition.

A *gallium scan* is used to determine if any inflammatory conditions exist within the lungs or if abscesses, adhesions, or tumors are present. Clients receive an intravenous injection of gallium, a radioisotope, and then have scans taken at various intervals up to 48 hours after the gallium injection. The scan shows gallium uptake by the lung tissues.

A *PET scan* also uses radioisotopes with advanced technology that allows the examiner to differentiate normal and abnormal tissue and view metabolic changes within the lung tissue. This scan can evaluate malignancies by showing blood flow and other functioning of organs and tissues.

Bronchoscopy

Bronchoscopy is used to diagnose, treat, or evaluate lung disease; obtain a biopsy of a lesion or tumor; obtain a sputum specimen; perform aggressive pulmonary cleansing; or remove a foreign body. Bronchoscopy allows for direct visualization of the larynx, trachea, and bronchi. Fiberoptic bronchoscopy uses a flexible fiberoptic bronchoscope, which allows for more thorough visualization of the smaller and more peripheral airways. The primary provider introduces the bronchoscope through the nose or mouth or through a tracheostomy or artificial airway. Rigid bronchoscopy uses a hollow metal tube with a light at the end for removing foreign bodies or diseased tissue or visualizing sources of massive bleeding. Figure 19-6 depicts fiberoptic and rigid bronchoscopy.

Bronchoscopy is very frightening to clients, who require thorough explanations throughout the procedure. For at least 6 hours before the bronchoscopy, the client must abstain from food or drink to decrease the risk of aspiration. Risk is increased because the client receives local anesthesia, which suppresses the swallow, cough, and gag reflexes.

The client receives medications before the procedure—usually atropine to dry secretions and a sedative or narcotic to depress the vagus nerve. This consideration is important because if the vagus nerve is stimulated during the bronchoscopy, hypotension, bradycardia, or arrhythmias may occur. Other potential complications include bronchospasm or laryngospasm secondary to edema, hypoxemia, bleeding, perforation, aspiration, cardiac arrhythmias, and infection. Nursing Care Plan 19-1 provides more information about nursing care.

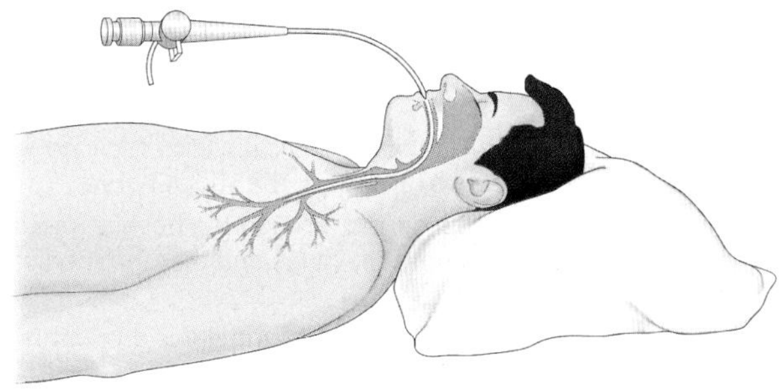

Fiberoptic bronchoscopy

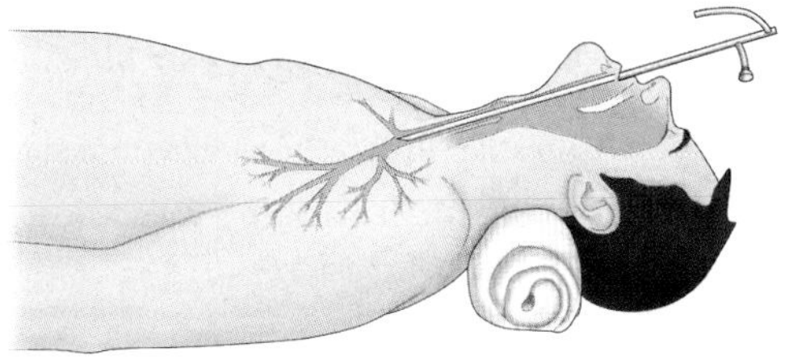

Rigid bronchoscopy

Figure 19-6 Endoscopic bronchoscopy permits visualization of bronchial structures. The bronchoscope is advanced into bronchial structures orally. Bronchoscopy permits the clinician not only to diagnose but also to treat various lung problems. (Reprinted with permission from Hinkle, J. L., & Cheever, K. H. (2014). *Brunner & Suddarth's textbook of medical-surgical nursing* (13th ed.). Wolters Kluwer Health/Lippincott Williams & Wilkins.)

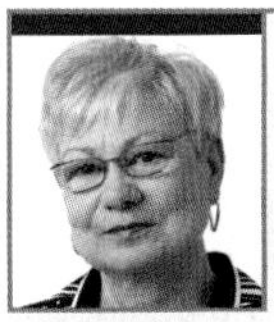

Clinical Scenario A 64-year-old client tells the nurse that she has been experiencing increased shortness of breath with frequent cough over the last 16 hours. She is 6 days postoperative for abdominal surgery. Other tests have been inconclusive, and the primary provider has ordered a bronchoscopy. **What are important considerations for the nurse when caring for a client who is having a diagnostic bronchoscopy? See Nursing Care Plan 19-1.**

NURSING CARE PLAN 19-1 The Client Undergoing a Bronchoscopy

Assessment

- Assess level of anxiety and understanding of the procedure.
- Obtain baseline vital signs.
- Assess lung sounds.
- Ask client if they wear dentures and when they last ate or drank.
- Check record to ensure that the consent form is signed and witnessed.

Nursing Diagnosis. **Fear** related to lack of knowledge about what to expect during and after procedure

Expected Outcome. Client will exhibit coping behaviors and follow instructions.

Interventions	Rationales
Acknowledge client's fear.	*Validating fear communicates acceptance.* *Acknowledging misconceptions provides a starting point.*
Provide simple explanations about the procedure after determining what the client knows and their misconceptions.	*Adults learn more readily when teaching is based on their previous knowledge and experience. Understanding helps to alleviate fear.*

(*continued*)

NURSING CARE PLAN 19-1 The Client Undergoing a Bronchoscopy (*continued*)

Inform client that they will receive medications to alleviate anxiety, reduce secretions, and block the vagus nerve.	*Information reduces fear and anxiety.*
Explain that a tube will be inserted through the nose or mouth and down the throat and into the lungs and that the medication will assist the client.	*Thorough explanations reinforce understanding and reduce fear.*
Tell client that after the procedure, food and fluids are withheld until the cough reflex returns.	*Preoperative sedation and local anesthesia impair the cough reflex and swallowing for several hours.*
Inform client that the throat will be irritated and sore for a few days and that they may cough up blood-tinged mucus.	*Knowledge about expected signs and symptoms reduces fear after the procedure.*

Evaluation of Expected Outcome

Client tolerates procedure without untoward effects, follows instructions, and states that fear is minimal.

Nursing Diagnosis. **Aspiration Risk** related to diminished gag reflex

Expected Outcomes. (1) Client will maintain a patent airway. (2) Risk of aspiration will decrease.

Interventions	Rationales
Assess cough and gag reflexes.	*Depressed cough or gag reflex increases risk of aspiration.*
Keep client NPO until the gag reflex returns (usually 2–8 hours).	*NPO status reduces the risk of aspiration.*
Keep suction equipment available.	*If the client aspirates, suctioning helps to maintain a patent airway.*
Place client in semi-Fowler's position with the head to one side.	*Proper positioning decreases the risk of aspiration.*
Encourage client to expectorate secretions frequently into an emesis basin.	*Expectoration reduces the risk of aspiration.*
After the gag reflex returns, offer sips of water or ice chips initially, then progress the diet to soft foods.	*Beginning with sips of water or ice chips ensures that the gag reflex has returned. The client can most easily swallow soft foods.*

Evaluation of Expected Outcomes

Airway remains patent. Client does not experience aspiration.

Nursing Diagnosis. **Risk for Pneumothorax, arrhythmia, and bronchospasm**

Expected Outcome. The nurse will manage and minimize potential complications.

Interventions	Rationales
Monitor vital signs and respiratory status, comparing against baseline assessment data.	*Comparison helps the nurse determine if the client is experiencing any respiratory distress.*
Observe for symmetric chest movements.	*Decreased or asymmetric chest expansion is a sign of pneumothorax.*
Report hemoptysis, stridor, or dyspnea immediately.	*These findings indicate respiratory distress and probable pneumothorax.*

Evaluation of Expected Outcome

Client experiences no postprocedure complications.

Laryngoscopy

Laryngoscopy provides direct visualization of the larynx using a laryngoscope. It is done to diagnose lesions, evaluate laryngeal function, and determine any inflammation. Primary providers also may dilate laryngeal strictures and biopsy lesions. Refer to the preceding section on bronchoscopy and to Nursing Care Plan 19-1 for more information.

Mediastinoscopy

Mediastinoscopy provides visualization of the mediastinum and is done under local or general anesthesia. The primary provider makes an incision above the sternum and inserts a mediastinoscope. With this procedure, the primary provider can visualize lymph nodes and obtain biopsy samples. Possible complications include arrhythmias, myocardial infarction, pneumothorax, and bleeding.

Thoracoscopy

Thoracoscopy allows for examination of the pleural cavity. Small incisions are made into the pleural cavity through an intercostal space. An endoscope is inserted to visualize a specific area (Fig. 19-7). The location selected is based on other clinical and diagnostic findings. If fluid is present, the examiner aspirates it and sends it for culture and cellular studies. Biopsies also may be done. A chest tube may be inserted following the procedure (see Chapter 21). Thoracoscopy is done to evaluate pleural effusions and pleural diseases and for staging of tumors. Future potential exists

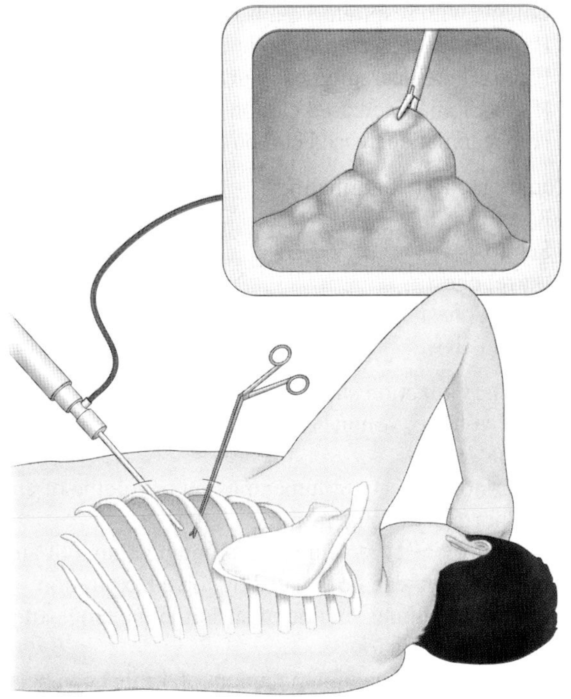

Figure 19-7 Endoscopic thoracoscopy. Like bronchoscopy, thoracoscopy uses fiberoptic instruments and video cameras to visualize thoracic structures. Unlike bronchoscopy, thoracoscopy usually requires the surgeon to make a small incision before inserting the endoscope. Thoracoscopy is used to excise tissue for biopsy, evaluate pleural disease, and stage tumor.

for laser treatment of pulmonary nodules and other growths. This technique is less invasive than thoracotomy procedures (see Chapter 21).

Thoracentesis

A small amount of fluid lies between the visceral and parietal pleurae. When excess fluid or air accumulates, the primary provider aspirates it from the pleural space by inserting a needle into the chest wall. This procedure, called **thoracentesis**, is performed with local anesthesia. Thoracentesis also may be used to obtain a sample of pleural fluid or a biopsy specimen from the pleural wall for diagnostic purposes, such as a culture and sensitivity or microscopic examination. Bloody fluid usually suggests trauma. Purulent fluid is diagnostic for infection. Serous fluid may be associated with cancer, inflammatory conditions, or heart failure. When thoracentesis is done for therapeutic reasons, 1 to 2 L of fluid may be withdrawn to relieve respiratory distress. Medication may be instilled directly into the pleural space to treat infection.

Thoracentesis is done at the bedside or in a treatment or examining room. The client either sits at the side of the bed or examining table or is in a side-lying position on the unaffected side. If the client is sitting, a pillow is placed on a bedside table, and the client rests their arms and head on the pillow. The primary provider determines the site for aspiration by radiography and percussion. The site is cleaned and anesthetized with local anesthesia. A needle or small tube is inserted between the ribs and into the pleural space to withdraw fluid. When the procedure is complete, a small pressure dressing is applied. The client remains on bed rest and usually lies on the unaffected side for at least 1 hour to promote expansion of the lung on the affected side. A chest X-ray is done after the procedure to rule out a pneumothorax (also called collapsed lung; see Chapter 21). Complications that can follow a thoracentesis are pneumothorax, subcutaneous emphysema (air in subcutaneous tissue), infection, pulmonary edema, and cardiac distress. Nursing Guidelines 19-3 outlines the nurse's role in assisting with thoracentesis.

NURSING GUIDELINES 19-3

Assisting With Thoracentesis

- Explain the procedure to the client.
- Reassure the client that they will receive local anesthesia. Explain that the client will still experience a pressure-like pain when the needle pierces the pleura and when fluid is withdrawn.
- Assist client to an appropriate position (sitting with arms and head on padded table or in side-lying position on unaffected side).
- Instruct client not to move during the procedure, including no coughing or deep breathing.
- Provide comfort.
- Inform client about what is happening.
- Maintain asepsis.
- Monitor vital signs during the procedure—also monitor pulse oximetry if client is connected to it.
- During removal of fluid, monitor for respiratory distress, dyspnea, tachypnea, or hypotension.
- Apply small sterile pressure dressing to the site after the procedure.
- Position client on the unaffected side. Instruct client to stay in this position for at least 1 hour and to remain on bed rest for several hours.
- Check that a chest X-ray is done after the procedure.
- Record the amount, color, and other characteristics of fluid removed.
- Monitor for signs of increased respiratory rate, asymmetry in respiratory movement, syncope or vertigo, chest tightness, uncontrolled cough or cough that produces blood-tinged or frothy mucus (or both), tachycardia, and hypoxemia.

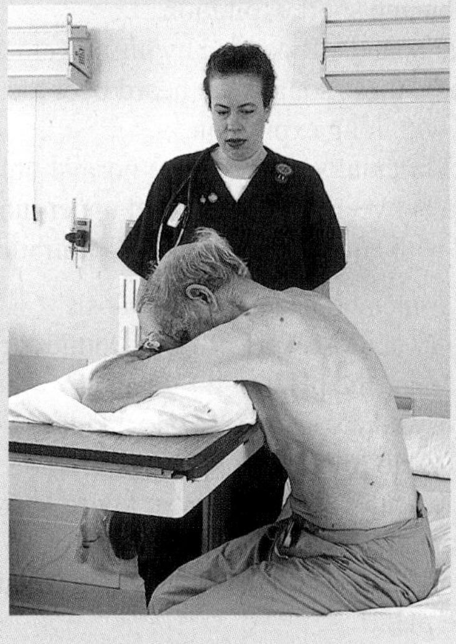

Client positioning for thoracentesis.

NURSING MANAGEMENT

In addition to the nursing management of individual tests, clients require informative and appropriate explanations of any diagnostic procedures they will experience. Nurses must remember that, for many of these clients, breathing may in some way be compromised. Energy levels may be decreased. For that reason, explanations should be brief yet complete and may need to be repeated. The nurse also must help ensure adequate rest periods before and after the procedures. After invasive procedures, the nurse must carefully assess for signs of respiratory distress, chest pain, blood-streaked sputum, and expectoration of blood. The client should be repeatedly informed about postprocedure expectations to help reduce anxiety and ensure the best possible recovery.

››› *Stop, Think, and Respond 19-2*

Why is it important that the client not take deep breaths or cough following a thoracentesis?

KEY POINTS

- Respiration: the exchange of oxygen and CO_2 between the atmospheric air and the blood and between the blood and the cells
- Ventilation: the actual movement of air in and out of the respiratory tract. Air must reach the alveoli for gas to be exchanged.
- Diffusion: the exchange of oxygen and CO_2 through the alveolar capillary membrane
- Perfusion: refers to blood supply to the lungs through which the lungs receive nutrients and oxygen. The two methods of perfusion are the bronchial and pulmonary circulation.
- Normal breath sounds
  - Vesicular sounds: Produced by air movement in bronchioles and alveoli, these sounds are heard over the lung fields; they are quiet and low pitched, with long inspiration and short expiration.
  - Bronchial sounds: Produced by air movement through the trachea, these sounds are heard over the trachea and are loud with long expiration.
  - Bronchovesicular sounds: These normal breath sounds are heard between the trachea and upper lungs; pitch is medium with equal inspiration and expiration.
- Respiratory–metabolic acidosis/alkalosis
  - Respiratory acidosis ($pH < 7.35$): kidneys retain more HCO_3 to raise the pH.
  - Respiratory alkalosis ($pH > 7.45$): kidneys excrete more HCO_3 to lower the pH.
  - Metabolic acidosis ($pH < 7.35$): lungs "blow off" CO_2 to raise the pH.
  - Metabolic alkalosis ($pH > 7.45$): lungs retain CO_2 to lower the pH.
- Problems with respiratory physiology
  - Hypoxia: decreased oxygen in inspired air
  - Hypoxemia: decreased oxygen in the blood
  - Hypercapnia: increased carbon dioxide in the blood
  - Hypocapnia: decreased carbon dioxide in the blood
- Common chest abnormalities
  - Kyphosis
  - Scoliosis
  - Barrel chest
  - Funnel chest
  - Pigeon chest
- Pulmonary function studies
  - Tidal volume: volume of air inhaled and exhaled with a normal breath
  - Inspiratory reserve volume: maximum volume of air that normally can be inspired
  - Expiratory reserve volume: maximum volume of air that normally can be exhaled by forced expiration
  - Residual volume: volume of air left in the lungs after maximal expiration
  - Vital capacity: maximum amount of air that can be expired after maximal inspiration
  - Forced vital capacity: amount of air exhaled forcefully and rapidly after maximal inspiration
  - Inspiratory capacity: maximum amount of air that can be inhaled after normal expiration
  - Functional residual capacity: amount of air left in the lungs after a normal expiration
  - Total lung capacity: total volume of air in the lungs when maximally inflated

CRITICAL THINKING EXERCISES

1. Lung disease can impact a client's quality of life. For what psychosocial issues may the client with lung disease be at risk?
2. Your client had a bronchoscopy and just returned back to your unit. What are the most important assessments that need to be made?
3. There are many respiratory diseases and conditions. What are common signs of respiratory disease?
4. What factors do you think contribute to lung disease?

NCLEX-STYLE REVIEW QUESTIONS PrepU

1. A nurse is auscultating the lung sounds of a client who came to the clinic for a physical examination. There is not any history of lung disease. What should the nurse expect to hear?
   1. Adventitious breath sounds
   2. Bronchial breath sounds
   3. Bronchovesicular breath sounds
   4. Vesicular breath sounds

2. A nurse is caring for a client who complains of shortness of breath and strange breath sounds when inhaling deeply. The nurse notes sibilant wheezes when auscultating the lung fields. Which of the following statements by the nurse is most correct?
   1. "Wheezes result from air between visceral and parietal pleurae."
   2. "Wheezes result from air collecting in the pleural cavity."
   3. "Wheezes result from air escaping through a pneumothorax."
   4. "Wheezes result from air passing through narrowed passages."

3. A nurse needs to obtain a sputum specimen from an adult client. Which nursing action will best facilitate obtaining the specimen?
   1. Ask the client to spit into the collection container.
   2. First have the client take deep breaths.
   3. Restrict the client's fluids for 4 hours.
   4. Wait until after the client has eaten to get the specimen.

4. The nurse is giving instructions to a client having pulmonary angiography. Which of the following statements is the best evidence that the client understands the nurse's instructions about what will take place during the diagnostic procedure? Select all that apply.
   1. "I may feel some pressure at the site."
   2. "I may have bleeding at the site following the procedure."
   3. "I will be able to go to the bathroom when I return from the test."
   4. "I will not be allowed to cough after the procedure."
   5. "I will sense a warm, flushed feeling and an urge to cough when the dye is injected."

5. A nurse, when caring for a client having a lung scan, recognizes that which of the following nursing interventions is most important during the procedure?
   1. Administer sedative or narcotic as per orders before the procedure.
   2. Aid the client to rest arms and head on a pillow during the procedure.
   3. Coach the client to hold their breath at times during the procedure.
   4. Reassure the client about the amount of radiation from the procedure.

20

Caring for Clients With Upper Respiratory Disorders

Words To Know

adenoidectomy
adenoiditis
aphonia
apnea
central sleep apnea
complex sleep apnea
coryza
deviated septum
epistaxis
hemoptysis
hypertrophied turbinates
laryngitis
laryngoscopy
laryngospasm
nasal polyps
obstructive sleep apnea
peritonsillar abscess
pharyngitis
polysomnography
rhinitis
rhinorrhea
sinusitis
stridor
tonsillectomy
tonsillitis
tracheostomy
tracheotomy

Learning Objectives

On completion of this chapter, you will be able to:

1. Describe nursing care for clients experiencing infectious or inflammatory upper respiratory disorders.
2. Discuss assessment data required to provide nursing care to clients with structural disorders of the upper airway.
3. Describe airway problems a client may experience following trauma or obstruction to the upper airway.
4. Identify risk factors that contribute to the development of laryngeal cancer.
5. Identify the earliest symptom of laryngeal cancer.
6. Discuss treatments for laryngeal cancer.
7. Describe measures used to promote alternative methods of communication for clients with a laryngectomy.
8. Discuss psychosocial issues that clients may experience following a laryngectomy.
9. Relate treatment modalities for clients experiencing short-term or long-term problems with airway management.
10. Identify possible reasons for and nursing management of a tracheostomy.
11. Explain why a client may require endotracheal intubation.

Disorders of the upper airway range from common colds to cancer. The severity depends on the nature of the disorder and the client's physiologic response. Most people experience common colds and sore throats and find them more inconvenient than serious. For others, even the most common disorders of the upper respiratory airway are of great concern because other physical problems compound their effects.

Gerontological Considerations

- Upper respiratory infections (URIs), including the common cold, may be potentially serious for older adults, especially when they have other diseases such as a chronic respiratory disorder or heart disease. Teach older adults to see a health care provider if cold symptoms are severe, do not resolve in 7 to 10 days, or if breathing is difficult.
- Teaching for older clients must include potential side effects of over-the-counter (OTC) medications such as antihistamines or cough suppressants. Antihistamines may increase dryness and contribute to confusion or dizziness (which increases fall risks). These OTC medications may

Gerontologic Considerations (continued)

also prevent effective airway clearance by cough production, especially in those who have weakened respiratory musculature. Specifically, pseudoephedrine side effects are potentially serious, and the following should be reported to a health care provider: low blood pressure, heart palpitations or rapid heart rate, chest tightness, confusion, hallucinations, visual changes, seizures, or other signs that could indicate an allergic reaction.

- Older adults must carefully weigh the potential risks and benefits of steroid use. The intended benefit of decreasing inflammation may be warranted in some situations. However, the potential risk of tissue thinning may contribute to gastrointestinal tract bleeding, or prolonged use may be a factor in the development of avascular necrosis of hip joints.
- Large neck circumference, obesity, and other comorbidities experienced by older adults increase the risk for sleep apnea.
- Older adults who experience sleep apnea should be carefully evaluated for fall risks owing to cardiopulmonary changes and the tendency to drift into short frequent daytime naps from which they may have difficulty being aroused.

INFECTIOUS AND INFLAMMATORY DISORDERS

The most common upper airway illnesses are infectious and inflammatory disorders. The average person experiences three to five URIs each year. For some individuals, URIs develop into bronchitis or pneumonia, which involves more serious symptoms and may require antibiotics or other treatments (see Chapter 21).

Rhinitis

Rhinitis is inflammation of the nasal mucous membranes. It is also referred to as the *common cold*, or **coryza**. Rhinitis may be acute, chronic, or allergic, depending on the cause. The most common cause is the rhinovirus, of which more than 100 strains exist. Colds are rapidly spread by inhalation of droplets and direct contact with contaminated articles (e.g., telephone receivers, doorknobs). Allergic rhinitis is a hypersensitive reaction to allergens, such as pollen, dust, animal dander, or food. Rhinitis is usually not a serious condition; however, it may lead to pneumonia and other more serious illnesses for debilitated, immunosuppressed, or older clients.

Symptoms associated with rhinitis include sneezing, nasal congestion, **rhinorrhea** (clear nasal discharge), sore throat, watery eyes, cough, low-grade fever, headache, aching muscles, and malaise. With the common cold, these symptoms continue for 5 to 14 days. A sustained elevated temperature suggests a bacterial infection or infection in the sinuses or ears. Symptoms of allergic rhinitis will persist as long as the client is exposed to the specific allergen.

For most clients, treatment for rhinitis is minimal. Unless specific bacteria are identified as the cause of the infection, antibiotics are not used. Clients may be advised to use antipyretics, such as acetaminophen or nonsteroidal analgesics, for fever. Decongestants such as pseudoephedrine may be recommended for severe nasal congestion. For clients experiencing a prolonged cough, antitussives may be ordered. Saline gargles are useful for a sore throat, as is saline spray for nasal congestion and prevention of crusting. For allergic rhinitis, antihistamines are often used. An example of a first-generation antihistamine is diphenhydramine (Benadryl). Newer antihistamines include loratadine (Claritin), fexofenadine (Allegra), and cetirizine (Zyrtec). Combined decongestants and antihistamines may also be helpful. An example of this is brompheniramine/pseudoephedrine (Dimetapp). Medications that desensitize or suppress immune responses, such as cromolyn (NasalCrom), or intranasal glucocorticosteroids, such as fluticasone (Flonase), may also be prescribed for allergic rhinitis (Drug Therapy Table 20-1).

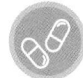

Pharmacologic Considerations

- Encourage clients to read labels carefully.

Second-generation antihistamines have less sedative effect. Antihistamines also dry out mucus, making it thicker and more likely to block nasal passages.

The nurse teaches the client simple measures to treat rhinitis (Client and Family Teaching 20-1). Teaching clients about URIs helps prevent them and minimizes potential complications. Maintaining a healthy lifestyle of adequate rest and sleep, proper diet, and moderate exercise is the best prevention (Nutrition Notes). Another important preventive factor is frequent hand washing, which greatly reduces the spread of infection.

Sinusitis

Sinusitis, also known as rhinosinusitis, is inflammation of the sinuses. It may be classified according to its duration as follows:

- *Acute sinusitis*: generally lasts less than 4 weeks
- *Subacute sinusitis*: does not get better with initial treatment and generally lasts 4 to 8 weeks
- *Chronic sinusitis*: occurs with repeated acute infections or inadequately treated infections—can last more than 12 weeks

Recurrent sinusitis refers to three or more episodes in 1 year. The maxillary sinus is affected most often. Sinusitis can lead to serious complications, such as infection of the middle ear or brain.

Pathophysiology and Etiology

The principal causes are the spread of an infection from the nasal passages to the sinuses and the blockage of normal sinus drainage (Fig. 20-1). The infection can be bacterial or viral, generally occurring after a URI or with allergic rhinitis. Interference with sinus drainage predisposes a client to sinusitis because trapped secretions readily become infected.

DRUG THERAPY TABLE 20-1 Agents to Treat Upper Respiratory Disorders

Category and Common Generic (Brand) Drugs	Intended Use	Common Side Effects	Safety Warnings for Nurses
Antihistamines			
First Generation Brompheniramine (Veltane) Chlorpheniramine (ChlorTrimeton) Clemastine (Dayhist) Diphenhydramine (Benadryl) Promethazine	Temporary relief of sneezing, itchy, watery eyes, and runny nose caused by hay fever or other respiratory allergies and the common cold Antiemetic, hypersensitivity reactions, motion sickness, sedation	Drowsiness, dry mouth, urinary hesitancy	• Increased fall risk due to sedative side effects • Often taken at home, teach to refrain from driving or using dangerous equipment when drowsy
Second Generation Azelastine (Astelin) Bilastine Cetirizine (Zyrtec) Desloratadine (Clarinex) Fexofenadine (Allegra) Loratadine (Claritin)	Seasonal or allergic rhinitis, chronic urticaria	Dizziness, dry mouth, nose, and throat	• Drying effect can potentiate nose bleeds • Contraindicated in clients with certain heart conditions
Decongestants			
Epinephrine (Adrenalin) Oxymetazoline (Zicam) Phenylephrine (Neo-Synephrine) Pseudoephedrine (Sudafed) *Antiinflammatory* Fluticasone (Flonase)	Reduce nasal congestion by vasoconstriction Reduce nasal congestion by reducing inflammation	Anxiety, restlessness, nervousness, dry mouth, nose, and throat Dry mouth, nose, and throat	• Do not use sustained-release products with those under 12 years of age • Interacts with HIV antiretroviral meds • Can limit growth, do not use with children under 4 years of age
Antitussives			
Opioid Antitussives Codeine *Nonopioid Antitussives* Benzonatate (Tessalon) Dextromethorphan (Pertussin) Diphenhydramine (ZzzQuil)	Suppression of nonproductive cough Symptomatic relief of cough	Sedation, dizziness, constipation	• Greater CNS depressant effect if taken with alcohol • Increase fluids and fiber
Expectorants			
Guaifenesin (Mucinex)	Relief of cough associated with respiratory tract infection (sinusitis, asthma, bronchitis, pharyngitis), especially when the cough is dry and nonproductive	Nausea, vomiting, dizziness, headache, rash	

CNS, central nervous system.
The drugs in column 1 indicate the drug that matches up with explanations in columns 2 through 4.

Client and Family Teaching 20-1 Treating Rhinitis

For all types of rhinitis:

- Rest as much as possible.
- Increase fluid intake to assist in liquefying secretions.
- Use a vaporizer to help liquefy secretions.
- Blow nose with mouth open slightly to equalize pressure.
- Wash hands frequently to avoid spreading infection.
- Use OTC medications as directed; be aware of possible side effects, especially interactions with food and alcohol.

For allergic rhinitis:

- Be tested for allergen sensitivity.
- Avoid specific allergens.
- Use antihistamines and decongestants as ordered.

Nutrition Notes

The Client With Rhinitis

There is strong evidence that vitamin C shortens the duration of colds. Consuming at least 200 mg of vitamin C per day did appear to reduce the duration of cold symptoms by an average of 8% in adults and 14% in children (Vitamin C, 2020).

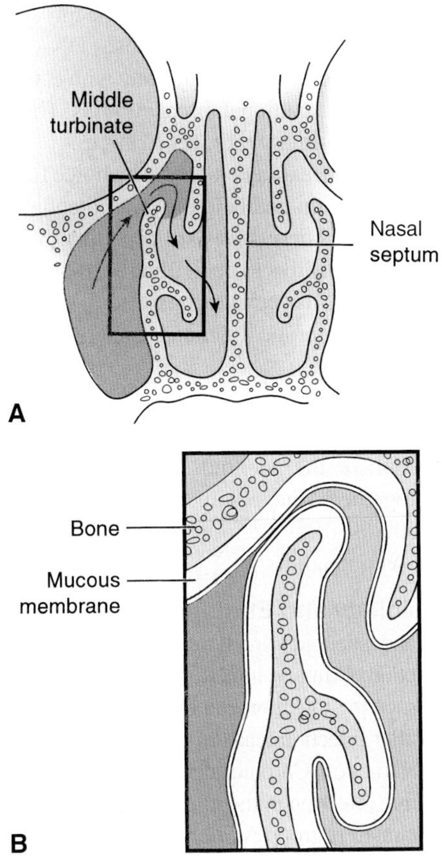

Figure 20-1 Edema can obstruct sinus drainage. **(A)** The maxillary sinuses normally drain through the openings that lie under the middle turbinates. The openings for the drainage are near the upper portion of the sinus. **(B)** Edema, which commonly accompanies upper respiratory infections, can obstruct the openings and prevent normal sinus drainage.

Other conditions that may interfere with sinus drainage include (Lane, n.d.):

- Structural abnormalities, such as nasal polyps or a deviated septum
- Enlarged adenoids
- Diving and swimming
- Tooth infections
- Trauma to the nose
- Foreign objects stuck in the nose
- Secondhand smoke

Measures that help reduce the incidence or severity of sinusitis include eating a well-balanced diet, getting plenty of rest, engaging in moderate exercise, avoiding allergens, and seeking medical attention promptly if a cold persists longer than 10 days or nasal discharge is green or dark yellow and foul smelling.

Assessment Findings

Signs and symptoms depend on which sinus is infected, including headache, fever, pain over the affected sinus, nasal congestion and discharge, postnasal drip causing a cough, pain and pressure around the eyes, and malaise. A nasal smear or material obtained from irrigation of the sinus for culture and sensitivity testing identifies the infectious microorganism and appropriate antibiotic therapy. Transillumination and X-rays of the sinuses may show a change in the shape of or fluid in the sinus cavity. A thorough history, including an allergy history, usually confirms the diagnosis. In some instances, nasal endoscopy may be done and/or imaging studies such as computed tomography (CT) or magnetic resonance imaging (MRI) may be also done.

Medical and Surgical Management

Medical management for acute sinusitis focuses on shrinking the nasal mucosa, relieving pain, and treating infection (Hinkle & Cheever, 2014). Acute sinusitis frequently responds to conservative treatment designed to help overcome the infection. Intranasal saline irrigation or lavage of the maxillary sinus may be done to remove accumulated exudate and promote drainage. Such irrigation is accomplished by insertion of a catheter through the normal opening under the middle concha. Antibiotic therapy is necessary for severe infections, but may not be prescribed for 10 to 14 days if symptoms are not severe. Vasoconstrictors, such as phenylephrine nose drops, may be recommended for short-term use to relieve nasal congestion and aid in sinus drainage. Nasal corticosteroids, such as mometasone (Nasonex), may be ordered for relief of sinus congestion. Nasal saline sprays or oral decongestants may be recommended.

Surgery may be indicated for chronic sinusitis. Functional endoscopic sinus surgery (FESS) helps provide an opening in the inferior meatus to promote drainage. Image-guided endoscopic surgery uses CT scanning with infrared lights to assure that placement of the surgical instruments is accurate and will not endanger the eyes, optic nerve, brain, or major arteries. More radical procedures, such as the Caldwell–Luc procedure and external sphenoethmoidectomy, are done to remove diseased tissue and provide an opening from the maxillary sinus into the inferior meatus of the nose for adequate drainage.

The nurse informs the client receiving medical treatment that the use of mouthwashes and humidification as well as increased fluid intake may loosen secretions and increase comfort. The nurse instructs the client to take nasal decongestants as recommended.

If the client has had sinus surgery, the nurse institutes standards for postoperative care (see Chapter 14) and observes the client for repeated swallowing, a finding that suggests possible hemorrhage. One risk of sinus surgery is damage to the optic nerve. Thus, the nurse assesses postoperative visual acuity by asking the client to identify the number of fingers displayed. The nurse monitors the client's temperature at least every 4 hours, assessing for pain over the involved sinuses, a finding that may indicate postoperative infection or impaired drainage. The nurse administers analgesics as indicated and applies ice compresses to involved sinuses to reduce pain and edema.

The postsurgical client will have nasal packing and a dressing under the nares ("moustache" dressing or "drip pad"). Because nasal packing forces the client to breathe through the mouth, the nurse encourages oral hygiene and gives ice chips or small sips of fluids frequently. Such measures alleviate the dryness caused by mouth breathing. The nurse instructs the client to change the drip pad as needed. In the first 24 hours, the client can expect to change this pad frequently. If bleeding is copious and/or continuous, the doctor must be notified. After 24 hours, the drainage normally decreases significantly. The client needs to report if excessive drainage persists. Postoperative client and family teaching includes telling the client not to blow the nose, lift objects more than 5 to 10 lb, or do the Valsalva maneuver for 10 to 14 days postoperatively. Airline travel must be avoided for 2 weeks. The nurse urges the client to remain in a warm environment and to avoid smoky or poorly ventilated areas.

››› *Stop, Think, and Respond 20-1*

A neighbor tells you that she is taking antibiotics for an acute sinus infection. She states that she has severe pain in her sinuses and wonders what she can do other than take analgesics. What advice might you give?

Pharyngitis

Pharyngitis, inflammation of the throat, is often associated with rhinitis and other URIs (Fig. 20-2). Viruses and bacteria cause pharyngitis. The most serious bacteria are the group A streptococci, which cause a condition commonly referred to as *strep throat*. Strep throat can lead to dangerous cardiac complications (endocarditis and rheumatic fever) and harmful renal complications (glomerulonephritis). Pharyngitis is highly contagious and spreads via inhalation of or direct contamination with droplets.

The incubation period for pharyngitis is 2 to 4 days. The first symptom is a sore throat, sometimes severe, with accompanying *dysphagia* (difficulty swallowing), fever, chills, headache, and malaise. Some clients exhibit a white or exudate patch over the tonsillar area and swollen glands. A throat culture reveals the specific causative bacteria. Rapid antigen tests can detect strep bacteria within minutes by determining that there are foreign substances (antigens) in the throat. If positive, treatment can begin right away. This test is not perfect, however, and may miss some strep infections. In this case, the primary health care provider may rely on the throat culture. In addition, there is a rapid DNA test that uses DNA technology to identify strep bacteria in less than a day with equal accuracy and in less time than traditional throat cultures. These tests are done in clinics and primary provider's offices.

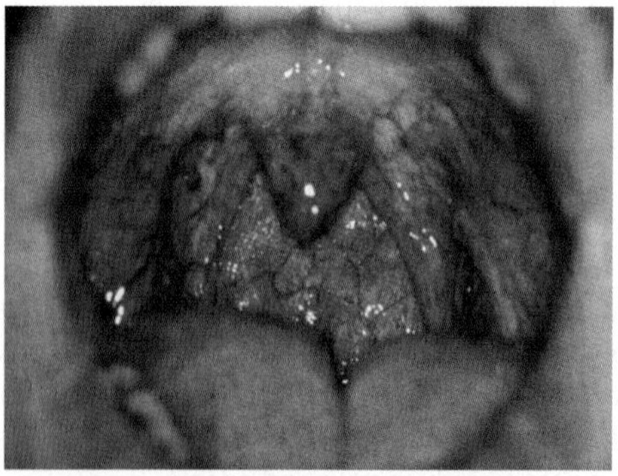

Figure 20-2 Pharyngitis—inflammation without exudate. (Reprinted with permission from Bickley, L. S. (2007). *Bates' guide to physical examination and history taking* (9th ed.). Lippincott Williams & Wilkins.)

Early antibiotic treatment is the best choice for pharyngitis to treat the infection and help prevent potential complications. Penicillin or its derivatives are generally the antibiotics of choice. Clients sensitive to penicillin receive erythromycin, a cephalosporin such as cephalexin (Keflex), or azithromycin (Zithromax). The antibiotic regimen is generally 5 to 14 days.

Tonsillitis and Adenoiditis

Tonsillitis is inflammation of the tonsils, and **adenoiditis** is inflammation of the adenoids. These conditions generally occur together—the common diagnosis is tonsillitis. Although both disorders are more common in children, they may also be seen in adults.

Pathophysiology and Etiology

The tonsils and adenoids are lymphatic tissues and common sites of infection. Primary infection may occur in the tonsils and adenoids, or the infection can be secondary to other URIs. Chronic tonsillar infection leads to enlargement and partial upper airway obstruction. Chronic adenoidal infection can result in acute or chronic infection in the middle ear (otitis media). If the causative organism is group A *Streptococcus*, prompt treatment is needed to prevent potential cardiac and renal complications.

Assessment Findings

Sore throat, difficulty or pain on swallowing, fever, and malaise are the most common symptoms. Enlarged adenoids may produce nasal obstruction, noisy breathing, snoring, and a nasal quality to the voice. Visual examination reveals enlarged and reddened tonsils. White patches may appear on the tonsils if group A streptococci are the cause. A throat culture and sensitivity test determines the causative microorganism and appropriate antibiotic therapy.

Medical and Surgical Management

Antibiotic therapy for bacterial tonsillitis, analgesics such as acetaminophen, and saline gargles may be used to treat the infection and associated discomfort. Chronic tonsillitis and adenoiditis may require **tonsillectomy**, operative removal of the tonsils, and **adenoidectomy**, operative removal of the adenoids. The criteria for performing these procedures are repeated episodes of tonsillitis (usually more than seven in a year or four to five times a year for 2 years in a row or three times a year for 3 years in a row), sleep disorders related to obstructed breathing, hypertrophy of the tonsils, enlarged obstructive adenoids, repeated purulent otitis media, hearing loss related to serous otitis media associated with enlarged tonsils and adenoids, and other conditions (e.g., asthma, rheumatic fever) exacerbated by tonsillitis. Tonsillectomy and adenoidectomy are generally done as outpatient procedures. Recovery time is generally at least 10 days to 2 weeks or longer, especially for adults. (See the "Nursing Process" section for related nursing care of this client.)

››› Stop, Think, and Respond 20-2

What is the most serious complication of a tonsillectomy? Why?

Concept Mastery Alert

Positioning After Tonsillectomy and Adenoidectomy

A standard of care to prevent aspiration for clients entering the postanesthesia care unit (PACU) is to place the client lying on either side with an emesis basin to catch drainage. Positioning the client in a semi-Fowler position is not recommended, as this does not provide an easy exit for secretions because the client is recovering from anesthesia.

Client and Family Teaching 20-2
Tonsillectomy and Adenoidectomy

The nurse ensures that the client and family members can manage self-care at home by communicating the following points:

- Report any signs of bleeding to the primary provider—this is particularly important in the first 12 to 24 hours and then 7 to 10 days after surgery as the throat heals.
- Gently gargle with warm saline or an alkaline mouthwash to assist in removing thick mucus.
- Maintain a liquid and very soft diet for several days after surgery—avoid spicy foods and rough-textured foods.
- Also, avoid milk and milk products if the client does not tolerate them well.

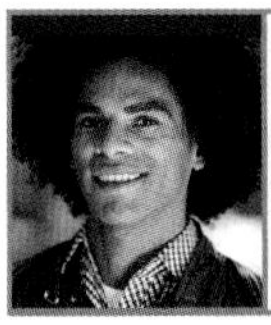

Clinical Scenario Over the past 6 months, a young adult was seen in a clinic with repeated fevers of at least 38.5°C, enlarged and painful lymph nodes in the neck, white patches on the tonsils, and positive strep tests. The client is scheduled for a tonsillectomy today. What are the essential considerations for the nurse in planning for this client's postoperative care? See the following Nursing Process section.

NURSING PROCESS FOR THE CLIENT UNDERGOING TONSILLECTOMY AND ADENOIDECTOMY

Assessment

Assess the client's understanding of the procedure and obtain baseline vital signs. Ask if the client wears dentures and when the client last had food or drink. Pay special attention to laboratory results for hematocrit, platelet count, and clotting time because of the high risk for postoperative hemorrhage. Ask the client about bleeding tendencies and recent use of aspirin, nonsteroidal antiinflammatory drugs (NSAIDs), or other medications that prolong bleeding time. Some herbal supplements such as feverfew or ginkgo may also prolong bleeding, so it is also important to ask about the use of these supplements.

Diagnosis, Planning, and Interventions

Following surgery, implement the postoperative standards described in Chapter 14. Additional nursing care is discussed as follows and in Client and Family Teaching 20-2.

Aspiration Risk: Related to impaired swallowing from throat surgery and reduced gag reflex secondary to anesthesia

Expected Outcomes: (1) Client will maintain a patent airway with clear breath sounds. (2) Client will expectorate secretions and vomitus as needed.

- After surgery, position client, until alert, on either side with emesis basin to catch drainage or vomitus. *Retained secretions/vomitus can obstruct airway and cause aspiration.*
- Assess gag reflex and ability to swallow. *A depressed gag reflex and inability to swallow increase the risk for aspiration.*
- Elevate head of bed 45° when client is fully awake. *This position decreases surgical edema and increases lung expansion.*
- Monitor for respiratory rate, rhythm, and effort at least every hour. *Increased respiratory rate or decreased breath sounds or both indicate an increased respiratory effort, possibly related to a partially obstructed airway or aspiration or both.*
- Auscultate breath sounds for crackles at least every hour. *Aspiration of small amounts may occur without evidence of coughing or respiratory distress.*
- Encourage client to spit secretions/vomitus into the emesis basin. *Removal of secretions/vomitus promotes a clear airway and prevents aspiration.*
- Assess for lethargy, behavior changes, or disorientation. *Decreased level of consciousness indicates poor air exchange.*
- Have oral suction equipment available. *Prompt oral suctioning removes secretions/vomitus from the mouth, preventing aspiration.*

Altered Tissue Integrity Risk: Related to injury to the suture line

Expected Outcome: Client will maintain an intact suture line.

(continued)

NURSING PROCESS FOR THE CLIENT UNDERGOING TONSILLECTOMY AND ADENOIDECTOMY (continued)

- Monitor client for bloody drainage from mouth or frequent swallowing. *These findings indicate increased bleeding from suture site and require immediate attention.*
- Instruct client not to cough, clear throat, blow nose, or use a straw in the first few postoperative days. *These actions increase pressure on the suture line and may cause disruption and bleeding.*
- Instruct client to avoid carbonated fluids and fluids high in citrus content. *Such fluids are caustic to the surgical site and may traumatize tissue, disrupting the suture line.*
- Encourage client to first try ice chips, then small sips of cold fluids, and then popsicles and full liquids as tolerated. Gradual introduction of increasingly thick fluids provides client with an opportunity to slowly try swallowing, without disrupting the suture line.
- Add soft food, such as gelatin and sherbet, as tolerated, after the first 24 hours postoperatively. As the diet advances, small amounts of soft foods are less likely to traumatize the suture line.

Acute Pain: Related to the surgical incision in the throat
Expected Outcome: Client will acknowledge relief from pain medications and demonstrate improved ability to swallow.

- Anticipate the need for pain relief, medicating client as ordered. *Early treatment of pain assists to decrease its intensity.*
- Apply ice collar as ordered. *Cold reduces swelling and inflammation in the soft tissues surrounding the surgical incision. The ice pack will help to control bleeding, reduce edema and inflammation, and block pain receptors.*
- Encourage client to gently gargle with warm saline three to four times daily. *Gentle gargling cleanses the surgical site and helps reduce inflammation and pain, remove thick mucus, and improve swallowing.*

Evaluation of Expected Outcomes

Client maintains a clear airway, can expectorate secretions and vomitus, and experiences minimal postoperative bleeding. The suture line remains intact. Client reports relief of pain and ability to swallow effectively.

Peritonsillar Abscess

A **peritonsillar abscess** is an abscess that develops in the connective tissue between the capsule of the tonsil and the constrictor muscle of the pharynx. It may follow a severe streptococcal or staphylococcal tonsillar infection. Clients with a peritonsillar abscess experience difficulty and pain with swallowing, fever, malaise, ear pain, and difficulty talking. On visual examination, the affected side is red and swollen, as is the posterior pharynx. Drainage from the abscess is cultured to identify the microorganism. Sensitivity studies determine the appropriate antibiotic therapy.

Immediate treatment of a peritonsillar abscess is recommended to prevent the spread of the causative microorganism to the bloodstream or adjacent structures. Penicillin or another antibiotic is given immediately after a culture is obtained and before results of the culture and sensitivity tests are known. Needle aspiration (preferred because it is less invasive and less painful) or surgical incision and drainage of the abscess are done if the abscess partially blocks the oropharynx. A local anesthetic is sprayed or painted on the surface of the abscess, and the contents are evacuated. Repeated episodes may necessitate a tonsillectomy.

Nursing management of the client undergoing needle aspiration or incision and drainage of an abscess includes placing the client in a semi-Fowler position to prevent aspiration. An ice collar may be ordered to reduce swelling and pain. Clients may have topical anesthetic agents and throat irrigations with warm saline or alkaline solutions every 1 to 2 hours. They may also use similar solutions or mouthwash for gentle gargling. The nurse instructs the client to be upright and to expectorate in a forward direction over a sink or basin. The nurse encourages the client to drink fluids that are cool or at room temperature and observes the client for signs of respiratory obstruction (e.g., dyspnea, restlessness, or cyanosis) or excessive bleeding.

Laryngitis

Laryngitis is inflammation and swelling of the mucous membrane that lines the larynx. Edema of the vocal cords frequently accompanies laryngeal inflammation. Laryngitis may follow a URI and results from spread of the infection to the larynx. Other causes include excessive or improper use of the voice, allergies, and smoking.

Hoarseness, inability to speak above a whisper, and/or **aphonia** (complete loss of voice) are the usual symptoms. Clients also complain of throat irritation and a dry, nonproductive cough. The diagnosis is based on the symptoms. If hoarseness persists more than 2 weeks, the larynx is examined (**laryngoscopy**). Persistent hoarseness is a sign of laryngeal cancer and, thus, merits prompt investigation. Treatment involves voice rest and treatment or removal of the cause. Antibiotic therapy may be used if a bacterial infection is the cause. If smoking is the cause, the nurse encourages smoking cessation and refers the client to a smoking-cessation program.

STRUCTURAL DISORDERS

Epistaxis

Pathophysiology and Etiology

Epistaxis, or nosebleed, is a common occurrence. It is usually not serious but can be frightening. Nosebleeds are the rupture of tiny capillaries in the nasal mucous membrane. They occur most commonly in the anterior septum, referred to as *Kiesselbach plexus*. Risk factors associated with nosebleeds include trauma, systemic infections such as rheumatic fever, local infections, dry nasal mucosa, hypertension, use of aspirin, nasal tumors, and blood dyscrasias. Epistaxis that results from hypertension or blood dyscrasias is likely to be severe and difficult to control. Those who abuse cocaine or other inhaled drugs may have frequent nosebleeds. Foreign bodies in the nose and deviated septum contribute to epistaxis, along with forceful nose-blowing and frequent or aggressive nose-picking.

Assessment Findings

Inspection of the nares using a nasal speculum and light reveals the area of bleeding. The examiner uses a tongue blade to check the back of the throat and a laryngeal mirror to view the area above and behind the uvula.

Medical and Surgical Management

The severity and location of the bleeding determine the treatment. One or a combination of the following therapies may be used:

- Direct continuous pressure to the nares for 5 to 10 minutes with the client sitting upright with head tilted forward to prevent swallowing and aspiration of blood
- Application of ice packs to the nose
- Cauterization with silver nitrate, electrocautery, or application of a topical vasoconstrictor such as 1:1000 epinephrine
- Nasal packing with a cotton tampon
- Pressure with a balloon-inflated catheter—inserted posteriorly for a minimum of 48 hours

Nursing Management

The nurse monitors vital signs and assesses for evidence of continued bleeding. The nurse may initiate measures to control bleeding, such as applying pressure and ice packs. Other treatments require a primary provider's order. The client experiencing epistaxis is usually anxious and requires reassurance. If underlying conditions are the cause, the nurse refers the client for medical follow-up. The nurse may also recommend humidification, use of a nasal lubricant to keep the mucous membranes moist, and avoidance of vigorous nose-blowing and nose-picking or other nose trauma. Client and Family Teaching 20-3 outlines teaching about the treatment of severe nosebleed.

Nasal Obstruction

Obstruction of the nasal passage interferes with air passage. Three primary conditions lead to nasal obstruction: a deviated septum, nasal polyps, and hypertrophied turbinates.

Client and Family Teaching 20-3
Epistaxis

The nurse instructs clients experiencing epistaxis to do the following:

- Apply pressure to the nares with two fingers. Breathe through the mouth and sit with the head tipped forward to prevent blood from running down the throat.
- Do not swallow blood; spit out any blood oozing from the area. Do not blow the nose. If blood has been swallowed, the client may see diarrhea and black, tarry stools for a few days.
- Do not attempt to remove nasal packing or to cut the string anchoring the packing.
- Take pain medications as ordered. Do not use aspirin or ibuprofen products until bleeding is controlled.
- Notify the primary provider if bleeding persists or if any respiratory problems develop.

Pathophysiology and Etiology

A **deviated septum** is an irregularity in the septum that results in nasal obstruction. The deviation may be a deflection from the midline in the form of lumps or sharp projections or a curvature in the shape of an "S." Marked deviation can result in complete obstruction of one nostril and interference with sinus drainage. A deviated septum may be congenital, but it often results from trauma.

Nasal polyps are grapelike swellings that arise from the nasal mucous membranes. They probably result from chronic irritation related to infection or allergic rhinitis. They obstruct nasal breathing and sinus drainage, ultimately leading to sinusitis. Most are benign and tend to recur when removed.

Hypertrophied turbinates are enlargements of the nasal conchae, three bones that project from the lateral wall of the nasal cavity. The hypertrophy, which results from chronic rhinitis, interferes with air passage and sinus drainage and eventually leads to sinusitis.

Assessment Findings

Symptoms include a history of sinusitis, difficulty breathing out of one nostril, frequent nosebleeds, and nasal discharge. Clients usually report difficulty breathing through one or both sides of the nose. Inspection with a nasal speculum reveals a left or right deviation of the nasal septum, the number and location of the polyps, or enlarged turbinates.

Medical and Surgical Management

A submucous surgical resection or septoplasty may be necessary to restore normal breathing and to permit adequate sinus drainage for the client with a deviated septum. This procedure involves an incision through the mucous membrane and removal of the portions of the septum that cause obstruction. After this procedure, both sides of the nasal cavity are packed with gauze, which remains in place for 24 to 48 hours. A moustache dressing or drip pad is applied to absorb any drainage.

Rhinoplasty, reconstruction of the nose, may also be done at the same time. This procedure enhances the client's appearance cosmetically and corrects any structural nasal deformities that interfere with air passage. The surgeon makes an incision inside the nostril and restructures the nasal bone and cartilage. As with septoplasty, the nasal cavity is packed with gauze, and the nose is taped. Application of a nasal splint maintains the shape and structure of the nose and reduces edema. The splint remains in place for at least 1 week.

Treatment for polyps includes a steroidal nasal spray to reduce inflammation or direct injection of steroids into the polyps. If nasal obstruction is severe, the surgeon performs a *polypectomy*, the removal of polyps with a nasal snare or laser under local anesthesia. The polyps are examined microscopically to rule out malignant disease.

Hypertrophied turbinates are often treated with the application of astringents or aerosolized corticosteroids to shrink them close to the nose. Occasionally, one of the turbinates may be surgically removed (*turbinectomy*).

Nursing Management

Surgery for correction of nasal obstruction is usually done on an outpatient basis. The nurse provides thorough explanations throughout the procedures to alleviate anxiety. It is particularly important to emphasize that nasal packing will be in place postoperatively, necessitating mouth breathing. The application of an ice pack will reduce pain and swelling.

Placing the client in a semi-Fowler position promotes drainage, reduces edema, and enhances breathing. The nurse inspects the nasal packing and dressings frequently for bleeding and asks the client to report excessive swallowing, which can indicate bleeding. Ongoing monitoring of vital signs is necessary, as is providing oral hygiene and saline mouth rinses (when permitted) to keep mucous membranes moist. The nurse tells the client that feeling or hearing a sucking noise when swallowing is normal and will resolve when the nasal packing is removed. Client and Family Teaching 20-4 lists additional teaching measures.

Client and Family Teaching 20-4
Surgery for Nasal Obstruction

Teaching measures for clients having surgery to relieve nasal obstruction include preparing the postoperative client for edema and discoloration around the eyes and nose that will disappear after a few weeks. The nurse also instructs the client to do the following to prevent bleeding:

- Do not bend over.
- Do not blow nose.
- If sneezing, keep mouth open.
- Avoid contact with nose or surrounding tissue.
- Keep head elevated with an extra pillow when lying down.
- Avoid heavy lifting.
- Do not use aspirin, ibuprofen, alcohol, or tobacco products.

TRAUMA AND OBSTRUCTION OF THE UPPER AIRWAY

Fractures of the Nose

A nasal fracture usually results from direct trauma. It causes swelling and edema of the soft tissues, external and internal bleeding, nasal deformity, and nasal obstruction. In severe nasal fractures, cerebrospinal fluid, which is colorless and clear, may drain from the nares. Drainage of cerebrospinal fluid suggests a fracture in the cribriform plate.

The diagnosis of a nasal fracture may be delayed because of significant swelling and bleeding. As soon as the swelling decreases, the examiner inspects the nose internally to rule out a fracture of the nasal septum or a septal hematoma. Both conditions require treatment to prevent destruction of the septal cartilage. If drainage of clear fluid is observed, a Dextrostix is used to determine the presence of glucose, which is diagnostic for cerebrospinal fluid. Radiography studies are done to ascertain any other facial fractures.

Medical and Surgical Management

If the fracture is a lateral displacement, pressure applied to the convex portion of the nose reduces the fracture. Cold compresses control the bleeding. If the fracture is more complex, surgery is done after the swelling subsides, usually after several days. The surgeon applies a splint postoperatively to maintain the alignment.

Nursing Management

Nursing management is similar to that for nasal obstruction. The nurse instructs the client to keep the head elevated and apply ice four times a day for 20 minutes to reduce the swelling and pain. They give analgesics as ordered to alleviate pain. Postoperatively, the nurse assesses the client for airway obstruction, respiratory difficulty (i.e., tachypnea, dyspnea), dysphagia, signs of infection, pupillary responses, level of consciousness, and periorbital edema. In addition, the nurse helps reduce the client's anxiety by answering questions and offering reassurance that the bruising and swelling will subside and sense of smell will return.

››› *Stop, Think, and Respond 20-3*

On your way to class, you see a woman suddenly slip on ice and fall on her face. As you approach, she gets to a sitting position. She is wearing a scarf. Blood is pouring from her nose, and your initial impression is that the nose appears deformed. What actions should you take?

Laryngeal Trauma and Laryngeal Obstruction

Pathophysiology and Etiology

Laryngeal trauma occurs during motor vehicle accidents when the neck strikes the steering wheel or other blunt trauma occurs in the neck region. Endoscopic and endotracheal intubations are other possible causes. Although uncommon, a fracture of the thyroid cartilage is also traumatic to the larynx.

Laryngeal obstruction is an extremely serious and often life-threatening condition. Some causes of upper airway obstruction include edema from an allergic reaction, severe head and neck injury, severe inflammation and edema of the throat, and aspiration of foreign bodies.

Assessment Findings

Signs and Symptoms

Laryngeal trauma causes neck swelling, bruising, and tenderness. If the tissues surrounding the larynx are greatly swollen, the client will exhibit **stridor**, a high-pitched, harsh sound during respiration, indicative of airway obstruction. The client also has dysphagia, hoarseness, cyanosis, and possible **hemoptysis** (expectoration of bloody sputum).

Total obstruction prevents the passage of air from the upper to the lower respiratory airway; choking clients will clutch their throats—the universal distress sign for choking. Unless total obstruction is relieved immediately, death occurs from respiratory arrest. Partial obstruction results in difficulty breathing.

Diagnostic Findings

Laryngoscopy reveals the extent of trauma and internal swelling. X-rays and oxygenation studies will be performed after a patent airway has been established.

Medical and Surgical Management

Maintenance of a patent airway is crucial. If the client has aspirated a foreign body, abdominal thrusts are initiated to force the object out of the upper respiratory passages (Nursing Guidelines 20-1). Allergic reactions resulting in severe inflammation and edema may be treated with epinephrine or a corticosteroid and, possibly, intubation. Severe obstruction requires an emergency **tracheostomy** (surgical opening into the trachea). See the "Nursing Process for the Client With Laryngeal Obstruction" section for related nursing care of this client.

Obstructive Sleep Apnea

Obstructive sleep apnea (OSA) is characterized by recurrent and frequent episodes of upper airway obstruction and reduced ventilation. **Apnea** (cessation of breathing) occurs as a result of upper airway obstruction, generally when the tongue collapses against the soft palate and, in turn, the soft palate collapses against the back of the throat. **Central sleep apnea** is not a result of obstruction but rather occurs because the brain fails to signal the muscles to breathe. It is not as common and is usually the result of specific medical conditions or medications. **Complex sleep apnea** is a combination of the two conditions. OSA is the most common and is the primary focus for this discussion.

Pathophysiology and Etiology

An estimated 22 million Americans have OSA (Sleep Apnea, 2021), with half of those affected classified as overweight. Sleep apnea affects 24% to 35% of men and 9% to 21% of women. Women are more likely to have sleep apnea after menopause. In general, as people age, they are at higher risk for sleep apnea, with 17% of men and 9% of women aged 50 to 70 years diagnosed with sleep apnea (Rakicevic, 2020). Other factors that may predispose people

NURSING GUIDELINES 20-1

Abdominal Thrusts for Dislodging an Airway Obstruction (Guidelines From the American Heart Association)

(Note: Hands crossed at the neck is the universal sign of choking.)

1. Stand behind the person who is choking.
2. Wrap both arms around the person's waist.
3. Tip the person forward slightly.
4. Grasp one fist with the other hand.
5. Press hard into the abdomen with a quick upward thrust (as if trying to lift the person up).
6. Initially perform five abdominal thrusts, if needed.
7. Continue to perform abdominal thrusts until the obstruction is cleared.
8. If the victim loses consciousness, quickly ease them to the ground.
9. Clear the airway if there is a visible blockage by reaching a hooked finger in the mouth and sweeping the cause of the blockage. Be careful not to push it back deeper into the airway (occurs easily in young children and is not generally advised).
10. Begin cardiopulmonary resuscitation (CPR) if the object remains lodged and the victim does not respond. The chest compressions used in CPR may dislodge the object. Recheck the mouth periodically.

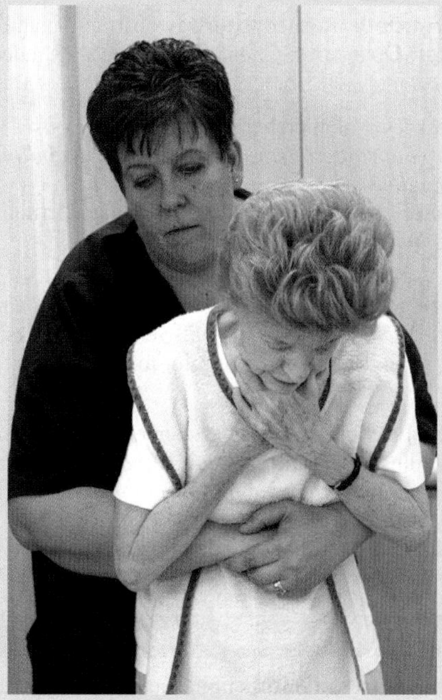

Abdominal thrusts on a conscious victim.

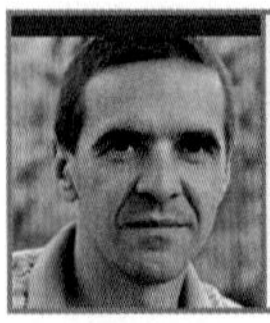

Clinical Scenario A client was seen in a clinic for a diagnostic procedure that required contrast. During the procedure, the client begins to complain of difficulty breathing and a feeling of fullness in the throat. **What actions by the nurse are essential to this client's care? See the following Nursing Process section.**

NURSING PROCESS FOR THE CLIENT WITH LARYNGEAL OBSTRUCTION

Assessment

Assess for air movement within the upper respiratory tract. Listen to lung sounds, monitor respiratory patterns, and look for signs of increased nasal swelling and bleeding and symptoms of laryngeal edema.

Diagnosis, Planning, and Intervention

Partial or total obstruction of the upper airway requires immediate recognition and intervention. When edema is the cause of partial upper airway obstruction, oxygen can be given until a primary provider is available to treat the client. Most likely procedures and protocols are in place to treat this emergency. Emergency drugs and a tracheostomy tray are available for immediate use. Other measures are as follows:

Altered Breathing Pattern: Related to partial obstruction of the upper airway secondary to edema
Expected Outcomes: (1) Client will maintain a patent airway. (2) Client will demonstrate improved breath sounds.

- Assess airway patency frequently until treatment is initiated. *Maintaining the airway is the highest priority.*
- Auscultate lungs for wheezing or decreased or absent breath sounds frequently until treatment is initiated and then as needed to assess client. *Wheezing may indicate increased airway resistance. Decreased or absent breath sounds indicate obstruction.*
- Discontinue administration of contrast agent. *Removing the potential cause of the airway obstruction reduces the client's reaction to the allergen and improves the client's response to treatment.*
- Administer subcutaneous epinephrine and a corticosteroid per orders and/or protocols. *These medications reduce the edema and relieve the obstruction.*
- Assess respiratory effort, including respiratory rate, depth, nasal flaring, and use of accessory muscles. *Increased respiratory effort indicates respiratory difficulties.*
- Assess vital signs and monitor for changes frequently or until the client demonstrates signs of improvement. *Increased work of breathing will increase respiratory rate and heart rate.*
- Monitor arterial blood gases (ABGs). *Increasing $PaCO_2$ and decreasing partial pressure of oxygen (PaO_2) indicate impending respiratory failure.*
- Position client in the semi-Fowler position. *This position promotes maximum lung expansion and improved air exchange.*
- Initiate CPR and prepare for possible airway intubation/tracheostomy if airway is completely obstructed. *Preparation for potential emergency assists to maintain the airway.*

Acute Anxiety: Related to airway obstruction and decreased ability to breathe
Expected Outcome: Client will demonstrate a decreased level of anxiety.

- Assess level of apprehension. *Anxiety increases with respiratory difficulties. Fear can interfere with ability to follow instructions.*
- Monitor for increased respiratory rate and irritability. *These signs indicate increased anxiety.*
- Provide brief explanations. *Increased anxiety impairs ability to focus.*
- Reassure client that they are safe—stay with client. *An anxious client will benefit from the nurse's calm and reassuring presence.*

Knowledge Deficiency: About allergic reaction related to administration of contrast agent
Expected Outcome: Client will verbalize understanding and need to report reaction to contrast agents and the need for alternative tests or prophylactic treatment prior to procedures.

- Teach the client to avoid the source of the allergic reaction by reading labels and asking if certain allergens are included in a treatment or procedure. *Avoiding sources of the allergen prevents future allergic reactions.*
- Explain the nature of the allergic reaction: causes, symptoms, and complications. *Having knowledge of the problem and its potential issues assists the client to avoid the problem and to seek immediate treatment.*
- Teach the client to inform all health care providers of the allergic reaction. *Informing health care providers is key to avoiding future exposure to the allergen or for prophylactic treatment prior to procedures.*

Evaluation of Expected Outcomes

The airway is free of obstruction, and breathing patterns improve. Client reports decreased anxiety and is able to verbalize knowledge and understanding of the allergic reaction, its cause and treatment, and the necessity to avoid future exposure by informing health care providers.

to sleep apnea are race or ethnicity (people who are African American, Hispanic or Latinx ethnicity, or Pacific Islander are more likely to develop sleep apnea), heredity, and having smaller airways, allergies, or other conditions that contribute to increased congestion (National Heart, Lung, and Blood Institute [NHLBI], 2021). Cigarette smokers are at increased risk, as are clients with any condition that reduces pharyngeal muscle tone: neuromuscular disease, use of sedative or hypnotic medications, and frequent and heavy intake of alcohol.

OSA results from a reduced diameter of the upper airway, which may develop when the upper airway collapses secondary to the normally reduced muscle tone during sleep. The repeated apneic spells have serious effects on the cardiopulmonary system. Clients with sleep apnea often have hypertension and are, therefore, at higher risk of cerebrovascular accident and myocardial infarction (MI) as well as heart arrhythmias and heart failure.

Assessment Findings

During sleep, clients with OSA snore loudly, with cessation of breathing for at least 10 seconds. These episodes may occur many times within 1 hour, from as few as 5 to 30 times and up to a total of several hundred per night. Clients awaken suddenly as the PaO_2 level drops, usually with a loud snort. Other symptoms include daytime fatigue, morning headache, inability to concentrate when awake, sore throat, enuresis, and erectile dysfunction. Partners may report that the client behaves differently and is not the same in personality and that the snoring progressively worsens. Box 20-1 reviews symptoms of sleep apnea.

Initial diagnosis is made according to the client's reported symptoms. These include symptoms of sleep apnea, such as loud snoring, gasping or snorting, morning headaches, or unusual tingling sensations or muscle jerking in the extremities. Sleep partners are sometimes better able to answer these questions. Clients may be asked to keep a sleep diary for a few weeks, recording how many hours of sleep a night, number of times waking up during the night and how long it takes to fall asleep, how rested clients feel when they wake up, and if they experience sleepiness during the day.

BOX 20-1 Symptoms of Sleep Apnea

- Loud snoring
- Stop in breathing during sleep (can be reported by another person)
- Gasping for air during sleep
- Awakening with a dry mouth
- Morning headache
- Difficulty staying asleep (insomnia)
- Excessive daytime sleepiness (hypersomnia)
- Difficulty paying attention while awake
- Irritability

From Mayo Clinic. (2021). *Sleep apnea*. https://www.mayoclinic.org/diseases-conditions/sleep-apnea/symptoms-causes/syc-20377631

To determine the nature of the sleep apnea, clients undergo **polysomnography**, which consists of tests that monitor the client's respiratory and cardiac status while asleep. Specifically, a polysomnogram records a client's brain activity, eye movement, muscle movement, respiratory, and heart rates; the amount of air that moves in and out of the lungs; and the oxygen concentration in the blood. Clients stay overnight at a sleep study lab and have electrodes and other monitors placed on their scalps, face, chest, and extremities. If OSA is diagnosed during the first half of the sleep study, clients will be placed on continuous positive airway pressure (CPAP) for the rest of the night to determine whether the sleep patterns improve.

Oximetry may be done to monitor and record oxygen levels while a client sleeps. With OSA, oxygen levels drop during sleep and rise when the client wakens. Health care providers may have clients do portable monitoring at home, which is a home version of polysomnography.

Medical and Surgical Management

Treatment for sleep apnea focuses on improving the quality of nighttime sleep and daytime wakefulness as well as reducing risks for cardiovascular problems. Depending on the severity of sleep apnea, clients may change their lifestyle, to include the following:

- Lose weight
- Exercise regularly
- Quit smoking
- Eliminate alcohol or other medications that depress respirations and contribute to an inability to maintain an open airway
- Use special pillows to keep clients in a side-lying position when sleeping
- Use allergy medications or saline nasal spray to reduce congestion and dryness

Another treatment is fitting the client for an oral appliance that assists in adjusting the lower jaw and tongue so that the airway remains open while the client is sleeping. A dentist or orthodontist fits the client for a custom-made oral appliance.

Additional treatment includes the use of noninvasive positive pressure ventilation (NPPV), which is the application of positive pressure via full-face mask, nasal mask, or cannula with supplemental oxygen to enhance ventilation. There are two commonly used types:

- *CPAP*: provides constant airway pressure during inspiration and expiration
- *Bilevel positive airway pressure (BiPAP)*: provides two levels of pressure: inspiratory and expiratory airway pressures

With this treatment, the client receives airway pressure either through their own inspirations or by machine-initiated inspirations. A set number of breaths are delivered. Clients are often not compliant because they do not like the continuous pressure of CPAP or the varying pressures of BiPAP or do not like using equipment and oxygen every night. In addition, these methods do not completely eliminate the problem. A newer technology referred to as *auto-titrating continuous positive airway pressure* (APAP) automatically adjusts airway pressure as needed. Side effects of positive pressure ventilation include dry mouth, rhinitis, and sinus congestion.

Surgical procedures may be done to relieve the obstruction. The most common surgery is *uvulopalatopharyngoplasty* (UPPP), a surgical procedure to remove tissues in the throat, including the uvula, palate, and pharynx, to relieve obstruction. Modified procedures can be done with laser (laser-UPPP) or with radiofrequency energy (radiofrequency ablation) to reduce snoring.

Jaw surgery involves maxillomandibular advancement, which involves moving the upper and lower parts of the jaw forward, in order to increase the space behind the tongue and soft palate, which decreases the obstruction. This is generally done by an oral surgeon. Complications may include bleeding, mouth numbness, infection, or problems with the temporomandibular joint.

For clients who experience mild OSA, a Pillar procedure may be performed. It involves the insertion of three small polyester rods into the soft palate. These rods become stiff and add support to soft palate tissue, reducing its collapse and, thus, decreasing snoring.

Tracheostomy is a successful treatment. Clients may reject this option, however, because of the trauma, the seemingly barbaric nature of the procedure, and the alteration that it creates in appearance. Tracheostomy also may be technically difficult if the client is markedly obese. If a client chooses to have a tracheostomy, they might plug it during the day.

Hypoglossal nerve stimulation therapy is an alternative surgical treatment for OSA. It was approved by the Food and Drug Administration in 2014. According to an article from the Mayo Clinic, a small impulse generator is implanted beneath the clavicle, and senses displacement of the tongue and adjusts its position, to decrease OSA (Airway, 2021).

Medication sometimes is prescribed for central sleep apnea, and clients take such drugs at bedtime. The goal is to increase the respiratory drive and improve upper airway muscle tone. An example of a medication for this purpose is protriptyline (Vivactil, Triptil). Clients may also use low-flow oxygen at night to relieve hypoxemia.

Nursing Management

Clients with sleep apnea are usually anxious and require reassurance and adequate instruction about their condition. The nurse provides thorough explanations of the disease process, polysomnography, and treatments referring clients to self-help groups or to appropriate counseling for weight loss or alcohol and substance abuse issues. The nurse collaborates with respiratory therapists to instruct the client in the use of CPAP or other NPPV and furnishes the client with information about sleep apnea and its potential complications if not treated.

LARYNGEAL CANCER

With early detection, cancer of the larynx has a high potential for cure. Preventive health measures focus on early consultation for persistent hoarseness and other changes in voice quality.

Pathophysiology and Etiology

In all, 12,620 new cases of laryngeal cancer (9,940 in men and 2,680 in women) were diagnosed in 2021 according to the American Cancer Society (2021). The rate of new cases of laryngeal cancer is falling by about 2% to 3% a year, most likely because fewer people are smoking (Laryngeal Cancer, 2021).

The cause of laryngeal cancer is unknown. Carcinogens such as tobacco, smokeless tobacco, secondhand smoke, alcohol, and industrial pollutants are associated with laryngeal cancer. In addition, chronic laryngitis, specific viruses such as the human papillomavirus (HPV), and acid reflux may be factors. As noted earlier, people over the age of 65 years and men more than women are at risk. Laryngeal cancer is more prevalent in African Americans and Whites. Most laryngeal malignancies are squamous cell carcinomas, that is, malignancies arising from the epithelial cells lining the larynx. The tumor may be located on the glottis (true vocal cords), above the glottis (supraglottis or false vocal cords), or below the glottis (subglottis).

Assessment Findings

Signs and Symptoms

Laryngeal cancers that start in the glottis generally cause persistent and progressive hoarseness (longer than 2 weeks), which is usually the earliest symptom. The hoarseness may be slight at first, and clients tend to ignore it. Cancers that start elsewhere in the larynx may not cause hoarseness until later and, therefore, may not be diagnosed as early. Later, the client notes a sensation of swelling or a lump in the throat or in the neck, followed by dysphagia and pain when talking. The client may also complain of burning in the throat when swallowing hot or citrus liquids. Weight loss often occurs owing to reduced calorie intake as a result of impaired swallowing and pain. If the malignant tissue is not removed promptly, symptoms of advancing carcinoma such as dyspnea, weakness, weight loss, enlarged cervical lymph nodes, pain, and anemia develop. Halitosis or bad breath is also characteristic of laryngeal cancer. Clients may complain of earaches.

Diagnostic Findings

Visual examination of the larynx (laryngoscopy) and fine-needle aspiration biopsy confirm the diagnosis and identify the type of malignancy. For clients who have difficulty swallowing, a barium swallow may be done. In addition, imaging tests such as X-rays, endoscopy, CT scanning, MRI, and positron emission tomography (PET) are used to detect metastasis and to determine tumor size. The primary provider also assesses the mobility of the vocal cords. Limited mobility indicates that the tumor growth is affecting the surrounding tissue, muscle, and airway.

Medical and Surgical Management

Treatment depends on factors such as the size of the lesion, the client's age, and metastasis. Medical treatment may include chemotherapy, which appears to have only minimal effects, and radiation therapy, either alone or with surgery.

TABLE 20-1 Descriptions of Laryngeal Surgery

SURGERY	DESCRIPTION	INDICATION	POSTOPERATIVE EXPECTATIONS
Vocal cord stripping	The affected cord is stripped of mucosa; may be treated with radiation therapy.	For very early-stage vocal cord lesions	Voice will be hoarse; extremely high cure rate
Cordectomy	Excision of a vocal cord, usually laser surgery.	For tumors confined to the middle third of the vocal cord	Voice quality depends on the amount of tissue removed
Laser microsurgery	Early-stage lesions are treated and removed with a laser process.	For early glottis cancers	Few side effects; slight hoarseness
Partial laryngectomy	The affected vocal cord and affected tissue around the cord are removed; other structures remain intact.	For early-stage laryngeal cancer when only one cord is involved	Voice will be hoarse; intact trachea; no problems with swallowing; high cure rate
Supraglottic laryngectomy	Hyoid bone, glottis, and false cords removed; radical neck dissection done on involved side; remaining structures left intact.	For supraglottic tumors	Voice will be hoarse; postoperative tracheostomy until glottic airway functions; nutrition administered through nasogastric tube until surgical sites heal; recurrence is possible.
Hemivertical laryngectomy	Thyroid cartilage of trachea is split at midline; one true cord and one false cord are removed along with arytenoid cartilage and half the thyroid cartilage.	When tumor extends beyond the vocal cord but is smaller than 1 cm	Client will have a tracheostomy and nasogastric tube after surgery until healed; voice will be hoarse and diminished; client will have an intact airway and the ability to swallow.
Total laryngectomy	Both vocal cords removed along with the hyoid bone, epiglottis, cricoid cartilage, and two or three rings of the trachea; the tongue, pharyngeal walls, and trachea remain intact; usually, a radical neck dissection is done on the affected side.	When the cancer extends beyond the vocal cords	Permanent tracheal stoma; prevents aspiration; no voice but ability to swallow remains. Metastasis to cervical lymph nodes is common.
Radical neck dissection	The neck is opened from the jaw to the clavicle from the midline to the interior border of the trapezius muscle. The following are removed: subcutaneous and soft tissue, sternocleidomastoid muscle, jugular vein, and the spinal accessory nerve that innervates the trapezius muscle—client's shoulder will droop after surgery as the trapezius muscle atrophies. A split-thickness skin graft is applied over the carotid artery.	When cancer has metastasized to cervical lymph nodes	Permanent tracheal stoma; no voice; ability to swallow remains. Client requires physical therapy for neck muscles along with a prescribed exercise program.

Surgical treatment (Table 20-1) includes laser surgery for early lesions or a partial or total laryngectomy. In more advanced cases, total laryngectomy may be the treatment of choice. If the disease has extended beyond the larynx, a radical neck dissection (removal of the lymph nodes, muscles, and adjacent tissues) is performed. Laser surgery may also be used to relieve obstruction in more advanced cases.

Chemotherapy and radiation therapy may be used in conjunction with a surgical procedure to treat throat cancers. Cetuximab (Erbitux) is a targeted drug therapy specifically used for laryngeal cancer. Other drugs are in trial stages.

A client with a total laryngectomy has a permanent tracheal *stoma* (opening) because the trachea is no longer connected to the nasopharynx. The larynx is severed from the trachea and removed completely. The only respiratory organs in use are the trachea, bronchi, and lungs. Air enters and leaves through the tracheostomy (Fig. 20-3). The client no longer feels air entering the nose. Because the anterior wall of the esophagus connects with the posterior wall of the larynx, it must be reconstructed. Tube feeding facilitates healing by preventing muscle activity and irritation of the esophagus (see Chapter 45).

Loss of the ability to speak normally is a devastating consequence of laryngeal surgery. Clients with a malignancy of the larynx require emotional support before and after surgery and help in understanding and choosing an alternative method of speech. Some methods of a laryngeal speech used after a laryngectomy include the following:

- *Esophageal speech*: requires regurgitation of swallowed air and formation of words with lips; voice quality will be lower pitched and gruff sounding but more natural.

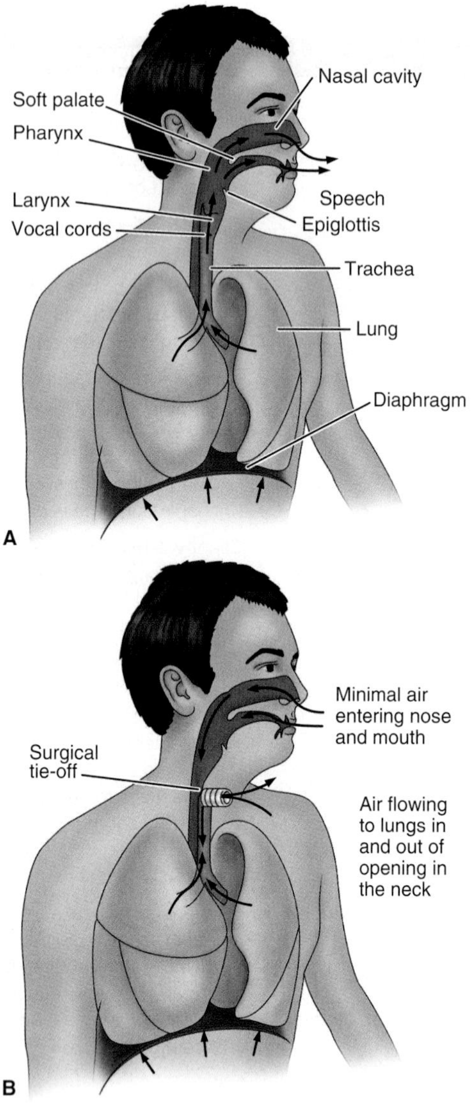

Figure 20-3 Total laryngectomy changes the airflow for breathing and speaking. **(A)** Normal airflow. **(B)** Airflow through a permanent tracheal stoma after total laryngectomy.

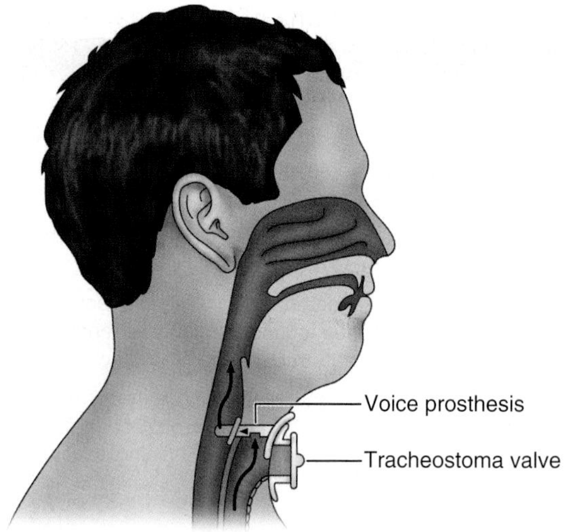

Figure 20-4 Schematic representation of tracheoesophageal puncture speech. Air travels from the lung through a puncture in the posterior wall of the trachea into the esophagus and out of the mouth. A voice prosthesis is fitted over the puncture site.

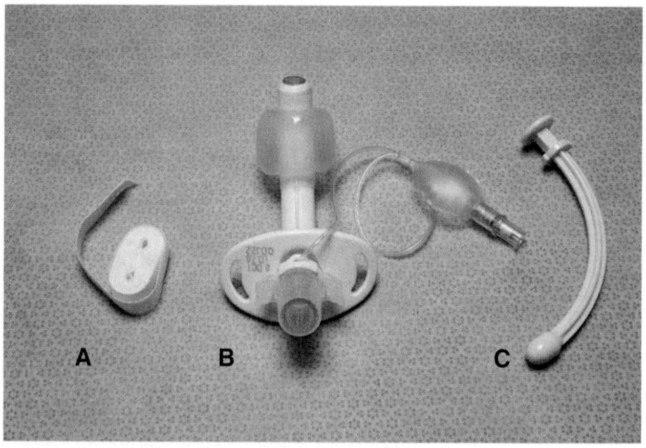

Figure 20-5 Cuffed tracheostomy components. **(A)** Tracheostomy ties. **(B)** Cuffed tracheostomy tube. The cuff at the lower end of the outer tracheostomy tube is inflated with air to provide a snug fit in the trachea. **(C)** Obturator is used to guide placement of tracheostomy tube.

- *Artificial (electric) larynx*: a throat vibrator held against the neck that projects sound into the mouth; words are formed with the mouth. The resulting voice sounds mechanical.
- *Tracheoesophageal puncture* (TEP): a surgical opening in the posterior wall of the trachea, followed by the insertion of a prosthesis such as a Blom-Singer device (Fig. 20-4). Air from the lungs is diverted through the opening in the posterior tracheal wall to the esophagus and out of the mouth. The client covers the stoma with their finger and forces air through the esophagus; this causes the walls of the throat to vibrate as the client speaks. It sounds more natural than an artificial larynx.

A speech pathologist works with the client to use an artificial speech device, learn esophageal speech, or speak clearly with a prosthesis. Clients having a partial laryngectomy also may require speech therapy.

››› *Stop, Think, and Respond 20-4*

Name three of the most common postoperative complications of laryngectomy.

TREATMENT MODALITIES FOR AIRWAY OBSTRUCTION OR AIRWAY MAINTENANCE

Clients with serious airway conditions require aggressive treatment to maintain an airway or relieve airway obstruction. This section discusses tracheostomy, tracheotomy, endotracheal intubation, and mechanical ventilation.

Tracheotomy and Tracheostomy

A **tracheotomy** is the surgical procedure that makes an opening into the trachea. A tracheostomy is a surgical opening into the trachea into which a tracheostomy or laryngectomy tube is inserted. A tracheostomy may be temporary or permanent. A permanent opening in the trachea is required for certain disorders, such as a laryngectomy for laryngeal cancer.

General Considerations

Tracheostomy tubes come in several sizes and differ from laryngectomy tubes in their length and diameter. A cuffed tracheostomy tube has a cuff on the lower end that is inflated with air to provide a snug fit (Fig. 20-5). The cuff prevents aspiration of liquids or escape of air when a mechanical ventilator is used. The primary provider specifies the amount of air to be injected into the cuff, usually to achieve a pressure between 20 and 25 mm H_2O. The amount of air determines the seating of the cuff in the trachea. The pressure in the cuff requires monitoring with a pressure gauge every 8 hours.

During the immediate postoperative period, the primary provider may change the tracheostomy tube every 3 to 5 days. To pass a tracheostomy tube into the tracheal opening, an obturator is placed in the tube to facilitate placement. Once the tracheostomy tube is in place, the obturator is removed. The outer tube is held snugly in place by tapes inserted into the openings on either side of it and tied at the side of the client's neck.

The respiratory passages react to the creation of the new opening with inflammation and excessive mucous secretion. Copious respiratory secretions are life-threatening. The client cannot be left unattended during the immediate postoperative period because the secretions make frequent suctioning necessary. In addition, inspired air passes directly into the trachea, bronchi, and lungs without becoming warmed and moistened by passing through the nose. Dry secretions can subsequently develop, which easily form crusts and can break off, obstruct the lower airway, and cause serious respiratory problems. Humidification by a mist collar is usually necessary to prevent drying and incrustation of the mucous membrane in the trachea and the main bronchus. The long- and short-term complications of tracheostomy include infection, bleeding, airway obstruction resulting from hardened secretions, aspiration, injury to the laryngeal nerve, erosion of the trachea, fistula formation between the esophagus and the trachea, and penetration of the posterior tracheal wall.

Nursing Management

After surgery, the nurse monitors vital signs, auscultates breath sounds, and assesses skin color, level of consciousness, and mental status. The nurse monitors for potential complications and checks airway patency frequently. Secretions can rapidly clog the inner lumen of the tracheostomy tube, resulting in severe respiratory difficulty or death by asphyxiation. If the airway is obstructed, the client becomes cyanotic, restless, and frightened.

To facilitate breathing during the immediate postoperative period, the nurse positions the client as ordered. When the client is fully awake and blood pressure is stable, the nurse elevates the head of the bed to about 45°. This position decreases edema and makes breathing easier.

NURSING GUIDELINES 20-2

Suctioning the Client With a Tracheostomy

- Use sterile equipment (e.g., gloves, suction catheter, normal saline) and aseptic technique for tracheal suctioning.
- Place client in Fowler position. Preoxygenate client for at least 1 to 2 minutes. Check that suction pressure is at a low setting.
- Open the suction kit, don gloves, lubricate a sterile 10- to 14-French disposable catheter with sterile saline, and insert it into the lumen of the tube.
- Do not apply suction while the catheter is inserted down the trachea because this irritates the lining of the trachea.
- Begin intermittent suctioning while slowly withdrawing and rotating the catheter. Do not suction for more than 10 seconds at a time.
- Allow client to rest and deep breathe before repeating if more suctioning is necessary.
- Discard the suction catheter after use.

The nurse inspects the tracheostomy carefully, ensuring that tapes are secure. If the tube is not tied securely, the client can cough it out, a serious occurrence if the edges of the trachea have not been sutured to the skin. This may be the case in a temporary tracheostomy. The nurse keeps a tracheal dilator at the bedside at all times. If the outer tube accidentally comes out, the nurse inserts the dilator to hold the edges of the stoma apart until the primary provider arrives to insert another tube. A tracheal tube must never be forced back in place. Use of force may compress the client's trachea (by pushing the tube alongside and compressing the trachea rather than inserting the tube into the stoma). Such action could cause respiratory arrest.

The nurse suctions the client to remove secretions that can obstruct the airway (Nursing Guidelines 20-2) but avoids unnecessary suctioning to decrease trauma to the airway. When explaining the procedure, the nurse tells the client that the suction catheter will be inserted for only a few seconds. Keeping an extra tracheostomy tube of the same size at the bedside is essential because an immediate change may be necessary if the tube becomes blocked with mucus that cannot be removed. The nurse provides routine tracheostomy care (Nursing Guidelines 20-3) and places a gauze dressing under the tube to absorb secretions. The hospital gown and bed linens must never cover the opening of the tracheostomy tube. Nursing Care Plan 20-1 describes additional care, and Evidence-Based Practice 20-1 describes research on tracheostomy safety considerations.

ENDOTRACHEAL INTUBATION AND MECHANICAL VENTILATION

An endotracheal tube (Fig. 20-6) is inserted through the mouth or the nose into the trachea to provide a patent airway for clients who cannot maintain an adequate airway on their own. Examples include those with respiratory difficulty, comatose clients, those undergoing general anesthesia, and clients with extensive edema of upper airway passages.

NURSING GUIDELINES 20-3

Providing Tracheostomy Care

- Maintain aseptic technique by washing hands before, during, and after the procedure.
- Position client in a supine or low Fowler position.
- Using a clean glove, remove the soiled stomal dressing and discard it, glove and all, in an appropriate receptacle.
- Open the tracheostomy kit without contaminating the contents. Don sterile gloves—keep the dominant hand sterile. Pour hydrogen peroxide and normal saline into respective containers.
- Unlock the inner cannula by turning it counterclockwise. Remove it and place in hydrogen peroxide. Clean the inside and outside of the cannula with pipe cleaners.
- Rinse the cleaned cannula with normal saline. Tap the cannula and wipe the excess solution with sterile gauze.
- Replace the inner cannula and turn it clockwise within the outer cannula.
- Clean around the stoma with an applicator moistened with normal saline.
- Place a sterile dressing around the tracheostomy tube. Change the tracheostomy ties by placing the new ones on first and removing the soiled ones last. Tie the new ends securely, but not tightly, at the side of the neck.

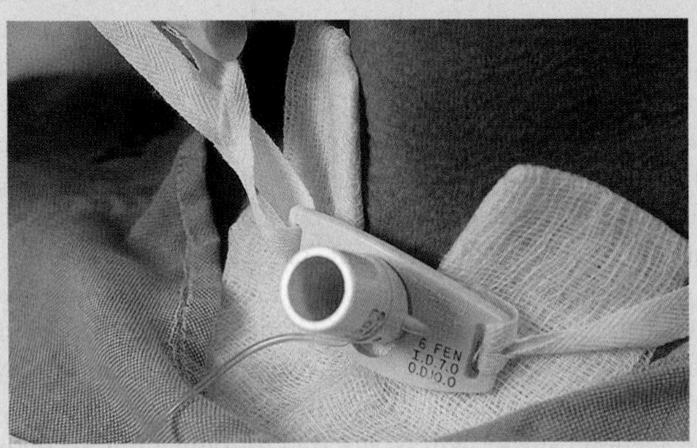

Securing a tracheostomy dressing.

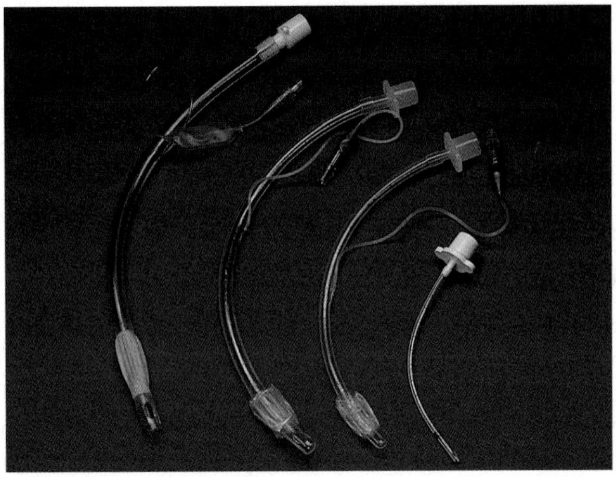

Figure 20-6 Endotracheal tubes.

Evidence-Based Practice 20-1

Tracheostomies

Clinical Question

Is there vital information that should remain at a client's bedside when a tracheostomy is present in case of medical emergencies?

Evidence

Tracheostomies occur as a common treatment in procedures that take place in the head and neck area. There is a National Tracheostomy Safety Project (NTSP) that occurred in 2013 to establish guidelines to manage tracheostomy medical emergencies (NTSP, n.d.). An audit was performed based on these guidelines to see if the following remain at the bedside: stoma information, contact information for emergencies, and if equipment is needed in emergencies based on NTSP guidelines (Darr, Siddiq, Jolly, & Spinou, 2016). The multicentered audit took place in a region in the United Kingdom over a 2-week period and included regular units and intensive care units (ICUs). A small sample of 34 stoma clients was in the audit. The results showed noncompliance across the units and ICU. Compliance in all three areas listed earlier was not consistent with each client audit. Complications can occur that leads to high levels of morbidity and mortality. It is important to follow emergency guidelines for client safety.

Nursing Implications

Nurses may not have clients frequently with tracheostomies. However, understanding the importance of assessment, emergency equipment, and emergency support is necessary. Nurses should review facility and unit policy and know where to get supplies and whom to contact for support.

References

Darr, A., Siddiq, S., Jolly, K., & Spinou, C. (2016). Neck stoma patients: Is vital information displayed at the bedside? *British Journal of Nursing, 25*(5), 242–247. https://doi.org/10.12968/bjon.2016.25.5.242

National Tracheostomy Safety Project. (n.d.). http://www.tracheostomy.org.uk/

General Considerations

An endotracheal tube can remain in place for up to 2 weeks. The cuff is inflated to provide a tight seal. The endotracheal tube is attached to a ventilator for control of respirations and ventilation of the lungs. Humidification is necessary because air going to the lungs through an endotracheal tube does not pass through the moist mucous membranes of the upper airway.

There are several modes of mechanical ventilation classified according to the manner in which they support ventilation. Two major classifications are negative pressure and positive pressure ventilators. Negative pressure ventilators exert negative pressure, a pulling or sucking force, on the external chest. Although widely used at one time for clients with chronic respiratory failure related to neuromuscular disease such as poliomyelitis or myasthenia gravis, this mode is rarely used now. Negative modes include iron lungs or respirator tanks, or pneumowrap and chest cuirass (a plastic shell-like apparatus that fits over the chest).

TABLE 20-2 Types of Positive Pressure Ventilators

TYPE OF POSITIVE PRESSURE VENTILATORS	HOW USED
Positive pressure ventilator—general information	Exerts positive pressure on airway to inflate lungs; expiration is passive Usually requires endotracheal or tracheal intubation
Pressure-cycled positive pressure ventilator	Inspiration ends when a preset pressure is reached; cycle means that ventilator cycles on, delivers flow of air until a certain pressure is reached, and then cycles off. Designed for short-term use because volume of air varies as client's airway resistance or compliance changes
Time-cycled positive pressure ventilator	Controls respiration after a preset time; length of inspiration and flow rate of air regulate volume the client receives; usually used on newborns and infants
Volume-cycled positive pressure ventilator	Delivers a preset volume of air with each inspiration; once volume is delivered, ventilator cycles off and client expires air passively. Provides consistent adequate breaths despite airway resistance or changes in compliance; most commonly used ventilator for adults
Airway pressure release ventilation (APRV)	Ventilator cycles between higher and lower pressure levels of CPAP. This helps to open alveoli and promotes better gas exchange. Clients require less sedation on and can maintain a cough reflex. Clients have potential for earlier removal (weaning) from the ventilator.
Noninvasive positive pressure ventilator (NIPPV)	Ventilation delivered by face masks or other nasal devices; does not require intubation of any kind; used for clients with sleep-related breathing disorders or other chronic respiratory disorders.
Continuous positive airway pressure (CPAP)	Provides positive pressure to airways throughout respiration. It is sometimes used for intubated clients being weaned from ventilators, or is used with masks to maintain alveoli patency. Clients must be able to breathe on their own for this modality.
Bilevel positive airway pressure (BiPAP)	Provides positive pressure support ventilation with independent control of inspiratory and expiratory pressures. Clients use a nasal or oral mask or a mouthpiece with a tight seal. The client initiates each inspiration or the machine will because it has a back-up mode, ensuring that the client receives a set number of breaths per minute. Clients with severe COPD or sleep apnea use this type of support ventilation.

COPD, chronic obstructive pulmonary disease.
Adapted from Hinkle, J. L., & Cheever, K. H. (2018). *Brunner & Suddarth's textbook of medical-surgical nursing* (14th ed.). Wolters Kluwer.

The second classification, positive pressure ventilators, are more commonly used. These types of ventilators inflate the lungs by exerting positive pressure, pushing air into the airway. Positive pressure ventilators generally require intubation and are used for clients with acute respiratory failure and primary lung disease, such as cystic fibrosis, or for clients who are comatose, are under general anesthesia, or have extensive upper airway edema. Complications related to mechanical ventilation include damage to the lungs, decreased lung expansion, and ventilator-associated pneumonia (VAP). Table 20-2 briefly describes types of positive pressure ventilators.

Accidental removal of an endotracheal tube must be prevented because this can result in laryngeal edema or **laryngospasm** (spasm of the laryngeal muscles, resulting in narrowing of the larynx) and subsequent respiratory arrest. The inflated cuff and placement of tape around the tube attached to the client's cheek secures the endotracheal tube. The proximal end of the tube is marked for determining whether downward displacement has occurred.

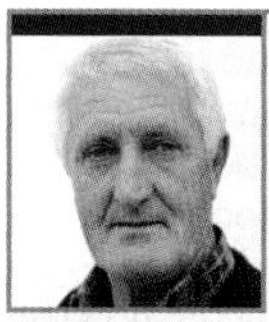

Clinical Scenario A 70-year-old client has a tracheostomy placed because he is on long-term mechanical ventilation. **What are the major considerations for the nurse when planning and providing nursing care to this client? See Nursing Care Plan 20-1.**

NURSING CARE PLAN 20-1 The Client With a Tracheostomy

Assessment

- Monitor for vital signs and auscultate breath sounds.
- Assess skin color, level of consciousness, and mental status.
- Monitor for potential complications.
- Assess frequently for a patent airway.
- Inspect tracheostomy frequently for placement and security of ties.

Nursing Diagnosis. **Safety, postsurgical procedure**

Expected Outcome. The nurse will prevent or manage complications of the tracheostomy.

Interventions	Rationales
Monitor for signs and symptoms of respiratory distress: difficulty breathing, diminished or absent breath sounds, use of accessory muscles, and asymmetric chest wall movements.	*Early recognition of signs and symptoms of respiratory distress prevents further complications.*

(continued)

NURSING CARE PLAN 20-1 The Client With a Tracheostomy (*continued*)

Assess for subcutaneous emphysema (air trapped in tissues) around the stoma, neck, and chest.	*Injury or trauma to the airway can cause air to leak into surrounding tissues. Severe subcutaneous emphysema indicates significant leaking and potential airway obstruction.*
Provide humidification.	*A tracheostomy bypasses the nose; thus, inspired air is not warmed or humidified. Increased warmth and humidity thin and help remove secretions.*
Keep tracheostomy ties secure but not too tight (one finger should slip easily under ties).	*Ties maintain tube placement without damaging underlying skin or causing discomfort.*
Monitor pulse oximetry or ABG results. Administer oxygen as needed.	*Such monitoring ensures adequate oxygenation.*

Evaluation of Expected Outcome

The nurse manages the client's care and prevents complications.

Nursing Diagnosis. **Ineffective Airway Clearance** related to increased secretions and possible occlusion of the inner cannula

Expected Outcome. Airway and tracheostomy tube will remain clear.

Interventions	Rationales
Provide warm, humidified air.	*Such air prevents drying and crusting of secretions.*
Suction as needed.	*Suctioning clears secretions.*
Maintain a patent airway. In cases of suspected obstruction, (1) suction the tracheostomy, (2) induce coughing, (3) change the inner cannula, and (4) position client to maximize respiratory effort.	*These measures remove thick secretions and possible mucus plugs and promote lung expansion.*

Evaluation of Expected Outcome

Client's airway and tracheostomy are patent.

Nursing Diagnosis. **Infection Risk** related to loss of upper airway protection

Expected Outcome. Risk for infection will be reduced.

Interventions	Rationales
Monitor stoma for erythema, exudate, or odor.	*Such findings may indicate infection.*
Assess skin around stoma and under tracheostomy ties for signs of breakdown.	*Intact skin prevents infection.*
Monitor white blood cell (WBC) count.	*Elevated WBCs may indicate infection.*
Provide routine tracheostomy care every 8 hours and as necessary. Maintain sterile technique.	*These measures prevent infection.*
Position client so that secretions do not pool around the stoma.	*Maintaining a clean and dry stoma prevents infection.*

Evaluation of Expected Outcome

Client does not have any signs or symptoms of infection.

Nursing Diagnosis. Altered Health Maintenance and Knowledge Deficiency related to lack of knowledge about tracheostomy care and home support.

Expected Outcome. Client or caregiver will demonstrate skills appropriate for tracheostomy care.

Interventions	Rationales
Assess client's and caregiver's ability to provide adequate home care.	*This assessment provides a baseline for teaching needs and referrals.*
Begin teaching skills one at a time.	*Step-by-step teaching provides time to absorb information.*
Teach client how to suction airway, clean tube, change dressing and ties, provide stoma care, and reinsert tracheostomy tube. Have client demonstrate skills.	*Demonstration of skills ensures that client or caregiver has adequate knowledge for home care.*
Teach client or caregiver to check for signs and symptoms of infection.	*Such measures prevent or enable early treatment of infection.*
Refer client and caregiver to support groups and home care services.	*Home care needs are planned for before discharge.*

Evaluation of Expected Outcome

Client or caregiver demonstrates adequate skill in tracheostomy care and is sufficiently independent for discharge home.

The intubated client has the endotracheal tube removed when the vital capacity is adequate and the client can breathe without assistance. Blood gas studies are also used as a guideline for removal. Depending on hospital policy, the removal of an endotracheal tube may be done by the nurse, the respiratory therapist, or the doctor. Before removing the tube, emergency equipment for respiratory support must be available. The pharynx must be suctioned before the cuff is deflated to prevent the aspiration of secretions during removal of the tube. The tube is usually removed with the client in semi-Fowler position. If laryngospasm occurs, air is administered by positive pressure. Reinsertion of the endotracheal tube by the health care provider or other trained personnel may be necessary if laryngospasm continues. Possible complications with the use of endotracheal intubation include ulceration and stricture of the trachea or larynx, atelectasis, and pneumonia.

Nursing Management

Major goals for the intubated client are to improve respirations, maintain a patent airway, and communicate needs to others. The nurse monitors vital signs periodically, depending on the client's condition and the reason for endotracheal tube insertion. Blood gas studies and pulse oximetry provide methods of ongoing evaluation of the client's respiratory status. The nurse reviews the results of these studies and reports changes to the primary provider.

The nurse observes the client at frequent intervals for response to respiratory support and complications associated with endotracheal intubation. They evaluate any change in mental status. Confusion may result from abnormal blood gas levels or electrolyte imbalances. Sudden restlessness or agitation may indicate obstruction of the endotracheal tube, which can be life-threatening. The nurse auscultates the lungs and observes the symmetric rise and fall of the chest every 30 to 60 minutes. If bilateral breath sounds cannot be detected, the nurse notifies the primary provider immediately.

Humidification is necessary to keep the inspired air moist. Clients with endotracheal intubation cannot cough, secretions are often thick and tenacious, and swallowing reflexes are depressed. An increase in $PaCO_2$ caused by blockage of the endotracheal tube or malfunctioning of the ventilator may occur secondary to secretions or because the client is biting on the tube. Keeping the airway patent at all times is absolutely necessary, using the same suctioning technique as for a tracheostomy. If the client is biting on the tube, a bite block or oral airway may be used to keep the tube patent.

The nurse changes the client's position every 2 hours to prevent atelectasis and gives oral care as needed to keep the mouth and lips free of crusts and mucus. The nurse suctions the oropharynx and mouth as needed and cleans the teeth with applicators. The nurse inspects the oral cavity frequently and reports any signs of oral bleeding to the primary provider.

The client may display anxiety or fear because of the tube, inability to speak, suctioning, and dependence on a machine for breathing. Each time suctioning is needed, the nurse reassures the client that the procedure takes only a short time. The client may attempt to remove or pull on the tube if they are awake or partially awake. Restraining the client may be necessary. The nurse should contact the primary provider if the client is extremely restless. Providing a "Magic Slate," wipe board, electronic device, or pencil and paper to the client enables communication, as does asking questions that the client can answer by shaking the head yes or no.

Once the endotracheal tube is removed, the nurse places the client in a high Fowler or semi-Fowler position to promote optimal chest and lung expansion. The posterior pharynx may be dry, and the voice may be hoarse. The nurse observes the client frequently for signs of laryngeal edema and increased respiratory distress. They immediately reports any sign of respiratory distress because reinsertion of the endotracheal tube may be necessary.

KEY POINTS

- Infectious and Inflammatory Disorders:
  - Rhinitis is inflammation of the nasal mucous membranes. It is also referred to as the *common cold*, or coryza.
  - Sinusitis, also known as rhinosinusitis, is inflammation of the sinuses.
  - Pharyngitis, inflammation of the throat, is often associated with rhinitis and other URIs.
  - Tonsillitis is inflammation of the tonsils, and adenoiditis is inflammation of the adenoids. These conditions generally occur together—the common diagnosis is tonsillitis.
  - Peritonsillar abscess is an abscess that develops in the connective tissue between the capsule of the tonsil and the constrictor muscle of the pharynx.
  - Laryngitis is inflammation and swelling of the mucous membrane that lines the larynx.
- Structural disorders:
  - Epistaxis, or nosebleeds: the rupture of tiny capillaries in the nasal mucous membrane
  - Nasal polyps: are grapelike swellings that arise from the nasal mucous membranes. They probably result from chronic irritation related to infection or allergic rhinitis and can obstruct nasal breathing and sinus drainage, ultimately leading to sinusitis.
  - Hypertrophied turbinates: enlargements of the nasal conchae, the three bones that project from the lateral wall of the nasal cavity, which results from chronic rhinitis, interferes with air passage and sinus drainage, and eventually leads to sinusitis
- Deviated septum is an irregularity in the septum that results in nasal obstruction.

- Trauma or obstruction:
  - Nasal fracture usually results from direct trauma, it causes swelling and edema of the soft tissues, external and internal bleeding, nasal deformity, and nasal obstruction.
  - Laryngeal trauma and laryngeal obstruction: neck swelling/bruising
  - OSA is characterized by recurrent and frequent episodes of upper airway obstruction and reduced ventilation.
  - Apnea (cessation of breathing) occurs as a result of upper airway obstruction, generally when the tongue collapses against the soft palate and, in turn, the soft palate collapses against the back of the throat.
- Laryngeal cancer: Most laryngeal malignancies are squamous cell carcinomas, that is, malignancies arising from the epithelial cells lining the larynx. The tumor may be located on the glottis (true vocal cords), above the glottis (supraglottis or false vocal cords), or below the glottis (subglottis).
- Tracheotomy is the surgical procedure that makes an opening into the trachea.
- Tracheostomy is a surgical opening into the trachea into which a tracheostomy or laryngectomy tube is inserted; a tracheostomy may be temporary or permanent.

CRITICAL THINKING EXERCISES

1. A client with severe pharyngitis is diagnosed with a group A streptococcal infection. The primary provider prescribes penicillin. What discharge instructions should you give the client?
2. The licensed practical nurse (LPN) is assigned to assist the registered nurse (RN) in the care of a client on a positive pressure ventilator. A primary nursing goal is for the client to maintain optimal gas exchange. What nursing actions would promote this?
3. Your client is scheduled for a total laryngectomy. What information must you share to help prepare the client for the postoperative period?
4. A client arrives at the emergency department with uncontrolled epistaxis. What actions should the RN instruct the LPN to take?

NCLEX-STYLE REVIEW QUESTIONS PrepU

1. The nurse is reviewing what the client can expect when taking diphenhydramine, a decongestant. Which of the following statements by the client indicates that more teaching is needed?
   1. "I may experience a headache with this medication."
   2. "I might need something to help me sleep."
   3. "It is important that I increase my fluid intake."
   4. "My mouth will most likely be quite dry."
2. Of the following instructions, which is most important for the nurse to teach the client to help loosen secretions and increase comfort during medical treatment for sinusitis?
   1. Blow the nose frequently.
   2. Elevate the head of the bed by 45°.
   3. Engage in normal activity.
   4. Increase fluid intake.
3. The nurse is providing postoperative care for a client who has undergone tonsillectomy. In which position will the nurse place the head of the bed when the client is fully awake?
   1. Flat with the head elevated on a pillow
   2. Slightly raised at a 15° angle
   3. Raised at a 45° angle
   4. Raised at a 90° sitting position
4. A client was seen in the emergency department with severe epistaxis. After the primary provider places a nasal packing, the bleeding is controlled. What should the nurse include as part of the discharge instructions? Select all that apply.
   1. Call the primary provider if bleeding persists or becomes worse.
   2. Continue taking baby aspirin as ordered.
   3. Do not blow the nose.
   4. Keep nasal packing in place until seen for follow-up appointment.
   5. Swallow any oozing blood to avoid coughing.
5. The nurse is reviewing the record of a client who is being seen for possible laryngeal cancer. What initial complaint from the client does the nurse expect?
   1. The client has had difficulty swallowing hot liquids.
   2. The client has had enlarged lymph nodes in the neck.
   3. The client has had generalized discomfort in the neck.
   4. The client has had persistent hoarseness for the last month.
6. A nurse identified Ineffective Airway Clearance related to a malignant mass in the client's airway. Which of the following interventions has the highest priority?
   1. Elevate the client's head of the bed.
   2. Encourage the client to deep breathe and cough every 2 hours.
   3. Place a nasal cannula with 2 L of oxygen.
   4. Provide emergency tracheostomy equipment at the bedside.

WANT TO KNOW MORE? There are a wide variety of online resources available on thePoint to enhance learning and understanding of this chapter.

Go to **thePoint.lww.com/activate** and use the activation code found in the front of this text to unlock these online resources.

21 Caring for Clients With Lower Respiratory Disorders

Words To Know

acute bronchitis
asbestosis
asthma
atelectasis
bronchiectasis
chronic bronchitis
chronic obstructive pulmonary disease
community-acquired pneumonia
cystic fibrosis
emphysema
empyema
flail chest
health care–associated pneumonia
hemoptysis
hospital-acquired pneumonia
influenza
lobectomy
lung abscess
orthopnea
pleural effusion
pleurisy
pneumoconiosis
pneumonectomy
pneumonia
pneumothorax
pulmonary contusion
pulmonary edema
pulmonary embolism
pulmonary hypertension
restrictive lung disease
segmental resection
septicemia
silicosis
subcutaneous emphysema
thoracotomy
tracheitis
tracheobronchitis
tuberculosis
ventilator-associated pneumonia
wedge resection

Learning Objectives

On completion of this chapter, you will be able to:

1. Describe infectious and inflammatory disorders of the lower respiratory airway.
2. Identify critical assessments needed for a client with an infectious disorder of the lower respiratory airway.
3. Define disorders classified as obstructive pulmonary disease.
4. Discuss strategies for preventing and managing occupational lung diseases.
5. Describe the pathophysiology of pulmonary hypertension.
6. List risk factors associated with the development of a pulmonary embolism.
7. Discuss conditions that may lead to acute respiratory distress syndrome.
8. Differentiate acute and chronic respiratory failure.
9. Explain the difficulties associated with early diagnosis of lung cancer.
10. Describe nursing assessments required for a client who experiences trauma to the chest.
11. Explain the purpose of chest tubes after thoracic surgery.
12. Describe preoperative and postoperative nursing management for clients undergoing thoracic care.

Various problems and disorders can compromise the ability of the lower respiratory tract to perform its primary functions of gas exchange and ventilation. If untreated, many of these disorders can lead to respiratory failure. Other disorders become chronic and affect the client's quality of life.

Gerontologic Considerations

- Older adults are at greater risk for pneumonia and may experience a higher acuity owing to concomitant health problems, such as heart disease and diabetes.
- Vaccination against pneumococcal pneumonia is recommended for clients older than 50 years with a chronic or debilitating illness, those over age 65, and residents in long-term care facilities.

(continued)

Gerontologic Considerations (*continued*)

- Current guidelines recommend a booster dose if the initial immunization was 5 or more years ago. Older adults should also be advised to receive an annual influenza immunization.
- Although the incidence of tuberculosis (TB) is decreasing, the rate is highest in the United States in adults aged 65 years or over. Globally, the rates are increasing in those who also have HIV, and tests are improving to identify a shift from latent to active disease status.
- Increasing accurate diagnosis of latent TB infection and improving treatment regimens for older adults involve all health care providers.
- Vascular changes of aging and chronic vascular diseases cause alterations in arterial and venous lumen, increasing the risk of deep vein thrombosis (DVT). The nurse should assess the older client's history of cardiovascular disease, level of activity, hydration status, and constricting clothing such as tight-fitting hose or socks.
- Changes associated with aging or chronic conditions may increase older adults' risk for falls. Falls may cause fracture of one or more ribs, increasing susceptibility to pneumonia from decreased lung expansion.

INFECTIOUS AND INFLAMMATORY DISORDERS

Infectious and inflammatory disorders of the lower airway are medically more serious than those of the upper airway. Inflammation and infection in the alveoli and bronchioles impair gas exchange. In addition, clients may experience greater difficulty in maintaining a clear airway secondary to retained secretions.

Acute Bronchitis

Pathophysiology and Etiology

Inflammation of the mucus membranes that line the major bronchi and their branches characterizes **acute bronchitis**. If the inflammatory process involves the trachea, it is referred to as **tracheobronchitis**. Typically, acute bronchitis begins as an upper respiratory infection (URI); the inflammatory process then extends to the tracheobronchial tree. The secretory cells of the mucosa produce increased mucopurulent sputum.

Viral infections most commonly give rise to acute bronchitis. Clients with viral URIs are more vulnerable to secondary bacterial infections, which then may lead to acute bronchitis. Sputum cultures identify the causative bacterial organisms, the most common of which are *Haemophilus influenzae*, *Streptococcus pneumoniae*, and *Mycoplasma pneumoniae*. Fungal organisms such as *Aspergillus* may be identified as the cause of acute bronchitis. Chemical irritation from noxious fumes, gases, and air contaminants also may induce acute bronchitis. A potential complication is bronchial asthma.

Assessment Findings

Signs and symptoms initially include fever; chills; malaise; headache; and a dry, irritating, and nonproductive cough. Later, the cough produces mucopurulent sputum, which may be blood streaked if the airway mucosa becomes irritated with severe tracheobronchitis and coughing. Clients experience paroxysmal attacks of coughing and may report wheezing. Laryngitis and sinusitis complicate the symptoms. Moist, inspiratory crackles may be heard on chest auscultation. A sputum sample is collected for culture and sensitivity testing to rule out bacterial infection. A chest X-ray also may be done to detect additional pathology, such as pneumonia.

Medical Management

Acute bronchitis usually is self-limiting, lasting for several days. Suggested treatment is bed rest, antipyretics, expectorants, antitussives (drugs used to alleviate coughing), and increased fluids. Humidifiers assist in keeping mucus membranes moist because dry air aggravates the cough. If secondary bacterial invasion occurs, the previously mild infection becomes more serious and usually is accompanied by a persistent cough and thick, purulent sputum. Secondary infections usually subside as the bronchitis subsides, but they may persist for several weeks. When a secondary infection is evident, the primary provider orders a broad-spectrum antibiotic when sputum culture results are available.

Nursing Management

The nurse auscultates breath sounds and monitors vital signs every 4 hours, especially if the client has a fever. The nurse encourages the client to cough and deep breathe every 2 hours while awake and to expectorate rather than swallow sputum. Humidification of surrounding air loosens bronchial secretions. The nurse changes the bedding and the client's clothes if they become damp with perspiration and offers fluids frequently. The nurse, in an effort to prevent the spread of infection, teaches the client to wash the hands frequently, particularly when handling secretions and soiled tissues; cover the mouth when sneezing and coughing; discard soiled tissues in a plastic bag; and avoid sharing eating utensils and personal articles with others.

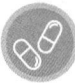

Pharmacologic Considerations

- The use of nonprescription cough medicines may cause more harm than good. Coughing is the body's mechanism to clear respiratory passages of mucus; using cough suppressants to depress the cough reflex may cause a pooling of secretions, leading to further problems. Encourage clients with lower respiratory illness to check with their health care providers before using nonprescription cough preparations.

Pneumonia

Pneumonia is an inflammatory process affecting the bronchioles and alveoli. Although it usually is associated with an acute infection, pneumonia also can result from radiation therapy, chemical ingestion or inhalation, or aspiration of foreign bodies or gastric contents. Pneumonia, when combined with influenza, ranks as the eighth leading cause of death in the United States (American Lung Association, 2015).

Pathophysiology and Etiology

There are four classifications for pneumonia (Table 21-1): community-acquired pneumonia, health care–associated pneumonia/hospital-acquired pneumonia, pneumonia in the immunocompromised host, and pneumonia from aspiration.

Community-Acquired Pneumonia

Community-acquired pneumonia (CAP) is the most common type of pneumonia. The client contracted the illness in

TABLE 21-1 Types of Pneumonia

TYPE	ORGANISM RESPONSIBLE	COMMON CLINICAL MANIFESTATIONS	USUAL TREATMENT
Community-Acquired Pneumonia (CAP)			
Streptococcal pneumonia (pneumococcal) *Haemophilus* influenza Legionnaires' disease Mycoplasmal pneumonia Viral pneumonia Chlamydial pneumonia	*Streptococcus pneumoniae* *Haemophilus influenzae* *Legionella pneumophila* *Mycoplasma pneumoniae* Influenza virus types A and B, adenovirus, parainfluenza, cytomegalovirus, coronavirus *Chlamydia pneumoniae*	Abrupt or insidious onset; one or more lobes involved; flulike symptoms; lobar infiltrates seen on X-ray; pleuritic and/or chest pain; often begins with a URI	Penicillins or alternative antibiotics such as cefotaxime, cephalosporin, erythromycin, or others Treated based on symptoms
Hospital-Acquired (HAP) and Health Care–Associated (HCAP) Pneumonias			
Pseudomonas pneumonia Staphylococcal pneumonia *Klebsiella* pneumonia	*Pseudomonas aeruginosa* *Staphylococcus aureus* *Klebsiella pneumoniae*	Diffuse consolidation on chest X-ray; fever; chills; productive cough; bacteremia; cyanosis; hypoxemia; clients have toxic appearance; can get lung abscesses	Antibiotics; antipseudomonal agents such as piperacillin; rifampin or gentamicin; third-generation cephalosporins
Pneumonia in the Immunocompromised Host			
Pneumocystis pneumonia	*Pneumocystis carinii*	Pulmonary infiltrates on chest X-ray, cough, dyspnea, hemoptysis, fever, night sweats, weight loss	Trimethoprim-sulfamethoxazole (TMP-SMZ), amphotericin B, rifampin, streptomycin
Fungal pneumonia	*Aspergillus fumigatus*	Cough, hemoptysis, infiltrates, fungus ball on chest X-ray	Voriconazole (Vfend) for invasive disease, amphotericin B, or caspofungin (Cancidas)
Tuberculosis	*Mycobacterium tuberculosis*	Weight loss, fever, night sweats, cough, sputum production, hemoptysis, nonspecific lower lobe infiltrate, pleural effusion on chest X-ray	Isoniazid (INH) + rifampin (Rifadin) + ethambutol (Myambutol) + pyrazinamide (PZA)—refer to section on tuberculosis
Atypical Pneumonia			
Caused by ("atypical") pathogens *Legionella,* *Mycoplasma,* *Chlamydia,* *coronavirus*	*Legionella,* *Mycoplasma,* *Chlamydia,* *SARS-CoV-2*	Headache, low-grade fever, cough, and malaise Pneumonia that affects both lungs as opposed to just one Lungs that had a characteristic "ground-glass" appearance via CT scan Abnormalities in some laboratory tests, particularly those assessing liver function Fever, chills, cough, which may or may not be productive Shortness of breath Chest pain that happens when you breathe deeply or cough Fatigue	Macrolide, doxycycline, fluoroquinolone + corticosteroid Supportive care, oxygen therapy

CT, computed tomography; SARS, severe acute respiratory syndrome; URI, upper respiratory infection.
From BMJ Best Practice. (n.d.). *Atypical pneumonia (non-COVID-19)—Treatment algorithm.* https://bestpractice.bmj.com/topics/en-us/18/treatment-algorithm; Adapted from Hinkle, J. L., & Cheever, K. H. (2018). *Brunner & Suddarth's textbook of medical-surgical nursing* (14th ed.). Wolters Kluwer; Healthline. (n.d.). *Coronavirus and pneumonia: COVID-19 pneumonia symptoms, treatment.* https://www.healthline.com/health/coronavirus-pneumonia

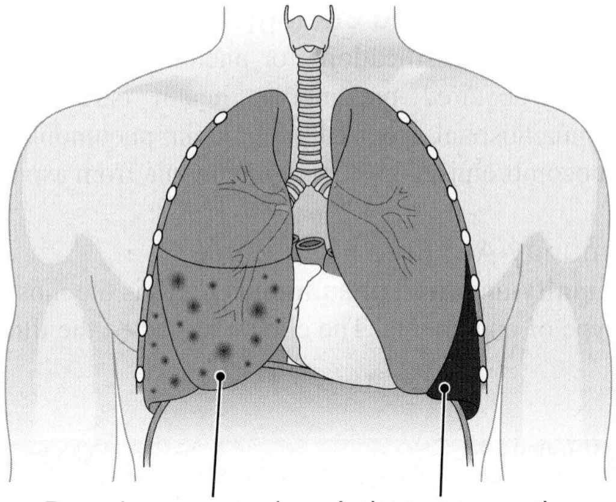

Figure 21-1 Types and subtypes of pneumonia. Reprinted with permission from Cohen, B. J. (2003). *Medical Terminology: An illustrated guide* (4th ed.). Lippincott Williams & Wilkins.

a community setting or within 48 hours of admission to a health care facility. The typical causes (see Fig. 21-1) are:

- *Bacteria*: the most common causative bacterial organism is *S. pneumoniae*. Others include *Pneumocystis jiroveci*, *Staphylococcus aureus*, and *Klebsiella pneumoniae*. This type of pneumonia is often referred to as *typical pneumonias*. *S. pneumoniae* is the most common bacterial cause of pneumonia. It spreads from the upper respiratory tract to the bronchi and lobes of the lower respiratory tract. *Mycobacterium tuberculosis* also may cause pneumonia.
- *Atypical bacteria*: also cause pneumonia, referred to as *atypical pneumonias*. An example of this type includes *M. pneumoniae*. This type of pneumonia is sometimes called "walking pneumonia" because the symptoms tend to be less severe. It spreads from person to person through infected respiratory droplets. Another example includes *Legionella pneumophila* (the causative agent of Legionnaires' disease). Box 21-1 provides brief overviews of atypical pneumonias.
- *Viruses*: also cause pneumonia, but more commonly in infants and children. However, the viruses that cause colds and influenza (*H. influenzae*) in adults can lead to viral pneumonias.
- *Fungi*: although not common, pneumonias caused by fungi can occur in immunocompromised clients or in clients with chronic health problems. Opportunistic fungal infections (those that take advantage of a host's compromised immune system) are the most usual causes of this type of pneumonia. Clients inhale aerosolized spores that are present because their habitat (soil or bird droppings) was disturbed. Once the lower respiratory tract is infected in immunocompromised individuals, it is very difficult to manage the infection as it spreads throughout the body.

Health Care–Associated Pneumonia

Health care–associated pneumonia (HCAP) is diagnosed in clients who generally reside in long-term care facilities or who are on dialysis in outpatient centers. HCAP may also include clients who were hospitalized within 90 days of being diagnosed with pneumonia. A common feature of HCAP is that the bacteria are more resistant to antibiotics (multidrug resistance [MDR]). This feature makes treatment a challenge.

Categories included with HCAP include the following:

- Immunocompromised clients who have underlying conditions that require immunosuppressant medications, such as clients with AIDS and long-term mechanically ventilated clients.
- Aspiration pneumonia can occur when a person inhales a foreign body such as food or drink or gastric contents during vomiting or regurgitation. Generally, pneumonia occurs with aspiration of infected material from the upper

BOX 21-1 Atypical Pneumonias

Mycoplasma pneumoniae

Is the most common cause of atypical pneumonia
Develops gradually, with a prolonged clinical course
Spreads by person-to-person contact via infected respiratory droplets
Usually a milder form of pneumonia—is rarely fatal

Chlamydia pneumoniae

Is a common cause of atypical pneumonia and URIs
Spreads by person-to-person contact via infected respiratory droplets
Requires long-term treatment with broad-spectrum antibiotics

Legionella pneumophila

Was first described at an American Legion convention in Philadelphia, Pennsylvania
Is a fastidious bacterium that resides in aquatic environments
Outbreaks traced to air conditioners, humidifiers, hot water tanks, and decorative fountains
Spreads by inhalation of mist or vapor water droplets containing the bacteria
Is rapid growing, causing inflammation and fibrin formation within the alveoli, and is often complicated by empyema
Symptoms include fever, cough, and chest pain, with a mortality rate of around 10%

Coronavirus—COVID-19– SARS-CoV-2

Coronavirus was first discovered in December 2019 in Wuhan, a central city in China. The causal agent was not identified until January 7, 2020; it is spread by SARS-CoV-2, which is spread by human-to-human transmission through droplets, contact, and fomites.
In the early stages of pneumonia, clients showed acute respiratory infection symptoms. Some clients quickly developed acute respiratory failure and others developed serious complications.
Treatment: supportive care is provided to the clients, including oxygen therapy, antibiotic treatment, antifungal treatment, and extracorporeal membrane oxygenation.
Currently, chloroquine and remdesivir are under phase three clinical trials (SARS, 2020).

SARS, severe acute respiratory syndrome; URI, upper respiratory infection.

respiratory tract—usually bacterial. However, the nature of what is aspirated can impair normal lung defenses and lead to a pneumonia.

Hospital-Acquired Pneumonia

Hospital-acquired pneumonia (HAP) (formerly referred to as "nosocomial pneumonia") occurs more than 48 hours after admission to a hospital; that is, it was not present when the client was admitted. Often, these clients have MDR because of a history of chronic illness or they are acutely ill when admitted and have prolonged hospitalizations. The latter increases potential exposure to bacteria or other pathogens through invasive procedures and improper technique, such as with ineffective handwashing by health care providers. HAP can have a high mortality rate, because of the virulent nature of the infection, the MDR involved, and the client's condition (Centers for Disease Control and Prevention [CDC], 2016b). Causative organisms include *Escherichia coli*, *K. pneumoniae*, *Pseudomonas aeruginosa*, and *H. influenza*, as well as methicillin-resistant *Staphylococcus aureus* (MRSA).

Ventilator-associated pneumonia (VAP) is pneumonia that occurs 48 hours or more after endotracheal intubation. In reality, it is a subset of HAP, because intubation and mechanical ventilation are the most common types of HAP in clients who are critically ill (Tedja & Gordon, 2013).

There is overlap with the various classifications of pneumonia. In addition, other types of pneumonia can include the following:

- *Radiation pneumonia* results from damage to the normal lung mucosa during radiation therapy for breast or lung cancer.
- *Chemical pneumonia* results from ingestion of kerosene or inhalation of volatile hydrocarbons (kerosene, gasoline, or other chemicals), which may occur in industrial settings.
- Hypoventilation of lung tissue over a prolonged period can occur when a client is bedridden and breathing with only part of the lungs. Bronchial secretions subsequently accumulate, which may lead to *hypostatic pneumonia*.

See Table 21-1 for a review of different types of pneumonias.

Pneumonia is also categorized according to its presenting symptoms. Bronchopneumonia means that the infection is patchy, diffuse, and scattered throughout both lungs. Lobar pneumonia means that the inflammation is confined to one or more lobes of the lung (Fig. 21-2).

Organisms that cause pneumonia reach the alveoli by inhalation of droplets, aspiration of organisms from the upper airway, or, less commonly, seeding from the bloodstream. When organisms reach the alveoli, the inflammatory reaction is intense, producing an exudate that impairs gas exchange. Capillaries surrounding the alveoli become engorged and cause the alveoli to collapse (**atelectasis**), further impairing gas exchange and interfering with ventilation. White blood cells (WBCs) move into the area to destroy the pathogens, filling the interstitial spaces. If untreated, consolidation occurs as the inflammation and exudate increase. Hypoxemia results from the inability of the lungs to oxygenate blood from the heart. Bronchitis, **tracheitis** (inflammation of the trachea), and spots of *necrosis* (death of tissue) in the lung may follow.

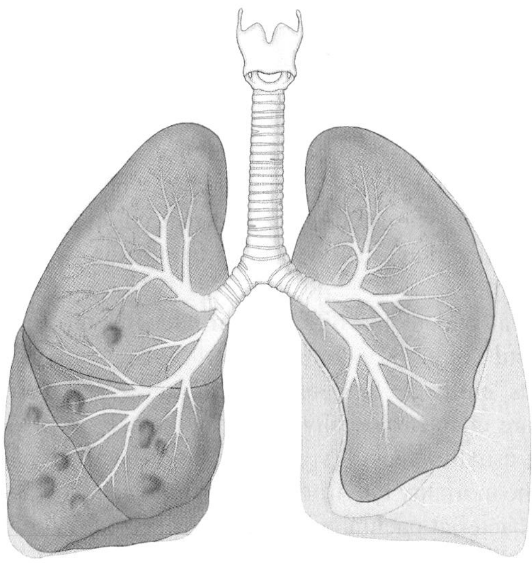

Figure 21-2 Distribution of lung involvement in bronchopneumonia and lobar pneumonia.

In atypical pneumonias, the exudate infiltrates the interstitial spaces rather than the alveoli directly. The pneumonia is more scattered, as described for bronchopneumonia. As the inflammatory process continues, it increasingly interferes with gas exchange between the bloodstream and lungs. Increased carbon dioxide (CO_2) in the blood stimulates the respiratory center, causing more rapid and shallow breathing.

Without an interruption of any type of pneumonia, the client becomes increasingly ill. If the circulatory system cannot compensate for the burden of decreased gas exchange, the client is at risk for heart failure. Death from pneumonia is most common in older adults and those weakened by acute or chronic diseases or disorders (e.g., HIV, AIDS, cancer, lung disease) or prolonged periods of inactivity. Complications of pneumonia include congestive heart failure (CHF), empyema (collection of pus in the pleural cavity), pleurisy (inflammation of the pleura), **septicemia** (infective microorganisms in the blood), atelectasis, hypotension, and shock. In addition, septicemia may lead to a secondary focus of infection, such as endocarditis (inflammation of the endocardium), pericarditis (inflammation of the pericardium), and purulent arthritis. Otitis media (infection of the middle ear), bronchitis, or sinusitis also may complicate recovery, especially from atypical pneumonia.

Assessment Findings

Signs and Symptoms

Symptoms vary for the different types of pneumonia. The onset of bacterial pneumonia is sudden. The client experiences fever, chills, a productive cough, and discomfort in the chest wall muscles from coughing. There also is general malaise. The sputum may be rust colored. Breathing causes pain; thus, the client tries to breathe as shallowly as possible.

Viral pneumonia differs from bacterial pneumonia in that results of blood cultures are sterile, sputum may be more copious, chills are less common, and pulse and respiratory rates are characteristically slow. The course of viral pneumonia usually is less severe than that of bacterial pneumonia. The mortality rate from viral pneumonia is low but rises when bacterial pneumonia occurs as a secondary infection. Many clients with viral pneumonia are weak and ill for a longer period than those with successfully treated bacterial pneumonia.

Diagnostic Findings

Auscultation of the chest reveals wheezing, crackles, and decreased breath sounds. The nail beds, lips, and oral mucosa may be cyanotic. Sputum culture and sensitivity studies can help to identify the infectious microorganism and effective antibiotics for treatment in cases of bacterial pneumonia. A chest X-ray shows areas of infiltrates and consolidation. A complete blood count discloses an elevated WBC count. Blood cultures also may be done to detect any microorganisms in the blood. A bronchoscopy may be done to obtain a sputum specimen for clients who have severe or chronic infection, are immunocompromised, or are on mechanical ventilation. A computed tomography (CT) scan may be done for clients with prolonged pneumonia to get a more definitive image of the lungs.

Medical Management

Medical management involves prompt initiation of antibiotic therapy for bacterial pneumonia, hydration to thin secretions, supplemental oxygen to alleviate hypoxemia, bed rest, chest physical therapy and postural drainage (techniques that involve manual pounding or clapping to loosen secretions and positioning of the client to drain and remove secretions from specific areas of the lungs), bronchodilators, analgesics, antipyretics, and cough expectorants or suppressants, depending on the nature of the client's cough. If a client is hospitalized, treatment is more vigorous, depending on the potential or actual complications. Fluid and electrolyte replacement sometimes is necessary secondary to fever, dehydration, and inadequate nutrition. If the client experiences severe respiratory difficulty and thick, copious secretions, they may require intubation along with mechanical ventilation.

Nursing Management

The nurse auscultates lung sounds and monitors the client for signs of respiratory difficulty. They check oxygenation status with pulse oximetry and monitor arterial blood gases (ABGs). Assessments of cough and sputum production also are necessary.

The nurse places the client in semi-Fowler position to aid breathing and increase the amount of air taken with each breath. Increased fluid intake is important to encourage because it helps to loosen secretions and replace fluids lost through fever and increased respiratory rate. The nurse monitors fluid intake and output, skin turgor, vital signs, and serum electrolytes, administering antipyretics as indicated and ordered.

Identifying clients at risk for pneumonia provides a means to practice preventive nursing care. Box 21-2 identifies strategies to implement for clients who are at risk for pneumonia. In addition, nurses encourage at-risk and older adult clients to receive vaccination against pneumococcal and influenza infections. Because the nursing care of clients with infectious lung disorders is similar regardless of the etiology, refer to the Nursing Process for the Client With Pulmonary Tuberculosis for additional interventions.

Pleurisy

Pleurisy or *pleuritis* refers to acute inflammation of the parietal and visceral pleurae. During the acute phase, the pleurae are inflamed, thick, and swollen; and an exudate forms from fibrin and lymph. Eventually, the pleurae become rigid. During inspiration, the inflamed pleurae rub together, causing severe, sharp pain.

Pathophysiology and Etiology

Pleurisy usually is a consequence of a primary condition, such as pneumonia or other pulmonary infections. The inflammatory process spreads from the lungs to the parietal pleura. Pleurisy also may develop with TB, lung cancer, cardiac and renal diseases, systemic infections, or pulmonary embolism (PE).

BOX 21-2 Preventing Pneumonia

- Promote coughing and expectoration of secretions if client experiences increased mucus production.
- Change position frequently if client is immobilized for any reason.
- Encourage deep-breathing and coughing exercises at least every 2 hours.
- Administer chest physical therapy as indicated.
- Suction client if they cannot expectorate.
- Prevent aspiration in clients at risk.
- Prevent infections.
- Cleanse respiratory equipment on a routine basis.
- Promote frequent oral hygiene.
- Administer sedatives and opioids carefully to avoid respiratory depression.
- Encourage client to stop smoking and reduce alcohol intake.

Assessment Findings

Respirations become shallow secondary to excruciating pain. Pleural fluid accumulates as the inflammatory process worsens. The pain decreases as the fluid increases because the fluid separates the pleurae. The client develops a dry cough, fatigues easily, and experiences dyspnea. A *friction rub* (coarse sounds heard during inspiration and early expiration) is heard during auscultation early in the disease process. As fluid accumulates, the pleural friction rub disappears. Decreased ventilation may result in atelectasis, hypoxemia, and hypercapnia.

Chest radiography and chest CT scan show changes in the affected area. Microscopic examination of sputum and a sputum culture may reveal pathogenic microorganisms. If a thoracentesis (removal of fluid from the chest; see Chapter 19) is performed, a pleural fluid specimen is sent to the laboratory for bacterial culture analysis. Occasionally, the primary provider may perform a pleural biopsy.

Medical Management

The underlying condition dictates the treatment. Analgesic and antipyretic drugs provide relief from pain and fever. A nonsteroidal anti inflammatory drug (NSAID) such as indomethacin (Indocin) provides analgesia and promotes more effective coughing. Antibiotics will be prescribed for bacterial infections. Thoracentesis may be done for pleural effusion, depending on the size of the effusion.

Nursing Management

The client has considerable pain with inspiration; sneezing and coughing make the pain worse. The nurse instructs the client to take analgesic medications as prescribed. Heat or cold applications may provide some topical comfort. The nurse teaches the client to splint the chest wall by turning onto the affected side. The client also can splint the chest wall with their hands or a pillow when coughing. Providing emotional support is essential—the client is very anxious and needs reassurance.

Pleural Effusion

Pleural effusion is an abnormal collection of fluid between the visceral and parietal pleurae (Fig. 21-3). Under normal conditions, approximately 5 to 15 mL of fluid between the pleurae prevent friction during pleural surface movement. Pleural effusion may be a complication of pneumonia, lung cancer, TB, PE, and CHF. The amount of accumulated fluid may be so large that the lung partially collapses on the affected side. As a consequence, pressure is placed on the heart and other organs of the mediastinum.

Assessment Findings

Fever, pain, and dyspnea are the most common symptoms. Chest percussion reveals dullness over the involved area. The examiner may note diminished or absent breath sounds over the involved area when auscultating the lungs and also may hear a friction rub. Chest radiography, ultrasound, and a CT scan will show fluid in the involved area. Thoracentesis is sometimes done to remove pleural fluid for analysis and examination for malignant cells.

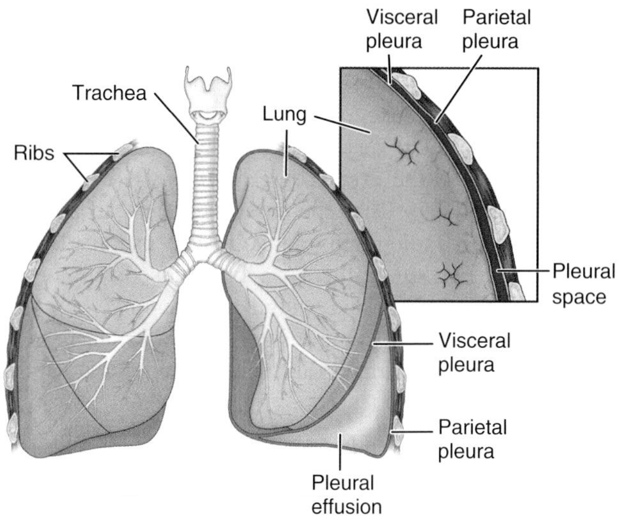

Figure 21-3 In pleural effusion, an abnormal volume of fluid collects in the pleural space.

Medical Management

The main goal of treatment is to eliminate the cause and relieve discomfort. Treatment includes antibiotics, analgesics, cardiotonic drugs to control CHF (when present), thoracentesis to remove excess pleural fluid, insertion of a chest tube to promote drainage over a longer period, and surgery for cancer when present.

Nursing Management

If thoracentesis is needed, the nurse prepares the client for this procedure (see Nursing Guidelines 19-3). The client usually is frightened; thus, the nurse must provide support. If a client has a chest tube, the nurse monitors the function of the drainage system and the amount and nature of the drainage (see discussion later in this chapter).

Lung Abscess

A **lung abscess** is a localized area of pus formation in the lung parenchyma. It can be differentiated as acute (less than 6 weeks) and chronic (more than 6 weeks). As the abscess increases, the tissue becomes necrotic. Later, the affected area collapses and creates a cavity. The infection can then extend into one or both bronchi and the pleural cavity.

Pathophysiology and Etiology

A lung abscess may develop from aspiration, bacterial pneumonia, or mechanical obstruction of the bronchi, such as with a tumor. Other causes include necrosis of lung tissue after an infection and necrotic lesions resulting from inhalation of dust particles. Clients with an impaired cough reflex or altered immune function are at risk for lung abscesses.

Assessment Findings

Signs and symptoms include chills, fever, weight loss, chest pain, and a productive cough. Sputum may be purulent or blood streaked. Finger clubbing may occur in chronic cases. Chest auscultation reveals dull or absent breath sounds in the area of the abscess, with possible pleural friction rub. Chest percussion detects an area of dullness. Chest radiography and CT scan usually locate the abscess. For some clients, a bronchoscopy may be done. Results of blood and sputum cultures may be positive for pathogens. In some instances, thoracentesis may be done, with the aspirated fluid sent to the laboratory for culture and sensitivity tests.

Medical and Surgical Management

Postural drainage and antibiotics assist in controlling the infection. Occasionally, a lobectomy is performed to remove the abscess and surrounding lung tissue.

Nursing Management

The nurse monitors the client for possible adverse effects of antibiotics. They administer chest physical therapy as indicated and encourage the client to deep breathe and cough frequently. A diet high in protein and calories is pivotal. The nurse provides emotional support while being honest with the client that the lung abscess may take a long time to resolve.

Empyema

Empyema is a general term used to denote pus in a body cavity. It usually refers, however, to pus or infected fluid in the pleural cavity (*thoracic empyema*). Empyema may follow chest trauma, such as a stab or gunshot wound, or a preexisting disease, such as pneumonia or TB, or a lung abscess. The pus-filled area may become walled off and enclosed by a thick membrane.

Assessment Findings

Fever, chest pain, dyspnea, anorexia, and malaise may accompany empyema. Chest auscultation reveals diminished or absent breath sounds over the affected area. The affected lung area is distinguished on a chest radiograph.

Medical and Surgical Management

Needle aspiration of purulent fluid by thoracentesis may be necessary to identify the microorganisms, remove pus or fluid, and select appropriate antibiotic therapy. Closed drainage may be used to empty the empyemic cavity. Tube **thoracotomy** (surgical opening of the thorax) is performed, and one or more large chest tubes are inserted, which are then connected to an underwater-seal drainage bottle. Open chest drainage, which may necessitate the removal of a section of one or more ribs, may be used when pus is thick and the walls of the empyemic cavity are strong enough to keep the lung from collapsing while the chest is opened. One or more tubes may be placed in the opening to promote drainage. The wound is then covered by a large absorbent dressing, which is changed as necessary. The drainage of pus results in a drop in temperature and general symptomatic improvement.

Inadequately treated empyema may become chronic. A thick coating forms over the lung, preventing its expansion. *Decortication* (removal of the coating) and evacuation of the pleural space allow the lung to reexpand.

Nursing Management

Empyema takes a long time to resolve. The client requires emotional support during treatment. The nurse teaches the client to do breathing exercises as prescribed.

Influenza

Influenza (flu) is an acute respiratory disease of relatively short duration. The major strains of the flu virus are A, B, and C; the strains are related yet distinct from one another. Each virus can mutate and produce variants within the given strain. The variants are called *subtypes*. The subtypes for type A influenza viruses are currently referred to as *influenza A (H1N1)* and *A (H3N2)*. Influenza A and B generally cause the seasonal epidemics. Influenza C causes milder respiratory illness and not an epidemic (Influenza, 2019).

Viruses that cause influenza are transmitted through the respiratory tract. It is generally thought that it is spread via droplets when people talk, cough, and sneeze. People nearby inhale the drops or touch them on a surface or on their skin and then touch their own mouth and nose. People are contagious for 1 day before they feel ill and up to 5 to 7 days after they get sick. The incubation period is between 1 and 4 days.

Flu chiefly occurs in epidemics, although sporadic cases appear between them. Because the viruses change, antibodies produced by those who have had one case of flu are not effective against new subtypes, and a different antibody must be produced annually or during major epidemics. Most clients recover. Fatalities usually are related to secondary bacterial complications, especially among pregnant women, older adults or debilitated clients, and those with chronic conditions such as cardiac disease and emphysema.

During a flu epidemic, the death rate from pneumonia and cardiovascular disease rises. According to the CDC, each year, 5% to 20% of the population in the United States are diagnosed with influenza. Generally, deaths occur in people who are 65 years and older. Complications include tracheobronchitis, bacterial pneumonia, and cardiovascular disease. Staphylococcal pneumonia is the most serious complication.

Table 21-2 lists signs and symptoms of flu that form the basis for diagnosis. Additional diagnostic studies, such as chest radiography and sputum analysis, may be performed to rule out other diseases.

Nursing management focuses on prevention. Annual flu vaccinations are recommended for health care providers and people at high risk for complications or

TABLE 21-2 Signs and Symptoms of Influenza

INCUBATION PERIOD	1–4 DAYS
Onset	Sudden Abrupt onset of fever and chills Severe headache Muscle aches
Progression	Anorexia Weakness, apathy, malaise Respiratory symptoms: Sneezing Sore throat, laryngitis Dry cough Nasal discharge—rhinitis Conjunctival irritation
Duration	Fever may persist for 3 days; other symptoms usually continue for 7–10 days. Cough may persist longer.
Period of contagion	One day before symptoms begin through 5 days after the onset of illness

for those exposed to many different people daily. Each year, a new vaccine is developed from three (trivalent) or four (quadrivalent) different virus strains that are predicted to be present in the coming flu season. Usually the flu vaccine is trivalent, protecting against an influenza A (H1N1), another influenza A (H3N2), and an influenza B strain. If it is quadrivalent, another influenza B strain is added. The standard flu vaccine is made from inactivated influenza vaccine and is administered intramuscularly. Another form of vaccine is called FluMist, which is a live, attenuated influenza vaccine administered intranasally. It is approved for healthy children aged 2 to 5 years who do not have a history of asthma and wheezing and for healthy persons between the ages of 5 and 49 years who are not pregnant. FluMist is not recommended for the following groups:

- People with underlying medical conditions such as diabetes or renal dysfunction
- People with known or suspected immunodeficiency diseases or those receiving immunosuppressive therapy
- People with a history of Guillain–Barré syndrome
- Children or adolescents who regularly take aspirin
- Pregnant women
- People with a hypersensitivity to eggs
- Children less than 2 years of age
- Adults 50 years and older

Clients admitted to the hospital with flu need to be isolated from clients who do not have it. Nurses must maintain airborne transmission precautions when caring for those clients. If a community is experiencing an epidemic, hospitals and other health care facilities usually develop policies regarding visitation and admissions. Box 21-3 provides information on preventing an influenza outbreak in a health care facility. The CDC (2016c) recommends three strategies: take time to get the flu vaccine; take ordinary preventive actions to stop the spread of germs, such as handwashing and covering nose and mouth when sneezing; and take antiviral drugs if prescribed.

BOX 21-3 Prevention Strategies for Seasonal Influenza in Health Care Settings

To prevent outbreaks of influenza, health care settings take the following precautions in addition to standard precautions:

- Promote and administer seasonal influenza vaccine.
- Take steps to minimize potential exposures:
  - Before clients enter the health care setting ask if they have any respiratory symptoms, such as cough, runny nose, fever.
  - Minimize elective visits by clients who are symptomatic.
  - Assure that all persons with respiratory symptoms adhere to respiratory hygiene, cough etiquette, and hand hygiene.
  - Monitor and manage health care providers who are ill.
- Adhere to standard precautions.
- Adhere to droplet precautions.
- Use caution when performing aerosol-generating procedures, such as bronchoscopy or sputum induction.
- Manage visitor access and movement within the facility.
- Monitor influenza activity.
- Implement environmental infection control.
- Implement engineering controls, such as installing partitions in triage areas.
- Train and educate health care providers.
- Administer antiviral treatment and prophylaxis of clients and health care providers when appropriate.

Adapted from Centers for Disease Control and Prevention. (2018). *Prevention strategies for seasonal influenza in healthcare settings*. https://www.cdc.gov/flu/professionals/infectioncontrol/healthcaresettings.htm

Pulmonary Tuberculosis

Pulmonary **tuberculosis** (TB) is a bacterial infectious disease primarily caused by *M. tuberculosis*. TB essentially affects the lungs, but it may also affect the kidneys and other organs. TB continues to be a worldwide health problem. About one-third of the world's population has been infected by TB, although they do not necessarily have active disease. It is among the top 10 causes of death from a single infectious agent (the first is HIV infection) (World Health Organization [WHO], 2020). In the United States, as in much of the world, new cases of TB are slowly declining. Asian countries have the largest number of new cases. TB declined by 2%, less than halfway from the milestone goal of the "End TB Strategy milestone" (Tuberculosis, 2020). The WHO has a Sustainable Development Goal of ending the TB epidemic by 2030.

Pathophysiology and Etiology

Tubercle bacilli are Gram-positive, rod-shaped, acid-fast, and aerobic. Although they can live in the dark for months as spores in particles of dried sputum, exposure to direct sunlight, heat, or ultraviolet light destroys them in a few hours. They are difficult to kill with ordinary disinfectants and are destroyed by pasteurization, a process widely used in milk and milk products to prevent the spread of TB.

TB is transmitted most commonly through the inhalation of droplets produced by coughing, sneezing, and spitting from a person with active disease. Brief contact usually does not result in infection. In contrast to the number of people who have been infected with tubercle bacilli, only a small proportion ever becomes ill. Many factors predispose a client to the development of TB, including inadequate health care, malnutrition, overcrowding, and poor housing.

TB is classified as latent TB infection and active disease. In clients with latent TB, the bacteria are present but their bodies prevent the bacteria from multiplying. These clients do not have symptoms, are not ill, and are not contagious. TB bacteria become active if they are able to multiply. These clients are sick and contagious (CDC, 2014). The classification of TB is based on the client's history, physical examination, skin test, chest X-ray, and microbiologic tests. Refer to Table 21-3 for more information.

TB is characterized by stages of early infection (or *primary* TB), latency, and potential for recurrence after the primary disease (called *secondary TB*). The bacilli may remain dormant for many years and then reactivate, producing clinical symptoms of TB.

Early Infection

Tubercle bacilli, when inhaled, pass through the bronchial system and implant on the bronchioles or alveoli. Initially, the host has no resistance to this infection. *Phagocytes* (neutrophils and macrophages) engulf the bacilli, which continue to multiply. The bacilli also spread through the lymphatic channels to the regional lymph nodes and subsequently to the circulating blood and distant organs. Eventually, the cellular immune response limits further multiplication and dissemination of the bacilli.

Immune Activation

When immune activation occurs (usually a full response occurs within 2 weeks), a characteristic tissue reaction results in the formation of a granuloma, referred to as the *Ghon tubercle*, from epithelial cells merging with the macrophages. Lymphocytes surround the Ghon tubercle, of which the central portion undergoes necrosis. This caseous necrosis has a cheesy appearance and may liquefy and slough into the connecting bronchus, producing a cavity. It also may enter the tracheobronchial system, promoting airborne transmission of infectious particles.

Healing of the Primary Lesion

Healing of the primary lesion occurs through resolution, fibrosis, and calcification. The granulation tissue of the primary lesion becomes more fibrous and creates a scar around the tubercle. This is referred to as the *Ghon complex* and is visible on radiography.

TABLE 21-3 Classification System for Tuberculosis (TB)

CLASS	TYPE	DESCRIPTION
0	No exposure to TB Not infected	No history of exposure, negative reaction to the tuberculin skin test
1	Exposure to TB No evidence of infection	History of exposure, negative reaction to a tuberculin skin test (given at least 10 weeks after exposure)
2	TB infection No TB disease	Positive reaction to the tuberculin skin test, negative bacteriologic examinations (if done), no clinical or X-ray evidence of TB disease
3	Current TB disease	Meets current laboratory criteria (e.g., a positive culture) *or* criteria for current clinical case definition
4	Previous TB disease (not current)	Medical history of TB disease, *or* Abnormal but stable X-ray findings for a person who has a positive reaction to the tuberculin skin test, negative bacteriologic examinations (if done), and no clinical or X-ray evidence of current TB disease
5	TB suspected	Signs and symptoms of TB disease, but evaluation not complete (diagnosis pending)

From Centers for Disease Control and Prevention. Tuberculosis guidelines. (2020). https://www.cdc.gov/tb/publications/guidelines/infectioncontrol.htm

Latent Period

As the lesion heals, the infection enters a latent period that can persist for many years or even an entire lifetime without producing clinical symptoms. If the immune response has been inadequate, however, the affected person eventually will develop clinical disease. Clients at particular risk are those with HIV infection or diabetes and those on chemotherapy or long-term steroids. Only a small percentage of those infected with TB actually develop clinical symptoms.

Active Tuberculosis

Secondary TB usually involves reactivation of the initial infection. The person already has had an immune response, and thus the lesions that form tend to remain in the lungs. The course of this phase usually is as follows:

- Acute local inflammation and necrosis occur.
- Infected lung tissue becomes ulcerated.
- Tubercles cluster together and become surrounded by inflammation.
- Exudate fills the surrounding alveoli.
- The client develops bronchopneumonia.
- TB tissue becomes caseous and ulcerates into the bronchus.
- Cavities form.
- Ulcerations heal, with scar tissue left around cavities.
- Pleurae thicken and retract.

The course of TB becomes a cyclical one of inflammation, bronchopneumonia, ulceration, cavitation, and scarring. The TB gradually spreads throughout the lung fields and into the rest of the respiratory structures as well as to other organs through the lymph system. A client may experience periods of exacerbation, followed by remissions.

Assessment Findings

Signs and Symptoms

The onset of TB is insidious, and early symptoms vary. An infected person may be asymptomatic until the disease is advanced. As symptoms develop, they often are vague and can be overlooked, particularly because they are systemic. Fatigue, anorexia, weight loss, and a slight, nonproductive cough are all symptoms attributable to overwork, excessive smoking, or poor eating habits. They also, however, are early symptoms of TB. Low-grade fever, particularly in the late afternoon, and night sweats are common as the disease progresses. The cough typically becomes productive of mucopurulent and blood-streaked sputum. Marked weakness, wasting, **hemoptysis** (expectoration of blood or bloody sputum), and dyspnea are characteristics of later stages. Chest pain may result from spread of the infection to the pleurae.

Diagnostic Findings

Diagnostic tests chiefly consist of the Mantoux tuberculin skin test (TST), chest radiography, CT scan, magnetic resonance imaging (MRI), and analysis of sputum and other body fluids. The Mantoux test determines if a client has been infected with *M. tuberculosis* (Nursing Guidelines 21-1). A positive TST result is evidence that a TB infection has existed at some time somewhere in the body but does not necessarily indicate active disease. The chief value of TSTs lies in case finding. All long-term care facilities are required to test each resident on admission for TB.

The QuantiFERON-TB Gold (QFT-G) test (an interferon-gamma release assay [IGRA]) was approved in 2005 for testing for TB. Another IGRA is called the T-SPOT

NURSING GUIDELINES 21-1

Performing a Mantoux Test

- Draw up 0.1 mL of intermediate-strength purified protein derivative (PPD) in a tuberculin syringe (½-inch 26- to 27-gauge needle).
- Prepare the injection site on the inner aspect of the forearm, approximately halfway between the elbow and wrist.
- Hold the syringe bevel up, almost parallel to the forearm.
- Inject the PPD to form a pronounced wheal, which indicates proper intradermal injection (Fig. A). The wheal should be 6 to 10 mm in diameter if correctly done.
- Record the site, name of PPD, strength, lot number, and date and time of test.
- Read the test site 48 to 72 hours after injection by palpating the site for induration. If induration is present, measure it at its greatest width (Fig. B). Erythema (redness) without induration is not significant. If erythema is present with induration, read the induration only. Interpret the test results as follows:
    - Up to 4-mm induration is considered not significant; no follow-up needed.
    - Greater than 5-mm induration may be significant in clients who are considered to be at risk; for example, if the client is aware of contact with someone with active TB, this reaction is seen as significant.
    - 10-mm or greater induration—considered significant; it indicates past exposure to *M. tuberculosis* or vaccination with bacillus Calmette-Guérin (BCG).

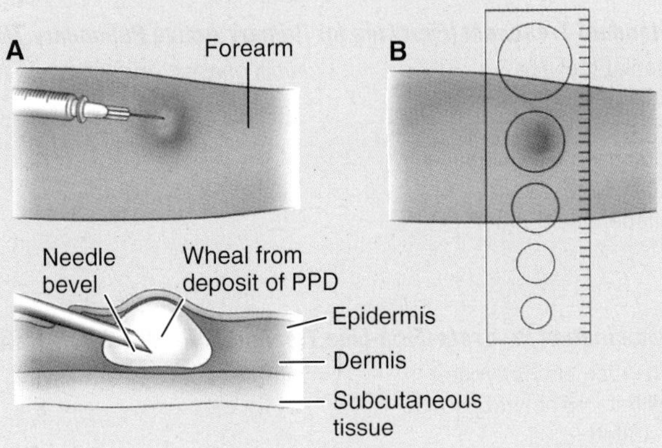

TB test (T-Spot). Similar to the TST, it measures a client's immune reactivity to *M. tuberculosis*. Results are available in less than 24 hours. Unlike the TST, the results are not impacted by previous vaccination with BCG, a vaccine for TB used in many countries but not in the United States. With the TST, clients will have a false-positive result if they had BCG, but with IGRA tests, the results are not affected. The IGRA is conducted by obtaining a small blood sample that is mixed with antigens and incubated for 16 to 24 hours. Results are presented as

- Positive: *M. tuberculosis* infection is likely.
- Negative: *M. tuberculosis* infection is unlikely.
- Indeterminate: Test did not provide useful information; repeat test, give the TST, or do nothing.

The IGRA may be used in all situations in which TST is used. As with the TST, the IGRA only indicates that a person has been infected with TB. It does not indicate anything about active disease or progression of disease.

A chest X-ray may be done, particularly if there is a positive TST or IGRA. It may demonstrate white spots in the lungs, indicating walled-off TB bacteria, or lung changes related to active disease. Microscopic examination of sputum and other body fluids identifies the bacilli and is ordered when TB is suspected, during and after a course of drug therapy for TB, and after surgical removal of a diseased lobe of the lung. The client is instructed to cough deeply so that the specimen does not consist mainly of saliva. Most clients find that it is easier to raise sputum when they first awaken. It may be necessary to collect specimens on several consecutive days (see Nursing Guidelines 19-2).

Gastric lavage, gastric aspiration, or bronchoscopy may be used to determine the presence of the tubercle bacilli, particularly when a client has had difficulty raising a sputum specimen for examination. Tubercle bacilli may reach the stomach from the lungs when the client raises sputum but swallows rather than expectorates it. When invasion of other body areas by tubercle bacilli is suspected, specimens are obtained to confirm the diagnosis.

Medical and Surgical Management

In many cases, drugs have speeded recovery and provided a chance to arrest TB in clients with advanced lesions; however, they do not guarantee a cure. Their usefulness lies in their ability to retard the growth and multiplication of tubercle bacilli, thus giving the body a chance to overcome the disease. Two factors make drug therapy less than ideal: drug toxicity and the tendency of the tubercle bacilli to develop drug resistance. Combined therapy with two or more drugs decreases the likelihood of drug resistance, increases the tuberculostatic action of the drugs, and lessens the risk for toxic drug reactions (Drug Therapy Table 21-1).

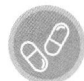

Pharmacologic Considerations

■ Latent treatment is used for those infected but do not have the disease. Five percent to 10% of these individuals will eventually present with active disease if not treated. Clients are typically treated for 6 to 9 months with isoniazid (INH) on a daily or biweekly schedule. To increase adherence and prevent drug resistance, less frequent protocols are being tested, such as a rifapentine/INH combination taken weekly for 12 weeks.

DRUG THERAPY TABLE 21-1 Drug Regimen for Tuberculosis (TB)

Category and Common Generic (Brand) Drugs	Length of Drug Therapy	Common Side Effects	Safety Warnings for Nurses
Latent Treatment (Prophylaxis)			
Isoniazid (INH) INH/rifapentine[a]	For those showing positive test, not active TB (latent TB) for 6–9 months Used in latent TB protocol for 12 weeks	Nausea, vomiting, epigastric distress, rash	• Effectiveness severely reduced when taken with food
Standard Treatment (First Line for Primary Active Pulmonary TB)			
Isoniazid (INH) Ethambutol (Myambutol) Pyrazinamide Rifabutin (Mycobutin) Rifampin (Rifadin) Rifapentine (Priftin)[a]	*Initial phase*: 2 months; *continuing phase*: 4–7 months	Nausea, vomiting, epigastric distress, myalgia, rash	• Effectiveness severely reduced when taken with food • Hepatotoxic at routine doses, monitor liver enzymes frequently • Peripheral neuropathy frequently occurs
Combination Products (First-Line Treatment) for Better Adherence			
INH/rifampin (Rifamate) INH/rifampin/pyrazinamide (Rifater)	Same as active treatment	Same as drugs for latent and standard treatment	

DRUG THERAPY TABLE 21-1 Drug Regimen for Tuberculosis (TB) (*continued*)

Category and Common Generic (Brand) Drugs	Length of Drug Therapy	Common Side Effects	Safety Warnings for Nurses
Retreatment and Multidrug-Resistant Treatment (MDR-TB) (Secondary TB)			
Aminosalicylate (Paser) Capreomycin (Capastat) Cycloserine (Seromycin) Ethionamide (Trecator)	Retreatment: use all with antibiotic up to 24 months	Nausea, vomiting, diarrhea, headache	• First priority of direct observation therapy (DOT) should go to MDR-TB clients • Dosing intervals may be increased when end-stage renal disease (ESRD) is present
Food and Drug Administration Fast Track Drug for MDR-TB			
Bedaquiline (Sirturo)	Only use in DOT setting for MDR-TB	Nausea, vomiting, hemoptysis, headache	• Sudden cardiac death has occurred, monitor for prolonged QT interval on electrocardiogram

[a]Taken with pyridoxine (vitamin B6) to prevent peripheral neuropathy.
The drugs in column 1 indicate the drug that matches up with explanations in columns 2 through 4.

Resistance of the bacilli to drugs is an important factor in the lack of response to medical treatment. Drug therapy usually is carried out while the client is at home. Regular visits to the primary provider's office or clinic for follow-up care are necessary for assessment of response to therapy. Culture and sensitivity tests may be performed, and the adverse effects of the drugs are evaluated.

When the disease is located primarily in one section of the lung, that portion may be removed by **segmental resection** (removal of a lobe segment) or **wedge resection** (removal of a wedge of diseased tissue). If the diseased area is larger, **lobectomy** (removal of a lobe) may be performed. In some cases, the lung is so diseased that **pneumonectomy** (removal of an entire lung) is necessary (Box 21-4).

BOX 21-4 Types of Lung Resections and Procedures

Lobectomy: single lobe of lung removed
Bilobectomy: two lobes of lung removed
Sleeve resection: cancerous lobe(s) removed and a segment of the main bronchus resected
Pneumonectomy: removal of entire lung
Segmentectomy (segmental resection): segment of lung removed
Wedge resection: removal of small, pie-shaped area of the segment
Chest wall resection with removal of cancerous lung tissue: for cancers that have invaded the chest wall

Adapted from Hinkle, J. L., & Cheever, K. H. (2018). *Brunner & Suddarth's textbook of medical-surgical nursing* (14th ed.). Wolters Kluwer.

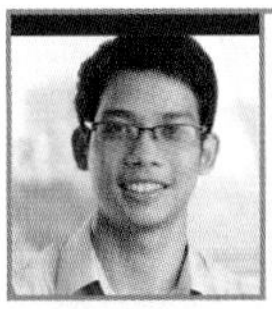

Clinical Scenario A male client who recently emigrated from Vietnam is seen in an international clinic. He complains of a cough productive of blood-tinged mucus, a 5-kg weight loss in the last 4 to 6 weeks, poor appetite, chest pain with respirations, and night sweats. Other relatives are being treated for TB. An IGRA test done the previous day is positive for TB exposure. Plans are made to admit the client to rehydrate him, do further diagnostic tests, and begin medical treatment for TB. **What are the important aspects to focus on when caring for a client with TB? See the following Nursing Process section.**

NURSING PROCESS FOR THE CLIENT WITH PULMONARY TUBERCULOSIS

Assessment

Assess breath sounds, breathing patterns, and overall respiratory status. Ask the client about any pain or discomfort experienced with breathing. Inspect the client's sputum for color, viscosity, amount, and signs of blood. Clients with primary TB may have complaints related to fatigue, weakness, anorexia, weight loss, or night sweats. Clients with secondary TB may report chest pain and a cough that produces mucopurulent or blood-tinged mucus or blood. They also may report a low-grade fever.

Diagnosis, Planning, and Interventions

Antitubercular drug regimens extend for long periods and without interruption because healing is slow and interrupted treatment increases drug resistance. The primary focus of nursing management is encouraging the client to adhere to the prescribed medication regimen and teaching.

(*continued*)

NURSING PROCESS FOR THE CLIENT WITH PULMONARY TUBERCULOSIS (continued)

Instruct the client to take medications exactly as prescribed, closely observing the time interval between each dose. Clients must not skip doses or take more than the amount prescribed. Clients need to complete the entire course of drug therapy to control infection. Continuous therapy is essential because lapses in taking the prescribed drugs can result in reactivation of the infection. Advise clients to notify the primary provider if symptoms worsen or sudden chest pain or dyspnea develops. Clients should also drink plenty of fluids, discontinue smoking immediately, and avoid exposure to secondhand smoke. They need to eat a balanced diet with ample protein and calories to promote healing and maintain weight.

Other nursing care includes the following diagnoses, outcomes, and interventions.

Ineffective Airway Clearance: Related to pain with coughing, inability to cough, and abnormal respirations
Expected Outcome: Client will effectively clear secretions.

- Assess cough, noting the attributes of the secretions: color, consistency, amount, and presence of blood. *Coughing usually becomes more frequent with increased expectorant; hemoptysis occurs in advanced TB.*
- Encourage client to drink 3 to 4 L/day. *This amount liquefies and thins secretions and facilitates expectoration.*
- Humidify inspired air. *Humidified air maintains moisture to assist in liquefying secretions.*
- Encourage deep breathing and coughing every 2 hours while awake. *These measures promote lung expansion and mobilization of secretions.*
- Place client in semi-Fowler position. *This position improves breathing and assists client to expectorate mucus.*
- Provide instructions about postural drainage. *Postural drainage facilitates airway drainage and clearance.*

Acute Pain: Related to chest expansion secondary to lung infection/inflammation
Expected Outcome: Client will manage pain with analgesics and use of splinting techniques when coughing.

- Assess pain level. *This information provides a baseline for treatment and evaluation.*
- Evaluate effectiveness of pain relief measures. *Such evaluation helps the nurse to determine if measures are effective or other therapies are necessary.*
- Administer analgesics as indicated. *Proper pain assessment and appropriate analgesic administration provide more effective pain control.*
- Instruct client in splinting techniques for use during coughing. *Proper splinting decreases pain and facilitates expectoration of secretions.*

Activity Intolerance: Related to general weakness, respiratory difficulties, fever, and severity of illness
Expected Outcome: Client will demonstrate increased activity tolerance.

- Encourage rest periods, particularly before meals. Space the timing of activities of daily living (ADLs) and exercise. *Rest reduces fatigue, and spacing activities allows the client to preserve energy.*
- Prioritize necessary tasks, eliminating nonessential tasks. *Prioritization of tasks promotes rest.*
- Assist client with activities as required. *Giving assistance reduces client's energy expenditure but allows choices.*
- Keep equipment (e.g., telephone, tissues, wastebasket, bedside commode) close to client. *Keeping needed items close by reduces energy expenditure.*
- Encourage active range-of-motion (ROM) exercises three times a day. *Active ROM exercises maintain muscle strength and joint ROM.*

RC: Side Effects of Medication Therapy: Hepatitis, neurologic changes, gastrointestinal (GI) upset
Expected Outcome: Nurse will assist client to minimize side effects of medications.

- Instruct client to take medication 1 hour before or 2 hours after meals. *Food interferes with medication absorption.*
- Instruct clients taking INH to avoid foods with tyramine and histamine (e.g., tuna, aged cheese, red wine, soy sauce, yeast extracts). *INH, when combined with these foods, may cause lightheadedness, flushing, hypotension, headache, and other symptoms.*
- Ask if client is taking any beta-blockers or oral anticoagulants. *Rifampin increases the metabolism of beta-blockers and oral anticoagulants. Dosages may need to be adjusted or medications changed.*
- Inform the client who wears contact lenses that rifampin may color them. *The client may prefer to wear glasses while taking rifampin.*
- Monitor for side effects related to medication regimen. For hepatitis, check liver enzymes. For kidney function, check blood urea nitrogen and serum creatinine levels. For neurologic changes, look for hearing loss and neuritis. Also check for skin rash. *Early identification of side effects promotes prompt treatment of side effects and adjustments in medications.*

Evaluation of Expected Outcomes

The client manages secretions with effective coughing, increased fluid intake, and appropriate postural drainage. The client reports adequate pain relief and can tolerate increased amounts of time out of bed and perform most ADLs. The client adheres to treatment regimen and schedules tests for liver and kidney function.

>>> *Stop, Think, and Respond 21-1*

A client diagnosed with TB lives in a four-room apartment with his wife. What precautions must the couple follow?

OBSTRUCTIVE PULMONARY DISEASES

Obstructive pulmonary disease describes conditions in which expiratory airflow is limited. **Chronic obstructive pulmonary disease** (COPD) is an umbrella term for chronic lung diseases that have limited airflow in and out of the lungs. Symptoms of COPD include chronic cough and expectoration, dyspnea, shortness of breath, wheezing, and impaired expiratory airflow. Bronchiectasis, atelectasis, chronic bronchitis, and emphysema, although not categorized as COPD, involve chronic impairment of airflow. Asthma also is an obstructive disorder in that it is more episodic and usually more acute than COPD, secondary to narrowed airways because of bronchospasm, inflammation, and increased airway secretions. Sleep apnea syndrome also can have obstructive causes (see Chapter 20). Cystic fibrosis (CF) has obstructive characteristics and is included in this section.

Bronchiectasis

Bronchiectasis is characterized by chronic infection and irreversible dilatation of the bronchi and bronchioles, as a result of destruction of muscle and elastic connective tissue. Causes include bronchial obstruction by tumor or foreign body, injury to the airway, congenital abnormalities, genetic disorders, exposure to toxic gases, and chronic pulmonary infections. When clearance of the airway is impeded, an infection can develop in the walls of the bronchus or bronchioles. The structure of the wall tissue subsequently changes, resulting in formation of saccular dilatations, which collect purulent material. Airway clearance is further impaired, and the purulent material remains, causing more dilatation, structural damage, and more infection.

Assessment Findings

Clients with bronchiectasis experience a chronic cough with expectoration of copious amounts of purulent sputum and possible hemoptysis. The coughing worsens when the client changes position. The amount of sputum produced during one paroxysm varies with the stage of the disease, but it can be several ounces. In addition to a chronic cough, clients experience fatigue, weight loss, anorexia, and dyspnea. The client's fingers may be clubbed secondary to respiratory insufficiency. Clients have repeated pulmonary infections.

CT scans, which show bronchial dilatation, provide an early and definitive diagnosis and differentiate bronchiectasis from bronchitis. Chest radiography and bronchoscopy may also be done to demonstrate the increased size of the bronchioles, possible areas of atelectasis, and changes in the pulmonary tissue. Sputum culture and sensitivity tests identify causative microorganisms and effective antibiotics to control the infection. Pulmonary function studies also may be done.

Medical Management

Treatment of bronchiectasis includes drainage of purulent material from the bronchi; antibiotics, bronchodilators, and mucolytics to improve breathing and help raise secretions; humidification to loosen secretions; bronchoscopy to remove purulent sputum; and surgical removal (rarely done) if bronchiectasis is confined to a small area. Treatment is aimed at preventing complications, such as respiratory failure and atelectasis.

Nursing Management

Nursing management focuses on instructing the client in postural drainage techniques, which helps clients mobilize and expectorate secretions. The positions for the client to assume depend on the site or lobe to be drained. Figure 21-4 shows positions that drain specific segments of all lobes of the lungs. The client remains in each position for 10 to 15 minutes. Chest percussion and vibration may be performed during this time. When complete, the client coughs and expectorates the secretions. This procedure may be repeated. The nurse provides oral hygiene after treatment.

>>> *Stop, Think, and Respond 21-2*

Your client with acute bronchitis smokes two packs of cigarettes per day. What would you advise this client?

Atelectasis

Clients with obstructive lung disease are at greater risk for developing atelectasis, the collapse of alveoli (Fig. 21-5). Atelectasis may involve a small portion of the lung or an entire lobe. When alveoli collapse, they cannot perform their function of gas exchange. Atelectasis occurs secondary to aspiration of food or vomitus, a mucus plug, fluid or air in the thoracic cavity, compression on tissue by tumors, an enlarged heart, an aneurysm, or enlarged lymph nodes in the chest. Clients who are ill may experience atelectasis when on prolonged bed rest, when unable to breathe deeply or cough and raise secretions, or both.

Assessment Findings

The amount of involved lung tissue determines the extent of the symptoms. Small areas of atelectasis may cause few symptoms. With larger areas, cyanosis, fever, pain, dyspnea, increased pulse and respiratory rates, and increased pulmonary secretions may be seen. Although crackling may be auscultated over the affected areas, usually, breath sounds are absent. A chest X-ray reveals dense shadows, indicating collapsed lung tissue. Sometimes, the X-ray results are inconclusive. CT scans demonstrate lung inflation and volumes, and if there is a tumor or other cause of obstruction. ABG and pulse oximetry results may be abnormal. A bronchoscopy may be done to determine if there is an obstructive cause, such as a tumor or foreign body.

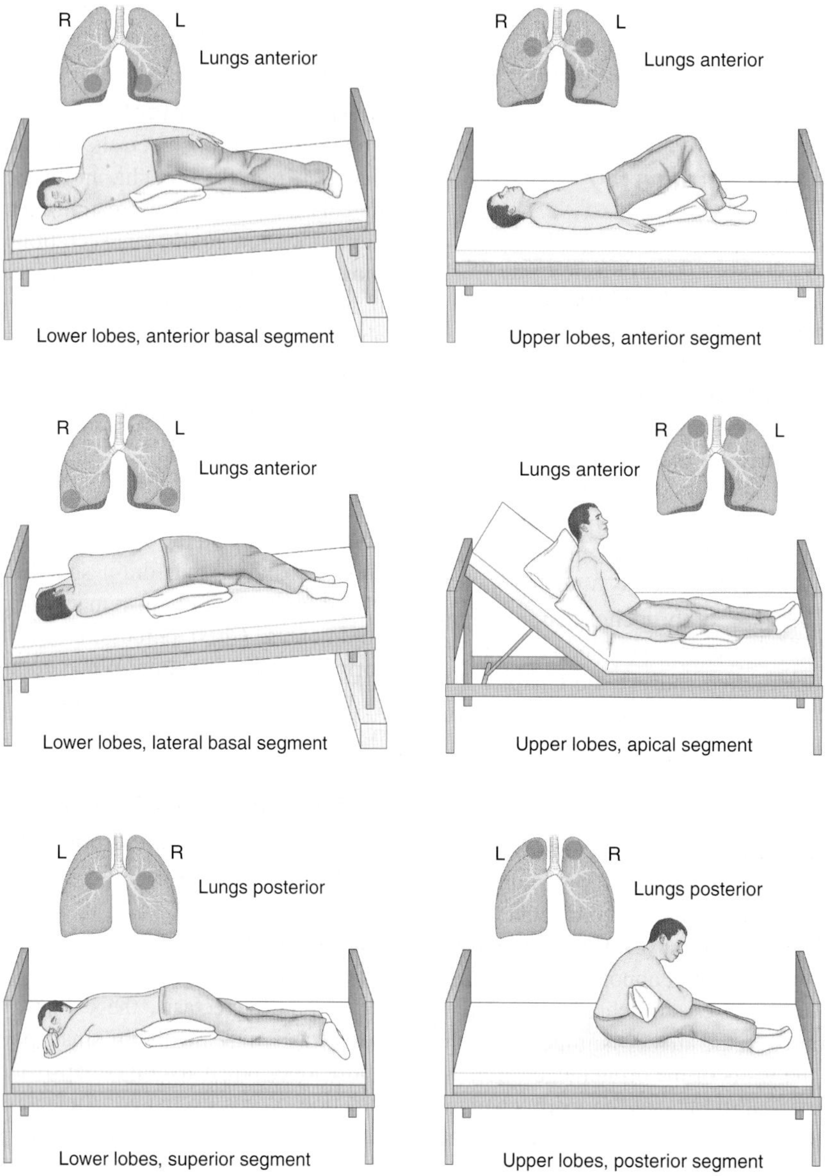

Figure 21-4 Lung areas to be drained and the best postural drainage positions for them.

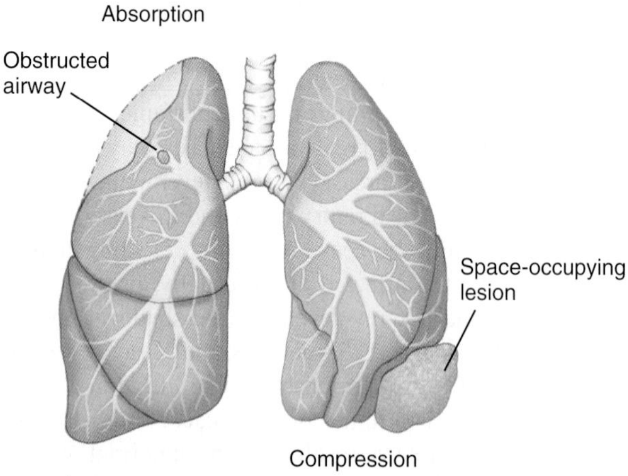

Figure 21-5 Atelectasis caused by airway obstruction and absorption of air from the involved lung area on the left and by compression of lung tissue on the right.

Medical Management

Treatment includes improving ventilation, suctioning, chest percussion, and deep breathing and coughing to raise secretions. Bronchodilators and humidification assist in loosening and removing secretions. Oxygen is administered for dyspnea. Removal of the cause of atelectasis helps to correct the condition.

Nursing Management

Nursing care focuses on preventing atelectasis (Box 21-5), especially when the client is at risk because of failure to aerate the lungs properly. Postoperative deep breathing and coughing can prevent atelectasis. If atelectasis occurs, the nurse encourages the client to take deep breaths and cough at frequent intervals and instructs the client in the use of an incentive spirometer (Client and Family Teaching 21-1).

BOX 21-5 Preventing Atelectasis

- Change client's position frequently, especially from supine to upright position, to promote ventilation and prevent secretions from accumulating.
- Encourage early mobilization from bed to chair, followed by early ambulation.
- Encourage appropriate deep breathing and coughing to mobilize secretions and prevent them from accumulating.
- Teach/reinforce appropriate technique for incentive spirometry.
- Administer prescribed opioids and sedatives judiciously to prevent respiratory depression.
- Perform postural drainage and chest percussion if indicated.
- Institute suctioning to remove tracheobronchial secretions if indicated.

Adapted from Hinkle, J. L., & Cheever, K. H. (2018). *Brunner & Suddarth's textbook of medical-surgical nursing* (14th ed.). Wolters Kluwer.

Chronic Bronchitis

Chronic bronchitis is a prolonged (or extended) inflammation of the bronchi, accompanied by a chronic cough and excessive production of mucus for at least 3 months each year for 2 consecutive years. This serious health problem develops gradually and may go untreated for many years until the disease is well established.

Client and Family Teaching 21-1
Using an Incentive Spirometer

The nurse instructs the client as follows:

1. Sit upright unless contraindicated.
2. Mark the goal for inhalation.
3. Exhale normally.
4. Place mouthpiece in mouth, sealing lips around it.
5. Inhale slowly until predetermined volume has been reached.
6. Hold breath for 2 to 6 seconds.
7. Exhale normally.
8. Repeat the exercise 10 to 20 times per hour while awake or as ordered.
9. Do not rush during the procedure. Slow down if dizziness is experienced.

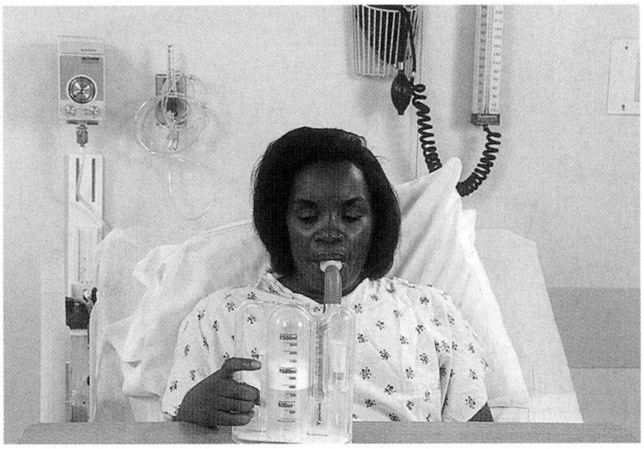

Pathophysiology and Etiology

Chronic bronchitis is characterized by hypersecretion of mucus and recurrent or chronic respiratory tract infections. As the infection progresses, the ability of the cilia that line the airway to propel secretions upward becomes significantly altered. Secretions remain in the lungs and form plugs in the smaller bronchi. These plugs become areas for bacterial growth and chronic infection, which increases mucus secretion and eventually causes areas of focal tissue death. Airway obstruction results from the bronchial inflammation (Fig. 21-6).

Multiple factors are associated with chronic bronchitis. Its development may be insidious or follow a long history of bronchial asthma or an acute respiratory tract infection, such as influenza or pneumonia. Air pollution and smoking are significant factors.

Chronic bronchitis may develop at any age, but it appears most commonly in middle age after years of untreated, low-grade bronchitis. Diagnosis is based on evaluation of the duration of symptoms, determination of how the disease process began, and history of occupational health hazards, pulmonary disease, and smoking.

Assessment Findings

Signs and Symptoms

The earliest symptom is a chronic cough productive of thick, white mucus, especially when rising in the morning and in the evening. Bronchospasm may occur during severe bouts of coughing. Acute respiratory infections are frequent during the winter months and may persist for at least several weeks. As the disease progresses, the sputum may become yellow, purulent, copious, and blood streaked after paroxysms of coughing. Expiration is prolonged secondary to obstructed air passages. Cyanosis secondary to hypoxemia may be noted, especially after severe coughing. Dyspnea begins with exertion but progresses to occurring with minimal activity and later occurs at rest. Right-sided heart failure results from tachycardia in response to hypoxemia, which causes edema in the extremities.

Diagnostic Findings

The progression and history of symptoms determine the diagnostic studies needed. Initially, results of the physical examination, chest radiography, and pulmonary function tests may be normal. As the disease progresses, these findings become increasingly abnormal. Chest radiography shows signs of fluid overload and consolidation in the lungs.

As right-sided failure develops, the heart enlarges. Pulmonary function test results demonstrate decreased vital capacity and forced expiratory volume and increased residual volume and total lung capacity. Diagnostic studies such as bronchoscopy, microscopic examination of the sputum for malignant cells, and lung scan may be necessary to rule out cancer, bronchiectasis, TB, or other diseases in which cough is a predominant feature.

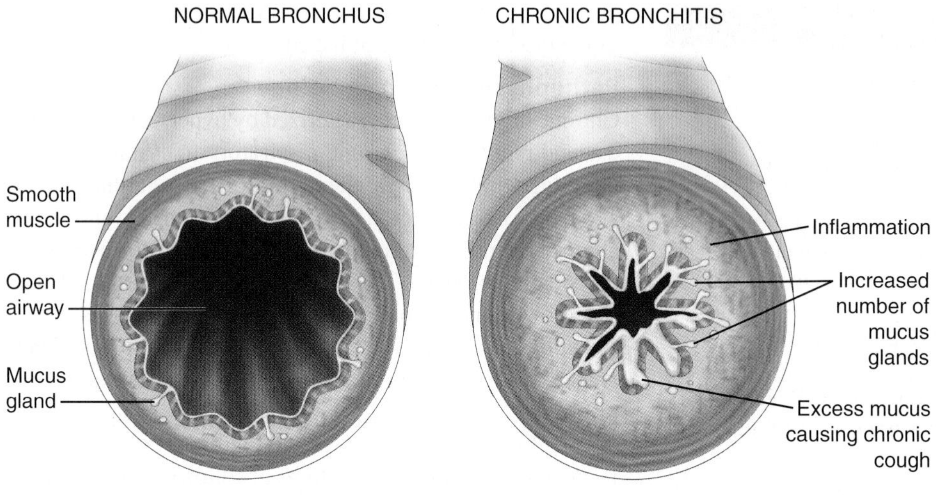

Figure 21-6 Pathophysiology of chronic bronchitis as compared with normal bronchus. The bronchus in chronic bronchitis is narrowed and has impaired airflow due to multiple mechanisms: inflammation, excess mucus production, and potential smooth muscle constriction (bronchospasm).

Medical Management

Treatment goals are to prevent recurrent irritation of the bronchial mucosa by infection or chemical agents, maintain the function of the bronchioles, and assist in the removal of secretions. Treatment includes smoking cessation, bronchodilators to reduce airway obstruction and bronchospasm, increased fluid intake, maintenance of a well-balanced diet, postural drainage to remove bronchial secretions, steroid therapy if other treatment is ineffective, change in occupation if work involves exposure to dust and chemical irritants, filtration of incoming air to reduce sputum production and cough, and antibiotic therapy.

Nursing Management

Nursing management focuses on educating clients in managing their disease. The nurse helps clients identify ways to eliminate environmental irritants. Such measures include smoking cessation, occupational counseling, monitoring air quality and pollution levels, and avoiding cold air and wind exposure that can cause bronchospasm.

Preventing infection is another important aspect of care. The nurse instructs clients to avoid others with respiratory tract infections and to receive pneumonia and flu immunizations. The nurse also teaches the client to monitor sputum for signs of infection and demonstrates the proper use of aerosolized bronchodilators and corticosteroids.

Metered-dose inhalers (MDIs) are pressurized devices that contain an aerosolized powder of specific medications. When the client pushes on the pressurized canister, an exact amount of medication is delivered via inhalation. Clients need instruction regarding the use of an MDI (Client and Family Teaching 21-2). It may be difficult for clients to coordinate the equipment and the need to inhale forcibly as the medication is released. For that reason, spacers (holding chambers) are added to hold the medication, allowing the client to inhale slowly and deeply and with more control to receive the full dose of the inhaled medication. There are also other types of inhalers specific to particular medications; each requires thorough client instruction.

Client and Family Teaching 21-2
Using a Metered-Dose Inhaler (MDI)

The nurse provides the following instructions:

1. Attach the stem of the canister into the hole of the mouthpiece so that the inhaler looks like an "L." If a spacer is used, attach the spacer to the mouthpiece on one end and to the MDI on the other end.
2. Shake the canister to distribute the drug in its pressurized chamber.
3. Exhale slowly through pursed lips.
4. Seal lips around the mouthpiece or hold inhaler a few inches from mouth.
5. Compress the canister between thumb and fingers and slowly inhale; if not using a spacer, you must compress the canister and inhale at the same time.
6. Release the pressure on the canister but continue inhaling as much as possible. Inhalation should be for 5 to 7 seconds in order to breathe in completely.
7. Withdraw the mouthpiece.
8. Hold breath for 10 seconds (count to 10 slowly) to allow the medication to reach the airways of the lungs.
9. Exhale slowly through pursed lips.
10. If second dose is required, wait for a few seconds before repeating procedure.

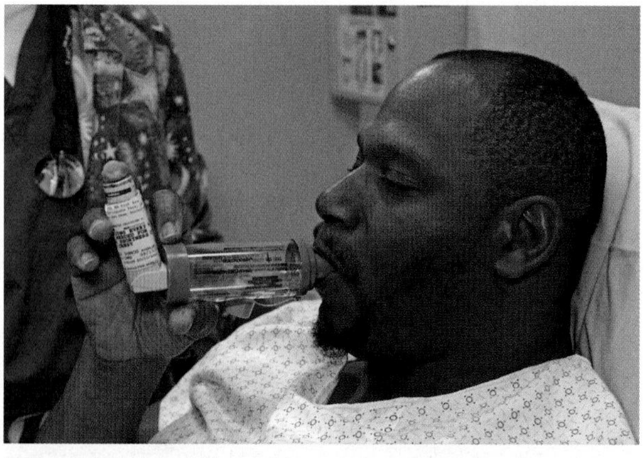

Metered-dose inhaler with spacer.

The nurse instructs the client in postural drainage techniques and measures to improve overall health, such as eating a well-balanced diet, getting plenty of rest, and engaging in moderate aerobic activity. For clients with lung disease, dyspnea, not heart rate, should determine the amount of aerobic activity. In other words, clients should exercise at the pace and for the length of time they can tolerate without dyspnea. Refer to nursing management of emphysema for nursing diagnoses and additional interventions.

Emphysema

Emphysema is a chronic disease characterized by abnormal distention of the alveoli. The alveolar walls and capillary beds also show marked destruction. This process of destruction occurs over a long period. By the time of diagnosis, damage to the lungs usually is permanent. Emphysema is a common cause of disability and the most common obstructive lung disorder.

Pathophysiology and Etiology

In emphysema, the alveoli lose elasticity, trapping air that the client normally would expire. On microscopic examination, the alveolar walls are broken down, forming one large sac instead of multiple, small air spaces. The capillary beds, previously located within the alveolar walls, are destroyed, and fibrous scarring replaces much of the tissue. Formation of fibrous tissue and destruction of the alveoli prevent the proper exchange of O_2 and CO_2 during respiration.

As the disease progresses, large air sacs (bullae, blebs) may be seen over the lung surface. These sacs can rupture, allowing air to enter the thorax (**pneumothorax**) with each respiration. In this case, emergency thoracentesis is performed to remove the air from the thoracic cavity. A chest tube may be inserted to keep additional air from entering. Recurrent episodes of pneumothorax may require surgery to correct the problem (see section on Thoracic Surgery).

Assessment Findings

Signs and Symptoms

Shortness of breath with minimal activity is called *exertional dyspnea* and often is the first symptom of emphysema. As the disease progresses, breathlessness occurs even at rest. A chronic cough invariably is present and productive of mucopurulent sputum. Inspiration is difficult because of the rigid chest cage, and the chest is characteristically barrel shaped (Fig. 21-7).

The client uses the accessory muscles of respiration (muscles in the jaw and neck and intercostal muscles) to maintain normal ventilation. Expiration is prolonged, difficult, and often accompanied by wheezing. In advanced emphysema, respiratory function is markedly impaired. Clients with advanced emphysema characteristically appear drawn, anxious,

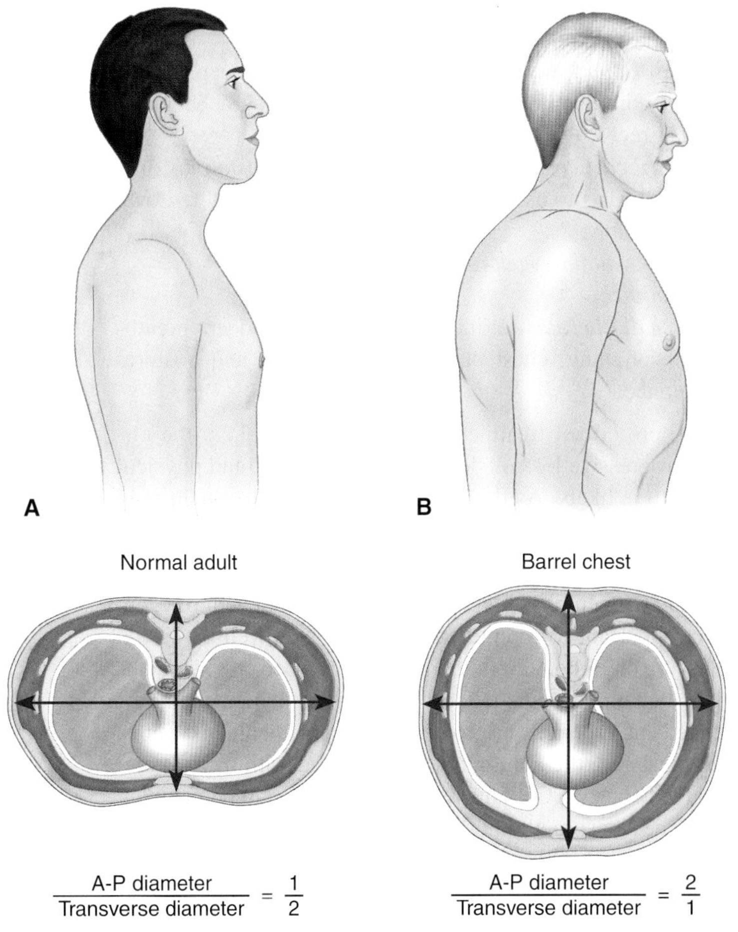

Figure 21-7 Characteristics of normal chest wall and chest wall in emphysema. **(A)** The normal chest wall and its cross-section. **(B)** The barrel-shaped chest of emphysema and its cross-section. A-P, Anterior-Posterior.

and pale. They speak in short, jerky sentences. When sitting up, they often lean slightly forward and are markedly short of breath. The neck veins may distend during expiration.

In advanced emphysema, memory loss, drowsiness, confusion, and loss of judgment may result from the markedly reduced oxygen that reaches the brain and the increased CO_2 in the blood. If the disorder goes untreated, the CO_2 content in the blood may reach toxic levels, resulting in lethargy, stupor, and, eventually, coma. This condition is called *carbon dioxide narcosis*. Lung auscultation reveals decreased breath sounds, wheezing, and crackles. Heart sounds are diminished or muffled. Visual inspection shows a barrel-chested person breathing through pursed lips and using the accessory muscles of respiration.

Diagnostic Findings

Chest radiography, fluoroscopy, and CT scanning demonstrate hyperinflated lung fields. Results of pulmonary function studies show a marked decrease in overall function, including increased total lung capacity and residual volume and decreased vital capacity and forced expiratory volume. ABG analysis usually reveals hypoxemia and respiratory acidosis.

Medical Management

The goals of medical management include improving the client's quality of life, slowing the disease progression, and treating the obstructed airways. Treatment includes the following measures:

- *Bronchodilators* to dilate airways by decreasing edema and spasms and improving gas exchange
- *Aerosol therapy* with nebulized aerosols for deep inhalation of bronchodilators and mucolytics in the tracheobronchial tree
- *Inhaled corticosteroid drugs and oral corticosteroids* on a limited basis to assist with bronchodilatation and removal of secretions
- *Supplemental oxygen* may be prescribed.
- *Antibiotics*
- *Physical therapy* to increase ventilation—deep breathing, coughing, chest percussion, vibration, and postural drainage

If the prescribed treatment regimen does not help the client, progressive loss of sleep, appetite, weight, and physical strength is likely. As the disease progresses, the client may need to curtail physical activities.

Nursing Management

Clients with emphysema may require supplemental oxygen. It is important to monitor oxygen levels as well as partial pressure of carbon dioxide ($PaCO_2$) levels because some clients with emphysema tend to have chronic hypercapnia (elevated $PaCO_2$). For this group, when supplemental oxygen is administered, the hemoglobin is saturated with oxygen and unable to carry CO_2. This results in increased hypercapnia.

The safest method of oxygen administration is by nasal catheter or cannula, with the oxygen flow rate set at no more than 2 to 3 L/min. If the client's color improves but their level of consciousness decreases, the nurse discontinues oxygen administration and notifies the primary provider; the client may be approaching a state of respiratory arrest.

Therapeutic breathing exercises effectively use the diaphragm (diaphragmatic breathing), thus relieving the compensatory burden on the muscles of the upper thorax. The nurse teaches the client to let the abdomen rise when taking a deep breath and to contract the abdominal muscles when exhaling. Clients can feel the correct way to do this by placing one hand on the chest and the other on the abdomen: during abdominal breathing, the chest should remain quiet and the abdomen should rise and fall with each breath.

Other exercises include blowing out candles at various distances and blowing a small object, such as a pencil or piece of chalk, along a tabletop. The nurse encourages the client to exhale more completely by taking a deep breath and then bending the body forward at the waist while exhaling as fully as possible. Pursed-lip breathing (i.e., breathing with the lips pursed or puckered on expiration) helps to control the respiratory rate and depth and slows expiration. This maneuver may decrease dyspnea and, in turn, reduce the anxiety that often is associated with breathing difficulties.

In addition, client education is aimed at helping clients adjust to their current level of disability and to the potential for increased disability in the future. The primary goal is to prevent or delay the progression of emphysema. Clients who are motivated will profit more from available treatments and make the best use of their remaining pulmonary function. Client and Family Teaching 21-3 outlines strategies to slow disease progression. Refer also to Nutrition Notes 21-1.

Client and Family Teaching 21-3
Following a Treatment Regimen for Emphysema

The nurse teaches the client strategies to slow the disease progression:

- Success of treatment depends on strict adherence to the treatment regimen.
- Take medication exactly as prescribed. Observe the time intervals between medications.
- Do not skip doses or take more than what is prescribed.
- Maintain close medical supervision.
- Contact the primary provider if adverse drug effects occur, drugs fail to relieve symptoms, new symptoms appear, symptoms become more severe, or signs or symptoms of respiratory infection develop.
- Drink extra fluids as indicated, unless fluids are restricted.
- Avoid respiratory irritants and people with respiratory infections.
- Eat a well-balanced diet.
- Perform breathing exercises as prescribed.
- Take frequent rests during the day. Space activities to prevent fatigue and shortness of breath.
- Avoid dry-heated areas that can aggravate symptoms.
- Humidify inspired air during the winter months.

Nutrition Notes 21-1

Client With Emphysema

- Malnutrition among clients with emphysema is multifactorial.
  - Shortness of breath and difficulty breathing impair the ability to chew and swallow.
  - Inadequate oxygenation of GI cells causes anorexia and gastric ulceration.
  - Slowed peristalsis and digestion contribute to loss of appetite.
  - Labored breathing increases calorie requirements.
  - Eating is not a priority among clients who are anxious about breathing.
- To correct malnutrition, a high-protein, high-calorie diet is indicated, but an excessive calorie intake is avoided because it increases respiratory stress by increasing carbon dioxide output.
- Small, frequent feedings of nutrient-dense foods help maximize intake and lessen fatigue; concentrated liquid supplements are beneficial.
- Encourage ample fluid intake. Fluids consumed between meals instead of with meals are less likely to interfere with food intake.
- Clients who are obese with emphysema are encouraged to lose weight to improve breathing.

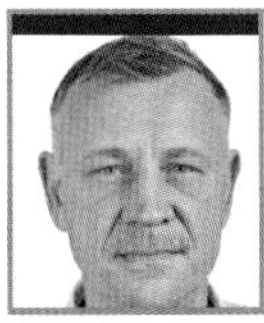

Clinical Scenario A 64-year-old client has been treated for COPD for 1 year. They are admitted for increased dyspnea and marked decrease in physical activity. The client's partner reports that the client is fearful, irritable, unable to sleep, and has not had any food or fluids for 12 hours. In caring for this client, what are the nurse's major concerns? See the following Nursing Process section.

NURSING PROCESS FOR THE CLIENT WITH OBSTRUCTIVE PULMONARY DISEASE

Assessment

Assess the client's respiratory status, including respiratory effort, rate, and pattern. Determine whether the client has diminished breath sounds and prolonged expiration. Observe for evidence of dyspnea at rest as well as accentuated accessory neck muscles and barrel-shaped chest. Ask the client about tolerance for activity and check the characteristics of secretions: consistency, quantity, color, or odor. Other important assessment data are the client's ability to expectorate secretions, signs and symptoms of infection, and what the client does to relieve pulmonary symptoms.

Diagnosis, Planning, and Interventions

Ineffective Airway Clearance: Related to bronchoconstriction, increased mucus production, and ineffective cough
Expected Outcome: Client will maintain a patent airway and adequate airway clearance.

- Auscultate breath sounds at least every 8 hours. *Findings may indicate airway obstruction secondary to mucus plug, increasing airway resistance, or fluid in larger airways.*
- Encourage client to cough and clear secretions; suction as needed. *These measures promote airway clearance and improve ventilation.*
- Perform postural drainage with percussion and vibration twice a day as indicated. *Postural drainage assists in mobilizing secretions for expectoration.*
- Observe for dyspnea, restlessness, increased anxiety, or use of accessory muscles. *Such findings indicate possible airway obstruction or ineffective clearance of secretions.*
- Increase fluid intake to 3 L/day if not contraindicated. (Right- or left-sided cardiac failure is a contraindication.) Humidify inspired air. *These measures keep secretions moist and easier to expectorate.*
- Instruct client in early signs of infection: increased sputum production, changes in sputum color and consistency, fever, increased coughing, and increased dyspnea. *Early recognition prevents an infection from progressing to a potentially lethal process.*
- Administer bronchodilators by nebulizer or MDI as indicated. *Bronchodilators open airways, facilitating breathing and expectoration of secretions.*
- Teach and encourage the use of diaphragmatic and pursed-lip breathing. *These techniques improve ventilation and mobilize secretions.*

Impaired Gas Exchange: Related to prolonged expiration, loss of lung tissue elasticity, and atelectasis
Expected Outcome: Client will maintain optimal gas exchange.

- Promote more effective breathing patterns through optimal positioning, pursed-lip breathing, and use of abdominal muscles. *High Fowler position promotes better lung expansion; turning side to side promotes aeration of lung lobes; pursed-lip breathing and other methods open airways and provide for better exhalation.*
- Administer oxygen as prescribed. *Clients with COPD chronically retain CO_2 and depend on hypoxic drive as the stimulus for breathing; accurate oxygen administration is essential for preventing cessation of breathing.*
- Monitor level of consciousness and mental status. *Problems with mentation indicate inadequate oxygenation.*
- Monitor results of ABGs and pulse oximetry. *Changes in these findings indicate respiratory deterioration and provide an opportunity for early interventions.*

(continued)

NURSING PROCESS FOR THE CLIENT WITH OBSTRUCTIVE PULMONARY DISEASE (continued)

RC: Atelectasis
Expected Outcome: Nurse will manage and minimize atelectasis.

- Instruct client to do deep-breathing and coughing exercises, incentive spirometry, or both. *These techniques promote lung expansion.*
- Encourage client to use abdominal muscles when breathing. *Diaphragmatic breathing promotes lung expansion.*

Evaluation of Expected Outcomes

The client's airway is free of secretions; breath sounds are clear. ABG and pulse oximetry results are within baseline values, and client remains alert and responsive. The client has no signs or symptoms of atelectasis and demonstrates the ability to do pulmonary exercises and abdominal breathing as instructed.

Asthma

Asthma is a chronic but usually reversible obstructive disease of the lower airway. Inflammation of the airway and hyperresponsiveness of the airway to internal or external stimuli characterize asthma. The incidence of asthma is increasing, particularly in children and adolescents. Asthma affects about 25 million people in the United States (National Heart, Lung, and Blood Institute, 2014a). Asthma may be fatal, but for most people, it causes disruptions in school and work attendance and affects choices in careers and activities.

Pathophysiology and Etiology

The chronic inflammation associated with asthma is related to airway hyperresponsiveness in response to a "trigger"—an allergen or irritant. Common allergens include pollens, dust, molds, spores, and animal dander. Irritants in the air, such as cigarette smoke or other types of smoke, strong fumes, vapors, or odors, and chemicals can cause an asthmatic response in sensitive individuals. Respiratory infections such as influenza, colds, and sinus infections can also cause asthmatic symptoms. Other causes of asthma include:

- Exercise
- Weather changes
- Emotional upsets
- Medication sensitivity

Asthma results from increasing airway obstruction caused by bronchospasm and bronchoconstriction, inflammation and edema of the lining of the bronchi and bronchioles, and production of thick mucus that can plug the airway (Fig. 21-8). The airways in people with asthma are hyperreactive in response to stimuli. Asthma causes the immunoglobulin E (IgE) inflammatory response (see Chapter 33). These antibodies attach to mast cells within the lungs. Reexposure to the antigen causes the antigen to attach to the antibody, releasing mast cell products such as histamine. The manifestations of asthma become evident as this occurs.

Because alveoli cannot expel air, they hyperinflate and trap air in the lungs. The client breathes faster, blowing off excess CO_2. Although the client tries to force the air out, the narrowed airway makes it difficult. Wheezing usually is audible with expiration, resulting from air being forced out of the narrowed airway. Other pathophysiologic changes include interference with gas exchange, poor perfusion, possible atelectasis, and respiratory failure if inadequately treated.

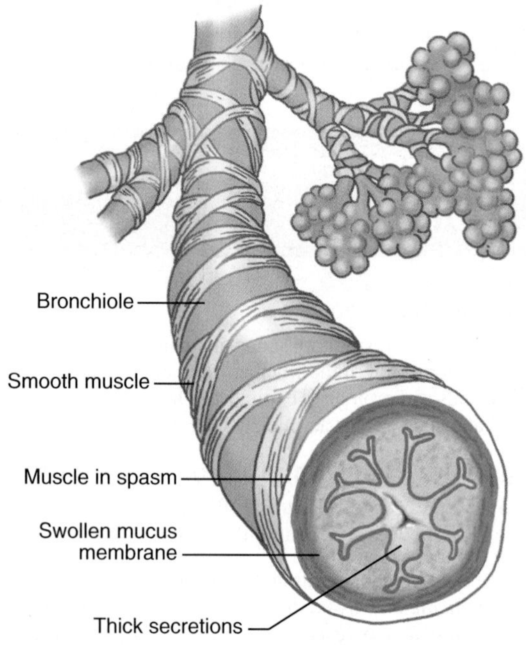

Figure 21-8 Bronchial asthma. Muscle spasms, mucosal edema, and thick secretions obstruct the bronchiole on expiration.

Asthma may develop at any age (Evidence-Based Practice 21-1). There appears to be a significant relationship between bronchiolitis (inflammation of the bronchioles) in the first year of life and development of asthma in early childhood. Asthma may be limited to occasional attacks, with the client symptom-free between attacks.

Assessment Findings

Signs and Symptoms

Asthma is typified by paroxysms of shortness of breath, wheezing, and coughing and the production of thick, tenacious sputum. Duration of acute episodes varies; it may

Evidence-Based Practice 21-1

Asthma and Older Adults

Clinical Question

Should special considerations be taken in older adults with a diagnosis of asthma?

Evidence

Asthma in the older adult population requires excellent nursing assessment and skills. As people age and health declines, this can lead to less independence, isolation, and decreased income. These changes may affect health access and transportation. Physiologic aging changes with the vertebrae and lung function can increase the risk of infection in older adults. When a diagnosis is made of asthma in an older adult, a comprehensive approach is suggested owing to complex health problems and interrelated disease processes. Care providers will need a full history and work with the client on resources and managing all disease processes. As people age, their symptoms and triggers to asthma can alter and this can cause confusion for the client and some symptoms may be missed.

Asthma treatment in an older adult focuses on reduction of symptoms and maintaining a good quality of life. The treatment includes medications that the older adult may forget or not take owing to cost, confusion, anxiety, and poor education. If an inhaler is prescribed, it is very important that the nurse complete a thorough medication teaching with the client for the prescribed device. It is important for the nurse to create and review an asthma action plan with the client and make sure that there is a clear understanding of worsening symptoms. Older adults may have many chronic illnesses and are taking multiple medications for these health conditions. Some asthma medications can react with those other treatments, causing unpleasant side effects. In addition, other medications may actually worsen asthma symptoms (Asthma, 2021). It is important to also educate the family or caregiver of the plan, medication, and symptoms.

Nursing Implications

Nurses need excellent assessment skills to assess physical, family, and psychosocial symptoms and histories of older adult clients with asthma. It is important to know the proper education of medications, symptoms, and triggers so that all important client–family education is completed.

Reference

Asthma and Allergy Foundation of America. (2021). *Asthma in older adults*. https://asthmaandallergies.org/asthma-allergies/asthma-in-older-adults/

be brief (less than 1 day) or extended (lasting for several weeks).

Most clients are aware of the wheezing and report it as one of their symptoms. Every breath becomes an effort. During an acute episode, the work of breathing greatly increases and the client may suffer from a sensation of suffocation. The client frequently assumes a classic sitting position, with the body leaning slightly forward and the arms at shoulder height. This position facilitates chest expansion and more effective excursions of the diaphragm. Because life depends on the power to breathe, fear and anxiety often accompany and also intensify the symptoms.

Marked prolongation of the expiratory phase of respiration accompanies the effort to move trapped air. Coughing commences with the onset of the attack but is ineffective in the early stage. Only as the attack begins to subside can the client expectorate large quantities of thick, stringy mucus. The skin usually is pale. During a severe attack, the nurse may observe cyanosis of the client's lips and nail beds. Perspiration typically is profuse during an acute attack. After spontaneous or drug-induced remission of the episode, examination of the lungs commonly shows normal findings. Sometimes an acute attack intensifies and progresses to status asthmaticus (persistent state of asthma), which can be life-threatening.

Diagnostic Findings

Chest auscultation reveals expiratory and sometimes inspiratory wheezes and diminished breath sounds. Results of pulmonary function studies, especially of forced expiratory volume, may be abnormal, with total lung capacity and functional residual volume increased secondary to trapped air. The forced expiratory volume and forced vital capacity are decreased. During acute attacks, blood gases show hypoxemia. The $PaCO_2$ level may be elevated if the asthma becomes worse, but usually, the $PaCO_2$ level is decreased because of the rapid respiratory rate. A normal $PaCO_2$ level in the latter part of an asthma attack may indicate impending respiratory failure.

Medical Management

Symptomatic treatment is given at the time of the attack. Long-term care involves measures to treat as well as to prevent further attacks. An effort must be made to determine the cause. If the history and diagnostic tests indicate allergy as a causative factor, treatment includes avoidance of the allergen, desensitization, or antihistamine therapy. Oxygen usually is not necessary during an acute attack because most clients are actively hyperventilating. Oxygen may be necessary if cyanosis occurs.

Pharmacologic management may be classified as quick relief (rescue) and long acting (maintenance). Quick-relief medications treat acute episodes of asthma, whereas long-acting therapy is a daily regimen designed to prevent and control symptoms. Many medications are taken through MDIs. Drug Therapy Table 21-2 lists medications used for both types of therapy. Refer also to Nutrition Notes 21-2.

Humidification of inspired air is valuable because dehydration of the respiratory mucus membrane may lead to asthmatic attacks. Use of steam or cool vapor humidifiers also has proved effective. Liquefaction of the secretions promotes more effective clearing of the airways and a rapid return to normal. Air conditioners may filter offending allergens as well as control temperature and humidity.

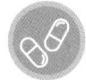

Pharmacologic Considerations

- Quick-relief drugs include bronchodilators called short-acting beta-2 agonists (SABAs). Long-acting drugs include inhalers of long-acting beta-2 agonists (LABAs), inhaled corticosteroids, mast cell stabilizers, or leukotriene modifiers.

DRUG THERAPY TABLE 21-2 Drug Therapy for Asthma

Category and Common Generic (Brand) Drugs	Intended Use	Common Side Effects	Safety Warnings for Nurses
Quick-Relief (Rescue) Therapy			
Bronchodilators—Short-Acting Beta-2 Agonists (SABAs—Adrenergics)			
Albuterol (Ventolin) Ephedrine Epinephrine (Adrenalin) Metaproterenol	Treat and prevent acute bronchospasm	Tachycardia, nervousness, anxiety, pain, dizziness, rhinitis, cough	• Inhalers not to be used for maintenance therapy
Cholinergic Blocking Drug (Anticholinergics)			
Aclidinium (Tudorza) Ipratropium (Atrovent) Tiotropium (Spiriva) Umeclidinium (Incruse)	Prevention of bronchospasm associated with chronic obstructive pulmonary disease, chronic bronchitis, and emphysema	Headache, cough, sinus irritation and stuffiness, jaw/tooth pain, urinary retention	
Long-Acting (Maintenance) Therapy			
Inhaled Corticosteroids (ICS)			
Beclomethasone (QVAR) Budesonide Ciclesonide (Alvesco) Fluticasone (Flovent)	Long-term treatment and prevention of bronchospasm by reducing inflammation of bronchi	Hoarseness, dry mouth, cough, and sore throat	• Inhalers affective for rescue therapy • Used after bronchodilator • Rinse mouth after use to prevent fungal infections • Symptoms worsen when medication stopped suddenly
Long-Acting Beta-2 Agonists (LABAs—Adrenergics)			
Arformoterol (Brovana) Formoterol (Foradil) Indacaterol (Arcapta) Salmeterol (Serevent)	Long-term treatment and prevention of bronchospasm by relaxing smooth muscle of bronchi	Palpations, tachycardia, dizziness, nervousness	• Inhalers not affective for rescue therapy • Use 15 minutes before activity for exercise-induced breathlessness (EIB) • Fatalities from acute asthma have occurred when using the drug
ICS/LABA Combination Inhalers			
Budesonide/formoterol (Symbicort) Fluticasone/salmeterol (Advair)			
Mast Cell Stabilizer			
Cromolyn (Gastrocrom)	Prevention of bronchospasm, and EIB Prevention and treatment of allergic rhinitis	Cough, wheeze, unusual taste, dizziness, headache, nausea, dry and irritated throat	• Symptoms worsen when medication is stopped suddenly
Leukotriene Modifiers and Immunomodulators (MAB)			
Montelukast (Singulair) Roflumilast (Daliresp) Zafirlukast (Accolate) Zileuton (Zyflo) Mepolizumab (Nucala) Omalizumab (Xolair)	Prophylaxis and treatment of chronic asthma by reducing inflammation	Headache, influenza-like symptoms	• Not affective for rescue therapy • Symptoms worsen when medication is stopped suddenly • Monitor liver enzymes while taking drug
Xanthine Derivatives			
Aminophylline Theophylline (Theochron)	Symptomatic relief or prevention of bronchial asthma and reversible bronchospasm by bronchodilatation	Nervousness, headache, insomnia	• Serum drug levels must be monitored for effect • Hold drug with nausea/vomiting (toxicity sign)

The drugs in column 1 indicate the drug that matches up with explanations in columns 2 through 4.

Nutrition Notes 21-2

Client With Asthma

- Encourage clients with asthma to consume adequate calories and protein to optimize health and resist infection.
- Large meals may aggravate asthma by distending the stomach and providing a high carbohydrate load, yielding increased CO_2 production when metabolized; small, frequent meals are generally better tolerated.
- Certain vitamins and minerals are important for immune function, especially vitamins A, C, B_6, and the mineral zinc, and should be liberally consumed but never in excess of 10 times the recommended dietary intake (RDI).
- Food allergens that may trigger asthma include milk, eggs, seafood, and fish.

Nursing Management

During asthma attacks, clients are extremely anxious. The nurse provides reassurance that someone will remain with the client during the acute phase. The nurse administers oxygen if indicated and puts the client in a sitting position. Rest and adequate fluid intake are important. Increasing fluid intake makes secretions less tenacious and replaces the fluids lost through perspiration. Thus, the nurse keeps fluids within easy reach and encourages the client to drink them. The nurse checks the intravenous (IV) site frequently for signs of extravasation. This monitoring is especially important during an acute attack because restlessness can result in catheter dislodgment. The nurse observes for adverse drug effects, especially when the client is receiving epinephrine or other adrenergic agents, which may cause palpitations, nervousness, trembling, pallor, and insomnia.

Clients with asthma must demonstrate understanding of the following (Hinkle & Cheever, 2017):

- Asthma as a chronic inflammatory disease
- Role of inflammation and bronchoconstriction
- Action and purpose of medications
- How to avoid triggers for asthma attacks
- Use of MDIs and other inhalers
- Use of peak flow monitoring
- When and how to obtain medical assistance

The nurse assesses the client's level of understanding of these topics and provides education as needed.

The nurse determines whether the client has a peak flow meter and obtains one for the client if needed. The peak flow meter measures the highest airflow during forced expiration. The nurse instructs the client in using the peak flow meter to monitor the degree of asthma control (Client and Family Teaching 21-4). The client can use the peak flow meter to assess the effectiveness of medication or breathing status. The nurse tells the client to seek care if readings fall below baseline, teaches the correct use of inhalers, and also helps the client to

Client and Family Teaching 21-4
Using a Peak Flow Meter

To determine peak flow, the nurse instructs the client as follows:

- Sit upright in bed or chair or stand and inhale as deeply as possible.
- Form a tight seal around the mouthpiece with lips.
- Exhale forcefully and quickly.
- Note the reading.

Repeat these steps two more times; write the highest of the three numbers in the asthma record.

After 2 to 3 weeks of asthma therapy, determine your best or usual individual peak flow.

Monitor the peak flow readings according to three zones:

- Green zone: 80% to 100% of your best or usual peak flow; indicates asthma is under good control
- Yellow zone: 50% to 80% of your best or usual peak flow; indicates the asthma symptoms are getting worse
- Red zone: less than 50% of your best or usual peak flow; indicates increasingly dangerous condition

Depending on the zone, take actions as instructed by health care providers.

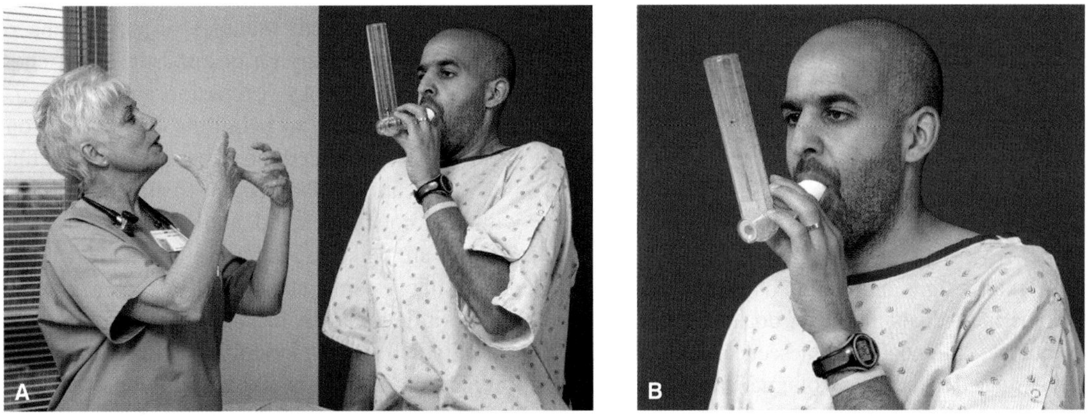

Reprinted with permission from Hinkle, J. L., & Cheever, K. H. (2018). *Brunner & Suddarth's textbook of medical-surgical nursing* (14th ed., p. 662). Wolters Kluwer.

identify triggering events such as dust, smoking, emotional upset, or exposure to irritants such as cleaning fluids or insecticides. The nurse teaches the client relaxation techniques and therapeutic breathing techniques, as discussed previously in the section on the nursing management of emphysema.

»» Stop, Think, and Respond 21-3

Your client has asthma caused by extrinsic factors, particularly dust. How can this client reduce asthma attacks?

Cystic Fibrosis

Cystic fibrosis (CF) is an inherited multisystem disorder that affects infants, children, and young adults. It obstructs the lungs, leading to major lung infections, as well as obstructing the pancreas. In the past, children with CF did not survive much beyond adolescence. Although CF remains a serious childhood disease, new treatments and therapies are enabling clients with CF to live longer and are improving their lives in terms of quality and productivity.

Pathophysiology and Etiology

CF results from a defective autosomal recessive gene. A person with CF inherits a defective copy of the CF gene from both parents. A person who is a carrier has one normal copy of the gene and one defective copy. When two carriers give birth to a child, the child has a 25% chance of having CF, a 50% chance of being a carrier but not having CF, and a 25% chance of not being a carrier and not having CF. The genetic mutation causes dysfunction of the exocrine glands, involving the mucus-secreting and eccrine sweat glands. Resulting major abnormalities include the following:

- Faulty transport of sodium and chloride in cells lining organs, such as the lungs and pancreas, to their outer surfaces
- Production of abnormally thick, sticky mucus in many organs, especially the lungs and pancreas
- Altered electrolyte balance in the sweat glands

The genetic defect causes inadequate synthesis of a protein (CF gene product) referred to as the *CF transmembrane conductance regulator* (CFTR). CFTR molecules are located in the cells lining the ducts of the exocrine glands, particularly the lungs, pancreas, intestine, and sweat ducts. Clients with CF cannot synthesize adequate CFTR to regulate the combination of water and electrolytes with exocrine secretions and mucus. Subsequently, thick, viscous secretions and protein plugs eventually block the ducts of the exocrine glands. Eventually, ducts may become fibrotic and convert into cysts.

Assessment Findings

Signs and Symptoms

Clients usually exhibit signs and symptoms in infancy or early childhood. Some individuals, however, do not have signs of the disease until late childhood or adolescence. Clinical manifestations differ related to the degree of organ involvement and the progression of the disease. The three major reasons to suspect CF in children are respiratory symptoms; failure to thrive; and foul-smelling, bulky, greasy stools. In newborns, the first clinical sign may be a meconium ileus (impacted meconium in the intestines). Another sign may be salty-tasting skin.

Respiratory symptoms become very common and include frequent respiratory infections, ranging from URIs with increased cough and purulent sputum to the production of thick, tenacious mucus. Finger clubbing is common. Hemoptysis also may occur as blood vessels are damaged in the lungs, secondary to frequent coughing and constant efforts to clear mucus.

Children also experience malabsorption of fats and fat-soluble vitamins, secondary to impaired pancreatic function. They have difficulty gaining weight. Risk for bowel obstruction, cholecystitis, and cirrhosis is increased.

Diagnostic Findings

The standard and most reliable diagnostic test for CF is the pilocarpine iontophoresis sweat test. Up to 20 years of age, levels higher than 60 mEq/L are diagnostic, and those between 50 and 60 mEq/L are highly suggestive for CF. In addition, a genetic test to determine disease and/or carrier should also be done. In many states, newborn testing for CF is available.

Chest radiography demonstrates widespread consolidation, fibrotic changes, and overaerated lungs. Some clients also have areas of collapse. Pulmonary function tests assist in determining current function as well as progression of the disease.

Radiographic studies of the GI system show fibrous abnormalities. In 80% of those with CF, tests for pancreatic enzymes in duodenal contents fail to show evidence of trypsin. Feces show steatorrhea (fat in stools).

Medical and Surgical Management

Treatment depends on the stage of the disease and the extent of organ involvement; it aims at relieving the symptoms. A medication called ivacaftor (Kalydeco, a CFTR modulator) is given to clients 2 years and older with a specific gene mutation. This medication assists the defective protein to work at the cell surface so that sodium and fluid move into the airways to thin thick mucus, making it easier to mobilize and cough up secretions. Another CFTR modulator is a combination of ivacaftor and lumacaftor (Orkambi) and is given when the child with a specific mutation turns 12 years of age. It moves the defective CFTR protein to the appropriate place on the cell membrane and increases the activity of the protein in order to thin the thick mucus (Cystic Fibrosis, 2021). Respiratory treatment includes promoting the removal of the thick sputum through postural drainage, chest physical therapy with vigorous percussion and vibration, breathing exercises, hydration to help thin secretions, bronchodilator medications, nebulized mist treatments with saline or mucolytic medications, and prompt treatment of lung infections with antibiotics. Inhaled antibiotics, such as tobramycin (TOBI), are being used successfully and have the benefit of decreasing systemic absorption. For some clients, ibuprofen, an anti-inflammatory, has been instrumental in slowing the rate at which lung function decreases; other clients are benefiting from azithromycin, an antibiotic that preserves and improves lung function (Cystic Fibrosis, 2021).

When the digestive system is involved, clients take pancreatic enzyme replacements (such as Pancreaze) with all meals and snacks to aid with the absorption of protein, fat, and fat-soluble vitamins. Clients also take multivitamins and fat-soluble vitamin supplements and follow a high-protein, high-calorie diet. A liberal sodium intake is recommended to replace sodium lost through sweat.

Clients with end-stage lung disease sometimes receive a lung transplant. In some cases, clients may receive a liver transplant as well. If successful, the transplants greatly extend the client's life.

Other new treatments are in various stages of implementation and investigation. These include mucus-thinning drugs that reduce lung infections, NSAIDs, inhaled antibiotics, drugs to stimulate cells to secrete chloride and thin mucus, and gene therapy. The potential for clients with CF to live longer increases every year. Current research is focused on treating not only the symptoms but also the causes of CF and finding a cure (Cystic Fibrosis, 2021).

Nursing Management

Nursing care of clients with CF focuses on preventing complications and promoting as normal a lifestyle as possible. It is important that the client prevent respiratory infections by avoiding people with colds or flulike symptoms, particularly in the fall and winter months. Strict adherence to a vigorous pulmonary toilet (cleansing) is essential for the client with CF who has significant respiratory involvement. Components include chest physical therapy (including postural drainage, percussion, and vibration) two to four times daily, deep-breathing and coughing exercises, nebulized treatments, and medications. New methods such as high-frequency chest wall oscillation (HFCWO) through the use of an inflatable vest may better clear secretions from the lungs. Attached to an air-pulse generator, the vest rapidly inflates and deflates to gently compress and release the chest wall, creating cough-like forces and increasing airflow in the lungs. In a 10- to 30-minute session, the airflow moves mucus toward larger airways where the client can clear them by coughing, huffing, or suctioning.

Clients also need to recognize early signs and symptoms of infection, which include low-grade temperature, increased mucus production, increased cough, and change in color of secretions (white to yellow to greenish). Clients must begin antibiotics as soon as infection occurs to prevent the infection from getting worse. Preventing or minimizing infection prevents or slows lung damage. Some clients are on prophylactic antibiotic therapy to decrease the occurrence of infections. This form of treatment is not common because of the threat of developing antibiotic-resistant infections, which can be deadly for clients with CF. Clients may be taught to administer IV antibiotics at home.

For the client with CF who has significant GI involvement, the nurse must review the client's diet. Collaboration with dietitians can ensure that the client has a diet high in calories, with appropriate amounts of carbohydrates, fats, and proteins. It is essential for the client to take their pancreatic enzymes (Creon or Pancreaze), which aid in the digestion of carbohydrates, fats, and proteins. The nurse reminds the client to take the pancreatic enzymes before or during all meals and snacks.

Young adults with CF usually are very knowledgeable about their condition. Nurses must respect their knowledge and allow them to determine their schedule for treatments and procedures. The nurse provides support for clients' efforts in self-care, referring the client as requested to other health care professionals such as dietitians and respiratory and physical therapists.

OCCUPATIONAL LUNG DISEASES

Exposure to organic and inorganic dusts and noxious gases over a long period can cause chronic lung disorders. **Pneumoconiosis** refers to a fibrous inflammation or chronic induration of the lungs after prolonged exposure to dust or gases. It specifically refers to diseases caused by the inhalation of silica (**silicosis**), coal dust (black lung disease, miners' disease), or asbestos (**asbestosis**). The resulting effect is referred to as **restrictive lung disease**, which means that the lungs have decreased volume and inability to expand completely. Although these conditions are not malignant, they may increase the client's risk for development of malignancies. Table 21-4 describes these specific conditions in more detail.

The primary focus is prevention, with frequent examination of those who work in areas of highly concentrated dust or gases. Laws require work areas to be safe in terms of dust control, ventilation, protective masks, hoods, industrial respirators, and other protection. Workers are encouraged to practice healthy behaviors, such as quitting smoking (Box 21-6).

Dyspnea and cough are the most common symptoms of occupational lung diseases. Those exposed to coal dust may expectorate black-streaked sputum. The diagnosis is based on the history of exposure to dust or gases in the workplace. A chest X-ray may reveal fibrotic changes in the lungs. The results of pulmonary function studies usually are abnormal.

Treatment typically is conservative because the disease is widespread rather than localized. Surgery seldom is of value. Infections, when they occur, are treated with antibiotics. Other treatment modalities include oxygen therapy if severe dyspnea is present, improved nutrition, and adequate rest. Many people with advanced disease are permanently disabled.

Nursing management of clients with occupational lung diseases is basically the same as for clients with emphysema. Many clients require a great deal of emotional support because these diseases may result in permanent disability at a relatively young age.

PULMONARY CIRCULATORY DISORDERS

Pulmonary Hypertension

Pulmonary hypertension (PH) refers to continuous high pressure in the pulmonary arteries and results from heart disease, lung disease, or both. It does not become clinically apparent until the client is quite ill. Diagnosis is difficult without invasive testing. Clients with PH experience difficulty breathing and usually present as quite ill.

TABLE 21-4 Occupational Lung Diseases

OCCUPATIONAL LUNG DISEASE	PATHOPHYSIOLOGY AND ETIOLOGY	SIGNS AND SYMPTOMS
Coal miners' pneumoconiosis	Referred to as *black lung disease*, this condition is caused by inhalation of coal dust and other dusts. Initially, lungs clear particles by phagocytosis and transport out of the lungs. When dust inhalation becomes too great, macrophages collect in the bronchioles, leading to clogging of the airways with dusts, macrophages, and fibroblasts. This results in local emphysema and eventually massive blackened lung lesions. Coal macules eventually form, seen as black dots on radiography.	Chronic cough—sputum production Dyspnea Large amounts of sputum containing black fluid (melanoptysis) Respiratory failure
Silicosis	This illness results from inhalation of silica dust and is seen in workers involved with mining, quarrying, stone cutting, and tunnel building. Silica particles inhaled into the lungs cause nodular lesions that enlarge and form dense masses over time. The results are loss of lung volume and restrictive and obstructive lung disease.	Shortness of breath Hypoxemia Obstruction of airflow Right-sided heart failure Edema
Asbestosis	This illness results from inhalation of asbestos dust. Laws restrict asbestos use, but old materials still contain asbestos. Asbestos fibers enter the alveoli and cause fibrous tissue to form around them. Pleura also have fibrous changes and plaque formation. Results are restrictive lung disease, decreased lung volume, and decreased gas exchange.	Dyspnea Chest pain Hypoxemia Anorexia and weight loss Respiratory failure

Note: The primary focus is prevention, with frequent examination of those who work in areas of highly concentrated dust or gases. Laws require work areas to be safe in terms of dust control, ventilation, protective masks, hoods, industrial respirators, and other protection. Workers are encouraged to practice healthy behaviors, such as quitting smoking (Box 21-6).

Pathophysiology and Etiology

Resistance to blood flow in the pulmonary circulation causes PH. The pressure in the pulmonary arteries increases, which, in turn, increases the workload of the right ventricle. Normal pulmonary arterial pressure is approximately 25/10 mm Hg. In PH, the pressure rises above 40/15 mm Hg and can be higher as the disease progresses. The WHO has divided PH into five categories based on the cause of the condition (National Heart, Lung, and Blood Institute, 2011d). Box 21-7 provides a brief overview of these categories. Complex mechanisms cause PH. In early PH, the inner lining of the pulmonary arteries thickens and hypertrophies, followed by increased pressure in the pulmonary arteries and vascular bed (Fig. 21-9). In late pulmonary arterial hypertension, alveolar destruction causes increased resistance and pressure in the pulmonary vascular bed. The increased resistance and pressure in the pulmonary vascular bed results in PH. Consequently, strain is placed on the right ventricle, resulting in enlargement and possible failure. Hepatic congestion may also occur.

BOX 21-6 Preventing Occupational Lung Diseases

- Do not smoke. Smoking increases the risk for occupational lung diseases.
- Wear appropriate protective equipment, such as face masks, when around airborne irritants and dusts.
- Schedule lung function evaluation with spirometry as often as recommended to monitor lung function.
- Get educated about the risks of lung diseases.
- Pay attention to risk evaluation of the workplace to identify risks for lung disease.

Assessment Findings

The most common symptoms of PH are dyspnea on exertion at first and then at rest, as well as weakness. Additional symptoms are those of the underlying cardiac or respiratory disease: chest pain, fatigue and weakness, **orthopnea** (difficulty breathing while lying flat), and dizziness. The client will show signs of right-sided heart failure (see Chapter 28), which include peripheral edema, ascites, distended neck veins, liver engorgement, crackles, and heart murmur.

An electrocardiogram (ECG) may show right ventricular hypertrophy or failure. Results of ABG analysis are abnormal. Cardiac catheterization demonstrates elevated pulmonary arterial pressures. The results of pulmonary function studies show an increased residual volume but a decreased forced expiratory volume. Echocardiography may show various abnormalities, such as left ventricular dysfunction and tricuspid valve insufficiency. A ventilation–perfusion (V–Q) scan or pulmonary angiography may be done to determine any defects in the pulmonary vessels, such as a PE.

Medical Management

Treatment of PH includes the administration of vasodilators and anticoagulants and management of the underlying cardiac or respiratory disease. Oxygen therapy commonly is used to increase pulmonary arterial oxygenation. If right-sided heart failure is present, other treatments include medications such as digitalis to improve cardiac function, rest, and diuretics. PH has a poor prognosis; therefore, some affected clients are considered candidates for lung or heart–lung transplantation.

Nursing Management

Nursing management focuses on recognizing signs and symptoms of respiratory distress. The nurse can reduce the body's need for oxygen by preventing fatigue, assisting with ADLs, and administering oxygen, when needed.

BOX 21-7 Types of Pulmonary Hypertension

Note: Group 1 is called pulmonary arterial hypertension (PAH) and groups 2 through 5 are called pulmonary hypertension. However, together, all groups are called pulmonary hypertension.

Group 1 PAH

- Unknown cause (idiopathic PAH)
- A genetic mutation passed down through families (heritable PAH)
- Use of some prescription diet drugs or illegal drugs such as methamphetamines—and other drugs
- Heart problems present at birth (congenital heart disease)
- Other conditions, such as connective tissue disorders (scleroderma, lupus, others), HIV infection or chronic liver disease (cirrhosis)

Group 2 Pulmonary hypertension caused by left-sided heart disease

- Left-sided heart valve disease, such as mitral valve or aortic valve disease
- Failure of the lower left heart chamber (left ventricle)

Group 3 Pulmonary hypertension caused by lung disease

- Chronic obstructive pulmonary disease (COPD)
- Pulmonary fibrosis, a condition that causes scarring in the tissue between the lungs' air sacs (interstitium)
- Obstructive sleep apnea
- Long-term exposure to high altitudes in people who may be at higher risk of pulmonary hypertension

Group 4 Pulmonary hypertension caused by chronic blood clots

- Chronic blood clots in the lungs (pulmonary emboli)
- Other clotting disorders

Group 5 Pulmonary hypertension triggered by other health conditions

- Blood disorders, including polycythemia vera and essential thrombocythemia
- Inflammatory disorders such as sarcoidosis and vasculitis
- Metabolic disorders, including glycogen storage disease
- Kidney disease
- Tumors pressing against pulmonary arteries

Mayo Clinic. (2021). *Pulmonary hypertension*. https://www.mayoclinic.org/diseases-conditions/pulmonary-hypertension/symptoms-causes/syc-20350697. Used with permission of Mayo Foundation for Medical Education and Research. All rights reserved.

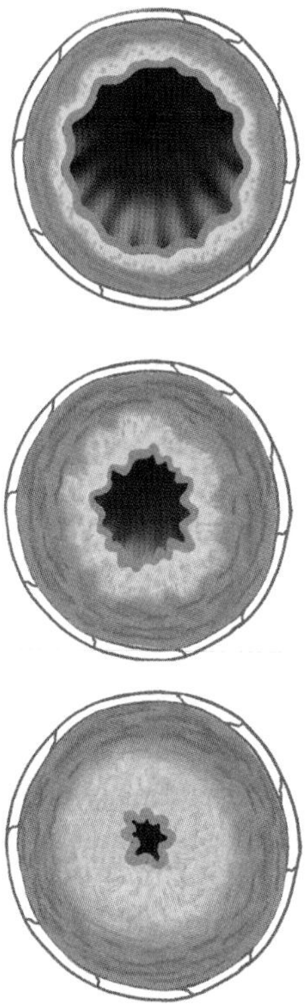

A. Normal. Pulmonary arteriole is normally thin and distensible.

B. Pulmonary hypertension (early). Mild pulmonary hypertension is characterized by thickening of the medial (muscular) layer.

C. Pulmonary hypertension (late). Severe pulmonary hypertension exhibits extensive intimal fibrosis and medial thickening.

Figure 21-9 Progression of pulmonary hypertension.

Pulmonary Embolism

Pulmonary embolism (PE) involves the obstruction of one of the pulmonary arteries or its branches. The blockage is the result of a thrombus (blood clot) that forms in the venous system or right side of the heart. The majority of pulmonary emboli travel from the lower extremity veins (DVT) to the pulmonary arteries. For this reason, this condition is frequently referred to as venous thromboembolism, which involves both a DVT and PE.

Pathophysiology and Etiology

An embolus is any foreign substance such as a blood clot, air, or particle of fat that travels in the venous blood flowing to the lungs. The clot moves to and completely or partially occludes one of the pulmonary arteries, decreasing or totally obstructing blood flow. This causes gas exchange impairment and disrupts the V–Q ratio. Eventually infarction (necrosis or death) occurs in the lung tissue distal to the clot. Scar tissue later replaces the infarcted area. It is not unusual for clients to have multiple pulmonary emboli.

Clots usually form in the deep veins of the lower extremities or pelvis and become the source for pulmonary emboli. Emboli also may arise from the endocardium of the right ventricle when that side of the heart is the site of a myocardial infarction (MI) or endocarditis. A fat embolus usually occurs after a fracture of a long bone, especially the femur. Other conditions that cause pulmonary emboli include recent surgery, prolonged bed rest, long journeys, trauma, postpartum state, heart valve malfunction (particularly in older adults), dehydration, and debilitating diseases. Family history is a significant factor—a client with a family member who had blood clots is more likely to have clots and pulmonary emboli. Clients who smoke, are overweight, and/or take estrogen replacement are at higher risk for pulmonary emboli. Three conditions, referred to as *Virchow triad*, predispose a person to clot formation: venostasis, disruption of the vessel lining, and hypercoagulability.

Assessment Findings

When a small area of the lung is involved, signs and symptoms usually are less severe and include pain, tachycardia, and dyspnea. The client may also have fever, cough, and blood-streaked sputum. Larger areas of involvement produce more pronounced signs and symptoms, such as severe dyspnea, wheezing, severe pain, cyanosis, tachycardia, irregular heart rate, diaphoresis, restlessness, and shock. Sudden death may follow a massive pulmonary infarction when a large embolism occludes a main section of the pulmonary artery.

A chest X-ray may show an area of atelectasis. An ECG rules out a cardiac disorder such as MI, which produces some of the same symptoms. In addition, pulse oximetry and ABGs will be measured. A lung scan, V–Q· scan, CT scan, or pulmonary angiography is performed to detect the involved lung tissue. Ultrasonography may also be done to confirm the presence of lower extremity DVT (see Chapter 23). A blood test called D-dimer assay is used to detect the presence of a protein when blood clots break down somewhere in the body. If positive, it is not definitive for a pulmonary embolus, but it does indicate that further tests are necessary.

Medical and Surgical Management

Treatment of a PE depends on the size of the area involved and the client's symptoms. PE often presents as an emergency. The treatment goal is to dissolve or lyse the clot, in order to restore cardiopulmonary function. Pharmacologic therapy (Hinkle & Cheever, 2014) includes the following:

- *Anticoagulant therapy*: includes the early use of IV heparin for the initial phase, or the use of newer anticoagulants, such as fondaparinux (Arixtra). Maintenance therapy may overlap IV heparin and oral anticoagulants such as warfarin for several days. Newer anticoagulants, such as fondaparinux, may be given orally and do not have to be overlapped with IV anticoagulants.
- *Thrombolytic therapy*: these medications are used to dissolve clots. The most commonly used thrombolytic is tissue plasminogen activator (tPA) for massive PE. Thrombolytics can cause sudden and problematic bleeding and are only used for clients in life-threatening situations, such as those clients experiencing severe hypotension or hypoxemia.

Other measures used to treat symptoms of pulmonary emboli include complete bed rest, oxygen, and analgesics.

Surgical management may be done to remove a clot. PE can be removed using transvenous catheters or by surgical removal while the client is on cardiopulmonary bypass to support circulation. The insertion of an inferior vena cava (IVC) filter serves as a screen to allow blood to flow but to prevent clots to pass. The primary purpose is to prevent recurrent episodes of PE.

Nursing Management

The best management of pulmonary emboli is through prevention of DVT (Box 21-8). When determining the client's potential for DVT, it is important to note the client's ability to engage in activities such as leg exercises and ambulation. Clients on bed rest are encouraged to do active and/or passive leg exercises. Primary providers may order clients to wear elastic compression stockings or use intermittent compression systems such as Venodyne. In addition, the nurse assesses the client for signs of localized calf tenderness, swelling, increased warmth, or prominence of superficial veins in one or both lower extremities and history of DVT, all of which may indicate the presence of DVT (see Chapter 23).

PE almost always occurs suddenly, and death can follow within 1 hour for a massive PE. Early recognition of this problem is essential for stabilizing cardiopulmonary function. The nurse starts an IV infusion as soon as possible to establish a patent vein before shock becomes profound. They administer vasopressors such as dopamine or dobutamine as ordered to treat hypotension. The nurse provides oxygen for dyspnea and analgesics for pain and apprehension. Close monitoring of vital signs is necessary, as is observing the client at frequent intervals for changes. The nurse institutes continuous ECG monitoring because right ventricular failure is a common problem.

Areas for the nurse to monitor include fluid intake and output, electrolyte determinations, and ABGs. The nurse assesses the client for cyanosis, cough with or without hemoptysis, diaphoresis, and respiratory difficulty. They monitor blood coagulation studies (e.g., partial thromboplastin time, prothrombin time) when anticoagulant or thrombolytic therapy is instituted.

The nurse assesses the client for evidence of bleeding and relief of associated symptoms. Because clients with pulmonary emboli are discharged on oral anticoagulants, they require instruction related to checking for signs of occult bleeding, taking medication exactly as prescribed, reporting missed or extra doses, and keeping all appointments for follow-up blood tests and office visits.

BOX 21-8 Preventing the Formation of Pulmonary Emboli

- Help client practice active and passive leg exercises.
- Instruct client to pump muscles (tense and relax) to improve circulation in lower extremities.
- Assist client to ambulate as early as possible after a procedure.
- Teach client to:
  - Wear compression hose as directed.
  - Avoid constrictive clothing.
  - Avoid sitting for long periods or with legs crossed.
  - Drink fluids liberally unless contraindicated.
  - When traveling, move lower legs and feet while sitting, change positions as able, do not cross legs, and ambulate if able.

››› *Stop, Think, and Respond 21-4*

A 54-year-old woman recently experienced thrombophlebitis in her left calf, probably related to prolonged bed rest after a motor vehicle collision. The thrombophlebitis resolved without complications. She is no longer taking anticoagulants. She expresses concerns about having clots in the future. What should she do?

Pulmonary Edema

Pulmonary edema is the accumulation of fluid in the interstitium and alveoli of the lungs, interfering with respiration. It is usually an emergency situation. Pulmonary congestion results when the right side of the heart delivers more blood to the pulmonary circulation than the left side of the heart can handle. The fluid escapes the capillary walls and fills the airways. A client with pulmonary edema experiences dyspnea, breathlessness, and a feeling of suffocation; in addition, they exhibit cool, moist, and cyanotic extremities. The overall skin color is cyanotic and gray. The client has a continual cough productive of blood-tinged, frothy fluid. This condition requires emergency treatment. (See Chapter 28 for a discussion of cardiogenic pulmonary edema.)

RESPIRATORY FAILURE

Respiratory failure describes the inability to exchange sufficient amounts of oxygen and CO_2 for the body's needs. Even when the body is at rest, basic respiratory needs cannot be met. The ABG values that define respiratory failure include ABG results of a PaO_2 less than 50 mm Hg, a $PaCO_2$ greater than 50 mm Hg, and a pH less than 7.3.

Respiratory failure is classified as acute or chronic. Acute respiratory failure occurs suddenly in a client who previously had normal lung function. In chronic respiratory failure, the loss of lung function is progressive, usually irreversible, and associated with chronic lung disease or other disease.

Pathophysiology and Etiology

Table 21-5 describes precipitating factors that can result in respiratory failure. Acute respiratory failure is a life-threatening condition in which alveolar ventilation cannot maintain the body's need for oxygen supply and CO_2 removal. The result is a fall in arterial oxygen (hypoxemia) and a rise in arterial CO_2 (hypercapnia) detected by ABG analysis. Ventilatory failure develops when the alveoli cannot adequately expand, when neurologic control of respirations is impaired, or when traumatic injury to the chest wall occurs.

The most common diseases leading to chronic respiratory failure are COPD and neuromuscular disorders. The underlying disease accounts for the pathology that is seen when the respiratory system fails. Gas exchange dysfunction occurs over a long period. Symptoms of acute respiratory failure are not apparent in chronic respiratory failure because the client experiences chronic respiratory acidosis over a long period. Refer to the section on COPD for discussion of diagnostic findings, medical management, and nursing management of chronic respiratory failure.

Assessment Findings

Apprehension, restlessness, fatigue, headache, dyspnea, wheezing, cyanosis, and use of the accessory muscles of respiration are seen in clients with impending respiratory failure. If the disorder remains untreated or if treatment fails to relieve respiratory distress, confusion, sleepiness, loss of consciousness, tachypnea, cyanosis, cardiac dysrhythmias and tachycardia, hypotension, CHF, respiratory acidosis, and respiratory arrest occur.

The client's symptoms, history (e.g., surgery, known neurologic disorder), and ABG results form the basis for a diagnosis of respiratory failure. Additional tests include chest radiography and serum electrolyte determinations.

TABLE 21-5 Factors That Precipitate Respiratory Failure

PRECIPITATING FACTOR	EXAMPLE
Pulmonary infection—especially with chronic obstructive pulmonary disease	Bacterial, viral, or fungal pneumonia
Trauma	Motor vehicle collision Gunshot/knife wound Burns
Infection	Sepsis Wound infection
Cardiovascular event	Myocardial infarction Aortic aneurysm Pulmonary embolism
Allergic reaction	Transfusion reaction Drug allergy Bee sting or other venom
Pulmonary aspiration	Vomitus Near drowning
Surgical procedure	Abdominal or thoracic surgery
Drug/alcohol reaction	Overdose of barbiturates, narcotics, or alcohol Reaction to anesthesia
Mechanical factor	Pneumothorax Pleural effusion Abdominal distention
Iatrogenic factor	Endotracheal intubation Failure to clear tracheobronchial secretions
Neuromuscular disorders	Guillain–Barré syndrome Multiple sclerosis Muscular dystrophy Amyotrophic lateral sclerosis Spinal cord injuries Cerebrovascular accident

Medical Management

Treatment of respiratory failure focuses on maintaining a patent airway (in cases of upper respiratory airway obstruction) by inserting an artificial airway, such as an endotracheal or a tracheostomy tube. Additional treatments include administration of humidified oxygen by nasal cannula, Venturi mask, or rebreather masks (Fig. 21-10). Respiratory failure is managed with mechanical ventilation using intermittent positive pressure ventilation. When possible, the underlying cause of respiratory failure is treated.

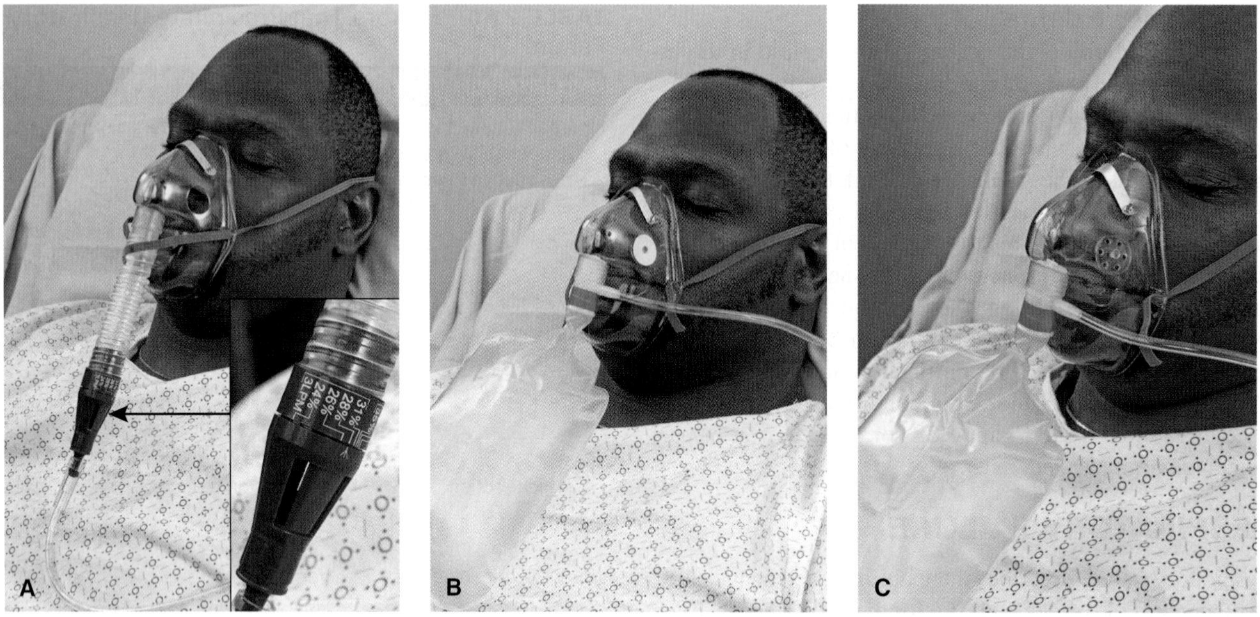

Figure 21-10 Types of oxygen masks. **(A)** Venturi mask. **(B)** Nonrebreather mask. **(C)** Partial rebreather mask.

Nursing Management

Because symptoms often occur suddenly, recognition is important. The nurse must notify the primary provider immediately and obtain emergency resuscitative equipment. Assessment and monitoring of respirations and vital signs are necessary at frequent intervals. The nurse must pay particular attention to respiratory rate and depth, signs of cyanosis, other signs and symptoms of respiratory distress, and the client's response to treatment. The nurse monitors ABG results and pulse oximetry findings and implements strategies to prevent respiratory complications, such as turning and range-of-motion (ROM) exercises. The nurse provides explanations to the client and initiates measures to relieve anxiety.

ACUTE RESPIRATORY DISTRESS SYNDROME

Acute respiratory distress syndrome (ARDS) is a clinical condition that occurs following other clinical conditions. The less severe form of this condition is referred to as acute lung injury (ALI). ARDS and ALI are not primary diseases. When it occurs, ARDS can lead to respiratory failure and death. It is referred to as *noncardiogenic pulmonary edema* (pulmonary edema not caused by a cardiac disorder—occurs without left-sided heart failure). Sudden and progressive pulmonary edema, increasing bilateral infiltrates seen on chest radiography, severe hypoxemia, and progressive loss of lung compliance characterize ARDS.

Pathophysiology and Etiology

Factors associated with the development of ARDS include aspiration related to near drowning or vomiting; drug or alcohol ingestion/overdose; hematologic disorders such as disseminated intravascular coagulation or massive transfusions; direct damage to the lungs through prolonged smoke inhalation or other corrosive substances; pneumonia or localized lung infection; metabolic disorders such as pancreatitis or uremia; shock; trauma such as chest contusions, multiple fractures, or head injury; any major surgery; embolism; and septicemia. The mortality rate with ARDS is high, particularly if the underlying cause cannot be treated or is inadequately treated.

The body responds to injury by reducing blood flow to the lungs, resulting in platelet clumping. The platelets release substances such as histamine, bradykinin, and serotonin, causing localized inflammation of the alveolar membranes. Increased permeability of the alveolar capillary membrane subsequently ensues. Fluid then enters the alveoli and causes pulmonary edema. The excess fluid in the alveoli and decreased blood flow through the capillaries surrounding them cause many of the alveoli to collapse (microatelectasis). Gas exchange decreases, resulting in respiratory and metabolic acidosis. ARDS also causes decreased surfactant production, which contributes to alveolar collapse. The lungs become stiff or noncompliant. Decreased functional residual capacity, severe hypoxia, and hypocapnia result. See Figure 21-11 for a depiction of the pathogenesis and pathophysiology of ARDS.

Assessment Findings

Severe respiratory distress develops within 8 to 48 hours after the onset of illness or injury. In the early stages, few definite symptoms may be seen. As the condition progresses, the following signs appear: increased respiratory rate; shallow, labored respirations; cyanosis; use of accessory muscles; respiratory distress unrelieved with oxygen administration; anxiety; restlessness; and mental confusion, agitation, and drowsiness with cerebral anoxia.

Diagnosis is made according to the following criteria: evidence of acute respiratory failure, bilateral infiltrates on chest radiography, and hypoxemia as evidenced by PaO_2 less

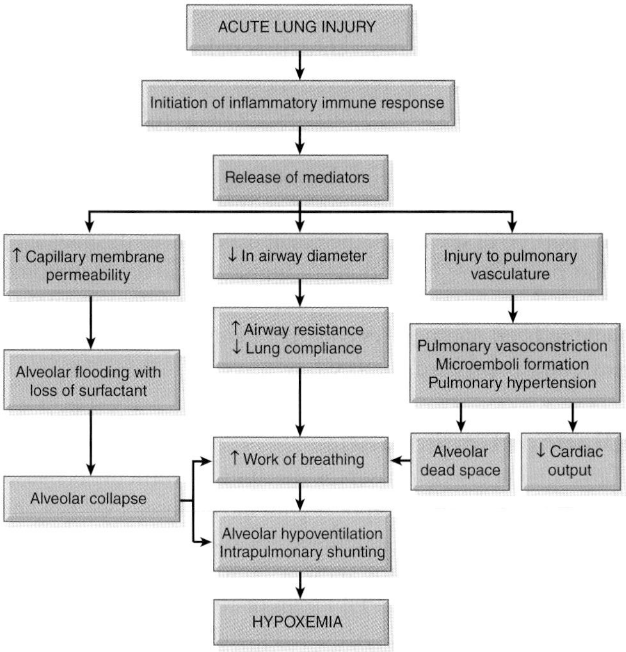

Figure 21-11 Pathogenesis and pathophysiology of acute respiratory distress syndrome.

than 50 mm Hg with supplemental oxygen of 50% to 60%. Chest X-rays reveal increased infiltrates bilaterally. There is no evidence of left-sided heart failure (see Chapter 28), such as increased size of the left ventricle.

Medical Management

The initial cause of ARDS must be diagnosed and treated. The client receives humidified oxygen. Insertion of an endotracheal or a tracheostomy tube ensures maintenance of a patent airway. Mechanical ventilation usually is necessary using positive end-expiratory pressure (PEEP), which provides pressures to the airway that are higher than atmospheric pressures. Mechanical ventilators usually raise airway pressure during inspiration and let it fall to atmospheric or zero pressure during expiration (intermittent positive pressure ventilation). When PEEP is used, positive airway pressure is maintained on inspiration, expiration, and at the end of expiration (continuous positive pressure ventilation). The client's pulmonary status, determined by ABG findings and pulse oximetry results, dictates the oxygen concentration and ventilator settings. Complications associated with the use of PEEP include pneumothorax and pneumomediastinum (air in the mediastinal space).

Hypotension results in systemic hypovolemia. Although the client experiences pulmonary edema, the rest of the circulatory volume is decreased. Pulmonary artery pressure monitors the client's fluid status and assists in determining the careful administration of IV fluids. Colloids such as albumin are used to help pull fluids in from the interstitium to the capillaries. Adequate nutritional support is essential (Nutrition Notes 21-3). Usually, the first choice is enteral feedings, but total parenteral nutrition may be necessary.

Nutrition Notes 21-3

The Client With Respiratory Failure or Distress

- Although adequate protein and calories are important to support lung function, overfeeding is avoided because it causes overproduction of CO_2 and increases respiratory workload.
- Specially designed enteral formulas are available for clients with respiratory failure or distress; they are high in fat and low in carbohydrates to reduce CO_2 production, although studies have not definitively confirmed their effectiveness in reducing respiratory distress.

Nursing Management

Nursing management focuses on promotion of oxygenation and ventilation and prevention of complications. Assessing and monitoring a client's respiratory status is essential. Potential complications include deteriorating respiratory status, infection, renal failure, and cardiac complications. The client is also anxious and requires explanations and support. In addition, if the client is on a ventilator, verbal communication is impaired. The nurse provides alternative methods for the client to communicate.

MALIGNANT DISORDERS

Tumors and growths affecting the respiratory system usually are malignant. Malignancies may be primary in that they arise from the lungs or mediastinum, or they can be secondary metastatic growths from other sites. Treatment of primary or secondary cancers usually does not stop progression of the disease (see Chapter 18). Disability, debilitation, and death are common outcomes from respiratory malignancies.

Lung Cancer

Lung cancer is a very common cancer, particularly among cigarette smokers and those regularly exposed to secondhand smoke. It remains the primary cause of cancer-related deaths among men and women in the United States (American Cancer Society, 2021), with more Americans dying each year from lung cancer than from breast, prostate, and colorectal cancers combined. The incidence of lung cancer has markedly increased since the early 1980s related to the following:

- More accurate methods of diagnosis
- The growing population of aging people
- The continued popularity of cigarette smoking
- Increased air pollution
- Increased exposure to industrial pollutants

The American Cancer Society (2021) published the following statistics related to lung cancer:

- Lung cancer (both small cell and non–small cell) is the second most common cancer in both men and women (not counting skin cancer).
- For 2021, about 235,760 new cases of lung cancer and about 131,880 deaths from lung cancer are predicted.
- Lung cancer occurs primarily in older adults, the average age at the time of diagnosis being 70 years.

Pathophysiology and Etiology

The exact mechanism for the development of lung cancer is unknown; however, the link between irritants and lung cancer is well established. Prolonged exposure to carcinogens more than likely will produce cancerous cells. Smokers who quit reduce their risk of lung cancer to that of nonsmokers within 10 to 15 years.

Lung cancers are grouped in three overall categories: *non–small cell lung carcinomas* (NSCLCs), which include epidermoid or squamous cell carcinomas, large cell or undifferentiated type, and adenocarcinoma; *small cell lung carcinomas* (SCLCs), formerly referred to as oat cell carcinomas, and lung carcinoid tumors, also known as neuroendocrine tumors (rare). Many tumors begin in the bronchus and spread to the lung tissue, regional lymph nodes, and other sites such as the brain and bone. Many tumors have more than one type of cancer cell, referred to as *mixed small cell/large cell cancer*. Table 21-6 differentiates between the major cell types of lung cancer.

The transformation of an epithelial cell in the airway initiates the growth of a lung cancer lesion. As the tumor grows, it partially obstructs the lumen of an airway or completely obstructs it, resulting in airway collapse distal to the tumor. The tumor may hemorrhage, causing hemoptysis.

Assessment Findings

Signs and Symptoms

The cell type of the lung cancer, size and location of the tumor, and degree and location of metastasis determine the presenting signs and symptoms. A cough productive of mucopurulent or blood-streaked sputum is a cardinal sign of lung cancer. The cough may be slight at first and attributed to smoking or other causes. The cough can be new or noticed by a client as different from a chronic cough. As the disease advances, the client may report dyspnea, fatigue, anorexia, and weight loss. Chest pain occurs later in the disease. Hemoptysis is common. Some clients exhibit recurring fevers and frequent respiratory infections before lung cancer is diagnosed.

If pleural effusion occurs from tumor spread to the outside portion of the lungs, the client experiences dyspnea and chest pain. Other indications of tumor spread are symptoms related to pressure on nerves and blood vessels. Symptoms include head and neck edema, pericardial effusion, hoarseness, and vocal cord paralysis.

Diagnostic Findings

Early diagnosis of cancer of the lung is difficult because symptoms often do not appear until the disease is well established. The sputum is examined for malignant cells. Chest X-rays may or may not show a tumor. A CT or positron emission tomography (PET) scan or MRI is done if results from the chest radiograph are inconclusive, or to further delineate the tumor area.

Sputum cytology may be done on coughed-up specimens. Bronchoscopy may be done to obtain bronchial washings and a tissue sample for biopsy. Fine needle aspiration under fluoroscopy or CT guidance may be done to aspirate cells from a specific area that is not accessible by bronchoscopy. A lung scan also may locate the tumor. A bone scan detects metastasis to the bone. The results of a lymph node biopsy may be positive for malignant changes if the lung tumor has metastasized. Mediastinoscopy provides a direct view of the mediastinal area and possible visualization of tumors that extend into the mediastinal space.

TABLE 21-6 Differentiation of Lung Cancers

CELL TYPE	PATHOLOGY	METASTASIS
Non–Small Cell Lung Carcinomas (NSCLCs)		
Account for 84% of all lung cancers		
Epidermoid or squamous cell carcinomas (most common type of NSCLC in men)	These slow-growing tumors form in the lining of the bronchial tubes; they spread into the bronchial lumen, causing obstruction.	Well-differentiated epidermoid cells typically metastasize in the thorax, whereas poorly differentiated epidermoid cells metastasize to the small bowel.
Large cell (undifferentiated) carcinomas (found near the bronchial surface)	These arise in peripheral bronchi and do not have well-defined growth patterns. They usually are diagnosed first as a bulky tumor mass.	These metastasize rapidly, usually to the CNS.
Adenocarcinomas (arise from glands in the lungs that produce mucus; most common type of NSCLC in women and in people who have not smoked)	These occur in the peripheral lung tissue and lead to patchy growth throughout the lung fields. They typically invade the pleura, leading to malignant pleural effusion.	Early metastasis occurs to the brain, other lung tissue, bone, liver, and adrenal glands.
Small Cell Lung Carcinomas		
Account for 13% of all lung cancers		
Formerly referred to as *oat cell carcinoma*	This most malignant form of lung cancer arises from the bronchi; the cells grow quickly and form large tumors.	Metastasis is early via infiltration along the bronchial wall into the bloodstream and lymphatics to the mediastinum, liver, bone, bone marrow, CNS, adrenal glands, pancreas, and other endocrine organs.

CNS, central nervous system.

Medical and Surgical Management

The client's prognosis is poor unless the tumor is discovered in its early stages and treatment begins immediately. Because lung cancer produces few early symptoms, its mortality rate is high. Metastasis to the mediastinal and cervical lymph nodes, liver, brain, spinal cord, bone, and opposite lung is common.

Treatment depends on several factors. One major consideration is the classification and staging of the tumor. After classification of the tumor, the stage of the disease is determined. Staging refers to the extent and location of the tumor and the absence or presence and extent of metastasis (see Chapter 18). Other factors that determine treatment are the client's age and physical condition and other diseases or disorders, such as renal disease and CHF.

Surgical removal of the tumor offers the only possibility of cure and usually is successful only in the early stages of the disease. The type of lung resection (see Box 21-4) depends on the tumor's size and location. Lymph nodes may also be excised to check for cancer.

Radiation therapy may help to slow the spread of the disease and provide symptomatic relief by reducing tumor size, thus easing the pressure exerted by the tumor on adjacent structures. In turn, pain, cough, dyspnea, and hemoptysis may be relieved. In a small percentage of cases, radiation may be curative, but for most, it is palliative. Complications associated with the use of radiation therapy include esophagitis, fibrosis of lung tissue, and pneumonitis.

Chemotherapy may be used alone or with radiation therapy and surgery. The principal effects of chemotherapy are to slow tumor growth and reduce tumor size and accompanying pressure on adjacent structures. Chemotherapy is also used to treat metastatic lesions. Most chemotherapeutic regimens use a combination of drugs rather than a single agent and, although not curative, often make the client more comfortable.

New treatments in various stages of development include the following (LungCancer.org, 2021):

Immunotherapy known as an immune checkpoint inhibitor: Cemiplimab-rwlc (Advanced Lung Cancer, 2021)

- New chemotherapy regimens
- Targeted therapies that include monoclonal antibodies (target-specific cancer proteins), antiangiogenesis agents (to counter the tumor's ability to create new blood supplies), and growth factor inhibitors (to block the effects of growth factors)
- Photodynamic therapy that is a combination treatment with chemicals and light
- Lung cancer vaccines to stimulate an effective immune response
- Gene therapy—designed to correct genetic changes made by the cancer

Nursing Management

Management of clients with lung cancer is essentially the same as that for any client with a malignant disease. See Chapter 18 for the nursing management of a client with cancer and Chapter 14 for perioperative care.

Mediastinal Tumors

Tumors of the mediastinum in adults often are malignant and metastatic. They are designated as anterior, middle, or posterior according to their location on the mediastinum. The cause of these tumors is not known. Mediastinal tumors may be asymptomatic initially. When symptoms occur, they include chest pain, chest wall bulging, difficulty swallowing, dyspnea, and orthopnea. Symptoms are related to pressure of the tumor on other chest structures. Chest radiography, CT scan, MRI, mediastinoscopy, and biopsy of the lesion identify the tumor. Malignant tumors of the mediastinum almost always are inoperable but may respond to radiation therapy and chemotherapy. Benign tumors are operable.

>>> *Stop, Think, and Respond 21-5*

Your 65-year-old neighbor tells you that he smoked for 25 years but quit 5 years ago. He has been experiencing a productive cough for 3 weeks. Occasionally he sees blood in the sputum. What can you advise him?

TRAUMA

All chest injuries are serious or potentially serious. A client with a chest injury must be observed for dyspnea, cyanosis, chest pain, weak and rapid pulse, and hypotension—all signs and symptoms of respiratory distress. Clients with a chest injury need to be examined by a primary provider as soon as possible.

Fractured Ribs

Fractured ribs are a common injury and may result from a hard fall or a blow to the chest. Fractured ribs usually are not considered serious unless accompanied by other injuries.

Pathophysiology and Etiology

Automobile and household accidents are frequent causes of fractured ribs. Rib fractures are painful but not generally life-threatening. When a client experiences a fractured rib, other structures may be injured as well. For example, the sharp end of the broken rib may tear the lung or thoracic blood vessels. If the injury involves fractured ribs without complications, the client usually may return home after emergency treatment.

Flail chest occurs when two or more adjacent ribs fracture in multiple places (two or more) and the fragments are free floating (Fig. 21-12). This affects the stability of the chest wall and results in impairment of chest wall movement. A paradoxical movement develops: with inspiration, the chest expands, but the free-floating segments move inward instead of outward. On expiration, the free-floating segments move outward, interfering with exhalation. These movements affect intrathoracic pressures, significantly decreasing the movement of air. Many pathophysiologic phenomena occur as a result: increased dead space, reduced gas exchange, decreased lung compliance, retained airway secretions, atelectasis, and hypoxemia.

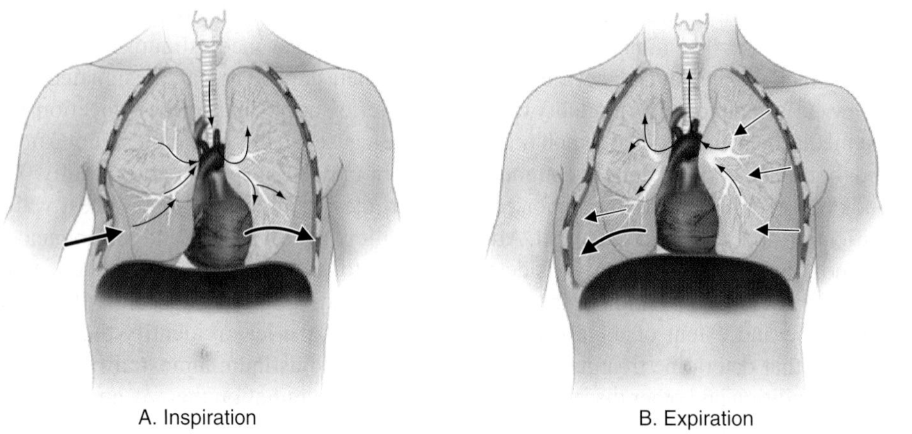

Figure 21-12 Flail chest is caused by a free-floating segment of rib cage resulting from multiple rib fractures. **(A)** Paradoxical movement on inspiration occurs when the flail rib segment is sucked inward and the mediastinal structures shift to the unaffected side. The amount of air drawn into the affected lung is reduced. **(B)** On expiration, the flail segment bulges outward and the mediastinal structures shift back to the affected side.

Assessment Findings

Symptoms consist primarily of obvious trauma and severe pain on inspiration and expiration. The client experiences shortness of breath. With flail chest, the client has hypotension and inadequate tissue perfusion secondary to decreased cardiac output. Respiratory acidosis occurs because of increased CO_2. Chest X-rays (usually from several angles) are necessary to confirm the diagnosis.

Medical Management

Supporting the chest with an elastic bandage or a rib belt assists in immobilizing the rib fractures. These measures, however, can lead to decreased lung expansion followed by pulmonary complications such as pneumonia and atelectasis. Therefore, the use of these devices usually is limited to multiple rib fractures. Analgesics such as codeine may be prescribed for pain. Sometimes a regional nerve block is used to relieve pain.

Management of flail chest includes supporting ventilation, clearing lung secretions, and managing pain. Other treatment depends on the severity of the flail chest. If a **pulmonary contusion** (crushing bruise of the lung) also exists, fluids are restricted because of the damage to the pulmonary capillary bed. Antibiotics are given to prevent infection, which is common after this type of injury. Endotracheal intubation and mechanical ventilation may be necessary if a client's respiratory status is greatly compromised.

Nursing Management

With fractured ribs, the nurse may apply the immobilization device after the primary provider examines the client. In such a case, the nurse instructs the client about the application and removal of the rib belt or elastic bandage, stressing the importance of taking deep breaths every 1 to 2 hours, even though breathing is painful. Nurses plan and implement care of clients with more severe injuries based on respiratory needs. The nurse assesses and monitors the client for signs of respiratory distress, infection, and increased pain.

Blast Injuries

Compression of the chest by an explosion can seriously damage the lungs by rupturing the alveoli. Death often results from hemorrhage and asphyxiation. Severe respiratory distress with outward evidence of chest trauma is apparent. **Subcutaneous emphysema** (air in subcutaneous tissues) is a common finding because the lungs or air passages have sustained an injury. This condition resembles a superficial swelling. Crepitation (a crackling sound) is heard or felt upon palpation and may be caused by air leaking around the chest wound. Diagnosis is based on symptoms and physical examination. Additional diagnostic tests, such as chest radiography and lung scan, may be necessary to identify foreign objects or air in the chest.

Treatment includes complete bed rest and oxygen administration. Thoracentesis to remove air or fluid may be necessary. Some clients may require surgery and the insertion of chest tubes if severe injury to lung tissue has occurred or if pneumothorax is present. When a client has suffered a blast injury, the most important nursing task is immediate recognition of respiratory distress. Victims of a blast injury are closely observed for early signs of respiratory distress.

Penetrating Wounds

Gunshot and stab wounds are common types of penetrating wounds to the lungs. Penetrating wounds potentially affect cardiopulmonary function and may be life-threatening.

Pathophysiology and Etiology

Penetrating wounds are classified according to the velocity of the cause. Stab wounds from weapons such as knives or switchblades usually are low velocity because they involve a small area. Gunshot wounds may be low, medium, or high velocity depending on the caliber of the gun, the distance from which the gun was fired, and the nature of the ammunition.

Any type of penetrating wound to the chest is serious because of the opening into the thorax. On inspiration, the thorax normally is at negative pressure. The penetrating wound creates continuous and direct communication with the outside,

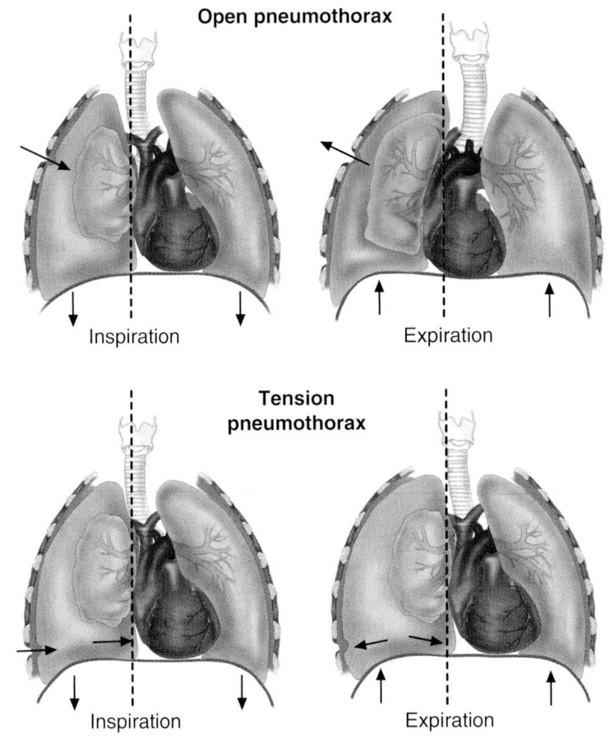

Figure 21-13 In open or communicating pneumothorax (*top*), air enters the chest during inspiration and exits during expiration. In tension pneumothorax (*bottom*), air enters but does not leave the chest. As pressure increases, the heart, great vessels, and unaffected lung are compressed, while the mediastinal structures and trachea shift toward the opposite side of the chest.

which is at positive pressure. Thus, air enters the thoracic cavity, causing an open pneumothorax (Fig. 21-13). If not recognized and treated promptly, death may occur. If the wound is large, a sucking noise may be heard as air enters and leaves the chest cavity. Depending on the size of the wound, it takes seconds to hours before the lung collapses as the pressure in the thorax reaches atmospheric pressure. Many chest injuries involve both pneumothorax and *hemothorax*, the collection of blood in the pleural cavity. Subcutaneous emphysema also may be present. Other possible trauma includes hemorrhage, lung contusion, damage to surrounding tissues, fractured ribs or other bones, and injury to the heart, blood vessels, or both.

Assessment Findings

Clients exhibit various signs and symptoms depending on the location and extent of the penetrating wound; dyspnea, pain, and bleeding are common. Clients are at risk for respiratory distress and shock. It also is important that the client be thoroughly examined to ascertain if other injuries are present, such as more penetrating wounds, particularly in the abdominal area.

Diagnosis is based on the history of injury, physical examination, and auscultation of the lungs. Radiographs show the degree of lung collapse and the amount of air or blood in the thoracic cavity. The client's cardiopulmonary status is assessed through ABG analysis, pulse oximetry, and ECGs. CT scans or MRI may be necessary depending on the extent of the injuries.

Medical and Surgical Management

Airway management is the first concern. Once an airway is established, then other treatment begins. Thoracentesis is done to remove air and blood from the pleural space. A chest tube is inserted and attached to an underwater-seal drainage system. A thoracotomy may be required to repair the injury. Foreign bodies that entered the chest, such as a bullet or a knife, are surgically removed. Their presence in the wound may prevent or slow the entrance of air. Removal before the victim is transported to the hospital may result in continuous sucking of air into the chest, collapse of the lung, compression of the heart and opposite lung, and death. Surgical intervention may be necessary if there is bleeding from the chest tube or indications of injury to other organs or blood vessels.

Emergency treatment of pneumothorax caused by a penetrating wound includes the application of a tight pressure dressing over the injury site to prevent more air from entering the thorax. Immediate evaluation of the client's respiratory status is imperative. Oxygen is given until the primary provider examines and treats the injury. IV fluids, colloid solutions, or blood is administered to treat or prevent shock. An indwelling catheter is inserted to monitor urine output. A nasogastric tube is placed to prevent aspiration of stomach contents and to decompress the GI tract.

Nursing Management

Care of a client with a penetrating chest wound is similar to that of a client who has thoracic surgery. Refer to the nursing management of a client undergoing thoracic surgery in the next section.

THORACIC SURGERY

A thoracotomy is a surgical opening in the chest wall. It may be done to

- Remove fluid, blood, or air from the thorax.
- Remove tumors of the lung, bronchus, or chest wall.
- Remove all or a portion of a lung (see Box 21-4).
- Repair or revise structures contained in the thorax, such as open heart surgery or repair of a thoracic aneurysm.
- Repair trauma to the chest or chest wall, such as penetrating chest wounds or crushing chest injuries.
- Sample a lesion for biopsy.
- Remove foreign objects such as a bullet or metal fragments.

A thoracentesis may be done as an emergency procedure to remove blood, fluid, or air from the chest. In some instances, it is necessary to perform a thoracotomy to insert chest tubes (tube thoracotomy) to remove air or fluid from the chest during the preoperative period.

Preoperative Nursing Management

Preparing clients for thoracic surgery includes assessment of vital signs and breath sounds, particularly noting the presence or absence of breath sounds in any area of the chest. The client's condition dictates the extent of the assessment and obtaining a history. If the surgery is an emergency, physical assessment may be limited to a general statement of the client's condition, a list of emergency measures and treatments done, and vital signs (see Chapter 14).

Postoperative Nursing Management

The opening of the thoracic cavity requires special postoperative nursing measures. A significant issue is the interference with normal pressures in the thoracic cavity. When the chest is opened, air from the atmosphere rushes in, owing to the negative pressure that exists in the thoracic cavity on inspiration. The entrance of air under atmospheric pressure causes the lungs to collapse and no longer expand or contract. The anesthesiologist ventilates the client during surgery.

After thoracic surgery, draining secretions, air, and blood from the thoracic cavity is necessary to allow the lungs to expand. A catheter placed in the pleural space provides a drainage route through a closed or underwater-seal drainage system (Fig. 21-14). Sometimes two chest catheters are placed—one anteriorly and one posteriorly. The anterior catheter (usually the upper one) removes air; the posterior catheter removes fluid.

Chest tubes are securely connected to an underwater-seal drainage system. The tube coming from the client always must be under water. A break in the system (e.g., loose or disconnected fittings) allows air to first enter the tubing and then the pleural space, further collapsing the lung. When chest tubes are inserted at the end of the surgical procedure, they are connected to an underwater-seal drainage system. All connections are taped carefully to minimize the possibility of air entering the closed system.

When caring for a client with chest tubes, the nurse should be aware of the following:

- Fluctuation of the fluid in the water-seal chamber is initially present with each respiration. Fluctuations cease when the lung reexpands. The time for lung reexpansion varies. Fluctuations also may cease if
  - The chest tube is clogged.
  - The wall suction unit malfunctions.
  - A kink or dependent loop develops in the tubing.
- Bubbling in the water-seal chamber occurs in the early postoperative period. If bubbling is excessive, the nurse checks the system for leaks. If leaks are not apparent, the nurse notifies the primary provider.
- Bloody drainage is normal, but drainage should not be bright red or copious.
- The drainage tube(s) must remain patent to allow fluids to escape from the pleural space.
- Clogging of the catheter with clots or kinking causes drainage to stop. The lung cannot expand, and the heart and great vessels may shift (mediastinal shift) to the opposite side. The nurse must be alert to the proper functioning of the drainage system. Malfunctions need immediate correction.
- If a break or major leak occurs in the system, the nurse clamps the chest tube immediately with hemostats kept at the bedside. They notify the primary provider if this occurs.

Immediate postoperative care includes following the standards outlined in Chapter 14. It is also essential that the nurse check the underwater-seal drainage system, noting the amount and color of drainage and any bubbling or fluctuation. The nurse assesses dressings for drainage and firm adherence to the skin, inspecting the skin around the dressings for signs of subcutaneous emphysema. The nurse assesses the client's color, neurologic status, and heart rate and rhythm; monitors respiratory rate, depth, and rhythm; and auscultates the chest for normal and abnormal breath sounds. They also assess levels of pain and anxiety. Nursing Care Plan 21-1 and Client and Family Teaching 21-5 describe additional nursing management.

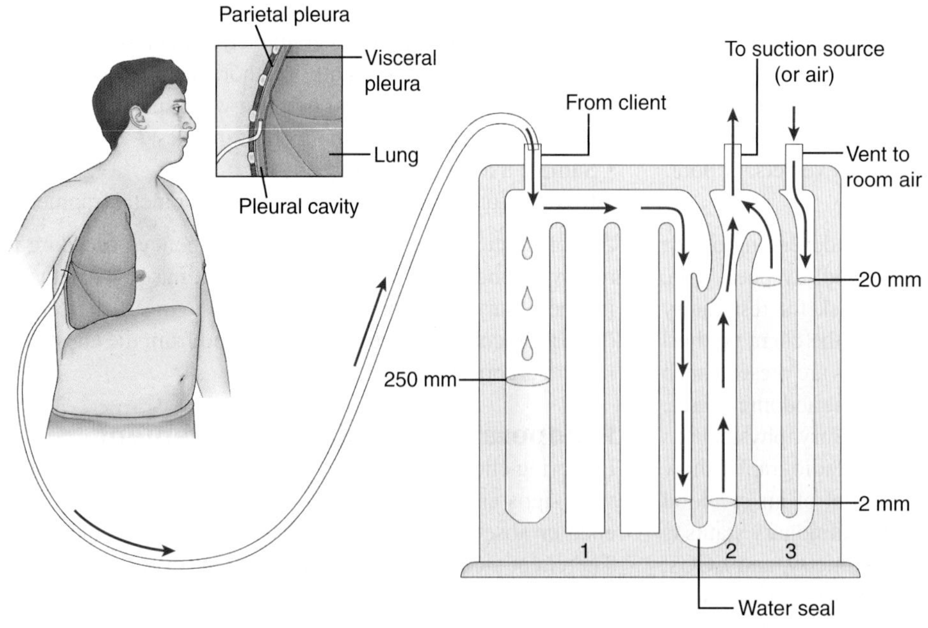

Figure 21-14 Chest drainage system. Chest catheter placed in right pleural space and attached to Pleur-Evac system with three chambers: **(1)** drainage collection chamber from client, **(2)** the water-seal chamber, and **(3)** the suction control chamber attached to source of suction and vented to room air.

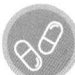

Pharmacologic Considerations

■ When administering a narcotic to a client who has had thoracic surgery, count the respiratory rate before and 20 to 30 minutes after the client receives the medication. If the respiratory rate is below 10 breaths/min at either time, notify the primary provider immediately.

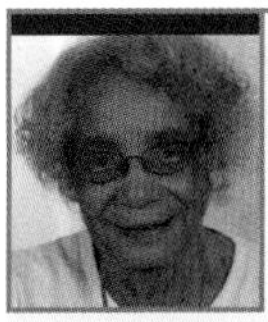

Clinical Scenario A 70-year-old client with a tumor in the left upper lobe of the lungs has a left upper lobectomy to remove the tumor. **What are essential nursing considerations for this client in the first 24 to 48 postoperative hours? See Nursing Care Plan 21-1.**

NURSING CARE PLAN 21-1 The Client Recovering From Thoracic Surgery

Assessment

- Assess respirations: rate, depth, rhythm, and use of accessory muscles.
- Observe skin color, particularly for signs of cyanosis.
- Auscultate breath sounds at least every 4 hours.
- Evaluate mental status.
- Monitor heart rate and rhythm.
- Monitor results of ABGs, pulse oximetry, and other blood tests.
- Assess dressings and incisions for drainage or adherence.
- Check the chest tube drainage system.
- Assess level of pain.

Nursing Diagnosis. **Impaired Gas Exchange** related to decreased lung expansion, impaired lung function, and surgical procedure

Expected Outcome. Client will maintain optimal gas exchange.

Interventions	Rationales
Monitor vital signs every 15 minutes for at least 2 hours after return from postanesthesia care unit and then less frequently as condition stabilizes.	*Such information provides baseline data and early indications of problems.*
Reinforce preoperative instructions about deep breathing, coughing, and incentive spirometry. Remind client to do these exercises every 1 to 2 hours.	*These exercises expand the alveoli, which prevents atelectasis.*
Position client with the head of the bed elevated 30 to 40 degrees initially. When the client can tolerate it, position them on the nonoperative side.	*Such positioning promotes lung expansion and drainage from operative side.*

Evaluation of Expected Outcomes

Client demonstrates improved gas exchange as evidenced by results of ABGs and pulse oximetry and improved efforts with incentive spirometry.

Nursing Diagnosis. **Acute Pain** related to surgical incision and presence of drainage tubes

Expected Outcome. Client will demonstrate relief of pain and discomfort.

Interventions	Rationales
Assess client's pain in terms of location and severity.	*Determining client's pain is essential to promote the client's comfort. A postoperative client cannot always convey pain in the immediate postoperative period, so the nurse must use all assessments to determine level and quality of pain.*
Administer pain medications as ordered and needed.	*Providing pain medication at regular intervals promotes comfort and prevents pain from becoming too intense.*
Position client within restrictions of surgery for comfort. A semi-Fowler position is usually the best positioning in the early postoperative period.	*A semi-Fowler position avoids the surgical site in the early postoperative period and promotes comfort.*

Evaluation of Expected Outcome

Client's pain is managed as evidenced by client's ability to rest and be calm with no agitation or distress.

Nursing Diagnosis. **Activity Intolerance** related to arm on affected side related to incisional pain, edema, and decreased strength

Expected Outcome. Client will demonstrate effective ROM on affected side.

Interventions	Rationales
Assess ROM in affected upper extremity within 24 hours by having the client raise arm laterally.	*This assessment provides baseline data about ROM. During thoracotomy, chest muscles are incised, making ROM difficult after surgery.*
Perform passive ROM exercises on affected arm four times a day.	*These exercises increase mobility and promote renewed strength of affected arm.*

(continued)

NURSING CARE PLAN 21-1 The Client Recovering From Thoracic Surgery (*continued*)

Encourage client to use affected arm in ADLs.	*Gradual use of arm promotes movement of it.*
Instruct client to move arms, slowly increasing movement and exercise as tolerated.	*These measures promote mobility and begin to increase strength on affected side.*
Increase exercise level after removal of chest tubes.	*Removal of chest tubes decreases discomfort and assists client to move more freely.*
Collaborate with physical therapists to plan therapy; reinforce instructions regarding exercise and discharge.	*A full exercise plan will help client gain full ROM of affected upper extremity.*

Evaluation of Expected Outcome

Client demonstrates increased ROM and better ability to perform ADLs independently.

Nursing Diagnosis. **Dehydration: risk of,** related to surgical procedure, drains, and pain

Expected Outcome. Client will maintain adequate fluid volume.

Interventions	Rationales
Monitor and record intake and output hourly.	*Such monitoring provides ongoing information about client's fluid status.*
Assess skin turgor and mucus membranes for signs of dehydration.	*These assessments provide baseline data about fluid status.*
Monitor and document vital signs.	*Tachycardia can occur with hypovolemia to maintain adequate cardiac output. Pulse may be weak with hypovolemia. Hypotension occurs with hypovolemia.*
Report urine output less than 30 mL/hour for two consecutive hours.	*Urine output of less than 30 mL/hour for two or more hours indicates dehydration.*
Monitor serum electrolyte and urine osmolality levels, reporting abnormal values.	*Elevated hemoglobin, blood urea nitrogen, and urine specific gravity suggest fluid deficit.*
Administer parenteral fluids as ordered and maintain an accurate record of IV intake.	*Parenteral fluids prevent dehydration.*
Encourage client to drink at least 30 mL every hour.	*This amount promotes adequate fluid intake.*

Evaluation of Expected Outcome

Client is adequately hydrated as evidenced by urine output greater than 30 mL/hour, stable blood pressure and pulse, and normal skin turgor.

Nursing Diagnosis. **Bleeding risk; hemorrhage**

Expected Outcome. Nurse will manage and minimize blood loss.

Interventions	Rationales
Monitor and record vital signs.	*Monitoring vital signs provides baseline data and information about changes in a client's status.*
Assess chest tube drainage and dressings for signs of bleeding.	*Bloody drainage from chest tubes may occur initially but should decrease. Increased blood in chest tubes, on dressings, or both indicates a bleeding problem that requires immediate intervention.*
Anticipate or prepare client for return to surgery if bleeding is secondary to surgical procedure.	*These measures are necessary to resolve the problem.*
Increase parenteral fluids as ordered.	*Increased parenteral fluid maintains an adequate circulating volume until bleeding stops.*
Administer blood products as ordered.	*Blood products replace lost blood and volume.*

Evaluation of Expected Outcome

Nurse ensures the management of bleeding and its complications.

Client and Family Teaching 21-5
Care After Thoracic Surgery

The nurse develops a teaching plan that includes instructions given by the primary provider as well as the following guidelines:

1. Continue to perform arm exercises to prevent stiffness and pain.
2. Eat a well-balanced diet, or follow the recommended diet.
3. Take rest periods throughout the day until fatigue decreases.
4. Practice breathing exercises and take frequent deep breaths.
5. Contact the primary provider if breathing is difficult; drainage, excessive redness, or pain develops around the incision; fever develops; or pain occurs elsewhere in the body.
6. Avoid infection or irritants.
7. Increase activities slowly and avoid fatigue.
8. Take drugs as prescribed and do not omit, increase, or decrease doses.

KEY POINTS

- Acute bronchitis: inflammation of the mucus membranes that line the major bronchi and their branches
- Pneumonia: an inflammatory process affecting the bronchioles and alveoli, and it usually is associated with an acute infection. Pneumonia also can result from radiation therapy, chemical ingestion or inhalation, or aspiration of foreign bodies or gastric contents.
- Types of pneumonia
  - community-acquired pneumonia
  - health care–associated pneumonia/hospital-acquired pneumonia
  - pneumonia in the immunocompromised host
  - pneumonia from aspiration
- Pleurisy or *pleuritis:* refers to acute inflammation of the parietal and visceral pleurae.
- Pleural effusion: an abnormal collection of fluid between the visceral and parietal pleurae. Pleural effusion may be a complication of pneumonia, lung cancer, TB, PE, and CHF. The amount of accumulated fluid may be so large that the lung partially collapses on the affected side.
- Lung abscess: a localized area of pus formation in the lung parenchyma
- Empyema: refers to pus or infected fluid in the pleural cavity.
- Influenza (flu): is an acute respiratory disease of relatively short duration. Each virus can mutate and produce variants within the given strain.
- Pulmonary TB: is a bacterial infectious disease primarily caused by *M. tuberculosis*. TB essentially affects the lungs, but it may also affect the kidneys and other organs.
  - Define disorders classified as obstructive pulmonary disease.
- COPD is a term for chronic lung diseases that have limited airflow in and out of the lungs.
  - Bronchiectasis: characterized by chronic infection and irreversible dilatation of the bronchi and bronchioles, as a result of destruction of muscle and elastic connective tissue
  - Atelectasis: may involve a small portion of the lung or an entire lobe. When alveoli collapse, they cannot perform their function of gas exchange.
  - Chronic bronchitis: a prolonged (or extended) inflammation of the bronchi, accompanied by a chronic cough and excessive production of mucus for at least 3 months each year for 2 consecutive years
  - Emphysema: a chronic disease characterized by abnormal distention of the alveoli. The alveolar walls and capillary beds also show marked destruction.
  - Asthma: a chronic but usually reversible obstructive disease of the lower airway. Inflammation of the airway and hyperresponsiveness of the airway to internal or external stimuli characterize asthma.
  - CF is an inherited multisystem disorder that affects infants, children, and young adults. It obstructs the lungs, leading to major lung infections, as well as obstructing the pancreas. Most children diagnosed with CF do not survive past adolescence.
- Occupational lung diseases/restrictive lung disease
  - Pneumoconiosis refers to a fibrous inflammation or chronic induration of the lungs after prolonged exposure to dust or gases. It is caused by the inhalation of silica (**silicosis**), coal dust (black lung disease, miners' disease), or asbestos (**asbestosis**).
- Pulmonary circulatory disorders
  - PH: refers to continuous high pressure in the pulmonary arteries and results from heart disease, lung disease, or both.
  - PE: the obstruction of one of the pulmonary arteries or its branches, the blockage is the result of a thrombus (blood clot) that forms in the venous system or right side of the heart. Most pulmonary emboli travel from the lower extremity veins (DVT) to the pulmonary arteries.
  - Pulmonary edema is the accumulation of fluid in the interstitium and alveoli of the lungs, interfering with respiration. Pulmonary congestion results when the right side of the heart delivers more blood to the pulmonary circulation than the left side of the heart can handle.
- Respiratory failure: the inability to exchange sufficient amounts of oxygen and CO_2 for the body's needs
  - Acute respiratory failure occurs suddenly in a client who previously had normal lung function.
  - Chronic respiratory failure, the loss of lung function, is progressive, usually irreversible, and associated with chronic lung disease or other disease.

- ARDS: a clinical condition that occurs following other clinical conditions. ARDS can lead to respiratory failure and death; also known as *noncardiogenic pulmonary edema* (pulmonary edema not caused by a cardiac disorder—occurs without left-sided heart failure).
- Lung cancer
  - NSCLCs: include epidermoid or squamous cell carcinomas, large cell or undifferentiated type, and adenocarcinoma
  - SCLCs: formerly referred to as oat cell carcinomas, are lung carcinoid tumors, also known as neuroendocrine tumors (rare). Many tumors begin in the bronchus and spread to the lung tissue, regional lymph nodes, and other sites such as the brain and bone.
  - Mixed small cell/large cell cancer: tumors have more than one type of cancer cell.
- Mediastinal tumors: are designated as anterior, middle, or posterior according to their location on the mediastinum, and in adults often are malignant and metastatic.
- Chest trauma
  - Fractured ribs: are a common injury and may result from a hard fall or a blow to the chest.
  - Flail chest: occurs when two or more adjacent ribs fracture in multiple places (two or more) and the fragments are free floating.
  - Blast injuries: compression of the chest by an explosion can seriously damage the lungs by rupturing the alveoli. Death often results from hemorrhage and asphyxiation.
  - Penetrating wounds: Gunshot and stab wounds are common types of penetrating wounds to the lungs. Penetrating wounds potentially affect cardiopulmonary function and may be life-threatening.
- Subcutaneous emphysema: air in subcutaneous tissues
- Thoracentesis: an emergency procedure to remove blood, fluid, or air from the chest
- Thoracotomy: a surgical procedure to gain access into the pleural space of the chest

CRITICAL THINKING EXERCISES

1. A client who underwent cholecystectomy (removal of the gallbladder) 2 days ago presses their call button. As you enter their room, they tell you that they are having trouble breathing and have chest pain. What brief questions would you ask the client before you call the primary provider?

2. A client has a history of asthma. They arrive at the outpatient clinic and state that their chest feels tight and that they cannot "catch my breath." The nurse notes that this client is having trouble speaking. Immediate care of this client includes fluids, administration of bronchodilators, and relief of anxiety. When the client is stabilized and able to be discharged, the nurse wants to assure that the client can take steps to help prevent future asthmatic attacks. What information from the client does the nurse need to better provide appropriate discharge teaching?

3. A client who has AIDS develops pleurisy. Their primary provider instructs them to perform deep-breathing and coughing exercises every 2 hours. What can you do to ease the client's pain and discomfort when they are performing these exercises?

4. A client who has bronchiectasis in their left lower lobe attends a pulmonary disease clinic. Their primary provider instructs them to perform postural drainage by lying laterally on the bed, leaning from the waist, and lowering their head close to the floor. Two weeks later, the client tells you that they cannot tolerate this postural drainage position. Can you think of another way to perform postural drainage for the left lower lobe that may cause less discomfort?

NCLEX-STYLE REVIEW QUESTIONS PrepU

1. The nurse admits an older adult client to the emergency department. Vital signs are temperature, 38.9°C; pulse rate, 88 beats/min; respiratory rate, 32 breaths/min; and blood pressure, 160/86 mm Hg. Upon physical examination, the client is having difficulty breathing. Which of the following would be most appropriate for the nurse to do next?
   1. Apply a pulse oximeter to the client's finger.
   2. Help the client perform postural drainage.
   3. Instruct the client to take slow, deep breaths.
   4. Suction the client's pharynx of secretions.

2. The nurse is caring for a client with TB. A sputum sample is ordered for the next 3 consecutive days. What time is it best for the nurse to schedule the collection of sputum?
   1. At bedtime
   2. Before a meal
   3. Following breakfast
   4. Upon arising in the morning

3. The nurse receives a call from a client with emphysema. Which of the client's symptoms requires immediate attention from the nurse?
   1. The client reports that the last oral temperature was 37.2°C.
   2. The client reports that the mucus is much thicker and harder to clear.
   3. The client reports that oxygen is on at least 18 hours/day at 2 L/min.
   4. The client reports that shortness of breath increases with minimal activity.

4. A client with moderately controlled asthma needs to use a peak flow meter. Which of the following statements by the nurse best explains the purpose of a peak flow meter?
   1. A peak flow meter measures the amount of forced inspiration.
   2. A peak flow meter measures the depth of forced inhalation.
   3. A peak flow meter measures the highest flow with forced expiration.
   4. A peak flow meter measures the residual volume after exhalation.

5. The licensed practical nurse (LPN) notes that the registered nurse (RN), in the care plan for a client who transferred from intensive care unit (ICU) 2 days postoperative thoracic surgery, selected "Impaired Gas Exchange related to decreased lung expansion, impaired lung function, and surgical procedure." Which interventions are of primary importance for the care of this client? Select all that apply.

1. Assess the client's dressings and incisions for increased drainage.
2. Monitor client's temperature at least every 4 hours.
3. Remind the client to breathe deeply and cough at least every 2 hours.
4. Reposition the client so that the head is elevated 30 to 40 degrees.
5. Thirty minutes after administering pain medication, ask the client to rate the pain on a scale of 1 to 10.

UNIT 6
Caring for Clients With Cardiovascular Disorders

22 Introduction to the Cardiovascular System

Words To Know

angiocardiography
aortic valve
aortography
arteries
arteriography
arterioles
atria
atrioventricular (AV) valves
baroreceptors
bicuspid valve
capillaries
cardiac catheterization
cardiac cycle
cardiac output
chemoreceptors
conduction system
coronary arteries
coronary veins
coronary ostia
depolarization
diastole
echocardiography
electrocardiography
endocardium
epicardium
exercise electrocardiography
inferior vena cava
magnetic resonance imaging
mediastinum
mitral valve
myocardium
pericardium
polarization
pulmonary artery
pulmonic valve
pulse deficit
refractory period
repolarization
sarcopenia
septum

Learning Objectives

On completion of this chapter, you will be able to:

1. Describe the normal anatomy and physiology of the cardiovascular system.
2. Identify and describe focus assessment criteria when caring for a client with cardiovascular problems.
3. List common diagnostic tests used to evaluate the client with suspected heart disease.
4. Discuss the nursing management of a client undergoing cardiovascular diagnostic tests.

The function of the cardiovascular system is to supply body cells and tissues with oxygen-rich blood and eliminate carbon dioxide (CO_2) and cellular wastes. Damage to and disease within the cardiovascular system greatly jeopardize a person's health. In fact, heart disease is the leading cause of death for adults in the United States. Many advanced treatments have been and are being created to reduce deaths from heart disease. Human heart transplantation and the temporary use of the total artificial heart as a bridge to transplant or permanent heart replacement are realities (Harrington, 2015). Nevertheless, the primary focus remains on preserving the natural heart by preventing heart disease.

Gerontologic Considerations

■ Changes in cardiovascular structure and function in older adults are related to genetic risk factors, lifestyle/environmental influences (e.g., smoking, inadequate nutrition, lack of exercise), and changes from the aging process itself.

■ Include age, lifestyle, environmental risk factors, and family history during an assessment. Early identification of risk factors facilitates early preventive efforts before actual damage occurs. (Teaching of potential benefits can increase motivation for early and midlife health behaviors.)

■ **Sarcopenia** refers to changes in composition of muscle tissue that can occur in aging as the result of deconditioning. Muscle fiber reduction and replacement with fatty tissue

Words To Know (*continued*)
stroke volume
superior vena cava
systole
telemetry
transesophageal echocardiography
tricuspid valve
veins
ventricles
venules

Gerontologic Considerations (*continued*)

decrease the strength of muscle contraction and thus can decrease cardiac output. Sarcopenic changes can be reduced to maintain or improve cardiac function through exercise that causes the heart muscle to work harder (i.e., brisk walking, swimming, dancing, etc.), if not contraindicated.

- The aging heart requires more time to return to baseline levels after stress. This inability to handle stress results from decreased cardiac output and contractile strength and delayed conduction in the heart.
- Age-related changes in the conductive system include a decrease in the number of pacemaker cells and changes in their shape. An increase in fat deposits, collagen, and elastic fibers in the sinoatrial (SA) node leads to a higher risk for cardiac arrhythmias.
- Abnormal rhythms are difficult to treat in the older adult because organs can be further compromised by the lack of adequate blood supply if other chronic conditions exist.
- The older adult who has renal impairment or is chronically dehydrated is at increased risk for complications during and after diagnostic studies requiring the use of a contrast medium because the iodinated contrast is nephrotoxic. Interventions to hydrate should be considered prior to the test.

ANATOMY AND PHYSIOLOGY

The cardiovascular system consists of the heart, the major blood vessels that empty into or exit directly from the heart, and a vast network of smaller peripheral blood vessels. The heart itself is about the size of a person's fist. It lies below and slightly to the left of the midline of the sternum in the **mediastinum**, a portion of the thoracic cavity that also contains the trachea and major blood vessels. The upper portion of the heart is the base, and the tip is the apex.

Heart Chambers

The heart is a four-chambered muscular pump (Fig. 22-1). The upper chambers, the right and left **atria** (singular, *atrium*), are the receiving chambers for blood. The lower chambers, the right and left **ventricles**, are the heart's major pumping chambers. A thick **septum**, or wall, separates the right side of the heart from the left side. The right atrium receives deoxygenated blood from the venous system, and the right ventricle pumps that blood to the lungs to be oxygenated. The left atrium receives oxygenated blood from the lungs, and the left ventricle pumps that blood to all the cells and tissues of the body. Therefore, the heart is a double pump—the right side facilitates pulmonary circulation, and the left side is responsible for systemic circulation.

Cardiac Tissue Layers

Three distinct layers of tissue make up the heart wall. The outer layer is the **epicardium**, which is composed of fibrous and loose connective tissue. The middle layer, the **myocardium**, consists of muscle tissue and is the force behind the heart's pumping action. The inner layer, the **endocardium**, is composed of a thin, smooth layer of endothelial cells. Folds of endocardium form the heart valves. The endocardium is in direct contact with the blood that passes through the heart.

The **pericardium** is a saclike structure that surrounds and supports the heart. Two membranous layers form the pericardium. The outer tougher layer is called the *parietal pericardium*. The inner serous layer is called the *visceral pericardium* (also called the *epicardium*), which adheres to the heart itself. The density of the parietal pericardium safeguards the heart from invasion by infectious microorganisms. Serous fluid fills the pericardial space between the two layers, lubricating the heart and reducing friction with each heartbeat (Fig. 22-2).

Heart Valves

The valves of the heart are membranous structures that ensure that blood passes through the heart in a one-way, forward direction. In a normal heart, the valves do not allow

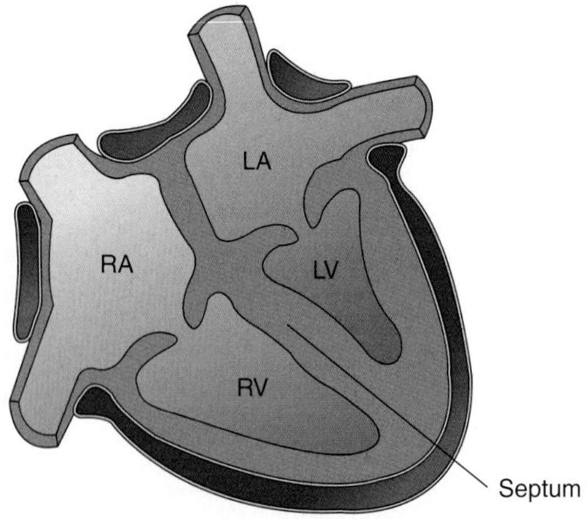

Figure 22-1 Cross-section of the heart showing the four chambers. LA, left atrium; LV, left ventricle; RA, right atrium; RV, right ventricle.

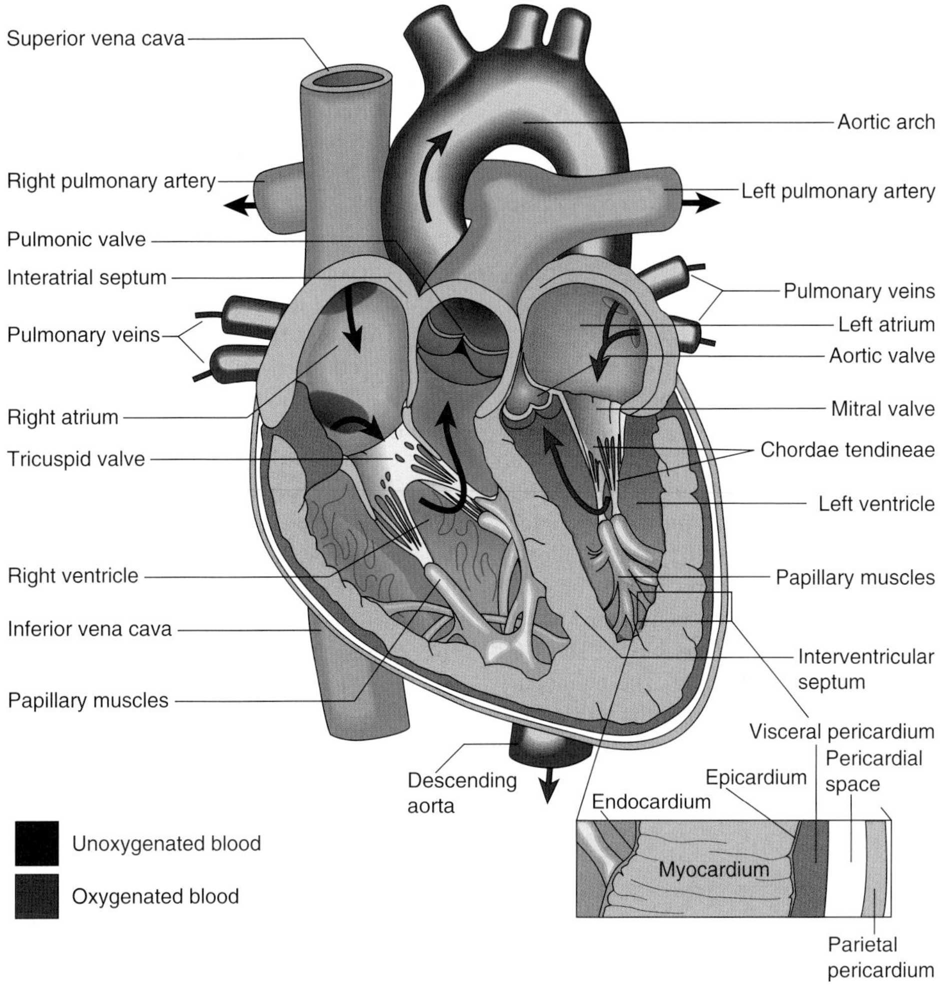

Figure 22-2 Structure of the heart. *Arrows* show the course of blood flow through the heart chambers.

blood to backflow, or regurgitate, into the chamber from which it has come.

The two **atrioventricular (AV) valves** separate the atria from the ventricles. They prevent blood from returning to the atria when the ventricles contract. These valves are cusped, or leaflike. The valve between the right atrium and the right ventricle is the **tricuspid valve**. The word *tricuspid* signifies that the valve has three cusps. The valve between the left atrium and the left ventricle is the **bicuspid (two-cusped) valve**, also known as the **mitral valve**.

Attached to the tricuspid and mitral valves are cordlike structures known as *chordae tendineae*, which in turn attach to *papillary muscles*, two major muscular projections from the ventricles. When the ventricles contract, the papillary muscles also contract, applying tension to the AV valves. The contraction of the papillary muscles and the firm support of the chordae tendineae prevent eversion of the valves and regurgitation of blood back into the atria.

The other two valves, called the *semilunar valves* because they resemble portions of the moon, prevent blood from flowing back into the ventricles after the heart contracts. The valves are named for the blood vessel into which the blood is deposited. The valve between the right ventricle and pulmonary artery is the **pulmonic** (or pulmonary) **valve**. The valve between the left ventricle and aorta is the **aortic valve**. Contraction of the ventricles forces blood into the pulmonary artery and aorta. Relaxation follows, and the fall in pressure in the ventricles causes the pulmonic and aortic valves to close, preventing backflow into the ventricles.

››› *Stop, Think, and Respond 22-1*

Where are the following cardiac valves located—(A) mitral valve, (B) tricuspid valve, and (C) pulmonic valve?

Arteries and Veins

Arteries carry oxygenated blood from the heart, and **veins** return deoxygenated blood to the heart. The smallest arteries are called **arterioles**, and the smallest veins are called **venules**. Arteries and arterioles are elastic and dilate or constrict to accommodate changes in blood flow. Veins have thinner walls than arteries because venous pressure is lower than arterial pressure. Despite being thinner, veins have larger diameters than corresponding arteries.

Arterioles branch into **capillaries**, which are microscopic vessels that form a connecting network between arterioles and venules. Capillaries are one cell-layer thick and in direct contact with the cells of all tissues. This complex circulatory network delivers oxygen and metabolic substances to the cells. After this exchange, the venules and veins transport blood back to the heart.

Heart contraction moves blood from the heart into arteries and arterioles; skeletal muscle contraction compresses veins and propels blood back to the heart. Closure of successive sets of valves in veins keeps the blood from pooling under the influence of gravity.

Cardiopulmonary Circulation

The largest veins, the **inferior vena cava** and **superior vena cava**, bring venous (deoxygenated) blood from all areas of the body into the right atrium. The right atrium fills with blood, and the tricuspid valve opens. Blood then travels into the right ventricle and is pumped into the **pulmonary artery** (the only artery in an adult that carries deoxygenated blood). The pulmonary artery branches to deliver venous blood to the right and left lungs. The lungs exchange the oxygen in inspired air for the CO_2 in the venous blood. The CO_2 is transferred into the alveoli and exhaled. The pulmonary veins then bring the oxygenated blood into the left atrium. The oxygenated blood flows out of the left atrium through the bicuspid, or mitral, valve and into the left ventricle. The left ventricle then pumps the blood through the aorta to all the body's cells and tissues.

››› *Stop, Think, and Respond 22-2*

Give the next location of blood when it is in the following structures: (A) right ventricle, (B) inferior vena cava, (C) left ventricle, and (D) pulmonary veins.

Blood Supply to the Heart

The left and right **coronary arteries** supply oxygenated blood to cardiac muscle (Fig. 22-3). The openings to the coronary arteries called the **coronary ostia** (singular, *ostium*) lie at the base of the aorta. When the left ventricle is filling with blood, the coronary ostia dilate and fill with blood. Thus, the myocardium is the first tissue of the body to receive oxygen-rich blood with each heartbeat.

After having distributed oxygenated blood to the myocardial cells, the **coronary veins** carry away the CO_2 produced by cellular metabolism. The coronary veins empty into the coronary sinus in the right atrium. The blood then mixes with blood from the inferior and superior venae cavae and is recirculated to the lungs.

Cardiac Cycle

The term **cardiac cycle** refers to the sequence of electrical and mechanical events in the atria and ventricles that result in a heartbeat (Fig. 22-4). First, the atria fill and then contract simultaneously to fill the resting, relaxed ventricles (**diastole**) with blood. When the pressure from accumulating blood increases in the ventricles, they contract (**systole**), and after a brief pause, the cycle begins again. The contraction of the left ventricle can be felt as a wavelike impulse (the pulse) in peripheral arteries. The pause between pulsations is ventricular diastole.

Concept Mastery Alert

Cardiac Cycle

During the cardiac cycle, the majority of the blood flowing to coronary arteries to fill the ventricles is supplied during *diastole*. When the ventricles are filled, they contract, which is called *systole*.

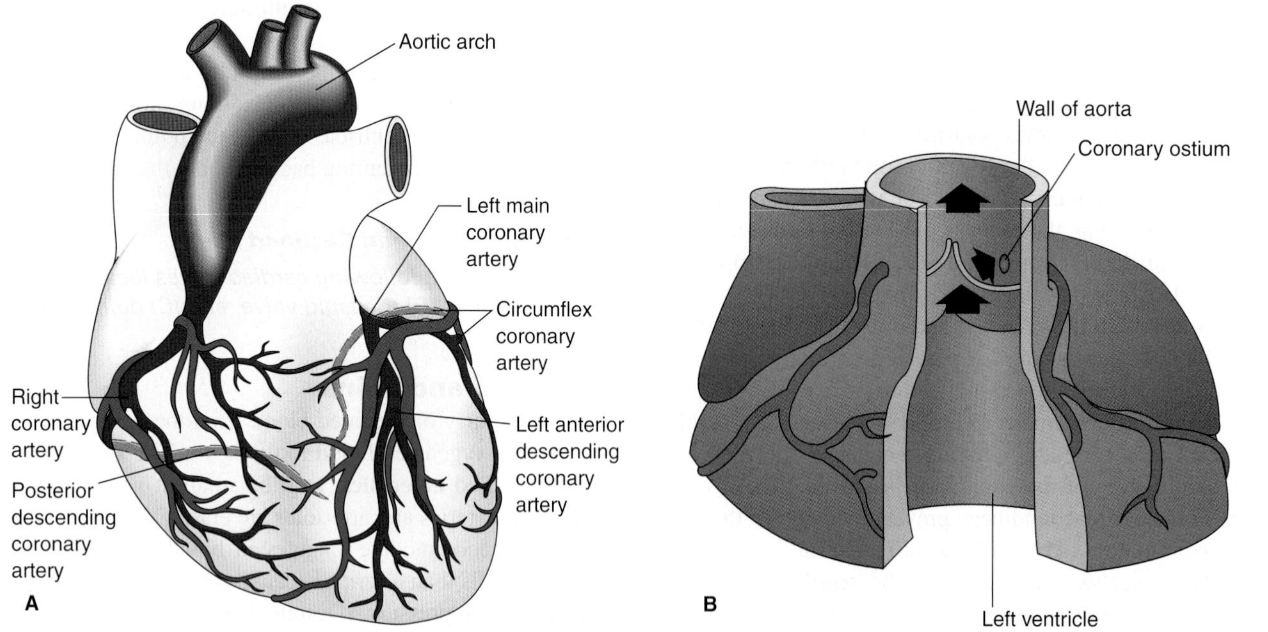

Figure 22-3 **(A)** Coronary arteries (*red vessels*) arise from the aorta and encircle the heart; coronary veins (*blue vessels*) run beside corresponding arteries and enter the main venous supply to the right atrium. **(B)** The orifices of the coronary arteries lie just beyond the aortic valve.

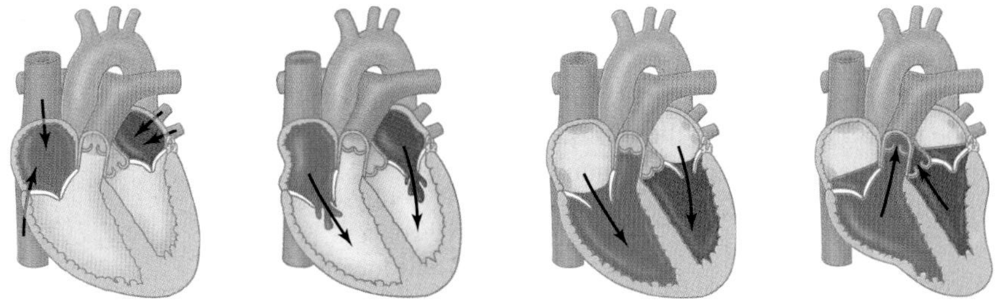

Figure 22-4 The sequence in the cardiac cycle begins when **(A)** blood from the venae cavae and pulmonary veins fills the atria. Near the end of atrial filling, an electrical stimulus causes **(B)** the atria to contract, allowing the atrial blood to fill the ventricles **(C)** when the atrioventricular valves open. A continuation of electrical stimulation causes ventricular contraction leading to the ejection of blood **(D)** through the pulmonic and aortic valves. After a brief pause, the cycle repeats.

Conduction System

The **conduction system**, which plays a role in the cardiac cycle, sustains the electrical activity of the heart. It consists of the SA node, AV node, bundle of His, bundle branches, and Purkinje fibers (Fig. 22-5).

The *SA node* is an area of nerve tissue located in the posterior wall of the right atrium. The SA node is called the *pacemaker of the heart* because it initiates the electrical impulses. Normally, it produces between 60 and 100 impulses per minute; the average is approximately 72 impulses per minute. Other areas in the conduction pathway may initiate an electrical impulse if the SA node malfunctions, but they do so at rates slower than the SA node.

In the normal sequence of events, the cardiac impulse starts in the SA node. It spreads throughout the atria over intranodal and interatrial pathways. The waves of stimulation through the heart resemble the rings that a pebble makes when dropped into a pond. Once the cells in the atria are excited, they contract in unison. When the impulse reaches the *AV node*, it is delayed a few hundredths of a second. While the ventricles fill with blood, the impulse travels from the AV node to the *bundle of His*, to the *right and left bundle branches*, and eventually to the *Purkinje fibers*. Then, both ventricles contract.

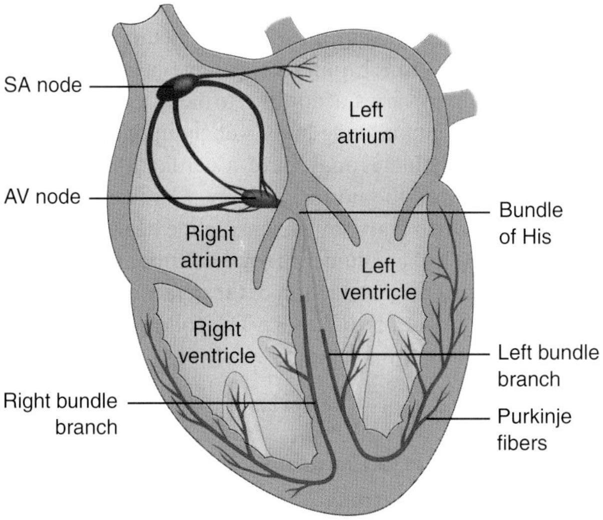

Figure 22-5 Electrical conduction system of the heart. AV, atrioventricular; SA, sinoatrial.

During diastole, while the myocardial cells are at rest and before an impulse is generated, the cells are in a polarized state (**polarization**). Positive ions predominate outside myocardial cell membranes; negative ions predominate inside. When an electrical impulse is initiated, it spreads from cell membrane to cell membrane, causing a transfer of ions. The positive ions move inside the myocardial cell membranes, and the negative ions move outside. This process, which corresponds with cardiac muscle contraction, is called **depolarization**. It occurs first in the atria and then in the ventricles. Once depolarization has occurred, the ions realign themselves in their original position and wait for another electrical impulse. This process is called **repolarization**. Another normal cardiac impulse cannot be carried out until the ions are again in polarized alignment. The time during which the cells are resistant to electrical stimulation is called the **refractory period**.

Depolarization and repolarization produce electrical changes. Because body tissues conduct current easily, this electrical activity can be detected by electrodes placed on the external surface of the body. The detection of the energy is recorded by a machine known as the *electrocardiogram* (ECG) (discussed later in this chapter).

>>> ***Stop, Think, and Respond 22-3***

Which part of the conduction system is known as the natural pacemaker because it initiates electrical impulses in normal heart conduction?

Regulation of Heart Rate

Heart rate fluctuates according to stimulation from the autonomic nervous system, baroreceptors, and chemoreceptors. The autonomic nervous system affects heart rate through sympathetic and parasympathetic nervous system innervation. When released by sympathetic nerve fibers, adrenergic neurotransmitters such as norepinephrine and epinephrine excite the SA node in the conduction system, increasing heart rate. These same neurotransmitters also stimulate beta-adrenergic receptors in the atria and ventricles, increasing the force of myocardial contraction. Conversely, the heart rate slows when parasympathetic nerve fibers from the cardiac branches of the vagus nerve release the cholinergic neurotransmitter acetylcholine. Parasympathetic neurostimulation, however, usually does not affect the force of contraction.

Responses to **baroreceptors**, pressure-sensitive nerve endings in the walls of the atria and major blood vessels (e.g., vena cava, arch of the aorta, and carotid arteries), also affect the heart rate. The main function of baroreceptors is to sense the pressure from blood as it stretches vascular tissues containing the baroreceptors. If blood pressure (BP) decreases in the areas of the baroreceptors, such as when a person rises quickly from a lying or standing position, the baroreceptors send impulses to the brain stem to increase heart rate. An almost immediate reflexive response of accelerated heart contractions follows. The heart rate increases to compensate for the drop in BP. When the BP is stabilized, the heart rate returns to within a normal range.

Chemoreceptors, structures that are sensitive to the pH and CO_2 and oxygen levels of blood, are located in the carotid bodies, aortic bodies, and medulla of the brain (Fig. 22-6). They regulate sympathetic stimulation or inhibition. A fall in pH, rise in CO_2, and decrease in oxygen levels in the blood result in increased heart contraction. The heart rate returns to a more usual parameter when pH and CO_2 levels become normalized. Box 22-1 highlights additional factors that alter heart rate.

BOX 22-1 Factors That Alter Heart Rate

Increase Heart Rate
Exercise
Fever
Hyperthyroidism
Hypoxia
Dehydration
Shock and hemorrhage
Anxiety
Caffeine
Drugs: central nervous system stimulants (cocaine, methylphenidate [Ritalin], methamphetamine), adrenergic drugs (epinephrine, isoproterenol [Isuprel]), anticholinergic drugs (atropine, glycopyrrolate [Robinul])
Alcohol withdrawal

Decrease Heart Rate
Rest
Hypothermia
Hypothyroidism
Athletic conditioning
Drugs: cardiac glycosides (digoxin [Lanoxin]), central nervous system depressants (morphine), calcium channel blockers (verapamil [Calan], nifedipine [Procardia]), beta-adrenergic blockers (atenolol [Tenormin], metoprolol [Lopressor], propranolol [Inderal]), Corlanor

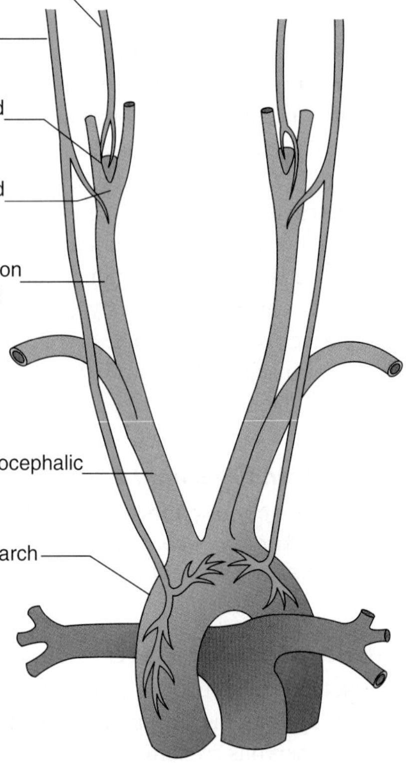

Figure 22-6 Location and innervation of the aortic arch and carotid sinus baroreceptors and the carotid body chemoreceptors. Chemoreceptors regulate sympathetic stimulation or inhibition. (Reprinted with permission from Chaffee, E. E., & Lytle, I. M. (1980). *Basic physiology and anatomy* (4th ed.). J. B. Lippincott.)

››› *Stop, Think, and Respond 22-4*

What effect will each of the following have on heart rate—(A) anxiety, (B) fever, (C) hypothyroidism, (D) caffeine, and (E) athletic conditioning?

Cardiac Output

Cardiac output is the amount of blood pumped out of the left ventricle each minute. In a healthy adult, cardiac output ranges from 4 to 8 L/min (the average is approximately 5 L/min). Volume varies according to body size. The heart adjusts cardiac output to the body's changing needs. During active exercise, athletes may have a cardiac output that is five to seven times the normal amount. Cardiac output can be increased in two ways: by increasing the heart rate and by increasing the stroke volume. **Stroke volume** is the amount of blood pumped per contraction of the heart. The stroke volume averages about 65 to 70 mL. The following formula is used to calculate cardiac output:

$$\text{Cardiac output} = \text{heart rate} \times \text{stroke volume}$$

››› *Stop, Think, and Respond 22-5*

If a person's heart rate is 72 beats/min and if the stroke volume is 65 mL/stroke, what is the cardiac output?

ASSESSMENT OF THE CARDIOVASCULAR SYSTEM

History

The initial assessment includes the client's (or family member's) description of the symptoms the client experienced before and during admission. The history also includes the client's past medical history and family medical history. The family medical history is important because many cardiac disorders have a familial or genetic predisposition. If close blood relatives are no longer living, it is important to ask about the cause of death, age at death, and relationship to the client.

The nurse asks the client to identify prescription and nonprescription drugs and herbal substances and nutritional substances that they are taking. Adverse effects or drug interactions can contribute to cardiac symptoms. Use of illicit drugs, such as cocaine and methamphetamine, is also significant to the cardiac history. Drug and food allergies are noted because future diagnostic procedures may involve the administration of drugs or substances, such as radiopaque dyes.

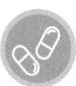

Pharmacologic Considerations

- When assessing the medication history, be sure to ask specifically about nonprescription medications and herbal or nutritional supplements. Clients may not think of these items as medications, yet they can also impact BP, pulse, or cardiac function.

Physical Examination

General Appearance

An appraisal of the client's general appearance may suggest problems that require further exploration. The client's nonverbal behavior and body position may indicate that they are anxious, depressed, in pain, or uncomfortable.

Pain

Poor circulation, a common problem in clients with cardiovascular disorders, causes ischemia (reduced blood supply) to body organs. A classical sign of ischemia is pain, which results from a lack of oxygen in the tissue. Chest pain is a manifestation of ischemia to the heart muscle. Leg pain, especially with activity, can indicate inadequate oxygenation to leg muscles.

When pain is present, the nurse evaluates it carefully. Obtaining as much information as possible is essential. Prompt management of pain is extremely important (see Chapter 11).

Vital Signs

Temperature

Fever is characteristic in some types of heart disease. It can accompany the inflammatory response when myocardial cells are damaged after an acute myocardial infarction (MI; heart attack) or infections such as rheumatic fever and bacterial endocarditis.

Pulse

When taking a client's pulse, the nurse notes its rate, rhythm, and quality. Pulse rhythm is the pattern of the pulsations and the pauses between them. A normal pulse is felt regularly with a similar length of pause. The pulse quality refers to its palpated volume. Pulse volume is described as feeling full, weak, or thready, meaning barely palpable. The nurse also determines any pulse deficit by counting the heart rate through auscultation at the apex while a second nurse simultaneously palpates and counts the radial pulse for a full minute. The difference, if any, is the **pulse deficit**.

Respiratory Rate

The nurse counts the respiratory rate for 60 seconds. They observe the character of the respirations, noting whether the client's breathing is effortless or labored (dyspneic), deep or shallow, noisy or quiet. The use of accessory muscles (neck or abdominal muscles) during respiration is an indication that the client is having difficulty breathing.

Blood Pressure

Cardiac disorders often are associated with changes in BP. If the client is not acutely ill, the nurse takes the BP with the client in the lying, sitting, and standing positions (orthostatic vital signs; Nursing Guidelines 22-1). These baseline determinations are necessary to monitor the effects of cardiovascular diseases and drugs that can alter the BP during position changes. To ensure an accurate assessment, the nurse selects the cuff width most appropriate for the diameter of the client's arm (Evidence-Based Practice 22-1).

NURSING GUIDELINES 22-1

Assessing Blood Pressure and Pulse for Postural Changes

- Have the client lie down for at least 3 minutes.
- Assess the client's BP and pulse.
- Assist the client to a sitting position.
- Be prepared to steady or assist the client should they become dizzy or faint.
- Reassess the BP and pulse within 30 seconds after the client sits.
- Repeat the assessments with the client standing.
- Determine the difference in systolic and diastolic BPs in the upright position from that recorded in the previous position.
- Determine the difference in the heart rate from that recorded in the previous position.
- Conclude that the client manifests postural changes if the BP is lower than 10 mm Hg from the previous measurement and the heart rate increases 10% or more from the previous measurement.

Evidence-Based Practice 22-1

Guidelines for Treating Hypertension

Clinical Question

What are the latest guidelines in treating a diagnosis of hypertension?

Evidence

The International Society of Hypertension (ISH), in 2020, identified the process to treat clients with the diagnosis of hypertension. Typically, clients can be nervous or anxious when having BP taken in the acute care or clinic settings. The new guidelines encourage the treatment of hypertension to include home monitoring or ambulatory monitoring for a 24-hour period. Once an accurate diagnosis of hypertension is met, then the ISH guidelines are followed for the antihypertensive drug therapy treatment. Stage 1: Adults with an elevated BP or stage 1 hypertension who have lower risk factors for cardiovascular disease should be managed with nonpharmacologic therapy and have a repeat BP evaluation within 3 to 6 months. Adults with stage 1 hypertension who have more risk factors should be managed initially with a combination of nonpharmacologic and antihypertensive drug therapy and have a repeat BP evaluation in 1 month. Stage 2: Adults with stage 2 hypertension should have a combination of nonpharmacologic and antihypertensive drug therapy initiated and have a repeat BP evaluation in 1 month. For adults with a very high average BP (e.g., systolic BP ≥ 180 mm Hg or diastolic BP ≥ 110 mm Hg), evaluation followed by prompt antihypertensive drug treatment is recommended. For adults with a normal BP, repeat evaluation every year is reasonable.

Nursing Implications

Nurses should review BP technique and make sure that they are accurate in taking BP and instructing clients on how to take accurate BP at home. Nurses may use the ISH guidelines as a resource for instructing clients on techniques. It is important that the BP results are accurate to ensure that the best treatment for hypertension is used. The following BP information is from the *2020 ISH Global Hypertension Practice Guidelines*:

Category	Systolic (mm Hg)	Diastolic (mm Hg)
Normal BP	<130	<85
High-normal BP	130–139	85–89
Grade 1 hypertension	140–159	90–99
Grade 2 hypertension	≥160	≥100

Reference

Clinical Practice Guidelines. (2020). *2020 International Society of Hypertension Global Hypertension Practice Guidelines*. https://www.ahajournals.org/doi/pdf/10.1161/HYPERTENSIONAHA.120.15026

The nurse takes the BP in both arms on admission and at least once daily thereafter, making sure to report a marked difference in pressure between the left and right arms. When charting, the nurse identifies the arm used to measure the BP and the client's position at the time it was measured. The nurse questions the client about dizziness or lightheadedness when changing positions, such as rising from a sitting or lying position. These symptoms may indicate postural (or orthostatic) hypotension.

Cardiac Rhythm

The electrical activity that produces the heart rhythm can be observed continuously with bedside cardiac monitoring. Electrodes are attached to the chest and connected to a machine that displays the cardiac rhythm on an oscilloscope. The components of an ECG are discussed later in this chapter. A paper strip of the cardiac rhythm can be printed and attached to the client's record.

A cardiac monitor reveals the heart's electrical but not its mechanical activity. The health care provider must palpate a peripheral pulse or auscultate the apical heart rate to obtain this information. Comparing the heart rate and rhythm with the information displayed on the monitor is important because the ECG pattern may appear normal in some clients even when mechanical function is abnormal.

Cardiac **telemetry** sends ECG information over radio waves to a monitor that is distant from the client. Paramedics use telemetry to communicate information to health care providers in the hospital emergency department. Telemetry also may be used when a client's condition is stable enough to allow transfer from a critical care unit but still requires continuous monitoring. When telemetry is used, the electrodes are attached to a battery pack, which is secured inside a pocket on the client's hospital gown or clothing.

Heart Sounds

Normal Heart Sounds

Auscultation of the heart requires familiarization with normal and abnormal heart sounds. The first heart sound ("lub"), referred to as S_1, is the closing of the mitral and tricuspid valves. S_1 is heard loudest over the apex of the heart and occurs nearly simultaneously with the palpated pulse. The second heart sound ("dub"), referred to as S_2, is the closing of the aortic and **pulmonic valves**. S_2 is heard loudest with the stethoscope in the aortic area, which is at the second intercostal space to the right of the sternum (Fig. 22-7).

Abnormal Heart Sounds

All other heart sounds are abnormal and take considerable practice to recognize. A sound that follows S_1 and S_2 is called an S_3 heart sound, or a ventricular gallop. When these three sounds are heard together, some say the cadence sounds like "Ken-tuck-y" or "lub-dub-dee." An S_3, although normal in children, often is an indication of heart failure in an adult. An extra sound just before S_1 is an S_4 heart sound, or atrial gallop. Some say this sound resembles the word "Ten-nes-see" or "lub-lub-dub." An S_4 sound often is associated with hypertensive heart disease.

In addition to heart sounds, auscultation may reveal other abnormal sounds, such as murmurs and clicks caused by turbulent blood flow through diseased heart valves. A friction rub may cause a rough, grating, or scratchy sound that is indicative of pericarditis (inflammation of the pericardium).

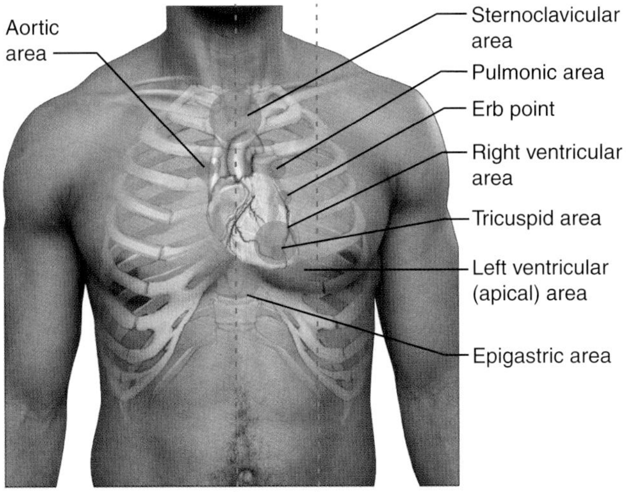

Figure 22-7 Areas assessed when evaluating heart function. Heart sounds can be auscultated in the aortic area, pulmonic area, Erb point, tricuspid area, and apical area.

Peripheral Pulses

The nurse palpates the radial arteries and other peripheral pulses during the physical assessment (Fig. 22-8). They record the presence or absence of these pulses and their strength.

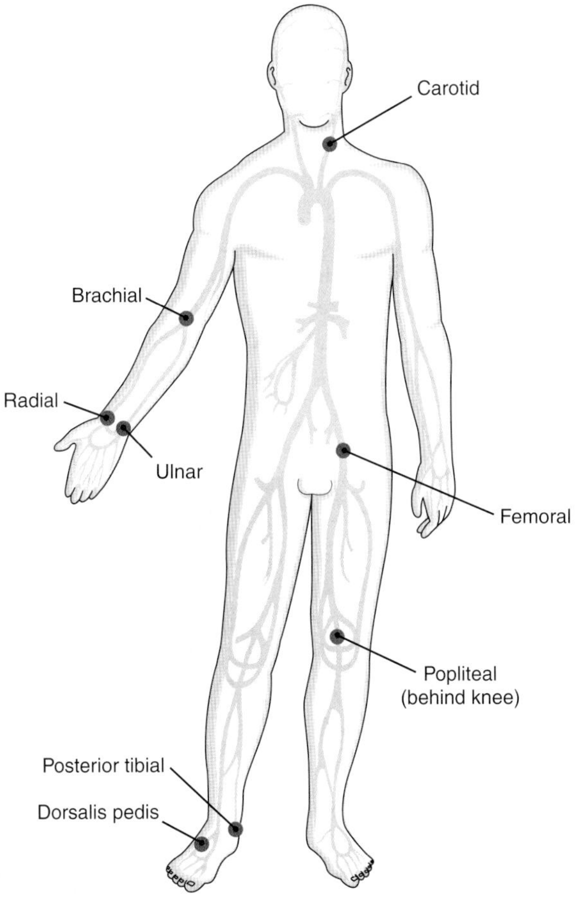

Figure 22-8 Peripheral pulses can be assessed where arteries can be palpated over bones. (Reprinted with permission from Houser, H. J., & Sesser, J. R. (2016). *Lippincott Williams & Wilkins' medical assisting exam review for CMA, RMA & CMAS Certification* (4th ed.). Wolters Kluwer.)

Skin

Many clients with cardiac disorders exhibit changes in skin color (e.g., cyanosis, pallor). A good light is necessary when assessing skin color. Cyanosis can be detected by carefully noting color changes in the oral mucous membranes as well as in the lips, earlobes, skin, and nail beds. In clients who are light skinned, extreme pallor is easy to detect because the skin appears almost bloodless. In clients who are dark skinned, a grayish cast to the skin usually indicates pallor.

The nurse inspects the arms and legs for variations in skin color and temperature and compares their bilateral findings with other areas of the body. Sparse hair growth on the legs and thick toenails can indicate poor circulation. The nurse also notes any varicosities (enlargement of veins) that are observed in lower extremities.

Peripheral Edema

Edema occurs when blood is not pumped efficiently or plasma protein levels are inadequate to maintain osmotic pressure. When blood has nowhere else to go, the extra fluid enters the tissues. Particular areas for examination are the dependent parts of the body, such as the feet and ankles. Other areas prone to edema are the fingers, hands, and over the sacrum. To assess for edema, the examiner gently presses their fingers into the skin and then quickly releases. If the marks of the fingers remain, the effect is termed *pitting edema*. Edema is evaluated on a scale of +1 to +4, depending on the depth of the pit and the amount of time it takes the pit to disappear (see Chapter 16). The higher the number, the more pronounced is the edema.

Weight

Weight gain can indicate edema. A rapid gain in weight often means that edema is increasing. Weight loss often reflects the loss of excess fluid from the tissues and is used to evaluate the effectiveness of drug therapy, especially diuretics. If weight is recorded daily, the nurse weighs the client at the same time, with the same amount of clothing, using the same scale, each day. The weight is recorded as accurately as possible.

Jugular Veins

If the right side of the heart fails to pump efficiently, blood becomes congested in the neck veins. With the client sitting at a 45-degree angle, the client turns their head to the left or right so the nurse can inspect the external jugular vein (Fig. 22-9). Distention of this vein usually indicates increased fluid volume and pressure in the right side of the heart (see Chapter 28).

Lung Sounds

If the left side of the heart fails to pump efficiently, blood backs up into the pulmonary veins and lung tissue. The nurse auscultates the lungs for abnormal and normal breath sounds. With left-sided heart failure, auscultation reveals a crackling sound and possibly wheezes and gurgles. Wet lung sounds are accompanied by dyspnea and an effort to sit up to breathe. If uncorrected, left-sided heart failure is followed by right-sided heart failure because the circulatory system is a continuous loop.

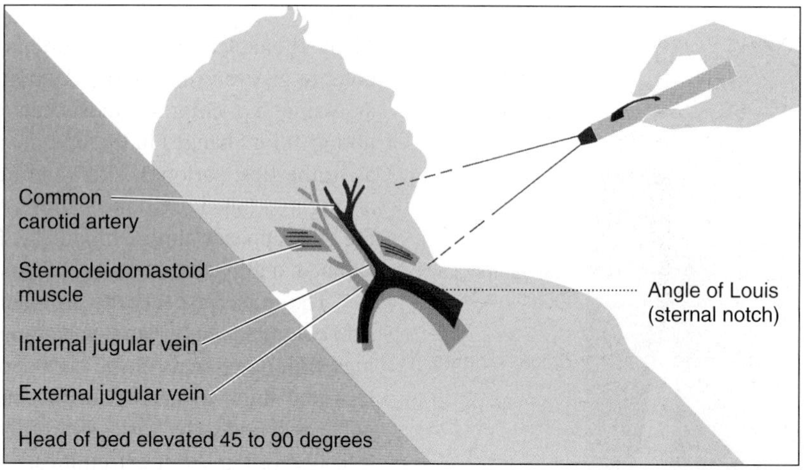

Figure 22-9 Assessing for jugular vein distention. (Reprinted with permission from Lippincott Williams & Wilkins. (2009). *Assessment. An incredibly visual pocket guide.* Wolters Kluwer Health/Lippincott Williams & Wilkins.)

Sputum

Clients with cardiac disease may have a productive or nonproductive cough. The nurse notes the type and frequency of the cough and the amount and appearance of the sputum. These findings can be important in diagnosing heart failure or other pulmonary complications.

Mental Status

Some clients with cardiac disorders may be alert and oriented; others may be alert, confused, or disoriented. Confusion or disorientation can result from a decrease in the oxygen supply to the brain (cerebral ischemia) as a result of poor circulation. Chest pain and impaired breathing can create anxiety. The nurse reports extremes of emotion or disturbances in thought processes to the primary provider because such effects could interfere with the client's safety, diagnostic testing, and prescribed therapy.

Diagnostic Tests

Laboratory Tests

Various general laboratory tests are used in the diagnosis of heart disease and in monitoring the client's progress. Laboratory tests may be performed daily or every few days. They may be used to monitor the results of therapy. Blood chemistries, such as fasting blood glucose and serum electrolyte, cholesterol, and triglyceride levels, may be used as part of the diagnostic process. Analysis of serum enzymes and isoenzymes may also be ordered. Serum cholesterol and lipid tests and isoenzyme analyses are discussed in more detail in Chapter 25. When tissues and cells break down, are damaged, or die, large quantities of certain enzymes are released into the bloodstream. Enzymes can therefore be elevated in response to cardiac or other organ damage.

Radiography and Radionuclide Studies

Chest radiography and fluoroscopy determine the size and position of the heart and condition of the lungs. These studies are also used to guide the insertion and confirm the placement of cardiac catheters, internal pacemaker wires, and internal cardiac defibrillators. Computed tomography (CT) scanning and magnetic resonance imaging are used to determine heart size and detect lung involvement.

Radionuclides are radioactive chemical elements that are injected into and travel through the bloodstream. Their use sometimes is referred to as *nuclear cardiology*. The radionuclide technetium-99m is used to detect areas of myocardial damage. The radionuclide thallium-201 is used to diagnose ischemic heart disease during a stress test.

Magnetic Resonance Imaging

Magnetic resonance imaging (MRI) is a diagnostic tool used to identify disorders that affect many different structures in the body without performing surgery (Fig. 22-10). The principle underlying MRI is that many elements within the human body, such as hydrogen, are magnetic. The MRI machine's magnetic field excites the hydrogen atoms, creating a radio signal. The radio signal is converted to an image on a computer monitor. Because magnetism is used, clients undergoing an MRI are not exposed to radiation as would occur with tests involving X-rays. Ferrous-based materials, nickel alloys, and most stainless steel materials are not

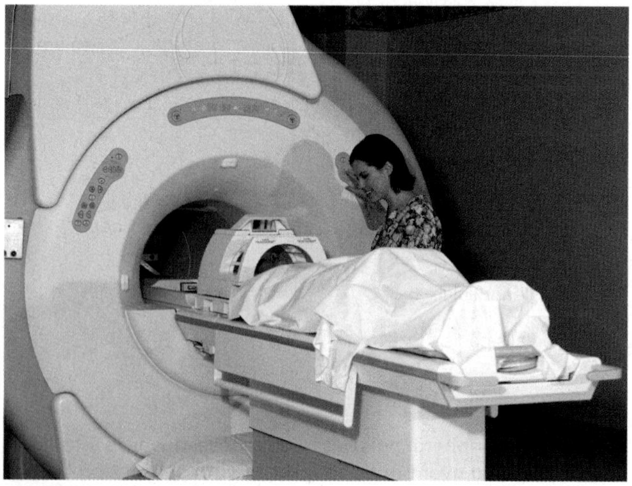

Figure 22-10 A client undergoing closed magnetic resonance imaging.

BOX 22-2 Metal Devices That Pose Contraindications in Magnetic Resonance Imaging (MRI)

Within the Body
Wound staples
Implanted pacemaker[a]
Implanted cardiac defibrillator[a]
Artificial heart valve or stents
Metallic pins, screws, plates[b]
Implanted drug delivery device
Aneurysm clips
Transdermal patches[c]
Implanted brain/spinal nerve stimulator
Tattooed eyeliner

On the Body (Must Be Removed)
Watch
Jewelry
Hearing aid
Hair clips or pins
Pocket knife
Keys
Credit cards or bank cards
Body piercings
Removable dental work

[a]Allen-Dicker (2017) reports that cardiac implantable devices are safe, but may require specialized preparation of the MRI machine.
[b]MRIs can be done on clients with metal joint implants, but it requires that the radiologist use a metal artifact reduction sequence (MARS) to avoid radiologic distortion of the image.
[c]Remove before MRI

compatible with an MRI because they may be pulled toward the magnetic source. Therefore, an MRI is prohibited on clients with various metal devices within their body. External metal objects such as body piercings, some types of hearing aids, and the like must be removed (Box 22-2). Nonferromagnetic materials are either safe or identified as "MR-conditional," but when questionable, the safety of various items can be checked by consulting lists provided by the Food and Drug Administration (Shellock, 2016).

Health care providers are now using MRI to diagnose cardiac disorders. Cardiovascular MRI scanning can provide data about cardiac anatomy, function, blood flow, metabolism, and circulatory perfusion with a single examination. The image of blood within the heart appears white; dense tissues such as cardiac muscle and the valves are dark gray. Advantages of a cardiac MRI include (1) the ability to observe the heart's structure, function, and blood circulation in three dimensions rather than observe only the electrical changes that occur with a stress ECG, which is discussed later, and (2) the elimination of exposure to radiation.

Preparation for a cardiac MRI includes attaching ECG leads, starting intravenous (IV) infusions in one or two sites for the purpose of instilling fluids; medication, such as adenosine (Adenocard), to accelerate the heart rate; and *contrast medium*, a radiopaque substance that fills hollow structures, to help the primary provider observe the heart in "real time."

The technician conducting the MRI informs the client that the machine produces loud knocking sounds during the test. To muffle the sounds, the technician can provide headphones and earplugs to the client. Some clients become claustrophobic when enclosed within the MRI scanning chamber and can receive medication to relieve their anxiety; however, they must remain conscious to follow instructions regarding brief periods of breath holding during the test. An open MRI, in which the client lies quietly on a table with a coil covering the part of the body that requires imaging, is now an alternative (Fig. 22-11). Besides relieving a client's distress, an open MRI also eliminates noise, provides additional body space for those who are obese, and allows the radiologist to access the client if an injection or insertion of a tube is necessary.

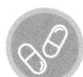

Pharmacologic Considerations

- When a client's heart cannot tolerate physical exercise, medications may be used for stress testing. Dipyridamole, adenosine (both can lead to bronchospasm), and dobutamine may be used to chemically stress the heart.
- Often, cardiac meds are held for 24 hours before the test; be sure and instruct the client regarding medications as they are ordered for testing.
- Although only 30% of scans use a contrast medium, check the medical record for history of kidney failure or reduced function; gadolinium-based contrast medium has been associated with nephrogenic system fibrosis.

Echocardiography

Echocardiography uses ultrasound waves to determine the functioning of the left ventricle and to detect cardiac tumors, congenital defects, and changes in the tissue layers of the heart. High-frequency sound waves, which the human ear cannot hear, pass through the chest wall (transthoracic) and are displayed on an oscilloscope. The image is recorded and kept as a permanent record. This technique is also known as transthoracic echocardiography.

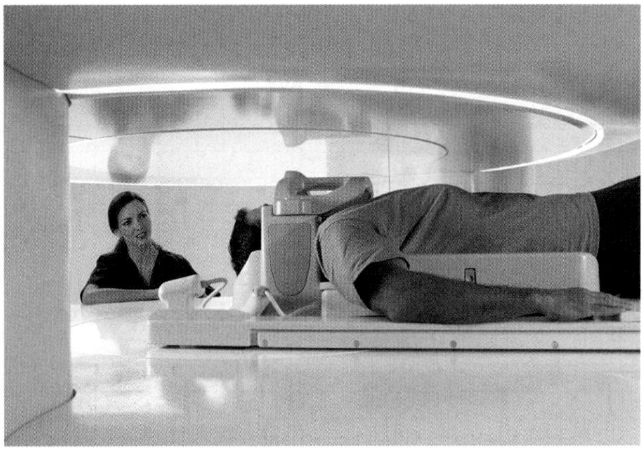

Figure 22-11 An open magnetic resonance imaging relieves anxiety experienced by those who are claustrophobic or obese. (Courtesy of Hitachi Medical Systems America, Inc., Twinsburg, OH.)

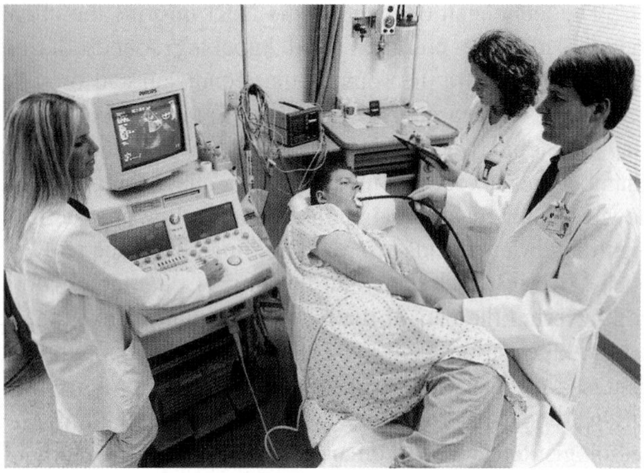

Figure 22-12 In transesophageal echocardiography, an ultrasound transducer mounted on a flexible tube is passed into the esophagus. When the transducer is at the level of the posterior heart, it transmits an image of the heart and its internal structures.

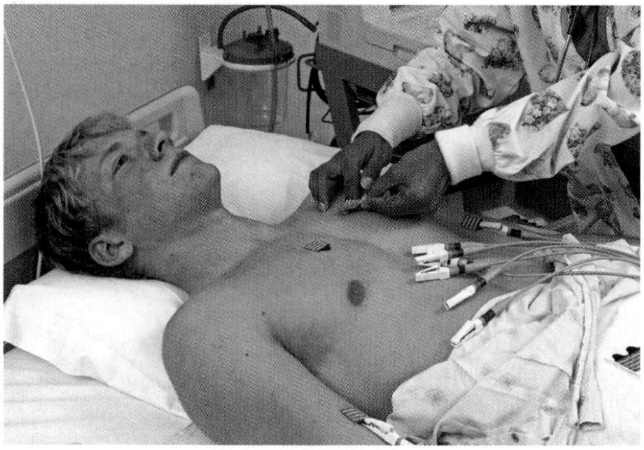

Figure 22-13 The nurse attaches electrodes to the client's chest and limbs before an electrocardiograph.

A second ultrasound technique is **transesophageal echocardiography** (TEE), which, as the name implies, involves passing a tube with a small transducer internally from the mouth to the esophagus (Fig. 22-12). The transducer can obtain images of the posterior heart and its internal structures from the esophagus, which lies behind the heart. TEE provides superior views that are not possible using standard transthoracic echocardiography. It is also an adjunct for assessing intraoperative complications in the heart during cardiothoracic surgery. Clients whose chests are rotund or who are obese are candidates for TEE. Because the throat is anesthetized locally, the nurse cautions the client to avoid eating or drinking until sensation and the gag reflex return, which may take 1 hour or longer after removal of the tube containing the transducer.

Electrocardiography

Electrocardiography is the graphic recording of the electrical currents generated by the heart muscle. The test performed during electrocardiography is called an ECG. During an ECG, color-coded electrodes matched to corresponding lead wires connect the client to the recording machine. The electrodes are coated with conductive gel and applied to the skin surface of the wrists, ankles, and chest (Fig. 22-13). A computerized ECG machine immediately interprets the tracings, or rhythm strips, which serve as a screening device. A primary provider later interprets the rhythm strips to aid in diagnosing heart disease (Fig. 22-14).

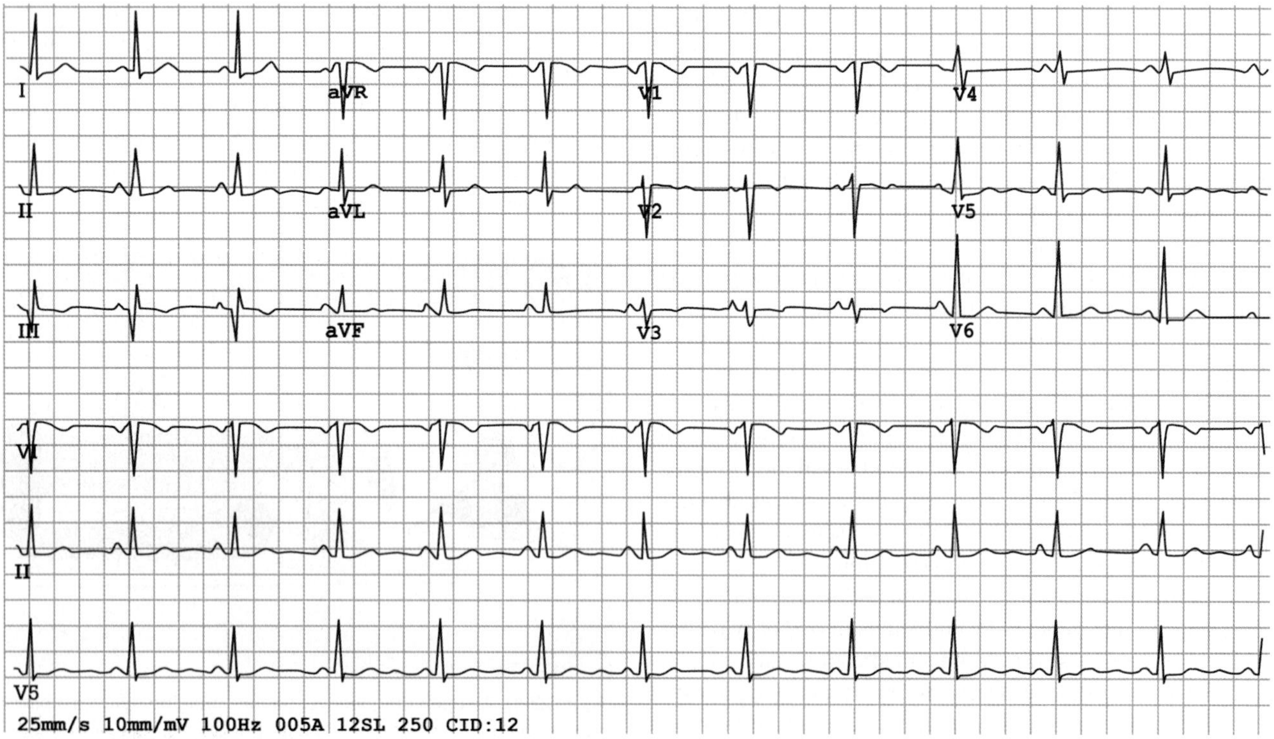

Figure 22-14 Normal 12-lead electrocardiograph configuration. (Source: shutterstock.com/ Inna Ogando)

Resting ECG is performed as a baseline before doing an exercise ECG. Exercise ECG is more diagnostic than resting ECG because it demonstrates how the heart functions when subjected to activity.

Ambulatory Electrocardiography

Ambulatory ECG, or Holter monitoring, is the recording of an ambulatory client's cardiac rate and rhythm over 24 to 48 hours as the client performs daily activities. The Holter monitor, which is worn on a belt or carried on a strap about the neck, consists of a tape recorder connected to ECG leads attached to the client's chest (Fig. 22-15). During the test period, the client keeps a diary of activities and associated symptoms. At the end of the recording period, the monitor is returned to the hospital or primary provider and the tape is analyzed. The client's written notes are compared with the recorded information. Ambulatory ECG helps to detect dysrhythmias (rhythm abnormalities) and myocardial ischemia that occur sporadically during activity or rest.

Exercise Electrocardiography

During **exercise electrocardiography**, also known as a stress test, the electrical activity of the heart is assessed with an ECG monitor while the client walks on a treadmill, pedals a stationary bicycle, or climbs up and down stairs (Fig. 22-16). The speed of the treadmill, the force required to pedal the bicycle, or the pace of stair climbing is gradually increased. The goal is to increase the heart's workload to reach a predetermined target heart rate. The client's heart rate and rhythm are monitored continuously, and ECG waveforms are recorded periodically. The client's BP and respiratory rate also are assessed. The client is instructed to report the onset of chest pain, dizziness, leg cramps, or weakness. The stress test is aborted if the client develops chest pain, severe dyspnea, elevated BP, confusion, or arrhythmias. The primary provider interprets ECG tracings obtained during the test. Radionuclides also may be used during a stress test to provide additional information.

Drug-Induced Stress Testing

Drugs may be used to stress the heart for clients with sedentary lifestyles or those with a physical disability, such as severe arthritis, that interferes with exercise testing. Drugs such as adenosine (Adenocard), dipyridamole (Persantine), or dobutamine (Dobutrex) may be administered singularly or in combination by the IV route. The drugs dilate the coronary arteries, similar to the vasodilation that occurs when a person exercises to increase the heart muscle's blood supply. When thallium, a radionuclide, is injected a few minutes later, a scan of the heart can detect compromised blood flow, which indicates coronary artery disease or evidence of well-perfused heart muscle.

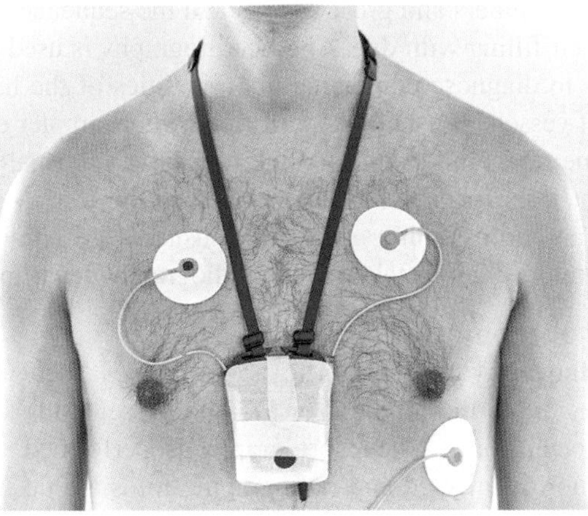

Figure 22-15 Ambulatory electrocardiography records the client's cardiac rate and rhythm during regular daily activities. (Source: shutterstock.com/marako85)

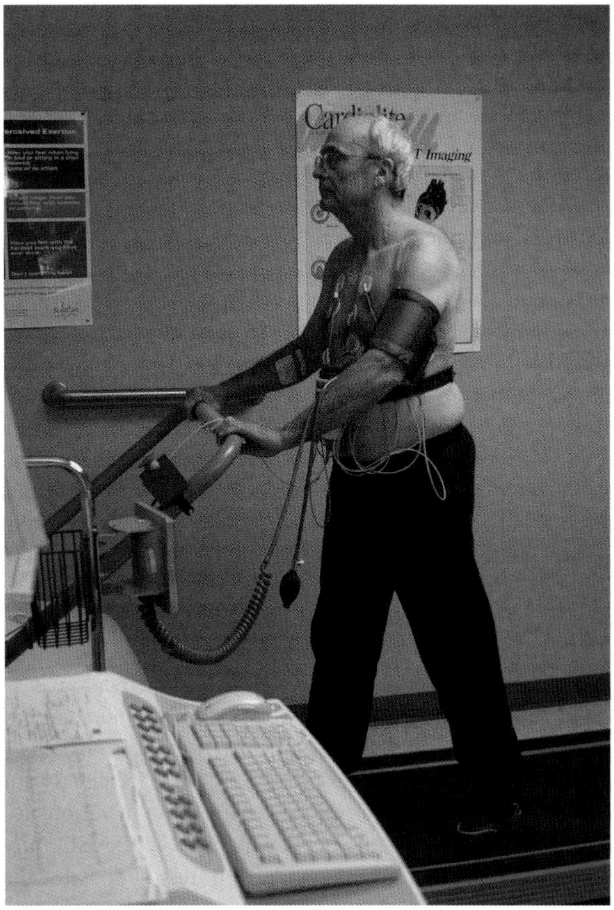

Figure 22-16 Treadmill exercise stress test. (Photo by Ken Timby.)

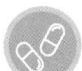

Pharmacologic Considerations

- Often, medications are held for 24 hours before procedures. Confer with the primary provider regarding medications for chronic conditions; this is especially important for those who take heart, hypertension, or diabetes medications.

Cardiac Catheterization

Cardiac catheterization is a diagnostic test performed in an operative setting. It can be done for a variety of purposes. In this procedure, a long, flexible catheter is inserted from a peripheral blood vessel in the groin, arm, or neck into one of the great vessels (inferior or superior vena cava which is attached to the heart) and then into the heart. Cardiac catheterization may be carried out on the left side of the heart by way of an artery or on the right side by way of a vein.

Before the procedure, the client needs to consult the primary provider about which prescribed medications to take or omit the day of the cardiac catheterization. Food and fluids usually are withheld; however, if the test is late in the day, light food may be permitted. Allergies must be identified; those of primary concern before a cardiac catheterization are iodine, shellfish, radiographic dye, and latex. IV fluids are administered before the test to maintain hydration and to administer any necessary medications. A sedative may be administered before the test. For a diagnostic cardiac catheterization, conscious sedation using midazolam (Versed) may be used. Conscious sedation allows the client to be sleepy and comfortable, but sufficiently awake to respond to questions and positional changes. A local anesthetic is administered at the site where the catheter is inserted. General anesthesia is reserved for a cardiac catheterization that will involve cardiac surgery. After the test, the catheter is removed and the site is covered with a pressure dressing to control bleeding. The usual length of stay following cardiac catheterization is at least 5 to 9 hours or overnight. After the test, the nurse monitors BP and pulse frequently to detect complications. They also check the dressing over the insertion site frequently for signs of bleeding. The nurse palpates the pulse in various locations and checks the color and temperature in the extremity to confirm that blood is circulating well. Instructions for the client and family include the following:

- Keep the extremity straight for several hours and avoid movement.
- Report any warm, wet feeling that may indicate oozing blood, numbness, tingling, or sharp pain in the extremity.
- Drink a large volume of fluid to relieve thirst and promote the excretion of the dye.
- Follow discharge instructions for home care (Client and Family Teaching 22-1).

Client and Family Teaching 22-1
Discharge Instructions for Clients Having Cardiac Catheterization

The nurse instructs the client as follows:

- Rest for the next 3 days and avoid heavy lifting, strenuous activity, or sports during this time.
- Do not drive or climb stairs for the next 24 hours.
- Do not take a tub bath until the puncture site is healed.
- Change the bandage in 24 hours; continue changing the bandage until a crust or scab forms over the puncture site.
- You may experience some soreness at the puncture site; however, if it becomes worse, notify your primary provider.
- If pain or swelling of the puncture site occurs, notify your primary provider.
- If the puncture site begins to bleed, hold pressure over the site and call 911 or another emergency services number.

Arteriography

Coronary Arteriography

The most common use of a left-sided cardiac catheterization is to determine the degree of blockage of the coronary arteries by performing arteriography while the catheter is in place. An **arteriography** is a diagnostic procedure that involves instilling contrast medium into an artery. In this case, it is instilled into the catheter and deposited into each coronary artery. Occlusive heart disease is indicated if one or more coronary arteries appear narrow or do not fill. Clients with coronary artery disease who are considered candidates for invasive treatment procedures must undergo cardiac catheterization and coronary arteriography.

After removal of the catheter, the nurse inspects the insertion site for bleeding, tenderness, hematoma formation, and inflammation. The client remains on bed rest for the rest of the day. They must avoid flexion, or bending, of the arm or leg used for catheter insertion. Vascular assessments distal to the insertion site continue at frequent intervals. Absent distal peripheral pulses, cool toes, and pale or cyanotic arms and legs indicate arterial occlusion, usually from a blood clot. These signs as well as a rapid or irregular pulse rate indicate a medical emergency that the nurse must report immediately to the primary provider.

Peripheral Arteriography

Peripheral arteriography is used to diagnose occlusive arterial disease in smaller arteries. Contrast medium is injected into an artery, and radiographic films are taken. After the procedure, the chance for bleeding is greater than after a venipuncture; therefore, a pressure dressing is applied and client activity is restricted for about 12 hours. The nurse observes the client for bleeding and cardiac arrhythmias and assesses the adequacy of peripheral circulation by frequently checking the peripheral pulses.

Angiocardiography

In **angiocardiography**, a radiopaque contrast medium is injected into a vein, and its course through the heart is recorded by a series of radiographic pictures taken in rapid succession. The pictures reveal the size and shape of the heart chambers and great vessels and the sequence and time of their filling with dye. Angiocardiography is used particularly to diagnose congenital abnormalities of the heart and great vessels. It usually is performed when simpler diagnostic measures fail to provide the necessary information. The client fasts for at least 3 hours before the test. A sedative and an antihistaminic medication usually are administered before the client is taken to the radiography department.

Aortography

Aortography detects aortic abnormalities such as aneurysms (abnormal dilation of a blood vessel wall) and arterial occlusions. When aortography is performed, contrast medium is injected and radiographic films are taken of the abdominal aorta and major arteries in the legs. Distribution of the contrast medium also may be observed as it circulates to other vessels, such as the renal arteries.

KEY POINTS

- The normal anatomy and physiology of the cardiovascular system.
  - Heart chambers:
    - Right and left atria
    - Right and left ventricles
  - Cardiac tissue:
    - Epicardium: outer layer
    - Myocardium: middle layer, composed of muscle tissue
    - Endocardium: inner layer, it has direct contact with the blood that passes through the heart
    - Pericardium: is a saclike structure that surrounds and supports the heart
  - Heart valves:
    - Two AV valves: separate the atria from the ventricles
    - Tricuspid valve: valve between the right atrium and the right
    - **Bicuspid valve**/mitral valve: valve between the left atrium and left ventricle
  - Arteries and ventricles:
    - Arteries: carry oxygenated blood from the heart
    - Veins: return deoxygenated blood to the heart
  - Cardiopulmonary circulation:
    - Largest veins: inferior vena cava and superior vena cava, bring venous (deoxygenated) blood from all areas of the body into the right atrium
    - Pulmonary artery (the only artery in an adult that carries deoxygenated blood): The pulmonary artery branches to deliver venous blood to the right and left lungs.
  - Blood supply to the heart:
    - Left and right coronary arteries supply oxygenated blood to cardiac muscle.
  - Cardiac cycle:
    - Diastole: the majority of the blood supply flowing to coronary arteries to fill the ventricles
    - Systole: when the ventricles are filled, they contract.
- Conduction system (sustains the electrical system of the heart):
  - SA node
  - AV node
  - Bundle of His
  - Bundle branches
  - Purkinje fibers
- Regulation of the heart rate:
  - Baroreceptors: the function is to sense the pressure from blood as it stretches vascular tissues
  - Chemoreceptors: structures that are sensitive to the pH and CO_2 and oxygen levels of blood are located in the carotid bodies, aortic bodies, and medulla of the brain.
- Cardiac output:
  - Cardiac output: the amount of blood pumped out of the left ventricle each minute
  - Stroke volume: the amount of blood pumped per contraction of the heart
- Focus assessment criteria for a client with cardiovascular problems:
  - Client history
  - General examination/physical appearance
  - Pain
  - Vital signs
  - Cardiac rhythm
  - Heart sounds
  - Peripheral pulses
  - Skin
  - Peripheral edema
  - Weight
  - Jugular veins
  - Lung sounds
  - Sputum
  - Mental status
  - Diagnostic tests used for heart disease
  - Lab tests
  - Radiography and radionuclide studies
  - Magnetic resonance imaging
  - Echocardiography
  - Electrocardiography
  - Cardiac catheterization
  - Arteriography

CRITICAL THINKING EXERCISES

1. During admission, the nurse notes that the client has an irregular pulse rate. What aspect of cardiac anatomy and physiology is most likely contributing to the assessment data?
2. The function of which heart chamber is most important to maintain? Explain your answer.
3. What are the consequences that may occur if cardiac output is decreased below normal?
4. What information is important for the nurse to communicate to a client who is scheduled for a cardiac diagnostic test?

NCLEX-STYLE REVIEW QUESTIONS PrepU

1. When a client comes to the emergency department complaining of chest pain, what question is most important for the nurse to ask initially?
   1. "When did your pain begin?"
   2. "Have you had this type of pain before?"
   3. "Do you have any food or drug allergies?"
   4. "Do you have pain in any other place?"

2. A hospitalized client takes an antihypertensive medication and complains of being lightheaded when getting out of bed. What nursing intervention is most appropriate at this time?
   1. Notify the client's primary provider.
   2. Take the client's BP while lying, sitting, and standing.
   3. Ask the client if this has happened before.
   4. Hold the client's medication until the client feels better.
3. When assessing heart sounds, place an "X" in the anatomic area that is best for auscultating an S_1 heart sound.

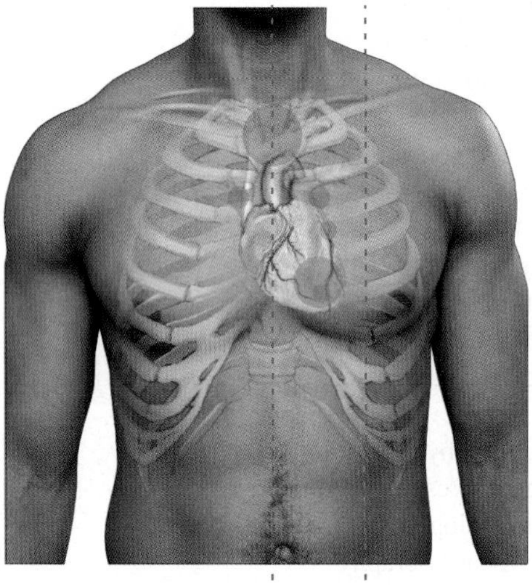

4. What are indications that a client may have cardiac disease? Select all that apply.
   1. Significant weight loss
   2. Chest pain on exertion
   3. Hypertension
   4. Father died at age 48 years
   5. Presence of S_2 heart sound
5. What client is most important for the nurse to assess for complications following a cardiac catheterization?
   1. A 75-year-old with chronic kidney disease
   2. A 50-year-old with occasional numbness and tingling in hands
   3. A 25-year-old who has a persistent cough
   4. A 38-year-old with a family history of diabetes

WANT TO KNOW MORE? There are a wide variety of online resources available on thePoint to enhance learning and understanding of this chapter.

Go to **thePoint.lww.com/activate** and use the activation code found in the front of this text to unlock these online resources.

23

Caring for Clients With Infectious and Inflammatory Disorders of the Heart and Blood Vessels

Words To Know

Buerger disease
cardiac tamponade
cardiomyopathy
chorea
decortication
deep vein thrombosis
effusion
emboli
impedance plethysmography
infective endocarditis
intermittent claudication
Janeway lesions
murmur
myocardial disarray
myocarditis
myofibrils
Osler nodes
pericardiectomy
pericardiocentesis
pericardiostomy
pericarditis
petechiae
polyarthritis
postphlebitic syndrome
precordial pain
pulmonary embolus
pulsus paradoxus
rheumatic carditis
Roth spots
sequelae
splinter hemorrhages
sympathectomy
syncope
thrombectomy
thromboangiitis obliterans
thrombophlebitis
vegetations
vena caval filter
vena caval plication
venography
ventriculomyomectomy
Virchow triad

Learning Objectives

On completion of this chapter, you will be able to:

1. Identify three organisms that cause infectious conditions of the heart.
2. List four inflammatory conditions of the heart.
3. Describe treatment for inflammatory and infectious heart disorders.
4. Discuss the nursing management of clients with infectious or inflammatory heart disorders.
5. Name three types of cardiomyopathy.
6. Differentiate between thrombophlebitis and thromboangiitis obliterans.
7. List three interventions that reduce the risk of thrombophlebitis.
8. Discuss the nursing management of clients with inflammatory disorders of peripheral blood vessels.

The body uses many defense mechanisms to combat the effects of trauma, disease, and microorganisms. The inflammatory response, skin and mucous membranes, and immune system work together to protect all systems of the body, including the cardiovascular system. Despite these protective mechanisms, infectious and inflammatory disorders may compromise the heart and blood vessels.

Gerontological Considerations

■ A decline in immune system function that occurs with age may lead to increased risk for infectious or inflammatory disorders of the cardiovascular system. Decreased inflammatory and immune responses may also prolong recovery from cardiovascular trauma, disease, or microorganisms.

- Rheumatic heart disease may occur in an older adult who had rheumatic fever at an earlier age or from an acute episode later in life.
- Circulatory changes can also occur from growth of vegetation at cardiac valves that affect closure following infections or dental work. Assess for shortness of breath or activity intolerance.

■ The prevalence of infective endocarditis among older adults has increased due, in part, to the increased number of prosthetic valve replacements and an increase in hospital-acquired bacteremia.

■ Encourage older clients who are inactive to move every hour during the day to promote circulation. Such movement is especially important during long car or airplane trips and can be as simple as flexion and extension of the foot. In addition, caution regarding prolonged crossing of legs or ankles that can reduce circulatory flow.

INFECTIOUS AND INFLAMMATORY DISORDERS OF THE HEART

Rheumatic Fever and Rheumatic Carditis

Rheumatic fever is a systemic inflammatory disease that sometimes follows a group A streptococcal infection of the throat. **Rheumatic carditis** refers to the inflammatory cardiac manifestations of rheumatic fever in either the acute or later stage. Cardiac structures that are usually affected include the heart valves (particularly the mitral valve), endocardium, myocardium, and pericardium.

Pathophysiology and Etiology

The inflammatory symptoms of rheumatic carditis are believed to be induced by antibodies originally formed to destroy the group A beta-hemolytic streptococcal microorganisms. The antibodies, however, "mistakenly" cross-react against the proteins in the connective tissue of the heart, joints, skin, and nervous system (Fig. 23-1). This cross-reaction causes valvular damage and *pancarditis*, inflammation of all layers of the heart (endocardium, myocardium, and pericardium).

As the antibody response ensues, white blood cells (WBCs) migrate to the endocardium, causing inflammatory debris to accumulate as **vegetations** around the valve leaflets (Fig. 23-2). When the inflammatory process is resolved, fibrinous tissue replaces the damaged structures. The fibrinous tissue fuses or thickens valve leaflets and shortens the chordae tendineae; thus, the valves may lose their ability to open fully or close tightly (see Chapter 24). The fibrinous replacements also cause surface irregularities around the valves, making them prone to future colonization by blood-borne bacteria.

The antibodies also attack cardiac myosin, the muscle protein in myocardial tissue. Because myosin is instrumental in cardiac muscle contraction, rheumatic carditis may cause weakened heart contractions and heart failure (see Chapter 28). If the pericardium is involved, it becomes tough and leathery from accumulated fibrinous fluid that interferes with the heart's ability to stretch and fill with blood. Tachydysrhythmias, fast abnormal heart rhythms, develop to compensate for the decreased cardiac output (the volume of blood ejected from the left ventricle per minute). After the acute episode, most clients recover, but valvular changes remain.

Assessment Findings

Signs and Symptoms

Acute rheumatic fever, a precursor to other pathologies, is most common in children aged 2 to 3 weeks after a streptococcal infection. The **sequelae**, conditions that are a consequence of a disease, include carditis (inflammation of the layers of the heart), **polyarthritis** (inflammation of more than one joint), rash, subcutaneous nodules, and **chorea**, characterized by jerky involuntary movements and an inability to use skeletal muscles in a coordinated manner. Adults do not exhibit the same degree and range of symptoms as young children.

A mild fever, if untreated, continues for several weeks. The heart rate is rapid, and the rhythm may be abnormal. A red, spotty rash referred to as *erythema marginatum* appears on the trunk but disappears rapidly, leaving irregular circles on the skin. Several joints, most commonly the knees, ankles, hips, and shoulders, become swollen, warm, red, and painful. The involvement migrates among joints. Sometimes, marble-sized nodules appear around the joints. Central nervous system manifestations result in chorea. Cardiac complications may develop: a heart murmur suggests valve damage; a pericardial friction rub indicates pericarditis; and heart failure develops if the myocardium fails to compensate for functional demands (Fig. 23-3).

Diagnostic Findings

No laboratory test is specific for the diagnosis of rheumatic fever. The results of laboratory tests such as an antistreptolysin O titer, erythrocyte sedimentation rate (ESR), and C-reactive protein are elevated, indicating an inflammatory process involving the streptococcal organism. Specific cardiac tests such as electrocardiography (ECG) and echocardiography may show structural changes in the valves, size of the heart, and the heart's ability to contract.

Medical and Surgical Management

Intravenous (IV) antibiotics are given. Penicillin (such as amoxicillin, penicillin G, and penicillin V) is the drug of choice for treating a group A streptococci infection unless contraindicated because of an allergy. For clients who are allergic to the penicillin family of antibiotics, another antibiotic such as azithromycin (Zithromax), clarithromycin (Biaxin), or clindamycin (Cleocin) may be prescribed. Cephalosporins such as cephalexin (Keflex) or cefadroxil (Duricef) may be prescribed if the client has not had a previous severe allergic reaction to penicillin. Bed rest may be indicated, depending on the client's condition. Aspirin is used to control the formation of blood clots around heart valves. Nonsteroidal drugs such as naproxen (Naprosyn, Aleve) and steroids are used to suppress the inflammatory response.

Concurrent treatment of rheumatic carditis depends on the extent of heart involvement. If minor, no treatment may be given; if heart failure or life-threatening arrhythmias occur, extensive treatment is necessary. Surgery may be required to treat constrictive pericarditis and damage to heart valves. The American Heart Association (2016) simplified the guidelines for prophylactic antibiotic therapy before invasive procedures, previously believed to predispose the body to bacteremia and recurrence of endocarditis (Box 23-1). Prophylactic antibiotics are no longer recommended for those having procedures involving the reproductive, urinary, or gastrointestinal (GI) tracts.

Nursing Management

The nurse administers prescribed drug therapy and monitors for therapeutic and adverse effects. They plan diversional activities that require minimal activity, such as reading and putting puzzles together, to reduce the work of the myocardium and counteract the boredom of bed rest. Focused cardiac assessments help to track the progression or improvement of

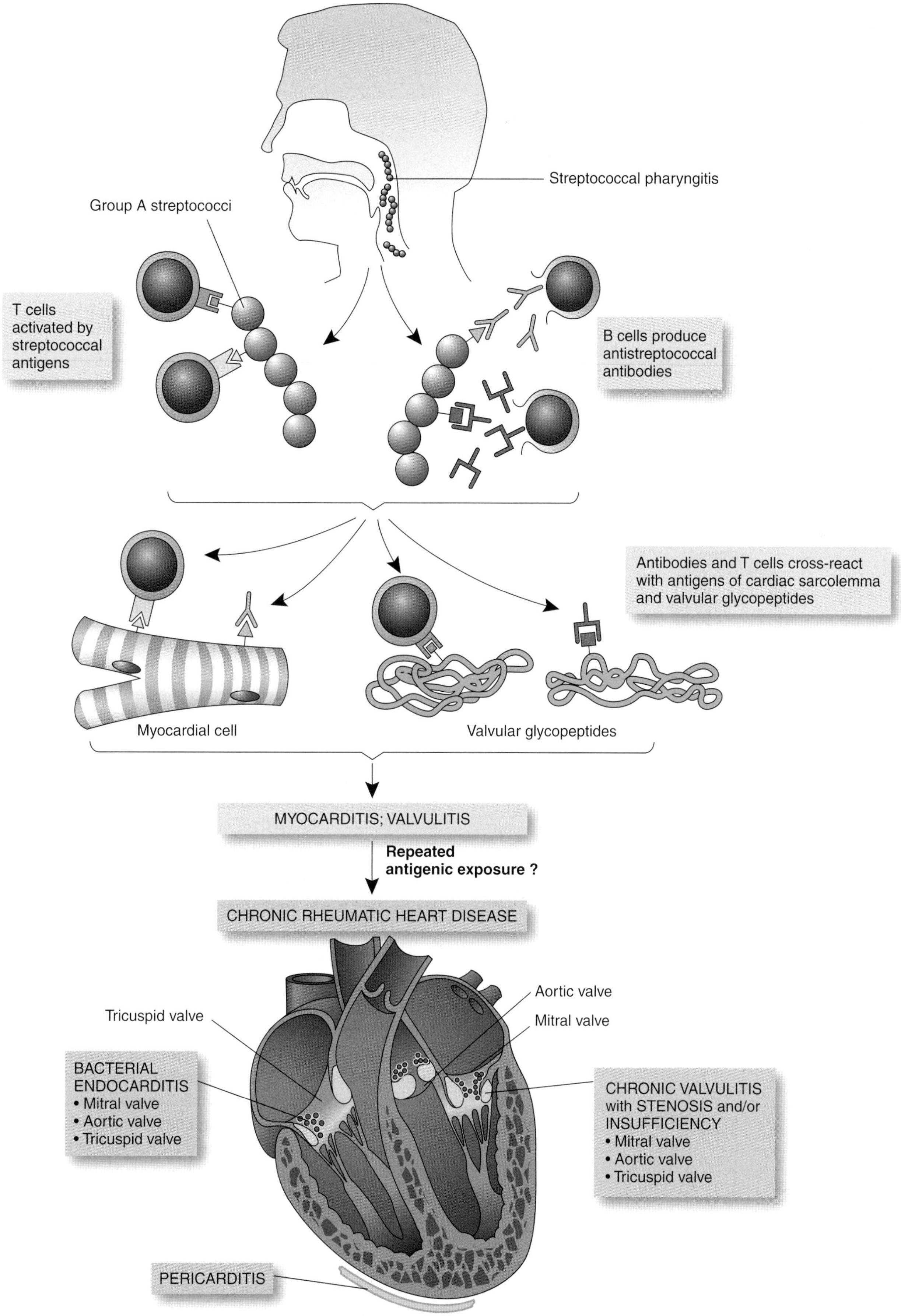

Figure 23-1 Rheumatic carditis after group A streptococcal pharyngitis. (Reprinted with permission from Rubin, E., & Strayer, D. S. (2014). *Rubin's pathology: Clinicopathologic foundations of medicine* (7th ed.). Wolters Kluwer.)

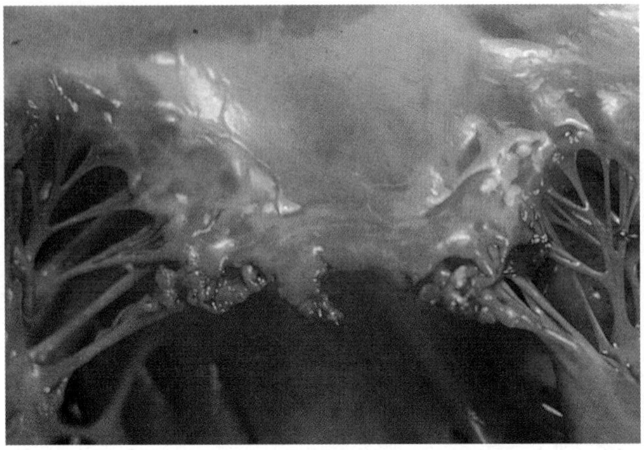

Figure 23-2 The mitral valve shows destructive vegetations. (Reprinted with permission from Rubin, E., & Strayer, D. S. (2014). *Rubin's pathology: Clinicopathologic foundations of medicine* (7th ed.). Wolters Kluwer.)

heart involvement. Clients with a history of rheumatic fever are susceptible to infective endocarditis (discussed next). Additional nursing management depends on assessment data. Nutrition Notes describes nutrition considerations.

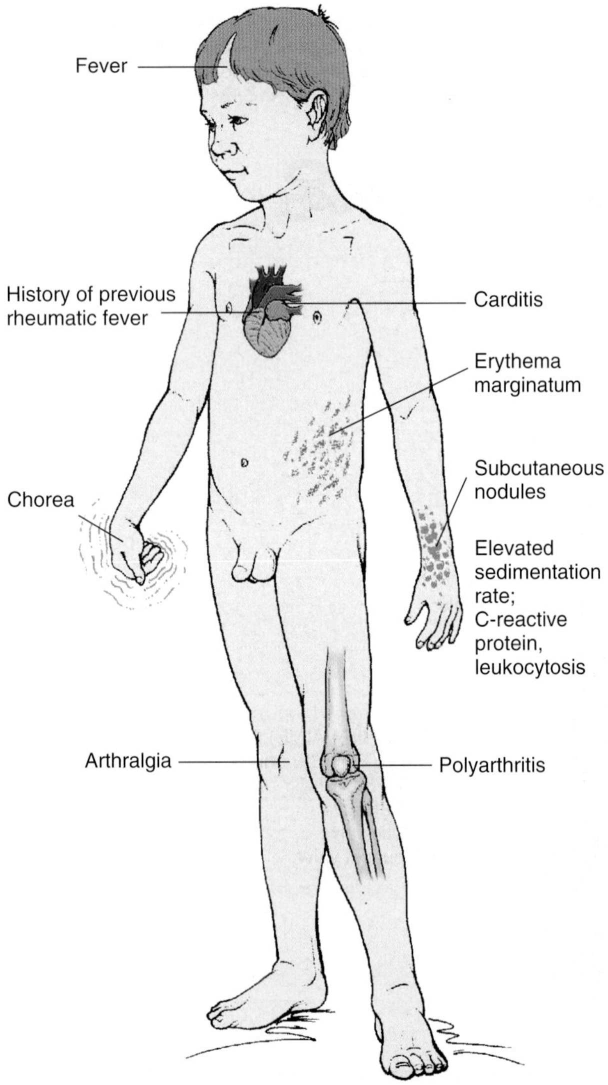

Figure 23-3 Manifestations of rheumatic fever.

BOX 23-1 High-Risk Procedures for Clients With a History of Rheumatic Carditis or Infective Endocarditis

Prophylactic antibiotic therapy is recommended before dental procedures for clients with:

- a prosthetic heart valve
- a history of endocarditis
- congenital heart defects that have not been fully repaired
- congenital heart defects repaired with prosthetic material for 6 months after the repair
- repaired congenital heart defects with residual defects

From American Heart Association. (2016). *Infective endocarditis.* Retrieved April 28, 2016, from http://www.heart.org/HEARTORG / Conditions/CongenitalHeartDefects/TheImpactofCongenitalHeartDefects/Infective-Endocarditis_UCM_307108_Article.jsp#.VyJOy2fmqM8

Concept Mastery Alert

Myocarditis Diagnosis

Although an echocardiography can reveal information about the heart that may be indicative of myocarditis, the most definitive diagnostic technique is myocardial biopsy.

Nutrition Notes

The Client With Rheumatic Carditis

- A full liquid diet is used in the initial treatment of rheumatic heart disease and is progressed as tolerated.
- Sodium is restricted if the client has edema or is treated with steroids.
- Anorexia and weight loss are common side effects of infections; calories and protein should be increased as needed to replenish losses.
- Fever increases fluid requirements.
- Encourage small, frequent feedings to maximize intake.

››› *Stop, Think, and Respond 23-1*

What information is important to give parents whose children develop a severe sore throat?

Infective Endocarditis

Infective endocarditis (formerly called *bacterial endocarditis*) is an inflammation of the inner layer of heart tissue as a result of an infectious microorganism (Fig. 23-4). Although clients with rheumatic carditis may develop endocarditis, it is initially considered an autoimmune response—not an infection—because no microorganism can be isolated from blood or other cultured specimens. Subsequent to the initial rheumatic carditis, however, the valvular changes increase the client's susceptibility to endocardial colonization by pathogens. In addition to clients who have recovered from rheumatic carditis, other susceptible clients include those who have nonrheumatic valve disease or artificial heart valves, repaired congenital heart defects, a prolapsed mitral valve, or hypertrophic cardiomyopathy (discussed later); IV drug users; and immunosuppressed clients with central venous catheters.

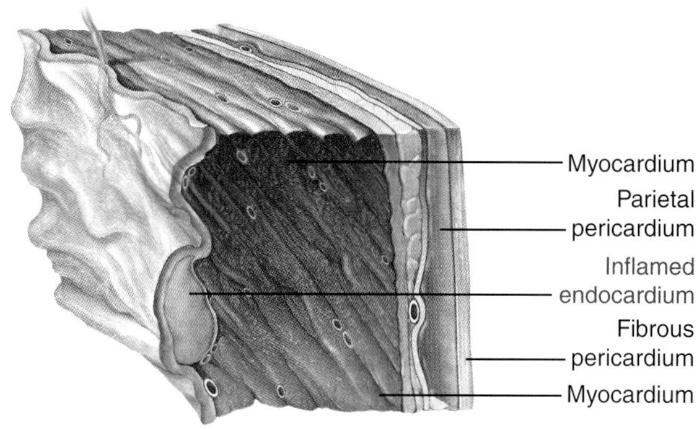

Figure 23-4 Tissue changes in endocarditis.

Pathophysiology and Etiology

The microorganisms that cause infective endocarditis include bacteria and fungi (Table 23-1). Streptococci and staphylococci are the bacteria most frequently responsible for this disorder. They are found abundantly on the skin and mucous membranes of the mouth, nose, throat, and other cavities.

Most pathogens find their way into the bloodstream through trauma caused by invasive procedures involving mucous membranes or other tissues that harbor microorganisms. Although anyone can contract endocarditis, clients with a history of rheumatic carditis are especially susceptible. Prolonged IV therapy, insertion of cardiac pacemakers, cardiac catheterization, tracheal intubation, cardiac surgery, genitourinary instrumentation (Foley catheters and cystoscopy), and IV drug abuse create portals of entry for the causative microorganisms.

Once the microorganisms migrate to the endocardial surface, they attach to the vegetations composed of fibrin and platelets surrounding the heart valves, chordae tendineae, and papillary muscles. The microorganisms bury themselves in the vegetative mass, making them difficult to destroy with natural defenses or antibiotic therapy. The cycle continues with layer upon layer of embedded microorganisms and fibrin/platelet deposits.

The endocardium on the left side of the heart is affected more often than on the right. The mitral valve is the most common location of vegetations and microbial deposits. If the valve leaflets erode and slough, blood leaks between the heart chambers, diminishing the heart's efficiency as a pump. Heart failure is often a consequence. The vegetations can break off to form **emboli**, mobile masses of fibrin and clusters of platelets that circulate in the bloodstream. Emboli may occlude small blood vessels and interfere with an organ's blood supply.

Assessment Findings

Signs and Symptoms

Infective endocarditis can have an acute onset (less than 1 week) from a previously healthy state. The client presents with fever, chills, muscle aches in the lower back and thighs, and joint pain. Subacute infections progress more insidiously over weeks to months with more vague manifestations, such as headache, malaise, fatigue, and sleep disturbances. As the condition advances, purplish, painful nodules called **Osler nodes** may appear on the pads of the fingers and toes. Black longitudinal lines called **splinter hemorrhages** can be seen in the nails. There may be small, painless, red-blue macular lesions known as **Janeway lesions** on the palms of the hands and soles of the feet (Vyas, 2014). **Roth spots**, white areas in the retina surrounded by areas of hemorrhage, may be detected. The spleen may be enlarged, and tenderness may be noted on abdominal palpation. A heart murmur may be present from malfunctioning valves. **Petechiae**, tiny, reddish hemorrhagic spots on the skin and mucous membranes, are signs of embolization.

TABLE 23-1 Microorganisms That Cause Endocarditis

MICROORGANISMS	DESCRIPTION
Streptococci Group A beta-hemolytic *Streptococcus bovis* *Streptococcus viridans*	• Account for 55% of cases of endocarditis • Attack normal or damaged heart valves and may cause rapid destruction • Related to GI malignancy • Tend to affect previously damaged heart valves
Staphylococci *Staphylococcus aureus* *Staphylococcus faecalis* *Staphylococcus epidermidis*	• Cause 30% of cases of endocarditis • Virulent strain with high mortality rate • Associated with dental procedures and valve replacements • Cause both acute and subacute infections
Enterococci *Enterococcus faecalis* and *Enterococcus faecium*	• Associated with urologic instrumentation in men, bacteremia, respiratory tract infections, pneumonia, sinusitis, otitis media, and epiglottitis • Normal inhabitants of the GI tract, anterior urethra, and occasionally the mouth
HACEK Group *Haemophilus parainfluenzae* and *Haemophilus aphrophilus* *Aggregatibacter actinomycetemcomitans* *Cardiobacterium hominis* *Eikenella corrodens* *Kingella kingae*	• Relatively resistant to single antibiotics; require combination of antibiotic therapy for a minimum of 4 weeks • Slow-growing Gram-negative bacilli • Require culture for 2 weeks or longer when initial culture is negative • Cause subacute presentations • Associated with very large vegetations
Fungi *Candida*	• Increased incidence in IV drug users • Risk increased with improper use of antibiotics and steroids
Gram-negative bacteria *Escherichia coli* *Klebsiella* species *Pseudomonas* species	• May travel from GI or genitourinary tract • Increased risk in older adults

GI, gastrointestinal; IV, intravenous.

Pronounced weakness, anorexia, and weight loss are common. Symptoms can change suddenly if embolization or heart failure occurs. Emboli to the brain cause cerebrovascular accidents (see Chapter 38); emboli to the kidneys cause flank pain and renal failure (see Chapter 58); pulmonary emboli result in sudden chest pain and dyspnea (see Chapter 21). Clients with heart failure present with dyspnea, hypotension, and peripheral or pulmonary edema.

Diagnostic Findings

Anemia and slight leukocytosis are common findings. A series of three blood cultures collected over 1 to 24 hours usually identifies the microorganism circulating in the blood. Some cultured specimens require incubation for 3 weeks or more to identify accurately the infecting species. Occasionally, the vegetations also can be cultured. Transesophageal echocardiography is more likely than transthoracic echocardiography to reveal the vegetations, altered valvular function, and impaired pumping quality of the ventricles. ECGs may reveal abnormalities in heart rhythm if the vegetations involve a valve close to conduction tissue.

Medical and Surgical Management

High doses of an IV antibiotic to which the organism is susceptible are prescribed initially (Drug Therapy Table 23-1). Antibiotic therapy extends at least 2 to 6 weeks. It is resumed if the infection recurs after discontinuation of the drug. Bed rest is ordered initially. When the client begins to improve, bathroom privileges and increased activity are allowed. If a heart valve has been severely damaged and drug therapy does not adequately support the heart in failure, valve replacement may be necessary (see Chapters 24 and 29).

Nursing Management

Many clients cannot appreciate the danger of the disease without seeing external signs of the damage. The nurse gently but firmly reminds the client to limit activity. The nurse continually assesses for changes in weight, pulse rate, and rhythm, noting and reporting new symptoms. The nurse administers prescribed antibiotics around the clock to sustain therapeutic blood levels of the medication at all times. They inform clients that periodic antibiotic therapy is a lifelong necessity because they will be vulnerable to the disease for the rest of their lives.

Client and Family Teaching 23-1 provides appropriate health information for clients who have infectious or inflammatory heart disorders.

>>> *Stop, Think, and Respond 23-2*

If a client asks why they have been advised to take an antibiotic such as penicillin before having dental work done, what information is appropriate to provide?

Myocarditis

Pathophysiology and Etiology

Myocarditis is an inflammation of the myocardium (the muscle layer of the heart; Fig. 23-5). A viral, bacterial, fungal, or parasitic infection causes most cases; a viral origin is most common in the United States. The usual viral agents

DRUG THERAPY TABLE 23-1 Agents Used to Treat Endocarditis

Category and Common Generic (Brand) Drugs	Intended Use	Common Side Effects	Safety Warnings for Nurses
Penicillin Family Penicillin G (Pfizerpen) Ampicillin Nafcillin	Kill susceptible microorganisms by interfering with bacterial cell wall development	Glossitis, stomatitis, gastritis, furry tongue, nausea, vomiting, diarrhea, rash, fever, pain at injection site	Monitor for anaphylactic reaction Monitor IV infusion for phlebitis
Cephalosporins Ceftriaxone (Rocephin)	Kill susceptible microorganisms by interfering with bacterial cell wall development	Nausea, vomiting, diarrhea, headache	May show allergy if allergic to penicillin Avoid alcohol intake Monitor for nephrotoxicity
Vancomycin (Vancocin)	Kills susceptible Gram-positive microorganisms not responding to treatment with other antibiotics	Nausea, chills, fever, urticaria	Monitor for ototoxicity and nephrotoxicity Increased bleeding risk when client is on anticoagulant therapy Hypotensive alert with rapid IV infusion
Aminoglycoside Gentamicin	Kills susceptible Gram-negative microorganisms by interfering with protein synthesis	Dizziness, vertigo, nausea, vomiting	Monitor for ototoxicity and nephrotoxicity Do not use if client has Parkinson disease
Daptomycin (Cubicin)	Kills *Staphylococcus aureus* microorganisms by interfering with protein synthesis	Nausea, diarrhea, constipation, rash, vein irritation	Monitor cardiac enzymes if taken with statin drugs Increased bleeding risk when client is on anticoagulant therapy
Rifampin (Rifadin)	Kills susceptible microorganisms by inhibiting RNA polymerase activity in bacterial cell	Headache, drowsiness, fatigue, dizziness, heartburn, epigastric distress	Must be taken on empty stomach Will turn body fluids orange Monitor liver enzymes Monitor for pancytopenia

Client and Family Teaching 23-1
Infectious and Inflammatory Heart Disorders

The nurse provides the following instructions:

- Continue regular follow-up care because there will always be a risk for a recurrence.
- If there is a history of rheumatic fever, congenital valve disorders, or prosthetic valve replacements, see a primary provider if fever, malaise, or other symptoms of infection occur.
- There may be a need for antibiotics just before, and for a short time after, an event that might cause bacteremia, such as dental surgery.
- If an antibiotic is prescribed, take the full dose for the full-time because noncompliance with the drug regimen can hinder the complete destruction of the pathogen.

are coxsackie viruses A and B, influenza A and B viruses, measles, adenovirus, mumps, rubella, rubeola, Epstein–Barr virus, cytomegalovirus, and COVID-19 (webmd.com). The myocardium also can become inflamed from the toxins of microorganisms, chronic alcohol and cocaine abuse, radiation therapy, or autoimmune disorders. Clients with bulimia who use syrup of ipecac to facilitate purging can develop myocardial damage similar to viral myocarditis.

Whatever the damaging agent, an inflammatory response causes the cardiac muscle tissue to swell, which interferes with the myocardium's ability to stretch and recoil. Cardiac output is reduced and blood circulation is impaired, predisposing the client to heart failure (see Chapter 28). The myocardium becomes ischemic from a reduced supply of oxygenated blood, creating a potential for tachycardia and arrhythmias. Cardiomyopathy, evidenced as atypical changes in the myocardial wall, may develop as a complication of myocarditis and other disorders.

Assessment Findings

Signs and Symptoms

Clients may complain of sharp stabbing or squeezing chest discomfort that resembles a myocardial infarction (MI); however, sitting up relieves the pain. Accompanying manifestations include a low-grade fever, tachycardia, arrhythmias, dyspnea, malaise, fatigue, and anorexia. The skin may be pale or cyanotic. If the heart's pumping activity becomes impaired, neck vein distention, ascites, and peripheral edema may be noted, indicating right-sided heart failure. Crackles may be heard in the lungs if the left side fails. An S_3 galloping rhythm or a pericardial friction rub may be heard.

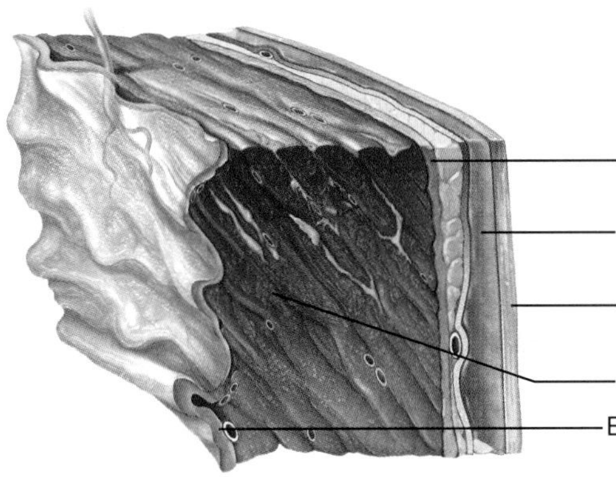

Figure 23-5 Tissue changes in myocarditis.

Diagnostic Findings

Serum electrolyte levels and thyroid function studies help rule out other causes for the client's symptoms. The WBC count is slightly elevated. C-reactive protein, a nonspecific antigen–antibody test, is elevated in inflammatory conditions. Cardiac isoenzyme levels are elevated, and ECG results may be abnormal. Chest radiography shows overall heart enlargement and fluid infiltration in the lungs. Echocardiography demonstrates structural and functional abnormalities in the ventricles, such as impaired motion of the ventricular wall and reduced ejection of blood from the heart. Radionuclide studies reveal areas where the myocardial wall is enlarged, thickened, or scarred. A myocardial biopsy may be done to obtain a definitive diagnosis.

Medical and Surgical Management

Management aims at treating the underlying cause and preventing complications. Antibiotics are prescribed if the infecting microorganism is bacterial. Bed rest, a sodium-restricted diet, and cardiotonic drugs (digitalis and related drugs) are prescribed to prevent or treat heart failure. In severe cases of cardiomyopathy, a heart transplant is necessary.

Nursing Management

The nurse monitors the client's cardiopulmonary status to assess for possible complications such as heart failure or arrhythmias. Assessments include vital signs, daily weights, intake and output, heart and lung sounds, pulse oximetry measurements, and determining the presence of dependent edema. The nurse also maintains the client on bed rest to reduce cardiac workload and promote healing. If the client has a fever, the nurse administers a prescribed antipyretic along with independent nursing measures, such as minimizing layers of bed linens, promoting air circulation and evaporation of perspiration, and offering oral fluids. Administering supplemental oxygen relieves tachycardia that may develop from hypoxemia. The nurse elevates the client's head to promote maximal breathing potential and uses a bedside cardiac monitor or telemetry unit to assess heart rhythm (see Chapter 26). The nurse uses cardiac rhythm analyses to determine whether and when antiarrhythmic medications are necessary or the client's response to their use.

Cardiomyopathy

Cardiomyopathy is a chronic condition characterized by structural changes in the heart muscle. The three major types of cardiomyopathies are (1) dilated cardiomyopathy, (2) hypertrophic cardiomyopathy, and (3) restrictive cardiomyopathy (Table 23-2; Fig. 23-6). The International Society and Federation of Cardiology and the World Health Organization added two other types of cardiomyopathy to the list: arrhythmogenic right ventricular cardiomyopathy, which is inherited, and peripartum cardiomyopathy, which develops in women shortly before or after giving birth (Porth, 2014). The following discussion focuses on dilated, hypertrophic, and restrictive cardiomyopathies.

TABLE 23-2 Types of Cardiomyopathy

TYPE	CAUSES	DESCRIPTION	TREATMENT
Dilated	Viral myocarditis Autoimmune response Chemicals (e.g., chronic alcohol ingestion)	The cavity of the heart is stretched (dilated).	Drug therapy to minimize symptoms and prevent complications Abstinence from alcohol Salt restriction Weight loss Possible heart transplantation
Hypertrophic	Hereditary Unknown	The muscle of the left ventricle and septum thickens, causing heart enlargement.	Drug therapy to reduce heart rate and force of contraction Antiarrhythmic drugs Artificial pacemaker Alcohol ablation: injection of alcohol into an artery supplying the extra tissue to destroy excess heart muscle (currently experimental) Ventriculomyotomy, a surgical procedure to reduce muscle tissue
Restrictive	Deposits of amyloid scleroderma, a connective tissue disorder Granulomatous tumors Hemochromatosis, iron stores in tissue Scar tissue that forms after a myocardial infarction	Heart muscle stiffens, which interferes with its ability to stretch and fill with blood.	No specific treatment; drugs such as diuretics and antihypertensives used to control symptoms

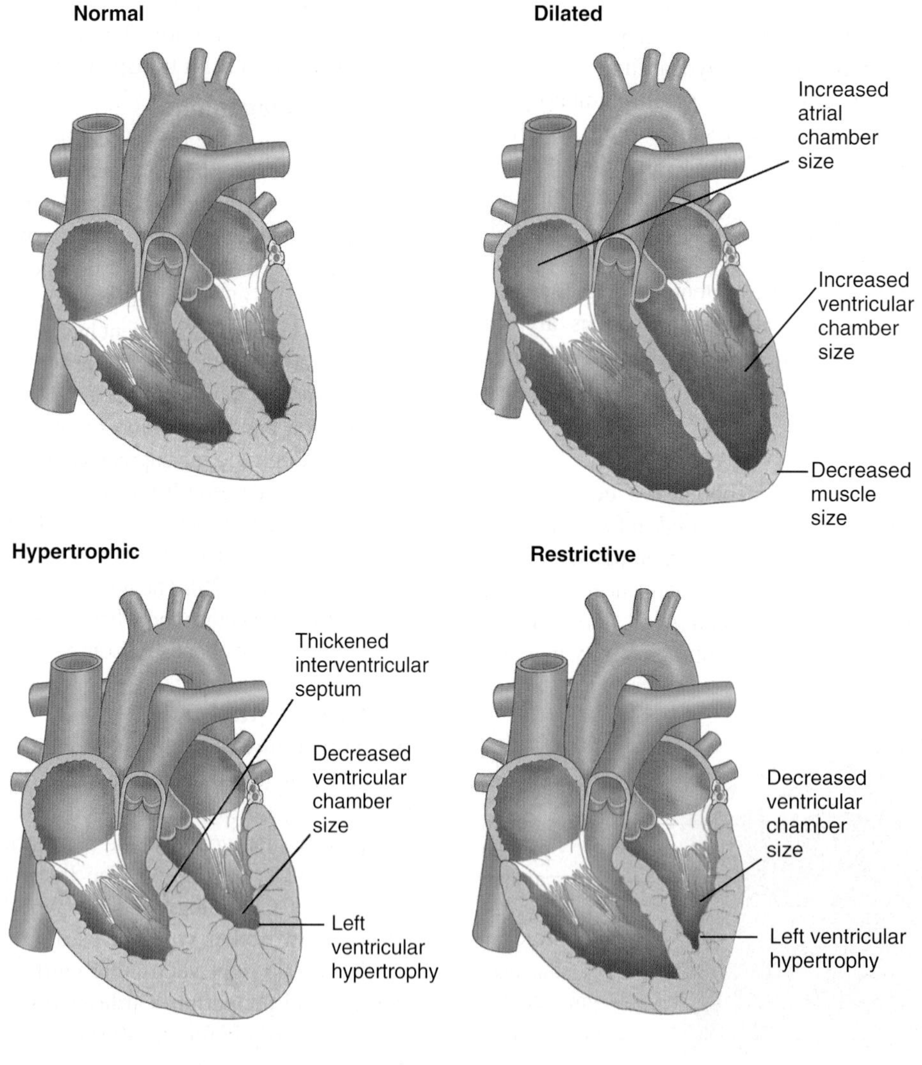

Figure 23-6 Types of cardiomyopathies: dilated, hypertrophic, and restrictive.

Pathophysiology and Etiology

In some cases, cardiomyopathy develops without explanation. In others, cardiomyopathy accompanies or follows another medical problem, such as myocarditis, connective tissue disorders such as systemic lupus erythematosus, muscular dystrophy, chronic alcoholism, or cancer chemotherapy.

Regardless of the cause, the heart muscle loses its ability to pump blood efficiently. When a client's medical history includes disorders that are bacterial or viral in origin, a family history of early cardiac deaths, or any of several other conditions that correlate with heart involvement, the possibility of cardiomyopathy is considered. Some affected clients remain in stable condition for a long period before they develop disabling symptoms; others may be unaware of their condition until they experience a potentially fatal cardiac event such as a sudden dysrhythmia or heart failure.

Assessment Findings

Signs and Symptoms

The manifestations of cardiomyopathy vary slightly according to the type that develops. *Dilated cardiomyopathy*, the most common type, is accompanied by dyspnea on exertion and when lying down. The client experiences fatigue and leg swelling and may also have palpitations and chest pain.

Hypertrophic cardiomyopathy is associated with **syncope** (sudden loss of consciousness, "fainting") or near-syncope episodes, which the client may describe as "graying out." Clients may also feel fatigued, become short of breath, and develop chest pain. Many are asymptomatic, however; and the disorder is not discovered until the affected person becomes acutely ill after strenuous exercise or dies.

Restrictive cardiomyopathy, which is the least common type in the United States but more common in tropical locales of Africa, India, South and Central America, and Asia, has symptoms of exertional dyspnea, dependent edema in the legs, ascites (fluid in the abdomen), and hepatomegaly (enlarged liver).

A heart **murmur**, which is an atypical heart sound, may be the first abnormal sign detected in any type. Forceful heart contractions may be palpated over the left chest wall.

Diagnostic Findings

Cardiomyopathy sometimes is detected among asymptomatic clients during other diagnostic tests. For example, chest radiography may show heart enlargement. An exercise, chemical, or ambulatory echocardiography provides evidence of abnormal cardiac rhythm. Definitive diagnosis is determined by performing an echocardiogram, cardiac magnetic resonance imaging (MRI), and cardiac catheterization. Cardiac catheterization detects elevated pressures in the ventricles of the heart. In some cases, an endomyocardial biopsy is performed to obtain a specimen of heart tissue for microscopic examination. The biopsy may reveal **myocardial disarray** (Fig. 23-7), an alteration in the usual alignment of **myofibrils**, the contractile component of muscle tissue. The result is a lack of coordination during systole (ventricular contraction) and impaired diastole (ventricular relaxation; Porth, 2014). Radionuclide studies show the heart muscle's inability to contract efficiently when stressed during exercise.

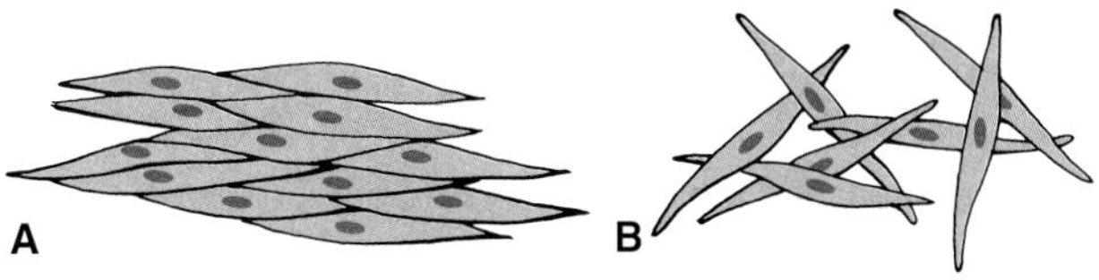

Figure 23-7 (A) Normal muscle structure. **(B)** Myocardial disarray.

Medical and Surgical Management

Treatment depends on the type of cardiomyopathy (see Table 23-2). In general, diuretics, cardiac glycosides such as digitalis, and antihypertensives are prescribed to promote effective heart contraction and adequate cardiac output. Antiarrhythmics are used to manage abnormally conducted heart impulses. Anticoagulants are administered to prevent the formation of blood clots that may develop when blood pools in the heart chambers. Anti-inflammatory agents such as corticosteroids are used in select clients to control cardiomyopathy caused by autoimmune connective tissue disorders. Dietary sodium is restricted to reduce fluid retention.

Drug therapy sometimes is accompanied by placement of an artificial pacemaker or implanted automatic defibrillator (see Chapter 26). Clients with hypertrophic cardiomyopathy may experience relief of symptoms when a **ventriculomyomectomy**, removal of thickened myocardial muscle from the septum, is performed. This surgical procedure enlarges the left ventricular chamber and allows a greater ejection of blood with each heart contraction. The mitral valve also may be replaced at the same time as the ventriculomyomectomy to correct the leakage of blood from the left atrium into the left ventricle (see Chapter 24). When there are no other alternatives for supporting the heart's pumping function, the client may become a candidate for an implanted left ventricular assist device (LVAD), artificial heart, or heart transplantation (see Chapter 29).

Nursing Management

The nurse obtains a comprehensive medical and family history and asks the client to describe any symptoms. Outpatients may be attached to an ambulatory cardiac monitor; nurses teach such clients to keep a journal of their symptoms. The nurse performs a physical examination that includes taking vital signs, auscultating heart and lung sounds, and checking for peripheral edema and abdominal enlargement. They are especially alert for an irregular pulse, tachycardia, or reduced levels of oxygen saturation (SpO_2) on pulse oximetry, which may occur during postural changes or exercise. The nurse advocates for cardiac monitoring either at the bedside or by telemetry.

Oxygen is administered either continuously or when dyspnea or arrhythmias develop. The nurse administers prescribed medications and collects data to evaluate their effectiveness. For example, if the client receives a diuretic, the nurse monitors intake and output, assesses weight, and checks for dependent edema regularly. The nurse ensures that the client's activity level is reduced and sequences any activity that is slightly exertional between periods of rest.

The nurse supports the client emotionally as they cope with a chronic, perhaps life-threatening illness. The nurse helps the client identify realistic limitations yet avoid

Client and Family Teaching 23-2 Cardiomyopathy

The nurse teaches the client with cardiomyopathy as follows:

- Achieve a healthy weight by following dietary instructions, limiting sodium to reduce fluid retention, and avoiding beverages containing caffeine, which contributes to tachycardia.
- Stop using tobacco products because nicotine is a vasoconstrictor and cardiac stimulant.
- Stay within your level of exercise tolerance or stop activity immediately if dyspnea or chest pain develops.
- Restrict driving or operating equipment if syncope is a common symptom.
- Keep appointments for medical follow-up to evaluate the status of the disease and symptom control.
- Receive the pneumonia vaccine and yearly influenza vaccinations to avoid pulmonary complications that may compromise cardiopulmonary function.
- For female clients, seek co-consultation with a cardiologist and an obstetrician if pregnancy is desired.

becoming a self-restricted invalid as a consequence of fear. Depending on the type of cardiomyopathy, the nurse may encourage family members to undergo diagnostic testing to determine whether they also have the same disorder. Client and Family Teaching 23-2 outlines teaching plan components.

Pericarditis

Pericarditis is an inflammation of the pericardium (Fig. 23-8). It can be a primary condition (developing independently of any other condition) or a secondary condition (developing because of another condition). The inflammation can occur with or without **effusion**, the accumulation of fluid between two layers of tissue.

Pathophysiology and Etiology

Pericarditis is usually secondary to endocarditis, myocarditis, chest trauma, or MI (heart attack) or develops after cardiac surgery. Other contributing causes include tuberculosis, malignant tumors, uremia, and connective tissue disorders. When the pericardial cells become inflamed, their membranes become more permeable and intracellular fluid leaks into the interstitial spaces. The exudate or effusion can be serous, resembling clear serum; fibrinous, like thick, congealed liquid; purulent, containing pus; or sanguineous, containing blood.

Pericardial fluid accumulation results in **cardiac tamponade**, acute compression of the heart. The pericardial fluid occupies space the heart needs to accommodate filling with blood. The impaired filling is reflected by a condition called *pulsus paradoxus* or *paradoxical pulse*. **Pulsus paradoxus** is a difference of 10 mm Hg or more between the first Korotkoff sound heralding systolic blood pressure (BP) heard during expiration and the first that is heard during inspiration. Normally, the difference between the two is 4 to 5 mm Hg. The technique for detecting pulsus paradoxus is described in Nursing Guidelines 23-1. Pulsus paradoxus develops because of a greater reduction in the volume capacity of the left ventricle during inspiration combined with an impaired ability of the left ventricle to expand because of the rigid pericardium. The smaller capacity reduces the stroke volume from the left ventricle. As cardiac tamponade progresses, stroke volume is diminished, cardiac output is compromised, and death may result if the condition continues uncorrected.

Assessment Findings

Signs and Symptoms

The typical signs and symptoms that accompany an inflammatory response, such as fever and malaise, are present. The client is dyspneic or complains of heaviness in the chest. One chief characteristic is **precordial pain** (pain in the anterior chest overlying the heart). It may be slight or severe and can be mistaken for esophagitis, indigestion, pleurisy, or MI. Moving and breathing deeply worsen the pain; sitting upright and leaning forward relieve it. In contrast, the pain of acute MI remains unchanged, regardless of position, movement, or breathing. A pericardial friction rub, a scratchy, high-pitched sound, is a diagnostic sign. Heart sounds are difficult to hear because the accumulating fluid muffles them. Respiratory symptoms occur as the enlarged heart crowds the airway passages and lung tissue and respirations become rapid and labored. Hypotension is severe, and pulse quality is weak.

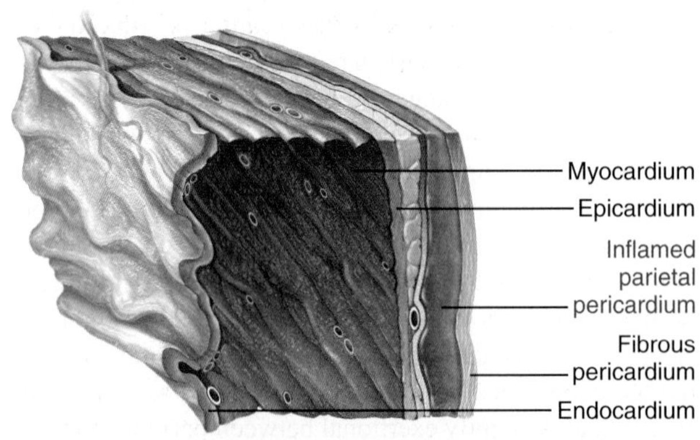

Figure 23-8 Tissue changes in pericarditis. Normally, the epicardium and pericardium slide over each other easily because they are lubricated by a small amount of fluid. Thicker material replaces this fluid in pericarditis.

NURSING GUIDELINES 23-1

Assessment of Pulsus Paradoxus

- Advise client to breathe normally throughout the assessment.
- Inflate BP cuff 20 mm Hg above systolic pressure.
- Deflate the cuff slowly, noting that sounds are audible during expiration, but not during inspiration.
- Note when the first BP sound (Korotkoff) is heard.
- Continue to deflate the cuff until BP sounds are heard during both inspiration and expiration.
- Measure the difference in millimeters of mercury between the first BP sound heard during expiration and the first BP sound heard during both inspiration and expiration.

Diagnostic Findings

The ST segment of the ECG is elevated, but cardiac isoenzyme levels are normal (see Chapter 25). The heart may appear enlarged on chest radiography. Echocardiography demonstrates a wide gap between the pericardium and the epicardium, indicating that the space is filled with fluid. Hemodynamic monitoring values are abnormal (see Chapter 29). Pericardial fluid may be cultured, but if the cause of the pericarditis is nonbacterial, the test results are often nondiagnostic. Because of the inflammatory nature of pericarditis, the WBC count and ESR are often elevated.

Medical and Surgical Management

An MI (see Chapter 25) must be ruled out. Treatment of pericarditis depends on the underlying cause. Rest, analgesics, antipyretics, nonsteroidal anti-inflammatory drugs (NSAIDs), and sometimes corticosteroids are prescribed. **Pericardiocentesis**, needle aspiration of fluid from between the visceral and parietal pericardium, may be necessary when cardiac output is severely reduced (Fig. 23-9). A small drainage catheter can be left in place. Needle aspiration is hazardous because the needle can puncture the myocardium, a branch of a coronary artery, or the pleura.

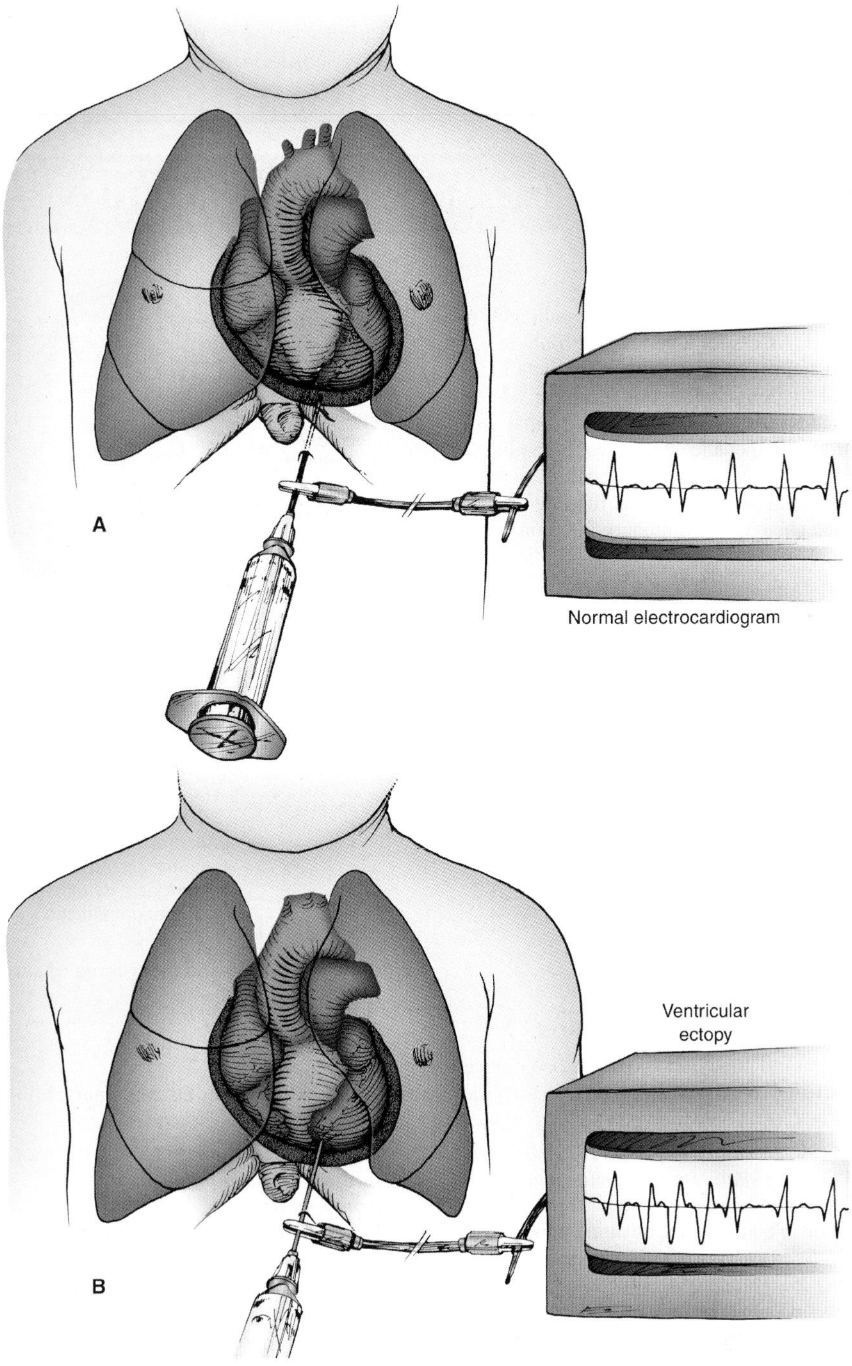

Figure 23-9 Pericardiocentesis, with syringe and needle to which ECG has been attached. **(A)** Normal electrocardiogram. **(B)** Ventricular ectopy. (Reprinted with permission from Bachur, R. G., Shaw, K. N., Chamberlain, J., Lavelle, J., Nagler, J., & Shook, J. E. (2021). *Fleisher & Ludwig's textbook of pediatric emergency medicine* (8th ed.). Wolters Kluwer. Figure 130.26.)

When pericardiocentesis and catheter drainage are inadequate, a **pericardiostomy**, a surgical opening or window, is made in the pericardium to allow the fluid to drain. Surgical treatment for constrictive pericarditis involves removing the pericardium (**pericardiectomy**) or removing the surface layer of the pericardium (**decortication**) to allow more adequate filling and contraction of the heart chambers.

››› *Stop, Think, and Respond 23-3*

While caring for a client with pericarditis, you measure the client's BP and hear the first Korotkoff sound during expiration at 110 mm Hg. The sounds continue throughout auscultation, and you note that when the manometer is at 98 mm Hg, you hear sounds during both inspiration and expiration. Is this client manifesting pulsus paradoxus?

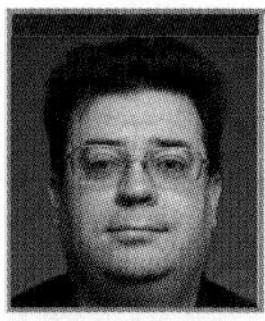

Clinical Scenario A client comes to the emergency department with nonradiating chest pain that is aggravated by breathing deeply and lying down. Vital signs are essentially normal; however, the BP is in the lower ranges of normal. There is no history of cardiovascular risk factors or disease. Lung sounds are clear in all lobes, but there is a grating friction rub detected when auscultating heart sounds. **The client is admitted for diagnostic and treatment purposes. How would you manage the care of this client? See the following Nursing Process section.**

NURSING PROCESS FOR THE CLIENT WITH PERICARDITIS

Assessment

Ask the client about the incidence and nature of the pain and what worsens or relieves it. Assess for a pericardial friction rub by auscultating heart sounds while the client briefly holds their breath; a pericardial friction rub does not disappear when the breath is held. Note additional signs and symptoms that may further suggest cardiac tamponade and decreased cardiac output, such as muffled heart sounds, pulsus paradoxus, jugular neck vein distention, persistent cough, dyspnea, fainting or near fainting, anxiety, and changes in pulmonary function (Fig. 23-10).

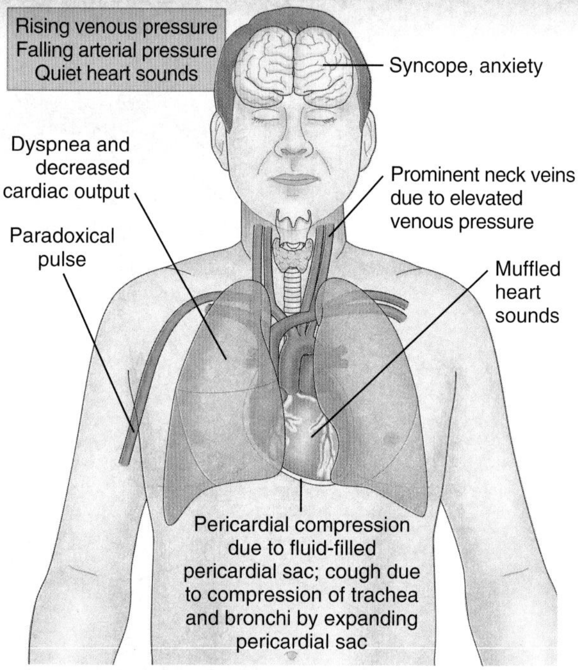

Figure 23-10 Signs and symptoms of cardiac tamponade.

Diagnosis, Planning, and Interventions

Pain: Related to pericardial inflammation and decreased myocardial perfusion
Expected Outcomes: Client will be free of pain or pain will be tolerable 30 minutes after nursing intervention.

- Assess pain status as often as vital signs. *Pain is considered the fifth vital sign. Whenever pain exists, the nurse must implement interventions targeted for its relief.*
- Assist client to a position of comfort such as sitting upright and leaning forward. *Only the outer layer of the lower parietal pericardium is sensitive to pain (Porth, 2014); some of the pain of pericarditis results from inflammation of the surrounding structures. Sitting up and leaning forward positions the stretched pericardium away from the pleura, which relieves discomfort.*
- Administer anti-inflammatory drugs and analgesics as prescribed. *Reduced inflammation and pain transmission promote comfort.*
- Reassure the client that pericardial pain does not indicate an MI. *Anxiety increases heart rate and force of heart contraction, which contribute to pain. Clarifying the reality and significance of the pain may reduce the workload of the heart and acuity of discomfort.*

NURSING PROCESS FOR THE CLIENT WITH PERICARDITIS (continued)

Decreased Cardiac Output: Related to inability of the heart muscle to stretch completely, fill with appropriate amount of blood, and eject a sufficient volume during ventricular systole
Expected Outcomes: Client will (1) maintain normal arterial BP, (2) remain alert, (3) be free of chest pain, and (4) eliminate at least 35 mL of urine per hour.

- Monitor vital signs every 4 hours and as needed. *Hypotension and tachycardia are signs of decreased cardiac output.*
- Measure urine output every hour unless output is greater than 35 mL/hour. *The kidneys cannot form urine when the renal arterial blood supply is reduced secondary to decreased cardiac output. An output of at least 35 mL/hour is necessary to eliminate nitrogen wastes and other toxic substances.*
- Monitor for cardiac arrhythmias. *Hypoxemia is a leading cause of arrhythmias. Inadequate cardiac output creates a potential for myocardial ischemia and disturbances in electrical conduction.*
- Assess orientation. *Confusion and disorientation are signs of compromised cerebral arterial blood flow secondary to decreased cardiac output.*
- Instruct the client to report chest pain. *It is a consequence of inadequate blood supply to the myocardium.*
- Maintain bed rest. *Activity increases the demand for myocardial oxygenation, which depends on cardiac output.*
- Administer supplemental oxygen as prescribed. *Giving more than the 20% oxygen that is present in room air helps to reduce hypoxemia that results from inadequate cardiac output.*
- Provide six small meals a day; avoid gas-forming foods. *Abdominal distention crowds the thoracic cavity and compresses the space the heart needs to fill with blood and the lungs need to fill with air.*
- Restrict caffeine and sodium. *Caffeine increases heart rate and sodium increases circulating blood volume, both of which increase myocardial work and the need for cardiac output.*
- Collaborate with the primary provider regarding a stool softener. *Bearing down during bowel movements interferes with cardiac filling and output. Stool softeners promote ease of eliminating stool.*
- Administer prescribed medications such as sedatives, anxiolytics, vasodilators, diuretics, and antiarrhythmics. *Reducing anxiety, keeping the client calm and quiet, reducing BP and volume, and facilitating normal heart conduction help avoid exceeding the heart's ability to eject an adequate cardiac output.*

RC of Cardiac Tamponade

Expected Outcome: The nurse will monitor for, manage, and minimize cardiac tamponade if it develops.

- Monitor for tachycardia, pulsus paradoxus, neck vein distention, cough, syncope, and muffled heart sounds every 4 hours and as needed. *This cluster of signs and symptoms accompanies cardiac tamponade, which interferes with filling volumes. Blood that cannot enter the heart accumulates in both venous and pulmonary circulation.*
- Have an emergency pericardiocentesis tray available. *Removing fluid from between the parietal and visceral pericardium relieves cardiac tamponade.*
- Reinforce the primary provider's explanation of a pericardiocentesis and witness the client's signature on a consent form. *Pericardiocentesis is an invasive procedure that requires informed consent from the client if they are alert or from whomever has durable power of attorney for health care.*
- Obtain baseline vital signs before pericardiocentesis. *They are used for comparison during and after the pericardiocentesis.*
- Measure, describe, and record the amount of pericardial fluid removed. *Documentation is a record of the client's care and outcomes of treatment.*
- Label all specimens for laboratory analysis and send them promptly to the laboratory. *Accurate information and prompt delivery facilitate diagnosis and appropriate treatment.*
- Cover the site of the pericardiocentesis with a sterile dressing and inspect the dressing for bleeding or leaking fluid. *Compromising the skin and underlying tissue creates a potential for blood and fluid loss as well as an entry site for microorganisms.*
- Reinforce the dressing if it becomes moist. *Moist gauze acts as a wick and pulls microorganisms from the skin surface toward the puncture wound and deeper tissue.*
- Continue to monitor vital signs until they are stable. *Continued assessments help identify complications so they can be treated early or validate a favorable response to therapy.*

Evaluation of Expected Outcomes

The client states pain is relieved. Vital signs are stable, and cardiac rhythm is normal. The client is alert and oriented. Urine output exceeds 35 mL/hour. Cardiac tamponade is managed.

INFLAMMATORY DISORDERS OF THE PERIPHERAL BLOOD VESSELS

Thrombophlebitis

Thrombophlebitis is an inflammation of a vein accompanied by clot or thrombus formation. Although clots can form in any blood vessel, the veins deep in the lower extremities are most commonly affected. In such cases, the condition is referred to as **deep vein thrombosis** (DVT). Thrombi that form in or above the popliteal vein of the leg are at high risk for migration toward the pulmonary circulation; these cases are referred to as a **pulmonary embolus** (PE).

Pathophysiology and Etiology

When the inner lining of a vein is irritated or injured, platelets clump together, forming a clot (Fig. 23-11). The clot interferes with blood flow, causing congestion of venous blood distal to the blood clot. Sometimes, collateral vessels recirculate the blood blocked by the clot. Accumulated waste products in the blocked vessel irritate the vein wall, initiating an inflammatory response. The increased permeability of cells and the convergence of leukocytes and lymphocytes cause the area to swell, redden, and feel warm and tender.

Pharmacologic Considerations

- Medications that can irritate vessels are called *vesicants*. Ask the clinical pharmacologist whether the drug is a vesicant infusion whenever you are about to inject a drug if you are not familiar with its properties.

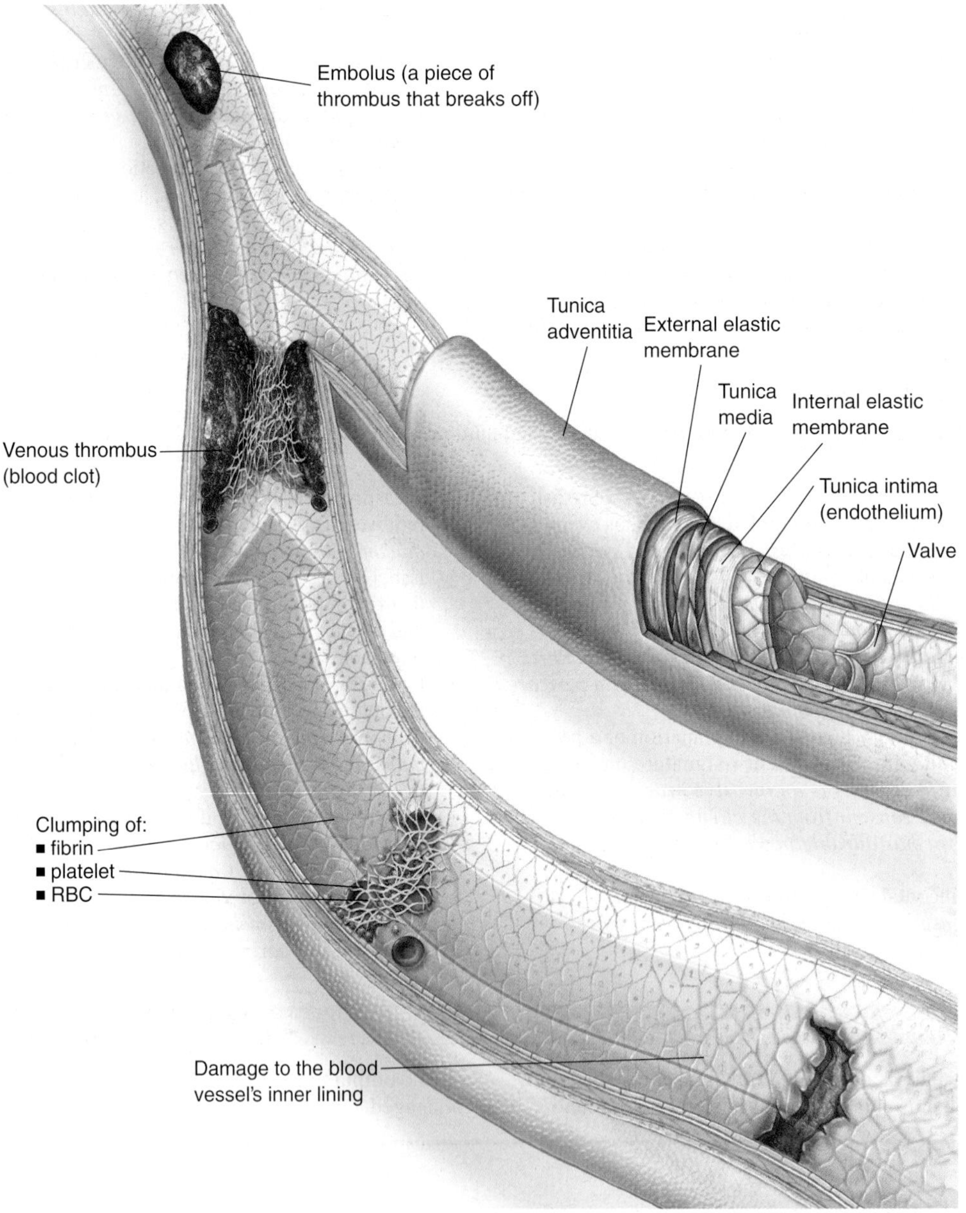

Figure 23-11 Deep vein thrombosis with a clot that may be accompanied by an embolus. (Reprinted with permission from Lippincott Williams & Wilkins. (2010). *Cardiovascular care made incredibly visual!* (2nd ed.). Wolters Kluwer Health/Lippincott Williams & Wilkins.)

The development of a PE may complicate thrombophlebitis if the clot in the extremity becomes mobile and moves in the venous circulation to the lungs (see Chapter 21). Despite appropriate and successful treatment of thrombophlebitis, some clients experience a vascular complication referred to as **postphlebitic syndrome** for up to 5 years after the initial episode. For example, valvular impairment in the affected vein may follow the original thrombotic event. The incompetent valves are less efficient at returning venous blood to the heart. When venous pressure increases because of pooled blood, some fluid leaks from capillaries into subcutaneous tissue, causing leg ulcers.

Venous stasis (slowed circulation), altered blood coagulation, and trauma to the vein, referred to as **Virchow triad**, predispose clients to thrombosis and thrombophlebitis. Factors that contribute to clot formation include inactivity, reduced cardiac output, compression of the veins in the pelvis or legs, and injury. Some IV drugs and chemicals also irritate the vein. Thrombi are prone to form in arm, subclavian, or jugular veins cannulated for extended IV use. Older adults with heart and blood vessel disease are susceptible to thrombophlebitis because of impaired mobility, reduced activity, and compromised circulation. Risk for clot formation is increased among women who take oral contraceptives, although the exact trigger is not known. Women who take oral contraceptives and smoke are at even higher risk.

Assessment Findings

Signs and Symptoms

Clients with thrombophlebitis often complain of discomfort such as calf pain in the affected extremity. Heat, redness, and swelling develop along the length of the affected vein. Capillary refill takes less than 2 seconds because of venous congestion. The client often has a fever, malaise, fatigue, and anorexia.

Diagnostic Tests

Most cases of thrombophlebitis are diagnosed according to clinical findings alone. Doppler ultrasound is a noninvasive diagnostic technique for imaging blood flow through cardiovascular structures that may detect an area of venous obstruction. The results of Doppler ultrasound sometimes are difficult to interpret because there are so many collateral vessels, and deep veins are especially difficult to assess.

Venography, using radiopaque dye instilled into the venous system, indicates a filling defect in the area of the clot. It is important to assess the client's allergy history prior to a venography because some are hypersensitive to the dye. Following a venography, the vein is flushed, and the client is instructed to drink extra fluids to promote dye excretion.

Impedance plethysmography (IPG) is the preferred test for diagnosing clots in deep veins. During IPG, a sensor records blood volume in the arm or leg before and after inflating a BP cuff to stop venous blood flow. If a clot is present, the blood volumes are nearly the same because the clot impairs venous return.

Medical and Surgical Management

Traditionally, clients with a thrombus in a lower extremity were placed on bed rest; the rationale being that restricting mobility would prevent the thrombus from breaking free and floating in the circulation (embolus). However, limiting movement can also contribute to the stasis of blood. More and more studies indicate that early ambulation may actually be beneficial when combined with compression bandaging and anticoagulant therapy (MayoClinic, 2021; Hematology Advisor, 2020; Evidence-Based Practice 23-1).

Anticoagulant therapy with heparin, oral anticoagulants, or drugs that prevent platelet aggregation (clustering) are prescribed to decrease the incidence of future clot formation (Drug Therapy Table 23-2). With the advent of low-molecular-weight heparins such as enoxaparin (Lovenox), some clients with thrombophlebitis in which the thrombi are small are not hospitalized but treated at home. People with repeated episodes may be placed on oral anticoagulant therapy for 3 to 6 months. Continuous warm, wet packs are ordered to improve circulation, ease pain, and decrease inflammation.

Evidence-Based Practice 23-1

Bed Rest Versus Early Ambulation for Deep Vein Thrombosis

Clinical Question

Is bed rest or early ambulation better in the management of DVT?

Evidence

DVT has been a concern for clients over centuries and also a concern of doctors and surgeons. Traditionally, the treatment for prevention was to put the client on complete bed rest. A recent study looked at bed rest compared to early ambulation for treatment. The authors did a meta-analysis that looked at 13 studies through literature focusing on pulmonary embolism, DVT and fatal complications related to DVT, and pain and swelling (Moore, 2020). The results concluded that there was not a higher incidence of complication with early ambulation over bed rest for treatment. However, the study did conclude that clients with early ambulation had a reduction in acute pain in the affected limb, which led to improved client outcomes.

Nursing Implications

Nurses can use results from their study to educate clients on DVT prevention and work with the health care team on the evidence-based approach to early ambulation to achieve better client outcomes.

Reference

Moore, V. (2020). *Deep vein thrombosis incidence and pulmonary embolism risk stratification.* https://www.hematologyadvisor.com/home/topics/thrombotic-disorders/dvt-incidendence-pulomany-embolism-risk-stratification/

DRUG THERAPY TABLE 23-2 Anticoagulants

Category and Common Generic (Brand) Drugs	Intended Use	Common Side Effects	Safety Warnings for Nurses
Parenteral Anticoagulants			
Heparin	Thrombosis/embolism, diagnosis and treatment of disseminated intravascular coagulation (DIC), prophylaxis of DVT, clotting prevention by blocking conversion of prothrombin/fibrinogen to form clots in vessels	Bleeding, chills, fever, urticaria, local irritation, erythema, mild pain, hematoma, or bruising at the injection site	Typical dose in thousand unit increments Monitor aPTT frequently to maintain blood level Monitor for bleeding of injection sites, orifices, wounds
Low-Molecular-Weight Heparins Enoxaparin (Lovenox) Dalteparin (Fragmin) Fondaparinux (Arixtra)	DVT and presurgical prophylaxis, PE treatment, unstable angina/non–Q-wave MI by inhibiting clot formation through clotting factors	Bleeding, bruising, rash, fever, erythema, and irritation at site of injection	Does not require frequent lab monitoring Nutrition teaching for foods to avoid with high vitamin K diet
Misc. Agents Desirudin (Iprivask)	DVT prophylaxis	Bleeding at subcutaneous injection site	Packaged in latex Monitor for bleeding of injection sites, orifices, wounds
Oral Anticoagulants			
Warfarin (Coumadin, Jantoven)	Prophylaxis/treatment of venous thrombosis by inhibiting vitamin K–dependent clotting factors	Bleeding, fatigue, dizziness, abdominal cramping	INR must be monitored at regular intervals Dietary vitamin K decrease blood levels
Misc. Agents Apixaban (Eliquis) Dabigatran (Pradaxa) Edoxaban (Savaysa) Rivaroxaban (Xarelto)	Stroke and embolism prevention nonvalve atrial fibrillation, after hip/knee replacement	Bleeding	Not for use if impaired creatinine clearance or hepatic issues Grapefruit will increase drug blood levels Thrombosis risk increases if drug therapy is stopped[b]
Antiplatelet Agents			
Salicylates Aspirin (Ecotrin, Ascriptin)	Stroke prevention in men (and women older than 65 years only) by inhibiting platelet aggregation and clotting	Nausea, vomiting, epigastric distress	Monitor for tinnitus, indicates toxicity Should not be taken as pain reliever when on anticoagulant therapy
Aggregate Inhibitors Clopidogrel (Plavix) Eptifibatide (Integrilin) Prasugrel (Effient) Ticagrelor (Brilinta) Vorapaxar (Zontivity)	Thrombus prevention in recent MI, stroke, and acute coronary syndrome by inhibiting platelet aggregation and clotting	Diarrhea, nausea, vomiting	Monitor for bleeding of injection sites, orifices, wounds

aPTT, activated partial thromboplastin time; DVT, deep vein thrombosis; INR, international normalized ratio.
The drugs in column 1 indicate the drug that matches up with explanations in columns 2 through 4.

Surgical intervention may be necessary when a clot occludes a large vein or the danger of a PE arises. **Thrombectomy**, the surgical removal of a clot, is performed if the clot interferes with venous drainage from a large vein, such as the femoral vein. With danger of PE, surgery on the inferior vena cava may be necessary to reduce the possibility of a clot traveling from the legs to the lungs. Several surgical procedures may be performed on the vena cava: ligation, insertion of a vena caval filter, or plication. A **vena caval filter** (Fig. 23-12) is an umbrella-like filter inserted to trap emboli before they reach the heart and lungs. A **vena caval plication** is a procedure that changes the lumen of the vena cava from a single channel to several small channels through the use of a

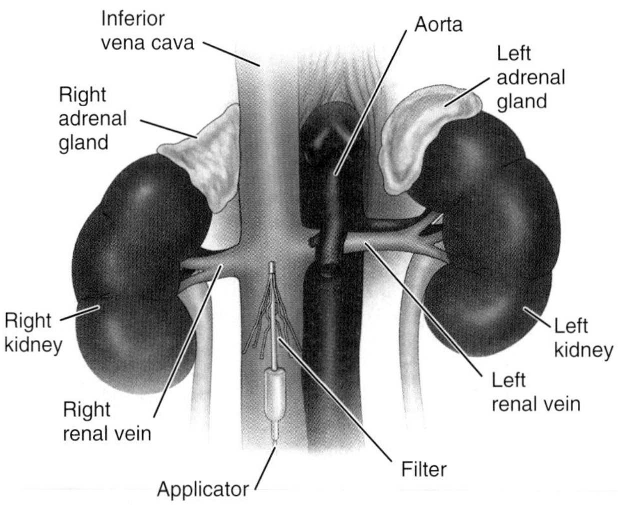

Figure 23-12 A permanently implanted vena caval filter is an umbrella-like filter that allows blood to circulate to the lungs but traps blood clots before they enter the pulmonary circulation. The filter is inserted with an applicator; the applicator is withdrawn when the filter fixes itself to the wall of the inferior vena cava.

suture or Teflon clip. Although vena caval filters are relatively safe and effective, migration and fracture of the filter can occur. When this complication develops, the freed fragment can advance into the right ventricular wall and diaphragm. Endovascular or open surgical extraction may be required.

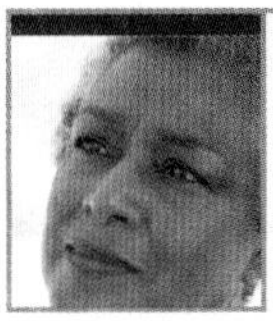

Clinical Scenario Three days after being discharged following an abdominal hysterectomy, the client calls her primary provider to report swelling in her left lower extremity accompanied by tenderness. The primary provider suspects the client has developed a thrombus with secondary inflammation of the vein and advises the client to go to the hospital for subsequent admission. What nursing assessments and nursing care are indicated? See the following Nursing Process section.

NURSING PROCESS FOR THE CLIENT WITH THROMBOPHLEBITIS

Assessment

Determine whether the client has a history of blood clots or other risk factors that predispose to thrombus formation, such as cardiovascular disorders or recent surgery, especially repair of a hip fracture or hip joint replacement; self-imposed inactivity as a result of obesity or sedentary lifestyle; immobility from a medical condition, pain, or treatment regimen; current use of an oral contraceptive; use of tobacco products; dehydration that may decrease the fluid volume of blood; or recent trauma to an extremity.

Assess if movement in the affected extremity causes or aggravates pain. Inspect the color, temperature, and capillary refill of extremities and measure the circumference of the leg (or arm) at various areas; compare the findings with the unaffected extremity (Fig. 23-13). Regularly check for a low-grade fever. Consult with the client about chest pain and dyspnea, which are hallmarks of PE, a complication of thrombophlebitis. If drug therapy is prescribed, monitor the laboratory test results associated with anticoagulant therapy.

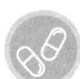

Pharmacologic Considerations

- Clients receiving warfarin for the first time often require daily adjustment of the dose, which is based on the daily prothrombin time (PT)/international normalized ratio (INR) results. If the PT exceeds 1.2 to 1.5 times the control value or the INR ratio exceeds 3, the primary health care provider is notified before the drug is given. A daily PT/INR is performed until it stabilizes and when any other drug is added to or removed from the client's drug regimen. After the INR has stabilized, it is monitored every 4 to 6 weeks.

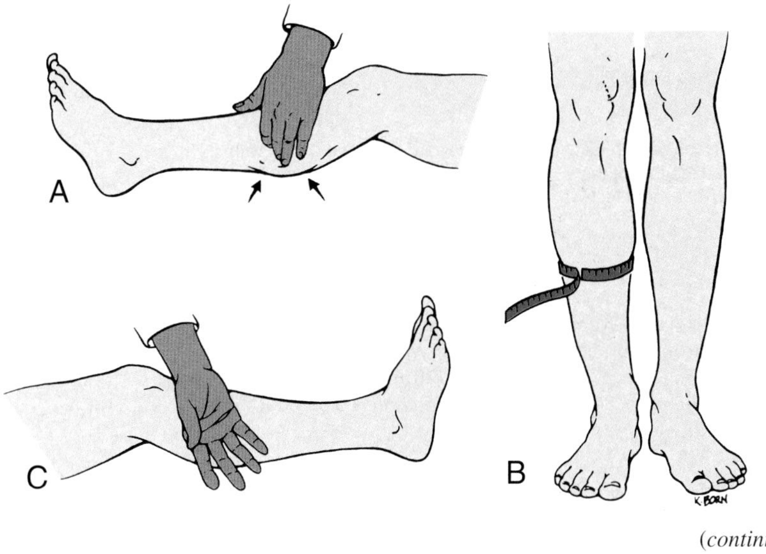

Figure 23-13 Nursing assessment for deep vein thrombosis includes checking for **(A)** pain and tenderness in the calf of the affected extremity, **(B)** larger calf circumference of the affected extremity caused by edema, and **(C)** greater localized warmth than on unaffected extremity.

(continued)

NURSING PROCESS FOR THE CLIENT WITH THROMBOPHLEBITIS (continued)

Diagnosis, Planning, and Interventions

An important role is to prevent venous stasis and thrombophlebitis by promoting activity and exercise for at-risk clients (Fig. 23-14). Ankle-pumping exercises are imperative for clients on bed rest. For inactive clients, apply knee- or thigh-high elastic stockings or use a pneumatic venous compression device that alternately inflates and deflates to support vein walls and promote venous circulation (Fig. 23-15). Assist the client to change positions frequently and avoid restricting venous blood flow from prolonged sitting or bending the bed at the knees (Client and Family Teaching 23-3).

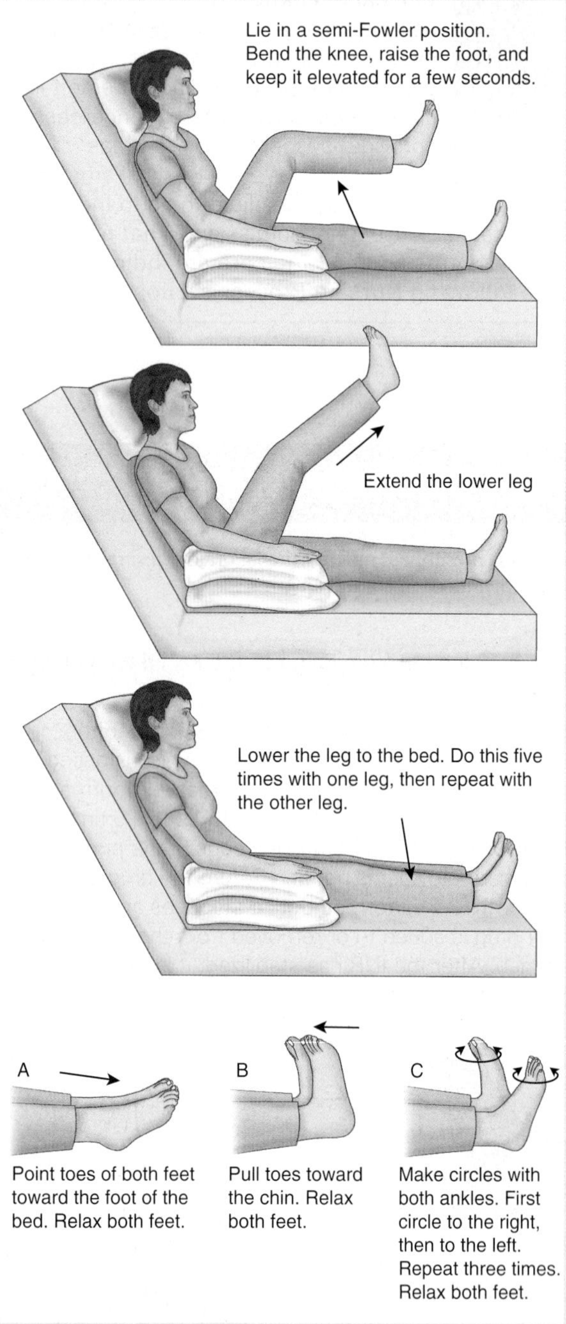
Lie in a semi-Fowler position.
Bend the knee, raise the foot, and keep it elevated for a few seconds.
Extend the lower leg
Lower the leg to the bed. Do this five times with one leg, then repeat with the other leg.
A
B
C
Point toes of both feet toward the foot of the bed. Relax both feet.
Pull toes toward the chin. Relax both feet.
Make circles with both ankles. First circle to the right, then to the left. Repeat three times. Relax both feet.

Figure 23-14 Leg exercises to increase venous return and prevent thrombophlebitis. (Reprinted with permission from Taylor, C. R., Lynn, P. & Bartlett, J. L. (2019). *Fundamentals of nursing: The art and science of person-centered care* (9th ed.). Wolters Kluwer.)

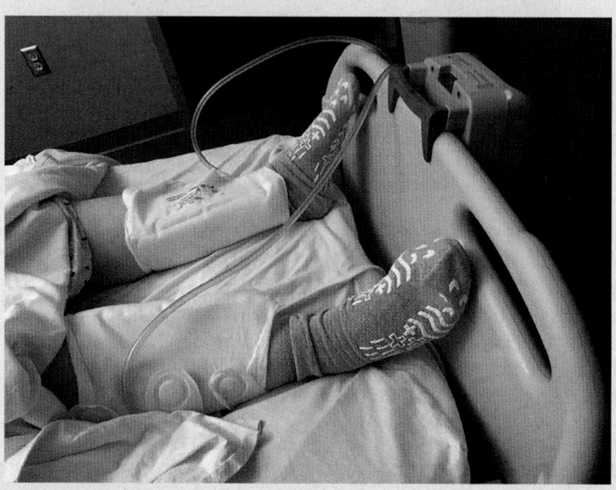

Figure 23-15 Pneumatic compression device. (shutterstock.com/Vogtguy)

Pharmacologic Considerations

- To prevent thrombus formation, an injectable anticoagulant, such as a low-molecular-weight heparin like dalteparin or fondaparinux as opposed to unfractionated heparin, is administered after some major surgical procedures. Low-molecular-weight heparins have several advantages: they can be given once a day; they do not require laboratory monitoring; and they facilitate home treatment following a hospital discharge. These medications support standard nursing postoperative care and are not a substitute for ambulation or other activities to promote venous circulation.

Client and Family Teaching 23-3 Thrombophlebitis

The nurse teaches clients with thrombophlebitis and their families the following:

- Take measures to prevent recurrences: avoid prolonged sitting and crossing the legs at the knee, perform active movement, elevate the legs periodically, wear support hose, and drink fluids liberally.
- Take long-term anticoagulant therapy exactly as prescribed.
- Keep appointments for the ordered laboratory tests to determine the effectiveness of therapy.
- Watch for and report signs that indicate impaired clotting: nosebleeds, bleeding gums, rectal bleeding, easy bruising, and prolonged oozing from minor cuts.

Additional nursing management includes the following:

Acute Pain: Related to venous inflammation

Expected Outcome: Discomfort will be relieved or reduced to a tolerable level.

NURSING PROCESS FOR THE CLIENT WITH THROMBOPHLEBITIS (continued)

- Administer prescribed nonnarcotic analgesics and anti-inflammatory agents. *Nonnarcotic agents inhibit prostaglandin, a chemical that sensitizes nerve receptors that transmit pain. Relief of inflammation interferes with the release of cellular chemicals that contribute to pain and localized swelling.*
- Support and handle the extremity gently. *Movement and muscle contraction increase pain.*

Ineffective Peripheral Tissue Perfusion: Related to localized swelling secondary to the inflammatory response and edema associated with third spacing
Expected Outcomes: Client's venous circulation will be adequate as evidenced by (1) reduced localized edema, (2) capillary refill less than 3 seconds in the toes of the affected extremity, and (3) skin color in affected extremity that is similar to that of the unaffected extremity.

- Instruct client to ambulate as soon and as much as possible; some suggest within 48 to 72 hours of having a DVT confirmed, and perform active leg exercises at least five times each waking hour. *Exercise prevents venous stasis by promoting venous circulation, relieves swelling, and reduces pain. Promoting venous blood flow prevents the formation of thrombi and subsequent potential for emboli in the unaffected extremity.*
- Apply an elastic compression bandage or stocking from the foot to the thigh; remove for 20 minutes and reapply twice a day or whenever it becomes loose. *Pressure from compression promotes the movement of fluid trapped in the interstitial space to vascular and lymphatic circulation, thus reducing lower extremity edema.*
- Elevate the affected extremity 20 degrees or more in a straight plane on pillows (do not bend the knees). *Elevation relieves swelling by promoting venous circulation; bending the knees interferes with venous circulation and may increase the size of the existing clot or contribute to the formation of additional thrombi.*
- Apply warm, moist compresses to the area of discomfort or apply an aquathermia pad over protected skin at a setting of approximately 105 °F (40.5 °C). Remove compresses and reapply after 20 minutes or sooner if cooling occurs. Remove the aquathermia pad every 2 hours for 20 minutes to assess the skin. *Warmth dilates blood vessels, improves circulation, and relieves swelling, all of which relieve discomfort. Moist heat is more comforting than dry heat. Skin assessments are standard care to avoid injury.*
- Promote a liberal intake (2000 to 2500 mL/24 hours) of oral fluid unless contraindicated. *Adequate fluid volume dilutes blood cells in plasma and reduces the risk for platelet aggregation.*

RC of Pulmonary Embolus

Expected Outcome: The nurse monitors for, manages, and minimizes complications such as a PE.

- Administer prescribed anticoagulant therapy. *Depending on the prescribed drugs, medications that alter clotting factors or interfere with platelet aggregation prevent additional thrombi and subsequent emboli.*
- Monitor for dyspnea, tachypnea, cough, hypotension, abnormal lung sounds, or chest pain. *Abnormal results of focus assessments indicate cardiopulmonary complications such as a PE.*
- Elevate the head if dyspnea develops. *Head elevation lowers abdominal organs away from the diaphragm and facilitates increased inspiration of higher lung volumes to compensate for impaired oxygenation in the pulmonary circulation.*
- Prepare to administer oxygen by cannula or mask if dyspnea and chest pain occur. *Raising oxygen levels above 20% compensates for impaired oxygenation at the alveolar-capillary level.*
- Prepare to start an IV and administer prescribed parenteral narcotic analgesia and emergency medications by the IV route. *Drug therapy helps relieve severe chest pain and improve BP.*

RC of Bleeding

Expected Outcome: The nurse monitors for, manages, and minimizes blood loss.

- Monitor laboratory test findings that reflect coagulation status such as partial thromboplastin time (PTT), PT, and INR; report values that exceed therapeutic levels. *With the exception of low-molecular-weight heparin, doses of anticoagulant drug therapy are adjusted according to laboratory test results.*
- Calculate dosages of anticoagulants carefully and administer drug therapy as prescribed. *Unfractionated heparin may be administered by IV infusion; the dose is often titrated according to PTT and may require periodic rate adjustments during the infusion. Oral and subcutaneous dosages of anticoagulants (except low-molecular-weight heparin) may be changed daily.*
- Keep antidotes for overdose of anticoagulants (protamine sulfate for unfractionated heparin and vitamin K [phytonadione, AquaMEPHYTON] for warfarin) available. *In extreme cases, it may be prudent to quickly reverse the effects of anticoagulant therapy.*
- Observe the client for blood in the urine or stool, easy bruising, bleeding gums, and excessive bleeding from minor cuts or scratches. *These findings are signs of impaired clotting and suggest that the client could easily bleed internally.*
- Provide the client with a soft-bristled toothbrush for oral hygiene; advise using an electric razor for shaving. *Reducing the potential for skin and soft-tissue trauma decreases the possibility of bleeding.*

(continued)

NURSING PROCESS FOR THE CLIENT WITH THROMBOPHLEBITIS (continued)

- Test stools, emesis, urine, and nasogastric drainage for blood. *Hemoccult testing may detect blood that is not obvious to the naked eye.*
- Protect the client from falls or other trauma. *An injury, even though ordinarily minor, may precipitate excessive or prolonged bleeding if the client is receiving anticoagulant therapy.*
- Perform neurologic assessments every 1 to 2 hours if the client experiences a head injury (see Chapters 36 and 39). *Changes in the level of consciousness, size and response of pupils to light, and verbal responses suggest intracranial bleeding.*
- Apply direct pressure to the site of external bleeding. *Pressure compresses vascular walls and decreases blood flow, providing time for an initial clot to form.*
- Place an ice pack at the site of prolonged oozing of blood. *Ice causes vasoconstriction and decreases the volume of blood loss.*
- Be prepared to administer IV fluid, blood, or blood products. *Parenteral fluids replace lost fluid volume; blood and blood products replace cells and fluid.*

Evaluation of Expected Outcomes

Expected outcomes include reduced or eliminated pain. Venous circulation improves, and adequate blood flow to the heart is maintained; both extremities are comparable in size, temperature, and color. If a PE develops, it is managed successfully. Bleeding is prevented or controlled.

Buerger Disease (Thromboangiitis Obliterans)

Buerger disease, also known as **thromboangiitis obliterans**, is an inflammation of blood vessels associated with clot formation and fibrosis of the blood vessel wall. It affects primarily the small arteries and veins of the legs. It occasionally involves the arms.

Pathophysiology and Etiology

The cause of Buerger disease, which is rare, is far more common in men than in women, predominantly among those who smoke cigarettes or use smokeless tobacco. The onset is usually during young adulthood. The affected arteries are prone to spasms that constrict the arterial lumen. Inflammatory lesions are found in isolated segments intermixed among healthy areas of the same vessel. The lesions occlude blood flow through the vessel during exercise and at rest. Skin and soft-tissue cells experience degrees of hypoxia and anoxia. Some cells die. The necrotic (dead) tissues slough, forming ulcerations. The extent may be so severe that gangrene results. Thrombophlebitis may also be present.

Assessment Findings

The client notes that one or both feet are always cold and may report numbness, burning, and tingling in some areas of the feet. **Intermittent claudication**, leg cramps after exercise, is a common symptom. Pain occurs at rest when circulation has been seriously impaired. The symptoms usually fluctuate in severity; remissions often follow attacks of acute distress.

Cyanosis and redness of the feet and legs sometimes occur. The skin is frequently a mottled purplish red and appears thin and shiny, with sparse hair growth. Shallow, dry leg ulcers in various stages of healing may be seen. Black gangrenous areas may develop on the toes and heels (Fig. 23-16). The nails are thick. Peripheral pulses are present during rest but diminish or disappear with activity. Capillary refill is prolonged. Doppler ultrasound, IPG, and angiography help evaluate the location and extent of vessel destruction.

Medical and Surgical Management

Tobacco in any form is restricted. Buerger–Allen exercises are ordered to stimulate and promote collateral circulation. Walking and active foot exercises are allowed as long as they do not cause pain. Analgesics are prescribed to ease discomfort. If leg ulcers develop, treatment may include moist dressings that are changed when the gauze becomes damp and topical antiseptics or antibiotic ointments.

Sympathectomy, the surgical interruption or suppression of some portion of the sympathetic nerve pathway, is performed to relieve vasospasm. If ulcerations occur, wound debridement (removal of necrotic tissue) and skin grafting may be required. If circulation becomes so impaired that gangrene results, amputation is necessary.

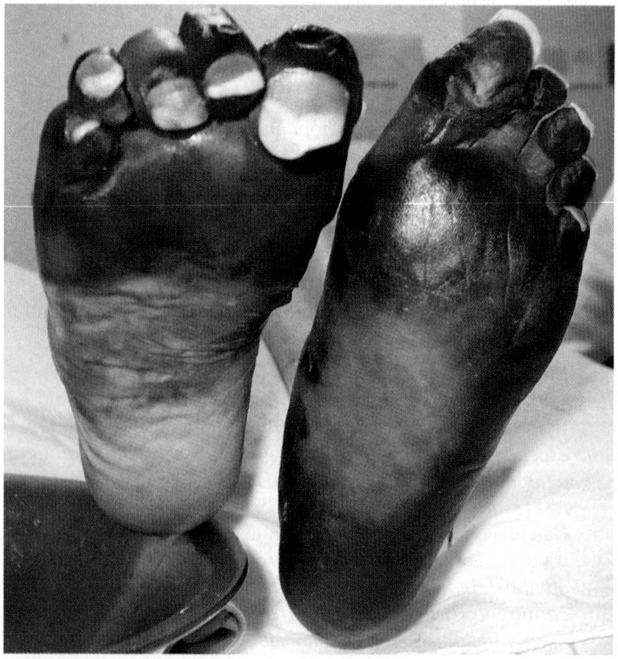

Figure 23-16 Thromboangiitis obliterans accompanied by gangrene.

Nursing Management

The nurse takes a thorough history, which includes a smoking history, and a review of symptoms and how long they have been present. The history also includes the client's description of the type and degree of pain and factors that increase or decrease it. The nurse examines the affected areas for redness, swelling, and other color changes, such as cyanosis and mottling. They inspect the nails and skin for changes and note the skin temperature above and below the affected area. The nurse also monitors the presence and quality of peripheral pulses and assesses capillary refill time.

The nurse instructs and supervises the client about Buerger–Allen leg exercises (Client and Family Teaching 23-4). When the client is not performing exercises, they must keep the legs horizontal or dependent. Elevating the legs increases ischemia and, therefore, contributes to pain. The nurse carries out meticulous wound care if leg or foot ulcers exist.

Client and Family Teaching 23-4
Performing Buerger–Allen Exercises

The nurse teaches the client to

1. Lie flat in bed, with both legs elevated above the level of the heart for 2 or 3 minutes.
2. Sit on the edge of the bed with the legs dependent, or lower than the head, for 3 minutes.
3. Exercise the feet and toes by moving them up, down, inward, and outward.
4. Return to the first position and hold it for about 5 minutes.
5. Repeat the exercises several times during one exercise period and perform them periodically throughout the day.

Hospitalization for acute problems or complications may occur, but the client must carry out most care at home. The nurse teaches the client self-care techniques and stresses the importance of smoking cessation and performing prescribed exercises consistently. Self-care includes avoiding caffeine, tobacco products, and over-the-counter drugs that cause vasoconstriction, such as nasal decongestants, and inspecting the fingernails, toenails, and skin on the arms and legs daily. The nurse teaches the client to clean the arms and legs daily, prevent trauma to the extremities, wear properly fitting shoes and stockings (or socks), and avoid prolonged exposure to the cold. When cold weather is unavoidable, the nurse advises the client to wear thick socks or insulated boots and gloves to protect against exposure to low temperatures.

KEY POINTS

- Two organisms that cause infectious conditions of the heart:
  - Streptococci
  - Staphylococci
- Inflammatory conditions of the heart:
  - Rheumatic fever and rheumatic carditis
  - Infective endocarditis
  - Myocarditis
  - Cardiomyopathy
    - Dilated: the cavity of the heart is stretched (dilated)
    - Hypertrophic: the muscle of the left ventricle and septum thickens, causing heart enlargement
    - Restrictive: heart muscle stiffens, which interferes with its ability to stretch and fill with blood
  - Pericarditis
- Inflammatory disorders of the peripheral blood vessels
  - Thrombophlebitis: is an inflammation of a vein accompanied by clot or thrombus formation. The veins deep in the lower extremities are most commonly affected.
  - Thromboangiitis obliterans/Buerger disease: is an inflammation of blood vessels associated with clot formation and fibrosis of the blood vessel wall. It affects primarily the small arteries and veins of the legs and can occasionally involve the arms.
- Anticoagulant treatment
  - Parenteral anticoagulants:
    - Heparin
  - Low-molecular-weight heparins:
    - Lovenox
    - Arixtra
  - Oral anticoagulants:
    - Warfarin
    - Eliquis
    - Pradaxa
    - Xarelto
  - Antiplatelet agents:
    - Aspirin: Ecotrin, Ascriptin
    - Plavix
    - Brilinta
    - Integrilin

CRITICAL THINKING EXERCISES

1. Of the three major inflammatory disorders of the heart—endocarditis, myocarditis, and pericarditis—which has the fewest long-term effects? Support your answer.
2. A client complains of intermittent claudication, pain when the legs are elevated, and cold, numb feet. The nurse notes several dry ulcerations of the feet. Does the client suffer from venous or arterial insufficiency? What additional assessment data must the nurse collect? What lifestyle habits might predispose the client to this disorder?
3. What health teaching is important for a client with a history of thrombophlebitis?
4. Which category of anticoagulant drug therapy would a client be most able to manage independently?

NCLEX-STYLE REVIEW QUESTIONS PrepU

1. When auscultating the chest of a client with pericarditis, what will the nurse most likely hear?
   1. A grating friction rub
   2. S_1 and S_2 heart sounds
   3. Expiratory wheezing
   4. A bounding apical pulse

2. What question asked by the nurse is most important initially when obtaining the medical history of a client with endocarditis?
   1. "Have you recently been treated for strep throat?"
   2. "Have you recently had flu-like symptoms?"
   3. "Do you have any skin rashes?"
   4. "Have you had any recent cuts or bruises?"

3. What nursing interventions should a nurse perform when a client with cardiomyopathy receives a loop diuretic? Select all that apply.
   1. Monitor intake and output.
   2. Administer oxygen.
   3. Assess daily weight.
   4. Check for dependent edema.
   5. Maintain strict bed rest.
   6. Encourage foods containing potassium.

4. When the nurse checks the PTT laboratory result of a client who has been receiving a daily subcutaneous dose of heparin, it is 100 seconds. Based on a normal PTT value of 60 to 70 seconds, which of the following can the nurse expect when the lab result is reported to the primary provider?
   1. The primary provider will order the same daily dose of heparin because the client's PTT level is within a therapeutic range.
   2. The primary provider will order a higher dose of heparin because the client is not adequately anticoagulated.
   3. The primary provider will order to withhold today's dose of heparin because the client's ability to clot is dangerously impaired.
   4. The primary provider will order protamine sulfate to counteract the effect of the heparin.

5. After having received instructions regarding thrombophlebitis, which statement made by the client indicates a need for further teaching?
   1. "When I go back to work, I need to change my position often."
   2. "I will need to take anticoagulants for a while."
   3. "I will notify the nurse if I have any trouble breathing."
   4. "When I feel cramping in my calf, I should rub it until the pain goes away."

WANT TO KNOW MORE? There are a wide variety of online resources available on thePoint to enhance learning and understanding of this chapter.

Go to **thePoint.lww.com/activate** and use the activation code found in the front of this text to unlock these online resources.

24 Caring for Clients With Valvular Disorders of the Heart

Words To Know

aortic regurgitation
aortic stenosis
arrhythmia
balloon valvuloplasty
commissures
dysrhythmia
mitral regurgitation
mitral stenosis
mitral valve prolapse
mitral valve prolapse syndrome
point of maximum impulse
transcatheter aortic valve replacement (TAVR)
valvular incompetence
valvular regurgitation
water-hammer pulse

Learning Objectives

On completion of this chapter, you will be able to:

1. List five disorders that commonly affect heart valves.
2. Discuss assessment findings common among clients with valvular disorders.
3. Name three diagnostic tests used to confirm valvular disorders.
4. Identify consequences of valvular disorders.
5. Name five categories of drugs used to treat valvular disorders.
6. Give two examples of treatments other than drug therapy to correct valvular disorders.
7. Discuss nursing management of clients with valvular disorders.

Each heart structure helps to maintain normal cardiac function. The four cardiac valves—aortic, mitral, tricuspid, and pulmonic—promote the forward circulation of blood to sustain adequate cardiac output (Fig. 24-1). The structure and function of cardiac valves can be affected by malformations at birth, inflammatory and infectious disorders (see Chapter 23), age-related degeneration, structural damage after myocardial infarction (MI), or injury during an intracardiac procedure. The aortic and mitral valves, located on the left side of the heart, where fluid pressures are higher than on the right side, are most commonly affected. Less common are disorders involving the pulmonic and tricuspid valves. This chapter provides information on common valvular disorders and the medical and nursing management of clients who are affected.

Gerontologic Considerations

- Age-related effects, such as stiffening of the aorta and calcification and fibrotic thickening of the mitral and aortic valves, contribute to development of symptoms (e.g., increased systolic blood pressure [BP], dangerous arrhythmias [erratic heart rhythms or rates that are too fast or slow] sometimes referred to as *dysrhythmias*) and complications (e.g., increased myocardial oxygen demand, heart failure, and alterations in cardiac output) in the older adult with valvular heart disease.
- Older adults may experience a decreased thirst sensation, increasing the risk for dehydration and volume depletion, which may result in fatigue and weakness that can be confused with symptoms of valvular disease.
- Older adults may require lower doses of cardiac glycosides than younger clients because of age-related metabolic changes. The more medications older adults take, the more likely they are to have dangerous interactions. For older adults taking beta-blockers, monitor the heart rate and BP closely; the adverse effects of bradycardia and hypotension can cause confusion and falls.

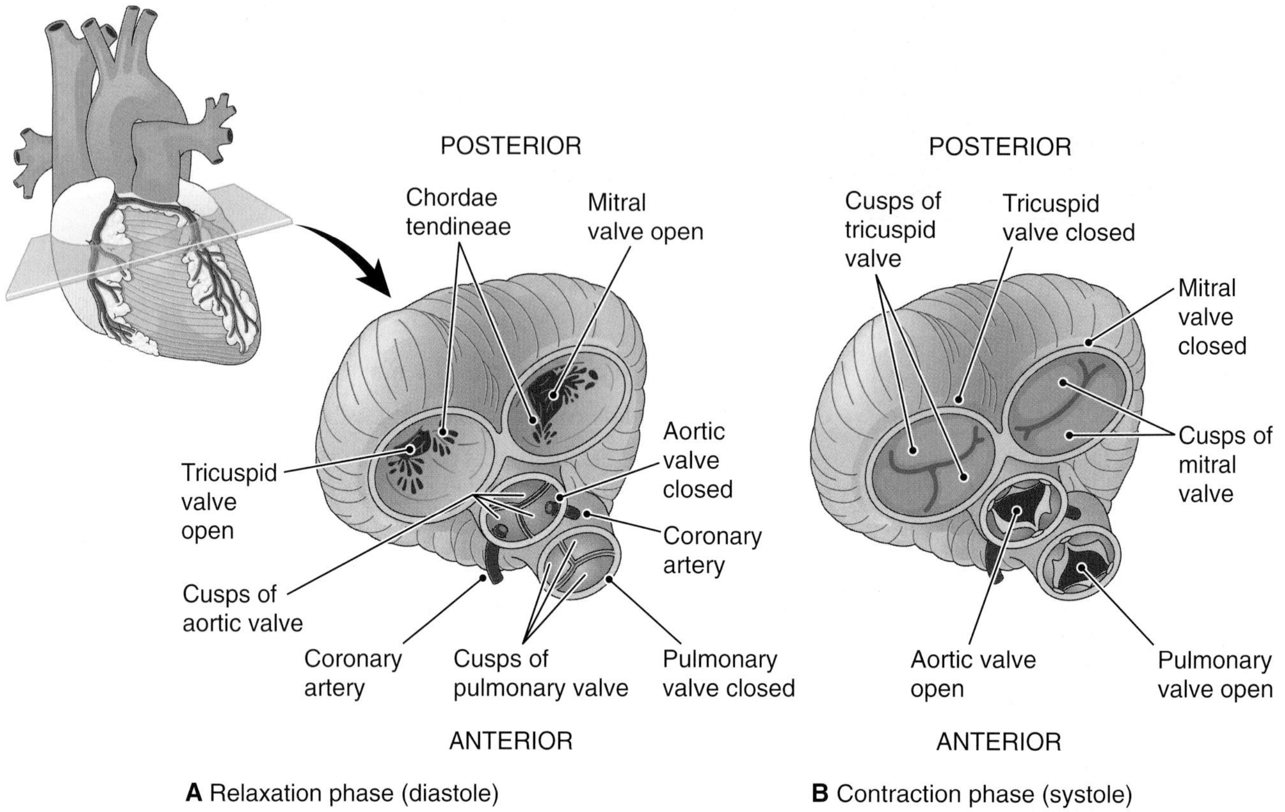

Figure 24-1 Valves of the heart. **(A)** During diastole, the tricuspid and mitral valves are open and allow blood to flow freely from the atria to the ventricles. The aortic and pulmonary valves are closed. **(B)** When the ventricles contract (systole), the tricuspid and mitral valves close, preventing blood from returning to the atria. The pulmonary and aortic valves open as blood is ejected from the ventricles. (Adapted from Cohen, B. J., & Hull, K. (2014). *Memmler's structure and function of the human body* (11th ed.). Wolters Kluwer.)

DISORDERS OF THE AORTIC VALVE

The aortic valve has three cusps, or leaflets, and each cusp is described as a *semilunar* valve because each cusp appears like a half-moon. The left ventricle pumps blood from the heart through the aortic valve. When the left ventricle contracts, a nondiseased aortic valve opens to allow the unrestricted passage of oxygenated blood into the arterial vascular system. The coronary arteries supplying the myocardium are the first blood vessels perfused. After ejection of left ventricular blood, the aortic valve closes tightly to prevent backflow of blood. Two valvular conditions interfere with unidirectional blood flow from the left side of the heart: aortic stenosis and aortic regurgitation.

Aortic Stenosis

Stenosis means *narrowing*. **Aortic stenosis** is a narrowing of the opening in the aortic valve when the valve cusps become stiff and rigid. It is a common valvular disorder in the United States, especially among older adults.

Pathophysiology and Etiology

In older adults without predisposing cardiac conditions, narrowing of the aortic valve is an age-related degenerative change from progressive calcium deposits in valve cells. In young adults, aortic stenosis usually is a later consequence of a congenital defect in which the valve has two instead of three cusps. At birth and throughout childhood, this defect does not produce symptoms. Symptoms appear after several decades, when the same calcification process that affects older adults causes the valves to harden. In others, aortic stenosis results directly from valvular damage related to rheumatic carditis and infective endocarditis (see Chapter 23).

The stiff, calcified valve cannot open properly and needs more force to push blood through its narrowed opening (Fig. 24-2). The muscular wall of the left ventricle enlarges

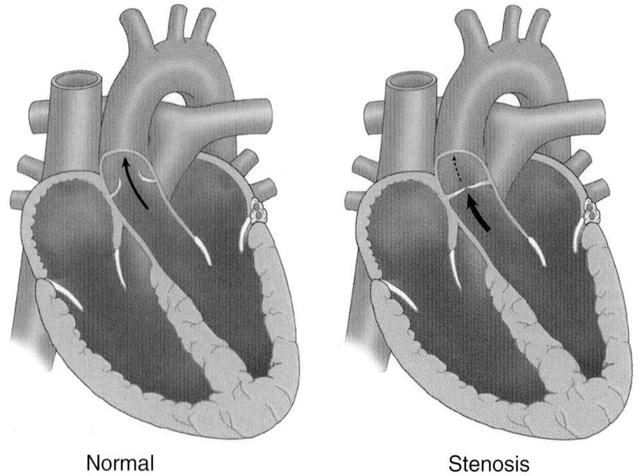

Figure 24-2 Aortic stenosis. Because blood cannot completely pass through the narrowed valve opening, blood pools in the left ventricle and cardiac output is reduced.

and thickens (*hypertrophies*) in response. The blood volume passing through the narrowed valve eventually becomes insufficient to nourish the myocardium and other organs. Exercise or any circumstance that increases heart rate can cause myocardial ischemia, affecting the heart's ability to contract effectively. Left-sided heart failure (see Chapter 28) may develop because the heart cannot fully empty during systole and becomes more fatigued as it tries to overcome the resistance created by the narrowed valve. Should the adult with aortic stenosis develop coronary artery disease (CAD) and MI (see Chapter 25), the infarct may enlarge. Risk of mortality thus increases because of the valve's compromised ability to perfuse the myocardium with oxygen.

Assessment Findings

Signs and Symptoms

A client with aortic stenosis may be asymptomatic for several decades. When symptoms develop, they include dizziness, fainting, and angina because of insufficient cardiac output. At first, the client experiences dyspnea and fatigue during activity. With ventricular enlargement, heart pulsations are displaced laterally or distally on the chest wall from the usual **point of maximum impulse** (PMI) at the fifth intercostal space medial to the left midclavicular line. The carotid pulse feels weak because of a low stroke volume.

The S_2 heart sound is split; that is, there is a definite separation between the sounds of the aortic valve and pulmonic valve closing. Usually, these sounds occur in unison or are so closely timed that they seem as one. While listening at the second intercostal space to the right and left of the sternum, the S_1 and split S_2 sounds like "lub-t-dub." The split persists throughout inspiration and expiration and does not disappear when the client sits up during auscultation. This finding distinguishes the split S_2 from a normal, physiologic splitting. Sometimes, auscultation identifies other abnormal sounds (e.g., systolic murmur, click). Box 24-1 explains grading of heart murmurs.

Diagnostic Findings

Ventricular enlargement is evident on a chest radiograph. An echocardiogram validates ventricular thickening and diminished transvalvular size. On an electrocardiogram (ECG), the height of the R wave may be increased, reflecting the large mass and force of contracting muscle. During left-sided cardiac catheterization, the pressure of blood in the left ventricle is higher than usual.

BOX 24-1 Heart Murmur Grades

- Grade I: faint murmur, barely audible
- Grade II: soft murmur
- Grade III: easily audible but without a palpable thrill
- Grade IV: easily audible murmur with a palpable thrill
- Grade V: loud murmur, audible with stethoscope lightly touching the chest
- Grade VI: loudest murmur, audible with stethoscope not touching the chest

From Thomas, S. L., Heaton, J., Makaryus, A. N. (2020). *Physiology, cardiovascular murmurs*. StatPearls [Internet]. StatPearls Publishing. https://www.ncbi.nlm.nih.gov/books/NBK525958/

Medical and Surgical Management

Medical treatment may begin while the client is asymptomatic and focuses on maintaining adequate cardiac output by supporting the heart's pumping activity. Digitalis, an antidysrhythmic drug particularly for atrial fibrillation with rapid ventricular response (see Chapter 26), and a diuretic may be prescribed. Sodium is restricted. Antibiotics are prescribed for clients with artificial heart valves, history of a heart valve infection, or congenital heart defects, to prevent recurrences of infective endocarditis, which can compound valvular damage. Nitrates or beta-adrenergic blockers are beneficial for relieving chest pain.

Additional treatment eventually becomes critical because survival is jeopardized once symptoms develop. Surgery may be needed to correct a damaged or leaky valve that causes a heart murmur.

Other treatment options are available depending on the client's risk factors. **Balloon valvuloplasty** is an invasive, nonsurgical procedure to enlarge a narrowed valve opening for clients whose conditions are too unstable for immediate surgery yet whose symptoms cannot be adequately controlled more conservatively. With this treatment option, a catheter with a deflated balloon is threaded through a peripheral blood vessel into the heart until the tip is located in the stenotic valve. When in position, the balloon is inflated to stretch the opening. **Annuloplasty** is a procedure that has the surgeon tightening the tissue around the valve by implanting an artificial ring. This allows the leaflets to come together and close the abnormal opening through the valve.

Aortic valve replacement eventually becomes necessary to sustain life and relieve recurring symptoms. Traditionally, this has been performed via a transthoracic incision. There are two optional sources for replacement valves: (1) tissue valves, harvested from pigs (porcine), cows (bovine), or human cadavers; or (2) manufactured mechanical prostheses, made from metal (see Chapter 29). The latter require lifelong anticoagulant therapy to reduce the risk of blood clots forming, but tend to last longer than the tissue valves.

Until recently, 30% to 40% of high-risk older adults were not candidates for replacement of the aortic valve using conventional, open heart surgery. **Transcatheter aortic valve replacement** (TAVR), or transcatheter aortic valve implantation (TAVI) are less invasive approaches. While visualizing the heart with transesophageal cardiography, a catheter is inserted in the femoral artery (or in some cases, the apex of the heart) and advanced to the stenotic valve. When the catheter traverses the aortic valve, the diseased leaflets are opened via an inflated balloon (balloon valvuloplasty). Once opened, a self-expanding stent is positioned to hold the valve leaflets out of the way. A porcine tissue replacement valve mounted within the framework of the stent then functions to restore blood flow into the aorta (Fig. 24-3). As with any procedure, there continue to be risks, but TAVI has improved the quality of life for

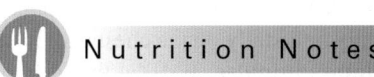

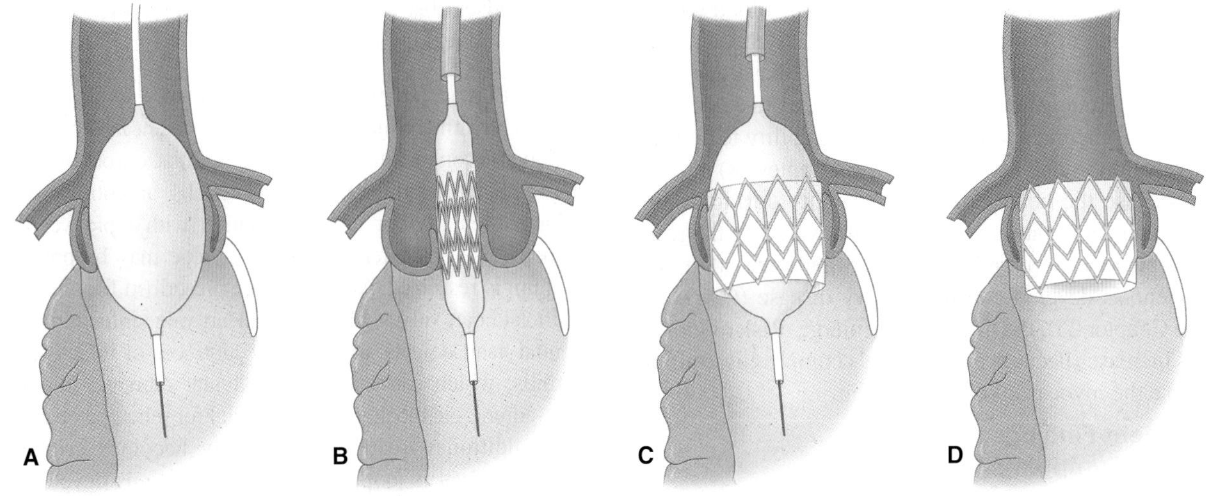

Figure 24-3 Sequence in transcatheter aortic valve implantation: **(A)** the stenotic valve is opened with a balloon; **(B)** the balloon is deflated and a stent is positioned within the valve; **(C)** the stent expands to hold the valve leaflets open; and **(D)** the bioprosthetic replacement valve is implanted.

those who previously faced their inoperable condition with a poor prognosis and ultimate death.

Nursing Management

The nurse monitors subjective and objective symptoms and explains the purposes and techniques of diagnostic tests. They administer prescribed medications and monitor for therapeutic or adverse responses and institute measures to ensure adequate cardiac output and tissue oxygenation. The nurse assists the client to adhere to dietary modifications to reduce fluid volumes and the work placed on the heart (Nutrition Notes).

Aortic Regurgitation

Aortic regurgitation occurs when the aortic valve does not close tightly and blood can leak backward. The valve's inability to close tightly is a condition called **valvular incompetence**.

Pathophysiology and Etiology

Valvular incompetence can result from damage to the valve cusps or papillary muscles. It may be a consequence of various disorders such as rheumatic carditis, endocarditis, syphilis, age-related stretching of the proximal aorta, and systemic inflammatory conditions. In 1997, the incidence of aortic and mitral regurgitation increased as a result of the use of fenfluramine (Pondimin) with phentermine (known as Fen-Phen), fenfluramine alone, and dexfenfluramine (Redux) alone for weight loss.

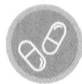

Pharmacologic Considerations

- Some of these drugs are no longer on the market, yet it does not mean they have no effect. Be sure and ask about historical use of medications, as your client may have taken the drug when it was available.

Nutrition Notes

The Client With a Valvular Heart Disorder

- Clients with valvular disorders often need to limit sodium intake because decreasing the volume of blood decreases cardiac workload.
- Because approximately 75% of sodium in the typical American diet comes from processed foods, encourage clients to substitute homemade foods for convenience products and commercially prepared items. Foods to avoid include canned fish, meat, poultry, soup, vegetables, and vegetable juices; smoked and processed meats; sauerkraut; commercial mixes; instant rice and pasta mixes; casserole mixes; frozen dinners, entrees, pizzas, and vegetables with sauces; most fast foods; condiments such as catsup, relish, pickles, barbecue sauce, soy sauce, and Worcestershire sauce; and seasoning salts.
- Salt substitutes replace sodium with potassium or other minerals and may taste bitter. Low-sodium salt substitutes may contain up to half as much sodium as regular table salt. Clients should not use either type without a primary provider's approval.
- Clients with valvular disorders may need to restrict fluid because volume affects cardiac emptying. Foods that liquefy at room temperature (e.g., ice cream, ice milk, gelatin, ice pops, sherbet) are counted as liquids when fluid intake is restricted.

When blood is pumped through the incompetent aortic valve, some leaks backward (**valvular regurgitation**) into the left ventricle. This backflow reduces cardiac output and causes fluid overload in the left ventricle, which becomes chronically stretched, hindering its ability to pump effectively (see Chapter 28). High fluid pressure in the left ventricle causes the mitral valve to shut early, which interferes with left atrial emptying. The blood in the left atrium backs up into the pulmonary circulation. Left ventricular enlargement increases the heart's need for oxygen. When the coronary arteries cannot supply the heart muscle with enough oxygen because of decreased cardiac output, the myocardium becomes ischemic and the client experiences angina. Dizziness, dyspnea on exertion, confusion, and left ventricular failure may develop.

Assessment Findings

Signs and Symptoms

The client remains asymptomatic as long as the left ventricle can sustain adequate circulation. Tachycardia is one of the first signs of cardiac compensation. When valve damage affects the left ventricle, the client becomes aware of forceful heart contractions (palpitations). At first, palpitations occur only when lying flat or on the left side. In later stages, the client experiences dyspnea and chest pain.

During physical examination, skin may be flushed and moist, especially in the upper body. The radial pulse may be very strong, with quick, sharp beats followed by a sudden collapse of force, a characteristic called a **water-hammer pulse** or *Corrigan pulse*. Often, pulse pressure is wide because systolic BP tends to be extremely high, whereas diastolic BP usually remains low or normal. The enlarged heart displaces the PMI. The chest may heave or rock from the forceful contractions of the enlarged left ventricle. A heart murmur, caused by the turbulence of blood falling back through the dilated aortic valve, also may be heard.

Diagnostic Findings

Cardiac catheterization reveals high left ventricular pressure and backward movement of blood. A chest radiograph reveals heart enlargement, and the aortic valve appears dilated. The ECG shows tall R waves; depressed ST segments indicate myocardial ischemia. A radionuclide scan comparing blood flow through the heart at rest and during exercise reveals the severity of the disease. Standard or transesophageal echocardiography provides images of atypical valvular and myocardial function. A computed tomography (CT) or magnetic resonance imaging (MRI) scan may be performed if the echocardiographic images are inconclusive.

Medical and Surgical Management

Because aortic regurgitation is mild and only slowly progressive in most people, clients are sustained with cardiac glycosides (Drug Therapy Table 24-1) or beta-blockers and

DRUG THERAPY TABLE 24-1 Agents to Treat Valvular Heart Disorders

Category and Common Generic (Brand) Drugs	Intended Use	Common Side Effects	Safety Warnings for Nurses
Antibiotics			
Penicillin family Penicillin G (Pfizerpen) Ampicillin Nafcillin	Kill susceptible microorganisms by interfering with bacterial cell wall development	Glossitis, stomatitis, gastritis, furry tongue, nausea, vomiting, diarrhea, rash, fever, pain at injection site	Monitor for anaphylactic reaction Monitor IV infusion for phlebitis
Anticoagulants			
Warfarin (Coumadin, Jantoven)	Prophylaxis/treatment of venous thrombosis by inhibiting vitamin K–dependent clotting factors	Bleeding, fatigue, dizziness, abdominal cramping	INR must be monitored at regular intervals Dietary vitamin K decreases blood levels
Direct-acting oral anticoagulants (DOACs) Apixaban (Eliquis), rivaroxaban (Xarelto), dabigatran (Pradaxa	Prophylaxis/treatment of venous thrombosis by inhibiting Factor Xa and/or inhibiting thrombin	Bleeding, stomach upset	Continuous blood testing is not needed, no dietary restrictions
Salicylates Aspirin (Ecotrin, Ascriptin)	Stroke prevention in men (and women older than 65 years only) by inhibiting platelet aggregation and clotting	Nausea, vomiting, epigastric distress	Tinnitus (ringing in ears) can indicate overmedication use Should not be taken as pain reliever when on anticoagulant therapy
Antiplatelets			
Aggregate Inhibitors Clopidogrel (Plavix) Eptifibatide (Integrilin) Prasugrel (Effient) Ticagrelor (Brilinta) Vorapaxar (Zontivity)	Thrombus prevention by inhibiting platelet aggregation and clotting	Diarrhea, nausea, vomiting	Monitor for bleeding of injection sites, orifices, wounds Do not use PPI with these drugs Do not take aspirin or NSAIDs as pain reliever

(*continued*)

DRUG THERAPY TABLE 24-1 Agents to Treat Valvular Heart Disorders (*continued*)

Category and Common Generic (Brand) Drugs	Intended Use	Common Side Effects	Safety Warnings for Nurses
Cardiac Glycosides			
Digoxin (Lanoxin)	Increases cardiac output by slowing heart rate (negative chronotropic action) and increasing force of contraction (positive inotropic action)	Fatigue, generalized muscle weakness	Monitor potassium, hypokalemia increases serum blood levels Monitor for toxicity, GI distress, muscle fatigue, CNS disturbances, cardiac changes Drug is usually held if heart rate is less than 60 bpm or more than 120 bpm
Antiarrhythmics			
Class I (fast channel) Propafenone (Rythmol) Quinidine *Class II (beta-blockers)* Propranolol (Inderal) *Class III (K^+ channel blockers)* Dofetilide (Tikosyn) Dronedarone (Multaq) Ibutilide (Corvert) Sotalol (Betapace) *Class IV (Ca^{++} channel blockers)* Verapamil (Calan)	Reduce atrial fibrillation by altering the action potential of cardiac cells and interfere with heart's electrical excitability	Headache, nausea, vomiting	When given IV, constant cardiac monitor is required Monitor for new or worsening arrhythmias Drug is usually held if heart rate is less than 60 bpm or more than 120 bpm No grapefruit with Class III drugs Initially, monitor blood every 2–3 weeks for agranulocytosis Monitor for toxicity when quinidine is used
ACE Inhibitors (ACEI)			
Quinapril (Accupril)	Suppression of the renin–angiotensin–aldosterone system reduces water and sodium retention which lessens blood pressure	Dizziness, dry cough	Increased fall risk owing to hypotensive side effects Do not use if impaired renal function, or dialysis Monitor for lower blood glucose in clients with diabetes Interaction with herbal: St. John's wort Perimenopausal women need to use effective birth control

diuretics. When taken appropriately, prophylactic antibiotics prevent recurrences of infective endocarditis. Clients are advised to modify their lifestyle to avoid excessive demands on the heart, such as those that may result from strenuous exercise and emotional stress.

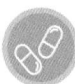

Pharmacologic Considerations

- Nonselective beta-blockers can aggravate chronic obstructive pulmonary disease and contribute to hyperglycemia in insulin-dependent adults. Some diuretics deplete potassium, causing hypokalemia.
- Before administering beta-blockers, take the client's apical pulse. If the heart rate is less than 60 beats/min, withhold the drug and notify the primary health care provider.
- Closely monitor clients taking beta-blockers for signs and symptoms of overdosage: bradycardia, severe dizziness, drowsiness, and bluish discoloration of the palms, fingernails, or both. Notify the primary health care provider immediately if these symptoms appear.

When a client becomes symptomatic, replacement of the diseased aortic valve is considered (see Chapter 29). The less the heart damage that occurs before surgery, the better the outcome. If the aorta is diseased, the procedure is more involved because repair involves a vascular graft.

Nursing Management

The nurse prepares the client for diagnostic procedures and monitors responses, reporting changes in heart rate and rhythm, dyspnea, chest pain, and loss of consciousness to the primary provider immediately. The nurse administers prescribed medications and evaluates the client's response. Ensuring that physical activity is balanced according to the client's tolerance is important. Before discharge, the nurse explains the need for antibiotic therapy before medical and dental procedures and teaches how to assess BP regularly as well as methods to control hypertension.

>>> Stop, Think, and Respond 24-1

A client with an aortic valvular disorder experiences chest pain while performing bathing and hygiene. What nursing actions are appropriate?

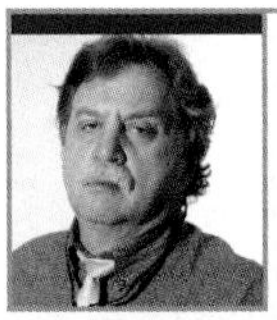

Clinical Scenario A 62-year-old man who may have a past history of rheumatic fever has been followed by his primary provider for a grade 3 heart murmur for the past 3 years. The client has become progressively breathless and fatigued with everyday activities. He has experienced some syncopal episodes recently. After undergoing an echocardiogram, the client was found to have some cardiac enlargement and aortic valve stenosis. He is admitted for further diagnostic evaluation and potential for correcting the valvular problem.
What type of data does the nurse need to gather? See Nursing Care Plan 24-1.

NURSING CARE PLAN 24-1 The Client With a Valvular Disorder

Assessment

Determine the following:

- Vital signs, noting tachycardia, rapid respirations, dyspnea, hypotension, or hypertension
- Any episodes of dizziness or fainting with or without confusion
- Chest pain and its characteristics
- Normal or abnormal lung and heart sounds
- Fluid intake and output
- Current weight and fluctuations during treatment
- Level of activity tolerance
- Social aspects (e.g., occupational activities) as they relate to physical energy requirements
- Knowledge of medical condition and current and future treatment protocols

Nursing Analysis. **Hypotension risk** related to diminished cardiac muscle contractility, tachycardia, and hypertension

Expected Outcome. Blood pressure will be adequate as evidenced by cardiovascular assessment, and blood pressure within clients normal limits.

Interventions	Rationales
Monitor cardiac rhythm and rate.	*Rapid heart rate and tachyarrhythmias compromise cardiac output.*
Measure urine output every 8 hours or more often if less than 500 mL/day.	*Renal output reflects the heart's ability to perfuse the renal arteries.*
Maintain client on bed rest.	*Rest lowers heart rate, which increases diastolic filling volume.*
Reduce anxiety by responding to requests for attention or assistance.	*Relief of anxiety reduces tachycardia.*
Provide substitutes for dietary sources of caffeine and sodium.	*Caffeine increases heart rate and promotes vasoconstriction; sodium contributes to fluid retention.*
Promote ease in eliminating stool through such measures as increasing fiber and administering a prescribed stool softener.	*Bearing down to eliminate stool interferes with cardiac filling; reduced cardiac filling decreases cardiac output.*
Reduce any fever by changing to lighter or fewer bed linens, assisting with tepid sponge baths, or administering prescribed antipyretics.	*Increased heart rate accompanies fever and adds to the heart's workload, which may compromise cardiac output.*

Evaluation of Expected Outcome

Client's heart rate, BP, and urine output are within normal ranges. The client's sensorium is clear.

Nursing Analysis. **Activity Intolerance** related to decreased cardiac output

Expected Outcome. Client will tolerate activity without dyspnea or heart rate above 100 beats/min.

Interventions	Rationales
Provide complete or partial assistance with activities of daily living.	*Activity taxes endurance and results in increased heart rate and BP.*
Allow adequate time for client to perform self-care.	*Activity that is done without urgency is less physically demanding.*
Intersperse periods of activity with rest.	*Rest helps the heart recover from demands that increase its rate or force of contraction.*

Evaluation of Expected Outcome

Client manages self-care and moderate activity without becoming breathless, hypotensive, or tachycardic.

Nursing Analysis. **Acute Pain** related to myocardial ischemia

Expected Outcome. Pain will be reduced to client's self-described tolerance level within 30 minutes of a nursing intervention

Interventions	Rationales
Provide rest immediately.	*Rest slows the heart rate and decreases the myocardium's need for oxygen.*

(continued)

NURSING CARE PLAN 24-1 The Client With a Valvular Disorder (*continued*)

Administer oxygen temporarily.	*Increasing inhaled oxygen concentration promotes myocardial cellular oxygenation.*
Give prescribed short-acting nitrate or analgesic	*Nitrates cause vasodilatation and increase blood flow from the coronary arteries to the myocardium; analgesics block the transmission or perception of pain.*

Evaluation of Expected Outcome

Client is free of pain.

Nursing Analysis. **Infection Risk** related to increased susceptibility secondary to previous endocardial inflammatory or infectious disorders

Expected Outcome. Client will remain free of infection as evidenced by normal temperature and white blood cell count.

Interventions	Rationales
Reassign care of client if designated caregiver has infectious symptoms, or have caregiver don protective garments (e.g., face mask) and change them frequently.	*Reducing exposure to microorganisms associated with infective endocarditis minimizes the potential for infection and repeated valvular damage.*
Perform conscientious hand hygiene.	*Hand hygiene is the single most effective method to reduce infectious microorganisms.*
Follow aseptic principles when changing dressings covering impaired skin and vascular insertion sites.	*Impaired skin is an entrance site for microorganisms that may lead to bacteremia and repeated valvular damage.*

Evaluation of Expected Outcome

Client does not acquire a nosocomial infection.

RC of Heart Failure

Expected Outcome. The nurse will monitor for, manage, and minimize heart failure.

Interventions	Rationales
Auscultate lung and heart sounds at least once per shift or more often if abnormal sounds are evident.	*Crackles, rhonchi (gurgles), and an S_3 heart sound are signs of cardiopulmonary complications such as left-sided congestive heart failure.*
Weigh client daily at the same time, with similar clothing, on the same scale.	*A weight gain of 2 lb or more in 24 hours suggests fluid retention equal to 1 L.*
Support compliance with prescribed sodium and fluid restrictions.	*Such restrictions decrease the work and sustain the ability of the heart to contract efficiently.*

Evaluation of Expected Outcome

The nurse documents appropriate assessment findings, reports critical information to the primary provider, and implements prescribed interventions.

Nursing Analysis. **Knowledge Deficiency** related to insufficient knowledge of self-care

Expected Outcome. Client will accurately describe discharge instructions.

Interventions	Rationales
Completely explain all treatments.	*Client cannot implement interventions that are not explained.*
Advise client to consult the primary provider about prophylactic antibiotic therapy before dental or invasive treatments.	*Prophylactic antibiotics reduce the potential for recurrent endocarditis and additional valvular damage.*
Caution against lifting heavy objects or straining at stool.	*Bearing down with forced expiration through a closed glottis (Valsalva maneuver) increases BP, which predisposes the client to heart failure.*
Teach client to recognize signs and symptoms of heart failure (see Chapter 28) and to report them immediately.	*Early intervention facilitates an improved prognosis if a complication develops.*
Advise client to avoid caffeine and over-the-counter medications that contain cardiac stimulants (e.g., decongestants).	*They cause tachycardia and vasoconstriction, increasing the risk for myocardial ischemia, tachyarrhythmias, and heart failure.*
Instruct client to avoid strenuous exercise and competitive sports.	*Activity beyond tolerance and competition increase heart rate, BP, and cardiac risks.*

Evaluation of Expected Outcome

Client accurately describes their disorder, methods for controlling symptoms, and precautions that reduce the risk for complications.

DISORDERS OF THE MITRAL VALVE

The mitral valve, which lies between the left atrium and left ventricle, is a bicuspid valve. The two cusps are attached on the ventricular surface to strands of fibrous tissue called *chordae tendineae*, which are projections from papillary muscles (see Fig. 22-2, Chapter 22). The papillary muscles contract in unison with the ventricle, pull on the chordae tendineae, and prevent the cusps from ballooning into the left atrium. The functions of the mitral valve are to open widely to allow oxygenated blood to fill the left ventricle and close tightly to prevent blood from reentering the left atrium after the left ventricle is filled. As long as the mitral valve remains structurally sound, blood exits the left ventricle through the aortic valve, where the aorta receives a 50- to 70-mL bolus of oxygenated blood referred to as the *stroke volume*. The valve may become rigid (stenotic), incompetent (inadequate closure), or prolapsed (floppy). Mitral valve prolapse is the most commonly diagnosed valvular disorder.

Mitral Stenosis

Pathophysiology and Etiology

Mitral stenosis means that the valve does not open properly to facilitate filling of the left ventricle (Fig. 24-4). It is primarily a *sequela* (a condition that follows a disease) of rheumatic carditis (see Chapter 23). Mitral stenosis worsens with each recurrence of endocarditis. The inflammation causes the cusps to stick together and form a thick, rigid, calcified scar at the **commissures**, the area where the cusps contact each other and the chordae tendineae fuse and shorten. The mitral valve cannot open completely, leading to incomplete emptying of the left atrium. Pooled blood from incomplete emptying contributes to clot formation, which puts the client at risk for arterial emboli. The left atrium enlarges because it has to contract more forcibly to empty. Pressure from overfilling is conveyed backward through the blood vessels to the lungs, creating pulmonary hypertension and the potential for pulmonary edema (see Chapter 21). Pulmonary hypertension increases the work of the right ventricle as it pumps against the high pressure in the pulmonary vascular system.

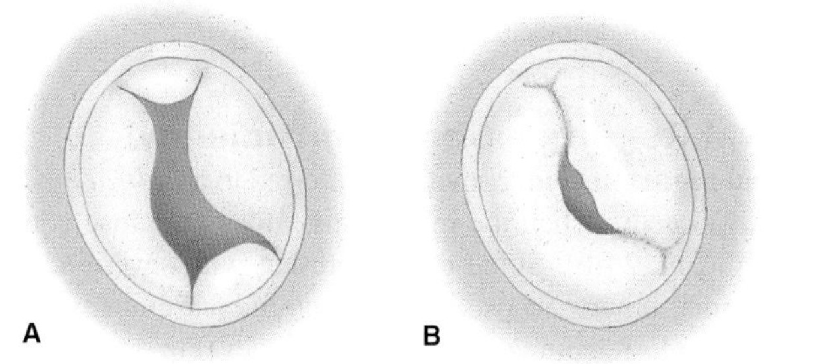

Figure 24-4 **(A)** The normal mitral valve opens widely to allow blood to pass from the left atrium to the left ventricle. **(B)** Following what is generally an infectious process, the mitral valve leaflets become fused with scar tissue, causing a partially obstructed pathway for the passage of blood.

Because blood flows in a circuit, the disease on the left side of the heart eventually affects the right side. The right ventricle may enlarge in response to its increased workload. When the contraction of the right ventricle can no longer overcome the pulmonary resistance, right-sided heart failure develops. Excess blood accumulates in the venous circulation, the liver becomes congested, and edema occurs in the legs.

Assessment Findings

Signs and Symptoms

It may take 20 to 40 years for a client who has had rheumatic fever to develop mitral stenosis. The normal valve opening is 4 to 5 cm^2; symptoms develop when the valve area is less than 2.5 cm^2. At that time, clients report fatigue and dyspnea after slight exertion. Symptoms become disabling approximately 10 years after onset; they are accentuated when unusual demands are placed on the heart (e.g., fever, emotional stress, pregnancy). Later, clients experience heart palpitations caused by *tachyarrhythmias* (rapid arrhythmias). With the onset of pulmonary hypertension, clients may become more dyspneic at night and must sleep in a sitting position. They may develop a cough productive of pink, frothy sputum. Crackles heard in the bases of the lungs are a sign of pulmonary congestion.

Changes in heart sounds may be the earliest indication of mitral valve stenosis. S_1 may be extremely loud if the cusps are fused or muffled or absent if the cusps have calcified and are immobile. A murmur, described as sounding like a rumbling underground train, can be heard at the heart's apex, especially when the client assumes a left lateral position. The systolic BP is low from reduced cardiac output. If backward pressure through the pulmonary circulation is sufficient to affect the right ventricle, the client's face is flushed, neck vein distention is evident, the liver is enlarged, and there is peripheral edema.

> *Concept Mastery Alert*
>
> **Pulmonary Hypertension**
>
> Low systolic pressure is associated with pulmonary hypertension. A productive cough with pink-tinged frothy sputum can indicate a progression of the disorder and a need for treatment.

Diagnostic Findings

A chest radiograph reveals an enlarged left atrium and mitral valve calcification. In advanced stages, evidence of fluid congestion in the lungs (pulmonary edema) is found. A standard or esophageal echocardiogram demonstrates decreased movement of the mitral valve cusps and changes in the size of the atrial chamber. On ECG, the P wave is notched, showing that the left atrium takes longer to depolarize than the right atrium because of its increased size.

Medical and Surgical Management

Antibiotic therapy is prescribed to prevent future episodes of infective endocarditis. Preventing or relieving the symptoms of heart failure is essential. A daily aspirin, dipyridamole (Persantine), or other oral anticoagulant may be ordered to avoid clot formation.

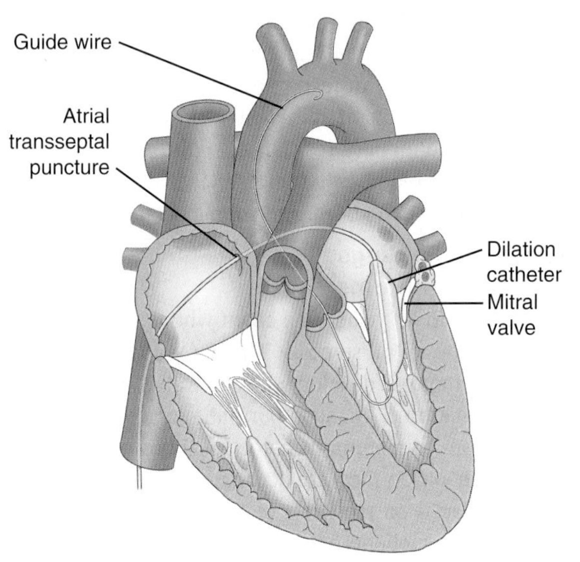

Figure 24-5 Balloon valvuloplasty. Cross-section of heart illustrating dilation catheter placed through an atrial transseptal puncture and across the mitral valve. The guide wire extends from the aortic valve into the aorta for catheter support.

Arrhythmias (abnormal electrical impulse transmission through the conduction system), such as *atrial fibrillation* (quivering of the atrial muscle with insufficient force to pump blood), are treated with drugs or cardioversion. Cardioversion stops the heart momentarily to allow the sinoatrial node to reestablish itself as the pacemaker.

Commissurotomy is a surgical technique to separate the fused valve leaflets (see Chapter 29). However, not all clients with mitral stenosis are suitable candidates for surgery. Those whose condition is so slight that it does not cause symptoms or so severe or of such long duration that profound changes in the heart and lungs have occurred usually are excluded. The earlier surgery is performed, the greater is the likelihood that it will relieve the symptoms.

Percutaneous balloon valvuloplasty, also called *valvotomy*, is a nonsurgical alternative. When percutaneous balloon valvuloplasty is performed, a catheter with an uninflated balloon is passed through the femoral vein and threaded into the right atrium. The septum is then punctured between the right and left atria. When the catheter is in the mitral valve, it is inflated (Fig. 24-5). Clients often are discharged on the same day as the procedure. The atrial puncture allows some blood to shunt from the left atrium to the right, but the opening usually closes within 6 months. Complications, although rare, include mitral regurgitation (discussed next); residual atrial septal defect; perforation of the left ventricle; embolization; and MI.

Management of the client after percutaneous balloon valvuloplasty includes the following:

- Echocardiogram within 72 hours to detect mitral regurgitation, left ventricular dysfunction, or pronounced atrial septal defect
- Oral anticoagulation therapy within 1 to 2 days for clients who have a history of atrial fibrillation or instituted for others if atrial fibrillation develops in the future
- Prophylactic antibiotic protocols to prevent infective endocarditis
- Yearly medical follow-up that includes echocardiography, chest radiography, and ECG

Nursing Management

The nurse monitors the client's physical condition, prepares them for diagnostic testing, and provides posttreatment care. Discharge teaching includes information regarding drug therapy, activity modification, signs and symptoms of complications, and when to contact the primary provider (Evidence-Based Practice 24-1). (See Nursing Care Plan 24-1 for additional discussion.)

Evidence-Based Practice 24-1

Identifying Client Learning Needs Related to Cardiovascular Disease

Clinical Question

Can the support of the nurse with communication on cardiovascular risk affect the client?

Evidence

As the study was done with approximately 18 clients, this included the nurse giving support on cardiovascular risk for primary prevention. The study was led by nurses providing communication, positive attitude, encouragement, and helping clients set small goals to name a few. The clients were interviewed after communication and support as a client–nurse relationship developed. The study concluded that nurse risk communication with positive encouragement was positive for clients. They reported the clients feeling positive even when goals were not met because the nurses continued to be supportive and communicated positively (Loon et al., 2014).

Nursing Implications

Nurses need training in how to be supportive for healthy lifestyles with clients and foster the ability to reinforce habits, behaviors, and communicate client risks. Providing client understanding and encouragement even when goals are not met may be an important factor in clients following primary prevention behaviors.

Reference
Loon, M. K., van Dijk-de Vries, A., van der Weijden, T., Elwyn, G., & Widdershoven, G. A. (2014). Ethical issues in cardiovascular risk management: Patients need nurses' support. *Nursing Ethics, 21*(5), 540–553. https://doi.org/10.1177/0969733013505313

Mitral Regurgitation (Insufficiency)

Mitral regurgitation, sometimes referred to as *mitral insufficiency*, occurs when the mitral valve does not close completely (Fig. 24-6). Some clients present with severe acute symptoms; others, whose heart muscle increases in size to compensate, remain asymptomatic or develop symptoms gradually over many years.

Pathophysiology and Etiology

Mitral regurgitation is associated with rheumatic carditis and mitral valve prolapse (discussed next). It also is linked with damage to the papillary muscles, impaired myocardial

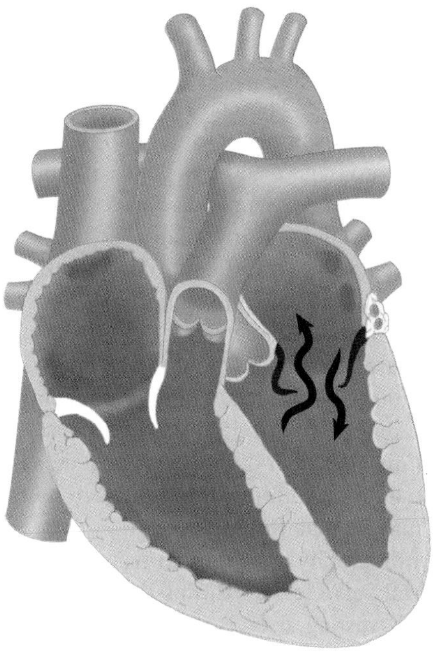

Figure 24-6 Mitral regurgitation (insufficiency). The incompetent atrioventricular valve allows blood to return to the left atrium.

function after MI, connective tissue disorders, stretching of the valve opening from an enlarged left ventricle, and malfunction of a replaced valve. It also can develop after balloon valvuloplasty. Use of the weight loss drugs identified in the discussion of aortic regurgitation also has been associated with mitral valve regurgitation.

When the mitral valve becomes incompetent (i.e., does not close completely), blood flows backward into the left atrium during ventricular systole and leaks into the left ventricle during atrial diastole. The heart usually can compensate for a small amount of blood that is regurgitated backward and forward by increasing the size of the left ventricle and left atria. The larger size facilitates ejection of blood from the heart, in which case pulmonary congestion does not occur. If the regurgitation occurs rapidly, however, the heart is less able to compensate. Forward output from the left ventricle is diminished, and the client develops signs of cardiogenic shock (see Chapter 17). Accumulation of blood in the left atrium results in pulmonary congestion.

Assessment Findings

Signs and Symptoms

The client typically experiences chronic fatigue and dyspnea on exertion. Heart palpitations may occur caused by the forceful contraction of the left ventricle as it attempts to empty the excess blood from its chamber. The S_1 heart sound is diminished because of incomplete closure of the mitral valve. An S_3 heart sound, if heard, is an early sign of impending heart failure. Hypertension may develop when reduced cardiac output triggers the renin–angiotensin–aldosterone cycle (see Chapter 16). Tachycardia is a compensatory mechanism when stroke volume decreases. A loud, blowing murmur often is heard throughout ventricular systole at the heart's apex. If pulmonary congestion occurs, the client develops shortness of breath and moist lung sounds typical of left ventricular failure (see Chapter 28).

Diagnostic Findings

Standard transthoracic or transesophageal echocardiography is the best technique to identify structural changes in the mitral valve. Chest radiography shows enlarged chambers on the left side of the heart. Radionuclide angiography, an imaging procedure using an intravenously injected radioactive substance, shows the heart's chambers in motion and provides information on the volume of regurgitated blood. Echocardiography reflects cardiac enlargement, papillary muscle or chordae tendineae dysfunction, and factors that contribute to various associated arrhythmias (e.g., atrial fibrillation).

Medical and Surgical Management

Asymptomatic clients are monitored through physical examination and annual echocardiograms. Exercise is not limited until mild symptoms develop. An angiotensin-converting enzyme (ACE) inhibitor such as quinapril (Accupril), an angiotensin receptor blocker (ARB) such as losartan (Cozaar), or a nitrate such as isosorbide dinitrate (Isordil) reduces afterload, preserving the left ventricle's ability to eject blood effectively. Digitalis, calcium channel blockers, beta-blockers (Carvedilol), or other antiarrhythmic drugs control tachycardia. Some clients are given drugs to prevent intracardiac thrombi, a common complication of blood stasis that accompanies atrial fibrillation. Prophylactic antibiotics are prescribed to prevent recurrences of infective endocarditis. An intra-aortic balloon pump, which provides counterpulsation to the contraction of the left ventricle, can be used in an emergency to stabilize a client in left ventricular failure (see Chapter 28).

Surgery to correct mitral regurgitation includes *annuloplasty*, repair of the valve leaflets and their fibrous ring. The implantation of a biologic or mechanical prosthetic valve to restore unidirectional blood flow may accompany annuloplasty. Annuloplasty and valve replacement are discussed in Chapter 29.

Nursing Management

The nurse closely monitors BP, heart rate and rhythm, heart sounds, and lung sounds. If sodium is restricted, the nurse works with the client and dietitian to find palatable seasonings and foods and weighs the client to determine changes in fluid volume. They administer medications to treat symptoms and report signs of left- or right-sided heart failure immediately. The nurse emphasizes the need for prophylactic antibiotics and periodic health assessments. Refer to Nursing Care Plan 24-1 for more specific interventions.

Mitral Valve Prolapse

In **mitral valve prolapse**, the valve cusps enlarge, become floppy, and bulge backward into the left atrium (Fig. 24-7). Mitral regurgitation may occur, but not in all cases. Mitral

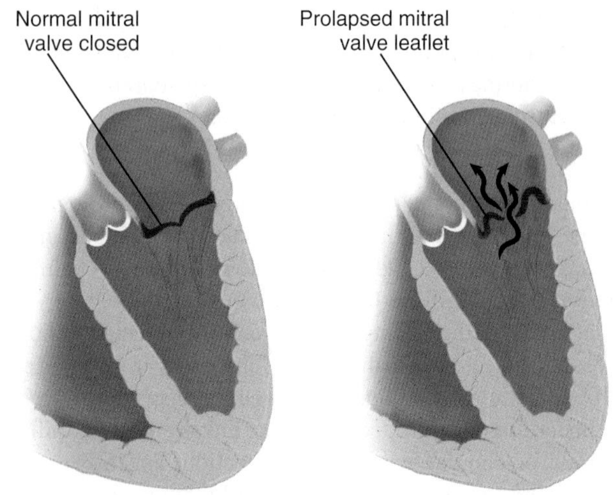

Figure 24-7 In mitral valve prolapse, the floppy valve leaflets bulge backward into the left atrium. This may allow blood to regurgitate, or move in retrograde fashion, from the left ventricle to the left atrium.

valve prolapse is the leading cause of mitral regurgitation. It is more common in young women than men. Despite its high incidence, it is considered to be a benign disease for most affected people.

Pathophysiology and Etiology

The cause of mitral valve prolapse is not completely understood, and it often is classified as idiopathic (having no known cause). It also has been suggested that the tissue changes result from an inherited connective tissue disorder that affects the mitral valve and other connective tissues in the body. It has been observed that some clients develop mitral valve prolapse in association with CAD, although there is speculation that no etiologic relationship actually exists. There is, however, strong evidence that mitral valve prolapse accompanies the valvular changes of rheumatic carditis, and structural changes predispose the valve to further damage if infective endocarditis develops.

Some people develop **mitral valve prolapse syndrome**, symptoms that cannot be attributed to valvular disease alone. It is associated with autonomic nervous system dysfunction. This association may explain why some clients have increased levels of catecholamines (i.e., epinephrine, norepinephrine), abnormal catecholamine regulation, and decreased intravascular volume, which causes symptoms that mimic severe anxiety (tachycardia, palpitations, breathlessness, dizziness). Decreased circulatory volume may contribute to the client's symptomatology by triggering an abnormal renin–angiotensin–aldosterone response (see Chapter 16). Changes in the mitral valve tissue layers cause the cusps to distend. The billowing cusps stretch the papillary muscles as they balloon backward into the left atrium. The stretching of the papillary muscles causes local ischemia and atypical chest pain. As the papillary muscles provide less support to the mitral valve, valvular incompetence occurs. The left atrium and ventricle eventually may enlarge and subsequently progress to heart failure.

Assessment Findings

Many clients with mitral valve prolapse are asymptomatic. When symptoms are present, they include chest pain, palpitations, and fatigue. The chest pain differs from that of angina: Its onset does not correlate with physical exertion, its duration is prolonged, and it is not easily relieved. Some clients also experience symptoms that resemble anxiety or panic, such as a rapid and irregular heart rate, shortness of breath, light-headedness, difficulty concentrating, and fear that the symptoms indicate impending death. Auscultation of heart sounds reveals a characteristic "click" during ventricular systole caused by tightening of the chordae tendineae. A systolic murmur is associated with mitral regurgitation. The presumptive diagnosis of mitral valve prolapse is strong if the murmur disappears or diminishes when the client squats during auscultation. Additional symptoms of mitral regurgitation also may be manifested.

Echocardiography shows abnormal movement of one or more mitral valve leaflets during systole. The electrocardiogram ECG (resting, exercise, chemical, or ambulatory) is essentially normal, eliminating MI as a cause for the chest pain. ECG, however, may detect other causes.

Medical and Surgical Management

Many clients with mitral valve prolapse require no treatment. Such drugs as digitalis, beta-blockers, and calcium channel blockers control tachydysrhythmias; all but digitalis also control hypertension. Medications to reduce or inhibit platelet aggregation in cases where mitral valve prolapse is accompanied by atrial fibrillation include a single, daily, low-dose aspirin, warfarin (Coumadin), clopidogrel (Plavix), to prevent thrombus formation. If symptoms become severe, valve replacement is indicated.

Antianxiety medication may be prescribed to prevent symptoms related to the sympathetic nervous system among those with mitral valve prolapse syndrome. Such clients also are advised to avoid caffeine to prevent tachycardia and heart palpitations. To compensate for symptoms associated with hypovolemia, liberal fluid and adequate sodium intake is recommended. Because alcohol can suppress antidiuretic hormone (ADH), leading to loss of extracellular fluid, clients with mitral valve prolapse syndrome are advised to restrict or eliminate its use.

Pharmacologic Considerations

- Dabigatran, rivaroxaban, and apixaban do not require close monitoring. Dosing for these drugs is not dependent upon international normalized ratio (INR) blood levels; therefore, frequent blood testing is not required when taking these medications compared to other anticoagulants.
- How dehydrating is an alcoholic drink? A "shot" of alcohol produces an additional 120 mL of urine. That means one 8-ounce beer will make a person urinate about 14 ounces of fluid.

Nursing Management

One measure to relieve chest pain is to have the client lie flat with the legs elevated and supported against a wall or couch at a 90-degree angle for 3 to 5 minutes to facilitate volume changes in the heart. Other recommendations include increasing activity when tachycardia occurs to eliminate the initiation of extra, ineffective beats; make up for reduced cardiac output; and lower levels of catecholamines. To relax or decrease shortness of breath, the nurse instructs the client to breathe deeply and slowly and then exhale through pursed lips. Client teaching also includes instructions to avoid caffeinated beverages and over-the-counter medications that contain stimulating chemicals to avoid contributing to an already rapid heart rate. If hypertension is not a problem, the nurse encourages the client to drink adequate fluids and continue moderate use of salt to maintain intravascular fluid volume. Alcohol is discouraged, however, because of its dehydrating effects and because withdrawal after chronic use can cause cardiac stimulation. The nurse warns clients who are prescribed minor tranquilizers not to stop the medication abruptly or they may experience stimulating withdrawal symptoms. Additional nursing management depends on other assessment data. (See Nursing Care Plan 24-1.)

>>> ***Stop, Think, and Respond 24-2***

Explain why clients with valvular disorders may need exercise modifications.

KEY POINTS

- Four cardiac valves: promote the forward circulation of blood to sustain adequate cardiac output
  - Aortic: (semilunar valve) has three cusps. The left ventricle pumps blood from the heart through the aortic valve. When the left ventricle contracts, the aortic valve opens to allow the unrestricted passage of oxygenated blood into the arterial vascular system.
  - Mitral: lies between the left atrium and left ventricle, it is a bicuspid valve. It opens to allow oxygenated blood to fill the left ventricle and closes tightly to prevent blood from reentering the left atrium after the left ventricle is filled.
  - Tricuspid: is located between the right atrium and right ventricle. Its role is to make sure blood flows in a forward direction from the right atrium to the ventricle.
  - Pulmonic: is located in the right ventricle of the heart. It prevents regurgitation of deoxygenated blood from the pulmonary artery back to the right ventricle. It is a semilunar valve with three cusps.
- Disorders that commonly affect heart valves:
  - **Stenosis** is a narrowing of the opening in the aortic valve when the valve cusps become stiff and rigid. **Treatment:** stenosis that causes any symptoms (particularly shortness of breath on exertion, angina, or fainting), or if the valve begins to fail, then it is replaced. Replacement of the abnormal valve is the best treatment for nearly everyone, and the prognosis after valve replacement is excellent.
  - **Regurgitation** occurs when the aortic valve does not close tightly, and blood can leak backward. **Treatment**: Sometimes valve repair or replacement. If regurgitation is mild, no specific treatment may be required. However, the regurgitation may gradually worsen, so echocardiography is done periodically to help determine whether surgery becomes necessary. Surgery must be done before the heart muscle becomes permanently weakened.
  - **Valve prolapse**, the valve cusps enlarge, become floppy, and bulge backward into the left atrium. **Treatment**: Sometimes beta-blockers. Most people with valve prolapse do not need treatment. If the heart is beating too fast, a beta-blocker may be taken to slow the heart rate and to reduce palpitations and other symptoms

CRITICAL THINKING EXERCISES

1. Compare and contrast stenosis and regurgitation of the aortic and mitral valves.
2. You are assisting a newly admitted client with a diagnosis of mitral stenosis into his hospital room. The person in the next bed is diagnosed with tracheobronchitis, has a humidifier at the bedside, and receives frequent aerosol breathing treatments. What is the potential problem? What measures are appropriate to correct it?
3. What effect would the administration of a vasodilator, such as nitroglycerin, have on a client with aortic stenosis?
4. Explain why angina, syncope, and exertional dyspnea are common symptoms of aortic stenosis.

NCLEX-STYLE REVIEW QUESTIONS PrepU

1. Arrange the following valves in the order that blood circulates from the right to the left side of the heart:
   1. Aortic valve
   2. Pulmonic valve
   3. Mitral valve
   4. Tricuspid valve
2. A client with aortic stenosis is most at risk for which one of the following problems?
   1. Falls
   2. Impaired skin
   3. Muscle atrophy
   4. Dehydration

3. For which assessment should the nurse withhold a beta-blocker such as atenolol (Tenormin) when caring for a client with a valvular disorder of the heart?
  1. The client's systolic BP is 150 mm Hg.
  2. The client's heart rate is 56 beats/min.
  3. The client has an S_2 heart sound.
  4. The client's heart rhythm is irregular.

4. What topics would the nurse include in teaching the client with aortic regurgitation? Select all that apply.
  1. An exercise plan for weight loss
  2. Reasons for antibiotic therapy
  3. Elevate the legs to relieve chest pain
  4. Assess BP regularly
  5. Methods to control hypertension

5. When taking a history from a client with mitral valve prolapse, what assessment data characterize the chest pain the client experiences? Select all that apply.
  1. Chest pain occurs without exertion.
  2. Chest pain radiates to the jaw.
  3. Chest pain is prolonged in duration.
  4. Chest pain is aggravated by stress.
  5. Chest pain is easily relieved by rest.

6. What is the nurse most likely to detect when assessing the chest of a client diagnosed with mitral valve prolapse?
  1. A clicking sound during systole
  2. Heart rate less than 60 beats/min
  3. Moist breath sounds on inspiration
  4. Respiratory rate less than 12 breaths/min

WANT TO KNOW MORE? There are a wide variety of online resources available on thePoint to enhance learning and understanding of this chapter.

Go to thePoint.lww.com/activate and use the activation code found in the front of this text to unlock these online resources.

25 Caring for Clients With Disorders of Coronary and Peripheral Blood Vessels

Words To Know

acute coronary syndrome
aneurysm
angina pectoris
angiogenesis
ankle-brachial index
arteriosclerosis
atherectomy
atheroma
atherosclerosis
bruit
cardiac rehabilitation
cholesterol
collateral circulation
coronary artery disease
coronary occlusion
coronary stent
coronary thrombosis
critical limb ischemia
electron beam computed tomography
embolus
enhanced external counterpulsation
high-density lipoprotein
homocysteine
hyperlipidemia
infarct
intermittent claudication
ischemia
isoenzyme
laser angioplasty
lipid profile
low-density lipoprotein
myocardial infarction
percutaneous transluminal coronary angioplasty
peripheral vascular disease
phlebothrombosis
phytoestrogens
plaque
subendocardial infarction
thrombolytic agents
thrombophlebitis
thrombosis
thrombus
topical hyperbaric oxygen
transmural infarction
transmyocardial revascularization

Learning Objectives

On completion of this chapter, you will be able to:

1. Distinguish between arteriosclerosis and atherosclerosis.
2. List risk factors associated with coronary artery disease and discuss which can be modified.
3. Describe the symptoms, diagnosis, treatment, and nursing management of coronary artery disease.
4. Discuss the symptoms, diagnosis, treatment, and nursing management of myocardial infarction.
5. Discuss the symptoms, diagnosis, treatment, and nursing management of peripheral vascular diseases such as peripheral artery disease, Raynaud syndrome, thrombosis, phlebothrombosis, embolism, and venous insufficiency.
6. Discuss the symptoms, diagnosis, and treatment of varicose veins.
7. Describe nursing management of clients undergoing surgery for varicose veins.
8. Discuss the symptoms, diagnosis, treatment, and nursing management of clients with an aortic aneurysm.

Cardiovascular disease (CVD) is the leading cause of death in the United States. Occlusive disorders of the coronary arteries and resulting complications are largely responsible for cardiac deaths. Occlusive disorders of peripheral blood vessels also contribute to morbidity and mortality. The most common causes of occlusive vascular diseases are arteriosclerosis, atherosclerosis, clot formation, and vascular spasm. Venous insufficiency and valvular incompetence also foster peripheral vascular disorders. This chapter discusses a variety of conditions that affect the coronary arteries and peripheral blood vessels.

Gerontologic Considerations

- The incidence of arteriosclerosis and other vascular disorders increases with age. General physiologic changes of aging predispose clients to vascular occlusive disease, especially as a result of atherosclerotic plaque formation. In addition, atherosclerosis is the most common cause of peripheral arterial problems in older adults.
- Older adults are more sensitive to the hypotensive effects of nitrates and calcium channel blockers, probably because of impaired venous valves, diminished baroreceptor reflex, and decreased vascular volume. Therefore, these drugs are used with caution.

(continued)

Words To Know (*continued*)
varicose veins
vein ligation
vein stripping
venous insufficiency
venous reflux
venous stasis ulcer

Gerontologic Considerations (*continued*)

- Assessing for orthostatic blood pressure (BP) changes following meals can help identify risk for postprandial hypotension. During digestion, blood flow diverts to the gastrointestinal tract. Peripheral vascular valve closure may be sluggish in older adults, allowing gravity to pull blood volume to the lower extremities, resulting in decreased cerebral blood flow and increased potential for falls.
- Symptoms of myocardial infarction (MI) in older adults can include dyspnea, confusion, syncope, epigastric distress, nausea, heartburn, or indigestion. These symptoms may be unrecognized as significant by older adults, family members, or health care providers, thus causing a delay in treatment.
- Many older adults have peripheral vascular insufficiency that is manifested in weak or absent pedal pulses; cold, clammy feet; thickened toenails; and shiny skin on the lower extremities.
- Discourage older adults from using electric heating devices; burns are more likely to occur because of decreased temperature perception resulting from impaired circulation. Thermal underwear, socks, gloves, and blankets are alternatives to electric blankets and heating pads.

ARTERIOSCLEROSIS

Arteriosclerosis refers to the loss of elasticity or hardening of the arteries that accompanies the aging process. As cells in arterial tissue layers degenerate with age, calcium is deposited in the cytoplasm. The calcium causes the arteries to lose elasticity. As the left ventricle contracts, sending oxygenated blood from the heart, the rigid arterial vessels fail to stretch. The potential result is a reduced volume of oxygenated blood delivered to organs such as the myocardium, brain, kidneys, and extremities.

ATHEROSCLEROSIS

Atherosclerosis is a condition in which the lumen of arteries fills with fatty deposits called **plaque**. The plaque is chiefly composed of **cholesterol**, a fatty (lipid) substance. Atherosclerosis is a more modifiable contributor than arteriosclerosis to vascular disease. Therefore, it is the focus of attention and research into the mechanisms that contribute to plaque formation and its reduction to decrease vascular disease.

Pathophysiology and Etiology

Areas of atherosclerotic research include determining the mechanisms by which lipids are formed and metabolized and the roles that body fat, obesity, and infectious and inflammatory processes may play in contributing to higher risk factors for vascular diseases.

Hyperlipidemia

Hyperlipidemia, or high levels of blood fat, triggers atherosclerotic changes. Factors such as gender, heredity, diet, diseases such as metabolic syndrome (see Chapter 51), and inactivity individually or collectively contribute to hyperlipidemia. For example, some clients are genetically predisposed to produce cells with reduced numbers of receptors for binding with cholesterol; therefore, they are more likely to develop high lipid levels (Evidence-Based Practice 25-1). Clients who consume a high-fat diet may saturate all available cholesterol receptors, which also results in hyperlipidemia. Obese people with metabolic syndrome who are prone to diabetes tend to have lower levels of *leptin*, which regulates energy metabolism, and *adiponectin* a protein with anti-inflammatory effects (López-Jaramillo et al., 2014). Above-normal cholesterol levels also have been linked to a byproduct of methionine, an amino acid present in meat, called **homocysteine**. High levels of homocysteine are also implicated in thickening, narrowing, and scarring of arterial walls.

Infection

A current hypothesis is that atherosclerosis is linked to prior infections with *Chlamydia pneumoniae*, a bacterium that commonly causes respiratory infections (Anderson, 2016). Research has shown that *C. pneumoniae* can infect smooth muscle and endothelial cells of arterial walls. Some evidence suggests that *C. pneumoniae* either accelerates the atherosclerotic process or destabilizes one that already exists, leading to an area of local inflammation. The results of blood tests such as highly sensitive C-reactive protein (hs-CRP) levels and white blood cell (WBC) counts, which reflect inflammation and infection, are elevated among clients hospitalized for coronary events. An elevated high-sensitivity C-reactive protein, also called ultrasensitive CRP, level (Box 25-1) recently has been added as a predictive cardiac risk factor especially for women.

Recently conducted large clinical trials support the *C. pneumoniae* hypothesis and also suggest a connection between atheromatous plaque formation and other infectious microorganisms such as *Helicobacter pylori*, herpes simplex virus, and cytomegalovirus (Charakida & Tousoulis, 2013). However, studies have not shown that antibiotic therapy plays a significant role in secondary prevention or improving long-term outcomes.

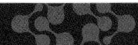

Evidence-Based Practice 25-1

Risk for Cardiovascular Disease in Postmenopausal Women

Clinical Question

Are women more at risk for CVD after menopause?

Evidence

The updated 2019 American College of Cardiology (ACC)/American Heart Association (AHA) Guideline on the Primary Prevention of CVD highlights the concern of an increase in CVD risk for women, which includes early menopause and preeclampsia (*American Journal of Preventative Cardiology*, 2020). "Additionally, other female-specific risk factors including early menarche, polycystic ovarian syndrome, multi-parity, other adverse pregnancy outcomes, and hormone therapy also influence women's CVD risk throughout their lifespan" (Elder, Sharma, Gulati, & Michos, 2020). "CVD risk accelerates after menopause due to withdrawal of endogenous estradiol levels, which can worsen many traditional CVD risk factors including body fat distribution, impairment of glucose tolerance, adverse changes in lipid profile, elevations in BP, endothelial dysfunction and increased sympathetic tone, which all have detrimental effects on arterial/cardiovascular function" (Rosano, Vitale, Marazzi, & Volterrani, 2007).

Nursing Implications

Nurses can use this evidence in their assessment and education practice with women populations that are of menopause age. Knowing the risk for women, good assessment skills, reporting BP findings, educating the client about risks, and monitoring signs and symptoms are important aspects of care.

Reference
Elder, P., Sharma, G., Gulati, M., & Michos, E. D. (2020). Identification of female-specific risk enhancers throughout the lifespan of women to improve cardiovascular disease prevention. *American Journal of Preventive Cardiology, 2*, 100028. https://doi.org/10.1016/j.ajpc.2020.100028Rosano, G. M., Vitale, C., Marazzi, G., & Volterrani, M. (2007). Menopause and cardiovascular disease: The evidence. *Climacteric, 10* (Suppl 1), 19–24. https://doi.org/10.1080/13697130601114917

Inflammation

2019 ACC/AHA Guideline on the Primary Prevention of CVD indicates a relationship between body fat and the production of inflammatory and thrombotic (clot-facilitating) proteins. Researchers are finding that fatty tissue releases proinflammatory proteins: interleukin 6, tumor necrosis factor-alpha, and a third protein known as plasminogen activator inhibitor-1. The first pair of proteins is believed to promote the buildup of atherosclerotic plaque in blood vessels. The third interferes with the body's ability to dissolve blood clots that form within the vessels. This information suggests that decreasing obesity and body fat stores via exercise, dietary modification, or developing drugs that target proinflammatory proteins may reduce risk factors for heart disease.

BOX 25-1 Cardiac Risk Based on Highly Sensitive C-Reactive Protein Test

HS-CRP (MG/L)	RISK FOR CARDIOVASCULAR DISEASE
Less than 1.0	Low
1.0–2.9	Intermediate
Greater than 3.0	High

The Centers for Disease Control and Prevention recommend checking two separate hs-CRP levels approximately 2 weeks apart and using the average of the two measurements.

Effect of Multiple Factors

Currently, it is safe to assume that multiple factors contribute to arteriovascular disease. A client with elevated lipid levels who also has other risk factors (cigarette smoking, stressful lifestyle, obesity, diabetes mellitus, hypertension, or previous infection with *C. pneumoniae* or other microorganisms) is predisposed to the accelerated accumulation of fatty plaque beneath the intimal layer of the arteries.

When lipids accumulate, they are deposited under the endothelial cells of the tunica intima. The enlarging lesion elevates the endothelium of the artery wall and narrows the lumen (Fig. 25-1). Atherosclerotic vessels cannot produce endothelial-derived relaxing factors, which impairs the ability of the artery to dilate. As the subendothelial **atheroma** enlarges, the intimal layer may split and expose the lesion. As blood flows through the vessel, platelets become trapped in the roughened wall and initiate the clotting cascade. When the clot develops in a coronary artery, the resulting condition is called **coronary thrombosis**.

OCCLUSIVE DISORDERS OF CORONARY BLOOD VESSELS

Coronary occlusion is the closing of a coronary artery, which reduces or totally interrupts blood supply to the distal muscle area. Coronary artery disease (CAD) precedes coronary occlusion, which, if untreated, leads to **myocardial infarction** (MI), which laypersons refer to as a heart attack. Symptoms usually do not occur until at least 60% of the arterial lumen is occluded.

Coronary Artery Disease

CAD refers to arteriosclerotic and atherosclerotic changes in the coronary arteries supplying the myocardium. It may not be diagnosed until clients are in late middle age or older, but the vascular changes most likely begin much earlier. Although CAD occurs 10 to 15 years earlier in men than in women, the incidence rises in postmenopausal women

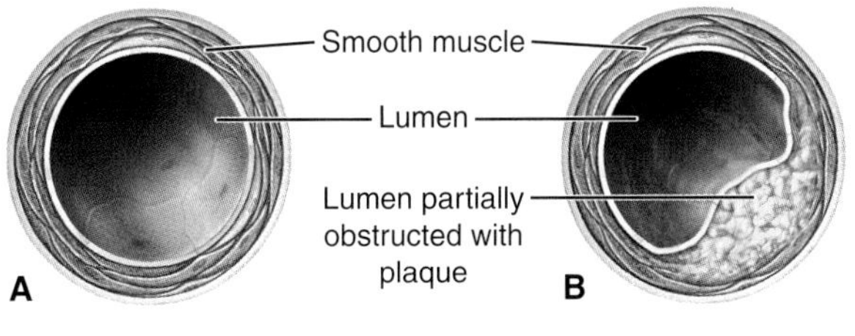

Figure 25-1 (A) Cross-section of a normal artery in which the lumen is fully patent or open. **(B)** Cross-section of an atherosclerotic artery.

BOX 25-2 Risk Factors for Coronary Artery Disease

Inherited	
Male sex	Genetic predisposition
Diabetes mellitus	Hypertension
Increased lipid levels	
Behavioral	
Smoking	Competitive, aggressive personality
Sedentary lifestyle	
Obesity	High-fat diet

and becomes similar to that in men thereafter. Women with a family history of cardiac disease show symptoms 7 years earlier than women with no family history. In a presentation at the AHA Scientific Session in Orlando, Florida, William Herzog, a cardiologist on staff at Johns Hopkins Hospital, reported that women who smoke are symptomatic 9 years earlier than nonsmokers who are women and 4 years earlier than smokers who are men, suggesting that women who smoke have a greater gender susceptibility to CAD.

Pathophysiology and Etiology

CAD results from many factors rather than a single cause. Several inherited and behavioral risk factors contribute to the development of CAD (Box 25-2).

At rest, ample blood flow may be maintained despite considerable CAD. The condition may go unrecognized, particularly among those with a sedentary lifestyle. During situations that increase myocardial oxygen demand (i.e., exercise, emotional stress), however, the compromised coronary arteries cannot adequately oxygenate the myocardium. When the myocardial tissue becomes *ischemic* (deprived of oxygen), clinical manifestations of CAD, such as **angina pectoris** (chest pain of cardiac origin), occur. Death of heart muscle does not accompany angina.

Assessment Findings

Signs and Symptoms

In mild CAD, clients are asymptomatic or complain of fatigue. The classical symptom is chest pain (angina pectoris) or discomfort during activity or stress. Such pain or discomfort typically is manifested as sudden pain or pressure that may be centered over the heart (precordial) or under the sternum (substernal). The pain may radiate to the shoulders and arms, especially on the left side, or to the jaw, neck, or teeth (Fig. 25-2). Some clients, especially women, experience more atypical symptoms such as nausea, fatigue, and dizziness, which are often overlooked as significant for heart disease and consequently go misdiagnosed. Some describe discomfort other than pain, such as indigestion or a burning, squeezing, or crushing tightness in the upper chest or throat. Table 25-1 highlights various types of angina. The AHA now suggests the term **acute coronary syndrome** to describe any group of clinical symptoms compatible with acute myocardial **ischemia** (impaired oxygenation).

Some clients show signs suggesting hyperlipidemia. They may be obese and hypertensive. A person who is obese with an apple-shaped body (carries most weight in the abdomen) is at higher risk for CAD than one with a pear-shaped body (carries most weight below the hips). The pulse may be high at rest and become irregular with exercise. An opaque

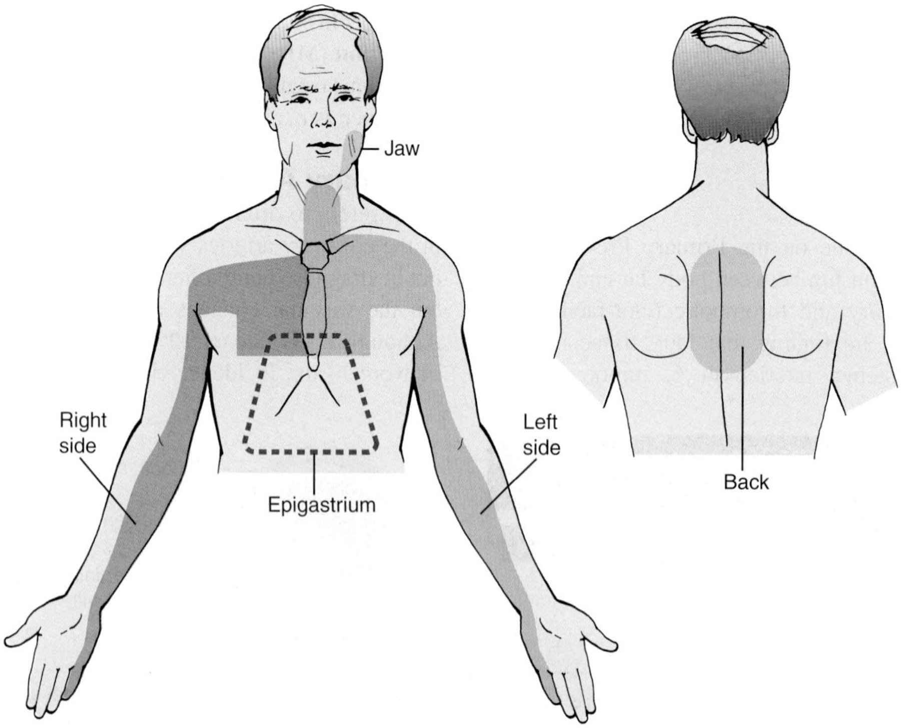

Figure 25-2 Pain patterns with myocardial ischemia. *Blue* indicates usual distribution of pain with myocardial ischemia.

TABLE 25-1 Types of Angina

	STABLE ANGINA	UNSTABLE ANGINA	VARIANT (PRINZMETAL) ANGINA	MICROVASCULAR ANGINA (CARDIAC SYNDROME X)
Causes	75% coronary occlusion that accompanies exertion Elevated heart rate or BP Eating a large meal	Progressive worsening of stable angina, with more than 90% coronary occlusion	Arterial spasm in normal or diseased coronary arteries	Constriction of myocardial capillaries too small for standard cardiac tests to detect
Symptoms	Chest pain that lasts 15 minutes or less and may radiate Similar pain severity, frequency, and duration with each episode	Chest pain of increased frequency, severity, and duration poorly relieved by rest or oral nitrates Client at risk of MI within 18 months of angina's onset	Chest pain that occurs at rest (usually between 12 and 8 a.m.), is sporadic over 3–6 months, and diminishes over time; ST elevation rather than depression on ECG	Prolonged chest pain that accompanies exercise and is not always relieved by medication
Treatment	Rest, sublingual nitrates, antihypertensives, lifestyle changes	Sedation, IV nitroglycerin, oxygen, antihypertensives, anticoagulant or antiplatelet therapy, revascularization procedures	Nitrates or calcium channel blockers	Heart-healthy habits and trials with medications like a nitrate, beta-blocker, or calcium channel blocker

BP, blood pressure; ECG, electrocardiogram; IV, intravenous; MI, myocardial infarction.

white ring about the periphery of the cornea, called *arcus senilis* (Fig. 25-3), results from a deposit of fat granules but may be apparent only in older adults. *Xanthelasma*, a raised yellow plaque on the skin of the upper and lower eyelids (Fig. 25-4), suggests lipid accumulation. Although research is ongoing, some cardiologists indicate a relationship between a diagonal crease in the earlobe and the risk for CAD (Fig. 25-5; www.heathline.com).

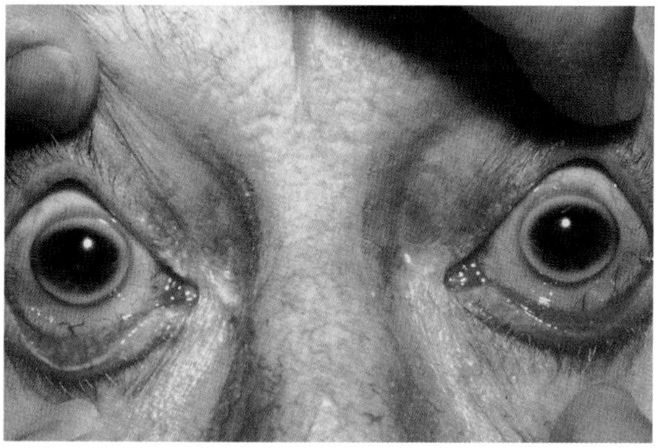

Figure 25-3 Arcus senilis, an opaque ring in the periphery of the cornea, is a sign of systemic fat deposits. (Courtesy of Patrick J. Saine, CRA.)

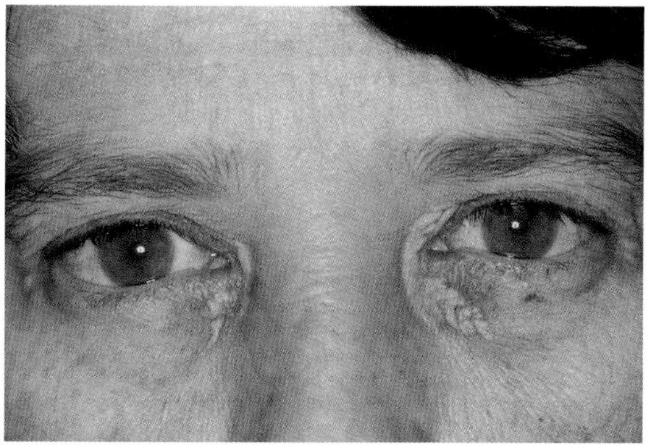

Figure 25-4 Xanthelasma, yellowish plaques about the eyelids, is a sign of lipid accumulation. (Courtesy of Patrick J. Saine, CRA.)

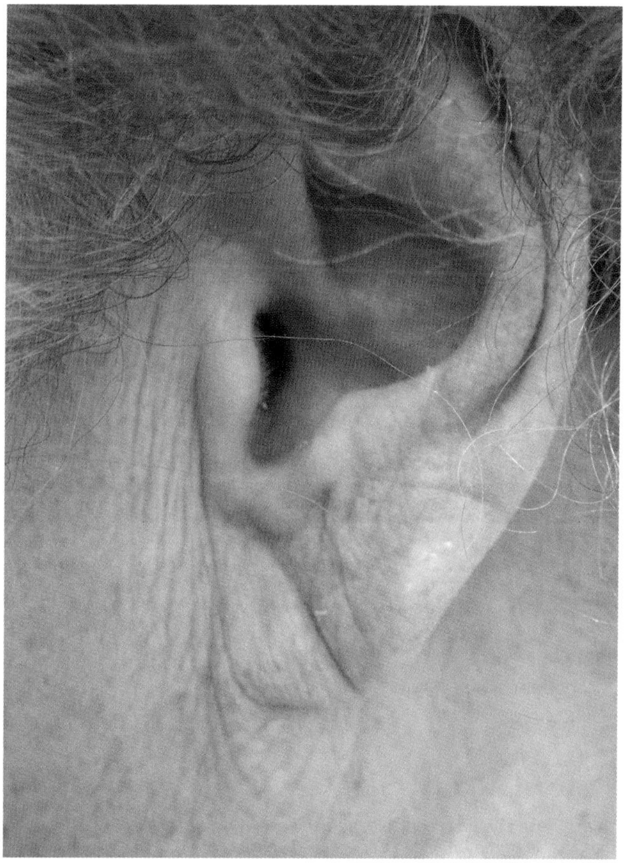

Figure 25-5 The presence of a bilateral diagonal earlobe crease is associated with coronary artery disease. (Photo by Ken Timby.)

Diagnostic Findings

Diagnosis of CAD is a composite of lipid profile studies and electron beam computed tomography (EBCT; discussed later) as well as exercise electrocardiography, cardiac catheterization, and arteriography, all of which are discussed in Chapter 22. Electrocardiogram (ECG) or stress testing may reveal ST-segment depression, arrhythmias, or exercise-induced hypertension. A nuclear stress test using a radionuclide such as thallium may be injected intravenously during and a few hours after exercise electrocardiography followed by a heart scan. Narrowing of one or more coronary arteries is documented during coronary arteriography.

Lipid Profile Studies A **lipid profile** is a group of tests that measure various blood fats. It is one indicator of a person's risk for cardiac and vascular disease. A lipid profile generally consists of measuring total serum cholesterol, low-density lipoprotein (LDL) cholesterol, high-density lipoprotein (HDL) cholesterol, and triglycerides. Cardiac risk increases when the level of total serum cholesterol is elevated. Another risk factor is an elevation of triglycerides, which are chains of fatty acids.

Proteins transport lipids (cholesterol) in the blood. **Low-density lipoprotein** (LDL) has a lower ratio of protein to cholesterol; **high-density lipoprotein** (HDL) is just the opposite—it has a higher ratio of protein to cholesterol. In clients with CAD, the level of LDL, which sometimes is referred to as "bad cholesterol" because it sticks to arteries, exceeds recommended amounts. The level of HDL, called "good cholesterol" because it carries cholesterol to the liver for removal, is lower than desirable (Table 25-2).

Cardiac risk can be estimated by dividing the total serum cholesterol level by the HDL level; a result greater than 5 suggests a potential for CAD. Depending on an assessment of risk factors, treatment for hyperlipidemia may begin when the LDL level ranges between 100 mg/dL and 130 mg/dL, with the goal being a level below 100 mg/dL.

››› *Stop, Think, and Respond 25-1*

Although the recommended total cholesterol level is below 200 mg/dL, determine which client has the lowest cardiac risk by dividing total cholesterol level by HDL level and explain your answer.

- *Client A: Total cholesterol level is 224 mg/dL; HDL level is 38 mg/dL.*
- *Client B: Total cholesterol level is 198 mg/dL; HDL level is 35 mg/dL.*
- *Client C: Total cholesterol level is 210 mg/dL; HDL level is 55 mg/dL.*

Electron Beam Computed Tomography **Electron beam computed tomography** (EBCT) is a radiologic test that produces X-rays of the coronary arteries using an electron beam. This noninvasive test can scan the heart in 1/20th of a second using 10 times less exposure to radiation than that of mechanical computed tomography (CT) machines. EBCT also produces much clearer images for diagnostic purposes. The advantage of EBCT is that it can detect and quantify calcified plaque in the coronary arteries before clients who do not fit the usual cardiac risk profile are symptomatic. There is a high degree of correlation between the amount of calcium plaque identified by EBCT and the future risk of MI. If the test results demonstrate the existence of heart disease, treatment interventions are instituted earlier than with conventional diagnostic regimens. The efficacy of treatment or the need to modify it is evaluated by repeating the test at 1-year or longer intervals.

Medical and Surgical Management

The first line of defense for managing CAD consists of lifestyle changes such as smoking cessation, weight loss, stress management, and exercise. Blood glucose is kept regulated. When these methods are inadequate, drug therapy and other noninvasive, nonsurgical, or surgical interventions are indicated.

TABLE 25-2 Cardiac Risk Associated With Blood Fat Levels

	TOTAL CHOLESTEROL	HDL CHOLESTEROL	LDL CHOLESTEROL	TRIGLYCERIDES
Good	Less than 200 (but the lower the better)	Ideal is 60 or higher; 40 or higher for men and 50 or higher for women is acceptable	Less than 100; below 70 if coronary artery disease is present	Less than 149; ideal is <100
Borderline to moderately elevated	200–239	n/a	130–159	150–199
High	240 or higher	60 or higher	160 or higher; 190 considered very high	200 or higher; 500 considered very high
Low	n/a	Less than 40	n/a	n/a

Note: These are the acceptable, borderline, and high measurements for adults, according to the 2018 guidelines on blood cholesterol management published in the *Journal of the American College of Cardiology* (JACC).
All values are in milligrams per deciliter (mg/dL) and are based on fasting measurements.
HDL, high-density lipoprotein; LDL, low-density lipoprotein.
Healthline. (n.d.). *The recommended cholesterol levels by age.* https://www.healthline.com/health/high-cholesterol/levels-by-age#

Drug Therapy

Drug therapy includes medications that produce arterial vasodilation, such as nitrates (e.g., nitroglycerin, isosorbide dinitrate). Beta-adrenergic blockers, which decrease consumption of myocardial oxygen by reducing heart rate, also are used. Calcium channel blockers may be used as well, although research has shown that they may be less beneficial than beta-adrenergic blockers (Drug Therapy Table 25-1). Drugs such as

DRUG THERAPY TABLE 25-1 Agents Used to Treat Coronary Artery Disease and Myocardial Infarction

Category and Common Generic (Brand) Drugs	Intended Use	Common Side Effects	Safety Warnings for Nurses
Vasodilators			
Isosorbide (Isordil) Nitroglycerin (Nitrostat)	Relieve chest pain by dilating coronary arteries, helps to reestablish blood flow around thrombus	Headache, dizziness, orthostatic hypotension, tachycardia, flushing	• Increased fall risk due to hypotensive side effects • Do not use with head trauma client • Do not use with erectile dysfunction drugs
Beta-Adrenergic Blockers			
Atenolol (Tenormin) Metoprolol (Lopressor) Propranolol (Inderal) Timolol	Reduce heart rate and decrease consumption of oxygen by myocardium, helps to prevent angina attacks	Headache, dizziness, nausea, vomiting	• When given IV, constant cardiac monitoring is required • Drug is usually held if heart rate <60–120> • Initially, monitor blood every 2–3 weeks for agranulocytosis
Thrombolytics			
Alteplase (Activase) Reteplase (Retavase) Tenecteplase (TNKase)	Reestablish blood flow to ischemic areas by dissolving thrombi	Cardiac dysrhythmias, hypotension, bleeding at venous or arterial access sites, nausea, vomiting	• Monitor increased bleeding when used with anticoagulant • Do not use in client with stroke/bleeding history • Monitor for bleeding of injection sites, orifices, wounds
Anticoagulants and Antiplatelet Agents			
Heparin	Thrombosis/embolism, diagnosis and treatment by blocking the conversion of prothrombin/fibrinogen to form clots in vessels	Bleeding, chills, fever, urticaria, local irritation, erythema, mild pain, hematoma, or bruising at the injection site	• Typical dose in thousand unit increments • Monitor aPTT frequently to maintain blood level • Monitor for bleeding of injection sites, orifices, wounds • Antidote Protamine should be readily available
Clopidogrel (Plavix)	Thrombus prevention by inhibiting platelet aggregation and clotting	Dizziness, skin rash, chest pain, constipation	• Do not use PPI with this drug • Do not take aspirin or NSAIDs as a pain reliever • Monitor for bleeding of injection sites, orifices, wounds
Salicylates Aspirin (Ecotrin, Ascriptin)	MI prevention by inhibiting platelet aggregation and clotting	Nausea, vomiting, epigastric distress	• Monitor for tinnitus, indicates toxicity • Should not be taken as a pain reliever when on anticoagulant therapy
Calcium Channel Blockers			
Amlodipine (Norvasc) Diltiazem (Cardizem) Nifedipine (Procardia) Verapamil (Calan)	Relieve angina by dilating arteries, improving myocardium blood supply, and reduces myocardial oxygen demand	Hypotension, dizziness, nausea, dry cough	• When given IV, constant cardiac monitoring is required • Drug is usually held if heart rate <60–120> • No grapefruit • Initially, monitor blood every 2–3 weeks for agranulocytosis
HMG-CoA Reductase Inhibitors (Statins)			
Atorvastatin (Lipitor) Rosuvastatin (Crestor) Simvastatin (Zocor)	Inhibit the manufacture of cholesterol which increases the integrity of vessels following cardiac procedures	Dizziness, headache, constipation	• Wear protective clothing and sunscreen due to photosensitivity • Monitor enzymes if preexisting hepatic disease • No grapefruit • Unusual muscle pain may indicate rhabdomyolysis • Women need to use effective birth control
Diuretics			
Furosemide (Lasix)	Decrease work of the heart by promoting excretion of sodium and water, thus reducing circulating blood volume	Dizziness, dehydration, nausea, diarrhea, nocturia, polyuria, orthostatic hypotension	• Monitor serum potassium • Increased fall risk owing to hypotensive side effects • Encourage fluids to prevent dehydration

aPTT, activated partial thromboplastin time; HMG-CoA, 3-hydroxy-3-methylglutaryl coenzyme A; IV, intravenous; MI, myocardial infarction; NSAIDs, nonsteroidal anti-inflammatory drugs; PPI, proton pump inhibitors angiotensin-converting enzyme inhibitors and diuretics, as well as stress management, are used to control hypertension. Nicotinic acid (niacin) in pharmacologic doses (i.e., not the dosage in multivitamins) helps increase HDL and lower LDL. Daily intake of food sources or supplements of folate or folic acid, vitamin B_6 (pyridoxine), and vitamin B_{12} (cyanocobalamin) reduce homocysteine levels; however, available evidence is not sufficient to recommend folate and other vitamin B supplements as a means to reduce CVD risk, according to the AHA.

Pharmacologic Considerations

- Ubiquinone, also known as coenzyme Q10 (CoQ10), is a *nutraceutical* (dietary supplement that provides health benefits). CoQ10 is an antioxidant synthesized from food sources to produce mitochondrial ATP production in all cells, but especially in muscle tissue. The administration of cholesterol-lowering drugs like "statins" inhibits the formation of CoQ10. When depleted, those taking a statin may experience myalgia (muscle pain). Supplementing 100 to 200 mg of CoQ10 daily while taking a statin medication is believed to decrease the incidence of muscle pain.

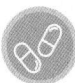

Pharmacologic Considerations

- Sublingual nitroglycerin is placed under the tongue for acute relief of angina pectoris. A transdermal nitroglycerin patch is for the prevention of angina pectoris. Nitroglycerin transdermal patches are typically applied for 12 to 14 hours, and then removed for the same amount of time.
- When removing a patch, close the adhesive edges together, preventing accidental exposure to others. Teach clients to dispose of patches away from children and pets.

If weight loss, diet, and exercise are not successful in lowering elevated cholesterol and triglyceride levels, drugs may be used to prevent further plaque formation. Lipid-lowering drugs such as 3-hydroxy-3-methylglutaryl coenzyme A (HMG-CoA) reductase inhibitors, known as *statins*, and bile acid sequestrants may be prescribed. Fibric acid agents such as gemfibrozil (Lopid) are used to decrease triglycerides. Some primary providers advise taking one aspirin (325 mg) or low-dose aspirin (81 mg) tablet daily to prevent thrombi from developing. Because soy products are classified as **phytoestrogens**, plant sources of estrogen, some clients are increasing consumption of soy as a cardioprotective strategy, although evidence of benefits from soy protein is minimal.

Reverse Lipid Transport

Reverse lipid transport is a new form of treatment. Researchers have developed synthetic HDL (ApoA-I Milano), an investigational drug, using recombinant DNA techniques from a variant protein obtained from the genes of a group of people living in Milan, Italy. Those people with the variant form of apolipoprotein A-1, a component of HDL, have a low rate of CVD. Research participants in recent clinical trials demonstrated a rapid decrease of plaque in diseased arteries, suggesting that the substance has the potential to reverse CAD (Kallend et al., 2015). Research and development continue with recombinant versions of ApoA-I Milano.

Another approach in reverse lipid transport that is under study is HDL selective delipidation, a procedure in which plasma is withdrawn, processed in such a way as to modify the HDL into "super HDL," and reinfused into the client to reverse plaque formation (Schaefer, 2010).

››› Stop, Think, and Respond 25-2

If a person with a family history of CAD asked how to reduce the risk of developing a similar problem, what information might you provide?

Enhanced External Counterpulsation

Enhanced external counterpulsation (EECP) may be used as an adjunct to drug therapy and lifestyle modifications. This fairly new, noninvasive, and nonsurgical approach helps relieve angina. It requires 1- to 2-hour sessions in the primary provider's office, 5 days a week for approximately 7 weeks. During EECP, the client puts on a pressure suit with pneumatic cuffs at the upper and lower thighs and calves. The cuffs are connected to a cardiac monitor and are sequentially inflated in a wavelike fashion from the calves to the upper thighs during ventricular diastole (resting; Fig. 25-6). The cuff pulsation, which has been compared to a "strong hug," moves blood toward the heart. Because the coronary arteries fill during ventricular diastole when the aortic valve closes, cuff inflation increases perfusion of the coronary arteries with oxygenated blood. When the cuffs deflate during ventricular systole (contraction), the left ventricle's work is reduced because there is less resistance. A number of randomized control studies have found that EECP promotes the development of **collateral circulation**, accessory vascular pathways for blood, through **angiogenesis** (formation of new blood vessels), reduces inflammatory activity, and improves endothelial function (Choudary, 2015; Wu et al., 2012).

Advantages of EECP are that it reduces the frequency of angina and improves exercise tolerance. Disadvantages are that EECP is time-consuming and few primary providers offer or refer clients for it. Some believe that lack of interest from primary providers is related to the fact that third-party payers can better reimburse them for other less time-consuming treatment modalities.

Invasive Perfusion Techniques

Invasive nonsurgical procedures that can reopen narrowed coronary arteries include percutaneous transluminal coronary angioplasty (PTCA), coronary stent, and atherectomy. Surgical procedures include coronary artery bypass graft (CABG) and transmyocardial revascularization (TMR).

Percutaneous Transluminal Coronary Angioplasty For clients who fit specific criteria, **percutaneous transluminal coronary angioplasty** (PTCA), sometimes referred to as *balloon angioplasty*, is performed. In PTCA, which uses sedation and local anesthesia, a balloon-tipped catheter is inserted through the skin and threaded from a peripheral artery into the diseased coronary artery (Fig. 25-7). While passage

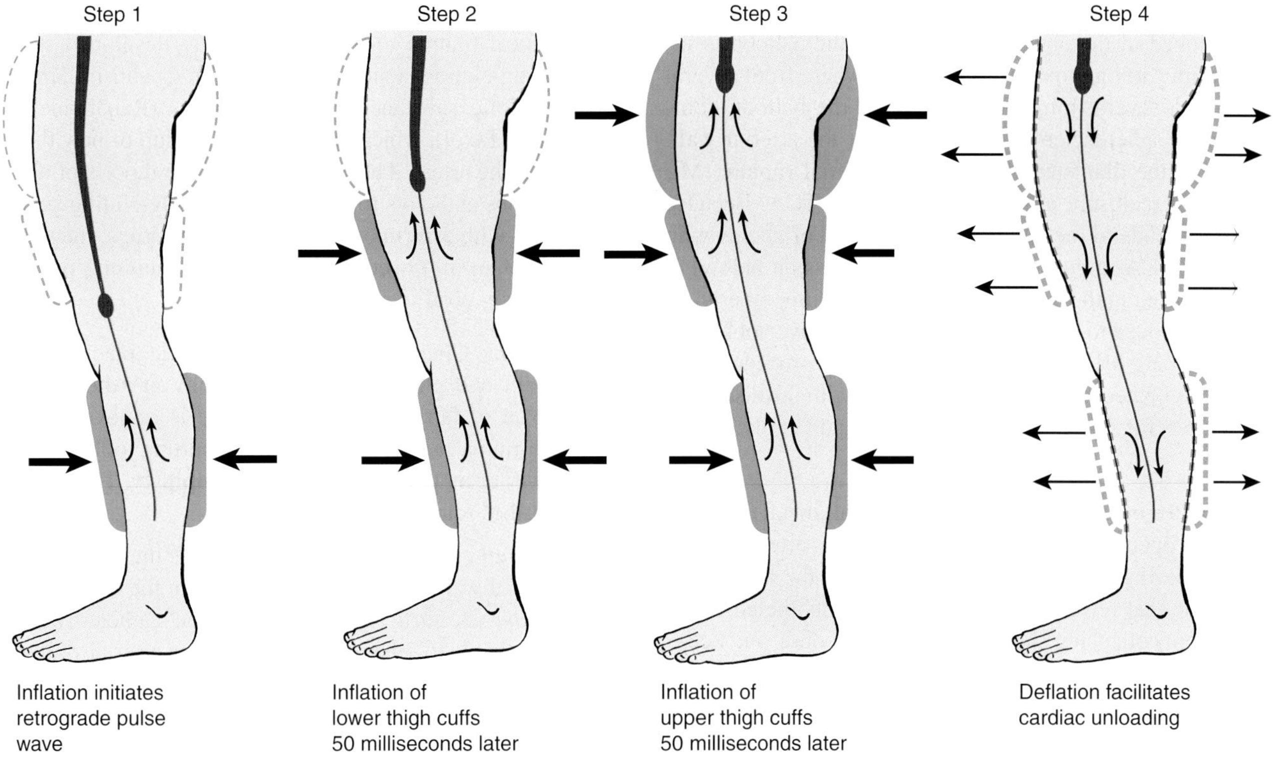

Figure 25-6 Inflation and deflation sequence of enhanced external counterpulsation.

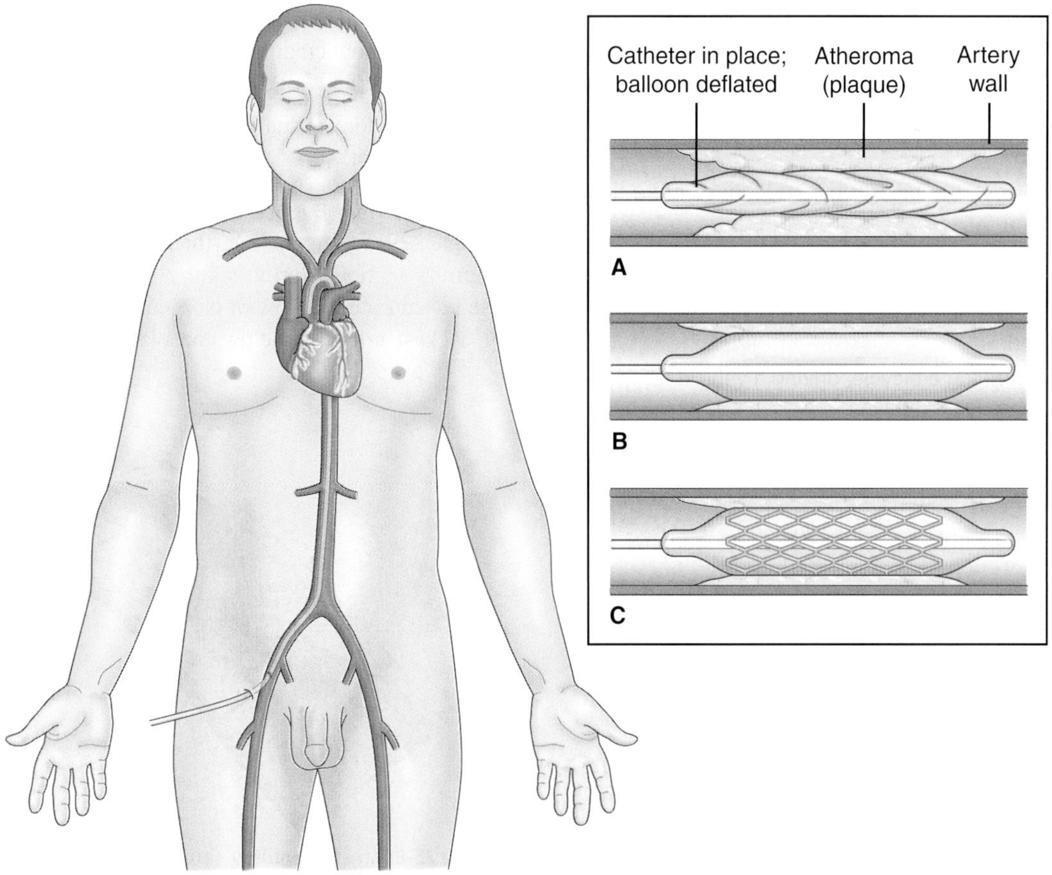

Figure 25-7 Percutaneous transluminal coronary angioplasty (PTCA). **(A)** A balloon-tipped catheter is passed into the affected coronary artery and placed within the area of the atheroma (plaque). **(B)** The balloon is then rapidly inflated and deflated with controlled pressure to compress the atheroma. **(C)** A stent is placed to maintain patency of the artery, and the balloon is removed.

of the catheter is monitored under fluoroscopy, the catheter is positioned in the area of stenosis, and the balloon is inflated with carbon dioxide (CO_2) for anywhere from several seconds to several minutes. Inflation of the balloon compresses the atherosclerotic plaque against the arterial wall, increasing the diameter of the artery. Arterial rupture, MI, and abrupt reclosure are complications of PTCA. Because the artery tends to reocclude in 40% to 50% of clients who undergo PTCA, a coronary stent (see discussion below) is usually placed in the artery during the procedure; otherwise, PTCA may need to be repeated. Clients who have not had an accompanying MI but have had PTCA or any procedure that uses a percutaneous catheter are provided with the discharge instructions for self-care shown in Client and Family Teaching 25-1.

Coronary Stent A **coronary stent** is a small metal coil with meshlike openings placed in the coronary artery during PTCA (see Fig. 25-7C). The stent prevents the buildup of new tissue that reforms in the artery, prevents the coronary artery from collapsing shortly after the procedure, and keeps the lumen open for a longer period than traditional PTCA alone. The stent remains permanently in the enlarged artery, and endothelial tissue is incorporated into the mesh within 4 to 6 weeks. Restenosis usually is a problem even with the placement of a stent. Restenosis does not necessarily result from an accelerated atherosclerotic process but from an overgrowth of cells accompanying the inflammation caused by the local trauma to the tissue. Newly developed stents called drug-eluting stents are coated with an anti-inflammatory/antibiotic substance, either sirolimus (Rapamune) or paclitaxel (Taxol), which prevents the buildup of new tissue that clogs the artery. There have been some reports of allergic reactions and clots forming with the drug-eluting stents; but, along with aspirin or other antiplatelet drugs, they continue to be an improved technique for maintaining patency of previously obstructed arteries.

Client and Family Teaching 25-1 Self-Care Following Percutaneous Transluminal Coronary Angioplasty

The nurse provides the following instructions before the client is discharged:

- Avoid lifting more than 10 lb for at least 3 days if the groin was used for catheter insertion. Avoid lifting more than 1 lb for at least 3 days if a site in the upper extremity was used.
- Refrain from riding a bicycle, driving a vehicle, or mowing the lawn for at least 3 days.
- Refrain from sexual activity for 1 week.
- Shower rather than bathe until the cutaneous catheterization site heals.
- Clean the site with soap and water; eliminate any dressing.
- Relieve discomfort at the site with a mild analgesic such as acetaminophen (Tylenol); numbness at the site is temporary and not unusual.
- Expect to see a bruise, which may last 1 to 3 weeks, at the catheter insertion site.
- Report any signs of bleeding, infection, or impaired circulation: fever, swelling, redness, bloody or purulent drainage, acute pain in the extremity, and cold or pale skin.
- Notify the cardiologist immediately if there is pain or tightness in the chest, which could indicate obstructed blood flow through the coronary artery.

Atherectomy Clients whose atherosclerotic plaque is no longer soft and pliable may benefit from an **atherectomy** or removal of fatty plaque. The plaque is removed by either inserting a cardiac catheter with a cutting tool at the tip (Fig. 25-8) or by performing **laser angioplasty**. The following describes four atherectomy options:

- *Directional coronary atherectomy* shaves the plaque from the arterial wall and stores the particles in the catheter.
- *Transluminal extraction* uses a cardiac catheter with a spinning blade to separate plaque from the arterial wall and removes the debris with a vacuum attachment.
- *Percutaneous transluminal catheter rotational ablation* uses a rotating bur that spins at 200,000 revolutions/min. Because the particles of freed plaque are smaller than red blood cells, phagocytes and the lymphatic system remove them.
- *Laser angioplasty* uses short pulses of light that vaporize plaque without creating heat that is intense enough to damage the arterial wall.

Atherectomy usually is followed by PTCA and placement of a stent.

Coronary Artery Bypass Graft Surgery CABG surgery (see Chapter 29) is a technique for revascularizing the myocardium. A section from a healthy leg vein or chest artery is used to reroute the flow of oxygenated blood from the aorta or a chest artery to below the obstruction in the diseased

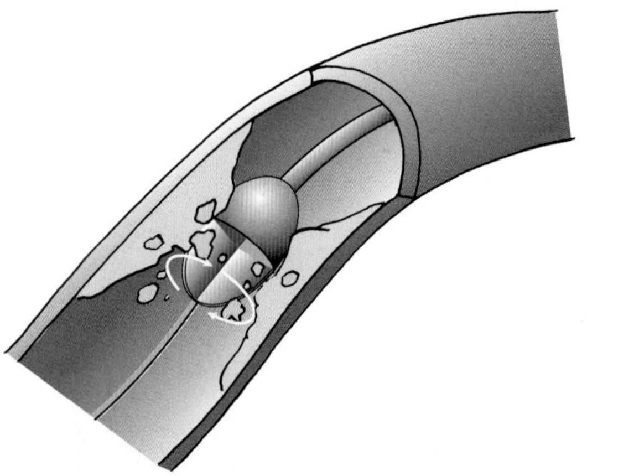

Figure 25-8 An atherectomy catheter removes plaque with either a circular blade or an abrasive material. This type of catheter is effective when plaque is hardened. Soft plaque can be compressed by a balloon catheter.

coronary artery. More than one graft may be necessary if several coronary arteries are occluded. The procedure is performed through a 10- to 12-inch midsternal incision, which is closed with wire, staples, or sutures. The heart is stopped during traditional CABG surgery, but blood is circulated through a heart–lung machine so that oxygen continues to be delivered to cells, tissues, and organs while CO_2 is removed. When the vascular reconnections are completed, heart function is restored. The client remains on a ventilator for approximately 24 hours. It may be several weeks before the client can return to work. Results after CABG surgery tend to last longer than PTCA, stenting, or atherectomy. Chapter 29 provides information about minimally invasive direct coronary artery bypass, an alternative to traditional CABG surgery.

Transmyocardial Revascularization A **transmyocardial revascularization** (TMR) laser procedure, which improves oxygenation of myocardial tissue, may improve quality of life for clients with chest pain that does not respond to medication and who are not candidates for CABG surgery. TMR may be performed for the following reasons:

- The occluded coronary arteries are too narrow or distal to permit catheter insertion.
- There are so many occlusions that risks from a lengthy surgical procedure are unreasonable.
- The client has end-stage (seriously advanced) CAD, which increases the potential for life-threatening complications or death.

To access the heart, a thoracotomy incision is made between ribs on the left side of the chest. While the heart is visualized with transesophageal echocardiography, the laser probe is aimed at the beating heart. The probe makes 15 to 40 channels that are 1-mm deep and 1-cm apart from the epicardium, through the ischemic myocardium, to the endocardium. The channels that the laser creates allow the ischemic myocardium to absorb the oxygenated blood that seeps into the area (Fig. 25-9). Therefore, the myocardium receives oxygen not from a coronary artery but from the blood that seeps into the space between the cells. There are other hypotheses for the mechanism by which TMR relieves the client's symptoms. Some believe that it disrupts the myocardial nerve supply, which suppresses the ability to perceive anginal pain. Others suggest that the trauma stimulates the growth of new blood vessels, which results in additional collateral blood supply to the heart muscle.

Clients remain in the hospital for up to 1 week. Activity is restricted for several weeks to allow a safe period of healing. Because TMR relieves symptoms only, cardiac rehabilitation requires clients to continue to modify risk factors that caused CAD. Such modification means the client must eliminate smoking; follow a heart-healthy diet; and incorporate regular, moderate exercise. Variations in TMR also are being implemented. Sometimes, TMR is performed with a percutaneously inserted catheter.

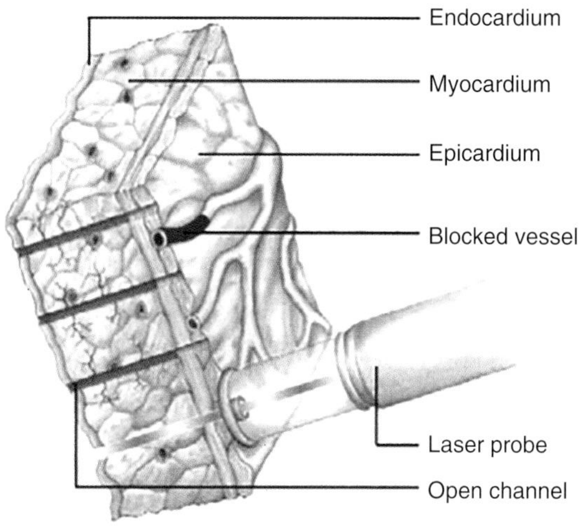

Figure 25-9 Transmyocardial revascularization uses a laser to puncture 1-mm holes in the myocardial to the inner areas of the heart. The holes heal in a matter of minutes but leave the channel open allowing blood to reach the myocardial muscle and stimulate angiogenesis. (Reprinted with permission from Lippincott's Nursing Advisor 2009. Lippincott Williams & Wilkins.)

Nursing Management

The nurse assesses the characteristics of chest pain and administers prescribed drugs that dilate the coronary arteries or reduce the work of the heart. They encourage rest and administer oxygen to improve the available oxygen supply to the heart muscle. If drugs, rest, and oxygen do not relieve the pain, the nurse notifies the primary provider.

The nurse helps clients learn how to reduce modifiable CAD risk factors, which can improve not only cardiac health but also overall well-being. They explain that balancing caloric intake with physical activity to achieve or maintain a healthy body weight can significantly reduce risks. The nurse arranges a consultation with a dietitian and provides written material about a heart-healthy diet (see Nutrition Notes). They refer clients to smoking cessation programs and discuss medications that can help (see Chapter 71).

The nurse teaches about the administration and side effects of antianginal drugs (Client and Family Teaching 25-2). They emphasize that severe, unrelieved chest pain indicates a need to be examined by a primary provider without delay. The nurse advises the client to report changes in the usual pattern of angina, such as increased frequency or severity or occurrence with rest or during sleep.

Nutrition Notes

The Client at Risk for Cardiovascular Disease

- A healthy diet and lifestyle forms the cornerstone of CVD prevention and treatment. The following recommendations for risk reduction are appropriate for all people over the age of 2 years; they may be intensified for clients with established CVD.
- Attain or maintain healthy weight by balancing calorie intake with physical activity. Excess body weight increases

LDL cholesterol levels, blood glucose levels, and BP and lowers HDL levels.

- Consume an overall healthy diet rich in a variety of fruits and vegetables. Fruits and vegetables are rich in vitamins, minerals, and fiber and low in calories.
- Select whole grains for at least half of all grain choices. Whole grains are rich sources of fiber; soluble fiber helps lower LDL cholesterol, and insoluble fibers are associated with lower CVD risk.
- Eat fatty fish at least twice a week. Fatty fish such as salmon, swordfish, and king mackerel provide omega-3 fatty acids that are associated with a reduced risk of both sudden death and death from CAD. Limit the intake of saturated fat, trans fat, and cholesterol by choosing lean meats, using plant proteins, choosing fat-free dairy products, and limiting the intake of partially hydrogenated fats found in stick margarines, shortenings, and commercially baked products. Diets low in saturated fat, trans fat, and cholesterol lower CVD risk mostly by lowering LDL cholesterol.
- Limit food and beverages high in added sugars, such as desserts, candy, and carbonated beverages. Added sugars contain empty calories devoid of nutrients.
- Limit salt intake by eating and preparing foods with little or no salt. Compare sodium in foods like soup, bread, and frozen meals, and choose the foods with lower numbers. Add spices or herbs to season food without adding salt. Generally, as salt intake increases, so does BP.
- Drink alcohol in moderation, if at all. Moderate alcohol intake (less than 1 drink/day for women, 2 drinks/day for men) increases HDL cholesterol levels, but it is not recommended that people begin drinking for the purpose of reducing their risk of CVD.
- Antioxidant supplements, such as those containing vitamins C and E, beta carotene, and selenium, are not recommended because clinical trials have failed to confirm beneficial effects from their use. People are urged to consume dietary sources of antioxidants, such as fruits, vegetables, whole grains, and vegetable oils.

The nurse informs clients about diagnostic tests or treatment procedures. The nurse who prepares the client for invasive, nonsurgical procedures performed with a percutaneous catheter cleanses and removes hair from skin insertion sites (one for the coronary catheter and the other for an arterial line through which BP will be directly monitored). The nurse withholds anticoagulant therapy before the procedure to decrease the chance of hemorrhage. They monitor all vascular sites for bleeding after a procedure and assesses distal pulses. The nurse also observes mental status because cerebral emboli can occur. They monitor urine output and administer analgesics for discomfort. Any of the following data are reported immediately: severe chest pain; abnormal heart rate or rhythm; mental confusion or loss of consciousness; hypotension; urine output of less than 30 to 50 mL/hour; or a cold, pulseless extremity. (See Chapter 29 for the Nursing Process for the Client Undergoing Cardiac or Vascular Surgery.)

Client and Family Teaching 25-2
Use of Short-Acting Nitroglycerin

The nurse discusses the following points with clients who are prescribed short-acting nitroglycerin and their families.

For Sublingual Nitroglycerin:

- Sit down and rest before self-administering nitroglycerin. Decreased activity may relieve chest pain; sitting will prevent injury should the nitroglycerin lower BP and cause fainting.
- Place one nitroglycerin tablet under the tongue if 2 to 3 minutes of rest fails to relieve pain.
- Expect to feel dizzy or flushed or to develop a headache.
- Let the tablet dissolve slowly; there should be slight tingling or burning under the tongue.
- Take a second nitroglycerin tablet in 5 minutes if chest pain is still present.
- Take a third nitroglycerin tablet in 5 more minutes if chest pain is still present.
- Call 911 if chest pain continues; do not drive to an emergency department. Discuss the chest pain with the primary provider if self-management relieved it or its usual characteristics changed.
- Keep a few nitroglycerin tablets in a dark, dry container with you at all times; consult with the pharmacist about a sealed metal container that you can wear around the neck.
- Do not place other medications in the container with the nitroglycerin.
- Replace nitroglycerin tablets every 6 months or after any container has been opened six times.

For Nitroglycerin Spray:

- Assume a sitting position.
- Hold the canister upright.
- Spray the nitroglycerin onto the tongue without inhaling.
- Close the mouth immediately afterward.
- Expect to feel dizzy or flushed or to develop a headache.
- Repeat spraying every 5 minutes for a second and third time if chest pain is unrelieved.
- Call 911 if chest pain continues.
- Discuss the chest pain with the primary provider if self-management relieved it or its usual characteristics changed.
- Expect a new canister of nitroglycerin to deliver approximately 200 doses.
- Check the amount of nitroglycerin in the canister by floating it in a bowl of water; the higher the canister floats, the less medication it contains. Obtain a reserve canister when the present canister shows signs of becoming empty.

Myocardial Infarction

An **infarct** is an area of tissue that dies (*necrosis*) from inadequate oxygenation. An MI, or heart attack, occurs when there is prolonged total occlusion of coronary arterial blood flow. The larger the necrotic area is, the more serious the damage. An infarct that extends through the full thickness of the myocardial wall is called a **transmural infarction** or Q-wave MI. A partial-thickness infarct is called a **subendocardial infarction** or a non-Q-wave MI. Each coronary artery supplies oxygenated blood to a different area of the myocardium. The location of the infarction depends on the area where the blood supply to the myocardium is interrupted by the respective occluded coronary artery (Fig. 25-10).

Pathophysiology and Etiology

The most common cause of MI is **coronary thrombosis**, the consequence of a blood clot located within a coronary artery. **Thrombosis** usually is secondary to arteriosclerotic and atherosclerotic changes. Arterial spasms also may cause an MI. Once an area of the myocardium has been damaged and destroyed, the cells in that area lose their special functions of automaticity, excitability, conductivity, contractility, and rhythmicity. Thus, arrhythmias and heart failure are common consequences (see Chapters 26 and 28).

Injury to the myocardium triggers the inflammatory response. Proinflammatory chemicals disrupt the permeability of cell membranes (see Chapter 12). The damaged cells release serum cardiac markers (intracellular enzymes) and electrolytes into the extracellular fluid. Loss of intracellular potassium and accumulation of lactic acid from anaerobic cellular metabolism affect depolarization and repolarization of myocardial cells. Dangerous arrhythmias can develop during this time because the affected areas are electrically unstable.

The infarction process can take up to 6 hours. There are three zones of tissue damage:

- The first zone consists of a central area of necrotic (dead) myocardial cells.
- The second zone of injured cells, which may live if blood supply to the area is restored, surrounds the first zone.
- The third zone is the ischemic area that will probably survive.

Thrombolytic drugs called clot busters are given during this 6-hour window of opportunity to reestablish blood flow and save as much myocardial tissue as possible.

Leukocytosis and slightly elevated body temperature follow in 3 to 7 days. New capillaries begin to grow to establish collateral circulation to the infarcted area; however, it takes 2 or 3 weeks before such flow is significant. A "cardiac patch" of collagen fibers begins to form within the first 2 weeks of the infarct, but it takes as long as 3 months for the scar to grow firm. The scar tissue is less effective than the myocardium it is replacing; it does not stretch and contract like the original tissue. Lack of resiliency impairs the heart's ability to pump effectively. Consequently, cardiomyopathy (see Chapter 23) and heart failure (see Chapter 28) are always lifelong, potential complications.

Complications

Arrhythmias

The term **arrhythmia** (sometimes called a **dysrhythmia**) refers to changes from the normal sequence of cardiac impulses resulting in erratic heart rhythms or rates that are too

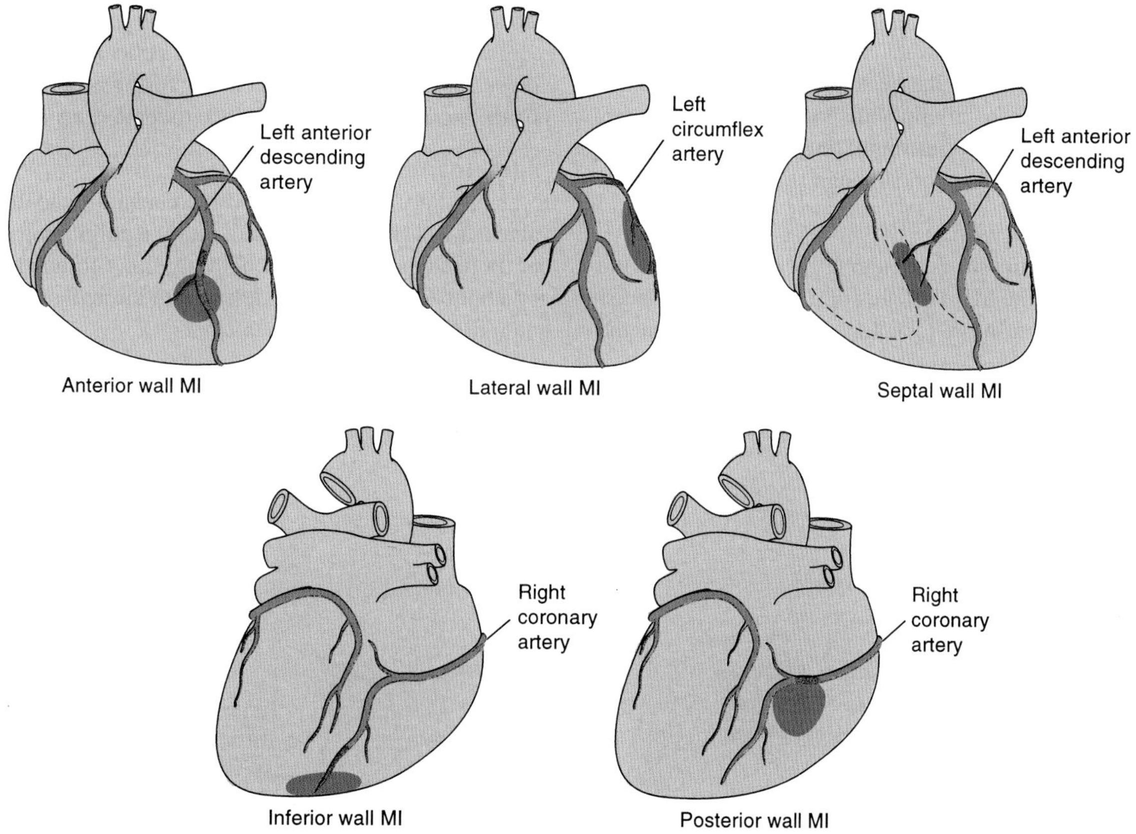

Figure 25-10 Zones of myocardial infarction (MI) based on the artery that becomes occluded.

fast or slow. Any number of arrhythmias (see Chapter 26) may occur during the acute phase. More than 50% of deaths from MI occur within 72 hours for this reason. Some abnormal rhythms can be fatal within a few minutes. Early detection and treatment reduce the fatality rate.

If a client experiences cardiac arrest (asystole), neurologic damage may occur. Neurologic outcomes can be improved by preventing hyperthermia. The AHA and others (Adler, 2014) indicate that maintaining an induced hypothermic state (89.6°F to 93.2°F) for 12 to 24 hours after resuscitation reduces the brain's oxygen requirements. The best method for facilitating hypothermia is the application of several cooling gel pads at strategic locations on the body; the pads are connected to a temperature management console (Fig. 25-11). In rural areas where this type of equipment is unavailable, hypothermia can be induced using an external hypothermia blanket or ice packs or administering cold saline through a peripheral intravenous (IV) catheter or endovascular cooling catheter.

Cardiogenic Shock

Cardiogenic shock, which has a high mortality rate, occurs when 40% of the left ventricle has lost the ability to pump effectively (see Chapter 17). The onset may be sudden or the condition may develop over hours or days. The sooner shock is detected (monitoring with a pulmonary artery catheter) and treatment is instituted, the better the client's chances of survival. This complication has been successfully treated with medications, ventricular assist devices, and an intra-aortic balloon pump (see Chapter 28).

Ventricular Rupture

Ventricular rupture occurs when a soft necrotic area from a transmural or interventricular septal MI ruptures. Dyspnea, rapid right-sided heart failure, and shock result. *Hemopericardium* (blood in the pericardium) and cardiac tamponade follow. The prognosis is poor, although survival is possible.

Ventricular Aneurysm

A ventricular **aneurysm** is a bulging of the portion of the heart affected by the MI. This area of poorly contractile tissue predisposes the heart to failure. Blood trapped in the projection tends to form thrombi, which may be released into the arterial circulation, or the aneurysm may burst, resulting in hemorrhage and death.

Arterial Embolism

Clots can form in the cavity of the ventricular aneurysm (mural thrombi), or tissue debris can break free. If clots enter the systemic arterial circulation, they may occlude a peripheral artery. Symptoms depend on the location of the affected artery. Arteriotomy (opening of an artery) and embolectomy (removal of an embolus) may be necessary; a client who has recently had an MI, however, is at poor surgical risk.

Venous Thrombosis

Venous thrombosis arises mostly in the veins of the lower extremities and pelvis. The use of antiembolism stockings and regular performance of foot and leg exercises help to prevent thrombus formation. Antiplatelet medications and anticoagulants also are prescribed.

Pulmonary Embolism

Most pulmonary emboli arise from venous thrombi in the lower extremities and pelvis (see Chapter 21). They may also arise from the right ventricle after an MI. The onset of a pulmonary embolism usually is sudden, with chest pain, dyspnea, and cyanosis being the first symptoms. The sputum may be tinged with blood. Treatment depends on the size of the infarcted area, the age and condition of the client, and the seriousness (or extent) of the MI.

Pericarditis

Pericarditis may be mild or severe. The mild form may not require treatment (see Chapter 23). If pericardial effusion develops, the client is observed closely for signs of cardiac tamponade; pericardiocentesis is done to remove excess fluid.

Mitral Insufficiency

If the papillary muscles are involved in an MI and the mitral valve leaflets are compromised, mitral regurgitation may occur. In this condition, blood not only flows forward into the aorta but backward into the left atrium through an incompetent mitral valve (see Chapter 24).

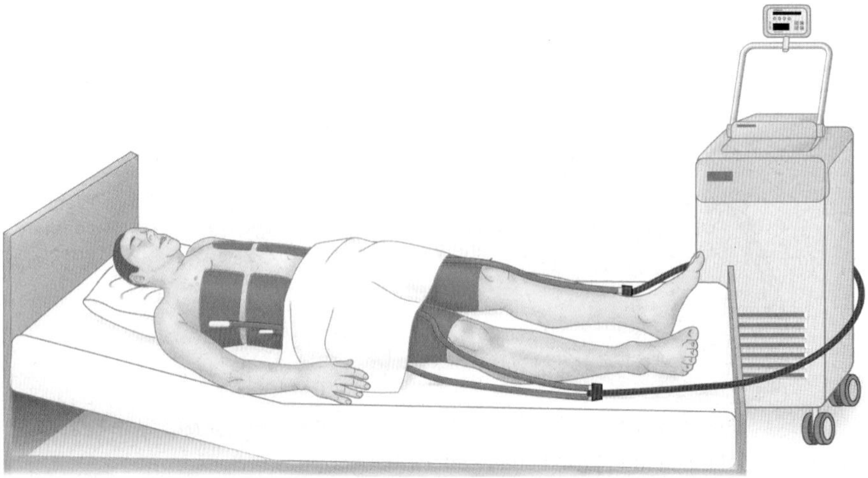

Figure 25-11 Hypothermia is induced using gel pads attached to a cooling system.

Assessment Findings

Signs and Symptoms

Symptoms vary between men and women. Men typically experience sudden, severe chest pain, which usually is substernal and may radiate to the shoulder, arm, teeth, jaw, or throat. Women more often than men have more vague symptoms, such as unexplained fatigue, abdominal pain, and shortness of breath, which often leads to misdiagnosis of women in emergency departments (www.diseasefix.com/). Most clients are aware of the seriousness of their symptoms and are apprehensive. When chest pain is experienced, it is more severe and lasts longer than anginal pain. Some clients describe it as squeezing or crushing. Unlike anginal pain, rest and sublingual nitrates do not relieve MI pain. If untreated, it may last for several hours or 1 or 2 days. Finally, it becomes sore or achy before disappearing entirely. A few clients, such as older adults and diabetics, experience little or no pain and may never know that they had an MI until an ECG detects it weeks, months, or years later. Clients appear pale and diaphoretic. They may experience nausea and vomiting or be hypotensive and faint. Pulse is rapid and weak and may be irregular. Signs of left-sided heart failure (dyspnea, cyanosis, cough) may appear if left ventricular pumping is sufficiently impaired.

Concept Mastery Alert

Cardiac Biomarkers

Myoglobin is a cardiac biomarker for MI and can be detected prior to the detection of troponin I and T.

Diagnostic Findings

Serum Enzymes and Isoenzymes. Laboratory tests to diagnose MI include a series of serum cardiac markers, substances that are released by damaged myocardial cells during an infarct (Table 25-3). When tissues and cells break down, are damaged, or die, great quantities of certain enzymes are released into the bloodstream. Enzymes are complex proteins produced by living cells that function as catalysts, substances capable of producing chemical changes without being changed themselves. An **isoenzyme** is one of several forms of the same enzyme that may exist in cells and is capable of being identified separately from others. The following serum cardiac markers are measured initially and every 8 hours for 24 hours to determine elevated levels:

- Myoglobin, a biomarker that rises in 2 to 3 hours after heart damage
- Troponin and subunits known as troponin T and troponin I, enzymes in myocardial contractile tissue
- Creatine kinase (CK), formerly creatine phosphokinase, and its cardiospecific isoenzyme CK-MB
- Lactate dehydrogenase (LDH) and isoenzymes LDH_1 and LDH_2
- Aspartate aminotransferase (AST), formerly called serum glutamic oxaloacetic transaminase (SGOT)

Troponin is present only in myocardial tissue; therefore, it is the gold standard for determining heart damage in the early stages of an MI. The other enzymes can be elevated in response to cardiac or other organ damage. Therefore, the isoenzymes CK-MB, LDH_1, and LDH_2 are evaluated for their cardiac specificity.

Miscellaneous Laboratory and Diagnostic Tests

The WBC count, C-reactive protein, and erythrocyte sedimentation rate increase on about the third day following MI because of the inflammatory response that the injured myocardial cells triggered. Blood glucose level may be elevated because of the body's response to a major stressor. After an MI, characteristic changes appear on the ECG within 2 to 12 hours. They may, however, take as long as 3 days to develop. These changes include T-wave inversion, ST-segment elevation, and a Q wave (Fig. 25-12).

Medical Management

Treatment is directed toward reducing tissue hypoxia, relieving pain, treating shock (if present), and alleviating arrhythmias if they occur. Because women younger than 55 years are seven times more likely to be misdiagnosed than men of similar age, they are erroneously discharged and have a higher mortality rate following an MI (Doshi, 2015).

Thrombolytic Therapy

The goal for administering **thrombolytic agents**, IV drugs that dissolve blood clots, is a "door-to-needle" time of 30 minutes, but no more than 90 minutes. Drugs such as streptokinase and recombinant tissue plasminogen activator (tPA) dissolve the thrombus occluding the coronary artery, restoring the circulation of oxygenated blood to the myocardium. If administered within the first 2 hours after the onset of symptoms, an MI can be greatly minimized. Even if the client is seen within 12 to 24 hours of the onset of the occlusion, reestablishing coronary artery blood flow can reduce the zone of necrosis. A thrombolytic can be administered within the specified timelines unless the client

TABLE 25-3 Serum Cardiac Markers After an Acute Myocardial Infarction (MI)

CARDIAC MARKER	CHARACTERISTICS
Myoglobin	Present as early as 2 hours after MI; peaks in 3–15 hours; returns to normal in 20–24 hours
Troponin T	Rises 3–4 hours after MI; peaks in 4–6 hours; returns to normal in several weeks
Troponin I	Rises 4–6 hours after MI; peaks in 14–18 hours; returns to normal in 6–7 days
Creatine kinase (CK-MB)	Rises 4–12 hours after MI; peaks in 24 hours; returns to normal in 3–4 days
Aspartate aminotransferase (AST)	Increases 6–12 hours after MI; peaks in 36 hours; returns to normal in 3–4 days
Lactate dehydrogenase (LDH_1 and LDH_2)	Rises 24–48 hours after MI; peaks in 3–6 days; returns to normal in 7–14 days An LDH_1:LDH_2 ratio greater than 1.0 indicates myocardial damage.

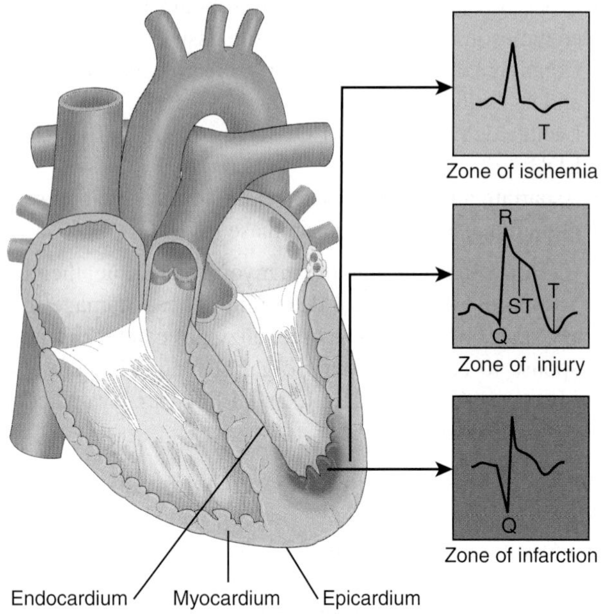

Figure 25-12 Characteristic electrocardiogram (ECG) changes after a myocardial infarction (MI). T-wave inversion, ST-segment elevation, and sometimes a Q wave are evidence of myocardial ischemia, injury, and infarction, respectively.

is disqualified on the basis of criteria that identify possible concomitant risks for neurologic complications and bleeding (Box 25-3).

BOX 25-3 Contraindications for Thrombolytic Therapy

Absolute Contraindications

- Any prior intracranial hemorrhage
- Structural cerebral vascular lesion
- Malignant intracranial neoplasm
- Ischemic stroke within past 3 months
- Suspected aortic dissection
- Active bleeding (excluding menses)
- Significant closed head or facial trauma within past 3 months
- Intracranial or intraspinal surgery within 2 months
- Severe uncontrolled hypertension (unresponsive to emergency therapy)
- For streptokinase, prior treatment within the previous 6 months

Relative Contraindications

- History of chronic, severe, poorly controlled hypertension
- Uncontrolled hypertension as evidenced by systolic BP more than 180 mm Hg or diastolic BP more than 110 mm Hg
- Ischemic stroke in less than 3 months ago, dementia, or other intracranial pathology not covered in absolute contraindications
- Traumatic or prolonged CPR or major surgery within past 3 weeks
- Internal bleeding within past 2–4 weeks
- Noncompressible vascular punctures
- Pregnancy
- Active peptic ulcer
- Current use of anticoagulant that has produced an elevated international normalized ratio (INR) higher than 1.7 or a prothrombin time (PT) longer than 15 seconds

Content modified with permission from Medscape Drugs & Diseases (https://emedicine.medscape.com/), Thrombolytic Therapy, 2017, available at: https://emedicine.medscape.com/article/811234-overview. Data for this content were sourced from O'Gara, P. T., Kushner, F. G., Ascheim, D. D., et al; for the American College of Cardiology Foundation/American Heart Association Task Force on Practice Guidelines. (2013). 2013 ACCF/AHA guideline for the management of ST-elevation myocardial infarction: a report of the American College of Cardiology Foundation/American Heart Association Task Force on Practice Guidelines. *Circulation, 127*(4):e362-e425. https://www.ahajournals.org/doi/full/10.1161/CIR.0b013e3182742cf6.

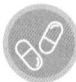

Pharmacologic Considerations

■ Aminocaproic acid (Amicar) is suggested as an antidote to control excessive bleeding when thrombolytics are administered. Aminocaproic acid binds to plasminogen and prevents its conversion to plasmin. Although this drug is theoretically beneficial, the action of most thrombolytics is generally complete by the time the drug can be administered (Jang & Nelson, 2012).

■ Hemorrhage associated with thrombolytics may be controlled by infusing platelets, fresh frozen plasma (FFP), or cryoprecipitate—the latter of the two contain concentrated clotting factors. Frozen blood products take 30 minutes to thaw. FFP must be obtained from an ABO compatible blood type; it is preferred for platelets and cryoprecipitate as well (Hassan, 2015).

Depending on how stable the client's condition is, PTCA or CABG may follow thrombolytic therapy after the risk for bleeding has been reduced. Clients who are not candidates for thrombolytic therapy should undergo PTCA within 90 minutes from the time they are assessed in the emergency department; delaying for 2 to 3 hours postinfarct correlates with a higher incidence of 1-year mortality (Kushner, 2013).

Symptomatic Treatment

An IV infusion is initiated to provide fluid while eating is restricted. The IV route also is used to administer parenteral medications. Drug therapy includes analgesics for pain, nitrates or other vasodilating drugs to improve blood flow, diuretics to reduce circulating blood volume, sedatives to promote rest and reduce anxiety, anticoagulants to prevent additional thrombus formation, and drugs to treat arrhythmias (see Drug Therapy Table 25-1). Oxygen is ordered to treat or prevent hypoxemia. Complete bed rest is prescribed initially but not recommended for uncomplicated MIs after the first 12 hours. Activity is adjusted according to the extent of the MI, complications, and response to therapy. When chest pain is controlled, a clear liquid diet is allowed and progressed to a heart-healthy diet thereafter (see Nutrition Notes). Clients who regularly consumed caffeine before an MI and consumed three to five cups of coffee per day afterward did not affect their mortality (Ding et al., 2014; Mukamal et al., 2009). A stool softener is prescribed to prevent increased BP from straining with the passage of stool. Permanent smoking cessation is imperative. The intra-aortic balloon pump may be used for clients who develop severe left ventricular failure (see Chapter 28).

Surgical Management

CABG surgery (see Chapter 29) is done to revascularize the myocardium surgically. In clients who are experiencing cardiogenic shock, a ventricular assist device may be implanted or cardiomyoplasty (a procedure for grafting skeletal muscle to the heart) or an alternative called a heart wrap may be used (see Chapter 28).

Cardiac Rehabilitation

After a significant cardiac event such as an MI or heart surgery, clients are encouraged to participate in a medically supervised **cardiac rehabilitation** program, which combines exercise and educational activities to speed recovery and reduce or prevent recurring episodes. Cardiac rehabilitation usually begins before discharge but continues on an outpatient basis. The plan is designed according to the client's unique needs. Some clients may achieve the goals of therapy by meeting two to three times a week for 1 hour or more over a few weeks. Other clients may require therapy for 3 to 4 months. Activities and educational topics include the following:

- Gradual exercise that increases according to the client's tolerance
- Establishment of physical limitations such as the maximum amount the client can lift
- Recognition and management of depression
- Medication regimen: importance of drug therapy, dose, time taken, adverse drug effects
- Smoking cessation
- When and how to resume sexual activity (Client and Family Teaching 25-3)
- Diet modifications, how to read food labels, what food labels indicate
- How to monitor pulse rate and BP
- Symptoms to report to a primary provider as soon as possible
- How to avoid or minimize stressors
- Importance of continued medical supervision

Nursing Management

The detailed nursing management of a client experiencing an acute MI is discussed in Nursing Care Plan 25-1. Instructions for performing cardiopulmonary resuscitation (CPR) (also discussed in the Nursing Care Plan) are presented in Nursing Guidelines 25-1.

Client and Family Teaching 25-3
Sexual Guidelines After Myocardial Infarction

The nurse provides the following information to the client:

- Check with primary provider before resuming sexual activity; those with an "uncomplicated" heart attack (no heart failure, shock, severe arrhythmias, or residual chest pain) may resume sex in about 1 week or when able to perform mild or moderate activity such as walking up two flights of stairs without experiencing angina.
- Avoid sex with anyone other than your usual partner.
- Avoid positions that require supporting your own weight.
- Get adequate rest before sexual intercourse.
- For women, apply an over-the-counter estrogen cream or other friction-reducing substance on or in the vagina to promote lubrication.
- Have sex in the same environment as before the MI.
- Postpone sex for 2 to 3 hours after eating a heavy meal or consuming alcohol.
- Use a short-acting nitrate, if the primary provider approves, before intercourse; avoid combining a medication for erectile dysfunction with a nitrate.
- Begin with moderate sexual foreplay.
- Use medium water temperatures when bathing or showering before or after sexual activity.

Adapted from Reiley, R. (2013). *How to have sex after a heart attack: Go slow, have therapy and DON'T go "on top."* http://www.dailymail.co.uk/health/article-2381351/How -sex-heart-attack-Go-slow-therapy-DONT-top.html
Rettner. R. (2013). Sex after a heart attack? Here's how and when. http://www.livescience.com-heart-attack-safe -sex-guidelines.html

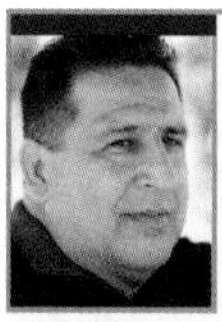

Clinical Scenario After experiencing severe ongoing chest pain radiating down the left arm for an hour, a client with no previous history of cardiac disease arrives by ambulance at the emergency department. The client's wife has already given the client two 325-mg tablets of aspirin, which the client has chewed and swallowed. The client is anxious, nauseous, and diaphoretic. Stat cardiac enzymes and resting ECG are ordered. Based on the results of diagnostic tests, administration of thrombolytic therapy is anticipated. What focused nursing assessments and subsequent nursing care are appropriate? See Nursing Care Plan 25-1.

NURSING CARE PLAN 25-1 The Client With Acute Myocardial Infarction

Assessment

Determine the following:

- Client's description of pain: location, type, duration, intensity using a scale of 0 to 10, and whether it radiates to other areas
- Vital signs every 30 minutes until stable and then every 4 hours and as needed (p.r.n.)
- Presence of nausea, vomiting, diaphoresis, anxiety
- Oxygen saturation level with a pulse oximeter
- Cardiac rhythm via cardiac monitor or ECG
- Heart and lung sounds
- Presence and quality of peripheral pulses
- Results of serum cardiac markers
- A thorough history to establish baseline data about disorders such as diabetes mellitus, hypertension, recent streptococcal infection, or allergic reaction to streptokinase, and findings that may disqualify the client from thrombolytic therapy
- Drug history for prescribed, over-the-counter, and herbal products

(continued)

NURSING CARE PLAN 25-1 The Client With Acute Myocardial Infarction (*continued*)

Nursing Diagnosis. Acute Pain related to diminished myocardial oxygenation

Expected Outcome. Pain will be within client's identified comfort level within 30 minutes.

Interventions	Rationales
Administer oxygen at 2 L/min by nasal cannula or as prescribed.	*Supplemental oxygen raises hemoglobin saturation and oxygen in plasma. Adequate myocardial oxygen diminishes angina.*
Administer prescribed sublingual or spray nitroglycerin every 5 minutes, up to three doses, if pain is unrelieved.	*Nitroglycerin dilates blood vessels, improving blood flow through coronary arteries, and lowers BP, which decreases cardiac afterload.*
Administer prescribed IV morphine sulfate.	*Morphine reduces pain perception and anxiety. Reduced anxiety decreases heart rate and BP, alleviating the heart's demand for oxygenation.*

Evaluation of Expected Outcome

Pain is eliminated or reduced to a tolerable level.

Nursing Diagnosis. Anxiety or Fear related to perception of impending doom, concern over actual/potential lifestyle changes, worry concerning family situation

Expected Outcome. Client will report decreased anxiety and fear.

Interventions	Rationales
Allow client to express fears and anxiety.	*Sharing feelings with a supportive person tends to relieve or reduce emotional distress.*
Explain all procedures before performing them.	*Information eliminates the element of surprise or misinterpretation of nursing activities.*
Carry out procedures in a calm, relaxed manner.	*A client who senses confidence in the nurse may experience less apprehension.*
Promote uninterrupted blocks of time for rest, sleep, or visits with family members.	*Physical rest and support from others promote the ability to cope.*
Check client frequently, and answer call lights promptly.	*Knowing that help is quickly available can relieve fear.*
Acknowledge grief over perceived or actual changes in lifestyle.	*Dealing with reality facilitates grieving.*
Administer prescribed sedatives and anxiolytic drugs as indicated.	*They block sympathetic nervous system responses, which reduce anxiety and fear.*

Evaluation of Expected Outcome

Anxiety is reduced as evidenced by normal heart rate and BP, no nervous activity, and self-reported tolerance of stressors.

RC of Hemorrhage. Related to thrombolytic therapy

Expected Outcome. The nurse will monitor to detect, manage, and minimize bleeding.

Interventions	Rationales
Observe closely for bleeding during thrombolytic therapy and until sufficient half-lives reduce pharmacodynamic effects.	*The client is at risk for bleeding when thrombolytic drugs change plasminogen to plasmin.*
Check for blood in stool or urine, bruising, epistaxis, abdominal pain, or altered neurologic status.	*Thrombolytic drugs dissolve blood clots and interfere with their formation.*
Avoid intramuscular, IV, and arterial punctures during therapy and until the risk for excessive bleeding has subsided.	*Controlling bleeding may be difficult while an active level of thrombolytic drug remains in the bloodstream.*
Keep client on bed rest; pad the side rails if agency policy mandates.	*Trauma can cause excessive blood loss.*
Be prepared to administer platelets, fresh frozen plasma (FFP), or cryoprecipitate.	*Platelets contain thrombocytes from pooled blood donations. FFP and cryoprecipitate contain concentrated clotting factors.*

Evaluation of Expected Outcome

Client shows no evidence of bleeding.

RC for Arrhythmias. Related to reperfusion of myocardium with thrombolytic therapy and instability of the conduction system

Expected Outcome. The nurse will monitor to detect, manage, and minimize arrhythmias.

NURSING CARE PLAN 25-1 **The Client With Acute Myocardial Infarction (*continued*)**

Interventions	Rationales
Place client on a cardiac monitor and closely observe for dangerous arrhythmias.	*A cardiac monitor continuously displays heart rate and rhythm; it sounds an alarm to call attention to an arrhythmic event.*
Be prepared to perform CPR if a life-threatening arrhythmia or asystole occurs.	*CPR provides basic life support (see* Nursing Guidelines 25-1*).*
Assist with endotracheal intubation, defibrillation, and administration of antiarrhythmic drugs.	*Advanced cardiac life support may resuscitate a client.*

Evaluation of Expected Outcome

Arrhythmias are controlled.

NURSING GUIDELINES 25-1

Performing Cardiopulmonary Resuscitation

- Attempt to arouse client by shaking and calling their name.
- Notify emergency personnel if client is unresponsive or not breathing normally.
- Delegate someone to obtain an automated external defibrillator (AED) if one is available.
- Feel for a carotid pulse. If absent, administer chest compressions at a rate of 100 to 120 per minute.
- Open airway, if trained to do so, with head tilt, chin lift, or jaw thrust.
- Continue chest compressions and rescue breathing in a ratio of 30 compressions to two breaths for one or two rescuers for adults and children who have reached puberty; 30 compressions to two breaths for one rescuer of children age 1 year up to puberty and infants less than 1 year; if there are two rescuers for children and infants, administer 15 chest compressions to two breaths.
- Use the AED as soon as it is available after beginning resuscitation.
- Check effectiveness of CPR or AED after five cycles (2 minutes) of compressions and breaths (pupils responding to light, pulse at carotid artery, improved skin color).
- Continue CPR if client remains unresponsive between or in lieu of defibrillation if an AED is not available.
- Do not interrupt CPR for more than 10 seconds.

Highlights of the 2019 Focused Updates to the American Heart Association Guidelines for Cardiopulmonary Resuscitation and Emergency Cardiovascular Care. https://cpr.heart.org/-/media/cpr-files/resus-science/ecc-digital-digest/highlights-update.pdf?la=en

OCCLUSIVE DISORDERS OF PERIPHERAL BLOOD VESSELS

Peripheral vascular disease (PVD) is a general term for disorders that affect blood vessels distant from the large central blood vessels supplying the myocardium or that circulate blood directly in and out of the heart. PVD includes disorders that affect arteries or veins. Common peripheral vascular disorders, which reduce blood flow by various mechanisms, include peripheral artery disease (PAD), Raynaud syndrome, thrombosis, phlebothrombosis, and embolism.

Peripheral Artery Disease

More than 9 million people in the United States have PAD, a condition that affects primarily the blood vessels that supply oxygen to lower limbs, which is the focus of this discussion. The same pathologic process, however, can affect the carotid, renal, and mesenteric arteries as well.

Men are affected more than women by PAD in the lower extremities. As the disorder worsens, some affected individuals may develop **critical limb ischemia**, a complication characterized by open sores or infections that do not resolve, become gangrenous, and threaten the viability of the limb, making amputation necessary.

Pathophysiology and Etiology

When blood flow through arteries distal to the aortic arch becomes restricted, individuals experience manifestations of ischemia in the tissues where circulation is impaired. The primary cause is atherosclerosis, which—like its counterpathology, CAD—is secondary to obesity, hypertension, hyperlipidemia, diabetes mellitus, chronic smoking, and, in some cases, a family history of PAD or other atherosclerotic diseases. Hyperhomocysteinemia (increased blood level of homocysteine, an amino acid formed from protein-rich food containing methionine) is higher among those with PAD. Other than identifying it as a risk factor for PAD, however, the role of hyperhomocysteinemia in the disease and the effect of controlling its level have not been sufficiently explored (Andras et al., 2013; Ganguly & Alam, 2015).

Assessment Findings

Signs and Symptoms

Clients with PAD experience **intermittent claudication**, or pain and cramping in thigh, calf, or buttock muscles during activity such as walking or climbing stairs. The discomfort is relieved after resting for several minutes. One or both lower limbs feel cold to the touch. Upon exertion, many describe feeling numbness in the affected leg(s) accompanied by heaviness and fatigue. Some develop skin lesions that are slow to heal. Hair and toenail growth is slow. The skin over the leg(s) appears red in a dependent position but returns to normal color in one minute when elevated. Pulses in the lower extremities are difficult to palpate.

Diagnostic Findings

The tentative diagnosis begins with taking a history of the client's symptoms and examining the lower extremities. Blood tests that reveal elevated total cholesterol, high LDL, above-normal triglyceride, and increased homocysteine contribute to the diagnosis.

One of the simplest tests involves measuring the **ankle-brachial index**, a comparison of the systolic pressure in the brachial artery with that in the posterior tibial artery using Doppler ultrasound at rest or after exercise (Fig. 25-13). The severity of the disorder is determined by dividing the systolic BP in the ankle by the systolic pressure in the arm. When the *quotient* (result of the division) is 0.9 or less, the data support a diagnosis of PAD.

Clients may also undergo angiography using a CT scan or magnetic resonance imaging. Invasive angiography using a contrast agent may be used to detect the specific location of blocked arteries or determine improvement after endovascular procedures.

Medical and Surgical Management

Clients are encouraged to lose weight, exercise daily, and cease smoking. Diabetics must strive to keep their blood sugar levels under control. Several classes of drugs, such as antihypertensive, lipid-lowering, antiplatelet, and antithrombotic medications, help to slow the progression of symptoms and reduce the risk of complications. Percutaneous and surgical revascularization procedures are performed when clients develop advanced disease.

Nursing Management

The nurse explains the rationale for lifestyle changes in diet, exercise, and adherence to medication self-administration. The action, dosage, administration schedule, and side effects of each drug are explained as well as any blood tests that are required for monitoring safety. The nurse palpates and compares lower extremity peripheral pulses bilaterally. The skin on the extremities is assessed, and the nurse teaches the client to notify the primary provider if cyanosis, skin lesions, or gangrene is detected. The nurse sets an example for daily skin and foot care, including washing and drying the feet well, applying moisturizing lotion, changing cotton socks daily, and wearing supportive shoes. Regular attention by a podiatrist is recommended for thick nails that are difficult

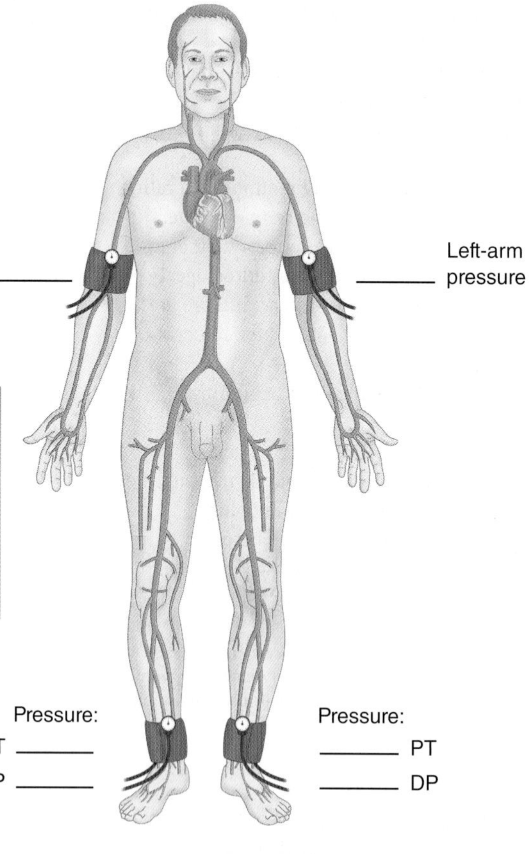

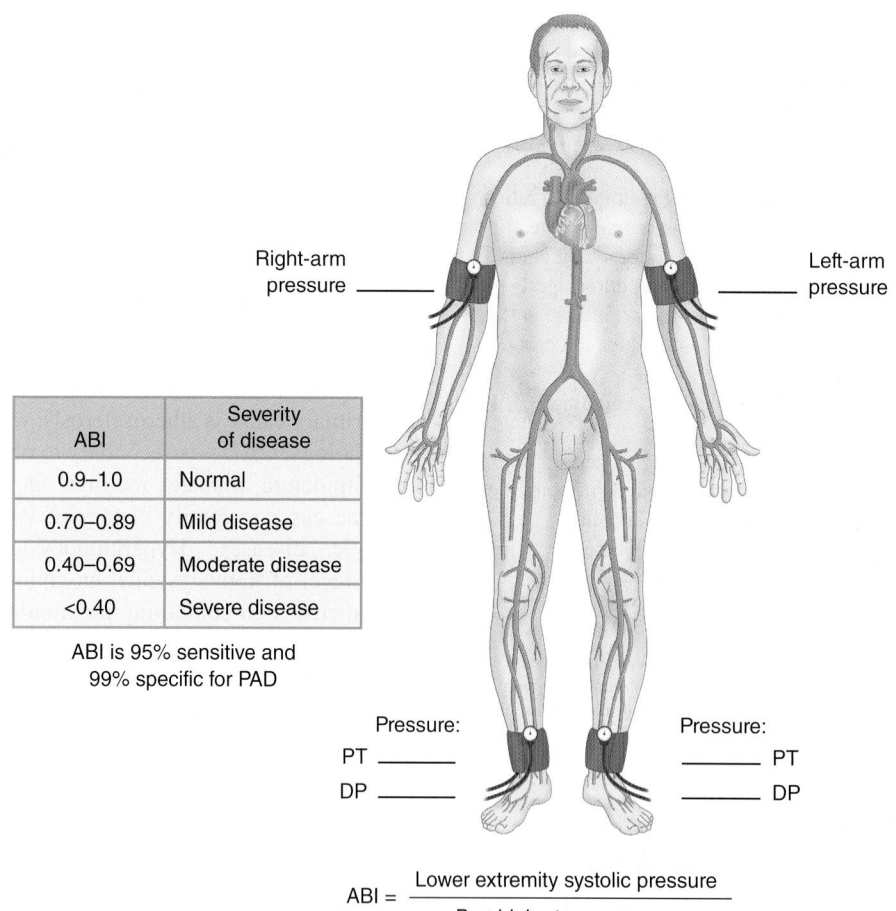

ABI	Severity of disease
0.9–1.0	Normal
0.70–0.89	Mild disease
0.40–0.69	Moderate disease
<0.40	Severe disease

ABI is 95% sensitive and 99% specific for PAD

$$\text{ABI} = \frac{\text{Lower extremity systolic pressure}}{\text{Brachial artery pressure}}$$

Figure 25-13 Ankle-brachial index (ABI) measurement to detect peripheral artery disease (PAD). ABI, ankle brachial index; DP, dorsalis pedis artery; PT, posterior tibial artery.

to trim, corns, calluses, or blisters that may form. The nurse stresses the danger of applying direct heat to the lower extremities and shows the client how to avoid positions that interfere with blood flow, such as crossing the legs at the knee. Besides the prescribed exercise regimen, the nurse recommends sedentary exercises such as extending the knees and ankle pumping and rotation to promote circulation, followed by periods of rest.

Raynaud Syndrome

Raynaud syndrome is characterized by periodic constriction of the arteries that supply the extremities. The disorder is most common in young women.

Pathophysiology and Etiology

Raynaud syndrome is characterized by brief spasms of the arteries and arterioles in the fingers (most common site), toes, nose, ears, or chin. The spasms last approximately 15 minutes and cause temporary ischemia (impaired oxygenation) to the tissues. The vessels then dilate widely, apparently to compensate for the restriction. Patchy areas of necrosis occur with prolonged ischemia.

The underlying cause of Raynaud syndrome is not entirely clear. In some clients, it seems *idiopathic* (no explainable reason); in others, it is secondary to connective tissue diseases, such as scleroderma, systemic lupus erythematosus, or rheumatoid arthritis (see Chapter 63).

The anatomy of the arteries and arterioles is normal. One theory explaining the vasospasms is impaired release of *prostaglandins* (chemicals stored in cellular membranes). Some prostaglandins cause vasoconstriction; others cause vasodilation. The type that accompanies an inflammatory response causes vasodilation.

Assessment Findings

Signs and Symptoms

Attacks are intermittent and of varying frequency but are especially common after exposure to cold. When the condition occurs in the hands, they become cold, blanched, and wet with perspiration. Numbness and tingling also may occur. The client may note awkwardness and fumbling, especially when attempting fine movements. After the initial pallor, the hands, especially the fingers, become deeply cyanotic and begin to ache. The hallmark symptoms of arterial insufficiency include ischemia, pain, and paresthesia. Placing the affected part in warm water or going to a warm area can relieve an attack. Eventually, the vasospasm is relieved, and blood rushes to the affected part. The skin in the deprived areas becomes flushed, swollen, and warm, and the person has a sensation of throbbing pain.

In the early stages of the disease, the hands usually appear normal between attacks. The disease does not necessarily progress to cause severe disability. Symptoms often are mild and may even improve spontaneously. When the disease is severe and of long-standing, cyanosis of the fingers persists between attacks and skin changes gradually develop. Painful ulcers and superficial gangrene may appear at the fingertips. The fingers are especially vulnerable to infection. Healing of even minor lesions often is slow and uncertain.

Diagnostic Findings

No specific laboratory studies can confirm Raynaud syndrome. Diagnosis is made by a history of the symptoms and examination of the involved part. Laboratory blood tests are ordered to confirm or rule out an accompanying connective tissue disorder (see Chapter 63).

Medical and Surgical Management

Treatment involves avoiding factors that precipitate attacks. Smoking is contraindicated because it causes vasoconstriction. Drug therapy with peripheral vasodilators, such as isoxsuprine (Vasodilan), may be attempted, but results usually are less favorable than desired. Other drugs, such as nifedipine (Procardia), are being used investigationally. An IV infusion of prostaglandin E may provide temporary relief. *Sympathectomy* (cutting peripheral sympathetic nerves) may be performed; however, because of disappointing results, the procedure is performed less frequently than in the past. Gangrenous areas are amputated.

Nursing Management

Once an episode of pain occurs, there are several ways that the attack can be aborted. If warming the hands in water is impossible, the nurse encourages the client to imagine warming them in some way such as holding them near a roaring fire. The mind can alter the physiology of blood flow. Another technique is to teach clients to imitate the exercise snow skiers use called the McIntyre maneuver: while standing, clients swing their arms behind and then in front of their bodies at a rate of about 180 times per minute. The swinging motion distributes blood to the distal areas of the fingers.

Teaching for clients with Raynaud syndrome and their family members is important. The nurse instructs clients to avoid situations that contribute to ischemic episodes, explaining that injuries may heal slowly. If clients smoke, they must stop because nicotine causes vasoconstriction and increases the frequency of episodes. The nurse advises clients to wear wool socks and mittens during cold weather. Clients should avoid over-the-counter decongestants, cold remedies, and drugs for symptomatic relief of hay fever because of their vasoconstrictive qualities. The nurse advises clients to wear work gloves during household chores such as gardening and washing dishes to prevent accidental injury. Client teaching also includes information about how to perform nail care to avoid injury, such as soaking the hands or feet before trimming nails, trimming nails straight across, and seeing a podiatrist for the treatment of corns or calluses. If a sympathectomy is done, the nurse emphasizes that the areas of altered sympathetic stimuli no longer perspire and explains that applying cream to prevent excessive skin dryness may be helpful.

Thrombosis, Phlebothrombosis, and Embolism

A **thrombus** is a stationary clot. **Thrombosis** is a state in which a thrombus has formed in a blood vessel. **Thrombophlebitis** is an inflammation of a vein accompanied by clot or thrombus formation (see Chapter 23). **Phlebothrombosis** is the development of a clot within a vein without inflammation. Phlebothrombosis and thrombophlebitis have similar symptoms and treatment. An **embolus** is a moving mass (clot) of particles, either solid or gas, in the bloodstream.

Pathophysiology and Etiology

Thrombosis in the venous system most often occurs in the lower extremities and usually is associated with disorders or circumstances that cause venous stasis (inactivity, immobility, or trauma to a blood vessel). Orthopedic surgical procedures increase the incidence of deep vein thrombosis (DVT) of the lower extremities. Atherosclerosis, endocarditis, pooling of blood in a ventricular aneurysm, and arrhythmias such as atrial fibrillation can precipitate arterial thrombosis and subsequent embolization. When a thrombus forms or an embolus reaches a blood vessel too small to permit its passage, blood flow is partly or totally occluded.

Assessment Findings

Signs and Symptoms

When an arterial clot is present, symptoms arise from ischemia to the tissues that depend on the obstructed vessel for their oxygenated blood supply. With total occlusion, the extremity suddenly becomes white, cold, and extremely painful. Arterial pulsations are absent below the obstructed area. Numbness, tingling, or cramping also may be present, and surrounding blood vessels spasm. Loss of sensation and ability to move the part follows. Symptoms of shock frequently result if a large vessel is obstructed. When a small vessel is occluded, symptoms of ischemia, such as pallor and coldness, occur but are less severe. Unless blood flow is restored, gangrene develops (see Fig. 23-16).

Clients with phlebothrombosis may have few, if any, symptoms because inflammation is absent. Signs and symptoms of DVT usually include mild fever and pain, swelling, and tenderness of the affected extremity. A thrombus may become a mobile embolus and lodge in a distal blood vessel, such as the pulmonary capillaries, causing symptoms related to the organ to which circulation has become impaired. (See discussions of pulmonary embolism in Chapter 21 and cerebral embolism in Chapter 38.)

Diagnostic Findings

Arteriography or venography (also called *phlebography*) using a contrast dye identifies the point of obstruction. Doppler ultrasonography is used to detect abnormalities in peripheral blood flow. Plethysmography measures volume changes in the venous or arterial system.

Medical and Surgical Treatment

Treatment depends on whether an artery or a vein is occluded and the degree of occlusion (partial or complete).

Arterial Occlusive Disease

If an artery is completely occluded, treatment cannot be delayed. The primary provider may order an immediate IV bolus of heparin followed by a continuous infusion or multiple high doses of heparin administered subcutaneously to prevent the development of further clots or the extension of those already present. An attempt may be made to improve circulation by administering vasodilating drugs. A sympathetic nerve block (injection of a local anesthetic into the sympathetic ganglia) may relieve vasospasm. Opioids may relieve pain and ease the client's apprehension. A thrombolytic agent may be prescribed if the client has experienced a pulmonary embolism or the embolus is occluding a large arterial vessel. If circulation to the extremity cannot be restored, a thrombectomy, embolectomy, *endarterectomy* (removal of the lining of an artery), or CABG is necessary. Nursing management of thrombectomy, embolectomy, endarterectomy, and CABG is discussed in Chapter 29.

Venous Occlusive Disease

Venous thrombosis is treated with bed rest, elevation of the extremity, local heat, analgesics for pain, and intermittent subcutaneous injections or continuous IV heparin therapy followed by oral anticoagulants once the heparin has achieved a therapeutic effect. DVT may necessitate surgical removal of the clot (*thrombectomy*).

Nursing Management

The nurse obtains a history of symptoms and identifies characteristics of the pain. The nurse examines the extremities and compares skin color, temperature, capillary refill time, and tissue integrity; they also measure each calf. The nurse palpates peripheral pulses or uses a Doppler ultrasound device if pulses cannot be palpated. They mark the location of each peripheral artery with a soft-tipped pen to facilitate its relocation. The nurse immediately reports any change in the quality of a peripheral pulse or its sudden absence. Outlining any color change (line of demarcation) above or below the occluded area with a soft-tipped pen is useful to establish a baseline for future comparison.

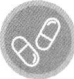

Pharmacologic Considerations

- The most common test used to monitor heparin is activated partial thromboplastin time (aPTT) or partial thromboplastin time (PTT). PTT and aPTT are the same; however, in aPTT, an activator is added that speeds up the clotting time and results in a narrower reference range. The aPTT is considered a more sensitive version of the PTT. The dose is adjusted to attain a therapeutic range of 1.5 to 2.5 times the normal. When oral anticoagulant therapy begins, so does the importance of monitoring prothrombin time (PT) and international normalized ratio (INR). Therapeutic PT levels are 1.5 to 2.5 times the control value and the normal range for INR is 2.0 to 3.0. Monitoring continues monthly while the oral anticoagulant is taken.

The nurse monitors the client's response to anticoagulation therapy. If heparin is administered, the nurse assesses IV infusions hourly. They monitor aPTT, PT, and INR when concurrent oral anticoagulation is prescribed. These values help determine therapeutic response and daily dosage. The nurse is alert for signs of bleeding and keeps protamine sulfate on hand for reversing heparin and vitamin K on hand for reversing oral anticoagulants. Additional nursing management is directed at increasing arterial or venous blood flow, relieving pain, and preventing complications.

Thorough teaching before discharge is essential. To prevent a recurrence of thrombosis, phlebothrombosis, or embolism, the nurse informs clients to avoid prolonged periods of inactivity (especially sitting), elevate the legs periodically, and walk or do isometric leg exercises frequently if sitting is unavoidable. They recommend wearing antiembolism stockings to prevent venous stasis (especially if the client has venous leg ulcers). The nurse instructs the client to apply these stockings before assuming a dependent position or after elevating the extremities for several minutes. The client needs to remove and reapply antiembolism stockings twice a day or as recommended by the primary provider. The nurse informs those who must take continued anticoagulants to observe for signs of unusual bleeding and keep appointments for laboratory tests.

Venous Insufficiency

Venous insufficiency is a peripheral vascular disorder in which the flow of venous blood is impaired through deep or superficial veins (or both). The condition usually affects the lower extremities, most often the medial aspect of the leg or around the ankle.

Pathophysiology and Etiology

Venous insufficiency may be a consequence of varicose veins (discussed later) or valvular damage from a previous venous thrombosis. When the forward movement of venous blood is affected, venous congestion develops from the accumulating blood volume. Increased hydrostatic fluid pressure causes fluid to leave the veins and enter interstitial spaces. Localized edema is evident; the skin becomes shiny and hard. The fluid-filled space acts as a barrier between the cells in the surrounding tissue and their capillary blood supply. Consequently, cells are subjected to accumulating amounts of CO_2. As unoxygenated cells die, they release inflammatory chemicals that cause *dermatitis* or inflammation of the dermis layer of skin. The skin becomes red and "hot." Hemoglobin from blood cells also escapes into the extravascular space, causing the tissue to appear dark brown, deep purple, or black. Serous fluid oozes from the skin when there is no outlet for vascular or lymphatic circulation. Eventually, the skin becomes impaired. A lesion referred to as a **venous stasis ulcer** forms (Fig. 25-14). Without adequate circulation, healing is retarded. Some ulcers may be present for years. The skin is fragile and easily retraumatized in the process of healing. Secondary infections often occur in the ulceration.

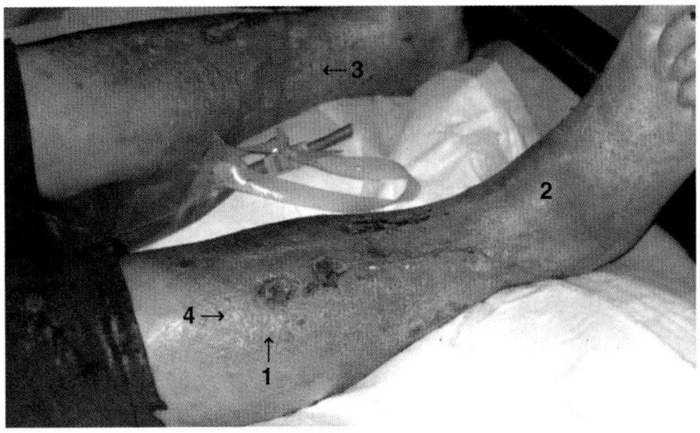

Figure 25-14 Multiple shallow ulcers from venous stasis. (From Sussman, C., & Bates-Jensen, B. M. (2011). *Wound care: A collaborative practice manual for health professionals* (4th ed.). Wolters Kluwer Health/Lippincott Williams & Wilkins. Copyright © B.M. Bates-Jensen.)

Assessment Findings

Signs and Symptoms

The foot or feet appear swollen. Testing for pitting is difficult because the congested fluid cannot be displaced. Superficial veins are dilated and obvious during inspection. Skin color is not uniform; there usually is a red or darkly pigmented area. If a lesion is present, its margin usually is irregular. Serous fluid may have collected in a pocket beneath the skin, or the area has beads of fluid on its surface that return after being wiped away. If an infection is present, the drainage may change from clear to opaque. Most clients report moderate pain. Pedal and tibial pulses may be difficult to palpate because of the congestion of venous fluid.

Diagnostic Findings

Doppler ultrasound demonstrates a reversed direction of blood flow, indicating valvular incompetence in superficial or deep veins. *Photoplethysmography*, a diagnostic test for venous pathology, measures light that is not absorbed by hemoglobin and consequently is reflected to the machine. When clients with venous insufficiency undergo photoplethysmography during exercise and rest, light reflection is greater during rest, showing that the client has decreased oxygen-bound hemoglobin and an increased volume of **venous reflux** (downward flow of venous blood). Air plethysmography measures venous pressure by filling a cuff with air after it is applied to the calf while the client is supine with the legs elevated. When the client stands, the pressure is measured again and venous pressure increases, indicating an increased volume of venous reflux.

Medical and Surgical Management

A major goal of therapy is to promote venous circulation. This is accomplished by applying elastic compression stockings, such as *Jobst* stockings, that maintain venous pressure at 40 mm Hg. The client wears the stockings at all times except when lying down. Because older adults may have difficulty applying elastic compression stockings, the primary provider may apply a nonelastic gauze dressing soaked in zinc paste and glycerin known as an *Unna boot*. Pneumatic compression pump therapy, similar to EECP, also may be implemented. The compression pump promotes venous blood flow more efficiently than compression stockings but is more expensive and time-consuming. Furthermore, it interferes with performance of daily activities during its use. Mild analgesics are recommended for pain. Vascular surgery can be performed in which the valves in larger veins are repaired or incompetent valves are bypassed using a length of vein with healthy valves from elsewhere in the body.

A stasis ulcer is managed by keeping the skin and ulcer clean with soap and water or a diluted solution of a disinfectant such as Hibiclens. Necrotic tissue is debrided. Any infection is treated by applying Silvadene, an antibacterial cream, or an antibiotic ointment. The wound is covered with an occlusive transparent dressing such as Tegaderm that traps moisture, which speeds healing. Chronic, nonhealing skin lesions also are treated with **topical hyperbaric oxygen** (THBO) therapy. This approach delivers oxygen above atmospheric pressure directly to the wound rather than to the full body as with other disorders such as carbon monoxide poisoning. Oxygen accelerates the healing process. THBO is applied by covering the area with an inflatable boot that confines the oxygen at low hyperbaric pressure at the wound site. The boot remains in place for approximately 90 minutes a day for 4 consecutive days. The treatment is repeated after 3 days of nontreatment in a cycle over 8 to 10 weeks.

Nursing Management

The nurse assesses the appearance of the extremities and the quality of circulation. If an ulcer is present, they measure it and describe its appearance. If the client has pain, the nurse asks the client to rate it and administers an analgesic if warranted. The nurse measures the diameter of the calf and ankle and the length of the leg from heel to knee to obtain accurately fitting compression stockings. They help apply the stockings each morning before the client lowers the legs to the floor and implements wound care according to primary provider directives.

The nurse teaches the client to do the following:

- Purchase more than one pair of compression stockings so one pair is worn while the other pair is laundered.
- Dry elastic stockings by laying them flat rather than hanging them, which stretches elastic.
- Lose weight if necessary.
- Elevate the legs periodically for at least 15 to 20 minutes.
- Walk or do isometric calf muscle pumps hourly to promote venous circulation.
- Raise the foot of the bed to promote venous circulation during sleep.
- Avoid morning showers or sitting in front of a fire because heat dilates blood vessels and contributes to venous congestion.
- Wear shoes with laces rather than slippers or sandals to reduce pooling of blood in the feet.

DISORDERS OF BLOOD VESSEL WALLS

Varicose Veins

Varicose veins or varicosities are dilated, tortuous veins. Both men and women suffer equally from this disorder. The saphenous leg veins commonly are affected because they lack support from surrounding muscles. Varicose veins also may occur in other body parts, such as the rectum (hemorrhoids) and esophagus (esophageal varices). Varicose veins may be accompanied by a smaller variation called spider veins, which appear closer to the surface of the skin.

Pathophysiology and Etiology

Varicose veins have a familial tendency. The valves of the veins become incompetent in early adulthood, resulting in varicosities. In others, anything that constricts or interferes with venous return contributes to the formation of varicose veins. Prolonged standing compromises venous return as blood pools distally with gravity. Obesity and pressure on blood vessels from an enlarging fetus, liver, or abdominal tumor contribute to venous congestion. Thrombophlebitis may lead to varicose veins because the inflammatory process may damage vein valves.

Normally, the action of leg muscles during movement and exercise aids venous return (Fig. 25-15). When valves in veins become incompetent, blood accumulates rather than being propelled efficiently to the heart. The congestion stretches the veins. Over time, they cannot recoil and remain chronically distended. Venous hypertension then forces some fluid to move into the interstitial spaces of surrounding tissue. Venous congestion and local edema may diminish arterial blood flow, impairing cellular nutrition. Even minor skin or soft tissue injuries easily become infected and ulcerated. The healing of such lesions is slow and uncertain.

Assessment Findings

Signs and Symptoms

Often, the condition first manifests itself when other factors impair venous return. The legs feel heavy and tired,

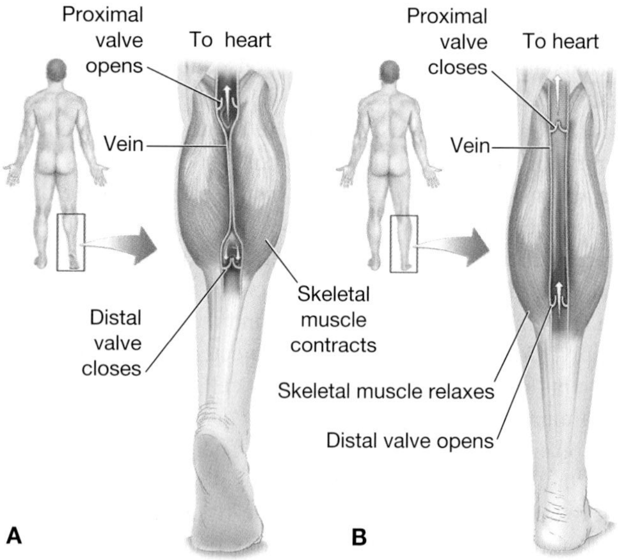

Figure 25-15 The skeletal muscle pumps and promotes blood flow in the deep and superficial calf vessels. Most perforating veins lie below the knee. Muscle contraction **(A)** propels blood in the deep veins toward the heart; closure of the venous valves prevents backflow. When the calf muscle is relaxed **(B)**, blood moves from the superficial to the deep veins. (Reprinted with permission from Wingerd, B. (2013). *The human body: Concepts of anatomy and physiology* (3rd ed.). Wolters Kluwer Health/Lippincott Williams & Wilkins.)

particularly after prolonged standing. The client may say that activity or elevation of the legs relieves the discomfort. The leg veins look distended and tortuous and can be seen under the skin as dark blue or purple, snakelike elevations. The feet, ankles, and legs may appear swollen. The skin may be slightly darker in the areas of impaired circulation. There may be signs of skin ulcerations in various stages of healing. Capillary refill may be abnormal.

Diagnostic Findings

The Brodie–Trendelenburg test is performed for diagnostic purposes. The client lies flat and elevates the affected leg to empty the veins. A tourniquet is then applied to the upper thigh, and the client is asked to stand. If blood flows from the upper part of the leg into the superficial veins when the tourniquet is released, the valves of the superficial veins are considered incompetent. Ultrasonography and venography are also used to detect impaired blood flow.

Medical and Surgical Management

Treatment of mild varicose veins includes exercising (walking, swimming), losing weight (if needed), wearing elastic support stockings, and avoiding prolonged periods of sitting or standing. Defective smaller veins may be occluded using skin surface laser treatments. Deeper varicose veins may be sclerosed or occluded by injecting a chemical that sets up inflammation in the vein wall. Endovascular radiofrequency, in which a catheter with a heated probe is inserted into the vein, is another alternative. Eventually, adhesions form, and blood flow must find an alternate route through collateral veins.

Surgical treatment for severe or multiple varicose veins consists of vein ligation with or without vein stripping. A **vein ligation** is a procedure in which the affected veins are ligated (tied off) above and below the area of incompetent valves, but the dysfunctional vein remains. For better results, a **vein stripping** is performed; in this procedure, the ligated veins are severed and removed. The entire great saphenous vein, which extends from the groin to the ankle, or the small saphenous vein may be removed.

Nursing Management

The nurse assesses the skin, distal circulation, and peripheral edema, asking the client to rate the level of discomfort and ability to do active and isometric leg exercises. (See Chapter 14 for routine perioperative care.)

When a surgical approach is used, the client returns with a gauze dressing covered by elastic roller bandages on the operative leg(s). The nurse monitors for swelling in the operative leg(s) and its effect on circulation. The nurse removes and rewraps the roller bandage to facilitate blood flow and inspects the dressing for signs of active bleeding. In the immediate postoperative period, the nurse elevates the foot of the bed to aid venous circulation to the heart and reminds the client to alternately contract and relax the lower leg muscles. If active exercise is inadequate, the nurse consults with the primary provider about using pneumatic venous compression stockings, which cover the leg from foot to thigh and periodically inflate and release air, simulating isometric muscle contraction. The nurse helps the client ambulate as soon as possible to promote venous circulation, reduce edema, and prevent venous thrombosis. When bleeding is no longer a problem, the nurse applies elastic antiembolism stockings in place of the elastic roller bandage and provides adequate fluid to decrease potential thrombosis.

When teaching the client and family, the nurse identifies factors that impair venous circulation: wearing elastic girdles or tight belts, using round garters or rolling and twisting nylon stockings, standing or sitting for prolonged periods, and sitting with the knees crossed. The nurse describes appropriate foot and nail care to facilitate tissue integrity, explaining that any open areas on the feet or lower legs require examination and treatment by the primary provider. The nurse recommends active or isometric exercises and elevation of the extremities frequently during the day. They demonstrate how to apply and remove elastic support stockings and refers the client to the dietitian if weight loss is indicated.

Aneurysms

An **aneurysm** is the stretching and bulging of an arterial wall. Aneurysms of the aorta (aortic arch, thoracic, abdominal) are the most common, but aneurysms can be found in other arteries, such as those in the legs and brain.

Pathophysiology and Etiology

Arteriosclerosis, hypertension, trauma, or a congenital weakness can affect the elasticity of the *tunica media* (middle layer of the artery wall), causing part of the vessel to bulge. Once formed, some aneurysms lay down layers of clots, blocking the vessel until blood flow stops. Most aneurysms enlarge until they rupture. Loss of a large volume of arterial blood leads to shock and death if not controlled. Some aneurysms tear and leak blood into surrounding cavities, such as the thorax or abdomen. Blood in a dissecting aneurysm is unavailable to arteries that branch off the aorta. When blood flow decreases or stops, tissue necrosis occurs.

Assessment Findings

Signs and Symptoms

Many aneurysms go unnoticed until found during physical examination or the client has a massive hemorrhage. Some cause pain, discomfort, and symptoms related to pressure on nearby structures. For example, a thoracic aortic aneurysm can cause bronchial obstruction, *dysphagia* (difficulty swallowing), and dyspnea. An abdominal aortic aneurysm can produce nausea and vomiting from pressure exerted on the intestines, or it may cause severe back pain from pressure on the vertebrae or spinal nerves. Most clients are hypertensive. A pulsating mass may be felt or even seen around the umbilicus or to the left of midline over the abdomen. A **bruit** (purring or blowing sound) can be auscultated over the mass. Circulation to tissue may be impaired.

Symptoms of a dissecting aneurysm vary and depend on whether a branching artery has been occluded or a tear has occurred in the aortic wall. Many clients become suddenly and acutely ill. Difference in the BPs of the left and right arms may be marked, or the BPs of the left and right legs may be unequal. Severe pain and signs of shock usually are present, but symptoms can be less severe in some instances. Because symptoms vary, diagnosis may be difficult.

Diagnostic Findings

Radiographs can demonstrate aneurysms when the arterial wall contains calcium deposits. Aortography identifies the size and exact location of the aneurysm.

Medical and Surgical Management

Medical treatment includes administering antihypertensive drugs to keep BP within normal range. Aneurysms are treated surgically whenever possible; no other cure exists. They are repaired by bypass or replacement grafting (see Chapter 29). A dissecting or ruptured aneurysm is a surgical emergency.

Nursing Management

The nurse helps control hypertension by keeping activity and stress to a minimum. The client should avoid straining during bowel movements, coughing, and holding the breath while changing positions. The nurse monitors BP, pulse, hourly urine output, skin color, level of consciousness, and characteristics of pain for signs of hemorrhage or dissection. They prepare the client for diagnostic testing and surgical interventions. Afterward, the nurse monitors for shock and adequate tissue perfusion. (See Chapter 29 for nursing management of a client undergoing cardiovascular surgery.)

KEY POINTS

- Arteriosclerosis: refers to the loss of elasticity or hardening of the arteries that accompanies the aging process.
- Atherosclerosis: a condition in which the lumen of arteries fill with fatty deposits called plaque
- Hyperlipidemia: high levels of blood fat triggers atherosclerotic changes. Factors such as gender, heredity, diet, diseases such as metabolic syndrome, and inactivity individually or collectively contribute to hyperlipidemia.
- Modifiable risk factors:
  - Smoking
  - Sedentary lifestyle
  - Obesity
  - Competitive, aggressive personality
  - High-fat diet
- Nonmodifiable risk factors:
  - Male sex
  - Diabetes mellitus
  - Increased lipid levels
  - Genetic predisposition
  - Hypertension
- CAD: arteriosclerotic and atherosclerotic changes in the coronary arteries supplying the myocardium
- Types of angina:
  - Stable angina
  - Unstable angina
  - Variant (Prinzmetal) angina
  - Microvascular angina (cardiac syndrome X)
- Proteins that transport lipids (cholesterol)
  - LDL has a lower ratio of protein to cholesterol. Or "bad cholesterol" because it sticks to arteries, exceeds recommended amounts (less than 100 mg/dL).
  - HDL has a higher ratio of protein to cholesterol. Or "good cholesterol" because it carries cholesterol to the liver for removal, is lower than desirable (more than 60 mg/dL).
- Drug therapy
  - Nitrates (e.g., nitroglycerin, isosorbide dinitrate): cause arterial vasodilation.
  - Beta-adrenergic blockers: decrease consumption of myocardial oxygen by reducing heart rate.
  - Calcium channel blockers: decrease consumption of myocardial oxygen by reducing heart rate.
  - Angiotensin-converting enzyme inhibitors: cause blood vessels to enlarge or dilate and reduces BP.
  - Diuretics: decrease work of heart by promoting excretion of sodium and water.
  - Nicotinic acid (niacin): in pharmacologic doses helps increase HDL and lower LDL.
- PTCA, or *balloon angioplasty:* uses sedation and local anesthesia, a balloon-tipped catheter is inserted through the skin and threaded from a peripheral artery into the diseased coronary artery. The catheter is positioned in the area of stenosis, and the balloon is inflated with CO_2 for anywhere from several seconds to several minutes. Inflation of the balloon compresses the atherosclerotic plaque against the arterial wall, increasing the diameter of the artery.
- Coronary stent: a small metal coil with meshlike openings placed in the coronary artery during PTCA. The stent prevents the buildup of new tissue that reforms in the artery, prevents the coronary artery from collapsing shortly after the procedure, and keeps the lumen open for a longer period.
- Atherectomy, or removal of fatty plaque: plaque is removed by either inserting a cardiac catheter with a cutting tool at the tip or by performing laser angioplasty.
- Cardiac markers:
  - Myoglobin
  - Troponin T
  - Troponin I
  - CK-MB (creatine kinase)
  - AST
  - LDH_1
  - LDH_2
- PVD is a general term for disorders that affect blood vessels distant from the large central blood vessels supplying the myocardium or that circulate blood directly in and out of the heart.
- PAD is a condition that affects primarily the blood vessels that supply oxygen to lower limbs. Can affect the carotid, renal, and mesenteric arteries.

- Raynaud syndrome: characterized by periodic constriction of the arteries that supply the extremities. The disorder is most common in young women.
- Thrombus is a stationary clot.
- Thrombosis is a state in which a thrombus has formed in a blood vessel.
- Thrombophlebitis is an inflammation of a vein accompanied by a clot or thrombus formation.
- Phlebothrombosis is the development of a clot within a vein without inflammation.
- Venous insufficiency: a peripheral vascular disorder in which the flow of venous blood is impaired through deep or superficial veins (or both). The condition usually affects the lower extremities, most often the medial aspect of the leg or around the ankle.
- Varicose veins or varicosities: dilated, tortuous veins, found mainly in the saphenous veins. May occur in other body parts, such as the rectum (hemorrhoids) and esophagus (esophageal varices). Varicose veins may be accompanied by a smaller variation called spider veins, which appear closer to the surface of the skin.
- Aneurysm: is the stretching and bulging of an arterial wall. Aneurysms of the aorta (aortic arch, thoracic, abdominal) are the most common, but aneurysms can be found in other arteries, such as those in the legs and brain.

CRITICAL THINKING EXERCISES

1. A client presents in the emergency department complaining of substernal chest pain. They have a history of angina. What assessment criteria will help you differentiate between an anginal attack and an MI? What diagnostic tests will confirm an MI?
2. What are some possible reasons women are often misdiagnosed and erroneously treated at the time of an MI?
3. A client with Raynaud syndrome relates that they have difficulty reducing attacks during the winter. What client teaching is indicated? How can the client reduce the ischemic episodes?
4. A client who has had ligation of varicose veins returns to their room after surgery. What assessments are a priority? How can you teach the client to reduce the incidence of further varicose vein formation?

NCLEX-STYLE REVIEW QUESTIONS PrepU

1. A client's lipid panel indicates an LDL of 182 mg/dL. What is an accurate analysis of the laboratory result?
   1. The client's LDL is desirable because it is less than 200 mg/dL.
   2. The client's LDL is optimal; lifestyle habits should be continued.
   3. The client's LDL is high; lifestyle changes should be encouraged.
   4. The client's LDL is borderline optimal; regular reassessment is recommended.
2. A client is given a prescription for sublingual nitroglycerin to be taken when chest pain develops. What nursing instructions are appropriate? Select all that apply.
   1. Place the tablet in the pouch between your cheek and gum.
   2. You may feel dizzy within minutes of taking the medication.
   3. Experiencing a headache is a sign of nitroglycerin toxicity.
   4. Take another tablet in 5 minutes if chest pain is unrelieved.
   5. Keep the tablets in a tightly closed container.
   6. Replace your supply of nitroglycerin tablets at least every month.
3. The nurse advises a client recovering from an MI to decrease dietary fat and salt. What choices would the nurse encourage in the client's diet? Select all that apply.
   1. Oatmeal rather than cold cereal.
   2. Egg substitute rather than scrambled eggs.
   3. Pepperoni pizza rather than sausage pizza.
   4. Soy sauce rather than table salt.
   5. Frozen yogurt rather than ice cream.
   6. Baked salmon rather than steak.
4. What discharge instructions for self-care should the nurse provide to a client who has undergone a PTCA? Select all that apply.
   1. Take tub baths to promote healing at the catheter insertion site.
   2. Clean the catheter insertion site with soap and water each day.
   3. Replace the dressing over the catheter insertion site daily.
   4. Refrain from driving for at least 3 days after the procedure.
   5. Resume sexual activity after the procedure at any time.
   6. Perform at-home exercises in lieu of a cardiac rehabilitation program.
5. A client with venous stasis in the lower extremities complains to the nurse that the elastic compression stockings are "too tight." What response by the nurse is most appropriate?
   1. "I'll remove them and remeasure your extremities."
   2. "I will call the doctor about discontinuing them."
   3. "Do you feel numbness and tingling in your toes?"
   4. "I'll request a larger pair of stockings."

WANT TO KNOW MORE? There are a wide variety of online resources available on thePoint to enhance learning and understanding of this chapter.

Go to thePoint.lww.com/activate and use the activation code found in the front of this text to unlock these online resources.

26 Caring for Clients With Cardiac Arrhythmias

Words To Know

arrhythmia
asystole
atrial fibrillation
atrial flutter
automated external defibrillator
bigeminy
cardiac rhythm
chemical cardioversion
couplets
defibrillation
demand (synchronous) mode pacemakers
ectopic pacemaker site
elective electrical cardioversion
electrophysiology study
fixed-rate (asynchronous) mode pacemakers
heart block
implantable cardioverter defibrillator
implanted pacemaker
Maze procedure
multifocal PVCs
pacemaker
premature atrial contraction
premature ventricular contraction
radiofrequency catheter ablation
R-on-T phenomenon
sinus bradycardia
sinus tachycardia
supraventricular tachycardia
surgical ablation
tachyarrhythmias
transcutaneous pacemaker
transvenous pacemaker
ventricular fibrillation
ventricular tachycardia
wireless intracardiac pacemaker

Learning Objectives

On completion of this chapter, you will be able to:

1. Name and describe common cardiac arrhythmias.
2. Identify medications to control or eliminate arrhythmias.
3. Explain the purpose and advantages of elective cardioversion.
4. Explain when defibrillation is used to treat arrhythmias.
5. Discuss the purpose for implanting an automatic internal cardiac defibrillator.
6. Name various types of artificial pacemakers and the purpose for their use.
7. Describe nursing management of the client with an arrhythmia treated by drug therapy, elective cardioversion, defibrillation, or pacemaker insertion.

Cardiac rhythm refers to the pattern (or pace) of the heartbeat. The conduction system of the heart and the inherent rhythmicity of cardiac muscle produce a rhythm pattern, which greatly influences the heart's ability to pump blood effectively. Basic cardiac conduction and electrocardiogram (ECG) waveforms are discussed in Chapter 22. The usual cardiac rhythm is called *normal sinus rhythm* (Box 26-1; Fig. 26-1). An ECG is used to identify normal and abnormal cardiac rhythms.

Gerontologic Considerations

- In older adults with atrial fibrillation, the incidence and complications of stroke increase. Prompt identification facilitates client and family education and conversion to normal sinus rhythm.
- Age increases the risk for arrhythmias as a result of a decreased number of cells in the sinoatrial (SA) node and altered function of the cells from accumulated fat and calcium. In older adults, stress, exercise, or illness may cause arrhythmias and other cardiac disorders such as heart failure and myocardial ischemia. (Age-related changes in the cardiac conduction system are identified in Chapter 22.)

This chapter gives a comprehensive overview of various arrhythmias. An **arrhythmia** (also called a *dysrhythmia*) is a conduction disorder that results in an abnormally slow or rapid heart rate or one that does not proceed through the conduction system in the usual manner. Cardiac output, the volume of blood ejected from the heart per minute, may be greatly compromised when a rhythm disturbance develops.

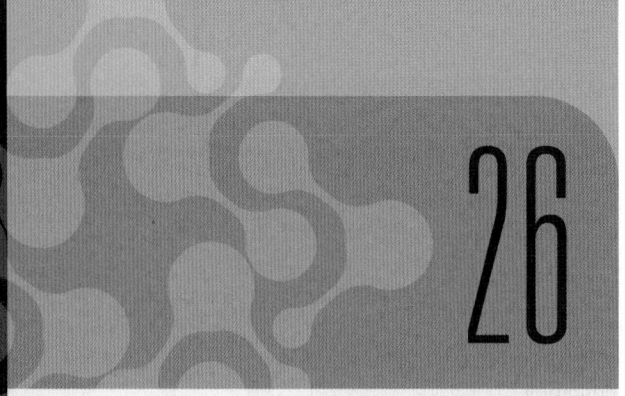

BOX 26-1 Characteristics of Normal Sinus Rhythm

- Heart rate is between 60 and 100 beats/min.
- The SA node initiates the impulse (upright P wave before each QRS complex).
- Impulse travels to the AV node in 0.12–0.2 second (the PR interval).
- The ventricles depolarize in 0.12 second or less (the QRS complex).
- Each impulse occurs regularly (evenly spaced).

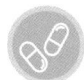

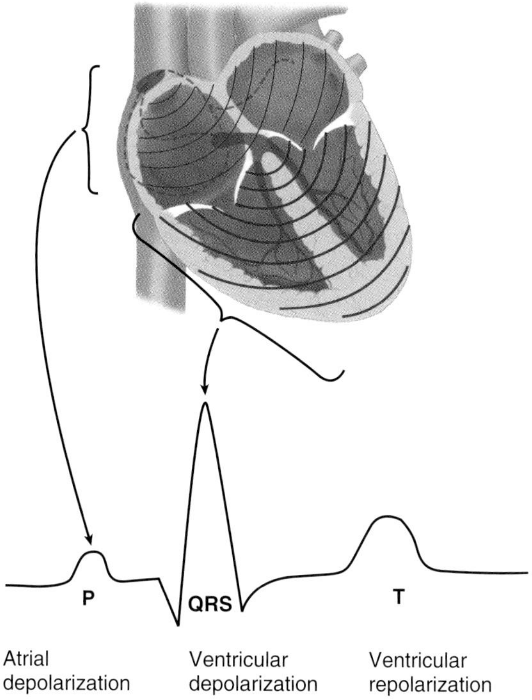

Figure 26-1 Normal conduction and electrocardiogram (ECG) waveforms.

Some arrhythmias do not require treatment; others require immediate intervention because they are potentially fatal. The most common cause of an arrhythmia is ischemic heart disease (see Chapter 25). Drug therapy, electrolyte disturbances, metabolic acidosis, hypothermia, and degenerative age-related changes are other conditions that cause arrhythmias.

>>> *Stop, Think, and Respond 26-1*

Describe the characteristics of normal sinus rhythm.

CARDIAC ARRHYTHMIAS

Cardiac arrhythmias may originate in the atria, atrioventricular (AV) node, or ventricles.

Arrhythmias Originating in the Atria

Examples of arrhythmias originating in the sinus node of the right atrium include sinus bradycardia and sinus tachycardia. Atrial arrhythmias that develop in sites outside the sinus node, yet within the atria, include premature atrial contractions, supraventricular tachycardia, atrial flutter, and atrial fibrillation.

Sinus Bradycardia

Sinus bradycardia is an arrhythmia that proceeds normally through the conduction pathway but at a slower-than-usual rate (≤60 beats/min; Fig. 26-2). Healthy athletes and others who are physically fit often have heart rates below 60 beats/min; however, it reflects a well-toned heart conditioned through regular exercise. A heart rate slower than 60 beats/min is pathologic in clients with heart disorders, increased intracranial pressure, hypothyroidism, or digitalis toxicity. The danger in sinus bradycardia is that the slow rate may be insufficient to maintain cardiac output. Atropine sulfate, a cholinergic blocking agent, is given intravenously to increase a dangerously slow heart rate.

Sinus Tachycardia

Sinus tachycardia is an arrhythmia that proceeds normally through the conduction pathway but at a faster-than-usual rate (100 to 150 beats/min; see Fig. 26-2). It occurs in clients with healthy hearts as a physiologic response to strenuous exercise, or anxiety and fear, pain, fever, hyperthyroidism, hemorrhage, shock, or hypoxemia.

Pharmacologic Considerations

- Atropine 0.5 mg IV may be given every 3 to 5 minutes to increase the heart rate, until a maximum dose of 3.0 mg. Other agents used include dopamine or epinephrine.

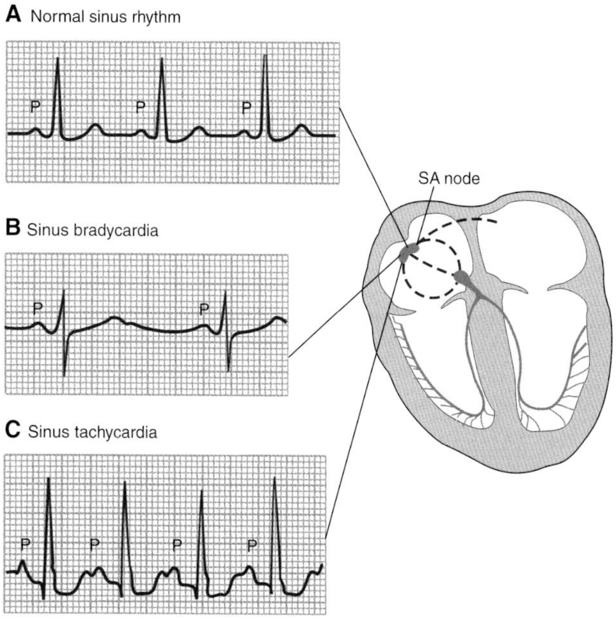

Figure 26-2 **(A)** In sinus rhythm, the sinoatrial (SA) node initiates impulses (P waves) at 60 to 100 times/min. **(B)** In sinus bradycardia, the SA node initiates impulses at 40 to 60 times/min. **(C)** In sinus tachycardia, the SA node initiates impulses at 100 to 150 times/min.

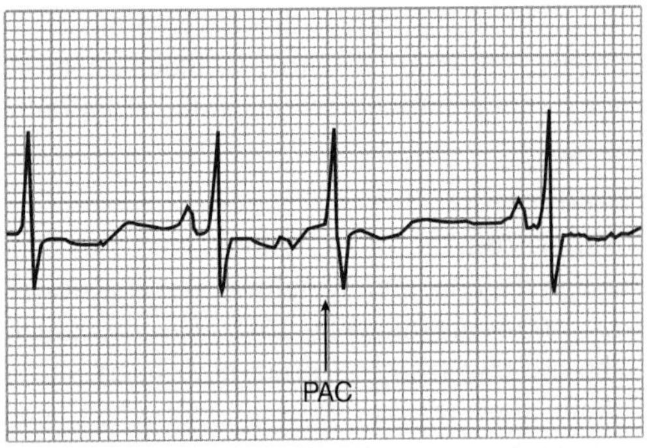

Figure 26-3 Normal sinus rhythm with one premature atrial contraction (PAC).

Premature Atrial Contractions

Occasionally, neural tissue in the atrial conduction system initiates an early electrical impulse called a **premature atrial contraction** (PAC), which is identified by an irregularity in the underlying rhythm (Fig. 26-3). The P wave of the waveform may look similar to other conducted impulses or may differ slightly because it is initiated somewhere in the atrium other than the sinoatrial (SA) node. PACs can occur for various reasons: consumption of caffeine, use of nicotine or other sympathetic nervous system stimulants, or in response to heart disease or metabolic disorders such as hyperthyroidism. When PACs are isolated or infrequent, there is no cause for alarm. Eliminating the cause usually controls PACs. Occasionally, the **ectopic pacemaker site**, one that initiates an electrical impulse independently of the SA node, can lead to more serious arrhythmias such as supraventricular tachycardia.

Supraventricular Tachycardia

Supraventricular tachycardia (SVT) is an arrhythmia in which the heart rate has a consistent rhythm but beats at a dangerously high rate (≥150 beats/min). Diastole is shortened and the heart does not have sufficient time to fill. Cardiac output drops dangerously low and heart failure can occur, especially in clients with preexisting heart disease or damage. Clients with coronary artery disease (CAD) and SVT can develop chest pain because coronary blood flow cannot meet the increased need of the myocardium for oxygen imposed by the fast rate. Besides tachycardia and angina, hypotension, syncope, and reduced renal output are signs and symptoms of low cardiac output and impending heart failure. Digitalis, adrenergic blockers, and calcium channel blockers are used to slow the heart rate.

Atrial Flutter

Atrial flutter (Fig. 26-4) is a disorder in which a single atrial impulse outside the SA node causes the atria to contract at an exceedingly rapid rate (200 to 400 contractions/min). The AV node conducts only some impulses to the ventricle, resulting in a ventricular rate that is slower than the atrial rate. The atrial waves in atrial flutter have a characteristic sawtooth pattern.

Atrial Fibrillation

In **atrial fibrillation**, several areas in the right atrium initiate impulses resulting in disorganized, rapid activity. The atria quiver rather than contract (Fig. 26-5, Evidence-Based Practice 26-1). The ventricles respond to the atrial stimulus

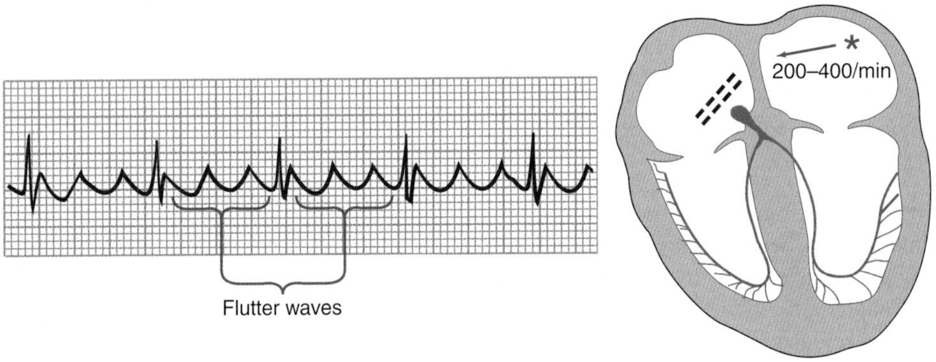

Figure 26-4 Atrial flutter produces sawtooth flutter waves. Most of the atrial impulses are not conducted to the ventricles.

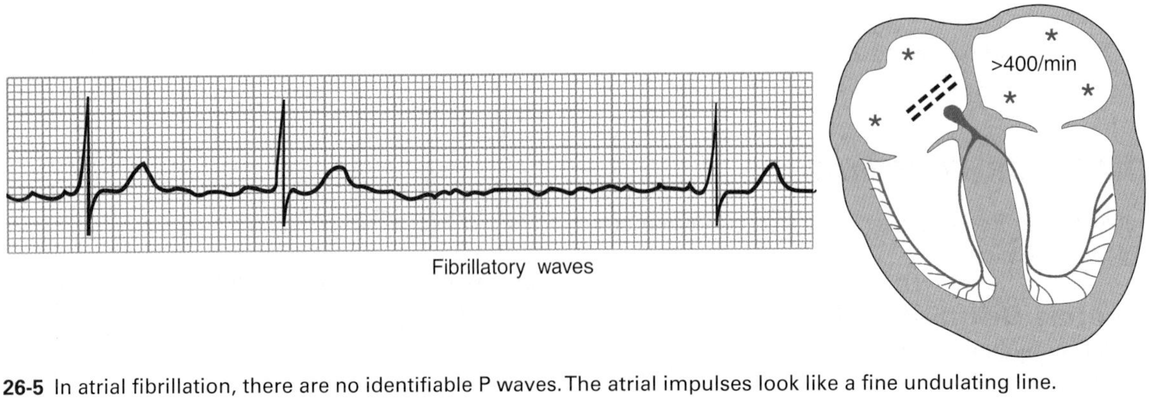

Figure 26-5 In atrial fibrillation, there are no identifiable P waves. The atrial impulses look like a fine undulating line.

Evidence-Based Practice 26-1

Atrial Fibrillation

Clinical Question

What is the management after atrial fibrillation?

Evidence

Atrial fibrillation (AF) can be the biggest cause of strokes. "The Framingham study has shown that during a follow up period of 30 years, clients with nonvalvular AF had a more than fivefold risk of stroke and the risk of stroke attributed to stroke increased with age" (Cantillon & Amuthan, 2018).

Treatment of AF varies with the type of stroke, the age and medical health of the client. Invasive and noninvasive treatment attempts to restore the heart rate to within normal limits. As the population ages and treatment options continue to improve, "AF therapy for AF may be personalized to improve treatment outcomes. Further research into the underlying molecular and genetic causes of AF may lead to novel methods of disease prevention" (Cantillon & Amuthan, 2018).

Nursing Implications

This review indicates a strong need for close monitoring of older adult clients. This is important for prevention and early diagnosis. Nurses can use this evidence in their education when planning care for older adult clients in inpatient and outpatient settings. Close monitoring and assessments of older adult clients may be the best prevention for the occurrence of a severe stroke.

Reference

Cantillon, D. J., & Amuthan, R. *Atrial fibrillation.* http://www.clevelandclinicmeded.com/medicalpubs/diseasemanagement/cardiology/atrial-fibrillation/

randomly, causing an irregular ventricular heart rate, which may be too infrequent to maintain adequate cardiac output. One of the chief complications of atrial fibrillation is the formation of blood clots within the atria that may become stroke-causing emboli if they enter the circulation.

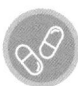

Pharmacologic Considerations

- Ongoing anticoagulant therapy is prescribed for those with atrial fibrillation. Living conditions of the client may determine which type of drug is used. Warfarin (Coumadin) is a low-cost drug commonly prescribed, but it requires frequent serum-level monitoring and some dietary restrictions. Should a person on anticoagulants live far away from medical services, they now have an alternative. Dabigatran (Pradaxa), rivaroxaban (Xarelto), and apixaban (Eliquis) are newer anticoagulants that do not require frequent laboratory testing.

Ibutilide (Corvert) is an antiarrhythmic drug used to convert new-onset atrial fibrillation into sinus rhythm; flecainide (Tambocor) and propafenone (Rythmol) also are used to treat and prevent atrial fibrillation. Use of drugs to eliminate an arrhythmia is referred to as **chemical cardioversion.** Atrial fibrillation also is treated with elective cardioversion (discussed later) or digitalis if the ventricular rate is not too slow. Some individuals with atrial fibrillation continue to experience chronic atrial fibrillation or episodic events.

Clients with atrial fibrillation who are not candidates for cardioversion and fail to respond to conventional measures may be candidates for a surgical intervention referred to as the **Maze procedure** or **surgical ablation.** During the Maze procedure, the surgeon restores the normal conduction pathway in the atria by eliminating the rapid firing of ectopic pacemaker sites using scar-forming techniques. The traditional approach requires an open-chest incision, but a newer minimally invasive method, referred to as a *Mini Maze*, has been developed using a closed-chest approach and application of catheter-directed energy at the tissue creating abnormal electrical impulses.

Arrhythmias Originating in the Atrioventricular Node: Heart Block

Heart block refers to disorders in the conduction pathway that interfere with the transmission of impulses from the SA node through the AV node to the ventricles. Heart block may be first degree, second degree, or third degree (also called *complete heart block*). In first- and second-degree heart block, the impulse is delayed. In complete heart block (Fig. 26-6), the atrial impulse never gets through, and the ventricles develop their own rhythm independent of the atrial rhythm. In complete heart block, the ventricular rate is slow (30 to 40 beats/min). Pacemaker insertion (discussed later) is the treatment for complete heart block.

››› *Stop, Think, and Respond 26-2*

Discuss the consequences of a slow heart rate and low cardiac output.

Arrhythmias Originating in the Ventricles

Ventricular arrhythmias include premature ventricular contractions, ventricular tachycardia, and ventricular fibrillation.

Premature Ventricular Contractions

Premature ventricular contraction (PVC) is a ventricular contraction that occurs early and independently in the cardiac cycle before the SA node initiates an electrical impulse. No P wave precedes the wide, bizarre-looking QRS complex (Fig. 26-7). If the heart rate is very slow, the ventricles can repolarize after a PVC in sufficient time to receive the atrial stimulus precisely when it is due. PVCs often cause a flip-flop sensation in the chest, sometimes described as "fluttering." Associated signs and symptoms include pallor, nervousness, sweating, and faintness. Many people experience occasional PVCs, which usually are harmless. They may be related to anxiety, stress, fatigue, alcohol withdrawal, or tobacco use. Although PVCs normally are not associated with a specific heart disorder, those whom they frequently trouble should consult a primary provider. A thorough examination is important to ensure no heart disease exists.

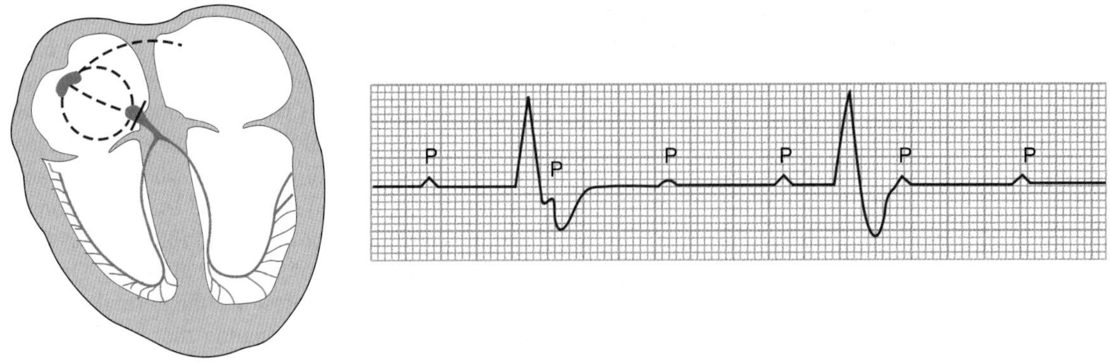

Figure 26-6 In heart block, sinoatrial (SA)-initiated impulses are delayed at the atrioventricular (AV) node or fail to progress altogether. In this example of complete heart block, the ventricles are beating independently of the atria.

In the presence of acute heart injury, such as after cardiac surgery or with acute myocardial infarction (MI), PVCs in certain patterns suggest myocardial irritability and are precursors of lethal arrhythmias (Fig. 26-8):

- Six or more PVCs per minute
- Runs of **bigeminy** (every other beat is a PVC)
- Two PVCs in a row (**couplets**)
- Runs of PVCs (three or more in a row)
- **Multifocal PVCs** (originating from more than one location)
- A PVC whose R wave falls on the T wave of the preceding complex (**R-on-T phenomenon**)

When dangerous PVCs occur, the client is given an intravenous (IV) bolus of lidocaine (Xylocaine) followed by a continuous IV infusion of the drug.

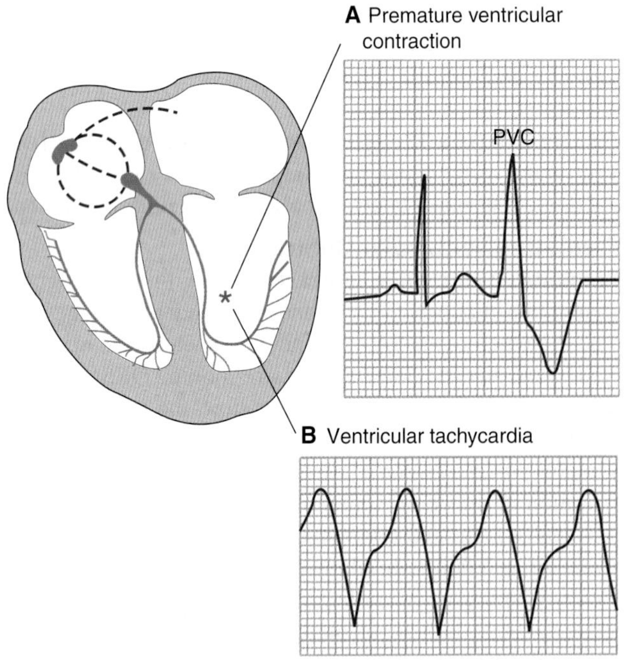

Figure 26-7 **(A)** An area outside the normal conduction pathway in the ventricles initiates a premature ventricular contraction (PVC). **(B)** Continuous generation of impulses results in ventricular tachycardia.

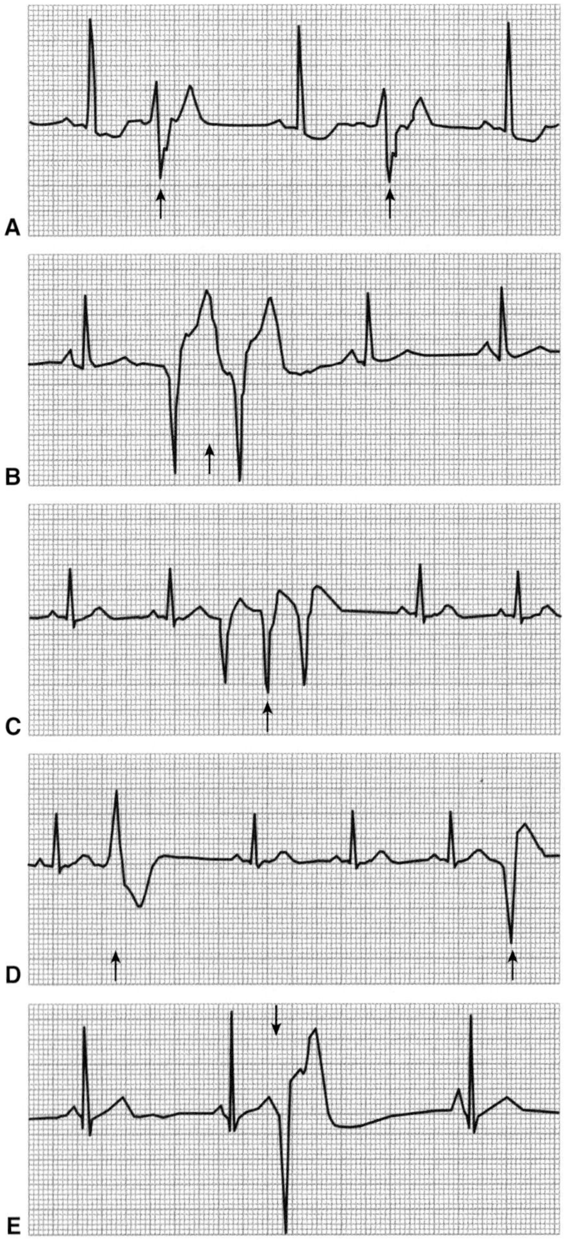

Figure 26-8 Dangerous forms of premature ventricular contractions (PVCs): **(A)** bigeminy, **(B)** couplets, **(C)** run, **(D)** multifocal, and **(E)** R-on-T phenomenon.

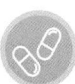

Pharmacologic Considerations

- Watch for toxicity with lidocaine infusions. Symptoms of lidocaine toxicity progress in the following predictable pattern: beginning with numbness of the tongue, lightheadedness, and visual disturbances, then progressing to muscle twitching, unconsciousness, and seizures, and then to coma, respiratory arrest, and cardiovascular depression.

Ventricular Tachycardia

Ventricular tachycardia is caused by a single, irritable focus in the ventricle that initiates and then continues the same repetitive pattern (see Fig. 26-7). The ventricles beat very fast (150 to 250 beats/min), and cardiac output is decreased. Depending on how long the arrhythmia is present, the client may lose consciousness and become pulseless. Ventricular tachycardia sometimes ends abruptly without intervention but often requires defibrillation. It may progress to ventricular fibrillation.

Ventricular Fibrillation

Ventricular fibrillation (Fig. 26-9) is the rhythm of a dying heart. PVCs or ventricular tachycardia can precipitate it. The ventricles do not contract effectively, and there is no cardiac output. Ventricular fibrillation is an indication for cardiopulmonary resuscitation (CPR) and immediate defibrillation.

Pathophysiology and Etiology of Cardiac Arrhythmias

Many clinical states predispose clients to arrhythmias. One of the most common causes of serious arrhythmias is myocardial ischemia, lack of oxygenated blood to the heart muscle, which can occur secondary to CAD congestive heart failure, inadequate ventilation, and shock. The conduction system also is susceptible to disturbances from anxiety, pain, endocrine disorders, electrolyte imbalances, valvular heart disease, placement of invasive catheters in the heart, and drug effects. Because of the altered rate and rhythm, all arrhythmias affect the heart's pumping action and cardiac output to some degree.

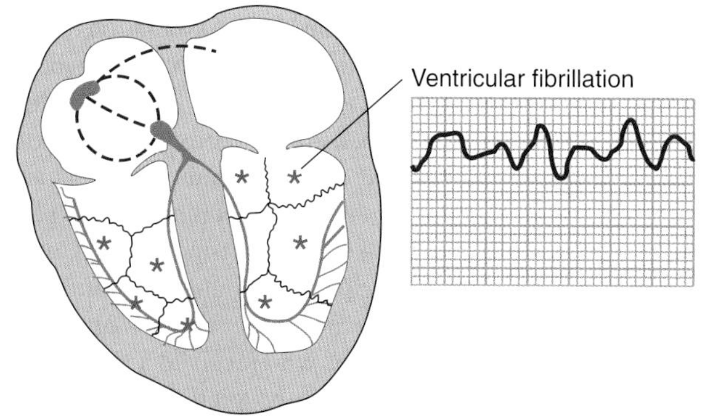

Figure 26-9 During ventricular fibrillation, the ventricles quiver, as shown by a wavy line.

Assessment Findings

Signs and Symptoms

A client whose arrhythmia causes decreased cardiac output is likely to feel weak and tired, experience anginal pain, or faint. Some clients with **tachyarrhythmias** (abnormally fast rhythms) describe palpitations or flutterings in their chest. blood pressure (BP) usually is low. Pulse is irregular or difficult to palpate; the rate is unusually fast or slow. The apical and radial pulse rates may differ. The skin may be pale and cool. The client may be disoriented and confused if the brain is not adequately oxygenated, or there may be loss of consciousness and even clinical death.

Diagnostic Findings

A monitor rhythm strip or 12-lead ECG can identify arrhythmias. Electrophysiology studies can locate their origin. An **electrophysiology study** is a procedure that enables the primary provider to examine the electrical activity of the heart; produce actual arrhythmias by stimulating structures in the conduction pathway; determine the best method for preventing further arrhythmic episodes; and, in some cases, eradicate tissue in the area of the heart that is producing the arrhythmia.

The test is performed by passing three flexible wire electrode catheters into veins in the neck and groin. The catheters are then advanced into the heart in each of the following locations: right atrium, bundle of His, and right ventricle. The electrode catheters monitor and record the heart's rhythm. The primary provider can use these same catheters to reproduce the abnormal heart rhythm that the client usually experiences by stimulating areas in the conduction system. When the arrhythmia is produced, the primary provider uses several drugs to evaluate each one's efficacy at restoring normal heart rhythm. The outcome of the trial drugs helps determine how to relieve the client's symptoms medically. The normal heart rhythm also may be restored with electrical shocks. With the catheters in place, the primary provider may use the opportunity to prevent the arrhythmia from ever reoccurring by delivering electricity to the area that originates the arrhythmia. The electricity destroys the pathogenic tissue with a *procedure called radiofrequency catheter ablation*, discussed later in this chapter.

Preparation, management, and recovery for the client undergoing an electrophysiology study are similar to those for a client undergoing a heart catheterization (see Chapter 22). Usually, the client is monitored for a full day and discharged the following day if no bleeding or vascular complications occur.

Medical and Surgical Management

Some arrhythmias are not life-threatening and may not require treatment. Many are treated with drug therapy and electrical modalities such as elective electrical cardioversion, defibrillation, or temporary or permanent pacing (Table 26-1).

TABLE 26-1 Characteristics and Treatment of Selected Arrhythmias

ARRHYTHMIA	RHYTHM	ATRIAL RATE (BEATS/MINUTE)	VENTRICULAR RATE (BEATS/MINUTE)	TREATMENT
Sinus bradycardia	Regular	<60	<60	None unless symptomatic; atropine
Sinus tachycardia	Regular	100–150	100–150	None unless symptomatic; treat underlying disease
Premature atrial contraction	Irregular	60–100	60–100	None or treat underlying cause, if known
Supraventricular tachycardia	Regular	150–250	150–250	Valsalva maneuver, unilateral carotid massage, immersion of face in ice water, administration of IV adenosine, cardioversion, radiofrequency ablation
Atrial flutter	Usually regular	250–350	75–175	Cardioversion, digitalis, quinidine, propranolol, verapamil
Atrial fibrillation	Grossly irregular	400–600	100–160	Digitalis, quinidine, cardioversion, verapamil, ibutilide, flecainide, amiodarone, anticoagulant
First-degree AV block	Regular	60–100	60–100	None unless symptomatic
Second-degree AV block	Regular	60–100	30–100	Pacemaker
Complete heart block	Regular	60–100	<40	Pacemaker
Ventricular tachycardia	Regular	60–100[a]	150–300	Lidocaine, procainamide, bretylium, cardioversion, defibrillation if pulseless
Ventricular fibrillation	Chaotic	60–100[a]	400–600	Defibrillation preceded by or followed with epinephrine

AV, atrioventricular; IV, intravenous.
[a]Rate may not be distinguishable.

Drug Therapy

Oral and IV antiarrhythmic drugs are used to treat clients with arrhythmias; however, not all clients require medication. Usually, long-term antiarrhythmic drug therapy is based on the degree of hemodynamic compromise and the potential for the client to develop a life-threatening arrhythmia. During resuscitation efforts, one or more of the various drugs used in cardiac emergencies is administered (Drug Therapy Table 26-1).

Elective Electrical Cardioversion

Elective electrical cardioversion is a nonemergency procedure done by a primary provider to stop rapid, but not necessarily life-threatening, atrial arrhythmias. It is similar to defibrillation (Table 26-2). One difference is that the machine that delivers the electrical stimulation waits to discharge until it senses the appearance of an R wave. By doing so, the machine prevents disrupting the heart during the critical period of ventricular repolarization.

The client is sedated for the procedure. Electrodes lubricated with a special gel or moist saline pads are applied to the chest wall. When the discharge buttons on the paddles (Fig. 26-10) are depressed and the heart is in ventricular depolarization, the electrical energy is released. The electrical current completely depolarizes the entire myocardium. As the heart repolarizes, ideally, the normal pacemaker regains control and restores continued normal conduction through the heart.

Defibrillation

The only treatment for a life-threatening ventricular arrhythmia is immediate **defibrillation**, which has exactly the same effect as cardioversion except that defibrillation is used when there is no functional ventricular contraction. Without defibrillation, the client will die. A defibrillator discharges its electrical energy when the discharge button is depressed. It is used during pulseless ventricular tachycardia, ventricular fibrillation, and **asystole** (cardiac arrest) when no identifiable R wave is present.

Automated External Defibrillator

An **automated external defibrillator** (AED) analyzes the heart's rhythm to determine if defibrillation is needed and, if so, allows the user to administer electrical energy to stop the arrhythmia and allow the heart to reestablish an effective rhythm (Fig. 26-11). The American Heart Association recommends public access defibrillation—that is, that AEDs be located in public places such as worksites and locations where large numbers of people gather. AEDs currently are carried on some airplanes and police cars. Nontraditional rescuers, those other than emergency medical technicians and paramedics, are encouraged to take the Heartsaver AED Course to learn how to provide defibrillation in out-of-hospital locations as soon as possible after a person becomes unresponsive. Sixty-six percent of victims who received a shock from AED from a bystander survived to hospital discharge (Cardiac Arrest, 2018). Survival decreases 7% to 10% with every minute that defibrillation is delayed (Defibrillation, 2020).

DRUG THERAPY TABLE 26-1 Antiarrhythmics

Category and Common Generic (Brand) Drugs	Intended Use	Common Side Effects	Safety Warnings for Nurses
Class I: Sodium (or Fast) Channel Blockers			
Class I A (moderate block) Disopyramide (Norpace) Quinidine (generic only)	Ventricular arrhythmias, prevent recurrent paroxysmal atrial fibrillation	Dry mouth, constipation, urinary hesitancy, nausea, fatigue, dizziness, headache, rash, hypotension	When given IV, constant cardiac monitoring is required Monitor for ringing in the ears Monitor for toxicity when quinidine is used Monitor immune system with chronic use
Class I B (weak block) Lidocaine (Xylocaine) Mexiletine (Mexitil) Phenytoin (Dilantin)	Ventricular tachyarrhythmias	Lightheadedness, nervousness, bradycardia, hypotension	Cardiac monitoring Do not use during and immediately after MI
Class I C (pronounced block) Flecainide (Tambocor) Propafenone (Rythmol)	Prevent paroxysmal atrial fibrillation, ventricular tachyarrhythmias	Dizziness, headache, faintness, unsteadiness	Monitor for new or worsening arrhythmias Do not give immediately after MI
Class II (Beta-Blockers or Beta-Adrenergic Blockers)			
Atenolol (Tenormin) Metoprolol (Lopressor) Propranolol (Inderal) Timolol (Blocadren)	Prevents recurrence of tachyarrhythmias	Nausea, vomiting, bradycardia, dizziness, hypotension	When given IV, constant cardiac monitoring is required Drug is usually held if heart rate <60 and >120 Initially, monitor blood every 2–3 weeks for agranulocytosis
Class III (Potassium Channel Blockers)			
Amiodarone (Cordarone, Pacerone) Dofetilide (Tikosyn) Dronedarone (Multaq) Ibutilide (Corvert) Sotalol (Betapace)	Conversion of atrial fibrillation/flutter to normal sinus rhythm	Malaise, fatigue, tremor, nausea, vomiting, constipation	Can harm kidneys, check creatinine clearance
Class IV (Calcium Channel Blockers)			
Diltiazem (Cardizem) Verapamil (Calan)	Prevents recurrence of supraventricular tachycardia	Hypotension, dizziness, nausea, dry cough	When given IV, constant cardiac monitoring is required Drug is usually held if heart rate 60–120 No grapefruit Initially, monitor blood every 2–3 weeks for agranulocytosis
Class V			
Adenosine (Adenocard)	Stops supraventricular tachycardia, cardiac stress testing	Flushing, headache	Use cautiously in the elderly

IV, intravenous; MI, myocardial infarction.

TABLE 26-2 Comparison of Cardioversion and Defibrillation

CARDIOVERSION	DEFIBRILLATION
Scheduled procedure 1 to several days in advance	Emergency procedure performed during resuscitation
Used to eliminate atrial arrhythmias (e.g., atrial flutter, atrial fibrillation, supraventricular tachycardia)	Used to eliminate ventricular arrhythmias (e.g., ventricular fibrillation, asystole)
Client sedated before procedure	Client not sedated but unresponsive
Uses less electrical energy (50–100 joules) than defibrillation, but higher levels can be administered if initial outcome is unsuccessful	Uses more electrical energy (200–360 joules) than cardioversion
Delivers electrical energy when the machine senses the R wave of the ECG	Delivers electrical energy whenever the buttons on the paddles are pressed

ECG, electrocardiogram.

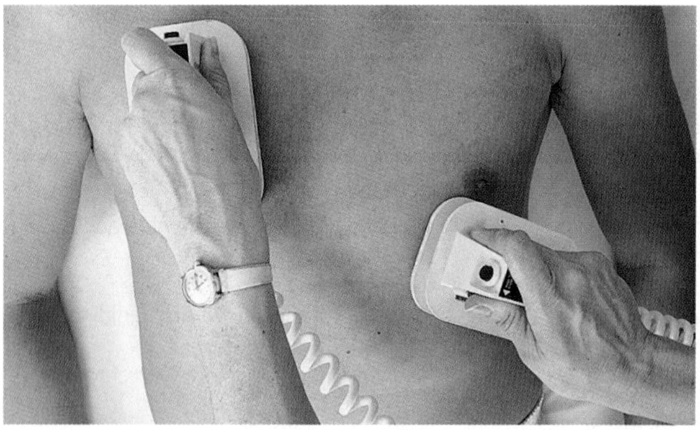

Figure 26-10 Standard paddle placement for cardioversion or defibrillation.

Concept Mastery Alert

Medication for Cardioversion

Prior to cardioversion, a sedative such as diazepam (Valium) is used. To increase a dangerously slow heart rate, atropine may be used.

Implantable Cardioverter Defibrillator

An **implantable cardioverter defibrillator** (ICD) is an internal electrical device used for selected clients with recurrent life-threatening tachydysrhythmias. Candidates for an ICD include those who (1) have survived at least one episode of cardiac arrest from a ventricular dysrhythmia, (2) experience recurrent episodes of ventricular tachycardia, or (3) are at risk for sudden cardiac death because of structural heart disease such as cardiomyopathy (see Chapter 23) with poor ventricular function.

An ICD consists of a generator with a battery and one (sometimes two) electrical lead that resembles a wire (Fig. 26-12). The generator is placed in a pocket under the skin near the clavicle, and the lead wire is inserted transvenously through the subclavian or cephalic vein to the apex or septum of the right ventricle. The lead senses the cardiac rhythm, which it transmits to the generator. The generator, which is programmed for various responses depending on the sensed rhythm, delivers an electrical shock through the lead to restore a life-sustaining cardiac rhythm, records the data, and then resets itself. A conscious client perceives the defibrillating shock as a thump or "kick" to the chest. ICDs also can pace the heart to obliterate a tachydysrhythmia and perform low-energy cardioversion. Various studies have confirmed that ICDs reduce death rates among at-risk clients.

The ICD is checked every 3 to 4 months. The stored information can be retrieved by passing an electromagnetic wand over the implanted generator. The ICD can be reprogrammed in the same way. ICDs can deliver approximately 200 to 250 discharges and last for approximately 3 to 6 years before the battery requires replacement. Although ICDs are highly safe, some forms of electrical interference may adversely affect their function. Clients are instructed to avoid devices with a magnetic field. Examples include magnetic resonance imaging devices, extracorporeal shock wave lithotripsy machines (see Chapter 58), electrocautery and diathermy devices, peripheral nerve stimulators, large industrial electrical motors, and arc welding equipment. Also, electrical signals from digital cellular telephones can mimic an abnormal heart rhythm, activating the ICD if placed close to the device (Cell phone, 2020).

Most power tools and microwave ovens have shields or are grounded, making them safe. Occasionally, however, devices that use radiofrequency signals have affected ICDs. A hand search is preferable to a scan with a metal detector at airports. Placing a donut magnet over the generator deactivates the device and should be done only if equipment is available to use an external defibrillator.

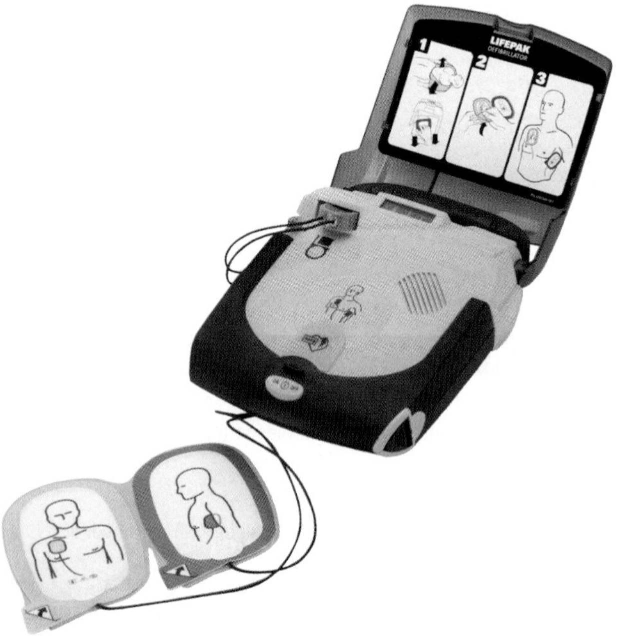

Figure 26-11 An automated external defibrillator commonly located in various public facilities. (Courtesy of Physio-Control, Inc.)

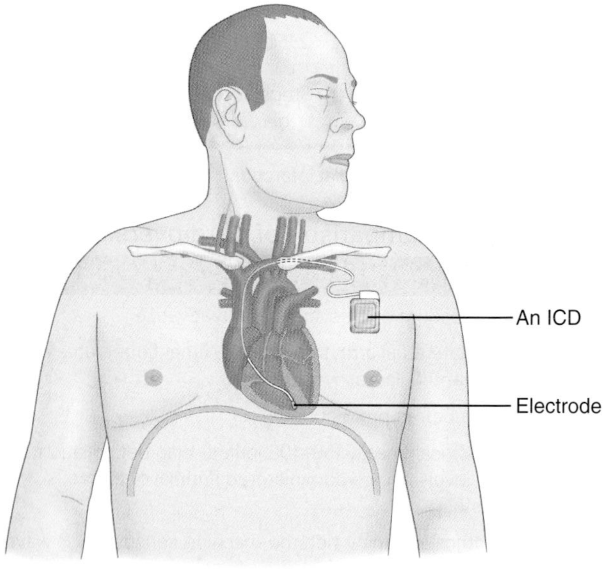

Figure 26-12 An implanted cardioverter defibrillator (ICD).

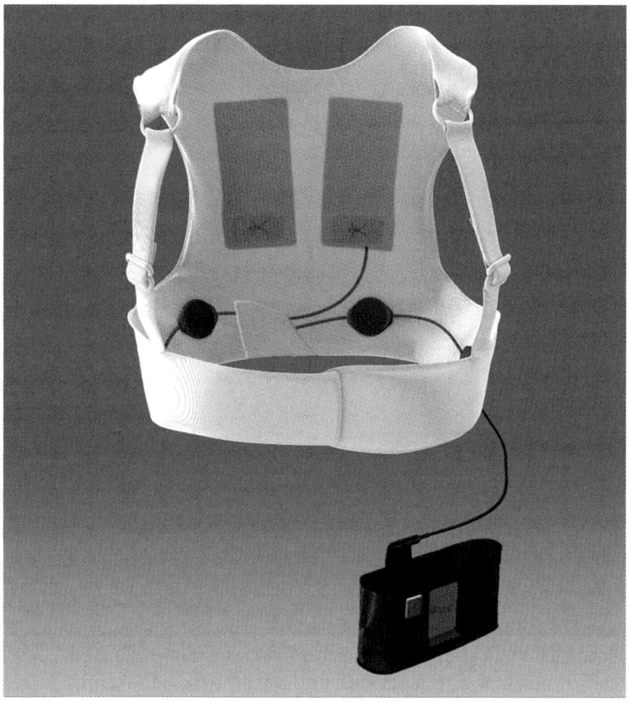

Figure 26-13 A wearable cardioverter defibrillator monitors a client for dangerous arrhythmias and shocks the heart to restore a normal rhythm. (Courtesy of ZOLL LifeVest.)

Clients with ICDs are advised to carry information about the device on their person, including the names of primary providers involved in their care. Driving usually is restricted for 1 week for those whose ICDs were implanted for primary prevention; driving is restricted for 6 months following a previous cardiac arrest or ventricular dysrhythmia (Mayo Clinic Staff, 2015). Furthermore, clients are told to report episodes in which they sense ICD activity evidenced by feeling a light thump or kick to the chest. If the ICD discharges repeatedly or the client is symptomatic, immediate assessment by a cardiologist or electrophysiologist is warranted. The ICD may need to be reprogrammed, additional therapy with antiarrhythmic drugs may be initiated, or current medications may be adjusted.

Wearable cardiac defibrillators, worn outside the body, are now available (Fig. 26-13). The device is designed for temporary use by clients at high risk for sudden cardiac arrest following an MI, those awaiting myocardial revascularization surgery, and those with cardiomyopathy and heart failure until such time that the primary provider can suggest further definitive treatment.

Stop, Think, and Respond 26-3

Explain why ventricular dysrhythmias are more serious than most atrial dysrhythmias.

Pacemakers

A **pacemaker** provides an electrical stimulus to the heart muscle to treat an ineffective slow rhythm. Pacemakers function in either a demand (synchronous) or fixed-rate (asynchronous) mode. **Demand (synchronous) mode pacemakers** self-activate when the client's pulse falls below a certain level. Thus, if the pacemaker is set at 72 beats/min, it will not activate until the client's natural heart rate falls below 72 beats/min. **Fixed-rate (asynchronous) mode pacemakers** produce an electrical stimulus at a preset rate (usually 72 to 80 beats/min) despite the client's natural rhythm. This type is used less frequently than the demand (synchronous) mode pacemaker.

Pacemakers can be categorized into two broad divisions: temporary or permanent. Temporary pacing is done under urgent or emergency circumstances. A permanent pacemaker is implanted when the client has a chronic ineffective slow cardiac rhythm that requires long-term electrical support.

Temporary Pacemakers

The three types of temporary pacemakers are transcutaneous, transvenous, and transthoracic. An external **transcutaneous pacemaker** is an emergency measure for maintaining adequate heart rate. It uses disposable, self-adhering leads (wires) applied to the chest (Fig. 26-14). The heart rate is paced from an external generator. Use of a transcutaneous pacemaker is temporary until either a transvenous or a permanent pacemaker can be placed or the client is stabilized with medication.

A **transvenous pacemaker** is a temporary pulse-generating device that sometimes is necessary to manage transient bradyarrhythmias such as those that occur during acute MIs or after coronary artery bypass graft surgery or to override tachyarrhythmias. The electrical lead is introduced through the subclavian, external or internal jugular, or cephalic vein and threaded first into the right atrium, and then into the right ventricle (Fig. 26-15). It may be inserted at the bedside. Fluoroscopy and a cardiac monitor are used to determine the correct placement of the tip of the pacemaker lead.

The leads of a *transthoracic pacemaker* are inserted during open heart surgery. They extend from the chest incision. If the client requires cardiac pacing during postoperative recovery, the leads are connected to a temporary pacing unit.

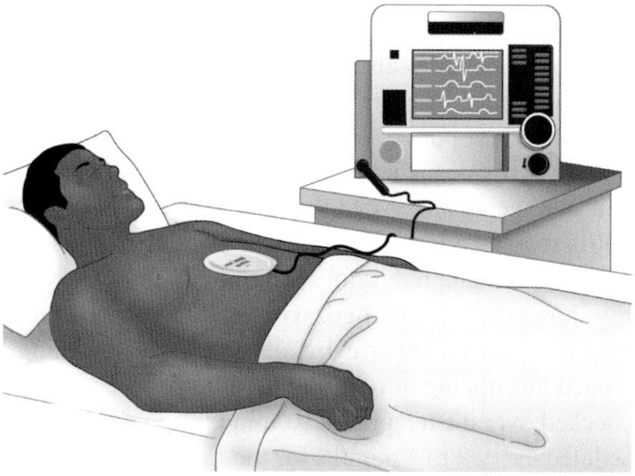

Figure 26-14 Transcutaneous pacemaker with electrode pads connected to the anterior and posterior chest walls.

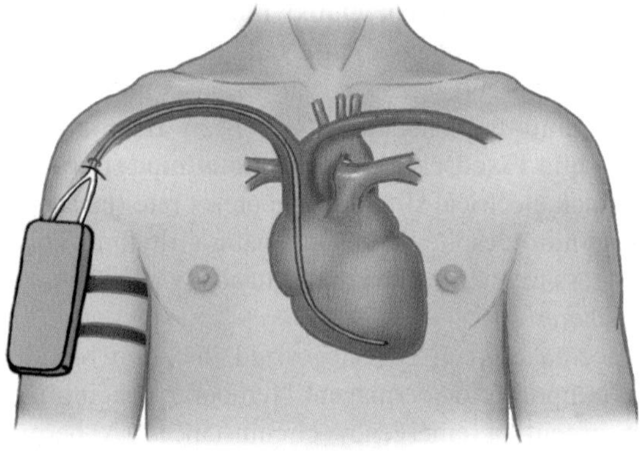

Figure 26-15 A transvenous pacemaker.

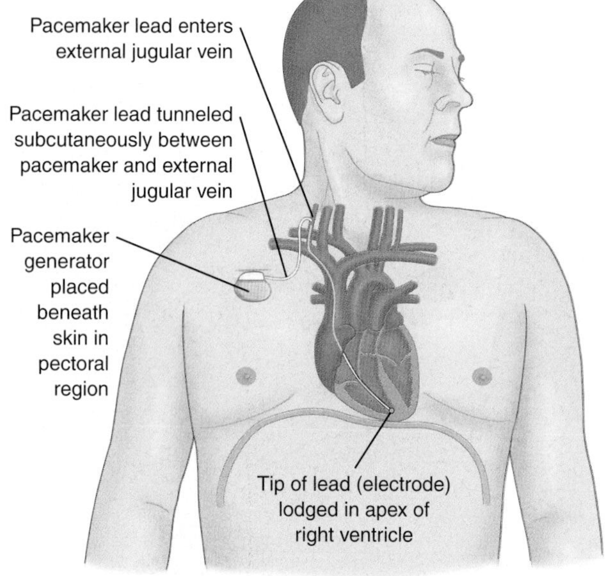

Figure 26-16 A permanent pacemaker uses an implanted transvenous pacing electrode and pacemaker generator.

Permanent (Implanted) Pacemaker

An **implanted pacemaker** is a totally implanted electrical device used to manage a chronic bradyarrhythmia. It consists of a battery-powered generator that controls the heart rate and one or more leads (wires) that connect the heart to the generator.

The most frequent indication for inserting a permanent pacemaker is complete or second-degree heart block accompanied by a slow ventricular rate. Occasionally, permanent pacing is used to treat certain tachyarrhythmias that do not respond to treatment or whose treatment results in bradycardia.

The lead of an implanted pacemaker is inserted transvenously, and the pacing threshold, voltage, and rate are set. One type of pacemaker has leads in both the right atrium and right ventricle (dual chamber); the lead of a single-chamber pacemaker is in either the right atrium or right ventricle. The implantable pacemaker generator, which is about the size of a half-dollar coin and three times as thick, is then positioned under the skin below the right or left clavicle, preferably on the client's nondominant side (Fig. 26-16). The small incision is closed with sutures. PVCs are more frequent during the early postimplantation period, and drug therapy may be ordered to suppress this arrhythmia.

Power for the pacemaker is provided by mercury, lithium, or nuclear-powered (plutonium) batteries. The mercury battery has the shortest life, 5 to 7 years; the nuclear-powered battery has the longest, 6 to 15 years (Chen, 2014). Externally charged batteries also are used. Pacemaker batteries do not fail suddenly. The primary provider regularly monitors the status of their power. When the battery is nearing its end, the entire generator is replaced and the leads are connected to the new generator. After the pacemaker is inserted, the client is reassessed in 3 months and every 6 months thereafter. If the client redevelops original symptoms or suddenly shows dyspnea, vertigo, syncope, unexplained fatigue, edema in upper or lower extremities, muscle twitching, or extended hiccupping develops in the interim, the pacemaker is checked over the telephone. Routine telephone checks are scheduled every 2 to 4 months for the first 3 years and every month thereafter. If a problem develops, the pacemaker is reprogrammed with an external wand just like the ICD.

Wireless Intracardiac Pacemaker. The miniaturized **wireless intracardiac pacemaker** which is about the size of a large capsule, has a self-contained battery, electronics, and electrodes. The wireless pacemaker is inserted nonsurgically with a catheter that extends from the femoral vein to the right ventricle (Fig. 26-17). Once the catheter reaches the right ventricle, the pacemaker is implanted in the heart muscle with a coiled spring-like device on its distal end and is disengaged from the vascular catheter. Besides eliminating the skin pouch that contains a traditional pacemaker and its potential for an incisional infection, there are no wires that can fracture over time. The battery that powers the wireless

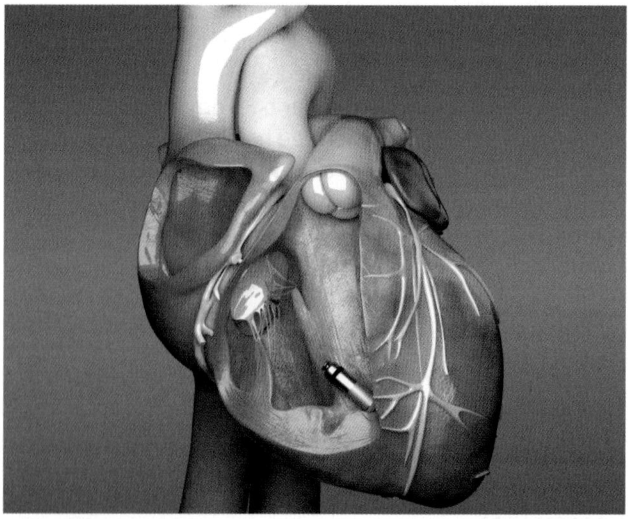

Figure 26-17 A wireless pacemaker attached to a catheter is threaded through the femoral vein into the right ventricle where the pacemaker is released and becomes implanted. (Reproduced with permission of Medtronic.)

pacemaker is projected to last 8 to 10 years and is retrieved and replaced using the same technique as its insertion.

Radiofrequency Catheter Ablation

Radiofrequency catheter ablation is a procedure in which a heated catheter tip destroys arrhythmia-producing tissue. A catheter is threaded transvenously into the heart, initially for electrophysiology studies. Once the location of the arrhythmia-generating tissue is identified, electrical energy is sent to the catheter tip (Fig. 26-18). The heat destroys the errant tissue, allowing impulse conduction to travel over appropriate pathways. Accompanying risks include bleeding from the insertion site, perforation of the catheterized vein, and vascular complications such as thrombus formation. When the catheter is in the heart itself, it may pierce the myocardium, leading to pericardial tamponade. It is also possible for the heated tip to obliterate normal conductive tissue, requiring a permanent pacemaker to ensure heart contraction.

Nursing Management

Clients with symptomatic arrhythmias require careful monitoring and documentation of symptoms. Clients with serious arrhythmias are potentially unstable, making frequent rhythm analyses important. Administering and monitoring the effects of antiarrhythmic drugs are key nursing responsibilities. Drugs given to restore or control cardiac rhythm are powerful, and their therapeutic levels often are close to toxic levels. Many of these drugs cause unwanted side effects and are contraindicated in certain conditions. The nurse assists with medical procedures that help to restore normal sinus rhythm and manages postprocedural care. The nurse also provides health teaching that promotes the client's ability to maintain safe self-management after discharge. Clients with cardiac risk factors should avoid drinking more than 6 oz of beer or wine per day; during alcohol withdrawal, catecholamines are released and may cause dangerous arrhythmias.

Elective Electrical Cardioversion

Prior to electrical cardioversion, the client may be anticoagulated to reduce the risk of thrombus formation and embolization. When the partial thromboplastin time (PTT) or international normalized ratio (INR) is within a therapeutic range, the nurse prepares the client for electrical cardioversion. This preparation is similar to preparing a client for a surgical procedure, making sure to verify that a consent form has been signed. Food and oral fluids are restricted. The nurse ensures a patent IV line and consults the primary provider to determine if scheduled drugs are to be temporarily withheld or additional drugs to decrease anxiety are to be administered. The primary provider may order a sedative 30 to 60 minutes before the procedure. Digitalis and diuretics are withheld for 24 to 72 hours before cardioversion; it is believed that the presence of these drugs in myocardial cells decreases the ability to restore normal conduction and increases the chances of a fatal arrhythmia developing after cardioversion.

The nurse places the cardioverter in the client's room and checks that emergency equipment such as an oral airway, oxygen, suction, and emergency drugs are on hand. Just before the procedure, the nurse assists the client with bladder or bowel elimination. They administer an IV tranquilizer, usually diazepam (Valium) or midazolam (Versed), as prescribed and insert an oral airway once the client is sedated. The desired response to elective cardioversion is a normal sinus rhythm, normal or adequate BP, and strong peripheral

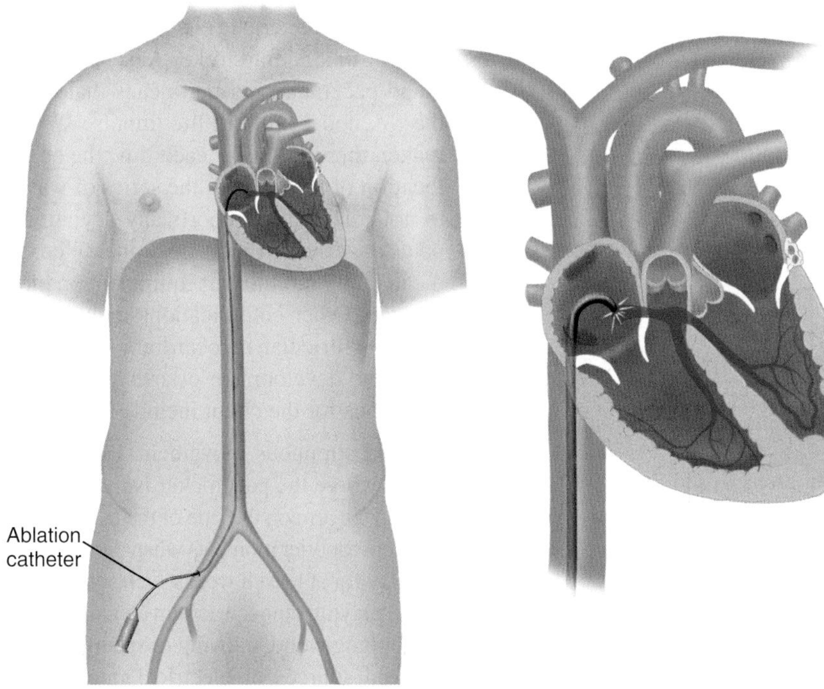

Figure 26-18 A catheter is guided to the heart, and radiofrequency catheter ablation destroys the defective conducting tissue.

pulses in all extremities. After cardioversion, the nurse monitors vital signs every 15 minutes for the first 1 or 2 hours and then as ordered. They observe the cardiac monitor to evaluate heart rate and rhythm continuously and compare ECG changes with those before the procedure.

Nursing Care and Defibrillation

Defibrillation is instituted as soon as possible after a dangerous arrhythmia is detected. Until such time, the nurse administers CPR to maintain oxygenation and circulation of blood. Defibrillation is performed by a nurse or other health care team member who is trained in the use of the defibrillator (Nursing Guidelines 26-1).

Nursing Care and Pacemakers

Transcutaneous Pacemaker

When initiating the use of a transcutaneous pacemaker, the nurse

- Attaches the anterior electrode patch to the left side of the chest, halfway between the xiphoid process to below the left nipple
- Adheres the posterior electrode patch to the left posterior chest beneath the scapula and lateral to the spine
- Adjusts the rate knob beginning at 40 beats/min in increments of 10 until reaching the rate prescribed by the primary provider or established by agency policy
- Regulates the current knob, which has a capacity starting at zero and advancing to 120 milliamps, until capturing is observed—that is, a QRS complex follows each spike of the pacemaker; capturing usually occurs between 50 and 100 milliamps
- Selects the demand mode, which programs the pacemaker to produce an electrical stimulus whenever the heart rate falls below a preset rate but remains inactive when the client's heart beats naturally at an adequate rate
- Palpates the pulse and observes the client's response

Transvenous Pacemaker

The nurse keeps resuscitation equipment close by because the tip of the pacemaker lead can mechanically provoke ventricular fibrillation. Once the pacemaker lead is inserted, the nurse attaches the external end to the external pacemaker unit, which is held securely to the client's forearm by means of tape or other anchoring device. The nurse positions the unit so that no tension is on the pacemaker lead. They check the connection several times each day because an improper connection or displacement of the wire from the terminal results in pacemaker malfunction. If the client is confused or restless and movement disturbs the external pacemaker or its lead, the nurse notifies the primary provider. Only grounded electrical equipment is used in the room. This means that all electrical plugs must have three prongs.

If the client is on a cardiac monitor, an alarm sounds if the client's heart rate drops below the lowest level programmed on the alarm system. The drop in heart rate may result from battery failure, internal dislodgment of the pacemaker lead, or a break in the pacemaker lead. The battery of an external pacemaker is easily replaced; the nurse keeps one or more spare batteries readily available. The nurse reports dislodgment of the pacemaker lead or a broken wire to the primary provider immediately so that the pacemaker can be repositioned or replaced by a new one.

Permanent Pacemaker

The nurse places the client with an internal pacemaker on a cardiac monitor and examines the rhythm strip for the pacemaker's characteristic electrical artifact or "spike," identified by a thin, straight stroke. Absence of the spike with a demand pacemaker setting means that the natural pacemaker, the SA node, initiates the impulse. With a fixed-rate pacemaker, there is a spike each time the heart is stimulated. The location of the spike in the series of waveforms is important to note. The nurse reports any deviation from the expected pattern. Absence of the spike in a fixed-rate pacemaker may mean faulty monitoring equipment or, more seriously, failure to pace. Other complications include infection, perforation of the ventricular myocardium by the tip of the pacemaker lead, and development of arrhythmias. Postimplantation instructions for the client include the following:

- Avoid strenuous movement, especially of the arm on the side where the pacemaker is inserted.
- Keep the arm on the side of the pacemaker lower than the head except for brief moments when dressing or performing hygiene.
- Delay for at least 8 weeks such activities as swimming, bowling, playing tennis, vacuum cleaning, carrying heavy objects, chopping wood, mowing or raking, and shoveling snow.
- Avoid sources of electrical interference similar to those problematic for people with ICDs.

NURSING GUIDELINES 26-1

Performing Defibrillation

When performing defibrillation, the nurse

- Determines that there is no breathing or pulse
- Checks the ECG rhythm
- Facilitates CPR until the client is prepared for defibrillation
- Applies gel or saline pads to the skin of the upper right chest near the sternum and apical area
- Charges the paddles to 200 joules of energy while stating "Charging"
- Selects the nonsynchronized mode on the defibrillator (the synchronized mode is used for cardioversion)
- Places the paddles on the chest over the gel or pads with firm pressure
- Shouts "All clear" to ensure that no one is in contact with the client or the bed
- Presses the discharge buttons on each paddle with the thumbs while stating "Shocking now"
- Evaluates the postdefibrillation cardiac rhythm
- Repeats defibrillation using 200 joules one more time and 360 joules for subsequent defibrillation attempts if there is no improvement in the cardiac rhythm
- Continues CPR as IV medications are administered and between defibrillation attempts

Client and Family Teaching 26-1 highlights maintenance and care instructions for clients with permanent pacemakers.

Client and Family Teaching 26-1
Permanent Pacemakers

The nurse instructs clients with permanent pacemakers and their families as follows:

- Maintain follow-up care.
- Report if the suture line becomes inflamed or sore.
- Avoid injury to the area where the pacemaker is inserted.
- Follow the primary provider's advice regarding lifting, sports, and exercise.
- Palpate the pulse and count the rate for a full minute daily or when feeling ill.
- Obtain and wear a MedicAlert bracelet or tag identifying that a pacemaker is implanted.
- Be cautious of situations that can cause pacemaker malfunction: gravitational force during airplane departures or landings, bumpy car rides, high-tension wires, shortwave radio transmissions, telephone transformers, and nuclear magnetic resonance imaging. Move to another location and check the pulse rate if dizziness or palpitations occur.
- Request hand scanning during airport security checks; some pacemakers trigger alarms.
- Maintain at least 6 inches between a cellular phone and the pacemaker generator or 12 inches if the cellular phone transmits over 3 watts.
- Check with the primary provider concerning transtelephonic pacemaker checks or when a pacemaker battery change will be necessary in the future.

KEY POINTS

- Common cardiac arrhythmias:
  - Arrhythmias originating in the atria:
    - Sinus bradycardia: an arrhythmia that proceeds normally through the conduction pathway but at a slower-than-usual rate (≤60 beats/min)
    - Sinus tachycardia: an arrhythmia that proceeds normally through the conduction pathway but at a faster-than-usual rate (100 to 150 beats/min)
    - Premature atrial contraction (PAC): the P wave of the waveform may look similar to other conducted impulses or may differ slightly because it is initiated somewhere in the atrium other than the sinoatrial (SA) node.
    - Supraventricular tachycardia (SVT): an arrhythmia in which the heart rate has a consistent rhythm but beats at a dangerously high rate (≥150 beats/min)
    - Atrial flutter: is a disorder in which a single atrial impulse outside the SA node causes the atria to contract at an exceedingly rapid rate (200 to 400 contractions/min)
    - Atrial fibrillation: several areas in the right atrium initiate impulses, resulting in disorganized, rapid activity.
  - Arrhythmias originating in the atrioventricular node:
    - Heart block: refers to disorders in the conduction pathway that interfere with the transmission of impulses from the SA node through the AV node to the ventricles
  - Arrhythmias originating in the ventricles:
    - Premature ventricular contraction (PVC) is a ventricular contraction that occurs early and independently in the cardiac cycle before the SA node initiates an electrical impulse.
    - Ventricular tachycardia: 150 to 250 beats per minute, caused by a single, irritable focus in the ventricle that initiates and then continues the same repetitive pattern
    - Ventricular fibrillation: the rhythm of a dying heart; PVCs or ventricular tachycardia can precipitate it. The ventricles do not contract effectively, and there is no cardiac output.
- Pacemaker: provides an electrical stimulus to the heart muscle (to treat an ineffective slow rhythm)
  - Demand (synchronous) mode pacemakers: self-activate when the client's pulse falls below a certain level
  - Fixed-rate (asynchronous) mode pacemakers: produce an electrical stimulus at a preset rate (usually 72 to 80 beats/min) despite the client's natural rhythm
- Temporary pacemaker: used until either a transvenous or permanent pacemaker can be placed or the client is stabilized with medication
- Permanent pacemaker: permanently embedded under the skin, the client must be monitored, and the battery should be changed every 8 to 10 years.
- Implantable cardioverter defibrillator (ICD): an internal electrical device used for selected clients with recurrent life-threatening tachydysrhythmias

CRITICAL THINKING EXERCISES

1. A client for whom an antiarrhythmic drug has been prescribed returns for a follow-up examination. How would you determine if the client has followed the drug therapy regimen?
2. What information is essential to document when helping to resuscitate a client who has experienced a cardiac arrest?
3. Describe similarities and differences between an implanted pacemaker and an ICD.
4. Many individuals purchase and self-medicate with ubiquinone (Coenzyme Q10, CQ10, CoQ, vitamin Q10) as a form of complementary or alternative therapy. It accounted for more than $519 million in sales in the United States in 2011 (ConsumerLab.com, 2013). Discuss the use of this substance in relation to cardiovascular disease.

NCLEX-STYLE REVIEW QUESTIONS PrepU

1. Atropine sulfate 0.5 mg is prescribed. The supplied dosage is 0.4 mg/mL. Calculate the volume to administer. Record your answer to the nearest decimal.

   ____

2. What evidence indicates to the nurse that a client with an arrhythmia has insufficient cardiac output? Select all that apply.
   1. Hypotension
   2. Confusion
   3. Decreased urine output
   4. Labored respirations
   5. Thready pulse
   6. Flushed skin
3. When a client develops ventricular fibrillation, what nursing action is most appropriate initially?
   1. Performing immediate defibrillation
   2. Preparing the client for pacemaker insertion
   3. Assessing the client for electrolyte imbalance
   4. Taking temperature, pulse, and BP
4. What nursing intervention is required when caring for a client undergoing elective electrical cardioversion?
   1. Restrict food and fluids before the procedure.
   2. Continue to administer digitalis daily.
   3. Perform CPR until cardioversion is successful.
   4. Monitor the pulse pressure every 15 minutes.
5. What intervention is essential when caring for a client with a transvenous pacemaker?
   1. Keep the resuscitation equipment at a distance.
   2. Use only grounded electrical equipment in the room.
   3. Check the connection of the unit once a day.
   4. Monitor the client's vital signs every 15 minutes.

WANT TO KNOW MORE? There are a wide variety of online resources available on thePoint to enhance learning and understanding of this chapter.

Go to **thePoint.lww.com/activate** and use the activation code found in the front of this text to unlock these online resources.

27 Caring for Clients With Hypertension

Words To Know

accelerated hypertension
aldosterone
angiotensin-converting enzyme
angiotensin II
angiotensinogen
central aortic systolic pressure
diastolic blood pressure
essential hypertension
hypernatremia
hypertension
hypertensive cardiovascular disease
hypertensive heart disease
hypertensive vascular disease
malignant hypertension
natriuretic factor
papilledema
prehypertension
renin
renin–angiotensin–aldosterone system
secondary hypertension
stage 1 hypertension
stage 2 hypertension
systolic blood pressure
white coat hypertension

Learning Objectives

On completion of this chapter, you will be able to:

1. Identify the two physiologic components that create blood pressure.
2. List factors that influence blood pressure.
3. List three structures that physiologically control arterial pressure.
4. Explain systolic and diastolic arterial pressure.
5. Discuss the potential value in assessing central aortic systolic pressure.
6. Define hypertension and identify groups at risk for it.
7. Differentiate essential and secondary hypertension.
8. Identify causes of secondary hypertension.
9. List consequences of chronic hypertension.
10. Discuss the assessment findings in hypertension.
11. Discuss the medical and nursing management of the client with hypertension.
12. Differentiate between accelerated and malignant hypertension.
13. Identify potential complications of uncontrolled malignant hypertension.
14. Discuss the medical and nursing management of the client with malignant hypertension.

This chapter provides information about the physiology that underlies normal blood pressure (BP); the ranges in normal and abnormal BP measurements; the consequences of sustained, elevated BP or hypertension; and medical and nursing interventions that help to lower BP measurements to healthier levels.

Gerontologic Considerations

■ BP changes in older adults may go undiagnosed during changes in life situations or with gradual progression of other changes associated with aging or chronic disease progression. Older adults should be encouraged to have BP checks by a health care provider at least every 6 months, and keep written documentation of dates, BP levels, and all updates of medications with time and dose.

■ The American Heart Association recommendation for monitoring and recording BP levels at home is helpful for those with white coat syndrome, risk factors for hypertension, or who are diagnosed with prehypertension or hypertension.

(continued)

Gerontologic Considerations (*continued*)

- Medication teaching must include (1) continued adherence to the regimen when BP levels have decreased to target levels and (2) discussion of side effects, including changes in sexual functioning, with the health care provider rather than suddenly stopping BP medications.
- Older adults are at increased risk for development of hypokalemia from potassium-wasting diuretic drugs. Lower doses of potassium-wasting diuretics or the use of potassium-sparing diuretics can control hypertension and minimize the risk of hypokalemia. Awareness of symptoms of hypokalemia is essential.
- Older adults may be at higher risk for postprandial hypotension owing to increased amount of blood for digestion resulting in reduced volume available for circulation. BP should be checked following meals in the lying, sitting, and standing positions. Recommend voiding prior to eating, then rest after eating to reduce risk. Some may benefit from increasing fluid before meals.

PHYSIOLOGY OF BLOOD PRESSURE

BP is the force produced by the volume of blood in arterial walls. It is represented by the formula:

$$BP = CO \text{ (cardiac output)} \times PR \text{ (peripheral resistance)}$$

Blood pressure is regulated by a variety of neural, hormonal, and chemical mechanisms that either raise or lower BP. The sympathetic and parasympathetic nervous systems adjust BP by facilitating vasoconstriction or vasodilation, respectively. They do so by altering the diameter of vascular smooth muscle.

Baroreceptors and chemoreceptors, neurons in the right atrium and carotid artery above the aorta, stimulate the brain when there is a decrease in BP or changes occur in the blood levels of oxygen and carbon dioxide.

Hormones also play a role in BP regulation via the renin–angiotensin–aldosterone system and natriuretic peptides (see Chapter 16 and later discussion). The former raises BP by causing vasoconstriction and retention of sodium ions; natriuretic peptides have the opposite effect.

Chemicals such as alcohol, nicotine, and nitric oxide (NO) also affect BP. The consumption of alcohol inhibits the vasomotor center in the brain causing vasodilation and also inhibits the release of antidiuretic hormone (ADH) resulting in lowered BP and decreased circulating blood volume.

MEASURING BLOOD PRESSURE

The measured BP reflects the ability of the arteries to stretch and fill with blood, the efficiency of the heart as a pump, and the volume of circulating blood. BP is affected by age, body size, diet, activity, emotions, pain, position, gender, time of day, and disease states. Studies of healthy persons show that BP can fluctuate within a wide range and remain normal. Thus, obtaining several measurements for comparison is important.

When measured with a standard sphygmomanometer and stethoscope, arterial BP at the brachial artery during systole and diastole is expressed as a fraction. The top number is the systolic BP; the bottom number is the diastolic BP. Normal BP for adults ranges from 100/60 to 119/79 mm Hg. The autonomic nervous system, the kidneys, and various endocrine glands regulate arterial pressure. BP tends to increase with age, most likely from arteriosclerotic and atherosclerotic changes in blood vessels or other effects of chronic diseases such as diabetes and renal dysfunction. Screening of BP is an important method for identifying people at risk for heart failure, renal failure, and stroke. Those at highest risk are older adults, African Americans, and clients with diabetes mellitus.

Systolic Blood Pressure

Systolic blood pressure is determined by the force and volume of blood that the left ventricle ejects during systole and the ability of the arterial system to distend at the time of ventricular contraction. The arterial walls are normally elastic and yield to the force and volume of ventricular contraction. In older clients, systolic BP may be elevated because of loss of arterial elasticity (arteriosclerosis). Narrowing of the arterioles, either from arteriosclerosis or from some other mechanism causing vasoconstriction, increases peripheral resistance, which in turn increases systolic BP. This resistance can be compared to the narrowing of a tube, such as the stem of a balloon. The narrower the lumen, the greater is the pressure needed to move a substance through it.

Diastolic Blood Pressure

Diastolic blood pressure reflects arterial pressure during ventricular relaxation. It depends on the resistance of the arterioles and the diastolic filling times. If arterioles are resistant (constricted), blood is under greater pressure.

Central Aortic Systolic Pressure

Central aortic systolic pressure (CASP), the pressure of blood at the root of the aorta as blood is pumped from the left ventricle, can be lower by as much as 30 mm Hg than the corresponding brachial arm systolic pressure. The inference is that some clients are diagnosed and treated for hypertension prematurely based on the measurement of brachial arm pressure.

CASP has been measured invasively by passing a catheter from the femoral artery to the aorta. But now, CASP can be measured simply, noninvasively, and inexpensively with a U.S. Food and Drug Administration (FDA)–approved device called a *CASPro computerized monitor*. This device uses dual connections, with a wrist sensor positioned over the radial artery and a cuff attached to the upper arm like a traditional sphygmomanometer (Fig. 27-1). The measured BP with this device is 99% as accurate as that measured with a vascular catheter.

Some feel that CASP is the better predictor of future vascular and cerebral complications such as heart or kidney

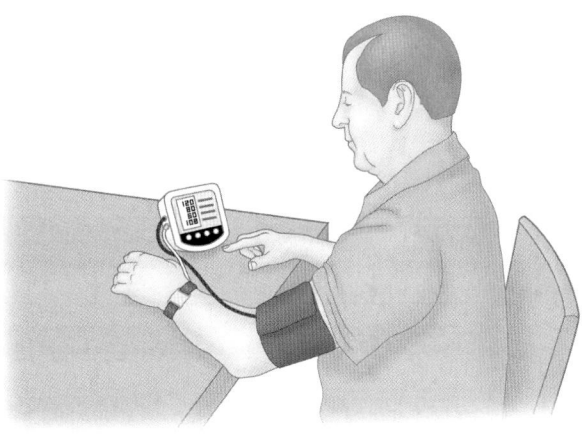

Figure 27-1 The noninvasive central aortic systolic pressure (CASP) monitoring system consists of a wrist sensor and a blood pressure cuff connection that transmit data to a computer where software calculates the CASP within minutes.

failure and stroke, especially in older adults with arteriosclerosis. Critics remain skeptical about the widespread use of a CASP monitoring system based on the cost of the equipment, its potential reimbursement by third-party payers, and training a technician to use it. At the present time, the majority of practitioners are relying on conventional brachial arm pressure measurements (Black & Townsend, 2015).

HYPERTENSIVE DISEASE

Approximately 70 million people, or one in three adults, in the United States have high BP, with only 52% having their BP under control (Centers for Disease Control and Prevention, 2016). Because hypertension places people at risk for heart disease, heart failure (see Chapter 28), stroke, kidney disease, and the potential for blindness (Fig. 27-2), health care providers have revised guidelines for identifying it.

What once was considered normal BP measurements, a systolic pressure of 120 mm Hg and diastolic pressure of 80 mm Hg, are now the lower ranges of prehypertension (Table 27-1). According to the National Heart, Lung, and Blood Institute (2015), **prehypertension** is defined as a systolic BP of 120 to 139 mm Hg or a diastolic BP between 80 and 89 mm Hg.

The term **hypertension**, sustained elevations in systolic or diastolic BP that exceed **prehypertension** levels, is now subdivided into two categories. **Stage 1 hypertension** is defined as a systolic BP of 140 to 159 mm Hg or a diastolic BP between 90 and 99 mm Hg. **Stage 2 hypertension** is systolic BP that equals or exceeds 160 mm Hg or a diastolic pressure that equals or exceeds 100 mm Hg. The parameters defining hypertension were neither addressed nor changed by the Eighth Joint National Committee on Prevention, Detection, Evaluation, and Treatment of High Blood Pressure in their 2014 report, but recommendations for pharmacologic treatment were identified according to age, race, and the presence or absence of diabetes and chronic kidney disease.

When elevated BP causes a cardiac abnormality, the term **hypertensive heart disease** is used. When vascular damage is present without heart involvement, the term **hypertensive vascular disease** is used. When both heart disease and vascular damage accompany hypertension, the appropriate term is **hypertensive cardiovascular disease**.

Essential and Secondary Hypertension

Hypertension is further divided into two main categories: essential (primary; idiopathic) and secondary. **Essential hypertension**, about 95% of cases, is sustained elevated BP with no known cause. **Secondary hypertension** is elevated BP that results from or is secondary to some other disorder.

Some people experience **white coat hypertension**, a term describing elevated BP that develops during evaluation by health care providers who traditionally have worn a white coat (Fig. 27-3). This type of hypertension most likely results from anxiety that is accompanied by a surge of epinephrine and norepinephrine, powerful neurohormones that cause vasoconstriction. To confirm or exclude this phenomenon, the BP is measured a second time before the client leaves the agency. In cases of white coat hypertension, this subsequent measurement is likely to be normal. If the client remains hypertensive, he or she is advised to check BP regularly either at home with the help of a family member, at a public service location in the community (e.g., pharmacy), or at the office of the primary provider. The client is advised to bring the record of BP measurements to his or her medical appointments.

Pathophysiology and Etiology

The exact cause of essential hypertension is unknown. BP often increases with age; hypertension may run in families. Essential hypertension affects African Americans at a higher rate than it does other ethnic groups. Obesity, inactivity, smoking, excessive alcohol intake, and ineffective stress management are risk factors.

Research into specific factors that contribute to the development of essential hypertension continues. For instance, it is well documented that **hypernatremia** (elevated serum sodium level) increases blood volume, which raises BP. A low serum potassium level, however, actually may cause sodium retention as the kidneys try to maintain a balanced number of cations (positively charged electrolytes) in body fluid. Scientists are also investigating the role of calcium in hypertension because serum calcium levels are low in some hypertensive clients.

Essential hypertension may also develop from alterations in other body chemicals. Defects in BP regulation may result from an impairment in the **renin–angiotensin–aldosterone system** (see Chapter 16). **Renin** is a chemical that the kidneys release to raise BP and increase vascular fluid volume in response to renal hypoperfusion. Renin causes the conversion of **angiotensinogen**, a protein, into angiotensin I which is then converted with an enzyme, **angiotensin-converting enzyme** found in the lungs, into

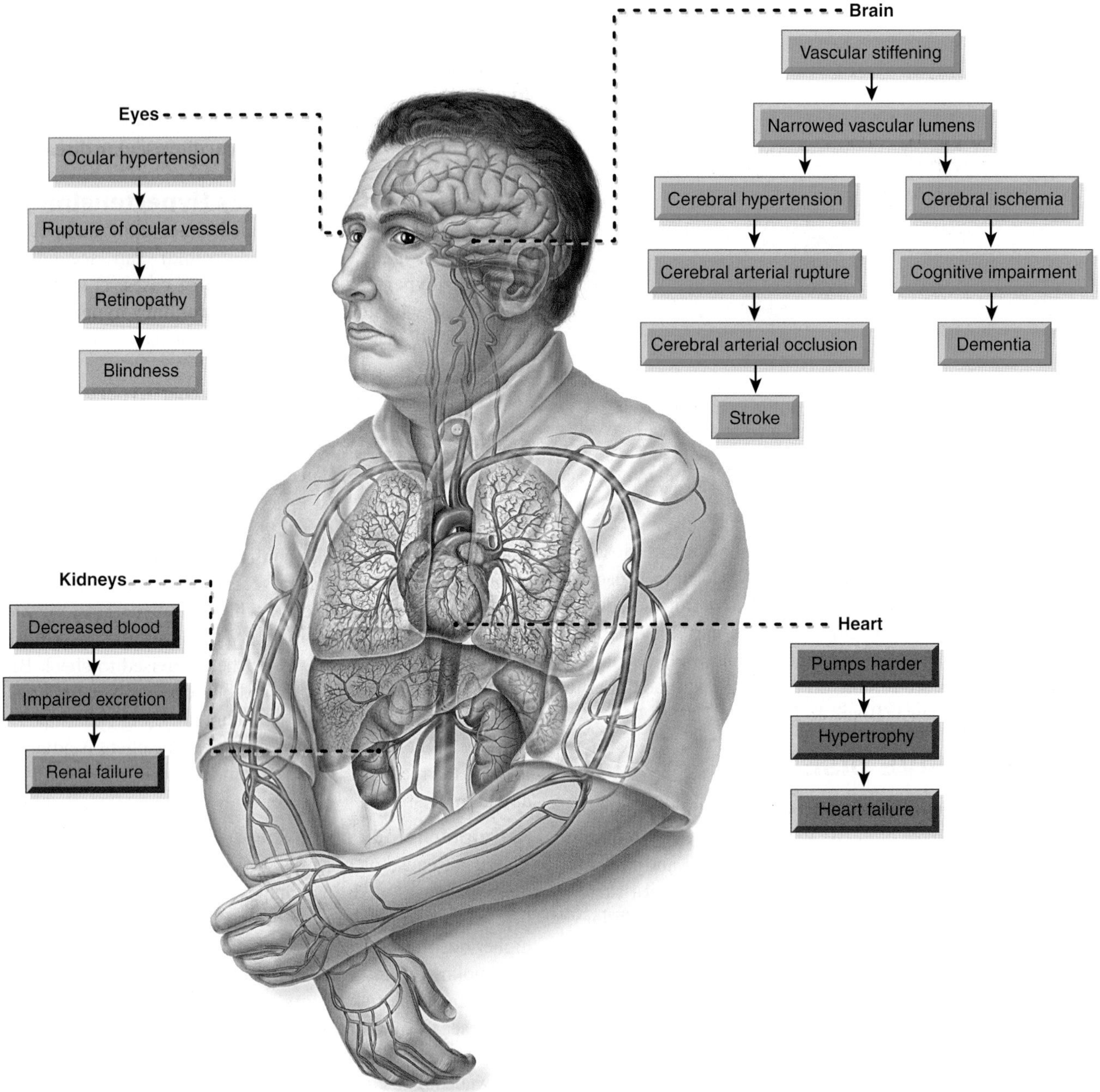

Figure 27-2 Effects of hypertension on target organs. (Modified from Anatomical Chart Company. (2016). *Hypertension*. Lippincott Williams & Wilkins.)

TABLE 27-1 Classification of Blood Pressure in Adults 18 Years or Older

BP CLASSIFICATION	SYSTOLIC BP (mm Hg)		DIASTOLIC BP (mm Hg)
Normal	Less than 120	and	Less than 80
Elevated	120–129	or	Less than 80
High Blood Pressure (hypertension) stage 1	130–139	or	80–89
High Blood Pressure (hypertension) stage 2	140 or higher	or	90 or higher
Hypertensive Crisis (consult your doctor immediately)	Higher than 180	and/or	Higher than 120

From American Heart Association. (2021). *Understanding blood pressure readings*. https://www.heart.org/en/health-topics/high-blood-pressure/understanding-blood-pressure-readings

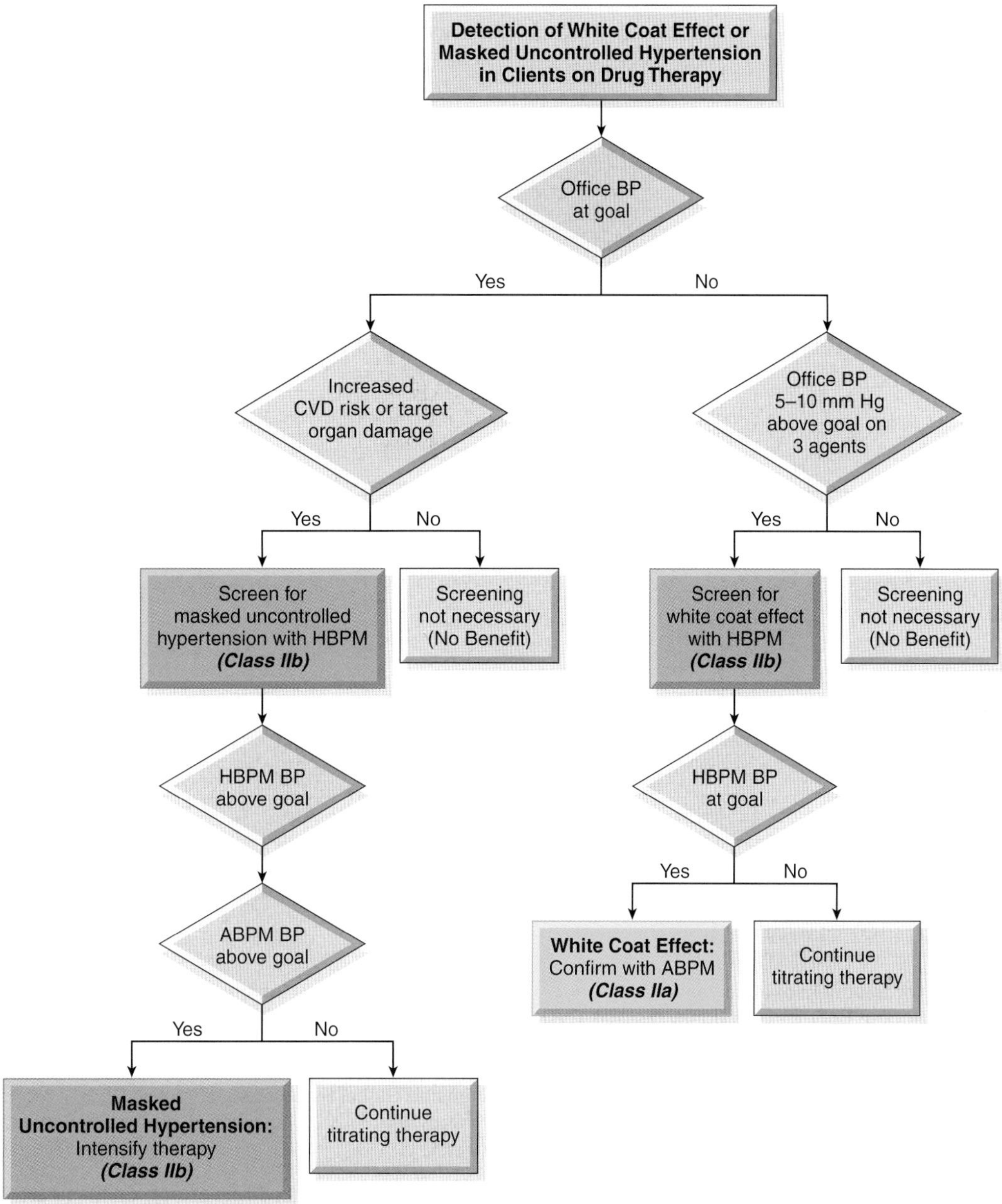

Figure 27-3 Guidelines for treatment of white coat syndrome. (Reprinted from Whelton, P. K., Carey, R. M., Aronow, W. S., Casey, D. E., Jr, Collins, K. J., Dennison Himmelfarb, C., DePalma, S. M., Gidding, S., Jamerson, K. A., Jones, D. W., MacLaughlin, E. J., Muntner, P., Ovbiagele, B., Smith, S. C., Jr, Spencer, C. C., Stafford, R. S., Taler, S. J., Thomas, R. J., Williams, K. A., Sr, Williamson, J. D., ... Wright, J. T., Jr (2018). 2017 ACC/AHA/AAPA/ABC/ACPM/AGS/APhA/ASH/ASPC/NMA/PCNA guideline for the prevention, detection, evaluation, and management of high blood pressure in adults: A report of the American College of Cardiology/American Heart Association Task Force on Clinical Practice Guidelines. *Journal of the American College of Cardiology*, 71(19), e127–e248. https://doi.org/10.1016/j.jacc.2017.11.006. Copyright © 2018 by the American College of Cardiology Foundation. With permission.)

angiotensin II, a powerful vasoconstrictor. Angiotensin II stimulates the secretion of **aldosterone**, an adrenal hormone that causes salt and water to be reabsorbed increasing BP. Hypertension is controlled using drugs that inhibit angiotensin-converting enzyme, block the receptors for angiotensin II, or are antagonists of aldosterone.

For people with a heightened stress response, hypertension may be correlated with a higher-than-usual release of catecholamines, such as epinephrine and norepinephrine, which elevate BP. Last, some researchers theorize that a deficiency of **natriuretic factor**, a hormone produced by the heart, results in an elevation of BP because its role is to promote the excretion of sodium by the kidneys (see Chapter 16).

Secondary hypertension may accompany any primary condition that affects fluid volume or renal function or causes arterial vasoconstriction. Predisposing conditions include kidney disease, pheochromocytoma (a benign tumor of the adrenal medulla), hyperaldosteronism (increased secretion of mineralocorticoid by the adrenal cortex), atherosclerosis, use of cocaine or other cardiac stimulants (e.g., weight-control drugs, caffeine), and use of oral contraceptives.

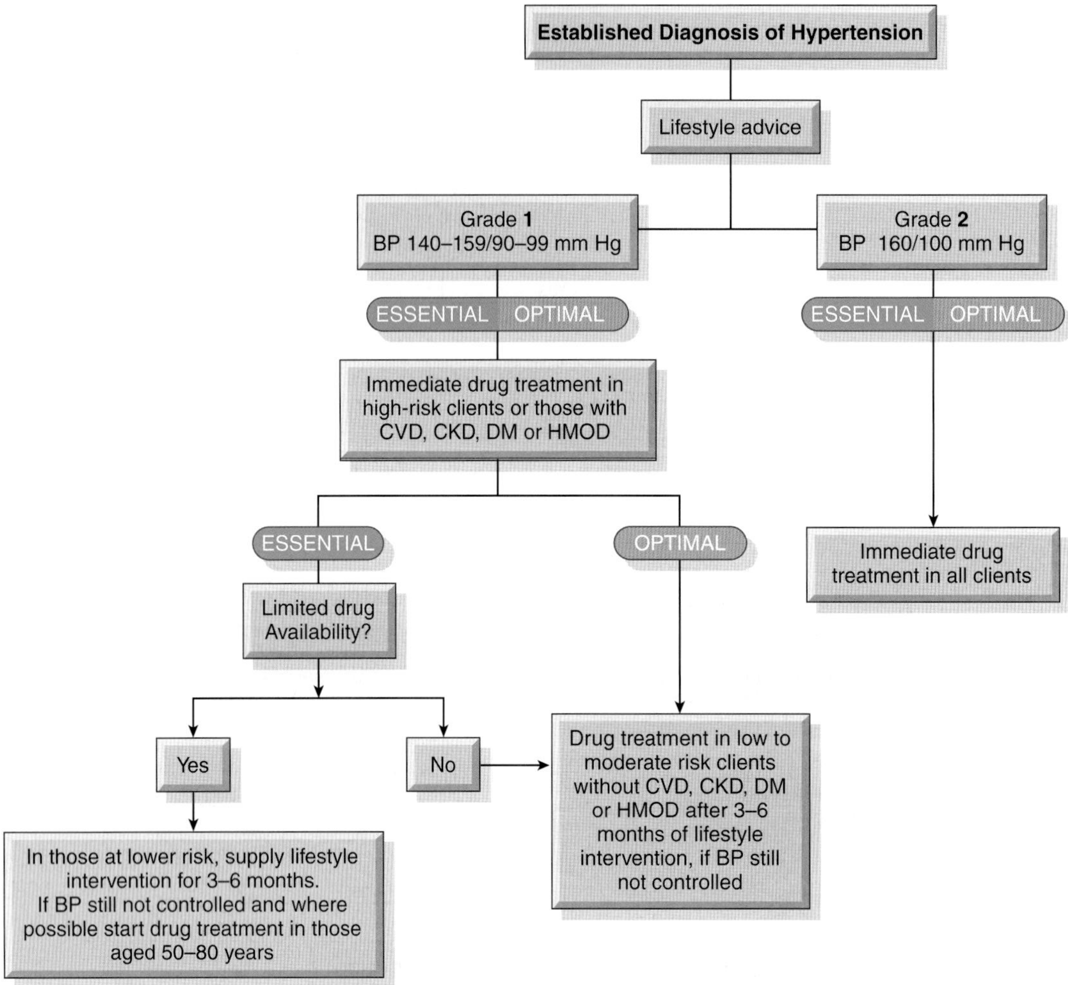

Figure 27-4 Algorithm for treatment of hypertension. ACEI, angiotensin-converting enzyme inhibitor; ARB, angiotensin receptor blocker; CCB, calcium channel blocker; CKD, chronic kidney disease; CVD, cardiovascular disease; DBP, diastolic blood pressure; DM, diabetes mellitus; HMOD, hypertension-mediated organ damage; SBP, systolic blood pressure. (Reprinted with permission from Unger, T., Borghi, C., Charchar, F., Khan, N. A., Poulter, N. R., Prabhakaran, D., Ramirez, A., Schlaich, M., Stergiou, G. S., Tomaszewski, M., Wainford, R. D., Williams, B., & Schutte, A. E. (2020). 2020 International Society of Hypertension Global Hypertension Practice Guidelines. *Hypertension, 75*(6), 1334–1357. https://doi.org/10.1161/HYPERTENSIONAHA.120.15026. Copyright © 2020 American Heart Association, Inc.)

Pharmacologic Considerations

■ Specific medications may contribute to malignant hypertension. Drugs thought to cause this condition include cocaine, amphetamines, monoamine oxidase inhibitors (MAOIs) used for depression, and oral contraceptives. Include a drug history in your basic assessment.

Regardless of whether a person has essential or secondary hypertension, the accompanying organ damage and complications are the same. Hypertension causes the heart to work harder to pump against the increased resistance. Consequently, the size of the heart muscle increases. When the heart no longer can pump adequately to meet the body's metabolic needs, heart failure occurs (see Chapter 28). The extra work and the greater mass increase the heart's need for oxygen. If the myocardium does not receive sufficient oxygenated blood, myocardial ischemia occurs and the client experiences angina.

In addition to its direct effects on the heart, high BP damages the arterial vascular system. It accelerates atherosclerosis. Furthermore, the increased resistance of the arterioles to the flow of blood causes serious complications in other body organs, including the eyes, brain, heart, and kidneys. Hemorrhage of tiny arteries in the retina may cause marked visual disturbances or blindness. A cerebrovascular accident (stroke) may result from hemorrhage or occlusion of a blood vessel in the brain. Myocardial infarction (MI) may result from occlusion of a branch of a coronary artery. Impaired circulation to the kidneys may result in renal failure.

Assessment Findings

Signs and Symptoms

Clients with hypertension may be asymptomatic. The onset of hypertension considered "the silent killer," often is gradual. It can exist for years but be discovered only during a routine physical examination or when the client experiences a major complication. As the BP becomes elevated, clients may identify symptoms such as a throbbing or pounding headache, dizziness, fatigue, insomnia, nervousness, nosebleeds, and blurred vision. Angina or dyspnea may be the first clue to hypertensive heart disease.

The most obvious finding during a physical assessment is a sustained elevation of one or both BP measurements. The pulse may feel like it is bounding from the force of ventricular contraction. Clients may be overweight. They may have a flushed face from engorgement of superficial blood vessels. Peripheral edema may be present. An ophthalmic examination may reveal vascular changes in the eyes, retinal hemorrhages, or edema of the optic nerves known as **papilledema**.

Diagnostic Findings

Diagnostic tests are performed to determine the extent of organ damage. Electrocardiography, echocardiography, and chest radiography may reveal an enlarged left ventricle. A multiple gated acquisition (MUGA) scan, a test that detects how well or inefficiently the heart pumps, can detect heart failure that may be associated with hypertension (see Chapter 28). Blood tests may show elevated blood urea nitrogen and serum creatinine levels, indicating impaired renal function, findings that excretory urography (intravenous pyelography [IVP]) may further validate. Fluorescein angiography, an ophthalmologic test using intravenous (IV) dye, often reveals leaking retinal blood vessels.

If the cause of hypertension is a renal vascular problem, renal arteriography demonstrates narrowing of the renal artery. If the cause is related to dysfunction of the adrenal gland, a 24-hour collected urine specimen detects elevated catecholamines. Blood studies reveal elevated cholesterol and triglyceride levels, indicating that atherosclerosis is an underlying factor.

Medical Management

The primary objective of therapy for hypertension is to lower the BP and prevent major complications. Nonpharmacologic interventions are used for all clients whether they are hypertensive or not. These same measures are continued once hypertension has been detected (Fig. 27-4). Examples of lifestyle changes include weight reduction, decreased sodium intake (Box 27-1), moderate exercise, and reduced contributing factors (e.g., smoking, alcohol use) that may return the BP to normal levels. Table 27-2 identifies the potential benefits that are possible with lifestyle changes alone.

Pharmacologic treatment recommendations depend on the client's age, race, presence or absence of diabetes and chronic kidney disease, and the stage of the client's hypertension. Some have questioned the new

BOX 27-1 Recommendations for Limiting Sodium

- Consume less than 2300 mg of sodium per day or no more than 1500 mg if you are 51 years or older; are African American; or have hypertension, diabetes, or chronic kidney disease. One teaspoon of table salt equals 2300 mg of sodium.
- Because the sodium content of prepared foods can vary greatly among different brands, read nutrition facts labels to compare the sodium content. Any food that provides more than 20% of the daily value of sodium in one serving is considered very high in sodium.
- Prepare food from "scratch" without adding salt as opposed to purchasing premade, convenience, or packaged foods, which usually are highly salted.
- Substitute unsalted, no salt, sodium-free, low sodium, or reduced sodium products for regular salted products.
- Choose fresh or plain, frozen vegetables. If canned vegetables are chosen, drain and rinse before eating.
- Avoid or limit consumption of hot dogs, ham, bacon, and processed meat products, which often contain sodium nitrate as a preservative.
- Substitute healthy snacks such as fresh or dried fruit for those that are salted.
- Experiment with seasonings such as lemon, garlic, and onion powder as alternatives to salt.
- Eliminate or restrict items that contain significant sodium such as pickles, green olives, sauerkraut, mustard, catsup, barbecue sauce, pizza sauce, canned soup, and packaged mixes.

TABLE 27-2 Lifestyle Changes to Prevent High Blood Pressure

Preventing high blood pressure means having a healthy lifestyle. This means:

Eating healthy.	To help control your blood pressure, you should reduce the amount of sodium (salt) that you eat. Eating foods that are lower in fat, as well as plenty of fruits, vegetables, and whole grains, can help with eating a heart healthy diet. The DASH diet eating plan can help with meal planning, for a diet that aids lowering your blood pressure.
Regular exercise.	Regular exercise can help you support a healthy weight and lower your blood pressure. The recommendation is to get moderate-intensity aerobic exercise at least 2 and a half hours per week. Aerobic exercise, such as brisk walking, is any exercise in which your heart beats harder and you use more oxygen than usual.
Healthy weight.	*Obesity* or being overweight can increase your risk for high blood pressure. Maintaining a healthy weight can help you control high blood pressure and reduce your risk for other health problems.
Limit alcohol.	Restricting your *alcohol* intake can help in reducing blood pressure. Alcohol also adds extra calories, which may cause weight gain. Men should have no more than two drinks per day, and women only one.
Not smoking.	Cigarette smoking increases your blood pressure and puts you at higher risk for cardiovascular disease. If you do not smoke, do not start. If you do smoke, discuss options to *quit* smoking with your health care provider.
Manage stress.	Learning how to manage stress can improve your emotional and physical health and lower high blood pressure. Stress management practices include exercising, listening to music, focusing on something calm or peaceful, and meditating.

Adapted from Medline Plus. (January 2021). *How to prevent high blood pressure.* https://medlineplus.gov/howtopreventhighbloodpressure.html

guidelines that recommend waiting to treat hypertension among older African Americans until later because waiting places those clients who are already at risk for complications for premature harm. Table 27-2 identifies the potential benefits that are possible with lifestyle changes alone.

Currently, it is believed that in persons older than 60 years of age, reducing the systolic pressure below 150 mm Hg is more important than decreasing the diastolic BP. Once the systolic BP is controlled below 150 mm Hg, a reduction in the diastolic BP generally follows. In clients with higher risk for hypertensive complications, as in clients with diabetes or chronic kidney disease, the goal is to reduce BP to <140/90 mm Hg.

Clients who require drug therapy may be treated initially with one drug, usually a thiazide diuretic. However, most people with hypertension will need two or more antihypertensive medications to reduce their BP to target level (Drug Therapy Table 27-1). If the BP remains elevated with two-drug combinations, a third or fourth antihypertensive agent may be added. Secondary hypertension often resolves by treating its cause. When additional clinical conditions are accompanied by complications of hypertension, other drug therapy is indicated (Table 27-3).

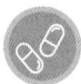

Pharmacologic Considerations

- All drugs used to reduce BP can produce dizziness and syncope when rising to a sitting or standing position. Teach clients how to reduce symptoms of hypotension as they adjust to their medications.
- Monitor angiotensin-converting enzyme (ACE) inhibitors cautiously in clients with renal or hepatic impairment and older adults. A sudden drop in BP may occur during the first 1 to 3 hours after the initial dose of an ACE inhibitor; administration of IV normal saline may manage the hypotensive episode.
- ACE inhibitors may cause a persistent cough until the medication is discontinued.
- A bothersome dry cough is associated with angiotensin-converting enzyme inhibitors (ACEIs). Many mechanisms of action are suggested, from bradykinin stimulation of the vagal nerve to increased prostaglandins. Remedies range from the addition of cromolyn, baclofen, or a local anesthetic such as sulindac and low-dose aspirin (NSAIDs).
- Fetal toxicity is associated with ACEIs. A pregnancy test should always be conducted before medication is prescribed for any woman of childbearing age.

DRUG THERAPY TABLE 27.1 Antihypertensive Agents

Category and Common Generic (Brand) Drugs	Intended Use	Common Side Effects	Safety Warnings for Nurses
Diuretics			
Furosemide (Lasix) Chlorothiazide (Diuril)	Decrease work of heart by promoting excretion of sodium and water, thus reducing circulating blood volume	Dizziness, dehydration, nausea, diarrhea, nocturia, polyuria, orthostatic hypotension	• Monitor serum potassium • Increased fall risk owing to hypotensive side effects • Encourage fluids to prevent dehydration
ACE inhibitors (ACEI)			
Benazepril (Lotensin) Captopril (Capoten) Enalapril (Vasotec) Fosinopril (Monopril) Lisinopril (Prinivil) Quinapril (Accupril)	Suppression of the renin–angiotensin–aldosterone system reduces water and sodium retention which lessens blood pressure	Dizziness, headache, fatigue, dry cough	• Increased fall risk owing to hypotensive side effects • Do not use if impaired renal function, or dialysis • Monitor for lower blood glucose in clients with diabetes • Interaction with herbal: St. John's wort • Perimenopausal women need to use effective birth control
Calcium Channel Blockers			
Amlodipine (Norvasc) Diltiazem (Cardizem) Felodipine (Plendil) Nifedipine (Procardia) Verapamil (Calan)	Relieve angina by dilating arteries, improving myocardium blood supply and reduces myocardial oxygen demand	Hypotension, dizziness, nausea, dry cough	• When given IV, constant cardiac monitoring is required • Drug is usually held if heart rate <60–120> • No grapefruit • Initially, monitor blood every 2–3 weeks for agranulocytosis

DRUG THERAPY TABLE 27.1 Antihypertensive Agents (*continued*)

Category and Common Generic (Brand) Drugs	Intended Use	Common Side Effects	Safety Warnings for Nurses
Beta-Adrenergic Blockers			
Atenolol (Tenormin) Metoprolol (Lopressor) Nadolol (Corgard) Propranolol (Inderal)	Reduce heart rate and decrease consumption of oxygen by myocardium, helps to prevent anginal attacks	Headache, dizziness, nausea, vomiting	• When given IV, constant cardiac monitoring is required • Drug is usually held if heart rate <60–120> • Initially, monitor blood every 2–3 weeks for agranulocytosis
Anti-Adrenergic Blockers			
Clonidine (Catapres) Prazosin (Minipress)	Relax smooth muscle of vascular system	Dry mouth, sedation, dizziness, headache	• Symptoms worsen when medication is stopped suddenly
Alpha/Beta-Adrenergic Blockers			
Carvedilol (Coreg) Labetalol (Trandate)	Relax smooth muscle of vascular system	Sedation, dizziness, headache	• Symptoms worsen when medication is stopped suddenly
Angiotensin II Receptor Antagonists			
Azilsartan (Edarbi) Candesartan (Atacand) Eprosartan (Teveten) Irbesartan (Avapro) Losartan (Cozaar) Olmesartan (Benicar) Telmisartan (Micardis) Valsartan (Diovan)	Inhibit the pressor effect of angiotensin II, suppressing the negative feedback loop of RAAS to reduce hypertension	Dizziness, fainting, diarrhea	• Perimenopausal women need to use effective birth control
Selective Aldosterone Receptor Antagonist			
Eplerenone (Inspra)	Blocks aldosterone which reduces blood pressure	Hyperkalemia	• Monitor serum potassium and renal function at day 3, week 1, monthly × 3, 4 × yearly while taking drug
Direct Renin Inhibitor			
Aliskiren (Tekturna)	Suppress the negative feedback loop of RAAS to reduce hypertension	Diarrhea, URI symptoms	• Perimenopausal women need to use effective birth control

RAAS, Renin–angiotensin–aldosterone system.

TABLE 27-3 Compelling Indications for Antihypertensive Drug Classes

INDICATIONS	RECOMMENDED DRUGS[a]					
	DIURETIC	BB	ACEI	ARB	CCB	ALDOANT
Heart failure	X	X	X	X		X
Postmyocardial infarction		X	X			X
High risk for coronary disease	X	X	X		X	
Diabetes	X	X	X	X	X	
Chronic kidney disease			X	X		
Prevention of recurrent stroke	X	X				

[a]Drug abbreviations: BB, beta blocker; ACEI, angiotensin-converting enzyme inhibitor; ARB, angiotensin receptor blocker; CCB, calcium channel blocker; Aldo ALDOANT, aldosterone antagonist; X indicates appropriate uses for drug.
From Koracevic, G., Micic, S., Stojanovic, M., Lovic, D., Simic, D., Colic, M., Koracevic, M., Stojkovic, A., & Paunovic, M. (2021). Compelling indications should be listed for individual beta-blockers (due to diversity), not for the whole class. *Current Vascular Pharmacology, 19*(4), 343–346. https://doi.org/10.2174/1570161118666200518113833

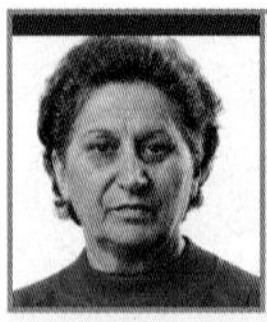

Clinical Scenario The nurse measures a BP of 158/94 mm Hg during a 58-year-old female client's appointment for a routine pelvic examination and mammogram. The client has a family history of hypertension. Her mother died of a stroke at the age of 72 years. The nurse schedules an appointment to track the trend in the client's BP at 1-week intervals for 2 weeks to determine if the client has essential or white coat hypertension. **What steps in the nursing process will the nurse follow when a client's data suggest a diagnosis of stage 1 hypertension? See the following Nursing Process section and Evidence-Based Practice 27-1.**

NURSING PROCESS FOR THE CLIENT WITH HYPERTENSION

Assessment

Take the BP accurately (Box 27-2) in both arms initially with the client in a supine, sitting, and then standing position, using an appropriately sized cuff (Table 27-4). Thereafter, use the same arm and place the client in the same position each time a reading is taken. Ask questions to determine if the client is following the treatment regimen. Perform additional cardiac assessments (see Chapter 22) depending on the client's medical history and current symptoms.

BOX 27-2 Factors That Affect Accuracy When Assessing Blood Pressure

- Failure to allow the client to sit quietly for 5 minutes prior to assessment
- Smoking or drinking coffee within 30 minutes of assessment
- Neglecting to position the arm and BP cuff at heart level
- Using an improperly calibrated sphygmomanometer
- Applying an incorrectly sized cuff
- Deflating the cuff too rapidly
- Talking with the client during the assessment
- Rounding the pressure measurement up or down
- Limiting the assessment to one measurement at the beginning of the interaction
- Ignoring signs of client anxiety

Adapted from Vidt, D. G., Lang, R. S., Seballos, R. J., Misra-Hebert, A., Campbell, J., & Bena, J. F. (2010). Taking blood pressure: too important to trust to humans? *Cleveland Clinic journal of medicine, 77*(10), 683–688.

Diagnosis, Planning, and Interventions

Teach the client about nonpharmacologic and pharmacologic methods for restoring and maintaining BP at or below goal levels as well as techniques for self-management (Client and Family Teaching 27-1; Evidence-Based Practice 27-1). Collaborate with a dietitian to provide information on dietary modifications such as Dietary Approaches to Stop Hypertension, also referred to as the *DASH diet* (Nutrition Notes).

TABLE 27-4 Recommended Bladder Dimensions for Blood Pressure Cuffs

		RECOMMENDED CUFF SIZE	
ARM CIRCUMFERENCE (cm)[a]	CUFF NAME	WIDTH (cm)	LENGTH (cm)
22–26	Small adult	12	22
27–34	Adult	16	30
35–44	Large adult	16	36
45–52	Adult thigh	16	42

[a]To convert cm to inches, multiply by 0.39.
heart.org.

Risk for Decreased Cardiac Output: Related to excessive or prolonged systemic vascular resistance
Expected Outcome: Client will maintain an adequate cardiac output as evidenced by reduced BP to normal or goal levels, heart rate between 60 and 100 beats/min, effortless breathing, clear lung sounds, alert mental status, and urine output that approximates or slightly exceeds intake.

- Promote physical rest. *Rest decreases BP and reduces the resistance that the heart must overcome to eject blood.*
- Relieve emotional stress. *Reduced stress decreases production of neurotransmitters that constrict peripheral arterioles.*
- Instruct client to avoid bearing down against a closed glottis (Valsalva maneuver). *Straining or bearing down against a closed glottis momentarily increases BP.*
- Encourage adherence to treatment with salt/sodium restrictions. *Doing so decreases blood volume and improves the potential for greater cardiac output.*
- Recommend smoking cessation. *Nicotine raises heart rate, constricts arterioles, and reduces the heart's ability to eject blood.*
- Enforce prescribed fluid restrictions. *Reduced oral fluid ultimately decreases circulating blood volume and systemic vascular resistance.*
- Help client reduce or eliminate caffeine and tobacco. *Caffeine and nicotine increases heart rate and causes vasoconstriction.*
- Administer prescribed antihypertensives. *They use various mechanisms to control BP, including increasing urine elimination, blocking production of angiotensin, and dilating blood vessels.*

NURSING PROCESS FOR THE CLIENT WITH HYPERTENSION (continued)

Injury Risk: Related to syncope and dizziness secondary to side effect of antihypertensive drugs
Expected Outcome: The client will be injury free.

- Monitor postural changes in BP by assessing client while he or she is lying, sitting, and standing. *A 20-mm Hg fall in systolic BP or a 10-mm Hg fall in diastolic BP within 1 to 3 minutes of assuming an upright position indicates postural hypotension (Mayo Clinic Staff, 2014). Assessment validates whether the drop in BP is significant.*
- As appropriate, ensure the signal cord is within the client's reach and advise him or her to use it whenever getting out of bed. *Nursing personnel can prevent injury if they assist clients.*
- Encourage client to rise slowly from a sitting or lying position. *Gradual changes in position provide time for the heart to increase its rate of contraction to resupply oxygen to the brain.*
- Help client to sit or lie down if he or she is dizzy. *The support of a chair or bed reduces the potential for falling.*

Evaluation of Expected Outcomes

Expected outcomes are that adequate cardiac output is maintained or improved when systolic BP is below 140 or 130 mm Hg for those with diabetes or chronic kidney disease or diastolic BP is below 90 or 80 mm Hg for those with diabetes or chronic kidney disease. The client does not experience syncope or fall from postural changes in BP.

Client and Family Teaching 27-1
Hypertension

The nurse instructs as follows:

- Adhere to the treatment regimen even if you have few, if any, symptoms and feel well. Hypertension is a chronic condition requiring lifelong management and treatment.
- Learn to regularly monitor BP using a home sphygmomanometer or arrange for monitoring by a community agency that provides this service at no or low cost.
- Keep a log of BP measurements for follow-up visits.
- Comply with the treatment regimen involving diet, exercise, and drug therapy.
- Consult cookbooks published or endorsed by the American Heart Association, American Diabetes Association, or other reliable sources for "heart smart" recipes.
- Follow directions for medications; never increase, decrease, or omit a prescribed drug unless first conferring with the primary care provider.
- Report adverse effects from medications to the prescribing provider. Get medical approval before taking nonprescription drugs. Inform all primary providers and dentists of medications that you are taking.
- Avoid tobacco and beverages containing caffeine or alcohol unless permitted by the provider.

Evidence-Based Practice 27-1

Preventing Hypertension

Clinical Question

What are preventable methods for hypertension?

Evidence

Hypertension is very common and can be a risk factor for such types of disease as: myocardial infarction, stroke, kidney failure, and possible death. Prevention and early diagnoses is the key in treatment according to an article by Santosa et al., 2020. The article reviewed research and random trials to recommend guidelines. The panel found that besides the standard guidelines, management of hypertension should be individualized for the client and health promotion needs.

Nursing Implications

This review indicates a strong need for the nursing process to include monitoring, prevention, and education. Nurses can use this evidence in their education when planning care for clients and teaching the client and families about health promotion. Close monitoring and assessments of clients may be the best prevention and an opportunity to provide education. Nursing should reinforce diet, exercise, and medication as prescribed by the health care provider.

Reference
Santosa, A., Zhang, Y., Weinehall, L., Zhao, G., Wang, N., Zhao, Q., Wang, W., & Ng, N. (2020). Gender differences and determinants of prevalence, awareness, treatment and control of hypertension among adults in China and Sweden. *BMC Public Health, 20*(4), 1. https://doi.org/10.1186/s12889-020-09862-4

Nutrition Notes

The Client With Hypertension

- Losing weight without reducing sodium intake lowers BP even if the client does not attain ideal weight and regardless of the degree of excess weight. Ideally, body mass index (BMI) should be <25 kg/m^2. Preventing weight gain in those with a normal weight is vitally important. Generally, even a loss of 10% of body weight will result in significant positive change.
- The DASH diet, a total diet approach to preventing or treating hypertension, has been shown to significantly lower BP in both normotensive and hypertensive people and in all major risk groups. The diet is rich in fruit, vegetables, and low-fat dairy products and emphasizes whole grains, poultry, fish, and nuts. Fat, red meat, sweets, and sugar-containing beverages are restricted. Nutritionally, the diet is high in potassium, magnesium, calcium, and fiber and slightly high in protein. The diet's effectiveness likely comes from several factors, not just one food or nutrient.
- Subsequent studies have shown that lowering the sodium content of a DASH diet further improves its effectiveness in lowering BP. Although the relationship between sodium and BP is direct and progressive, the benefits of lowering sodium intake are generally greater in African Americans; middle-aged and older adults; and those with hypertension, diabetes, or chronic kidney disease. While 1.5 g/day of sodium may be ideal, 2.3 g/day is a more realistic goal.
- The DASH eating plan contains the following:
  - 6 to 8 servings of grains, with whole grains recommended for most grain choices
  - 4 to 5 servings of vegetables
  - 4 to 5 servings of fruit
  - 2 to 3 servings of low-fat or nonfat dairy products
  - 6 oz. or less of lean meat, poultry, and fish
  - 4 to 5 servings of nuts per week
  - 2 to 3 servings of added fat per day
  - 5 or fewer servings of sweets and added sugars per week

>>> *Stop, Think, and Respond 27-1*

A neighbor asks you to take her BP. The measurement is 160/90 mm Hg. What questions will you ask? What recommendations will you make for follow-up?

Accelerated and Malignant Hypertension

Accelerated hypertension and **malignant hypertension** are more serious forms of elevated BP that develop in clients with either essential or secondary hypertension. Accelerated hypertension is considered a hypertensive crisis. It is manifested by markedly elevated BP accompanied by hemorrhages and exudates in the eyes. If untreated, accelerated hypertension may progress to malignant hypertension, which describes dangerously elevated BP accompanied by papilledema.

Pathophysiology and Etiology

Accelerated hypertension and malignant hypertension occur in clients with undiagnosed hypertension or in those who fail to maintain follow-up or adhere to medical therapy. Accelerated hypertension and malignant hypertension usually have abrupt onset; if untreated, severe symptoms and complications follow rapidly. Malignant hypertension is fatal unless BP is quickly reduced. Even with intensive treatment, the kidneys, brain, and heart may be permanently damaged.

Consequences are life-threatening when the BP in the vascular system becomes extremely elevated. Some arterial blood vessels already may have ruptured or will soon. Retinal hemorrhages can lead to blindness. A stroke occurs if vessels in the brain rupture and bleed. If an aneurysm has developed in the aorta from chronic hypertension, it may burst and cause hemorrhage and shock. Cardiac effects include left ventricular failure with pulmonary edema or MI. Renal failure also may be forthcoming if the pressure is not reduced.

Assessment Findings

Signs and Symptoms

Some clients may present with confusion, headache, visual disturbances, seizures, and, possibly, coma. The sudden, marked rise in BP may cause chest pain, dyspnea, and moist lung sounds. Renal failure is evidenced by less than 30 mL/hour of urine. The onset of sudden, severe back pain accompanied by hypotension (abnormally low BP) indicates that an aortic aneurysm is dissecting or has ruptured (see Chapter 25).

Systolic BP is 160 mm Hg or higher, diastolic BP is 100 mm Hg or higher, or both. The optic disk (nerve) appears to bulge forward into the posterior chamber from swelling of the brain. The retinal blood vessels are obscured where they radiate from the bulging disk, making identification of their continuous pathway difficult. The retinas may show flame-shaped hemorrhages or fluffy white exudates.

Diagnostic Findings

Diagnostic studies that may reveal abnormalities include computed tomography scan, positron emission tomography scan, and magnetic resonance imaging. Reduced BP is a priority, and these neurologic tests may be postponed while emergency treatment measures are instituted.

Medical Management

In true hypertensive emergencies, the goal is to lower the BP within 1 to 2 hours by using potent IV drugs, such as diazoxide (Hyperstat IV), nitroprusside (Nitropress), nitroglycerin, or labetalol (Normodyne). If the client's condition is not extremely critical, other alternative antihypertensive drugs such as nifedipine (Procardia), verapamil (Isoptin), captopril (Capoten), and prazosin (Minipress) are prescribed for oral administration. Oxygen is ordered to reduce hypoxia-induced tachycardia.

Nursing Management

The nurse implements medical orders promptly to ensure that BP is lowered as quickly and safely as possible. He or she mixes drugs with IV solution after carefully calculating the dosage. The nurse administers the medicated solution with an infusion pump or controller and titrates the rate of infusion according to the client's response and the parameters set by the primary provider. He or she checks the site and progress of the infusion at least hourly. The nurse applies an automatic BP recording machine to the arm to measure the BP every few minutes or assesses the BP directly if using an arterial catheter. The nurse reports a systolic BP of 160 mm Hg or higher or a diastolic BP of 115 mm Hg or higher immediately. While awaiting medical orders, the nurse restricts client activity and monitors the client closely for neurologic, cardiac, and renal complications. He or she keeps emergency equipment and drugs ready in case complications develop. See Nursing Process for the Client with Hypertension for additional nursing management.

KEY POINTS

- Central aortic systolic pressure (CASP): the pressure of blood at the root of the aorta as blood is pumped from the left ventricle. Measured by a CASPro computerized monitor.
- Essential hypertension: about 95% of cases, is sustained elevated BP with no known cause.
- Secondary hypertension: is elevated BP that results from or is secondary to some other disorder.
- High blood pressure prevention
  - Eating a healthy diet
  - Getting regular exercise
  - Being at a healthy weight
  - Limiting alcohol
  - Not smoking
  - Managing stress
- Health problems caused by hypertension
  - Stroke
  - Cognitive decline
  - Vision
  - Heart attack
  - Heart failure
  - Peripheral artery disease
  - Kidney disease/failure
  - Sexual dysfunction
  - Pregnancy-related complications
- Malignant hypertension: is extremely high blood pressure that develops rapidly and causes some type of organ damage. Usually, the Blood Pressure reading is greater than 180/120 mm Hg; it is considered a medical emergency.

CRITICAL THINKING EXERCISES

1. On admission, a client's BP is 210/112 mm Hg in a supine position. What additional data would be pertinent to collect before reporting the finding to the nurse in charge and primary provider?
2. To which community resources in your locale would you refer a client with hypertension for support or care after discharge?
3. A nurse takes a BP on an obese client using an adult-sized cuff. What error in BP measurement is likely to result?
4. What response is appropriate when a client with hypertension divulges that they do not take prescribed antihypertensive medications because they do not experience any symptoms?

NCLEX-STYLE REVIEW QUESTIONS PrepU

1. At a community center, the nurse instructs men and women about the signs and symptoms of hypertension. Of the following people who are present at the discussion, whose BP is most important for the nurse to assess?
   1. A 75-year-old African American man
   2. A 50-year-old executive who lifts weights
   3. A 35-year-old woman who weighs 120 lb
   4. A 60-year-old man with atrial fibrillation
2. While getting a blood pressure assessment, a client asks the nurse why it is important to control hypertension. What nursing response is most accurate?
   1. Sustained hypertension predisposes to narrowing of the cardiac valves.
   2. Sustained hypertension decreases the life span of many blood cells.
   3. Sustained hypertension leads to the formation of venous blood clots.
   4. Sustained hypertension compromises blood flow to many vital organs.
3. When obtaining a health history from a client, what finding is most suggestive that the client is hypertensive?
   1. The client experiences occasional heart palpitations.
   2. The client has observed blood in urine.
   3. The client has had unexplained nosebleeds.
   4. The client has difficulty sleeping all night.
4. A client diagnosed with hypertension begins drug therapy using an antihypertensive agent. The nurse knows that the teaching has been successful when the client restates which of the following?
   1. "Antihypertensive drugs can lead to hypotension, resulting in falls."
   2. "Blurred vision is a common side effect of antihypertensive therapy."
   3. "Fatigue and weakness are manifestations of antihypertensive medications."
   4. "Antihypertensives can contribute to muscle weakness and joint instability."

5. The hypertensive client's primary provider recommends following a low-sodium diet. What is the best evidence that the client understands the dietary restriction?
   1. The client avoids seasoning with onion powder.
   2. The client uses maple syrup instead of sugar.
   3. The client eliminates the use of soy sauce.
   4. The client drinks skim rather than whole milk.

WANT TO KNOW MORE? There are a wide variety of online resources available on thePoint to enhance learning and understanding of this chapter.

Go to **thePoint.lww.com/activate** and use the activation code found in the front of this text to unlock these online resources.

28

Caring for Clients With Heart Failure

Words To Know

acute heart failure
acute pulmonary edema
afterload
aldosterone
Beta-type natriuretic peptide
cardiac resynchronization therapy
cardiogenic pulmonary edema
cardiomyoplasty
chronic heart failure
congestive heart failure
cor pulmonale
destination therapy
ejection fraction
heart failure
inotropic medications
intra-aortic balloon pump
left-sided heart failure
multiple gated acquisition (MUGA) scan
myocardial oxygen demand
orthopneic position
phlebostatic axis
preload
pulmonary vascular bed
refractory heart failure
right-sided heart failure
surgical ventricular restoration
total artificial heart
tripod position
ventricular assist device
ventricular remodeling

Learning Objectives

On completion of this chapter, you will be able to:

1. Discuss the pathophysiology and etiology of heart failure.
2. Distinguish between acute and chronic heart failure.
3. Identify differences between left-sided and right-sided heart failure.
4. Describe the symptoms, diagnosis, and treatment of left-sided and right-sided heart failure.
5. Discuss the medical and nursing management of clients with heart failure.
6. Discuss the pathophysiology, etiology, symptoms, diagnosis, and treatment of pulmonary edema.
7. Discuss the medical and nursing management of clients with pulmonary edema.

The heart is a double pump: the right side pumps deoxygenated blood to the lungs for oxygenation, and the left side pumps oxygen-rich blood into the systemic circulation (see Chapter 22). This process provides a continuous supply of oxygen and nutrients for cellular metabolism and a mechanism to eliminate carbon dioxide (CO_2) and metabolic wastes. Disturbances in one part of the heart, if they are severe or sustained, eventually affect the entire circulation. This chapter discusses the pathophysiology of heart failure and the medical and nursing management for clients who develop it.

Gerontologic Considerations

- Age-related vascular changes can contribute to heart failure by interfering with the blood supply to the heart muscle, thus causing the heart to become fatigued. Various levels of compensation may be required owing to a variety of factors that contribute to narrow and inflexible vessels.
- Early symptoms of heart failure in older adults can present differently than in younger adults, and include fatigue, confusion, anxiety, dyspnea on exertion, worsening renal function, or other comorbidities.
- Age-related changes in the gastrointestinal and hepatic systems may alter drug metabolism, necessitating careful monitoring for therapeutic or adverse effects of cardiac medications, including symptoms of toxicity. Older adults are at increased risk for toxicity because of the decreased ability of the kidneys to excrete drugs.
- The Beers criteria, a list of potentially inappropriate medications to be avoided in older adults owing to their reduced kidney function and potential drug–drug interactions can be helpful to determine potentially beneficial versus potentially harmful medications for older adults (American Geriatrics Society, 2019).

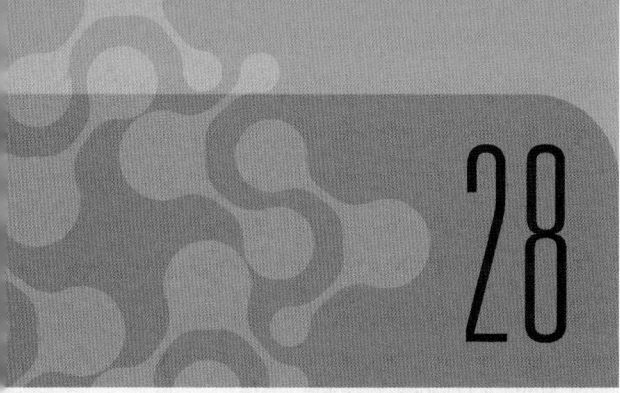

HEART FAILURE

Heart failure is the inability of the heart to pump sufficient blood to meet the body's metabolic needs. An estimate of the heart's efficiency as a pump is its **ejection fraction**, the percentage of blood the left ventricle ejects when it contracts. Normally, a healthy heart ejects 55% or more of the blood that fills the left ventricle during diastole. As the heart fails, the amount of ejected blood decreases (Table 28-1). The heart's ejection fraction is measured using an echocardiogram (see Chapter 22) or multiple gated acquisition scan (discussed later). The term **congestive heart failure** (CHF) describes the accumulation of blood and fluid in organs and tissues from impaired circulation.

Types of Heart Failure

One way to classify heart failure is by how it develops: acute or chronic. Another way to classify it is by location: right sided or left sided.

Acute and Chronic Heart Failure

Acute heart failure is a sudden change in the heart's ability to contract. It can cause life-threatening symptoms and pulmonary edema (discussed later). **Chronic heart failure** occurs when the heart's ability to pump effectively is gradually compromised and its impaired contractility remains prolonged. The New York Heart Association (NYHA) further classifies chronic heart failure based on the amount of activity restriction it imposes; their four functional stages of chronic heart failure are as follows (Heart Failure Society of America, 2016):

- Class I (Mild): Ordinary physical activity does not cause undue fatigue, palpitations, or dyspnea. The client does not experience any limitation of activity.
- Class II (Mild): The client is comfortable at rest, but ordinary physical activity results in fatigue, heart palpitations, or dyspnea.
- Class III (Moderate): There is marked limitation of physical activity. The client is comfortable at rest, but less than ordinary activity causes fatigue, heart palpitations, or dyspnea.
- Class IV (Severe): The client is unable to carry out any physical activity without discomfort. Symptoms of cardiac insufficiency occur at rest. Discomfort is increased if any physical activity is undertaken.

The American Heart Association and the American College of Cardiology also use criteria to describe four stages of heart failure. The scale ranges from Stage A, in which there are no current symptoms but the client has one or more risk factors (such as hypertension or diabetes) that predispose to heart failure, to Stage D, in which there is advanced structural heart disease and marked symptoms at rest despite maximal medical therapy. The two classification systems differ in that there is no comparable class in the NYHA classification for Stage A (Hobbs & Boyle, 2014).

TABLE 28-1 Assessment of Left Ventricular Ejection Fraction

EJECTION FRACTION (%)	EVALUATION OF FUNCTION
>55	Normal
45–55	Mildly reduced
35–45	Moderately reduced
<35	Severely reduced

Left-Sided and Right-Sided Heart Failure

Because the heart is a double pump, it is possible for either the left or right ventricle (or both) to become impaired. The terms *left-sided* (left ventricular) *heart failure* and *right-sided* (right ventricular) *heart failure* describe the location of the pumping dysfunction. **Left-sided heart failure** results from various conditions that impair the left ventricle's ability to eject blood into the aorta. **Right-sided heart failure** occurs when the right ventricle fails to eject its diastolic filling volume into the pulmonary artery, causing congestion of blood in the venous vascular system. The major cause of right-sided heart failure is left-sided heart failure. Chronic obstructive pulmonary disease (COPD) also contributes to the development of right-sided heart failure.

Pathophysiology and Etiology

Two mechanisms can cause heart failure. The primary reason for failure of either the left or right ventricle is inability of the heart muscle to contract because of direct damage to the muscular wall. Myocardial infarction (MI) usually affects the pumping ability of the left or right ventricle and frequently contributes to acute heart failure. Acute heart failure may immediately follow an MI or develop some time after the initial episode. The second mechanism occurs when the pumping chambers enlarge and weaken, as in cardiomyopathy and hypertension, making it impossible for the ventricles to eject all the blood they receive.

Left-Sided Heart Failure

When the left ventricle fails, the heart muscle cannot contract forcefully enough to expel blood into the systemic circulation (cardiac output). Blood subsequently becomes congested in the left ventricle, left atrium, and finally the pulmonary vasculature. The fluid accumulates and creates congestion in the **pulmonary vascular bed** (the capillary network surrounding the alveoli). Increased pulmonary vascular bed pressure causes fluid to move from the pulmonary capillaries into the alveoli. Gas exchange is impaired, cells become hypoxic (a state of insufficient oxygen), and CO_2 accumulates in the blood.

Hypertension, tachyarrhythmias, valvular disease, cardiomyopathy, and renal failure can contribute to chronic heart failure. These conditions reduce cardiac output by

- Increasing afterload or systemic vascular resistance. **Afterload**, the force that the ventricle must overcome to empty its diastolic volume, increases with arterial hypertension, aortic stenosis, pulmonary hypertension, or excessive blood volume from renal failure.

- Reducing ventricular ejection volume because diastole, during which the ventricle fills with blood (**preload**), is shortened as a result of tachyarrhythmia.
- Causing a loss of elasticity in the muscle as a result of cardiomyopathy.

Right-Sided Heart Failure

When right ventricular failure develops, the right ventricle cannot forcefully contract and push the blood into the pulmonary artery. As a result, congestion of blood and backflow accumulate first in the right ventricle; then in the right atrium; the superior and inferior vena cavae; and, subsequently, the venous vasculature. MIs that affect the right ventricle also can cause right ventricular failure.

Clients with chronic respiratory disorders tend to develop right-sided failure as a consequence of cor pulmonale. **Cor pulmonale** is a condition in which the heart (*cor*) is affected secondarily by lung damage (*pulmonale*). Pulmonary disease impairs exchange of oxygen and CO_2 in the alveoli, leading to increased CO_2 in the blood. By an unknown mechanism, pulmonary arterial vasoconstriction occurs. Prolonged pulmonary arterial vasoconstriction results in *pulmonary hypertension* (elevated pressure in the pulmonary arterial system; see Chapter 21). With pulmonary hypertension, the right ventricle is forced to pump against a high pressure gradient. Subsequently, the right ventricle enlarges and weakens under the increased workload, leading to failure. When the right ventricle fails to empty completely, blood is trapped in the venous vascular system. Eventually, the fluid is forced to move in retrograde fashion into the interstitial spaces and cells of other organs and tissues of the body.

Compensatory Mechanisms

The body can compensate for changes in heart function that occur over time (Fig. 28-1). When cardiac output falls, the body uses certain compensatory mechanisms designed to increase stroke volume and maintain blood pressure (BP). These compensatory mechanisms can temporarily improve the client's cardiac output but ultimately fail when contractility is further compromised.

As cardiac output falls, the client becomes hypotensive. The low BP stimulates the sympathetic nervous system to release catecholamines (e.g., epinephrine, norepinephrine) to raise heart rate and BP. The increased force and contraction of the heart maintain the client's BP but increase **myocardial oxygen demand** (the amount of oxygen the heart needs to perform its work). Epinephrine also causes blood vessels to constrict in an effort to raise BP. As the sympathetic nervous system is stimulated, the body shunts more blood to the vital organs of the brain and heart, decreasing blood supply to the kidneys. The kidneys secrete renin in response to decreased blood flow, which initiates the renin–angiotensin–aldosterone system (RAAS). Renin activates angiotensin. Angiotensin causes vasoconstriction and increases BP. Angiotensin also stimulates the adrenal gland to secrete **aldosterone**, a hormone that causes retention of sodium and water to increase BP by increasing the amount of blood returning to the heart. Sensing an increase in fluid pressure within the heart, the ventricles secrete a neurohormone known as **Beta-type natriuretic peptide** (BNP). BNP is cardioprotective. Its function is to decrease BP by increasing the excretion of sodium and water and promoting arterial

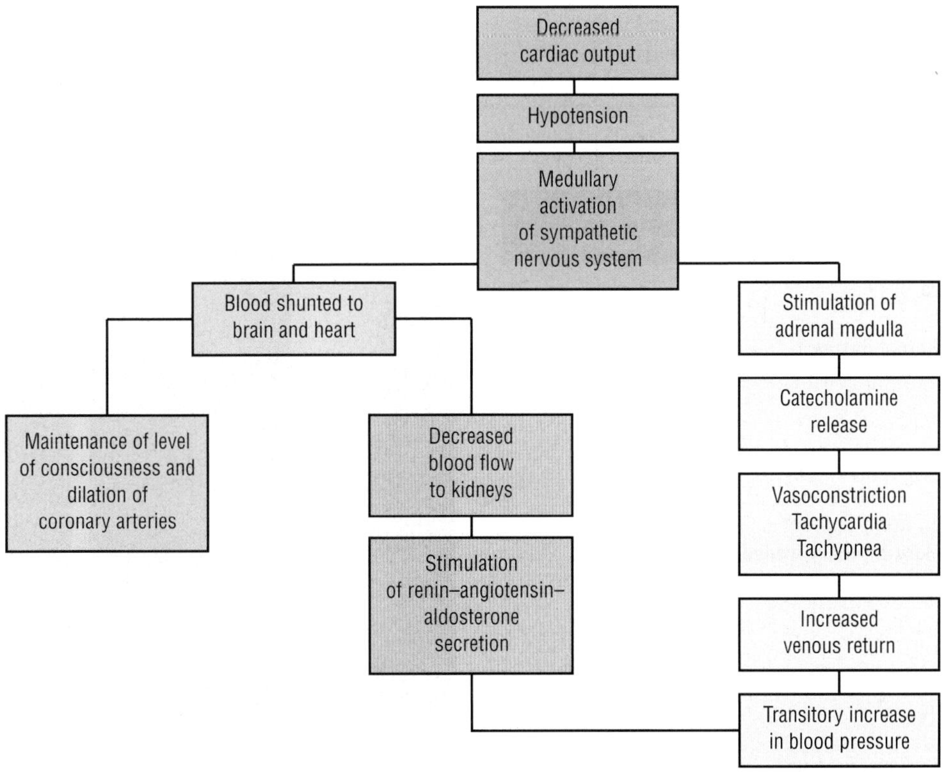

Figure 28-1 Compensatory mechanisms of the sympathetic nervous system. Decreased cardiac output triggers a series of compensatory mechanisms in the body in an effort to maintain level of consciousness and blood pressure.

dilation. It achieves its effects by counteracting renin, angiotensin, and aldosterone.

Ultimately, if compensatory mechanisms fail to restore homeostasis, the client's status is compromised by increased blood volume that the heart must pump and overwhelming the resistance the heart must overcome from arterial constriction. As cardiac output falls, the body's cells become deprived of oxygen and switch from aerobic metabolism to less efficient anaerobic metabolism. Anaerobic metabolism results in an accumulation of lactic acid, which lowers blood pH and can eventually cause metabolic acidosis.

Assessment Findings

Signs and Symptoms

The severity of symptoms depends on the body's ability to adjust to the decreased cardiac output. Initial signs and symptoms reflect the ventricle of the heart that is experiencing dysfunction. Usually, when a client has chronic heart failure, they develop signs and symptoms of both right-sided and left-sided heart failure. Box 28-1 highlights the clinical differences between left-sided and right-sided heart failure.

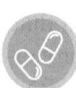

Pharmacologic Considerations

- Ask about history of cancer treatment during the intake assessment. Cardiac toxicity may develop in cancer survivors who were treated with chest radiation or chemotherapy drugs such as doxorubicin (Adriamycin) and vincristine (Oncovin). Chemo-protective agents such as dexrazoxane (Zinecard) are now used to reduce cardiac adverse effects.

BOX 28-1 Signs and Symptoms of Left and Right Ventricular Failure

Left-Sided Failure
- Fatigue
- Paroxysmal nocturnal dyspnea
- Orthopnea
- Hypoxia
- Crackles
- Cyanosis
- S_3 heart sound
- Cough with pink, frothy sputum
- Elevated pulmonary capillary wedge pressure

Right-Sided Failure
- Weakness
- Ascites
- Weight gain
- Nausea, vomiting
- Arrhythmias
- Elevated central venous pressure
- Jugular vein distention

Left-Sided Heart Failure

Left-sided heart failure produces hypoxemia as a result of reduced cardiac output of arterial blood and respiratory symptoms. Many clients notice unusual fatigue with activity. Some find exertional dyspnea (effort at breathing when active) to be the first symptom. Inability to breathe unless sitting upright (orthopnea) or being awakened by breathlessness (paroxysmal nocturnal dyspnea) may prompt the client to use several pillows in bed or to sleep in a chair or recliner. Pulse may be rapid or irregular. BP may be elevated from sympathetic nervous system stimulation. A cough, hemoptysis (blood-streaked sputum), and moist crackles on auscultation are typical respiratory findings. Urine output is diminished. If acute, left-sided heart failure with pulmonary edema develops, the client suddenly becomes hypoxic, restless, and confused.

Right-Sided Heart Failure

The client with right-sided heart failure may have a history of gradual, unexplained weight gain from fluid retention. *Dependent pitting edema* (excess fluid volume in the interstitial space in body areas affected by gravity) in the feet and ankles can be observed by pressing into tissue over a bone for 5 seconds and then releasing the pressure. The pressure forces fluid into the underlying tissue causing an indentation that slowly disappears. (Fig. 28-2). This type of edema may seem to disappear overnight but really is temporarily redistributed by gravity to other tissues, such as the sacral area. Fluid may distend the abdomen (ascites), and the liver may be enlarged (hepatomegaly). Jugular veins often are distended from increased central venous pressure (Nursing Guidelines 28-1). Enlarged abdominal organs often restrict ventilation, creating dyspnea. Clients may observe that rings, shoes, or clothing have become tight. Accumulation of blood in abdominal organs may cause anorexia, nausea, and flatulence. (Also see Evidence-Based Practice 28-1.)

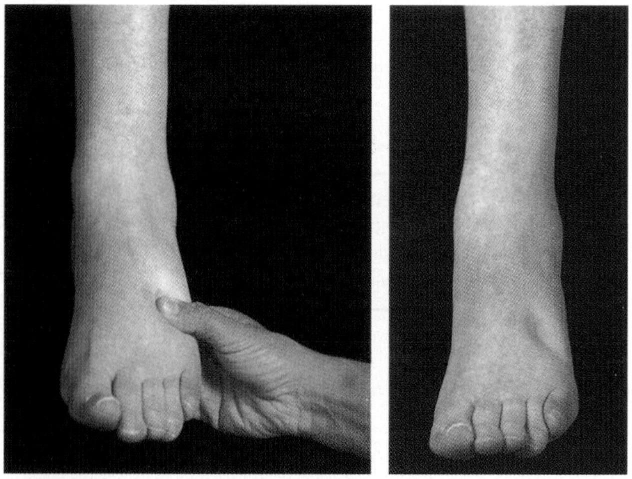

Figure 28-2 Assessing for pitting edema. (Reprinted with permission from Bickley, L. S., Szilagyi, P. G., & Hoffman, R. M. (2017). *Bates' guide to physical examination and history taking* (12th ed.). Wolters Kluwer.)

NURSING GUIDELINES 28-1

Estimating Central Venous Pressure

Central venous pressure (CVP) is the pressure produced by venous blood in the right atrium. CVP measurement and monitoring are discussed in Chapter 29. To estimate CVP, the nurse measures the height of jugular vein distention:

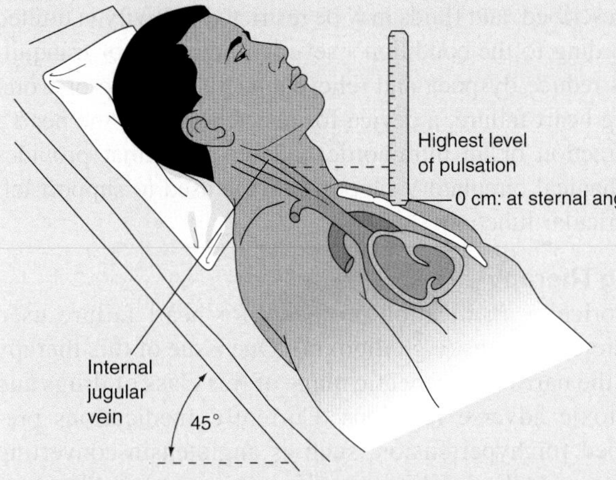

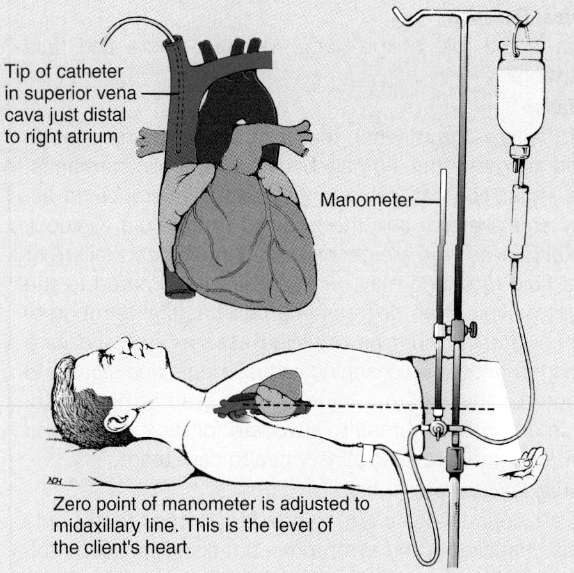

Reprinted with permission from Nettina, S. M. (2001). *The Lippincott Manual of Nursing Practice* (7th ed.). Lippincott Williams & Wilkins.

1. Obtain a centimeter ruler.
2. Help client to lie flat.
3. Slowly elevate head of bed to 45°.
4. Locate the sternal angle by placing two fingers at the sternal notch and sliding them down the sternum until they reach a bony prominence.
5. Estimate venous pressure by measuring the vertical distance from the sternal angle (0 cm) to the level of jugular vein distention (cm above 0).
6. Add 5 cm to the ruler measurement to estimate CVP. CVP is elevated more than 12 to 15 cm H_2O in clients who have right ventricular heart failure.

A more accurate measurement of CVP is obtained by using a water manometer in the following manner:

1. Place the zero on the water manometer at the client's **phlebostatic axis** which is at the 4th intercostal space in the midaxillary line.
2. Turn the stopcock off to the client so fluid from the IV solution fills the water manometer (A) to 10 or 20 cm above normal; normal CVP pressure is 5 to 10 cm of H_2O.
3. Turn the stopcock off to the IV solution (B) allowing the fluid in the manometer to fall by gravity as it enters the client's venous circulation.
4. Read the cm level when the fluid stops or at the lowest number if it fluctuates slightly as the client breathes.
5. Turn the stopcock off to the manometer (C) to resume the infusion of IV solution to the client.

>>> Stop, Think, and Respond 28-1

Which type of heart failure is evidenced by the following assessment findings?

- *Client A has swollen ankles. His clothes fit poorly, and he has purchased larger pants and shirts. When he is weighed, he remarks that he has gained 10 lb in the last month, but his diet has not changed. He says he feels "full," can't eat as much as usual, and "works hard" to breathe.*
- *Client B becomes breathless while changing into a gown before the assessment. She reports sleeping better when sitting up in a recliner. Her cough is "wet." She is tachycardic and says she has noticed less frequent urination.*

Diagnostic Findings

Left-Sided Heart Failure

Chest radiography shows cardiac enlargement and fluid accumulation in the lungs. An echocardiogram can reveal the increased size of the left ventricle and ineffective pumping of the heart. A **multiple gated acquisition (MUGA) scan**, also called a *gated blood pool scan*, measures a decrease in the ejection fraction. An MUGA scan is the most accurate noninvasive test that measures the left ventricle's ejection fraction during rest and activity. When an MUGA scan is performed, the client receives an injection with an intravenous (IV) radioisotope that concentrates within the red blood cells in approximately 20 to 30 minutes. A gamma camera can identify the cells once they are radioactive. The client is then attached to a cardiac monitor, and the gamma camera takes images as the blood passes through the heart and major blood vessels. The client must lie very still at intermittent times during the 45-minute test. Diuretics are contraindicated the morning of a test to avoid any interruptions for urination. Clients also are medicated to relieve a cough that may cause movement during the test. Although allergic reactions to the IV chemical can occur, they are rare.

Evidence-Based Practice 28-1

Heart Failure and Fluid Retention

Clinical Question

What is the role of the nurse in heart failure and fluid retention?

Evidence

Heart failure occurs when the heart cannot pump enough blood to meet the human body's metabolic demands. This imbalance can cause a decreased tolerance to activity and exercise and the body to retain fluid (Colucci, 2020). Clients who are decompensating in heart failure or have fluid retention may end up being readmitted to the hospital, which can decrease certain hospital reimbursements. Nurses must have skilled assessment and care management to see changing assessments and signs and symptoms that treatments are not missed or given late. It is important for nurses to advocate for their clients and work with the inter-disciplinary health care team.

Nursing Implications

This article indicates a strong need for nurses to not only assess the clients and symptoms, but also assess the tolerance a client has with activity. It is also helpful to take a thorough history and make a note of previous hospital admissions to assess for hypervolemia. This data will be useful for the care team and plan of care during stay (Colucci, 2020).

Reference

Colucci, W. S. (2020). *Treatment of acute decompensated heart failure: Specific therapies.* https://www.uptodate.com/contents/treatment-of-acute-decompensated-heart-failure-specific-therapies

At first, arterial blood gas (ABG) analysis may reveal respiratory alkalosis as a result of rapid, shallow breathing. Later, there is a shift to metabolic acidosis as gas exchange becomes more impaired. Serum sodium levels may be elevated. Elevated blood urea nitrogen indicates impaired renal perfusion. If the client is seriously ill, a pulmonary artery catheter may be inserted for hemodynamic monitoring. Cardiac output can be measured with the pulmonary artery catheter. Cardiac output is diminished in left-sided heart failure, and pulmonary artery pressure and pulmonary capillary wedge pressure measurements are elevated. The BNP levels are above 100 picograms/mL (pg/mL) (a picogram is a billionth of a gram; Box 28-2).

Right-Sided Heart Failure

A chest radiograph, electrocardiogram (ECG), and echocardiography reveal right ventricular enlargement. A lung scan and pulmonary arteriography can confirm cor pulmonale. Liver enzymes are elevated if the liver is impaired.

BOX 28-2 Significance of BNP Levels

$<$100 pg/mL indicates no heart failure
100–300 pg/mL suggests heart failure is present
$>$300–599 pg/mL indicates mild heart failure
$>$600–899 pg/mL indicates moderate heart failure
$\geq$900 pg/mL indicates severe heart failure

Medical Management

Medical management of both left-sided and right-sided heart failure is directed at reducing the heart's workload and improving cardiac output primarily through dietary modifications, drug therapy, and lifestyle changes. A low-sodium diet is prescribed, and fluids may be restricted. Activity is limited according to the condition's severity. Sedatives or tranquilizers reduce dyspnea and relieve anxiety. In acute or worsening heart failure, a device for resynchronizing the heart's contraction or an intra-aortic balloon pump that provides mechanical circulatory support may be used to support left ventricular function.

Drug Therapy

Historically, medication protocols for heart failure used cardiotonic drugs (e.g., digoxin). One issue of this therapy was the narrow therapeutic range of this class of drugs and the toxic adverse reactions. Currently, medications prescribed for hypertension, such as angiotensin-converting enzyme (ACE) inhibitors, angiotensin receptor blockers (ARB), diuretics, and beta (β)-blockers are the mainstay of heart failure drug therapy. However, digoxin use continues:

- For older clients maintained on the drug for many years
- For people who continue to experience symptoms after using the first choice drugs
- In some cases, to treat atrial fibrillation (which is also decreasing) (Freeman et al., 2014)

A newer cardiotonic replacing digoxin—ivabradine—blocks the If (funny) channel and inhibits the pacing of the S-A node of the heart (Drug Therapy Table 28-1). This, in turn, slows the heart rate and allows blood to fill the heart chamber. Recent studies demonstrate the use of a combination drug sacubitril/valsartan which reduces mortality and hospitalization owing to heart failure better than ACE inhibitors alone. Sacubitril (neprilysin inhibitor) interferes with an enzyme that metabolizes endogenous vasodilators while valsartan (angiotensin receptor blocker) works better than other ACE inhibitors.

Diuretic therapy helps reduce the heart's workload by decreasing the exertion required to overcome afterload. Thiazide diuretics such as hydrochlorothiazide (HydroDIURIL) can manage many cases of mild heart failure. Severe heart failure usually requires a loop diuretic such as furosemide (Lasix). These drugs increase sodium excretion and therefore water excretion, but they also increase potassium excretion. If a client becomes hypokalemic, digitalis toxicity is more likely; it is evidenced by loss of appetite; nausea or vomiting; rapid, slow, or irregular heart rate; or sudden disturbance in color vision. Low serum potassium levels and signs of digitalis toxicity must be reported to the primary provider. The blood level of digitalis is measured if there is a question concerning its concentration.

DRUG THERAPY TABLE 28-1 Agents to Treat Heart Failure

Category and Common Generic (Brand) Drugs	Intended Use	Common Side Effects	Safety Warnings for Nurses
ACE Inhibitors (ACEI)			
Captopril (Capoten) Enalapril (Vasotec) Lisinopril (Prinivil)	Suppression of the renin–angiotensin– aldosterone system (RAAS) reduces water and sodium retention which lessens blood pressure, relaxes blood vessels lessening heart workload	Dizziness, headache, fatigue, dry cough	• Increased fall risk owing to hypotensive side effects • Do not use if impaired renal function, or dialysis • Monitor for lower blood glucose in clients with diabetes • Interaction with herbal: St. John's wort • Perimenopausal women need to use effective birth control
Angiotensin II Receptor Antagonists (ARB)			
Losartan (Cozaar) Valsartan (Diovan)	Inhibit the pressor effect of angiotensin II, suppressing the negative feedback loop of RAAS relaxes blood vessels lessening heart workload	Dizziness, fainting, diarrhea	• Perimenopausal women need to use effective birth control
Beta-Adrenergic Blockers			
Bisoprolol (Zebeta) Carvedilolol (Coreg) Metoprolol (Lopressor)	Reduce heart rate and decrease consumption of oxygen by myocardium	Headache, dizziness, nausea, vomiting	• When given as IV, constant cardiac monitoring is required • Drug is usually held if heart rate <60 and >120 • Initially, monitor blood every 2–3 weeks for agranulocytosis
Diuretics			
Furosemide (Lasix) Chlorothiazide (Diuril)	Decrease work of heart by promoting excretion of sodium and water, thus reducing circulating blood volume	Dizziness, dehydration, nausea, diarrhea, nocturia, polyuria, orthostatic hypotension	• Monitor serum potassium • Increased fall risk owing to hypotensive side effects • Encourage fluids to prevent dehydration
Selective Aldosterone Receptor Antagonist			
Eplerenone (Inspra) Spironolactone (Aldactone)	Blocks aldosterone which reduces BP	Hyperkalemia	• Monitor serum potassium and renal function at day 3, week 1, monthly $\times$ 3, 4 $\times$ yearly while taking drug • Gynecomastia in males
Cardiac Glycosides			
Digoxin (Lanoxin)	Increases cardiac output by slowing heart rate (negative chronotropic action) and increasing force of contraction (positive inotropic action)	Fatigue, generalized muscle weakness	• Monitor potassium, hypokalemia increases serum blood levels • Monitor for toxicity, GI distress, muscle fatigue, CNS disturbances, cardiac changes • Drug is usually held if heart rate <60 and >120
Vasodilators			
Isosorbide (Isordil) Nitroglycerin (Nitrostat)	By dilating coronary arteries, improves heart pumping action and maintains blood pressure in severe heart failure	Headache, dizziness, orthostatic hypotension, tachycardia, flushing	• Increased fall risk owing to hypotensive side effects • Do not use with head trauma client • Do not use with erectile dysfunction drugs

(*continued*)

DRUG THERAPY TABLE 28-1 Agents to Treat Heart Failure (*continued*)

Category and Common Generic (Brand) Drugs	Intended Use	Common Side Effects	Safety Warnings for Nurses
Miscellaneous Drugs			
Inotropic Dobutamine (Dobutrex)	Improves heart pumping action and maintains BP in severe heart failure	Hypotension, PVCs	• Monitor serum potassium for hypokalemia
Nesiritide (Natrecor)	Adjuvant to diuretic therapy in smooth muscle relaxation to lower vessel pressure	Headache, hypotension, nausea	• Angioedema
Ivabradine (Corlanor)	Reduces heart rate by inhibiting electrical impulses of the S-A node	Dizziness, hypotension, rash, itching	• Perimenopausal women need to use effective birth control • May see bright, flashing light
Angiotensin receptor-neprilysin inhibitors Sacubirtil/valsartan (Entresto)	Protects and reduces RAAS to lower pressure and workload of heart	Dizziness, hypotension, cough, hyperkalemia	• Perimenopausal women need to use effective birth control • Angioedema • Not to be taken if diabetic

RAAS, renin–angiotensin–aldosterone system
The drugs in column 1 indicate the drug that matches up with explanations in columns 2 through 4.

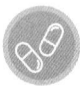

Pharmacologic Considerations

■ Digitalis preparations are potent and may cause various toxic effects. The margin between a therapeutic and toxic effect is narrow. Observe clients for signs of digitalis toxicity throughout client care. Teach the client about the signs and symptoms of electrolyte and water loss and the importance of adhering to the prescribed medication schedule. Also instruct the client to eat foods high in potassium or take a prescribed potassium supplement to decrease the risk for digitalis toxicity.

Vasodilators also reduce afterload. Clients with a history of heart failure may receive a drug such as an angiotensin-converting enzyme (ACE) inhibitor (e.g., captopril [Capoten]), an angiotensin receptor blocker (ARB) such as irbesartan (Avapro), or some other category of drug that causes vasodilatation. ACE inhibitors such as captopril, fosinopril (Monopril), enalapril (Vasotec), and ramipril (Altace) may also be used to treat heart failure in clients who have not responded to digitalis and diuretics.

>>> *Stop, Think, and Respond 28-2*

A client with a possible bowel obstruction has a history of chronic heart failure. He has been taking digoxin (Lanoxin) at home. What nursing actions are appropriate?

Cardiac Resynchronization Therapy

Cardiac resynchronization therapy (CRT) is a new technique that restores synchrony in the contractions of the right and left ventricles. CRT is used primarily for clients whose heart failure is caused by dilated cardiomyopathy (see Chapter 23). It is achieved with a biventricular pacemaker. The biventricular pacemaker is inserted transvenously similarly to a traditional pacemaker, with electrical leads in the right atrium and right ventricle and the battery placed beneath the skin of the chest (see Chapter 26). It has an additional internal third lead, however, that is placed outside the left ventricle. The dual ventricular leads stimulate the right and left ventricles to contract at the same time. When the ventricles contract simultaneously, the force of contraction improves, and more blood is ejected with each heartbeat.

Concept Mastery Alert

Cardiac Resynchronization

The purpose of a biventricular pacemaker is resynchronization of the heart. This intervention is used to treat advanced heart failure that does not respond to medication. The purpose of defibrillation is to stop a life-threatening ventricular dysrhythmia.

Intra-aortic Balloon Pump

If cardiogenic shock (see Chapter 17) accompanies acute left ventricular heart failure, an **intra-aortic balloon pump** (IABP) may be used. An IABP acts as a secondary mechanical circulatory pump to temporarily supplement the ineffectual contraction of the left ventricle. It is inserted as a catheter into the left femoral artery and threaded up to the descending aortic arch (Fig. 28-3). The IABP is connected to a machine that inflates the balloon portion during ventricular diastole and deflates during systole, a process known as *counterpulsation*. Inflation of the IABP increases coronary artery, renal artery, and myocardial perfusion. Deflation actually keeps the aorta distended so that cardiac output is improved; the

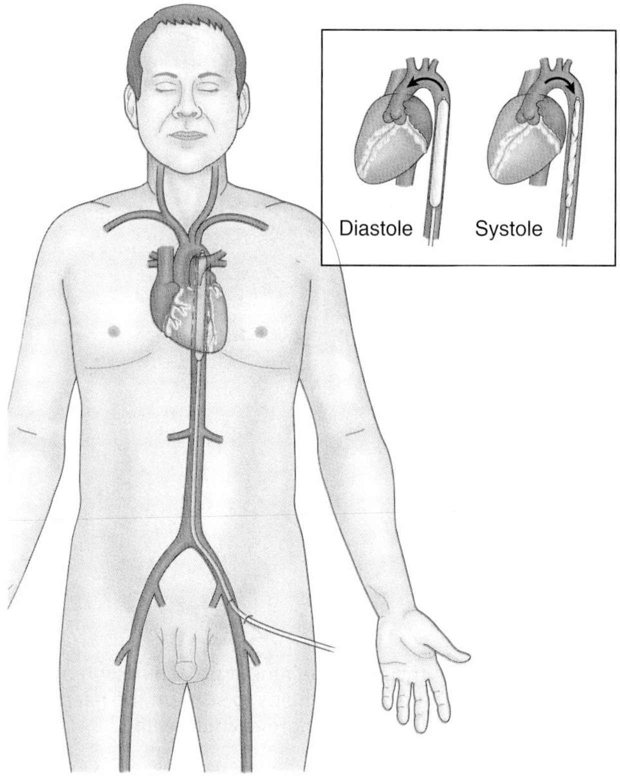

Figure 28-3 The intra-aortic balloon pump (IABP).

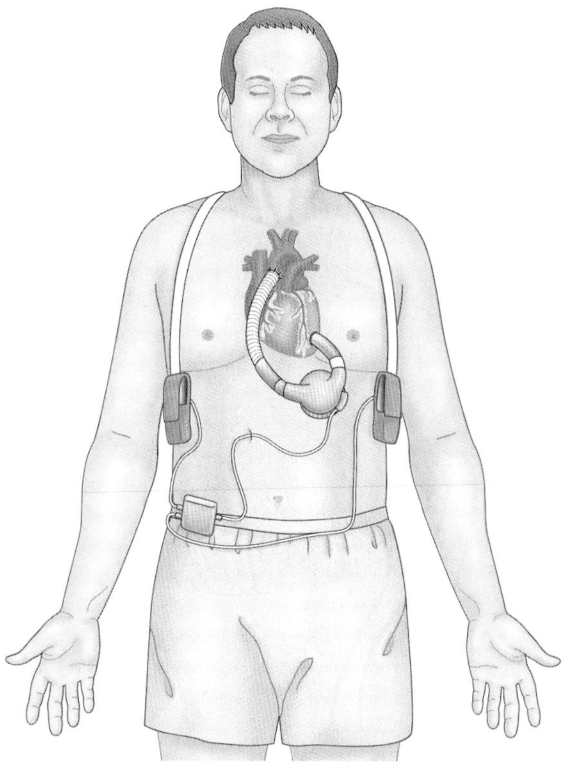

Figure 28-4 The left ventricular assist device (LVAD) pump weighs 1.5 lb. It is implanted below the diaphragm; its battery pack is carried outside the body. Tubes connect the pump to the left ventricle and aorta.

work of the left ventricle is decreased, and peripheral organs are more adequately perfused with oxygenated blood. The IABP is intended for only a few days' use.

Surgical Management

When medical treatment alone is unsuccessful, clients may require surgical treatment options such as the insertion of a ventricular assist device, cardiomyoplasty, or an implantable artificial heart. Human heart transplantation is discussed in Chapter 29.

Ventricular Assist Device

There are approximately 870,000 people who develop heart failure each year. Of those, 50,000 to 100,000 usually in the New York Heart Association class III or IV have refractory heart failure (Texas Heart Institute, 2015). **Refractory heart failure** refers to symptoms of heart failure that persist despite maximum medical therapy with proven efficacy for managing heart failure. Many with refractory heart failure experience disease progression, repeated hospitalizations, and may ultimately succumb to their disease.

Some clients with refractory heart failure who meet specific criteria are candidates for interventional therapies like a **ventricular assist device** (VAD), an auxiliary heart pump that supplements the heart's ability to eject blood. If the VAD supports left ventricular function, it is referred to as a *left ventricular assist device* or LVAD. VADs may be used for one of three purposes: (1) a bridge to recovery, (2) a bridge to transplant, or (3) **destination therapy** (mechanical circulatory support when there is no option for a heart transplant).

When a VAD is implanted, the natural heart remains in place and continues to function at whatever capacity is possible. Most VADs use an outflow and inflow cannula to carry blood from the left ventricle into the aorta (Fig. 28-4). They are battery operated through an external power source worn about the waist. By assisting the weak, ineffective left ventricle, VADs maintain cardiac output at normal volumes. Some VADs act as a double-assist device that can be used for left-sided, right-sided, or biventricular heart failure. The trend is to develop miniaturized devices; one current model weighs only 3.25 oz. Companies are now working on LVADs that can be implanted with less invasive surgery with a potential survival rate of 2 years with fewer complications such as bleeding, strokes, and a decline in cognitive function (Shah & Brisco, 2015; O'Riordan, 2015). Clients can easily manage smaller models, making it possible for some to return home and continue a functional life or await heart transplantation.

Cardiomyoplasty

Cardiomyoplasty is a surgical procedure in which the client's own chest muscle (latissimus dorsi) is grafted to the aorta and wrapped around the heart. An electrical stimulator placed in a subcutaneous pouch triggers skeletal muscle contraction (Fig. 28-5). The contraction acts as a counterpulsation mechanism similar to the IABP. It augments the ineffective myocardial muscle contraction.

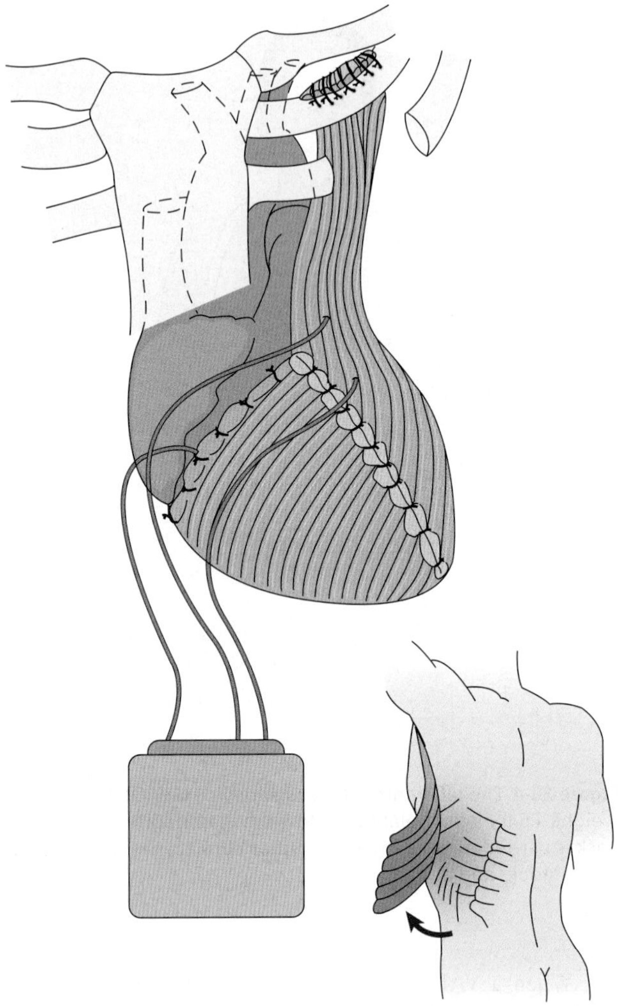

Figure 28-5 In cardiomyoplasty, the latissimus dorsi muscle is dissected and wrapped around the heart itself.

A ventricular containment procedure, sometimes referred to as a *heart wrap*, may be performed. In this procedure, a polyethylene/polyester support mesh device (Fig. 28-6), which some have likened to pantyhose, serves as an alternative to the cardiomyoplasty procedure. The heart wrap is pulled over the heart and sutured in place. The wrap supports the heart and reverses **ventricular remodeling**, a condition in which there are changes in the size, shape, structure, and physiology of the heart after myocardial injury. This procedure may be an alternative to a cardiac transplant.

Ventricular Restoration

A procedure known as **surgical ventricular restoration** (SVR) decreases the size of the heart to a near normal size and shape by removing dysfunctional heart muscle that does not contract properly. Once the adynamic (nonfunctioning) area is removed, the ventricle is repaired with a patch (Fig. 28-7). Other procedures such as mitral valve replacement or coronary artery bypass graft can be performed while the heart and chest are still open. In the cases that were studied, 91% were free of CHF after surgery, with an ejection fraction that increased from 30% to 40% (Johns Hopkins Medicine, n.d.).

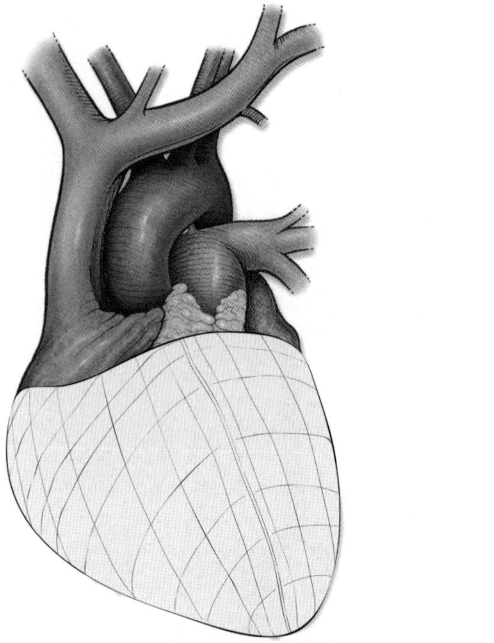

Figure 28-6 In a ventricular containment procedure, wrapping the heart with a synthetic mesh helps to support the heart, restore its functional size, and improve contractility.

Total Artificial Heart

A **total artificial heart** (TAH) is an electrically powered pump that circulates blood into the pulmonary artery and the aorta, thus replacing the functions of both the right and left ventricles. It is considered an extension of LVADs, which only support a failing left ventricle. TAHs are targeted for clients who are unlikely to live more than a month without further interventions. Currently, there are two TAH models, SynCardia's CardioWest TAH and Abiomed's AbioCor TAH, that are available as a bridge to transplant or destination therapy (Fig. 28-8). When implanted, the TAH replaces the functioning of both ventricles of the diseased heart, including the four heart valves. Although both TAHs achieve similar outcomes, there are several differences (Box 28-3). As technology in developing artificial hearts improves, they may eventually become an alternative to human heart transplantation (see Chapter 29).

Nursing Management

Most clients can manage chronic heart failure at home. Many medications, lifestyle changes, and diet restrictions (Nutrition Notes) are involved to control heart failure. During times of acute illness, usual methods may not control symptoms, and the client may require hospitalization for additional treatment. The home health nurse, the nurse in an extended or intermediate care facility, and nurses in acute care settings administer prescribed medications and monitor for therapeutic and adverse effects. They implement interventions that promote the heart's ability to eject as much blood as possible, monitor for signs of excess fluid volume and evidence of electrolyte imbalance, promote oxygenation, balance activity according to the client's tolerance, and support family members who may be the usual primary caregivers (Client and Family Teaching 28-1).

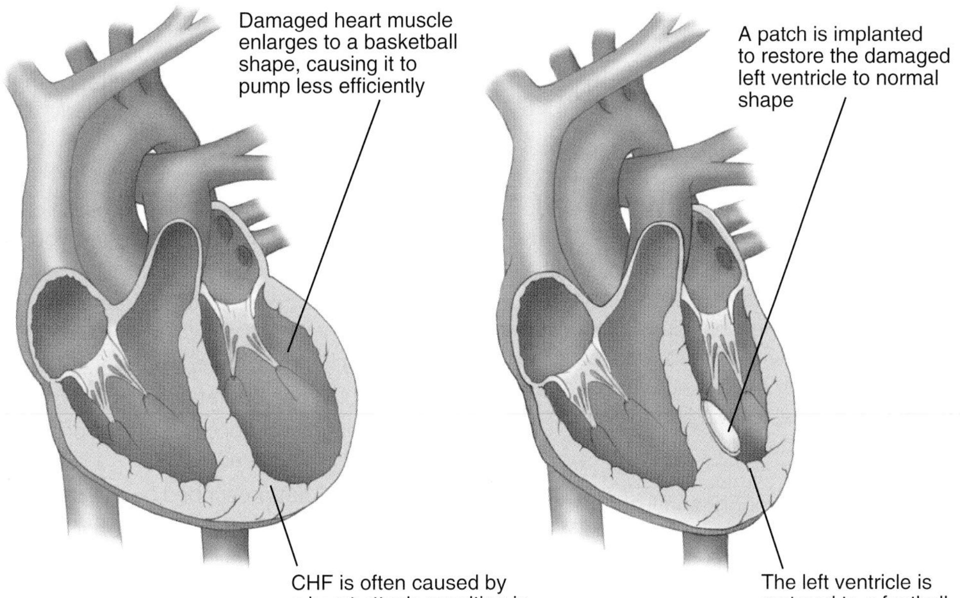

Dilated heart in congestive heart failure
Restored heart after surgery
Damaged heart muscle enlarges to a basketball shape, causing it to pump less efficiently
A patch is implanted to restore the damaged left ventricle to normal shape
CHF is often caused by a heart attack, resulting in scar tissue around the left ventricle
The left ventricle is restored to a football shape, resulting in improved function

Figure 28-7 Surgical ventricular restoration remodels the heart by removing nonfunctioning heart muscle and patching the defect. CHF, congestive heart failure.

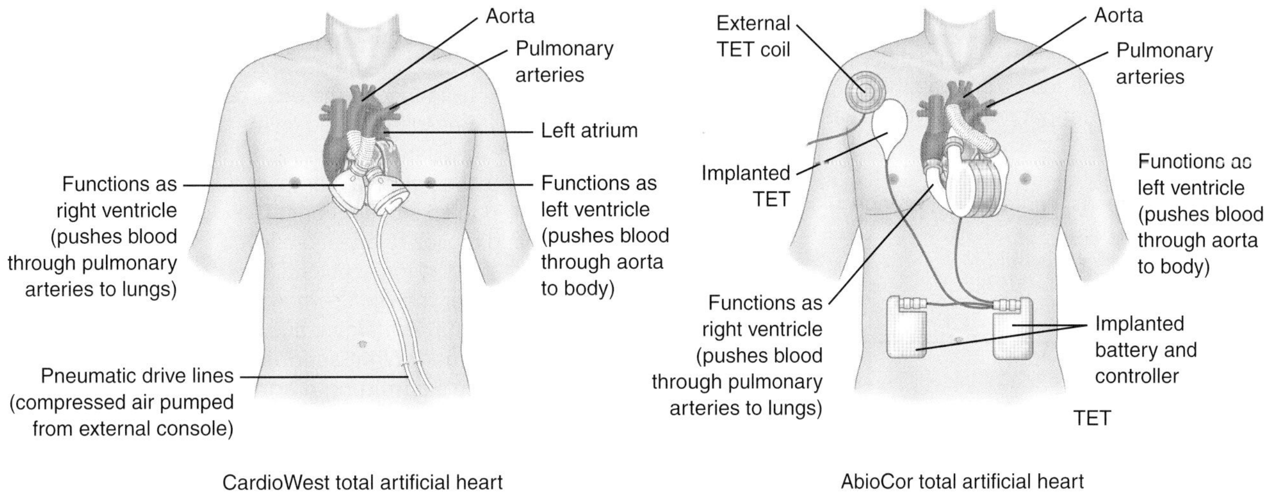

Aorta
Pulmonary arteries
Left atrium
Functions as right ventricle (pushes blood through pulmonary arteries to lungs)
Functions as left ventricle (pushes blood through aorta to body)
Pneumatic drive lines (compressed air pumped from external console)
CardioWest total artificial heart
External TET coil
Aorta
Pulmonary arteries
Implanted TET
Functions as left ventricle (pushes blood through aorta to body)
Functions as right ventricle (pushes blood through pulmonary arteries to lungs)
Implanted battery and controller
TET
AbioCor total artificial heart

Figure 28-8 Examples of total artificial hearts. (*Left*) CardioWest TAH with internal lines that extend externally through the abdomen; (*Right*) AbioCor TAH, which is totally contained within the chest. TET, transcutaneous energy transmission.

BOX 28-3 Total Artificial Heart (TAH) Differences

SynCardia TAH
- Replaces the entire heart
- Tubes extend through the abdomen outside the body
- Must protect tubes from getting wet
- Higher risk of infection
- Pumps blood simultaneously into right and left circulation
- Powered by an external portable power source
- Status must be checked by visit to a healthcare provider

AbioCor TAH
- Replaces only the ventricles
- Completely contained inside the chest
- Can shower or swim
- Lower potential for infection
- Pumps blood out of one ventricle at a time
- Internal battery charged by radiofrequency through the skin (transcutaneous energy transmission [TET])
- Can be checked remotely via a computer with Internet access

Nutrition Notes

The Client With Heart Failure

- Clients with symptomatic heart failure may need to limit their sodium intake to 2 g/day or less. General guidelines are as follows:
  - Eliminate processed and prepared foods and beverages high in sodium; use fresh, frozen, and canned low-sodium products.
  - Do not use salt in cooking or at the table.
- Encourage clients to read Nutrition Facts Labels; most foods eaten should provide <300 mg sodium per serving. Foods that fall under these guidelines include the following:
  - Most breads; many ready-to-eat cereals, cooked cereals, pasta, rice, and other starches cooked without salt
  - Fresh and frozen vegetables; low-sodium or sodium-free canned vegetables and soups
  - Fresh and canned fruit
  - Low-fat and nonfat milk and yogurt; small amounts of low-fat natural cheese
  - Fresh and frozen meats; low-sodium canned tuna, dried peas and beans, eggs
  - Baked goods made without baking soda, angel food cake
  - Tub or liquid margarine; vegetable oils
- Dyspnea and nausea related to enlarged abdominal organs interfere with appetite and intake. Provide five to six small meals of soft or easily chewed foods. Encourage the client to rest after eating and to avoid spicy, gas-forming, and high-fiber foods to lessen heartburn and flatulence.
- Clients taking potassium-wasting diuretics should consume potassium-rich foods, such as:
  - Potatoes, sweet potatoes, winter squash, tomatoes, tomato juice
  - Milk, yogurt
  - Dates, bananas, cantaloupes, orange juice, prunes, raisins, prune juice
  - Dry beans, peas, lentils
  - Peanut butter
  - Bran cereals

Client and Family Teaching 28-1
Heart Failure

The nurse instructs about the disease process, meaning of the term *failure*, signs and symptoms of impending CHF (weight gain, ankle swelling, fatigue, dyspnea), and importance of taking all medications regularly. They also cover the following points:

- Measure pulse and BP daily.
- Check weight at the same time each day using the same scale; consult a primary provider if you gain more than 2 lb in 24 hours.
- Schedule rest periods to reduce or eliminate fatigue and dyspnea.
- Increase activities such as walking when able to do so without dyspnea or fatigue.
- Identify and avoid occasions that produce stress. Elevate the legs while sitting.
- Follow the diet prescribed by the primary provider.
- Avoid extreme heat, cold, or humidity.
- Report a heart rate less than 60 or more than 120 beats/min before taking digitalis.
- Contact the primary provider if symptoms return or swelling in the legs, ankles, or feet suddenly increases.
- Maintain follow-up care.

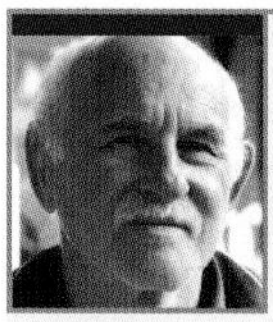

Clinical Scenario A 70-year-old male arrives on the nursing unit after being examined in the emergency department. Because a pulse oximeter measured his oxygen saturation at 87%, he is receiving oxygen and was given a loop diuretic before being transferred to an inpatient unit. The client is short of breath and replies to questions in one word or short sentences owing to dyspnea. The client wants to sit in the chair rather than lie down in bed. The client's radial pulse rate is 100 beats/min, and his respiratory rate is 32 breaths/min. **What actions does a nurse take when a client's admitting diagnosis is heart failure? See the following Nursing Process section.**

NURSING PROCESS FOR THE CLIENT WITH HEART FAILURE

Assessment

During the initial interview, elicit the client's history of symptoms and medications. Perform an initial physical assessment to establish baseline data. Observe for dyspnea; auscultate apical heart rate and count radial heart rate; measure BP; observe for distended neck veins; and note any signs of peripheral edema, lethargy, or confusion during a head-to-toe assessment. Obtain an admission weight and thereafter weigh the client daily on the same scale, at about the same time of day, with the client wearing similar clothing. Note laboratory test results of serum electrolytes because drug therapy with certain diuretics depletes potassium blood levels. Initiate intake and output measurements and evaluate fluid volumes at least every 8 hours. Measure abdominal girth to determine if the client is developing ascites or responding to therapeutic measures. Note respiratory difficulties during activity and rest. Question the client about nocturnal dyspnea (asking how many pillows the client normally uses for sleep) and listen for crackles on auscultation of lungs. While auscultating the chest, listen for S_1 and S_2 heart sounds that are heard as "lub-dub." S_3 or S_4 heart sounds are abnormal when they are present in adults. An S_3 appears after the S_2 heart sound. It sounds like "lub-dub-**dub**" or the cadence of sounds in "Ken-tuck-y." The S_4 heart sound is heard just before S_1. It sounds like "**lub**-lub-dub" or the syllables in "**Ten**-nes-see." Monitor oxygenation status with pulse oximetry or review the results of ABG studies.

NURSING PROCESS FOR THE CLIENT WITH HEART FAILURE (continued)

Analysis, Planning, and Interventions

Fluid Overload Risk: Related to ineffective ventricular contraction, tachycardia, reduced stroke volume, hypertension, and increased vascular volume

Expected Outcome: Client will have increased cardiac output as evidenced by heart rate between 60 and 100 beats/min, urinary output between 1500 and 3000 mL/day, systolic BP below 120 mm Hg, diastolic BP below 80 mm Hg, and no mental confusion.

- Assess apical heart rate before administering a cardiac glycoside (digitalis) or other drug that slows heart rate. *Cardiac output is related to heart rate and stroke volume. Withhold a cardiac glycoside until the primary provider is consulted when the heart rate is less than 60 or more than 120 beats/min.*
- Administer prescribed medications such as cardiac glycosides (digitalis), diuretics, and antihypertensives. *Cardiac glycosides slow heart rate and increase force of contraction. Diuretics decrease afterload by reducing circulating fluid volume. Antihypertensives promote vasodilation, thus reducing afterload. One or a combination of these drugs reduces the workload of the left ventricle.*
- Promote rest. *Rest reduces heart contraction (ventricular work). Increasing diastole helps increase the volume in the ventricles (preload) and the ejected volume (stroke volume).*
- Avoid activities that involve the Valsalva maneuver, such as straining with bowel elimination or using the arms to pull and reposition oneself. *The Valsalva maneuver increases intrathoracic pressure, reduces right atrial filling, triggers tachycardia, and increases BP.*
- Prepare client or assist with procedures that improve cardiac output, such as the insertion of a biventricular pacemaker, cardiomyoplasty, LVAD, IABP, or artificial mechanical heart. *Improving the heart's force of contraction or stroke volume improves cardiac output.*

Fluid Overload: Related to reduced renal function secondary to increased antidiuretic hormone and aldosterone production and reduced cardiac output

Expected Outcome: Fluid volume will be reduced as evidenced by reduced weight and peripheral edema, normal BP measurements, increased urine output, and no adventitious lung sounds.

- Administer prescribed diuretic. *Diuretics promote the excretion of sodium and water.*
- Provide sodium-restricted diet as prescribed. *Sodium attracts water; reduced sodium decreases water retention.*
- Apportion oral fluid according to prescribed limitations. *Limiting oral fluid intake reduces circulating volume.*

Impaired Gas Exchange: Related to pulmonary congestion secondary to left ventricular dysfunction

Expected Outcome: Client will maintain adequate gas exchange as evidenced by clear lung sounds, decreased work of breathing, pulse oximeter reading above 90%, partial pressure of arterial oxygen (PaO_2) between 80 and 100 mm Hg, partial pressure of arterial CO_2 ($PaCO_2$) between 35 and 45 mm Hg, and blood pH between 7.35 and 7.45.

- Maintain client in a high-Fowler's, semi-Fowler's, or **orthopneic position** also called a **tripod position**, a sitting position in which the client leans on several pillows on the overbed table. *Elevating the upper body maximizes lung expansion by decreasing pressure on the diaphragm.*
- Administer supplemental oxygen therapy as prescribed to maintain the pulse oximetry level (oxygen saturation [SpO_2]) at or above 90%. *If SpO_2 is at or above 90%, PaO_2 usually is high enough to maintain plasma levels of oxygen in less-than-critical ranges.*
- Avoid gas-forming foods. *Gas that accumulates in the intestine increases the volume in the abdominal cavity. Expansion of the intestine can crowd the diaphragm and interfere with inspired volumes of air.*
- Offer small, frequent feedings. *Preventing stomach distention increases the space in the thoracic cavity for lung expansion.*
- Limit physical activity. *Activity requires increased oxygen for cellular metabolism.*

Activity Intolerance: Related to hypoxemia secondary to decreased cardiac output and pulmonary congestion

Expected Outcome: Client will tolerate activity associated with daily living without becoming breathless, hypertensive, or tachycardic.

- Space activities of daily living (ADLs) between periods of rest. *Rest reduces oxygen deficits.*
- Keep personal items within easy reach. *Reduced exertion decreases oxygen expenditure.*
- Gradually increase activity and self-care as condition improves. *Tolerance for activity increases after a therapeutic response to the treatment regimen.*

RC of Hypokalemia: Related to excretion of potassium secondary to loop diuretic therapy

Expected Outcome: The nurse will monitor for evidence of hypokalemia and prevent or manage low serum potassium levels.

- Monitor for clinical signs of hypokalemia: fatigue, muscle weakness, and abnormal sensations such as tingling or numbness. *Potassium is necessary for normal nerve and muscle activity; neuromuscular changes, anorexia, nausea, and vomiting are signs of a low potassium level.*
- Observe the ECG, cardiac monitor, or cardiac rhythm strip for a U wave or cardiac arrhythmia. *A U wave is associated with hypokalemia. The heart is a muscle that may develop an arrhythmia if the potassium level is not within normal range. U waves may also appear with electrolyte imbalances, other than hypokalemia, enlarged heart muscle, and drugs such as digoxin, phenothiazines, and some antiarrhythmics such as procainamide and amiodarone.*
- Provide foods and beverages that are good sources of potassium, such as bananas and orange juice, within the client's dietary and fluid restrictions. *Dietary intake of foods and beverages that are rich in potassium affects serum potassium levels (see* Nutrition Notes*).*
- Administer a prescribed potassium supplement. *It ensures potassium replacement.*

Evaluation of Expected Outcomes

Expected outcomes are that BP and heart rate return to baseline, with no evidence of excess peripheral fluid. Respirations are unlabored, and lungs are clear. Fluid intake approximates output. The client can participate in ADLs within their level of tolerance. Serum potassium level remains within or is restored to normal range.

CARDIOGENIC PULMONARY EDEMA

Pulmonary edema is fluid accumulation in the lungs, which interferes with gas exchange in the alveoli. It represents an acute emergency and is a frequent complication of left-sided heart failure. Cardiac arrhythmias and cardiac or respiratory arrest are associated complications. The following discussion focuses on cardiogenic pulmonary edema, which develops as a result of heart disease in general and heart failure more specifically. Noncardiogenic pulmonary edema, also referred to as *acute respiratory distress syndrome*, develops when a pulmonary embolism, infection, or blast injury alters the pulmonary capillary membrane; it is discussed in Chapter 21.

Pathophysiology and Etiology

In **cardiogenic pulmonary edema**, the left ventricle becomes incapable of maintaining sufficient output of blood with each contraction. The right ventricle continues to pump blood toward the lungs, however, and the left ventricle has difficulty emptying. There is retrograde fluid accumulation in the left atrium and pulmonary veins. The pulmonary capillaries and alveoli become engorged with blood. The lungs rapidly fill with fluid, and acute respiratory distress develops. As CO_2 accumulates, respiratory rate and depth increase. Without treatment, hyperventilation becomes insufficient to prevent respiratory acidosis. Metabolic acidosis follows.

Assessment Findings

Clients with **acute pulmonary edema** exhibit sudden dyspnea, wheezing, orthopnea, restlessness, cough (often productive of pink, frothy sputum), cyanosis, tachycardia, and severe apprehension. Respirations sound moist or gurgling. If a pulmonary artery catheter is in place, the pulmonary artery and pulmonary capillary wedge pressures are elevated, and cardiac output is reduced. While the body responds with arterial vasoconstriction, it may temporarily sustain adequate BP; however, the client eventually becomes hypotensive, and peripheral pulses disappear. Chest radiographs show pulmonary infiltration with fluid. ABGs indicate severe hypoxemia (low PaO_2), hypercapnia (high $PaCO_2$), and a pH below 7.35.

Medical Management

Because pulmonary edema can be fatal, lung congestion needs to be relieved as quickly as possible. Supplemental oxygen or mechanical ventilation is used to support breathing. **Inotropic medications**, which improve myocardial contractility, are administered to relieve symptoms. If the cause of heart failure and pulmonary edema can be corrected surgically (e.g., a mitral valve disorder), the client is supported medically while being prepared for surgery.

Oxygenation

To facilitate gas exchange, oxygen is administered. A mask rather than nasal cannula is needed to deliver the maximum percentages of oxygen. If respiratory failure occurs, the client is intubated and oxygen is administered under continuous positive airway pressure or with mechanical ventilation with positive end-expiratory pressure.

Drug Therapy

Inotropic agents, such as dopamine (Intropin), dobutamine (Dobutrex), and in amrinone (Inocor), or digitalis, are administered by IV to improve the force of ventricular contraction and improve renal perfusion. To reduce myocardial oxygen consumption, drugs that reduce venous return to the heart (diuretics) and promote vasodilatation (nitrates, ACE inhibitors, calcium channel blockers) are prescribed. IV morphine sulfate often is given to lessen anxiety. Morphine seems to help relieve respiratory symptoms by depressing higher cerebral centers, thus relieving anxiety and slowing respiratory rate. Morphine also promotes muscle relaxation and reduces the work of breathing.

Invasive Measures

If the client does not respond to drug therapy and oxygenation, additional interventions such as the insertion of an IABP, biventricular pacemaker, or LVAD are used to sustain life. Cardiomyoplasty, use of an artificial heart, and subsequent heart transplantation are further treatments.

Nursing Management

Effective resolution of pulmonary edema requires both medical and nursing management. The nursing diagnoses, interventions, and expected outcomes for clients with pulmonary edema are similar to those for clients experiencing heart failure. Clients with pulmonary edema need close assessment in an intensive care unit.

The nurse establishes an IV line immediately (if one is not already in place) for medication administration. Because of the severity of symptoms and respiratory compromise, the nurse administers IV diuretics and inotropic agents and monitors the therapeutic and adverse effects of medication therapy. Bedside ECG monitoring is standard, as are continuous pulse oximetry and automatic BP and pulse measurements approximately every 15 to 30 minutes. Critically ill clients who are hemodynamically unstable may have a pulmonary artery catheter inserted to measure the pressure readings in the heart chambers and to estimate cardiac output. A urinary catheter is inserted to evaluate response to diuretics. The nurse assesses for proper placement/adherence of electrodes and ascertains that electronic monitoring equipment is functioning properly.

The client receives oxygenation to maintain normal blood gases. If the client requires mechanical ventilation, the nurse suctions the airway as needed, provides frequent mouth care, and establishes an alternative method for verbal communication.

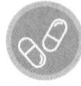

Pharmacologic Considerations

- Typically, clients are monitored for hypokalemia when diuretics are used for rapid diuresis. Be aware that ACE inhibitors are potassium sparing, and therefore symptoms of hyperkalemia should be monitored if these drugs are administered, too.

KEY POINTS

- Heart failure: the inability of the heart to pump sufficient blood to meet the body's metabolic needs.
  - Normal ejection fraction: >55%
- Congestive heart failure (CHF): the accumulation of blood and fluid in organs and tissues from impaired circulation.
- Heart failure
  - Acute heart failure: a sudden change in the heart's ability to contract.
  - Chronic heart failure: the heart's ability to pump effectively is gradually compromised and its impaired contractility remains prolonged.
  - Left-sided heart failure: results from various conditions that impair the left ventricle's ability to eject blood into the aorta.
  - Right-sided heart failure: the right ventricle fails to eject its diastolic filling volume into the pulmonary artery, causing congestion of blood in the venous vascular system.
- Afterload: the force that the ventricle must overcome to empty its diastolic volume.
- Preload: is the amount of ventricular stretch at the end of diastole, during which the ventricle fills with blood
- Cor pulmonale: a condition in which the heart (*cor*) is affected secondarily by lung damage (*pulmonale*).
- Beta-type natriuretic peptide (BNP) test: is a blood test that measures levels of a protein called BNP that is made by your heart and blood vessels. BNP levels are higher than normal when you have heart failure.
- Multiple gated acquisition (MUGA) scan (*gated blood pool scan*): measures a decrease in the ejection fraction
- Cardiogenic pulmonary edema: fluid accumulation in the lungs, which interferes with gas exchange in the alveoli, it is a frequent complication of left-sided heart failure and is considered a medical emergency.

CRITICAL THINKING EXERCISES

1. Discuss how the care of a client with right-sided heart failure differs from the care of a client with left-sided heart failure.
2. A client diagnosed with heart failure presents with the following assessment data: temperature, 99.1°F; pulse, 100 beats/min; respirations, 42 breaths/min; BP, 110/50 mm Hg; crackles in both lung bases; nausea; pulse oximeter reading of 89%; and enlarged, soft abdomen. What assessment findings need immediate attention? Why?
3. While making a home visit to evaluate the status of a client who is being treated for heart failure, what assessment data suggest that the client's treatment regimen is effective?
4. A client with heart failure is on a low-sodium diet. While reviewing the modifications in the client's diet before discharge, what information indicates that the client understands the foods that should be avoided or limited for sodium restriction?

NCLEX-STYLE REVIEW QUESTIONS PrepU

1. What instruction is most important for the nurse to include in the teaching plan for a client with right-sided heart failure?
   1. Count pulse rate every hour.
   2. Eat three meals per day.
   3. Maintain bed rest.
   4. Elevate the legs while sitting.
2. Prior to giving a client the morning dose of digoxin (Lanoxin), the nurse determines that the apical pulse is less than 55 beats/min. What nursing action is the priority?
   1. Call the primary provider and report the finding.
   2. Hold the drug and assess for toxic effects.
   3. Take the client's blood pressure.
   4. Recheck the pulse in 30 minutes.
3. A client with chronic heart failure takes a daily thiazide diuretic. The client asks the nurse why it is important to consume potassium-rich foods on a daily basis. What is the most accurate response?
   1. Consuming potassium-rich foods replaces what is lost in your urine.
   2. Potassium promotes the excretion of excess fluid by your kidneys.
   3. Potassium improves the therapeutic action of your diuretic.
   4. Your thiazide diuretic may cause significant hypocalcemia.
4. A client comes to the clinic complaining of shortness of breath, pink-tinged sputum, and a cough. The nurse suspects left-sided heart failure. What assessment finding further confirms the diagnosis?
   1. Moist crackles in the lung fields
   2. Bradycardia less than 60 beats/min
   3. Blood pressure 90/60 mm Hg
   4. Increased excretion of urine
5. A client with left-sided heart failure is admitted to the hospital for treatment. What nursing intervention is the first action the nurse should take?
   1. Administer 3 L oxygen per nasal cannula.
   2. Give a loading dose of digoxin (Lanoxin).
   3. Draw blood for baseline electrolytes.
   4. Assess for distended neck veins.Increased fall risk owing to hypotensive side effects

WANT TO KNOW MORE? There are a wide variety of online resources available on thePoint to enhance learning and understanding of this chapter.

Go to thePoint.lww.com/activate and use the activation code found in the front of this text to unlock these online resources.

29 Caring for Clients Undergoing Cardiovascular Surgery

Words To Know

annuloplasty
cardiac index
cardiac tamponade
cardioplegia
cardiopulmonary bypass
central venous pressure
commissurotomy
coronary artery bypass
drug-eluting stent
embolectomy
endarterectomy
extracorporeal circulation
hemodynamic monitoring
hybrid revascularization
left ventricular end-diastolic pressure
myocardial revascularization
nomogram
pulmonary capillary wedge pressure
thrombectomy
valvuloplasty

Learning Objectives

On completion of this chapter, you will be able to:

1. Describe the purpose of cardiopulmonary bypass and its disadvantages.
2. Name indications for cardiac surgery.
3. Describe how coronary artery blood flow is surgically restored.
4. Name four surgical procedures for revascularizing the myocardium.
5. Identify techniques to correct valvular disorders.
6. Describe two methods for controlling bleeding from heart trauma.
7. List five problems associated with heart transplantation.
8. List three types of surgery performed on central or peripheral blood vessels.
9. Discuss the medical and nursing management of clients undergoing cardiovascular surgery.

Cardiovascular surgery is performed to correct and treat various cardiac and vascular disorders discussed in earlier chapters in this unit. This chapter describes the operative procedures and management of clients undergoing surgery to revascularize the myocardium, repair or replace cardiac valves, repair a ventricular aneurysm, remove heart tumors, manage heart trauma, and replace the heart with one that is artificial or from a human donor.

Gerontologic Considerations

- Older adults often experience delirium (an abrupt change in cognition) following cardiac surgery. Symptoms may be either hyperactive (distractibility, disorientation, excessive talkativeness, restlessness, etc.) or hypoactive (stupor, drowsiness, difficulty in engaging). There may be several causative factors, including cardiopulmonary bypass, sensitivity to drugs, or cerebral ischemia from compromised blood flow or volume. Identifying and then minimizing or eliminating the causes of delirium after cardiac surgery is critical.
- Older adults may have comorbidities such as diabetes, heart failure, cardiac arrhythmias, hypertension, poor renal function, and/or frailty. Potential risks and benefits of cardiovascular surgery and clarification of client/family expectations must be discussed prior to surgery. Astute monitoring is required before, during, and following surgery for complications, client motivation for rehabilitative care, and potential for postoperative depression if expectations were not met.

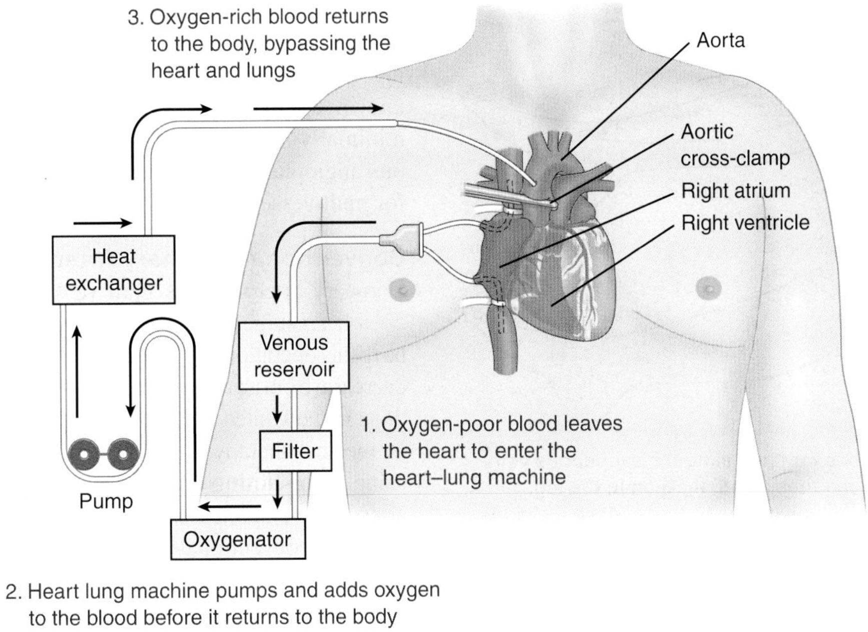
3. Oxygen-rich blood returns to the body, bypassing the heart and lungs
Aorta
Aortic cross-clamp
Right atrium
Right ventricle
Heat exchanger
Venous reservoir
Filter
Pump
Oxygenator
1. Oxygen-poor blood leaves the heart to enter the heart–lung machine
2. Heart lung machine pumps and adds oxygen to the blood before it returns to the body

Figure 29-1 The cardiopulmonary bypass system. Cannulae are placed into the superior and inferior venae cavae to divert blood from the body and into the bypass system. The pump creates a vacuum and pulls blood into the venous reservoir. The filter clears the blood of air bubbles, clots, and particulates. The blood then passes through the oxygenator, to the pump, and to the heat exchanger, which regulates the blood's temperature. The blood is then returned to the body.

CARDIAC SURGICAL PROCEDURES

Before the 1950s, few attempts at cardiac surgery were made. Initially, hypothermia and crude mechanisms for oxygenating blood outside the body were used. In the 1960s, the technique for mechanically circulating and oxygenating blood outside the body, called **extracorporeal circulation** or **cardiopulmonary bypass**, was developed (Fig. 29-1). Removing blood from the venae cavae, circulating it through an oxygenator, and returning it to the aorta or femoral artery provides a nearly bloodless area while the beating heart is stopped.

Although most forms of cardiac surgery use cardiopulmonary bypass, some new surgical techniques have eliminated its use. Surgery on the beating heart without cardiopulmonary bypass reduces the potential for negative "pump" consequences (Box 29-1).

Myocardial Revascularization

Myocardial revascularization refers to surgical techniques that improve the delivery of oxygenated blood to the myocardium for clients who have coronary artery disease (CAD). These techniques are used when less invasive methods such as an atherectomy or percutaneous transluminal coronary angioplasty (PTCA) are not treatment options (see Chapter 25). (Chapter 25 also discusses transmyocardial revascularization [TMR].) **Coronary artery bypass** surgery improves myocardial oxygenation by bypassing or detouring around the occluded portion of one or more coronary arteries with a relocated blood vessel. A coronary artery bypass is performed when (1) the client has multiple coronary artery occlusions, (2) the atheromas are calcified and noncompressible, or (3) the anatomic location of the occlusion(s) interferes with the safe insertion of a coronary artery catheter.

The saphenous vein in the leg is the vessel most often used for grafting in coronary artery bypass. It is harvested either by making a long incision on the medial aspect of the leg or by removing the vein endoscopically through one to three small (1-inch) leg incisions (Fig. 29-2). An endoscopically removed vein is the preferred method for harvesting the saphenous vein because it provides several advantages: (1) better cosmetic appearance postoperatively, (2) less muscle and tissue damage, (3) less postoperative pain, (4) fewer wound infections, (5) decreased length of hospitalization, (6) fewer hospital readmissions. There is no difference in the rate of revascularization between the two harvesting approaches. The mortality rate is 20% less when the vein

BOX 29-1 Disadvantages of Cardiopulmonary Bypass

- Long operative period (6 hours)
- Necessity for anticoagulation
- Hypotension
- Need for postoperative blood replacement
- Overall decline in mental function, perhaps because of an inflammatory response triggered by blood circulating through plastic tubing or gaseous bubbles in the circulated blood
- Risk for stroke, arrhythmias, and renal failure

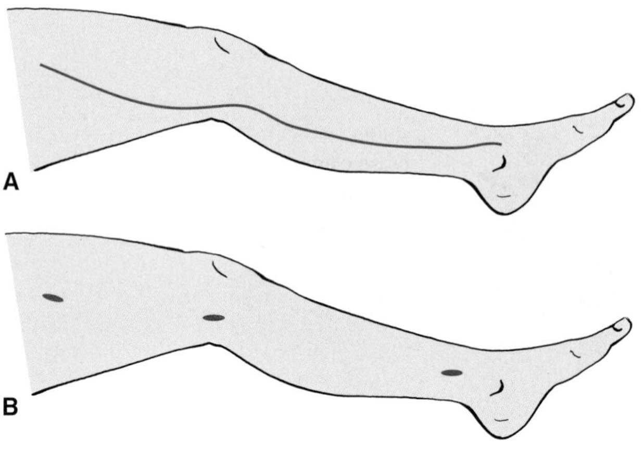

Figure 29-2 Two methods for harvesting the saphenous vein. **(A)** Traditional surgery requires a long incision in the leg. **(B)** Endoscopic removal involves one to three 1-inch incisions.

is harvested endoscopically (Dacey, 2012). Alternative harvesting vessels for grafting include the following:

- The internal mammary and internal thoracic arteries in the chest
- The basilic and cephalic veins in the arm
- The radial artery in the arm
- The gastroepiploic artery from the stomach, in some cases

Although used less often than the saphenous vein, internal mammary artery (IMA) grafts have 90% or greater patency, which results in better survival rates, fewer reoperations, and fewer cardiac events for up to 10 years after surgery. Grafts using the saphenous vein tend to develop thromboses and progressive atherosclerosis that compromises long-term patency.

Techniques for performing coronary bypass surgery include conventional coronary artery bypass graft (CABG), off-pump coronary artery bypass (OPCAB), minimally invasive direct coronary artery bypass (MIDCAB), and port access coronary artery bypass (PACAB), also known as TECAB, which stands for totally endoscopic coronary artery bypass. Table 29-1 compares these methods for performing myocardial revascularization. An additional approach known as **hybrid revascularization**, which combines a minimally invasive surgical procedure as well as percutaneous angioplasty with placement of a stent (see Chapter 25) for multivessel disease, is currently being done.

Conventional Coronary Artery Bypass Graft

Coronary artery bypass graft (CABG) is the most common open-heart surgery in the United States. "About 395,000 people have this operation every year" (Surgeries, 2019). This is a slight decrease from statistics in 2015 showing more than 500,000 done in the United States. This has been attributed to advances in medical therapy and percutaneous coronary interventions using **drug-eluting stents**, scaffolding that keeps a coronary artery open and releases a drug that prevents reocclusion.

The conventional technique involves a long (approximately 8- to 12-inch) midchest incision, use of a cardiopulmonary bypass machine, and **cardioplegia** (stopping the heart) during surgery. During CABG, the surgeon attaches one end of a vessel such as a harvested portion of the saphenous vein or other distant vessel to the aorta and the other end below the occlusion in the coronary artery (Fig. 29-3). One or several occluded arteries can be bypassed during the surgical procedure, which is referred to as a *double*, *triple*, or *quadruple* bypass depending on the number of grafts required.

Pharmacologic Considerations

■ Drug-eluting stents help to reduce tissue regeneration. In turn, this helps to reduce fibrosis and reocclusion in the artery. Drugs used include everolimus, paclitaxel, sirolimus, and zotarolimus, agents that prevent cell growth. Revascularization was significantly lower with drug-eluding stents than with the bare metal stent (Kalyanasundaram, 2020).

TABLE 29-1 Comparison of Surgical Myocardial Revascularization Techniques

	CONVENTIONAL CABG	MIDCAB	PACAB	OPCAB
Length of incision (inches)	8–12	4	(3) $\frac{1}{3}$ (1) 1	8–10
Duration of hospitalization (days)	7–10	4–6	3–4	6–10
Time for full recovery (weeks)	6–10	2–4	2–3	4–6
Maximum number of grafted arteries	5	1–2	4	4
Years in clinical practice (years)	60	18	19	10 in the United States
Cost	$60,000	~40% less than conventional CABG	~15% less than conventional CABG	~25% less than conventional CABG
Operation on beating heart	No	Yes	No	Yes
Use of cardiopulmonary bypass	Yes	No	Yes	No
Time in surgery (hours)	3–6	2–3	2	2–5
Operative mortality rate (%)	2.9	1.5	1.0	0.8

From Kalyanasundaram, A. (2020). *Comparison of coronary artery bypass grafting (CABG) and percutaneous coronary intervention (PCI)*. https://emedicine.medscape.com/article/164682-overview

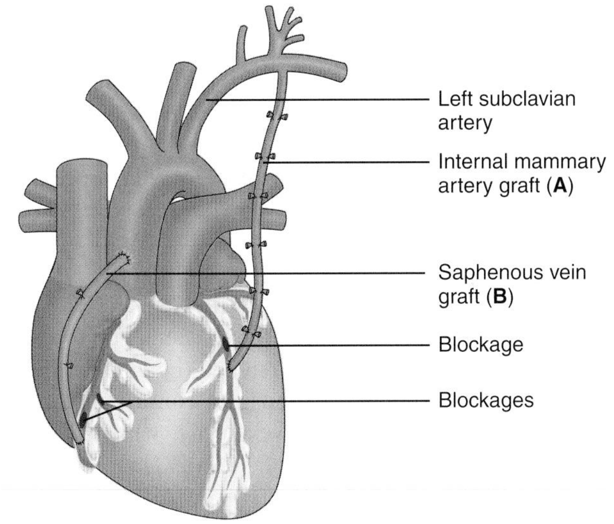

Figure 29-3 Coronary artery bypass grafts using **(A)** internal mammary artery and **(B)** saphenous vein.

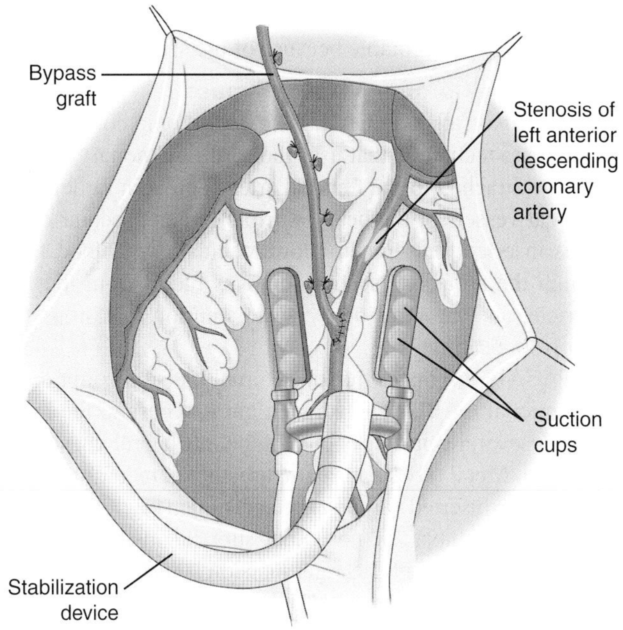

Figure 29-4 Example of stabilizer device used for off-pump coronary artery bypass (OPCAB).

As an alternative, the distal end of the IMA or internal thoracic artery (ITA) can be reattached below the occlusion on the anterior surface of the heart while leaving the proximal end in its natural location. The advantages of using chest arteries versus a vein graft is that doing so avoids making an operative leg incision to harvest a vein, and the IMA and IUTA arteries are less likely to spasm and develop thromboses. The disadvantage is that the portion of the chest arteries available for graft use is shorter than other graft vessels. The shorter length may be insufficient to bypass the occluded vessel(s).

Off-Pump Coronary Artery Bypass

OPCAB, which began being performed in the United States at the turn of the 21st century, is very similar to conventional CABG except that it does not involve the use of a cardiopulmonary bypass machine. Instead, the surgeon keeps the heart beating at a slow rate (about 40 beats/min) with drugs such as adenosine (Adenocard) and esmolol (Brevibloc). The OPCAB chest incision is approximately 8 to 10 inches, somewhat shorter than in a conventional CABG procedure. Instruments that lift and stabilize the heart facilitate the surgeon's ability to graft vessels on the anterior, lateral, and posterior walls of the beating heart (Fig. 29-4). Advocates note that OPCAB has a reduced mortality rate, fewer perioperative complications than conventional CABG likely owing to elimination of cardiopulmonary bypass, and decreased postoperative recovery time in the hospital.

Minimally Invasive Direct Coronary Artery Bypass

A MIDCAB is another example of a "beating heart" procedure. It is called *minimally invasive* because the incision, which is made between the ribs, is only about 3 to 5 inches long. Because the incision is small, the surgeon uses an endoscope to view the heart while grafting the vessels. Some surgeons are performing robotically assisted coronary artery bypass. The robotic instrument is placed inside the chest cavity and acts like a miniature set of hands (Fig. 29-5).

This type of procedure is limited to grafting only one or two vessels on the anterior surface of the heart in clients who are not obese or whose coronary arteries are not heavily calcified. Despite these limitations, the MIDCAB procedure shortens the surgical time and postoperative recovery period,

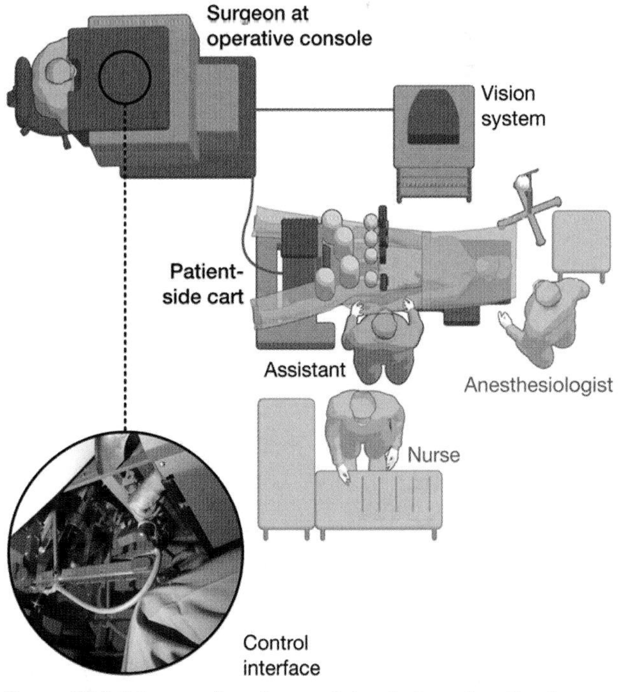

Figure 29-5 When performing a minimally invasive direct coronary artery bypass (MIDCAB) procedure, robotic arms and a small camera, which magnifies the operative area 10 times the normal vision, are inserted into tiny incisions. The surgeon sits at a remote console and controls the robotic arms.

eliminates the risks of cardiopulmonary bypass, and is cosmetically more acceptable because of the smaller scar.

Port Access Coronary Artery Bypass

PACAB, also called TECAB, is an endoscopic coronary artery bypass technique that uses the cardiopulmonary bypass machine attached to the femoral artery and vein rather than the great vessels of the heart. A triple lumen vascular catheter is inserted: one lumen allows occlusion of blood flow through the aorta, the second removes blood from the left ventricle, and the third delivers the solution that stops the heart from beating.

PACAB eliminates the long sternal incision common in conventional CABG. The surgeon gains access to the heart through several small incisions on the left lateral chest near the axilla. Metal tubes approximately the diameter of a pencil are then inserted through the incisions (Fig. 29-6). It is through these tubes, or ports that surgical instruments are inserted. Another slightly larger incision is made in the chest to insert a video camera attached to an endoscope called a *thoracoscope*. The surgeon uses the image from the video camera and transesophageal echocardiography to visualize the operative area after the heart is stopped. A robotic hand is used to manipulate the surgical instruments that are inserted through the ports.

PACAB has shortened the operative procedure from 3-to-6 hours to 2 hours and has reduced mortality rates from complications. Clients stay in the hospital only 2 to 3 days after the procedure, compared with 7 to 10 days after conventional CABG. Full recovery is much faster as well.

Cardiac Stents

A cardiac stent is used to treat narrowed or blocked coronary arteries. It can also be used to improve blood flow immediately following a heart attack. Cardiac stents are expandable coils made of metal mesh (Cardiac Stent, 2021). Angioplasty (unblocking of an artery) with stenting is usually recommended for clients who have only one or two blocked arteries, which are not 100% occluded. A drug-eluting stent (DES) is sometimes used during the procedure. It is coated with medication to lower your risk of restenosis (Cardiac Stent, 2021).

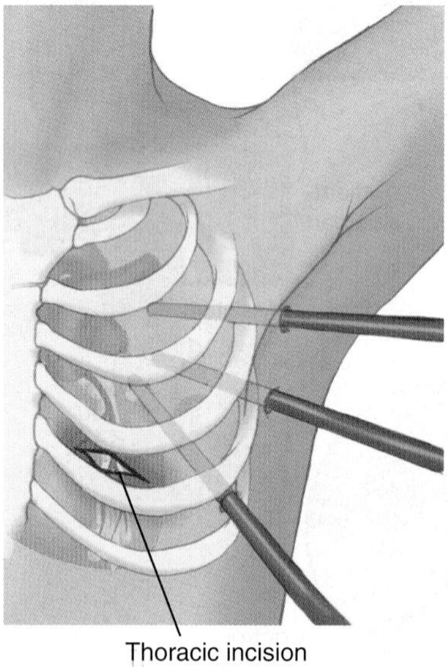

Figure 29-6 In a port access coronary artery bypass (PACAB) technique, the surgeon makes three small incisions in the chest near the axilla. They insert surgical instruments through the ports and an endoscope through a larger incision. The surgeon then views the surgical field.

Valve Repairs or Replacements

Heart valves need surgical repair or replacement if they become narrowed (stenosed) or stretched (incompetent; see Chapter 24). One method of repair is **commissurotomy** (opening adhesions in the valve cusps), which is done without direct visualization of the valve. This procedure is performed by means of a thoracotomy (chest incision). The surgeon places a purse-string suture in the wall of the heart, makes an incision, and inserts their finger or a metal dilator into the narrowed valve, stretching its opening. The surgeon then pulls the purse-string suture tight to prevent blood from escaping. Other less-invasive techniques are *balloon valvuloplasty* and transcatheter valve implantation, which use a balloon catheter to stretch the stenosed valve (see Chapter 24). Cardiopulmonary bypass is not required for minimally invasive techniques but it usually is kept available for immediate use if complications develop or direct visualization is required to repair the valve.

Other methods of repair include **valvuloplasty** (valve repair) and **annuloplasty** (repair of the fibrous ring that encircles the valve), procedures that surgically tighten an incompetent valve (Fig. 29-7).

If a valve cannot be repaired and needs to be replaced, the diseased valve can be excised and replaced with a mechanical valve, a bioprosthetic valve, a valve harvested from pigs or cows, or human tissue from a cadaver, or the client's own autologous tissue (Fig. 29-8; Table 29-2).

Surgeons use an open-chest incisional approach or a minimally invasive approach. One example of a minimally invasive approach is a transcatheter aortic valve replacement (TAVR) for clients who are older adults and potentially cannot tolerate an open-chest procedure because of multisystem disease (see Chapter 24). Minimally invasive valve replacement surgeries are performed through a mini-sternotomy, parasternal incision, or a port access approach. Although cardiopulmonary bypass is required, proponents of the minimally invasive approaches to valve replacement cite the following advantages:

- Less surgical trauma
- Decreased blood loss
- Less mechanical ventilation
- Reduced postoperative pain
- Faster mobility
- Shortened hospital stay
- Reduced perioperative costs
- Improved cosmetic appearance

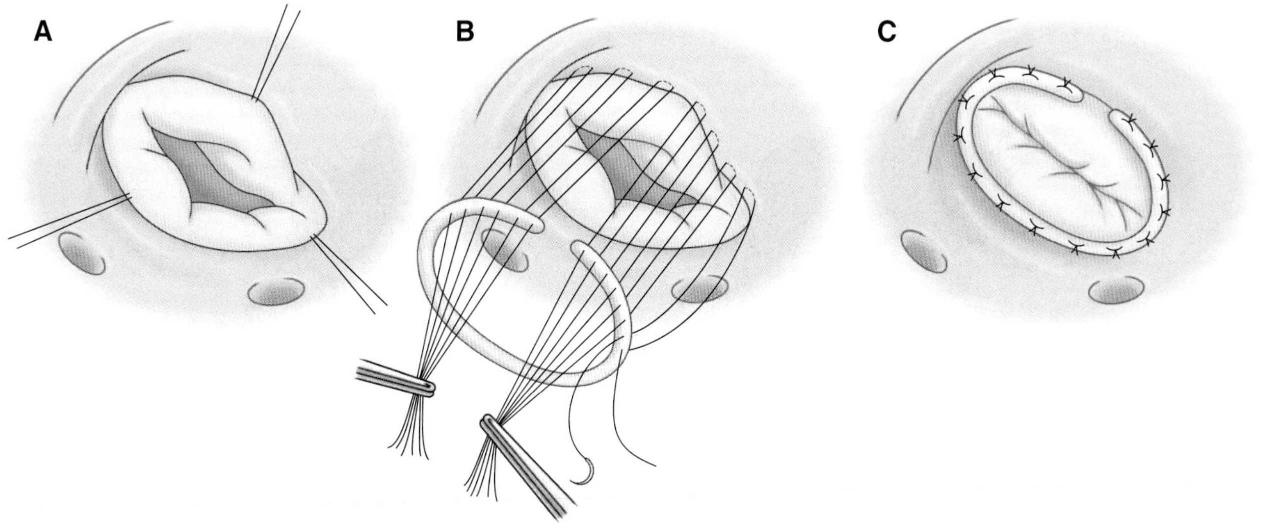

Figure 29-7 Annuloplasty ring insertion. **(A)** Mitral valve regurgitation; leaflets do not close. **(B)** Insertion of an annuloplasty ring. **(C)** Completed valvuloplasty; leaflets close.

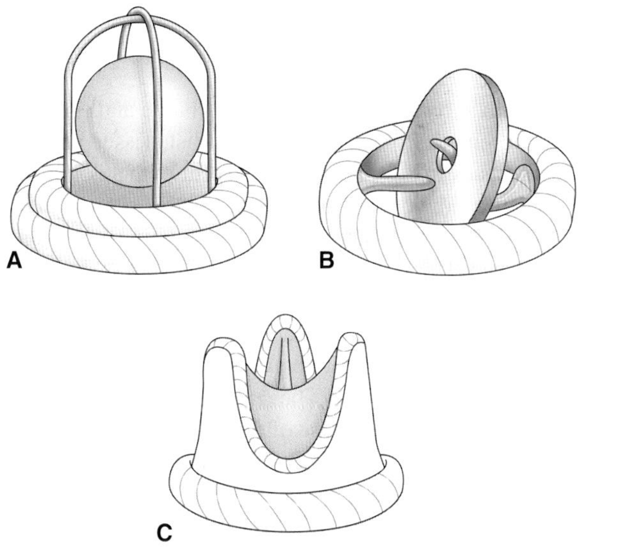

Figure 29-8 Common mechanical and biologic valve replacements. **(A)** Caged-ball valve (Starr-Edwards, mechanical). **(B)** Tilting-disk valve (Medtronic Hall, mechanical). **(C)** Porcine heterograft valve (Carpentier-Edwards, biologic).

Repair of Ventricular Aneurysm

An aneurysm of the ventricular wall develops when an infarcted area of myocardium balloons outward. Thrombi commonly form in the crater of the bulging tissue. A ventricular aneurysm is the most lethal complication among clients who survive the acute stage of a myocardial infarction (MI). Because the motion of the myocardium may rupture the aneurysm, an emergency procedure may be performed to suture the weakened area (Fig. 29-9). If waiting is possible, the stretched tissue is excised 4 to 8 weeks after the MI when scar tissue has formed. If surgery is performed too early, it is difficult to differentiate healthy from necrotic tissue, and sutures placed in necrotic tissue usually are not retained.

Removal of Heart Tumors

Primary tumors of the heart, both benign and malignant, are rare. The clinical course and operative procedure depend on the type of tumor and its location in the heart. Benign tumors typically extend from a pedicle or stem, making their removal uncomplicated. Malignant tumors are more difficult to remove, and the prognosis is extremely poor.

TABLE 29-2 Types of Heart Valves

	MATERIAL	ADVANTAGES	DISADVANTAGES
Mechanical	Man-made from carbon, stainless steel, Dacron	Durable Lasts 20 years Lifelong	Risk for thrombi and emboli Anticoagulation necessary Risk for bleeding Sudden malfunction
Bioprosthetic	Natural tissue mounted on a metallic or polymer stent or unstented	Low potential for thrombi No anticoagulation necessary Gradual malfunction	Xenografts less durable than allografts Prone to deterioration and calcification
Xenograft	Porcine (pig) valve or bovine (cow) pericardium	Highly available Less expensive	Lasts 7–10 years
Allograft (also known as homograft)	Human cadaver	Lasts 10–15 years Better blood flow characteristics	Less available Expensive
Autograft	Tissue from client's own pulmonic valve or pulmonary artery	Viable for 20+ years	More difficult to insert surgically

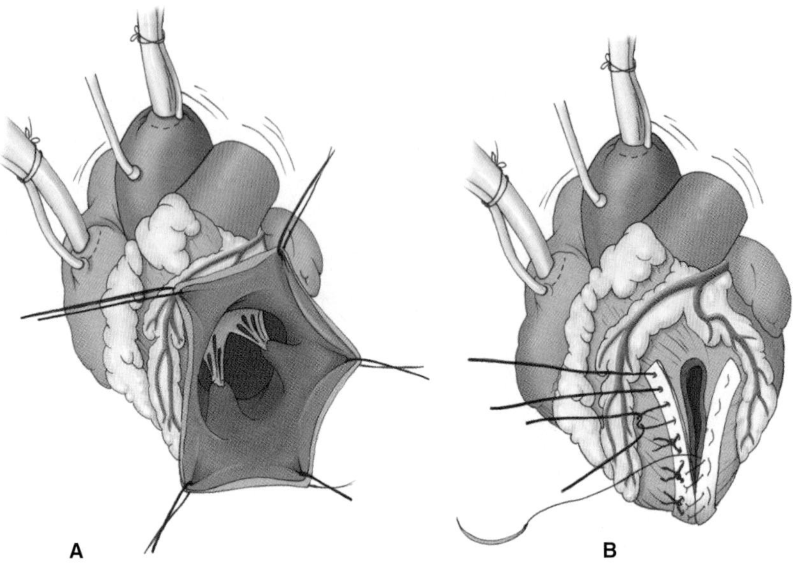

Figure 29-9 Surgical repair of a ventricular aneurysm. **(A)** The ventricle is opened and the nonfunctioning tissue from the aneurysm is differentiated from normal myocardium. **(B)** Healthy tissue from the endocardium through the epicardium is approximated.

Repair of Heart Trauma

A nonpenetrating injury of the chest, such as being crushed against a steering wheel, may cause bruising and bleeding of the heart. Because the pericardium encloses the heart, **cardiac tamponade** (compression of the heart with accumulating blood) can result. Sometimes, traumatic cardiac tamponade is treated conservatively with bed rest. The inactivity and increased pressure from blood in the pericardium may stop the bleeding. The client may need to have the blood aspirated from the pericardial sac, in which case pericardiocentesis is performed (see Chapter 23). One aspiration is sufficient in most cases, but if bleeding continues, open thoracotomy is indicated to control blood loss.

A penetrating injury, such as a stab wound, also causes blood to leak into the pericardium. A pericardial tear often seals with a clot, whereas a myocardial tear continues to bleed. Large tears necessitate surgery. If the wound is severe enough to cause immediate shock from hemorrhage, the prognosis is poor.

Heart Transplantation

In adults, heart transplantation is indicated for cardiomyopathy (see Chapter 23), end-stage CAD (see Chapter 25), and end-stage heart failure (see Chapter 28). In newborns and infants, heart transplantation is indicated for a severe congenital cardiac defect. It is performed only when other treatment modalities fail or are unavailable. Although more than **3,000** people receive a heart transplant each year, there were nearly 3,500 awaiting a heart transplant in 2020 (Organ Procurement and Transplantation Network, 2021).

In 1984, Congress passed the National Organ Transplant Act, which outlaws the sale of human organs. The United Network for Organ Sharing (UNOS) is the official organization that maintains a computerized database with which to match organs with recipients (Box 29-2). Once a client is certified as a candidate for transplantation, their name and tissue type are placed on a computerized recipient list. Tissue and blood typing is necessary to match the recipient with a donor.

When a donor heart becomes available, it must be removed from the donor and transplanted within 6 hours of being harvested. There are two methods of heart transplantation. The most common method is an orthotopic heart transplant, in which the recipient's failing heart is removed leaving the back half of both atria. The front part of the donor heart is sutured to the back recipient's atria. The donor's aorta and pulmonary arteries are connected to those of the recipient (Fig. 29-10).

The heterotropic method for transplanting a heart is rarely performed. With the heterotropic method, the recipient's heart is left in place to act as support for the transplanted donor heart and to allow heart function if a life-threatening rejection should occur. With double organs within the chest, the lungs are compressed, and there is difficulty in obtaining an endomyocardial biopsy to detect organ rejection.

Transplant Problems and Complications

Many problems are associated with heart transplantation, including the scarcity of donor organs and high cost. There are a number of complications that may arise from transplantations; for example, tissue rejection, postoperative infection, progressive cardiovascular problems, and potential for postoperative psychosis.

Scarcity of Donors

There are multiple reasons that contribute to the scarcity of donor hearts:

- The ideal donor is young, fit, healthy, and dies suddenly, but most people do not fit that description.
- Few possess documented consent for organ donation; next of kin are reluctant to donate organs when the client appears to be alive with machines that provide life-support.

BOX 29-2 United Network for Organ Sharing Criteria for Thoracic Organ Donation

Those adults who are 18 years old and awaiting heart transplantation are assigned a status code that corresponds to their medical urgency.

Status 1A Criteria

- Person who is admitted to a transplant hospital or an affiliated Veteran's Administration (VA) hospital and who has at least one of the following devices or therapies:
  - Mechanical circulatory support such as a total artificial heart (TAH), intra-aortic balloon pump (IABP), extracorporeal membrane oxygenation (ECMO)
  - Continuous mechanical ventilation
  - Requires continuous intravenous infusion of a single intravenous inotrope or multiple intravenous inotropes, and requires continuous hemodynamic monitoring of left ventricular filling pressures
- Not currently hospitalized
- Has at least one circulatory support device in place such as left ventricular assist device (LVAD), right ventricular assist device (RVAD), or left and right ventricular assist device (BiVAD)
- Has mechanical circulatory support with a significant device-related complication such as thromboembolism, device infection, mechanical failure, or life-threatening ventricular arrhythmias.

Status 1B Criteria

- A person who has at least one of the following devices or therapies in place:
  - Left or right implanted ventricular assist device
  - Continuous infusion of intravenous inotropes or
  - Justification of an exceptional case based on recommendation of their transplant primary provider and approval of the Regional Review Board and Thoracic Organ Transplantation Committee.

Status 2 Criteria

- Person who meets neither Status 1A nor 1B criteria, but is suitable for transplant.
- The Thoracic Committee (2016) is proposing two changes to the adult heart allocation system:
- Additional urgency stratifications based on relative waiting list mortality rates for all adult heart candidates, and
- Modifying the geographic sharing scheme to provide the most medically urgent candidates access to donors from a broader geographic area (https://optn.transplant.hrsa.gov/governance/public-comment/adult-heart-allocation-changes-2016)

Adapted from United Network of Organ Sharing. (2020). *Policy 6: Allocation of heart and lungs.* https://optn.transplant.hrsa.gov/media/1200/optn_policies.pdf

- There are no financial incentives to donate a heart or other organ.
- Some primary providers delay discussing organ donation with the family of potential donors while they attempt more and more sophisticated measures to keep dying clients alive while the quality of organs decline.
- Stringent criteria for donated organs results in the rejection of marginal hearts from older donors with various comorbidities that could lower the risk of death among potential recipients as compared to prolonging the wait for a higher quality heart.
- A false belief that organ donation will interfere with a traditional open casket funeral.
- Some medical conditions, such as diabetes and high blood pressure, can put a person at increased risk for organ failure, especially kidney and heart failure. "Underrepresented groups, including Black and Hispanic Americans, suffer higher rates of these conditions, that is one reason why minorities make up nearly six out of 10 people on the national waiting list for lifesaving organ transplants. Twenty people die each day, waiting for a transplant that doesn't arrive in time" (Organ donation, 2020).
- Some cultures and religions advance a belief that a person should die with all organs intact

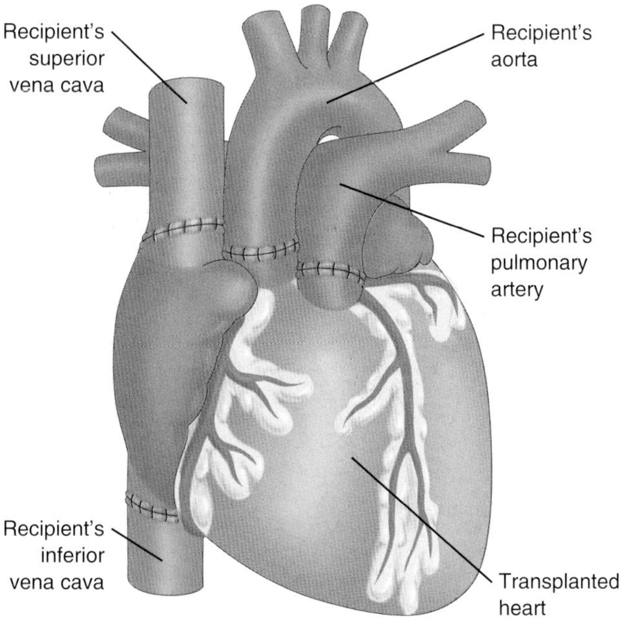

Figure 29-10 Orthotopic method of heart transplantation. Note the suture lines indicating the attachment of the donor heart.

Despite the scarcity of donor hearts, only one in three potential donor hearts is accepted for transplant.

High Cost

Estimates for the cost of a heart transplant—including the preheart transplant evaluation, the initial surgery, drugs, post-surgery care, and follow-up tests—is approximately 1.4 to 1.5 million dollars (organ transplants, 2020). Insurance carriers, Medicare, or Medicaid assume most of this financial burden.

Rejection

Despite matching the organ donor and recipient as closely as possible, the recipient's immune system has the potential to detect the donor heart as "foreign" and attempt to destroy it. There are three types of rejection that may occur: hyperacute, acute, and chronic rejection. *Hyperacute rejection* is rare. It occurs within a few minutes of the transplant when the donor organ and recipient are extremely mismatched. *Acute rejection* occurs from 1 week to 3 months after the transplant; almost all transplant recipients experience acute rejection to some degree. *Chronic rejection* may occur at any time over the remaining lifetime of a recipient, causing varying degrees of damage to the donor heart.

Clinical signs and symptoms of rejection include some of the following (Columbia University Medical Center, Department of Surgery, 2021):

- Fever over 100°F (38°C)
- Flulike symptoms such as chills, aches, headaches, dizziness, nausea, and vomiting
- Shortness of breath
- New chest tenderness/pain
- Weight gain over 2 lb for 2 days in a row, or a total of 5 lb in a week
- Fatigue and malaise
- Elevated blood pressure (BP)

Rejection has traditionally been validated by performing an endomyocardial biopsy. This test involves inserting a catheter into a neck vein and threading it into the right ventricle. Then the pathway is used for advancing an instrument called a *biotome*, which obtains a sample of tissue approximately the size of a pin. Biopsies are performed weekly for the first 3 to 6 weeks after surgery, every 3 months for the first year, and then yearly unless the client becomes symptomatic. A cell-free DNA test is a blood test that has recently been developed to detect heart transplant rejection by identifying genetic material being destroyed by the immune system. The test identifies acute rejection weeks to months before the findings of an endometrial biopsy. It can replace endometrial biopsies that are uncomfortable, expensive, and time-consuming.

To prevent and manage tissue rejection, recipients are given immunosuppressive drugs such as cyclosporine (Sandimmune), azathioprine (Imuran), prednisone (Meticorten), tacrolimus (Prograf), or mycophenolate (CellCept). Although these drugs help prevent rejection, their side effects increase the risk for infection, fluid retention, hypertension, and diabetes.

Pharmacologic Considerations

■ Reducing threat of organ rejection requires life-long commitment to a specific drug protocol. *Transplant360TM* is a program to support clients in issues related to transplant such as staying motivated to continue taking antirejection drugs as prescribed. Reminder apps and other suggestions are offered at their website, https://www.donoralliance.org/newsroom/donation-essentials/preventing-organ-and-tissue-rejection/

Infection

As a result of taking immunosuppressive drugs, clients are at risk for bacterial, viral, and fungal infection. If there are signs and symptoms of infection, which may resemble those of tissue rejection, neutropenic precautions consisting of standard precautions and scrupulous hand hygiene are taken because an infection can be life-threatening. In addition to antirejection medications, clients are treated with antibiotics, antivirals, and antifungals depending on the type of acquired infection.

Cardiovascular Disease

The transplanted heart beats faster than the client's natural heart, averaging about 100 to 110 beats/min, because nerves that affect heart rate have been severed. The new heart also takes longer to increase the heart rate in response to exercise. CAD is a common problem among heart transplant recipients; however, they do not experience angina because the transplanted heart's nerve supply is no longer intact. The rate for survival following a heart transplant is more than 85% after 1 year and about 69% after 5 years for adults (Heart transplant, 2020).

CENTRAL OR PERIPHERAL VASCULAR SURGICAL PROCEDURES

Vascular Grafts

Just as grafts are used to bypass a diseased section of a coronary blood vessel, vascular grafts are used to bypass or replace diseased sections of major blood vessels such as the ascending aorta, descending aorta, and femoral or popliteal arteries. The replacement graft may be made of synthetic fiber, such as Dacron or Teflon, or may be human tissue harvested from cadavers. A clamp is placed above and below the affected area, and the diseased blood vessel is removed. The replacement graft is then sewn in place, and the clamps are removed (Fig. 29-11). Depending on the area involved, cardiopulmonary bypass may be necessary.

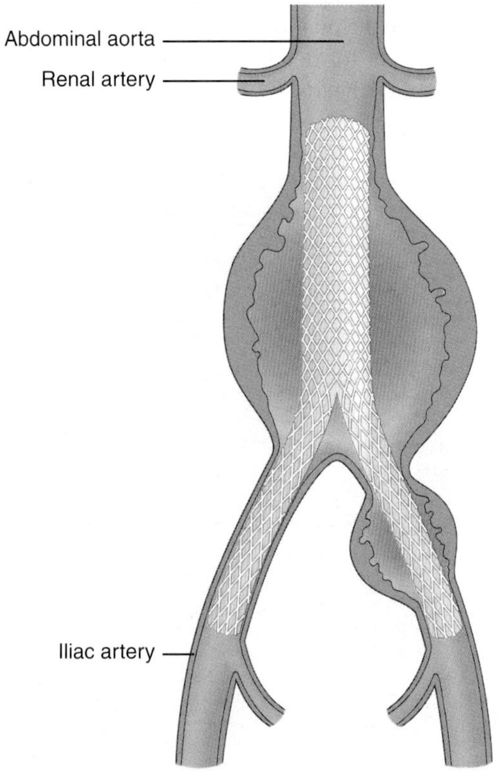

Figure 29-11 Surgical repair of an abdominal aortic aneurysm using a synthetic graft.

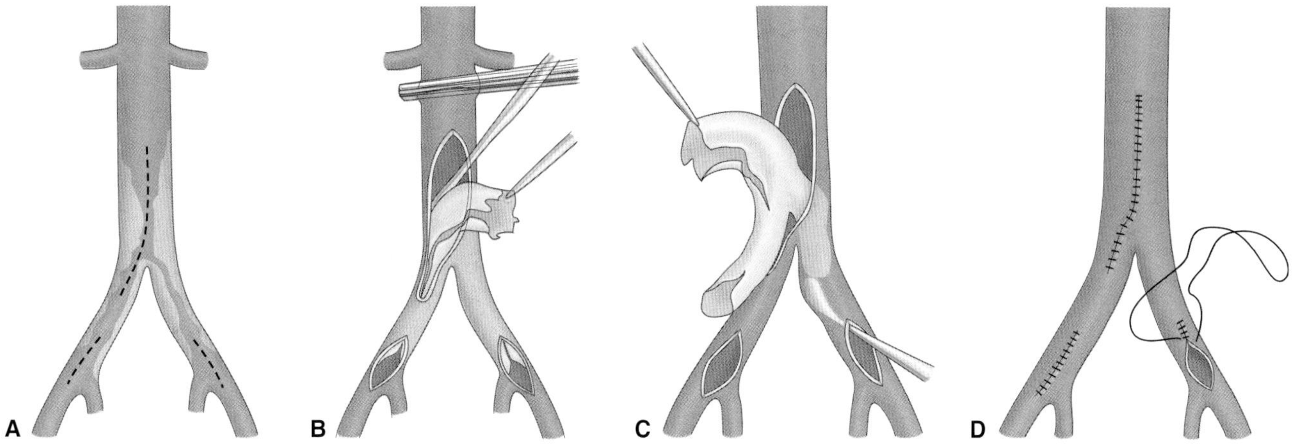

Figure 29-12 In an aortoiliac endarterectomy, the vascular surgeon **(A)** identifies the diseased area, **(B)** clamps off blood supply to the vessel, **(C)** removes the plaque, and **(D)** sutures the vessel shut, after which blood flow is restored. (Adapted from Rutherford, R. B. (2005). *Vascular surgery* (6th ed., Vols.1 and 2). Copyright © 2005 Elsevier. With permission.)

Embolectomy and Thrombectomy

When thrombi or emboli occlude a major vessel, a **thrombectomy** (removal of a thrombus) or **embolectomy** (removal of an embolus) is performed. The vessel is opened above the clot, the clot is removed, and the vessel is sutured closed. This type of surgery may be an emergency because complete occlusion results in loss of blood supply to an area.

Endarterectomy

Endarterectomy is the resection and removal of the lining of an artery (see Chapter 38). This type of surgery is performed to remove obstructive atherosclerotic plaques from the aorta, carotid, femoral, or popliteal arteries (Fig. 29-12).

NURSING MANAGEMENT FOR THE CLIENT UNDERGOING CARDIOVASCULAR SURGERY

The nurse manages the care of the client undergoing cardiovascular surgery throughout the perioperative and rehabilitation phases. Clients who undergo cardiovascular surgery are cared for in an intensive care unit during the immediate postoperative period because of their unstable condition and the need for nurses with expertise in managing complex monitoring equipment.

Concept Mastery Alert

Endarterectomy

Endarterectomy is performed on the aorta or peripheral arteries, whereas a conventional coronary artery bypass graft (CABG) is performed on a coronary artery.

Hemodynamic Monitoring

Hemodynamic monitoring is used to assess the volume and pressure of blood in the heart and vascular system by means of a surgically inserted catheter. Such monitoring is used to assess cardiac function and circulatory status, detect fluid imbalances, adjust fluid infusion rates, and evaluate the client's response to therapeutic measures, such as drug therapy. Methods for hemodynamic monitoring include direct BP monitoring, central venous pressure (CVP) monitoring, and pulmonary artery pressure monitoring.

Direct Blood Pressure Monitoring

Direct BP monitoring requires the placement of a catheter in a peripheral artery. The artery most commonly used is the radial artery. The brachial and femoral arteries also may be used. The catheter tip contains a sensor that measures and transmits the fluid pressure to a transducer, which electronically converts the data to a visual waveform. A monitor continuously displays the waveform and indicates the client's systolic, diastolic, and mean arterial pressures. This type of equipment eliminates the need to auscultate the BP. Direct BP monitoring may be used in clients with severe and sustained hypertension or hypotension and during and after cardiac surgery. A three-way stopcock can be attached to the tubing to allow the nurse periodically to draw arterial blood samples for blood gas analysis (Fig. 29-13).

Central Venous Pressure Monitoring

Right atrial pressure, or **central venous pressure** (CVP), is the pressure produced by venous blood in the right atrium. Normal CVP is 2 to 7 mm Hg. This measurement is used to detect an excess or a deficit in venous blood volume.

To monitor CVP, a catheter is inserted into a large vein, usually the jugular or subclavian vein in the neck, and advanced into the superior vena cava (see Chapter 28). The catheter's proximal end is connected to a three-way stopcock, which controls the direction in which intravenous (IV) fluid flows. The catheter is attached to a transducer that connects to a computer used to analyze hemodynamic data.

When measuring CVP, the nurse makes sure that the transducer is at the level of the client's right atrium; otherwise, an incorrect reading is obtained. The client is positioned supine or with the head slightly elevated but in exactly the same position as during previous measurements. Between CVP measurements, the head of the bed

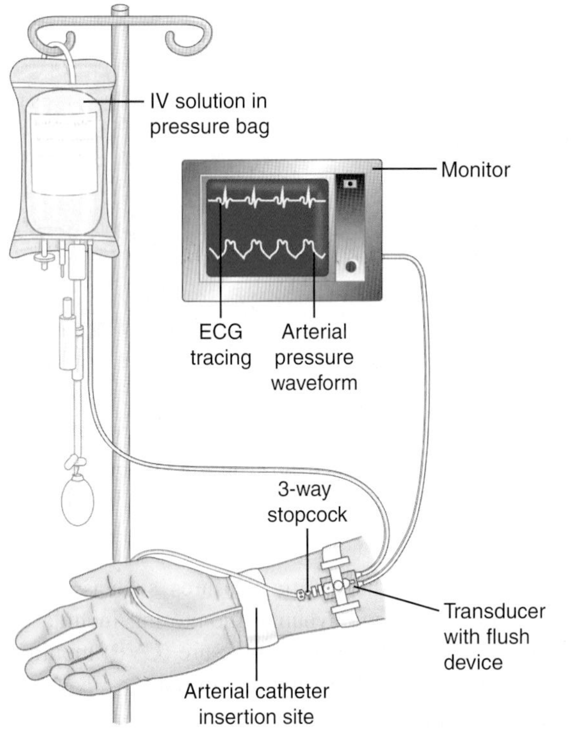

Figure 29-13 Example of a direct blood pressure monitoring system. The catheter is inserted in the radial artery. A three-way stopcock is used for drawing arterial blood samples.

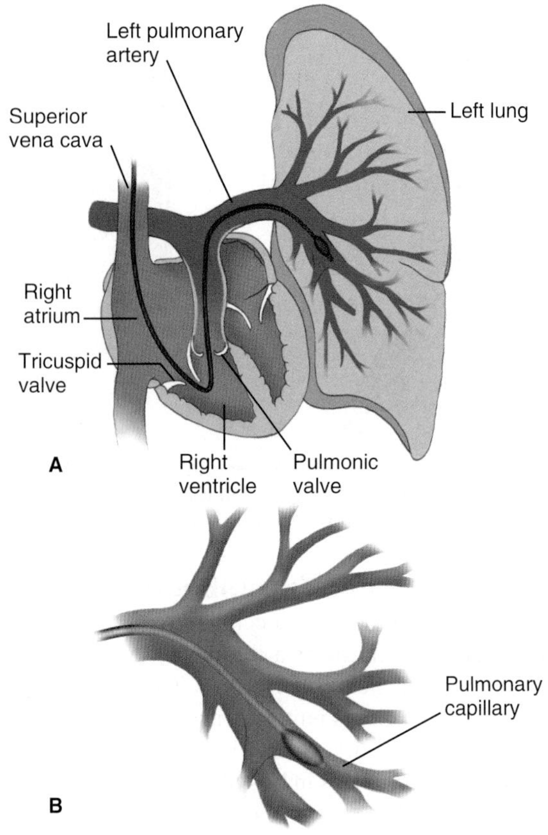

Figure 29-14 Fluid status can be monitored with a pulmonary artery catheter. **(A)** Location of the catheter in the heart. The catheter enters the right atrium through the superior vena cava. The balloon is then inflated, allowing the catheter to follow the blood flow through the tricuspid valve, right ventricle, pulmonic valve, and main pulmonary artery. Waveform and pressure readings are noted during insertion to identify the location of the catheter within the heart. The balloon is deflated once the catheter is in the pulmonary artery and properly secured. **(B)** Pulmonary capillary wedge pressure (PCWP). The catheter floats into a distal branch of the pulmonary artery when the balloon is inflated and becomes "wedged." The wedged catheter occludes blood flow from behind, and the tip of the lumen records pressures in front of the catheter. The balloon is then deflated, allowing the catheter to flow back into the main pulmonary artery.

can be raised or lowered. The primary provider orders the frequency of CVP measurements; however, the nurse may obtain measurements any time they suspect a change in the client's fluid status.

Pulmonary Artery Pressure Monitoring

By inserting a multilumen catheter into a peripheral vein with a distal tip in the pulmonary artery, pressures and cardiac output can be measured to assess left ventricular function (see Fig. 17-3). When in place, the pulmonary artery catheter can measure both pulmonary artery pressure and right atrial pressure or CVP. Pulmonary artery pressure monitoring aids in the early treatment of fluid imbalances prevents left-sided heart failure or promotes its early correction, and helps monitor the client's response to treatment.

The pulmonary artery catheter is advanced through the right side of the heart until the distal tip rests in the right or left pulmonary artery. When the small balloon at the tip of the catheter is inflated, the balloon floats forward, eventually wedging in a pulmonary capillary (Fig. 29-14). As the balloon blocks the flow of blood through the capillary, the catheter tip that protrudes from the inflated balloon senses the fluid pressure ahead of it. **Pulmonary capillary wedge pressure** is the retrograde pressure from the fluid on the left side of the heart at the end of left ventricular diastole. Sometimes, this is abbreviated as LVEDP, for **left ventricular end-diastolic pressure**. The balloon must be deflated immediately after the pressure is measured to avoid pulmonary infarction from prolonged blockage of capillary blood flow.

To measure cardiac output, a syringe with 5 to 10 mL of 5% dextrose in water solution (D_5W) is pushed through a port of the catheter. In the past, iced injectate was used; but with the newer computers, injectate at room temperature may be used. A computerized probe measures the temperature change as the fluid exits the catheter in the heart. The computer then calculates the rate of temperature change with the speed at which the fluid traveled through the heart. A solution that is quite warm after its instillation indicates impairment of the heart's pump function. If the solution remains close to the instillation temperature, the heart's pump function is working optimally. The computer converts the electronic data into numerical equivalents for cardiac output.

The nurse repeats the assessment three to four times in succession and takes the average of the data. Using a formula, the nurse can calculate the **cardiac index**, which reflects the cardiac output in relation to the particular client's body size. The cardiac index is computed by dividing the cardiac output by the client's body surface area. Body surface area is obtained from a **nomogram**, a chart based on height and weight.

Because there are serious potential risks involved with a pulmonary artery catheter, it is used less and less often. In lieu of a pulmonary artery catheter, a minimally invasive hemodynamic monitoring system may be used. It is attached to a client's arterial line in the radial artery to obtain continuous hemodynamic measurements.

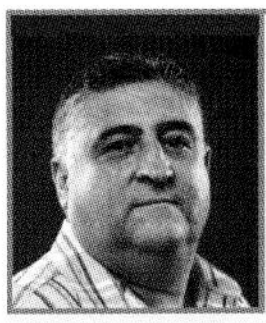

Clinical Scenario A 68-year-old hypertensive male has been experiencing unstable angina and is scheduled for a coronary arteriogram. During the procedure, the cardiologist identified over 50% stenosis of the left main coronary artery as well as narrowing in the left circumflex artery and the right coronary artery. He is scheduled for conventional triple CABG surgery, which will involve a median sternotomy and grafts from the saphenous vein and IMA. **What actions does a nurse take when a client is scheduled for CABG surgery? See the following Nursing Process section.**

NURSING PROCESS FOR THE CLIENT UNDERGOING CARDIAC OR VASCULAR SURGERY

Assessment

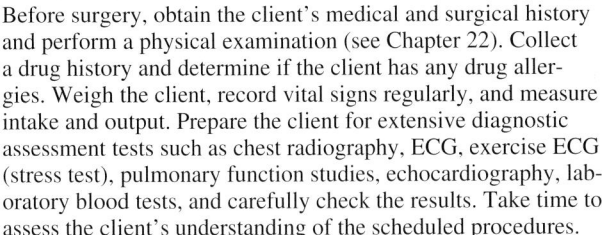

Before surgery, obtain the client's medical and surgical history and perform a physical examination (see Chapter 22). Collect a drug history and determine if the client has any drug allergies. Weigh the client, record vital signs regularly, and measure intake and output. Prepare the client for extensive diagnostic assessment tests such as chest radiography, ECG, exercise ECG (stress test), pulmonary function studies, echocardiography, laboratory blood tests, and carefully check the results. Take time to assess the client's understanding of the scheduled procedures.

After cardiothoracic surgery, the anesthetist and other members of the operating team send many clients directly from the operating room to the intensive care unit. Obtain a comprehensive surgical report from the anesthetist or anesthesiologist and check all invasive monitoring devices. Systematically assess for signs and symptoms of potential complications, such as hemorrhage and shock, thrombus or embolus formation, cerebral anoxia, cardiac arrhythmias, fluid overload, electrolyte imbalance, respiratory failure, and cardiac tamponade.

Palpate the peripheral pulses or use a Doppler ultrasound device if the pulses are not palpable. Check for inadequate tissue perfusion, such as a weak or absent pulse, cold or cyanotic extremity, or skin mottling. Assess BP and pulse rates in both arms after surgery. Inspect IV sites and monitor the rates of infusing solutions. Calculate urine output and other fluid intake hourly. Perform a neurologic assessment every 30 minutes, including evaluation of level of consciousness, size of pupils and their reaction to light, movement in both arms and legs, verbal response, and status of orientation. Figure 29-15 illustrates postoperative monitoring following cardiovascular surgery.

Analysis, Planning, and Interventions

Knowledge Deficiency: Related to unfamiliarity with diagnostic tests, preoperative preparations, and postoperative care
Expected Outcome: Client and family will understand the purpose, preparation, and aftercare of tests and surgery.

- Assess client and family's knowledge concerning procedures. *Teaching builds on a foundation of knowledge.*
- Provide both verbal and written information concerning the surgical procedure and aftercare using language the client can understand. *Using terms the client can easily understand and giving both auditory and visual information enhance the learning process.*
- Ask the client or family member to explain the surgical procedure before signing the consent form. *The ability to paraphrase information validates that the client understands and is capable of giving informed consent.*
- Explain coughing, deep breathing, and leg exercises. Teach the use of an incentive spirometer and splinting the incision with a pillow when coughing. *The standard of care for all clients undergoing general anesthesia is to preoperatively teach techniques that prevent postoperative pneumonia and stasis of venous circulation.*
- Promote a relaxed environment conducive to asking questions. *Demonstrating personal interest and encouraging verbal interaction promotes free communication.*
- Clarify misconceptions concerning surgery. *The nurse is obligated to ensure that the client's knowledge and perceptions are accurate.*

Acute Anxiety: Related to potential surgical outcome
Expected Outcome: The client's anxiety will be reduced to a mild level or one the client indicates is tolerable as a result of developing realistic expectations concerning surgery.

- Listen and encourage the client to express concerns about the surgery and its outcome. *Verbalizing what may be real or imagined often lifts the mental burden that a client experiences.*
- Provide clear information about the surgical procedure and aftercare in short, simple explanations. *Anxiety interferes with the ability to attend to, concentrate on, and process information, especially if it is extensive or complex.*
- Acknowledge emotions and expressions of fear. *Empathetic acceptance of fears decreases anxiety.*
- Demonstrate competence when performing skills. *Sensing that the nurse is knowledgeable and competent relieves the client's insecurity.*
- Provide instruction on presurgical medications such as anxiolytics to be taken before surgery especially at home the day/night before procedure. *Clients who are relaxed and calm when anxiolytics are given require a smaller dose of anesthetic for induction.*

(continued)

NURSING PROCESS FOR THE CLIENT UNDERGOING CARDIAC OR VASCULAR SURGERY (continued)

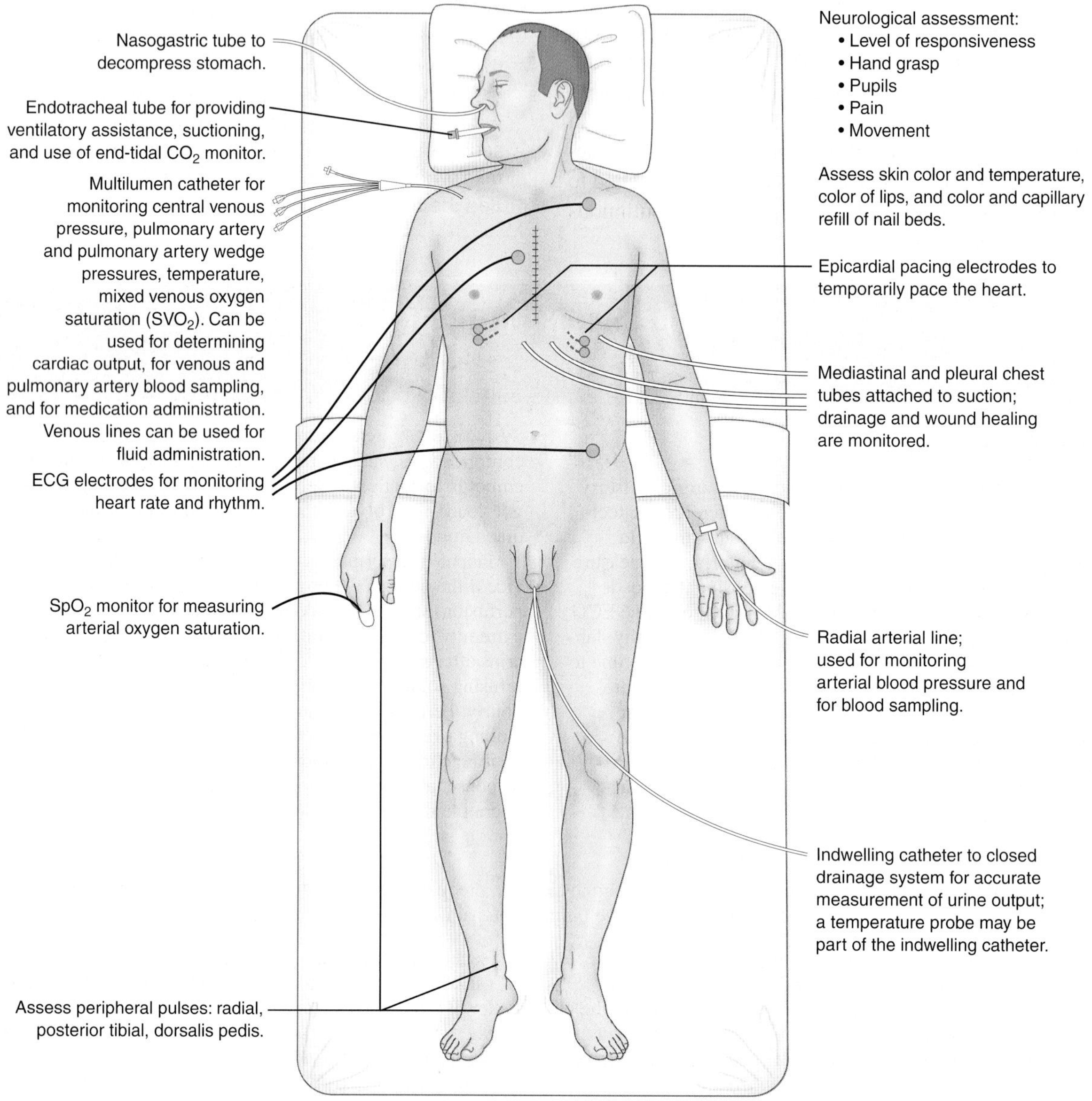

Nasogastric tube to decompress stomach.
Endotracheal tube for providing ventilatory assistance, suctioning, and use of end-tidal CO_2 monitor.
Multilumen catheter for monitoring central venous pressure, pulmonary artery and pulmonary artery wedge pressures, temperature, mixed venous oxygen saturation (SVO_2). Can be used for determining cardiac output, for venous and pulmonary artery blood sampling, and for medication administration. Venous lines can be used for fluid administration.
ECG electrodes for monitoring heart rate and rhythm.
SpO_2 monitor for measuring arterial oxygen saturation.
Assess peripheral pulses: radial, posterior tibial, dorsalis pedis.
Neurological assessment:
• Level of responsiveness
• Hand grasp
• Pupils
• Pain
• Movement
Assess skin color and temperature, color of lips, and color and capillary refill of nail beds.
Epicardial pacing electrodes to temporarily pace the heart.
Mediastinal and pleural chest tubes attached to suction; drainage and wound healing are monitored.
Radial arterial line; used for monitoring arterial blood pressure and for blood sampling.
Indwelling catheter to closed drainage system for accurate measurement of urine output; a temperature probe may be part of the indwelling catheter.

Figure 29-15 Postoperative monitoring of the client following cardiovascular surgery.

Acute Pain: Related to surgical trauma to skin and operative tissue
Expected Outcome: Pain will be reduced to a tolerable level within 30 minutes of a nursing intervention.

- Assess the location, intensity, and quality of pain when assessing vital signs. *Pain assessment is the fifth vital sign. Pain beyond the client's tolerance requires immediate intervention.*
- Demonstrate how to self-administer narcotic analgesia with a patient-controlled analgesia (PCA) pump. *Small, frequent self-administrations of an opioid drug control acute pain within consistently tolerable levels.*
- Administer narcotic analgesics promptly as prescribed if PCA is not used. *Pain is more easily controlled by giving analgesic medication before the pain becomes severe.*
- Administer nonopioid analgesics between prescribed doses of opioid analgesics. *Nonopioids have a different mechanism of action and are not likely to cause respiratory depression or depressed level of consciousness if given concurrently with opioids.*

Ineffective Airway Clearance Risk: Related to ineffective cough secondary to pain and accumulated secretions in response to artificial airway
Expected Outcome: Client will have a patent airway as evidenced by noiseless respirations and clear lung sounds.

NURSING PROCESS FOR THE CLIENT UNDERGOING CARDIAC OR VASCULAR SURGERY (continued)

- Assess lung sounds every 4 hours or as often as indicated by the client's condition. *Early detection of problems allows for swift intervention.*
- Promote deep breathing and coughing every hour while the client is awake after extubation. Suction when respirations are noisy. *Coughing is a natural method for clearing the airway. Suctioning uses negative pressure to remove mucus from the airway.*
- *Administer prescribed analgesics. Analgesia relieves incisional pain and facilitates deep breathing and coughing.*
- Instruct client to press a pillow against the chest when deep breathing, coughing, and performing active exercise. *Splinting promotes comfort and decreases the potential for dehiscence.*
- Encourage oral fluids to the extent allowed when extubated; humidify oxygen. *Hydration and humidification liquefy mucous secretions, making them easier to expectorate.*

Impaired Gas Exchange: Related to retained secretions, hypoventilation secondary to pain, displacement of chest tubes
Expected Outcome: Client maintains adequate gas exchange as evidenced by arterial blood gases (ABGs) within normal limits, $SpO_2 \geq 90\%$, and no dyspnea or tachycardia.

- Assess lung sounds, heart rate, level of consciousness, pulse oximetry, and ABG results as often as necessary. *Any abnormal findings are indicators of developing hypoxemia.*
- Notify primary provider if oxygen saturation remains below 90%. *This finding indicates that the client requires supplemental oxygenation.*
- Administer oxygen as prescribed. *Supplemental oxygen prevents hypoxemia or relieves oxygen deficits.*
- Elevate head of bed as much as possible. *Elevation of the head facilitates maximum chest/lung expansion, promotes comfort, and decreases the work of breathing.*
- Hyperoxygenate with 100% oxygen before suctioning; do not suction for more than 10 to 15 seconds. *Suctioning removes oxygen and can cause hypoxemia, myocardial ischemia, and arrhythmia. Hyperoxygenation saturates the blood and hemoglobin to compensate for temporary removal during suctioning.*
- Promote rest and administer prescribed sedatives. *Rest reduces oxygen consumption; sedatives promote rest and are sympathetic antagonists.*
- Inspect chest tubes frequently to ensure that they are not kinked or compressed. *Obstructed chest tubes interfere with removal of air and blood from the pleura, which interferes with lung expansion.*

Risk for fluid overload: Related to impaired ventricular contraction
Expected Outcomes: Client will maintain an adequate cardiac output as evidenced by stable vital signs; alertness; adequate urine output; and no arrhythmias, chest pain, dyspnea, confusion, or dizziness. Cardiac output readings are within normal limits.

- Assess hemodynamics with direct BP monitoring by arterial line or a pulmonary artery catheter that provides cardiac output measurements, vital signs, heart and lung sounds, intake and output, pulse rhythm and quality, mental status, and signs of peripheral edema as often as necessary. *Focused assessments that reflect the heart's ability to circulate intravascular fluid are an indication of an adequate or inadequate cardiac output.*
- Administer IV fluids and blood replacement at the rate prescribed. *Parenteral fluids increase the intravascular volume to facilitate an adequate cardiac output.*
- Administer prescribed inotropic medications. *Inotropes increase the force of heart contraction.*
- Administer prescribed vasodilators or diuretics. *They decrease afterload and promote optimum cardiac output.*
- Administer prescribed antiarrhythmics. *They promote normal conduction, depolarization, and repolarization of myocardial tissue to ensure normal cardiac output.*
- Be prepared to use a transcutaneous or transvenous pacemaker. *A temporary pacemaker ensures a heart rate that is compatible with life.*

Infection Risk: Related to impaired skin
Expected Outcome: Client will remain free of infection.

- Assess sternal and leg incisions for redness, warmth, swelling, or purulent drainage. *Focused assessments that reflect the inflammatory process signify a possible infection.*
- Practice conscientious hand hygiene. *Hand hygiene is the single most important method for preventing infection.*
- Change moist or loose dressings. Use aseptic technique when changing dressings, IV tubing, bags, or other equipment. *Sterile technique prevents the transmission of microorganisms to impaired tissue. Dry, intact dressings are a barrier to microorganisms in the environment.*
- Administer prescribed antibiotic therapy. *Antibiotics are administered prophylactically and must be given on time to maintain therapeutic blood levels.*
- Implement infection control precautions for the immunosuppressed client. *They reduce the potential for exposing such clients to infectious microorganisms.*

RC of Hemorrhage

Expected Outcome: The nurse will monitor for, manage, and minimize hemorrhage.

- Assess the following as often as necessary: incisional drainage; sites used for cardiopulmonary bypass cannulation; volume and color of chest tube drainage; BP and pulse rate; urinary output; mental status; partial thromboplastin time, prothrombin time, and international normalized ratio; presence of occult blood in stool; bruising; bleeding gums; and hemodynamic measurements. *Abnormal findings of such focused assessments are indicators of bleeding.*
- Report to the primary provider a cluster of symptoms that suggest significant blood loss. *The nurse works collaboratively to manage complications.*
- Be prepared to administer parenteral fluids, blood replacement, fresh frozen plasma, or antidotes for anticoagulants. *Fluids, blood, and blood products increase blood volume. Fresh frozen plasma replaces clotting factors. Antagonists of anticoagulants restore endogenous clotting mechanisms.*
- Apply direct pressure to bleeding sites. *Pressure promotes stasis of blood.*

(continued)

NURSING PROCESS FOR THE CLIENT UNDERGOING CARDIAC OR VASCULAR SURGERY (continued)

Altered Tissue Perfusion: Peripheral: Related to compromised collateral circulation in extremity used to harvest donor vein, cannulation of peripheral artery and vein for cardiopulmonary bypass, venous stasis secondary to inactivity
Expected Outcome: Client's donor extremities will be adequately perfused with oxygenated blood; venous blood circulation will be adequate.

- Assess peripheral pulses, dependent edema, capillary refill, skin color and temperature, urinary output, and mental status as often as necessary. *Focused assessment of these data reflects the status of peripheral blood flow.*
- Position extremity above level of heart. *Gravity promotes venous return to the heart. Reducing edema facilitates potential space for arterial circulation.*
- Encourage leg exercises every hour while awake. *Contraction of skeletal leg muscles propels venous blood toward the heart.*
- Apply elastic stockings or use a mechanical compression device. *Elastic stockings support valves in the leg veins to prevent venous stasis. Mechanical compression devices apply pressure to the tissues of the legs to propel venous blood.*
- Assist the client to ambulate several times a day. *Walking contracts leg muscles that promote venous blood return.*
- Ensure that the client avoids prolonged sitting or crossing the legs at the knee. *Gravity and pressure on veins contribute to venous stasis.*
- Encourage oral fluids within prescribed limits. *Adequate fluid volume decreases the potential for hemoconcentration and thrombus formation.*

Evaluation of Expected Outcomes

Expected outcomes for the client undergoing cardiovascular surgery are that they understand the treatment and recovery regimen and can cope with the anxiety created by the change in health status and surgical experience. Pain is controlled or eliminated; the airway is patent. The client ventilates adequately to maintain adequate gas diffusion; cardiac output is sufficient to maintain vital signs and renal output within normal ranges. There is no evidence of wound infection, and no significant bleeding develops. The extremities are warm and nonedematous, reflecting adequate arterial and venous circulation. Client and Family Teaching 29-1 offers discharge instructions after cardiac surgery. Also see Evidence-Based Practice 29-1 for research on postoperative cardiac clients.

Client and Family Teaching 29-1
Discharge Instructions After Cardiothoracic Surgery

The nurse teaches the following points:

- It may take several weeks for a normal appetite to return.
- Increase fruits, fiber, and liquids to relieve constipation or use an occasional mild laxative.
- Depression is normal and temporary.
- You may have some slight problem with memory, but it should not be severe.
- A painless lump, if felt at the top of the chest incision, will disappear given time.
- There may be an occasional "grating" sound in the chest until the sternum heals.
- There may be some numbness in the chest if the IMA was used as a graft.
- After 1 week, the adhesive strips that cross the incision can be removed.
- Wait to take a tub bath until all incisions are healed; take showers until then.
- Report any redness, drainage, or tenderness from any incision.
- Loose, nonconstricting clothing promotes comfort and avoids interfering with circulation.
- Refrain from lifting, pushing, or pulling anything that weighs more than 10 lb until the primary provider relieves the restriction (approximately 6 to 12 weeks).
- Do not drive or sit in a seat behind an airbag for 4 weeks.
- Sexual relations usually can be resumed in 2 to 4 weeks depending on your comfort level and tolerance for activity; climbing two flights of stairs without dyspnea or chest pain is a common guideline.
- Perform exercises as taught; report if swelling of the legs increases.
- Continue to wear support hose or elastic stockings during the day and remove them at night.
- Check your weight daily and report if you gain more than 2 lb in 24 hours.
- Count your pulse rate at the wrist or neck and report a rate that exceeds 150 beats/min.
- Contact the primary provider if you have difficulty breathing without a logical reason.
- If chest pain develops, rest; if the chest pain is unrelieved, take nitroglycerin as prescribed, and report the event to the primary provider regardless of whether it was relieved.
- Avoid crowds if you are taking an immunosuppressive drug.

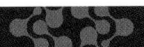

Evidence-Based Practice 29-1

Postoperative Cardiac Clients

Clinical Question

What are the three main risk factors for post cardiac nosocomial infections?

Evidence

A big risk to clients postoperatively is the development of a nosocomial infection. In a study published in the Journal of Clinical Anesthesia, May 2021, they reviewed potential risk factors and the mortality rates for clients within the first few weeks after cardiac surgery. The three main risk factors for the development of a nosocomial infection were identified: cardiopulmonary bypass time, kidney failure, and emergency surgery. For clients who developed a nosocomial infection the mortality rate was 18% higher than for those clients who did not acquire a nosocomial infection (Nosocomial Infections, 2021). The main infections were pneumonia, urinary tract infection, bacteremia, and wound infection.

The information from this study suggests that infection prevention following cardiac surgery must be prioritized to improve client outcomes.

Nursing Implications

This article indicates a strong need for nurses to assess the clients and symptoms of the above-stated risk factors. Nurses should record and monitor vital signs, perform a thorough respiratory assessment and notify the health care provider if deterioration occurs, and monitor labs and intake and output. The importance of this assessment data could lead to early diagnosis and treatment of nosocomial infections

Reference
de la Varga-Martínez, O., Gómez-Sánchez, E., FeMuñoz, M., Lorenzo, M., Gómez-Pesquera, E., Poves-Álvarez, R., Tamayo, E., & Heredia-Rodríguez, M. (2021). Impact of nosocomial infections on patient mortality following cardiac surgery. *Journal of Clinical Anesthesia, 69*(5/2021). https://doi.org/10.1016/j.jclinane.2020.110104

>>> *Stop, Think, and Respond 29-1*

A client has been in the intensive care unit for the past 4 days after CABG surgery. Normally alert and oriented, the client is very confused, restless, and agitated. What could be possible reasons for this new-onset confusion? What other data will you need to collect? What can you do to help the client right now?

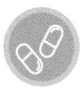

Pharmacologic Considerations

- Opioids must be given with caution in older adults owing to changes in absorption, distribution, metabolism, and excretion. Change in cognition is an early symptom of adverse reaction that can occur prior to respiratory depression.

KEY POINTS

- Cardiopulmonary bypass: removes blood from the venae cavae, circulating it through an oxygenator, and returning it to the aorta or femoral artery provides a nearly bloodless area while the beating heart is stopped.
- Coronary artery bypass is performed when:
  - The client has multiple coronary artery occlusions.
  - The atheromas are calcified and noncompressible.
  - The anatomic location of the occlusion(s) interferes with the safe insertion of a coronary artery catheter.
- Coronary artery bypass surgery types:
  - Conventional (CABG)
  - Minimally invasive direct coronary artery bypass (MIDCAB)
  - Off-pump coronary artery bypass (OPCAB)
  - Port access coronary artery bypass (PACAB)
  - Totally endoscopic coronary artery bypass (TECAB)
- Heart valves repair or replacement: needed if they become narrowed (stenosed) or stretched (incompetent)
  - Commissurotomy: opening adhesions in the valve cusps, done without direct visualization of the valve
  - Balloon valvuloplasty: uses a balloon catheter to stretch the stenosed valve
  - Transcatheter valve implantation (TAVI/TAVR): minimally invasive procedure by which a new valve is inserted without removing the old, damaged valve, the new valve is placed inside the diseased valve.
- Heart valves:
  - Mechanical: man-made from carbon, stainless steel, Dacron
  - Bioprosthetic: natural tissue mounted on a metallic or polymer stent or unstented
  - Xenograft: porcine (pig) valve or bovine (cow) pericardium
  - Allograft (also known as homograft): human cadaver
  - Autograft: tissue from client's own pulmonic valve or pulmonary artery
- Heart transplantation: indicated for cardiomyopathy, end-stage CAD and end-stage heart failure
- Percutaneous coronary interventions (PTCA/PCA): uses drug-eluting stents that keep a coronary artery open and release a drug that prevents reocclusion.
- Right atrial pressure, or central venous pressure (CVP), is the pressure produced by venous blood in the right atrium.
- Pulmonary artery pressure monitoring: the pulmonary artery catheter can measure both pulmonary artery pressure and right atrial pressure or CVP

CRITICAL THINKING EXERCISES

1. A client has been told that the primary provider advises myocardial revascularization. The client tells you that the thought of a long midchest incision and leg incision are very frightening. What information would you offer this person?

2. While caring for a client who is recovering from CABG surgery, you gather the following data: the client has leg pain, which the client rates as 8 on a scale of 1 to 10; the respiratory rate is 30 breaths/min at rest; there is dried blood on the thoracic dressing; the client's throat is sore after being weaned from mechanical ventilation; and the client is concerned because there has been no bowel movement in 3 days. Which assessment finding is the major concern at this time?
3. What teaching would you provide if you see a client with a conventional CABG using a saphenous vein graft sitting in a chair with the legs crossed at the knee?
4. If one of your family members requires myocardial revascularization, discuss the type of procedure for which you would advocate and the reasons for that choice.

NCLEX-STYLE REVIEW QUESTIONS PrepU

1. A client with 90% occlusion of the left anterior descending artery is anxious about undergoing conventional CABG surgery. What is the best nursing approach for relieving the client's anxiety?
   1. Explain to the client how CABG surgery is performed.
   2. Listen to the client verbalize feelings about the surgery.
   3. Reassure the client how well others have done after surgery.
   4. Avoid discussing the surgical procedure until the client is relaxed.
2. A client is recovering from cardiovascular surgery and has decreased cardiac output. The nurse reviews the client's care plan, which states that an expected outcome is to maintain adequate cardiac output. Which sign or symptom best demonstrates the expected outcome?
   1. The client's urine output is 25 mL/kg/hour.
   2. The client has fixed, dilated pupils.
   3. The client has frequent palpitations.
   4. The client's vital signs are within normal limits.
3. A client returns to the intensive care unit after a coronary artery bypass graft in which the saphenous vein was removed. During the immediate postoperative period, which one of the following nursing interventions is most important?
   1. Inspect the IV site and infusion rate.
   2. Assess the client for peripheral edema.
   3. Palpate the peripheral pulses.
   4. Administer an anticoagulant.
4. Immediately after open-chest cardiac surgery involving cardiopulmonary bypass, which of the following can be expected temporarily? Select all that apply.
   1. Numbness in the chest
   2. A pulsating sound over the sternum
   3. Emotional depression
   4. Memory loss or confusion
   5. Painful lump at the proximal incision
5. A client who has received a heart transplant is on high doses of immunosuppressant drugs. What health teaching is essential by the nurse at the time of discharge?
   1. Refrain from outdoor activity in cold weather.
   2. Avoid gatherings where there are crowds.
   3. Take an oral temperature twice a day.
   4. Space and pace physical activities.

WANT TO KNOW MORE? There are a wide variety of online resources available on thePoint to enhance learning and understanding of this chapter.

Go to thePoint.lww.com/activate and use the activation code found in the front of this text to unlock these online resources.

UNIT 7
Caring for Clients With Hematopoietic and Lymphatic Disorders

30 Introduction to the Hematopoietic and Lymphatic Systems

Words To Know

agranulocytes
albumin
basophils
B lymphocytes
bone marrow aspiration
eosinophils
erythrocytes
erythropoietin
fibrinogen
globulins
granulocytes
hematopoiesis
hemoglobin
hemolysis
hemostasis
leukocytes
leukocytosis
leukopenia
lymph
lymphatics
lymph nodes
lymphokine
lymphocytes
monocytes
neutrophils
phagocytosis
plasma
platelets
pluripotential stem cells
Schilling test
T lymphocytes

Learning Objectives

On completion of this chapter, you will be able to:

1. Define hematopoiesis.
2. Name the major structures in the hematopoietic system.
3. Name three types of blood cells produced by bone marrow, and discuss the function of each.
4. List at least five components of plasma.
5. Name three plasma proteins and explain the function of each.
6. Identify the four blood groups and discuss the importance of transfusing compatible types.
7. Explain the components and function of the lymphatic system and its role in hematopoiesis.
8. Describe the pertinent assessments of the hematopoietic and lymphatic systems when obtaining a health history and conducting a physical examination.
9. Name laboratory and diagnostic tests for disorders of the hematopoietic and lymphatic systems.
10. Discuss the nursing management of clients with hematopoietic or lymphatic disorders.

This chapter discusses the structures that are involved in **hematopoiesis**, the manufacture, and development of blood cells. It also considers the lymphatic system, which includes the thymus gland and spleen; this system assists in the maturation of certain **lymphocytes** (specific types of white blood cells).

Gerontologic Considerations

- The components of blood change only slightly with age. RBCs become slightly less flexible and fewer in number. Lymphocytes also decrease in number, causing a decreased resistance to infection.
- Decreased renal perfusion can result in inadequate erythropoietin production, resulting in decreased RBC production.
- Cellular and humoral immunity are affected by age-related changes in the lymphatic system, including decreases in primary antibody, T-Cell and B-cell responses, and antibody production. This results in an increased susceptibility of older adults to infections and malignancies, and indication for recommended adult immunizations.
- The Schilling test may pose a problem in older adults if proper collection of the 24-hour specimen is not possible as a result of cognitive problems or urinary incontinence. Recent research indicates that gastric pH levels vary in older adults, requiring individual consideration of appropriateness of the Schilling test to detect B12 deficiencies for older adults. However, the full Schilling test is indicated if other causes are suspected.

ANATOMY AND PHYSIOLOGY

Hematopoietic System

Bone Marrow

Bone marrow, the soft tissue that fills spaces in the interior of the long bones and spongy bones of the skeleton, manufactures blood cells. The two types of bone marrow are *red marrow* and *yellow marrow*. Red marrow is found in the ribs, sternum, skull, clavicles, vertebrae, proximal ends of the long bones, and iliac crest. It manufactures blood cells and hemoglobin. Yellow marrow consists of fat cells and connective tissue. It does not participate in the manufacture of blood cells; however, yellow bone marrow can form blood cells under conditions involving intense stimulation, such as after significant blood loss (hemorrhage). The lymphatic system also plays a role in hematopoiesis.

Blood

Blood consists of cells suspended in a fluid called **plasma** (Fig. 30-1). All blood cells are produced from undifferentiated precursors called **pluripotential stem cells** in the bone marrow (Fig. 30-2). Myeloid stem cells are converted to (1) **erythrocytes**, which are red blood cells (RBCs); (2) several types of **leukocytes**, or white blood cells (WBCs); and (3) **platelets**, also known as *thrombocytes* because they help control bleeding by forming a loose blood clot. Lymphoid stem cells are converted to lymphocytes, WBCs with immune functions. Each component of blood has specialized functions (Table 30-1).

Erythrocytes

Erythrocytes (or RBCs) are flexible, anuclear (lacking a nucleus), biconcave disks covered by a thin membrane through which oxygen (O_2) and carbon dioxide (CO_2) pass freely.

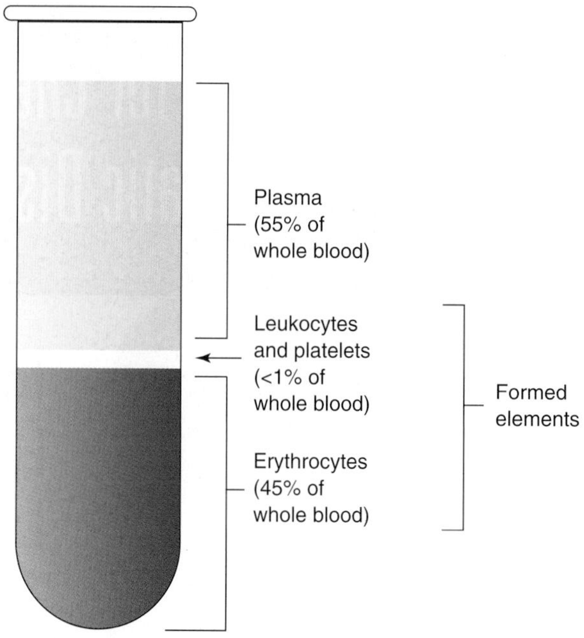

Figure 30-1 Components of blood.

The flexibility of erythrocytes allows them to change shape as they travel through capillaries. Their major function is to transport O_2 to and remove CO_2 from the tissues.

Production of erythrocytes is called *erythropoiesis*. The rate of erythrocyte production is regulated by **erythropoietin**, a hormone released by the kidneys. Erythrocytes arise from myeloid stem cells, which also require iron and B vitamins such as B_{12}, B_6, and folate to mature properly (Nutrition Notes). Immature erythrocytes, known collectively as *erythroblasts*, go through several intermediary

Nutrition Notes

Nutrients Involved in Red Blood Cell Formation

- Iron is the basic nutritional component of heme in hemoglobin.
- Protein is the building block of hemoglobin and the enzymes involved in red blood cell (RBC) production.
- Folic acid and vitamin B_{12} are essential for the maturation of RBCs.
- Vitamin C enhances the absorption of folic acid and iron.
- Vitamin B_6 serves as a coenzyme in hemoglobin formation.
- Copper (minute amount) is involved in the transfer of iron from storage to plasma.
- Vitamin E protects blood cells from vitamin E–deficient hemolytic anemia.
- Food sources rich in these nutrients are: lean red meats (iron); lean meats, eggs, dairy, and legumes (protein); animal products (B_{12}); dark leafy greens, beans and lentils, seeds and nuts (folic acid); citrus (vitamin C); fortified cereals, beef, and poultry (B_6); shellfish, grains, beans, and nuts (copper); and sunflower seeds, almonds, spinach, safflower oil, and asparagus (vitamin E).

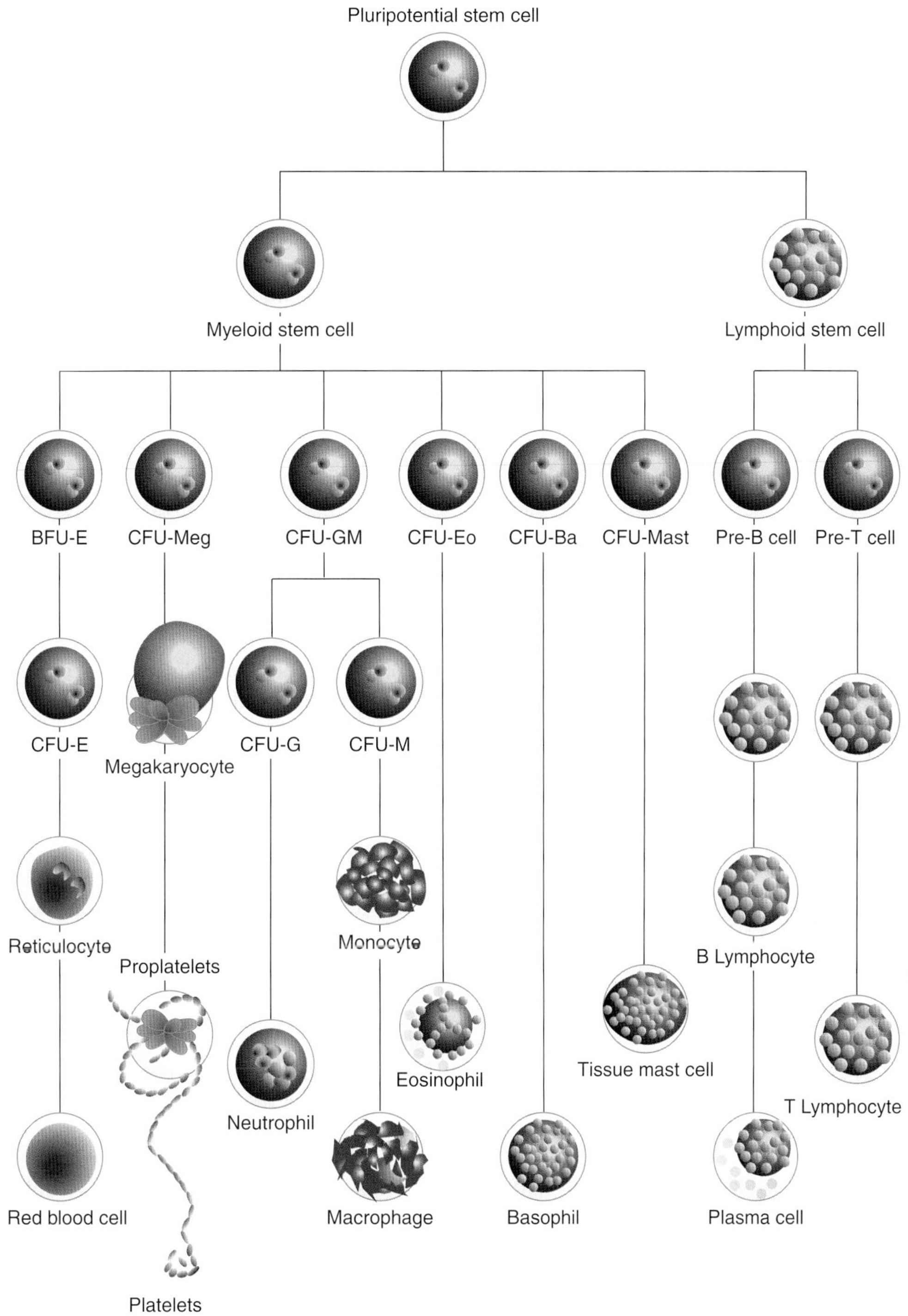

Figure 30-2 Hematopoiesis. All blood cells develop from pluripotential stem cells in the bone marrow. (Reprinted with permission from Smeltzer, S. C., Bare, B. G., Hinkle, J. L., & Cheever, K.H. (2010). *Brunner & Suddarth's textbook of medical-surgical nursing* (12th ed.). Wolters Kluwer Health/Lippincott Williams & Wilkins.)

stages of maturation before being released into the blood. In their immature state, erythroblasts contain a nucleus; the mature erythrocyte has no nucleus.

The normal number of erythrocytes varies with age, gender, and altitude and ranges between 3.6 and 5.4 million/mm^3. Infants have more erythrocytes than adults; women have fewer erythrocytes than men. People who live at high altitudes or engage in strenuous activity have an increased number of erythrocytes to maximize the transport of O_2 and CO_2.

TABLE 30-1 Functions of Blood Components

COMPONENT	FUNCTION
Blood Cells	
Erythrocytes (red blood cells)	Transport oxygen and carbon dioxide
Leukocytes (white blood cells)	Protect against infection
Platelets (thrombocytes)	Participate in clotting blood
Plasma	
Water	Circulates blood cells and noncellular components Contributes to blood pressure Relocates to other fluid compartments as needed
Plasma Proteins	
Albumin	Affects intravascular osmotic pressure
Fibrinogen	Participates in clotting blood
Globulin	Carries other protein substances, for example, those that are involved in inflammatory and immune responses
Clotting factors	Convert a loose blood clot to a stabilized blood clot
Nutrients	
Glucose	Provides source of immediate energy
Amino acids	Provide components for cell growth and repair
Lipids	Provide a reserve for cellular energy in the absence of glucose
Vitamins	Participate in essential physiologic functions
Electrolytes	Facilitate a variety of biochemical actions
Hormones	Perform multiple endocrine functions
Wastes (carbon dioxide, drug metabolites)	Prevent toxicity when biotransformed and excreted

The red color of blood is the result of **hemoglobin**, an iron-containing pigment attached to erythrocytes. The heme portion of the molecule freely binds with blood gases. As erythrocytes pass through the alveolar capillary membranes, the hemoglobin picks up oxygen from the alveoli and releases carbon dioxide (CO_2). The oxygen saturated hemoglobin is called *oxyhemoglobin;* it circulates through arteries, arterioles, and capillaries to all body cells. After hemoglobin releases O_2 for use by the cells, the blood becomes dark red; the hemoglobin is then called *reduced* (or *deoxygenated*) *hemoglobin* owing to the acquisition of carbon dioxide from cellular metabolism. In adults, the normal range of hemoglobin is 12.0 to 17.4 g/dL; the amount of hemoglobin can vary depending on the sex of the individual. Erythrocytes circulate in the blood for about 120 days, after which the spleen removes them; the liver removes severely damaged erythrocytes. When erythrocytes are destroyed, the iron component of hemoglobin is returned to the red marrow and reused. The residual pigment is stored in the liver as bilirubin and excreted in bile.

Leukocytes

Leukocytes (or WBCs) perform various protective functions such as engulfing invading microorganisms and cellular debris and manufacturing antibodies (see Chapter 33). They not only circulate in blood but also migrate from the blood into body tissues to search for and destroy potentially harmful substances.

The normal range of leukocytes is between 5,000 and 10,000/mm^3. An increased number of leukocytes is called **leukocytosis**; a decreased number is called **leukopenia.** Table 30-2 shows the differential leukocyte count. The lifespan of leukocytes is only 1 to 2 days; consequently, the demand for the production of WBCs is continuous. The need is even greater with an infection.

Leukocytes are divided into two categories; **granulocytes**, which contain cytoplasmic granules, and **agranulocytes** that do not contain granules (Fig. 30-3).

Granulocytes. Granulocytes, also called *polymorphonuclear leukocytes*, and are divided into three subgroups: neutrophils, basophils, and eosinophils. **Neutrophils** are a major component of the inflammatory response and defense against bacterial infection. Also called *microphages*, they protect the body by **phagocytosis,** the ingestion and digestion of bacteria and foreign substances (Fig. 30-4). Immature neutrophils, called *band cells*, circulate in peripheral blood.

Basophils are also capable of phagocytosis; they are active in allergic contact dermatitis (immediate hypersensitivity) and some delayed hypersensitivity reactions**. Eosinophils** phagocytize foreign material. Their numbers increase in allergies, some dermatologic disorders, and parasitic infections.

Agranulocytes. Agranulocytes are divided into two groups: *lymphocytes* and *monocytes*. **Lymphocytes** are divided into *B lymphocytes* (or B cells), which provide humoral immunity by producing antibodies (immunoglobulins), and *T lymphocytes* (or T cells), which provide cellular immunity (or cell-mediated response). **B lymphocytes** produce antibodies against foreign antigens, and **T lymphocytes** interact with foreign cells and release a substance called **lymphokine,** which enhances the actions of phagocytic

TABLE 30-2 Differential White Blood Cell (WBC) Count

	PERCENTAGE OF TOTAL WBCs	NUMERIC RANGE (mm^3)
Neutrophils	60–70	3,000–7,000
Basophils	0.5–1	25–100
Eosinophils	1–4	50–400
Lymphocytes	20–40	1,000–4,000
Monocytes	2–6	100–600

Leukocytes are divided into two categories: granulocytes, which contain cytoplasmic granules and agranulocytes, which do not contain granules (Fig. 30-3, p. 507).

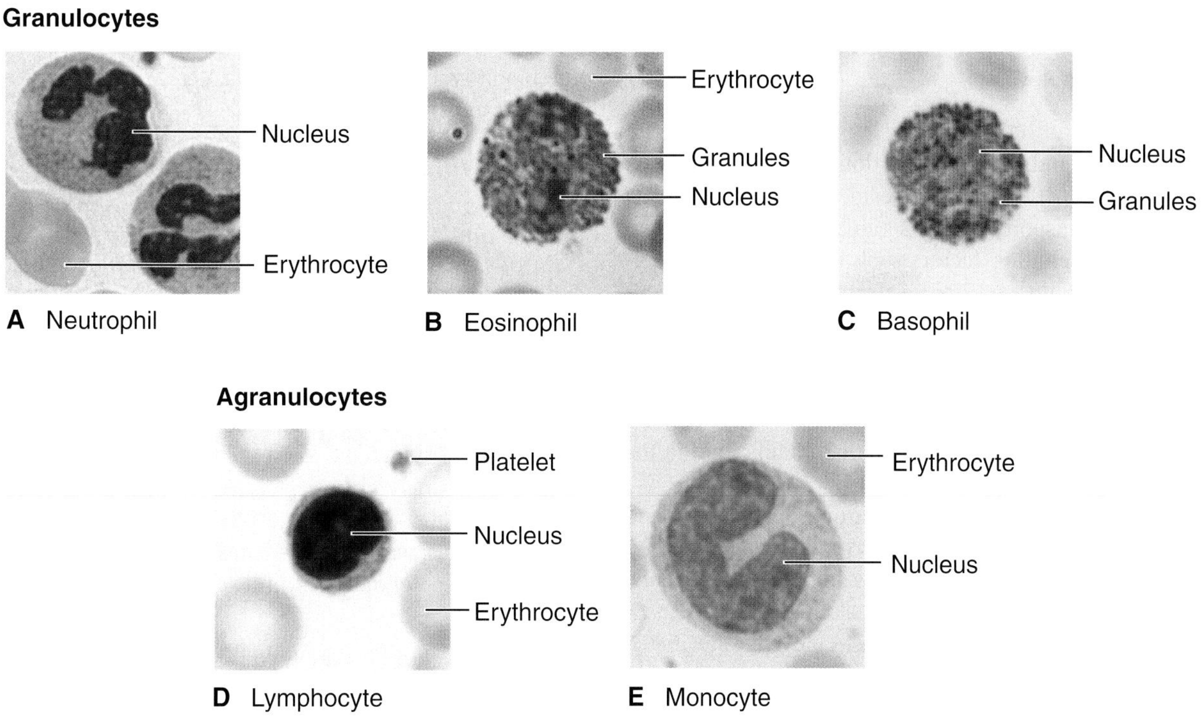

Figure 30-3 Categories of leukocytes (or white blood cells [WBCs]). *Granulocytes*: **(A)** neutrophil, **(B)** eosinophil, **(C)** basophil. *Agranulocytes*: **(D)** lymphocyte, **(E)** monocyte. (Reprinted with permission from Cohen, B. J., & Hull, K. L. (2012). *Memmler's the human body in health and disease* (12th ed.). Wolters Kluwer Health/Lippincott Williams & Wilkins.)

cells. Some lymphoid stem cells mature in the bone marrow, whereas others migrate to peripheral lymphoid tissue to complete their maturation.

Monocytes, also known as *macrophages* because they phagocytize large-sized debris, help combat severe infections and contribute to the immune response. They are antigen-presenting cells, which engulf microbial invaders and display the antigenic surface to T lymphocytes. T lymphocytes then engage B lymphocytes to make the appropriate antibody (see Chapter 34).

Platelets

Platelets (*thrombocytes*) are disklike, nonnucleated cell fragments with a lifespan of approximately 7.5 days. They are manufactured in the red bone marrow. Approximately two-thirds of the total 150,000 to 350,000/mm^3 platelets circulate in the blood and contribute to **hemostasis**, the control of bleeding. The remaining one-third are sequestered in the spleen, where they remain unless needed in cases of significant bleeding. When a blood vessel is injured, platelets migrate to the injury site. The platelets release a substance

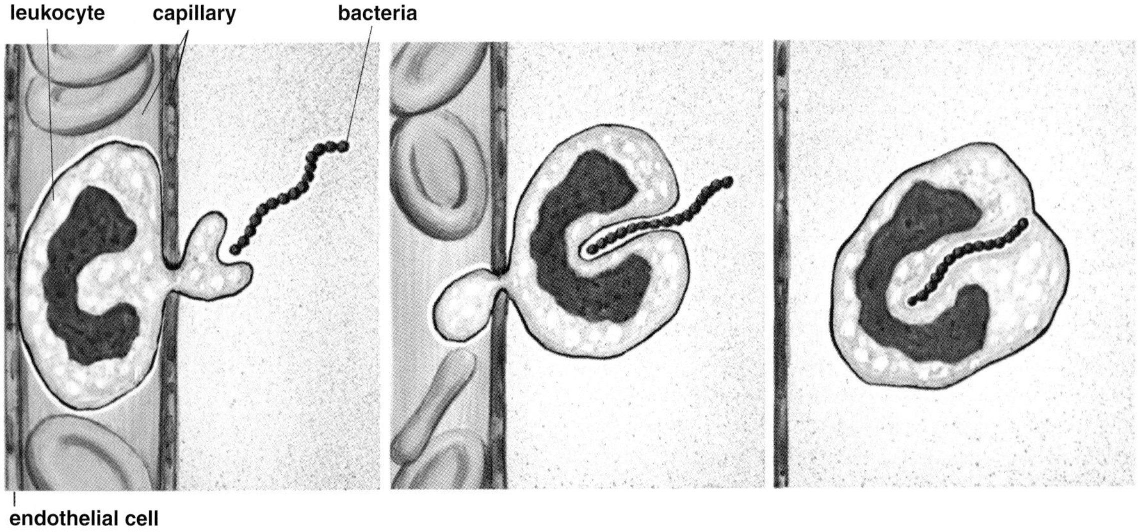

Figure 30-4 Phagocytosis. The cell membrane of the neutrophil surrounds and pinches off the bacterium or dead tissue. Enzymes within the cell destroy the foreign material. (Reprinted with permission from Smeltzer, S. C., Bare, B. G., Hinkle, J. L., & Cheever, K. H. (2010). *Brunner & Suddarth's textbook of medical-surgical nursing* (12th ed.). Wolters Kluwer Health/Lippincott Williams & Wilkins.)

known as glycoprotein IIb/IIIa, which causes the platelets to adhere (platelet aggregation) and form a plug, or clot, that occludes the injured vessel.

Plasma and Plasma Proteins

Plasma is the liquid, or serum, portion of blood. It consists of 90% water and 10% proteins. Besides blood cells, plasma contains and transports proteins (albumin, globulins, and fibrinogen) and clotting factors such as prothrombin, pigments, vitamins, glucose, lipids, electrolytes, minerals, enzymes, and hormones.

Albumin, which is formed in the liver, is the most abundant protein in plasma. Under normal conditions, albumin cannot pass through a capillary wall. Consequently, albumin helps maintain the osmotic pressure that retains fluid in the vascular compartment.

Globulins are divided into three groups: alpha, beta, and gamma. The gamma globulins are also called *immunoglobulins*. **Globulins** function primarily as immunologic agents; they prevent or modify some types of infectious diseases. Like albumin, they help maintain osmotic pressure in the vascular compartment.

Fibrinogen plays a key role in forming blood clots. It can be transformed from a liquid to fibrin, a solid that controls bleeding.

Blood Groups

There are four blood groups or types—A, B, AB, and O, which are determined by heredity. Blood type is ascertained by identifying the protein, or *antigen*, on the red cell membranes. Group A has A antigen, group B has B antigen, group AB has A and B antigen, and group O has no antigen. **Antibodies**, immunoglobulins in plasma that inactivate any substance that is nonself, react with incompatible RBC antigens. Therefore, people with type O blood are termed *universal donors* because they do not have antigens on the red cell membrane. Clients with all blood types can receive type O blood provided the Rh factor is compatible (discussed later). Those with type O blood, however, can only receive type O blood. People with type AB blood are considered universal recipients because both A and B antigens are present on the red cell membrane (see Chapter 13 and Table 13-4). Clients with type AB blood can receive blood from persons with any type of blood, but the Rh factor must be compatible.

The Rh factor is a specific protein on the RBC membrane. If the protein is present, the person is Rh positive. If the protein is absent, the person is Rh negative. When blood is transfused, donor blood must be both type and Rh compatible with the recipient's blood. The donor's blood is typed and labeled at the time of donation. When a blood transfusion is needed, the recipient's blood is typed and crossmatched (matched for compatibility with donor blood). Donor and recipient blood are considered compatible if there is no clumping or **hemolysis** (destruction of erythrocytes) when both samples are mixed in the laboratory. In an emergency, type O blood can be given to recipients with type A, B, AB, or O. People with Rh-positive blood can receive Rh-positive or Rh-negative blood because Rh negative indicates the Rh factor is missing. Those with Rh-negative blood, however, must never receive Rh-positive blood regardless of whether the blood type is compatible. Chapter 13 discusses various types of transfusion reactions.

››› *Stop, Think, and Respond 30-1*

When you go to the hospital's blood bank to obtain a unit of blood for a client with blood type A, Rh-positive blood, you receive a unit of blood that is blood type A, Rh negative. Is this unit of blood compatible? Explain your answer.

Lymphatic System

The lymphatic system includes the thymus gland, spleen, and a network of lymphatic vessels, lymph nodes, and lymph. This system of **lymphatics** circulates interstitial fluid and carries it to the veins (Fig. 30-5). Along the pathway, the lymphatic system filters and destroys pathogens and removes other potentially harmful substances.

Thymus Gland

The **thymus gland** is lymphoid tissue in the upper chest that contains undifferentiated stem cells released from bone marrow. Once the undifferentiated cells migrate to the thymus gland, they develop into *T lymphocytes*, so called because they are thymus derived (Fig. 30-6).

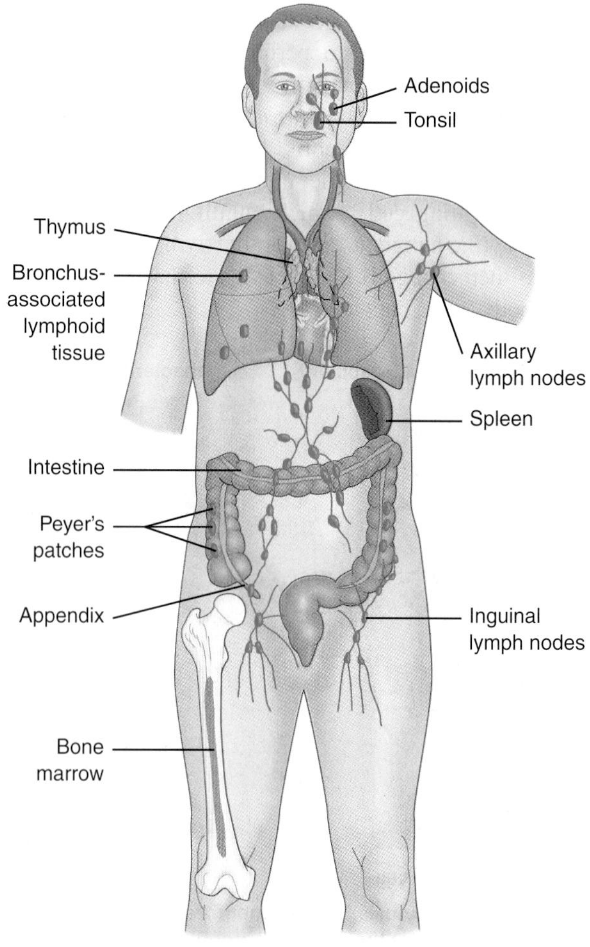

Figure 30-5 Central and peripheral lymphoid organs and tissues.

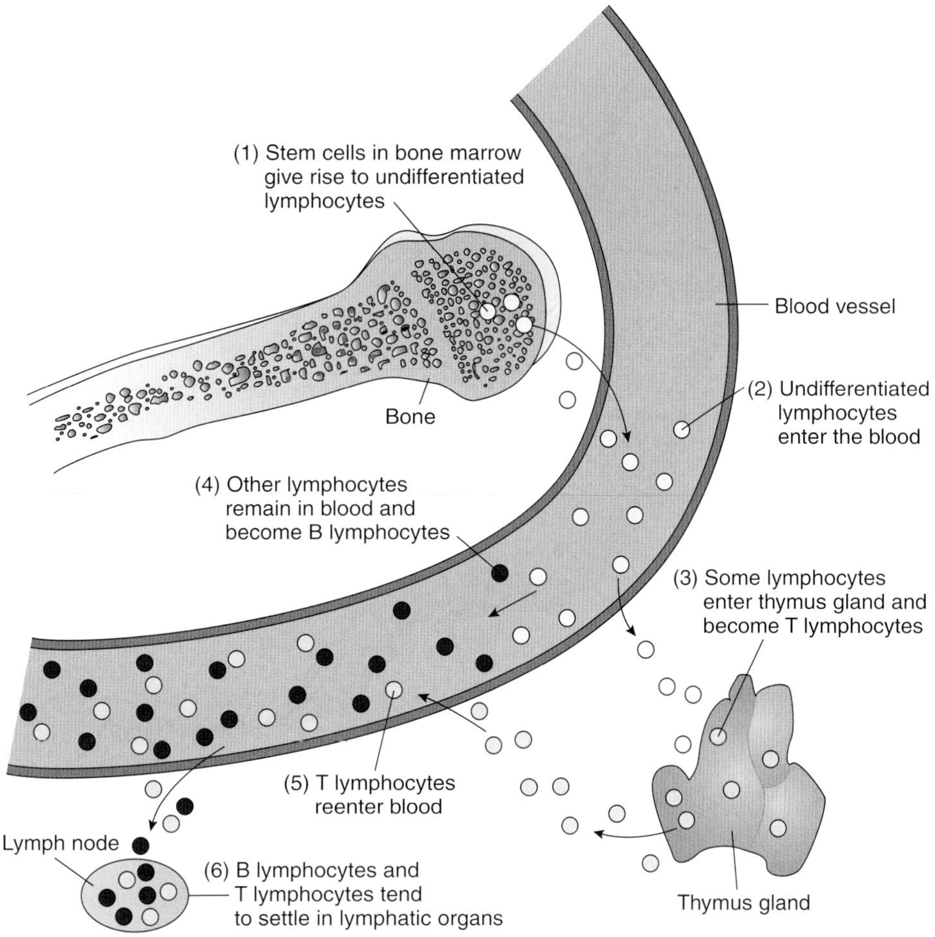
(1) Stem cells in bone marrow give rise to undifferentiated lymphocytes
Blood vessel
Bone
(2) Undifferentiated lymphocytes enter the blood
(4) Other lymphocytes remain in blood and become B lymphocytes
(3) Some lymphocytes enter thymus gland and become T lymphocytes
(5) T lymphocytes reenter blood
Lymph node
(6) B lymphocytes and T lymphocytes tend to settle in lymphatic organs
Thymus gland

Figure 30-6 Transformation of T and B lymphocytes.

Spleen

The spleen is the largest lymphatic structure. It lies in the abdomen beneath the diaphragm and behind the stomach. The **spleen** is a reservoir of blood and contains phagocytes that engulf damaged erythrocytes and foreign substances.

Lymph Nodes

Lymph nodes, glandular tissue along the lymphatic network, are clustered in the axilla, groin, neck, and large vessels of the thorax and abdomen. Lymphatic ducts, through which lymph flows, connect the nodes. The nodes contain both T and B lymphocytes (released from the bone marrow but do not reach the thymus gland) in the smaller nodules of each lymph node.

Lymph

Lymph is fluid with a composition similar to plasma. It flows through the lymphatic system by contraction of skeletal muscles. Lymph enters each node by way of the afferent lymph duct, passes through the node, and leaves by the efferent lymph duct (Fig. 30-7). As lymph passes through the node, macrophages attack and engulf foreign substances such as bacteria and viruses, abnormal body cells, and other debris.

ASSESSMENT

The nurse collects data by taking a health history, examining the client, and monitoring the results of laboratory tests.

History

The health history includes the client's description of signs and symptoms. If abnormalities are present, the nurse determines when the signs or symptoms began, their severity, and their frequency. In relation to the hematopoietic and lymphatic systems, it is important to establish if the client:

- Experiences prolonged bleeding from an obvious injury.
- Has unexplained blood loss, as in rectal bleeding, nosebleeds, bleeding gums, or vomiting blood.
- Feels fatigued with normal activities.
- Becomes dizzy or faints.
- Bruises easily.
- Is easily chilled.
- Has frequent infections.
- Feels discomfort in the axilla, groin, or neck.
- Has difficulty swallowing, with localized throat tenderness.

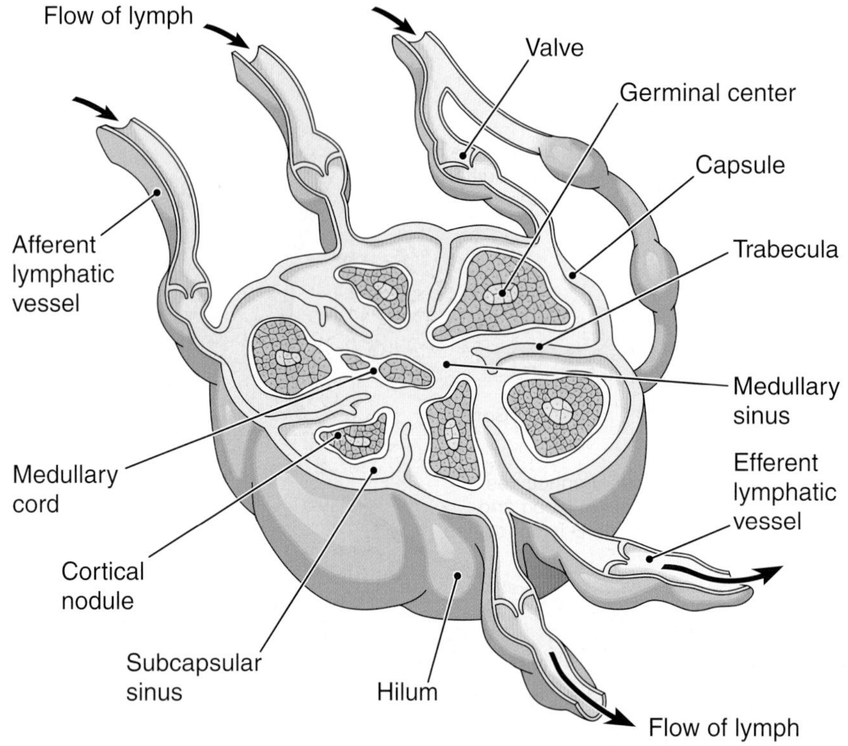

Figure 30-7 Structure of a lymph node. The lymph filters out bacteria that gain entry to the body. (Reprinted with permission from Cohen, B. J., & Hull, K. L. (2012). *Memmler's the human body in health and disease* (12th ed.). Wolters Kluwer Health/Lippincott Williams & Wilkins.)

- Has had surgery with lymph node removal or splenectomy, is undergoing treatment for cancer, or has renal failure—all of which may affect blood cell volume or lymphatic circulation.

The nurse obtains a dietary history because compromised nutrition interferes with the production of blood cells and hemoglobin (see Nutrition Notes).

The nurse takes a drug history of prescription and nonprescription medications. Some antibiotics and cancer drugs contribute to hematopoietic dysfunction. Aspirin and anticoagulants can contribute to bleeding and interfere with clot formation. Because industrial materials, environmental toxins, and household products also can affect blood-forming organs, the nurse explores any exposure to these agents.

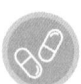

Pharmacologic Considerations

- Many pharmacologic agents affect the hematopoietic system, causing a decrease in various blood components. Closely monitor clients taking medications that depress the hematopoietic system, particularly thrombocytes and leukocytes, for signs of leukopenia (fever, sore throat, chills) and thrombocytopenia (unusual or easy bleeding; oozing from injection sites; bleeding gums; dark, tarry stools).
- The drug epoetin alfa (Epogen, Procrit) can be used to stimulate the production of RBCs. Filgrastim (Neupogen) and pegfilgrastim (Neulasta) promote proliferation of neutrophils.

The nurse also asks about foreign travel to countries where malaria or parasitic roundworms are common. The agent that causes malaria following the bite of an infected mosquito invades erythrocytes and causes anemia. Filariasis, also known as elephantiasis, is a consequence of a roundworm infection in which the lymphatic vessels become occluded (Fig. 30-8).

Physical Examination

Physical examination includes inspection of the skin with particular attention to color (e.g., normal, extreme redness,

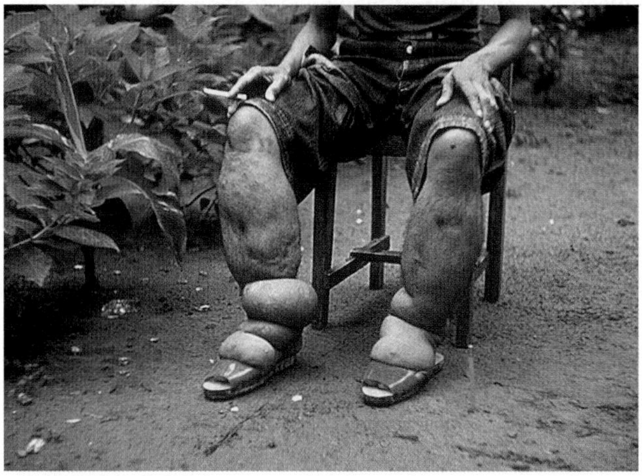

Figure 30-8 In filariasis, long, threadlike adult worms live in lymph nodes where they block the flow of lymph. Chronic filariasis leads to enlargement of legs and other structures—a condition known as elephantiasis. (Courtesy of the CDC.)

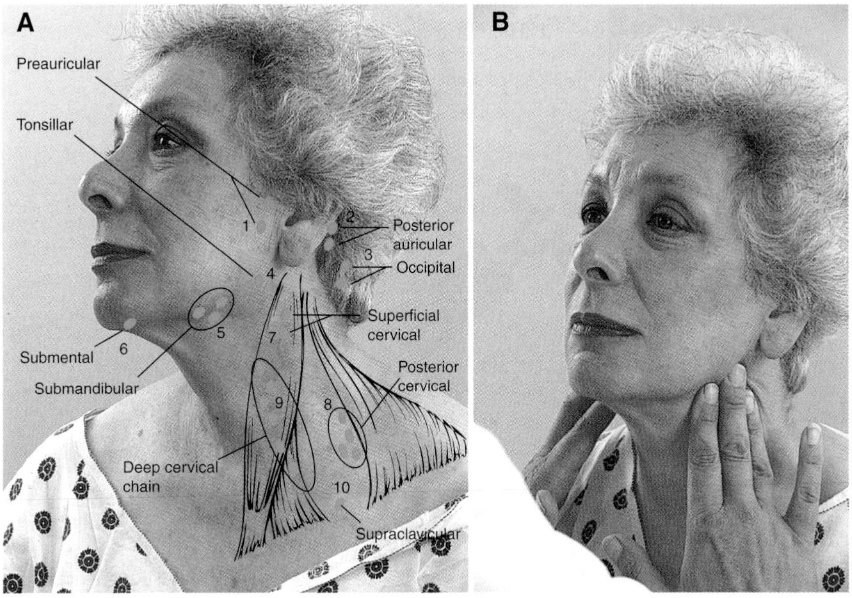

Figure 30-9 Assessment of cervical lymph nodes. **(A)** Locations of lymph nodes in the head and neck. **(B)** Palpation of tonsillar lymph nodes. (Photos by B. Proud.)

pallor), temperature, and ecchymosis or other lesions. A rapid pulse rate can indicate reduced erythrocytes or inadequate hemoglobin levels.

The nurse palpates the lymph nodes in the neck for tenderness or swelling and notes the size, location, and characteristics of symptomatic lymph nodes (Fig. 30-9). They examine the skin adjacent to the node for redness, streaking, and swelling.

Using a penlight and tongue blade, the nurse inspects the tonsils for size and appearance. If the tonsils are present, the nurse uses the following scale to document assessment findings related to size (Fig. 30-10):

- 1 = Tonsils are visible.
- 2 = Tonsils extend medially toward the uvula.
- 3 = Tonsils touch the uvula.
- 4 = Tonsils touch each other.

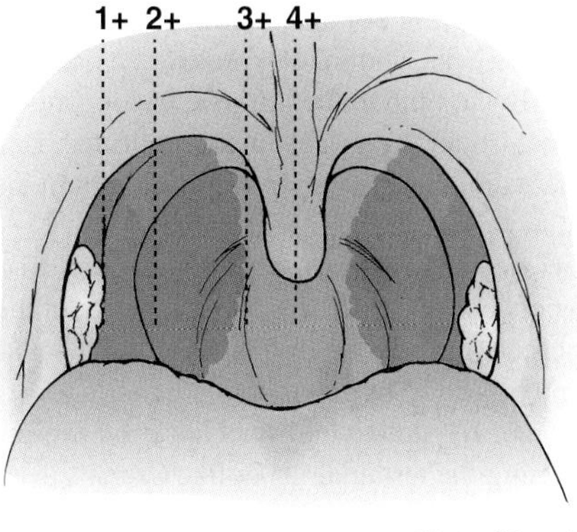

Figure 30-10 Assessing and grading tonsillitis. (Reprinted with permission from Weber, J. R. (2014). *Nurses' handbook of health assessment* (8th ed.). Wolters Kluwer Health/Lippincott Williams & Wilkins.)

Purulent exudate on the surface of the tonsils suggests tonsillitis.

The nurse examines the extremities to determine if they are of similar size—obstruction of lymphatic circulation can cause unilateral enlargement.

Diagnostic Tests

The nurse obtains a blood sample from a vein, finger, or earlobe. The blood sample is used to perform a complete blood count or to measure the hemoglobin. The primary provider may order other blood tests that reflect the client's clotting status, such as prothrombin time, fibrinogen level, activated partial thromboplastin time, D-dimer test for fibrin, fibrin degradation products, and factor assays.

A **bone marrow aspiration** is performed to determine the status of blood cell formation (Fig. 30-11). In this procedure, the primary provider applies local anesthesia and removes bone marrow from the posterior iliac crest or the sternum. The marrow is examined for the types and percentage of immature and maturing blood cells. The nurse assists the primary provider, supports the client during the procedure, and monitors the client's status afterward (Nursing Guidelines 30-1).

Lymphatic disorders are diagnosed using procedures such as lymph node biopsy, ultrasound of the spleen or selected lymph nodes, and lymphangiography (radiographic examination using contrast media). Additional diagnostic tests include radiography, computed tomography, bone scan, and magnetic resonance imaging. Although they are not specific for hematologic or lymphatic disorders, they are used to rule out other disorders or note changes in organs that have a direct or indirect relationship to a hematologic or lymphatic disorder.

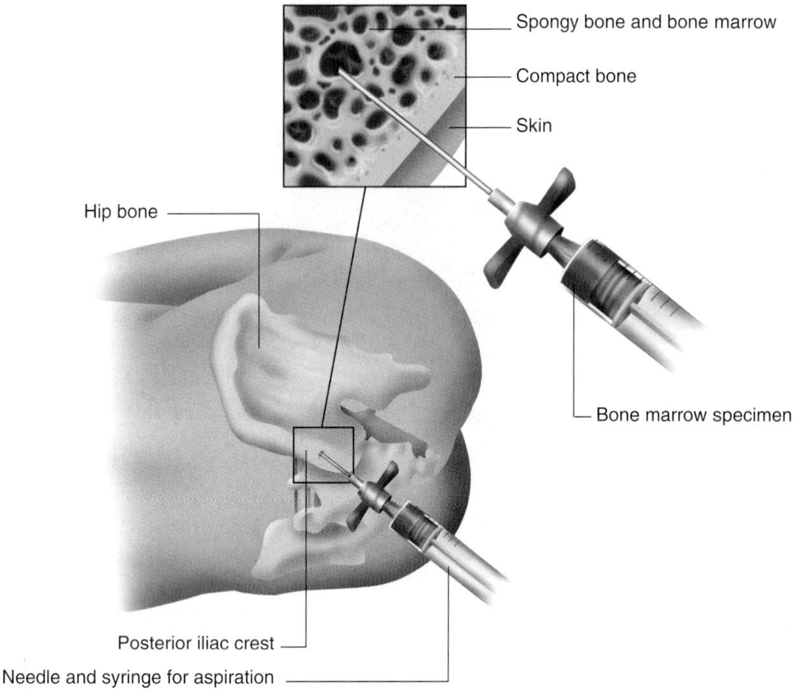

Figure 30-11 Bone marrow aspiration. (Reprinted with permission from Springhouse. (2009). *Lippincott's visual encyclopedia of clinical skills.* Wolters Kluwer Health/Lippincott Williams & Wilkins.)

NURSING GUIDELINES 30-1

Assisting With a Bone Marrow Aspiration

- Inform the client of the plan and approximate time for the bone marrow aspiration. Allow time to answer questions.
- Witness the client's signature on a consent form for the procedure as well as for conscious sedation.
- Check the client's medical record for history of allergies, especially to local anesthetics or latex, and the results of coagulation studies that may have been performed.
- Obtain a sterile bone marrow aspiration tray and the type and strength of local anesthetic according to the primary provider's orders.
- Determine the site from which the primary provider intends to obtain the sample of bone marrow, for example, iliac crest or sternum. The posterior superior iliac crest is the preferred site because no vital organs or blood vessels are nearby. Aspiration from the sternum involves the greatest risk but may be used because the site is near the surface, the bone is thin, and the marrow contains numerous cells (Gendron et al., 2019).
- Attach a pulse oximeter to the client's finger to monitor oxygenation that may be compromised when conscious sedation is used.
- Position the client on their back or side to facilitate access to the aspiration site.
- Cleanse, clip hair, and drape the skin at the test site.
- Suggest distraction techniques to avoid focusing on the pressure or discomfort associated with puncturing the bone that may take approximately 20 minutes.
- Administer analgesia for significant discomfort.
- Be prepared to place samples of the aspirate on slides and allow them to dry.
- Label the biopsy specimen once in preservative and ensure its delivery to the laboratory.
- Follow standard precautions when there is a potential for contact with blood from the client, equipment, and bedside environment.
- Apply direct pressure followed by a pressure dressing to the site after the needle has been withdrawn.
- Instruct the client to lie on the site for at least 10 minutes or longer.
- Limit the client's activity for approximately 30 minutes after the procedure.
- Monitor the puncture site frequently for continued bleeding; change or reinforce the dressing as needed.
- Report prolonged bleeding, unusual pain at the site that is unrelieved by analgesics, fever, and other signs of an infection such as swelling and purulent drainage.
- Delay bathing or showering for 24 hours.

A **Schilling test** is used to determine the etiology of vitamin B_{12} (cobalamin) deficiency causing pernicious anemia. The test is performed in four separate stages. In each stage oral radiolabeled vitamin B_{12} is administered. Radiolabeled means the substance has been tagged with a radioactive tracer. In the first and subsequent stages, the oral radiolabeled vitamin B_{12} is combined with an intramuscular injection of nonradiolabeled vitamin B_{12}, then oral intrinsic factor which is secreted by parietal cells in the stomach to aid absorption of the vitamin, next an antibiotic like tetracycline for 2 weeks, and finally, protease, a pancreatic enzyme that frees B_{12} to bind to the intrinsic factor. After each stage is completed, a 24-hour urine specimen is collected. Depending on whether the radiolabeled vitamin is low or high in the urine, the etiology may be one of the following:

- Dietary deficiency of vitamin B_{12} that often occurs among vegans who do not consume animal protein, a source of the vitamin,
- Deficiency of the intrinsic factor that may be due to having had a gastrectomy or gastric bypass,
- Malabsorption of B_{12} due to intestinal bacterial overgrowth or a disorder affecting the terminal ileum like Crohn's disease where a major portion of B_{12} is absorbed, or
- Deficiency of protease, common among those with pancreatitis, that interferes with the binding of free B_{12} to the intrinsic factor.

Once the etiology is determined, the treatment of the anemia is based on its cause. (Also see Evidence-Based Practice 30-1.)

Evidence-Based Practice 30-1

Anemia

Clinical Question

What is included in the nursing management of a client with anemia?

Evidence

Anemia is a decrease in the number of RBCs in the human body. This could be due to an underproduction, destruction of the cells, or trauma or loss of the cells. According to the National Heart, Lung, Blood Institute (2020), the signs and symptoms of anemia include: dizziness, shortness of breath, chest pain, headache, pale skin color, and decreased temperature in extremities. Clients with anemia are also at risk for arrhythmias, further weakened immune systems if they are immunocompromised, and possible organ damage (Warner & Kamran, 2020).

Nursing Implications

This article indicates a strong need for nurses to assess clients for symptoms of the above-stated risk factors. Nurses should record and monitor vital signs, perform a thorough respiratory assessment, monitor fluids, and review labs. Anemia can have an impact on other health issues, so a thorough assessment and monitoring of clients should occur.

Reference

National Heart, Lung, Blood Institute. (2020). *Anemia?* http://www.nhlbi.nih.gov/health/health-topics/topics/anemia/signs

Warner, M. J., & Kamran M. T. (2020). *Iron deficiency anemia.* StatPearls. StatPearls Publishing. https://www.ncbi.nlm.nih.gov/books/NBK448065/

NURSING MANAGEMENT

The nurse collects appropriate data to assist the primary provider in diagnosing hematologic or lymphatic disorders and the client's response to treatment. Before any diagnostic testing, the nurse determines the client's knowledge of the procedure and offers a description of the test routine, what tasks are necessary to participate in the test, and any potential for discomfort.

The nurse wears gloves when collecting specimens. After collection, they check the specimen for the correct label and immediately take it to the laboratory. When the test involves a puncture, the nurse assesses the area for excessive bleeding and applies pressure or a pressure dressing to the site as needed. The nurse monitors vital signs to assess the client's recovery, notifies the primary provider regarding adverse responses, and analyzes and reports test results promptly.

KEY POINTS

- Anatomy and physiology
  - Hematopoietic system
    - Bone marrow: soft tissue inside bones that manufactures blood cells
    - Blood: cells suspended in plasma. Consists of erythrocytes, leukocytes, platelets, plasma, and plasma proteins
    - Blood groups: four main types (A, B, AB, and O) with each having an Rh positive or Rh negative factor
  - Lymphatic system
    - Thymus gland: in upper chest
    - Spleen: in abdomen beneath the diaphragm, is a reservoir of blood
    - Lymph nodes: glandular tissue along the lymphatic network
    - Lymph: fluid with a composition similar to plasma
- Assessment should include:
  - History
  - Physical examination
  - Diagnostic test: as indicated and ordered, including blood tests such as complete blood count, prothrombin time, D-dimer, and fibrin degradation products
    - Bone marrow aspiration: to determine status of blood cell formation
    - Schilling test to determine cause of vitamin B12 deficiency
- Nursing management should include collecting appropriate data, assisting with any testing, monitoring client before, during, and after procedures.

CRITICAL THINKING EXERCISES

1. Describe the process of blood cell formation.
2. Describe the nurse's responsibilities when assisting with bone marrow aspiration.
3. Three clients have the following blood count values:
   Client A = 80,000/mm^3 platelets
   Client B = 2,400,000/mm^3 RBCs
   Client C = 24,500/mm^3 WBCs

   After notifying the primary provider, what precautions are appropriate?
4. A client reports feeling chronically fatigued and chilled when others feel comfortable. The client has a heart rate of 92 beats/min at rest and a blood pressure of 110/60 mm Hg. The skin, conjunctiva, and mucous membranes are pale. What additional information is important to obtain? What laboratory or diagnostic tests can the nurse anticipate the primary provider will order?

NCLEX-STYLE REVIEW QUESTIONS PrepU

1. A complete blood count indicates that a client is anemic. What disorder in the client's health history is most likely contributing to the reduction in red blood cells?
   1. Osteoarthritis
   2. Renal failure
   3. Emphysema
   4. Diabetes mellitus

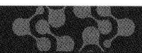

2. When the nurse reviews a client's complete blood cell count, what finding is most suggestive that a client is at risk for acquiring an infection?
1. Low number of platelets
2. Low number of erythrocytes
3. Low number of granulocytes
4. Low number of agranulocytes

3. A primary provider tells a client that her body is not making enough blood cells. After the primary provider leaves, the client appears very upset and states, "I do not even know how my body is supposed to make blood cells." What is the simplest, yet correct, instruction for the nurse to give the client at this time?
1. Complex mechanisms within the body make blood cells.
2. The bone marrow produces blood cells.
3. Blood cells originate from a healthy immune system.
4. The lymphatic system produces blood cells.

4. What blood type could be transfused into anyone if there is no time to perform a type and crossmatch of the recipient's blood?
1. AB, Rh positive
2. AB, Rh negative
3. O, Rh positive
4. O, Rh negative

5. After completion of a bone marrow aspiration, what is most important for the nurse to monitor?
1. Fluctuations in blood pressure
2. Bleeding from the puncture site
3. Changes in the client's pulse
4. Level of consciousness

WANT TO KNOW MORE? There are a wide variety of online resources available on thePoint to enhance learning and understanding of this chapter.

Go to **thePoint.lww.com/activate** and use the activation code found in the front of this text to unlock these online resources.

31 Caring for Clients With Disorders of the Hematopoietic System

Words To Know

acute chest syndrome
agranulocytosis
anemia
aplasia
aplastic anemia
blood dyscrasias
chelation therapy
coagulopathy
erythrocytosis
folic acid–deficiency anemia
graft-versus-host disease
heme
hemoglobin A (HbA)
hemoglobin F (HbF)
hemoglobin polymerization
hemoglobin S (HbS)
hemolytic anemia
hemophilia
leukemia
leukocytosis
leukopenia
multiple myeloma
osteoclasts
osteolytic tumors
pancytopenia
pernicious anemia
phlebotomy
polycythemia vera
purpura
sickle cell crisis
sickle cell disease
thalassemias
thrombocytopenia

Learning Objectives

On completion of this chapter, you will be able to:

1. List seven types of anemia, including examples of inherited types.
2. Identify nutritional deficiencies that can lead to anemia.
3. Discuss clinical problems that clients with any type of anemia experience.
4. Discuss factors that cause sickling of erythrocytes and related adverse effects.
5. List activities a person with sickle cell disease can do to reduce the potential for a sickle cell crisis.
6. Explain the term *erythrocytosis*, give one example of a characteristic disease, and list possible complications.
7. Explain how forms of leukemia are classified.
8. List clinical problems or nursing diagnoses common among clients with leukemia.
9. Explain how the bone marrow dysfunction of multiple myeloma has an effect on the skeletal system.
10. Differentiate agranulocytosis from leukopenia.
11. Explain the term *pancytopenia* and give an example of a disorder that represents this condition.
12. Discuss the meaning of *coagulopathy* and name two coagulopathies.
13. Discuss nursing responsibilities when managing the care of clients with coagulopathies.

This chapter discusses common **blood dyscrasias**, abnormalities in the numbers and types of blood cells, and coagulopathies, bleeding disorders that involve platelets or clotting factors. These disorders develop from various pathologic processes, some of which are life threatening. Despite their differences, many blood disorders have similar symptoms and require similar diagnostic tests.

Gerontologic Considerations

- Iron-deficiency anemia is unusual in older adults. Normally, the body does not eliminate excessive iron, causing total body iron stores to increase with age and necessitating maintenance of hydration. If an older adult is anemic, blood loss from the gastrointestinal (GI) or genitourinary tract is suspected.
- Iron-deficiency anemia can develop in older adults because of inadequate intake of iron for many reasons, including living on a fixed income, being unable to shop for food, and lacking energy or motivation to prepare complete meals. Thorough evaluation of dietary habits and education related to methods of preventing iron-deficiency anemia is needed in this client set.
- Pernicious anemia can cause memory loss, dementia, confusion, and depression. These neurological symptoms for clients experiencing cognitive changes should indicate a need for screening to prevent neurologic damage (National Heart, Lung, and Blood Institute, 2020).
- Decreased levels of gastric acidity can affect absorption of vitamin B_{12}, suggesting careful evaluation of older individuals and/or those who take antacid medications.
- Folic acid deficiency may play a role in depression, cognitive decline, and psychosis. Folic acid levels should be measured in older clients who exhibit signs of these symptoms (Khan & Jialal, 2020).
- Both acute and chronic leukemias are prevalent in older adults. Older adults with acute lymphoblastic leukemia have a poor prognosis owing to the lack of tolerance to pancytopenia that results from prolonged. Rates of both chronic lymphocytic leukemias (CLLs) and chronic myelogenous leukemia (CML) increase in adults aged 50 years and older.
- Individual comorbidities, level of functional reserve and preference should be considered for best management strategies for older adults with CLL.

ANEMIA

Erythrocytes are mature red blood cells (RBCs) to which hemoglobin is attached. Their function is to carry oxygen to cells and transport carbon dioxide (CO_2) to the lungs. **Anemia** is a term that refers to a deficiency of either erythrocytes or hemoglobin. Various terms are used to differentiate the features of erythrocytes and describe pathogenesis related to them (Table 31-1).

Most anemias result from (1) blood loss, (2) inadequate or abnormal erythrocyte production, or (3) destruction of normally formed RBCs. The most common types include hypovolemic anemia, iron-deficiency anemia, pernicious anemia, folic acid–deficiency anemia, sickle cell anemia, and hemolytic anemias. Although each form of anemia has unique manifestations, all share a common core of symptoms (Box 31-1).

TABLE 31-1 Terms Used to Describe Erythrocytes and Erythrocyte Pathology

DESCRIPTOR	MEANING
Normocytic	Normal cell size
Microcytic	Small cell size
Macrocytic	Large cell size
Megaloblastic	Large immature cell
Normochromic	Normal hemoglobin concentration
Hypochromic	Low hemoglobin concentration
Hyperchromic	High hemoglobin concentration
Aplastic	Decreased cell production
Hemolytic	Premature destruction
Pernicious	Potentially injurious

BOX 31-1 Clinical Manifestations of Anemia

Inadequate RBC Volume
Orthostatic hypotension
Thready pulses
Oliguria
Heart murmur

Compensatory Mechanisms for Lost RBC Function
Tachycardia
Tachypnea
Cool, clammy skin
Amenorrhea
Decreased RBC function
Dyspnea
Chest discomfort
Acidosis
Headache
Vertigo
Pallor
Constipation
Difficulty concentrating
Decreased bowel sounds

Hypovolemic Anemia

Hypovolemia is caused by a loss of blood volume, which results in fewer blood cells. Because erythrocytes are the most abundant type of blood cell, one consequence of blood loss is *hypovolemic anemia.*

Pathophysiology and Etiology

Hypovolemic anemia can occur as a consequence of a sudden loss of a large volume of blood or a gradual, chronic loss of small amounts of blood. An example of the former is trauma, such as a gunshot wound; an example of the latter is gastric bleeding from a peptic ulcer. When blood is lost, the bone marrow responds by increasing production of erythrocytes. As a result, the cells are smaller and contain less **heme**, the pigmented, iron-containing portion of

TABLE 31-2 Normal Complete Blood Count (CBC) Values

COMPONENT	ADULT MEN	ADULT WOMEN
Red Blood Cells (Erythrocytes) (million/mm^3)	4.6–6.2	4.2–5.4
Hematocrit (%)	40–54	38–47
Hemoglobin (g/dL)	13.5–18	12–16
Mean cell volume (MCV) (μg/m^3)	80–94	81–99
Mean cell hemoglobin (MCH) (pg/cell)	27–31	27–31
Mean cell hemoglobin concentration (MCHC) (g/dL)	32–36	32–36
Reticulocytes	0.5%–2.0% of RBCs	Slightly higher in females
White Blood Cells (Leukocytes) (per mm^3)	5000–13,000	5000–10,000
Neutrophils (per mm^3)	3000–7500	3000–7500
Eosinophils (per mm^3)	50–400	50–400
Basophils (per mm^3)	25–100	25–100
Monocytes (per mm^3)	100–500	100–500
Lymphocytes (per mm^3)	1500–4500	1500–4500
T lymphocytes	60%–80% of lymphocytes	60%–80% of lymphocytes
B lymphocytes	10%–20% of lymphocytes	10%–20% of lymphocytes
Platelets (per mm^3)	150,000–450,000	150,000–450,000

RBCs, red blood cells.

hemoglobin. Consequently, the RBCs are microcytic and hypochromic (see Table 31-1). If the formation of new RBCs cannot compensate for the loss, cellular function is compromised from an inadequate oxygen supply and accumulated CO_2.

Pharmacologic Considerations

- Low-dose aspirin, nonsteroidal anti-inflammatory drugs (NSAIDs), or a COX-2 inhibitor are all known to increase risk for GI bleeding. When taken with selective serotonin reuptake inhibitor (SSRI) antidepressants, the risk increases significantly. Corticosteroids, aldosterone antagonists and anticoagulants also increase the risk of GI bleeding with aspirin and NSAIDs, but not with a COX-2 inhibitor (Masclee et al., 2014).

Assessment Findings

Acute hypovolemic anemia from severe blood loss is evidenced by signs and symptoms of hypovolemic shock: extreme pallor, tachycardia, hypotension, reduced urine output, and altered consciousness (see Chapter 17). Symptoms of chronic hypovolemic anemia include pallor, fatigue, chills, postural hypotension, and rapid heart and respiratory rates.

Acute or chronic hypovolemic anemia is confirmed in the laboratory through a complete blood count (CBC), which demonstrates decreased erythrocytes, increased *reticulocytes* (erythrocytes in the process of maturation), and low hemoglobin and hematocrit levels (Table 31-2). Mean cell volume is lower than normal as a result of the smaller size of the erythrocytes. The mean cell hemoglobin concentration is below normal, reflecting the reduced hemoglobin level.

Medical Management

Treatment of sudden severe bleeding requires replacement of blood by transfusions. If blood loss is chronic (e.g., from bleeding uterine tumors, peptic ulcer disease, hemorrhoids), the underlying condition is treated. Depending on how much blood is lost, treatment includes blood transfusion or administration of oral, intravenous (IV), or intramuscular (IM) iron to help restore the body's hemoglobin. Oxygen therapy sometimes is necessary if the anemia is severe.

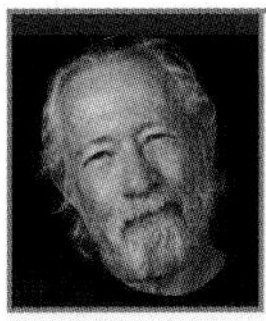

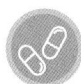

Clinical Scenario A 56-year-old client tells the nurse that they have felt "wiped out" for quite some time and feels chilled when others do not. The client says their fatigue has interfered with performing home maintenance. They report not having the energy to play golf and participate in other activities they enjoy. The client has osteoarthritis for which the client takes multiple daily doses of aspirin. The client has been vomiting bright red blood and has noticed that stools are of a dark color. The client's spouse is concerned about the vomiting and because the client has been fainting lately. **How might the nurse proceed to manage this client's care? See the following Nursing Process section.**

NURSING PROCESS FOR THE CLIENT WITH HYPOVOLEMIC ANEMIA

Assessment

Question the client to determine possible reasons for the presenting symptoms, obtain vital signs, review laboratory test results, prepare the client for diagnostic tests such as endoscopic examinations, and perform a physical examination to detect sources of bleeding.

Diagnosis, Planning, and Interventions

Activity Intolerance: Related to reduced cellular capacity to carry oxygen
Expected Outcomes: The client will (1) tolerate essential activity as evidenced by a heart rate below 100 beats/min and (2) have a respiratory rate less than 28 breaths/min.

- Limit the client's nonessential activities. *Demands for cellular oxygenation are controlled according to the available supply.*
- Distribute essential tasks over a long period. *Minimizing exertion promotes endurance.*
- Provide periods of rest. *Rest prevents acute hypoxemia.*
- Administer supplemental oxygen during periods of rapid breathing or tachycardia. *Short-term, periodic oxygen administration relieves brief episodes of hypoxemia.*

Hypovolemia

Expected Outcome: The nurse will monitor to detect hypovolemia and manage and minimize blood loss.

- Monitor the results of CBC, especially RBC count and hematocrit and hemoglobin levels. *Lower-than-normal RBCs and hemoglobin level reflect blood cell loss. The hematocrit level indicates the percentage of RBCs in the volume of whole blood.*
- Assess vital signs every 2 to 4 hours or more often if indicated. *Hypotension and tachycardia are signs of hypovolemia. Changes in vital signs indicate worsening, stabilization, or improvement in the client's condition.*
- Report systolic blood pressure (BP) below 90 mm Hg and heart rate above 100 beats/min. *The normal adult systolic BP is between 100 and 119 mm Hg. Decreasing BP reflects hypovolemia and shock. Tachycardia is a heart rate above 100 beats/min. A rapid heart rate indicates a compensatory mechanism to oxygenate cells.*
- Monitor intake and output accurately each shift or every hour. *Urine output is one indication of the circulating blood volume.*
- Report urine output less than 30 to 50 mL/hour. *Low urine volume reflects inadequate renal perfusion. The kidneys must excrete 30 to 50 mL/hour or 500 mL/24 hours to eliminate wastes sufficiently.*
- Use standard precautions to examine and test stool and body fluids for evidence of blood. *Blood may be occult (hidden) rather than obvious. Nurses commonly perform tests to detect blood in stool and body fluids.*
- In cases of traumatic hemorrhage, apply direct pressure to the bleeding site. Alternatively, apply pressure to a proximal artery. *Compression of blood vessels decreases blood loss.*
- If an IV solution is infusing, increase the rate of flow if the client is bleeding profusely. *A temporary increase in IV fluid administration compensates briefly for rapid blood loss.*
- Place the client in a modified Trendelenburg position if hypovolemic shock develops. *This position facilitates blood flow to the brain.*
- Notify the primary provider and be prepared to administer blood or blood products. *Crystalloid solutions do not contain blood cells (see* Chapter 13). *The most definitive management of hypovolemic anemia is to replace lost blood cells.*
- Supplement parenteral fluids with oral fluids, if possible. *Oral fluids contribute to intravascular fluid replacement.*
- Prepare the client with gastric bleeding for an endoscopy. *An upper endoscopic examination is necessary to diagnose and assess the source of bleeding.*

Impaired Gas Exchange

Expected Outcome: The nurse will monitor to detect hypoxemia and manage and minimize inadequate oxygenation related to impaired gas exchange.

- Monitor oxygen saturation continuously with a pulse oximeter. *It measures the percentage of oxygen bound to hemoglobin.*
- Report a sustained oxygen saturation value below 90%. *Normal oxygen saturation is 95% to 100%; clients become compromised when oxygen saturation falls below 90%.*
- Give oxygen per nasal cannula or simple mask to maintain oxygen saturation at or above 90%. *Supplemental oxygen delivers more than 21% oxygen present in room air.*

Thermal Injury Risk: Related to reduced oxygen for aerobic metabolism
Expected Outcome: Temperature will remain at 98.6°F plus or minus 1°F.

- Prevent drafts. *Air circulating over the body promotes heat loss by convection.*
- Provide additional layers of clothing or cover with warmed blankets. *Covering the client in layers of fabric keeps body heat from escaping.*
- Increase the room temperature and add humidity. *Warming the environment decreases heat loss from convection or conduction. The heat index increases when air contains moisture. Increasing environmental humidity reduces heat loss through evaporation.*
- Offer warm oral fluids. *They maintain or promote an increase in core body temperature.*

Knowledge Deficiency: Related to lack of awareness of aspirin side effects as manifested by chronic use of aspirin to control symptoms of osteoarthritis
Expected Outcome: The client will identify the potential for gastric bleeding from self-administration of aspirin and relate alternatives to avoid gastric irritation by the time of discharge.

NURSING PROCESS FOR THE CLIENT WITH HYPOVOLEMIC ANEMIA (continued)

- Explain that aspirin and other NSAIDs decrease the production of prostaglandins. *Prostaglandins, which are produced in the stomach, protect and restore gastric and duodenal mucosa. Gastric ulceration and bleeding are not appreciably reduced when these drugs are buffered or enteric-coated.*
- Prepare to teach the client about self-administration of medications such as a proton pump inhibitor, for example, omeprazole (Prilosec); an H_2-receptor antagonist such as famotidine (Pepcid). *Proton pump inhibitors reduce acid secretion from gastric parietal cells and the secondary release of pepsinogen. Raising the gastric pH to 6 or higher helps promote platelet aggregation and epithelial cell proliferation, which reduces bleeding and fosters mucosal healing. H_2 receptors such as famotidine (Pepcid) and cimetidine (Tagamet) may be compromised by client compliance because they are generally dosed twice or more daily.* Anticipate that the primary provider may prescribe a selective COX-2 inhibitor such as celecoxib (Celebrex) as an alternative to aspirin. *A COX-2 inhibitor spares COX-1, an enzyme known as cyclooxygenase, which facilitates prostaglandin production while relieving joint inflammation. A COX-2 inhibitor significantly lowers GI events and complications.*
- Advise the client to avoid combining an NSAID such as ibuprofen with aspirin, drinking alcohol, or ingesting other stomach-irritating substances when taking aspirin or NSAIDs. *The gastric mucosa is more susceptible to damage when gastric prostaglandin synthesis is suppressed or the mucosa is subjected to multiple inflammatory substances.*
- Tell the client to take aspirin or other NSAIDs with food or milk. *Taking these medications with food or milk decreases gastric irritation.*
- Recommend that the client inform any and all primary providers about a history of gastric bleeding related to aspirin or NSAID therapy. *Other drugs, such as corticosteroids, increase the risk for gastric distress and bleeding and should be used cautiously or not at all with aspirin or NSAIDs.*

Evaluation of Expected Outcomes

The client's BP and heart rate are within normal target ranges before, during, and after performing activities of daily living (ADLs). Blood volume is restored or blood loss is minimized; RBC count and hematocrit level are within normal ranges. The client has 90% or greater saturation of hemoglobin. Body temperature is within 97.6°F to 99.6°F. The client accurately paraphrases information about the side effects of anti-inflammatory medications and methods for minimizing GI complications. The client identifies the purpose for concomitantly prescribed drugs and the schedule for their self-administration.

Iron-Deficiency Anemia

Pathophysiology and Etiology

Iron-deficiency anemia develops when iron is insufficient to produce hemoglobin. Examples include when (1) heme cannot be recycled because of blood loss, (2) dietary intake of iron is insufficient, (3) absorption of iron from food is inadequate, and (4) the need for iron exceeds the reserves. Even those who consume a healthy diet absorb less than 10% of the iron in food. Clients whose nutrition is compromised by unhealthy dieting or who cannot afford to eat a healthy diet, lack knowledge about nutrition, or have malabsorption disorders are at great risk for iron-deficiency anemia. The need for iron increases during periods of rapid growth, pregnancy, and the female reproductive years when intermittent blood loss accompanies menses.

When iron deficiency develops, the iron stores in the body are depleted first, followed by reduced hemoglobin. The result is smaller (microcytic) and fewer RBCs, which leads to manifestations of anemia. Reduced hemoglobin, for whatever reason, compromises the oxygen-carrying capacity of RBCs. Without sufficient oxygen, cells must switch to anaerobic metabolism, which is less efficient than aerobic metabolism at producing energy and sustaining functions at the cellular level.

Assessment Findings

Most clients with iron-deficiency anemia have reduced energy, feel cold all the time, and experience fatigue and dyspnea with minor physical exertion. The heart rate usually is rapid even at rest. The CBC and hemoglobin, hematocrit, and serum iron levels are decreased. A blood smear reveals erythrocytes that are *microcytic* (smaller than normal) and *hypochromic* (lighter in color than normal). Other laboratory and diagnostic tests (e.g., stool examination for occult blood) reveal the source of blood loss.

Medical Management

Treatment aims at determining the cause and, when possible, eliminating it. Correction of a faulty diet by adding foods high in iron is an important aspect of treatment. In some instances, an oral supplement or parenteral administration of iron is prescribed. In severe cases, a blood transfusion is necessary, but transfusion is the most expensive and potentially dangerous method for replacing iron.

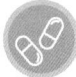

Pharmacologic Considerations

- Newer research suggests oral iron supplements be taken every other day (Moretti, 2015) because of the effect of iron on hepcidin, a hormone synthesized by the liver, that regulates iron absorption and distribution to the tissues. An excess of iron stimulates hepcidin and blocks dietary iron absorption. Iron deficiency suppresses hepcidin allowing increased absorption of dietary iron and replenishment of iron stores. Taking an oral iron supplement every other day rather than daily or twice daily promotes the efficacy of iron absorption.

Nursing Management

The nurse focuses on improving the client's nutritional intake of iron. The nurse takes a dietary history and collaborates with the dietitian to resolve dietary deficiencies (Nutrition Notes 31-1).

Nutrition Notes 31-1

The Client With Iron-Deficiency Anemia

- Heme iron is found in animal foods such as beef, pork, lamb, egg yolks, oysters, and the dark meat of poultry. It is well absorbed, and its rate of absorption is influenced only by need, not by other dietary factors.
- Adding three servings of lean meats per week in the context of a nutrient-rich diet is recommended to help correct iron-deficiency anemia.
- Nonheme iron is found in plant foods such as enriched and whole-grain breads, iron-fortified cereals, legumes, and nuts.
- Absorption of nonheme iron is greatly affected by other dietary factors. Vitamin C (citrus fruits and juices, strawberries, red peppers, tomatoes) and foods high in heme iron, such as beef, pork, lamb, or egg yolks, *enhance* the absorption of nonheme iron when eaten at the same time. Tea, coffee, and wheat bran *inhibit the* absorption of nonheme iron when eaten at the same time.
- To maximize nonheme iron absorption, the client should consume a rich source of vitamin C at every meal and avoid coffee and tea around and during mealtime.

In addition, they administer the prescribed oral or parenteral iron supplementation. If a client is taking an oral iron supplement, the nurse instructs as follows:

- Dilute liquid preparations of iron with another liquid such as juice and drink with a straw to avoid staining the teeth.
- Take iron on an empty stomach unless gastric upset occurs; then take with or immediately after meals.
- Avoid taking iron simultaneously with an antacid, which interferes with iron absorption.
- Check with the primary provider or pharmacist about combining iron with other prescribed or over-the-counter medications to determine appropriate absorption of each.
- Drink orange juice or take other forms of vitamin C with iron to promote its absorption.
- Expect iron to color stool dark green or black.
- Consult the prescribing primary provider if constipation or diarrhea develops.
- Keep medications containing iron out of the reach of small children, for whom an accidental poisoning may be fatal.

The nurse uses the Z-track technique to administer IM iron (Nursing Guidelines 31-1). For a review of blood transfusion, see Chapter 13. Discharge instructions include pacing activities to minimize fatigue and providing information about oral medications and medical follow-up to determine if the client's hemoglobin level stabilizes within normal limits.

>>> *Stop, Think, and Respond 31-1*

Why does the nurse use the Z-track technique to administer parenteral iron?

NURSING GUIDELINES 31-1

Administering an Intramuscular Injection by Z-Track Technique

1. Check the medical orders. Read and compare the label on the drug container with the medical order or medication administration record at least three times.
2. Ask the client's name and birthdate and check the client's identity using the identification bracelet.
3. Determine the client's understanding of the purpose and technique for the procedure.
4. Inspect the intramuscular site.
5. Obtain the necessary equipment.
6. Wash your hands.
7. Fill the syringe with the prescribed amount of drug and change the needle.
8. Draw up an additional 0.2 mL of air in the syringe.
9. Attach a needle that is at least 1½ to 2 inches long.
10. Don gloves.
11. Position the client to facilitate the injection site you intend to use.
12. Using the side of your hand, pull the tissue laterally about 1 inch (2.5 cm) until it is taut (see A). Swab the site with an alcohol pledget.
13. Insert the needle at a 90° angle while continuing to hold the tissue laterally (see B).
14. Steady the barrel of the syringe with the fingers and use the thumb to manipulate the plunger.
15. Aspirate for a blood return.
16. Instill the medication by depressing the plunger with the thumb.
17. Wait 10 seconds with the needle in place and the skin still held taut.
18. Withdraw the needle and immediately release the taut skin (see C).
19. Apply direct pressure to the injection site with a gauze square, but do not rub it.
20. Cover the injection site with a bandage or gauze square and tape.
21. Discard the syringe without recapping the needle.
22. Remove your gloves and wash your hands.
23. Document the medication administration.

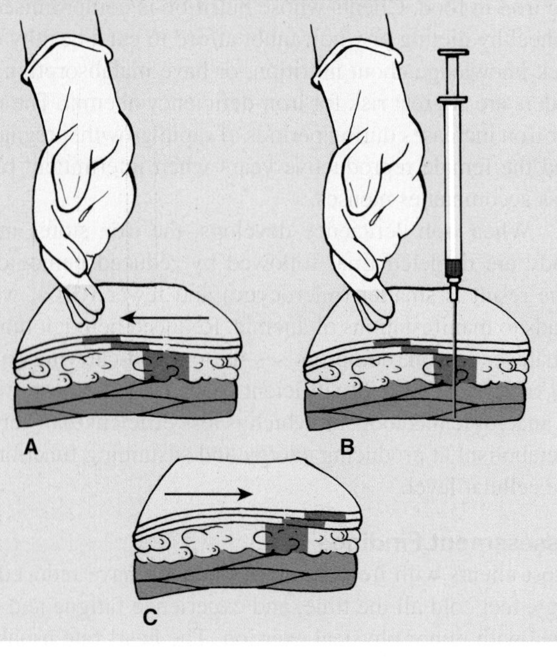

Sickle Cell Disease

Sickle cell disease is a type of anemia in which erythrocytes become sickle- or crescent-shaped when oxygen supply in the blood is inadequate (Fig. 31-1). This common genetic disorder, found primarily in African Americans and also in people from the Mediterranean and Middle Eastern countries, currently affects 1 in 355 African Americans in the United States (National Heart, Lung, and Blood Institute, 2020).

Pathophysiology and Etiology

Fetal **hemoglobin (HbF)** is present during intrauterine development through 6 months of age. **Hemoglobin A (HbA)**, a normal form of hemoglobin, eventually replaces HbF. In people with sickle cell anemia, instead of HbA, an abnormal form of hemoglobin, **hemoglobin S (HbS)**, replaces HbF. Under hypoxic conditions, HbS causes RBCs to assume a sickle shape.

Factors that cause deoxygenation in those affected, such as exposure to cold, dehydration, and infections, also cause **hemoglobin polymerization**, the formation of crystal-like rods that change the biconcave RBC into an irregular, brittle, sticky, sickle-shaped cell. Polymerization potentiates vascular occlusion with local tissue ischemia and cellular hypoxia. Although polymerization is reversible, if the process occurs repeatedly, it damages the membranes on the affected blood cells.

The person with sickle cell disease repeatedly suffers from two major problems: (1) episodes of **sickle cell crisis** from vascular occlusion, which develops rapidly under hypoxic conditions, and (2) chronic hemolytic anemia (see later discussion). During a sickle cell crisis, the sickle-shaped cells lodge in small blood vessels, where they block the flow of blood and oxygen to the affected tissue. The vascular occlusion induces severe pain in the ischemic tissue. Stroke is a common complication, even in young children.

The anemia results from the defective HbS molecule, which shortens the lifespan of affected erythrocytes and causes them to become hemolyzed (destroyed) prematurely.

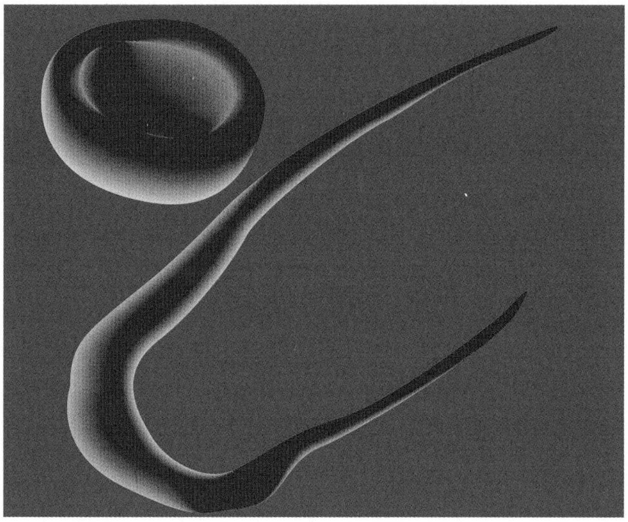

Figure 31-1 A normal spherical red blood cell and a sickle cell. (Reprinted with permission from Hinkle, J. L., & Cheever, K. H. (2018). *Brunner & Suddarth's textbook of medical-surgical nursing* (14th ed.). Wolters Kluwer.)

The spleen becomes enlarged, obstructed, and infarcted with the excess dead erythrocytes. The bone marrow enlarges to compensate for the continuous need to produce more erythrocytes. The persistent anemia causes tachycardia, dyspnea, cardiomegaly (enlargement of the heart), and arrhythmias. Liver dysfunction occurs in about 10% of those affected.

Once the spleen is damaged, risk of infection, especially pneumonia, increases. Hypoperfusion and hypoxia also leave the affected person susceptible to pathogens. One of the unique manifestations of sickle cell disease is **acute chest syndrome**, a type of pneumonia triggered by decreased hemoglobin and infiltrates in the lungs. Acute chest syndrome is characterized by respiratory symptoms such as coughing, wheezing, tachypnea, and chest pain.

Sickle cell disease is a hereditary disorder. To manifest this disorder, a person must inherit two defective genes, one from each parent, in which case all the hemoglobin is inherently abnormal. If the person inherits only one gene, they carry the sickle cell trait. The hemoglobin of those who have sickle cell trait is about 40%. Consequently, these people are at less risk for developing signs and symptoms than those who have two defective genes. Many more people have sickle cell trait than have sickle cell disease.

Assessment Findings

Signs and Symptoms

There is generally a family history of sickle cell disease as well as previous episodes of illness attributed to hemoglobinopathy (pathology affecting hemoglobin), such as a vaso-occlusive crisis and various infections during early childhood. The client's height and weight may be lower than expected as a result of anaerobic metabolism.

The reduced blood flow during sickle cell crisis leads to localized ischemia, severe pain, and possible tissue infarction (necrosis) if the oxygen supply is inadequate. Fever, pain, and swelling of one or more joints are common. Other symptoms depend on the blood vessels involved. Sickle cell crisis can lead to cerebrovascular accident (stroke), pulmonary infarction, shock, and renal failure.

Evidence of the accelerated rate of erythrocyte destruction is manifested by jaundice caused by *hyperbilirubinemia* (excess bilirubin pigment in the blood; Fig. 31-2). Secondary consequences include gallstones (see Chapter 47) or a predisposition to infection when the spleen becomes dysfunctional. Chronic leg ulcers develop from the blockage of the small blood vessels of the legs. Priapism (prolonged erection) occurs from delayed emptying of thick blood from the penis (see Chapter 55). Signs and symptoms of anemia also are present.

Diagnostic Findings

A sickle cell screening test called the *Sickledex test* determines the presence of abnormal HbS. Hemoglobin electrophoresis determines whether the person has sickle cell disease or carries the sickle cell trait. Hemoglobin levels tend to range between 7 and 10 g/dL in those with sickle cell disease. An increase in secretory phospholipase A is a predictor of acute chest syndrome.

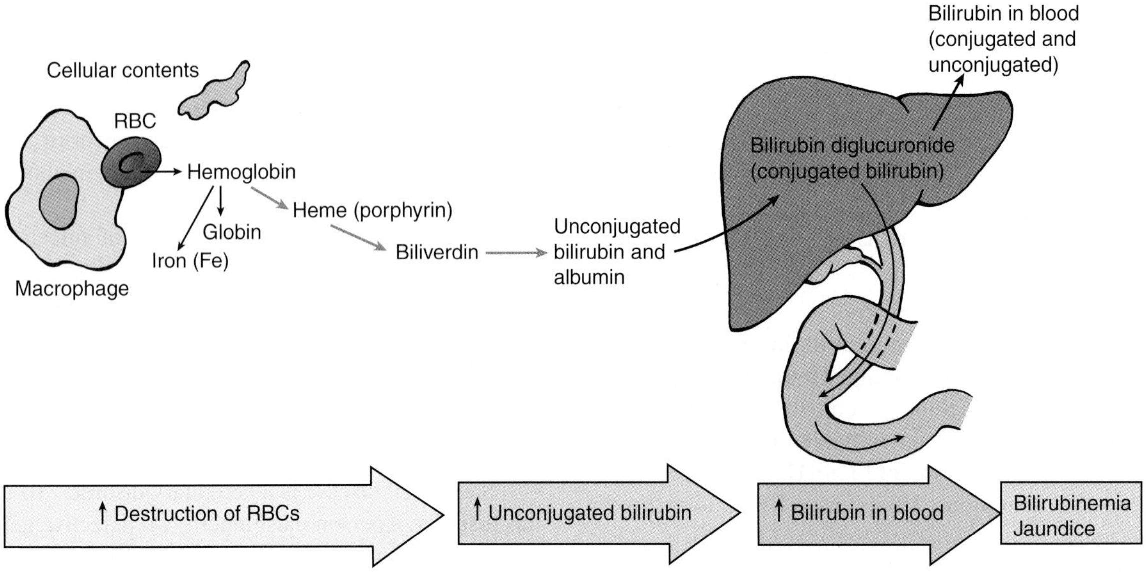

Figure 31-2 Hemolysis of red blood cells (RBCs) causes the release of heme, which becomes unconjugated bilirubin and must be conjugated in the liver for excretion into the bile. Increased amounts of bilirubin lead to bilirubinemia and jaundice.

Medical Management

Currently, treatment for most clients is supportive rather than curative (Client and Family Teaching 31-1). Regular blood transfusions decrease the risk of stroke and other complications of infarction. Transfused blood, however, increases blood viscosity (thickness), which can potentially do more harm than good. It can also result in sensitization to minor antigens in donor blood—especially when the source of the donor blood is from someone of different ethnic origin than the recipient. Voxelotor (Oxbryta) is an oral medication that prevents the cells from forming the sickle shape and clumping together. Crizanlizumab-tmca (Adakveo) is an intravenous treatment that is used to help reduce the number of episodes of pain crisis for clients with sickle cell anemia (National Heart, Lung, and Blood Institute, 2020). Treatment with hydroxyurea (Hydrea, Droxia), an anticancer agent, shows evidence that it decreases sickling by stimulating the production of HbF. Hydroxyurea is toxic to RBCs with defective hemoglobin. As a result of taking hydroxyurea, the body produces RBCs containing HbF, which has the ability to block the sickling action of RBCs. Drug-induced formation of HbF, which has a high affinity for oxygen, has several benefits: It promotes round, flexible blood cells that are less sticky so they move better through blood vessels,

Client and Family Teaching 31-1 Sickle Cell Anemia

The nurse teaches clients with sickle cell anemia and their families as follows:

- Keep all medical appointments to determine the best drugs and dosages and to detect any developing drug toxicities.
- Never exceed the recommended dosages of analgesics, especially narcotic analgesics, and avoid self-medicating with illegal substances.
- Consume a liberal amount of fluids.
- Dress warmly in cold temperatures.
- Avoid vigorous physical exercise and leg positions or clothing that cause vasoconstriction.
- Stop smoking or other use of nicotine.
- Avoid travel to places with high altitudes.
- Obtain immunizations for pneumococcal pneumonia and influenza caused by *Haemophilus influenzae.*
- See a primary provider at the first sign of infection.
- Be aware that pregnancy creates risks for maternal and fetal complications. Obtain genetic testing and counseling before conceiving children (CDC, n.d.).

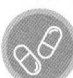

Pharmacologic Considerations

■ Special precautions should be taken by clients with sickle cell disease who use hydroxyurea daily to reduce severe acute pain episodes.
■ Wear gloves to minimize drug handling
■ Wash hands before and after administration
■ Do not open capsules/avoid touching the medication
■ Wipe spills with damp paper towel, and then wash area three separate times with detergent
■ Dose is based on weight; tell your health care provider if you gain/lose weight
■ Do not take if pregnancy is desired or suspected

thus decreasing organ damage, this medication may cause the client's WBC and/or platelet level to drop, and can rarely cause anemia (National Heart, Lung, and Blood Institute, 2020).

Inhaled nitric oxide—not nitrous oxide (laughing gas), a vasodilating agent—is believed to reduce sickling by promoting the binding of oxygen to hemoglobin. It is being used in the form of handheld inhalers to abort or relieve pain experienced during sickle cell crises.

Bone marrow transplantation has cured sickle cell disease primarily in children, but the process of destroying all the defective cells in an adult client's bone marrow tends to be more dangerous. Adults fare better with blood stem cell transplantation (see Chapter 18), in which a portion of the client's bone marrow is not totally destroyed. The procedure requires a compatible donor, generally a sibling. Production of stem cells in the donor is pharmacologically stimulated after which the stem cells are released into the donor's bloodstream and collected in bags, which are frozen. Once the recipient is prepared, the frozen stem cells are thawed and infused. Because the nondiseased stem cells mature and have a longer lifespan than the cells containing HbS, they gradually replace the diseased cells with healthy RBCs containing HbA. Clients must take medications to avoid rejecting the transplant. The procedure has approximately an 85% cure rate in children when the donor is related and matched regarding HLA (human leukocyte antigen) factors (National Heart, Lung, and Blood Institute, 2020).

Researchers continue to investigate the possibility of curing sickle cell disease with gene replacement therapy, but practical application of the technique is remote at this time. Those clients who are not cured with bone marrow or stem cell transplantations are subject to potentially life-threatening infections. Continuous antibiotic therapy is prescribed for some; every infection, no matter how minor, is treated promptly with antibiotics. Folic acid is prescribed to facilitate the replacement of hemolyzed erythrocytes.

During sickle cell crisis, clients are given narcotic analgesia on a scheduled basis or can self-administer it using an IV pump. As an alternative to narcotic analgesics, synthetics such as buprenorphine (Buprenex) and nalbuphine (Nubain) may be prescribed. Oxygen is given to relieve hypoxemia. The client must remain on complete bed rest, be hydrated with IV fluids, and may be given blood transfusions. An iron-chelating agent, such as deferoxamine (Desferal), is used to remove excess iron associated with multiple blood transfusions and erythrocyte destruction. (Also see Evidence Based Practice 31-1.)

››› *Stop, Think, and Respond 31-2*

What is the correlation between sickle cell anemia and stroke (cerebrovascular accident)?

Evidence-Based Practice 31-1

Sickle Cell Anemia and Drug Therapy for Stroke Prevention

Clinical Question

Are there other treatments available for children with sickle cell anemia to decrease the risk of a stroke?

Evidence

The National Institutes for Health performed a study with approximately 120 children with sickle cell anemia. They had two groups for treatment. One group received regular blood transfusions and the second group received a trial drug called hydroxyurea. Both treatments were aimed at changing the velocity of the blood to decrease the risk of strokes in children with sickle cell anemia. The treatment was to last over 2 years, but was stopped early owing to positive results. Normal children receiving multiple transfusions also need an iron-reduction treatment too so that their blood was not overloaded with iron. Because the drug hydroxyurea was so successful, the children receiving this drug would not need the iron reduction. The study contributed to the ongoing research regarding the treatment of sickle cell anemia (National Heart, Lung, Blood Institute, 2015).

Nursing Implications

This study indicates a strong need for nurses to assess the clients and symptoms of the above stated risk factors. Nurses need to be aware of new treatments and research and the effects new drugs have. They need to be supportive to clients and families undergoing new treatments and assist in educating them each step of the way.

Reference
National Heart, Lung, Blood Institute. (2015). *Study shows hydroxyurea as a viable option for some children who have sickle cell anemia.* http://www.nhlbi.nih.gov/news/press-releases/2015/study-shows-hydroxyurea-viable-option-some-children-who-have-sickle-cell

››› *Stop, Think, and Respond 31-3*

What are the differences between HbF, HbA, and HbS?

Hemolytic Anemia

The term **hemolytic anemia** is a generic term that refers to the consequence of a widely diverse group of conditions, some acquired, for example, with malaria; some hereditary (see sickle cell disease); and some idiopathic, in which there is chronic premature destruction of erythrocytes.

Pathophysiology and Etiology

Some examples of conditions that can produce hemolytic anemia are the use of cardiopulmonary bypass during surgery, arsenic or lead poisoning, invasion of erythrocytes by the malaria parasite, infectious agents, or toxins and exposure to hazardous chemicals. Other causes include the production of antibodies that destroy erythrocytes. Antibodies can be produced against antigens from another person, such as is seen in blood transfusion reactions, as well as against the body's own erythrocytes. As the number of destroyed blood cells increases, the potential for hyperbilirubinemia (excess bilirubin) and jaundice also increases.

Assessment Findings

Symptoms are similar to those associated with hypovolemic anemia. In more severe forms of hemolytic anemia, the client is jaundiced and the spleen is enlarged. In some cases, hemolysis is so extensive that it causes shock.

Microscopic examination reveals erythrocyte fragments. When an erythrocyte survival study is performed using radioactive chromium, the lifespan of erythrocytes is 10 days or less. Reaction on a direct Coombs test (direct antiglobulin test) is positive when the hemolytic anemia results from a transfusion reaction, use of certain drugs, or production of antibodies against the erythrocytes.

Medical and Surgical Management

Treatment includes removing the cause (when possible) and administering corticosteroids. In some cases, the steroid dose can be reduced and then discontinued after several weeks. Blood transfusions often are necessary. Splenectomy is performed if the client fails to respond to medical treatment.

Nursing Management

The nurse obtains a comprehensive health history to help determine the cause of the hemolysis. Until the cause is determined, the nurse provides supportive care to help the client meet basic needs. When the diagnosis is confirmed, they implement the medical regimen for treatment and prepare the client for discharge by teaching measures for self-care. The nurse arranges the plan for follow-up evaluations and shares the information with the client.

Thalassemias

Thalassemias are hereditary hemolytic anemias. They are divided into two major groups: alpha-thalassemias and beta-thalassemias. Alpha-thalassemias are found in people from Southeast Asia and Africa; beta-thalassemias are found in people from the Mediterranean islands and the Po Valley in Italy.

Assessment Findings

Clients with alpha-thalassemias typically are asymptomatic, as are those with minor forms of beta-thalassemia. Clients with Cooley anemia, a severe form of beta-thalassemia, exhibit symptoms of severe anemia and a bronzing of the skin caused by hemolysis of erythrocytes. Diagnosis is based on symptoms and the results of hemoglobin electrophoresis.

Medical Management

Treatment of the various forms of thalassemia is symptomatic. Clients usually require frequent transfusions. Repeated blood transfusions can lead to toxic levels of unexcreted iron, which becomes trapped in tissues and organs. Iron **chelation therapy**, a process in which heavy metals such as iron are pharmacologically removed from the blood to prevent organ damage and death, is necessary. Deferoxamine (Desferal) is administered intravenously or subcutaneously to bind with excess iron, facilitating urinary excretion; deferiprone (Ferriprox) and deferasirox (Exjade) are oral iron-chelating agents.

Nursing Management

When anemia is severe, the nurse places the client on bed rest and protects them from contact with those who have infections. When transfusions are necessary, the nurse closely monitors the rate of administration.

Pernicious Anemia

Pernicious anemia develops when a client lacks the intrinsic factor, which normally is present in stomach secretions, or fails to consume sufficient dietary sources of the extrinsic factor. Intrinsic factor is necessary for absorption of vitamin B_{12}. Vitamin B_{12}, the extrinsic factor in blood, is required for the maturation of erythrocytes. Dietary sources of vitamin B_{12} is found in animal products such as meat, eggs, fish, and milk. It is not present in plant foods, except those that have been fortified such as cereals, soy, nut, and rice milk.

Pathophysiology and Etiology

The production of intrinsic factor decreases with age and gastric mucosal atrophy. It also decreases secondary to surgical removal of the stomach, bariatric surgery, or small bowel resection, in which the ileum (site for vitamin B_{12} absorption) is removed. Without adequate vitamin B_{12}, for example, when there is an inadequate dietary intake as may occur among vegetarians or clients who cannot afford to purchase animal protein, erythrocytes remain in an immature form. If the condition is not recognized and treated promptly, degenerative changes in the nervous system develop. Sometimes, permanent damage occurs before treatment begins.

> *Concept Mastery Alert*
>
> The most common cause of iron deficiency in anemia in men and postmenopausal women is bleeding. Iron malabsorption is not as common in most people.

Assessment Findings

Signs and Symptoms

In addition to the usual symptoms of anemia, some clients with pernicious anemia develop stomatitis (inflammation of the mouth) and glossitis (inflammation of the tongue), digestive disturbances, and diarrhea. Anemia may be so severe that dyspnea occurs with minimal exertion. Jaundice, irritability, confusion, and depression are present when the disease is severe. Mental changes usually disappear with treatment. Numbness and tingling in the arms and legs and ataxia are common signs of neurologic involvement. Some affected clients lose vibratory and position senses.

Diagnostic Findings

Diagnosis is established by the client's history, symptoms, and blood and bone marrow studies. The Schilling test is used to confirm the diagnosis (see Chapter 30). Microscopic examination of a blood smear reveals many large, immature erythrocytes.

Medical Management

Vitamin B_{12} is given intramuscularly in a dose adequate to control the disease. Therapy must continue for life. The typical dose is 100 g IM daily for 2 weeks and then 100 g monthly. No toxic effects have been noted from the use of vitamin B_{12}. Oral vitamin B_{12} seldom is effective, except for short intervals. Iron therapy rarely is needed because mature erythrocytes are manufactured, and the hemoglobin level is normal when the condition is corrected. Clients with permanent neurologic deficits benefit from physical therapy.

Nursing Management

If glossitis and stomatitis are present, a soft, bland diet relieves the discomfort associated with eating. Most clients tolerate small, frequent meals better than three large meals. Meticulous oral care after eating is essential to remove particles of food that may irritate the oral mucosal lining and increase soreness. If a permanent neurologic deficit has occurred, the nurse encourages the client to move about as much as possible to prevent complications associated with immobility, such as contractures and pressure ulcer formation. Assistance with ambulation is necessary because some clients have difficulty walking and are prone to falling. If behavioral changes occur, close supervision is necessary. The nurse emphasizes the importance of lifelong administration of vitamin B_{12} or improving dietary consumption. The nurse teaches a family member of the client how to administer vitamin B_{12} injections or refers the client to a home health nursing service.

Folic Acid–Deficiency Anemia

Folic acid–deficiency anemia is characterized by immature erythrocytes.

Pathophysiology and Etiology

A folic acid deficiency commonly is related to an insufficient dietary intake of folate, vitamin B_9, found naturally in foods (Nutrition Notes 31-2). Folic acid is a synthetic form of folate that is found in supplements or fortified foods. Older adults and clients with alcoholism, intestinal disorders that affect food absorption, malignant disorders, and chronic illnesses often have a folic acid deficiency because of poor nutrition. Certain drugs, such as anticonvulsants and methotrexate, are folic acid antagonists and interfere with folic acid absorption. Because pregnant women and clients with chronic hemolytic anemias have increased folic acid requirements, they can experience a folic acid deficiency even when they follow a normal diet. Prolonged IV therapy and total parenteral nutrition also can result in a folic acid deficiency. Chronic alcoholism predisposes to folic acid deficiency; affected people tend to obtain most of their calories from alcohol, causing nutritional compromise.

Assessment Findings

Severe fatigue, a sore and beefy red tongue, dyspnea, nausea, anorexia, headaches, weakness, and light-headedness occur. Blood test results reveal low hemoglobin and hematocrit levels. The serum folate level is decreased. A Schilling test differentiates pernicious anemia and anemia caused by a folic acid deficiency.

Medical Management

Oral folic acid supplements (1 mg daily) are usually prescribed. Parenteral administration of folic acid is required for clients with an intestinal malabsorption disorder. A well-balanced diet that includes foods with high folate content is also recommended.

Nursing Management

The nurse encourages the client to eat foods high in folate; choose soft, bland foods; and perform good oral hygiene. If fatigue is a prominent symptom, the nurse plans adequate rest periods between activities.

> **Nutrition Notes 31-2**
>
> **The Client With Folic Acid–Deficiency Anemia**
>
> - *Folate* is the generic term for all forms of the family of molecules that can be converted to the acid form, folic acid. This includes three naturally occurring molecules of folate (food folate) and synthetic folic acid used in fortified foods and supplements.
> - Rich sources of food folate include fortified breads and cereals, green leafy vegetables, orange juice, and dried peas and beans.
> - Anemia resulting from folic acid deficiency is similar to that of vitamin B_{12} deficiency; both are classified as megaloblastic anemias. However, each has a different root cause and different physiologic outcomes. Neurologic symptoms resulting from B_{12} deficiency, if untreated, can be irreversible. Ascertaining the correct cause of megaloblastic anemia before treatment begins is imperative.

ERYTHROCYTOSIS

Polycythemia Vera

There are some conditions in which one of the primary characteristics is **erythrocytosis**, an increase in circulating erythrocytes. One of these conditions is **polycythemia vera,** which is characterized by a greater-than-normal number of erythrocytes, leukocytes, and platelets. For people who live at high altitudes, erythrocytosis is a normal phenomenon and usually requires no treatment.

Pathophysiology and Etiology

Polycythemia vera is associated with a rapid proliferation of blood cells produced by the bone marrow. The cause of this accelerated production is unknown. Polycythemia vera usually has an insidious onset and a prolonged course. Despite the abundance of erythrocytes, their lifespan is shorter. The dead erythrocytes release intracellular potassium, which can cause hyperkalemia, and increased uric acid, which causes goutlike joint symptoms (see Chapter 63). The oxygen-combining capacity of the erythrocytes is impaired, compromising cellular oxygenation. The increased number of erythrocytes makes the blood more viscous than normal and increases the likelihood for the development of thrombi in small blood vessels. Complications include hypertension, heart failure, stroke, tissue and organ infarction, and hemorrhage.

Assessment Findings

Signs and Symptoms

The face and lips are reddish purple. Fatigue, weakness, headache, pruritus, exertional dyspnea, and dizziness are common. Excessive bleeding after minor injuries, perhaps because of the engorgement of the capillaries and veins, occurs. Hemorrhoids develop. Splenomegaly (enlargement of the spleen) is common. The joints become swollen and painful because of elevated uric acid levels.

Diagnostic Findings

The blood cell count, especially erythrocytes, is elevated, with a similar rise in hemoglobin and hematocrit levels. The platelet and white blood cell (WBC) counts are increased. Levels of serum potassium and uric acid may be above normal.

Medical Management

Treatment involves measures to reduce the volume of circulating blood, lessen its viscosity, and curb the excessive production of erythrocytes. A **phlebotomy** (opening a vein to withdraw blood) is done several times a week; 500 mL of blood is removed each time. Anticoagulants are prescribed to reduce the potential for forming clots. Radiophosphorus and radiation therapy can be used to decrease the production of erythrocytes in the bone marrow. Antineoplastic drugs such as mechlorethamine (Mustargen) are given to curb excessive bone marrow activity.

Nursing Management

The nurse observes the client for complications and provides information about drug therapy and techniques to promote circulation and reduce potential thrombi formation. The plan of care includes the following measures:

- Advise the client to drink 3 quarts (or liters) of fluid per day. *Adequate hydration promotes venous return and ensures sufficient urine production.*
- Teach the client to avoid crossing the legs at the knee and wearing tight clothing. *Restricting blood circulation increases the risk for thrombus formation.*
- Encourage the client to be physically active, change positions frequently, and elevate the lower extremities as much as possible. *Movement and leg elevation promotes the circulation of venous blood.*
- Teach the client how to perform isometric exercises such as contracting and relaxing the quadriceps and gluteal muscles during periods of inactivity. *Contraction of skeletal muscles compresses the walls of veins and increases the circulation of venous blood as it returns to the heart.*
- Help the client apply and use thromboembolic stockings or support hose during waking hours. *Compression of veins promotes venous circulation and prevents the formation of thrombi.*
- Tell the client to rest immediately if chest pain develops. *Chest pain indicates myocardial ischemia. Rest reduces the work of the heart and may restore sufficient oxygenated blood flow to overcome the temporary deficiency.*

LEUKOCYTOSIS

Leukocytosis is an increased number of leukocytes above normal limits. Increased leukocytes generally serve as a protective mechanism in response to inflammation and healing, but in some disease conditions such as leukemia, the proliferation of leukocytes is not advantageous.

Leukemia

Leukemia refers to any malignant blood disorder in which proliferation of leukocytes, usually in an immature form, is unregulated. There often is an accompanying decrease in production of erythrocytes and platelets. There are four general types of leukemia, classified according to the bone marrow stem cell line that is dysfunctional (Table 31-3). Acute and chronic lymphocytic leukemias (CLLs) result from bone marrow dysfunction that affects lymphoid stem cells; the primary marrow dysfunction in acute and chronic myelogenous leukemia (CML) is in myeloid stem cells (Fig. 31-3).

Pathophysiology and Etiology

The cause of leukemia is unknown, although exposures to toxic chemicals and radiation, viruses, and certain drugs are known to precipitate the disorder. In some cases, there is a genetic correlation. Although the increase in leukocytes is rampant, there are many more immature than mature cells. Because of their immaturity, the leukocytes are ineffective at fighting infections. The rapid proliferation of leukocytes

TABLE 31-3 Types of Leukemia

TYPE	CELLULAR CHARACTERISTICS	AGE OF ONSET
Acute lymphocytic leukemia (ALL)	Increased immature lymphocytes Normal or decreased granulocytes Decreased erythrocytes Decreased platelets	Younger than 5 years; uncommon after 15 years
Chronic lymphocytic leukemia (CLL)	Same as above, but erythrocyte and platelet counts may be normal or low	Older than 40 years; most common type in adults
Acute myelogenous leukemia (AML)	Decrease in all myeloid formed cells: monocytes, granulocytes, erythrocytes, and platelets	Occurs in all age ranges
Chronic myelogenous leukemia (CML)	Same as above, but greater number of normal cells than in acute form	Older than 20 years, but incidence increases with age; genetic link in 90%–95% of cases

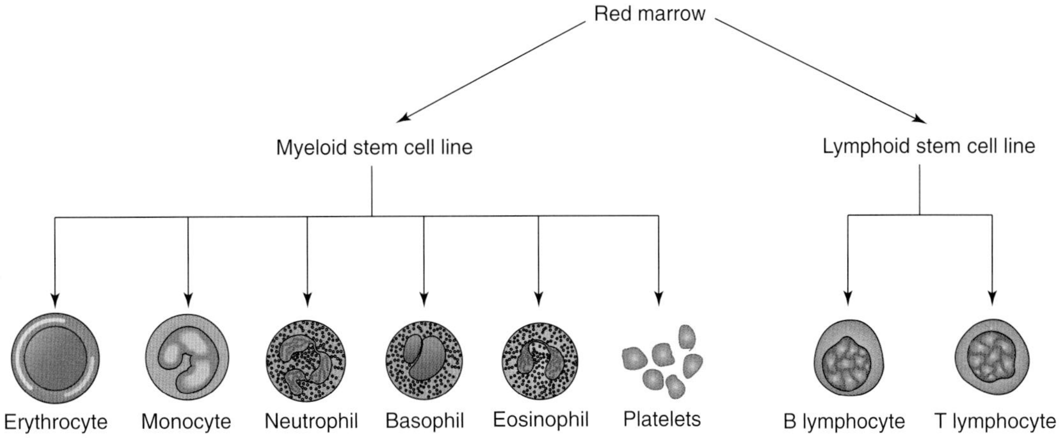

Figure 31-3 Maturation of myeloid and lymphoid stem cells. Leukemia is classified according to the bone marrow stem cell line that is dysfunctional.

results in a decreased production of erythrocytes and platelets. The client eventually develops severe anemia, and the reduction in platelets leads to bleeding. The excessive leukocytes infiltrate the spleen, liver, lymph nodes, and brain if unchecked.

Assessment Findings

Infections, fatigue from anemia, and easy bruising are hallmarks of leukemia. At the onset of leukemia, particularly in acute lymphocytic leukemia (ALL), a fever is present, the spleen and lymph nodes enlarge, and internal or external bleeding develops. Common sites of bleeding include the nose, mouth, and GI tract. The leukocyte count is low, normal, or high, but the number of normal leukocytes is decreased. Consequently, the number of erythrocytes and platelets decreases as well.

Medical Management

Drug therapy is the primary weapon for curing or promoting a remission of leukemia. Years of research has led to the development of successful drug protocols using one or combinations of antineoplastic drugs. The type of drug or combination of drugs depends on the form of leukemia. Treatment is most successful in young clients.

Erythrocyte and platelet transfusions are necessary to treat the anemia and decreased platelets. Antibiotics are given when secondary infections develop.

Bone marrow transplantation and stem cell transplantation have increased survival for some clients. The harvesting and use of adult (somatic) stem cells is different from the potential use of harvested embryonic stem cells (Table 31-4). Adult stem cells are classified as either *autologous* (from oneself),

TABLE 31-4 Comparison of Adult Stem Cells and Embryonic Stem Cells

	ADULT	EMBRYONIC
Source	Bone marrow, peripheral blood, umbilical cord blood	4–5-day-old embryo in the blastocyst stage
Donor	Client,relative, public	Female whose excess ova that have been fertilized *in vitro* (in a laboratory) are no longer needed for reproductive purposes
Characteristics	Unspecialized and differentiate usually into cells in the tissues where they reside	Unspecialized but have the potential to differentiate into various different body cells
Harvesting method	Aspiration of bone marrow, *apheresis* (separation of stem cells from differentiated cells) of peripheral blood, collection of blood from the umbilical cord and placenta at birth	Needle aspiration of inner cell mass within the blastocyst
Preservation	Combined with a preservative and frozen until needed	Cultured and *replated* (removal and reculturing) of proliferating cell mass for 6 months or more, then frozen when millions of cells have been grown
Use	Restore the bone marrow's ability to produce blood-forming cells destroyed by high doses of chemotherapy or radiation	Replace various body cells that are diseased or injured (heart muscle following a myocardial infarction, dopamine-producing cells for those with Parkinson disease, beta cells of those with diabetes mellitus, etc.)
Method of transplant	IV infusion	Currently restricted to laboratory research on animals to determine how unspecialized cells differentiate
Evidence of success	*Engraftment* (increased production) of blood cells in 2–4 weeks; recovery from disease for at least 5 years to confirm absence of cancer cells	

IV, intravenous.

syngeneic (from an identical twin), or *allogenic* (from another; see Chapter 18). Stem cells are harvested by removing them from peripheral blood, obtaining cells from bone marrow, or collecting cord blood from a newborn. Malignant stem cells are removed from an autologous specimen before transplantation. Toxic drugs or radiation are administered before transplantation, which renders the client extremely susceptible to infection. The client remains hospitalized for several weeks to observe if normal blood cells are eventually produced; to detect signs of **graft-versus-host disease**, in which the foreign donor cells destroy the recipient's tissues and organs; and to protect the client who is immunosuppressed from acquiring a life-threatening infection (see Chapter 12).

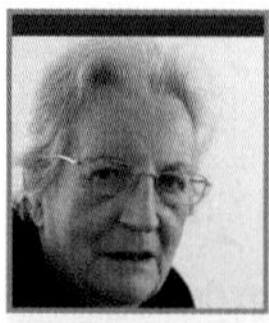

Clinical Scenario A 78-year-old client says, "I've been getting one respiratory infection after another, and I have been so tired lately. I don't have energy to do much of anything. I've noticed that I can feel the lymph nodes in my neck, which I never could do before. Look at all these bruises that appear without much cause. I'm worried that these may indicate some kind of disease." **How can the nurse use the nursing process to manage this client's care? See the following Nursing Process section.**

NURSING PROCESS FOR THE CLIENT WITH LEUKEMIA

Assessment

Begin the initial assessment by obtaining a history of symptoms. Look for a cluster of symptoms that includes weakness and fatigue, frequent infections, nosebleeds or other prolonged bleeding events, and joint pain. Also look for symptoms associated with leukocyte infiltration of the central nervous system, such as headache and confusion.

Examine the client's body for evidence of bruising. Palpate lymph nodes and the abdomen to detect enlargement and tenderness over the liver and spleen. Review laboratory test results, noting the numbers and types of blood cells. Calculate the absolute neutrophil count to determine the client's potential for infection (Box 31-2). In addition, assess the outcome of bone marrow aspiration.

Diagnosis, Planning, and Interventions

Infection Risk: Related to compromised immunity
Expected Outcome: Client will be free of infection as evidenced by normal temperature and no signs of an infectious disorder.

- Implement neutropenic precautions (Box 31-3). *They reduce exposure to pathogens that are dangerous when immunity is suppressed.*
- Ensure that any staff person, family member, or visitor who is ill temporarily discontinues direct contact with the client. *Eliminating direct contact with others who are infectious reduces the potential for transmitting microorganisms to the client.*
- Monitor temperature at least once per shift and continually assess for signs of infection, such as swelling and tenderness, which can appear in any area or organ of the body. *Progressive hyperthermia occurs in some types of infections, and fever (unrelated to drugs or blood products) occurs in most clients with leukemia. Early intervention is essential to prevent sepsis/septicemia in immunosuppressed persons. (Note: Septicemia may occur without fever.)*

Bleeding Risk:
Expected Outcome: The nurse will monitor for hemorrhage; if bleeding is detected, the nurse will manage and minimize it.

- Monitor the platelet count. *Suppression of bone marrow and platelet production places the client at risk for spontaneous and uncontrolled bleeding.*
- Inspect the skin for signs of bruising and petechiae; report melena, hematuria, or epistaxis (nosebleeds). *Fragile tissues and altered clotting mechanisms can result in hemorrhage after even minor trauma.*
- Handle client gently when assisting with care and encourage use of electric razors. *Trauma and microabrasions from razors can contribute to anemia from bleeding.*
- Apply prolonged pressure to needle sites or other sources of external bleeding. *Reduced platelet production results in a delayed clotting process.*
- Implement primary provider's orders for transfusions of blood and platelets. *Transfusion restores and normalizes the cell count and oxygen-carrying capacity of RBCs to correct anemia and prevent and treat hemorrhage.*

Activity Intolerance: Related to hypoxia.
Expected Outcomes: The client will (1) tolerate essential activity as evidenced by a heart rate below 100 beats/min and (2) have a respiratory rate less than 28 breaths/min.

- For interventions, see the discussion that accompanies anemia.

Altered Body Image Perception: Related to hair loss secondary to chemotherapy.
Expected Outcome: Client will cope with hair loss and changing body image.

- Provide opportunity for client to express feelings about hair loss and changing body image; offer suggestions such as scarves, turbans, baseball caps, or wigs. *Head coverings may increase self-esteem and foster more interactions with others.*

NURSING PROCESS FOR THE CLIENT WITH LEUKEMIA (continued)

Acute Anxiety and Fear: Related to unfamiliar experiences and unknown prognosis.
Expected Outcome: Anxiety and fear will be relieved as evidenced by the client's report of emotional comfort.

- Acknowledge your awareness of the client's anxieties and fears. *Open communication validates and communicates acceptance of the client's feelings.*
- Encourage the client to talk about the disorder and its potential and actual effects. *Vocalizing inner feelings helps identify each client's specific emotional response to the disease and treatment.*
- Explain the plan of care and all treatment procedures. *Explaining the purpose, goal, and plan of care promotes confidence that the health care team is dedicated to resolving the illness.*
- Give encouragement and emotional support, and foster hope without implying unrealistic expectations. *A positive attitude sends a message of caring and optimism. Fostering unrealistic hope is not helpful and may significantly decrease the trust that the client places in the health care provider.*
- Teach the client and family how to manage their disease and treatment regimen. *Knowledge empowers the client and family and contributes to a sense of control* (Client and Family Teaching 31-2).

Evaluation of Expected Outcomes

Expected outcomes include that the client does not acquire an infection, experiences little or no blood loss, and tolerates activity between periods of rest. The client adapts to changes in body image and copes with anxiety and fears.

Client and Family Teaching 31-2 Leukemia

If the client is to take medication at home, the nurse explains the dosage schedule because compliance is essential to treat the disease successfully. If untoward effects occur, the health care team will make every effort to control the symptoms while continuing chemotherapy. The nurse includes the following points in a teaching plan:

- Have frequent examinations of the blood and sometimes the bone marrow, which are necessary to monitor the results of therapy. (The nurse emphasizes the importance of these examinations to promote wellness rather than focusing on possible complications from drug therapy.)
- Take precautions to avoid physical injury.
- Avoid exposure to people who have infections (e.g., colds).
- Seek medical care promptly if excessive bleeding or bruising or symptoms of illness or infection occur.
- Obtain sufficient rest and eat an adequate diet to prevent secondary infections.
- When feeling well, continue usual activities unless the primary provider instructs otherwise.
- If sores in the mouth occur, contact the primary provider as soon as possible. Do not self-treat this problem.
- Contact the primary provider immediately about any of the following: severe nausea with prolonged vomiting, severe diarrhea, fever, chills, excessive bleeding or bruising, cough, chest pain, cloudy urine, rash, blood in the stool or urine, severe headache, extreme fatigue, increased respiratory rate or difficulty breathing, and rapid pulse rate.
- Follow the primary provider's recommendations to monitor temperature and weight.
- Keep all clinic or office appointments.

BOX 31-2 Calculating the Absolute Neutrophil Count

Step 1: Use the formula:

$$\text{ANC} = \frac{\%\text{Neutrophils} + \%\text{ Bands}}{100} \times \text{Total white blood cell count}$$

Step 2: Interpret results:

ANC of 999 to 500 = risk for infection
ANC of 499 to 100 = high risk for infection
ANC of 99 or less = almost certain development of infection

BOX 31-3 Neutropenic Precautions

To help prevent infection in clients with neutropenia:

- Place the client in a private room.
- Always wash hands before touching the client; encourage client to remind all staff and visitors to wash hands.
- Tell client to wash their hands before and after eating and after using the bathroom.
- Encourage the client to shower daily.
- Place a mask over client's mouth and nose if leaving the room; minimize time client spends in crowded areas.
- Ensure that no raw fruits or vegetables are served.
- Minimize invasive procedures (schedule all blood work to be drawn at one time of the day; discontinue invasive lines as soon as possible).
- Tell client not to handle cut flowers.

MULTIPLE MYELOMA

Multiple myeloma is a malignancy involving plasma cells, which are B-lymphocyte cells in bone marrow. The overall prognosis is poor but has dramatically improved recently with the advent of new drug treatments and stem cell transplants; the median survival rate is 53% after 5 years (American Cancer Society, 2020). Some people have survived for 10 to 20 years or more depending on the age of the client, stage of the cancer, whether treated with a bone marrow transplant, and complications.

Pathophysiology and Etiology

The exact triggering mechanism for the disorder is unknown. Multiple myeloma is associated with aging, recurrent infections, drug allergies, exposure to occupational toxins, and radiation. Onset before age 40 years is rare. The abnormal plasma cells proliferate in the bone marrow, where they release osteoclast-activating factor. This, in turn, causes the formation of **osteoclasts**, cells that break down and remove bone cells, which results in increased blood calcium and pathologic fractures. The plasma cells also form single or multiple **osteolytic tumors** (bone-destroying) that produce a "punched-out" or "honeycombed" appearance in bones such as the spine, ribs, skull, pelvis, femurs, clavicles, and scapulae. Weakened vertebrae lead to compression of the spine accompanied by significant pain.

The malignant plasma cells release two types of abnormal proteins. In the process of being excreted by the kidneys, *Bence Jones proteins* impair renal tubules, causing renal failure. The other protein, called *M-type globulin*, compromises production of functional immunoglobulins (also known as *antibodies*), thus interfering with an optimal immune response (see Chapter 33). The excess production of plasma cells reduces the formation of erythrocytes and platelets, causing anemia and increasing the risk of bleeding. In addition to infection, which may cause death, those with multiple myeloma experience bone pain, pathologic fractures, thrombotic complications such as clot formation in the deep veins of the legs, pulmonary embolism, and stroke caused by increased viscosity of the blood. CRAB (**c**alcium levels elevated, **r**enal insufficiency, **a**nemia, and **b**one lesions) is an acronym used to identify the combined pathologic effects.

Assessment Findings

Signs and Symptoms

The first symptom usually is vague pain in the pelvis, spine, or ribs. As the disease progresses, the pain becomes more severe and localized. The pain intensifies with activity and is relieved by rest. When tumors replace bone marrow, pathologic fractures develop. The client may have an unusually high incidence of infection, especially pneumonia, caused by decreased production of appropriate antibodies. The client may experience symptoms typically associated with anemia: weakness, fatigue, and chills. Bruising and nosebleeds are evidence of decreased platelets. Renal calculi (stones) may develop from hypercalcemia and renal failure.

Diagnostic Findings

Skeletal radiographic and pathology specimens reveal characteristic bone lesions (Fig. 31-4). Blood cell counts are abnormally low. Serum calcium levels are elevated from bone destruction. Urine samples are positive for Bence Jones protein. Bone marrow aspiration demonstrates increased atypical plasma cells. The uric acid level is elevated from cellular destruction.

Medical Management

Steroid therapy in combination with established anticancer drugs (Drug Therapy Table 31-1) and newer biologic drugs (immunomodulators, proteasome inhibitors, histone deacetylase (HADC) inhibitors, interferons, and monoclonal antibodies) remarkably induce remission, decrease the tumor mass, lessen bone pain, and stimulate killer T cells of the immune system.

Lenalidomide, pomalidomide, and thalidomide (the immunomodulators) are all associated with severe birth defects and are administered under strict supervision of a Risk Evaluation and Mitigation Strategy (REMS) program overseen by the U.S. Food and Drug Administration (FDA). Bisphosphonates are prescribed to increase bone density. Analgesics control pain; stronger narcotic analgesics are reserved for the terminal stages of the disease. Allopurinol (Zyloprim) is used to prevent uric acid crystallization and subsequent renal calculus formation. See Chapter 58 for a discussion of the management of renal failure.

Anemia is treated with erythropoietin (Epogen) or blood transfusions. Infections are managed with antibiotics. Back braces are necessary when the spine is involved, and body casts are used when involvement is extensive and causes pathologic fractures.

Autologous hematopoietic stem cell transplants, those that only produce blood cells, are now considered standard care for clients with multiple myeloma. However, the choice of drug therapy must be selectively considered if a transplant is anticipated so as not to eliminate this as an option later in the disease process. Another possibility is to harvest stem cells before starting stem cell–damaging drug therapy. Research shows that those who receive a bone marrow or stem cell transplant early in the disease have a slightly greater survival time than those who delayed a transplant.

Nursing Management

The nurse assesses the client frequently for pain, signs of infection, excessive fatigue, bleeding, thrombus formation, and changes in the quantity or quality of urine production. They administer prescribed analgesics for effective pain management. The nurse assists the client with ambulation

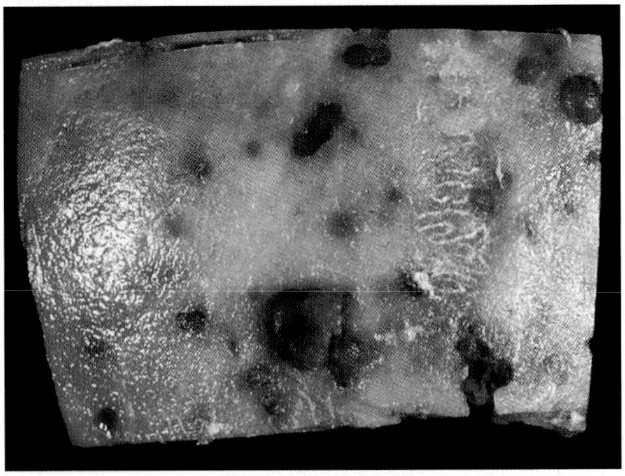

Figure 31-4 A segment of bone from a person with multiple myeloma reveals numerous punched-out, lytic lesions characteristic of this disease. (Reprinted with permission from Rubin, R., & Strayer, D. S. (2012). *Rubin's pathology: Clinicopathologic foundations of medicine* (6th ed.). Wolters Kluwer Health/Lippincott Williams & Wilkins.)

DRUG THERAPY TABLE 31-1 Treatment Options for Multiple Myeloma

Drug Category and Common Examples	Intended Use	Therapy-Related Side Effects
Chemotherapy **Cell Cycle–Specific Agents**		
Vinca Alkaloid: vincristine	Chemotherapy to kill or destroy cancerous cells	• Immediate: extravasation potential • During therapy cycles: alopecia, anemia, leukopenia, paresthesia, nausea, vomiting, constipation • Long term: fertility problems
Podophyllotoxins: etoposide		• During therapy cycles: anemia, leukopenia, thrombocytopenia, alopecia, nausea, vomiting
Cell Cycle–Nonspecific Agents		
Nitrogen Mustard Derivatives: Cyclophosphamide Melphalan (Alkeran)	Chemotherapy to kill or destroy cancerous cells	• During therapy cycles: anemia, leukopenia, thrombocytopenia, leukopenia, • Hemorrhagic cystitis, • Long term: fertility problems, • Secondary cancers
Antibiotics: doxorubicin (Doxil)		• Immediate: nausea, vomiting, extravasation potential • During therapy cycles: anemia, leukopenia, thrombocytopenia, vomiting, alopecia, skin erythema, cutaneous changes • Long term: pulmonary fibrosis
Ethyleneamines: bendamustine (Treanda)		• During therapy cycles: anemia, leukopenia, thrombocytopenia, nausea, vomiting, dizziness

Category and Common Generic (Brand) Drugs	Intended Use	Common Side Effects	Safety Warnings for Nurses
Adjuvant therapy (taken along with Chemotherapy agents)			
Corticosteroids: dexamethasone (Decadron) Prednisone (Deltasone)	Inhibit inflammatory immune response	Acne, water retention, weight gain, hair loss, increased appetite	• Give with food to decrease gastric irritation • Monitor for higher blood glucose in clients with diabetes • Abrupt withdrawal may precipitate Addison disease crisis
Immunomodulators—lenalidomide (Revlimid) Pomalidomide (Pomalyst) Thalidomide (Thalomid)	Prompt the body's immune system to attack cancerous cells	Drowsiness, fatigue, constipation	• Severe birth defects, only used through special programs • DVT, must take aspirin or warfarin • Monitor for neuropathy
Proteasome Inhibitors: Bortezomib (Velcade) Carfilzomib (Kyprolis) Ixazomib (Ninlaro)	Stop enzymes from breaking down proteins which helps control cell division	Nausea and vomiting, tiredness, diarrhea, constipation, fever, decreased appetite, and lowered blood counts	• Monitor blood serum for pancytopenia • Monitor for neuropathy, liver disease
HDAC Inhibitor: panobinostat (Farydak)	Interacts with genes inside cells	Nausea and vomiting, tiredness, diarrhea, constipation, fever, decreased appetite, and lowered blood counts	• Monitor for liver disease and heart dysrhythmias
Monoclonal antibodies: daratumumab (Darzalex), elotuzumab (Empliciti)	Attacks protein in cancerous cells	Flu-like symptoms	• Monitor for anaphylactic reaction during/immediately after injection
Bisphosphonates: pamidronate (Aredia), zoledronic acid (Zometa)	Reduce bone loss caused by the multiple myeloma cancer cells	Hypotension, confusion, anxiety, agitation, nausea, diarrhea, constipation, fatigue	• Dental check and repair before starting to reduce osteonecrosis of jaw bone
Interferon Alpha: Interferon alfa (Roferon)	Regulate the immune response	Flu-like symptoms, fatigue	• Monitor blood serum for pancytopenia

The drugs in column 1 indicate the drug that matches up with explanations in columns 2 through 4.

because immobility can worsen loss of calcium from the bone. They provide up to 4000 mL of fluid to prevent renal damage from hypercalcemia and precipitation of protein in the renal tubules. The nurse documents and reports signs suggestive of calculus formation in the kidney, ureters, or bladder (see Chapters 58 and 59).

Safety is paramount because any injury, no matter how slight, can result in a fracture. When pain is severe, the nurse delays position changes and bathing until an administered analgesic has reached its peak concentration level and the client is experiencing maximum pain relief. The nurse takes measures to reduce the potential for infection.

AGRANULOCYTOSIS

Agranulocytosis refers specifically to a decreased production of granulocytes, neutrophils, basophils, and eosinophils. This is opposed to **leukopenia**, which is a general reduction in all WBCs. Decreased granulocytes place the client at risk for infection.

Pathophysiology and Etiology

The most common cause of agranulocytosis is toxicity from drugs such as sulfonamides, chloramphenicol (Chloromycetin), antineoplastics, and some psychotropic medications.

Assessment Findings

Fatigue, fever, chills, headache, and opportunistic infections in the mouth, throat, nose, rectum, or vagina can develop.

Medical Management

Treatment includes removal of the cause, such as discontinuing the drug that is producing agranulocytosis. The prognosis is related to the condition's cause and severity. When the cause can be determined and promptly removed, the client usually recovers. Some clients improve after receiving filgrastim (Neupogen) or pegfilgrastim (Neulasta), drugs that supply human granulocyte colony-stimulating factor.

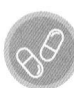

Pharmacologic Considerations

- Colony-stimulating factors help increase production of blood cells. When given after chemotherapy or radiation, these drugs help both RBCs and WBCs increase to minimize anemia, infection, and bleeding.

Nursing Management

The nurse determines the names of all drugs (prescription and nonprescription) the client has used in the past 6 to 12 months. Neutropenic precautions (refer to Box 31-3) are necessary if the leukocyte count is extremely low. Visitors or staff members with any type of infection are restricted from close client contact until the infection has cleared.

PANCYTOPENIA

Pancytopenia refers to conditions in which numbers of all marrow-produced blood cells are reduced.

Aplastic Anemia

Aplastic anemia is more than just a deficiency of erythrocytes, although rarely that is the case. Its name is derived from the word **aplasia**, which means failure to develop. Usually it is manifested by insufficient numbers of erythrocytes, leukocytes, and platelets, collectively described as *pancytopenia*.

Pathophysiology and Etiology

Aplastic anemia is a consequence of inadequate stem cell production in the bone marrow. In some cases, the cause of the disorder is never determined, but it may be autoimmune (self-destroying) in nature (see Chapter 34). In many cases, the bone marrow becomes dysfunctional from exposure to toxic chemicals, radiation, and drug therapy with anticancer drugs and some antibiotics. Clients with aplastic anemia are very ill, and the death rate is high if the bone marrow has been severely damaged.

Assessment Findings

Clients with aplastic anemia experience all the typical characteristics of anemia (weakness and fatigue). In addition, they have frequent opportunistic infections plus coagulation abnormalities that are manifested by unusual bleeding, small skin hemorrhages called *petechiae*, and *ecchymoses* (bruises). The spleen becomes enlarged with an accumulation of the client's blood cells destroyed by lymphocytes that failed to recognize them as normal cells, or with an accumulation of dead transfused blood cells. The blood cell count shows insufficient numbers of blood cells. A bone marrow aspiration confirms that the production of stem cells is suppressed.

Medical Management

In some instances, withdrawal of the causative agent allows the bone marrow to regenerate and assume normal function. Transfusions of whole blood, packed cells, and platelets are given to boost circulating blood cells. Antibiotics are administered to prevent or treat infection. High doses of corticosteroids that suppress the immune system are given in cases of an autoimmune connection. Bone marrow transplantation is considered if a matching donor can be found; otherwise, autologous stem cell transplantation is an alternative (see Chapter 18).

Nursing Management

The nurse assesses for signs of severe anemia, infection, and bleeding tendencies and makes every effort to prevent infection. If the leukocyte count is extremely low, the nurse implements special precautions to prevent infection, such as restricting visitors and locating the client in a laminar airflow room.

The nurse includes soft foods in the diet and modifies oral hygiene techniques to prevent bleeding from the gums. The nurse collaborates with the primary provider concerning alternative routes for drugs administered parenterally. If that is not possible, they apply additional pressure to any punctures from injections or sites where IV fluids are administered and discontinued. The nurse monitors the client closely during blood transfusions because the risk of a reaction increases with the repeated introduction of foreign cells from multiple blood donors.

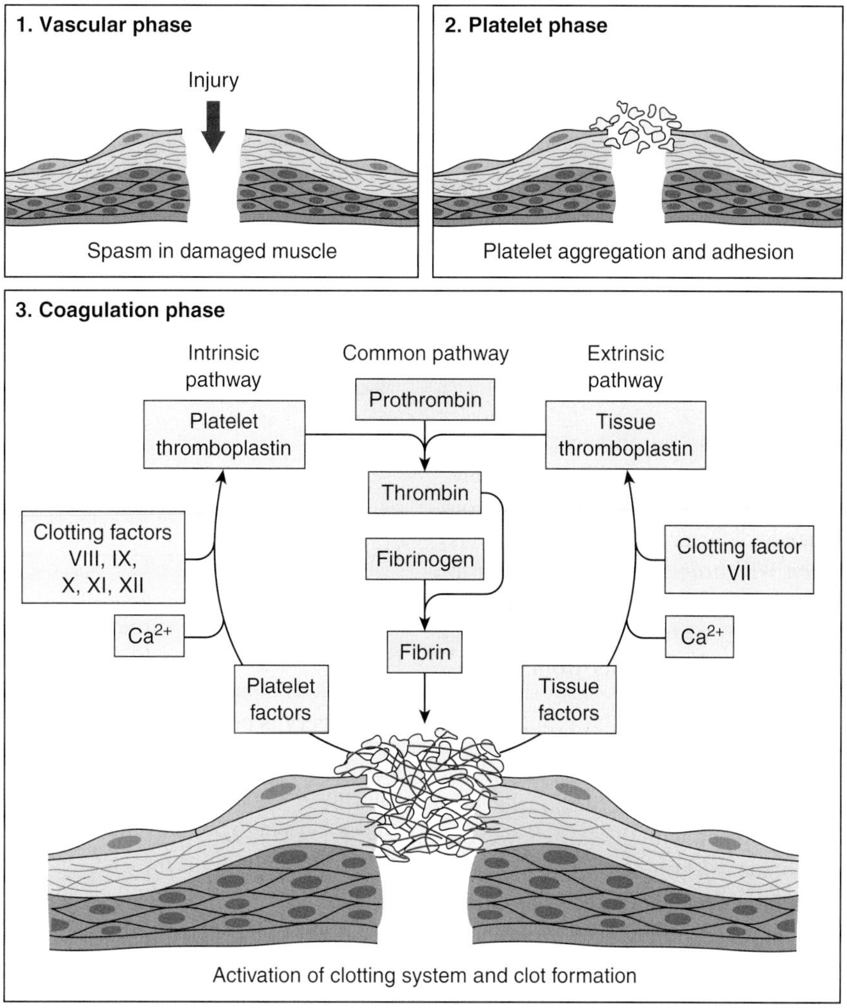

Figure 31-5 Activation of the clotting system and clot formation. Clotting factors are identified by name and Roman numeral or by Roman numeral alone. (Adapted from http://www.irvingcrowley.com/cls/clotting.gif.)

COAGULOPATHIES

The term **coagulopathy** refers to conditions in which a component that is necessary to control bleeding (Fig. 31-5) is missing or inadequate. Two common examples are thrombocytopenia and hemophilia. For information on disseminated intravascular coagulation, a condition in which hypercoagulation (excessive clot formation) is followed by diffuse bleeding as clotting factors are exhausted, refer to texts on trauma and critical care nursing.

Thrombocytopenia

Thrombocytopenia is a lower-than-normal number of platelets or thrombocytes.

Pathophysiology and Etiology

Thrombocytopenia occurs when the platelets manufactured by the bone marrow are decreased or platelet destruction by the spleen is increased. It accompanies leukemia and other malignant blood diseases and is caused by severe infections and certain drugs. Idiopathic thrombocytopenia purpura is thrombocytopenia without a known cause.

Assessment Findings

Thrombocytopenia is evidenced by **purpura**, small hemorrhages in the skin, mucous membranes, or subcutaneous tissues. Bleeding from other parts of the body, such as the nose, oral mucous membrane, and the GI tract, also occurs. Internal hemorrhage, which can be severe and even fatal, is possible.

Diagnosis is based on symptoms, a low platelet count, and abnormal bleeding and clotting times. In some instances, bone marrow aspiration is performed. A health history sometimes reveals agents that are associated with drug-induced thrombocytopenia, such as heparin.

Medical and Surgical Management

When possible, the cause is eliminated. Corticosteroids provide symptomatic relief until the platelet count returns to normal. Transfusions of platelets or whole blood are given in a hemorrhagic emergency. If spontaneous recovery does not occur, splenectomy is necessary to stop destruction of platelets in the spleen. Removal of the spleen results in a rise in the platelet count and relief of symptoms, but there is a lifelong potential for infection because the absent spleen cannot filter bacteria present in the blood.

Clients with idiopathic thrombocytopenia often recover spontaneously. If the cause can be removed or treated, the prognosis is good. Thrombocytopenia in conjunction with illnesses such as leukemia has a poor prognosis.

Nursing Management

Refer to nursing interventions for managing and minimizing bleeding and hemorrhage discussed with leukemia. If instituting corticosteroid therapy, the nurse observes the client for adverse drug effects. The dose and frequency of steroid medication are tapered before discontinuing it to avoid adrenal insufficiency or crisis (see Chapter 50).

Hemophilia

Hemophilia is a disorder involving an absence or reduction of a clotting factor. The three types of hemophilia are hemophilia A, B, and C. Hemophilia A, the most common type, results from a deficiency of factor VIII. In a less serious form of hemophilia A, *von Willebrand disease*, the amount and quality of factor VIII is diminished. Hemophilia B, or *Christmas disease*, is a deficiency of factor IX. Hemophilia C, also known as *Rosenthal disease*, results from a deficiency of factor XI.

Pathophysiology and Etiology

Hemophilia is inherited from mother to son as a sex-linked recessive characteristic. Daughters can inherit the trait but seldom develop the disease. Women with the trait, however, can transmit the disease to male offspring.

The severity of hemophilia depends on the type inherited. Bleeding typically is noted in infancy and childhood. Milder forms can go unrecognized for years. The disease considerably shortens life expectancy; many clients with hemophilia do not reach adulthood. Those with mild hemophilia may lead full and productive lives despite the illness. Human immunodeficiency virus (HIV) and hepatitis virus have been transmitted to clients with hemophilia through transfusion of blood and blood products. The testing of donated blood has markedly reduced the risk for acquiring blood-borne pathogens.

Assessment Findings

Persistent oozing and sometimes severe bleeding that occurs spontaneously or after an injury are manifestations of the disease. Bleeding in joints eventually damages the joints and leads to deformity and limitation of motion. Diagnosis is based on the history of symptoms and laboratory tests such as coagulant factor assay, which shows a deficiency of factor VIII, IX, or XI.

Medical Management

Treatment includes transfusions of fresh blood, frozen plasma, factor VIII concentrate, and anti-inhibitor coagulant complex for hemophilia A, factor IX concentrate for hemophilia B, factor XI for hemophilia C, and the application of thrombin or fibrin to the bleeding area. Other measures used to help control bleeding are the administration of fresh frozen plasma, aminocaproic acid (Amicar) that helps to hold a clot in place once it has formed, direct pressure over the bleeding site, and cold compresses or ice packs.

Client and Family Teaching 31-3
Hemophilia

The nurse explains the treatment regimen and educates the client and family as follows:

- Eliminate aspirin and NSAIDs because these drugs can increase bleeding tendencies.
- Avoid activities that can result in injury.
- Wear a MedicAlert bracelet and inform the dentist and others, when appropriate, of the condition.
- Notify the primary provider promptly if pain, discomfort, or obvious bleeding from the nose or rectum, in vomitus, or elsewhere occurs. Bleeding in internal organs or structures initially produces only vague symptoms.
- Use a soft toothbrush and rinse the mouth with warm water between and after meals.
- Support painful joints on pillows.

Relatively minor surgical procedures, such as tooth extraction, carry considerable risk and are best performed in a hospital. Transfusions usually are necessary even when minor surgery is performed.

Nursing Management

The nurse obtains a comprehensive health history that includes current symptoms and treatment for the bleeding disorder. They question the client about when the last episode occurred, its location (e.g., mouth, rectum, skin), duration, and what treatments, if any, were necessary. The nurse assesses the joints and mobility and inspects the skin for purpura or hemorrhagic areas. Before taking a BP, the nurse asks the client if the use of a BP cuff has ever produced bleeding under the skin or in the arm joints. The nurse takes the temperature over the temporal artery or tympanically to avoid oral or rectal injuries and checks the urine and stools for signs of bleeding.

Overall care includes preventing trauma, managing and minimizing bleeding episodes, reducing pain or discomfort, conserving energy, and helping the client learn ways to prevent further bleeding episodes. When the client requires transfusion of products such as whole blood, plasma, or antihemophilic factor for bleeding episodes, the nurse closely observes for signs that bleeding has been controlled. They keep the primary provider informed of the client's progress because additional treatment modalities often are necessary. Client and Family Teaching 31-3 provides information related to teaching about hemophilia.

KEY POINTS

- Anemia types
  - Hypovolemic: caused by loss of blood volume, can be sudden or gradual
    - Signs and symptoms: changes in vital signs noted, signs of shock with severe loss
    - Treatment: contain the loss, blood transfusions, surgical need for underlying issues

- Iron-deficiency: iron is insufficient to produce hemoglobin
  - Signs and symptoms: reduced energy, feel cold, has fatigue, dyspnea with minor exertion
  - Treatment: determine cause and eliminate it. Correct diet, add supplements
- Sickle cell disease: erythrocytes change shape to sickle/crescent when oxygen supply is inadequate
  - Signs and symptoms: family history, cells clog, reducing blood flow, causes severe pain, ischemia, fever, possible tissue infarction
  - Treatment: supportive, blood transfusions, medications to treat symptoms
- Hemolytic: generic term for anemia when caused by other conditions such as malaria
  - Signs and symptoms: similar to hypovolemic, may have jaundice and enlarged spleen
  - Treatment: remove the cause, administer steroids, blood transfusion
- Thalassemias: hereditary hemolytic anemias, alpha and beta types
  - Signs and symptoms: may be asymptomatic, may exhibit skin bronzing and severe anemia signs
  - Treatment: treat symptoms, determine cause
- Pernicious: lack of intrinsic factor or does not consume dietary sources of extrinsic faction necessary for absorption of vitamin B_{12}
  - Signs and symptoms: typical symptoms of anemia, stomatitis, digestive disturbances, diarrhea. Severe cases may show signs of jaundice, confusion, depression and mental changes
  - Treatment: Vitamin B_{12} intramuscularly
- Folic acid-deficiency: immature erythrocytes, commonly related to insufficient intake of folate
  - Signs and symptoms: severe fatigue, swollen tongue, dyspnea, nausea, anorexia, headaches, weakness
  - Treatment: folic acid supplements, diet

- Erythrocytosis
  - Polycythemia Vera: increase in circulating erythrocytes
    - Signs and symptoms: face and lips reddish purple, fatigue, weakness, headaches, pruritis, exertional dyspnea, dizziness
    - Treatment: reduce volume of circulating blood, chemotherapy agents to curb excessive bone marrow production

- Leukocytosis
  - Leukemia: malignant blood disorder, proliferation of leukocytes, usually immature
    - Acute lymphocytic leukemia (ALL)
    - Chronic lymphocytic leukemia (CLL)
    - Acute myelogenous leukemia (AML)
    - Chronic myelogenous leukemia (CML)
      - Signs and symptoms: fatigue, infections, easy bruising, fever, spleen and lymph nodes enlarged
      - Treatment: drug therapy using combinations of antineoplastic drugs, blood transfusions, bone marrow, and stem cell transplants
  - Multiple myeloma: malignancy of plasma cells
    - Signs and symptoms: vague pain in pelvis, spine or ribs, intensifies with activity, becomes more severe as disease progresses
    - Treatment: antineoplastic drugs, steroid therapy, stem cell transplants

- Agranulocytosis: decreased production of granulocytes, neutrophils, basophils, and eosinophils
  - Signs and symptoms: fever, chills, fatigue, headache, opportunistic infections
  - Treatment: removal of cause (discontinuing the causing drug if indicated)

- Pancytopenia: reduction of all marrow produced blood cells
  - Aplastic anemia: insufficient numbers of erythrocytes, leukocytes, and platelets
    - Signs and symptoms: typical anemia signs, frequent infections, unusual bleeding
    - Treatment: determine and remove causative agent, transfusions, antibiotics, corticosteroids, bone marrow transplantation
  - Thrombocytopenia: lower than normal number of platelets
    - Signs and symptoms: purpura small hemorrhages in the skin, mucus membranes, or subcutaneous tissues, bleeding from other areas
    - Treatment: eliminate cause, corticosteroid treatment, platelet transfusion or whole blood, splenectomy if indicated
  - Hemophilia: absence or reduction of clotting factor—three types A, B, and C
    - Signs and symptoms: persistent oozing and/or severe bleeding after an injury but may occur spontaneously
    - Treatment: blood transfusion, frozen plasma, clotting factors

CRITICAL THINKING EXERCISES

1. List hematopoietic disorders associated with anemia and an etiology for each.
2. When taking a dietary history from a client with anemia, the frequency and amount of consumption of what foods would be important to ascertain?
3. Discuss the problems that clients with anemia, leukemia, or thrombocytopenia share. What interventions can nurses use regardless of the particular disorder?
4. For what hematopoietic disorders would stem cell transplantation be appropriate?

NCLEX-STYLE REVIEW QUESTIONS PrepU

1. A client arrives at the emergency department after a motorcycle accident. Vital signs are T = 97.7°F; P = 122; R = 28; and BP = 96/54 mm Hg. The client has suffered profuse blood loss. From the clinical picture, what position is best for the nurse to place the client?
   1. Semi-Fowler
   2. Modified Trendelenburg
   3. Reverse Trendelenburg
   4. Lithotomy

2. The nurse must give an IM iron injection using a Z-track technique. Arrange the following actions in the correct sequence. Use all the options.
   1. Depress the plunger of the syringe.
   2. Release the taut skin.
   3. Insert the needle at a 90° angle.
   4. Wait 10 seconds with the needle in place.
   5. Pull the tissue laterally until it is taut.
   6. Add 0.2 mL of air to the filled syringe.

3. The nurse is assessing a client with anemia possibly resulting from malaria. What information would be most important to ascertain to assist the primary provider in making a correct diagnosis?
   1. Recent exposure to radiation
   2. Exercise routine
   3. Foreign travel
   4. Alcohol consumption

4. A client has been diagnosed with pernicious anemia. They say, "I'm worried because my grandmother died of the disease years ago." What nursing explanation is most accurate?
   1. "We have come a long way in furthering life expectancy."
   2. "We now give vitamin B_{12} to control the disease."
   3. "Regular blood transfusions keep the disease in remission."
   4. "Bone marrow transplant is the only cure for the disease."

5. A nurse must administer 0.2 mg of vitamin B_{12} subcutaneously to a client with pernicious anemia. Calculate the dosage from a vial that contains 100 µg/mL. Record your answer in a whole number.

________ mL

WANT TO KNOW MORE? There are a wide variety of online resources available on thePoint to enhance learning and understanding of this chapter.

Go to thePoint.lww.com/activate and use the activation code found in the front of this text to unlock these online resources.

32 Caring for Clients With Disorders of the Lymphatic System

Words To Know

complex decongestive physiotherapy
Epstein–Barr virus
Hodgkin disease
infectious mononucleosis
lymph nodes
lymphadenitis
lymphangitis
lymphatics
lymphedema
lymphoma
non-Hodgkin lymphomas
Reed–Sternberg cells
right lymphatic duct
thoracic duct

Learning Objectives

On completion of this chapter, you will be able to:

1. Explain the cause and characteristics of lymphedema.
2. Discuss the role of the nurse when managing the care of clients with lymphedema.
3. Describe nursing interventions that promote the resolution of lymphangitis and lymphadenitis.
4. Explain the nature and transmission of infectious mononucleosis.
5. List suggestions the nurse can offer to individuals who acquire infectious mononucleosis.
6. Define the term *lymphoma* and name two types.
7. Name the type of malignant cell diagnostic of Hodgkin disease.
8. List three forms of treatment used to cure or promote remission of lymphomas.
9. Name at least four problems that nurses address when caring for clients with Hodgkin disease and non-Hodgkin lymphoma.

As described in Chapter 30, the lymphatic system is a network of vessels, known as **lymphatics**, which transport *lymph*, the watery fluid derived from plasma that exits the walls of capillaries and enters interstitial spaces. The lymphatic vessels carry the lymph to and through **lymph nodes**, clusters of bean-sized structures located primarily in the neck, axilla, chest, abdomen, pelvis, and groin. The lymph nodes contain lymphocytes and macrophages, specialized immune defensive cells that trap, destroy, and remove infectious microorganisms, cellular debris, and cancer cells. The tonsils, thymus gland, and spleen are accessory lymphatic structures.

Most lymphatic fluid circulates with the help of skeletal muscle contraction and is returned to venous circulation through one of two ducts. The **thoracic duct**, located in the posterior abdominal cavity, collects lymph from all body areas except that which circulates above the right diaphragm and deposits the fluid into the left subclavian vein. The **right lymphatic duct** returns lymph from the right side of the head, neck, chest, and right arm and empties it into the right subclavian vein (Fig. 32-1).

Gerontologic Considerations

- The risk of lymphoma is increased in older adults, primarily because of the immunologic changes of aging and prolonged exposure to carcinogens.
- The etiology and presentation of Hodgkin disease differs among older adults and the incidence increases with age (Straus, 2017).
- Physical changes that accompany aging can impact the absorption, metabolism, distribution, and elimination of chemotherapeutic agents. Thus, older adults may require decreased dosing that may influence effectiveness of treatment. In addition, doxorubicin is not tolerated owing to its toxic effects on the kidneys. Although it is necessary to weigh the benefits of chemotherapy against the adverse reactions that may affect older adults, treatment modalities are not based on age alone.
- Nursing management for older adults with non-Hodgkin lymphomas must include assessment of the functional status of the cardiopulmonary, renal, and central nervous systems to assist the client and family in decision-making regarding the risks and benefits of chemotherapy. Advocating for the older client includes planning for end-of-life concerns.

Occlusive, inflammatory, infectious, and malignant disorders of the lymphatic system result in fluid distribution problems, tender and painful lymph node enlargement, compromised immune functions, or a combination of these. This chapter discusses such disorders.

OCCLUSIVE, INFLAMMATORY, AND INFECTIOUS DISORDERS

Lymphedema

Pathophysiology and Etiology

Lymphedema is an accumulation of lymphatic fluid that results from impaired lymph circulation. Primary lymphedema usually is congenitally acquired, although manifestations often do not appear until adolescence or early adulthood. It affects women more often than men. Secondary lymphedema develops (1) as a complication of other disorders, such as repeated bouts of phlebitis and streptococcal infection, burns, insect bites, and parasitic infections in tropical and subtropical countries; or (2) as a consequence of treatment, such as the removal of multiple lymph nodes at the time of a mastectomy (see Chapter 54) or radiation for cancer. Worldwide, the most common

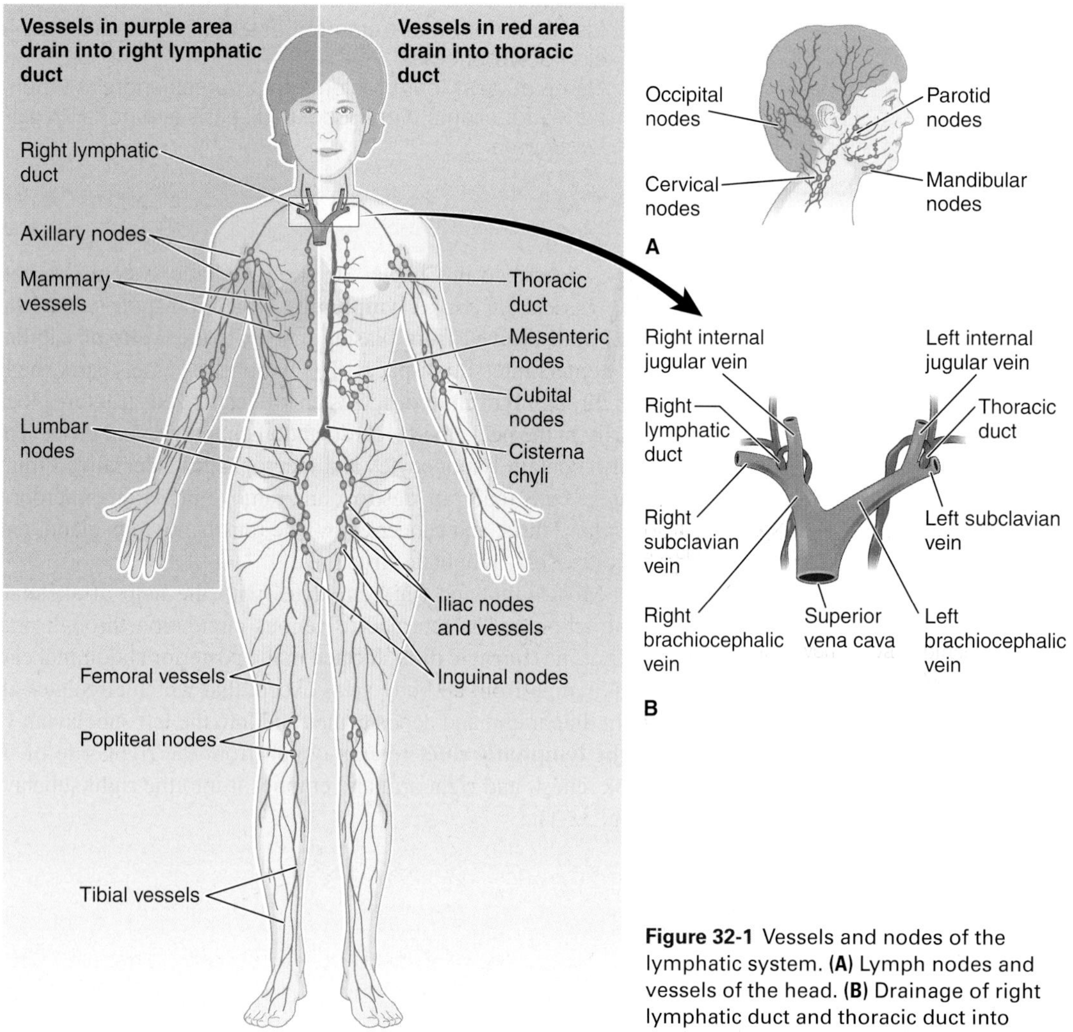

Figure 32-1 Vessels and nodes of the lymphatic system. **(A)** Lymph nodes and vessels of the head. **(B)** Drainage of right lymphatic duct and thoracic duct into subclavian veins.

cause of lymphedema is a parasitic worm; mosquitoes transmit the parasite, resulting in a condition known as elephantiasis (see Chapter 31).

Lymphedema is the result of an accumulation of lymph containing a large percentage of protein within lymphatic vessels. When the volume of the lymph exceeds the capacity of the vessels, the lymph enters the interstitial spaces within soft tissues. The trapped fluid attracts fibroblasts and collagen, eventually causing a nonpitting edema in the late stage that appears different from other types of edema. When massive, the resulting edema leads to chronic deformities in locations such as the arms, legs, and genitalia, with subsequent poor nutrition to tissues (Fig. 32-2).

Assessment Findings

The skin in the affected area swells, especially in a dependent position. The severity of lymphedema is identified according to a grading system (Box 32-1). Pitting is evident in the early stages, but the tissue remains soft. The skin eventually becomes firm, tight, and shiny. Eventually, elevation does not diminish the swelling. The skin also appears thickened, rough, and discolored; it is described as brawny (orange). Weeping, or oozing of fluid from the skin, may occur. Because tissue nutrition is impaired from the stagnation of lymphatic fluid, ulcers and infection can develop in the edematous area. The area can appear red and feel warm and painful. *Lymphangiography*, a special examination in which an intravenous (IV) dye and radiography are used to detect lymph node involvement, reveals the degree and extent of blockage in the lymph system.

Medical and Surgical Management

Treatment usually is symptomatic. In the early stages, the client elevates the affected part to promote lymphatic drainage and wears an elastic compression garment such as a stocking or sleeve (Fig. 32-3). A compression garment, which consists of multiple layers of elastic material with proximal to distal compression gradation, increases local tissue pressure, decreases stretching of the skin, assists muscles to propel lymphatic drainage, and prevents tissue refilling with an excess volume of lymph.

Many clients are referred for **complex decongestive physiotherapy**, which includes (1) distal-to-proximal massage of edematous areas to facilitate lymphatic drainage into collateral vessels, (2) application of compression dressings to relieve edema by reducing the excess volume of fluid in the interstitial space, (3) active exercise to promote lymphatic circulation and maintain functional use of the limb, and (4) care and maintenance of skin and nails that are vulnerable to secondary complications. A mechanical pulsating compression device or pneumatic device (Fig. 32-4) is applied to the arm and trunk. The alternating filling and emptying "milks" the lymph toward the duct, leading to venous drainage.

Sometimes, a microlymphatic surgical procedure in which veins and lymphatics are anastomosed (joined) may

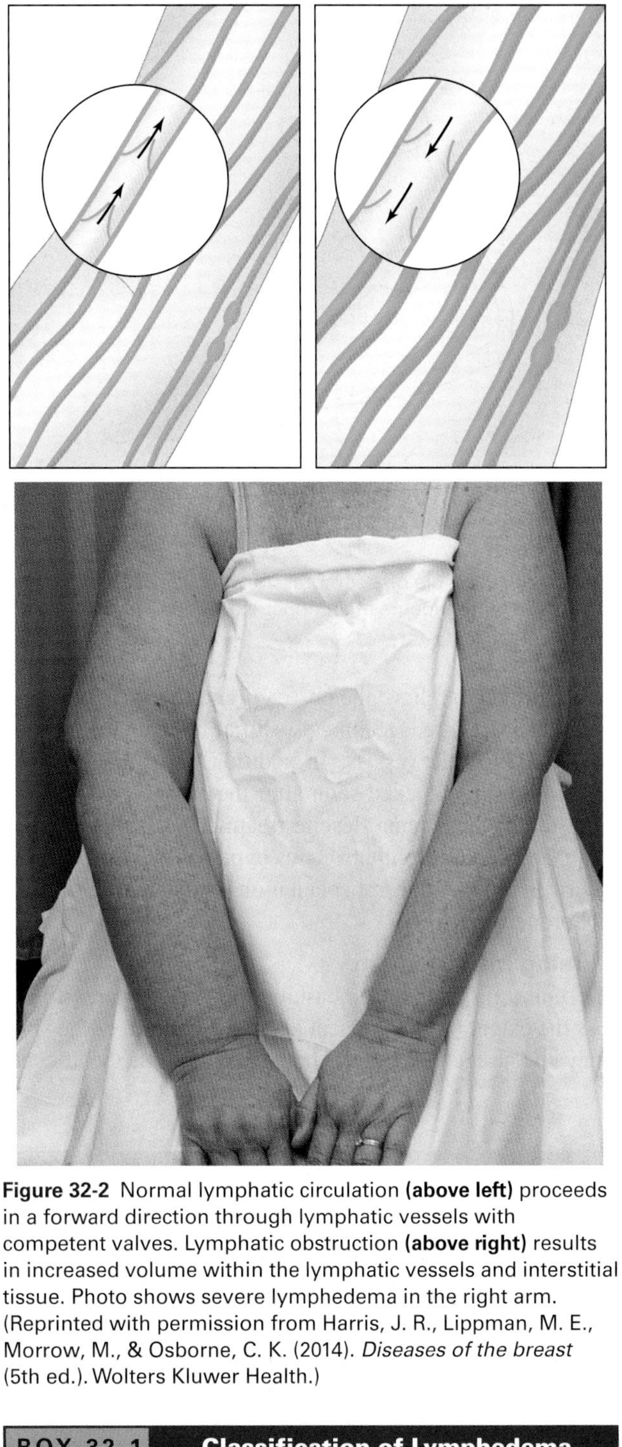

Figure 32-2 Normal lymphatic circulation **(above left)** proceeds in a forward direction through lymphatic vessels with competent valves. Lymphatic obstruction **(above right)** results in increased volume within the lymphatic vessels and interstitial tissue. Photo shows severe lymphedema in the right arm. (Reprinted with permission from Harris, J. R., Lippman, M. E., Morrow, M., & Osborne, C. K. (2014). *Diseases of the breast* (5th ed.). Wolters Kluwer Health.)

BOX 32-1 Classification of Lymphedema

Grade I (Mild): Circumference of affected limb is 2 cm, but not more than 4 cm larger than the unaffected limb; client is asymptomatic.

Grade II (Moderate): Circumference of affected limb is 4 cm, but not more than 8 cm larger than the unaffected limb; client experiences symptoms such as heaviness in the limb, pain, and limited movement.

Grade III (Severe): Circumference of affected limb is 8 cm greater than the unaffected limb, involves the entire limb, or is accompanied by infection or cellulitis (inflammation of connective tissue in or close to the skin).

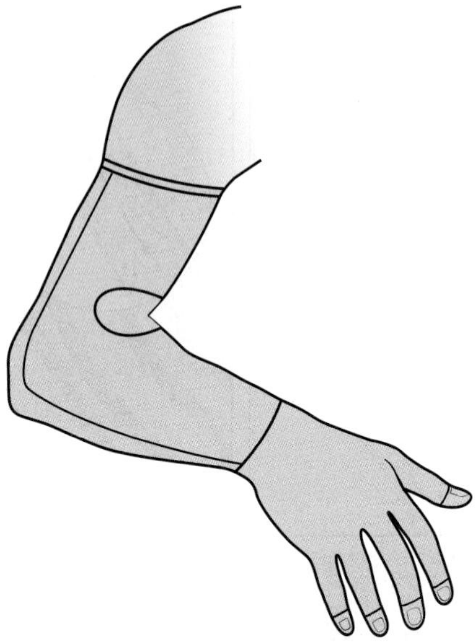

Figure 32-3 Example of a compression sleeve with glove used to manage lymphedema in an upper extremity.

be performed to relieve the obstruction of lymphatics. However, the procedure is technically difficult owing to the small size of lymphatic vessels. In addition, the joined vessels tend to become blocked soon after the surgery, resulting in persistent lymphedema despite treatment. Current surgical treatments include lymphovenous bypass procedure and vascularized lymph node transplantation procedure (Schaverien & Coroneos, 2019).

Nursing Management

The nurse inspects and measures the affected area to assess the extent of enlargement and the condition of the skin. They encourage the client to move and exercise the affected arm or leg to enhance the flow of lymph from the congested area. The nurse instructs the client to elevate the edematous extremities when sitting and teaches how to apply and use elastic garments and mechanical devices (Client and Family Teaching 32-1).

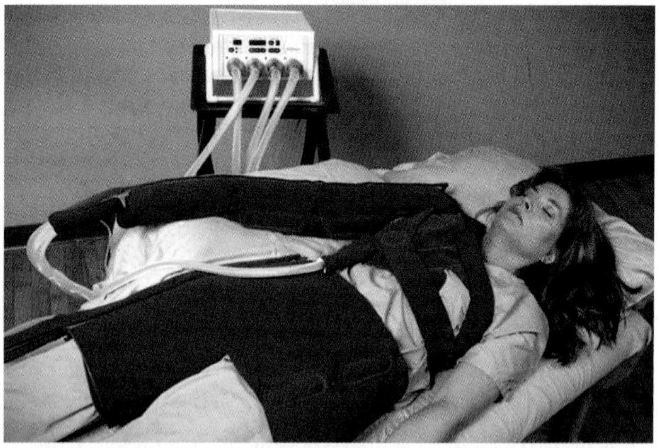

Figure 32-4 The Flexitouch is an example of a pneumatic device that simulates manual lymphatic drainage. This device is different than a traditional compression pump; it is a pneumatic device that has a light and variable pressure and works in two phases by treating the trunk first and then the affected extremity based on the principles of manual lymphatic drainage. (Used with permission from Tactile Medical.)

Client and Family Teaching 32-1
Use of a Compression Garment

When teaching the client about using a compression garment, the nurse instructs the client to

- Purchase two compression garments so that one can be worn while the other is washed and dried.
- Change the garment in the morning and again in the evening because the garment becomes stretched after 12 hours of being worn.
- Limit the time that the garment is *not* worn to no more than 30 to 60 minutes to prevent reaccumulation of tissue fluid and stretched skin.
- Follow the primary provider's direction for wearing the garment for shorter amounts of time after the limb has become remodeled, which may take 6 to 12 months or longer.
- Wash the removed garment in soap and water each day to prolong its elasticity and remove perspiration, bacteria, and dead skin cells.
- Use air drying out of direct sun to preserve the longevity of the garment.
- Remove the garment when swimming, if desired, as long as the extremity is submerged in water; if worn during swimming, rinse the garment to remove chlorinated or salt water before washing and drying.
- Replace a compression garment every 4 to 6 months.

Adapted from Boris, M., Weindorf, S., & Lasinski, B. B. (2012). *Lymphedema therapy.* http://www.lymphedema-therapy.com/FAQ.htm

Extensive emotional support is necessary when the edema is severe. The client's self-esteem often is decreased, which can lead to social withdrawal. The nurse supports the client's self-image by suggesting certain styles of clothing that conceal abnormal enlargement of an arm or leg. For information on client teaching, see the discussion that follows nursing management for clients after a mastectomy, in Chapter 54.

>>> ***Stop, Think, and Respond 32-1***

Why is a client at an increased risk for lymphedema after a mastectomy?

Lymphangitis and Lymphadenitis

Lymphangitis is inflammation of lymphatic vessels. When such inflammation affects the lymph nodes near the lymphatics, the condition is called **lymphadenitis**.

Pathophysiology and Etiology

An infectious agent, commonly a streptococcal microorganism, usually causes both lymphangitis and lymphadenitis. The lymph nodes and lymph vessels manifest typical signs of inflammation: redness, swelling, discomfort, and compromised function.

Assessment Findings

Red streaks follow the course of the lymph channels and extend up the arm or leg. Fever also may be present. When lymphadenitis is present, the lymph nodes along the lymphatic channels are enlarged and tender on palpation. Diagnosis is made by visual inspection and palpation.

Medical Management

A broad-spectrum antibiotic commonly is ordered.

Nursing Management

The nurse inspects the area and notes the client's response to antibiotic therapy. Assistance is given if the discomfort interferes with activities of daily living. Elevation reduces the swelling. Warmth promotes comfort and enhances circulation. The nurse notifies the primary provider if the affected area appears to enlarge, additional lymph nodes become involved, or body temperature remains elevated. In severe cases with persistent swelling, the nurse teaches the client how to apply an elastic sleeve or stocking.

Infectious Mononucleosis

Infectious mononucleosis is a viral disease that affects lymphoid tissues such as the tonsils and spleen. It can also involve other organs such as the brain, meninges, and liver.

Pathophysiology and Etiology

The **Epstein–Barr virus** causes infectious mononucleosis. The virus most commonly affects young adults, especially those in close living quarters, such as armed services housing and college dormitories. This contagious disorder spreads by direct contact with saliva and pharyngeal secretions from an infected person. It is transmitted by intimate kissing (not closed-mouth kissing); oral spraying during coughing, talking, or sneezing; or sharing food, cigarettes, or other items containing oral secretions. The incubation period can be as long as 30 to 50 days (Box 32-2).

At the time of infection, macrophages engulf the virus, resulting in a display of the antigen on the cell surface. Active production of T lymphocytes follows. The T lymphocytes trigger the production of B-cell lymphocytes and antibodies (refer to Fig. 33-1 in Chapter 33). They also infiltrate tissue, particularly the spleen, causing it to enlarge. An enlarged spleen may rupture if force is applied to the abdomen.

The symptoms generally resolve in approximately 2 to 6 weeks unless complications develop. One episode of infectious mononucleosis produces subsequent immunity; however, the virus remains in the body for the person's lifetime. The Epstein–Barr virus is believed to trigger Hodgkin lymphoma (discussed later in this chapter) in approximately 40% of people with this disease.

BOX 32-2 Characteristics of Infectious Mononucleosis

Usual age: 15–25 years

Incubation period: 30–50 days

Fever: irregular, usually about 2 weeks

Sore throat: marked, whitish-gray exudate

Adenopathy (enlargement of lymph nodes): most commonly anterior and posterior cervical chains; often generalized

Splenomegaly (enlargement of spleen): approximately 50%

Hepatomegaly (enlargement of liver): approximately 10%

››› *Stop, Think, and Respond 32-2*

What factors might make young adults particularly susceptible to acquiring infectious mononucleosis?

Assessment Findings

Signs and Symptoms

Fatigue, fever, sore throat, headache, and cervical lymph node enlargement typically occur. The tonsils ooze white or greenish-gray exudates (Fig. 32-5). Pharyngeal swelling can compromise swallowing and breathing. Some clients develop a faint red rash on their hands or abdomen. The liver and spleen may become enlarged. The symptoms persist for several weeks.

Diagnostic Findings

The leukocyte and differential cell counts demonstrate lymphocytosis. A positive slide agglutination test (Monospot, Monotest, Monosticon) is presumptive evidence that the Epstein–Barr virus is causing the symptoms. A rise in the Epstein–Barr virus antibody titer and a heterophil agglutination test result of 1:224 or greater is conclusive for infectious mononucleosis.

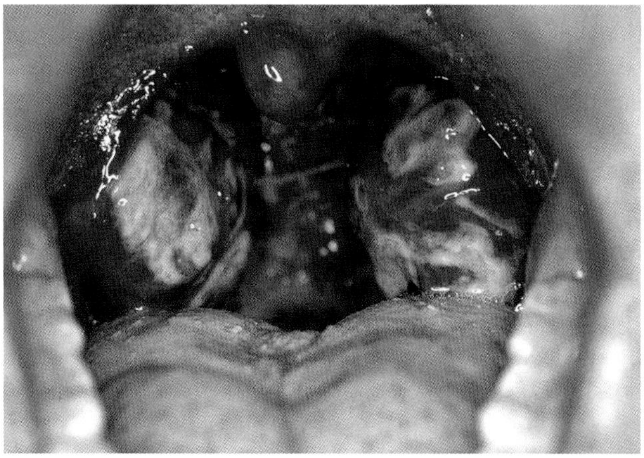

Figure 32-5 The throat of a person with infectious mononucleosis is red. The tonsils exude purulent drainage. The appearance can be mistaken for a streptococcal throat infection. (Copyright Dr. P. Marazzi/Science Source/Photo Researchers, Inc.)

Medical Management

The infection usually is self-limiting. Bed rest, analgesic and antipyretic therapy, and increased fluid intake are recommended. Corticosteroid therapy is prescribed to minimize severe pharyngeal inflammation or if complications such as hepatic involvement occur. If a bacterial infection such as sinusitis or streptococcal pharyngitis accompanies mononucleosis, an antibiotic is prescribed.

Nursing Management

The nurse inspects the client's throat for the extent of inflammation or edema, gently palpates the lymph nodes to detect swelling, and encourages fluids. Soft, bland foods; cool liquids; and gargling with warm salt water are best for clients with inflammation of the oral and pharyngeal mucosa. The nurse advises the client to rest as much as possible. If the client expresses concern over prolonged time off from work or school, the nurse listens and helps the client cope with the anxiety. Standard precautions are used when caring for a client with infectious mononucleosis because its transmission requires intimate contact with saliva; transmission as an airborne pathogen is unlikely. Although the virus remains dormant for the rest of a person's life, the possibility of infecting someone via blood transmission is low. A precautionary guideline is to withhold donating blood for at least 6 months after recovering from the illness. The transmission by blood transfusion is not considered to be a significant health hazard; a person can donate blood once the person is asymptomatic and has been released from further medical care (American Red Cross, 2016).

LYMPHOMAS

The term **lymphoma** applies to a group of cancers that affect the lymphatic system. The types of lymphoma are classified by the microscopic appearance of the malignant cells and how quickly the malignancy spreads. Two of the most common forms of lymphoma are **Hodgkin disease** and non-Hodgkin lymphoma (Table 32-1). AIDS-related lymphoma occurs in people who have been infected with the human immunodeficiency virus (HIV).

Hodgkin Disease

Hodgkin disease is a malignancy that produces enlargement of lymphoid tissue, the spleen, and the liver, with invasion of other tissues such as the bone marrow and lungs. It may appear in several forms: acute, localized, or latent with relapsing pyrexia (elevated temperature); splenomegaly (enlarged spleen); and as lymphogranulomatosis (multiple granular tumors or growths composed of lymphoid cells).

Pathophysiology and Etiology

Although the exact cause of Hodgkin disease is unknown, it appears that a virus, particularly the Epstein–Barr virus (the etiologic agent of infectious mononucleosis), causes mutations in some but not all lymphocytes, creating malignant cells known as *Reed–Sternberg cells.* **Reed–Sternberg cells** are nearly immortal, continue to reproduce prolifically, and, perhaps because of their somewhat similar appearance to normal lymphocytes, are somehow shielded from being destroyed by killer T cells. The virus also is believed to inactivate the immune system's ability to suppress tumor growth. The malignant cells release chemicals known as *cytokines* (see Chapter 33), causing inflammatory symptoms such as pain and fever. Some clients develop generalized itching and a skin rash because of the release of histamine from an atypical allergic/immune response.

The disease is more common in men than in women and most frequently occurs during late adolescence and young adulthood. Some clients survive 10 or more years; others die in 4 to 5 years. A cure is possible when the disease is localized to one section of the body. Clients who receive treatment usually have remissions that last for months or even years. Death results from respiratory obstruction, cachexia (state of ill health, malnutrition, and wasting), or secondary infections.

Assessment Findings

Signs and Symptoms

Early symptoms of Hodgkin disease include painless enlargement of one or more lymph nodes. The cervical lymph nodes are the first to be affected (Fig. 32-6). As the nodes enlarge, they press on adjacent structures, such as the esophagus or bronchi. As retroperitoneal nodes enlarge, there is a sense of fullness in the stomach and epigastric pain. Marked weight loss, anorexia, fatigue, and weakness occur.

TABLE 32-1 Comparison of Lymphomas

HODGKIN	NON-HODGKIN
Four subtypes	Thirty subtypes
Two peaks of onset: ages 15–40 years and older than age 55 years	Peaks after age 50 years
Reed–Sternberg cells	No Reed–Sternberg cells
Forty percent of affected clients test positive for Epstein–Barr virus	More common in industrial countries; common among clients with immunosuppression
B-cell origin	B- and T-cell origin
Usually starts in lymph nodes above the clavicle, commonly in the neck and chest; 15% are below the diaphragm; spreads downward from initial site	Common in abdomen, tonsils; can develop in areas other than lymph nodes (e.g., brain, nasal passages)
More orderly growth from one node to adjacent nodes; more curable	Less predictable growth; spreads to extranodal sites; less curable

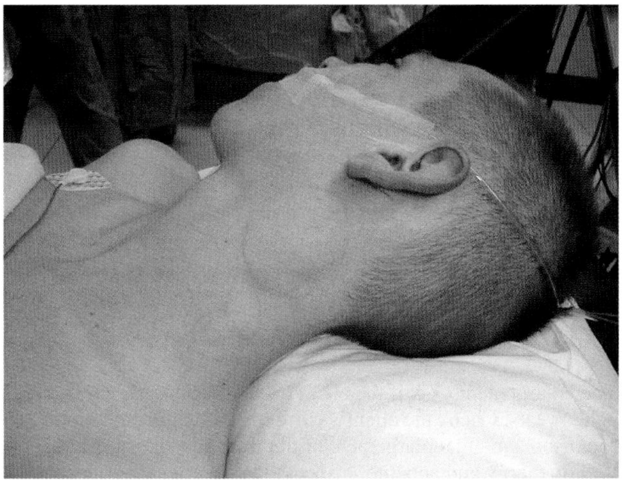

Figure 32-6 Fixed masses of cervical lymph nodes in Hodgkin lymphoma. (Photo courtesy of Mary L. Bradt, MD.)

Low-grade fever, pruritus, and night sweats are common. Sometimes, marked anemia and thrombocytopenia develop, causing a tendency to bleed. Resistance to infection is poor, and staphylococcal skin infections and respiratory tract infections often complicate the illness.

Diagnostic Findings

A complete blood count demonstrates low red blood cell count, elevated leukocytes, and a paradoxical decrease in lymphocytes. The Reed–Sternberg cells, characterized as giant multinucleated B lymphocytes, are microscopically identifiable in lymph node biopsies. Results of blood chemistry tests such as erythrocyte sedimentation rate are elevated, suggesting a current inflammatory process. Liver enzymes such as alkaline phosphatase are elevated. Computed tomography (CT), positron emission tomography (PET), and magnetic resonance imaging (MRI) demonstrate the size of lymph nodes and the spread of the disease in the thorax, abdomen, or pelvis. A bone marrow aspiration and lymph node biopsy may help to confirm the diagnosis or identify abnormalities of other blood cells. After diagnosis, the disease is staged from stage I to IV based on the number of positive lymph nodes and the involvement of other organs (Table 32-2). Staging helps determine treatment.

Stages I, II, III, and IV of adult Hodgkin disease are subclassified into A and B categories: B for those with defined general symptoms and A for those without B symptoms. The B designation is given to clients with any of the following symptoms:

- Unexplained loss of more than 10% of body weight in the 6 months before diagnosis
- Unexplained fever with temperatures above 100.4°F (38°C)
- Drenching night sweats (Note: The most significant B symptoms are fever and weight loss. Night sweats alone do not confer an adverse prognosis.)

Careful staging and treatment planning by a multidisciplinary team of cancer specialists is required to determine optimal treatment of clients with this disease.

TABLE 32-2 Stages of Hodgkin Disease

STAGE	INVOLVEMENT
I	Single lymph node region
II	Two or more lymph node regions on one side of the diaphragm
III	Lymph node regions on both sides of the diaphragm but extension is limited to the spleen
IV	Bilateral lymph nodes affected and extension includes spleen plus one or more of the following: bones, bone marrow, lungs, liver, skin, gastrointestinal structures, or other sites

Medical Management

Treatment of Hodgkin disease includes localized radiation to affected lymph nodes and chemotherapy with combinations of antineoplastic drugs (Table 32-3). Antibiotics are given to fight secondary infections. Transfusions are prescribed to control anemia. If resistance to treatment develops, autologous bone marrow or peripheral stem cells are harvested, followed by high doses of chemotherapy that destroy the bone marrow (see Chapters 18 and 31). Normal stem cells are separated from the malignant cells in the harvested specimen, and a transplant is performed.

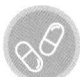

Pharmacologic Considerations

- Because young adults are most commonly diagnosed with Hodgkin disease, fertility is a big concern. Infertility is a side effect of chemotherapy agents used to treat this disease. Men should be told about sperm banking, and women should be counseled for menopausal symptom management before treatment is initiated.

TABLE 32-3 Drug Combinations for Hodgkin Lymphoma[a]

REGIMEN	DRUGS
ABVD	Doxorubicin (**A**driamycin), **b**leomycin, **v**inblastine, **d**acarbazine
BEACOPP	**B**leomycin, **e**toposide, doxorubicin (**A**driamycin), **c**yclophosphamide, vincristine (oncovin), **p**rocarbazine, **p**rednisone
Stanford V	Doxorubicin, vinblastine, mechlorethamine (nitrogen mustard), bleomycin, vincristine, etoposide, prednisone

Note. Chemotherapy is often given as a combination of drugs. Combinations usually work better than single drugs because different drugs kill cancer cells in different ways. The regimen of drugs is often times referred to by the abbreviation of the drugs (brand or generic names). The most common combination of agents in the United States is called ABVD. Other frequently used chemotherapy regimens for treating Hodgkin lymphoma are listed as well.
[a]Each of the drugs in these combinations is approved by the U.S. Food and Drug Administration to treat Hodgkin lymphoma.
American Cancer Society. (2020). *Chemotherapy for Hodgkin disease.* http://www.cancer.org/cancer/hodgkindisease/detailedguide/hodgkin-disease-treating-chemotherapy

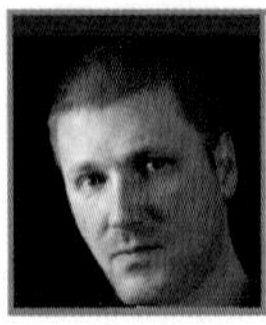

Clinical Scenario A 30-year-old male sees the occupational health nurse at his place of employment. He says, "Besides feeling tired all the time, I've felt a lump in my neck that has been getting larger over time. I've basically ignored it because it doesn't hurt; it just looks and feels strange." **How would the nurse use the nursing process to manage this client's care? See the following Nursing Process section.**

NURSING PROCESS FOR THE CLIENT WITH HODGKIN DISEASE

Assessment

Review the client's past history for infectious mononucleosis or symptoms resembling this disorder. Palpate enlarged lymph nodes and identify their location, size, and other notable characteristics, such as whether they are fixed or mobile. Inquire how long the client has noticed the enlarged lymph nodes and check for the presence and extent of tenderness in the area of lymph node enlargement. Ask if the client experiences fever, chills, or night sweats. Check the client's current weight and deviation from usual weight, enlargement of the liver and spleen, and level of energy and appetite. Inspect the appearance of the skin, ask about any itching, and discuss any additional symptoms caused by lymph node enlargement (e.g., coughing, breathlessness, nausea, vomiting).

Diagnosis, Planning, and Interventions

Client and Family Teaching 32-2 describes instructions for nurses to communicate to clients with Hodgkin disease. Other nursing care includes, but is not limited to, the following:

Ineffective Airway Clearance Risk and Impaired Gas Exchange: Related to compression of trachea secondary to enlarged cervical lymph nodes
Expected Outcome: Breathing will remain adequate to maintain blood oxygen saturation of 90% or greater.

- Assess respiratory status each shift and as needed. Note quality, rate, pattern, depth, flaring of nostrils, dyspnea on exertion, evidence of splinting, use of accessory muscles, and position for breathing. *Any deviation from quiet, effortless breathing indicates compromised ventilation.*
- Keep the neck in midline and place the client in high-Fowler position if respiratory distress develops. *This position avoids unnecessary pressure on the trachea and provides for increased lung expansion and improved air exchange.*
- Administer oxygen per primary provider's orders if blood saturation is consistently less than 90%. *Increasing the percentage of inhaled oxygen beyond 21% in the atmosphere reduces deficits in the blood oxygen level.*
- Place an endotracheal tube, laryngoscope, and bag-valve mask at the bedside for intubation. *Anticipation of the need for airway management ensures that medical intervention and emergency assistance are not delayed.*

Infection Risk: Related to immunosuppression secondary to impaired lymphocytes and drug or radiation therapy
Expected Outcome: Client will remain free of infection as evidenced by no fever and no symptoms of secondary infection.

- Restrict visitors or personnel with infections from contact with the client. *Reducing the number of organisms in the environment and restricting visitors and personnel with an infection reduce the transmission of pathogens to the client.*
- Practice conscientious hand hygiene and follow other principles of medical and surgical asepsis. *Cleaning hands and using aseptic techniques reduce the risk of transmitting pathogens from one location to another.*
- Institute infectious disease precautions if normal white blood cells are suppressed to dangerous limits. *Protective isolation techniques provide an environmental barrier against pathogens while a client is highly susceptible to disease.*

Altered Skin Integrity Risk: Related to pruritus, inadequate nutrition, and inactivity
Expected Outcome: Client's skin will remain intact throughout care.

- Use mild soap for bathing, rinse well, and pat dry. *Mild soap prevents excessive drying of the skin; patting instead of rubbing dry helps prevent friction, which can damage skin.*
- Apply ice to the skin for brief periods, give cool sponge baths, or provide cotton gloves if itching is intolerable. An oral or topical antipruritic medication often is necessary. *Cooling the skin reduces the sensation of itching, and cotton gloves reduce skin trauma from scratching with sharp fingernails. Antipruritic medications block the release of histamine.*
- Trim nails short to avoid scratching when itching occurs. *Trimming fingernails short prevents abrading the skin and providing an entrance for pathogens.*
- Change bedding as soon as possible if night sweats occur. *Wet bedding contributes to skin maceration.*
- Lift rather than pull the client across sheets when changing positions. *Lifting the client prevents shearing forces on the skin.*
- Support and protect bony prominences. *Areas where skin is stretched tautly over bony prominences create ischemia as a result of compressing skin capillaries between a hard surface (mattress) and the bone.*
- Collaborate with the primary provider to avoid drugs administered by the parenteral route. *Any breaks in skin integrity can provide an open route for the entrance of pathogens.*

NURSING PROCESS FOR THE CLIENT WITH HODGKIN DISEASE (continued)

Activity Intolerance and ADL Deficit: Related to anemia and generalized weakness from disease
Expected Outcome: Client will tolerate and perform essential activities as evidenced by heart and respiratory rates within normal limits.

- Divide care into manageable amounts. *Proportioning activities reduces energy expenditures.*
- Provide rest periods between activities. *Rest gives the body time to recover before the next demand for energy.*
- Perform priority activities first. *Client completes most important or necessary activities while energy levels are highest.*
- Assist the client with whatever activities of daily living are independently unmanageable. *Assistance reduces the client's energy expenditure.*

Evaluation of Expected Outcomes

Breathing is noiseless and effortless. The client shows no signs or symptoms of infection, the skin remains intact, and they can perform essential activities without compromising cardiorespiratory status.

Client and Family Teaching 32-2 Hodgkin Disease

The nurse instructs the client as follows:

- Keep appointments for medical follow-up.
- Take prescribed medications as directed. Report side effects to the primary provider.
- Avoid crowds or people who may have infectious diseases.
- Wash hands frequently.
- Avoid oral contact with germ-laden objects.
- Contact the primary provider if breathing becomes labored.
- Eat small amounts frequently or include a liquid nutritional supplement between meals and at bedtime (see Nutrition Notes).
- Reduce work schedule to avoid exhaustion. If that is not possible, rest frequently.
- Consult with an employer about sick leave considerations or a representative from the Social Security Administration about unemployment benefits and disability payments.
- Obtain a disability parking hanger to facilitate easy access to public buildings to lessen fatigue.

Non-Hodgkin Lymphomas

Non-Hodgkin lymphomas are a group of 30 subclassifications of malignant diseases that originate in lymph glands and other lymphoid tissue. Examples include lymphosarcoma, Burkitt lymphoma, and reticulum cell sarcoma. The incidence of non-Hodgkin lymphomas is six to seven times that of Hodgkin disease, and the number of cases continues to rise.

Pathophysiology and Etiology

No single definitive cause for non-Hodgkin lymphomas has been found, although a genetic link is strongly implicated in some types. An environmental trigger, such as a viral agent, chemical herbicides, pesticides, or hair dye, may induce the disease. The administration of immunosuppressive drugs to prevent transplant rejection also has been correlated with cases of non-Hodgkin lymphoma.

In non-Hodgkin lymphoma, chromosomal changes occur in the affected lymphocytes, and lymphoid tissue enlarges to accommodate the proliferative production of malignant cells. Non-Hodgkin lymphoma is classified as either (1) *indolent*, meaning that the client is relatively asymptomatic at diagnosis, and the disorder is relatively responsive to radiation and chemotherapy; or (2) *aggressive*, because the condition has a shorter onset with acute symptoms. Nevertheless, 30% to 60% of aggressive forms of non-Hodgkin lymphoma are curable with intensive treatment.

Assessment Findings

Symptoms of non-Hodgkin lymphoma depend on the site of lymph node involvement. Lymph node enlargement, which usually is diffuse rather than localized, occurs in cervical, axillary, and inguinal regions. The diagnosis and differentiation of the subtypes of non-Hodgkin lymphoma from Hodgkin disease depend on microscopic examination of lymphoid tissue biopsies. Additional tests are performed to determine the stage of the lymphoma.

Medical Management

Non-Hodgkin lymphoma is treated with radiation, chemotherapy, or both. The primary provider may adopt a "watch and wait" approach for clients with indolent forms of non-Hodgkin lymphoma, choosing to treat the client once the disease accelerates. Immunotherapy with monoclonal antibodies (MABs) and bone marrow transplants (BMTs) also is being used to cure lymphomas or extend the lives of clients with these diseases.

Monoclonal Antibody Therapy

Research continues on the use of biologic therapy (immunotherapy) with MABs to eliminate malignant cells and induce remission. With MABs, human cancer cells are injected into laboratory animals such as mice (see Chapter 18). The mice make lymphocytes that produce antibodies against the cancer cells. The mouse lymphocytes are harvested and fused with

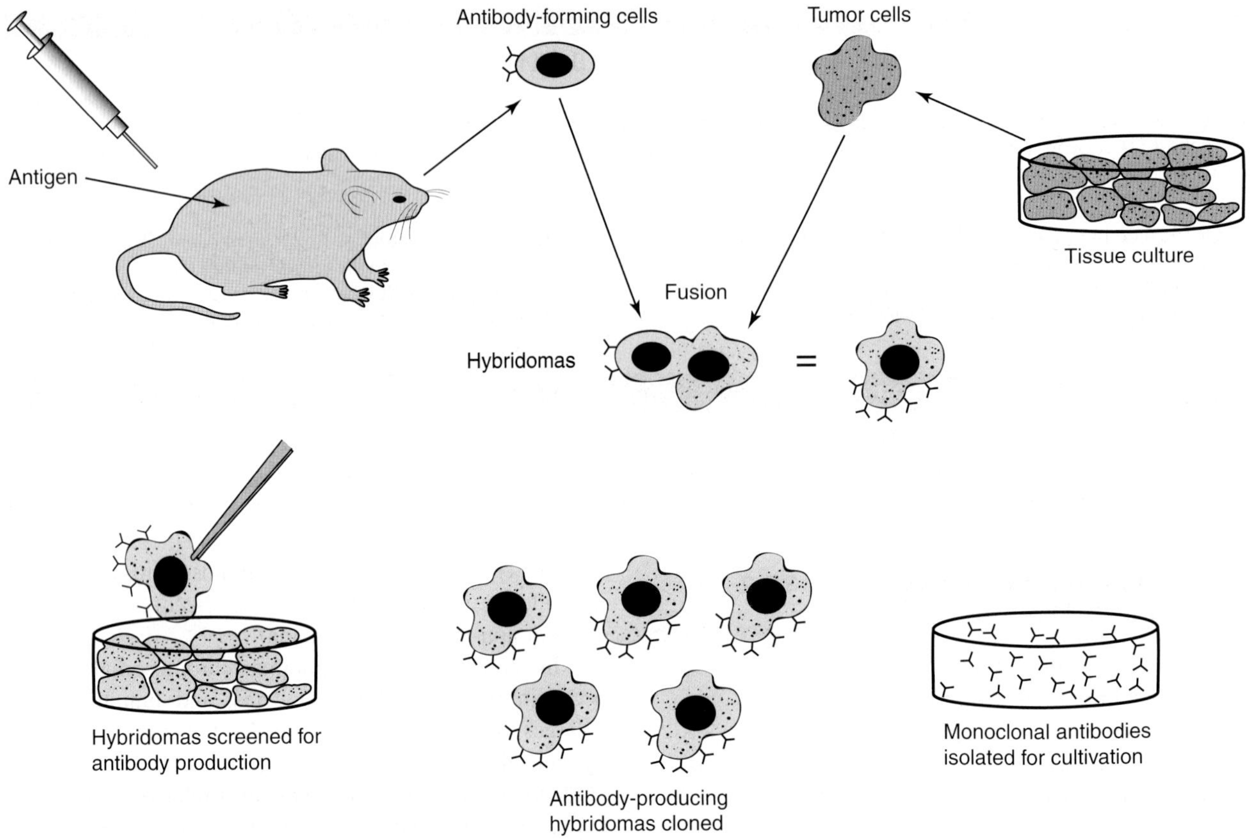

Figure 32-7 In monoclonal antibody (MAB) therapy, hybridomas, cloned cells that have been engineered to produce a specific antibody from sensitized mice, attack harmful proteins in the human body such as cancer cells.

a laboratory-grown cell, creating clones called hybridomas that, when administered to a client with cancer, continue to produce tumor-fighting antibodies (Fig. 32-7). The MABs are used alone or are bound to a chemotherapeutic or radioactive agent. The advantage of combining MABs with drugs or radiation is that they target and destroy cancer cells while sparing normal cells. MAB drugs approved for treating non-Hodgkin lymphoma include rituximab (Rituxan), ibritumomab and radioactive iodine (Zevalin), and ^{131}I Lym-1 (Oncolym).

Bone Marrow Transplant

Bone marrow and stem cell transplants (see Chapters 18 and 31) are considered a potential treatment modality when others are ineffective. Autologous (self-donated) bone marrow and peripheral blood stem cells are removed from the client with cancer and frozen. The donor cells are then infused with high doses of drugs and sometimes radiated to destroy all cancer cells. The same is done to the client, thus destroying most remaining bone marrow and stem cells. The frozen marrow and cells are thawed and transplanted into the client's vein, whereupon they recolonize the marrow with normal blood cells.

Instead of autologous transplants, some clients receive allogenic BMTs (i.e., marrow from a human donor), sometimes referred to as a *mini–bone marrow transplant* (mini-BMT). During a mini-BMT, the client is treated with moderate doses of drugs or mild total-body radiation to destroy as many cancer cells as possible and suppress the immune system to reduce the potential for destroying the donor cells. Consequently, when the client undergoes a mini-BMT, the possibility for rejection still exists. The phenomenon is referred to as *graft-versus-host disease* (GVHD) (see Chapter 18). Despite GVHD, allogenic BMTs have two advantages: (1) relapses of lymphoma are less frequent than with autologous transplants, and (2) they induce remissions when a relapse occurs.

Nursing Management

Nursing care is similar for all clients with lymphoma, whether they have non-Hodgkin lymphoma or Hodgkin disease (see Evidence-Based Practice 32-1). Because chemotherapy and radiation kill many cells, the nurse encourages clients to drink extra fluids (≥2500 mL/day) to facilitate excretion of the cells destroyed by therapy and compensate for fluids that are lost due to vomiting (Nutrition Notes).

Nutrition Notes

The Client With Hodgkin and Non-Hodgkin Disease

- Nausea and vomiting may accompany radiation and chemotherapy.
- Clients must maintain food and fluid intake.
- Offer clear liquids such as carbonated beverages and water, ice pops, and flavored gelatin until nausea subsides. Thereafter, small, frequent, low-fat meals help prevent nausea, improve nutritional intake, and reduce weight loss.

Evidence-Based Practice 32-1

Non-Hodgkin Lymphoma

Clinical Question

What support is available for clients if treatment for non-Hodgkin lymphoma ceases effectiveness?

Evidence

The odds of non-Hodgkin lymphoma returning or continuing to progress after being treated differs among clients. The response to treatment may be great at first; however, over time, the effect of treatments such as chemotherapy may be less effective. A client must make the personal decision to continue treatments when improvement or survival is unlikely. The client is able to choose to be supported through palliative care. Palliative care helps lessen or decrease symptoms such as pain or nausea and vomiting, to help clients feel the best they can. Palliative care can be offered along with medical interventions or might be the only treatment given based on the client's decision. The health care team works collaboratively with the client to make the best choices and support the client through the disease process. As progression continues, the client may also be referred for hospice care with a focus on comfort through this disease (American Cancer Society, 2018).

Nursing Implications

Clients with this disease process need support to have the best quality of life and comfort. Nurses may be part of a client's journey in this disease from diagnosis to comfort care near the end of the process. Client's needs, desires, and support are necessary throughout the process. Nurses can advocate for the client through these stages and provide compassion and support.

Reference

American Cancer Society. (2018). *Palliative and supportive care for non-Hodgkin lymphoma.* https://www.cancer.org/cancer/non-hodgkin-lymphoma/treating/palliative-care.html

KEY POINTS

- Occlusive, inflammatory, and infectious disorders
  - Lymphedema: accumulation of lymphatic fluid resulting from impaired lymph system
    - S&S: swelling, especially when dependent, skin thickened and rough
    - Treatment: symptomatic, elevate, pressure garments
  - Lymphangitis and lymphadenitis: inflammation of lymphatic vessels and nodes
    - S&S: red streaks following lymph channels, fever, swelling of lymph nodes
    - Treatment: antibiotics
  - Infectious mononucleosis: viral disease affects lymph tissues, tonsils spleen, can affect brain and liver
    - S&S: fatigue, fever, sore throat, headache, cervical lymph node enlargement
    - Treatment: bed rest, analgesic therapy, antipyretic therapy, increased fluid intake, corticosteroid therapy
- Lymphomas: group of cancer that affect lymphatic system
  - Hodgkin disease: malignancy that produces enlargement of lymphoid tissue, the spleen, and the liver with invasion of other tissues
    - S&S: painless enlargement of one or more lymph nodes, nodes enlarge and press on surrounding tissue. Weight loss, anorexia, fatigue, weakness, fever, pruritis, night sweats
    - Treatment: radiation of lymph nodes, chemotherapy, antibiotics to fight secondary infection, blood transfusions, bone marrow and/or stem cell transplants
  - Non-Hodgkin lymphomas: malignant diseases that originate in lymph glands, multiple types that include lymphosarcoma, Burkitt lymphoma, and reticulum cell sarcoma
    - S&S: depends on site, lymph node enlargement (diffuse to areas)
    - Treatment: radiation, chemotherapy, bone marrow transplants

CRITICAL THINKING EXERCISES

1. What are some differences between lymphedema and lymphoma?
2. What teaching is indicated for a person diagnosed with lymphedema?
3. What information can the nurse provide to parents who are concerned about their teenager who has acquired infectious mononucleosis?
4. Explain which lymphoma—Hodgkin disease or non-Hodgkin lymphoma—has the better prognosis and why.

NCLEX-STYLE REVIEW QUESTIONS PrepU

1. A college student diagnosed with infectious mononucleosis asks the school health nurse how the condition was acquired. The best answer by the nurse is that the virus is transmitted by what methods?
   1. Through microorganisms in infected blood
   2. Contact with the saliva of an infected person
   3. Consuming contaminated food or water
   4. The bite of an insect such as a mosquito
2. What nursing statements are accurate when teaching a client with infectious mononucleosis? Select all that apply.
   1. Take a mild analgesic for discomfort.
   2. Avoid contact sports temporarily.
   3. Continue usual activities of daily living.
   4. Antibiotic therapy can cure the infection.
   5. Tell others to avoid contact with your blood.
   6. The illness generally subsides in a week to 10 days.

3. A hospitalized client with Hodgkin disease is at risk for ineffective airway clearance and impaired gas exchange related to compression of the trachea by enlarged lymph nodes. What measure should the nurse take first to help ensure that breathing and blood oxygen saturation remain adequate?
   1. Administer oxygen per the primary provider's orders.
   2. Assess respiratory status during each shift.
   3. Place the client in semi- to high-Fowler position.
   4. Restrict visitors and unnecessary personnel.
4. When performing a physical assessment of the client in the early stages of Hodgkin disease, what is the most likely finding when the nurse palpates the client's lymph nodes?
   1. The lymph nodes are fixed and hard.
   2. The lymph nodes are enlarged and painless.
   3. The lymph nodes are small and firm.
   4. The lymph nodes are swollen and tender.
5. A primary provider orders a dose of vincristine (Oncovin) according to the client's body surface area (BSA) in square meter. The client is 65 inches tall and weighs 140 lb, which is 1.75 m^2. If the usual adult dose is 1.4 mg/m^2, what is the safe dose for this client? Record the answer in the nearest tenth. ______________ mg

WANT TO KNOW MORE? A wide variety of resources are available to enhance your learning and understanding of this chapter.

- Visit thePoint for resources such as:
  - NCLEX-Style Student Review Questions
  - Internet Resources
  - Journal Articles
  - Animations
  - Heart and Breath Sounds
  - Watch and Learn video clips
  - Practice and Learn video clips
  - Full text online
  - Documentation tool
- The Workbook for Introductory Medical-Surgical Nursing, 12th edition, sold separately, will help you review and apply essential content.
- PrepU is available to help students prepare for the NCLEX-PN examination.
- Lippincott CoursePoint combines digital text content and prepU for a fully integrated course solution that works the way you study and learn.
- Lippincott DocuCare presents ample opportunities to perform electronic health record keeping.

UNIT 8
Caring for Clients With Immune Disorders

33 Introduction to the Immune System

Words To Know

adenoids
anergy
antibodies
antigens
artificially acquired active immunity
B-cell lymphocytes
cell-mediated response
colony-stimulating factors
complement cascade
complement system
cytokines
cytotoxic T cells
effector T cells
helper T cells
histocompatibility markers
humoral response
immune response
immunocompetence
immunoglobulins
interferons
interleukins
lymph nodes
lymphatic system
lymphocytes
lymphoid tissues
lymphokines
macrophages
memory cells
microphages
monocytes
natural killer (NK) cells
naturally acquired active immunity
passive immunity
phagocytes
plasma cells
regulator T cells
spleen
stem cells
suppressor T cells
T-cell lymphocytes
thymus gland
tonsils
tumor necrosis factor

Learning Objectives

On completion of this chapter, you will be able to:

1. Explain the meaning of an immune response.
2. List two general components of the immune system.
3. Discuss the role of T-cell and B-cell lymphocytes.
4. Differentiate between an antigen and an antibody.
5. Name examples of lymphoid tissue.
6. List some cells and chemicals that enhance the function of the immune system.
7. Discuss the function of the complement cascade.
8. Name three types of immunity, describing how each develops.
9. Discuss techniques for detecting immune disorders.
10. Describe the role of the nurse when caring for a client with an immune disorder.

Although all humans have the same types of cells, each person's cells are unique and different from those of all others. Everyone's body cells are coded with distinct **histocompatibility** (tissue cell) **markers**. These markers act as a "fingerprint" that enables the immune system to differentiate self from nonself. When it detects a nonself substance, the immune system protects, defends, and destroys what it perceives as atypical or abnormal. Its primary targets are infectious, foreign, or cancerous cells. The **immune response**, a target-specific system of defense, primarily involves the **lymphocytes**, which are specialized cells that are located in blood and lymphoid tissue. An immune system that is overly active, as in allergic or autoimmune disorders (see Chapter 34), or one that is functioning poorly, as in AIDS (see Chapter 35), can be life threatening.

Gerontologic Considerations

- The body's number of T-cell lymphocytes decreases with age, which may be the result of gradual degeneration of the thymus gland. This change decreases the activity of the immune system, which increases the older client's risk for immunity-related problems.
- The amount of antibody produced in response to most foreign antigens decreases with age. Although vaccination against viral disorders is recommended, vaccines are less effective in older adults than in younger adults, probably because of the decreased immune response that occurs with age. The Centers for Disease Control and Prevention recommend annual seasonal influenza vaccine, pneumococcal polysaccharide vaccine (PPSV23; Pneumovax) for all adults 65 years or older or those who are at high risk, and shingles vaccine (Zostavax) for all over the age of 60.

ANATOMY AND PHYSIOLOGY

The immune system is a collection of specialized white blood cells and lymphoid tissues that maintain **immunocompetence**, the ability to cooperatively protect a person from external invaders and the body's own altered cells. The function of these structures is assisted and supported by the activities of natural killer cells, antibodies, and nonantibody proteins such as cytokines and the complement system (Fig. 33-1).

White Blood Cells

White blood cells (leukocytes) are produced in the bone marrow. Initially, all blood cells are nonspecific **stem cells** that later differentiate into various types of cells including lymphocytes, neutrophils, and monocytes (see Chapter 30). Figure 33-2 shows the development of various types of blood cells.

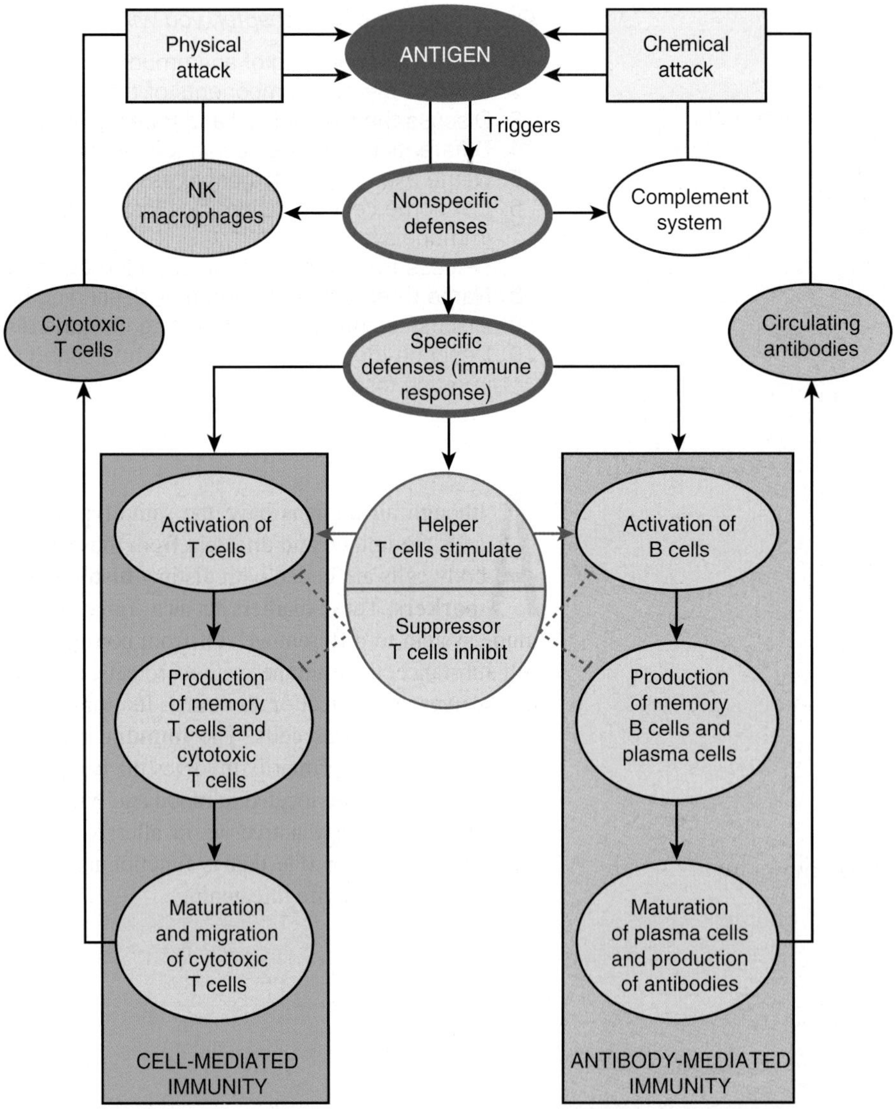

Figure 33-1 Schematic representation of the immune response. NK, natural killer.

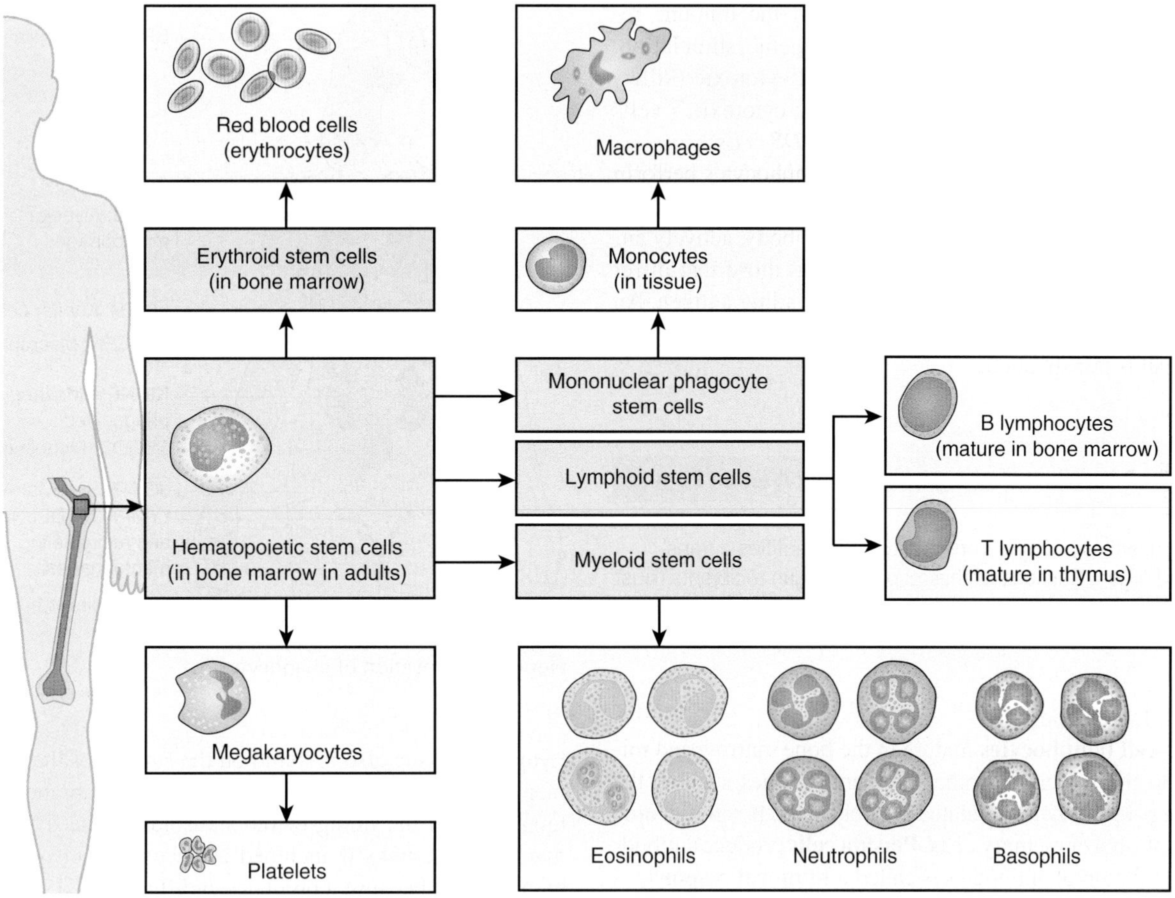

Figure 33-2 Origin of blood cells.

Lymphocytes

Lymphocytes, which are either T-cell or B-cell lymphocytes, comprise 20% to 30% of all leukocytes. T-cell and B-cell lymphocytes are the primary participants in the immune response. They distinguish harmful substances and ignore those natural and unique to a person. Table 33-1 identifies various types of lymphocytes and the roles they play in the immune response.

T-Cell Lymphocytes

The **T-cell lymphocytes** are manufactured in the bone marrow and travel to the thymus gland where they mature to become either regulator T cells or effector T cells. **Regulator T cells** are made up of helper and suppressor cells; **effector T cells** are killer (cytotoxic) cells. **Helper T cells** are especially important in fighting infection. They recognize **antigens**, which are protein markers on cells, and form additional T-cell clones that stimulate B-cell lymphocytes to produce antibodies against foreign antigens. **Antibodies** are chemical substances that destroy foreign agents such as microorganisms. Helper T cells are also called *T4 cells* or *CD4 cells*.

Cytotoxic T cells bind to invading cells, destroy the targeted invader by altering their cellular membrane and intracellular environment, and stimulate the release of chemicals called *lymphokines*. **Lymphokines**, a type of cytokine (discussed later in this chapter), attract neutrophils and monocytes to remove the debris. They also promote the maturation of more T cells when they detect antigens and direct B-cell lymphocytes to multiply and mature.

TABLE 33-1 Types and Functions of Lymphocytes

TYPE	FUNCTION
T Cells	
Regulator T Cells	
Helper T cells	Recognize antigens; stimulate B cells to produce antibodies
Suppressor T cells	Turn off the immune response
Effector T Cells	
Cytotoxic T cells	Bind to and destroy invader cells; stimulate the release of lymphokines
B Cells	
Plasma cells	Produce antibodies
Memory cells	Convert to plasma cells that will produce antibodies when reexposed to an antigen

Suppressor T cells limit or turn off the immune response in the absence of continued antigenic stimulation. The surface molecules of suppressor and cytotoxic (killer) T cells differ from those of helper T cells; cytotoxic T cells sometimes are referred to as *T8 cells* or *CD8 cells*.

The immune response that T-cell lymphocytes perform is called a *cell-mediated response*. A **cell-mediated response** occurs when T cells survey proteins in the body, actively analyze the surface features, and respond to those that differ from the host by directly attacking the invading antigen. An example of a cell-mediated response is one that occurs when an organ is transplanted.

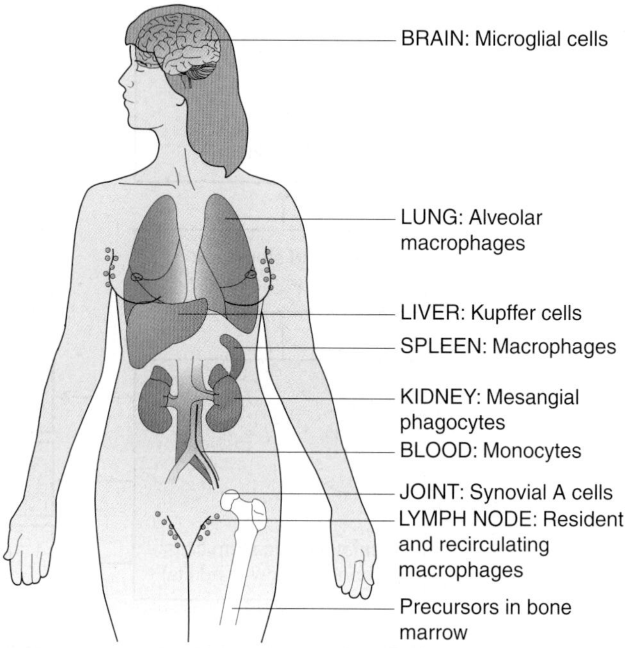

Figure 33-3 Location of phagocytes.

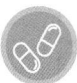

Pharmacologic Considerations

- "Nonself" is how the immune system identifies a transplanted organ. Because of this response, organ recipients must take antirejection drugs daily for the remainder of their lives.

B-Cell Lymphocytes

The **B-cell lymphocytes** mature in the bone marrow and migrate to the spleen and other lymphoid tissues such as the lymph nodes. When stimulated by T cells, the B cells become either plasma or memory cells. **Plasma cells** produce antibodies. Formation of antibodies is called a **humoral response**.

Memory cells convert to plasma cells on reexposure to a specific antigen. When activated, B cells accumulate in lymphoid tissues, which explains the phenomena of swollen and tender lymph nodes that accompany infectious disorders and an enlarged spleen in various immune disorders.

>>> *Stop, Think, and Respond 33-1*

Explain the difference between a cell-mediated response and a humoral response.

Neutrophils and Monocytes

Neutrophils and monocytes are **phagocytes**, cells that perform phagocytosis. *Phagocytosis* is the process of engulfing and digesting bacteria and foreign material (see Chapter 30). Phagocytes are stationary (fixed) or mobile. *Neutrophils*, also called **microphages** because they are small, are present in blood and migrate to tissue as necessary after a cell-mediated response. **Monocytes**, also called **macrophages** because they are large, are present in tissues such as the lungs, liver, lymph nodes, spleen, and peritoneum (Fig. 33-3). They also migrate after a cell-mediated response. The mononuclear phagocyte system consisting of monocytes and lymphocytes was formerly known as the *reticuloendothelial system*.

Lymphoid Tissues

Lymphoid tissues, such as the thymus gland, tonsils and adenoids, spleen, and lymph nodes, play a role in the immune response and prevention of infection (see Fig. 30-5). Lymphoid tissue also is found on the surface of the mucous membranes of the intestine, on alveolar membranes in the lungs, and in the lining of the sinusoids of the liver. Bone marrow sometimes is included as a component of the immune system because it produces undifferentiated stem cells.

Thymus Gland

The thymus gland is located in the neck below the thyroid gland. It extends into the thorax behind the top of the sternum. The thymus gland produces lymphocytes during fetal development. It may be the embryonic origin of other lymphoid structures such as the spleen and lymph nodes. After birth, the **thymus gland** programs T lymphocytes to become regulator or effector T cells. The thymus gland becomes smaller during adolescence but retains some activity throughout the life cycle.

Tonsils and Adenoids

The **tonsils** are located on either side of the soft palate of the oropharynx. The **adenoids** are located behind the nose on the posterior wall of the nasopharynx. These tissues filter bacteria from tissue fluid. Because they are exposed to pathogens in the oral and nasal passages, they can become infected and locally inflamed.

Spleen

The **spleen** has both hematopoietic and immune functions. It both acts as an emergency reservoir of blood and removes bacteria and old or damaged red blood cells from circulation.

Lymph Nodes

The **lymphatic system** consists of vessels similar to capillaries that drain tissue fluid, called *lymph*. At various areas in the body, the lymphatics converge and drain into larger structures called *lymph nodes*. The **lymph nodes** contain B lymphocytes and T lymphocytes and remove bacteria and other foreign particles from the lymph. Superficial lymph nodes in the axilla, groin, and neck are palpable when enlarged.

Natural Killer Cells

Natural killer (NK) cells are lymphocyte-like cells that circulate throughout the body looking for virus-infected cells and cancer cells. NK cells can identify atypical markers on the membranes of these cells without the help of T-cell or B-cell lymphocytes. Once identified, NK cells release potent chemicals that lethally alter the target cell's membrane, leading to its demise. Unfortunately, cancer cells can escape NK cell surveillance, which explains how cancer is able to become established and spread beyond its primary site.

Antibodies

Antibodies, proteins produced by B-lymphocyte plasma cells, are more correctly referred to as immunoglobulins (Igs). There are five types of immunoglobulins: IgA, IgD, IgE, IgG, and IgM. Each immunoglobulin has a separate role in ensuring the maintenance of a healthy state (Table 33-2).

Immunoglobulins bind with antigens and promote the destruction of invading cells in one of two ways. First, immunoglobulins may hinder antigens physically by (1) neutralizing their toxins; (2) linking them together in a process called *agglutination*; and (3) causing them to precipitate, or become solid. Second, antibodies can facilitate the destruction of antigens with other mechanisms—for example, those performed by nonantibody proteins such as the complement system and cytokines. (see Evidence-Based Practice 33-1.)

Nonantibody Proteins

Nonantibody proteins provide additional methods for disabling antigens and further protecting the body. There are two groups of nonantibody proteins. One group is referred to as the *complement system*, and the other is known collectively as *cytokines*.

Complement System

The **complement system** is made up of many different proteins that are activated in a chain reaction, known as the **complement cascade**, when an antibody binds with an antigen. Collectively, the complement proteins cooperate with antibodies to attract phagocytes, coat antigens to make them more recognizable for phagocytosis (a process known as *opsonization*). Collective complements insert themselves within the antigen's cell wall causing holes to form and the antigen's contents to leak resulting in its destruction (Fig. 33-4), and stimulate inflammation through the release of histamine from mast cells and basophils.

Cytokines

Cytokines are chemical messengers released by lymphocytes, monocytes, and macrophages. There are many subgroups of cytokines, including interleukins, interferons, tumor necrosis factor, and colony-stimulating factors.

Evidence-Based Practice 33-1

Sleep and the Immune System

Clinical Question

How does sleep affect the immune system?

Evidence

The sleep-and-wake cycle is a 24-hour rhythm that is connected to numerous functions of the body. The immune system also has an internal clock based on the release of certain proteins such as cytokines which can stimulate immunity. The sleep–wake cycle is a balance between the sleep cycle and the internal clock of the immune system. Sleep may be interrupted in numerous situations, including sickness, chronic diseases with pain and inflammation, and hospitalizations. Another example may be the ICU, with sleep disturbances that may include noise level, lights, client symptoms, medications, and equipment. In such situations, the sleep–wake cycle and the immune system are off balance, which may lead to sickness and infection in clients. Clients in intensive care units (ICUs) who have acute recovery needs may have their healing hampered by a lack of sleep (Physical Health, 2020)

Clients in the ICU or hospital may have their health affected owing to sleep disturbances. The nurse should keep noises at a low level and adjust lighting if needed to promote sleep. The nurse should also take note of medications that interfere with sleep patterns in clients. The nurse and health care team can work with the client to make sure that every opportunity is used to promote sleep and decrease the risk of illness.

Reference

Sleep Foundation. (2020). *How sleep affects immunity*. https://www.sleepfoundation.org/physical-health/how-sleep-affects-immunity

TABLE 33-2 Types of Immunoglobulins

TYPE	PERCENTAGE OF TOTAL (%)	LOCATION	FUNCTION
IgG	75	Intravascular and intercellular fluid	Neutralizes bacterial toxins; accelerates phagocytosis
IgA	15	Body secretions such as saliva, sweat, tears, mucus, bile, colostrum	Interferes with entry of pathogens through exposed structures or pathways
IgM	10	Intravascular serum	Agglutinates (clusters) antigens and lyses (dissolves) cell walls
IgD	0.2	Surface of lymphocytes	Binds to antigens; promotes secretion of other immunoglobulins
IgE	0.004	Surface of basophils and mast (connective tissue) cells	Promotes release of vasoactive chemicals such as histamine and bradykinin in allergic, hypersensitivity, and inflammatory reactions

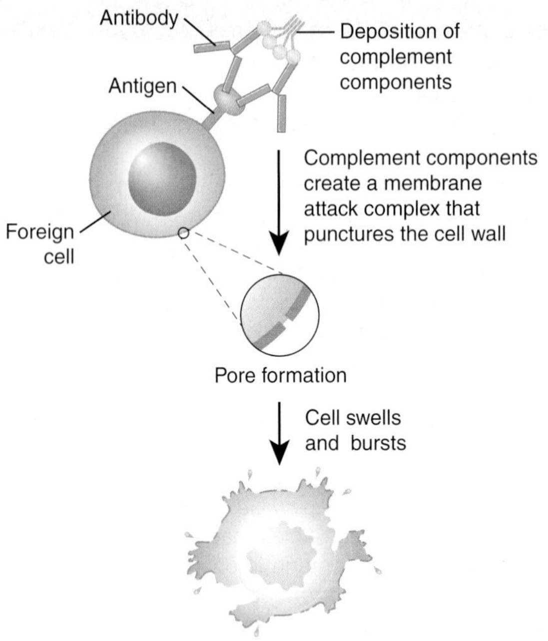

Figure 33-4 Pathway of the complement system. (Adapted from Harris, J. R., Lippman, M. E., Morrow, M., Osborne, C. K. (2004). *Diseases of the breast* (3rd ed). Lippincott Williams & Wilkins.)

Interleukins

Interleukins carry messages between leukocytes and tissues that form blood cells. Some interleukins enhance the immune response, whereas others suppress it (Martini & Bartholomew, 2016). Examples of interleukin activity include the following:

- Promotion of inflammation and fever
- Formation of scar tissue by fibroblasts
- Growth and activation of NK cells and additional T cells
- Production of mast cells
- Growth of B cells, formation of plasma cells, and production of antibodies
- Formation of new blood vessels, known as *angiogenesis*
- Stimulation of the anterior pituitary gland to secrete corticotrophin

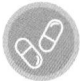

Pharmacologic Considerations

■ Manufactured interleukins are being used and studied for some types of cancer, autoimmune, and immunity disorders. Aldesleukin (Proleukin) is a manufactured interleukin currently used to treat malignant melanoma and metastatic renal tumors.

Interferons

Interferons are chemicals that primarily protect cells from viral invasion. They enable cells to resist viral infection and slow viral replication. They have been used as adjunctive therapy in the treatment of AIDS. Interferons have also been used to treat some forms of cancer such as leukemia because they stimulate NK-cell activity. Interferon is administered because digestive enzymes destroy its protein structure.

Tumor Necrosis Factor

When **tumor necrosis factor** (TNF), a type of cytokine, was first discovered, it showed promise as a means of shrinking tumors. Although TNF reduced tumors in laboratory animals, it caused toxic effects in humans. Experiments continue to determine if the antitumor effect can be achieved and the toxic side effects limited by injecting TNF directly into the tumor rather than administering it by a route through which it is systemically absorbed and distributed.

Research has found that TNF helps in cellular repair when administered in small doses. Excess amounts destroy healthy tissue. Consequently, TNF and drugs known as *TNF inhibitors* are being used to regulate various autoimmune (see Chapter 34) and inflammatory disorders.

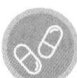

Pharmacologic Considerations

■ Tumor necrosis factor (TNF) inhibitors that are used to treat rheumatoid arthritis are called *disease-modifying anti-rheumatic drugs* or *Biologic DMARDs*. They work to stimulate the body's natural immune response. Biologic DMARDs include etanercept (Enbrel), adalimumab (Humira), infliximab (Remicade), certolizumab pegol (Cimzia), and golimumab (Simponi).

Colony-Stimulating Factors

Colony-stimulating factors (CSFs) are cytokines that prompt the bone marrow to produce, mature, and promote the functions of blood cells. CSFs enable stem cells in bone marrow to differentiate into specific types of cells such as leukocytes, erythrocytes, and platelets. Pharmacologic preparations of CSFs, such as epoetin alfa (Epogen), filgrastim (Neupogen), pegfilgrastim (Neulasta), and sargramostim (Leukine), are used to promote the natural production of blood cells in people whose own hematopoietic functions have become compromised. Consequently, clients with cancer who are receiving antineoplastic drugs may avoid interrupting treatment by reducing their risk of infection, clients who have undergone bone marrow transplantation may recover sooner, and those with chronic renal failure can avoid repeated blood transfusions to compensate for their anemia.

TYPES OF IMMUNITY

The three types of immunity are naturally acquired active immunity, artificially acquired active immunity, and passive immunity (Fig. 33-5). Both forms of active immunity require the person's own production of plasma and memory cells. Passive immunity occurs when ready-made antibodies are provided.

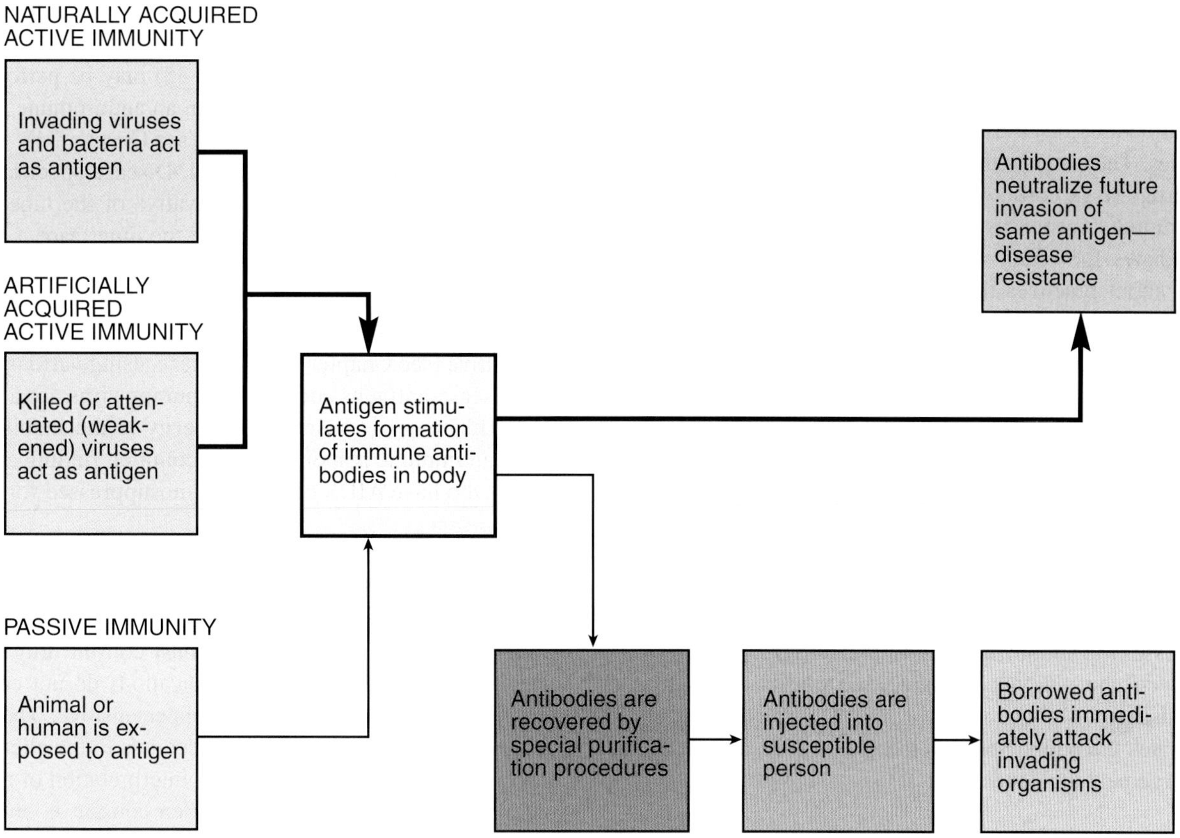

Figure 33-5 Active and passive immunity.

Naturally Acquired Active Immunity

Naturally acquired active immunity occurs as a direct result of infection by a specific microorganism. An example is the immunity to measles that develops after the initial infection. Not all invading microorganisms produce a response that gives lifelong immunity.

Artificially Acquired Active Immunity

Artificially acquired active immunity results from the administration of a killed or weakened microorganism or toxoid (attenuated toxin). The memory cells manufactured by the B lymphocytes and their subsequent replacements "remember" the killed or weakened antigen and recognize it if a future invasion occurs. Recommended immunization schedules are available on the Centers for Disease Control and Prevention website at http://www.cdc.gov. Immunizations that are not administered or completed during childhood are recommended for adults. Some immunizations, such as those for tetanus, influenza, and pneumonia, require readministration to maintain adequate immunity.

Passive Immunity

Passive immunity develops when ready-made antibodies are given to a susceptible person. The antibodies provide immediate but short-lived protection from the invading antigen. No memory cells are produced, and the level of the injected antibodies diminishes over a period of several weeks to a few months.

Ready-made antibodies are obtained from the serum of another organism, either animal or human. Immune serum globulin, also called *gamma globulin* or *immunoglobulin*, is recovered from pooled human plasma. Because the pool comprises plasma from more than one donor, the serum is likely to contain a variety of specific antibodies. Human immune serum is used for passive immunization against measles (rubella), pertussis (whooping cough), hepatitis B, chickenpox (varicella), and tetanus.

Newborns receive passive immunity to some diseases for which their mothers have manufactured antibodies. The circulating maternal antibodies cross the placenta and enter fetal circulation. As with other forms of passive immunity, infants are protected for only a few months after birth.

Concept Mastery Alert

Passive Immunity

With passive immunity, ready-made antibodies are given to provide temporary protection from an invading antigen. By contrast, with artificially acquired active immunity, memory cells are created that "remember" the antigen and trigger future antibody production.

››› *Stop, Think, and Respond 33-2*

Identify the type of immunity that develops from (1) receiving a vaccine for hepatitis B, (2) having chickenpox, and (3) receiving an injection of gamma globulin.

ASSESSMENT

History

The nurse obtains a history of immunizations, recent and past infectious diseases, and recent exposure to infectious diseases. They review the client's drug history because certain drugs (e.g., corticosteroids) suppress the inflammatory and immune responses (e.g., TNF inhibitors). The nurse investigates the client's allergy history and questions the client about practices that put them at risk for AIDS (see Chapter 35).

Physical Examination

The beginning of the physical examination is a general appraisal of the client's health. The nurse notes whether the client appears healthy, acutely or mildly ill, malnourished, extremely tired, or listless (nutrition can affect immune function; Nutrition Notes). The nurse records vital signs and weight. The nurse then performs the following:

- Examines the skin for rashes or lesions
- Assesses the abdomen for an enlarged liver or spleen
- Inspects the pharynx for large, red tonsils and purulent drainage
- Palpates the lymph nodes in the neck, axilla, and groin for enlargement and tenderness

Nutrition Notes

Nutrition and Immunocompetence

- Nutrients important in immune system functioning include amino acids such as arginine and glutamine; essential fatty acids and omega-3 fatty acids; the B vitamins, especially vitamin B_6 and folic acid; vitamins A, C, and E; and the minerals copper, iodine, and magnesium.
- Singly or combined, nutrient deficiencies have the potential to affect almost all aspects of immune system functioning. Excesses of certain nutrients, namely, iron, zinc, vitamin E, and polyunsaturated fatty acids, also can impair immune function. The exact amounts and proportions of nutrients needed for optimal immune system function in healthy people, however, are not yet known.
- Until more is known about nutrient interactions, the best dietary advice to maximize immune function in healthy people is to eat a balanced diet that is rich in fruits and vegetables, and adequate in protein.
- Several immune-enhancing tube-feeding formulas are available, such as Immun-Aid, Impact, Alitraq, Perative, Crucial, and Vivonex T.E.N. These formulas are enriched with glutamine and/or arginine, omega-3 fatty acids, and nucleotides. These added ingredients enhance the production of T lymphocytes and NK cells, resulting in increased cell-mediated immunity.

Diagnostic Tests

Laboratory tests are used to identify immune system disorders. They usually include a complete blood count (CBC) with differential. Protein electrophoresis screens for diseases associated with a deficiency or excess of immunoglobulins. T-cell and B-cell assays (or counts) and the enzyme-linked immunosorbent assay (see Chapter 35) may be performed. Additional tests are performed when an autoimmune or genetic immune disorder is suspected (see Chapter 34).

Skin tests may be administered. Disease-specific antigens, such as purified protein derivative of the tuberculin toxin, are injected intradermally on the inner aspect of the forearm. The injection area swells if the client has developed antibodies against the antigen (see Chapter 21). The client is not necessarily actively infectious if the test results are positive (see Chapter 21). Skin tests using various common disease antigens such as the mumps virus are administered if anergy is suspected. **Anergy** is the inability to mount an immune response. It is a common finding among clients who have AIDS or are immunosuppressed for other reasons.

Nursing Management

Clear identification of any substances to which the client is allergic is essential. The nurse must consult drug references to verify that prescribed medications do not contain substances to which the client is hypersensitive. They explain all diagnostic skin testing procedures to the client and inform the client when to return for interpretation of the results. The nurse ensures that a written consent is obtained before testing for human immunodeficiency virus (HIV) and keeps the results of HIV testing confidential. Standard precautions (see Chapter 12) are required whenever there is the potential for contact with blood or body fluids. The nurse should follow agency guidelines for controlling infectious diseases or protecting the client who is immunosuppressed. Client teaching includes information about immunizations and instructions regarding drug therapy prescribed for disorders involving the immune system.

KEY POINTS

- The complement system is made up of many different proteins that are activated in a chain reaction, known as the complement cascade, when an antibody binds with an antigen.
  - Antibody: a blood protein produced in response to and counteracting a specific antigen. Antibodies combine chemically with substances which the body recognizes as alien, such as bacteria, viruses, and foreign substances in the blood.
  - Antigen: a toxin or other foreign substance which induces an immune response in the body, especially the production of antibodies.
- Colony-stimulating factors (CSFs): cytokines that prompt the bone marrow to produce, mature, and promote the functions of blood cells. CSFs enable stem cells in bone marrow to differentiate into specific types of cells such as leukocytes, erythrocytes, and platelets.

- Immunity
  - Naturally acquired active immunity: a direct result of infection by a specific microorganism.
  - Artificially acquired active immunity: results from the administration of a killed or weakened microorganism or toxoid.
  - Passive immunity: develops when ready-made antibodies are given to a susceptible person. The antibodies provide immediate but short-lived protection from the invading antigen. Newborns receive passive immunity to some diseases for which their mothers have manufactured antibodies.

CRITICAL THINKING EXERCISES

1. How would you respond to a friend who tells you that their sister has an immune disorder and asks what this means?

2. Discuss the benefit of obtaining immunizations for common childhood diseases.

3. If someone you know has been exposed to hepatitis B, what would you recommend to prevent a subsequent infection?

4. Why are the tonsils and adenoids not being removed as aggressively as they were in the past?

NCLEX-STYLE REVIEW QUESTIONS PrepU

1. A client had a splenectomy following a serious motor vehicle accident. The parents ask the nurse if there are any special considerations following the surgical removal of the spleen. What is the most correct response?
   1. The client is susceptible to anemia because the spleen produces red blood cells.
   2. The client is susceptible to acidosis because the spleen maintains acid–base balance.
   3. The client is susceptible to bleeding because the spleen synthesizes vitamin K.
   4. The client is susceptible to infection because the spleen removes bacteria from the blood.

2. What type of immunity develops as a result of having an infection with a specific microorganism?
   1. Naturally acquired passive immunity
   2. Artificially acquired passive immunity
   3. Naturally acquired active immunity
   4. Artificially acquired active immunity

3. When a nurse administers drugs that suppress a client's immune system, what is the client most likely to develop?
   1. Allergic reactions
   2. Opportunistic infections
   3. Malignant cancers
   4. Acquired anemia

4. When the nurse cares for a client, what structures should the nurse examine to detect signs of an immune-related disorder? Select all that apply.
   1. The nurse collects a voided urine specimen.
   2. The nurse inspects the skin's appearance.
   3. The nurse auscultates the abdomen.
   4. The nurse palpates the client's neck.
   5. The nurse looks at the oral and nasopharynx.

5. A client is suspected of having an immune system disorder. What laboratory test would the nurse expect to be ordered during the initial blood studies?
   1. Blood chemistry
   2. Complete blood count (CBC)
   3. CBC with differential
   4. Liver enzyme studies

WANT TO KNOW MORE? There are a wide variety of online resources available on thePoint to enhance learning and understanding of this chapter.

Go to **thePoint.lww.com/activate** and use the activation code found in the front of this text to unlock these online resources.

34 Caring for Clients With Immune-Mediated Disorders

Words To Know

antigens
allergens
allergic disorder
alloimmunity
anaphylaxis
angioneurotic edema
autoantibodies
autoimmune disorders
chemotaxis
chronic fatigue syndrome
contactants
desensitization
exacerbations
fibromyalgia
histocompatible cells
immunoglobulin antibodies
induration
inhalants
injectants
intradermal injection test
mast cells
orthostatic intolerance
patch test
radioallergosorbent blood test
remission
scratch test
sensitization
sublingual-swallow immunotherapy
tilt-table test
urticaria

Learning Objectives

On completion of this chapter, you will be able to:

1. Describe an allergic disorder.
2. List five examples of allergic signs and symptoms.
3. Name four categories of allergens, and give an example of each.
4. Give four examples of allergic reactions, including two that are potentially life-threatening.
5. Describe diagnostic skin testing.
6. Name three methods for treating allergies.
7. Discuss the nursing management of a client with an allergic disorder.
8. Explain the meaning of autoimmune disorder, and give at least three examples of related diseases.
9. Discuss theories that explain the development of an autoimmune disorder.
10. Name three categories of drugs used in the treatment of autoimmune disorders.
11. Discuss the nursing management of a client with an autoimmune disorder.
12. Give two explanations for how chronic fatigue syndrome (CFS) develops.
13. List common symptoms experienced by people with chronic fatigue syndrome.
14. Name common nursing diagnoses, desired outcomes, and related nursing interventions for clients who have chronic fatigue syndrome.

The immune system sometimes responds aggressively and destructively to substances that may not always be potentially harmful. Two examples of such a response include allergic and autoimmune disorders. This chapter discusses allergic and autoimmune disorders and the appropriate nursing care for affected clients. It also explores chronic fatigue syndrome (CFS), which is a consequence of an immune-mediated disorder, and its nursing management.

Gerontologic Considerations

■ Adverse reactions to antihistamines, such as dizziness, sedation, and confusion, are more common in older adults, necessitating careful assessment and monitoring. Beers criteria, a reference that identifies prescription drug safety issues for older adults, is helpful for evaluating potential risks and benefits commonly experienced because of

Gerontologic Considerations (*continued*)

changes from aging (American Geriatrics Society, 2015). For example, older men with benign prostatic hypertrophy may experience difficulty voiding while taking antihistamines due to anticholinergic side effects.

- With age, cells within the body decrease in sensitivity, which interferes with recognition of self from foreign components. This change increases the risk of autoimmune disorders (e.g., systemic lupus erythematosus). As a person ages, higher levels of autoantibodies may be directed to endocrine glands, so attention to symptoms of hypothyroidism and hypopituitarism is important.
- Chronic fatigue and diminished energy are functional consequences of late-life depression.
- An older adult who reports CFS should be evaluated for depression.

ALLERGIC DISORDERS

An **allergic disorder** is characterized by a hyperimmune response to weak antigens that usually are harmless. The antigens that can cause an allergic response are called **allergens** (Table 34-1). Allergens gain entry to the host from the environment. Allergies can occur at any age, and the pattern of allergic response can vary in the same person during their life. For example, a person may suddenly develop an allergic reaction to a substance such as latex, even though they have had multiple prior contacts with latex and no past problems. On the other hand, an allergic response to one agent may gradually disappear or be replaced by sensitivity to another substance. The reason for these changes is unclear.

Types of Allergies

An allergic disorder is manifested in a variety of ways depending on the manner in which the allergen gains entry to the body and the intensity of the response. Organs and structures that are primarily involved in allergic reactions include the skin, respiratory passageways, gastrointestinal tract, blood, and vascular system (Table 34-2). Some types of allergic manifestations cause temporary, localized discomfort, whereas others are life-threatening.

TABLE 34-1 Common Allergens

ALLERGEN	EXAMPLES	COMMON REACTION
Ingestants	Food (peanuts, milk, wheat, eggs, fish), drugs (aspirin, sulfonamides, antibiotics, especially penicillin)	Gastroenteropathy, dermatitis, asthma, anaphylaxis, urticaria, angioedema, serum sickness
Inhalants	House dust and mites, insect excrement, animal products (dander, saliva, urine), pollens, spores	Allergic asthma, rhinitis, hypersensitivity pneumonitis
Contactants	Plant oils, topical medications, occupational chemicals, cosmetics, metals in jewelry and clothing fasteners, hair dyes, latex	Contact dermatitis, urticaria, or anaphylaxis (rare)
Injectants	Drugs, bee venom	Anaphylaxis, angioedema, acute urticaria

>>> *Stop, Think, and Respond 34-1*

List substances to which you or others you know are allergic and how the symptoms are managed.

Pathophysiology and Etiology

More than 50 million Americans have one or more allergic disorders, the fifth most common cause of chronic disorders in the United States (Allergy, 2018). The tendency to develop allergies can be inherited. Although members of the same family may have allergies, they may not all be sensitive to the same allergens. Allergy-prone individuals may react to more than one type of antigen. For example, the same person may be sensitive to ragweed pollen and eggs.

The first exposure to an allergen does not produce symptoms; rather, it causes sensitization. **Sensitization** is the process by which cellular and chemical events occur after a second or subsequent exposure to an allergen. Once

TABLE 34-2 Types of Allergies

ALLERGY TYPE	SIGNS AND SYMPTOMS	MEDICAL MANAGEMENT
Allergic rhinitis	Sneezing, itching, nasal congestion, watery nasal discharge, itching and redness of the eyes	Antihistamines, nasal decongestants, corticosteroid nasal spray, immunotherapy, allergen avoidance, eye drops
Contact dermatitis	Itching, burning, redness, rash on contact with substance	Allergen avoidance, wearing gloves, topical or oral antihistamines and corticosteroids
Dermatitis medicamentosa	Sudden generalized bright red rash, itching, fever, malaise, headache, arthralgias	Discontinuation of drug, antihistamines, and topical corticosteroids
Food allergy	Nausea, vomiting, diarrhea, abdominal cramping, malaise, itching, wheezing, rash, cough	Identification and avoidance of allergenic food Intubation, subcutaneous epinephrine, aminophylline in severe reactions
Urticaria	Itching, swelling, redness, wheals of superficial skin layers	Topical or oral antihistamines and corticosteroids
Angioedema	Itching, swelling, redness of deeper tissues and mucous membranes	Intubation, subcutaneous epinephrine, aminophylline

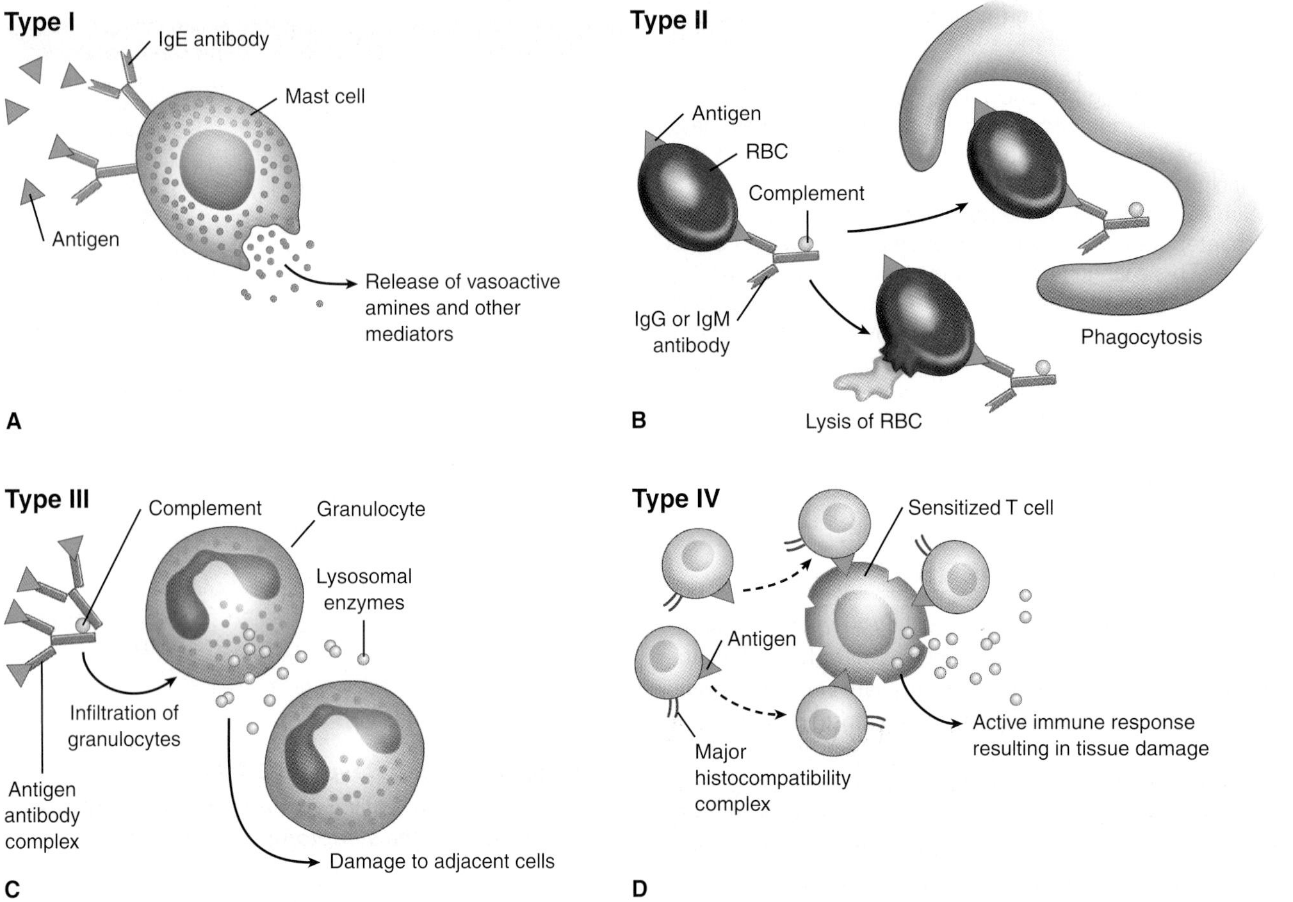

Figure 34-1 Types of hypersensitivity responses. **(A)** type I, atopic or anaphylactic; **(B)** type II, cytotoxic; **(C)** type III, immune complex; and **(D)** type IV, delayed. IgE, immunoglobulin E; IgG, immunoglobulin G; IgM, immunoglobulin M; RBC, red blood cell.

sensitization occurs, one of four types of hypersensitivity responses can occur (Fig. 34-1). These may be immediate or delayed, depending on the time it takes for the immune system to mount a response.

Immediate Hypersensitivity Responses: Types I, II, and III

An *immediate hypersensitivity response* is due to **immunoglobulin antibodies** (Refer to Chapter 33) interacting with allergens and occurs rapidly. There are three types of immediate hypersensitivity responses: type I, atopic or anaphylactic, which is mediated by immunoglobulin E (IgE) antibodies; type II, cytotoxic, which is mediated by immunoglobulin M or G (IgM or IgG) antibodies; and type III, immune complex, which is mediated by IgG antibodies. The first two types of responses occur within minutes; type III responses reach a peak within 6 hours after exposure to an allergen.

In type I, the most severe of the three immediate hypersensitivity responses, IgE antibodies attach to basophils or mast cells. **Mast cells** are constituents of connective tissue that contain granules of heparin, serotonin, bradykinin, and histamine (the most potent chemical of this group). With subsequent exposures to the allergen, mast cells and basophils release their vasoactive granules, causing various allergic and inflammatory manifestations.

Anaphylaxis is a rapid and profound type I hypersensitivity response. A massive release of histamine causes vasodilation; increased capillary permeability; **angioneurotic edema** (acute swelling of the face, neck, lips, larynx, hands, feet, genitals, and internal organs; Fig. 34-2); hypotension; and bronchoconstriction.

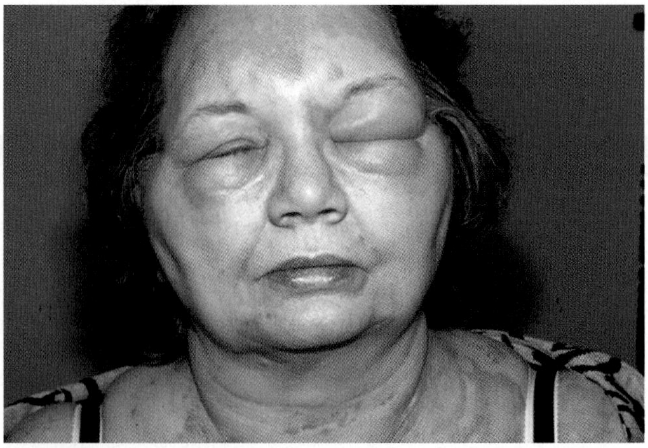

Figure 34-2 Angioneurotic edema manifested by swelling of the lips, eyelids, and tongue. Evidence of urticaria on the neck, shoulders, and chest. (Reprinted with permission from Goodheart, H. P. (2009). *Goodheart's photoguide to common skin disorders: Diagnosis and management* (3rd ed., p. 306). Wolters Kluwer Health/Lippincott Williams & Wilkins.).

Delayed Hypersensitivity Response: Type IV

A *delayed hypersensitivity response* is also termed a type IV hypersensitivity response. Antigens are initially phagocytized by macrophages. Sensitized T cells then produce cytokines that cause an inflammatory reaction. Antibody production is not a component of a delayed hypersensitivity response.

A delayed hypersensitivity response may develop over several hours or days, or it may reach maximum severity after repeated exposure. Examples of a delayed hypersensitivity response include a blood transfusion reaction that occurs days to weeks after blood administration, rejection of transplanted tissues, and reaction to a tuberculin skin test. Delayed hypersensitivity may also explain how people who have been in contact with latex multiple times without showing evidence of an allergy may develop an allergic reaction.

Suppression of the Allergic Response

The body suppresses the allergic response through various mechanisms. One method involves the release of *eosinophil chemotactic factor* (ECF), a chemical mediator, from mast cells. **Chemotaxis** refers to a process of attracting migratory cells to a particular area in the body. ECF attracts eosinophils, whose role is to suppress inflammation by degrading histamine and the other vasoactive chemicals. Epinephrine, a neurotransmitter, interferes with the release of vasoactive chemicals from mast cells. Corticosteroids, which are anti-inflammatory hormones produced by the adrenal cortex, block the synthesis of prostaglandins and leukotrienes, also known as *slow-reactive substance of anaphylaxis*. Both these substances contribute to vascular permeability and smooth muscle contraction.

>>> *Stop, Think, and Respond 34-2*

Look up the following medications in a drug reference or pharmacology text: diphenhydramine (Benadryl), epinephrine hydrochloride (Adrenalin Chloride), prednisone (Meticorten), montelukast (Singulair), and cromolyn (Intal, Crolom). Correlate their mechanisms of action with events that occur in an allergic reaction.

Assessment Findings

Signs and Symptoms

Manifestations of anaphylactic reactions include shock (see Chapter 17), laryngeal edema, wheezing, stridor, tachycardia, and generalized itching as well as hypotension, bronchospasm, and angioneurotic edema, as described previously. Less severe localized hypersensitivity responses can include watery eyes, increased nasal and bronchial secretions, sneezing, vomiting, and diarrhea. Additional symptoms include hives (**urticaria**), itching, and localized redness (e.g., in the conjunctiva of the eyes). Dark areas under the eyes, referred to as "allergic shiners," which are due to accumulation of blood around the orbit of the eye, may also be apparent. Figure 34-3 illustrates manifestations of allergic reactions.

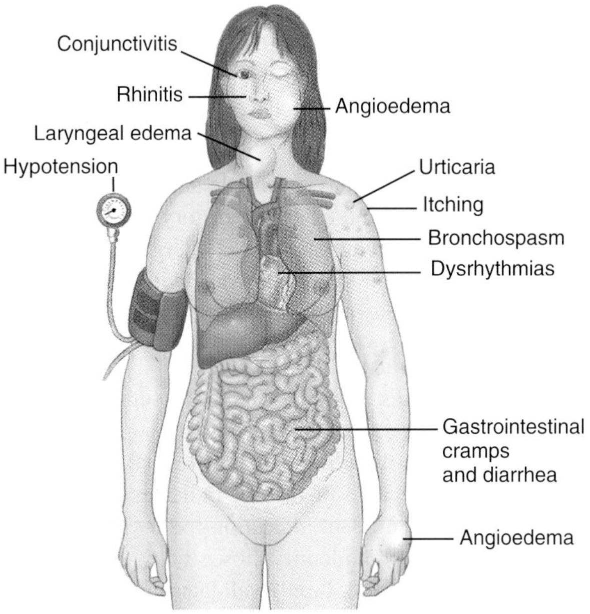

Figure 34-3 Manifestations of allergic reactions.

Clients often identify a cause-and-effect relationship between particular substances and their allergic symptoms. Clinical manifestations generally correlate with the manner in which the allergen enters the body. For example, **inhalants** (inhaled allergens) usually cause respiratory symptoms, including nasal congestion, runny nose, sneezing, coughing, dyspnea, and wheezing. Inhaled allergens often trigger asthma (see Chapter 21). **Contactants** cause skin reactions such as hives, which appear as vesicles filled with clear fluid surrounded by a margin of redness, rash, and localized itching. Cramping, vomiting, and diarrhea are associated with ingested food allergens (Nutrition Notes 34-1). **Injectants,**

Nutrition Notes 34-1

The Client With a Food Allergy

- Proteins in milk, egg whites, peanuts, wheat, and soybeans trigger approximately 90% of food allergies. Other common allergens are fish, shellfish, nuts, corn, and strawberries.
- Food allergies are more common in infants and children. Many infants outgrow food allergies. Food allergies may develop in adults with no history of food allergies. Food intolerances often produce symptoms similar to those of food allergies, such as nausea, vomiting, diarrhea, and cramping. The difference, however, is that no immune response is involved. With food intolerances (e.g., lactose intolerance caused by a deficiency of the digestive enzyme lactase), most people can eat a small amount of the offending food without adverse effects. With true food allergies, even a tiny amount of a food allergen produces symptoms.
- Food oils such as peanut or soybean oils are highly refined and therefore contain no allergenic proteins. However, cold pressed or flavored oils, such as various nut oils, may contain allergenic proteins that are capable of producing allergic reactions in sensitive clients.

such as bee venom, and some other allergens can produce systemic and potentially fatal effects, including shock and airway obstruction caused by laryngeal swelling. Clients exhibit the same reaction with each exposure to the allergen.

Diagnostic Findings

Diagnosis of an allergy may be simple and clear cut or may require multiple tests and extensive history taking. Diagnosis becomes difficult when a client is allergic to more than one substance or when symptoms vary with fatigue, emotional stress, or the seasons.

Radioallergosorbent Blood Test

Various abnormalities in blood test results suggest an allergic disorder. For example, the eosinophil count may be elevated. When the **radioallergosorbent test** (RAST), which measures IgE on a scale of 0 to 5, indicates a score of 2 or greater, it is a significant indication for an allergic disorder. The RAST does not identify those, if any, substances to which a person is allergic. It only validates that the person is potentially hypersensitive to antigenic substances.

Skin Tests

Specific allergens can be identified by skin testing with extracts of various substances (**antigens**), such as pollens, animal dander, food, dust, and stinging insects. The three methods of skin testing are the scratch or prick test, the patch test, and the intradermal injection test.

The **scratch** or prick **test** involves scratching the skin and applying a small amount of the liquid test antigen to the scratch. The tester applies one allergen per scratch over the client's forearm, upper arm, or back. The back is more sensitive than the arms. It also provides a larger area for testing because each substance being tested should be distributed at least 3 cm and preferably up to 5 cm (slightly more than 1 to 2 inches) from one another. Results from a scratch test are identifiable in as little as 20 minutes. If a raised wheal with localized erythema appears (Fig. 34-4), the tester measures its length and width in millimeters. The larger the reaction, the greater is the likelihood that the test allergen is the cause of symptoms in the tested person.

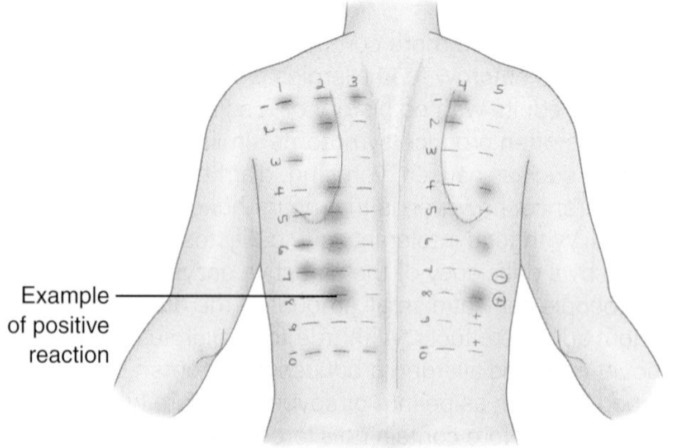

Figure 34-4 Results of an allergy scratch test.

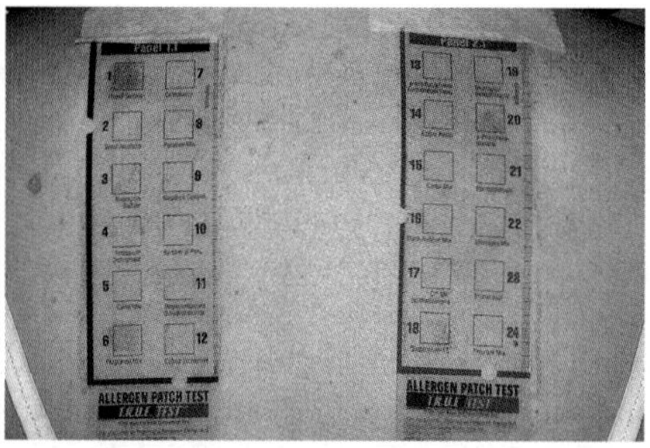

Figure 34-5 A patch test is used to identify contact allergens. A range of common substances is applied to the client to identify positive reactions.

The **patch test** is used to identify the offending substance in allergic contact dermatitis (Fig. 34-5). The tester applies a concentrated form of the substance to the skin and covers the area with an occlusive dressing. After 48 hours, the tester removes the dressing and examines the area for erythema, edema, and vesicles.

In the **intradermal injection test**, which usually is performed only when results of a scratch test are negative for allergies, the tester injects a dilute solution of an antigen intradermally. A positive reaction is based on the size of a raised wheal with localized erythema (redness) that forms where the antigen was injected (Fig. 34-6). In the case of a tuberculin skin test, only the area of **induration**, the hard, raised area—not including the reddened area—is measured. (See Nursing Guidelines in Chapter 21 for directions for administering and reading a tuberculin Mantoux skin test.)

Identification of Food Allergens

To identify food allergens, meticulous record keeping of symptoms and a food diary listing all foods and beverages consumed are necessary. Skin testing and a blood test for IgE antibodies provide more objective data. Elimination diets try to establish cause-and-effect relationships: The client completely avoids suspected foods for 1 to 2 weeks and then adds them back to the diet one at a time and in small amounts. That way, if symptoms develop, the offending food

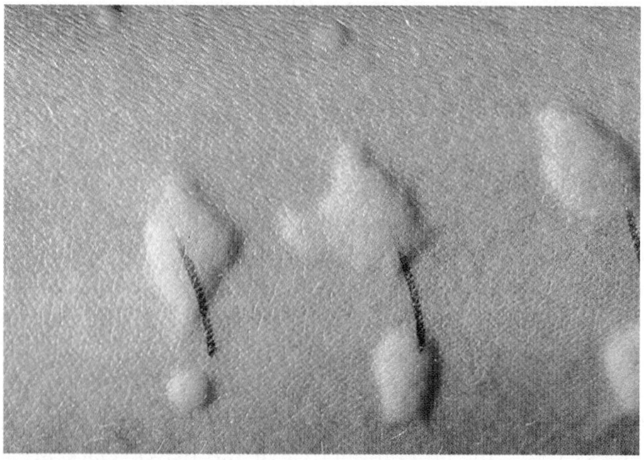

Figure 34-6 The wheal and localized erythema (redness) that appear after an intradermal skin test are measured to interpret the allergic response.

NURSING GUIDELINES 34-1

Identifying Food Allergens

- Have the client fast for 1 to 2 days, drinking only distilled water.
- Introduce hypoallergenic foods (e.g., rice, tapioca) one at a time.
- Introduce allergenic foods (e.g., wheat, peanuts) one at a time in small quantities.
- Observe client for allergic symptoms after introducing each new food.

can be identified. Because elimination studies are subjective, clients may experience symptoms based on their expectations, not from a true allergy. Clients who have experienced severe allergic reactions should not use elimination diets. Nursing Guidelines 34-1 explains the process of identifying food allergens in more detail.

Complications

Clients with inhalant allergies such as seasonal or allergic rhinitis (also known as *hay fever*) may develop nasal polyps from the chronic inflammation. They are also prone to sinus infections related to chronic nasal congestion. Secondary pulmonary infections such as bronchitis also occur. Asthma develops in some clients. The most severe complications among persons with allergies, regardless of type, are anaphylactic shock and angioneurotic edema which can be lethal without immediate medical interventions.

Medical Management

The treatment used to relieve allergic symptoms depends on the type of allergy. Besides avoiding the allergen if possible, many clients experience symptomatic relief with drug therapy (Drug Therapy Table 34-1).

Pharmacologic Considerations

- To protect against poison ivy, a skin allergen, clients can apply bentoquatam 5% (Ivy Block) to the skin 15 minutes prior to exposure and at least every 4 hours as long as risk of exposure continues. The cream forms a protective layer on top of the skin. The oral drug pentoxifylline (Trental) may decrease the rash slightly, but clients must take it before exposure.

DRUG THERAPY TABLE 34-1 Agents to Treat Allergic Disorders

Category and Common Generic (Brand) Drugs	Intended Use	Common Side Effects	Safety Warnings for Nurses
Antihistamines			
First Generation: Brompheniramine (Veltane) Chlorpheniramine (ChlorTrimeton) Clemastine (Dayhist) Diphenhydramine (Benadryl) Promethazine (Phenergan)	Temporary relief of sneezing, itchy, watery eyes, and runny nose caused by hay fever or other respiratory allergies and the common cold Antiemetic, hypersensitivity reactions, motion sickness, sedation	Drowsiness, dry mouth, urinary hesitancy	• Increased fall risk due to sedative side effects. • Teach to refrain from driving or using dangerous equipment when drowsy.
Second Generation: Azelastine (Astelin) Cetirizine (Zyrtec) Desloratadine (Clarinex) Fexofenadine (Allegra) Loratadine (Claritin) Levocetirizine (Xyzal)	Seasonal or allergic rhinitis, chronic urticaria	Dizziness, dry mouth, nose, and throat	• Drying effect can potentiate nose bleeds.
Nasal Decongestants			
Epinephrine (Adrenalin) Oxymetazoline (Zicam) Phenylephrine (Neo-Synephrine) Pseudoephedrine (Sudafed) *Anti-inflammatory:* Fluticasone (Flonase)	Reduce nasal congestion by vasoconstriction Reduce nasal congestion by reducing inflammation	Anxiety, restlessness, nervousness, dry mouth, nose, and throat Dry mouth, nose, and throat	• Avoid sustained-release products with those under 12 years of age. • May cause rebound effect (nasal congestion) if overused. • Contraindicated in clients with certain heart conditions such as hypertension. Combination with protease inhibitor category of HIV antivirals can result in steroid accumulation, adrenal suppression, and Cushing syndrome. Can limit growth; do not use with children under 4 years of age.

(continued)

DRUG THERAPY TABLE 34-1 Agents to Treat Allergic Disorders (*continued*)

Category and Common Generic (Brand) Drugs	Intended Use	Common Side Effects	Safety Warnings for Nurses
Corticosteroids			
Inhaled (ICS): Beclomethasone (QVAR) Budesonide (Symbicort) Ciclesonide (Alvesco) Fluticasone (Flovent)	Inhibit inflammatory immune response reducing inflammation of bronchi	Hoarseness, dry mouth, cough, and sore throat	• Low-dose corticosteroid inhalers effective for rescue therapy for mild persistent asthma when combined with Albuterol. • Rinse mouth after use to prevent fungal infections. • Symptoms worsen when medication is stopped suddenly.
Oral: Dexamethasone (Decadron) Prednisone (Deltasone)	Inhibit inflammatory immune response	Acne, water retention, weight gain, hair loss, increased appetite	• Administer with food to decrease gastric irritation. • Monitor for higher blood glucose in clients with diabetes. • Abrupt withdrawal may precipitate Addisonian crisis.
Bronchodilators—Short-Acting Beta-2 Agonists (SABAs—Adrenergics)			
Albuterol (Ventolin) Ephedrine Epinephrine (Adrenalin) Metaproterenol (Alupent)	Treat and prevent acute bronchospasm by relaxation of smooth muscle and constriction of blood vessels in lungs.	Tachycardia, nervousness, anxiety, pain, dizziness, rhinitis, cough	• Considered rescue inhalers; not to be used for maintenance therapy.
Cholinergic Blocking Drug (Anticholinergics)			
Aclidinium (Tudorza) Ipratropium (Atrovent) Tiotropium (Spiriva) Umeclindinium (Incruse)	Prevention of bronchospasm associated with chronic obstructive pulmonary disease, chronic bronchitis and emphysema	Headache, cough, sinus irritation and stuffiness, urinary retention	• Should not be used for treating sudden breathing problems. • Consult prescriber if urinary hesitancy, excessive dry mouth, blurred vision, or allergic symptoms develop.
Xanthine Derivatives			
Aminophylline (Truphylline) Theophylline (Theochron)	Symptomatic relief or prevention of bronchial asthma and reversible bronchospasm by bronchodilation	Nervousness, headache, insomnia	• Monitor serum drug levels. • Hold drug with nausea/vomiting (toxicity sign).
Leukotriene Modifiers and Immunomodulators (mab)			
Montelukast (Singulair) Roflumilast (Daliresp) Zafirlukast (Accolate) Zileuton (Zyflo) Mepolizumab (Nucala) Omalizumab (Xolair)	Prophylaxis and treatment of chronic asthma by reducing inflammation	Headache, influenza-like symptoms	• Not effective for rescue therapy. • Symptoms worsen when medication is stopped suddenly. • Monitor liver enzymes while taking drug; report yellowing of skin and eyes, dark urine, or clay-colored stools.

The drugs in column 1 indicate the drug that matches up with explanations in columns 2 through 4.

Desensitization is another option. **Desensitization** is a form of immunotherapy in which a person receives weekly or twice-weekly injections of dilute but increasingly higher concentrations of an allergen without interruption. Repeated exposure to the weak antigen promotes the production of IgG, an antibody that blocks IgE so it cannot stimulate mast cells. When the maximum dose is achieved after 2 to 4 months of treatment, maintenance injections are administered at longer intervals, usually every 2 to 4 weeks. It may take several years before a person treated with desensitization experiences significant relief. After a desensitization injection, the client is observed for 30 minutes to assess for allergic symptoms. Epinephrine (Adrenalin) is administered if a severe reaction occurs. Desensitization for poison ivy, oak, or sumac currently is unavailable.

Clients with severe allergies to bee venom are advised to carry an emergency kit that contains a premeasured dose of injectable epinephrine (Epipen). The syringe, when pressed to the skin, autoinjects the epinephrine. The lateral thigh is the site most commonly used for injection (Fig. 34-7).

››› *Stop, Think, and Respond 34-3*

List signs and symptoms that suggest a person who is undergoing desensitization needs epinephrine.

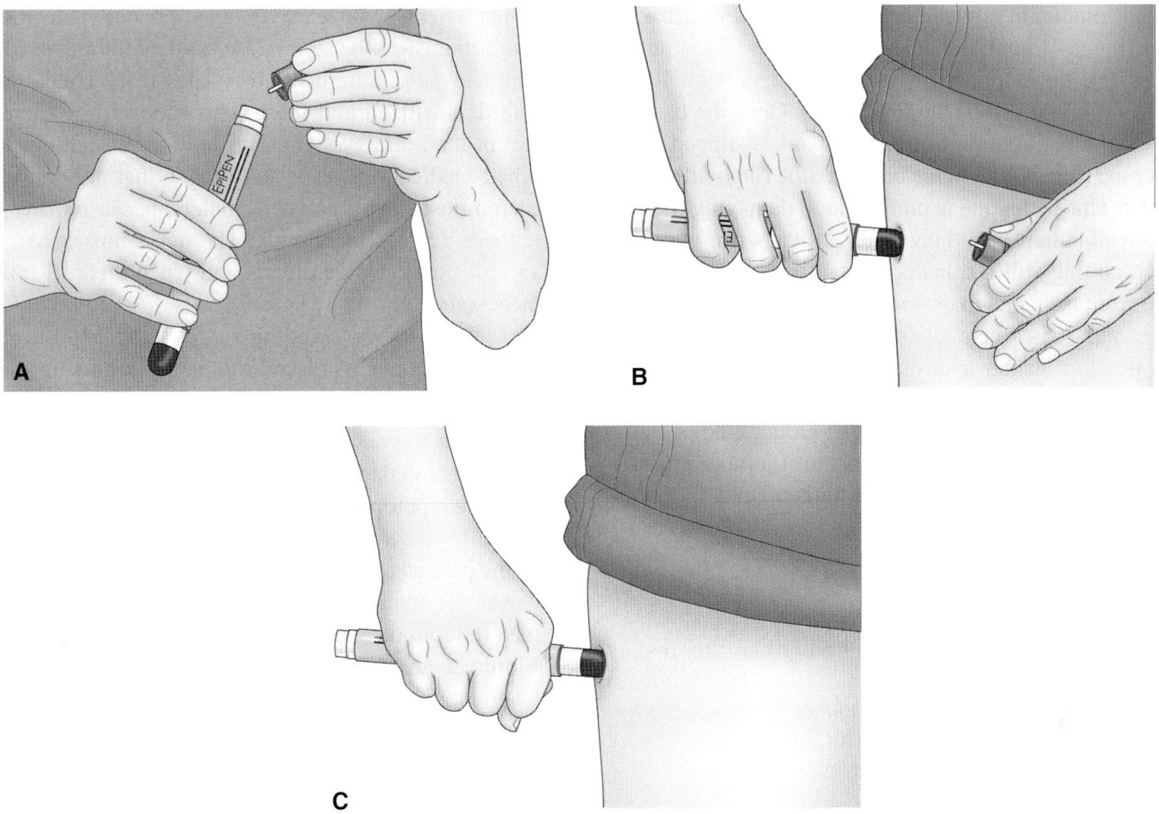

Figure 34-7 Self-injection of epinephrine to avoid anaphylactic reaction. **(A)** The client uncaps the Epipen, holding it with the injecting end upright. **(B)** The client positions the device at the middle portion of the thigh. **(C)** The client pushes the device into the thigh as far as possible. The Epipen autoinjects a premeasured dose of epinephrine into the subcutaneous tissue.

Recently, **sublingual-swallow immunotherapy** (SLIT) has been used for desensitization against allergens that cause allergic rhinitis. When SLIT is used, a self-administered solution or tablet containing grass and pollen allergens is placed under the tongue once a day during allergy season; a caregiver can administer SLIT for those who are too young for self-administration. These allergens do not generally produce a serious systemic allergic reaction because the sublingual mucosa has very few mast cells. The cells in the oral mucosa present the antigen to regulatory suppressor T cells that inhibit the inflammatory/allergic response. Consequently, a tolerance to the allergens develops. Repeated SLIT results in a reduction of symptoms associated with allergic rhinitis and asthma in children with hay fever. Children tend to prefer SLIT to desensitizing injections.

Nursing Management

The nurse asks each client about the existence of any allergies. If any are reported, the nurse flags the medical record and applies a wristband with the appropriate information. Throughout the client's care, the nurse observes for signs of an allergic reaction, especially when administering medications, applying substances such as tape or adhesive patches to the skin, using latex products (Box 34-1), or caring for a client receiving contrast media for diagnostic testing. If the nurse suspects a mild allergic reaction, they remove or withhold the offending substance and notifies the primary provider. If a client has an anaphylactic reaction, the nurse acts immediately to stop the client's exposure to the allergen, summons the code team, or calls the 911 operator, and provides life support.

BOX 34-1 Products That Contain Latex

Household Products

Carpet backing	Condoms/diaphragms
Feeding nipples	Computer mouse pads
Pacifiers	Buttons on electronic equipment
Elastic in clothing	Food handled with powdered latex gloves
Sports equipment	Handles on racquets, tools, and similar items
Balloons	
Erasers	
Toys	
Shoe soles	

Medical Products

Gloves	Tourniquets
Face masks	Electrode pads
Mattresses	Bulb syringes
Client-controlled analgesia	Syringe stoppers and medication vial stoppers
Sports equipment syringes	Adhesive tape
Ambu bags	Bandages
Stethoscopes	Injection ports
Blood pressure cuff tubing	Wound drains
Dental devices	
Urinary catheters	

Occasionally, the nurse needs to remove a ring from a swollen finger. If applying soap or oil to the finger proves unsuccessful, the nurse may wrap the finger with twine, dental floss, or narrow elastic (Fig. 34-8). Once the tissue is compressed, the proximal free end of twine is slipped under and over the ring. As the twine unwinds, the ring will slip off the finger. This technique is preferable to damaging the ring with a metal cutter. If nothing else facilitates ring removal, however, cutting still is a better option than allowing tissue damage from ischemia to develop.

The nurse instructs clients who are scheduled for diagnostic skin testing to avoid taking prescribed or over-the-counter antihistamines or cold preparations for at least 48 to 72 hours before testing. Doing so reduces the potential for false-negative test results. Clients must temporarily discontinue some medications for even longer.

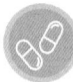

Pharmacologic Considerations

- In addition to antihistamines, other drugs can alter results of allergy skin testing; these include:
  - Topical glucocorticosteroids (stop for 3 weeks)
  - Tricyclic antidepressants (stop for 7 to 14 days)
  - Benzodiazepines (stop for 7 days)
  - H_2 blockers (stop for 2 days)
  - Omalizumab (Xolair; stop for 6 months)

The nurse assists the provider who performs diagnostic testing and helps document findings. Once the test is completed, the nurse monitors the client's response until it is safe for the person to return home.

For clients who elect to undergo desensitization, the nurse administers the serial doses and monitors the client for 30 minutes after administration. They teach clients who are being desensitized and those who choose drug therapy for relief of their allergy symptoms how to self-administer prescribed medications, especially those that are delivered by metered-dose or dry-powder inhalers, because many people use these devices incorrectly. The nurse must make clients aware of possible side effects and when medical follow-up is necessary.

Techniques for avoiding or reducing exposure in the client's home and work environment are nursing areas for health teaching. Some examples include the following:

- Insist that the environment be smoke free when a person manifests inhalant allergies or respiratory symptoms.
- Keep pets outdoors or at least in one confined area of the home.
- Bathe pets weekly or at frequent intervals.
- Cover the mattress and box springs with an impervious material to reduce dust mites.
- Eliminate area rugs.
- Contract with an exterminator if cockroaches or other vermin are present.
- Clean humidifiers and heating and cooling ducts to remove mold spores.

For other health teaching information, see Client and Family Teaching 34-1.

››› *Stop, Think, and Respond 34-4*

Discuss ways to avoid inhaled and ingested allergens.

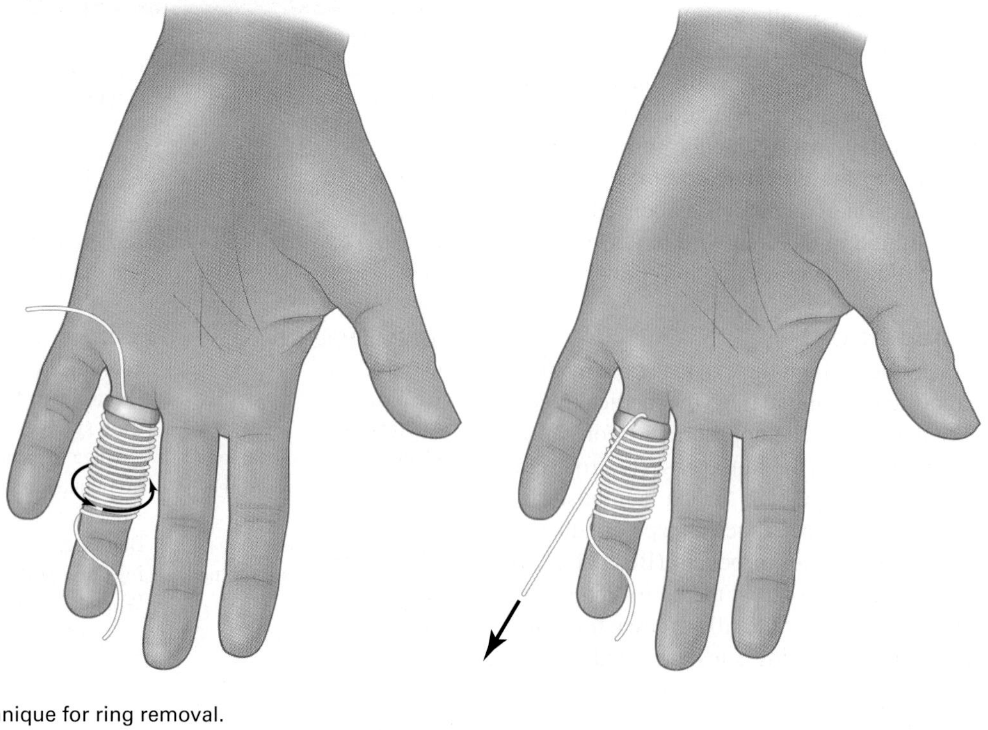

Figure 34-8 Technique for ring removal.

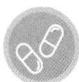

Pharmacologic Considerations

■ Closely observe a client with allergies each time a new drug is added to the therapeutic regimen. This includes drugs given by the nurse and drugs used for diagnostic studies, such as radiopaque dyes. Continue monitoring the client when a second dose of a new drug is given because reactions may follow the first sensitizing dose.
■ Many antihistamines cause drowsiness, although some newer antihistamines are less likely to do so. Advise the client not to drive a car, operate machinery, or perform tasks that require alertness when taking antihistamines that reduce alertness. Tell clients not to take antihistamines with alcohol or other central nervous system depressants because additive sedative effects can occur.
■ Advise clients with disorders of the lower respiratory tract not to take antihistamines. If, for example, these drugs are administered for asthma, a drying effect may occur, making secretions thicker and more difficult to expectorate.
■ Suggest that clients avoid the use of nonprescription eye preparations to reduce redness. An ophthalmologist should evaluate and treat itching and redness of the eyes because the symptoms may or may not be caused by an allergy.

Client and Family Teaching 34-1
Allergies

The nurse teaches clients who have allergic disorders and their family members the following guidelines:

- Never begin smoking, or quit if you are currently smoking and if your allergy causes respiratory symptoms.
- Understand that treatment for chronic allergic disorders, such as allergic rhinitis and food allergies, may extend over several years.
- Follow the medical regimen as instructed by the primary provider.
- Do not overuse nose drops or sprays for nasal congestion. Use only prescribed or recommended drugs and only in the dosage suggested by the primary provider.
- Keep a record of symptoms or lack of symptoms. Bring the record to the primary provider's office or clinic. The record will help the primary provider determine therapy.
- Keep a record of symptoms or absence of symptoms each time you add a new food to the diet. Add new foods to the diet slowly and one at a time.
- Avoid environmental substances that cause allergic reactions.
- Seek immediate medical attention if symptoms worsen or new symptoms occur.
- Carry identification, such as a Medic Alert card or bracelet, to inform healthcare providers of allergies, especially if you have a history of anaphylactic reactions.
- Do not miss an immunotherapy appointment; missed appointments may necessitate restarting the series of injections.
- Check prefilled syringes that contain epinephrine for an expiration date. You must refill the prescription and discard the old prescription on or immediately before this date. Keep the directions for use with the product.

Concept Mastery Alert

Medical Identification Bracelet

When educating the parents of a child diagnosed with a severe food allergy, the nurse should emphasize the importance of the child wearing a medical identification bracelet.

AUTOIMMUNE DISORDERS

Autoimmune disorders are those in which killer T cells and autoantibodies attack or destroy natural cells—those cells that are self. **Autoantibodies**, antibodies against self-antigens, are immunoglobulins. They target **histocompatible cells**, cells whose antigens match the individual's own genetic code.

Diseases are considered autoimmune disorders when they are characterized by unrelenting, progressive tissue damage without any verifiable etiology. Various specific disorders classified as autoimmune are discussed throughout this text. Refer to Chapter 37 for information on multiple sclerosis, Chapter 58 for discussion of acute glomerulonephritis, and Chapter 63 for coverage of rheumatoid arthritis and systemic lupus erythematosus. The term **alloimmunity** is used to describe an immune response that is waged against transplanted organs and tissues that carry nonself antigens. See Chapters 29 and 58 for more information.

Pathophysiology and Etiology

Several theories have been proposed to explain the cause of autoimmune disorders (Table 34-3). None appear to explain autoimmunity completely, which suggests that more than one mechanism is responsible.

In many autoimmune disorders, there tend to be a triggering event, such as an infection, trauma, or introduction of a drug or food that integrates itself into the membranes of the host's cells. One hypothesis is that the triggering event upsets the immune system's tolerance or recognition of self-antigens. A cause-and-effect relationship exists between some viral and bacterial infections (e.g., measles) and the development of a blood disorder called *thrombocytopenic purpura* (see Chapter 31). Another cause-and-effect relationship is found between streptococcal infections and disorders such as rheumatic heart disease (see Chapter 23). Despite such relationships, no scientific evidence has been found to support the hypothesis. It may be that the antigenic surface of the microorganism so closely resembles the person's histocompatible cell markers that the antibodies cannot differentiate between host and invader.

Some believe that certain people are genetically predisposed to autoimmune disorders. Theorists have proposed that the histocompatible cell markers, which are genetically inherited, act as receptors for disease-causing microorganisms, making certain cells more vulnerable than others. Another possibility is that some people inherit a trait for suppressor T-cell dysfunction. The role of suppressor T cells is to mediate immune responses. Without adequate suppressor T-cell function, killer T cells can destroy healthy cells, tissues, and organs without restraint. Consequently, genetic factors may also be a link in explaining why autoimmune disorders have a tendency to occur among blood relatives.

TABLE 34-3 Autoimmunity Theories

THEORY	HYPOTHESIS
Cross-antigen theory	Self-antigens that resemble foreign antigens cause T cells to misidentify natural cells and mount an immune attack.
Tissue injury theory	Infection, trauma, drugs, and radiation alter natural cells. Consequently, they no longer resemble self-antigens.
Viral mutation theory	Viruses alter T-cell receptors that are used to differentiate self from nonself.
Sequestered antigen theory	Some cells, like those of the thyroid, brain, and lens of the eye, are separated from lymphocytes during fetal development. When these cells enter circulation later because of trauma or infection, T cells do not recognize them as "self."
Diminished T-suppressor theory	Reduced numbers of suppressor cells or a shortened lifespan because of aging and atrophy of the thymus gland alter immunoregulation.
Genetic instruction theory	Genetic coding for antibody production is altered, which explains the familial pattern to some autoimmune disorders.

Another interesting phenomenon supports the sequestered antigen theory. Evidence has shown that when a person experiences trauma followed by inflammation to the iris, ciliary body, and choroid layer of one eye, the vision in the untraumatized eye also becomes affected. The term for this phenomenon is *sympathetic uveitis*. The explanation may be related to the fact that during fetal development, the cells and tissues of the eye are not exposed to the lymphatic drainage system. Therefore, the lymphocytes have never learned to recognize the histocompatible markers on these ocular cells as self. When trauma occurs and these cells are no longer sequestered, or hidden, from the lymphocytes, the immune system attacks what it perceives to be foreign.

Regardless of whether one or all of these theoretical etiologies is valid, the outcome is clear. The immune system fails to recognize histocompatible cells. Consequently, T and B cells mount a cell-mediated or humoral response (see Chapter 33). The attack may be localized to one organ or type of tissue or it may be systemic (Box 34-2). Cells, tissues, and organs under attack are damaged or destroyed.

Assessment Findings

Signs and Symptoms

Autoimmune disorders produce various signs and symptoms depending on the tissues and organs affected. The symptoms are characteristic of an acute inflammatory response. They develop as antibodies attack normal tissue mistakenly identified as nonself. In some cases, the inflammatory symptoms are episodic. Periods of acute flare-ups (known as **exacerbations**) alternate with periods of **remission** (asymptomatic periods). The duration of these periods is completely unpredictable. During acute exacerbations, clients often experience a low-grade fever, malaise, or fatigue. They may also lose weight.

BOX 34-2 Examples of Autoimmune Disorders

Organ Specific

Blood
Hemolytic anemia
Thrombocytopenic purpura

Central Nervous System
Multiple sclerosis
Guillain–Barré syndrome

Eye
Uveitis

Joint
Ankylosing spondylitis

Heart
Endocarditis

Muscles
Myasthenia gravis

Endocrine
Hashimoto thyroiditis
Type 1 diabetes mellitus

Gastrointestinal
Ulcerative colitis

Renal
Glomerulonephritis

Systemic
Systemic lupus erythematosus
Scleroderma
Rheumatoid arthritis
Sjögren syndrome

››› *Stop, Think, and Respond 34-5*

What could explain why autoimmune disorders have periods of remission and exacerbation?

Diagnostic Findings

Diagnostic testing varies depending on the autoimmune disorder. Overall, elevated circulating antibodies are the hallmark findings for autoimmune disorders. Some examples include elevated erythrocyte sedimentation rate, antistreptolysin O titer, antinuclear antibody titer, and rheumatoid factor.

Medical Management

Autoimmune disorders are rarely cured. The goal of therapy is to induce a remission or slow the immune system's destructive activities. Drug therapy using anti-inflammatory and immunosuppressive agents is the mainstay for alleviating symptoms (Drug Therapy Table 34-2). Some antineoplastic (cancer) drugs also are used for their immunosuppressant effects. Controlling or limiting side effects of the drugs, one of which is increased susceptibility to infection, is a major concern. Even with remission, most people must continue taking prescribed medications to avoid another acute exacerbation.

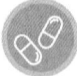

Pharmacologic Considerations

- When taking drugs to suppress the immune system, the client has an increased risk of infection, especially of the respiratory or urinary system. Observe such clients for signs and symptoms of infection such as fever, sore throat, productive cough, and dysuria.

DRUG THERAPY TABLE 34-2 Immunosuppressive Drugs for Autoimmune Disorders

Category and Common Generic (Brand) Drugs	Intended Use	Common Side Effects	Safety Warnings for Nurses
Anti-Inflammatory Glucocorticoids			
Dexamethasone, prednisone, methylprednisolone (Medrol)	Treat autoimmune disorders by suppressing inflammatory immune response	Acne, water retention, weight gain, hair loss, increased appetite	• Take with food to decrease gastric irritation. • Monitor for higher blood glucose in clients with diabetes. • Abrupt withdrawal may precipitate Addisonian crisis.
Cytotoxic Drugs			
Mercaptopurine azathioprine (Imuran) Lesser-used agents, reserved when disease is unresponsive: methotrexate, cyclosporine	Inhibit inflammatory immune of T and B cells (lymphocytes)	Increased vulnerability to infection, rash, nausea, vomiting, diarrhea	• Immune suppression increases susceptibility to infections. • Review lab test results for evidence of immune suppression. • Use barrier method birth control.
TNF-binding Proteins (Biologic Agents)			
Adalimumab (Humira) Certolizumab (Cimzia) Infliximab (Remicade) Natalizumab (Tysabri)	Neutralizing immune proteins reducing inflammation	Fever, chills, headache, muscle aches, diarrhea	• Immune suppression increases susceptibility to infections. • Review lab test results for immune suppression. • Special permission must be obtained for natalizumab therapy owing to its potential for pancytopenia.
Interferons			
Interferon Beta: Interferon beta 1a (Avonex)	Reduce relapse in multiple sclerosis by reducing number of inflammatory cells crossing the blood–brain barrier	Flu-like symptoms, fatigue, skin reaction at injection site	• Monitor laboratory test results for pancytopenia. • Monitor liver function tests to assess for adverse effect. Administer at bedtime to minimize flu-like side effects.

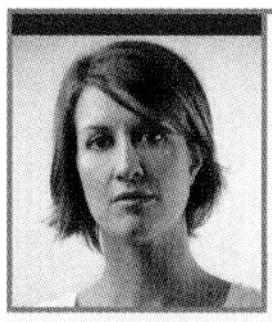

Clinical Scenario A 28-year-old woman is seen by a nurse. The client says that she is experiencing fatigue, joint pain, and stiffness in the joints at the base of her hands and wrists. She reports that she had a similar episode 3 months earlier, but the discomfort went away. Because she felt better, she did not make an appointment with her primary provider. However, the symptoms have returned again, and she is concerned about their significance. **Using the nursing process, what actions are appropriate if the nurse suspects that the client may have rheumatoid arthritis, an autoimmune disorder? See the following Nursing Process section.**

NURSING PROCESS FOR THE CLIENT WITH AN AUTOIMMUNE DISORDER

Assessment

Obtain a family history during the initial interview with the client and be alert to information about family members who have had chronic diseases with an inflammatory component that involve cardiac, urinary, neurologic, or connective tissues. During acute exacerbations, the client is quite ill; therefore, note elevated vital signs, a finding that suggests an infectious or inflammatory process. Examine the client for signs of localized inflammation and compromised body functions, such as changes in the skin, joints, gait, heart, and renal function. Ask about the client's level of energy because fatigue is common. Review laboratory test findings for evidence that correlates with an inflammatory process or immunologic changes typical of one of many autoimmune disorders. Teaching points for those with autoimmune disorders are discussed in Client and Family Teaching 34-2.

(continued)

NURSING PROCESS FOR THE CLIENT WITH AN AUTOIMMUNE DISORDER (continued)

Analysis, Planning, and Interventions

Activity Intolerance: Related to joint pain secondary to inflammation, malaise, and fatigue
Expected Outcome: The client will perform activities of daily living (ADLs) without extreme fatigue or discomfort.

- Encourage rest during periods of severe exacerbation and regular exercise during periods of remission. *Activity levels within a client's level of endurance promote well-being. Endurance is related to the frequency, duration, and intensity of activity.*
- Provide nonpharmacologic and pharmacologic pain management as ordered by the primary provider. *Nonpainful stimuli (e.g., massage, activity, heat, cold, imagery, pleasant sounds) can reduce or relieve pain. Analgesic anti-inflammatory medications block neurotransmitters that carry pain stimuli to the brain; narcotic analgesics dull the brain, making it less perceptive to pain transmission; corticosteroids suppress the immune response.*

Infection Risk: Related to immunosuppression secondary to drug therapy for the autoimmune disorder and generally poor physical condition
Expected Outcome: The client will be free of infection.

- Instruct the client about signs and symptoms of and the increased risk for infection. *Access to knowledge facilitates an active role in restoring health.*
- Instruct the client to report signs and symptoms of infection (e.g., cough, dyspnea, diarrhea, fever) immediately to the primary provider. *Early treatment promotes a shorter duration of illness and reduced complications.*
- Tell the client to avoid high-risk activities, such as being in crowds, during periods of immunosuppression. *Risk for infection increases with exposure to others who may have infectious disorders or whose hand washing and hygiene measures are less than adequate.*

Chronic Low Self-Esteem: Related to coping with chronic illness and physical changes associated with autoimmune disorders
Expected Outcome: The client will maintain a positive self-concept.

- Interact with and frequently show genuine interest in the client. *A person's concept of self is determined to a great extent by the responses of others. The client may interpret lack of interest and avoidance as rejection and being unworthy of attention.*
- Refer the client to community organizations and support groups. *Sharing problems and experiences with others who are similarly affected dispels the idea that a person's symptoms and feelings are unique. A person can more easily resolve and tolerate problems when they share the burden with others.*

Evaluation of Expected Outcomes

The client participates in self-care and ADLs without overwhelming fatigue. There is no evidence of *iatrogenic* (treatment-caused) infection. The client perceives themselves realistically, with more positive attributes than negative.

CHRONIC FATIGUE SYNDROME

Chronic fatigue syndrome (CFS), also called *chronic fatigue, chronic fatigue immune dysfunction syndrome* (CFIDS), and *myalgic encephalomyelitis* (ME), is a complex of symptoms primarily characterized by profound fatigue with no identifiable cause. The fatigue worsens with physical activity and does not improve with rest. The term *chronic* refers to the fact that the duration of fatigue has been unrelenting for 6 or more months. Some believe that CFS is somewhat like **fibromyalgia** because both conditions share many symptoms such as pain in fibrous tissues of the body such as muscles, ligaments, and tendons. Estimates are that as many as 2.5 million people in the United States have symptoms corresponding with CFS, but fewer than 80% have been diagnosed by a medical provider (Epidemiology, 2018) Most clients who seek treatment for their symptoms

Client and Family Teaching 34-2
Autoimmune Disorders

The nurse teaches clients who have autoimmune disorders and their family members the following guidelines:

- Notify a health care provider of any sign of infection such as cough, fever, severe diarrhea, mouth lesions, or sore throat.
- Notify a healthcare provider of any new side effects to prescribed medications.
- Do not stop taking any medications abruptly.
- Avoid crowds or people with infections if you are taking an immunosuppressant drug.
- Limit stress and use stress reduction techniques such as progressive relaxation or breathing exercises.
- Maintain close follow-up with a primary provider.

are White women 40 to 59 years of age. CFS also occurs at lower rates among children, adolescents, and men. Statistics for minorities may be low when taking into account their reduced access to the health care system. It is difficult to determine the duration of CFS or recovery rates because the disorder has a pattern of unsustained remissions followed by exacerbations. Some people with CFS improve but are not completely symptom free, while others continue to suffer, sometimes for decades. When the duration of symptoms is lengthy, the prognosis is less optimistic.

Pathophysiology and Etiology

No cause for CFS has yet been established, but those affected exhibit a deficiency in adenosine triphosphate (ATP), the source of cellular energy. Some believe that the disorder results from immune system dysregulation, in which the immune system remains activated for an extended period after an infectious triggering event. Although researchers have attempted to find a link between CFS and viral diseases, no single causal relationship has been found. Some hypothesize that T cells are activated initially in response to a virus, and that levels of proinflammatory cytokines, such as various interleukins and tumor necrosis factor, remain elevated (see Chapter 33). It is well documented that cytokines produce achy, flu-like symptoms accompanied by fever and malaise during the early stages of infections. People with CFS experience these same symptoms. The difference is that during infections, the symptoms are brief, but in CFS, they are relentlessly prolonged.

Evidence is mounting that CFS is caused by a combination of a genetic predisposition, a triggering event such as a viral or bacterial exposure and an atypical immune response (Osborne, 2016). It has been found that people with CFS produce a defective form of ribonuclease termed RNase L, an enzymatic protein induced by the cytokine interferon that has antiviral activity. The RNase L destroys the RNA in viruses as well as in normal cells. The RNase L attacks the wrong enemy, that is, normal body cells, and leaves the person subject to reactivation of viruses that should remain dormant. Thus, some believe that CFS should be called "chronic viral reactivation syndrome".

The fact that serum cortisol levels are low among those with CSF symptoms has led to another hypothesis. Some believe that CSF is a consequence of impaired activation of three neuroendocrine structures: the hypothalamus, pituitary gland, and adrenal glands. Collectively, these structures are sometimes referred to as the *HPA axis* (refer to Chapter 68). The adrenal glands secrete corticosterone (cortisol) which suppresses inflammation and immune activity. Downregulation of the HPA axis interferes with immune suppression and allows the hyperfunctioning immune processes to continue unabated.

Downregulation of the HPA axis also helps explain why those with CFS experience orthostatic intolerance. **Orthostatic intolerance** is a condition in which individuals experience hypotension accompanied by fatigue after standing for more than 10 minutes.

Assessment Findings

Signs and Symptoms

Many clients with CFS report having had a recent illness with flu-like symptoms or an upper respiratory infection. Despite having been uncomfortable, most clients do not describe their initial symptoms as being extraordinarily severe. In fact, the opposite is true. Thereafter, however, severe, ongoing fatigue has lasted for at least 6 months without any explanation. Even though the fatigue is constant, it worsens after physical activity. The fatigue is so debilitating that it usually interferes with a person's ability to work in or outside the home.

According to the Centers for Disease Control and Prevention (Symptoms of ME/CFS, 2021), in addition to fatigue, the client exhibits at least four or more of the following:

- Malaise that lasts more than 24 hours after an exertional activity
- Sore throat that is frequent or recurring
- Tender cervical or axillary lymph nodes
- Joint pain without swelling or redness
- Myalgia (muscle pain)
- Headaches of a new type, pattern, or severity
- Unrefreshing sleep
- Significant impairment of short-term memory or concentration
  - Digestive issues, like irritable bowel syndrome
  - Chills and night sweats
  - Allergies and sensitivities to foods, odors, chemicals, light, or noise
  - Shortness of breath
  - Irregular heartbeat

››› *Stop, Think, and Respond 34-6*

Discuss possible consequences among people who suffer unrelenting fatigue and pain.

Diagnostic Findings

Findings of the medical history and physical examination are unremarkable. Results from a battery of blood tests specific for diagnosing diseases associated with fatigue fail to reveal an explanation for the client's symptoms. The exhaustive medical workup excludes all diagnoses except CFS.

Currently, research is focused on measuring levels of RNase L in CFS. The knowledge that the enzyme is elevated in clients with CFS has not improved diagnosis of the disorder. Recent research at Cornell University found a correlation between intestinal bacteria and inflammatory microbial agents in blood that trigger an immune response, but it is unknown at this time if the results indicate a cause or a consequence of the disease.

A **tilt-table test**, one in which the client lies horizontally on a table whose incline is elevated to approximately 70° for 45 minutes, may be done. During the test, the blood pressure (BP) and pulse are monitored. The test tends to provoke hypotension in those eventually diagnosed with CFS and may be a diagnostic marker.

Medical Management

Treatment focuses on relieving the client's symptoms because nothing, as yet, holds promise for a cure. Without a disease-specific drug, most are treated with medications such as analgesics, antidepressants, and central nervous system stimulants that only manage their symptoms.

Without any definitive drug treatment, the client is advised to balance activity with rest. An employed client may need to resign from their job or negotiate for a less physically demanding position. The primary provider may prescribe a modest exercise program under the supervision of a physical therapist to avoid muscle atrophy that contributes to weakness. The client is to avoid overexertion at all costs.

Mild pain and fever are treated with aspirin, acetaminophen (Tylenol), or nonsteroidal anti-inflammatory agents such as ibuprofen (Motrin, Advil) or naproxen sodium (Naprosyn, Aleve). Even low doses of tricyclic antidepressants such as amitriptyline (Elavil), doxepin (Sinequan), or nortriptyline (Pamelor) can relieve pain and improve sleep.

Clients who experience orthostatic intolerance are advised to increase salt and water intake as long as doing so is not contraindicated by cardiac or renal disease. Some clients also experience greater BP stability when fludrocortisone (Florinef), a corticosteroid, is prescribed. An antihypotensive agent such as midodrine (ProAmatine) may be prescribed to increase vascular tone and elevate BP. Several adjunct and alternative therapies are suggested to treat clients with CFS holistically (Nutrition Notes 34-2).

Some clients benefit from cognitive therapy, a form of psychotherapy in which people learn skills to change distorted thoughts about themselves. For example, cognitive therapy may help a person with CFS who believes that they are a helpless victim of the disease to perceive themselves as capable of dealing with the fatigue. Some promote the use of acupuncture, Eastern exercise and meditation techniques such as yoga and tai chi, and phototherapy (see Chapters 9 and 69) contribute to well-being. Until more information is known about CFS, however, clients may fall victim to herbal and dietary claims that promise a cure. As long as alternative therapies are not dangerous, the client's right to incorporate unproven or nonstandardized methods is not challenged.

Nutrition Notes 34-2

The Client With Chronic Fatigue Syndrome

- Some studies suggest that people with CFS may be marginally deficient in various nutrients, including B vitamins, vitamin C, magnesium, zinc, and essential fatty acids. It is not known, however, whether nutrient deficiencies precede CFS or are a consequence of the disease process. Because the potential benefits outweigh potential risks, a multivitamin and mineral supplement may be prudent.
- An omega-3 fatty acid known as *eicosapentaenoic acid* (EPA) is thought to block the release of cytokines and prostaglandins and therefore may prevent or reduce inflammation and pain experienced with CFS and other inflammatory autoimmune disorders.
- Fish oils provide the only dietary source of EPA. Fatty fish, such as mackerel, sardines, herring, salmon, and tuna, are the best sources.
- Fish oil supplements usually are not recommended because no clearly prescribed guidelines on the optimal dose are available. Also, fish oil supplements have the potential to cause gastrointestinal upset, increased bleeding time, vitamins A and D toxicities, and decreased levels of various immune system components, the significance of which is uncertain.

Nursing Management

The nurse educates the client about their disease process and the limitations that it requires (see Client and Family Teaching 34-3, Nursing Care Plan 34-1, and Evidence-Based Practice 34-1).

Client and Family Teaching 34-3
Chronic Fatigue Syndrome

The nurse teaches clients who have CFS and their family members the following guidelines:

- When using over-the-counter analgesics, follow the recommended dosages and frequency for administration. Excess use can lead to increased potential for bleeding, liver, and kidney damage.
- Herbal products also have potential side effects and toxic effects; therefore, consult with the primary provider and keep them informed of any alternative therapeutic approaches you are using.
- Many companies make herbal and health-related supplements, but there is no standard among them for safe, effective dosages. Read and compare labels and ask the primary provider for their opinion on a product's efficacy.
- No scientific evidence has shown that vitamins or minerals alter the course of CFS; however, they are not harmful if taken in recommended dosages.
- When searching for a support group, be wary of organizations that:
  - Promise a cure for CFS
  - Use meetings as an opportunity to criticize specific primary provider or treatment programs
  - Advise abandoning standard treatment regimens
  - Recommend an untested, unresearched, unscientific approach for managing CFS
  - Press participants to discuss information of a personal nature
  - Charge unreasonable fees for membership
  - Do not tolerate differences of opinion among group participants
  - Sell health-related items for a profit
  - Rely on family and friends. A strong network of family and supportive friends is an important factor in coping with the chronicity of CFS.

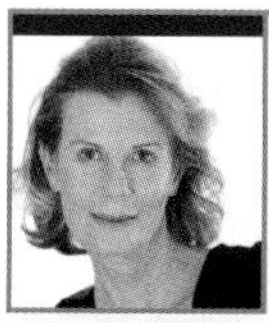

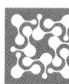

Clinical Scenario A 41-year-old woman tells the nurse, "I am so tired all the time. Although I have good intentions to accomplish things, I get overwhelmed by fatigue. Despite getting what I think should be sufficient sleep, I still don't have enough energy to get through the day. I even feel dizzy and nearly faint when I force myself to get some work done. My joints and muscles ache even though I haven't exerted myself." **How might the nurse plan to manage this client's care? See Nursing Care Plan 34-1.**

NURSING CARE PLAN 34-1 The Client With Chronic Fatigue Syndrome

Assessment

- Ask client to rate their energy level using a scale of 0 to 10, with 10 being the highest level. Have the client keep an energy diary to track periods during the day when energy levels are highest and lowest to determine any predictable pattern.
- Assess BP and pulse in resting and sitting positions to detect postural changes.
- Have client report their estimation of the quality of sleep.
- Determine client's pain level and location of discomfort.

Nursing Analysis. Fatigue related to dysregulation of energy secondary to CFS

Expected Outcome. Client's fatigue will be reduced sufficiently so that they can manage ADLs.

Interventions	Rationales
Have client identify ADLs of high priority. Determine ADLs that the client can delegate.	*Setting limits keeps physical and mental stress manageable. Delegation ensures completion of ADLs without the client expending personal energy.*
Help client perform one or more priority ADLs during a period of peak energy.	*Matching periods of activity with peaks in energy minimizes fatigue and avoids overexertion, which contributes to a relapse.*
Schedule 5- to 10-minute rest periods every hour or more.	*Relaxation can be more restorative than long naps.*
Assist client to perform gentle stretching exercises in a chair followed by low-grade active exercises recommended by the primary provider or physical therapist for 2–5 minutes daily.	*Stretching exercises promote blood circulation to muscles and ease the response to exercise.*
Increase exercise periods by ½–1 minute every 2–3 weeks according to client's response.	*Conditioning increases endurance.*

Evaluation of Expected Outcomes

Client performs hygiene and essential ADLs between periods of rest.

Nursing Diagnosis. Chronic pain related to unknown etiology.

Expected Outcome. Client's pain will be reduced to a tolerable level.

Interventions	Rationales
Apply a covered hot or cold pack to joints or muscles for 20 minutes; reapply after allowing the skin some recovery time.	*Heat improves circulation and relieves muscle spasm and pain. Cold prevents swelling, numbs sensation, and relieves pain.*
Encourage client to float in a pool or tub of tepid water (85°F) for 15 minutes as desired.	*Cool temperatures reduce metabolic processes, including the immune response. Submersion in water results in buoyancy, a feeling of weightlessness, and relaxation. Movement and exercise are easier to perform in water.*
Massage painful areas gently.	*Massage releases endorphins and enkephalins that inhibit neurotransmission of pain.*
Administer prescribed analgesics, corticosteroids, and antidepressants.	*Medications relieve pain through several physiologic mechanisms.*

Evaluation of Expected Outcome

The client's pain is reduced to a level of 5, which is within the client's tolerable range.

Nursing Diagnosis. Injury risk related to neurally mediated hypotension

Expected Outcome. The client will remain injury free.

Interventions	Rationales
Advise client to salt food liberally and to consume at least eight full glasses of fluid per day.	*Sodium attracts water. An adequate amount of fluid maintains circulating blood volume, reducing the potential for hypotension.*

Interventions	Rationales
Keep the signal for assistance within reach, and advise client to use it before attempting to ambulate.	*A nursing staff member may support the client in such a way as to break their fall and reduce or eliminate injury.*

(continued)

NURSING CARE PLAN 34-1 The Client With Chronic Fatigue Syndrome (*continued*)

Apply elastic stockings or thigh-high support hose before client lowers legs below the level of the heart.	*Elastic fibers compress vein walls and prevent pooling of blood in the extremities.*
Have client dangle and flex their lower limbs before getting out of bed.	*Muscle contraction promotes circulation of blood from distal body areas to the heart and brain. Adequate blood flow to the brain reduces hypotensive episodes.*
Instruct client to use a shower chair and avoid hot water when performing hygiene.	*Remaining seated reduces the potential for injury from a fall. Hot water causes vasodilation and a drop in BP.*
Administer prescribed antihypotensive or corticosteroid medications.	*Raising vascular tone and promoting sodium and water retention reduce the potential for low BP.*

Evaluation of Expected Outcome

Client's BP is within normal limits, and no fainting or injuries have occurred.

Evidence-Based Practice 34-1

Nursing Management of Fibromyalgia

Clinical Question

Why is the nursing role important in the management of fibromyalgia?

Evidence

Fibromyalgia is a condition that affects muscles, bones, and sleep. Clients who have this condition experience symptoms of muscle stiffness, fatigue, and muscle and bone pain. When a client experiences these symptoms every day, it begins to have an impact on their psychosocial well-being, and activities of daily living. The interventions that are possible with drug therapy are limited, so nursing has an important role in client care by offering therapeutic interventions (Ryan, 2013). Nurses can assess clients using a holistic view to find out what affects the client's pain and the management of their pain. The nurse can also help manage care by promoting exercise for comfort and health promotion, conducting medication reviews to make sure current drugs are effective, and suggesting behavioral measures to promote sleep. The cause of fibromyalgia is not known, but nurses can assist the client to manage their symptoms (Ryan, 2013).

Nursing Implications

This article describes the importance of the nursing role for clients with fibromyalgia, a disorder with no cure and little-to-no effective drug therapy. Teaching clients about exercise, sleep habits, and coping skills will be beneficial to the client in managing this condition. Nursing has an important role as a partner in the health care team by assessing the client's knowledge of the condition, current functional activity, and mood. The nurse encourages the client to identify problems associated with the condition from their own personal perspective. Offering methods for modifying activities of daily living and alternative coping skills may improve the client's quality of life.

Reference

Ryan, S. (2013). Care of patients with fibromyalgia: assessment and management. *Nursing Standard, 28*(13), 37–43. https://doi.org/10.7748/ns2013.11.28.13.37.e7722.

KEY POINTS

- Common allergens
  - Ingestants
  - Inhalants
  - Contactants
  - Injectants
- Allergies
  - Medication
  - Food
  - Environmental
- Immediate hypersensitivity
  - Type I, atopic or anaphylactic, which is mediated by immunoglobulin E (IgE) antibodies; response occurs within minutes.
  - Type II, cytotoxic, which is mediated by immunoglobulin M or G (IgM or IgG) antibodies: response within minutes.
  - Type III, immune complex, which is mediated by IgG antibodies: responses reach a peak within 6 hours after exposure to an allergen.
- Delayed hypersensitivity response: Type IV
  - Antibody production is not a component of a delayed hypersensitivity response. A delayed hypersensitivity response may develop over several hours or days, or it may reach maximum severity after repeated exposure (e.g., blood transfusions).
- Allergic response
  - Inhalants (inhaled allergens) usually cause respiratory symptoms, including nasal congestion, runny nose, sneezing, coughing, dyspnea, and wheezing. Inhaled allergens often trigger asthma.
  - Contactants: cause skin reactions such as hives, which appear as vesicles filled with clear fluid surrounded by a margin of redness, rash, and localized itching. Cramping, vomiting, and diarrhea are associated with ingested food allergens.
  - Injectants: (such as bee venom, and some other allergens) can produce systemic and potentially fatal effects, including shock and airway obstruction caused by laryngeal swelling.

- Diagnostic testing
  - Radioallergosorbent blood test (RAST), which measures IgE on a scale of 0 to 5, indicates a score of 2 or greater, it is a significant indication for an allergic disorder.
  - Scratch or prick test involves scratching the skin and applying a small amount of the liquid test antigen to the scratch. Results in 20 minutes or more.
  - Intradermal injection test: the tester injects a dilute solution of an antigen intradermally.
- Treating allergies
  - The treatment used to relieve allergic symptoms depends on the type of allergy. Besides avoiding the allergen if possible, many clients experience symptomatic relief with drug therapy.
  - Anaphylaxis: severe allergic reaction: medical emergency, signs and symptoms: angioneurotic edema, bronchospasms, hypotension
- Autoimmune disorders: diseases are considered autoimmune disorders when they are characterized by unrelenting, progressive tissue damage without any verifiable etiology.
- Chronic fatigue syndrome (CFS), also called *chronic fatigue*, *chronic fatigue immune dysfunction syndrome* (CFIDS), and *myalgic encephalomyelitis* (ME): a complex of symptoms primarily characterized by profound fatigue with no identifiable cause.
- Fibromyalgia: a condition that causes symptoms such as pain in fibrous tissues of the body such as muscles, ligaments, and tendons.

CRITICAL THINKING EXERCISES

1. A client reports having an allergy to aspirin. What additional information is needed to differentiate a true allergy from the drug's unwanted side effects?
2. A client complains about being delayed from going home for 30 minutes after receiving a desensitizing injection to control his allergies. How would you respond?
3. Explain why allergies, autoimmune diseases, and CFS are classified as immune-mediated disorders.
4. What teaching can you give to a client who seeks relief from symptoms of allergic rhinitis?

NCLEX-STYLE REVIEW QUESTIONS PrepU

1. A client who is symptomatic after having been stung by a bee is brought to the emergency department. Which of the following is the initial priority nursing assessment?
   1. Respiratory status
   2. Level of consciousness
   3. Heart rate
   4. Urinary output

2. What findings are likely to be evident when the nurse assesses a client with an allergy? Select all that apply.
   1. Rashes or lesions
   2. Nasal congestion
   3. Excess secretion of lymph
   4. Production of antibodies
   5. Itchy, red eyes
   6. Dyspnea

3. A nurse prepares to administer 0.2 mg of epinephrine subcutaneously to a client experiencing a severe allergic reaction. If the vial of epinephrine says it contains 1 mL of epinephrine that originally came from a 1:1000 dilution (e.g., 1 g of epinephrine in 1000 mL diluent), calculate the volume the nurse should administer. Record your answer to one decimal place.

   ____________mL

4. When the nurse provides teaching about an autoimmune disorder, what statement by the client demonstrates a correct understanding?
   1. "I will be cured of the autoimmune disorder."
   2. "I will need no more pharmacologic therapy."
   3. "I will be asymptomatic by avoiding immunologic triggers."
   4. "I will be in remission or have occasional exacerbations."

5. When all the nursing assessment findings are normal for an older adult client who reports being chronically fatigued, it is most appropriate for the nurse to further evaluate the client for which of the following?
   1. Depression
   2. Anxiety
   3. Fear
   4. Confusion

WANT TO KNOW MORE? There are a wide variety of online resources available on thePoint to enhance learning and understanding of this chapter.

Go to thePoint.lww.com/activate and use the activation code found in the front of this text to unlock these online resources.

35 Caring for Clients With HIV/AIDS

Words To Know

acquired immunodeficiency syndrome (AIDS)
acute retroviral syndrome
AIDS dementia complex
AIDS Drug Assistance Program (ADAP)
autologous blood
candidiasis
capsid
chemokines
codons
combination antiretroviral therapy (cART)
directed donor blood
distal sensory polyneuropathy (DSP)
drug cross-resistance
drug resistance
entry inhibitor
enzyme-linked immunosorbent assay
fusion inhibitor
genotype testing
human immunodeficiency virus (HIV)
integrase
integrase inhibitors
Kaposi sarcoma
opportunistic infections
phenotype testing
Pneumocystis pneumonia
polymerase chain reaction (PCR) test
preexposure prophylaxis (PrEP)
protease
protease inhibitor (PI)
reverse transcriptase
reverse transcriptase inhibitors
reverse transcription
safer-sex practices
salvage therapy
viatical settlement
viremia
Western Blot test

Learning Objectives

On completion of this chapter, you will be able to:

1. Explain the term acquired immunodeficiency syndrome (AIDS).
2. Identify the virus that causes AIDS.
3. Discuss the characteristics of a retrovirus.
4. Explain how human immunodeficiency virus (HIV) is transmitted.
5. Name at least four methods for preventing transmission of HIV.
6. List three criteria for diagnosing AIDS.
7. Discuss the pathophysiologic process of AIDS.
8. List at least five manifestations characteristic of acute retroviral syndrome.
9. Name two laboratory tests used to screen for HIV antibodies and one that confirms a diagnosis of AIDS.
10. Name two laboratory tests used to measure viral load and give two purposes for their use.
11. Identify categories of drugs that are used to treat individuals infected with HIV and give an example of a specific drug in each category.
12. Give the criterion for successful drug therapy for HIV/AIDS.
13. Discuss the nursing management of a client with AIDS, including client teaching.
14. Describe techniques for preventing HIV infection among health care providers who care for infected clients.
15. Discuss two ethical issues that affect health care providers in relation to clients with HIV infection.

Acquired immunodeficiency syndrome (AIDS) is an infectious and potentially life-threatening disorder that severely compromises the immune system. A pathogen known as the **human immunodeficiency virus (HIV)** causes AIDS. People can remain well, sometimes up to 10 years or longer, despite being infected with HIV, before the initial infection develops into AIDS. During this asymptomatic period, the infected person can infect others.

Gerontologic Considerations

■ Treatment advances have resulted in longer life spans for those who contracted HIV at an early age. HIV is now considered a chronic infection, and infected older adults and their health care providers must focus on interaction of HIV and changes with aging, including decreased immunity.
■ Older adults are more likely to be diagnosed later in the course of disease progression, with possible immune

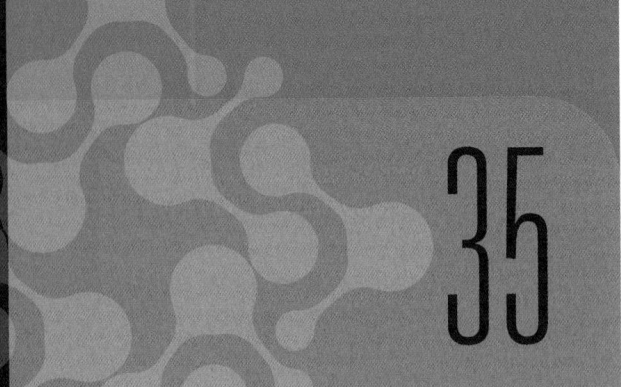

Gerontologic Considerations (*continued*)

system damage and earlier death. Efforts to increase older adults' awareness of risk factors, prevention, and provider's awareness of need for screening may increase earlier identification of infection.

- Data regarding rates of HIV/AIDS indicate cases and death in people older than 50 years remain high, with risk factors similar to other age groups. Early identification and treatment is imperative, with consideration for other possible comorbidities.
- An accurate sexual history in older adults is important, because sexual activity may continue throughout the life span.
- Antiretroviral treatment may accelerate physical changes associated with aging and damage to organ systems, which can increase morbidity and mortality.
- The dementia caused by AIDS may be mistaken for other dementias that may affect older adults and may occur concurrently.
- HIV education and prevention efforts in the United States have focused on increasing HIV prevention and surveillance of older adults. The goal of the National HIV/AIDS Strategy is to increase health care providers' awareness, discussions, education, regarding sexual activity, and support for older adults with HIV/AIDS (National HIV/AIDS Strategy).

An estimated 1.7 million individuals worldwide acquired HIV in 2019, marking a 23% decline in new HIV infections since 2010 (Epidemic, 2020). Even with the decrease in newly diagnosed people, and those who are infected living longer, HIV continues to spread easily from person to person, especially in particular parts of the world. In 2019, there were 20.7 million people with HIV (54% of total worldwide infection) in eastern and southern Africa (Epidemic, 2020).

There were approximately 38 million people across the globe with HIV/AIDS in 2019. Of these, 36.2 million were adults and 1.8 million were children (less than 15 years old; Epidemic, 2020). In the early history of HIV/AIDS, HIV occurred more often among gay men, but that exclusivity is no longer the case. Others who are at higher risk are intravenous (IV) drug users and prisoners. Infection of heterosexual women leads to transmission of HIV to newborns. To date, nurses are the largest group of health care providers to have occupationally acquired HIV infection; however, occupational HIV transmission is extremely rare (HIV Exposure, 2019).

In 2019, around 700,000 people died from AIDS-related illnesses worldwide, compared to 1.1 million people in 2010. AIDS-related mortality has declined by 39% since 2010 (AIDS statistics, 2020). The decrease is in part due to the number of people with HIV receiving treatment in resource-poor countries, and progress has been made in preventing mother-to-child transmission of HIV and keeping mothers alive (Global HIV/AIDS, 2020).

In 2019, a new approach was implemented by the U.S. government to eliminate new infections by:

- **Diagnosing** all individuals with HIV as early as possible.
- **Treating** people with HIV rapidly and effectively to achieve sustained viral suppression.
- **Preventing** new HIV transmissions by using proven interventions, including preexposure prophylaxis (PrEP) and syringe services programs (SSPs).
- **Responding** quickly to potential HIV outbreaks to get needed prevention and treatment services to people who need them.

HIV.gov. (2020). *U.S. Statistics*. https://www.hiv.gov/hiv-basics/overview/data-and-trends/statistics

HIV

It is speculated that HIV is an altered genetic form of simian (monkey) immunodeficiency virus (SIV). It is believed that the transformation allowed the virus to "jump" from chimpanzees to humans in Africa when humans slaughtered and consumed the meat of the chimpanzees.

Subtypes of HIV

Two HIV subtypes have been identified: HIV-1 and HIV-2. HIV-1 is composed of four groups identified as M, N, O, and P. Group M mutates easily and frequently, producing multiple substrains that are identified by letters from A through K, and circulating recombinant form (CRF), a hybrid virus formed by genetic material from various combined subtypes (AVERT Organization, 2016b). HIV-2 is the primary type of infection in Western Africa. It is less transmittable, and the interval between initial infection with HIV-2 and the development of AIDS is longer. HIV-1, Group M, subtype B is more prevalent in the United States and in the rest of the world, but the distribution of subtypes changes from time to time because of the diverse merging of populations.

Structural Characteristics

Viruses require a living host cell for survival and duplication. Like all viruses, HIV is genetically incomplete. A double layer of lipid material surrounds the incomplete HIV. A surface-binding glycoprotein called *gp120* has projections extending in all directions from the lipid bilayer; the purpose of *gp120* is to attach the virus to the T cell's receptor, called a *CD4 receptor*. Another binding protein, called *gp41*, which is composed of three stalks, is used to fuse the virus to the T cell's coreceptors, either CCR5 or CXCR4. The discovery of the mechanisms for attachment and fusion with coreceptors has led to the development of antiretroviral drugs called entry inhibitors (see later discussion).

The fusion of the virus and CD4 coreceptors provides a means by which the genetic contents within the **capsid**, the viral structure that encloses the single strands of ribonucleic acid (RNA) along with three important enzymes—reverse transcriptase, integrase, and protease—can combine with the genetic code of the helper T cell (National Institute of Allergy and Infectious Diseases, 2012; Fig. 35-1).

››› *Stop, Think, and Respond 35-1*

What is the role of helper T cells in the immune response?

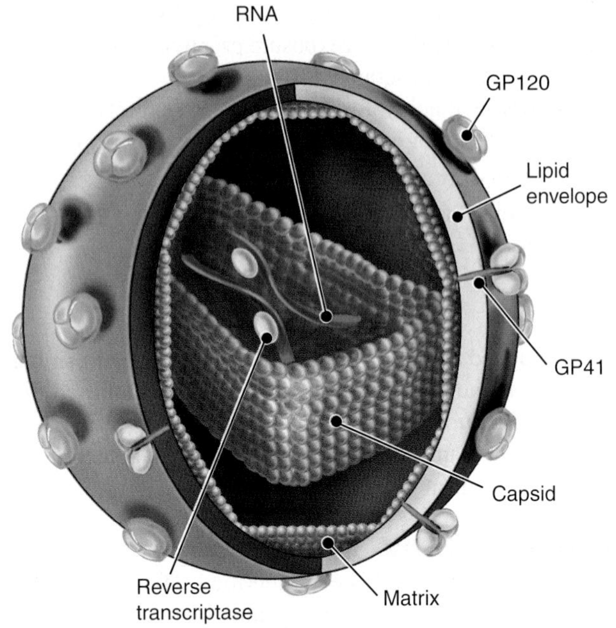

Figure 35-1 Structure of human immunodeficiency virus (HIV), a retrovirus. RNA, ribonucleic acid.

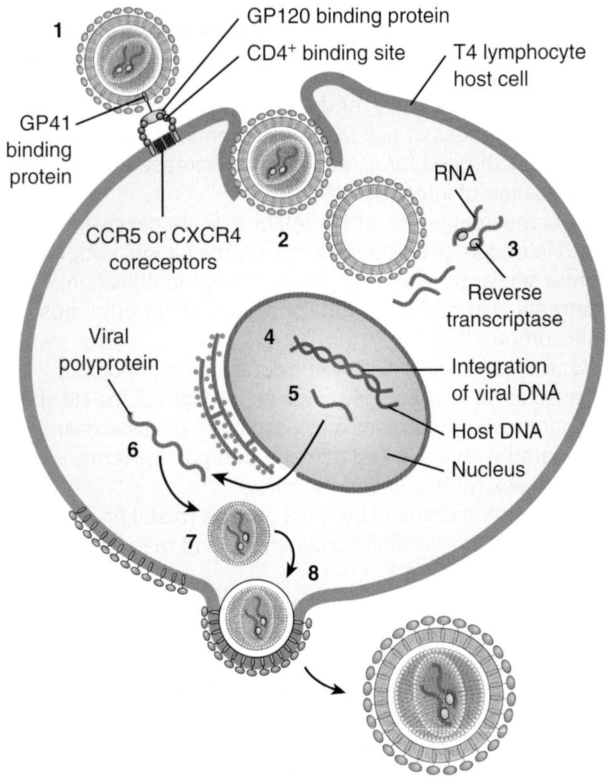

Figure 35-2 HIV replication. (1) To enter a T-cell lymphocyte, the human immunodeficiency virus (HIV) must attach to a CD4 receptor and additional coreceptors on the surface of the cell. (2) Internalization and uncoating of the virus with viral ribonucleic acid (RNA) and reverse transcriptase. (3) Reverse transcription, which produces a mirror image of the viral RNA and double-stranded deoxyribonucleic acid (DNA) molecule. (4) Integration of viral DNA into host DNA. (5) Transcription of inserted viral DNA to produce viral messenger RNA. (6) Conversion of viral messenger RNA to create viral polyprotein. (7) Cleavage of viral polyprotein into viral proteins that make up new virus. (8) Assembly and release of new virus from the host cell.

Replication

To replicate, which means to produce more copies, HIV becomes a parasite of helper T cells (also known as *T4* or *CD4 cells* because of their CD4 receptor; see Chapter 33). HIV alters the helper T cell's genetic code to make more viral particles. To do this, the enzyme **reverse transcriptase** copies the viral RNA into viral deoxyribonucleic acid (DNA); this process is called **reverse transcription**. A second viral enzyme, **integrase**, incorporates the reprogrammed viral DNA into the host cell's DNA.

The altered DNA tells the cell how to assemble amino acids to form protein substances, such as the virus. The transformed DNA provides the blueprint or cookbook for making clones of HIV along with the enzymes the virus needs to continue reinfecting additional cells.

The T cell's nucleus follows the pirated DNA's directions and forms long chains of viral particles enclosed within its membrane. **Protease**, the third viral enzyme, cuts the long chains, freeing the replicated viral particles into the cytoplasm of the cell. Some migrate to the cell wall and form buds. When the buds rupture, they release many copies of the virus that reinfect other helper T cells (Fig. 35-2).

More than 10 billion viral particles are released daily; most, but not all, are destroyed. Mutations occur frequently, complicating drug therapy and making production of a vaccine nearly impossible. In February 2005, a new strain of HIV, identified as 3-DCR HIV, was detected in a gay man in New York. Scientists consider 3-DCR highly virulent because it converts the initial HIV infection to full-blown AIDS in a matter of months; the new strain is highly drug resistant. The infected man also used methamphetamine, which scientists believe can accelerate the replication of the virus, especially in the brain. AIDS activists are warning people to avoid becoming complacent about the potential for acquiring HIV by stressing consistent condom use, avoiding illicit psychostimulants such as methamphetamine that promote disinhibition and hypersexuality, and adhering to antiretroviral drug therapy if they have been diagnosed with HIV.

Transmission

HIV is not transmitted by casual contact. There are only four known body fluids through which HIV is transmitted: blood, semen, vaginal secretions, and breast milk. HIV may be present in saliva, tears, and conjunctival secretions, but transmission of HIV through these fluids has not been implicated. HIV is not found in urine, stool, vomit, or sweat.

>>> *Stop, Think, and Respond 35-2*

How would you respond to those who avoid drinking from a common cup, such as those used in Christian church services, because they fear acquiring AIDS?

BOX 35-1 High-Risk Factors for HIV Infection

- Unprotected vaginal, anal, or oral sex
- Contact with blood and infectious body fluids during medical, surgical, dental, or nursing procedures
- Sharing intravenous needles or syringes
- Receiving nonautologous transfusions of blood or blood products before antibodies can be detected in the donated blood
- Receiving plasma or clotting factors that have not been heat treated
- Contact with infected blood on body piercing, tattoo, and dental equipment
- Transmission from infected mothers to infants during pregnancy, birth, or breastfeeding

Certain behaviors increase the risk of acquiring HIV from infectious body fluids (Box 35-1). Unprotected sexual intercourse and multiple sexual partners increase the risk of HIV infection and other sexually transmitted infections (STIs). Using a condom is one of the most effective ways to reduce the risk of HIV infection. Condoms are available for both men and women (Client and Family Teaching 35-1).

Before 1984, blood and blood products were a major source of HIV transmission. Since then, an HIV screening test known as nucleic acid testing (NAT) is performed on all blood and plasma donations. Although screening donated blood for HIV antibodies reduces the risk of transfusion-related infection with HIV, it is not flawless. Antibody screening cannot identify infected blood from donors who have yet to produce significant antibodies. The window of time between infection (entrance of HIV into the body) and production of antibodies is currently 2.93 days. The Verywell Health's website states that the risk for HIV infection in the United States from a blood transfusion is approximately 1 in 2 million units of blood. Another potential, but less common method of transmission is a puncture with an HIV-contaminated needle or other sharp object.

Prevention Strategies

The transmission of HIV is reduced or eliminated by adhering to the following guidelines:

- Abstain from sexual intercourse.
- Have mutually monogamous sex with an uninfected partner.
- Avoid casual sex with multiple partners.
- Use a condom and spermicide that contains nonoxynol-9 during sexual intercourse.
- Abstain from using IV drugs, especially psychostimulants such as methamphetamine, that contribute to disinhibition and hypersexuality.
- Use a new needle and syringe each time IV drugs are injected.
- Refrain from donating blood if engaged in high-risk behaviors.
- Bank **autologous blood** (self-donated) or **directed donor blood** (specified blood donors among relatives and friends) when preparing for nonemergency surgical procedures (Table 35-1).

Client and Family Teaching 35-1
Using a Condom

The nurse teaches the clients the following points:

Male Condom

- Purchase latex condoms, or vinyl if sensitive to latex.
- Select a strong condom and use lubricant liberally for anal intercourse.
- Do not store condoms where they are exposed to heat or light.
- Use a new condom each time you engage in sexual intercourse.
- Apply the condom after the penis is erect and before making any sexual contact with a partner.
- Leave a half inch between the tip of the penis and the bottom of the condom.
- Unroll the condom from the base of the penis.
- Expel any air bubbles that have formed.
- On withdrawal, hold the base of the condom and withdraw the penis before it becomes limp.
- When removing the condom, knot the open end and discard it in a lined waste container.

Female Condom

- Make sure that the purchased condom is labeled for female use; one brand available in the United States is called "FC 2."
- Distribute the coated lubricant over the outside by rubbing the outer surface.
- Observe that a reinforced ring is at the open end at the bottom.
- Compress the bottom ring to form an oval shape.
- Insert the compressed ring with the index finger into the vagina as far as the finger can reach.
- Ensure that the condom is not twisted and that the ring at the open end is externally visible.
- Guide the penis into the condom.
- Remain horizontal after intercourse.
- Remove the condom by squeezing the lower ring and twisting the polyurethane sheath.
- Knot the opening and dispose of the condom in a lined waste container; do not flush the condom in the toilet.

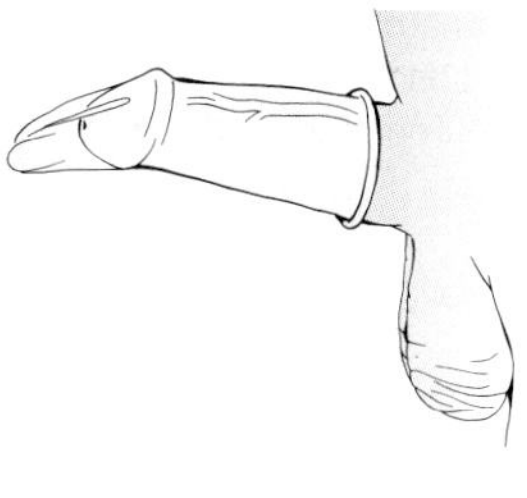
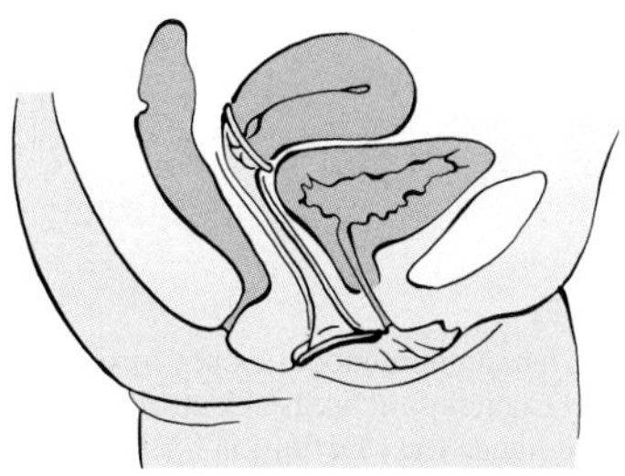

TABLE 35-1 Guidelines for Autologous and Directed Donor Blood Donation

AUTOLOGOUS DONATION	DIRECTED DONOR DONATION
Donor must weigh 95 lb.	Donor must weigh 110 lb.
Donor must be at least 14 years of age.	Donor must be at least 17 years of age.
Exceptions may be made in medical history.	Donor must meet volunteer donor medical history criteria.
Blood is used only for transfusion to donor.	Client's primary provider must be informed of directed donation. Blood may be transfused to others if not needed by client.
Blood type does not need to be known at time of donation.	Donors should be compatible with blood type of client.
Units that test positive for a disease (other than HIV) will be issued.	Units that test positive for HIV or hepatitis will not be used.
Donation frequency may not be greater than 1 unit every 56 days.	Donation frequency may not be greater than 1 unit every 56 days.
Additional fee to hospital or recipient may be charged for holding blood on reserve.	Additional fees may be charged to the recipient.

HIV, human immunodeficiency virus.

Some authorities believe that directed donor blood is no safer than blood collected from public donors. Nurses and other health care providers use standard precautions (see Chapter 12) when caring for all clients whose infectious status is unknown. Nurses must immediately report any needlestick or sharp injury to a supervisor. Postexposure protocols using antiretroviral medications can reduce the risk of HIV infection if initiated within 72 hours after a possible exposure. Prophylaxis requires self-administration of medications once or twice daily for 28 days. Because postexposure prophylaxis is not 100% effective, condoms should be used until an HIV infection can be ruled out. If infected, health care providers can continue to practice; however, they usually are restricted from performing procedures in which they may exchange blood with clients.

ACQUIRED IMMUNODEFICIENCY SYNDROME

AIDS is the end stage of HIV infection. Certain events establish the conversion of HIV infection to AIDS: (1) a markedly decreased T4-cell count from a normal level of 800 to 1200/mm^3 and (2) the development of certain cancers and **opportunistic infections**, infections that usually do not occur in individuals with a healthy immune system. In 1993, the Centers for Disease Control and Prevention (CDC) revised its classification system into two categories that constitute an AIDS diagnosis: (1) Category 1, 2, or 3 and (2) Category A, B, or C (Table 35-2).

TABLE 35-2 Classification for HIV Infection

CATEGORY 1	CATEGORY 2	CATEGORY 3
T4-cell count ≥500/mm^3	T4-cell count 200–499/mm^3	T4-cell count <200/mm^3
CATEGORY A	**CATEGORY B**	**CATEGORY C**
HIV positive with one or more of the following: • Asymptomatic • Persistent generalized lymphadenopathy (swollen lymph nodes) • Acute (primary) HIV infection with accompanying illness or history of acute HIV infection	HIV positive with conditions attributed to or complicated by HIV infection such as • Bacillary angiomatosis • Candidiasis (oral, vulvovaginal) persistent, frequent, or poorly responsive to therapy • Cervical dysplasia or carcinoma • Fever or diarrhea for more than 1 month • Hairy leukoplakia • Herpes zoster (at least two episodes) • Idiopathic thrombocytopenic purpura • Listeriosis • Pelvic inflammatory disease/tubo-ovarian abscess • Peripheral neuropathy	HIV positive with one or more of the following: • Candidiasis (bronchial, tracheal, lungs, or esophagus) • Cervical cancer (invasive) • Coccidioidomycosis (disseminated or extrapulmonary) • Cryptococcosis (extrapulmonary) • Cryptosporidiosis for more than 1 month • Cytomegalovirus (other than liver, spleen, or nodes) • Encephalopathy (HIV related) • Herpes simplex (for more than 1 month) or bronchitis, pneumonitis, esophagitis • Histoplasmosis (disseminated or extrapulmonary) • Isosporiasis (for more than 1 month) • Kaposi sarcoma • Lymphoma, Burkitt (or equivalent), immunoblastic (or equivalent), brain (primary) • *Mycobacterium avium* complex or *Mycobacterium kansasii*, disseminated or extrapulmonary • *Mycobacterium tuberculosis*, any site, pulmonary or extrapulmonary • *Mycobacterium*, other species • *Pneumocystis carinii* pneumonia • Pneumonia, recurrent • Progressive multifocal leukoencephalopathy • *Salmonella* septicemia, recurrent • Toxoplasmosis of brain • Wasting syndrome

HIV, human immunodeficiency virus.
From Centers for Disease Control and Prevention. Revised Surveillance Case Definition for HIV Infection—United States, 2014 from Revised Surveillance Case Definition for HIV Infection—United States, 2014 (cdc.gov)

>>> ***Stop, Think, and Respond 35-3***

What classification would be assigned to a person who is HIV positive with a T4-cell count of 350/mm^3 who develops Pneumocystis pneumonia?

Pathophysiology and Etiology

AIDS is transmitted from direct contact with the blood or body fluids of a person diagnosed with HIV or from indirect contact with infected blood or body fluids. When HIV infection occurs, it gradually impairs the ability of infected T4 cells to recognize foreign antigens (e.g., disease pathogens) and stimulate B-cell lymphocytes. Although massive numbers of viral particles are being released, infected T4 cells are destroyed by HIV itself and by killer T8-cell lymphocytes that no longer recognize the altered T4 cell's membrane as being self. Although new T4 cells are produced, the process is never as fast as replication of the virus. Eventually, T4 cells become significantly depleted, and immunodeficiency develops (Fig. 35-3). The person who has HIV may ultimately die from an opportunistic infection.

The rate of progression from HIV infection to AIDS is related to the concentration of virus in the blood, the subtype and strain of infecting HIV, and the status of coreceptors on the CD4 cells. If inherited abnormalities and mutations in CCR5 or CXCR4 coreceptors are blocked with **chemokines**, chemicals responsible for immune surveillance and immune cell recruitment, there is interference with HIV's entry into cells (Barmania & Pepper, 2013). HIV can be prevented from invading cells among individuals who have mutated forms of CCR5 coreceptors that are located inside rather than outside the CD4 cell. For some, the process of progression may take 10 years or more. Although most people infected with HIV die as a result of their disease or an opportunistic infection, a few are long-term survivors. Some explanations for long-term survival include the following:

- The infectious HIV is a weak strain.
- The amount of virus is kept low with stronger-than-normal killer T8 cells.
- Strict adherence to drug therapy and the combination of drugs used for treatment are highly effective.

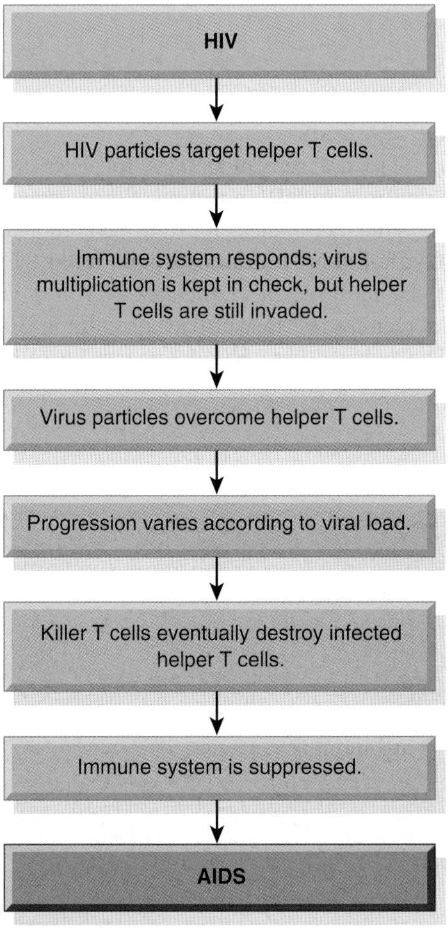

Figure 35-3 Progression of human immunodeficiency virus (HIV) infection and development of AIDS.

Assessment Findings

Signs and Symptoms

At the time HIV is acquired, one-third to more than one-half of those who are HIV positive develop **acute retroviral syndrome** (**viremia**), also called acute HIV syndrome, which often is mistaken for flu or some other common illness (Fig. 35-4). Some manifestations include fever; swollen and tender lymph nodes; pharyngitis; rash about the face, trunk, palms, and soles; muscle and joint pain; headache; nausea and vomiting; and diarrhea. In addition, there may be enlargement of the liver and spleen, weight loss, and neurologic symptoms such as visual changes or cognitive and motor involvement. However, admission of risk behaviors for HIV narrows the differential diagnosis. Although viral replication is rapid at this time, antibody tests cannot detect the infection.

Eventually, individuals with HIV may present with an opportunistic infection or a form of cancer that is atypical for the person's age and health history. For example, **Kaposi sarcoma**, a type of connective tissue cancer common among those with AIDS, may be noted (Fig. 35-5). Others who acquire Pneumocystis pneumonia (discussed later) have a nonproductive cough and shortness of breath. In women, gynecologic problems may be the focus of the chief complaint. Abnormal results of Papanicolaou tests, genital warts, pelvic inflammatory disease, and persistent vaginitis (see Chapters 53 and 56) may also correlate with HIV infection.

Testing Recommendations

The CDC recommends routine testing for the following populations (Cennimo, 2014):

- All persons aged 13 to 24 years
- All persons seeking treatment for an STI on each visit
- All persons initiating treatment for tuberculosis
- All persons with signs and symptoms or illnesses consistent with HIV infection

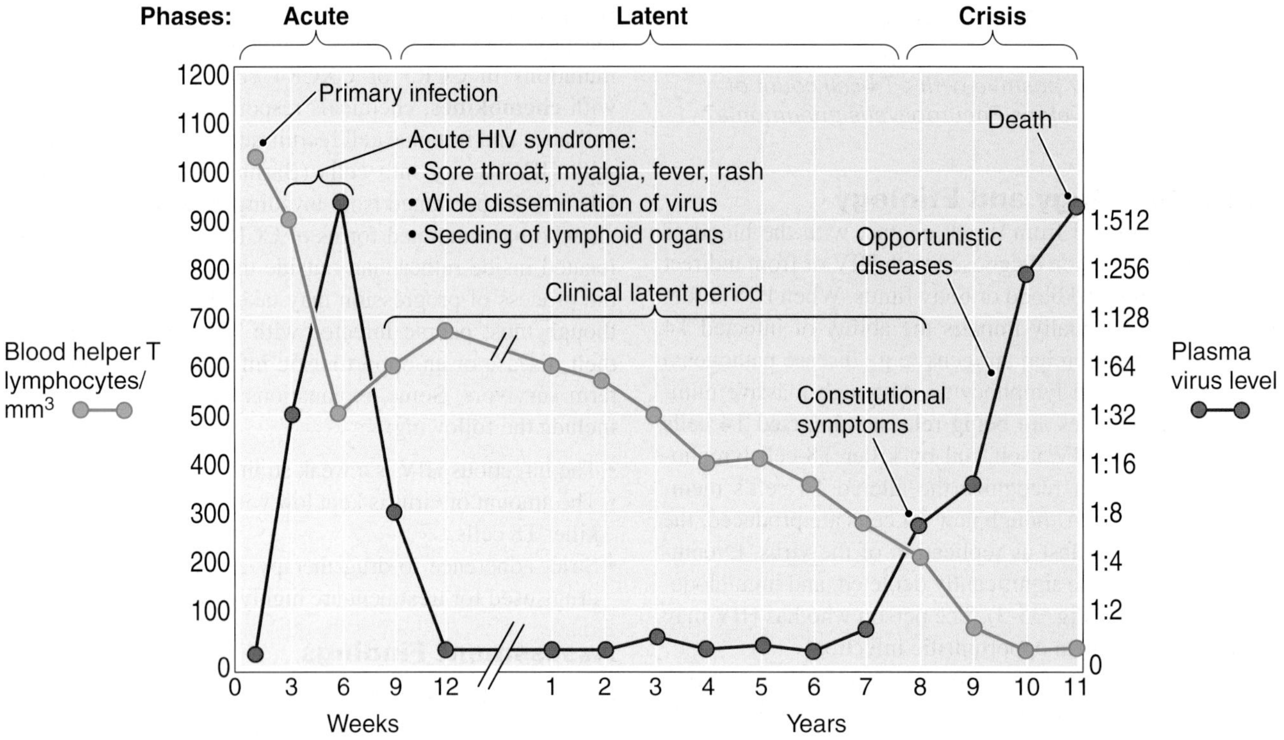

Figure 35-4 Phases of human immunodeficiency virus (HIV) infection and AIDS. During the initial diagnosis of HIV, a flu-like syndrome occurs. The virus level is high, and the helper T-cell count begins to fall. In the latent period, which may last for years, the helper T-cell count continues falling well below normal. During the crisis phase, the T-cell count is so depressed that opportunistic infections occur that are usually the cause of death.

Repeated HIV testing should be performed yearly among individuals at high risk for HIV infection such as:

- IV drug users and their sex partners
- Persons who exchange sex for money or drugs
- Partner of an HIV-infected person
- Person or partner who has more than one sexual partner since their last HIV test
- Persons starting a new sexual relationship regardless of a previous negative test result

HIV Screening Tests

Currently, there are screening tests for HIV as well as tests that confirm an HIV infection. Some screening tests detect only HIV antibodies, the most common of which is the **enzyme-linked immunosorbent assay** (ELISA or EIA) test. In addition, *the OraQuick HIV test* is a rapid antibody screening test that provides results in 30 minutes or less. The *home access HIV-1 test* can be self-obtained with a finger prick and mailed to a licensed laboratory. A

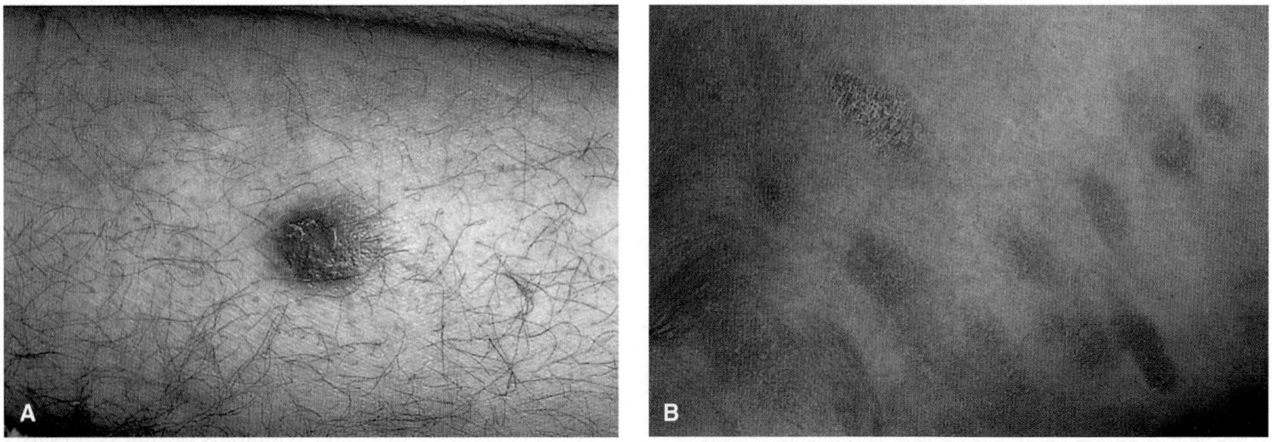

Figure 35-5 Kaposi sarcoma: **(A)** single lesion and **(B)** multiple lesions.

fourth-generation test is a combination test that detects HIV antibodies as well as a HIV antigen called p24. The antigen is present before antibodies develop. Because all screening tests can yield false-positive results, specimens are retested a second time and an additional test to confirm an HIV infection is obtained.

HIV Confirmational Tests

There are three tests that can be used to confirm previously positive screening tests. The **Western Blot test** is the gold standard. It determines antibodies to specific HIV antigens such as *p24*, *gp41*, and *gp120*. A reaction to at least two antigens indicates a positive result.

The *indirect fluorescent antibody (IFA) test* is used when the Western Blot test is not definitively positive. It mixes cells that are likely infected with HIV with immunoglobins and viewed using a fluorescent microscope. Although it can confirm HIV disease, it is expensive and subject to the examiner's interpretation.

Lastly, the **polymerase chain reaction (PCR) test**, also called an RNA test, is used to detect the HIV virus itself. The PCR test is quite expensive and generally reserved for diagnosing infants with HIV born to mothers with HIV.

Miscellaneous Tests

A total T-cell count, T4- and T8-cell counts, and T4/T8 ratio determine the status of T-cell lymphocytes. A T4-cell count of less than 500/mm^3 indicates immune suppression; a T4-cell count of 200/mm^3 or less is an indicator of AIDS.

It is now possible to measure a person's viral load, that is, the number of viral particles in the blood. It is used to guide drug therapy and follow the progression of the disease. Viral load tests and T4 cell counts may be performed every 2 to 3 months once it is determined that a person is HIV positive.

Other general laboratory and diagnostic tests are prescribed when opportunistic infections are involved. In addition, cancer screenings, especially Papanicolaou cervical tests for women (see Chapter 53), are recommended for those infected with HIV. Immunosuppression tends to facilitate the development of cancer and accelerate its progression.

Medical Management

People with HIV and AIDS are treated with antiretroviral drugs, adjunct drug therapy to boost the immune response, and supportive care during opportunistic infections. It usually is recommended that clients infected with HIV receive pneumococcal, hepatitis B, and yearly influenza vaccines. Additional medical management includes treating anorexia, diarrhea, weight loss, and side effects of antiretroviral medications. Research continues on developing an effective HIV vaccine or reducing the potential for infection with a microbicide (discussed later).

Antiretroviral Drug Therapy

The current recommendation is to initiate antiretroviral drug therapy regardless of the client's disease stage or CD4 T-cell lymphocyte count rather than wait until the cell count decreases significantly (National Institutes of Health, 2016a). The recommendation is based on the following rationale. Early treatment:

- restores normal CD4/CD8 cell counts
- improves immune function
- reduces viremia, the presence of viruses in the blood
- delays disease progression
- improves overall quality of life
- diminishes drug resistance
- lessens AIDS-defining illnesses and serious non-AIDS conditions
- decreases transmission of HIV to sex partners and prevalence in a community
- reduces perinatal transmission
- prolongs life

Besides treating adults and adolescents who are HIV positive, the World Health Organization (2013) also recommends providing antiretroviral drug therapy to all HIV-infected children under 5 years of age, infected pregnant women, and breastfeeding women.

Drug Regimens

At present, the majority of drugs used to manage clients who are infected with HIV target viral enzymes (Fig. 35-6). The combinations of antiretroviral drugs, referred to as a *drug cocktail*, are more effective than monotherapy (only one drug used for treatment). Some clients may take as many as four types of medications. **Combination antiretroviral therapy (cART)** has several benefits:

- Using different mechanisms, the combination of drugs suppresses replication of the virus.
- The drugs lower the viral load more quickly—sometimes to undetectable levels. Doing so ultimately slows the rate of disease progression, prevents opportunistic infections, and, in turn, lengthens survival.
- Combination therapy diminishes the rate of viral mutations and prolongs drug effectiveness.
- Using two or more drugs simultaneously reduces the chance that the virus will develop resistance or cross-resistance.
- A combination of drugs increases the numbers of healthy helper T-cell lymphocytes because it protects many from becoming infected.

The goal of antiretroviral therapy is to bring the viral load to a virtually undetectable level. This level is no more than 500 or 50 copies, depending on the sensitivity of the selected viral load test.

When drug therapy is begun, clients are generally prescribed a combination of three antiretroviral drugs: two nucleoside **reverse transcriptase inhibitors** (NRTIs), drugs that interfere with the ability of the virus to make a genetic blueprint, and a third drug from one of three other drug classes: a non-nucleoside reverse transcriptase inhibitor (NNRTI), an **integrase inhibitor** also called an integrase strand transfer inhibitor (INSTI), or a pharmacokinetic (PK)-enhanced **protease inhibitor (PI)**. The combination of drugs is selected on the basis of virologic efficacy, toxicity,

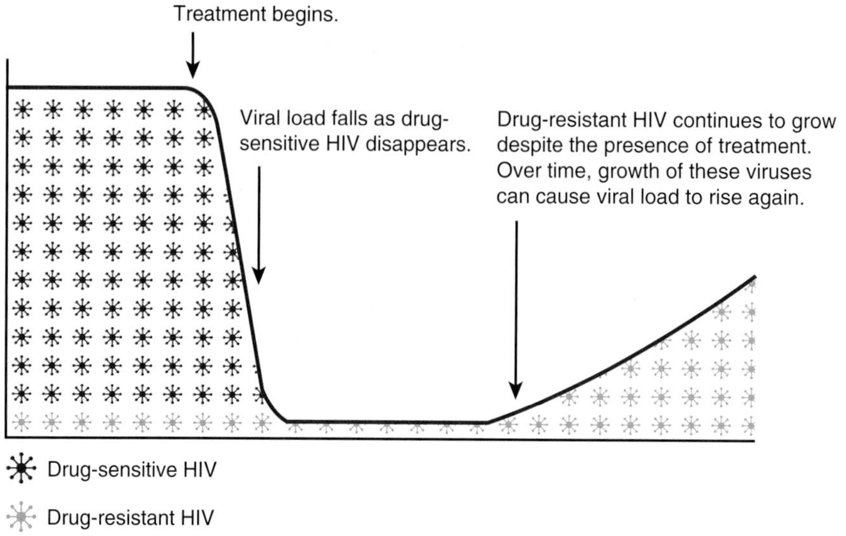

Treatment begins.
Viral load falls as drug-sensitive HIV disappears.
Drug-resistant HIV continues to grow despite the presence of treatment. Over time, growth of these viruses can cause viral load to rise again.
Drug-sensitive HIV
Drug-resistant HIV

Figure 35-6 The development of drug-resistant strains of human immunodeficiency virus (HIV).

pill burden, dosing frequency, potential for drug–drug interactions, development of drug resistance, coexisting conditions, and cost (National Institute of Health [NIH], 2016a). An **entry inhibitor**, also called CCR5 antagonist, and **fusion inhibitor** acting at the surface between the virus and CD4 cell wall are also available (Drug Therapy Table 35-1).

Entry and Fusion Inhibitors. An **entry inhibitor**, maraviroc (Selzentry), stops HIV from attaching to a CD4 T cell by

DRUG THERAPY TABLE 35-1 Drugs Used in HIV Therapy

Category and Common Generic (Brand) Drugs	Intended Use	Common Side Effects	Safety Warnings for Nurses
Antiretrovirals			
Nucleoside/nucleotide reverse transcriptase inhibitors (NRTIs)			
Abacavir (Ziagen) Didanosine (ddI) (Videx) Emtricitabine (Emtriva) Lamivudine (3TC) (Epivir) Stavudine (Zerit) Tenofovir disoproxil (Viread) Zidovudine (AZT) (Retrovir)	Treat HIV infection by blocking the reverse transcriptase enzyme so the HIV material cannot change into DNA in the new cell, and preventing new HIV copies from being created. • HIV infection, prevention of maternal–fetal HIV transmission	Headache, nausea, rash, vomiting, peripheral neuropathy, abdominal pain, diarrhea	• Monitor for pancreatitis and liver dysfunction.
Non-nucleoside reverse transcriptase inhibitors (NNRTIs)			
Delavirdine (Rescriptor) Efavirenz (Sustiva) Etravirine (Intelence) Nevirapine (Viramune) Rilpivirine (Edurant)	Treat HIV infection by latching on to the reverse transcriptase molecule to block the ability to make viral DNA	Headache, nausea, diarrhea	Flu-like symptoms may be a side effect of the drug or the underlying disease. St. John's wort can decrease antiviral effects.
Protease inhibitors			
Atazanavir (Reyataz) Darunavir (Prezista) Fosamprenavir (Lexiva) Indinavir (Crixivan) Nelfinavir (Viracept) Ritonavir (Norvir) Saquinavir (Invirase) Tipranavir (Aptivus)	Treat HIV infection by blocking the protease enzyme so new viral particles cannot mature; used as a pharmacokinetic enhancer	Nausea, rash, headache, diarrhea, constipation, peripheral and circumoral paresthesias, altered lipid profiles Hyperglycemia Changes in fat distribution from arms and legs to deposition on trunk and neck commonly referred to as "protease paunch"	• Do not give with ergot-based migraine headache medicines. • Do not give if sulfonamide drug allergy. • Monitor for kidney/bladder stones. • Monitor for liver dysfunction, intracranial bleeding. • Keep a record of blood sugar measurements; adjust diabetic medications accordingly. • Monitor cholesterol and triglyceride levels.

DRUG THERAPY TABLE 35-1 Drugs Used in HIV Therapy (*continued*)

Category and Common Generic (Brand) Drugs	Intended Use	Common Side Effects	Safety Warnings for Nurses
Entry (fusion) inhibitors			
Maraviroc (Selzentry) Enfuvirtide (Fuzeon)	Treat HIV infection by preventing the attachment or fusion of HIV to a host cell for initial entry	• Injection site reaction such as itching, swelling, redness, pain, tenderness • May cause dizziness	• Monitor for pneumonia and respiratory symptoms. • Ensure all particles are in solution, which may require standing up to 45 minutes after reconstitution • Caution to avoid activities requiring alertness until response to medication is known • Monitor for muscle pain or weakness moving arms and legs; dark red or brown urine.
Integrase inhibitors			
Elvitegravir (Vitekta) Raltegravir (Isentress) Dolutegravir (Tivicay)	Treat HIV infection by preventing enzymes from inserting HIV genetic material into the cell's DNA	Diarrhea, insomnia At risk for rhabdomyolysis and myopathy	
Combination agents	See separate drugs above		
Abacavir/dolutegravir/lamivudine (Triumeq) Atazanavir/cobicistat (Evotaz) Darunavir/cobicistat (Prezcobix) Elvitegravir/cobicistat/emtricitabine/tenofovir (Genvoya) Elvitegravir/cobicistat/emtricitabine/tenofovir disoproxil (Stribild)			
Antivirals			
Agents used to treat cytomegalovirus (CMV)-related infections			
Cidofovir (Vistide) Foscarnet (Foscavir) Ganciclovir (Cytovene) Valganciclovir (Valcyte)	Treat CMV retinitis; acyclovir-resistant HSV-1 and -2, by interfering with the ability of the virus to reproduce within a cell, CMV prevention in transplant recipients	Headache, seizures, nausea, vomiting, diarrhea, anemia, abnormal renal function test results	• Monitor for renal dysfunction, do not give with aminoglycosides. • Monitor for electrolyte depletion.
Antiherpes virus agents			
Acyclovir (Zovirax) Famciclovir (Famvir) Valacyclovir (Valtrex)	HSV, herpes zoster, varicella zoster, acute herpes zoster, HSV-2	Nausea, vomiting, diarrhea, fever, headache, dizziness, confusion, rashes, myalgia	• Monitor for hypersensitivity reactions, muscle pain. • Report difficulty in urination. • Use gloves when applying topical forms. • Advise against sexual contact while lesions are visible.
Pharmacokinetic enhancers			
Ritonavir (Norvir) (see above) Cobicistat	Inhibits enzymes to boost antiviral action	Jaundice signs	• May see sudden inflammatory response

The drugs in column 1 indicate the drug that matches up with explanations in columns 2 through 4.
DNA, deoxyribonucleic acid; HIV, human immunodeficiency virus; HSV, herpes simplex virus.

blocking a coreceptor on the cell's surface. In 2003, the U.S. Food and Drug Administration (FDA) approved the **fusion inhibitor** enfuvirtide (Fuzeon), the first drug in this category. Enfuvirtide acquired its brand name because it blocks the CXCR4 receptor known as *fusin*. Entry and fusion inhibitors are reserved for HIV-infected people who are resistant or developing resistance to NRTIs, NNRTIs, and PIs. People with less advanced HIV/AIDS may also benefit from the inclusion of maraviroc or enfuvirtide in their drug regimen.

Enfuvirtide and maraviroc work best when combined with at least one or two other antiretroviral drugs. Potential drug resistance remains a concern. The fear is that once subjected to a specific entry inhibitor, the virus may mutate so as to utilize the other receptor to gain entry. It is not likely that entry inhibitors will develop cross-resistance to other categories of antiretroviral drugs. The biggest disadvantage of enfuvirtide is that the medication requires self-injection twice daily, and nearly all users experience some type of reaction at the injection site. Use of entry inhibitors requires testing the person with HIV to determine which receptor the virus uses to gain access to the CD4 T cell.

Reverse Transcriptase Inhibitors. There are three approved categories of **reverse transcriptase inhibitors**: NRTIs, NNRTIs, and nucleotide analogues. Nucleosides are building blocks of DNA and RNA. By binding to viral DNA, NRTIs abort the terminal completion of gene copying.

Non-nucleoside drugs are molecularly similar to nucleoside analogues; however, NNRTIs bind directly to the reverse transcriptase enzyme, thus preventing transcription. They are effective only against HIV-1. The potent combination of drugs from these two classes cripples the ability of the virus to copy itself. Unfortunately, drug resistance develops very quickly if the client does not take the NNRTI as prescribed. If drug resistance develops to one NNRTI, cross-resistance usually develops to all others in this same class.

Researchers have developed a third reverse transcriptase inhibitor category, called a nucleotide analogue. Nucleotides are compounds that are part of a chain of substances in nucleic acids (i.e., DNA and RNA). Although nucleotide analogues are technically different from NRTIs and NNRTIs, they act similarly. The essential difference is that nucleotides activate immediately when they enter the CD4 cell. They become incorporated within the viral DNA and cause premature termination of viral DNA synthesis. This group of drugs adds yet another weapon to the arsenal being used to extend the lives of those with AIDS.

Integrase Inhibitors. **Integrase inhibitors**, also called INSTI, prevent the incorporation of viral DNA into the host cell's DNA by blocking the activity of the integrase enzyme. Preventing the integration of viral DNA with the host cell's DNA interferes with the ability of the infected cell to make copies of HIV. Raltegravir and others in this category have been combined with other types of anti-HIV drugs to prevent viral mutations. Integrase inhibitors may also be useful in **salvage therapy**, a treatment option for infected people with significant HIV drug resistance in whom possibilities for effective antiretroviral drug management are limited.

Protease Inhibitors. One or two PIs usually are used in combination with both NRTIs and NNRTIs. PIs interfere with the maturation of the viral copies. If viral copies do manage to escape from the host T4 cell, they usually are too immature to invade healthy T4 cells. Because PIs and reverse transcriptase inhibitors affect separate processes in the viral life cycle, the combination is most likely to control the virus.

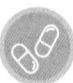

Pharmacologic Considerations

- Redistribution of body fat is a problem with PIs. Adipose tissue moves to the center of the body, and clients appear to have thinner arms and legs with a rounder abdomen or enlarged breasts. Sometimes body fat relocates to the area behind the neck (this is called a buffalo hump).

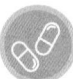

Pharmacologic Considerations

- Those taking PIs should be cautioned that there is an increased risk of adverse reactions (hypotension, visual disturbances, and prolonged penile erection) when the drug sildenafil (Viagra) is used.

Combination Antiretroviral Drugs. Because adherence to antiretroviral drug therapy decreases when a client must take multiple drugs at varying times in 24 hours, manufacturers are combining several drugs in one pill that can be taken once a day. Some examples include Atripla, which contains efavirenz, emtricitabine, and tenofovir; and Stribild, a combination of four HIV medications: emtricitabine, tenofovir, elvitegravir, and cobicistat. Cobicistat is not an antiretroviral drug. It is a PK enhancer. PK enhancers improve the effectiveness of PIs, thereby promoting a higher rate of viral suppression (Deeks, 2014).

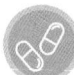

Pharmacologic Considerations

- Successful treatment outcomes rely on adherence to multiple drug regimens. Stribild (also known as the Quad pill) combines four antiretrovirals and cobicistat, an antiretroviral boosting agent. This agent inhibits liver enzymes from metabolizing the other drugs, which results in higher blood concentrations of drug with lower dosing, reducing adverse reactions.

Truvada, a combination of emtricitabine and tenofovir, is taken once a day. Truvada is being called the first HIV **preexposure prophylaxis (PrEP)** or prevention pill because when taken daily, it lowers an HIV-negative person's risk of acquiring the virus by 92% (CDC, 2016b). The drug, which contains two antiretrovirals, tenofovir (Viread) and emtricitabine (Emtriva), is targeted for those cases in which one sexual partner is HIV positive and the other is HIV negative, like monogamous sex partners, couples wishing to conceive a child, and those who work in the sex industry. It is recommended that those taking Truvada be tested for HIV every few months because the drug is not 100% effective, continue using condoms, and limit their sexual partners.

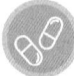

Pharmacologic Considerations

- The herbal supplement St. John's wort is one of the most popular herbal products in the United States. The herb is effective in treating mild depression. This supplement reduces the effectiveness of antiretroviral medications when taken together.

Drug Resistance

The development of **drug resistance**, ineffective response to a prescribed drug or drug category (**drug cross-resistance**) because of the survival and replication of exceptionally

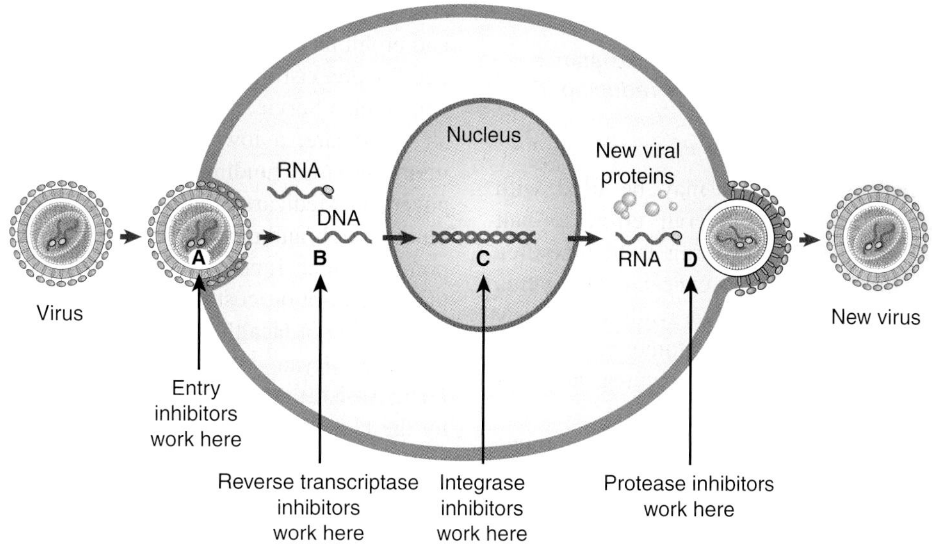

Figure 35-7 Current drug therapy interferes with human immunodeficiency virus (HIV) replication by **(A)** blocking the coreceptor and fusion of the viral protein on the surface of the T-cell lymphocyte, thus preventing the virus from entering the cell; **(B)** inhibiting the enzyme necessary for converting viral ribonucleic acid (RNA) to deoxyribonucleic acid (DNA); **(C)** preventing integration of viral RNA with host cell DNA; and **(D)** preventing virus particles from budding from the infected T cell.

virulent mutations, limits future alternative treatment options (Fig. 35-7).

Clients who neglect to take antiretroviral drugs as prescribed (i.e., every dose, at its designated time, with or without food as directed) risk development of drug resistance. When drug levels are not adequately maintained, viral replication and mutations increase (Fig. 35-8). In other words, clients who do not adhere to drug regimens are one cause of antiretroviral drug failure.

It is possible to detect drug resistance with two different blood tests. When **genotype testing** is done, the blood is examined for genetic changes in circulating HIV particles. Scientists now know to look for mutations in particular **codons**, sequences of DNA where mutations occur. With **phenotype testing**, a measured amount of antiviral drug is mixed with the virus until there is a quantity that prevents the virus from reproducing. The higher the dose of drug that eventually inhibits viral growth, the greater is the viral drug resistance.

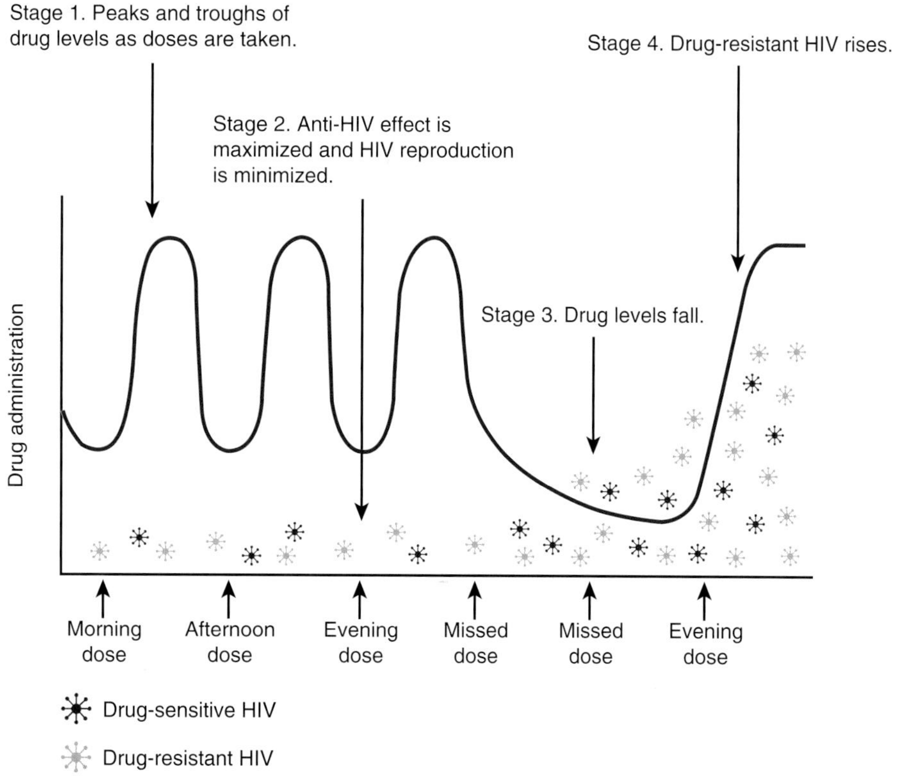

Figure 35-8 The effect of nonadherence to therapy on drug resistance. HIV, human immunodeficiency virus.

››› *Stop, Think, and Respond 35-4*

Explain the concept of antiretroviral drug resistance and cross-resistance and techniques for reducing its potential.

Adjunct Drug Therapy. Other drugs may be used with antiretroviral drug therapy in an overall effort to halt the progression of AIDS. One such drug is hydroxyurea (Hydrea), which usually is used to treat cancer. Hydroxyurea inhibits an enzyme that functions in DNA synthesis, thereby inhibiting or slowing the reproduction of tumor cells. When combined with antiretroviral drugs, hydroxyurea interferes with viral replication, increasing anti-HIV effects.

In addition, administration of endogenous immune substances known as *cytokines*, such as interferons and interleukin-2 (IL-2), may also be helpful (see Chapter 33). Interferons (Roferon-A and Betaseron) activate the cell's own defenses against viruses and are believed to increase blood levels of antiretroviral drugs like zidovudine (Retrovir). IL-2 stimulates the production of lymphocytes. The pharmaceutical counterpart of IL-2 (aldesleukin [Proleukin]) is used to increase the numbers of T4 helper and natural killer lymphocytes. Natural killer lymphocytes specifically target virus-infected cells and cancer cells; therefore, the use of IL-2 boosts the body's immune defenses against HIV.

Routes of Drug Delivery

Researchers are attempting to determine whether drugs used in HIV therapy may be delivered other than by the oral or parenteral route. The impetus to find alternative drug administration routes is related to the following:

- The oral route sometimes requires numerous medications taken around the clock, on a schedule that requires near-perfect adherence to the regimen.
- The oral route is associated with undesirable gastrointestinal side effects.
- The parenteral drugs require self-injection, which many people find objectionable.

Funding Drug Costs

Antiretroviral medications are very expensive, $500,000 or more per year in the United States, and nearly 30% of those with HIV are uninsured (Treatment cost, 2021). Take into account further that medications are only one portion of an infected person's total health care needs. With spiraling health care costs involving laboratory testing and treatment of opportunistic infections, the current expense is logically greater.

Medicaid, a state-based medical assistance program for low-income clients, is the largest source of public funding for HIV/AIDS care. Coverage varies from state to state, including criteria that must be met for antiretroviral drug coverage. Eligibility for Medicaid has expanded to include those with incomes at or below the federal poverty level with the health reforms within the Affordable Care Act (ACA). The ACA has created health insurance marketplaces in every state to help consumers with information about health plans and prohibits insurers from canceling or withdrawing coverage for preexisting conditions (U.S. Department of Health and Human Services, 2016a).

Medicare, a low-cost federal medical insurance program, provides funding for medications through its Part D coverage. Medicare enrollees are provided a 50% discount on covered brand name drugs while in the "donut hole," the point at which funding is temporarily withheld unless and until prescription costs reach a higher preset amount (U.S. Department of Health and Human Services, 2016b).

The Ryan White Program funds the **AIDS Drug Assistance Program (ADAP)**, which is administered by the U.S. Department of Health and Human Services. It is the third largest source of funding for HIV in the United States for individuals who do not have health insurance that pays for drug therapy.

In addition, some social agencies and pharmaceutical companies have drug assistance and compassionate need programs through which antiretroviral drugs are supplied to people who cannot afford them. Lastly, some may enroll in clinical trials testing new HIV medications that are not yet available by prescription.

HIV Vaccines

There are many different HIV vaccine trials in various stages of development and testing. They include the development of *preventive vaccines* for people who are HIV negative and *therapeutic vaccines* for people who are HIV positive to improve their immune system. Scripps research announced in early 2021 that it was close to finding a vaccine to prevent HIV. The research organization said it had success in the first clinical trial of a new approach against HIV, which involves vaccines that boost the body's ability to produce antibodies; however, a vaccine would probably not be available for another 5 to 10 years (Scripps, 2021).

Microbicide Trials

Researchers are developing microbicides, topical drugs that inhibit HIV transmission and other sexually transmitted pathogens by various means, such as increasing vaginal acidity, which is hostile to pathogens; using surfactant/detergents to inactivate the virus; or contain the antiretroviral drug dapivirine. Microbicide drugs are in clinical trials mostly in African countries because in these areas, men are culturally opposed to using condoms and HIV drug therapy is beyond the economic means of most people. A secondary goal is to create a microbicide that is also effective when instilled rectally to protect men who have sex with men. At last report in 2021, a vaginal ring containing dapivirine reduced the risk of HIV infection by 50% among women aged 25 years and older who used the ring consistently (Dapivirine, 2021).

Supportive Care of Opportunistic Infections

Clients with AIDS acquire many infectious disorders, some of which can cause death (Fig. 35-9). These infectious disorders and their comparative severity are uncommon in populations of relatively healthy people. The management of some common infectious conditions is discussed in the following sections.

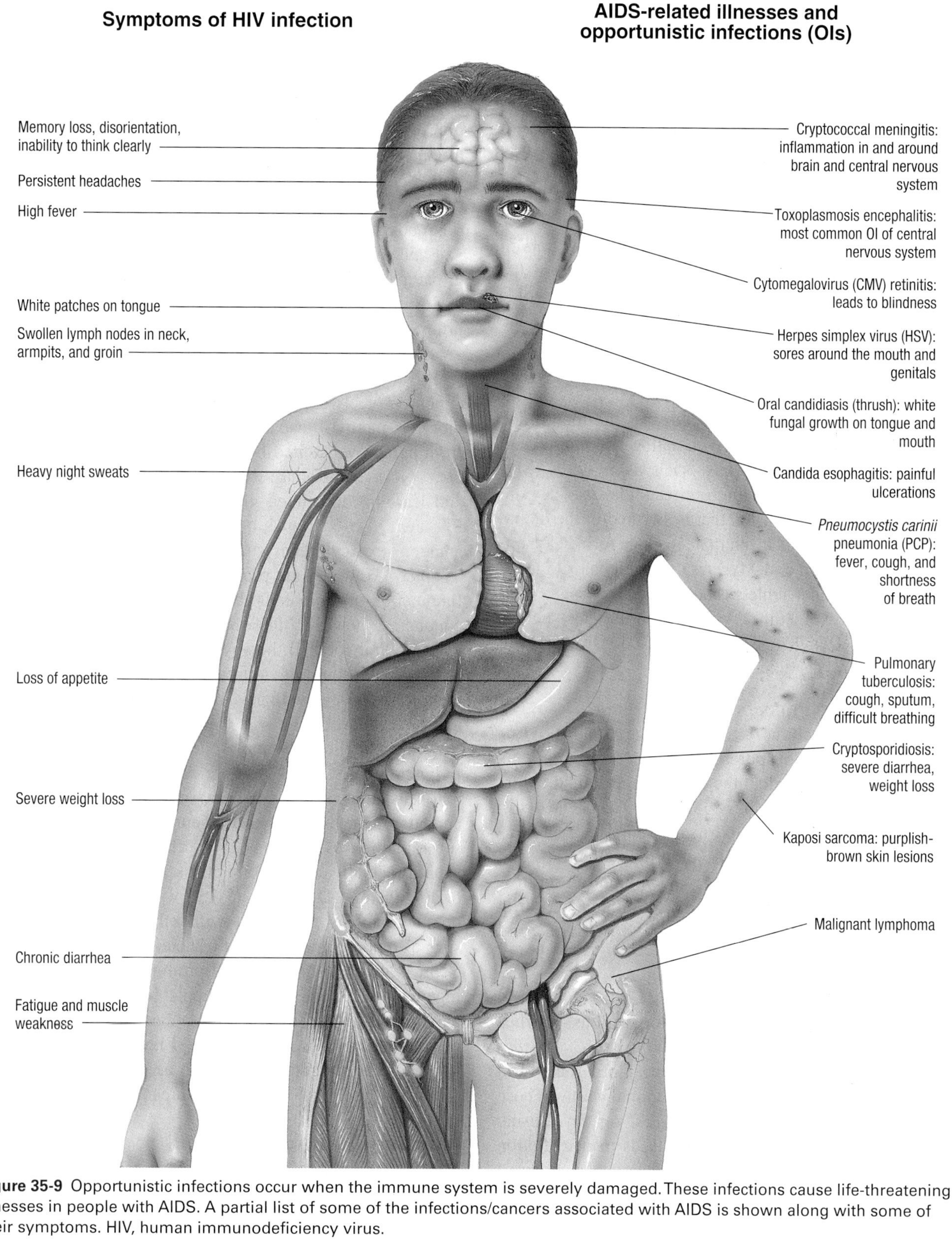

Figure 35-9 Opportunistic infections occur when the immune system is severely damaged. These infections cause life-threatening illnesses in people with AIDS. A partial list of some of the infections/cancers associated with AIDS is shown along with some of their symptoms. HIV, human immunodeficiency virus.

Pneumocystis Pneumonia

Clients infected with HIV are at particular risk for acquiring **Pneumocystis pneumonia**, a type of pneumonia caused by an organism called *Pneumocystis carinii*, which has been renamed *Pneumocystis jiroveci* to distinguish it as an organism that specifically infects humans rather than one that is common to other species of mammals. This type of pneumonia is rare among individuals with an intact immune system.

The pneumonia can become so severe as to result in respiratory failure. Mechanical ventilation may be necessary to sustain adequate pulmonary function. Aerosol therapy and deep suctioning often are necessary to clear the lungs of thick sputum. To prevent and treat *Pneumocystis pneumonia*, trimethoprim–sulfamethoxazole (Bactrim and Septra) is prescribed. Monthly aerosolized pentamidine isethionate (NebuPent) is also effective.

Candidiasis

Candidiasis is a yeast infection caused by the *Candida albicans* microorganism. Candidiasis may develop in the oral, pharyngeal, esophageal, or vaginal cavities or in folds of the skin. It often is called *thrush* when located in the mouth. Inspection of the mouth, throat, or vagina reveals areas of white plaque that may bleed when mobilized with a cotton-tipped swab.

When candidiasis affects structures of the mouth and throat, it can lead to problems with eating and subsequent weight loss. Topical antifungals, such as nystatin (Mycostatin), are useful for treating oral candidiasis. They are available in an oral suspension that is swished in the mouth and then swallowed or in an alternate lozenge form. Clotrimazole (Gyne-Lotrimin and Mycelex) and miconazole (Monistat) cream, vaginal tablets, and suppositories are used to treat vaginitis. Sometimes, systemic antifungals such as amphotericin B (Fungizone) or fluconazole (Diflucan) are required to control candidiasis.

Cytomegalovirus Infection

Opportunistic infections caused by cytomegalovirus (CMV) affect immunosuppressed people such as clients with AIDS. CMV can infect the choroid and retinal layers of the eye, leading to blindness. It can also cause ulcers in the esophagus, colitis and diarrhea, pneumonia, and encephalitis. Foscarnet (Foscavir), cidofovir (Vistide), and ganciclovir (Cytovene) are used in combination aggressively to treat acute CMV infections. Maintenance drug therapy follows to reduce the potential for future viral activation.

Cryptosporidiosis

Immunosuppressed clients may develop serious diarrhea as a result of infection with a protozoan called *Cryptosporidium*. The organism is spread by the fecal–oral route from contaminated water, food, or human or animal wastes. Those infected can lose from 10 to 20 L of fluid per day. Losing this massive amount of fluid quickly leads to dehydration and electrolyte imbalances. When diarrhea is accompanied by anorexia, nausea, and vomiting, weight is difficult to maintain.

Definitive diagnosis is made by examining the stool for ova and parasites and other cytologic examinations. Antibiotic therapy is then implemented. The macrolide family of antibiotics, such as azithromycin (Zithromax) or clarithromycin (Biaxin), or an antiprotozoal agent, such as paromomycin (Humatin), is used.

Management of AIDS-Related Complications

Besides AIDS-related cancers and opportunistic infections, clients may develop **AIDS dementia complex** (ADC), sometimes called HIV-associated neurocognitive disorders (HANDs). ADC, a neurologic condition, causes degeneration of the brain, especially in areas that affect mood, cognition, and motor functions. Clients exhibit forgetfulness, limited attention span, decreased ability to concentrate, and delusional thinking. Moods range from irritability to euphoria. A possible motor dysfunction is manifested by staggering gait and muscle incoordination, slowing of all movements, or paraplegia, which may be accompanied by incontinence.

Antiretroviral therapy can delay or prevent ADC. Other drugs, some of which are in clinical trials, may slow the progression of ADC once it manifests. One such drug is memantine (Namenda). It is believed that this medication performs a neuroprotective function (see Chapter 72). Memantine blocks *N*-methyl-D-aspartate (NMDA) receptors in the brain from being overexcited by a neurotransmitter called *glutamate*. Normal concentrations of glutamate enhance memory and learning; too much glutamate is lethal to brain cells. Research also continues on CPI-1189, an agent that is an antagonist of cytokines such as tumor necrosis factor (see Chapter 33), which are produced during *gp120*-induced inflammation of brain cells. Until more definitive studies are conducted, however, these drugs may be combined with antiretroviral cocktail therapy or with selegiline (Eldepryl), an anti-Parkinson drug, to treat motor and cognitive impairments of ADC, and with psychiatric drugs to moderate mood and activity levels.

Other clients may develop **distal sensory polyneuropathy (DSP)**, which is characterized by abnormal sensations, such as burning and numbness, in the feet and later in the hands. Because neuropathy is a side effect of several antiretroviral drugs, it is difficult to determine if the cause is actually destruction of the sensory peripheral nerves or drug therapy. DSP responds less well to drug therapy than do neuropathies associated with other primary disorders such as diabetes mellitus (see Chapter 51). Nevertheless, an effort is made to preserve and promote nerve function using vitamin B12 and thiamine supplementation. Neuropathic pain may also be amenable to treatment with tricyclic antidepressants such as amitriptyline (Elavil) and nortriptyline (Pamelor) or anticonvulsants such as gabapentin (Neurontin), carbamazepine (Tegretol), or pregabalin (Lyrica).

Nursing Management

The role of the nurse involves health teaching and counseling high-risk populations. The areas of emphasis include HIV prevention strategies such as sexual abstinence and **safer-sex practices**, sexual activities in which body fluids are not exchanged. The nurse encourages diagnostic screening for those whose behaviors place them at risk for HIV infection. They help interpret the results of diagnostic tests and monitor the need for continued follow-up in the months after potential exposure.

Concept Mastery Alert

AIDS Education

When educating clients with AIDS, the nurse should emphasize the importance of following safer-sex practices.

For clients with an established HIV status, the nurse explains the action of each antiretroviral drug and develops a schedule for the client's self-administration. This includes strong precautions about rigidly adhering to the dosage, time, and frequency of drug administration to avoid the development of drug resistance. Describing the side effects of drug therapy is essential, with the admonition to refrain from discontinuing any of the prescribed drugs without first consulting the prescribing primary provider (Evidence-Based Practice 35-1). The nurse makes appointments for laboratory tests for monitoring the effects of drug therapy.

Evidence-Based Practice 35-1

Self-Management Strategies for Clients With HIV/AIDS

Clinical Question

What type of self-management strategies are helpful in managing pain among HIV/AIDS clients?

Evidence

A qualitative study that reviewed approximately 25 interview studies of pain in HIV clients was completed (Merlin et al., 2015). Clients were interviewed to see what nonpharmacologic strategies supported them during the pain of their disease. The results found that things such as being with family, being involved in social functions, and participating in physical activities were therapeutic. The things clients reported that interfered with positive life experiences were adhering to medication schedules and being sedentary.

Nursing Implications

The strategies identified in the review of studies provide the nurse with resources to plan client care. Nurses can support and help manage pain in clients with HIV/AIDS, by encouraging clients to be involved in social and physical activities. These strategies can be inserted in care plans as nursing interventions for pain management.

Reference

Merlin, J. S., Walcott, M., Kerns, R., Bair, M. J., Burgio, K. L., & Turan, J. M. (2015). Pain self-management in HIV-infected individuals with chronic pain: A qualitative study. *Pain Medicine, 16*(4), 706–714. https://doi.org/10.1111/pme.12701.

Referral of HIV-positive clients to support groups and resources for information about new HIV drug development, clinical drug trials, ADAP, and progress on vaccine development are very important nursing interventions.

Reducing Occupational Risks

The nurse must observe standard precautions whenever there is a risk of exposure to blood and body fluids. They must follow the nursing guidelines for safe handling of needles and sharp instruments (Nursing Guidelines 35-1). The Occupational Safety and Health Administration (OSHA) also recommends the following when caring for all clients regardless of their infectious status:

- Transport specimens of body fluids in leak-proof containers.
- Clean, disinfect, or discard utility gloves used for cleaning.
- Remove barrier garments (e.g., face shields, glasses) as soon as possible after leaving a client's room.

If exposed to the blood of any client, the nurse should report the incident to the person in charge of employee health immediately. The nurse will be tested for HIV at regular intervals and treated with antiretrovirals, depending on the results of tests or the potential for infection. While awaiting the results of diagnostic tests, the nurse must follow the same sexual precautions as someone who has been diagnosed with AIDS.

NURSING GUIDELINES 35-1

Safe Handling of Needles and Sharp Instruments

- Do not become distracted when handling needles and sharp instruments. Concentrate on the task being performed.
- Use a clean tray to pass used or contaminated needles and sharp instruments to another person.
- Keep the container for disposal of needles and sharp instruments close by. When necessary, carry the container to the bedside.
- If a client is uncooperative, ask for assistance when obtaining blood specimens, handling body fluids and secretions, giving injections, or starting IV therapy.
- Do not leave uncapped or used needles unattended. Properly dispose of contaminated sharp instruments and needles as soon as they are used.

Client Teaching

For clients who are healthy enough to continue as outpatients, the nurse develops a teaching plan that includes the following guidelines:

- Understand that antiviral drugs do not cure HIV/AIDS but may slow its progression.
- Follow the medication schedule religiously; do not omit or increase the dose without primary provider's approval.
- Comply with the timing of antiviral medications around meals.
- Eat small, frequent, well-balanced meals; try to maintain or gain weight (Nutrition Notes).
- Drink plenty of water.
- Check weight weekly. Report progressive weight loss or loss of appetite to the primary provider.
- Avoid exposure to people with infections, including colds, sore throats, upper respiratory tract infections, and childhood diseases (e.g., mumps, chickenpox), and people who have recently been vaccinated. Avoid crowds.
- Notify the primary provider if signs of infection such as fever, sore throat, diarrhea, respiratory distress, and cough occur, or if signs of a skin, rectal, vaginal, or oral infection appear.

- Wear gloves and a mask when disposing of animal excreta, such as kitty litter, bird cage liners, and hamster shavings; wash hands thoroughly afterward.
- Wash all food before cooking; do not eat raw meat, fish, or vegetables or food that has not been completely cooked.
- Wash bedding and clothes in hot water and separate from the laundry of others, especially if the bedding and clothes are soiled with body secretions.
- Avoid smoking or exposure to secondhand smoke.
- Bathe or shower daily, wash hands before and after preparing food, clean the anal and perineal areas well after each bowel movement, and wash hands after voiding or defecating. Personal cleanliness is a must.
- When possible, avoid dry and dusty areas, excessive humidity, and extreme heat or cold. Wear clothing appropriate to the weather and temperature.
- Take frequent rest periods and space activities to prevent fatigue.
- Do not share IV needles, and do not donate blood.
- Inform health care providers of HIV-positive status.

Understanding Financial and Insurance Implications

Despite HIV-specific confidentiality laws, clients infected with AIDS fear that disclosure of their condition will affect employment, health insurance coverage, and even housing. An employer cannot cancel a client's currently active health insurance policy on the basis of AIDS. However, employers are more apt to dismiss a worker with a known HIV-positive status from employment to reduce future insurance premiums and death payments. The dismissal often is attributed to some reason not associated with HIV to avoid being charged with discrimination under the Americans with Disabilities Act.

Persons who are unemployed can apply for a continuation of the employer's health plan for 18 months at self-pay. Thereafter, they can extend their insurance for 11 more months if they meet the Social Security Administration's criteria for being disabled. Eventually, the person infected with HIV may need to obtain affordable health insurance through a health insurance marketplace. An AIDS caseworker often can help a person who is HIV positive with health insurance questions.

Discussing Viatical Settlements

A **viatical settlement** is an arrangement in which a terminally ill individual agrees to name a person as beneficiary to their life insurance in exchange for immediate cash. It is best to advise a person who is considering this option to work through an attorney or licensed insurance broker who will negotiate the value of the insurance policy with the potential purchaser. Other factors that the client must consider are whether the cash will cancel eligibility for food stamps or other forms of public assistance and that the cash will be considered earned income for tax purposes.

Nutrition Notes

The Client With HIV/AIDS

- There are no unanimously agreed-upon recommendations for calories or protein despite the universal goals of maintaining body weight and lean body mass in clients with HIV/AIDS. The registered dietitian should be consulted to create an individualized nutrition plan for each client.
- A Mediterranean diet that is low in saturated fat and refined sugar and high in fruit, vegetables, and whole grains may help improve the common metabolic abnormalities of hypertriglyceridemia and impaired glucose tolerance, a consequence of some antiretrovirals.
- Low blood levels and inadequate intakes of some vitamins and minerals are associated with faster HIV disease progression and mortality. Nutrient deficiencies may occur from poor intake, malabsorption, infections, or diet–medication interactions. Although food is the preferred source for nutrients, multivitamin and mineral supplements are usually recommended at levels of 100% to 200% of the daily reference intakes. Some evidence suggests that supplements of vitamin A, zinc, and iron can produce adverse outcomes by negatively impacting immune system functioning.
- Nutritional intervention may help alleviate symptoms that interfere with intake or nutrient use.
  - Clients with anorexia should be encouraged to eat small, frequent meals of easily digested food and liquids even when not hungry.
  - Clients with nausea and vomiting may tolerate a low-fat, high-carbohydrate, soft, or liquid diet better than large, high-fat meals.
  - Diarrhea and malabsorption may improve when clients avoid residue, lactose, fat, and caffeine.
  - Liquids should be encouraged to replace fluid and electrolyte losses.
  - Although eating may seem to trigger diarrhea, clients must understand that limiting food intake to control diarrhea only exacerbates wasting.
  - Gravies, sauces, and broth added to soft, nonirritating foods may promote ease of swallowing in clients with oral or esophageal ulcerations. Some clients may require a blenderized or liquid diet. Because temperature extremes (very hot or very cold) can irritate the mucosa, room temperature foods and liquids are recommended for clients with a sore mouth.
- Clients unable to consume an adequate oral diet may require tube feeding for supplemental or complete nutrition. Because many formulas have the potential to cause diarrhea, closely monitoring the client's tolerance is essential. Advera and Impact are commercial formulas designed for clients with impaired immune function.

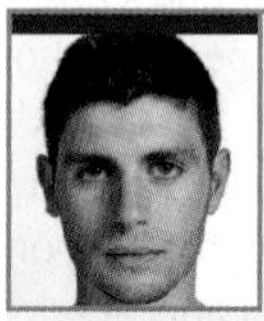

Clinical Scenario A 25-year-old client has come to the public health department asking to be tested for HIV. They tell the nurse that they have a fever, swollen glands, persistent diarrhea, and weight loss. Of primary concern is that the client had unprotected sex with other people and does not know their HIV status. How might the nurse proceed with this client or any other potentially HIV-positive client's care? See Nursing Care Plan 35-1.

NURSING CARE PLAN 35-1 The Client With HIV/AIDS

Assessment

- *Obtain a thorough history*, including risk factors for HIV infection. List all symptoms, exploring each thoroughly. Determine the client's past and current treatment medications. Inspect the oral mucous membranes and all skin surfaces for rashes, skin breakdown, and opportunistic infections such as herpes lesions. Look for Kaposi sarcoma, which appears as dark purple lesions that may be painful. Examine the arms and legs for edema. Auscultate the lungs for breath sounds. Question the client about coughing, sputum production, dyspnea, and orthopnea. Palpate the lymph nodes and abdomen for organ enlargement. Gather additional data based on the client's complaints or symptoms. Review results of recent laboratory and diagnostic tests.
- *Obtain vital signs and weight.* Question the client about weight loss and weight before they became symptomatic. Explore past and current dietary intake. Ask about factors that interfere with eating, such as difficulty swallowing, diarrhea, and oral discomfort.
- *Assess the client's mental status* (see Chapter 67) and *perform a neurologic assessment* (see Chapter 36). Look for peripheral neuropathies (sensation changes in extremities), which may be side effects of antiretroviral medications. Ask about any visual changes (e.g., floaters, spots, loss of peripheral vision).
- *Evaluate emotional status*, looking for signs of depression or anxiety.
- *Observe for signs of dehydration.* Examine the skin and mucous membranes for dryness. Evaluate skin turgor. Note additional findings such as decreased urine output, hypotension, and slow filling of hand veins. Look for indications of fluid and electrolyte deficit(s) such as excessive thirst, muscle weakness, cramping, nausea, vomiting, cardiac arrhythmia, shallow respirations, and headache.

Nursing Diagnosis. **Infection Risk** (opportunistic) related to immunodeficiency

Expected Outcome. Client will experience no secondary infections.

Interventions	Rationales
Follow practices of medical and surgical asepsis.	*Aseptic practices break the infection cycle by decreasing or eliminating infectious agents, their reservoirs, and vehicles for transmission.*
Use protective neutropenic precautions if T4-cell count is $\leq$500/mm^3.	*Keeping the immunosuppressed client in a separate environment and using precautions to limit the introduction of pathogens in that environment reduce the potential for transmission of a nosocomial infection.*
Promote hand hygiene especially before meals and after elimination.	*The fecal–oral route is a common mechanism for transfer of endogenous microorganisms from one body site to another, where they can become pathogenic. Hand hygiene is the best technique for reducing transmission of microorganisms.*
Facilitate adequate sleep and nutrition.	*Adequate sleep and nutrition reduce fatigue, stabilize mood, increase protein synthesis, maintain disease-fighting mechanisms of the immune system, promote cellular growth and repair, and improve capacity for learning and memory storage.*
Prohibit visitors who are ill and staff from contact with client.	*Microorganisms are transferred by one of the three routes: airborne, droplet, and contact.*

Evaluation of Expected Outcome

Client is free from secondary infections.

RC of ***Pneumocystis pneumonia***

Expected Outcome. Nurse will assess, manage, and minimize pneumonia.

Interventions	Rationales
Auscultate the lungs every 4 hours; monitor oxygen saturation at least once per shift.	*Diminished or wet lung sounds and arterial oxygen saturation (SpO_2) <90% indicate poor ventilation and oxygen diffusion.*
Assist with measures to clear respiratory secretions such as coughing, pharyngeal suctioning, aerosol treatments, and chest percussion.	*Clearing the airway promotes gas exchange.*
Give oxygen as medically prescribed if SpO_2 is $\leq$90%.	*Keeping SpO_2 above 90% ensures that oxygen in plasma (PaO_2) is between 80 and 100 mm Hg.*
Provide mechanical ventilation for acute respiratory failure (PaO_2 $\leq$ 50 mm Hg or $PaCO_2$ $\geq$ 50 mm Hg).	*Mechanical ventilation provides a prescribed rate of respiration, tidal volume, and supplemental oxygen when normal breathing is inadequate.*
Administer prescribed antimicrobials.	*Antimicrobials exert either bactericidal or bacteriostatic functions.*

Evaluation of Expected Outcome

Nurse ensures management of pneumonia and control of complications.

(*continued*)

NURSING CARE PLAN 35-1 The Client With HIV/AIDS (*continued*)

Nursing Diagnosis. **Hypovolemia** related to diarrhea secondary to viremia, opportunistic infection, and side effects of medication
Expected Outcome. Client's fluid intake and output will be balanced.

Interventions	Rationales
Keep a record of intake and output, measuring liquid feces.	*Measurements provide an objective account of fluid status.*
Offer oral fluids every hour while client is awake.	*Oral intake increases when the nurse encourages it.*
Withhold foods, especially caffeine, that are irritating until bowel function improves.	*Fibrous foods increase peristalsis and diarrhea; caffeine is a bowel stimulant and diuretic.*
Administer prescribed antidiarrheals.	*Antidiarrheals slow peristalsis, adsorbing gastrointestinal irritants and water.*
Report evidence of dehydration or electrolyte imbalance.	*Parenteral fluids and electrolyte additives are alternate ways to restore fluid and electrolyte balance when the oral route is inadequate.*

Evaluation of Expected Outcome

Client's fluid intake and output are at least 1500 mL/24 hours.

Nursing Diagnoses. **Risk for Activity Intolerance** and **ADL deficit** related to fatigue, weakness, and neurologic complications.

Expected Outcome. Client will tolerate activities of daily living (ADLs), maintain mobility, and perform self-care.

Interventions	Rationales
Prevent fatigue by spacing of activities between periods of rest.	*Aerobic metabolism, which provides greater energy yield than anaerobic metabolism, depends on cellular oxygen.*
Assist with ADLs.	*Assistance reduces energy expenditure.*
Place a commode at the bedside.	*Shortening distance between client and toilet conserves energy.*
Provide a walker for ambulatory assistance.	*Ambulatory aids promote movement and reduce the risk for injury.*

Evaluation of Expected Outcome

Client performs ADLs and self-care and maintains mobility.

Nursing Diagnosis. **Altered Skin Integrity Risk** related to impaired capillary blood flow secondary to immobility, skin infection, and rash

Expected Outcome. Client's skin will remain intact.

Interventions	Rationales
Change position every 2 hours.	*Relief of pressure ensures that capillary blood flow remains >32 mm Hg to keep tissues oxygenated.*
Keep skin clean and dry.	*Moist, soiled skin leads to maceration and bacterial growth.*
Apply skin moisturizer.	*Lubricated skin is more pliable and less likely to break down.*
Gently massage intact skin over bony prominences.	*Massage increases circulation and delivery of oxygen to tissues.*
Clean and dry perineal area after elimination.	*Ammonia from urine and stool debris erodes skin. Organisms in stool transmit yeast infections.*
Use lubricated wipes or a soft washcloth for cleansing.	*Rough textures injure skin.*

Evaluation of Expected Outcome

Client's skin is intact.

Nursing Diagnosis. **Dehydration** related to inflammation secondary to opportunistic infections

Expected Outcome. Client's mucous membranes will be pink, moist, and intact.

Interventions	Rationales
Provide meticulous oral care after and between meals.	*Oral hygiene removes bacteria and yeast from mouth.*
Avoid using mouthwashes that contain alcohol.	*Alcohol irritates inflamed tissue.*
Use mouth rinses with warm (not hot) plain water, normal saline solution, or water and hydrogen peroxide.	*Warmth increases circulation and promotes healing. Water, saline, and dilute peroxide do not irritate oral tissues.*
Use a soft toothbrush or foam swabs for oral care.	*Soft textures protect gums from injury and infection.*

Evaluation of Expected Outcome

Client's mucous membranes are normal.

NURSING CARE PLAN 35-1 The Client With HIV/AIDS (*continued*)

Nursing Diagnoses. **Grief** related to potentially poor prognosis

Expected Outcome. Client will control their time, make other personal choices, and develop a realistic perception of the immediate future

Interventions	Rationales
Give client choices whenever possible.	*Making choices reaffirms a sense of control.*
Help client formulate and achieve short-term goals to enjoy more frequent small successes.	*Accomplishment of goals enhances hope.*
Discourage client from abandoning traditional treatment for therapies that lack any evidence of effectiveness.	*Desperate clients may turn to unsubstantiated claims of a cure for AIDS.*

Evaluation of Expected Outcome

Client makes personal choices that give a sense of control without further damaging health and realistically perceives their future.

Nursing Diagnosis. **Death Anxiety** related to potential for early death; **Coping Impairment** related to stress of contending with an incurable disease

Expected Outcome. Client will work through grief, maintain social contacts with family and friends, and cope effectively with crises.

Interventions	Rationales
Be a role model of acceptance for family and friends.	*Learning occurs by example.*
Make an effort to touch the client.	*Touching demonstrates that casual contact does not transmit the disease.*
Avoid wearing gloves and other barrier garments unless absolutely necessary.	*Unnecessary use of barrier garments implies that the client is unfit to touch.*
Refer client to an AIDS support group.	*Groups confer acceptance, calm fear, and decrease isolation.*

Evaluation of Expected Outcome

Client deals with grief and crises with support of the nurse, family, and friends.

KEY POINTS

- AIDS: an infectious and potentially life-threatening disorder that severely compromises the immune system
- HIV: the pathogen that causes AIDS
- Body fluids through which HIV is transmitted:
  - Blood
  - Semen
  - Vaginal secretions
  - Breast milk
- AIDS is the end stage of HIV infection; AIDS develops when there is:
  - A markedly decreased T4-cell count from a normal level of 800 to 1200/mm^3
  - The development of certain cancers and opportunistic infections
- HIV diagnostic testing:
  - Western Blot test: is the gold standard, it determines antibodies to specific HIV antigens. A reaction to at least two antigens indicates a positive result.
  - IFA test: is used when the Western Blot test is not definitively positive. It mixes cells that are likely infected with HIV with immunoglobins and viewed using a fluorescent microscope. Although it can confirm HIV disease, it is expensive and subject to the examiner's interpretation.
  - PCR test, also called an RNA test: used to detect the HIV virus itself. The PCR test is quite expensive and generally reserved for diagnosing infants with HIV born to mothers with HIV.
- Antiretroviral drugs:
  - NRTIs: drugs that interfere with the ability of the virus to make a genetic blueprint.
  - NNRTIs: bind directly to the reverse transcriptase enzyme, thus preventing transcription.
  - Integrase inhibitor also called an INSTI: prevent the incorporation of viral DNA into the host cell's DNA by blocking the activity of the integrase enzyme.
  - PK-enhanced PIs: interfere with the maturation of the viral copies. If viral copies do manage to escape from the host T4 cell, they usually are too immature to invade healthy T4 cells.
  - Entry (fusion) inhibitors: stop HIV from attaching to a CD4 T cell by blocking a coreceptor on the cell's surface.
- Opportunistic infections:
  - Pneumocystis pneumonia
  - Candidiasis
  - CMV infection
  - Cryptosporidiosis

CRITICAL THINKING EXERCISES

1. What advice would you give adolescents to reduce their risk for becoming infected with HIV?
2. People may become complacent about reducing risks for HIV transmission because they believe that if they become infected, they will have a normal life expectancy with antiretroviral treatment. How would you respond?
3. A nurse on a medical unit sustains a needlestick injury. What actions should the nurse take? What are the responsibilities of the employing agency?
4. Besides implementing standard precautions, what other practices reduce the potential for HIV transmission among health care providers?

NCLEX-STYLE REVIEW QUESTIONS PrepU

1. A client makes an appointment with a primary provider because of weight loss and swollen lymph nodes in the axillae and groin. What situation places the client at highest risk for becoming HIV positive?
   1. The client is an IV drug user.
   2. The client drinks excessive amounts of alcohol.
   3. The client had cardiovascular surgery 6 months ago.
   4. The client went to Africa on vacation.
2. A nurse is obtaining a client's consent for receiving blood. The client asks if there is any way that HIV can be acquired from the transfusion. Which of the following statements would the nurse be most truthful and accurate in response?
   1. With any medical procedure, there are risks. You must weigh the risks against the benefits.
   2. The blood supply is safe because it is screened for HIV antibodies to ensure quality and safety.
   3. Antibody screening will not detect HIV in donated blood if sufficient antibodies have not yet been produced.
   4. Transmission of HIV through screened blood transfusions cannot occur.
3. A nursing assistant asks a nurse what causes death in a client with AIDS. Which of the following reasons is the nurse most correct in explaining from what a client with AIDS ultimately dies?
   1. An opportunistic infection
   2. A depleted white blood cell count
   3. Deterioration of the brain tissue
   4. A massive stroke or heart attack
4. The primary provider orders several laboratory tests for a client suspected of having AIDS. Which laboratory test is performed initially to diagnose antibodies to HIV?
   1. Venereal Disease Research Laboratory (VDRL) test
   2. T4-cell count
   3. Western Blot test
   4. ELISA test
5. A client who is HIV positive comes into the clinic with a suspected case of candidiasis. Which of the following signs and symptoms would the nurse observe in the client that would likely confirm a diagnosis of candidiasis?
   1. Excessive diarrhea
   2. Impaired breathing
   3. Red, swollen eyes
   4. White oral plaque

WANT TO KNOW MORE? There are a wide variety of online resources available on thePoint to enhance learning and understanding of this chapter.

Go to **thePoint.lww.com/activate** and use the activation code found in the front of this text to unlock these online resources.

UNIT 9
Caring for Clients With Neurologic Disorders

36 Introduction to the Nervous System

Words To Know

acetylcholine
acetylcholinesterase
arachnoid
autonomic nervous system
axons
brain scan
brain stem
cauda equina
central nervous system
cerebellum
cerebral angiography
cerebral cortex
cerebrum choroid plexus
computed tomography
corpus callosum
cranial nerves
decerebrate posturing
decorticate posturing
dendrites
dermatome
dopamine
dura mater
echoencephalography
electroencephalogram
electromyography
epinephrine
extrapyramidal fibers
flaccidity
frontal lobe
Glasgow Coma Scale
lumbar puncture
magnetic resonance imaging
medulla oblongata
meninges
midbrain
myelin
myelogram

Learning Objectives

On completion of this chapter, you will be able to:

1. Name the two anatomic divisions of the nervous system.
2. Name the three parts of the brain.
3. List the four lobes of the cerebrum.
4. Give two functions of the spinal cord.
5. Name and describe the function of the two parts of the autonomic nervous system.
6. Describe the methods used to assess motor and sensory function.
7. List six diagnostic procedures performed to detect neurologic disorders.
8. Discuss the nursing management of the client undergoing neurologic diagnostic testing.

The nervous system consists of the brain, spinal cord, and peripheral nerves. It is responsible for coordinating body functions and responding to changes in or stimuli from the internal and external environment. Changes in the functioning of the nervous system can profoundly affect the entire body.

Gerontologic Considerations

- When taking the health history of an older adult who has difficulty remembering recent or past events, symptoms, drug and medical history, and other necessary facts, obtain or confirm the information with a family member or friend.
- Diseases such as dementia often make it difficult to perform a neurologic assessment. With age, brain weight and the number of brain cells decrease and blood flow to the cerebrum is diminished.
- Although thought processes that involve life experience and judgment may be enhanced with age, older adults often experience short-term memory loss and a slower reaction time.

(continued)

Words To Know (*continued*)

neurilemma
neuron
neurotransmitters
norepinephrine
occipital lobe
parasympathetic nervous system
parietal lobe
peripheral nervous system
pia mater
pons
positron emission tomography
pyramidal motor pathways
single-photon emission computed tomography
spinal cord
spinal nerves
subarachnoid space
sympathetic nervous system
synapses
temporal lobe
ventricles

Gerontologic Considerations (*continued*)

- Older adults who have difficulty following directions during a physical examination or diagnostic test need brief instructions given one step at a time during the examination or test. The older person may respond better to mimicking, modeling of desired behaviors, in addition to verbal instructions.
- The possibility of drug toxicity or abrupt onset of delirium should always be considered when an older person has a change in mental status. The aging brain may develop various compensatory mechanisms. Mental exercises can help to retain vocabulary, special awareness, and problem-solving; physical exercise promotes circulation; and involvement in social or educational activities can help retain function.
- Pupillary response is more sluggish in older adults. When cataracts are present, there may be no pupillary response.
- Range of motion of the neck may be affected in older adults because of arthritic changes.

ANATOMY AND PHYSIOLOGY

The nervous system is divided into two anatomic divisions: the **central nervous system (CNS)** and the **peripheral nervous system (PNS)**. The basic structure of the nervous system is the nerve cell or **neuron** (Fig. 36-1). Neurons are either sensory or motor. *Sensory neurons* transmit impulses to the CNS and *motor neurons* transmit impulses from the CNS.

A neuron is composed of a cell body, a nucleus, and threadlike projections or fibers called dendrites and axons. **Dendrites** conduct impulses to the cell body and are called *afferent* ("to" or "toward") nerve fibers. **Axons** are nerve fibers that project and conduct impulses away from the cell body. They are therefore called *efferent* ("away from") nerve fibers. An axon is usually larger than the dendrites.

Neurons are separate units and not directly connected to one another. Impulses travel along the neurons, moving

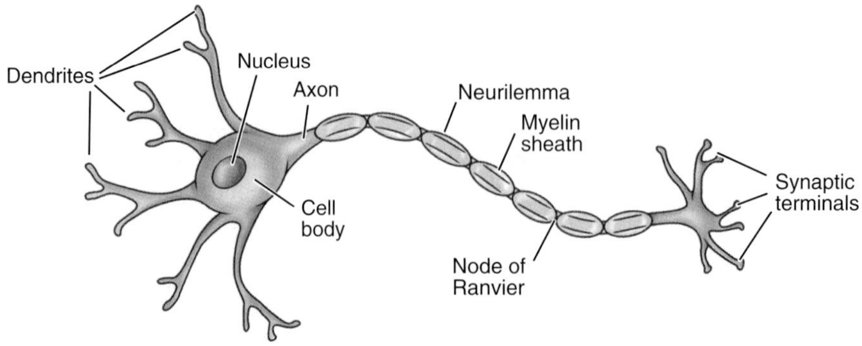

Figure 36-1 A neuron or nerve cell.

from one neuron to another by means of **synapses**, that is, junctions between the axon of one neuron and the dendrite of another. Substances called **neurotransmitters** (or neurohormones) accomplish the transmission of an impulse from one neuron to another (see Chapter 67). Neurotransmitters can either excite or inhibit neurons.

A fatty substance called **myelin** covers some axons in the CNS and PNS. A membranous sheath called the **neurilemma** covers the myelin of axons in peripheral nerves. Axons that are covered by myelin are called *myelinated*, white matter, or white nerve fibers. Axons that are not covered with myelin are called *unmyelinated*, gray matter, or gray nerve fibers.

Myelin serves as an insulating substance for the axon that confines the electrical conduction without allowing it to scatter. However, myelinated nerves are segmented with periodic gaps called the *nodes of Ranvier*. When impulses travel along the axons of myelinated nerves, they leap from node to node, a process called *saltatory conduction*, which is much faster than impulses traveling along the axons of unmyelinated nerves.

Central Nervous System

The CNS consists of the brain and spinal cord.

Brain

The brain is divided into three parts: the cerebrum, the cerebellum, and the brain stem. The **cerebrum** consists of two hemispheres connected by the **corpus callosum**, a band of white fibers that acts as a bridge for transmitting impulses between the left and right hemispheres. Each hemisphere has four lobes: **frontal**, **parietal**, **temporal**, and **occipital** (Fig. 36-2). The **cerebral cortex** is the surface of the cerebrum. It contains motor neurons, which are responsible for movement, and sensory neurons, which receive impulses from peripheral sensory neurons located throughout the body.

Motor tracts are pyramidal or extrapyramidal. **Pyramidal motor pathways** originate in the motor cortex of the cerebrum, cross over at the level of the medulla, and end in the brain stem and spinal cord. **Extrapyramidal fibers** originate in the motor cortex and project to the cerebellum and basal ganglia. They do not cross over because they connect to motor neurons in the spinal cord.

The **cerebellum**, which is located behind and below the cerebrum, controls and coordinates muscle movement. The **brain stem** consists of the midbrain, pons, and medulla oblongata. The **midbrain** connects the pons and cerebellum with the two cerebral hemispheres. The **pons** is located between the midbrain and medulla and connects the two hemispheres of the cerebellum with the brain stem, spinal cord, and cerebrum. The **medulla oblongata** lies below the pons and transmits motor impulses from the brain to the spinal cord and sensory impulses from peripheral

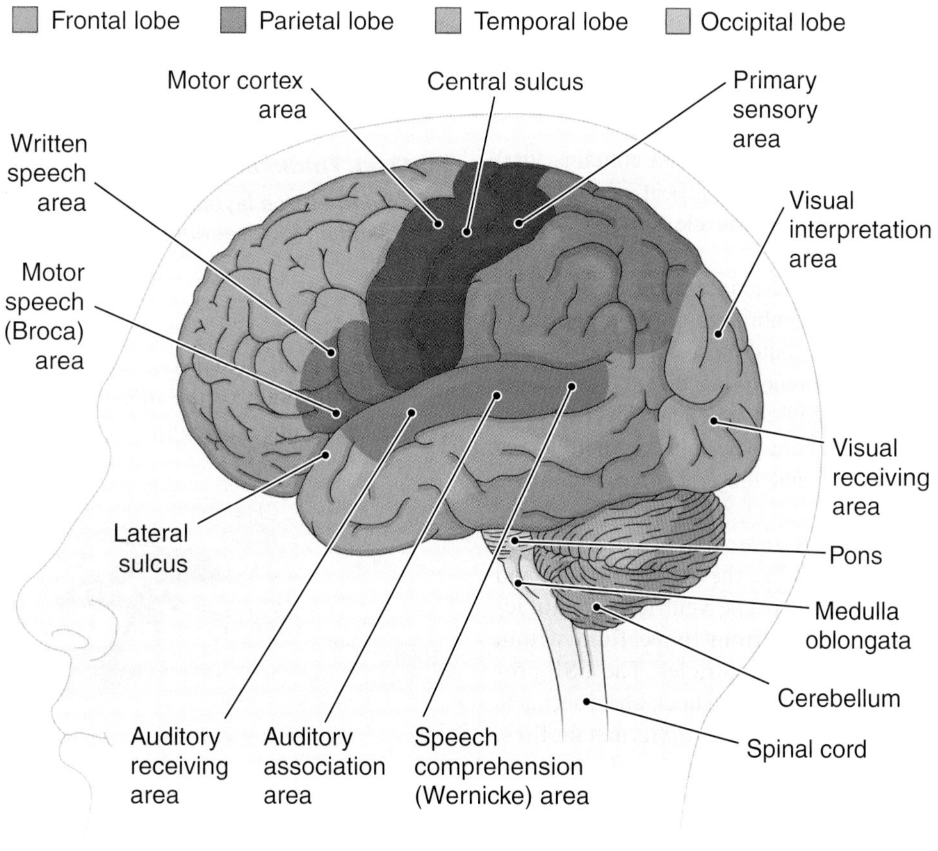

Figure 36-2 Lateral view of the brain showing the four lobes. The shaded areas show the regions of the cerebral cortex that are responsible for different functions.

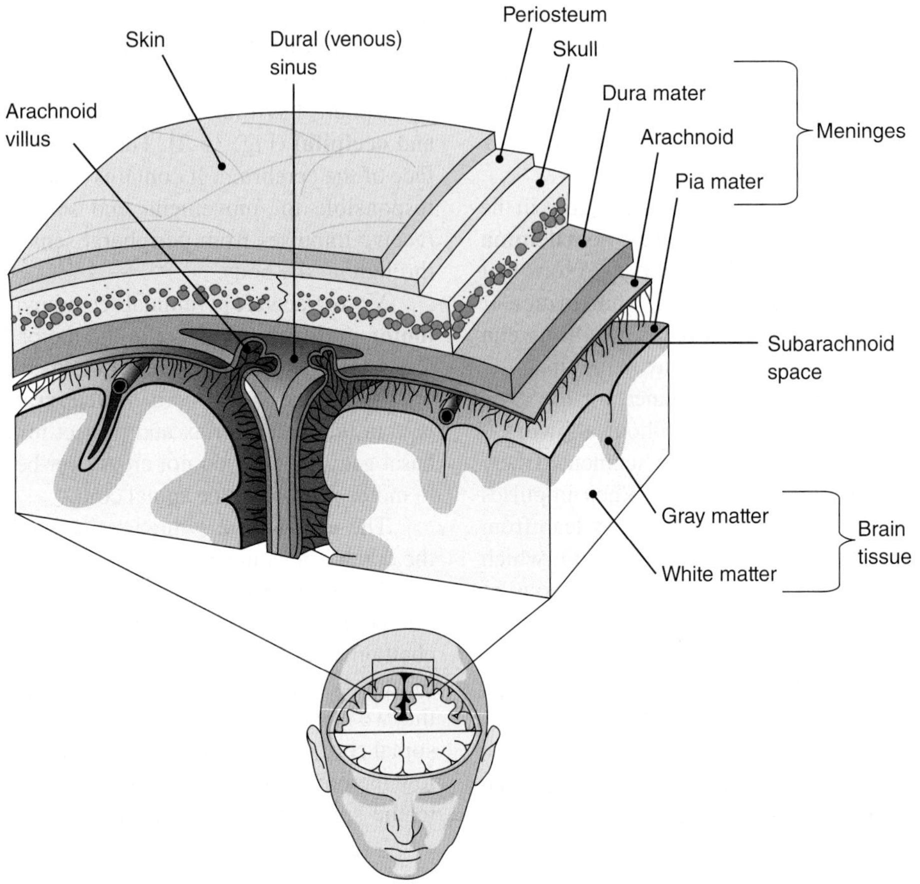

Figure 36-3 Frontal section of the top of the head showing the meninges of the central nervous system (pia mater, arachnoid, and dura mater) and related parts. (Reprinted with permission from Cohen, B. J., & Hull, K. L. (2015). *Memmler's the human body in health and disease* (13th ed.). Wolters Kluwer.)

sensory neurons to the brain. The medulla contains vital centers concerned with respiration, heartbeat, and vasomotor activity (the control of smooth muscle activity in blood vessel walls).

The brain is protected by the rigid bones of the skull and is covered by three membranes or **meninges**: (1) the **dura mater**, the tough, outermost covering; (2) the **arachnoid**, or middle membrane lying directly below the dura mater; and (3) the **pia mater**, a delicate layer that adheres to the brain and spinal cord. The **subarachnoid space** lies between the pia mater and the arachnoid membrane (Fig. 36-3).

Within the brain, there are four cavities called **ventricles**: two lateral ventricles, the third ventricle, and the fourth ventricle (Fig. 36-4). The ventricles manufacture cerebrospinal fluid (CSF) from tissue fluid within the **choroid plexus** that line the ventricles. The CSF protects the structures of the brain like a shock absorber; acts as a barrier to infectious organisms, toxic metabolites, and some drugs that enter the blood; floats the brain to reduce pressure at its base; and helps maintain relatively constant intracranial pressure. Once CSF is formed, it is circulated within the subarachnoid space of the brain and spinal cord to openings where it becomes reabsorbed into the venous system.

››› *Stop, Think, and Respond 36-1*

Name the three layers of meninges, starting below the skull and proceeding toward the surface of the brain.

Spinal Cord

The **spinal cord**, which is covered by the meninges, is a direct continuation of the medulla and is surrounded and protected by the *vertebrae* (or vertebral column). The

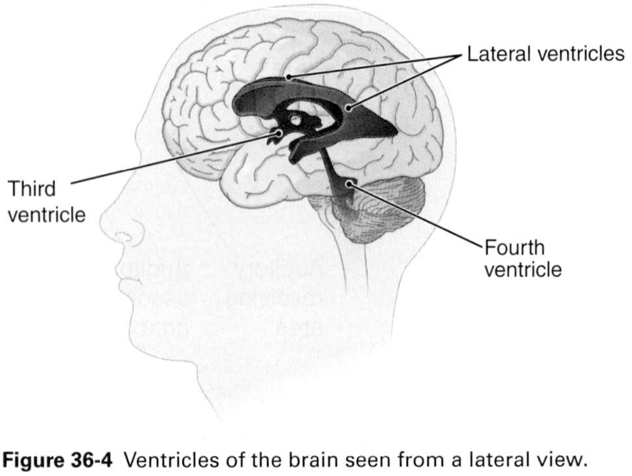

Figure 36-4 Ventricles of the brain seen from a lateral view.

spinal cord ends between the first and second lumbar vertebrae, where it divides into smaller sections called the **cauda equina.**

The spinal cord functions as a passageway for ascending sensory and descending motor neurons. Its two main functions are to provide centers for reflex action (Fig. 36-5) and to serve as a pathway for impulses to and from the brain. The sensory fibers enter the posterior (dorsal) portion of the cord, while the nerve fibers that transmit motor impulses run outward to the peripheral nerves from the anterior (ventral) portion of the cord.

Peripheral Nervous System

The PNS consists of all the sensory and motor nerves outside the CNS. The PNS includes the cranial, spinal, and sympathetic and parasympathetic nerves of the autonomic nervous system (ANS).

Cranial Nerves

The 12 pairs of **cranial nerves**, identified by Roman numerals, are as follows:

- *I*: *Olfactory nerve*: Sense of smell
- *II*: *Optic nerve*: Sight
- *III*: *Oculomotor nerve*: Contraction of iris and eye muscles
- *IV*: *Trochlear nerve*: Eye movement
- *V*: *Trigeminal nerve*: Sensory nerve to face, chewing
- *VI*: *Abducens nerve*: Eye movement
- *VII*: *Facial nerve*: Facial expression, taste, secretions of salivary and lacrimal glands
- *VIII*: *Vestibulocochlear (or auditory) nerve*: Hearing and balance
- *IX*: *Glossopharyngeal nerve*: Taste, sensory fibers of pharynx and tongue, swallowing, and secretions of parotid gland
- *X*: *Vagus nerve*: Motor fibers to glands producing digestive enzymes, heart rate, muscles of speech, gastrointestinal motility, respiration, swallowing, coughing, and vomiting reflex

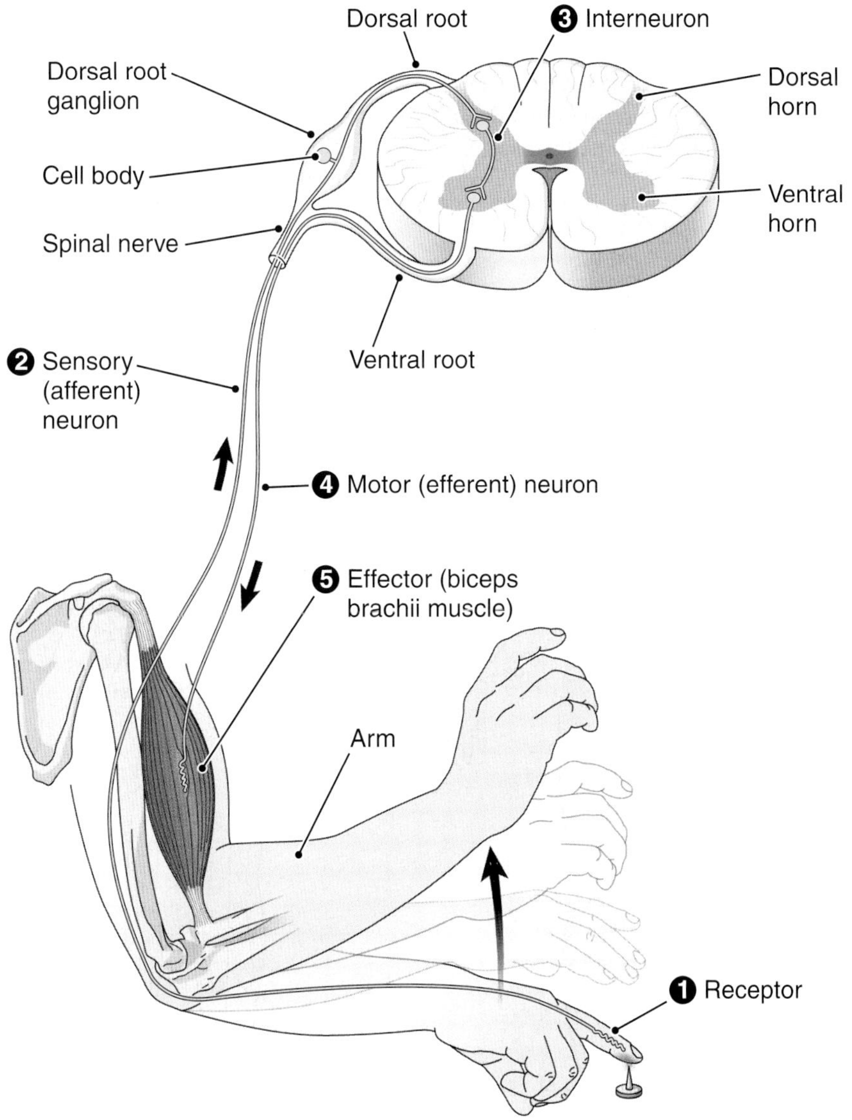

Figure 36-5 Reflex arc showing the pathway of impulses and cross section of the spinal cord. Numbers show the sequence of impulses through the spinal cord (*solid arrows*). (Reprinted with permission from Cohen, B. J., & Hull, K. L. (2018). *Memmler's the human body in health and disease* (14th ed.). Wolters Kluwer.)

- *XI*: *Accessory (or spinal accessory) nerve*: Head and shoulder movement
- *XII*: *Hypoglossal nerve*: Movement of the tongue

Spinal Nerves

There are 31 pairs of **spinal nerves**: 8 cervical, 12 thoracic, 5 lumbar, 5 sacral, and 1 coccygeal. Spinal nerves have two roots: dorsal and ventral. Dorsal nerve fibers are sensory and ventral nerve fibers are motor. Peripheral sensory nerve fibers in various areas of the body transmit impulses to the spinal nerves, which transmit impulses up the spinal cord to the brain. Motor impulses traveling from the brain and down the spinal cord leave by the ventral root and travel to areas of the body. Each spinal nerve root innervates a specific area or **dermatome** of the body surface (Fig. 36-6). Knowledge of the distribution of dermatomes is useful for identifying areas affected by certain viral infections such as shingles, anesthetizing localized areas of the body, and assessing and evaluating spinal injuries.

Autonomic Nervous System

The ANS consists of the sympathetic nervous system and the parasympathetic nervous system. It facilitates functions essential to survival. The two divisions of the ANS generally function antagonistically of each other; they maintain homeostasis by stimulating or inhibiting smooth muscles, cardiac muscle, and glands (Table 36-1).

Sympathetic Nervous System

The **sympathetic nervous system** is the division of the ANS that responds using a fight or flight response when there is a perceived or actual threat to survival. The neurotransmitters of the sympathetic nervous system, collectively known as *catecholamines*, are **epinephrine**, **norepinephrine**, and **dopamine**. The adrenal medulla produces and secretes epinephrine and norepinephrine. Norepinephrine is also produced at sympathetic nerve endings. Dopamine is a precursor (a substance that precedes another) of norepinephrine. Norepinephrine then becomes epinephrine. Stressful situations such as danger, intense emotion, and severe illness result in the release of catecholamines.

Parasympathetic Nervous System

The **parasympathetic nervous system** is the division of the ANS that works to conserve body energy and is partly responsible for slowing heart rate, digesting food, and eliminating body wastes. **Acetylcholine** is a neurotransmitter released at the nerve endings of parasympathetic nerve fibers, at some nerve endings in the sympathetic nervous system, and at nerve endings of skeletal muscles. Release of this neurotransmitter allows passage of a nerve impulse from the nerve fiber to the effector organ or structure, where the enzyme **acetylcholinesterase** inactivates acetylcholine.

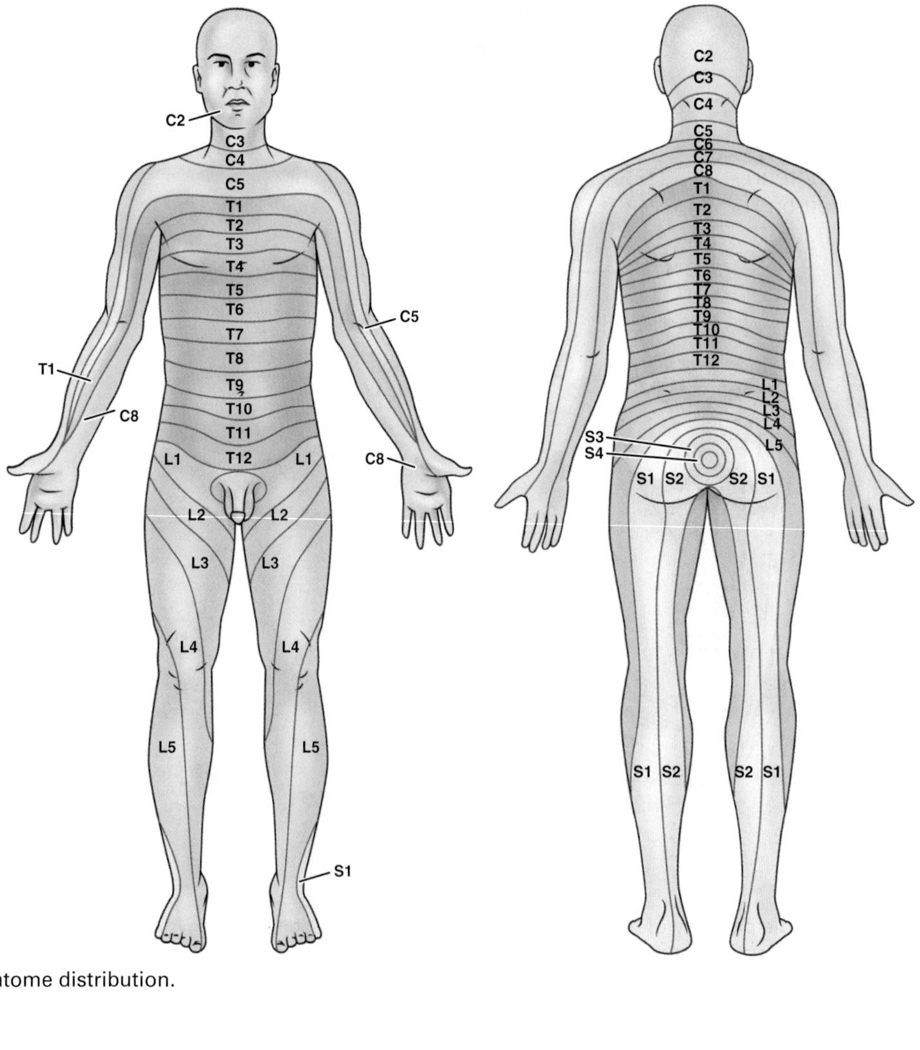

Figure 36-6 Dermatome distribution.

TABLE 36-1 Autonomic Effects of the Nervous System

STRUCTURE OR ACTIVITY	SYMPATHETIC EFFECTS	PARASYMPATHETIC EFFECTS
Pupil of the eye	Dilated	Constricted
Circulatory system		
Rate and force of heartbeat	Increased	Decreased
Blood vessels		
In heart muscle	Dilated	Constricted
In skeletal muscle	Dilated	[a]
In abdominal viscera and the skin	Constricted	[a]
Blood pressure	Increased	Decreased
Respiratory system		
Bronchioles	Dilated	Constricted
Rate of breathing	Increased	Decreased
Digestive system		
Peristaltic movements of digestive tube	Decreased	Increased
Muscular sphincters of digestive tube	Contracted	Relaxed
Secretion of salivary glands	Thick, viscid saliva	Thin, watery saliva
Secretions of stomach, intestine, and pancreas	[a]	Increased
Conversion of liver glycogen to glucose	Increased	[a]
Genitourinary system		
Urinary bladder		
Muscular walls	Relaxed	Contracted
Sphincters	Contracted	Relaxed
Muscles of the uterus	Contracted under some conditions; varies with menstrual cycle and pregnancy	Relaxed; variable
Blood vessels of external genitalia	[a]	Dilated
Integumentary system		
Secretion of sweat	Increased	[a]
Pilomotor muscles	Contracted (gooseflesh)	[a]
Adrenal medullae	Secretion of epinephrine and norepinephrine	[a]

[a]No direct effect.

ASSESSMENT

A neurologic assessment is performed to identify and locate disorders of the nervous system. The scope and extent of the neurologic examination often depend on the symptoms and the probable or actual diagnosis.

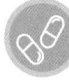

Pharmacologic Considerations

- The use of opioids or CNS depressants can affect the results of a neurologic assessment. Client assessment and history taking may be temporarily delayed until an opioid is metabolized.

History

A thorough history is essential. The nurse explores all symptoms and asks questions to clarify each symptom. The history must include a record of trauma (no matter how slight) to the head or body within the past 6 to 12 months, a drug history, an allergy history, and a family medical history. The nurse observes the client's speech pattern, mental status, intellectual functioning, reasoning ability, strength, and movement or lack thereof in all extremities.

Physical Examination

The physical examination consists of assessment of the cerebral, motor, and sensory activities. The nurse usually assesses a client's intellectual function and speech pattern during the history by noting responses to questions. Additional testing of intellectual function includes asking various questions that require mental tasks (see Chapter 67).

The nurse evaluates the client's body posture and any abnormal position of the head, neck, trunk, or extremities. If head trauma has occurred, the nurse examines the ears and nose for evidence of bleeding or other drainage. They carefully examine the head for bleeding, swelling, or wounds. The nurse does not move or manipulate the client's head during this part of the assessment, especially if there is a recent history of trauma.

Cranial Nerves

The experienced examiner evaluates all or some of the 12 cranial nerves (Table 36-2).

Motor Function

Assessment of motor function includes muscle movement, size, tone, strength, and coordination. The nurse inspects large muscle areas for evidence of atrophy and assesses opposing muscles for equality of size and strength. They ask the client to perform tasks such as

- Pushing the palm or sole against the examiner's palm
- Picking up small and large objects between the thumb and forefinger
- Grasping objects firmly
- Resisting removal of an object from the fist or fingers

To assess gait, movement, and balance, the nurse asks the client to walk away from the examiner, turn, and walk back. Other tests include climbing a small set of stairs, walking and turning abruptly, and walking heel to toe. In the Romberg test, the client stands with feet close together and eyes closed. If the client sways as if to fall, this is considered a positive Romberg test, indicating a problem with equilibrium. The examiner stands fairly close to the client during this test in case the client loses balance.

Tests that evaluate motor and cerebral function include doing the finger-to-nose test with eyes closed, writing words, and identifying common objects. The choice of tests depends on the original problem and the findings of diagnostic tests.

The nurse evaluates motor response in the comatose or unconscious client by administering a painful stimulus to

TABLE 36-2 Cranial Nerve Assessment

CRANIAL NERVE	ASSESSMENT TECHNIQUE	NORMAL FINDINGS
I—Olfactory	Ask client to occlude each nostril separately and close the eyes. Present familiar odors, such as vinegar, lemon, coffee, and ammonia.	Client identifies odors correctly.
II—Optic	Help client cover each eye separately; test visual acuity using a Snellen chart (see Chapter 42), newspaper, or Jaeger chart. Client and examiner cover an eye, and examiner moves an object from the periphery toward client's nose from superior, inferior, medial, and lateral positions while both fix their gaze straight ahead. Examiner then tests opposite eye. Inspect optic nerve with an ophthalmoscope.	Client names letters or reads words accurately. Client and examiner see object at the same time in the visual field. Optic nerve appears round and lighter than surrounding retina.
III—Oculomotor	In a darkened room, shine a bright light in each pupil; ask client to look at a near and far object (see Chapter 42). Ask client to follow an object you move in horizontal, vertical, and oblique directions (see Chapter 42).	Pupil constricts briskly in response to light and dilates when looking far away. Eye movement is coordinated in all directions.
IV—Trochlear	See assessment for motor function of oculomotor nerve.	Eyes move inferiorly and medially.
V—Trigeminal	Observe for jaw symmetry while client opens mouth. Instruct client to clamp jaws tightly together. Stroke forehead, cheeks, and jaw with a wisp of cotton, sharp object (e.g., pin), cold and warm objects, and a vibrating tuning fork. Touch each cornea with a wisp of cotton. Tap center of chin with a reflex hammer while client slightly opens the mouth.	Appearance is symmetric. The muscles contract bilaterally. Client shows bilateral sensitivity and correctly identifies sensory experience. Client blinks. Jaw closes suddenly and slightly.
VI—Abducens	See assessment for motor function of oculomotor nerve.	Client moves eyes in lateral directions.
VII—Facial	Ask client to wrinkle the forehead, smile, frown, raise eyebrows, look at ceiling, and whistle. Instruct client to close eyelids and resist examiner's efforts to open them. Apply sweet, sour, salty, and bitter flavors to both sides of the anterior tongue.	Facial movements are symmetrical. Both eyes equally resist efforts to open them. Client accurately identifies tastes.
VIII—Vestibulocochlear	Test hearing acuity and perform the Rinne and Weber tests with a tuning fork (see Chapter 43). Have client stand with both feet close together; note for swaying with eyes open and then shut.	Client repeats whispered words correctly; sound is lateralized equally and heard longer by air than by bone conduction. Client maintains balance or sways slightly.
IX—Glossopharyngeal	Touch palate with a tongue blade. Ask client to say "ah."	Blade elicits a gag response. Uvula remains in midline.
X—Vagus	Have client say "la, la, la."	Client speaks clearly and distinctly, with no hoarseness.
XI—Spinal accessory	Instruct client to shrug the shoulders as you apply resistance.	Client raises shoulders.
XII—Hypoglossal	Tell client to stick out the tongue.	Tongue remains in midline with no lateral deviation.

determine the client's response. An appropriate response is for the client to reach toward or withdraw from the stimulus. Clients with impaired cerebral function manifest abnormal posturing. **Decorticate posturing** (decorticate rigidity) is a position in which the arms are flexed, fists are clenched, and the legs are extended (Fig. 36-7A). **Decerebrate posturing** (decerebrate rigidity) is when the extremities are stiff and rigid (Fig. 36-7B). Decerebrate posturing is more serious than decorticate posturing. Even more ominous is **flaccidity**, when the client makes no motor response (Fig. 36-7C).

››› *Stop, Think, and Respond 36-2*

Which type of posturing is evidenced by (A) flexion of the arms, (B) extension of the arms, and (C) no movement of any extremities?

Sensory Function

The nurse evaluates the extremities for sensitivity to heat, cold, touch, and pain. They can use various objects such as cotton balls, tubes filled with hot or cold water, and sharp objects (that do not pierce the skin) to check sensation in the extremities.

Level of Consciousness

Depending on the client's symptoms, evaluation of the level of consciousness (LOC) is often necessary. The following classification of LOC applies to altered consciousness from any cause. Differentiating between each level can be difficult; some clients may show characteristics of two or more levels:

- *Conscious*: The client responds immediately, fully, and appropriately to visual, auditory, and other stimulation.
- *Somnolent or lethargic*: The client is drowsy or sleepy at inappropriate times but can be aroused, only to fall asleep again. Responses to questions and verbal commands are delayed or inappropriate. Speech is incoherent. Painful stimuli elicit a response.
- *Stuporous*: The client is aroused only by vigorous and repetitive physical, auditory, or visual stimulation. Stimulation results in one- or two-word answers or in motor activity or purposeful behavior directed toward avoiding further stimulation.
- *Semicomatose*: The client is unresponsive except to superficial, relatively mild painful stimuli to which the client makes some purposeful motor response (movement) to avoid further stimulation. Spontaneous motion is uncommon, but the client may groan or mutter.
- *Comatose*: The client responds only to very painful stimuli by fragmentary, delayed reflex withdrawal; in deeper stages, they lose all responsiveness. There is no spontaneous movement, and the respiratory rate is irregular.

The nurse assesses LOC at frequent intervals after injury to the head or neck, cranial surgery, a cerebrovascular accident (acute phase), a ruptured cerebral aneurysm, and other neurologic disorders. They make this assessment hourly unless the primary provider orders otherwise, or a change occurs in the client's condition.

Glasgow Coma Scale

The **Glasgow Coma Scale** (Box 36-1) is an objective assessment tool for evaluating LOC of a client. The scale consists of three parts: eye-opening response, best verbal response, and best motor response. To evaluate responses correctly, several verbal and motor responses are elicited, and the best response is recorded. The eye-opening response is determined by talking to the client and calling their name. If no response is noted (i.e., the eyes do not open spontaneously), a painful stimulus is applied and the response is noted. The

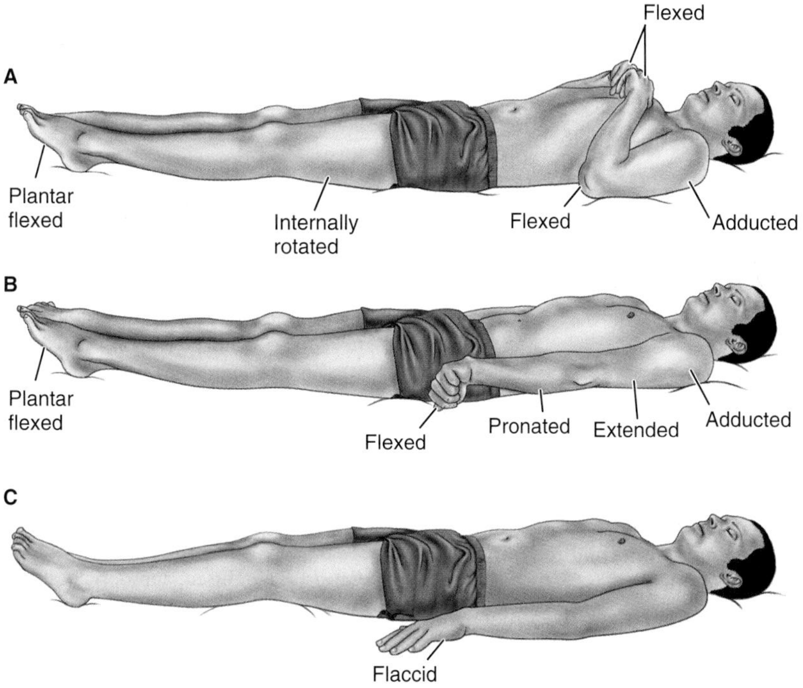

Figure 36-7 Abnormal posture response to stimuli: **(A)** decorticate posturing, **(B)** decerebrate posturing, and **(C)** flaccidity is when the client makes no motor response to stimuli.

BOX 36-1 Glasgow Coma Scale

The Glasgow Coma Scale is a tool for assessing a client's response to stimuli. A score of 10 or less indicates a need for emergency attention, and a score of 7 or less is generally interpreted as coma.

Eye-opening response	Spontaneous	4
	To voice	3
	To pain	2
	None	1
Best verbal response	Oriented	5
	Confused	4
	Inappropriate words	3
	Incomprehensible sounds	2
	None	1
Best motor response	Obeys command	6
	Localizes pain	5
	Withdraws (pain)	4
	Flexion (pain)	3
	Extension (pain)	2
	None	1
Total		3–15

Reprinted from Teasdale, G., & Jennett, B. (1974). Assessment of coma and impaired consciousness. A practical scale. *Lancet, 304*(7872), 81–84. Copyright © 1974 Elsevier. With permission. See at http://www.glasgowcomascale.org/.

verbal response is evaluated by a verbal reply to questions. The motor response is the ability of the client to follow commands, such as "Wiggle your toes" or "Move your left hand." If there is no response, a painful stimulus is used and the response is noted. The responses are assigned numbers, and the numbers are totaled. A normal response is 15. A score of 7 or less is considered coma. The evaluations are recorded on a flow sheet to quickly evaluate an increase or decrease in the LOC. Also see Evidence-Based Practice 36-1.

Rancho Los Amigos Scale

The Rancho Los Amigos Scale (Box 36-2) is another tool for assessing LOC. Some rehabilitation centers prefer this scale because it is a more flexible assessment tool for identifying variations in the client's status.

Pupils

The size and equality of the pupils and their reaction to light are an assessment of the third cranial (oculomotor) nerve (see Table 36-2). Pupil size (normal, pinpoint, dilated), equality (equal, unequal in size), and reaction to a bright light (normal, sluggish, no reaction, fixed) are noted (see Chapter 42). When the pupils are examined, any abnormal movement or position of one or both eyes is noted.

Unequal pupils (one pupil larger than the other), dilated or pinpoint pupils, and failure of the pupils to respond quickly to light are, in most instances, abnormal findings. Any sudden change in pupil size, equality, or reaction to light is an important neurologic finding and is reported to the primary provider at once.

Evidence-Based Practice 36-1

The Glasgow Coma Scale and Pupil Size

Clinical Question

What is the importance of pupil size in the Glasgow Coma Scale?

Evidence

Clients with intracranial pressure in the brain can show pupillary changes as the pressure increases. The Glasgow Coma Scale is an assessment tool that measures a client's response to stimulation. Pupil size and symmetry are assessed on the scale. In a study by Kerr and Bacon (2016) about the accuracy of nurses in critical care and neurology, pupil assessments were evaluated. The study found that nurse assessment of pupil diameters, recognizing anisocoria (unequal pupil size), and pupil reactivity were incorrect. Tools were provided for all nurses during the pupil assessment; however, it was observed that most nurses estimated instead of using the tools (Kerr & Bacon, 2016). A score of 10 or less may indicate emergency interventions, so proper assessment findings are needed.

Nursing Implications

This study observed nurses circumventing tool resources and making errors in assessment and Glasgow Coma Scale results. This assessment should be accurate in order to identify changes in the pupils early, so that interventions occur quickly and neurologic deterioration does not occur.

Reference
Kerr, R. G., & Bacon, A. M. (2016). Underestimation of pupil size by critical care and neurosurgical nurses. *American Journal of Critical Care, 25*(3), 213–219. https://doi.org/10.4037/ajcc2016554

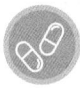

Pharmacologic Considerations

- Opioid use will cause the pupils to constrict and become pinpoint size. They will remain as such and not dilate in low-level light. The drug, not a neurologic disorder, causes the alteration.

BOX 36-2 Rancho Los Amigos Scale

Level I: No response to stimuli. Appears in deep sleep.
Level II: Generalized response. First reaction may be due to deep pain; has delayed, inconsistent responses.
Level III: Localized response. Inconsistent responses, but reacts in a more specific manner to stimulus; might follow simple command "squeeze my hand."
Level IV: Confused, agitated. Reacts to own inner confusion, fear, disorientation; excitable behavior, may be abusive.
Level V: Nonagitated, confused, inappropriate. Usually disoriented; follows tasks for 2–3 minutes but easily distracted by environment; frustrated.
Level VI: Confused, appropriate. Follows simple directions consistently. Memory and attention increasing; self-care tasks performed without help.
Level VII: Automatic, appropriate. If physically able, can carry out routine activities. Appears normal; needs supervision for safety.
Level VIII: Purposeful, alert, oriented. May have decreased abilities relative to premorbid state.

Neck

The neck is examined for stiffness or abnormal position. The presence of rigidity is checked by moving the head and chin toward the chest. This should never be done if a head or neck injury is suspected or known or trauma to any part of the body is evident.

Vital Signs

The blood pressure, pulse and respiratory rates, and temperature are closely monitored on all clients with a potential or actual neurologic disorder. The temperature often needs to be monitored every hour because CNS disorders can affect the temperature-regulating ability of the hypothalamus. A sudden increase or decrease in any of the vital signs indicates a change in the neurologic status, and the primary provider is notified immediately.

Diagnostic Tests

Imaging Procedures

Imaging procedures such as computed tomography (CT), magnetic resonance imaging (MRI), positron emission tomography (PET), and single-photon emission computed tomography (SPECT) are used in the diagnosis of neurologic disorders. Imaging procedures are particularly useful in the diagnosis of neurologic disorders such as brain tumors, Alzheimer's disease, intracranial bleeding or hemorrhage, and cerebral infections.

Computed Tomography

CT uses X-rays and computer analysis to produce three-dimensional views of thin cross sections, or "slices," of the body. A narrow X-ray beam rotates around the client, and a computer analyzes the results. CT is extremely sensitive to differences in tissue densities, allowing differentiation between intracranial tumors, cysts, edema, and hemorrhage. The client is exposed to the same amount of radiation as in a conventional X-ray.

A radiopaque dye may be used during a CT scan to emphasize or highlight a certain area. Use of a radiopaque dye decreases the safety of the procedure, primarily owing to the risk of an allergic reaction. Clients who are allergic to iodine should not receive radiopaque dyes that contain this substance. Seafood allergies suggest an allergy to iodine. A thorough allergy history is an essential assessment prior to a neurologic examination involving contrast media.

Magnetic Resonance Imaging

An MRI scan is based on the magnetic behavior of protons in body tissue. MRI uses radiofrequency waves to produce images of tissues of high-fat and high-water content such as soft tissue, veins, arteries, the brain, and spinal cord. Images are produced without contrast dye or radiation.

The client's whole body or a particular body part is imaged within a tunnel or under an open nontunneled machine containing a powerful magnet (Fig. 36-8). Open MRIs are used for those who are anxious, claustrophobic, or obese. The MRI lasts for 15 to 90 minutes; sedation is an option for those who cannot tolerate the length of the procedure or the feeling of being enclosed. A call button and an intercom are available for two-way communication. Clients should be prescreened for any internal device that contains magnetic metal materials, such as a cardiac pacemaker, implanted defibrillator, aneurysm clips, and the like, which may contraindicate using an MRI because metal interferes with the magnetic field. Clients with orthopedic metal implants can undergo an MRI because most are made of nonferromagnetic materials such as titanium, stainless steel, and ceramics.

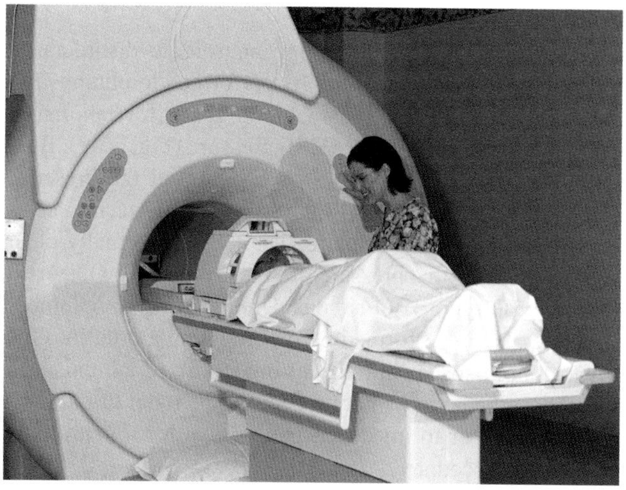

Figure 36-8 A technician discusses what the client should expect during magnetic resonance imaging.

Positron Emission Tomography

PET uses radioactive substances to examine metabolic activity of body structures. The client either inhales or is injected with a radioactive substance with positively charged particles that combine with negatively charged particles found normally in the body. The energy emitted when these combine is converted into color-coded images, indicating metabolic activity of the organ involved. The radioactive substances are short lived, resulting in minimal radiation exposure. PET is used less frequently than CT or MRI because the equipment is usually available only in major medical centers.

Single-Photon Emission Computed Tomography

SPECT is a noninvasive imaging tool with the advantage of providing information about the brain's function, whereas CT and MRI only image anatomic structures. SPECT provides information about the brain's cerebral blood flow and the status of receptors for neurotransmitters; it also identifies lesions before they are visible with other imaging techniques. Data from SPECT locate the site causing epileptic seizures, help diagnose Alzheimer's and Parkinson's diseases, and detect brain tumors and changes in blood flow that predict the potential or actual area of a stroke and offer prognosis for recovery.

SPECT obtains images of the brain after the client intravenously receives radiopharmaceuticals and radioisotopes approximately 1 hour before the test begins. Once the radioactive substances circulate, there is a scan of the brain. Colored cross sections of the brain images are evaluated for evidence of pathology. A potential risk of SPECT is the client's allergic reaction to the imaging material.

Lumbar Puncture

Changes in CSF occur in many neurologic disorders. A **lumbar puncture** (spinal tap) is performed to obtain samples of CSF from the subarachnoid space for laboratory examination and to measure CSF pressure (Fig. 36-9). Bacteriologic tests on specimens of CSF reveal the presence of pathogenic microorganisms. Strict aseptic technique is required during the procedure. The CSF is normally clear and colorless, with a pressure of 80 to 180 mm H_2O; a pressure over 200 mm H_2O is considered abnormal. A lumbar puncture also is performed before injecting a drug into the subarachnoid space (intrathecal injection); to administer a spinal anesthetic; to withdraw CSF for the relief of intracranial pressure; or to inject air, gas, or dye for a neurologic diagnostic procedure.

The design of the needle has been improved to decrease the occurrence of spinal headaches following a spinal tap. If the dura mater is accidentally punctured during the procedure, the chances of a spinal headache are higher (Spinal Headaches, 2020).

Sometimes, a cisternal puncture is performed to remove CSF. The back of the neck is shaved, the skin is washed with an antiseptic, and a needle is inserted just below the occipital bone of the skull. This procedure is performed more commonly on children. Headache appears to occur less frequently with cisternal puncture than with lumbar puncture.

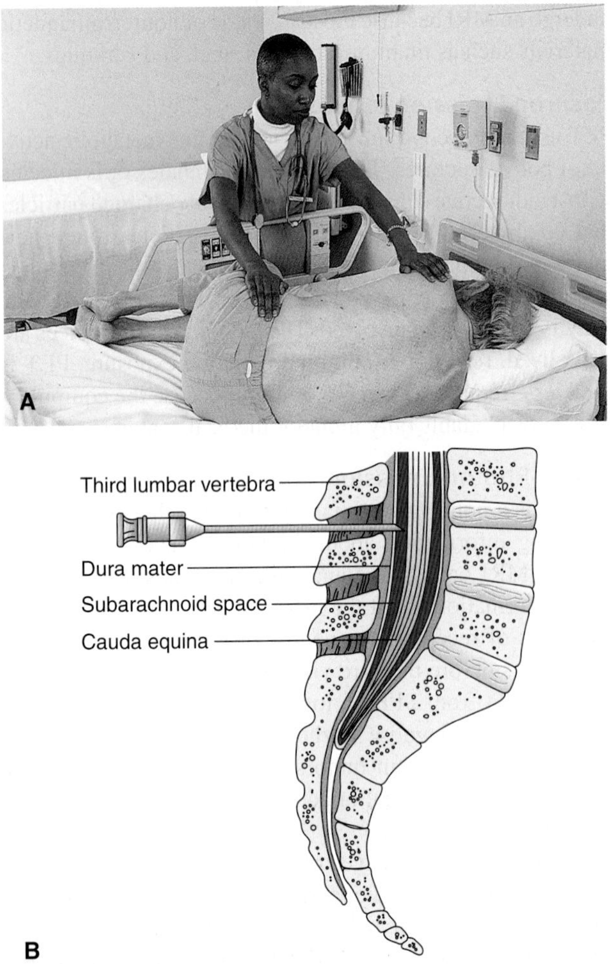

Figure 36-9 **(A)** Positioning of the client for lumbar puncture. **(B)** Insertion of the spinal needle into the subarachnoid space.

Contrast Studies

Cerebral Angiography

Contrast studies include **cerebral angiography**, which detects distortion of cerebral arteries and veins, indicating an aneurysm, a tumor, or other vascular abnormality. A radiopaque dye is injected into the right or left carotid artery, the brachial artery, or the femoral artery. A rapid sequence of radiographs is taken because the dye circulates through the cerebral arteries and veins.

Myelogram

For a **myelogram**, a radiopaque substance is injected into the spinal canal by means of a lumbar puncture. Radiographs are taken to demonstrate abnormalities of the spinal canal such as tumors or a ruptured intervertebral disk.

Electroencephalogram

An **electroencephalogram** (EEG) records the electrical impulses generated by the brain. Up to 25 electrodes are attached to the scalp with a type of skin adhesive, and electrical activity is recorded on a graph. Techniques such as rapid breathing or looking at a flashing light, known as *photic stimulation*, can induce a seizure during the EEG. In some cases, the primary provider may request that the client be deprived of sleep before an EEG. Sleep deprivation helps the client fall asleep naturally during the EEG. The electrical activity during sleep provides additional diagnostic information.

The nurse is responsible for preparing the client for the EEG as follows:

- Tell the client that they will not experience any electrical shock during the test, and that the source of the electrical energy is the client's neural activity within the brain.
- Withhold sedatives, coffee, tea, and soft drinks that contain caffeine for at least 8 hours before the test to avoid affecting the diagnostic findings.
- Allow the client to eat; a low blood glucose level can alter the EEG.
- Direct the client to shampoo their hair to remove oil and hair products. Clean hair facilitates and promotes maintenance of electrode attachment throughout the test.
- Awaken the client around midnight before the EEG to ensure sleep deprivation.

After the EEG is completed, the client who is sleep-deprived can rest and have the hair shampooed to remove the glue used to affix the electrodes to the scalp.

Brain Scan

A **brain scan** identifies tumors, hematomas in or around the brain, cerebral abscesses, cerebral infarctions, or displaced ventricles. A radioactive material is injected before the procedure. The length of this procedure varies from a few minutes to 1 hour. CT scans and MRI are replacing this procedure.

Electromyography

Electromyography (EMG) studies the changes in the electrical potential of muscles and the nerves supplying the muscles. An EMG is useful in determining the presence of neuromuscular disorders. Needle electrodes are placed into one or more skeletal muscles, and the results are recorded on an oscilloscope. Pain may occur at needle insertion sites, and muscle soreness may last for some time afterward.

Nerve Conduction Studies

Nerve conduction studies are performed by applying surface electrodes to the skin over locations of various nerves. When a mild electrical stimulus is administered, the speed with which the nerve impulse travels along the peripheral nerve is measured. These tests, which may be combined with EMG, aid in the diagnosis of nerve injury and compression or neurologic disorders affecting peripheral nerves such as carpal tunnel syndrome and the peripheral neuropathy experienced by clients with diabetes.

Echoencephalography

An **echoencephalography** is an ultrasound examination of the structures of the brain. This procedure is performed to detect abnormalities in the ventricles and the location of intracranial bleeding.

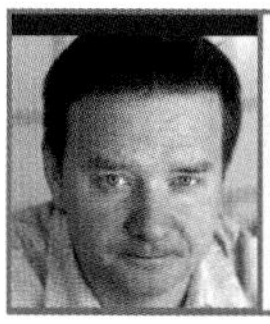

Clinical Scenario A 56-year-old client comes to the neurologic unit prior to undergoing an EEG and CT scan with contrast imaging. The client tells the nurse that he does not understand what these tests involve and what to expect during and after the examination. **What nursing actions are appropriate when caring for this client? See the following Nursing Process section.**

NURSING PROCESS FOR THE CLIENT UNDERGOING NEUROLOGIC TESTING

Assessment

Determine the client's understanding of the diagnostic procedures and answer any remaining questions. Check that a consent form has been signed and witnessed. Ask the client regarding any previous allergic reactions to radiographic dyes, iodine, or seafood because some contrast media contain iodine. Obtain the client's weight, baseline vital signs, and neurologic data such as LOC, pupil response, and muscle strength in all four extremities. Use the assessment findings for comparison when monitoring the client's condition during and after diagnostic testing. Closely observe the client for any mental or physical deviations from the baseline assessments.

Diagnosis, Planning, and Interventions

Prepare the client for neurologic diagnostic tests following agency policies. If the diagnostic test is performed at the bedside, bring necessary equipment to the room. Assist the primary provider and support the client during a test performed on the nursing unit. During and after the diagnostic test, monitor for adverse consequences and promote recovery after the test.
Diagnoses, expected outcomes, and interventions include, but are not limited to, the following:
Nursing problem: Knowledge Deficiency
Expected Outcome: Client will accurately describe the preparation, procedure, and aftercare that the scheduled diagnostic test involves.

- Clarify the primary provider's explanation. *Some clients have questions after the primary provider leaves the nursing unit or healthcare agency.*
- Answer the client's questions. *Clients have the right to information about their plan of care.*
- Describe the procedure to the client as well as what the procedure requires, such as positions to assume or the need to lie still during the procedure. *Specific information decreases anxiety and increases the client's trust and confidence in the nurse.*
- Discuss the preparation for the diagnostic test, which may include temporarily eliminating CNS depressants, such as barbiturates and minor tranquilizers, and CNS stimulants, such as caffeine, for several hours in the case of an EEG. *Drugs that affect neurologic function are sometimes withheld to ensure that factors other than the client's physiology do not affect the test results.*
- Explain that hair will be shampooed before an EEG. *Removing scalp and hair oil ensures that electrodes will remain in place until the EEG is completed.*
- Inform the client that they will need to shampoo the hair again after an EEG. *A second shampoo facilitates removing the adhesive used to secure the electrodes to the scalp.*
- Tell the client to expect some discomfort when undergoing a lumbar puncture, myelogram, EMG, or nerve conduction studies. *If the information about expected discomfort is not given, the client may assume that they are having an adverse reaction.*

RC of Allergic Reaction to Contrast Dye

Expected Outcome: The nurse will monitor to detect, manage, and minimize an allergic reaction.

- Report the allergy history to the primary provider. *Reporting helps the primary provider decide whether to cancel or modify the diagnostic test by administering a pretest antihistamine or substituting an alternative dye.*
- Identify allergy information prominently on the client's chart. *Documenting allergies on the chart provides a means for communicating the information to all healthcare workers.*

(continued)

NURSING PROCESS FOR THE CLIENT UNDERGOING NEUROLOGIC TESTING (continued)

- Attach an allergy band to the client's wrist when that is the agency's policy. *Some healthcare agencies require a second wristband that is of different color than the client identification band to alert personnel that the client has a history of one or more allergies.*
- Administer pretest antihistamines according to the primary provider's medical order. *Antihistamines block histamine receptors and reduce the manifestations of an allergic reaction.*
- Monitor client for severe hypotension, tachycardia, profuse diaphoresis, sudden change in LOC, dyspnea, and hives or itching. Notify the primary provider immediately of any such findings. *The most serious allergic reaction is anaphylaxis.*
- Obtain the emergency cart that contains drugs and resuscitation equipment; follow instructions for administering oxygen, intravenous fluids, drugs, and airway management depending on the client's symptoms. *Emergency measures are required to relieve anaphylaxis and other serious allergic reactions.*

RC of Meningeal Irritation or CNS Changes

Expected Outcome: The nurse will monitor to detect, manage, and minimize abnormal neurologic changes.

- Observe closely for any neurologic abnormalities, such as diminished LOC, weakness, numbness, paralysis in an extremity, unequal or unresponsive pupil reflexes, posturing, and speech disturbance. *Diagnostic tests pose potential risks for neurologic complications, which are characterized by changes in neurologic functions.*
- Assess for changes in vital signs, restlessness, vomiting, and mental changes in orientation and thought processes. *Rising intracranial pressure affects vital signs, stimulates the vomiting center in the brain, and alters the sensorium and cognition.*
- Report the onset of a headache and sudden or severe pain in any area of the body to the primary provider immediately. *Headache often accompanies increased intracranial pressure; pain of any kind requires further investigation and pain management.*
- Inspect injection sites, especially those made during a lumbar puncture, for signs of a hematoma (collection of blood). *Trauma at an injection site can result in bleeding; bloody drainage also may contain CSF.*
- Position the client flat for the time as directed by the primary provider after a lumbar puncture or myelogram. *Keeping the client in a recumbent position provides time for CSF to form and replace what has been lost and reduces the potential for a headache.*
- Encourage a liberal fluid intake. *A generous fluid intake helps restore the volume of CSF.*
- Keep the room dark and quiet after a lumbar puncture or myelogram. *Sensory stimulation tends to magnify discomfort.*
- Administer a prescribed analgesic or other medication if the client develops a headache. *An analgesic reduces the transmission or perception of pain stimuli.*

Evaluation of Expected Outcomes

Expected outcomes for the client are that they understand the preparation and performance involved in the neurologic procedure or diagnostic test and aftercare. Data concerning the client's allergy history are communicated appropriately. Interventions are implemented to control any allergic reaction. Measures to reduce the manifestation of complications are implemented successfully. Interventions to relieve discomfort are carried out.

KEY POINTS

- Two functions of the spinal cord:
  - Provides centers for reflex action
  - Serves as a pathway for impulses to and from the brain
- ANS: Facilitates functions essential to survival
  - Sympathetic nervous system
  - Parasympathetic nervous system
- Assessing motor function: Includes muscle movement, size, tone, strength, and coordination
- Assessing sensory function: Includes the extremities for sensitivity to heat, cold, touch, and pain
- Glasgow Coma Scale: An objective assessment tool for evaluating LOC of a client
- The Rancho Los Amigos Scale: A tool for assessing LOC; it is a more flexible assessment tool for identifying variations in the client's status
- Neurologic diagnostic testing:
  - Imaging procedures:
    - Computed tomography (CT)
    - Magnetic resonance imaging (MRI)
    - Positron emission tomography (PET)
    - Single-photon emission computed tomography (SPECT)
    - Lumbar puncture (spinal tap): Is performed to obtain samples of CSF from the subarachnoid space for laboratory examination and to measure CSF pressure
  - Contrast studies:
    - Cerebral angiography
    - Myelogram
    - Electroencephalogram
    - Brain scan
    - Electromyography

CRITICAL THINKING EXERCISES

1. Discuss appropriate nursing assessments when managing the care of clients with neurologic disorders.
2. A client with a neurologic disorder is being transferred from one nursing unit to another. What information is needed to plan the nursing care of the client?
3. Name any two neurologic tests and their potential complications. How can the nurse prevent, manage, and minimize them?
4. During an end-of-shift report, the nurse states that a client has a Glasgow Coma score of 6. Explain the significance of this score.

NCLEX-STYLE REVIEW QUESTIONS PrepU

1. When a nurse is asked to assist the primary provider with a diagnostic Romberg test, what nursing intervention is most appropriate to ensure client safety?
   1. Stand close to the client in case the client should begin to sway.
   2. Advise the client to use a handrail while ambulating to avoid falling.
   3. Use a gait belt to support the client during the test.
   4. Supply the client with a walker for stability if the client becomes unsteady.
2. What LOC is correct for a nurse to document when calling a client's name causes the client to awaken temporarily, followed by drifting back to sleep?
   1. Conscious
   2. Somnolent
   3. Stuporous
   4. Semicomatose
3. When a nurse uses the Glasgow Coma Scale to assess a client, what method should the nurse use to determine the "best verbal response" from the client?
   1. Ask the client to read aloud an item from the newspaper.
   2. Tell the client to repeat various random words.
   3. Note the client's reaction when using the client's name.
   4. Note the client's responses to general orientation questions.
4. Immediately following a lumbar puncture, a client asks to ambulate to the restroom. What nursing action is most correct?
   1. Explain that the client must temporarily lie flat and use a urinal.
   2. Provide a bedside commode and assist the client with its use.
   3. Instruct the client to remain still and insert a urinary catheter.
   4. Assist the client to the restroom and wait outside until finished.
5. A primary provider writes an order to administer 4 mg of sumatriptan subcutaneously stat for a client with a severe postprocedural headache following a lumbar puncture. The sumatriptan is in a single dose vial labeled 6 mg/0.5 mL. Calculate the volume of drug the nurse should administer. Round your answer to the nearest hundredth.______________

WANT TO KNOW MORE? There are a wide variety of online resources available on thePoint to enhance learning and understanding of this chapter.

Go to **thePoint.lww.com/activate** and use the activation code found in the front of this text to unlock these online resources.

37 Caring for Clients With Central and Peripheral Nervous System Disorders

Words To Know

amyotrophic lateral sclerosis
aura
automatisms
Bell palsy
bradykinesia
brain tumor
Brudzinski sign
Cheyne–Stokes respirations
choreiform movements
convulsion
Cushing triad
demyelinating disease
diplopia
encephalitis
epilepsy
facial reanimation
fasciculations
foramen magnum
gamma-knife radiosurgery
Guillain–Barré syndrome
Huntington disease
Kernig sign
meningitis
Monro–Kellie hypothesis
multiple sclerosis
neuralgia
nuchal rigidity
nystagmus
opisthotonos
papilledema
Parkinson disease
parkinsonism
photophobia
pill-rolling tremor
postictal phase
preictal phase
ptosis
seizure
status epilepticus
trigeminal neuralgia
widening pulse pressure

Learning Objectives

On completion of this chapter, you will be able to:

1. Name the three components within the cranium and explain the Monro–Kellie hypothesis.
2. Discuss at least four signs and symptoms and nursing care of the client with increased intracranial pressure.
3. Name four infectious or inflammatory diseases that affect the central or peripheral nervous system.
4. Discuss three neuromuscular disorders, common related problems, and nursing management.
5. Discuss the nursing management of clients with a cranial nerve disorder.
6. List the signs and symptoms of Parkinson disease.
7. Discuss the purpose of drug therapy and drugs commonly prescribed for Parkinson disease.
8. Describe signs and symptoms of Huntington disease and related nursing management.
9. Discuss the pathophysiology of seizure disorders and different types of seizures.
10. Discuss the nursing management of clients with seizure disorders.
11. Discuss the nursing management of clients with brain tumors.

Acute disorders of the central nervous system (CNS) and peripheral nervous system (PNS) are potentially life threatening. Chronic neurologic disorders, although not imminently fatal, profoundly affect a person's quality of life. This chapter discusses disorders in which components of the CNS or PNS are damaged, removed, or destroyed, which can result in neurologic deficits.

Gerontologic Considerations

- Older adults may not exhibit the typical signs and symptoms of meningitis; rather, they may display a change in mental status, slight to no fever, and no nuchal rigidity or headache.
- Mortality rates are high in older adults with this disease partly because of these atypical signs and symptoms. Contributing factors to death from meningitis are chronic illness and delays in diagnosis.
- Older adults with Parkinson disease are more susceptible to the complications of prolonged bed rest and immobility. These clients should be observed closely for such problems as hypostatic pneumonia, pressure ulcers, contractures, and deformities.

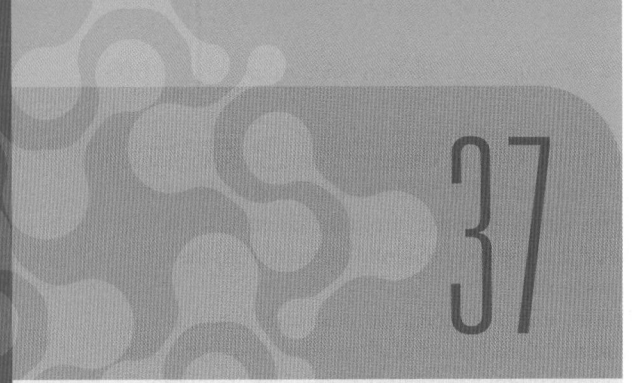

Gerontologic Considerations (*continued*)

- Physical/occupational therapy goals are individualized and may focus on maintaining comfort or function rather than achieving rehabilitation. Techniques can be taught to compensate for embarrassing or disabling symptoms such as shuffling, freezing gait, nuchal rigidity, and lack of control of swallowing to enable the older person to maintain self-esteem and social interactions.
- Older adults may experience primary brain tumors or cerebral metastasis from a primary neoplasm in another site. Early signs may be overlooked as changes associated with aging.

INCREASED INTRACRANIAL PRESSURE

Inside the cranium, there is (1) brain tissue, (2) blood, and (3) cerebrospinal fluid (CSF). The brain represents 80% of the cranial contents; the blood within the cranium contributes 10% of the total; and the CSF provides the remaining 10% (Fig. 37-1). According to the **Monro–Kellie hypothesis**, if one or more of these increases significantly without a decrease in either or both of the other two, intracranial pressure (ICP) becomes elevated. Examples of disorders that may lead to increased ICP include: brain tumors, traumatic brain injuries from concussions, ruptured cerebral aneurysms, stroke, obstructions in the circulation of CSF, and infectious disorders of the nervous system such as meningitis and encephalitis.

Pathophysiology and Etiology

Under normal circumstances, autoregulatory mechanisms keep brain tissue perfused with adequate oxygen and glucose. Dilation or constriction of cerebral blood vessels in response to changes in blood pressure (BP), blood oxygen levels, and blood pH maintains constant and consistent tissue perfusion. For example, increased $PaCO_2$ (carbon dioxide level in the blood), decreased blood pH, or decreased PaO_2 (oxygen level in the blood) causes cerebral blood vessels to dilate. Nevertheless, a delicate range of ICP helps maintain autoregulation. Ideally, ICP should remain at 5 to 15 mm Hg to ensure normal cerebral perfusion pressure of 70 to 100 mm Hg. Many conditions including brain tumors, swelling or bleeding within the brain from head trauma, and infectious and inflammatory disorders of the brain (e.g., meningitis, encephalitis) cause increased ICP.

When the intracranial volume (and therefore ICP) begins to increase, some initial compensation occurs. CSF production may decrease, or it may displace at a greater rate into venous circulation. However, as ICP continues to rise, vascular autoregulatory mechanisms can become compromised and fail. Hypotension and hypoxia lead to vasodilation, which contributes to increased ICP, compressing blood vessels, leading to cerebral ischemia.

If increased ICP continues to be unrecognized or untreated, the contents of the cranium are compressed further. Unrelieved pressure causes brain tissue to herniate or shift from normal locations intracranially and extracranially (Fig. 37-2). The **foramen magnum**, the opening in the lower part of the skull through which the upper part of the spinal cord connects with the brain, provides the only

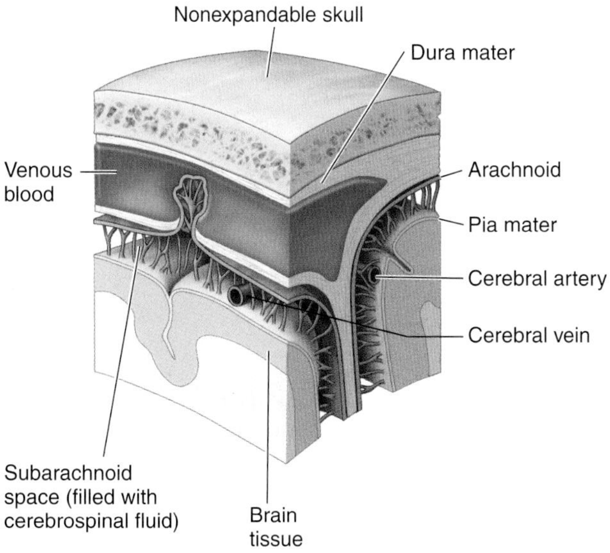

Figure 37-1 The components within the nonexpandable skull include solid brain tissue, blood, and cerebrospinal fluid. (Modified with permission from Moore, K. L., Agur, A. M. R., & Dalley, A. F. (2017). *Clinically oriented anatomy* (8th ed., p. 874). Wolters Kluwer.)

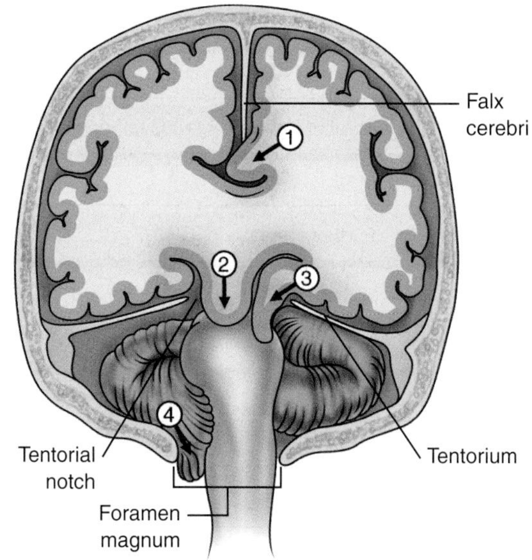

Figure 37-2 Major types of intracranial herniations. Supratentorial herniations (above the tentorium, a portion of dura mater that separates the cerebellum from the occipital lobes) include the following: **(1)** cingulate herniation under the falx cerebri, a fold of dura mater that separates the two cerebral hemispheres; **(2)** central (symmetrical) transtentorial herniation downward through the tentorial notch, an opening between the cerebellum and the brain stem; **(3)** uncal (portion of the temporal lobe) herniation laterally through the tentorial notch; **(4)** infratentorial (below the tentorium) herniation of a portion of the cerebellum known as the cerebral tonsils through the foramen magnum.

extracranial exit for brain tissue. If the brain stem herniates through the foramen magnum, respiration, heart rate, BP, and the functions of descending and ascending nerve fibers are affected. As increased ICP progresses, the consequences include impaired cellular activity, temporary or permanent neurologic dysfunction, or death (Fig. 37-3).

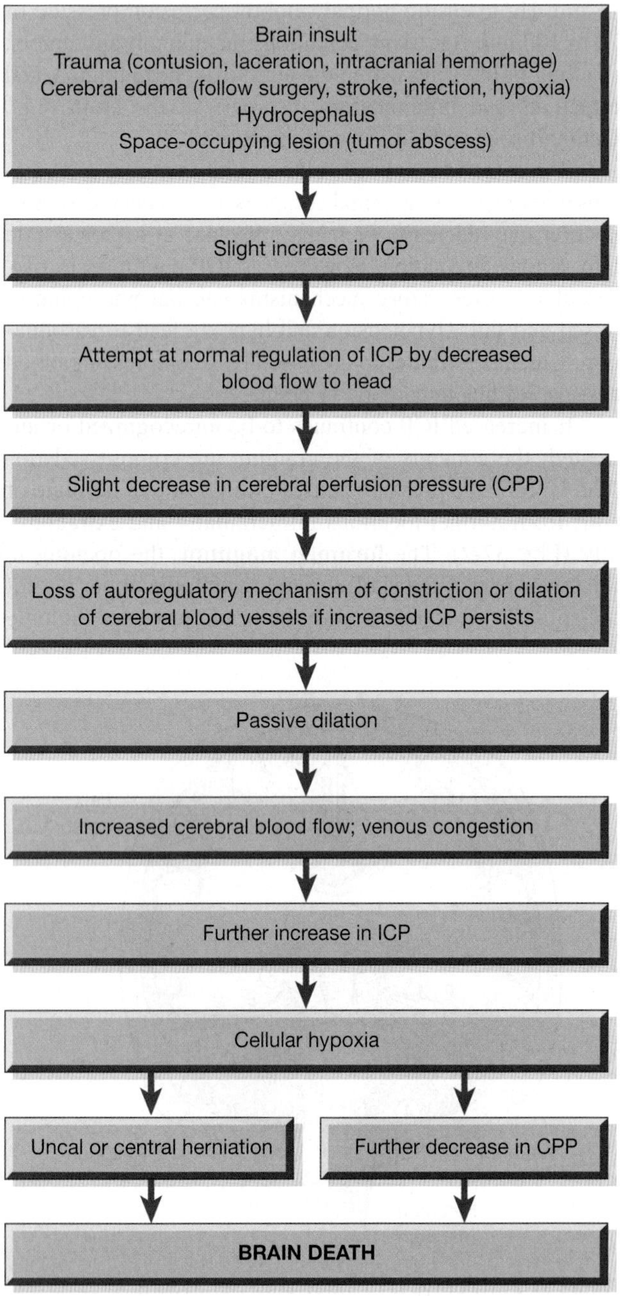

Figure 37-3 The brain compensates for increases in intracranial pressure (ICP) by autoregulation in the following ways: limiting blood flow to the head, increasing absorption or decreasing production of cerebrospinal fluid, withdrawing fluid from brain tissue and excreting it through the kidneys. When compensatory mechanisms become ineffective in reducing intracranial pressure, brain damage or death can result. (Reprinted with permission from Lippincott Williams & Wilkins. (2007). *Nurse's 5-Minute clinical consult: Diseases.* Lippincott Williams & Wilkins.)

Assessment Findings

Signs and Symptoms

The signs and symptoms of increased ICP (Box 37-1) can develop rapidly or slowly. When increased ICP develops slowly, subtle changes can be overlooked.

Decreasing level of consciousness (LOC) is one of the earliest signs of increased ICP. Clients may slip from alert and oriented to lethargic, stuporous, semicomatose, and, finally, comatose (see Chapter 36). Confusion, restlessness, and periodic disorientation often accompany decreasing LOC.

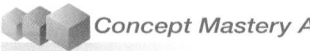

Concept Mastery Alert

Increased Intracranial Pressure

An assessment finding of lethargy in a client who has suffered multiple fractures (like the kind resulting from a motorcycle accident) is a significant indication that the client has early stages of ICP.

Headache is another symptom of increased ICP. More severe in the morning, headache increases with activities that elevate ICP, such as coughing, sneezing, or straining at stool. Rest or elevation of the head relieves the pain. A constant headache is a grave sign.

Vomiting, when associated with a neurologic condition, also suggests increasing ICP. Emesis commonly occurs without any forewarning of nausea.

Papilledema (swelling of the optic nerve) is caused by interference with venous drainage from the eye and is

BOX 37-1 Signs of Increased Intracranial Pressure

Early Signs

- Drowsiness; difficult to awaken
- Restlessness
- Confusion
- Irritability
- Glasgow Coma Scale ≥13
- Personality changes
- Sluggish or unequal pupil response
- Weakness in arms or legs
- Slow or slurred speech
- Dull headache, especially upon awakening
- Vomiting without nausea

Late Signs

- Unresponsive
- Glasgow Coma Scale ≤12
- Decreased response to painful stimuli
- Decorticate or decerebrate posturing
- Increased weakness or hemiparesis
- Dilated pupil(s)
- Seizures
- **Cushing triad**: bradycardia, elevated systolic blood pressure with wide pulse pressure, irregular breathing
- Loss of gag and corneal reflexes
- Periods of apnea

observed through examination with an ophthalmoscope. Pressure on the oculomotor nerve usually accompanies increased ICP and affects pupillary response to light. Normal pupillary response to strong light is rapid constriction. In increased ICP, the pupillary response is unequal. One pupil responds more sluggishly than the other or becomes fixed and dilated.

Changes in ICP are heralded by a body temperature that may rise or fall depending on the etiology of the increased ICP or its effect on the temperature-regulating center. This is accompanied by a series of changes in vital signs called **Cushing triad**. Cushing triad is characterized by (1) a pulse rate that increases initially but then decreases, (2) systolic BP that rises with a **widening pulse pressure** (the difference between the systolic and diastolic measurements), and (3) a respiratory rate that is irregular. Cushing triad occurs late in increased ICP. Later, **Cheyne–Stokes respirations** occur, consisting of shallow, rapid breathing followed by periods of apnea.

Decorticate or decerebrate posturing (see Chapter 36) develops spontaneously or in response to a painful stimulus when ICP is increased.

Diagnostic Findings

Diagnostic tests that determine the underlying cause of increased ICP include skull radiography, computed tomography (CT), magnetic resonance imaging (MRI), lumbar puncture, and cerebral angiography.

Medical and Surgical Management

Immediate treatment aims at decreasing ICP by relieving the cause if possible. The goals are to maintain BP, prevent hypoxia, and ensure cerebral perfusion. To maintain cerebral tissue perfusion and BP, the primary provider administers isotonic normal saline, lactated Ringer's, or hypertonic (3%) saline solutions. Hypotonic solutions and solutions containing glucose are avoided because they increase ICP. Providing supplemental oxygen to keep the arterial oxygen saturation (SaO_2) at 95% prevents hypoxia. Because increased $PaCO_2$ results in cerebral vasodilation, hyperventilation using a mechanical ventilator was used in the past to promote cerebral vasoconstriction and decrease the volume (and pressure) in the cranium. However, aggressive or prolonged hyperventilation can result in complications because it can exacerbate brain injury from cerebral vasoconstriction and cellular necrosis. The imminent possibility of brain herniation or an acute, sharp increase in ICP is the only justification for hyperventilation. Mild hyperventilation to maintain the $PaCO_2$ between 30 and 35 mm Hg can be used, but only when other measures are ineffective.

The client's head is maintained in midline at 30° of elevation to promote venous drainage of blood and CSF. Persistent hyperthermia caused by altered functioning of the hypothalamus may require measures such as administering acetaminophen (Tylenol) or applying a cooling blanket to maintain normothermia. Care must be taken to avoid hypothermia because shivering can increase ICP. The primary provider can control the client's seizures, which elevate ICP, by administering diazepam (Valium) and fosphenytoin (Cerebyx). Fosphenytoin, a parenterally administered anticonvulsant, is a *prodrug* (i.e., a drug that pharmacokinetically converts to another active compound). Fosphenytoin becomes phenytoin (Dilantin) when it is metabolized. It is indicated for short-term parenteral use when oral phenytoin is unavailable or less advantageous. The primary provider may prescribe a benzodiazepine such as midazolam (Versed) to sedate an agitated client because hyperactivity contributes to transient rises in ICP. Health care professionals currently question the use of barbiturate coma therapy because it lowers metabolic brain requirements, and the resultant sedation contributes to hypotension, pneumonia, hypoxia, and respiratory depression.

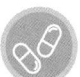

Pharmacologic Considerations

- With sudden ICP, check to see if the client has been taking an anticoagulant. Especially when head trauma is involved, a hematoma could be forming from anticoagulant therapy, causing cranial bleeding.

Monitoring devices (Fig. 37-4) are inserted to measure ICP and, in some cases, to withdraw CSF. These devices are connected to a transducer and a monitor that displays the pressure and a waveform to detect the status of ICP. Moderate elevation values range from 15 to 40 mm Hg, and high levels exceed 40 mm Hg. Although the ICP varies, a rise of 2 mm Hg from a previous measurement is cause for concern. Normal ICP below 20 mm Hg is desirable.

When the usual measures to reduce ICP are ineffective, sedation is, barbiturates and propofol are variably used with the goal of reducing elevated ICP and terminating seizure activity (Farrell & Bendo, 2018).

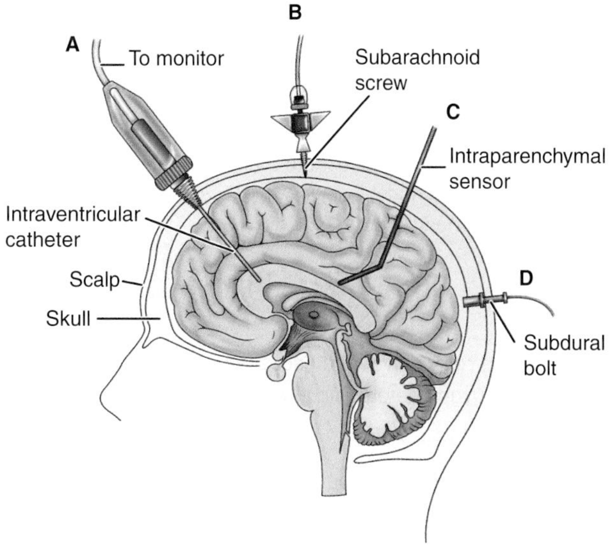

Figure 37-4 Techniques for monitoring intracranial pressure. **(A)** A fiber-optic, transducer-tipped device placed in the ventricle, **(B)** subarachnoid screw, **(C)** intraparenchymal sensor, or **(D)** subdural bolt. These devices connect to a pressure transducer and display system.

Depending on the degree and cause of increased ICP, the primary provider may order the insertion of an indwelling catheter, a nasogastric tube for gastric decompression or provision of tube feedings, a stool softener to prevent straining at stool, and a histamine antagonist such as famotidine (Pepcid) to prevent stress ulcers.

Emergency surgery is done to remove a blood clot if increased ICP results from a head injury with bleeding above or below the dura (see Chapter 39). Surgery is also performed to relieve pressure caused by a brain tumor.

Nursing Management

Nursing care of the client with increased ICP is presented in Nursing Care Plan 37-1.

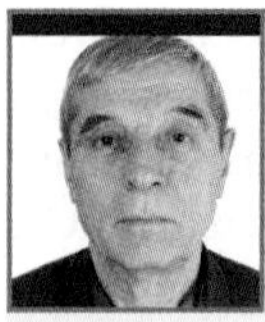

Clinical Scenario A 62-year-old man is admitted to the hospital after being evaluated in the emergency department following a fall from a ladder with a subsequent head injury while making home repairs. Upon arrival, the client was unconscious. Having regained consciousness, the client tells the assessing nurse that he has a headache and feels nauseous. There is a bruised, lacerated, and boggy area of tissue over the client's left temple. As time passes, his verbal responses are inappropriate and disorganized, and he becomes comatose. **What plan of care is appropriate during this client's extended period of recovery? See Nursing Care Plan 37-1.**

NURSING CARE PLAN 37-1 The Client With Increased Intracranial Pressure (IICP)

Assessment

- Gather from client or a witness, paramedic, or emergency medical technician the history of circumstances surrounding the altered neurologic state. Also, gather past medical history, concurrent health problems being treated, current medications, and allergy history.
- Assess LOC and vital signs.
- Assist with a head-to-toe physical examination.
- Perform complete neurologic assessments, including the Glasgow Coma Scale (GCS) or Ranchos Los Amigos Scale (see Chapter 36). Repeat these assessments every 30 to 60 minutes.
- Obtain current and daily weights and intake and output measurements.
- Study laboratory findings such as serum electrolyte and arterial blood gas levels.
- Evaluate the presence of bowel sounds and bowel elimination.
- Note evidence of any seizures.

Nursing Problem. **Altered Tissue Perfusion (Cerebral)** related to increased ICP as evidenced by decreased LOC, sluggish pupil response, papilledema, and posturing

Expected Outcomes. ICP will be less than 15 mm Hg, and the GCS will be 9 or greater.

Interventions	Rationales
Keep head of bed slightly elevated and the head in midline (straight). For clients with a basal skull fracture, keep bed flat.	*Head elevation promotes drainage of venous blood and CSF from the cranium.*
Limit movement, space essential nursing tasks, and reduce or eliminate environmental stimuli (e.g., loud noise, bright lights).	*Activities that increase BP, use of the Valsalva maneuver, impair blood circulation, or decrease oxygenation raise ICP.*
Avoid extreme hip flexion.	*It compresses femoral blood vessels and interferes with circulation.*
Keep client quiet. Change position with assistance and use a turning sheet. Avoid range-of-motion exercises until ICP approaches normal unless ordered otherwise by the primary provider.	*Activity increases ICP by raising BP. IICP predisposes to cerebral ischemia and cell damage.*
Administer reduced fluid volumes at an even rate for 24 hours. Give diuretics as prescribed; note client's response to therapy.	*Reduced fluid volume is one way to decrease the volume in the brain.*
Hyperventilate the mechanically ventilated client briefly according to medical orders.	*When carbon dioxide (CO_2) rises in the blood, cerebral blood vessels dilate as an autoregulatory mechanism to prevent cerebral ischemia; however, vasodilation increases volume in an already overloaded cranium. Hyperventilation reduces the intracerebral blood volume but is only used briefly when the client's condition is severely deteriorating.*
Suction the airway only when necessary.	*Suctioning stimulates coughing, which raises ICP.*
Give 100% oxygen before and after suctioning when it is required.	*Preoxygenation reduces the potential for hypoxemia; postoxygenation relieves any oxygen deficit. Keeping blood well oxygenated prevents cerebral ischemia.*
Keep suctioning brief, without exceeding 10–15 seconds per pass of the catheter.	*Prolonged suctioning contributes to hypoxemia and cerebral vasodilation.*
Administer a prescribed stool softener.	*It increases moisture in stool, making stool easy to pass and reducing the potential for the Valsalva maneuver.*
Ensure that a gastric tube used for decompression or nourishment remains patent.	*An obstructed gastric tube can contribute to gastric distention and vomiting. Elevated BP and ICP accompany vomiting.*
Administer prescribed medications if vomiting or persistent coughing occurs.	*Suppressing vomiting and coughing reduces the potential for IICP and cerebral ischemia.*

NURSING CARE PLAN 37-1 The Client With Increased Intracranial Pressure (IICP) (*continued*)

Evaluation of Expected Outcome

ICP returns to normal, and cerebral perfusion is maintained or restored.

Nursing Problem. **Altered Breathing Pattern and Ineffective Airway Clearance** related to diminished LOC and herniation of the brain stem secondary to increased ICP

Expected Outcomes. (1) Respiratory rate will be sufficient to maintain the oxygen saturation (SpO_2) above 90% and PaO_2 above 80 mm Hg. (2) Airway will be patent.

Interventions	Rationales
Attach a pulse oximeter to the finger, earlobe, bridge of the nose, or toe.	*A pulse oximeter measures the percentage of oxygen bound to hemoglobin.*
Insert an oral airway if client is comatose.	*It prevents the tongue from occluding the natural airway.*
Administer prescribed oxygen.	*Supplemental oxygen provides a greater percentage of oxygen than in room air.*
For mechanically ventilated clients, ensure that the ventilator delivers the prescribed tidal volume at the ordered rate.	*A mechanical ventilator supplements or controls the client's breathing.*
Suction when necessary to clear tracheal secretions or keep endotracheal tube patent.	*Artificial airways increase secretions, which reduce the volume of air within the airway.*

Evaluation of Expected Outcomes

Respirations are normal, airway is free of secretions, and lungs are clear to auscultation.

Nursing Problem. **Malnutrition Risk** related to inability to consume food orally secondary to decreased LOC or endotracheal intubation

Expected Outcome. Body weight will remain within 2 lb of preadmission.

Interventions	Rationales
Administer nutritional supplements by gastric tube or total parenteral nutrition (TPN) through a central venous catheter as medically prescribed.	*The enteral or parenteral route facilitates a means of providing essential nutrients and fluids.*

Evaluation of Expected Outcome

Nutritional needs are met with no evidence of aspiration.

Nursing Problem. **Infection Risk** related to impaired skin and tissue integrity secondary to surgery, invasive diagnostic or monitoring procedures, or original head injury

Expected Outcome. Client will be free of infection as evidenced by no fever, no purulent drainage from open areas of skin, and WBC count within normal limits.

Interventions	Rationales
Keep wounds clean and dry.	*Medical asepsis reduces transient pathogens.*
Use aseptic technique when handling any part of the intracranial monitoring device or changing a dressing applied after surgery.	*Surgical asepsis ensures that supplies and equipment are not contaminated with pathogens.*
Administer antibiotic therapy, if prescribed.	*Antibiotics inhibit the growth of or destroy susceptible microorganisms.*

Evaluation of Expected Outcome

Temperature is normal with no sign of infection.

RC of Hyperglycemia related to administration of TPN

Expected Outcome. The nurse will monitor to detect, manage, and minimize elevated blood glucose level.

Interventions	Rationales
Assess capillary blood glucose levels three times daily and at bedtime.	*Capillary blood glucose is a convenient bedside assessment that provides reliable measurements of current blood glucose level.*
Follow medical orders for administering insulin according to a sliding scale.	*Insulin helps lower blood sugar by facilitating its movement into body cells.*

Evaluation of Expected Outcome

Blood glucose level is within normal range or lowered with insulin therapy.

(*continued*)

NURSING CARE PLAN 37-1 The Client With Increased Intracranial Pressure (IICP) (*continued*)

RC of Stress Ulcer related to hyperacidity secondary to stress response

Expected Outcome. The nurse will monitor to detect, manage, and minimize the development of a peptic ulcer.

Interventions	Rationales
Check the pH of gastric secretions per shift.	*Obtaining a sample of gastric secretions and using a chemical strip for pH provide a quick means for monitoring the acidity of the stomach.*
Report a pH of less than 3.	*A pH above 3 helps to suppress the release of pepsin, which adds to the gastric pH created by hydrochloric acid.*
Administer prescribed drugs that protect the gastric mucosa, reduce histamine secretion, suppress the release of gastric secretions, or neutralize stomach acids.	*There are a variety of drugs whose mechanisms of action reduce the potential for developing a peptic ulcer.*

Evaluation of Expected Outcome

Gastric mucosa is intact.

Nursing Problem. Altered Skin Integrity Risk related to low capillary blood flow secondary to pressure and inactivity

Expected Outcome. Skin will remain intact.

Interventions	Rationales
Tilt or turn client from side to side every 2 hours.	*Maintaining intracapillary pressure above 32 mm Hg ensures that tissue can exchange oxygen and CO_2 at the cellular level.*
Avoid friction by using a lift sheet.	*Friction causes abrasions that impair skin integrity.*
Use a pressure-relieving mattress or mechanical bed for clients whose position cannot be readily changed.	*Specialty mattresses and beds are designed to intermittently reduce pressure on skin throughout the time a client is confined to bed.*
Keep skin clean and dry.	*Clean, dry skin prevents softening and erosion of epidermal cells.*

Evaluation of Expected Outcome

Skin is intact.

Nursing Diagnosis. Self-Care Deficit (total or specify type) related to diminished LOC as manifested by inability to follow directions and impaired neuromuscular function

Expected Outcome. Client's basic needs will be met.

Interventions	Rationales
Give client complete care, including bathing, oral care, nutrition, and elimination, until ICP is normal and client can resume these activities independently.	*The nurse manages needs that a client cannot perform until neurologic function returns.*

Evaluation of Expected Outcome

Basic needs are managed.

Nursing Diagnosis. Impaired Verbal Communication related to decreased LOC or endotracheal intubation as evidenced by an inability to speak

Expected Outcome. Client will communicate using body language, pantomime, or writing.

Interventions	Rationales
Look for grimacing or moaning.	*Sounds of distress are universal.*
Correct problems that may be causing discomfort, such as a wrinkled sheet or an object pressing on the skin.	*Astute assessment may determine the cause of discomfort and facilitate prompt intervention.*
Provide paper and pencil or a magic slate if client is alert but intubated.	*Written communication is an alternative to oral communication.*

Evaluation of Expected Outcome

Client communicates needs to others when conscious.

For additional suggestions for nursing management of a client undergoing surgery or who develops a neurologic deficit, see Chapter 40.

>>> *Stop, Think, and Respond 37-1*

What assessment findings suggest that ICP is increasing beyond the compensatory changes that result from autoregulation?

INFECTIOUS AND INFLAMMATORY DISORDERS OF THE NERVOUS SYSTEM

Four neurologic conditions have an infectious or inflammatory cause: meningitis, encephalitis, Guillain–Barré syndrome, and brain abscess (Fig. 37-5).

Meningitis

Meningitis is an inflammation of the meninges caused by various infectious microorganisms such as bacteria, viruses, fungi, or parasites. The inflammation often extends to the cerebral cortex. Depending on the causative organism, the client's condition may be mild and/or may rapidly become critical. Most adults with bacterial meningitis, the most serious form of meningitis, recover without permanent neurologic damage or dysfunction. When complications do occur, they are usually serious.

Pathophysiology and Etiology

The most highly contagious and potentially lethal form of meningitis is caused by either of two bacteria, meningococci (*Neisseria meningitidis*) and streptococci (*Streptococcus pneumoniae*). Meningococcal meningitis usually affects school-aged children, young adults, and people who are immunosuppressed. Viruses such as herpes simplex virus, mumps virus, and enteroviruses, which are common intestinal viruses, can cause viral meningitis, a milder form of the disease. Viral meningitis is more common in children and in older adults.

The infecting microorganisms circulate from blood and lymph to cerebral capillaries or by direct extension from infected areas such as the middle ear and the paranasal sinuses. When the pathogens arrive in the cerebral circulation, they travel to the subarachnoid space of the meninges where the inflammatory process begins. In virulent cases, cerebral edema and inappropriate secretion of antidiuretic hormone, which increases fluid volume, cause increased ICP. *Cerebral vasculitis*, inflammation of blood vessels in the brain, may be present, and cerebral blood flow may be decreased. The client may develop seizures, a brain abscess, neurologic changes, irreversible coma, and death from brain herniation. Neurologic sequelae in survivors include damage to the cranial nerves that facilitate vision and hearing.

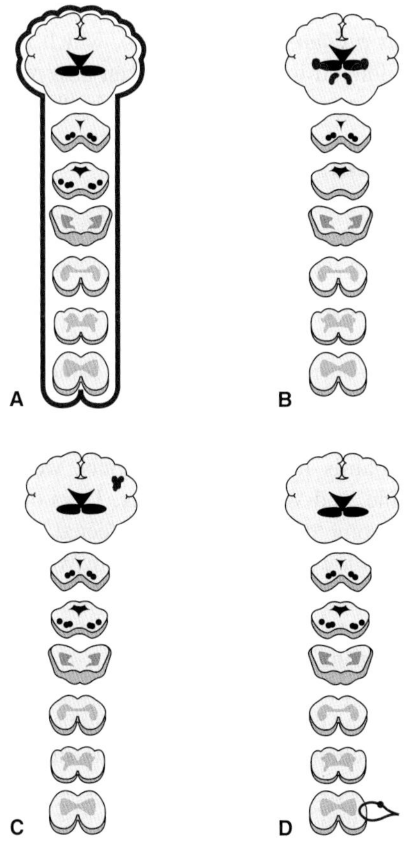

Figure 37-5 Sites of infectious and inflammatory disorders. **(A)** Meningitis, **(B)** encephalitis, **(C)** brain abscess, and **(D)** Guillain–Barré syndrome.

Assessment Findings

Signs and Symptoms

Classic symptoms include headache, fever, and **nuchal rigidity** (pain and stiffness of the neck, inability to place the chin on the chest). Nausea, vomiting, **photophobia** (aversion or sensitivity to light), restlessness, irritability, and seizures may also develop. Severe irritation of the meninges causes **opisthotonos**, an extreme hyperextension of the head and arching of the back. A positive **Kernig sign** (inability to extend the leg when the thigh is flexed on the abdomen) and a positive **Brudzinski sign** (flexion of the neck produces flexion of the knees and hips) are seen (Fig. 37-6).

The client with meningococcal meningitis may have multiple, small to large petechiae that spread over the body, giving the appearance of a rug burn. The petechiae intensify and coalesce (fuse together) to resemble purpura or ecchymoses due to a secondary disturbance in blood coagulation from thrombocytopenia or disseminated intravascular coagulation. Those with viral meningitis develop a nonspecific maculopapular rash.

Diagnostic Findings

A lumbar puncture is performed, and samples of CSF are obtained. If the meningitis is bacterial, the CSF appears cloudy. The CSF pressure is elevated, glucose concentration is decreased, protein levels are elevated, and white blood cell (WBC) and red blood cell counts are increased. Culture and sensitivity studies are performed to identify the specific causative bacteria. If meningitis is viral, the results of culture and sensitivity studies are negative. A CT scan, blood culture, complete blood cell count (CBC), and other laboratory tests are used to rule out other possible disorders.

Medical Management

Measures to manage and reduce ICP are used in the acute stage of infection. Taking precautions against diseases and

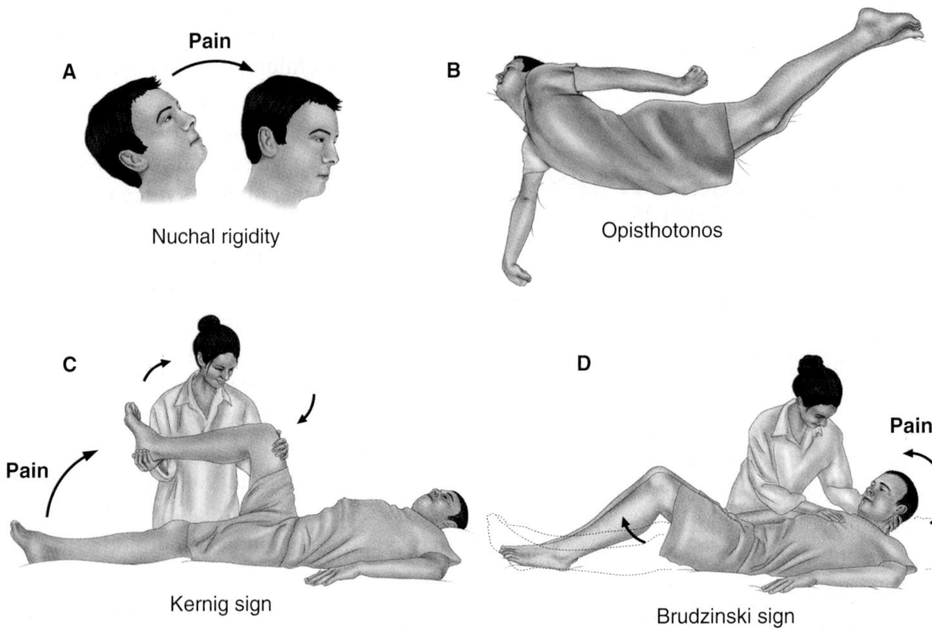

Figure 37-6 Signs of meningeal irritation. **(A)** Nuchal rigidity, **(B)** opisthotonos, **(C)** Kernig sign, and **(D)** Brudzinski sign.

hand hygiene are important in controlling the spread of infection. The local public health department is notified of all cases. Intravenous (IV) fluids and antimicrobial therapy are started immediately when bacterial meningitis is suspected. The appropriate antibiotic, usually penicillin, a cephalosporin, rifampin (Rifadin), vancomycin (Vancocin), or chloramphenicol (Chloromycetin), is determined when the causative microorganism is identified from the results of a sensitivity test. Drug therapy is continued after the acute phase of the illness to prevent recurrence. Anticonvulsants are necessary if seizures occur. Household members, contacts at daycare centers, roommates in a college dormitory, those living in the same military barracks, and anyone else directly exposed to an infected person's oral secretions are placed on one or two doses of prophylactic oral rifampin (Rifadin), ciprofloxacin (Cipro) azithromycin (Zithromax), or a single dose of intramuscular ceftriaxone (Rocephin).

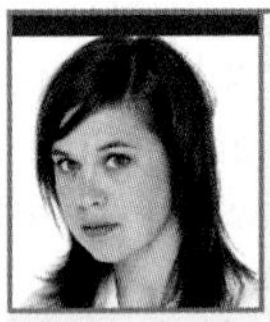

Clinical Scenario A 19-year-old college student comes to the campus health service. She tells the nurse, "I've had a headache for the past 24 hours that has become increasingly severe. I thought I might be getting the flu because I feel like I'm burning up, but it's probably something else because I've noticed a red rash on my arms. When I tried to pull a sweater over my head, I couldn't bend my neck like I've done before." **If there is a possibility that this college student has meningitis, how should the client's care be managed? If increased ICP develops, the nurse follows the care described in Nursing Care Plan 37-1.**

Many colleges and universities now recommend immunization for meningococcal meningitis (meningococcal polysaccharide vaccine [Menomune]). Immunization for *Haemophilus influenzae* type b (Hib), which is part of the series of childhood immunizations, can also reduce the acquisition of bacterial meningitis caused by that pathogen.

Encephalitis

Encephalitis is an inflammatory process affecting the CNS. It is characterized by swelling of the brain and pathologic changes in both the white and gray matter and surrounding meninges.

Pathophysiology and Etiology

Various causes of encephalitis exist, but the most common include vector-borne viral infections, complications from viral infection such as rubeola (measles), or neurotoxic effects associated with childhood vaccination. Viruses that cause encephalitis include the St. Louis, western equine, eastern equine, and West Nile viruses. Ticks or mosquitoes can transmit some of these viruses. Infected birds bitten by the common *culex* mosquito can transmit West Nile and St. Louis viruses. The virus remains in the mosquito's salivary glands, and the mosquito can inject the virus into humans and animals during blood feeding.

When encephalitis occurs, there is severe, diffuse inflammation of the brain. Nerve cell destruction can be extensive. Cerebral edema, neurologic deficits such as paralysis and speech changes, increased ICP, respiratory failure, seizure disorders, and shock can occur.

Assessment Findings

At the onset of viral encephalitis, symptoms include sudden fever, severe headache, stiff neck, vomiting, and drowsiness. During physical assessment, there may be evidence of insect bites. The client may disclose information about immunization or an activity such as recent camping that suggests possible exposure to mosquitoes, other vectors, or a neurotoxic substance. As the infection worsens, the client may develop tremors, seizures, spastic or flaccid paralysis, irritability, and muscle weakness. Lethargy, delirium, or coma develops. Incontinence and visual disturbances such as photophobia, involuntary eye movements, and double or blurred vision occur.

A lumbar puncture is performed. CSF pressure is elevated, but the fluid is clear. In some types of encephalitis, such as West Nile virus infection, blood or CSF shows a rise in immunoglobulin M (IgM) antibodies. Electroencephalography (EEG) reveals slow waveforms. The primary provider may order other diagnostic tests, such as MRI or CT scan, to rule out other etiologies of the symptoms.

Medical Management

Because no specific antiviral measure has been developed, treatment of viral encephalitis is supportive. The client's symptoms are managed with antipyretics, anticonvulsants, anti-inflammatory drugs, and analgesics.

Nursing Management

The nurse monitors vital signs and LOC frequently and compares findings with previous assessments. If urinary retention or urinary incontinence develops, the nurse consults the primary provider to discuss whether an indwelling urethral catheter is appropriate. The nurse measures fluid intake and output to detect signs of fluid volume deficit and electrolyte imbalances and assesses bowel elimination to determine if the client needs an enema or a stool softener.

Client and Family Teaching 37-1 lists measures for reducing potential bites from mosquitoes such as the *culex* species of mosquitoes that transmit West Nile virus and St. Louis encephalitis, anopheles mosquitoes that causes malaria, and the *Aedes aegypti* mosquitoes that transmit the Zika virus.

Client and Family Teaching 37-1 Measures to Control Exposure to Mosquitoes

- Pay attention to surveillance reports concerning the incidence of birds infected with West Nile virus or St. Louis virus in your community.
- Avoid being outdoors during peak mosquito biting times, such as early evening.
- Wear clothing that covers as much skin as possible when outdoors.
- Apply insect repellant containing permethrin or DEET (*N,N*-diethyl-*meta*-toluamide) to clothing and exposed skin.
- Repair or replace windows and door screens.
- Place netting around strollers and infant carriers.
- Empty outdoor items frequently that may hold standing water, such as pet dishes, birdbaths, flowerpots, and pool covers.
- Transport discarded tires to a location for waste management.
- Clear gutters of debris that may obstruct the drainage of rainwater.

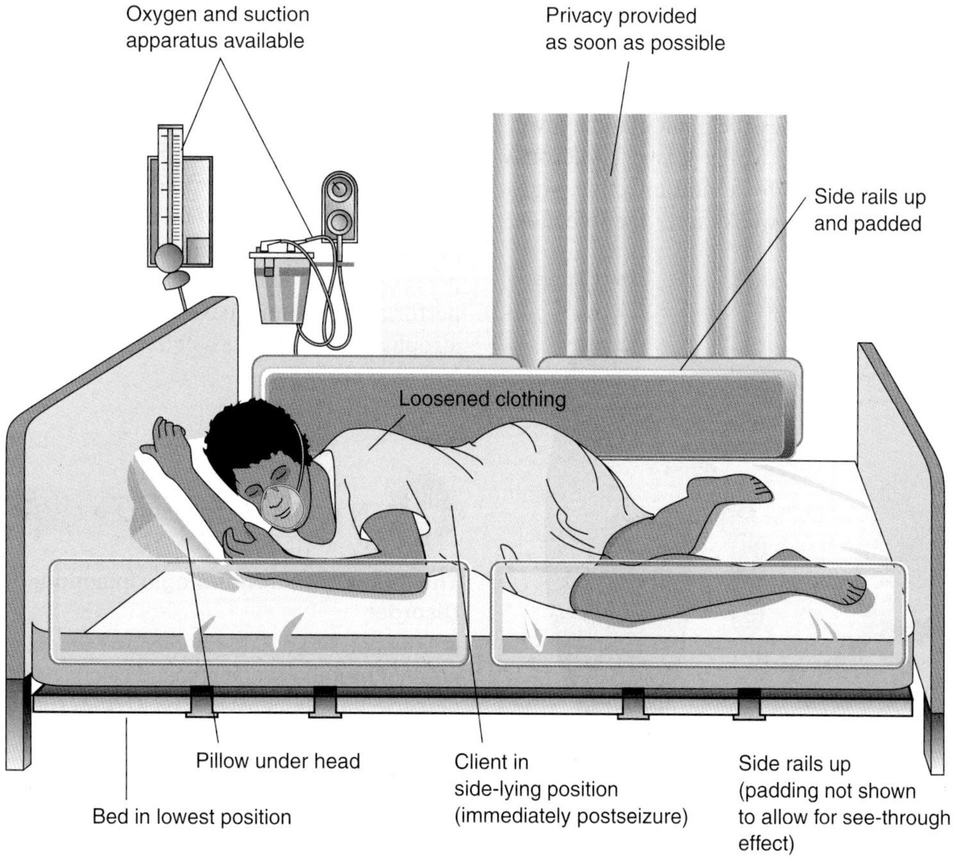

Figure 37-7 Environmental modifications for seizure precautions.

Guillain–Barré Syndrome

Guillain–Barré syndrome (acute postinfectious polyneuropathy, polyradiculoneuritis) affects the peripheral nerves and the spinal nerve roots. Most clients begin to show signs of recovery about 1 month after the progression of symptoms cease. Recovery may be slow and take 1 year or more. Death can occur from complications of immobility, such as pneumonia and infection.

Pathophysiology and Etiology

Although the exact cause of the disorder is unknown, Guillain–Barré syndrome (GBS) is believed to be an autoimmune reaction (see Chapter 34) that follows a primary disorder, especially one that is infectious. Many clients have a history of a recent viral infection, particularly of the respiratory tract. Others have a history of recent surgery or recent vaccination for a viral disease such as influenza. The syndrome also occurs in clients with malignant diseases and lupus erythematosus.

Antibodies attack the *Schwann cells* that make up the insulating myelin sheath surrounding the axons on nerves. The affected nerves become inflamed and edematous. As myelin becomes disrupted, nerve transmission becomes abnormal. Mild to severe ascending muscle weakness, tingling and numbness, or paralysis develops from the legs upward (Fig. 37-8). Overactivity or underactivity of the sympathetic or parasympathetic nervous system is evidenced by changes in BP as well as in heart rate and rhythm. Eventually, the myelin regenerates, function is restored, and recovery begins in reverse sequence from the upper body downward.

Types

Acute inflammatory demyelinating polyradiculoneuropathy (AIDP) is the most common form of GBS. Signs and symptoms include muscle weakness beginning in the lower extremities and moves upward. Miller Fisher syndrome (MFS) is thought to be triggered by a viral infection, signs and symptoms beginning 1 to 4 weeks after the infection. MFS generally begins with a weakness in the eye muscles and progresses downward.

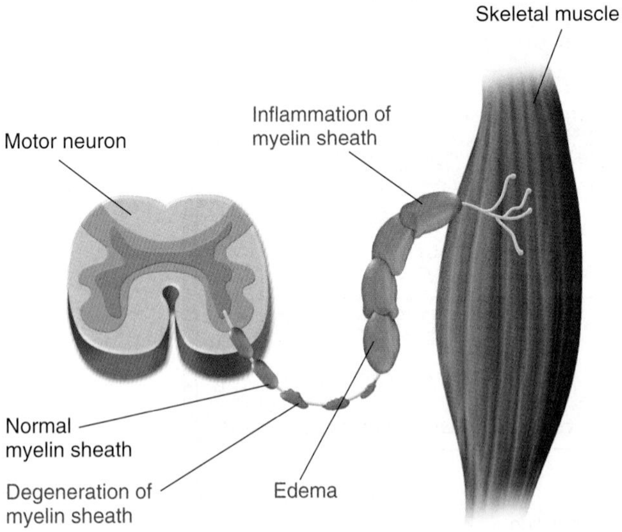

Figure 37-8 Peripheral nerve demyelination associated with Guillain–Barré syndrome. (From Anatomical Chart Co. (n.d.). *ACC atlas of pathophysiology*. Lippincott Williams & Wilkins.)

Assessment Findings

Although symptoms vary, weakness, numbness, and tingling in the arms and legs that the client may perceive as painful are often the first symptoms. The weakness is progressive and moves to upper areas of the body and affects the muscles of respiration. Paralysis may follow muscle weakness. If cranial nerve involvement develops, chewing, talking, and swallowing become difficult.

A lumbar puncture reveals elevated CSF protein levels and pressure. The results of electrophysiologic testing show marked slowing in the conduction of nerve impulses. Additional neurologic tests are performed to rule out other possible CNS disorders with similar symptoms.

Medical Management

Plasmapheresis, removal of plasma from the blood and reinfusion of the cellular components with saline, has been shown to shorten the course of the disease if performed within the first 2 weeks. Administration of IV immune globulin known as Gamimune N soon after symptoms manifest may enhance improvement. Otherwise, treatment is primarily supportive. For example, the primary provider may order gabapentin (Neurontin) or a tricyclic antidepressant such as amitriptyline (Elavil) or an opioid to relieve discomfort. If the respiratory muscles are involved, endotracheal intubation and mechanical ventilation become necessary. Difficulty chewing and swallowing necessitate the administration of IV fluids, gastric tube feedings, or total parenteral nutrition (TPN).

Nursing Management

The nurse observes the client closely for signs of respiratory distress using a spirometer to evaluate the client's ventilation capacity. To assess for pneumonia, the nurse checks vital signs and lung sounds frequently.

Because immobility incapacitates the client, the nurse provides meticulous skin care and changes the client's position every 2 hours. The nurse also helps the client perform active and passive exercises to prevent muscle atrophy. For further aspects of client care, see Nutrition Notes 37-1.

Nutrition Notes 37-1

The Client With a Neurologic Infectious/Inflammatory Disorder

- Infectious disorders often cause anorexia, altered nutrient metabolism, increased caloric needs, and a negative nitrogen balance, which may further compromise immune system functioning.
- To promote an adequate intake, small, frequent meals of nutrient- and calorie-dense foods are encouraged.
- High-protein liquid supplements can deliver a high nutrient load with a minimum amount of effort.

>>> ***Stop, Think, and Respond 37-2***

What infectious and inflammatory disorder of the nervous system that has been discussed is the easiest to prevent?

Brain Abscess

A brain abscess is a collection of purulent material in the brain. If untreated, it can be fatal.

Pathophysiology and Etiology

A brain abscess occurs from an infection in nearby structures such as the middle ear, sinuses, or teeth, or from an infection in other organs. A brain abscess can develop after intracranial surgery or head trauma. It can be secondary to such disorders as bacterial endocarditis, bacteremia, and pulmonary or abdominal infections.

A brain abscess produces neurologic changes according to its location. Because it occupies space in the cranium, increased ICP can develop. Complications include paralysis, mental deterioration, a seizure disorder, and visual disturbances.

Assessment Findings

Manifestations of a brain abscess include signs of increased ICP, fever, headache, and neurologic changes such as paralysis, seizures, muscle weakness, and lethargy.

Laboratory tests show an elevated WBC count. Analysis of CSF obtained by lumbar puncture helps confirm the diagnosis, but this procedure has a risk of herniation of the brain stem. A CT scan, MRI, and skull radiographs are safer techniques for diagnosing and locating the abscess.

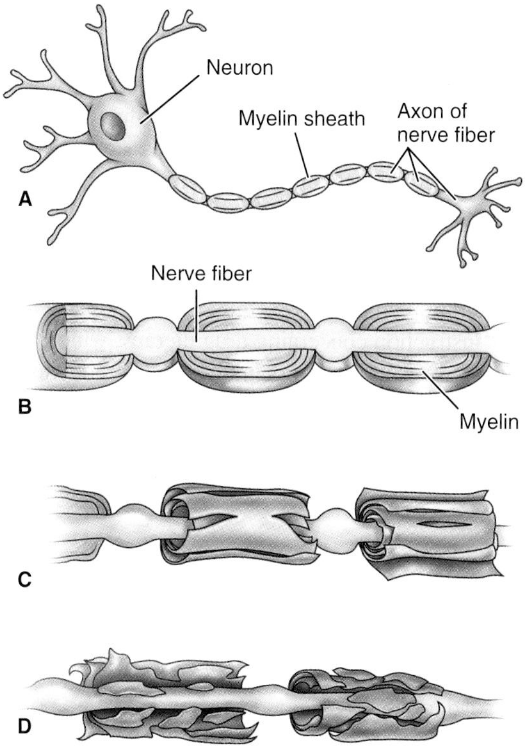

Figure 37-9 The process of demyelination. (**A**) and (**B**) depict a normal nerve cell and axon with myelin. (**C**) and (**D**) show the slow disintegration of myelin, which disrupts axon function.

Medical and Surgical Management

Antimicrobial therapy begins once the diagnosis is confirmed. A craniotomy, discussed later in this chapter, is typically performed to drain the abscess. Cerebral edema and seizures are treated with drug therapy. Additional treatment includes control of fever, mechanical ventilation, IV fluids, and nutritional support.

Nursing Management

The nurse assesses frequently for altered LOC, changes in sensory and motor functions, and signs of increased ICP, and monitors vital signs frequently. The nurse measures fluid intake and output because overhydration can lead to cerebral edema. See Nursing Care Plan 37-1 for the client with increased ICP for more detailed discussion.

NEUROMUSCULAR DISORDERS

A neuromuscular disorder involves the nervous system and indirectly affects the muscles. Some examples include multiple sclerosis (MS), myasthenia gravis, and amyotrophic lateral sclerosis (ALS)—all of which are chronic and progressively debilitating.

Multiple Sclerosis

Multiple sclerosis is a chronic, progressive disease of the peripheral nerves. Its onset is in young adulthood and early middle age. The incidence is greatest between 20 and 40 years of age, and it affects men and women approximately equally. MS is more common in northern temperate zones than in warm climates.

Pathophysiology and Etiology

MS is considered an autoimmune disorder that researchers believe is triggered by defective genes. Studies show that it is associated with an inflammation that affects genes involved in controlling the immune system (Jha, 2011; Rettner, 2016). Other research has shown a link between a distorted gene that causes vitamin D deficiency and MS (PR Newswire, 2012).

MS is characterized as a **demyelinating disease** because it causes permanent degeneration and destruction of myelin. Myelin acts as an insulator, enabling nerve impulses to pass along a nerve fiber. Loss of myelin and subsequent degeneration and atrophy of nerve axons interrupt transmission of impulses along these fibers (Fig. 37-9).

Many clients experience gradual and continuous worsening of their symptoms. A few have the disease in a mild form and do not experience increased severity of symptoms. For some, the symptoms subside during early phases of the illness (remission), and the client seems healthy for several months or even years. However, with each reappearance (exacerbation), the symptoms become more severe and last longer. Infections and emotional upsets precipitate exacerbations. Some people live a long time with MS, and survival for 20 years after the diagnosis is not unusual.

As the disease progresses, many complications such as pressure ulcers, cachexia, deformities, and contractures develop. Pneumonia, brought about by limited activity, shallow breathing, and general debility, is often the immediate cause of death.

Assessment Findings

Signs and Symptoms

Many clients first dismiss minor symptoms as a result of fatigue or strain. When they no longer can ignore symptoms, clients with MS report blurred vision, **diplopia** (double vision), **nystagmus** (involuntary movement of the eyeball), weakness, clumsiness, and numbness and tingling of an arm or a leg. An intention tremor and slurred, hesitant speech (scanning speech) may develop. Mood swings (emotional lability) are common.

Weakness of an arm or a leg progresses to ataxia (motor incoordination) or paraplegia (paralysis of both legs). Occasional bowel and bladder incontinence lead to total incontinence. Slight visual disturbances end in blindness. The illness impairs intellectual functioning late in its course. Loss of memory, difficulty concentrating, and impaired judgment occur.

Diagnostic Findings

Early diagnosis is difficult because symptoms are vague and, in some cases, temporary. A lumbar puncture and CSF analysis reveal an increased WBC count. Electrophoresis of the CSF, a technique for electrically separating and identifying proteins, demonstrates abnormal immunoglobulin G bands, described as oligoclonal bands. The bands appear separated rather than homogeneous, which is the normal finding. A CT scan and MRI may or may not disclose lesions in the brain's white matter.

Medical Management

There is no cure for MS, nor is there any single treatment that relieves all symptoms. The primary aim of treatment is to keep the client functional as long as possible. Current research for promoting nerve regeneration exists in four areas: (1) stimulating nearby oligodendrocytes (cells with projections that continue as myelin sheaths) to move to the diseased neurons and replace the damaged myelin, (2) identifying and reversing the inhibitors of remyelination, (3) producing growth factors that stimulate natural myelin repair, and (4) recruiting replacement cells such as cord blood and fetal stem cells to become myelin-producing cells (National Multiple Sclerosis Society, 2016a).

The first disease-modifying drugs that were used to treat MS were interferons, such as interferon beta-1a (Avonex), interferon beta-1b (Betaseron), and fingolimod (Gilenya). However, additional new drugs classified as immunosuppressives rather than immunomodulators, such as alemtuzumab (Lemtrada) and natalizumab (Tysabri), and an oral drug, teriflunomide (Aubagio), have been developed recently to inhibit neurodegeneration.

Another approach used in the management of MS is drug therapy with glatiramer acetate (Copaxone). This noninterferon/nonsteroidal medication reduces the frequency of exacerbations of MS. Glatiramer acetate changes harmful inflammatory T cells that destroy myelin into protective T cells that suppress myelin depletion. All drugs for MS have been shown to reduce relapse rates by 28% to 68% (National Multiple Sclerosis Society, 2016b).

Other drugs that may be used to treat symptoms that accompany MS include baclofen (Lioresal) and dantrolene (Dantrium) for muscle spasticity and rigidity, antibiotics for infection, and tranquilizers to alleviate mood swings. Oxybutynin (Ditropan) and botulinum toxin (Botox) are used to manage urinary incontinence, and bethanechol (Urecholine) is used to relieve urinary retention. The anti-inflammatory action of corticosteroids relieves symptoms and hastens remissions.

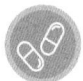

Pharmacologic Considerations

- There are serious issues with the following newer MS agents:
  - Teriflunomide (Aubagio) can cause birth defects. Women should be tested for pregnancy before starting this drug and use effective birth control while taking the drug. Men whose partners plan to become pregnant should not use this drug either.
  - Fingolimod (Gilenva) may cause progressive multifocal leukoencephalopathy (a rare but serious brain infection).

Nursing Management

The nurse assesses the client's current physical and emotional status to determine any new developments or changes in previously assessed conditions. The nurse identifies whether the client has visual problems and emphasizes that these may diminish when a remission occurs. The nurse also listens to the client's speech, which may be slurred and difficult to understand and recommends using a language board or other assistive device if communication is severely affected. Adaptive devices for self-care and feeding may be helpful if the client has hand tremors; the client's weight should be assessed regularly to ensure that there is no significant weight loss. Eventually, the client's food may require blenderization if swallowing is impaired (Nutrition Notes 37-2).

If ambulation is impaired, the client may find a wheelchair or other device to be useful temporarily. Safety is a real issue for clients as their mobility becomes less stable. The nurse may identify techniques for managing constipation with high-fiber food and fluids. Bladder elimination may be controlled with intermittent catheterization, inserting an indwelling catheter, or creation of a cystostomy. Skin care and position changes are implemented to avoid pressure sores. The nurse provides instruction concerning drug therapy, which often facilitates a remission of unknown duration or reduction in the rate of relapse. The nurse or family may be referred to a social

Nutrition Notes 37-2

The Client With a Neuromuscular Disorder

- Clients with muscle wasting benefit from an increased protein intake; commercial supplements (e.g., thickened liquids, fortified puddings, fortified gelatins) are tasty and easy options.
- Semisolid foods such as puddings and mashed potatoes are easier to swallow than thin liquids or a regular diet.
- Gastrostomy feedings are usually the best route for clients who require long-term enteral nutritional support.

worker to determine if the client qualifies for Social Security disability benefits. For additional nursing management, refer to the Nursing Process for the Client With a Chronic Neuromuscular Disorder, which appears later in this chapter.

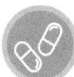

Pharmacologic Considerations

- All the disease-modifying drugs can decrease immune cells and infection protection. Therefore, be aware of increased risk for acquired infections, especially if the client is catheterized.

Myasthenia Gravis

Myasthenia gravis is a neuromuscular disorder characterized by severe weakness of one or more groups of skeletal muscles. Myasthenia gravis is more common in women, but it can affect both genders. The onset of the illness generally occurs during the young adult years.

Pathophysiology and Etiology

Although its exact cause is unknown, the disease is believed to be autoimmune in nature. It develops when antibodies, perhaps produced by the thymus gland, bind to and degrade acetylcholine receptors on the surface of skeletal muscles (Fig. 37-10). The outcome is extreme muscle weakness during activity. Strength is restored with rest.

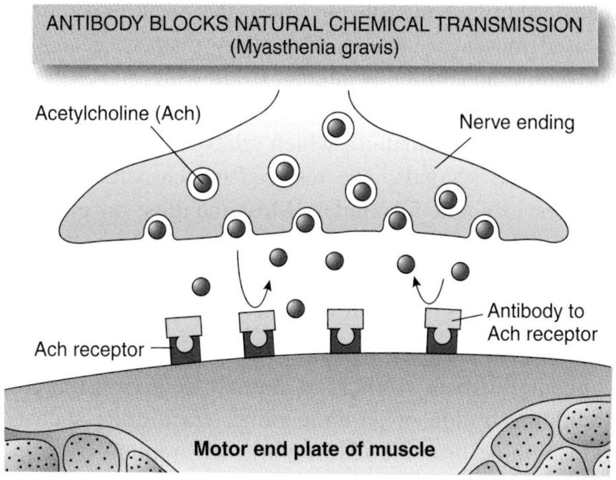

Figure 37-10 Inhibition of synaptic transmission of acetylcholine (Ach) in myasthenia gravis leads to profound muscle weakness. (Reprinted with permission from Rubin, E., Strayer, D. S., (Eds.). (2014). *Rubin's pathology: Clinicopathologic foundations of medicine* (7th ed.). Wolters Kluwer.)

Assessment Findings

Muscle weakness varies depending on the muscles affected. The most common manifestations are **ptosis** (drooping) of the eyelids (Fig. 37-11), difficulty chewing and swallowing, diplopia, voice weakness, masklike facial expression, and weakness of the extremities. The respiratory system is also

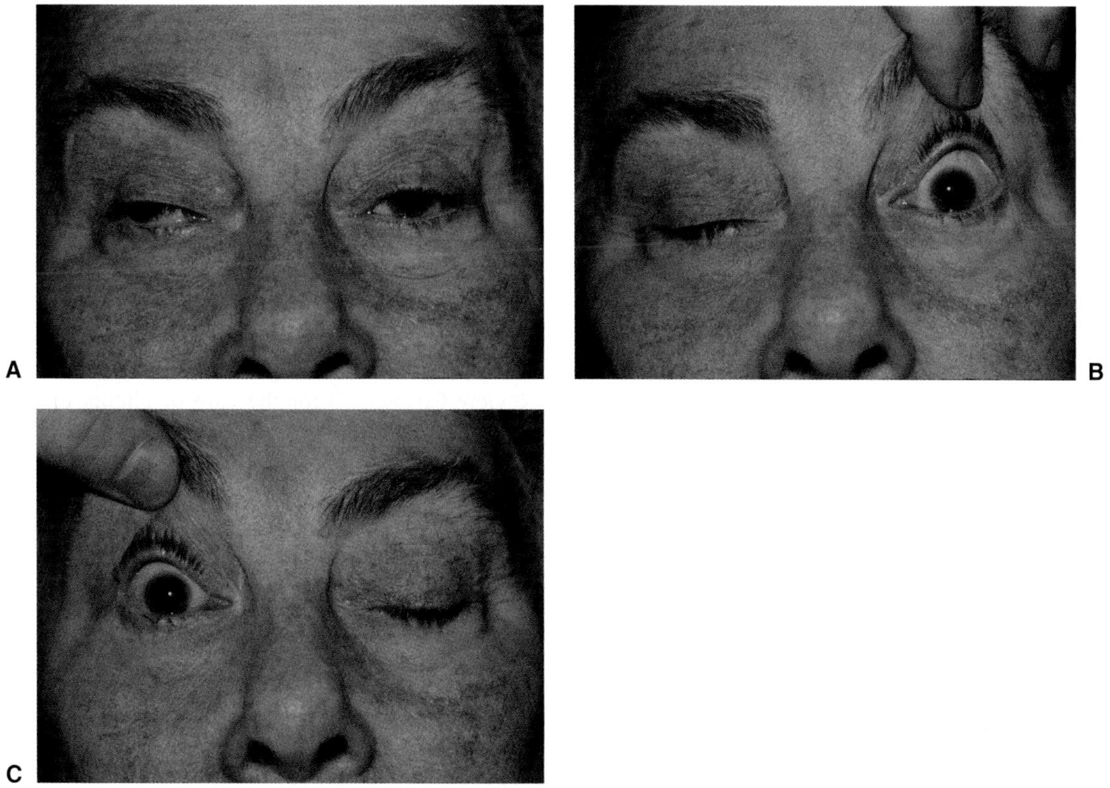

Figure 37-11 Enhancement of ptosis in a 61-year-old woman with myasthenia gravis. **(A)** The client has bilateral ptosis. Note also a right exotropia. **(B)** When the left eyelid is manually elevated, the right ptosis increases. **(C)** When the right eyelid is manually elevated, the left ptosis increases. (Reprinted with permission from Miller, N. R., Subramanian, P. S., & Patel, V. R. (2021). *Walsh and Hoyt's clinical neuro-ophthalmology: The essentials* (4th ed.). Wolters Kluwer.)

affected. During a myasthenic crisis, the client experiences increased muscle weakness, respiratory distress, decreased tidal volume, and difficulty talking, swallowing, and chewing.

Diagnostic confirmation is made by IV administration of edrophonium (Tensilon), which relieves muscular weakness in a few seconds. The restored muscle strength then dissipates in about 5 minutes. Most manifest an elevated acetylcholine receptor antibody titer. Chest radiography may show an enlargement of the thymus (thymoma). Electromyography measures the electrical potential of muscles.

Medical and Surgical Management

Treatment involves facilitating normal neurotransmission with administration of an anticholinesterase drug, such as pyridostigmine bromide (Mestinon), neostigmine (Prostigmin), or ambenonium chloride (Mytelase). The therapeutic effect prolongs the action of acetylcholine, which sustains muscle contraction. The dose of the drug is adjusted according to the client's response to therapy.

Other treatments include surgical removal of the thymus gland, prednisone or another type of immunosuppressant such as azathioprine (Imuran), and plasmapheresis three times a week for clients who do not respond to other methods of therapy. If myasthenic crisis with severe respiratory distress occurs, the client requires intubation and mechanical ventilation.

Nursing Management

The nurse provides periods of rest for the client to promote restoration of strength. In addition, the nurse supports ventilation by elevating the head of the bed and suctioning secretions that cause difficulty in swallowing for the client. The nurse also makes an effort to understand the client's efforts at communication during periods when the disease compromises intelligible speaking. The nurse demonstrates patience and empathy to help the client deal with changes in appearance, function, and lifestyle. The effects of drug therapy are observed, especially when first initiated or at times of stress. The nurse must administer medications at the exact intervals ordered to maintain therapeutic blood levels and prevent symptoms from returning. They observe for signs of drug overdose, such as abdominal cramps, clenched jaws, and muscle rigidity, which indicate that the dose is excessive. For more information, see Nursing Process for the Client with a Chronic Neuromuscular Disorder.

Amyotrophic Lateral Sclerosis

Amyotrophic lateral sclerosis (ALS), also known as *Lou Gehrig disease*, is a progressive and fatal neurologic disorder. The disease is more common in men than in women.

Pathophysiology and Etiology

The cause of ALS is unknown. The disease is characterized by degeneration of the motor neurons of the spinal cord and brain stem, which results in muscle weakness and wasting.

Assessment Findings

Progressive muscle weakness and wasting of the arms, legs, and trunk develop. The client experiences episodes of muscle **fasciculations** (twitching). If ALS affects the brain stem, speaking and swallowing become difficult. The client may display periods of inappropriate laughter and crying. Respiratory failure and total paralysis are seen in the terminal stage.

The disorder is difficult to diagnose in the early stages because no specific diagnostic tests are available for this disease. Electromyography validates weakness in the affected muscles.

Medical Management

There is no specific treatment, and death occurs several years after diagnosis in many cases. The client is encouraged to remain active as long as possible. Death usually results from respiratory arrest or overwhelming respiratory infection. Mechanical ventilation is necessary when ALS affects the muscles of respiration.

Clients are usually treated with riluzole (Rilutek), which slows the progression of ALS and delays the need for a tracheostomy. Trials are underway using stem cells. NurOwn is a proposed stem-cell-based treatment. "The therapy focuses on the cellular support system around a person with ALS' motor neurons. It aims to slow disease progression by replacing the damaged system with an enhanced one. Participants enrolled in NurOwn trials have their own stem cells harvested. These stem cells are then programmed to secrete neurotrophic factors (NTFs), aimed at promoting growth and survival of nerve cells when returned to the client's spinal cord" (Treatment and ALS Drugs, 2020).

Nursing Management

The nurse performs a comprehensive assessment and develops a plan of care on the basis of the client's identified problems. During the early stages of ALS, the nurse provides assistance with walking, bathing, shaving, and dressing. As ALS progresses, the client becomes totally dependent on the family or health care providers for care. The nurse teaches family members required skills, such as suctioning techniques, how to administer tube feedings, and catheter care. Client and Family Teaching 37-2 provides more information, as does Nursing Process for the Client With a Chronic Neuromuscular Disorder. Additional discussion on caring for clients with a neurologic deficit is covered in Chapter 40. Review Chapter 10 for the care of clients in the terminal phase of diseases.

Client and Family Teaching 37-2
Amyotrophic Lateral Sclerosis

The nurse reviews the following components with the client and family:

- Medication schedule, adverse effects of medications
- Dietary and feeding suggestions
- Agencies that can help with or give home care
- Sources of financial assistance
- Exercises to prevent muscle atrophy
- Positioning and good skin care
- Techniques for preventing skin breakdown

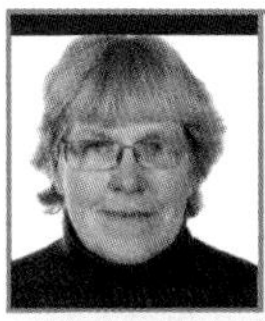

Clinical Scenario A 54-year-old woman tells the nurse, "I have been having trouble doing things I've always been able to do before, such as opening jars of food, holding onto an iron, or walking across the room. I seem to be weaker than I have ever been. Sometimes I choke on food." **If this client has a progressive neuromuscular disorder like ALS, what nursing measures are appropriate? See the following Nursing Process section.**

NURSING PROCESS FOR THE CLIENT WITH A CHRONIC NEUROMUSCULAR DISORDER

Assessment

Perform a thorough neurologic assessment. Evaluate pulmonary function, including respiratory rate, depth, and lung sounds, to determine the client's ability to ventilate. To detect early signs of infection, take the client's temperature regularly. Note the client's ability to chew and swallow effectively and observe for drooling, choking when swallowing liquids, and regurgitating fluids through the nose. Assess muscle strength and coordination as well as the client's response to physical activity. Measure intake and output to evaluate fluid status. Monitor the client's elimination patterns. As data accumulate, analyze the trends using the initial baseline for comparisons. In addition, monitor the client's and caregivers' ability to cope with the progressively debilitating nature of the disorder.

Diagnosis, Planning, and Interventions

Altered Breathing Pattern: Related to weakening of the muscles for respiration
Expected Outcome: Ventilation will be sufficient to maintain the SpO_2 above 90% and PaO_2 above 80 mm Hg.

- Place client in Fowler position and support the arms on pillows. *An upright position with the arms supported facilitates maximum chest expansion.*
- Eliminate foods that form intestinal gas or promote the expulsion of gas with a rectal tube. *Intestinal gas arises in the abdomen and places pressure on the diaphragm, which limits the volume of air that the client can inhale.*
- Encourage client to deep breathe several times an hour. *Frequent deep breaths increase tidal volumes, fill alveoli with air, and enhance gas exchange.*
- Notify the primary provider immediately if the client experiences inadequate ventilation. *Breathing is essential for life; medical interventions may be necessary.*

Ineffective Airway Clearance Risk: Related to weak or ineffective cough; **Impaired Swallowing, Risk for Imbalanced Nutrition (Less Than Body Requires), and Aspiration:** Related to muscular weakness
Expected Outcomes: (1) Airway will be patent. (2) Client will swallow food and fluids without aspiration. (3) Nutritional needs will be met.

- Help client to cough and raise respiratory secretions. *Coughing is a natural protective mechanism for clearing the airway.*
- Suction the oral cavity and airway. *If coughing is ineffective, applying negative pressure with a suction catheter can help clear secretions from the airway.*
- Offer liquids frequently in small amounts. *The client may be able to manage small volumes of liquids, but large volumes increase the risk for aspiration.*
- Consult with the dietitian on techniques for modifying the texture and consistency of foods. *Clients can best swallow smooth foods with texture. Commercial substances are available to thicken liquids to promote swallowing.*
- Provide rest before meals. *The client is more likely to have optimum energy to chew and swallow after rest. Fatigue interferes with attention and coordination.*
- Help client to sit upright when eating. *Sitting is the natural position for eating. It promotes movement of food from the mouth to the esophagus and stomach and reduces the potential for aspiration.*
- Place food in the posterior of the client's mouth. Flex the client's chin toward the chest when swallowing to facilitate passage of food into the esophagus. *Locating food posteriorly facilitates swallowing. Flexing the chin diverts food into the esophagus rather than the airway.*
- Feed client slowly. Wait to place more food in the client's mouth until they have swallowed the previous bolus. *Rushing or overloading the client's mouth increases the risk for airway obstruction or aspiration.*
- Consult with the primary provider about a plan for tube feedings or TPN. *These forms of nourishment may be necessary if oral nutritional intake becomes inadequate or dangerous.*

Impaired Physical Mobility, Bathing/Hygiene ADL Deficit, Feeding ADL Deficit, and Altered Skin Integrity Risk: Related to diminished muscle strength and inactivity
Expected Outcomes: (1) Client will be mobile and use muscles to the maximum extent possible. (2) Basic needs will be met. (3) Skin will remain intact.

- Encourage client to participate in self-care. *Attending to personal needs fosters a positive self-image.*
- Provide rest between bathing, shaving, performing oral care, eating, ambulating, toileting, and participating in diversional activities. *Rest provides time to recover from an activity. It builds stamina and endurance to proceed with additional tasks.*
- Complete whatever tasks the client cannot perform. *The nurse takes over further efforts at self-care when the client becomes fatigued or weak.*
- Change body position every 2 hours. *Changing position relieves pressure on capillaries that traverse over bony prominences. Relief of pressure reduces the potential for skin breakdown.*

(continued)

NURSING PROCESS FOR THE CLIENT WITH A CHRONIC NEUROMUSCULAR DISORDER (continued)

- Perform range-of-motion (ROM) exercises every 8 hours. *ROM exercises promote joint flexibility and muscle tone. They supplement or complement musculoskeletal activities the client actively performs.*
- Use a footboard and trochanter rolls to promote a neutral body position. *A neutral position keeps the body in good alignment and reduces the potential for contractures.*
- Consult with a physical or occupational therapist on techniques to facilitate client's independence and self-care. *They are experts in maintaining and regaining functional activities.*
- Use pressure-relieving devices when client is in bed or a wheelchair. *Relieving pressure prevents skin breakdown.*
- Keep bed dry and free of wrinkles. *Moisture softens the epidermis, making it vulnerable to breaking down. Wrinkles create pressure that interferes with blood circulation to cells and tissues.*
- Wash and dry the skin well. *Clean, dry skin decreases risk factors that can alter its integrity.*

Constipation: Related to inactivity and abdominal muscle weakness;
Functional Urinary Incontinence (specify type, such as total, functional, or reflex): Related to neuromuscular degeneration
Expected Outcomes: (1) Stool will be soft, and bowel elimination will occur at least every 3 days. (2) Urine elimination will be controlled.

- Consult with the primary provider about a regularly prescribed stool softener, bulk-forming laxative, or suppository. *Medications facilitate bowel elimination through various physical and chemical mechanisms.*
- Include soft fruit or fruit puree in the daily menu. *Fruits are a source of fructose; sugar (fructose) is a natural laxative. Fiber adds bulk to the stool and attracts moisture, making the stool softer and easier to pass.*
- Assist client to move as much as possible. *Activity promotes peristalsis, which propels stool toward the rectum.*
- Place client on a toilet or commode after meals, especially breakfast, or near the time of the client's usual bowel movement. *The gastrocolic reflex is more active after a meal. Most people have a bowel movement at about the same time each day.*
- Help client select clothing that facilitates toileting. *Clients are less likely to be incontinent if they can manipulate clothing to facilitate using a toilet or commode.*
- Assist client to the toilet regularly and frequently. *Clients can maintain continence if they receive some assistance getting to the bathroom and using toilet facilities.*
- Help client use incontinence garments or consult with the primary provider when client needs an indwelling or external catheter. *When efforts to maintain continence have been exhausted, measures to unobtrusively collect urine can maintain the client's dignity and reduce the potential for skin breakdown.*

Coping Impairment: Related to feelings of helplessness secondary to chronic illness
Expected Outcome: Client will cope effectively with situational stressors.

- Suggest joining a support group of people with a similar disorder or subscribing to the support group's newsletter. *Knowing that others experience similar problems facilitates coping. Clients acquire new coping strategies when others share their problem-solving approaches in person or in written communications.*
- Encourage client to express feelings. *Expressing frustration and other emotions relieves the client's personal emotional burden and fosters support.*
- Provide opportunities in which the client can make choices. *Making choices promotes a feeling of control, which fosters the ability to cope.*
- Facilitate client's network of social support, such as with family, neighbors, coworkers, and church members, through personal visits, telephone conversations, cards, and letters. *A network of supportive others decreases the burden of coping with an illness as an isolated individual.*
- Provide diversional activities that foster feelings of personal accomplishment. *Feeling useful, purposeful, and capable helps a client persevere in coping with adversity.*

Caregiver Fatigue: Related to unrelenting responsibility for client's care
Expected Outcome: Primary caregiver will cope with long-term care of client.

- Listen empathetically while caregiver expresses feelings about caring for the client. *Caregiver is likely to feel less guilty if they feel comfortable discussing the stressors involved with someone other than the client or another family member.*
- Help caregiver develop a list of surrogates who may provide regular periods of relief. *The caregiver's dedication will be prolonged if they experience intermittent periods when total responsibility is relieved.*
- Give caregivers permission to meet their own needs. *Unless encouraged to do so, caregivers suppress their own needs in deference to those for whom they care.*
- Identify available community resources and offer to facilitate a referral. *The caregiver may be unaware of service organizations whose missions are to provide help and support to clients and caregivers with particular disorders.*

Evaluation of Expected Outcomes

Respirations are of normal rate and depth. The airway is clear, and breathing is effortless. Nutrition is adequate to maintain body weight. The client regains mobility and attends to activities of daily living (ADLs) with minimal or no assistance. Skin is intact with no evidence of breakdown. Bowel elimination is regular; urinary incontinence is minimized or controlled. The client demonstrates effective coping skills. The caregiver continues their responsibilities but implements a plan for periodic relief or assistance.

CRANIAL NERVE DISORDERS

Trigeminal Neuralgia (Tic Douloureux)

Trigeminal neuralgia is a painful condition that involves the fifth cranial nerve (the trigeminal nerve or CN V), which has three major branches: mandibular, maxillary, and ophthalmic (Fig. 37-12). This sensory and motor nerve is important to chewing, facial movement, and sensation.

Pathophysiology and Etiology

The cause of the disorder is unknown. It has been suggested that it is related to compression of the trigeminal nerve root. For reasons not fully understood, the client experiences **neuralgia** (nerve pain) in one or more branches of the trigeminal nerve. The slightest stimulus (e.g., vibration of music, passing breeze, temperature change) over trigger points (areas that provoke the pain) can initiate an attack. The forehead over the eyebrow is a common trigger point when the ophthalmic branch of the nerve is affected.

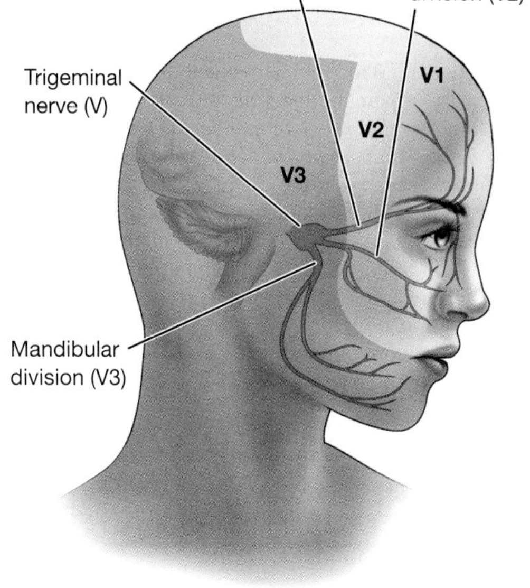

Figure 37-12 Areas innervated by the three branches of the trigeminal nerve. These are the areas that become painful in trigeminal neuralgia.

Assessment Findings

The client describes the pain as sudden, severe, and burning. The pain ends as quickly as it begins, usually lasting a few seconds to several minutes. The cycle repeats many times each day. During a spasm, the face twitches and the eyes tear.

Skull radiography, MRI, or CT are performed to rule out other pathologies, such as a brain tumor and intracranial bleeding. Ultimately, the diagnosis is based on the symptoms.

Medical Management

Medical treatment is primarily supportive and symptomatic rather than curative. Opioids are necessary. Anticonvulsants such as phenytoin (Dilantin) and carbamazepine (Tegretol) are used to reduce pain, but this approach is not always successful. The client is referred to a dentist because correction of dental malocclusion has relieved some cases of trigeminal neuralgia.

Surgical Management

If medical management is unsatisfactory, surgical intervention is an option. Surgical division of the sensory root of the trigeminal nerve provides permanent relief; however, some permanent loss of sensation accompanies this procedure. If the mandibular branch is severed, eating becomes a problem. The client may bite the tongue without realizing it, food may get caught in the mouth, and the jaw deviates toward the operative side. Until the client adjusts to the altered sensation, swallowing is difficult.

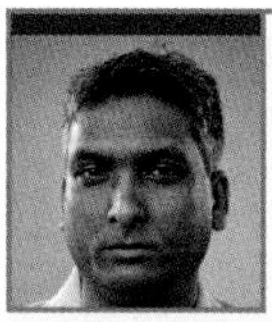

Clinical Scenario A 48-year-old man has been referred for a medical examination by his dentist whom the client consulted because of intermittent severe left facial pain. The pain is intensified when the client chews food and brushes his teeth. He tells the nurse, "The pain is getting progressively worse and it's hard to enjoy life. I don't even want to eat anymore." **How can the nurse help the client cope with his disorder? See the following Nursing Process section.**

NURSING PROCESS FOR THE CLIENT WITH TRIGEMINAL NEURALGIA

Assessment

Obtain a complete history and then carefully and gently examine the affected area. Ask the client to identify the location, pattern, and events associated with pain and document the information. Inspect the oral cavity for signs of injury. Weigh the client and assess the client's ability to eat food.

Diagnosis, Planning, and Interventions

Acute Pain: Related to stimulation over the trigeminal nerve as evidenced by client's description of localized discomfort
Expected Outcome: Pain will be relieved or reduced to a tolerable level.

(continued)

NURSING PROCESS FOR THE CLIENT WITH TRIGEMINAL NEURALGIA (continued)

- Use a scale from 0 to 10 to help client quantify the severity and intensity of pain, both before and after nursing intervention. *Using a scaled range of numbers is the standard for assessing pain. Pain is assessed before and at least 30 minutes after a nursing intervention.*
- Ask at what level the client can tolerate pain. *Pain may not be totally relieved, but asking the client to identify their tolerance level provides a realistic goal for achievement.*
- Administer prescribed drugs. *Medications relieve pain by various mechanisms.*
- Observe and record client's response. *If an intervention does not reduce pain to the client's level of tolerance, the nurse pursues additional measures and collaborates with the primary provider when nursing measures are unsuccessful.*
- Avoid drafts in the room. *Even slight stimulation of the trigeminal nerve can trigger pain.*
- Place a sign on the client's bed stating not to jar the bed or touch client's face in any way. *Sudden, unexpected movement can trigger pain.*
- Advise client to use protective measures such as shielding the face from wind and cold and avoiding shaving and situations or activities that cause pain. *The client can implement lifestyle changes to reduce or prevent pain from recurring* (Client and Family Teaching 37-3).

Evaluation of Expected Outcomes

Pain is alleviated or reduced to a level such that the client can continue functioning. The client cooperates with measures to avoid stimuli that trigger episodes of pain.

Client and Family Teaching 37-3 Trigeminal Neuralgia

The nurse instructs the client as follows:

- Inspect the mouth daily for breaks in the mucous membrane.
- Take small sips or bites of food and concentrate on chewing and swallowing if surgery has been performed.
- Chew on the opposite side.
- Avoid eating hot foods.
- Use mouth rinses after eating.
- Keep regular dental appointments because the warning pain of a cavity, abscess, or other dental problem may be mistaken for neuralgia.

Bell Palsy

Bell palsy involves the seventh cranial nerve (CN VII) that originates in the pons. At the location where the nerve exits the cranium, the nerve branches bilaterally into smaller fibers that supply the muscles for facial movement.

Pathophysiology and Etiology

The cause of Bell palsy is unknown, but a viral link is suspected. Inflammation occurs around one of the paired facial nerves, blocking motor impulses to muscles on one side of the face. Inflammation or ischemia leads to impaired neuromuscular function, which results in unilateral weakness and paralysis of facial muscles of the eyelids, cheek, and lip (Fig. 37-13). Most clients who recover begin to show improvement in a few weeks. Those whose paralysis is permanent fail to show improvement after 3 months or more.

Assessment Findings

Symptoms develop in a few hours or over 1 to 2 days. Facial pain, pain behind the ear, numbness, diminished blink reflex, ptosis of the eyelid, and tearing on the affected side occur. Speaking and chewing become difficult.

There are no specific diagnostic tests for this disorder; diagnosis is based on symptoms and visual examination of the face. Electromyography (EMG) is used to determine if

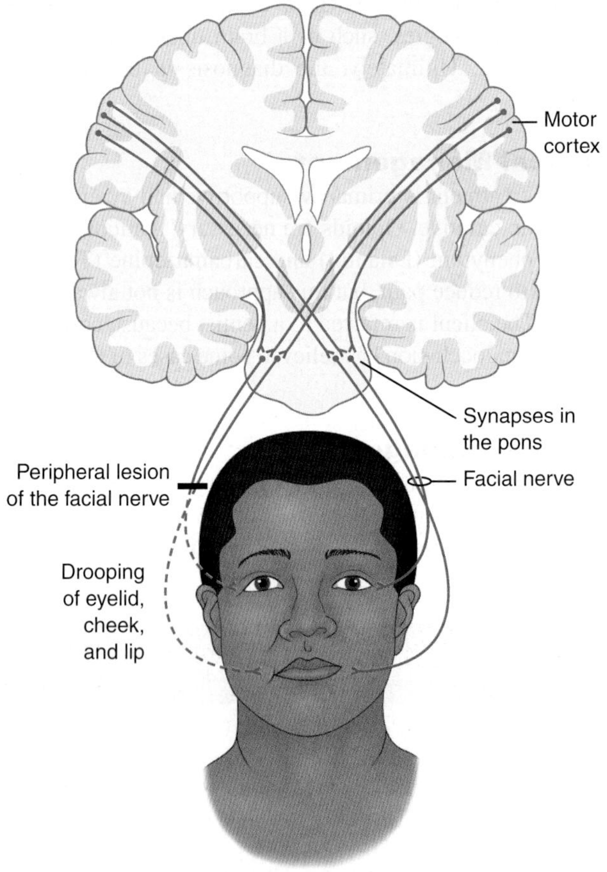

Figure 37-13 Weakness or paralysis of facial muscles associated with Bell palsy results in loss of tone causing the eyelid, cheek, and lip to droop.

there is any residual nerve and muscle activity. In some instances, an MRI or CT scan is performed to rule out other etiologies such as a brain tumor or stroke, which have comparable symptoms.

Medical Management

Short-term high-dose corticosteroid therapy with prednisone (Deltasone, Meticorten) is prescribed to reduce nerve inflammation and edema. The steroid may be combined with an antiviral such as acyclovir (Zovirax), famciclovir (Famvir), or valacyclovir (Valtrex) to inhibit viral replication and shorten the duration of symptoms. B-complex vitamins may also be beneficial. Various types of surgical reconstructive procedures referred to collectively as **facial reanimation** may be performed to improve facial movement and appearance. Examples include repair of the facial nerve, connecting another nerve to the facial nerve, transferring muscles to allow movement of the face, and other cosmetic procedures such as a brow lift, face lift, and eyelid reconstruction (Pames, 2016; Taylor, 2015).

Nursing Management

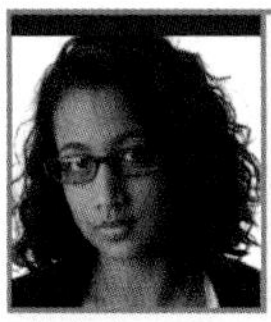

Clinical Scenario A 28-year-old woman makes an appointment with the nurse practitioner after being treated for a sinus infection 2 days ago. At the present time, she has developed an asymmetrical smile, numbness on the left side of her face, and drooping left eyelid and corner of her mouth. Although the client seems to have symptoms that accompany a stroke, that is ruled out. **What nursing interventions are appropriate when caring for this client or anyone with Bell palsy? See the following Nursing Process section.**

NURSING PROCESS FOR THE CLIENT WITH BELL PALSY

Assessment

Obtain the client's history, noting any recent illness that suggests a viral infection. Perform a physical examination to determine which side of the face is involved and the appearance of affected structures. Note whether the client has any speech impairment, is able to close the eyelids, and is able to chew and swallow food.

Diagnosis, Planning, and Interventions

Corneal Injury Risk: Related to diminished blink reflex
Expected Outcome: The eye will remain free of ulceration and infection as evidenced by no redness, drainage, or blurry vision.

- Cover the eye with an eye patch. *An eye patch keeps the eyelid closed and protects the eye surface from environmental debris.*
- Apply a protective eye shield at night. *An eye shield ensures that the client does not scratch or injure the eye during sleep.*
- Inspect the eye daily for signs of inflammation and infection. *Early treatment facilitates a quick resolution and minimizes potential impairment of vision.*
- Irrigate the eye with normal saline. *Irrigation flushes debris and microorganisms from the surface and conjunctival folds.*
- Instill prescribed antibiotic ophthalmic ointment. *Antibiotic therapy inhibits the growth of or destroys pathogens.*

Impaired Oral Mucous Membranes: Related to loss of sensation in the mouth, paralysis of chewing muscles as manifested by trauma to the cheeks, gums, teeth, or tongue
Expected Outcome: Oral mucous membrane and structures in the mouth will heal.

- Provide supplies for oral hygiene before and after meals. *Keeping the mouth clean promotes healing.*
- Check client's mouth after eating. *Client may be unaware that oral trauma has occurred.*
- Remove food particles that remain by using mouth rinses, cotton-tipped applicators, or a pulsating oral irrigator. *Physical measures are necessary in some cases to clear the cheek, buccal areas, and teeth of food residue. Retained food interferes with healing.*
- Ensure that food and beverages are not too hot to avoid burning oral mucous membranes. *Extremes in temperatures contribute to thermal injury in the mouth.*
- Encourage biannual dental examinations. *A client with residual paralysis requires regular dental examinations and care to ensure optimum oral health.*

Impaired Verbal Communication: Related to hemiparalysis of facial muscles and pain
Expected Outcome: Client will communicate verbally and understandably.

- Instruct client to speak slowly and in short sentences. *Slowing the rate of speech enables the client to coordinate the use of their teeth, tongue, and lips while speaking.*
- Provide a pad of paper and a pencil to facilitate communication during severe pain. *Written communication is an acceptable substitute for temporarily impaired oral communication.*

Evaluation of Expected Outcomes

The client understands the techniques for instilling ophthalmic ointment and applying an eye patch and eye shield. There is no redness, swelling of orbital tissue, or drainage that suggests an infection. Vision in the affected eye remains unaffected. The client's mouth is free of retained debris. The soft tissue structures in the mouth are pink, moist, and intact. Teeth are in good repair. The client satisfactorily communicates with spoken words.

EXTRAPYRAMIDAL DISORDERS

Extrapyramidal disorders have their origin in the motor cortex and surrounding areas of the cerebellum and basal ganglia. Two examples of extrapyramidal disorders are Parkinson disease and Huntington disease. One of their primary characteristics is abnormal movement.

Parkinson Disease

Parkinson disease usually begins after 50 years of age. It primarily affects the basal ganglia and connections in the substantia nigra and corpus striatum (Fig. 37-14). The term **parkinsonism** is used to describe the cluster of Parkinson-like symptoms that develops from several etiologies.

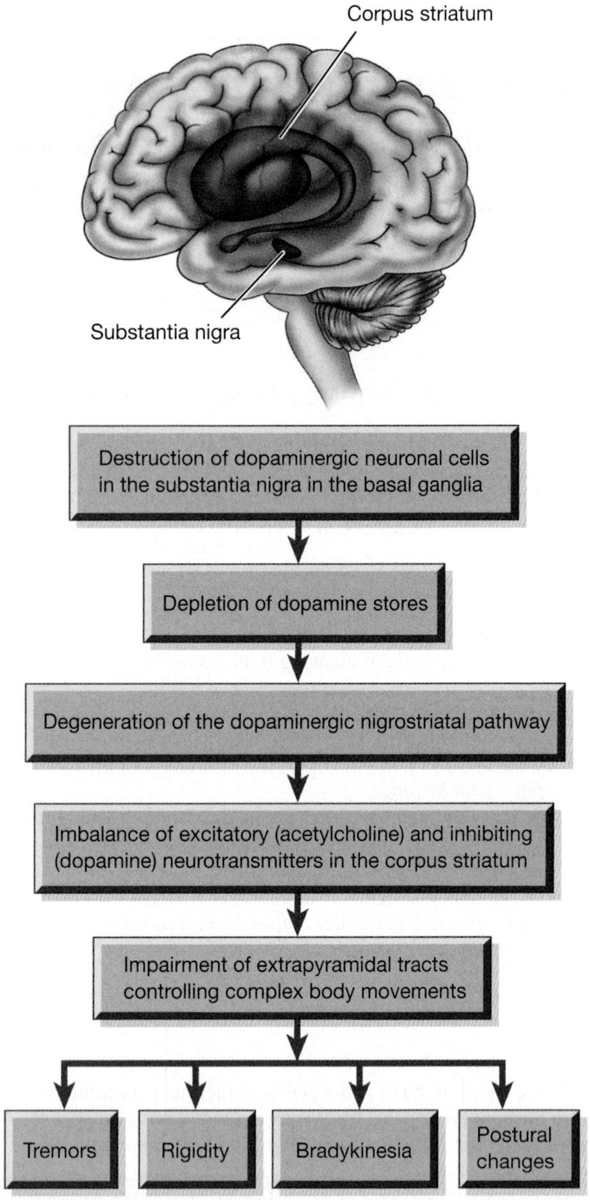

Figure 37-14 Nuclei in the substantia nigra protect fibers to the corpus striatum where the nerve fibers carry dopamine. Loss of dopamine from nerve cells is thought to cause symptoms of Parkinson disease. (Adapted with permission from Hinkle, J. L., & Cheever, K. H. (2018). *Brunner & Suddarth's textbook of medical-surgical nursing* (14th ed.). Wolters Kluwer.)

Pathophysiology and Etiology

Parkinson disease and parkinsonism result from a deficiency of the neurotransmitter dopamine. In the absence of dopamine, another area of the brain, known as the *globus pallidus*, which responds to acetylcholine, becomes overactive. The imbalance between dopamine and acetylcholine results in a movement disorder that characterizes Parkinson disease.

In most cases of Parkinson disease, no cause can be found for dopamine depletion. The symptoms of parkinsonism have been associated with exposure to environmental toxins such as insecticides and herbicides and self-administration of an illegal synthetic form of heroin known as MPTP; symptoms also can occur as sequelae of chronic traumatic encephalopathy from repeated blows to the head, and encephalitis. Phenothiazines, a category of antipsychotic drugs and other dopamine receptor-blocking antipsychotic drugs used to treat schizophrenia, also produce what is referred to as *pseudoparkinsonism* because the symptoms are reversible when the drug is discontinued.

Manifestations of the disorder progress so slowly that years may elapse between the first symptom and diagnosis. The symptoms initially are unilateral, but eventually, whether quickly or slowly, become bilateral.

Assessment Findings

Signs and Symptoms

Early signs include stiffness, referred to as *rigidity*, and a **pill-rolling tremor** (a circular movement of the fingers and wrist as if manipulating a small object or pill within the palm) in one or both hands. The hand tremor is obvious at rest and typically decreases when movement is voluntary, such as picking up an object.

Bradykinesia, slowness in performing spontaneous movements, develops. Clients have a masklike expression, stooped posture, hypophonia (low volume of speech), and difficulty swallowing saliva and food. Weight loss occurs (Nutrition Notes 37-3). A shuffling gait is apparent, and the client has difficulty turning or redirecting forward motion. Arms are rigid while walking (Fig. 37-15).

Nutrition Notes 37-3

The Client With Parkinson Disease

- Unintentional weight loss is a common occurrence and may increase the risk for morbidity and mortality. Weight loss may be due to increased energy expenditure related to tremor; due to impaired intake related to diminished sense of smell, dysphagia, or depression; or from medication side effects such as dry mouth, nausea, anorexia, fatigue, or anxiety. Strategies to prevent or treat unintentional weight loss may include small, frequent meals, providing semisolid foods to facilitate swallowing, and increasing the calorie density of foods served by added sauces, gravies, etc.
- Foods high in fiber, such as crushed bran added to hot cereal and fiber-fortified supplements, help prevent constipation when consumed with adequate fluids. Prunes and prune juice stimulate peristalsis.
- Clients taking levodopa should avoid high intake of protein (meat, fish, poultry, and dairy foods) because protein decreases its effectiveness. However, a high-protein diet may be needed for clients who experience unintentional weight loss.

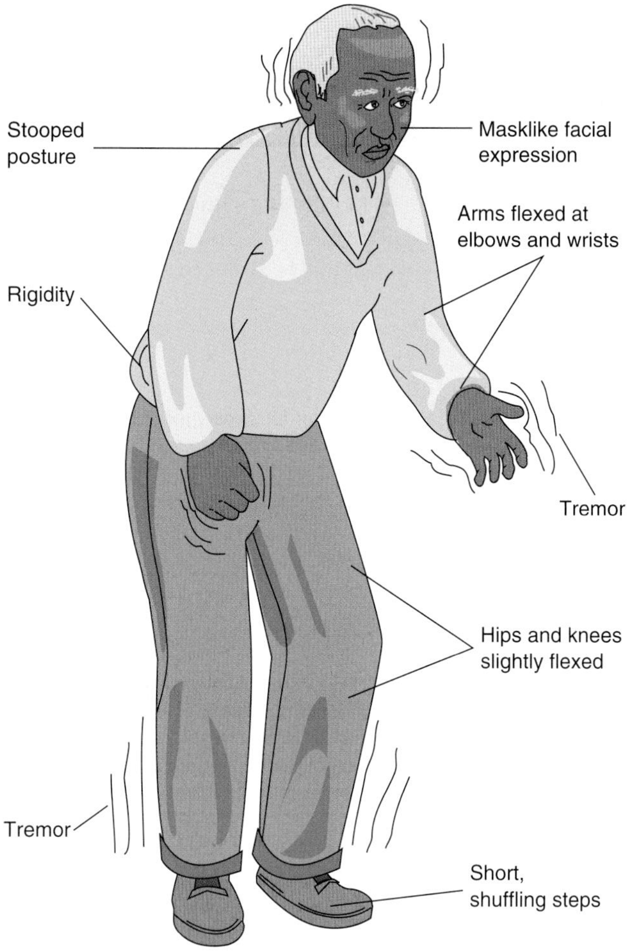

Figure 37-15 Typical manifestations of Parkinson disease.

In late stages, the disease affects the jaw, tongue, and larynx; speech is slurred; and chewing and swallowing become difficult. Rigidity can lead to contractures. Salivation increases, accompanied by drooling. There is a high risk for aspiration. In a small percentage of clients, the eyes roll upward or downward and stay there involuntarily (oculogyric crises) for several hours or even a few days.

Diagnostic Findings

Diagnosis is based on typical symptoms and a neurologic examination. There are no specific tests for this disorder.

Medical Management

Treatment aims at prolonging independence. Drugs such as selegiline (Eldepryl), which has neuroprotective properties; dopaminergics such as levodopa (Larodopa) or levodopa-carbidopa (Sinemet); amantadine (Symmetrel); dopamine agonists such as bromocriptine (Parlodel); apomorphine (Apokyn), the newest approved drug; and anticholinergics such as benztropine (Cogentin) are prescribed (Drug Therapy Table 37-1). Their sequence of use is based on the stage of the disorder and the decreasing effectiveness of the medication initially prescribed. Rehabilitation measures such as physical therapy, occupational therapy, client and family education, and counseling are used concurrently with drug therapy.

Surgical Management

Some clients with Parkinson disease have obtained relief of symptoms through deep brain stimulation (DBS). DBS involves the implantation of a neurostimulator that works like a pacemaker for the brain (Fig. 37-16). The neurostimulator

DRUG THERAPY TABLE 37-1 Antiparkinson Agents

Category and Common Generic (Brand) Drugs	Intended Use	Common Side Effects	Safety Warnings for Nurses
Dopaminergic Drugs			
Amantadine Bromocriptine (Parlodel) Carbidopa (Lodosyn) Carbidopa/levodopa (Sinemet)	Parkinson disease/drug-induced extrapyramidal symptoms; Combination replaces dopamine; allows lower doses of levodopa Alternative for levodopa when levodopa has decreased efficacy Allows separate dosing of carbidopa and levodopa	Lightheadedness, dizziness, insomnia, confusion, nausea, constipation, dry mouth, orthostatic hypotension	• Do not give with monoamine oxidase inhibitor antidepressants • May be used to decrease side effects Pyridoxine (vitamin B_6). • Do not discontinue abruptly for it can cause parkinsonian crisis
Dopaminergic Agonists			
Rasagiline (Azilect) Selegiline (Eldepryl, Emsam, Zelapar)	Agonist for levodopa/carbidopa in Parkinson disease	Headache, arthralgia, dyspepsia, flu-like syndrome	• Do not use with meperidine pain reliever
Dopamine Receptor Agonists, Nonergot			
Apomorphine (Apokyn) Pramipexole (Mirapex) Ropinirole (Requip)	Parkinson disease "off" episode Stimulates dopamine receptors Relieves tremor and movement disorders of Parkinson disease	Dizziness, somnolence, insomnia, hallucinations, confusion, nausea, dyspepsia, syncope	• Do not discontinue the drug abruptly • Older adults tend to experience hallucinations

(continued)

DRUG THERAPY TABLE 37-1 Antiparkinson Agents (*continued*)

Category and Common Generic (Brand) Drugs	Intended Use	Common Side Effects	Safety Warnings for Nurses
Catechol-O-methyltransferase (COMT) Inhibitors			
Entacapone (Comtan) Tolcapone (Tasmar)	Inhibits COMT, an enzyme that breaks down dopamine As adjunct to levodopa/carbidopa in Parkinson disease; Parkinson disease when refractory to levodopa/carbidopa	Dyskinesia, hyperkinesia, nausea, diarrhea, urine discoloration	• Monitor liver function
Cholinergic Blocking Drugs (Anticholinergics)			
Benztropine (Cogentin) Diphenhydramine (Benadryl) Trihexyphenidyl (Artane)	Parkinson disease, drug-induced extrapyramidal symptoms	Dry mouth, blurred vision, dizziness, nausea, nervousness, skin rash, urinary retention, dysuria, tachycardia, muscle weakness, disorientation, confusion	• Monitor for urinary retention, blockage
Combination Drugs			
Carbidopa, levodopa, entacapone (Stalevo)	Dizziness, lightheadedness when rising, nausea, vomiting, loss of appetite, dry mouth, flatulence	When combined with carbidopa and levodopa, it slows the breakdown of levodopa reducing the "wearing off" effect	• Monitor for behavioral and mood changes, altered kidney or liver function Consult primary provider about regular prostate screening, evidence of skin cancer, and increased eye pressure. Do not discontinue abruptly Consult primary provider if breastfeeding

The drugs in column 1 indicate that the drug matches with the explanations in the columns 2 through 4. (This article was published in Pagana, K. D., & Pagana, T. J. (2021). *Mosby's diagnostic and laboratory test reference* (15th ed.). Mosby.)

sends electrical impulses from a battery implanted under the skin near the clavicle to the globus pallidus, thalamus, or subthalamic nucleus. The electrical stimulus blocks abnormal nerve signals that cause the parkinsonian tremor. DBS eliminates the tremor in approximately 65% of people who have an implanted stimulator. Current research is attempting to produce a similar effect by attaching electrodes to the surface of the brain rather than by implanting a stimulator within the brain.

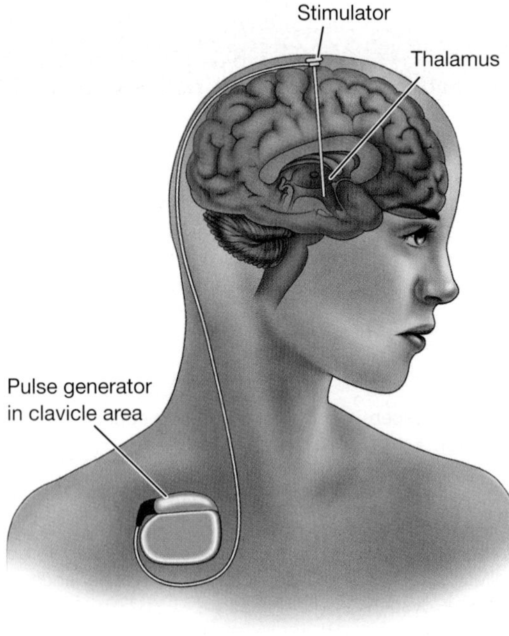

Figure 37-16 Deep brain stimulation with the use of a pulse generator.

Many areas of research are being conducted to find additional methods for managing Parkinson disease. Several clinical trials have shown that transplants of fetal dopamine neurons can survive transplantation and some clients saw their motor symptoms improved. "This discovery has the potential to significantly affect the development of next-generation cell-based therapies, which involve injecting healthy cells into brain regions already affected by the disease. Researchers believe the approach may help relieve motor symptoms such as tremor and balance issues" (Silva, 2019).

Gene therapy is still highly experimental. Currently, there are efforts to manipulate a gene for glutamic acid decarboxylase. This enzyme is key in the production of the inhibitory neurotransmitter gamma-aminobutyric acid (GABA). Researchers think that increasing GABA may inhibit the neurostimulating effects from the globus pallidus similar to the effect achieved with the deep brain stimulator.

Still another research approach for Parkinson disease is to enhance glial cell–derived neurotrophic factor (GDNF). This substance stimulates growth of dopamine-producing neurons. Finding a technique that improves the delivery of GDNF to the specific target areas in the brain has been the main obstacle of this project.

Nursing Management

Clients with parkinsonism are admitted to the hospital because of the debilitating effects of the disease. Others are cared for in extended care facilities when they can no longer be managed at home in a chronic state. One of the biggest nursing challenges is managing the client's drug therapy. Levodopa is associated with periods of "breakthrough" or "end-of-dose wearing off" in which symptoms are exacerbated when a consistent drug level is not maintained. The nurse must administer the drugs closely to the schedule the client previously established at home. Over time, clients may decreasingly respond to their standard drug therapy and have more frequent "off episodes" of hypomobility in which they may be unable to rise from a chair, speak, or walk. The drugs apomorphine (Apokyn and Stalevo) help in relieving this phenomenon. Drugs administered for parkinsonism can cause a wide variety of adverse effects such as involuntary movements, which require dose adjustments. The nurse works with physical and occupational therapists to increase the client's level of activity, optimize their gait, improve balance and coordination, and use adaptive equipment to perform ADLs.

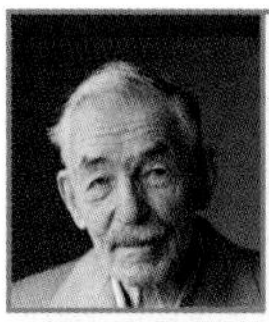

Clinical Scenario A 67-year-old client who was diagnosed several years ago with Parkinson disease has become progressively worse. He is experiencing the following signs and symptoms: a resting hand tremor that began on one side and is now occurring in the opposite hand; slowed movement with short steps and occasional freezing, which the client describes as "stuck in one place"; lack of arm swinging during ambulation; expressionless face; soft, raspy voice; and occasional difficulty swallowing. **What nursing care is appropriate for this client? Nursing Care Plan 37-2 provides more discussion of management of the client with an extrapyramidal disorder such as Parkinson disease or Huntington disease.**

NURSING CARE PLAN 37-2 The Client With an Extrapyramidal Disorder

Assessment

Determine the following:

- Year of current diagnosis
- Concurrent medical disorders
- Weight and vital signs
- Any unilateral or bilateral hand tremor
- Gait and balance
- Use of assistive ambulatory devices
- Ability to swallow
- Quality of speech
- Bowel and urinary elimination patterns
- Mental and emotional status
- Drug therapy, time and frequency of medication administration

Nursing Diagnoses. **Fall Risk** and **Bathing/Hygiene ADL Deficit** related to muscle rigidity, tremors, choreiform movements, and dementia as evidenced by inability to complete all or some ADLs

Expected Outcomes. (1) Client will be physically active. (2) Client will perform self-care to the level at which they are capable.

Interventions	Rationales
Assist client with walking and physical activities.	*Client is at risk for falls and injuries if activities are not assisted or supervised.*
Increase the type and amount of activity gradually.	*Client will have more strength and coordination once response to medications has improved.*
Minimize fatigue by providing rest periods.	*Rest relieves fatigue and restores stamina and endurance.*
Promote involvement in self-care activities within the client's individual capacity.	*Matching self-care involvement to client's functional level promotes dignity and improves self-image.*
Allow ample time to perform ADLs.	*Given sufficient time, client is more likely to pace themselves to complete ADLs semi-independently.*
Modify clothing and self-care supplies to promote independence.	*Clothing that is easily put on and taken off and aids for holding a toothbrush, fork, and so forth facilitate ability to perform self-care.*
Assist client but only when client cannot perform certain tasks.	*Too much assistance cultivates dependence on the nurse.*

Evaluation of Expected Outcomes

Client is active in their immediate environment and uses assistive devices as necessary.
Client attends to self-care as much as symptoms allow.

Nursing Problem. **Aspiration Risk**

Expected Outcomes. (1) Client will swallow food and liquids taken in orally. (2) Client's airway will be free of food or liquids.

Interventions	Rationales
Place client in a sitting position.	*Sitting, the natural position for eating and drinking, helps propel food toward the stomach.*
Keep suction equipment at the bedside; use it when the client chokes.	*Mechanical suctioning uses negative pressure to pull liquids and solids from the airway.*
Decrease environmental distractions.	*Reducing distractions helps client focus attention on chewing and swallowing.*

(continued)

NURSING CARE PLAN 37-2 The Client With an Extrapyramidal Disorder (*continued*)

Cut food into small pieces. Incorporate mashed potatoes or other pasty foods.	*A large bolus of food is more likely to cause a complete obstruction if aspirated. Foods like mashed potatoes bind in a soft bolus that is swallowed more easily.*
Thicken liquids with gelatin, cornstarch, applesauce, mashed bananas, ice cream, or a commercial thickener.	*Thickeners provide a consistency that the tongue can easily manipulate against the palate.*
Position client's chin on the chest during swallowing.	*This position decreases the potential for food to enter the airway.*
Stroke client's throat as they swallow or instruct client to swallow several times in a row.	*Stimulating swallowing with stroking or repeated swallowing efforts moves food from the oropharynx to the esophagus.*

Evaluation of Expected Outcomes

Client can swallow food and fluids without choking.
Client's lungs remain clear of food and liquids.

Nursing Diagnosis. **Impaired Verbal Communication** related to soft voice or inability to articulate words

Expected Outcome. Client will communicate needs, feelings, and ideas.

Interventions	Rationales
Reduce environmental noise.	*A quiet environment helps others hear what the client says.*
Listen closely to what the client tries to say.	*Attention and patience facilitate understanding.*
Ask client to speak slowly.	*Altering the rate of speech improves clarity.*
Anticipate client's needs.	*Doing so reduces client's frustration with having to ask for help.*

Evaluation of Expected Outcome

Client's verbalizations are heard and understood.

Nursing Diagnoses. **Acute Anxiety** and **Coping Impairment** related to awareness of diminished physical and mental capacities as manifested by periods of agitation, frustration, emotional irritability, and anger

Expected Outcomes. (1) Client will relax and feel secure. (2) Client will accept the gradual loss of physical or mental attributes and will allow others to help without opposition.

Interventions	Rationales
Help client to realistically determine tasks that are feasible and those that are not.	*A sense of control reduces anxiety.*
Suggest taking a break when the client cannot accomplish an activity.	*A break can help the client to regather physical and emotional resources to complete the task successfully.*
Offer support and encouragement when client succeeds.	*Deserved praise elevates self-esteem and encourages client to persevere.*
Help client focus on remaining strengths rather than deficits.	*Focusing on strengths promotes a more positive attitude.*
Provide information about support groups whose mission is to provide assistance to clients with similar problems.	*Clients are more likely to cope when they have an available network of support.*

Evaluation of Expected Outcomes

Client feels relaxed and in control.
Client implements strategies that facilitate coping with their disability.

Nursing Diagnosis. **Risk for Loneliness** related to depression and perceived potential for rejection secondary to altered physical appearance or cognitive function

Expected Outcome. Client will maintain social contacts.

Interventions	Rationales
Have client identify persons whose company they enjoy and activities they share.	*Naming or listing specific people reinforces that client has a circle of friends.*
Encourage client to interact with a few of the designated people for short periods in a place where client feels secure and comfortable, such as their home.	*Taking the initiative for contacting friends promotes reestablishing social relationships.* *Visiting at home shields the client from potential unwanted attention from strangers.*
Encourage client to participate in social activities outside the home.	*When client feels more accepted, they may extend socialization beyond the home.*
Refer client to and encourage joining a support group.	*Such groups promote bonding with new acquaintances.*

Evaluation of Expected Outcome

Client reestablishes social contacts with previous friends and develops friendships with new acquaintances.

Huntington Disease

Huntington disease is a hereditary disorder of the CNS.

Pathophysiology and Etiology

Huntington disease is an extrapyramidal disorder that is transmitted genetically and inherited by people of both genders. The basal ganglia and portions of the cerebral cortex degenerate. In the early stages, clients can participate in most physical activities. However, as the disease progresses, hallucinations, delusions, impaired judgment, and increased intensity of abnormal movements develop.

Assessment Findings

Symptoms develop slowly and include mental apathy and emotional disturbances, **choreiform movements** (uncontrollable writhing and twisting of the body), grimacing, difficulty chewing and swallowing, speech difficulty, intellectual decline, and loss of bowel and bladder control. Severe depression is common and can lead to suicide.

Diagnosis is based on symptoms as well as a family history of the disorder. Positron emission tomography shows CNS changes, but there is no specific diagnostic test for the disorder. Genetic testing can predict which family members will develop the disease, but not all blood relatives choose to undergo testing.

Medical Management

Treatment is supportive because there is no specific therapy or cure. Tranquilizers and antiparkinson drugs relieve the choreiform movements in some clients. No drugs are available to halt the mental deterioration. Because this disorder is inherited, genetic counseling before a pregnancy is advised.

Nursing Management

Nursing management aims at meeting client and family needs, such as preventing complications as well as encouraging counseling. The stage of the disease determines the scope of nursing care. The client eventually becomes totally dependent on others. Pneumonia, contractures, infections, aspiration of food or fluids, falls, and pressure ulcers are complications. The nurse prevents them by assessing the client frequently and updating the plan of care (see Nursing Care Plan 37-2).

The nurse encourages the client to lead as normal a life as possible, emphasizing the importance of exercise and self-care and explaining the medical regimen to the client and family. The nurse demonstrates how to facilitate tasks such as using both hands to hold a drinking glass, using a straw to drink, and wearing slip-on shoes.

All the disease-modifying drugs can decrease immune cells and infection protection. Therefore, be aware of increased risk for acquired infections, especially if the client is catheterized.

SEIZURE DISORDERS

The terms *seizure disorder* and *convulsive disorder* are used interchangeably, but they are not necessarily synonymous. A **seizure** is a brief episode of abnormal electrical activity in the brain. A **convulsion**, one manifestation of a seizure, is characterized by spasmodic contractions of muscles. **Epilepsy** is a chronic recurrent pattern of seizures.

Pathophysiology and Etiology

Seizure disorders are classified as idiopathic (no known cause) or acquired. Causes of acquired seizures include high fever, electrolyte imbalances, uremia, hypoglycemia, hypoxia, brain tumor, drug abuse, and alcohol withdrawal. Once the cause is removed, the seizures cease. The known causes of epilepsy include brain injury at birth, head injuries, and inborn errors of metabolism. In some clients, the cause of epilepsy is never determined.

Seizures represent abnormal motor, sensory, or psychic neural activity. The abnormal neural activity occurs alone or in combination from discharges in one or more specific areas of the cerebral cortex. Each type of seizure disorder is characterized by a specific pattern of events.

Types of Seizures

Seizures are divided into two general categories: partial and generalized (Box 37-2).

Partial Seizures

Partial, or focal, seizures begin in a specific area of the cerebral cortex. They can progress to generalized seizures. The two subcategories of partial seizures are those with elementary (or simple) symptoms and those with complex symptoms. A client who has a partial seizure with elementary symptoms usually does not lose consciousness, and the seizure lasts less than 1 minute. Partial elementary seizures with motor symptoms are accompanied by uncontrolled jerking movements of a body part, such as a finger, mouth, hand, or foot. Partial elementary seizures with sensory symptoms are accompanied by hallucinatory sights, sounds,

BOX 37-2 International Classification of Seizures

I. Partial (Focal) Seizures
- A. Partial seizures (no loss of consciousness)
  1. Motor symptoms
  2. Special sensory symptoms
  3. Autonomic symptoms
  4. Psychic symptoms
- B. Complex partial seizures (with loss of consciousness)
  1. Begins as a partial seizure and progresses to complex partial with loss of consciousness
  2. Loss of consciousness at onset of seizure

II. Generalized Seizures
- A. Absence seizures
- B. Myoclonic seizures
- C. Clonic seizures
- D. Tonic seizures
- E. Tonic-clonic seizures
- F. Atonic seizures

III. Unclassified Seizures

All seizures that do not fit into other classifications

and odors; mumbling; and the use of nonsense words. The terms *Jacksonian*, *focal motor*, and *focal sensory* describe partial elementary seizures.

A client who has a partial seizure with complex symptoms may have several sensory or motor manifestations, which also last less than 1 minute. After the seizure, the client is often confused. Complex partial seizures are manifested by automatic repetitive movements (**automatisms**) that are not appropriate, such as lip smacking and picking at clothing or objects. The terms *psychomotor* and *psychosensory* are used to describe complex partial seizures.

Generalized Seizures

Generalized seizures involve the entire brain. The client loses consciousness, and the seizure may last from several seconds to several minutes. Types of generalized seizures include absence seizures, myoclonic seizures, tonic-clonic seizures, and atonic seizures.

Absence Seizures

Absence seizures, formerly referred to as *petit mal seizures*, are more common in children. They are characterized by a brief loss of consciousness or cognition during which physical activity ceases. The person stares blankly; the eyelids flutter; the lips move; and slight movement of the head, arms, and legs occurs. These seizures typically last for a few seconds, and the person seldom falls to the ground. Because of their brief duration and relative lack of prominent movements, these seizures often go unnoticed. People with absence seizures can have them many times a day. Before diagnosis, many children with absence seizures are misidentified as having a learning disability because during their lapse of attention they miss instructions or explanations provided by teachers, which compromises their academic success.

Myoclonic Seizures

These seizures are characterized by sudden, excessive jerking of the arms, legs, or entire body. In some instances, the muscle activity is so severe that the client falls to the ground. These seizures are brief.

Tonic-Clonic Seizures

Formerly referred to as *grand mal seizures*, tonic-clonic seizures are characterized by a sequence of events that begins with a **preictal** (or prodromal) **phase**. The preictal phase is the time immediately before a seizure and consists of vague emotional changes, such as depression, anxiety, and nervousness. This phase lasts for minutes or hours and is followed by an **aura**, a sensation that occurs immediately before the seizure. The aura is sensory (i.e., a hallucinatory odor or sound) or a sensation of weakness or numbness. In clients who experience an aura, the aura almost always is the same.

The aura is followed by the epileptic cry, which is caused by spasm of the respiratory muscles and muscles of the throat and glottis. This cry immediately precedes loss of consciousness and the ensuing tonic and clonic phases of the seizure. In the tonic phase, the muscles contract rigidly; in the clonic phase, the muscles alternate between contraction and relaxation, resulting in jerking movements and thrashing of the arms and legs. The skin becomes cyanotic, and breathing is spasmodic. Saliva mixes with air, resulting in frothing at the mouth. The jaws are tightly clenched, and biting of the tongue and inner cheek may occur. Urinary or fecal incontinence is common. The clonic phase lasts for 1 minute or more, gradually subsides, and is followed by the **postictal phase**, the period following the seizure. The manifestations of this phase include headache, fatigue, deep sleep, confusion, nausea, and muscle soreness.

Status epilepticus is marked by a series of tonic-clonic seizures in which the client does not regain consciousness between seizures. If this extremely dangerous condition is not terminated, death can occur. Status epilepticus occurs spontaneously in acute neurologic disorders or for no known reason; it can be precipitated by the abrupt discontinuation of anticonvulsant medication. Because of this, anticonvulsants must be withdrawn gradually.

Atonic Seizures

Atonic (loss of muscle tone) seizures affect the muscles. The person loses consciousness briefly and falls to the ground. Recovery is rapid. An akinetic (loss of movement) seizure is similar because muscle tone is lost briefly. The client may or may not fall, and recovery is rapid.

Assessment Findings

The client's motor, sensory, and neurologic functions are normal except at the time of a seizure. Identification of seizure activity and type of seizure often depends on a witness's description of the client's actions during the seizure.

A neurologic examination and EEG are performed. Other laboratory or diagnostic studies, such as a CT scan, MRI, serology, and serum electrolyte levels, are used to confirm the diagnosis and to determine the cause of the seizure disorder. When epilepsy is suspected, a series of EEGs is required if the first results are normal.

Medical Management

Once a diagnosis of a seizure disorder is confirmed, one or more anticonvulsant drugs are used to control the seizures. Examples of anticonvulsants are phenytoin (Dilantin), phenobarbital, carbamazepine (Tegretol), ethosuximide (Zarontin), valproic acid (Depakene), felbamate (Felbatol), gabapentin (Neurontin), and fosphenytoin injection (Cerebyx; Drug Therapy Table 37-2). IV lorazepam (Ativan), diazepam (Valium), or midazolam (Versed) are administered initially to terminate status epilepticus. Alternative drugs include IV fosphenytoin, valproic acid, or levetiracetam (Keppra). If the seizure continues for 40 minutes or more, doses of thiopental (Pentothal) or propofol (Diprivan) may be required.

Pharmacologic Considerations

- Closely monitor side effects. Up to 25% of clients treated for seizures will stop or alter medication prescription due to unpleasant side effects.

DRUG THERAPY TABLE 37-2 Agents to Control Seizures

Massachusetts General Hospital and Harvard Medical School researchers are exploring an association between the use of antiepileptics by pregnant women and an increased incidence of birth defects. The Epilepsy Foundation has established the N. American AED Pregnancy Registry for women to gain information about the safety of AED's while pregnant and maintaining seizure control. For more information, visit: http://www.epilepsy.com

Category and Common Generic (Brand) Drugs	Intended Use	Common Side Effects	Safety Warnings for Nurses
Antileptics			
Hydantoins Ethotoin (Peganone) Fosphenytoin (Cerebyx) Phenytoin (Dilantin)	Tonic-clonic seizures, status epilepticus; used to stabilize neuronal membrane	Ataxia, CNS depression, headache, hypotension, nystagmus, mental confusion, slurred speech, dizziness, drowsiness, nausea, vomiting, gingival hyperplasia, rash	• Do not discontinue the drug abruptly • Monitor liver function • High rate of failure when hormonal birth control is used • Monitor serum drug levels
Carboxylic Acid Derivatives Valproic acid (Depakote, Depakene)	Epilepsy, migraine headache, mania; used to increase GABA	Headache, somnolence, dizziness, tremor, nausea, vomiting, diplopia	• Avoid alcohol use • Monitor platelets and ammonia levels
Succinimides Ethosuximide (Zarontin) Methsuximide (Celontin)	Focal seizures, reduces frequency; depresses the motor cortex	Drowsiness, ataxia, dizziness, nausea, vomiting, urinary frequency, pruritus, urticaria, gingival hyperplasia	• Do not discontinue the drug abruptly
Oxazolidinediones Trimethadione (Tridione)	Epilepsy; decrease synaptic transmission of nerve impulses	Dizziness, drowsiness, nausea, vomiting, photosensitivity, personality changes, increased irritability, headache, fatigue	• Monitor blood cell counts for blood dyscrasias • Fetal risks when taken during pregnancy • Report skin rash, signs of infection, or bleeding
Benzodiazepines			
Clonazepam (Klonopin) Clobazam (Onfi) Clorazepate (Tranxene) Diazepam (Valium) Lorazepam (Ativan)	Seizure disorders, panic disorders, anxiety disorders, alcohol withdrawal, decrease postsynaptic excitement	Drowsiness, depression, ataxia, anorexia, diarrhea, constipation, dry mouth, palpitations, visual disturbances, rash	• Instruct clients to avoid alcohol • Avoid tasks that require alertness and motor skills until response to drug is established
Nonspecified Preparations			
Acetazolamide (Diamox)	Reduces seizure activity by inhibiting carbonic anhydrase	Drowsiness, dizziness, nausea, diarrhea, constipation, visual disturbances	• Monitor for potassium loss • Avoid concurrent use with sulfonamides and thiazide diuretics • Ensure adequate fluid intake
Carbamazepine (Tegretol, Carbatrol, Epitol, Equetro)	Epilepsy, bipolar disorder, trigeminal/postherpetic neuralgia	Dizziness, nausea, drowsiness, unsteady gait, aplastic anemia and other blood cell abnormalities, Stevens Johnson syndrome	• High rate of failure when hormonal birth control is used • Monitor white blood cell count
Oxcarbazepine (Trileptal) Primidone (Mysoline) Zonisamide (Zonegran)	Epilepsy	Headache, dizziness, fatigue, somnolence, ataxia, diplopia, nausea, vomiting, abdominal pain	• High rate of failure when hormonal birth control is used
Brivaracetam (Briviact) Eslicarbazepine (Aptiom) Ezogabine (Potiga) Lacosamide (Vimpat) Tiagabine (Gabitril)	Focal seizures	Dizziness, drowsiness, headache, nausea, vomiting	• Monitor for urinary retention • Monitor sodium levels

(continued)

DRUG THERAPY TABLE 37-2 Agents to Control Seizures (*continued*)

Category and Common Generic (Brand) Drugs	Intended Use	Common Side Effects	Safety Warnings for Nurses
Felbamate (Felbatol)	Focal seizures in clients who fail other drug therapy first	Insomnia, headache, anxiety, acne, rash, dyspepsia, vomiting, constipation, diarrhea, upper respiratory tract infection, fatigue, rhinitis, aplastic anemia, hepatic disorders	• Be alert for signs of acute liver failure • High rate of failure when hormonal birth control is used
Gabapentin (Gralise, Neurontin) Gabapentin enacarbil (Horizant)	Focal seizures (adults), postherpetic neuralgia; restless leg syndrome	Somnolence, dizziness, ataxia	• Antacids decrease drug absorption; separate doses by 2 hours • Concentration and coordination may be impaired • Avoid abrupt discontinuation • Do not breastfeed while taking drug
Lamotrigine (Lamictal)	Focal seizures (used with other antiepileptics), bipolar disorder	Dizziness, insomnia, somnolence, ataxia, nausea, vomiting, diplopia, headache	• Be alert for skin disorders such as Stevens–Johnson syndrome
Levetiracetam (Keppra)	Focal seizures, tonic-clonic seizures, bipolar disorder, migraine headache	Headache, dizziness, asthenia, somnolence, infection	• Monitor complete blood cell count and liver function tests • Dosage should be decreased if there is renal impairment • Taper dose if discontinued • Avoid if pregnant or breastfeeding
Perampanel (Fycompa)	Focal seizures, tonic-clonic seizures (used with other antiepileptics)	Dizziness, somnolence, fatigue, irritability	• Reduces hormonal contraceptives • Not recommended during pregnancy • Avoid alcohol • Taper dose when discontinued
Pregabalin (Lyrica)	Focal seizures (adults), neuropathic pain, postherpetic neuralgia	Dizziness, somnolence	• Dosage reduction with renal dysfunction • Monitor diabetics for potential hypoglycemia • Withhold drug and notify primary provider if muscle pain in shoulders, thighs, or lower back develops • Monitor for weight gain, peripheral edema, or signs and symptoms of heart failure
Topiramate (Topamax)	Focal/tonic-clonic seizures, migraine headache	Fatigue, concentration problems, somnolence, anorexia	• Dosage is increased gradually until reaching maintenance dose • Encourage at least 6–8 full glasses of water per day • Advise barrier rather than hormonal contraception • Be aware that motor and speech may be impaired • Avoid if breastfeeding • Monitor renal and hepatic function
Vigabatrin (Sabril)	Focal seizures, infantile spasms	Somnolence, fatigue, dizziness, headache, weight gain, upper respiratory infection symptoms, permanent vision loss	• Vision testing every 3 months recommended • Report symptoms of depression, changes in mood, or emergence of suicidal thoughts

The drugs in column 1 indicate the drug that matches up with explanations in columns 2 through 4.

TABLE 37-1 Anticonvulsant Drug Monitoring

	THERAPEUTIC LEVEL (mcg/mL)	TOXIC LEVEL (mcg/mL)
Carbamazepine	5–12	>12
Ethosuximide	40–100	>100
Phenobarbital	10–30	>40
Phenytoin	10–20	>30
Valproic acid	50–100	>100

Reprinted from Pagana, K. D., & Pagana, T. J. (2009). *Mosby's diagnostic and laboratory test reference* (9th ed.). St. Louis, MO: Mosby. Copyright © 2009 Elsevier. With permission.

Drug therapy controls the seizures or reduces their frequency or severity. The dose is adjusted over a period of several weeks. The drug is changed or another drug is added to the regimen to obtain optimum control. Blood levels of some anticonvulsant drugs are monitored for accurate dose adjustment and to prevent toxicity (Table 37-1). Serum levels also identify clients who are not taking the drug as ordered.

Pharmacologic Considerations

- Because seizure control uses a variety of medications with variable dosing, care during an emergency is of concern. Encourage clients to use cell phone emergency functions to list all drugs taken and current dosing, or carry a current dose list, to facilitate care when unable to respond.

Surgical Management

Seizures that are caused by a brain tumor, brain abscess, or other disorders often require surgical intervention. Surgery for epilepsy is not considered unless the client does not respond to drug therapy and seizures are frequent and severe. The area of the brain in which abnormal electrical discharges are present is identified (mapped). The surgeon must consider whether removal of the involved area would result in permanent neurologic dysfunction such as paralysis or loss of speech.

Nursing Management

The nurse asks if the client has a history of seizures, the type and pattern of the client's seizure activity, and the current treatment regimen. If the client has no history of seizure, the nurse identifies clients who may be seizure prone. For example, a person who has a high fever, has suffered a recent head injury, is withdrawing from alcohol, or is experiencing hypoglycemia or hypoxia is at risk for having a seizure. The nurse modifies the environment to promote safety if a seizure should occur, by placing suction, oral airway, and oxygen equipment at the bedside; padding the side rails and head board; and maintaining the bed in a low position. Prescribed anticonvulsant therapy is administered, and the nurse reinforces the importance of drug compliance following discharge. Nutrition Notes 37-4 provides additional information.

Nutrition Notes 37-4

The Client With a Seizure Disorder

- Anticonvulsants impair vitamin D metabolism, leading to calcium imbalance, rickets, or osteomalacia if supplemental vitamin D is not given.
- A high-fat diet, known as *ketogenic nutrition therapy*, is used as part of treatment in children whose seizures are not well controlled on available medications. Fat provides approximately 85% to 90% of the calories in this diet; protein and carbohydrates are severely limited. The high fat content simulates starvation, except that the fat burned for energy comes from food, not stored body fat. Mild dehydration helps concentrate blood ketones; it is not known how or why ketosis affects seizure activity.
- At this time, there is little evidence to support the use of ketogenic nutrition therapy in adults.

In the event that a seizure occurs, the nurse positions the client on their side and loosens restrictive clothing (see Fig. 37-7). The airway is kept patent, the client is suctioned, and oxygen is administered. The mouth is inspected for injuries to the tongue, teeth, and buccal cavity. If the client is incontinent, the nurse cleans the client and changes clothing and bed linen. Documentation includes the situation that preceded the seizure to assist in identifying any precipitating factors or aura, the duration of the seizure, parts of the body involved, vital signs, oxygen saturation, and capillary blood glucose level if indicated.

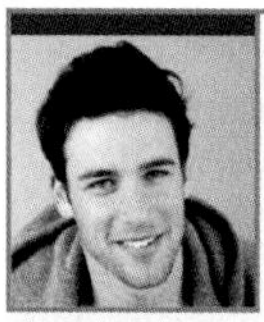

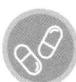

Clinical Scenario Since recovering from a head injury following a motorcycle accident, a 23-year-old client has been experiencing tonic-clonic seizures despite self-administering a prescribed anticonvulsant. He is accompanied by his wife, both of whom are concerned about his safety and employability in the future. The client's wife requests information on how to respond when the client has a seizure. What should the nurse include in this client's care? See the following Nursing Process section and Evidence Based Practice 37-1.

NURSING PROCESS FOR THE CLIENT WITH A SEIZURE DISORDER

Assessment

Obtain a complete history, including drug, allergy, and family history. Question the client regarding events or symptoms before and after the seizure. Acquire a description of the client's seizure(s) from an observer. Obtain information about any past head injury, neurologic infection such as meningitis, previous treatment for a seizure disorder, and whether the client takes medication as prescribed.

Note the characteristics of seizures if they occur while under your care. If the client's history is inconclusive and the type of seizure is unknown, it is important to provide a full, detailed description of the seizure (Box 37-3).

Diagnosis, Planning, and Interventions

The newly diagnosed client with seizures needs information about the specific type of disorder, the medications needed to control the seizures, and the precautions, if any, to take. Teach the client as follows:

- Take anticonvulsant medication as prescribed.
- Recognize adverse effects of the medication.
- Keep routine follow-up visits and laboratory appointments for blood level tests.
- Operate a motor vehicle or perform dangerous tasks only when seizures are controlled for at least 6 months.
- Wear a MedicAlert bracelet, tag, or other medical identification.
- Avoid situations known to trigger seizures, such as repetitively flashing or blinking lights, stress, or lack of sleep.

Other nursing care includes, but is not limited to, the following diagnoses, expected outcomes, and interventions:

Injury Risk: Related to uncontrolled movements and altered consciousness during seizure; **Risk for Impaired Oral Mucous Membranes:** Related to oral injury during a seizure and side effects of phenytoin drug therapy
Expected Outcomes: (1) Client will be free of injuries. (2) Oral mucous membranes and gingiva will remain unaltered.

- Use padded headgear on clients with atonic or akinetic seizures. *Loss of consciousness and falls are common with these types of seizures, increasing the potential for head injury.*
- Pad side rails with soft material. *Padding cushions the force on the client's skin and soft tissue when contact with metal side rails occurs during a seizure.*
- Protect client at the onset of the seizure by assisting the client to the floor or moving objects away from the client. *The nurse reduces the risk for serious injuries by modifying the environment and the client's location in the environment.*
- Loosen clothing about the neck. *Tight clothing can impair breathing.*
- Never forcibly restrain the client. *Physically restraining a client during a seizure increases the potential for injuries such as fractures.*
- Inspect the oral cavity and teeth after a generalized seizure. *The nurse assesses the mouth for signs of injury and reports injuries to the primary provider.*
- Apply ice to bleeding areas; if broken teeth are noted, notify the client's dentist. *Ice constricts blood vessels and reduces bleeding. The client's dentist may be able to reimplant broken teeth or minimize the outcome of the trauma with early interventions.*
- Promote oral hygiene after each meal and recommend dental checkups every 3 to 6 months. *Phenytoin (Dilantin) causes gingival hyperplasia (overgrowth of gum tissue); regular and frequent dental examinations facilitate the maintenance or restoration of teeth and gums.*

Chronic Anxiety: Related to unpredictability of seizures and social stigma as evidenced by uneasiness about resuming previous lifestyle activities at work and with social acquaintances
Expected Outcome: Anxiety will be reduced as evidenced by a resumption of social interactions.

- Help the client understand the disorder and treatment options. *Knowledge about the disorder and making choices promotes a sense of control.*
- Explain that a variety of drugs are available that can successfully reduce or control seizures. *Drug therapy prevents or reduces seizure activity.*
- Encourage the client to share information about the disorder with others. *Providing accurate information dispels fears and helps eliminate the misconception that people with seizure disorders have subnormal intelligence.*
- Suggest contacting the Epilepsy Foundation. *The Epilepsy Foundation provides counseling, low-cost prescription services, and referrals to agencies for vocational rehabilitation, job opportunities, personal and genetic counseling, and sheltered workshops.*

Evaluation of Expected Outcomes

Expected outcomes for the client are that there are fewer seizures or that they are completely controlled. The client remains safe from injury. The client's mouth and teeth are intact. The client who takes phenytoin understands the importance of regular dental examinations because of the potential for gingival hyperplasia. The client's anxiety is reduced to a tolerable level on a scale of 0 to 10. The client resolves to pursue employment in a safe environment, maintain social relationships, and participate in leisure activities. The client is aware of the services provided by the Epilepsy Foundation and how to contact this organization.

BOX 37-3 Seizure Assessment Data

- Onset—sudden or preceded by an aura
- Duration of seizure
- Behavior immediately before and after seizure
- Type of body movements
- Loss of consciousness—for how long
- Incontinence or not
- Seizure awareness afterward

Evidence-Based Practice 37-1

Management of Epilepsy

Clinical Question

What is the management of epilepsy in adults and children?

Evidence

A neurologic disorder known as epilepsy is usually a symptom of seizures that are recurring with possible underlying causes. The first line of treatment is medication. The National Institute for Health and Care Excellence (NICE) recently updated its treatment guidelines. The first time a client experiences a seizure and seeks medical care, they should be screened to rule out epilepsy. If a diagnosis is made, they should be seen within a 2-week time frame. The medications that are the first line of treatment vary on the basis of the type of seizure that occurs. The treatment may include a special diet and should include monitoring drug levels of the medication ordered (Nunes et al., 2012).

Nursing Implications

Nurses should obtain a thorough history and assessment. The nurse should educate the client and family on observing a seizure and when to call the health care provider. Medication teaching should also be reinforced.

Reference

Nunes, V. D., Sawyer, L., Neilson, J., Sarri, G., & Cross, J. H. (2012). Diagnosis and management of the epilepsies in adults and children: Summary of updated NICE guidance. *British Medical Journal (Clinical Research Edition), 344*, e281. https://doi.org/10.1136/bmj .e281

BRAIN TUMORS

A **brain tumor** is a growth of abnormal cells within the cranium. Brain tumors occur in all age groups. Some types are more common in people younger than 20 years of age; others more frequently affect older people.

Brain tumors are classified according to whether they are benign or malignant, the type of cells involved, and the site of the tumor. The most common types of adult brain tumors are (1) metastatic tumors from a primary site; (2) gliomas, which involve cells that support structures in the brain, including astrocytes, cells that protect neurons; oligodendrocytes, cells that make myelin; and ependymocytes, cells that line the pathways that carry CSF; and (3) meningiomas, tumors involving the meningeal coverings of the brain and spinal cord. About 50% of all brain tumors are malignant. However, a brain tumor, whether malignant or benign, can result in death.

Pathophysiology and Etiology

The cause of most brain tumors, which occur in various areas of the brain (Fig. 37-17), remains unknown. A small percentage is congenital, such as hemangioblastomas. Genetic factors are associated with two types of brain tumors: *astrocytoma*, a gliomal tumor in the frontal lobe, and *neurofibromatosis*. Other causative factors include viral infection, exposure to radiation, head trauma, and

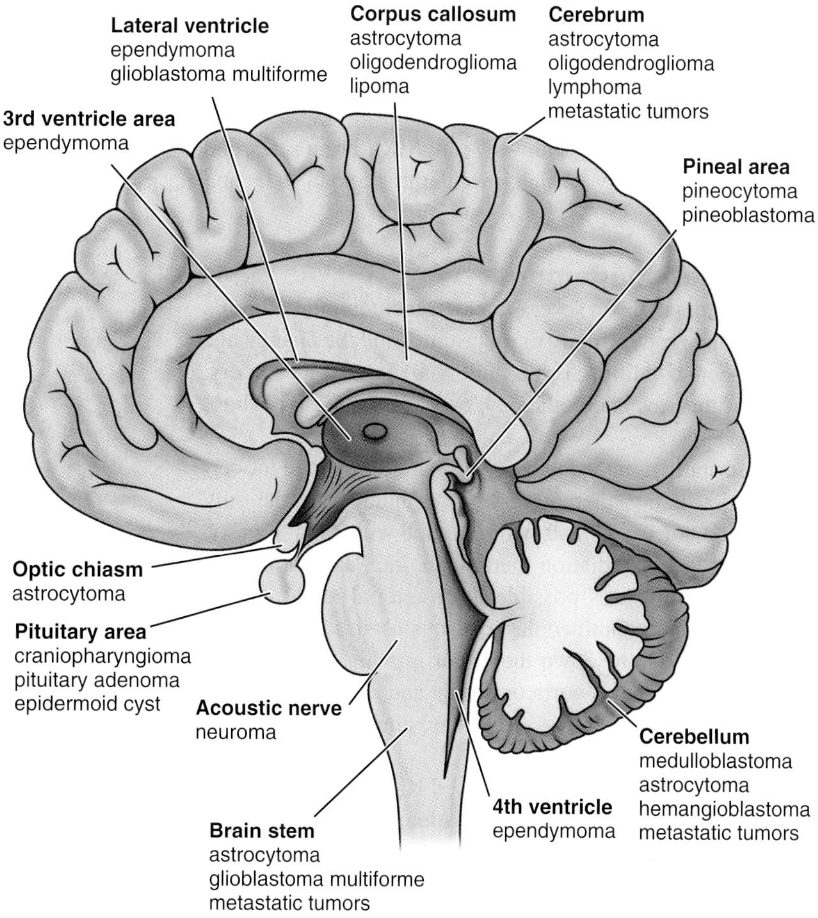

Figure 37-17 Common sites for a brain tumor.

immunosuppression. The brain is also the site of metastatic lesions from primary tumors, especially those of the lung and breast.

Tumors that arise from cerebral tissue, such as malignant gliomas and glioblastomas, and angiomas that involve cerebral blood vessels expand in the confines of the skull, encroach on brain tissue, and raise ICP. Extracerebral tumors, such as meningiomas, press on the brain tissue from within.

Assessment Findings

Signs and Symptoms

Because tumors take up space and block the flow and absorption of CSF, symptoms associated with increased ICP occur. The classic triad of headache, vomiting, and papilledema is common. Headache is most common early in the morning. It becomes increasingly severe and occurs more frequently as the tumor grows. Vomiting occurs without nausea or warning. Seizures also develop. Symptoms of disturbed neurologic function, such as behavioral and mood changes, speech difficulty, paralysis, and double vision, may be manifested depending on the tumor's location.

When the ICP is greatly increased, areas of the brain can herniate (see Fig. 37-2). If the brain stem is forced through the foramen magnum, the client is in grave danger because the vital centers that control respiration and heart rate are compressed. Respirations become deeper, labored, and noisy and then slow to only periodic. Unless the condition is relieved, the client dies of respiratory failure and cardiac arrest. Hyperthermia occurs as the temperature-regulating center in the brain is affected. Coma progressively deepens.

Diagnostic Findings

Diagnosis is confirmed with CT scan, MRI, brain scan, and cerebral angiography, which reveal the tumor's size and location.

Medical Management

Treatment depends on several factors, including the tumor's location and type (primary or metastatic) and the client's age and physical condition. Brain tumors are treated by surgery, radiation therapy, chemotherapy, or a combination of these methods.

Metastatic tumors and some primary tumors are inoperable, and radiation therapy and chemotherapy are the only treatment choices. Clients who cannot withstand surgery, chemotherapy, or radiation therapy are kept as comfortable and free from pain as possible. Intra-arterial or intrathecal administration of antineoplastic drugs is used to destroy the tumor or to slow down the tumor growth. Symptomatic drug therapy includes corticosteroids and osmotic diuretics to reduce cerebral edema, analgesics, anticonvulsants, and antibiotics.

Complications, such as increased ICP, paralysis, mental changes, infection, seizures, and prolonged immobility, are treated symptomatically.

Surgical Management

Surgery for an operable brain tumor involves a craniotomy (incision through the skull) or craniectomy (excision of part of the skull). A section of bone (bone flap) is removed to reach the brain (Fig. 37-18). After the tumor is removed, the dura is reapproximated (the cut edges are lined up and sewn together), the bone flap replaced, and the skin sutured. The bone flap is not reinserted when increasing ICP or tumor growth is expected.

The client's postoperative symptoms are determined by the location and function of any damaged or removed brain tissue. Brain tissue does not regenerate.

Another method of removing brain tumors uses a laser beam directed at the tumor site. This surgical technique enables the primary provider to reach tumors that previously were considered inoperable. Radioisotopes also are surgically inserted into the tumor. However, the cure rate for this procedure is about the same as for external radiation therapy.

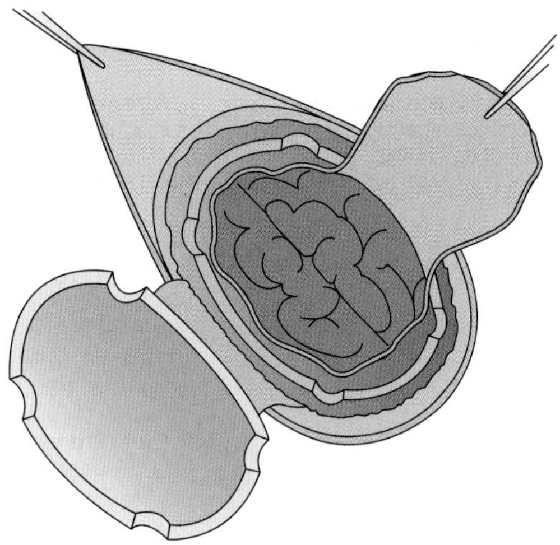

A Craniotomy

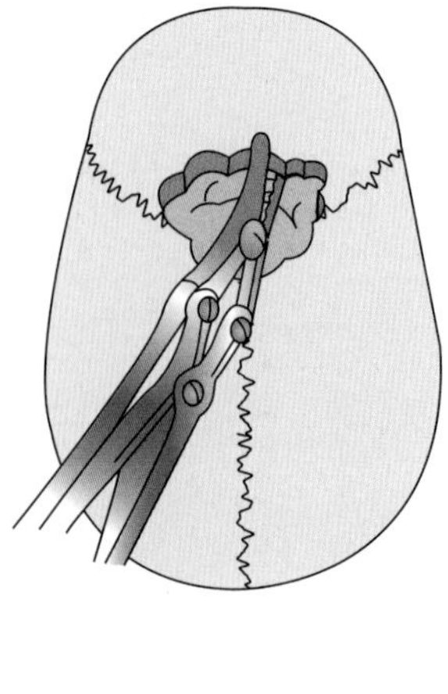

B Craniectomy

Figure 37-18 Neurosurgical techniques: **(A)** craniotomy and **(B)** craniectomy.

Gamma-Knife Radiosurgery

Gamma-knife radiosurgery is a noninvasive alternative for treating tumors deep within the brain or that conventional surgery can only partially remove. Removing these types of tumors through conventional surgery is difficult or generally impossible and can create the potential for damaging healthy brain tissue.

The gamma-knife targets the lesion without making an incision, thus eliminating the risk for surgical complications and dangers of prolonged general anesthesia. The gamma-knife directs gamma radiation from many computer-calculated directions to converge at a precise target area. Radiation is then delivered through holes in a helmet applied to the client's head. A box-shaped head frame attached to the scalp with screws holds the helmet in place and ensures that there is no head movement (Fig. 37-19). Treatment, done on an outpatient basis or as a 24-hour inpatient stay, involves more than one procedure. The duration of each treatment varies from 2 to 4 hours depending on the client's pathology. The client remains awake and experiences only a clicking sound, as the procedure commences and terminates. Over time, the brain tumor shrinks and disappears. Some clients develop a headache and minor nausea after a treatment. Temporary hair loss may occur if the radiated tumor is close to the surface of the skull.

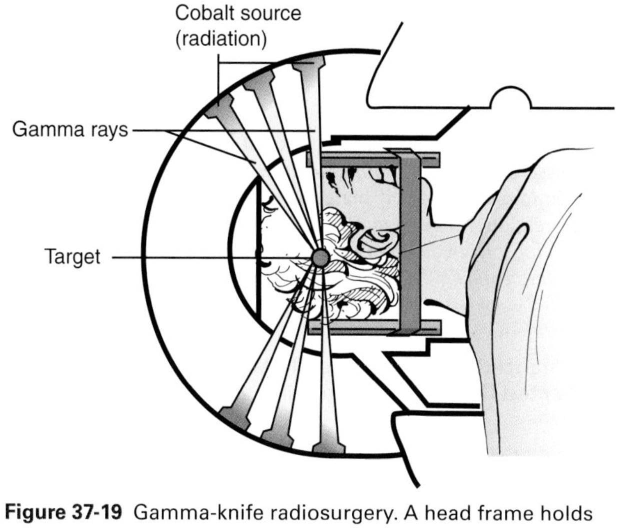

Figure 37-19 Gamma-knife radiosurgery. A head frame holds the head in place, and a plastic localizer is used during the pretreatment scans as a targeting landmark. Gamma rays converge on the targeted site of the tumor.

Nursing Management

Nursing management depends on the area of the brain affected, tumor type, treatment approach, and the client's signs and symptoms. If the tumor is inoperable or has expanded despite treatment, increased ICP is a major threat (see Nursing Care Plan 37-1). See Chapter 39 for the care of the client undergoing intracranial surgery. Clients who receive chemotherapy and radiation are supported through the adverse effects associated with antineoplastic drug administration and effects of radiation (see Chapter 18). The nurse clarifies the client's and family's questions concerning treatment modalities and directs the client to appropriate professionals to discuss treatment alternatives. The nurse explains hospice care and services to clients with brain tumors that no longer are at a stage where they can be cured.

Before the client is discharged, the nurse evaluates the client's and the family's immediate and long-term needs. The nurse develops an individualized teaching plan that addresses the following components:

- Medication regimen
- Appointments for chemotherapy or radiation therapy
- Adverse effects of chemotherapy or radiation and techniques for managing them
- Nutritional support
- Home care considerations
- Rehabilitation (exercises, physical therapy)
- Referrals to support services for physical, emotional, and financial assistance

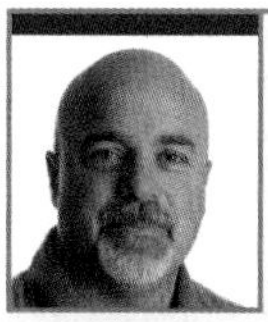

Clinical Scenario During an appointment for a routine gynecologic examination, the client tells the nurse, "I'm really concerned about my husband. He's been having persistent headaches. He is easily irritated and becomes angry over minor incidents, which is so unlike how he behaved 6 months ago. I've noticed that he stumbles and falls occasionally." The nurse suggests the client arrange an appointment for her husband with a neurologist for diagnostic and treatment purposes. Subsequently, a CT scan identifies an inoperable mass in the client's brain; a combination of radiation and chemotherapy will be used for palliation. **What might the client's care include from a nursing perspective as his condition worsens? See the following Nursing Process section.**

NURSING PROCESS FOR THE CLIENT WITH A BRAIN TUMOR

Assessment

Identify affected areas after a thorough history and neurologic examination. Perform a physical assessment and record the abnormal findings.

Diagnosis, Planning, and Interventions

Depending on the stage of the disease and the selected method(s) of treatment, the nurse's role includes, but is not limited to, the following:

Acute Pain: Related to increased ICP secondary to expansion of the tumor or a sequela of surgery
Expected Outcome: Pain will be controlled within client's level of tolerance.

(continued)

NURSING PROCESS FOR THE CLIENT WITH A BRAIN TUMOR (continued)

- Assess and monitor characteristics of pain every time you measure vital signs. *Pain assessment is the fifth vital sign.*
- Administer prescribed analgesia and monitor for respiratory depression. *Narcotic analgesics relieve pain, but tolerance develops. High doses of narcotic analgesics depress the respiratory center in the brain.*
- Give analgesia on a scheduled rather than an as-needed basis. *Regular administration of analgesia is most effective at controlling pain.*
- Advocate for client-controlled analgesia or transdermal analgesic patch. *Methods that facilitate frequent administration of small doses of IV analgesia or continuous absorption through the skin provide more continuous pain relief.*

Imbalanced Nutrition (Less Than Body Requirements): Related to nausea and vomiting or altered LOC
Expected Outcome: Nutritional and fluid needs are met as evidenced by maintenance of weight and intake above 2,000 mL.

- Administer prescribed antiemetics before meals. *A client is likely to consume adequate food without nausea or vomiting.*
- Determine client's food preferences and supply them. *Catering to likes and dislikes promotes a greater intake of food.*
- Give small, frequent servings of food or nourishing beverages. *Large servings tend to overwhelm a client. They may consume more food overall if smaller amounts are served several times a day. Liquid nutritional supplements provide extra calories and nutrients in an easily consumed form.*
- Collaborate with the primary provider concerning gastric tube feedings or TPN. *Enteral and parenteral routes for nutrition may be used when the oral route is no longer adequate.*

Impaired Oral Mucous Membranes: Related to fluid volume deficit, tissue damage secondary to chemotherapy or radiation as manifested by xerostomia (oral lesions)
Expected Outcome: Oral mucous membranes will be pink, moist, and intact.

- Relieve discomfort with a prescribed topical anesthetic. *It blocks sensory nerves and relieves local discomfort.*
- Provide meticulous mouth care. *The mouth contains many microorganisms that thrive on particles of food and sugar clinging to teeth. Increased microbial growth fosters the potential for dental decay and impaired tissue.*
- Offer mouth rinses of tap water or medicated solutions frequently. *Liquids keep the mouth moist and flush debris from the oral cavity.*

Grief: Related to uncertain future, physical, and social losses
Expected Outcome: Client and family members will express feelings and deal with potential losses while working through acceptance of the diagnosis.

- Give the opportunity to express feelings privately. *A person is more likely to be open and frank in an environment where others will not overhear intimate feelings.*
- Remain with client when emotions are overwhelming. *A supportive other helps client endure emotional pain and cope more effectively.*
- Help clarify any and all questions the client may have. *Honest and accurate information facilitates the client's right to self-determination.*
- Provide reassurance that the client will not be abandoned and that comfort and preservation of dignity are priorities of nursing care. *Most clients fear that they will be left alone when dying and will experience extreme pain or discomfort.*
- Assist client to complete unfinished business however they define it. *Taking care of tasks, accomplishing specific goals, or communicating feelings to significant others helps clients die more peacefully.*
- Refer client and family to the local hospice organization if the client is in the terminal stage. *Hospice organizations help client and family meet their physical and emotional needs.*

Evaluation of Expected Outcomes

The client reports that pain is relieved or resolved to a tolerable level. Nutritional intake is sufficient to maintain body weight. Oral mucosa is intact. The client and family progress through the grieving process and implement a plan for postdischarge care.

KEY POINTS

- Signs and symptoms of increased intracranial pressure:
  - Drowsiness
  - Difficult to awaken
  - Restlessness
  - Confusion
  - Irritability
- Infectious or inflammatory diseases of the CNS or PNS:
  - Meningitis: an inflammation of the meninges caused by various infectious microorganisms such as bacteria, viruses, fungi, or parasites
  - Encephalitis: an inflammatory process affecting the CNS
  - Guillain–Barré syndrome: (acute postinfectious polyneuropathy, polyradiculoneuritis) affects the peripheral nerves and the spinal nerve roots

- Brain abscess: a collection of purulent material in the brain
- Neuromuscular disorders:
  - Multiple sclerosis is a chronic, progressive disease of the peripheral nerves.
  - Myasthenia gravis is a neuromuscular disorder characterized by severe weakness of one or more groups of skeletal muscles.
  - Amyotrophic lateral sclerosis, also known as *Lou Gehrig disease*, is a progressive and fatal neurologic disorder.
- **Cranial Nerve Disorders:**
  - Trigeminal neuralgia is a painful condition that involves the fifth cranial nerve.
  - Bell palsy involves the seventh cranial nerve (CN VII), that affects facial movement.
- **Extrapyramidal Disorders:**
  - Parkinson disease primarily affects the basal ganglia and connections in the substantia nigra and corpus striatum and results from result from a deficiency of the neurotransmitter dopamine.
  - Huntington disease is a hereditary disorder of the CNS; it is transmitted genetically and inherited by people of both genders.
- Types of seizures:
  - Partial, or focal, seizures begin in a specific area of the cerebral cortex.
  - Generalized seizures involve the entire brain. The client loses consciousness, and the seizure may last from several seconds to several minutes.
  - Unclassified seizures: seizures that do not fit into other classifications

CRITICAL THINKING EXERCISES

1. When caring for a client with a seizure disorder, what nursing interventions are indicated?
2. What information can the nurse provide to a person who has recently been diagnosed with MS?
3. What discharge teaching is appropriate when discussing home care with the spouse of a client in the late stage of Parkinson disease?
4. An older female adult client with myasthenia gravis is concerned about the cost of medications under her Medicare prescription drug plan. She questions the necessity of neostigmine (Prostigmin) and pyridostigmine bromide (Mestinon). What information is important to provide this client to promote drug compliance following discharge?

NCLEX-STYLE REVIEW QUESTIONS PrepU

1. Based on the figure, place an X where the most dangerous and often fatal type of brain herniation can occur in clients with ICP.

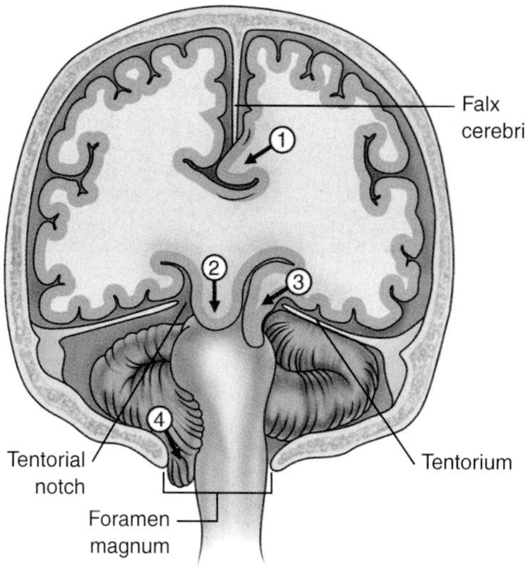

2. Because older adults often do not exhibit the typical signs and symptoms of meningitis, what assessment findings should the nurse be especially vigilant for in older clients with suspected meningitis? Select all that apply.
   1. Low-grade fever
   2. Nuchal rigidity
   3. Double vision
   4. Altered mental status
3. When the nurse selects the equipment to place in the room of a client who has been diagnosed with Guillain–Barré syndrome, what item is essential to managing the client's care?
   1. Supplemental oxygen
   2. Cardiac monitoring
   3. Nasogastric suction
   4. Intravenous therapy
4. To promote adequate nutrition and reduce the risk for aspiration when caring for a client with Parkinson or Huntington disease, what nursing measures are appropriate? Select all that apply.
   1. Modify the texture and consistency of food.
   2. Have the client flex the chin when swallowing.
   3. Encourage frequent sips of water while eating.
   4. Position the client in a sitting position.
   5. Allow ample time for consuming meals.
5. What nursing intervention is most appropriate for managing the care of a client experiencing a seizure?
   1. Restrain the client's involuntary movements.
   2. Suction client's mouth and pharynx during the seizure.
   3. Place client in supine position during the seizure.
   4. Provide oxygen during and after the seizure.

WANT TO KNOW MORE? There are a wide variety of online resources available on thePoint to enhance learning and understanding of this chapter.

Go to **thePoint.lww.com/activate** and use the activation code found in the front of this text to unlock these online resources.

38 Caring for Clients With Cerebrovascular Disorders

Words To Know

aneurysm
bruit
carotid endarterectomy
cephalalgia
cerebral infarction
cerebrovascular accident
collateral circulation
expressive aphasia
hemianopia
hemiplegia
receptive aphasia
transient ischemic attack

Learning Objectives

On completion of this chapter, you will be able to:

1. Identify three common types of headaches and their characteristics.
2. List the nursing techniques that supplement drug therapy in reducing or relieving headaches.
3. Explain the cause and significance of a transient ischemic attack (TIA).
4. Discuss the medical and surgical techniques used to reduce the potential for a cerebrovascular accident.
5. Differentiate between ischemic and hemorrhagic strokes.
6. Identify five manifestations of a cerebrovascular accident and discuss those that are unique to right-sided and left-sided infarctions.
7. Identify at least five nursing diagnoses common to the care of a client with a cerebrovascular accident and interventions for them.
8. Describe a cerebral aneurysm and the danger it presents.
9. Discuss appropriate nursing interventions when caring for a client with a cerebral aneurysm.

Cerebrovascular disorders are major medical problems that affect adults. Some, such as headaches, can disrupt a client's lifestyle, causing tremendous discomfort and anxiety. Others, such as a cerebrovascular accident (CVA) and transient ischemic attacks (TIAs), are life-threatening.

Gerontologic Considerations

■ Older adults may ignore the symptoms of a TIA, attributing them to part of the normal aging process. Careful documentation of history with sequence of symptoms can help identify etiology and health awareness or health behaviors.

■ A major risk factor for stroke is hypertension. Older adults who live on a limited income may choose to extend medications by taking them less frequently than prescribed or using one type of antihypertensive medication at a time if more than one is prescribed.

■ Client/family education must include a medication review, assessment of client's understanding about the purpose of the medication, and assessment of risks from not adhering to the recommended schedule.

■ Combination medications (e.g., diuretics combined with vasodilators) may be more expensive than single agents. Evaluation of the individual is critical to determine

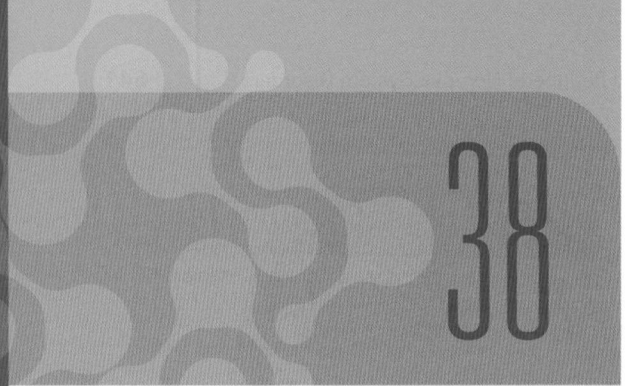

Gerontologic Considerations (continued)

if adherence is more influenced by cost or by difficulty remembering times for multiple doses.

- Additionally, health teaching should include the relationship of hidden dietary sodium, especially in prepared foods.
- Symptoms of decreased alertness, drowsiness, weakness, or falling may be attributed to other health concerns common in older persons. All clients with hypertension must be informed of these common symptoms of CVA to promote early access to care.
- Various evidence-based teaching techniques such as the teach-back method assist in increasing the effectiveness of health care teaching.
- The older adult is more susceptible to the complications of prolonged bed rest and inactivity such as hypostatic pneumonia, pressure ulcers, and contractures that may be involved in the rehabilitation period after a CVA.
- Health care providers should avoid stereotypes that suggest older persons may lack motivation or the ability to participate in rehabilitation efforts, or that the outcomes will not be positive. The health care provider may need to teach family and friends to encourage the person with a CVA during rehabilitation to provide motivation and support.
- Rehabilitation of the older client with a CVA is subject to more complications than rehabilitation of a younger adult. The nurse must work closely with the family and social service agencies to help the family assume the care of the client to the extent possible or to facilitate a transfer to a rehabilitation center or long-term care facility.

HEADACHE

Aching in the head is referred to as **cephalalgia.** This symptom accompanies many disorders such as meningitis, increased intracranial pressure (ICP), brain tumors, and sinusitis. When the duration is relatively brief, a headache is considered transient and benign. Although there are many types of headaches, *tension*, *migraine*, and *cluster* headaches are the most common (Table 38-1). Tension headaches, the most common of the three, occur when a person contracts the neck and facial muscles for a prolonged period of time. Migraine headaches, which are recurrent and severe and last for a day or more, have a vascular origin. Cluster headaches may be a variant of migraine headaches; they are episodic, recurring over 6 to 8 weeks, with only brief periods of recovery between multiple daily attacks.

Pathophysiology and Etiology

Tension Headaches

Neither the skull nor the brain itself contains sensory nerves. A vast network of sensory and motor nerves, however, is distributed throughout the scalp and facial muscles. During stressful conditions, people tend to contract muscles about the neck, face, and scalp, and a tension headache may develop. A tension headache also can develop when a person contracts the neck and facial muscles for a prolonged period. When the tensed muscles sensitize *nociceptors*, pain-relaying nerves in the head, the nociceptors transmit neurochemicals such as prostaglandin and substance P to the brain, which registers the presence and location of discomfort (see Chapter 11).

Migraine Headaches

Researchers are getting closer to finding what causes migraine headaches. They have targeted three sequential contributing cofactors: (1) changes in particular serotonin receptors that promote (2) dilation of cerebral blood vessels and pain intensification from (3) neurochemicals released from the trigeminal nerve (Fig. 38-1). Literature suggests that there are a variety of triggers that can cause migraines such as fluctuations in reproductive hormones, chemicals in certain foods, a food-related allergy, emotional stress, alcohol, caffeine, or drugs (Migraines, 2020; Box 38-1).

TABLE 38-1 Features of Common Headaches

FEATURE	CLUSTER HEADACHE	MIGRAINE HEADACHE	TENSION HEADACHE
Client's gender	Usually male	Usually female	Equally male/female
Age at onset	20–50 years	10–40 years	Any age
Frequency of attacks	1–8/day	1–8/month	Almost daily
Duration of attacks	30 minutes to 4 hours	4–72 hours	Gradual onset, steady
Intensity of pain	Excruciatingly relentless	Moderate to severe	Constant dull ache
Location of pain	Strictly unilateral	Unilateral or bilateral	Bilateral
Nasal congestion	70%	None	None
Droopy, teary eye	Common	Uncommon	Uncommon
Incidence of associated nausea and vomiting	Rare	Common	Rare
Incidence of attacks awakening client from sleep	Common	Rare	Rare
Characteristic behavior	Client cannot remain still during severe attack	Client prefers hibernation	Client prefers hibernation
Family history	7%	90%	Associated with stress
Treatment	Refer to primary provider	Refer to primary provider	Refer to primary provider

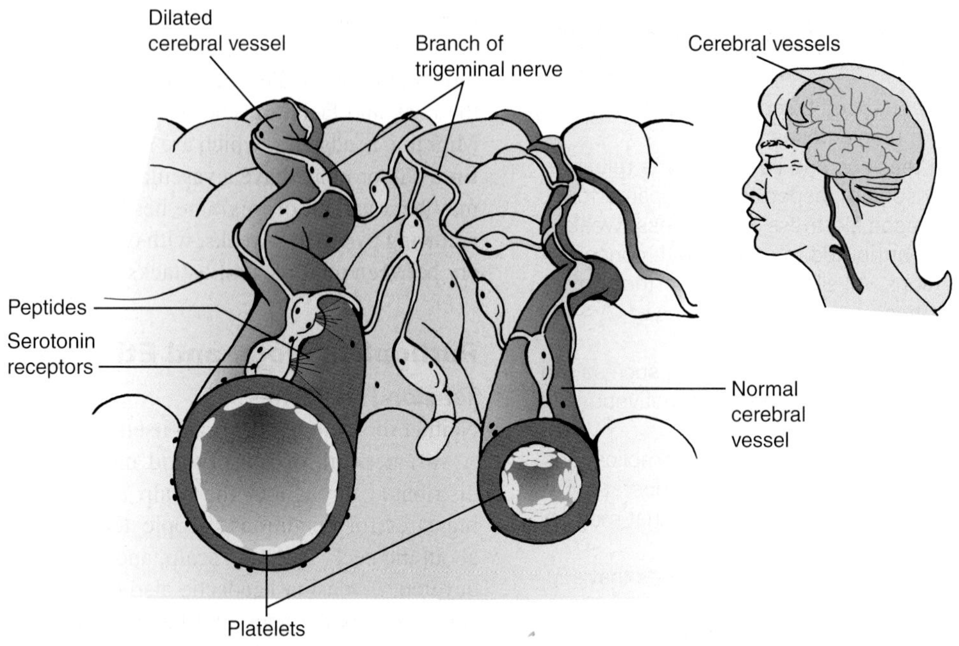

Figure 38-1 Chemical developments in migraine headaches. Cerebral blood vessels dilate in response to serotonin from platelets. Peptides released from the trigeminal nerve intensify pain.

Cluster Headaches

The cause of cluster headaches is unknown. Cluster headaches can be triggered by vasodilating agents such as nitroglycerin, histamine, and alcoholic beverages. A lower-than-normal level of the neurotransmitter serotonin may explain the mechanism by which serotonin-enhancing drugs provide relief. Acetylcholine, a parasympathetic neurotransmitter, also may play a role in cluster headaches.

BOX 38-1 Substances That Trigger Migraine Headaches

Foods
- Aged cheese
- Alcohol
- Bananas, figs, raisins
- Caffeine
- Citrus fruits
- Chocolate
- Dairy products
- Fermented or pickled food
- Nuts
- Onions
- Pea or lima bean pods
- Processed foods containing nitrites, sulfites, or monosodium glutamate (MSG)
- Saccharin or aspartame
- Yeast-containing products

Drugs
- Analgesic overuse
- Benzodiazepine withdrawal
- Cimetidine
- Decongestant overuse
- Estrogen replacement
- Fenfluramine
- Indomethacin
- Nifedipine
- Nitrates
- Oral contraceptives
- Reserpine
- Theophylline

Events
- Stress
- Menstruation; menopause
- Sleep changes; excess or loss
- Overexertion
- Hunger or fasting
- Odors, smoke, or perfume
- Strong glare or flashing lights

Assessment Findings

Symptoms vary from a mild ache to severe, disabling pain. Clients may describe a tension headache as pressure or steady constriction on both sides of the head. Some people correlate the onset of the headache with anxiety or emotional conflict.

Clients who have "classic" migraines may experience an *aura*, a sensory phenomenon that precedes the headache like seeing flashing lights or wavy lines for about 10 to 30 minutes. For others with the more "common" form of migraine, the prodromal period before the headache is marked by a change in mood, difficulty concentrating, or unusual fatigue. The client with a migraine describes the pain as "throbbing" or "bursting." Nausea and vomiting, vertigo, sensitivity to light, irritability, and fatigue accompany the headache.

A person with a cluster headache has pain on one side of the head, usually behind the eye, accompanied by nasal congestion, *rhinorrhea* (watery discharge from the nose), and tearing and redness of the eye. The pain is so severe that the person is not likely to lie still; rather they pace or thrash about.

Diagnosis is based on the pattern of headaches and the accompanying signs and symptoms. Persistent headaches require tests such as computed tomography (CT) scan, brain scan, head and neck radiographs, and angiography to rule out other neurologic disorders such as a brain tumor or intracerebral hemorrhage.

Medical Management

Transient tension headaches usually are relieved by rest, a mild analgesic, and stress management techniques such as relaxation or imaging (see Chapter 67). For severe, recurrent tension headaches, counseling and psychotherapy may help clients deal with emotional stressors in healthier ways. Antidepressants also help some clients.

Mild analgesics usually are ineffective for migraine headaches. Drug therapy with methysergide (Sansert) or topiramate (Topamax) may be prescribed to prevent migraines, or drugs such as sumatriptan (Imitrex) may be prescribed to interrupt migraines that have already developed (Drug Therapy Table 38-1). Prophylactic drug therapy may be necessary if migraine headaches occur several times a month and produce severe impairment or if acute attacks are not adequately relieved. Although this may not prevent all migraines, it may reduce the frequency, intensity, and duration of attacks. Antiemetics may control nausea and vomiting that accompany an acute migraine. Some clients learn to shorten or abort migraines with biofeedback techniques (see Chapter 67).

DRUG THERAPY TABLE 38-1 Drugs for Managing Headaches

Category and Common Generic (Brand) Drugs	Intended Use	Common Side Effects	Safety Warnings for Nurses
Migraine Prophylaxis			
Ergotamine derivatives Methysergide (Sansert)	Displaces serotonin on cranial artery receptors, promotes vasoconstriction	Insomnia, postural hypotension, nausea, vomiting, heartburn, abdominal pain, diarrhea, flushing, rash, edema	Increased fall risk owing to effects on blood pressure Dose must be titrated down when stopping drug Do not use when breastfeeding
Beta-adrenergic blocker Atenolol (Tenormin)	Blocks the beta receptors for norepinephrine and epinephrine, thereby preventing cerebral vasoconstriction	Hypotension, bradycardia, impotence, peripheral edema, depression, fatigue	Monitor pulse and blood pressure Withhold drug if pulse is <60 beats/min Teach to change positions slowly Contraindicated if breastfeeding
Antidepressants *Serotonin/norepinephrine and dopamine/norepinephrine reuptake inhibitors (SNRI/DNRI)* Duloxetine (Cymbalta) Venlafaxine (Effexor) *Tricyclics* Desipramine (Norpramin) Nortriptyline (Pamelor)	Used to treat migraine headaches, neuropathy, fibromyalgia	Dizziness, somnolence, dry mouth, nausea, flushing	Screen for suicidal ideation Dose must be titrated down when stopping drug Taking the herbal, St. John's wort can increase risk of Serotonin syndrome Overdoses may be fatal; ensure the client accurately understands self-administration
Antileptics Carbamazepine (Tegretol) Levetiracetam (Keppra) Topiramate (Topamax) Valproic acid (Depakote) *Calcium Channel Binders* Gabapentin (Neurontin) Pregabalin (Lyrica)	Migraine headache	Dizziness, somnolence, nausea, weight gain	Increased fall risk owing to sedative side effects Dose must be titrated down when stopping drug
Agents for Acute Migraines—Serotonin 5-HT Receptor Agonists			
Almotriptan (Axert) Eletriptan (Relpax) Frovatriptan (Frova) Naratriptan (Amerge) Rizatriptan (Maxalt) Sumatriptan (Alsuma, Imitrex, Sumavel) Zolmitriptan (Zomig)	Acute migraine headache pain	Headache, dizziness, fatigue, somnolence, nausea, dry mouth, flushing, hot/cold sensations, pain in chest or neck, paresthesias	If taking with selective serotonin reuptake inhibitor/serotonin and norepinephrine reuptake inhibitor (SSRI/SNRI) anti-depressant monitor for Serotonin syndrome Do not use injectable form if cloudy or yellow
Ergotamine derivatives Dihydroergotamine (DHE 45, Migranal) Ergotamine (Ergomar)	Cluster/vascular headache pain	Nausea, rhinitis, altered taste	Advise to take at first sign of headache Stress that maximum dose should not be exceeded Contraindicated during pregnancy

The drugs in column 1 indicate the drug that matches up with explanations in columns 2 through 4.

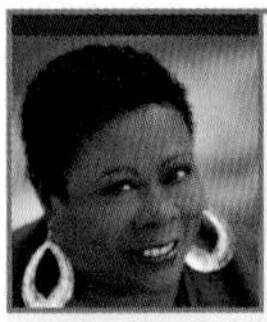

Clinical Scenario After unsuccessfully taking various over-the-counter analgesics to minimize or eliminate recurrent headaches, a 38-year-old client tells the nurse at an outpatient headache clinic, "I'm concerned because my headaches persistently occur sometimes once or twice a week. I feel like I've tried everything I can on my own; I'm a walking drug store. I'm hoping I can finally get something that will provide relief." **How can the nurse intervene to assist the client? See the following Nursing Process section.**

NURSING PROCESS FOR THE CLIENT WITH A HEADACHE

Assessment

Ask the client questions about the location, type of pain, and past history of the same type of headache because another disorder or problem may be occurring. Determine whether the pain is in one area or over the entire head; factors that appear to bring on, worsen, or relieve the headache; how long the pain lasts; and symptoms such as tearing, nasal congestion, nausea or vomiting, or sensitivity to light.

When assessing clients with chronic headaches or headaches that cause various symptoms, obtain a complete medical, allergy, and family history as well as a record of frequency and description of the pain, including its numeric intensity during an attack. Record vital signs to use as a baseline for comparison.

Diagnosis, Planning, and Interventions

The nurse reinforces the drug therapy regimen prescribed by the primary provider and instructs the client on self-administration of medications. The nurse teaches the client with migraines to take medication as soon as symptoms begin and to minimize noise and other pain-provoking stimuli (Client and Family Teaching 38-1, Evidence-Based Practice 38-1). In addition, the following nursing interventions are appropriate for clients with headache.

Acute pain: Related to muscle tension, changes in cerebral blood flow, or unknown etiology

Expected outcome: Headache will be reduced or eliminated within 30 minutes of a pain-relieving intervention.

- Eliminate environmental factors that intensify pain, such as bright light and noise. *Sensory stimuli decrease pain tolerance.*
- Administer prescribed medications as early as possible and note their effect. *Medications that relieve headaches are in many different categories with various mechanisms of action. If the medication is ineffective, collaborate with the primary provider to modify the method of treatment.*
- Seek someone who can provide a back massage to promote muscle relaxation. *Massage relaxes tense muscles, causes local dilation of blood vessels, and relieves headache. This approach is not likely to help a client with migraine or cluster headache.*
- Apply warm (or cool) cloths to the forehead or back of the neck. *Warmth promotes vasodilation; cool stimuli reduce blood flow.*
- Provide distraction with soft, soothing music, or suggest using a relaxation tape or one that provides guided imagery. *Reduced anxiety can relieve a tension headache; clients with migraine or cluster headaches are not receptive to this approach.*

Evaluation of Expected Outcomes

Head pain is reduced or eliminated. The client demonstrates understanding of the medication regimen and possible side effects. They identify ways to modify behavior to minimize pain.

Symptoms of cluster headaches are controlled with various drugs, including an ergotamine derivative such as dihydroergotamine (Migranal) or methysergide (Sansert). Some clients respond to corticosteroids such as triamcinolone (Aristocort) and prednisone (Deltasone), lithium carbonate (Eskalith), vasoconstricting drugs in the "triptan" group such as sumatriptan (Imitrex) and zolmitriptan (Zomig), anticonvulsants such as gabapentin (Neurontin) and divalproex (Depakote), and beta-adrenergic blockers such as atenolol (Tenormin) and propranolol (Inderal). Inhaled or injected drugs are preferred because they are absorbed more rapidly than those administered by the oral route (see Drug Therapy Table 38-1). Oxygen may be used during a headache to reduce the vasodilating compensatory response occurring in

Client and Family Teaching 38-1 Migraine Headaches

The nurse includes the following instructions:

- Follow the indications and dosage regimen for medication and notify the primary provider of any adverse drug effects.
- Identify and avoid factors that precipitate or intensify an attack. Keeping a food diary may help identify foods that trigger attacks.
- Keep a record of the attacks, including activities before the attack and environmental or emotional circumstances that appear to bring on the attack.
- Lie down in a darkened room and avoid noise and movement when an attack occurs, if that is possible.

the brain. For clients who do not respond to pharmacologic interventions, neurosurgical techniques such as rhizotomy may be the only hope for relief (see Chapter 11).

Evidence-Based Practice 38-1

Pharmacologic Compared With Alternative Therapies for Headache Management

Clinical Question

In clients with headaches, how does pharmacologic therapy compare with alternative therapies for pain management?

Evidence

Clients who suffer from headaches are looking for alternatives to traditional pharmacologic treatments (medication) for prevention and symptom control. Complementary and alternative medicine (CAM) has become an option that clients are exploring. Although there has been little research done in the United States, researchers in other countries have been studying this (Lieba-Samal et al., 2012; Rossi et al., 2006). Rossi and colleagues studied whether clients with chronic tension-type headaches (CTTH) considered and used CAM. Different types of CAM therapies such as chiropractic, massage therapy, acupuncture and acupressure, herbal therapy, and homeopathy were studied in Rossi's research. Of the 110 people who took part in the study, over 80% said they would think about using CAM therapies, and 41% said they felt that the therapies helped (Rossi et al., 2006). In another study of 114 clients, Lieba-Samal and associates also found that 80% of clients who suffered from various types of headaches were aware of at least one nonpharmacologic treatment and 75% had used at least one complementary or alternative treatment to treat their headaches (Lieba-Samal et al., 2012). In fact, more clients used complementary or alternative treatments than pharmacologic therapies (Lieba-Samal et al., 2012).

In a study done in 2019 reviewing 3 years of research they found that exercise, yoga, and tai chi (−3.6 migraine days, $P < 0.001$) showed improvements with a decrease in the number of migraine days and a decrease in severity, frequency, and impact of the migraine (Neurology Advisor, 2019).

Nursing Implications

CAM offers clients choices for treating their headache symptoms. Although CAM is provided by trained practitioners, CAM interventions offer nurses safe, easy, and inexpensive options to prevent headaches and help clients feel better. Interventions like deep breathing and guided imagery, use of pleasant music, warm or cold compresses, and adjusting room conditions (decreasing noise and brightness of lights) can be used to help clients avoid, delay, or supplement the use of traditional medications when they are suffering from headache symptoms. Communication and awareness is key, so talking to the client, family, and primary health care provider (or encouraging the client to alert their primary health care provider) when using CAM interventions is very important to helping clients get the best care and results.

References

Neurology Advisor. (2019). *Complementary and integrative treatments for migraine: An expert interview.* https://www.neurologyadvisor.com/topics/migraine-and-headache/complementary-and-integrative-treatments-for-migraine-expert-interview/

TRANSIENT ISCHEMIC ATTACKS

A **transient ischemic attack** (TIA) is a sudden, brief episode of neurologic impairment caused by a temporary interruption in cerebral blood flow. Symptoms may disappear within 1 hour; some continue for as long as 1 day. When the symptoms terminate, the client resumes their presymptomatic state. A TIA is a warning that a **cerebrovascular accident** (CVA; also known as *stroke*) can occur in the near future; one third of people who experience a TIA subsequently develop a stroke. The American Heart Association and the American Stroke Association advocate that the mnemonic FAST be used to evaluate if a person is in danger of having a stroke. FAST stands for: **F**—Face drooping especially on one side; **A**—Arm weakness; **S**—Slurred speech; **T**—Time to call 911.

Pathophysiology and Etiology

TIAs result from impaired blood circulation in the brain, which can be caused by atherosclerosis and arteriosclerosis, cardiac disease, or diabetes (see Chapters 25, 27, and 51). Circulation is impaired by atherosclerosis (buildup of fatty plaque) in cerebral blood vessels and the formation of thrombi and microemboli. The inelastic arterial system affected by arteriosclerosis restricts the volume of blood circulating through blood vessels. Arrhythmias and ineffective heart contraction are the catalysts for thrombi that can travel to cerebral vessels. Hypertension, which is associated with some of the previously mentioned etiologies, reduces the blood traveling to the brain and increases the potential for ruptured cerebral vessels from the elevated pressure. Smoking and other forms of tobacco use aggravate hypertension. Some medications, such as estrogens used for hormone replacement therapy and oral contraceptives, are thrombogenic. During the ischemic period, motor, sensory, and cognitive functions are temporarily affected.

Assessment Findings

Symptoms of a TIA include temporary light-headedness; confusion; speech disturbances; loss of vision; diplopia (double vision); variable changes in consciousness; and numbness, weakness, impaired muscle coordination, or paralysis on one side. The symptoms are short-lived.

A neurologic examination during an attack reveals neurologic deficits. Auscultation of the carotid artery may reveal a **bruit** (abnormal sound caused by blood flowing over the rough surface of one or both carotid arteries). Ultrasound examination of the carotid artery shows an irregular shape to the artery lining caused by atherosclerotic plaques. A carotid arteriogram shows narrowing of the carotid artery. A CT scan or magnetic resonance imaging (MRI) is used to rule out other neurologic disorders with similar manifestations, such as a brain tumor.

Medical and Surgical Management

Therapy for clients who have had a TIA and others who have a high potential for experiencing a CVA (stroke) is complex.

DRUG THERAPY TABLE 38-2 Drugs to Prevent or Treat Cerebrovascular Disorders

Category and Common Generic (Brand) Drugs	Intended Use	Common Side Effects	Safety Warnings for Nurses
Anticoagulants			
Heparin	Thrombosis/embolism, diagnosis and treatment by blocking conversion of prothrombin to thrombin and fibrinogen to fibrin in blood vessels	Bleeding, chills, fever, urticaria, local irritation, erythema, mild pain, hematoma or bruising at the injection site	Typical dose in thousand unit increments Monitor activated partial thromboplastin time (aPPT) frequently to maintain blood level Monitor for bleeding of injection sites, orifices, wounds Protamine sulfate should be readily available as an antidote
Warfarin (Coumadin, Jantoven)	Prophylaxis/treatment of venous thrombosis by inhibiting vitamin K-dependent clotting factors	Bleeding, fatigue, dizziness, abdominal cramping	international normalized ratio (INR) must be monitored at regular intervals Dietary vitamin K decreases blood levels; phytonadione (vitamin K) is used as an antidote for overdoses
Salicylates Aspirin (Ecotrin, Ascriptin)	Stroke prevention in men (and women older than 65 years only) by inhibiting platelet aggregation and clotting	Nausea, vomiting, epigastric distress	Monitor for tinnitus, indicates toxicity Should not be taken as pain reliever when on anticoagulant therapy
Miscellaneous agents Dabigatran (Pradaxa) Edoxaban (Savaysa) Rivaroxaban (Xarelto)	Stroke and embolism prevention nonvalve atrial fibrillation, post hip/knee replacement	Bleeding	Risk for thrombosis increases if drug therapy is stopped
Antiplatelets			
Aggregate inhibitors Clopidogrel (Plavix) Eptifibatide (Integrilin) Prasugrel (Effient) Ticagrelor (Brilinta) Vorapaxar (Zontivity)	Thrombus prevention by inhibiting platelet aggregation and clotting	Diarrhea, nausea, vomiting	Monitor for bleeding from injection sites, orifices, wounds The effect of aggregate inhibitors is diminished if combined with a proton pump inhibitor (PPI) such as omeprazole (Prilosec) Risk for bleeding increases if taken with aspirin or NSAIDs as pain reliever
Thrombolytics			
Alteplase (Activase) Reteplase (Retavase) Tenecteplase (TNKase)	Reestablish blood flow to ischemic areas by dissolving thrombi	Cardiac dysrhythmias, hypotension, bleeding at venous or arterial access sites, nausea, vomiting	Monitor for increased bleeding from injection sites, orifices, and wounds Contraindicated for clients with stroke/bleeding history

NSAID, nonsteroidal anti-inflammatory drug.
The drugs in column 1 indicate the drug that matches up with explanations in columns 2 through 4.

Clients must control their blood pressure (BP) with or without medications (see Chapter 27), lose excess weight, and stop tobacco and alcohol abuse. To manage atherosclerosis and the consequences of cardiac arrhythmias, especially atrial fibrillation (see Chapter 26), cholesterol-lowering drugs (see Chapter 25) and prophylactic anticoagulant or antiplatelet therapy are prescribed. Specific antiplatelet or anticoagulant medicines include daily aspirin, clopidogrel (Plavix), warfarin (Coumadin), dipyridamole (Persantine), and dabigatran etexilate (Pradaxa; Drug Therapy Table 38-2). Clients with diabetes are educated in techniques to control blood sugar within normal ranges with diet, exercise, and medications (see Chapter 51).

If narrowing of the carotid artery by atherosclerotic plaques is the cause of the TIAs, a **carotid endarterectomy** (surgical removal of atherosclerotic plaque) is a treatment option (Fig. 38-2). A percutaneous transluminal angioplasty, also called a balloon angioplasty, accompanied by placement of a stent (see Chapter 25), is performed to dilate the carotid artery and increase blood flow to the brain.

››› *Stop, Think, and Respond 38-1*

For a client who has had a TIA, what client teaching related to reducing risk factors for stroke is appropriate?

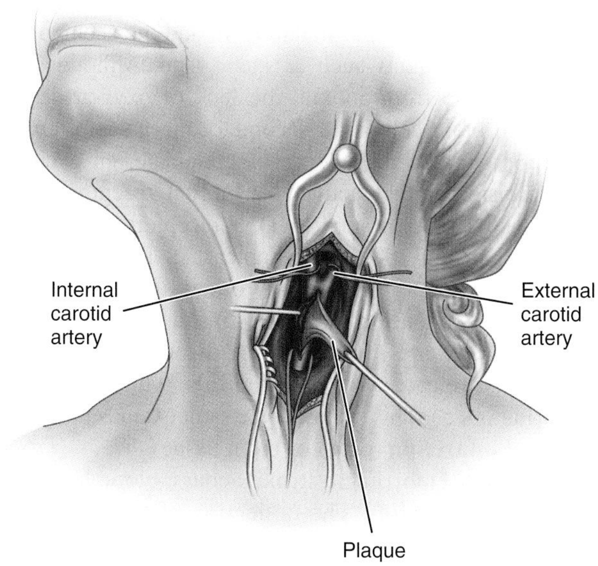

Figure 38-2 In endarterectomy, plaque—a potential source of emboli in transient ischemic attacks (TIAs) and cerebrovascular accidents (CVAs)—is surgically removed from the carotid artery.

Nursing Management

The nurse obtains a complete history of symptoms and medical, drug, and allergy histories. They weigh the client because obesity, hyperlipidemia, and atherosclerosis are related to cerebrovascular disease. The nurse checks the client's capillary blood sugar to help identify hyperglycemia associated with undiagnosed or uncontrolled diabetes mellitus. They measure vital signs and notes if the BP is at or greater than 140/90 mm Hg (refer to Chapter 27 for BP Classifications). The nurse asks the client about smoking habits. Although symptoms of a TIA usually are not permanent, the nurse performs a neurologic examination to identify the client's current status and establish a baseline for future comparisons. They document and report even subtle changes.

If the client undergoes carotid artery surgery, the nurse performs frequent neurologic checks to detect paralysis, confusion, facial asymmetry, or aphasia and monitors the heart rhythm because arrhythmias (see Chapter 26) can alter blood flow to the brain as well. Because it is possible for the neck to swell after surgery, the nurse observes the client closely for difficulty breathing or swallowing and hoarseness. The nurse places an airway at the bedside and is prepared for endotracheal intubation if an airway obstruction occurs.

The nurse teaches the client to

- Maintain hydration by drinking the equivalent of eight glasses of fluid a day unless contraindicated.
- Follow directions for drug therapy, including medications for controlling hypertension, hyperlipidemia, blood clotting, and diabetes.
- Monitor for signs of bruising or bleeding if antiplatelet or anticoagulant drugs are prescribed.
- Keep appointments for laboratory tests and medical follow-up to monitor the effectiveness of therapy.
- Report any future instances of sensory or motor impairment, or call 911 for emergency assistance.

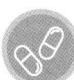

Pharmacologic Considerations

- Anticoagulant therapy—even daily low-dose aspirin—increases the risk of bleeding. Teach the client to monitor for cuts and bruises, in addition to using a soft-bristle toothbrush to reduce the risk of bleeding during care of teeth and gums.

CEREBROVASCULAR ACCIDENT (STROKE)

A CVA, or stroke, is a prolonged interruption in the flow of blood through one of the arteries supplying the brain. Stroke is the fifth leading cause of death among adult Americans. In 2018, 1 in every 6 deaths from cardiovascular disease was due to stroke (Stroke, 2020).

Brain and cerebral nerve cells are extremely sensitive to a lack of oxygen; if the brain is deprived of oxygenated blood for 3 to 7 minutes during a stroke, they both begin to die. Once these cells are destroyed, the outcome is irreversible. Although the site of the cellular damage is located in the brain, the consequences are widespread. About one third of stroke victims die; most survivors have permanent disabilities. Permanent neurologic deficits have a profound physical, emotional, and financial effect on the client and the family.

Pathophysiology and Etiology

There are two main types of stroke: *ischemic strokes* and *hemorrhagic strokes*. Ischemic strokes occur when a thrombus or embolus obstructs an artery carrying blood to the brain (Fig. 38-3); about 80% of strokes are the ischemic variety.

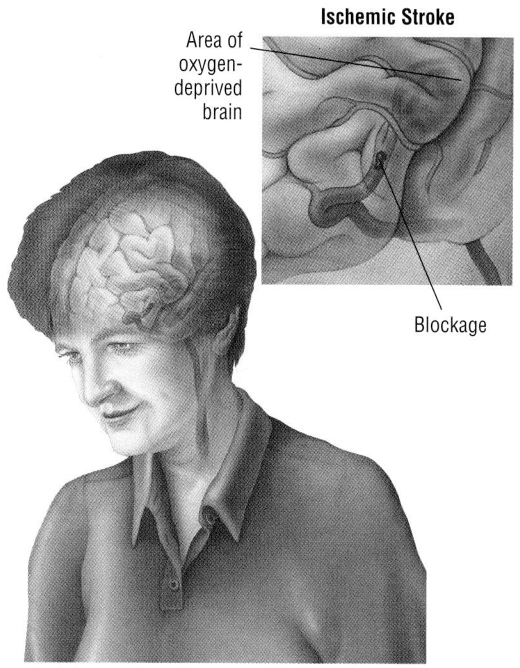

Figure 38-3 In ischemic stroke, arterial blood flow to part of the brain is blocked within a cerebral artery. A thrombotic stroke occurs when a clot forms in a blood vessel. An embolic stroke results when a clot travels to and lodges in a cerebral artery from another location. (From the Anatomical Chart Company.)

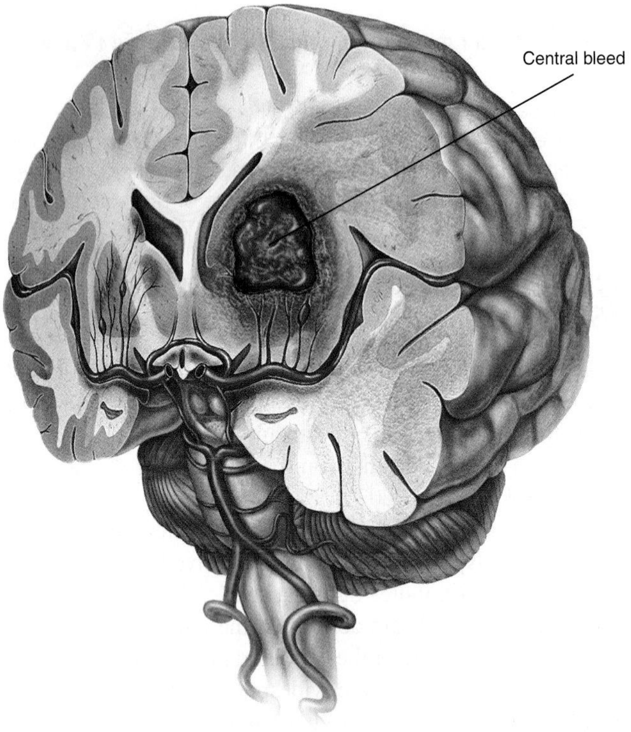

Figure 38-4 Intracerebral hemorrhage. (From the Anatomical Chart Company.)

Hemorrhagic strokes occur when a cerebral blood vessel ruptures and blood is released in brain tissue (Fig. 38-4).

When ischemic strokes occur, glucose and oxygen to brain cells are reduced. The reduced glucose quickly depletes the stores of adenosine triphosphate (ATP), resulting in anaerobic cellular metabolism and the accumulation of toxic by-products such as lactic acid. Although some brain cells die from anoxia, the lack of oxygen destroys additional brain cells by a secondary mechanism. Oxygen depletion triggers the release of glutamate, an excitatory neurotransmitter that activates neuronal receptors known as *N*-methyl-D-aspartate (NMDA) receptors (Bio-Techne, 2012; Teichberg, 2007; see Chapter 11). The receptors allow large amounts of calcium followed by glutamate to enter the cells. Once glutamate is inside the brain cells, it literally overexcites them, causing disordered enzyme activities that release toxic free radicals, which destroy the cells (Fig. 38-5). This secondary assault extends the zone of **cerebral infarction** (death of brain tissue).

When a hemorrhagic stroke occurs, blood leaks from intracerebral arteries. The collection of blood adds volume to the intracranial contents, resulting in elevated pressure (see Chapter 37). Hemorrhagic strokes are more common in particular areas of the brain such as the cerebellum, the structure that facilitates balance and coordination, and the brain stem, which controls breathing, BP, and heart rate.

Various factors increase the risk for a CVA. Some are controllable and some are uncontrollable (Box 38-2). Atherosclerosis and arteriosclerosis are major contributors to the formation of thromboemboli and subsequent CVAs. Common causes of cerebral hemorrhage are rupture of cerebral vessels (discussed later in this chapter), hemorrhagic disorders such as leukemia and aplastic anemia, severe hypertension, and brain tumors.

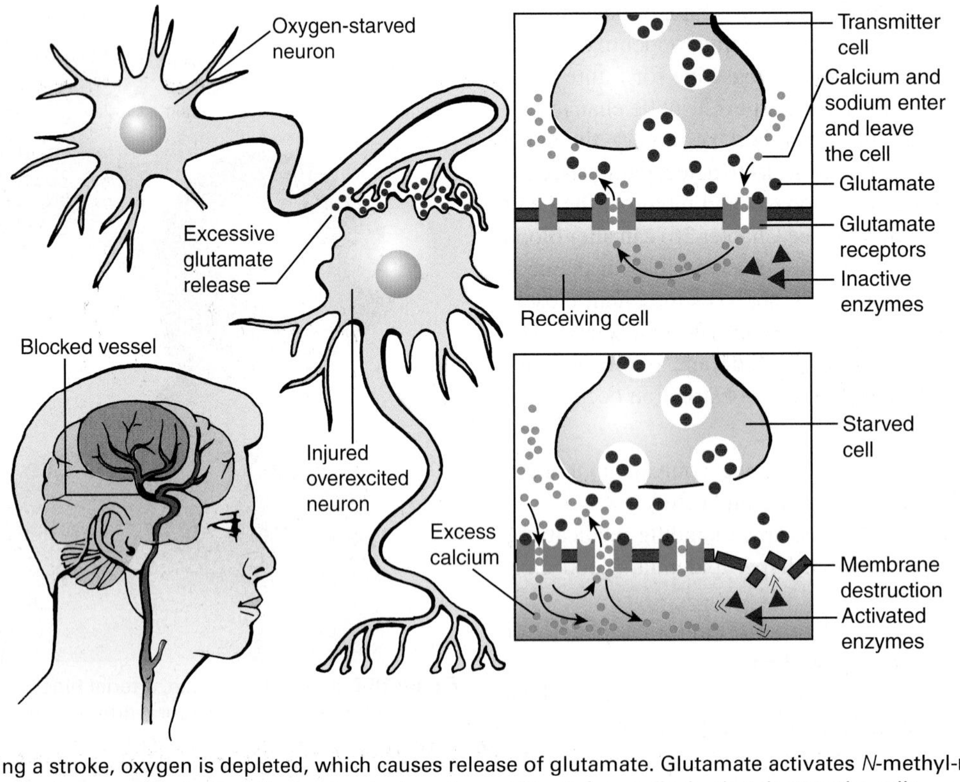

Figure 38-5 During a stroke, oxygen is depleted, which causes release of glutamate. Glutamate activates *N*-methyl-D-aspartate (NMDA) receptors and overexcites brain cells, leading to the release of toxic free radicals, that destroy the cells.

BOX 38-2 Risk Factors for Cerebrovascular Accident

Uncontrollable

- *Age*: Risk of CVA increases with each decade beyond age 55 years.
- *Sex*: Men have a slightly higher risk than women.
- *Race*: African Americans experience more CVAs than do other groups.
- *Genetics*: Those whose blood relatives have had a CVA are at increased risk.

Controllable

- *Hypertension*: 40% to 90% of clients with CVA have previous hypertension.
- *Atrial fibrillation*: 15% of those with atrial fibrillation, an arrhythmia associated with thromboembolic complications, develop a CVA.
- *Hyperlipidemia*: High blood cholesterol and low-density lipoprotein (LDL) levels increase the risk for atherosclerosis and CVA.
- *Diabetes*: Elevated blood glucose level increases triglycerides and accelerates their conversion to LDLs.
- *History of TIA or CVA*: 35% of clients who already have had a TIA will have a CVA within 5 years; after one CVA, 42% of men and 24% of women have another.
- *Smoking*: Nicotine is a vasoconstrictor.
- *Obesity*: It contributes to hypertension, hyperlipidemia, and diabetes.
- *Thrombogenic substances*: Stimulants such as herbal products derived from *ephedra* plants, estrogens, and oral contraceptives increase risk.
- *Valvular disease or replacement*: Thrombi and emboli form and break free from vegetations or valve replacements.

Assessment Findings

Signs and Symptoms

In some instances, clients experience one or more TIAs days, weeks, or years before a CVA, or there may be no warning and the symptoms develop suddenly. Signs of an impending stroke include the following:

- Numbness or weakness of one side of the face, an arm, or a leg
- Mental confusion
- Difficulty speaking or understanding
- Impaired walking or coordination
- Severe headache

Immediately after a large cerebral hemorrhage, the client is unconscious. Breathing is noisy and labored. The cheek on the side of the CVA blows out on exhalation. The eyes deviate toward the affected side of the brain. The pulse is slow, full, and bounding. Initially, BP is elevated. Temperature is elevated during the acute phase and persists for several days. The level of consciousness (LOC) ranges from lethargy and mental confusion to deep coma, which can persist for days or even weeks. The longer the coma, the poorer the prognosis and the less likely that consciousness will return.

Clinical manifestations following a stroke are highly variable and depend on the area of the cerebral cortex and the affected hemisphere (Box 38-3), the degree of blockage (total, partial), and the presence or absence of adequate **collateral circulation**, circulation formed by smaller blood vessels branching off from or near larger occluded vessels.

A common neurologic result of a CVA in the motor area of the cerebrum is **hemiplegia** (paralysis on one side of the body). Hemiplegia occurs on the side opposite the area of the brain that is affected because motor nerves cross over (decussate) at the level of the neck. For example, when the motor area on the right side of the brain incurs a CVA, hemiplegia develops on the left side of the body: There is left-sided hemiplegia when the CVA occurs in the right hemisphere of the brain. Immediately after the CVA, the affected side is flaccid. This progresses to spastic limbs. The arm typically is more severely affected than the leg.

Expressive aphasia, the inability to speak, or **receptive aphasia**, the inability to understand spoken and written language, can result depending on where the client's speech center is located in the brain. For most, the speech center is in the dominant hemisphere (i.e., if a person is right-handed, the speech center is in the left hemisphere). A right-handed person who has a CVA in the left brain usually develops aphasia, and vice versa for a left-handed person.

Confusion and emotional lability are characteristic symptoms of a CVA. Hemianopia on the affected side is another potential consequence. **Hemianopia** is the ability to see only half of the normal visual field (Fig. 38-6). When looking straight ahead, the client cannot see to the right (in left-sided stroke) or left (in right-sided stroke) with either eye. This condition is caused by damage to the visual area of the cerebral cortex or its connections to the brain stem (optic

BOX 38-3 Signs and Symptoms of Right-Sided Versus Left-Sided Hemiplegia

Right-Sided Hemiplegia (Stroke on Left Side of Brain)

Expressive aphasia
Receptive aphasia
Global aphasia
Intellectual impairment
Slow and cautious behavior
Defects in right visual fields
Short retention of information
Require frequent reminding to complete tasks
Difficulty with new learning
Problems with abstract thinking, such as conceptualizing and generalizing

Left-Sided Hemiplegia (Stroke on Right Side of Brain)

Spatial–perceptual defects
Disregard for the deficits on the affected side
Tendency to distractibility
Impulsive behavior; unaware of deficits
Poor judgment
Defects in left visual fields
Misjudging distances
Difficulty distinguishing upside down and right side up
Impairment of short-term memory
Neglect of left side of body; objects and people on left side

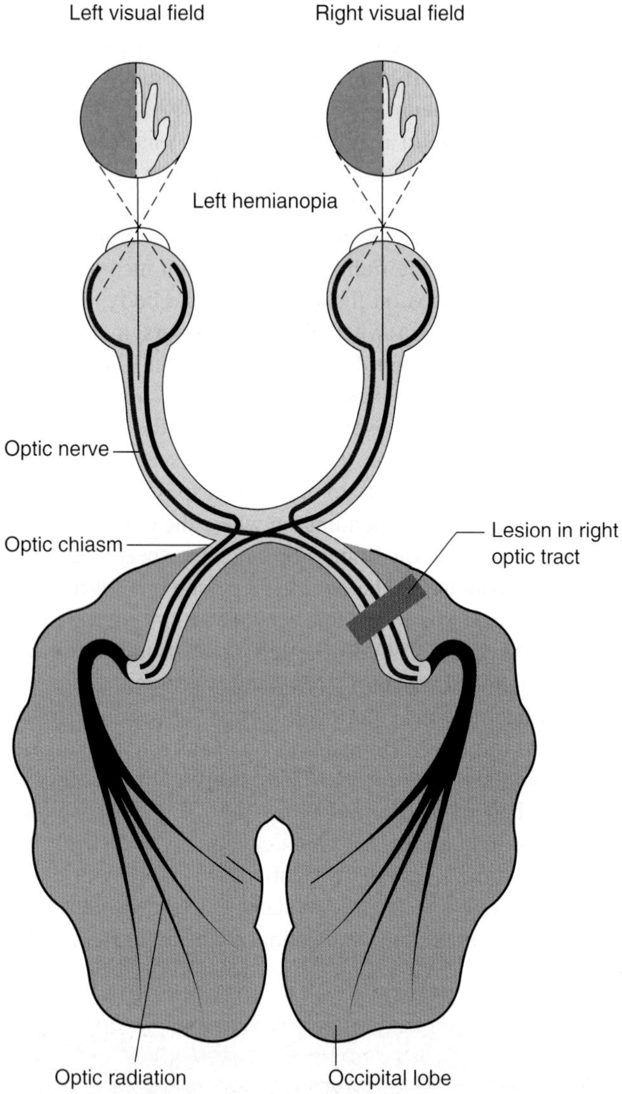

Figure 38-6 Hemianopia is a visual field defect in which a person experiences an inability to see the left or right half of an image. It develops when a stroke involves the visual pathway.

radiations). Neurologic deficits that result from a CVA may subside completely, partially, or not at all.

Diagnostic Findings

A CT scan or MRI differentiates a CVA from other disorders, such as a brain tumor or cerebral edema, and shows the size and location of the infarcted area. Transcranial Doppler ultrasonography determines the size of intracranial vessels and the direction of blood flow and locates the obstructed cerebral vessel. Single-photon emission computed tomography (SPECT) also identifies cerebral blood flow. An electroencephalogram (EEG) reveals reduced electrical activity in the involved area but is not a specific diagnostic test for a CVA. A lumbar puncture often is performed. If subarachnoid bleeding has occurred, the cerebrospinal fluid (CSF) will be bloody. Cerebral angiography shows displacement or blockage of cerebral vessels.

Medical and Surgical Management

A CVA is a medical emergency. Treatment varies and is directed toward relieving the cause, if known. Tissue plasminogen activator (TPA), a thrombolytic agent, has been found to limit neurologic deficits when given within 3 hours after the onset of an ischemic CVA (Box 38-4). It is contraindicated in hemorrhagic CVAs, as is anticoagulant therapy. Hypothermia is also being used to protect damaged cells by reducing their metabolic need for oxygen.

If atherosclerosis of the carotid artery is the cause, a carotid endarterectomy is considered. A ruptured cerebral aneurysm is treated surgically.

In many cases, treatment is supportive because medical or surgical interventions cannot repair damaged brain tissue. The best treatment available involves an intensive medical program aimed at rehabilitation and the prevention of future CVAs.

BOX 38-4 Inclusion and Exclusion Criteria for Therapy With Tissue Plasminogen Activator

Inclusion Criteria

- Clinical evidence of an ischemic attack
- Age >18 years
- Signed consent, if possible
- Onset of stroke within 3 hours of initiation of therapy (or from time client was last seen as "normal")
- Normal prothrombin and partial thromboplastin times

Exclusion Criteria

- Stroke or serious head trauma in past 3 months
- Major surgery or invasive procedure within past 14 days
- Gastrointestinal or urinary bleeding within past 21 days
- Puncture of noncompressible artery or biopsy of internal organ within past 7 days
- Seizure preceding or during stroke
- History of intracranial hemorrhage or known history of cerebral vascular malformations
- Pericarditis, endocarditis, septic emboli, recent pregnancy, or active inflammatory bowel disease

Nursing Management

Detailed nursing management for the client with a CVA is discussed in Nursing Care Plan 38-1. Client and family teaching also is essential, which focuses on the following points:

- Administer medications as directed and understand the potential side and adverse effects.
- Implement eating and swallowing techniques that reduce the potential for aspiration (Nutrition Notes).
- Perform the Heimlich maneuver to clear the airway if the client cannot speak or breathe after swallowing food (see Chapter 20).
- Continue follow-up care with the speech pathologist and dietitian.
- Contact community resources such as medical supply companies that rent or sell special care devices such as a hospital bed, bedside commode, walker, or tripod cane.
- Remove throw rugs, clutter, and electrical cords from the client's home environment to reduce the potential for falls.
- Perform regular exercises, change the client's position frequently, and apply braces or splints designed to maintain extremities in proper anatomic position.

Nutrition Notes

The Client With a CVA

■ When the client can resume oral intake after a CVA, individualize the diet according to their ability to chew and swallow. Semisolid and medium-consistency foods such as pudding, scrambled eggs, cooked cereals, and thickened liquids are easiest to swallow. Cold foods stimulate swallowing. The client should avoid tepid foods, because they are more difficult to locate in the mouth, and extremely hot foods, which can cause overreaction. The client should also avoid foods most likely to cause choking: peanut butter, bread, tart foods, dry or crisp foods, and chewy meats. Progress the texture as swallowing ability improves.

■ Clients with decreased salivation benefit from strategies to moisten their mouth, such as small sips of thickened liquids just prior to eating or bites containing gravies and sauces throughout the meal. Thinking of a specific food before eating stimulates salivation, such as eating dill pickles and sucking on lemon slices.

■ To minimize the volume of food needed, provide nutritionally dense foods such as thickened commercial beverages, fortified puddings, fortified cooked cereals, and scrambled eggs.

■ When a normal diet is resumed, encourage the client to eat "heart healthy"—less saturated and trans fats and more fruits, vegetables, and whole grains. Encourage overweight clients to lose weight to reduce cardiac workload. Sodium restriction is appropriate for clients with hypertension.

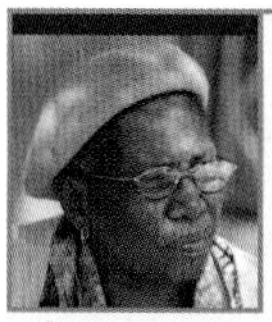

Clinical Scenario An older adult who lives with her daughter and son-in-law awoke with progressive weakness on her right side, and her speech was difficult to understand. She choked on water as she tried to swallow her usual medications. An ambulance was called, and the client was taken to the emergency department (ED). She was subsequently admitted to a nursing unit. The daughter pleads with the client's assigned nurse, "Please help my mother; I don't want her to die." **What assessments will help provide data to identify nursing care problems and what interventions are appropriate when the nurse proceeds to manage this client's care? See Nursing Care Plan 38-1.**

NURSING CARE PLAN 38-1 The Client With a CVA

Assessment

Determine the following:

- Time symptoms began
- Medical, drug, and allergy history from the family (or client if they can report)
- Vital signs and LOC
- Size and response of pupils to light
- Any musculoskeletal weakness or paralysis
- Capacity to speak or understand spoken language
- Changes in visual field
- Ability to swallow
- Any alteration in bladder or bowel control
- Integrity of the skin; evidence of soft tissue injury as a consequence of falling

Nursing Diagnoses. **Impaired Swallowing** related to hemiplegia; **Aspiration Risk** related to impaired swallowing; **Decreased Fluid Volume Risk** related to impaired swallowing; **Malnutrition Risk** related to impaired swallowing

Expected Outcomes. (1) Client will swallow without aspiration. (2) Fluid intake will be at least 2000 mL/24 hours without evidence of choking. (3) Client will consume sufficient calories to maintain admission weight.

Interventions	Rationales
Elevate client's head for eating or drinking; position client on their side at other times.	*Sitting and facing food or liquids raises client's awareness and attention; a side-lying position prevents aspiration if vomiting occurs or saliva accumulates in the mouth.*
Keep a suction machine at the bedside.	*Mechanical suctioning facilitates clearing the airway of saliva, food, and fluids.*
Limit distractions (e.g., turn off the television when the client eats or drinks).	*The client can better concentrate and follow nursing instructions when distracting stimuli are reduced.*
Use a thickening agent for watery substances; request viscous or pureed food from nutrition services.	*The tongue can more easily manipulate thickened liquids against the palate and oral pharynx.*
Request small, frequent nourishment from nutrition services rather than three large meals.	*Eating small amounts is less tiring, and the client may consume more on a daily basis.*
Offer or remind client to load the fork or spoon with a small amount of food.	*A small amount is easier to manage in the mouth and less likely to cause a complete airway obstruction.*
Place thickened liquids or pureed food on the unaffected side of the mouth.	*The client can feel and use the unaffected side of the mouth for chewing and swallowing.*
Lower client's chin to their chest when swallowing.	*Lowering the chin helps close the laryngopharynx and reduces the potential for aspiration.*

(continued)

NURSING CARE PLAN 38-1 The Client With a CVA (*continued*)

Encourage client to swallow several times.	*Several efforts at swallowing may be necessary to move food to the esophagus.*
Check the mouth for pocketed food before offering more.	*The client may be unaware of food that remains unswallowed.*
Instruct client to use the tongue to relocate pocketed food or apply gentle pressure on the cheek to reposition food.	*Physical manipulation helps reposition trapped food.*
Collaborate with the primary provider concerning gastric or enteral tube feedings if oral intake is inadequate.	*These routes can provide sufficient nutrients when oral intake is compromised.*

Evaluation of Expected Outcomes

The airway remains patent and lungs are clear to auscultation. There is an adequate intake of food and fluids.

Nursing Diagnoses. **Total Urinary Incontinence; Bowel Incontinence or Risk for Constipation** related to diminished LOC, confusion, and immobility

Expected Outcome. Urinary and bowel elimination will be controlled independently or with minimal assistance.

Interventions	Rationales
Maintain a record of bowel elimination.	*It provides data that can indicate if the client requires a stool softener, laxative, suppository, or enema.*
Place an elevated seat over the toilet.	*An elevated seat reduces the work of transferring to the toilet seat and back to a wheelchair.*
Assist client to the toilet every 2 hours while they are awake and after each meal.	*Positioning and environmental cues may help stimulate the client to eliminate. The gastrocolic reflex that promotes bowel evacuation is stronger soon after eating.*
Dress client in unrestricted clothing that facilitates elimination needs.	*Clothing that is easy to undo or lower reduces the potential for incontinence.*
Avoid negative comments if incontinence occurs; acknowledge client's success when they eliminate while on the toilet or commode.	*Criticism lowers self-confidence and self-esteem; praise encourages client to continue efforts at controlling elimination.*
Apply incontinence garments or place absorbent pads beneath client.	*Concealment of urine or stool preserves client's dignity.*
Collaborate with the primary provider concerning the insertion of an external or indwelling catheter.	*An external catheter is less likely to predispose to a urinary tract infection; a catheter helps keep the skin dry and reduces embarrassment of incontinence.*
Administer a prescribed suppository or low-volume enema when necessary.	*Chemical or mechanical stimulation increases intestinal contraction, which helps to evacuate the bowel.*

Evaluation of Expected Outcome

Bowel and urinary elimination are managed at the highest level the client can achieve.

Nursing Diagnoses. **Bathing/Hygiene deficit** related to hemiplegia; **Fall Risk** related to hemiplegia

Expected Outcomes. (1) Client will resume independent activities of daily living (ADLs). (2) Client will identify and care for paralyzed body parts. (3) Client will use assistive devices to achieve mobility.

Interventions	Rationales
Approach and place objects within client's field of vision.	*Client is likely to ignore objects and people that are located in areas where the visual field is impaired.*
Help reintegrate the weak side by reminding the client to look at it.	*Calling attention to the neglected side of the body helps the client recognize and accept that it exists.*
Set realistic goals for self-care.	*Unrealistic goals lead to frustration and discouragement.*
Consult with an occupational therapist (OT) or physical therapist (PT) regarding modifications in clothing, utensils, and assistive devices.	*Therapists have expertise in measures to accommodate for neurologic deficits.*
Attach a trapeze above the bed.	*Client can use a trapeze with one hand to independently facilitate position changes.*
Perform range-of-motion (ROM) exercises at least once each shift.	*ROM exercises maintain joint mobility and muscle tone.*
Support the affected arm in a sling when the client is upright.	*An arm sling improves posture and reduces musculoskeletal changes in the shoulder joint.*
Position client to avoid contractures (e.g., use a footboard, trochanter roll at the hip, rolled cloth in the paralyzed hand).	*Skeletal muscles tend to become permanently shortened unless efforts are made to maintain normal anatomic position.*
Consult the PT about devices to assist ambulation, such as a leg brace and walker.	*A brace promotes stability when standing and walking. A walker supports the client and facilitates ambulation.*

NURSING CARE PLAN 38-1 The Client With a CVA (*continued*)

Evaluation of Expected Outcomes

Client performs ADLs alone or with assistance; the client attends to bilateral body parts and learns to use assistive devices.

Nursing Diagnosis. **Altered Skin Integrity** related to pressure over bony prominences secondary to immobility

Expected Outcome. Skin will remain intact.

Interventions	Rationales
Keep skin clean and dry.	*Cleaning the skin removes transient bacteria.* *Drying the skin prevents maceration, a process in which skin is softened and easily eroded.*
Use a turning sheet and get assistance when changing client's position.	*A turning sheet prevents shearing, the movement of a layer of tissue in one direction as another moves in opposition.*
Massage skin areas that blanch when pressure is relieved.	*Massage improves blood flow to tissue, but it is contraindicated if tissue is already damaged as evidenced by a sustained redness when pressure is relieved.*
Use pressure-relieving devices or a therapeutic bed that alternately distributes the client's body weight.	*Tissue damage occurs unless intracapillary pressure is maintained at 32 mm Hg or more; relief of pressure at least every 2 hours reduces tissue hypoxia.*

Evaluation of Expected Outcome

Skin is intact; there is no evidence of pressure sores.

Nursing Diagnosis. **Impaired Verbal Communication** related to expressive aphasia

Expected Outcome. Client will make needs understood either verbally or nonverbally.

Interventions	Rationales
Ask questions requiring a "yes" or "no" and suggest the client respond by nodding the head.	*Nodding the head is a form of body language that communicates agreement or disagreement.*
Instruct client to speak slowly when attempting to communicate orally.	*If unpressured to quickly respond, the client may be able to formulate words and sentences more easily.*
Have client point to or write key words or phrases.	*Some clients retain the ability to read written language, although they may not be able to express themselves orally.*
Support and practice techniques used in speech therapy.	*Practicing new techniques helps to promote mastery.*

Evaluation of Expected Outcome

Client can communicate orally, in writing, or with techniques that facilitate nonverbal communication.

Nursing Diagnoses. **Risk Coping Impairment** related to diminished psychosocial resources to deal with multiple stressors

Expected Outcome. Client and family will cope with illness and changes in lifestyle.

Interventions	Rationales
Listen and try to identify clues to client's or family's future concerns.	*Identifying problems that require actions facilitates coping.*
Acknowledge personal strengths.	*Recognition of strengths promotes confidence in the ability to overcome current problems.*
Encourage individuals in the client's social network to collaborate on problem-solving.	*Successful outcomes are more likely when there is a team effort.*
Refer client and family to a discharge planner, social worker, or community social services for arranging extended care, home care, and respite care.	*The health team includes persons with expertise in assisting clients and their families with postdischarge issues.*

Evaluation of Expected Outcomes

Client and family cope with the client's neurologic deficits; referrals are made to services or facilities that can assist with long-term recovery.

The family pursues a plan for postdischarge management.

››› *Stop, Think, and Respond 38-2*

When a client with an evolving CVA arrives in the emergency department, her speech is difficult to understand, the left side of her face has a drooped appearance, and she cannot move her left arm and leg. Before this client becomes a candidate for TPA, what other information is important to gather?

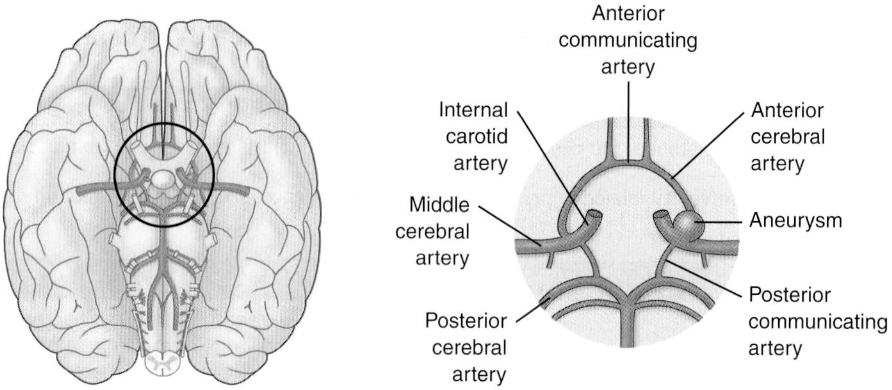

Figure 38-7 An intracranial aneurysm shown on the right may occur in any of the cerebral arteries that make up the circle of Willis.

CEREBRAL ANEURYSMS

An **aneurysm** is a weakening in the wall of a blood vessel. Most aneurysms occur in arteries where blood flow is under high pressure. Cerebral aneurysms usually occur in the circle of Willis, a ring of arteries that supply the brain (Fig. 38-7).

Pathophysiology and Etiology

Aneurysms develop at a weakened area in the blood vessel wall. The defect is congenital or secondary to hypertension and atherosclerosis. An aneurysm can affect cranial nerve function (see Chapter 36) as the aneurysm presses on these structures. For many, there is no prior warning that an aneurysm exists. Berry aneurysms, a type of congenital cerebral aneurysm, can rupture at any time without prior symptoms. The sudden cerebral hemorrhage causes immediate neurologic changes from increased ICP, interruption of oxygenated blood flow to the surrounding cells and tissues, and blood collecting in the subarachnoid space. Occasionally, there is a slow leakage of blood from an aneurysm, in which case symptoms are less severe.

Assessment Findings

Symptoms include sudden and severe headache, dizziness, nausea, and vomiting, usually followed by a rapid loss of consciousness. If the ruptured aneurysm produces a slow leak, a stiff neck, headache, visual disturbances, and intermittent nausea develop.

Medical Management

Conservative management is attempted until a decision is made regarding surgical repair of the aneurysm. Some aneurysms are considered inoperable because of anatomic location and only medical treatment is possible.

Complete bed rest, the prevention of rebleeding at the rupture site, and treatment of complications are primary goals. Absolute bed rest in a quiet area, preferably a private room, is essential. Visitors are restricted except for family members. The head of the bed is elevated to reduce ICP and cerebral edema. Hypertension is treated with antihypertensive agents.

Anticonvulsants are given to prevent seizures. Tranquilizers or barbiturates are used to keep the conscious client relaxed and quiet. Antipyretics are given to reduce a fever and thereby control the brain's metabolic need for oxygen. Increased ICP is managed with osmotic diuretics such as mannitol (Osmitrol) and, in some cases, a low-volume hypertonic solution.

Mechanical ventilation is necessary to support respirations and provide oxygenation if the client is unconscious. Aminocaproic acid (Amicar) is used to delay lysis (breaking up) of the blood clot because lysis results in rebleeding.

Concept Mastery Alert

Cerebral Aneurysm

An assessment finding of nausea is of great importance when prioritizing nursing care for a client with a cerebral aneurysm, because nausea needs to be controlled to prevent vomiting, which can greatly increase the ICP and subsequently rupture the aneurysm.

Cerebral angiography can reveal an unruptured aneurysm. The procedure is performed with caution because the added fluid pressure can increase the risk of rupturing the blood vessel, dislodge plaque-formed emboli, and cause ischemia from vasospasm. A CT scan and MRI are safer for locating the site of the aneurysm and determining the amount of blood in the subarachnoid space. A lumbar puncture reveals grossly bloody CSF when an aneurysm ruptures. The primary provider may identify the status and prognosis of the client based on criteria in the Hunt–Hess classification system (Table 38-2). As the grade increases, the prognosis becomes less optimistic.

Surgical Management

Surgical repair is attempted after the initial hemorrhage because the danger of further hemorrhage from the weakened aneurysm is great. The operation is not without hazard; manipulation of the small cerebral vessels can result in increased vasospasm or thrombosis and cerebral infarction. The risks of surgery are less serious than the dangers of recurrent hemorrhage from the aneurysm. Surgical approaches with a craniotomy include clipping (clamping) the aneurysm, inserting an endovascular stent, or filling the aneurysm with a coil with or without a stent in an attempt to prevent a potential rupture (Fig. 38-8).

TABLE 38-2 The Hunt–Hess Scale for Grading a Client With a Cerebral Aneurysm

CLASSIFICATION	CLINICAL CRITERIA
Grade I	Alert, oriented, asymptomatic
Grade II	Alert, oriented, headache, stiff neck
Grade III	Lethargic or confused, minor focal deficits such as hemiparesis (weakness on one side)
Grade IV	Stupor, moderate-to-severe focal deficits such as hemiplegia
Grade V	Comatose, severe neurologic deficits such as posturing (see Chapter 39)

Adapted from Hickey, J. V. (2019). *The clinical practice of neurological and neurosurgical nursing* (8th ed.). Wolters Kluwer.

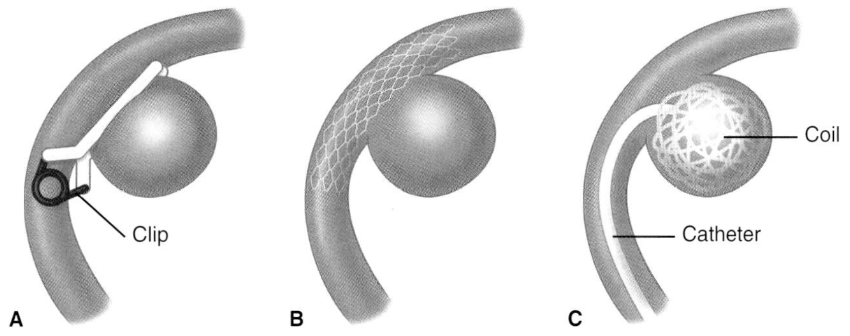

Figure 38-8 Three endovascular surgical methods for managing a cerebral aneurysm: **(A)** clip, **(B)** stent, **(C)** coil.

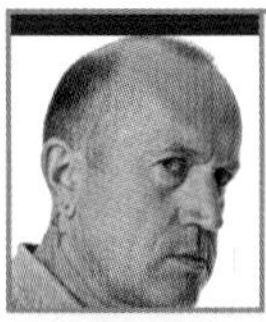

Clinical Scenario A 46-year-old male has had a headache for several days. The headache, which has worsened, is described by the client as "like my head is about to burst." The client tells the nurse, "I've felt dizzy and nauseous. Sometimes I have double vision, and I've had trouble verbalizing my thoughts. I thought I might be having a stroke because I've had some weakness on one side of my body." The client is admitted for diagnostic tests and definitive treatment. **How might the nurse contribute to the database and plan the nursing care for the client when test results reveal the client has a leaking cerebral aneurysm? See the following Nursing Process section.**

NURSING PROCESS FOR THE CLIENT WITH A CEREBRAL ANEURYSM

Assessment

Perform a neurologic examination, taking care to avoid disturbing the client. Measure vital signs frequently. If the client is conscious, ask only essential questions while gathering the client's history, limiting it primarily to the current onset of symptoms. Obtain a more complete history from the family.

Diagnosis, Planning, and Interventions

RC of Increased ICP: Related to bleeding in the brain
Expected Outcome: The nurse will monitor for, manage, and minimize increased ICP.

- Use the Glasgow Coma Scale (GCS) to assess neurologic status at least every hour (see Chapter 36). *The GCS is a systematic assessment tool for documenting neurologic function and identifying early clinical changes.*
- Report neurologic changes as soon as a trend indicates worsening of the client's condition. *Early collaboration with the primary provider facilitates implementing medically prescribed interventions that will reduce or eliminate more serious complications.*
- Keep client calm and physically still. *Activity or emotional distress elevates BP and ICP, which could cause or contribute to more bleeding.*
- Avoid any activities that cause a Valsalva maneuver such as coughing, straining at stool, and rough position changes. *Bearing down raises BP and increases the potential for rupture of the aneurysm or increased bleeding if the aneurysm is leaking or has already ruptured.*
- Follow the primary provider's orders for fluid restrictions and drug therapy for reducing hypertension, potential seizures, restlessness, and anxiety. *Interventions that reduce BP, large motor movements, and emotional stress help to reduce ICP.*
- Elevate client's head or follow the primary provider's directive for body position (some prefer that the client remain flat). *Head elevation helps venous blood and CSF drain from cerebral areas and reduces the volume in the cranium.*
- Limit visitors to the immediate family; suggest they take turns and stay briefly. *Although visitors' and family members' desires to interact with the client are well intentioned, the stimulation can increase ICP or trigger a seizure.*

(continued)

NURSING PROCESS FOR THE CLIENT WITH A CEREBRAL ANEURYSM (continued)

RC of Seizures: Related to increased ICP
Expected Outcome: The nurse will monitor to detect, manage, and minimize seizures.

- Institute seizure precautions (see Chapter 37). *Seizure precautions are used to prevent or minimize seizure-related injuries.*
- Implement anticonvulsant drug therapy as prescribed. *Anticonvulsants reduce excitation of neurons in the brain that result in seizure activity.*

Acute Pain (Headache): Related to increased ICP
Expected Outcome: Pain will be reduced or eliminated.

- Avoid administering opioid analgesics, except codeine. *Opioids interfere with accurate assessment of neurologic function because they constrict the pupils and depress LOC.*
- Reduce environmental stimuli, and use nursing interventions such as distraction, guided imagery, and soothing music. *Nonpharmacologic techniques for pain relief are based on blocking the brain's awareness of pain by substituting another form of sensory or cognitive stimulus.*
- Take care not to jar the bed or cause unnecessary activity. *Unexpected movement and physical activity tend to intensify the pain experience.*

ADL Deficit: Related to imposed rest and decreased LOC
Expected Outcome: Client's basic needs will be met.

- Perform only those ADLs for the client that are absolutely necessary. *Keeping the client quiet, which reduces the risk for life-threatening complications, takes greater precedence over bathing, ambulating, and the like.*
- Provide rest between necessary nursing tasks. *Limiting tasks to brief moments prevents overstimulating the client.*
- Feed client calorie-dense foods in small amounts at frequent intervals. *In this way, the client's hunger is managed without requiring a large intake of food at any one time.*

Altered Skin Integrity, Pressure Injury Risk: Related to imposed inactivity
Expected Outcomes: (1) Peripheral circulation will be maintained. (2) Skin will remain intact.

- Apply elastic stockings to lower extremities or use a pneumatic compression device. *Intermittent compression passively moves venous blood toward the heart in a way similar to active skeletal muscle contraction. Elastic stockings support the valves of veins in the lower extremities to prevent venous stasis.*
- Use pressure-relieving pads or a similar type of mattress. *Relieving pressure promotes the circulation of oxygenated blood through capillaries to peripheral cells and tissues and facilitates venous blood return.*

Evaluation of Expected Outcomes

The ICP is maintained within a safe range. The client does not manifest seizures. Their level of discomfort is tolerable. Essential needs for nutrition, hydration, ventilation, and elimination are met. Peripheral circulation is adequate; there are no signs of skin breakdown. For the client who undergoes a craniotomy, refer to Chapter 37.

Discharge teaching depends on the method of treatment and the recommendations of the primary provider. Usually, the nurse instructs clients to avoid heavy lifting, straining at stool, extreme emotional situations, and other work-related activities that could raise BP and increase ICP.

When the client must restrict their lifestyle, the changes are likely to cause financial, physical, and social hardships for the client and family. Referrals to a social service worker, counselor, or social service agency are appropriate.

KEY POINTS

- Three common types of headaches:
  - Tension headaches: muscles contracted about the neck, face, and scalp. A tension headache also can develop when a person contracts the neck and facial muscles for a prolonged period.
  - Migraine headaches: changes in particular serotonin receptors that promote dilation of cerebral blood vessels and pain intensification from neurochemicals released from the trigeminal nerve, may have triggers such as hormones, certain drugs or foods
  - Cluster headaches: The cause is unknown. Cluster headaches can be triggered by vasodilating agents such as nitroglycerin, histamine, and alcoholic beverages.
- TIA (transient ischemic attack): a sudden, brief episode of neurologic impairment caused by a temporary interruption in cerebral blood flow, symptoms may disappear within 1 hour; some continue for as long as 1 day.
- FAST be used to evaluate if a person is in danger of having a stroke. FAST stands for:
  - **F**—Face drooping especially on one side
  - **A**—Arm weakness
  - **S**—Slurred speech
  - **T**—Time to call 911

- CVA (cerebrovascular accident), or stroke, is a prolonged interruption in the flow of blood through one of the arteries supplying the brain.
- Ischemic strokes: occur when a thrombus or embolus obstructs an artery carrying blood to the brain
  - Hemorrhagic strokes occur when a cerebral blood vessel ruptures, and blood is released in brain tissue.
- A cerebral **aneurysm** is a weakening in the wall of a blood vessel in the brain.

CRITICAL THINKING EXERCISES

1. What suggestions could you give to someone who has migraine headaches to help reduce their severity?
2. A client is brought to the emergency department after being found unconscious at home. A CVA is the tentative diagnosis. The family is advocating for the administration of a thrombolytic agent. What factors may be contraindications to this form of treatment?
3. The family of a client who has had a stroke is concerned about postdischarge care. The client has left-sided paralysis, is incontinent, and has expressive aphasia. What help can you offer the family?
4. When assigned to care for a client with a leaking cerebral aneurysm, what nursing interventions are appropriate for reducing the potential for a serious intracranial bleed?

NCLEX-STYLE REVIEW QUESTIONS PrepU

1. A client arrives at the headache center for an initial evaluation. The client describes flashing lights in the field of vision before the headache begins. What nursing interpretation of the assessment data is most correct?
   1. The client is experiencing a premonition of a migraine headache.
   2. The client is experiencing an aura prior to a migraine headache.
   3. The client is experiencing a vasodilating response causing the headache.
   4. The client is experiencing intense photophobia prior to the onset of the headache.
2. What assessment finding suggests to a nurse that a client is having TIAs?
   1. Brief periods of photosensitivity
   2. Brief periods of mental depression
   3. Brief periods of unilateral weakness
   4. Brief periods of stabbing head pain
3. When providing a dietary tray to a client with right hemianopia, what is the best nursing action?
   1. Place the tray most convenient for staff, as the client will need to be assisted.
   2. Place the tray on the right side of the client to allow for self-feeding.
   3. Place the tray on the left side of the client to allow for self-feeding.
   4. Place the tray directly in front of the client to allow for self-feeding.
4. What nursing intervention is most appropriate to decrease the frustration experienced by a client with expressive aphasia?
   1. Use a picture or alphabet board with frequently needed topics.
   2. Ask the client to shake head yes or no to different options.
   3. Offer support by telling the client you know how frustrating this must be.
   4. Arrange for family to be present when attempting to communicate with the client.
5. When is it most important for the nurse to intervene while caring for a client with a leaking cerebral aneurysm?
   1. The client is not sleeping well.
   2. The client is constipated.
   3. The client has a diminished appetite.
   4. The client has a sore throat.

WANT TO KNOW MORE? There are a wide variety of online resources available on thePoint to enhance learning and understanding of this chapter.

Go to **thePoint.lww.com/activate** and use the activation code found in the front of this text to unlock these online resources.

39 Caring for Clients With Head and Spinal Cord Trauma

Words To Know

antegrade amnesia
autonomic dysreflexia
autoregulation
Battle sign
cerebral hematoma
chemonucleolysis
chronic traumatic encephalopathy
closed head injury
concussion
contrecoup injury
contusion
coup injury
craniectomy
cranioplasty
craniotomy
diskectomy
epidural hematoma
extramedullary lesions
functional electrical stimulation
halo sign
infratentorial
intermittent spasticity
intracerebral hematoma
intramedullary lesions
laminectomy
open head injury
otorrhea
paraplegia
paresthesia
periorbital ecchymosis
poikilothermia
rhinorrhea
spinal fusion
spinal shock
subdural hematoma
supratentorial
tentorium
tetraplegia
trephining
uncal herniation

Learning Objectives

On completion of this chapter, you will be able to:

1. Differentiate a concussion from a contusion.
2. Explain the cause and effects of chronic traumatic encephalopathy.
3. Identify differences between epidural, subdural, and intracerebral hematomas.
4. Discuss the nursing management of a client with a head injury.
5. Discuss the nursing management of a client undergoing intracranial surgery.
6. Explain spinal shock, listing four symptoms.
7. Discuss autonomic dysreflexia and at least five manifestations.
8. List possible long-term complications of spinal cord injury.
9. Describe the nursing management of a client with a spinal cord injury.
10. Identify the anatomic difference between intramedullary and extramedullary spinal nerve root compression.

Head and spinal cord trauma can result in permanent disability and dysfunction. This chapter discusses head injuries, which include lacerations, skull fractures, and bleeding and swelling within the brain and surrounding tissues. It also discusses spinal disorders caused by trauma and mechanical injury.

Gerontologic Considerations

■ Nurses should assess older adults for risk of falls and implement appropriate preventive interventions. However, if a fall occurs, the older adult should be assessed for skull fracture. Additionally, nurses should be aware of risk factors and signs of elder abuse, including physical shaking or blows that could lead to skull or spinal cord injury.

HEAD INJURIES

Injury to the head can cause concussions, contusions, hematomas, or skull fracture.

Concussion

Pathophysiology and Etiology

A **concussion** results from a blow to the head that jars the brain. It usually is a consequence of falling, striking the head against a hard surface such as a windshield, colliding with another person (e.g., between athletes), battering during boxing, or being a victim of violence. A concussion causes diffuse and microscopic injury to the brain. The force of the blow causes temporary neurologic impairment but no immediate evidence of serious damage to cerebral tissue. When concussions occur repetitively, even though the blows to the head may appear initially to have subclinical effects, they can result in **chronic traumatic encephalopathy** (CTE), a form of neurodegeneration. Cumulative and sustained concussions, such as those that are sports related, can result in long-term effects such as dementia, depression, Parkinson disease, and early-onset Alzheimer's (Chronic Traumatic Encephalopathy, 2019).

Assessment Findings

At the time the concussion occurs, the client may experience a brief lapse of consciousness, with temporary disorientation, headache, blurred or double vision, emotional irritability, and dizziness. A diagnosis is made clinically because there are no proven biomarkers that are evident in screening tests. Skull radiography, computed tomography (CT) scan, and magnetic resonance imaging (MRI) initially rule out a more serious head injury (e.g., skull fracture, intracranial bleeding) but may show reduced blood flow to the brain when performed later. In the years that follow, there may be behavioral changes, memory and cognitive dysfunction, movement disorders, and increased suicidality. Until large-scale studies produce cumulative data, the diagnosis of postconcussive CTE can only be confirmed by correlating the client's history and physical examination or on autopsy following death.

Medical Management

The client's activity is temporarily halted until the seriousness of the injury is determined. Mild analgesia (usually acetaminophen) relieves the headache. The client is observed over the course of their lifetime for neurologic complications.

Nursing Management

The nurse performs a neurologic assessment (see Chapter 36). If findings are normal and the client does not require hospitalization, the nurse instructs the family to watch the client closely for signs of increased intracranial pressure (ICP). Common signs of increased ICP include behavioral alterations, sleepiness, personality changes, vomiting, and speech or gait disturbances (see Chapter 37). The nurse instructs the client and family to contact a primary provider or return to the emergency department (ED) if any of these symptoms occur. For more information, see Evidence-Based Practice 39-1.

Contusion

A **contusion** is more serious than a concussion and leads to gross structural injury to the brain.

Pathophysiology and Etiology

A **contusion** results in bruising and, sometimes, hemorrhage of superficial cerebral tissue. When the head is struck directly, the injury to the brain is called a **coup injury**. Dual bruising can result if the force is strong enough to send the brain ricocheting to the opposite side of the skull, which is called a **contrecoup injury** (Fig. 39-1). Edema develops at the site of or in areas opposite to the injury. A skull fracture can accompany a contusion.

Evidence-Based Practice 39-1

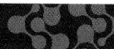

Concussions

Clinical Question

What is the current recommended management of concussions?

Evidence

There is now an official protocol for concussions for all ages and all contact sports that includes six steps with at least 24 hours between steps. All symptoms should completely disappear before progressing to subsequent steps. One organization's policy and procedure regarding a concussion protocol is:

- Education on concussion definition, signs and symptoms, and management
- Preseason baseline brain function test (ImPACT test or equivalent) of reaction time, memory, speed of mental processing, and other factors per individual player
- State law criteria for removing a player from activity
- Sideline assessment of the head injury (includes comparison to preseason ImPACT test or equivalent baseline results)
- School adjustments (shorter days, more breaks, extra time to finish assignments, etc.) during recovery
- Gradual return to activity via a gradual process of small increases in activity

Nursing Implications

Most concussion symptoms should disappear between 14 and 21 days. The consequences of concussions can be severe. The role of a nurse includes taking a good history and reporting findings to the health care provider. Once the diagnosis is confirmed, the nurse should explain the progressive steps and timelines in the protocol to the client and caregivers.

Reference
Cleveland Clinic. (2020). *Concussion*. https://my.clevelandclinic.org/health/diseases/15038-concussion/management-and-treatment

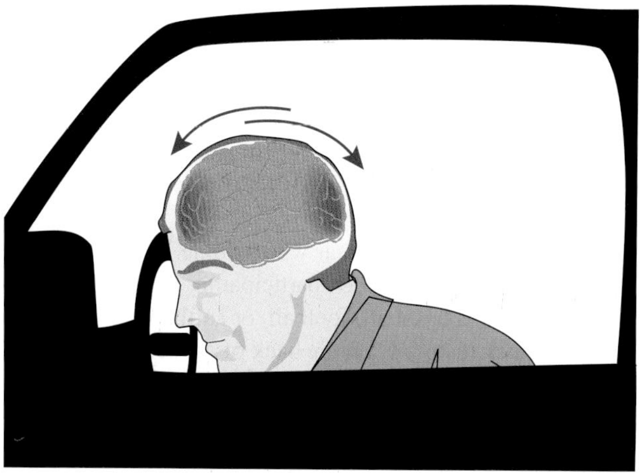

Figure 39-1 Coup injuries occur at the point of contact, and contrecoup injuries occur when the brain rebounds and hits the opposite side of the skull.

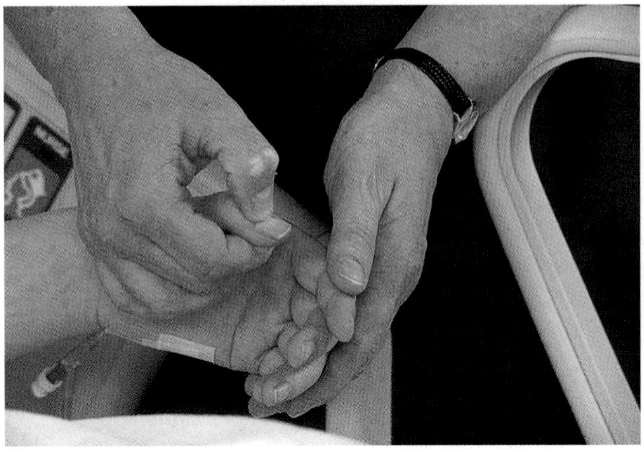

Figure 39-2 The nurse tests the client's motor response by assessing a reaction to a painful stimulus. (Photo by B. Proud.)

Assessment Findings

Signs and symptoms vary depending on the severity of the blow and the degree of head velocity. Clients exhibit hypotension, rapid and weak pulse, shallow respirations, loss of consciousness, and pale, clammy skin. Although unconscious, they usually respond to strong stimuli, such as pressure applied to the base of the nail (Fig. 39-2). On awakening, clients often have temporary **antegrade amnesia** (partial or complete inability to recall the recent past; memories from before the traumatic event remain intact). Permanent brain damage can impair intellect and gait and cause speech difficulty, seizures, and paralysis.

Skull radiography is performed to rule out or confirm skull fracture. CT or MRI detects bleeding or small hemorrhages in brain tissue, a shift in brain tissue, and edema at the injury site.

Medical Management

The unstable client's vital functions are supported with drug therapy and mechanical ventilation, if necessary.

Nursing Management

The nurse observes the client closely for changes in level of consciousness (LOC), signs of increased ICP (see Chapter 37), neurologic changes, respiratory distress, and changes in vital signs every 1 to 2 hours. If symptoms develop, the nurse reports them to the primary provider.

Prevention of health problems is a major component of nursing care. To reduce the potential for both minor and life-threatening head injuries, the nurse stresses the importance of the following:

- Using seatbelts for all passengers in automobiles
- Restraining infants in approved car seats located in the rear seats of automobiles
- Wearing protective headgear while riding bicycles or motorcycles, skiing, and when participating in contact sports such as hockey, baseball, football, or softball
- Raising neck restraints on the back of car seats
- Not driving under the influence of alcohol or drugs

Cerebral Hematomas

A **cerebral hematoma** is bleeding within the skull. The accumulation of blood forms an expanding lesion. People at high risk for cerebral hematomas are those receiving anticoagulant therapy or those with an underlying bleeding disorder, such as hemophilia, thrombocytopenia, leukemia, and aplastic anemia (see Chapter 31).

Pathophysiology and Etiology

Most hematomas result from head trauma or cerebral vascular disorders. The types of hematomas are epidural hematoma, subdural hematoma, and intracerebral hematoma (Fig. 39-3).

An **epidural hematoma** stems from arterial bleeding, usually from the middle meningeal artery, and blood accumulation above the dura. It is characterized by rapidly progressive neurologic deterioration. A **subdural hematoma** results from venous bleeding, with blood gradually accumulating in the space below the dura. Subdural hematomas are classified as acute, subacute, and chronic according to the rate of neurologic changes. Symptoms progressively worsen in a client with an acute subdural hematoma within the first 24 hours of the head injury. Clients with subacute and chronic subdural hematomas become symptomatic after 24 hours and up to 1 week later. An **intracerebral hematoma** is bleeding within the brain that results from an open or closed head injury or from a cerebrovascular condition such as a ruptured cerebral aneurysm (see Chapter 38).

Bleeding increases the volume of brain contents and ICP, which disrupts blood flow and causes the brain to become ischemic and hypoxic. Unrelieved increased ICP also causes the brain to shift to the lateral side (**uncal herniation**) or herniate downward through the foramen magnum. These developments affect the vital centers for respiration, heart

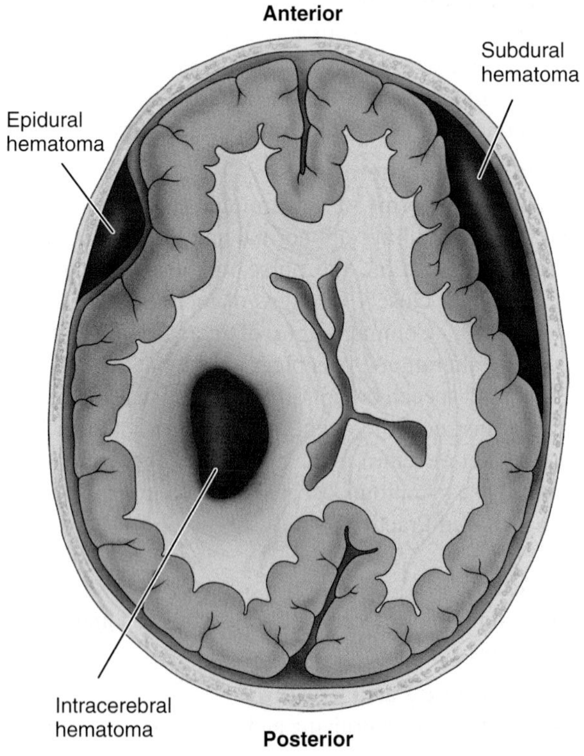

Figure 39-3 Location of epidural, subdural, and intracerebral hematomas.

TABLE 39-1 Differences in Cerebral Hematomas

TYPE	LOCATION	SIGNS AND SYMPTOMS
Epidural	Arterial blood collects between the skull and dura.	Client may be alert after initial unconsciousness but then becomes increasingly lethargic before lapsing into coma. Common symptoms are headache, ipsilateral (same side as injury) pupil changes, and contralateral (opposite side to injury) hemiparesis (weakness or paralysis).
Subdural	Venous blood collects between the dura and subarachnoid layers.	Deterioration in LOC is progressive. There are ipsilateral pupil changes, decreased extraocular muscle movement, and contralateral hemiparesis, with periodic episodes of memory lapse, confusion, drowsiness, and personality changes.
Intracerebral	Blood collects within the brain.	Client shows classic signs of increased ICP: headache, vomiting, seizures, posturing, hyperthermia, irregular breathing.

ICP, intracranial pressure; LOC, level of consciousness.

rate, and blood pressure, as well as cranial nerve functions. Death occurs if the symptoms are not recognized and the bleeding is not controlled.

Assessment Findings

The rapidity and severity of neurologic changes (Table 39-1) depend on the location, the rate of bleeding and size of the hematoma, and the effectiveness of **autoregulation**, the brain's ability to provide sufficient arterial blood flow despite rising ICP. MRI and CT scan show densities that indicate the location of the hematoma and shifts in cerebral tissue. ICP monitoring (see Chapter 37) provides direct and continuous data for evaluating the extent to which the lesion is expanding or responding to treatment.

Concept Mastery Alert

Epidural Hematoma

Deterioration in clients with epidural hematoma can be punctuated by periods of alertness. Therefore, if a client is initially unconscious, then regains consciousness, then lapses into a coma, it is indicative of an epidural hematoma. By contrast, symptoms in clients with acute subdural hematoma deteriorate progressively.

Medical Management

In some cases, the body walls off and absorbs a subdural hematoma with no treatment. However, a rapid change in LOC and signs of uncontrolled increased ICP indicate a surgical emergency.

Surgical Management

Surgery consists of drilling holes (*burr holes*) in the skull, known as **trephining,** relieving pressure (Fig. 39-4), removing the clot, and stopping the bleeding. If the source of bleeding cannot be located by means of burr holes, more invasive surgery is performed. Epidural hematomas require more prompt intervention because the rate of bleeding is greater from an arterial bleed than from a venous bleed.

Intracranial surgery consists of three possible procedures: craniotomy, craniectomy, and cranioplasty. A **craniotomy** is a surgical opening of the skull to gain access to structures beneath the cranial bones. It is performed to remove a blood clot or tumor, stop intracranial bleeding, or repair damaged brain tissues or blood vessels. A **craniectomy** is removal of a portion of cranial bone. **Cranioplasty** is the repair of a defect in a cranial bone (see Chapter 37). The portion of the bone removed during craniectomy may be implanted in the client's abdomen awaiting later replacement. As an alternative, a metal or plastic plate or wire mesh is used to replace the removed bone or to reinforce a defect in a cranial bone.

One of two surgical approaches is used to enter the brain above or below the **tentorium**, a double fold of dura mater that separates the cerebrum from the cerebellum. A **supratentorial** (above the tentorium) approach is made through a scalp incision at the site where a particular cerebral lobe requires surgical access. The **infratentorial** (below the tentorium) approach provides an opening to the midbrain and structures of the brain stem. The incision is made at the back of the head with the client in a sitting position (Fig. 39-5).

In cranial surgery, after several burr holes are made in the skull, a saw is used to cut a section of bone (bone flap). The bone flap is removed to provide a visual field for surgery. After surgery is completed, the bone flap usually is replaced.

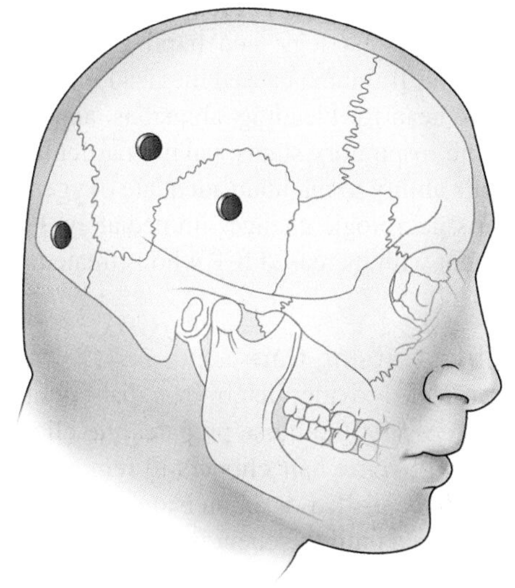

Figure 39-4 Neurosurgical procedures may require the use of burr holes to make a bone flap in the skull, aspirate a brain abscess, or evacuate a hematoma.

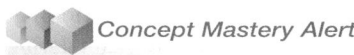

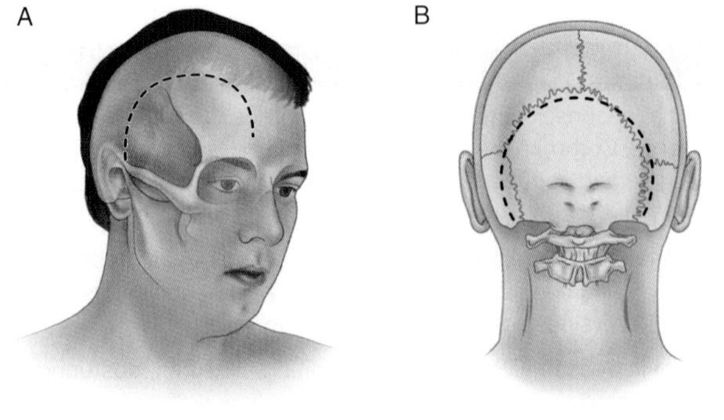

Figure 39-5 **(A)** A supratentorial incision is made behind the hairline on the side of pathology. **(B)** An infratentorial incision is a horseshoe-shaped incision around the occipital lobe.

In some instances, such as with an inoperable tumor, the bone flap is not replaced, allowing the tumor to expand, and thus reducing the rate at which ICP rises. Complications associated with intracranial surgery include cerebral edema, infection, neurogenic shock (see Chapter 17), fluid and electrolyte imbalances, venous thrombosis (especially in the arms and legs), increased ICP, seizures, leakage of cerebrospinal fluid (CSF), and stress ulcers and hemorrhage.

Pharmacologic Considerations

- The infusion nurse needs to monitor the administration of mannitol for crystal formation. Warming the solution may help dissolve the crystals and an in-line filter is recommended to use during the administration of 15%, 20%, and 25% solutions (Mannitol IV, 2020).

Nursing Management

The nurse regards a head injury, no matter how mild it appears, as an emergency. They obtain a history of the injury and perform a neurologic examination, paying particular attention to vital signs; LOC; presence or absence of movement in the arms and legs; and pupil size, equality, and reaction to light. If trauma caused the head injury, the nurse examines the head for bleeding, abrasions, and lacerations. They evaluate respiratory status, paying particular attention to the client's ability to maintain adequate oxygenation. The nurse reports neurologic changes immediately. For nursing care of a client with increased ICP who is treated medically, see Chapter 37.

Preoperative Nursing Care

Once the primary provider determines that operative intervention is necessary, the nurse prepares the client for surgery. They use electric hair clippers to remove hair where burr holes will be drilled or an incision will be made (this usually is deferred until the client is in the operating room). The nurse takes vital signs and maintains a record of continuing neurologic assessment findings. They administer prescribed medications, such as the anticonvulsant phenytoin (Dilantin) to reduce the risk of seizures before and after surgery, an osmotic diuretic, and corticosteroids. Preoperative sedation usually is omitted. Before surgery, the nurse restricts fluids to avoid intraoperative complications, reduce cerebral edema, and prevent postoperative vomiting. If indicated, the nurse inserts an indwelling urethral catheter and intravenous (IV) line. The nurse applies antiembolism stockings to prevent thrombophlebitis and deep vein thrombosis, which may develop from prolonged inactivity during neurosurgery.

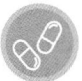

Pharmacologic Considerations

- Some medications (such as diazepam or phenytoin) can injure soft tissue if the IV solution is leaked out of the vein. Supplies and protocols for treatment should be readily available when these IV drugs are used.

Postoperative Nursing Care

After surgery, the nurse places the client in either a supine position with the head slightly elevated or a side-lying position on the unaffected side and performs postoperative and neurologic assessments every 15 to 30 minutes. The nurse maintains a neurologic flow sheet to compare trends in assessment findings. Edema around the eyes (periorbital edema) may make examination of the pupils difficult during the immediate postoperative period. Ecchymosis can also be present. The nurse removes antiembolism stockings briefly every 8 hours and reapplies them.

It is important to monitor the client's body temperature closely because hyperthermia increases brain metabolism, increasing the potential for brain damage. Therefore, elevated temperature must be relieved with antipyretic and other measures.

The nurse observes the client closely for increased ICP. They restrict fluids to control cerebral edema and to increase cerebral perfusion.

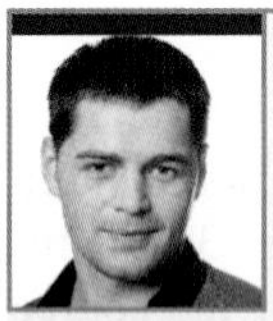

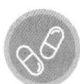

Clinical Scenario While on a skiing vacation, a 32-year-old client fell and struck their head on a tree. The client was found unconscious by members of the ski patrol. During transport to a medical center, the client could not be aroused, the scalp on the side of their head injury showed obvious swelling, and their pupillary response was sluggish and unequal. **What nursing care is appropriate for this client for whom emergency surgery is required? See Nursing Care Plan 39-1 and Client and Family Teaching 39-1.**

NURSING CARE PLAN 39-1 Care of the Client Undergoing Intracranial Surgery

Assessment

- Assess vital signs, LOC, verbal response, and understanding of oral communication.
- Determine the type and level of discomfort (e.g., headache, sensitivity to light).
- Assess current level of pain tolerance using a scale of 0 to 10.
- Evaluate orientation and level of pain to person, place, and time.
- Check cognitive function by determining ability to follow simple instructions or perform basic mathematical calculations.
- Check pupil size, equality, and response to light. Look for changes in visual field, blurred vision, or diplopia.
- Assess symmetry in facial appearance.
- Test mobility and strength in all four extremities.
- If client is unconscious, look for restlessness.
- Check appropriateness of mood.
- Ask about nausea, and look for evidence of vomiting.
- Monitor seizure activity and status of corneal blink and gag reflexes.
- Monitor urine production, and evaluate the sensation of thirst.

Nursing Analysis. **Altered Breathing Pattern** related to depressive effects of anesthesia and compression of medulla secondary to edema of the brain

Expected Outcome. Breathing will be sufficient to maintain an oxygen saturation (SpO_2) of at least 90% and a partial pressure of arterial oxygen (PaO_2) of at least 80 mm Hg.

Interventions	Rationales
Monitor SpO_2 with a pulse oximeter.	*SpO_2 of at least 90% indicates that PaO_2 is at least 80 mm Hg.*
Maintain a patent airway by keeping the head erect and in midline, inserting an oral or nasopharyngeal airway if necessary, and suctioning secretions.	*Neck flexion or rotation can compromise the diameter of the natural airway; an oral or pharyngeal airway prevents the tongue from obstructing the airway; suction removes secretions that reduce air exchange.*
Encourage client to deep breathe at least 10 times each hour or to use a bedside spirometer.	*Gas exchange depends on moving atmospheric air to the level of the alveoli and exhaling to remove carbon dioxide (CO_2).*
Avoid administering narcotic analgesia.	*Opioids depress respirations.*
Elevate the head of the bed.	*Elevating the head lowers abdominal organs away from the diaphragm, which helps improve inspired volume and reduce intracranial swelling.*
Report signs of hypoxemia; be prepared to administer supplemental oxygen or provide mechanical ventilation.	*Delivering oxygen at a greater concentration than room air increases oxygenation of blood; mechanical ventilation assists breathing.*

Evaluation of Expected Outcome

Client's airway is patent, and respirations are normal.

Nursing Analysis. **Altered (Cerebral) Tissue Perfusion** related to cerebral edema and bleeding within the cranium

Expected Outcome. ICP will be adequate to perfuse the brain as evidenced by normal neurologic signs and symptoms. Refer to Nursing Care Plan: The Client With Increased Intracranial Pressure in Chapter 37 for interventions.

Evaluation of Expected Outcome

Client shows neurologic stability.

Nursing Analysis. **Pain** related to chemicals released from traumatized tissue, swelling of cerebral tissue, and irritation of meninges

Expected Outcome. Pain will be reduced to client's preidentified level of tolerance within 30 minutes of intervention.

Interventions	Rationales
Assess presence, type, and level of pain whenever you assess vital signs and as needed.	*Pain assessment is the fifth vital sign.*
Reduce bright lights and noise.	*Annoying and disturbing sensory stimuli lower the pain threshold.*

(continued)

NURSING CARE PLAN 39-1 Care of the Client Undergoing Intracranial Surgery (*continued*)

Minimize activity when pain is acute.	*Movement and disturbed rest intensify pain.*
Administer prescribed analgesia.	*Nonopioid analgesia is preferred because it does not interfere with neurologic assessment findings.*

Evaluation of Expected Outcome

Client reports no pain or a tolerable level of pain.

Related Complication (RC) of Seizures

Expected Outcome. The nurse will monitor to detect, manage, and minimize seizure activity.

Interventions	Rationales
Observe client for changes in consciousness and involuntary muscle contraction.	*Seizures are categorized as generalized or partial; manifestations vary (see* Chapter 37*).*
Pad side rails; keep the bed in low position.	*Padding reduces the potential for trauma.* *Serious injury is less likely if a client falls from a bed in low position.*
Stay with the client if a seizure occurs; protect them from injury, suction secretions, and promote adequate ventilation.	*During a seizure, a client cannot protect themselves. Secretions accumulate, increasing the risk for aspiration. Contraction of the diaphragm and intercostal muscles can lead to hypoxia.*
Administer prescribed anticonvulsants.	*They decrease excitation of brain neurons.*

Evaluation of Expected Outcome

The nurse detects seizures and implements interventions to minimize their consequences.

Nursing Analysis. **Infection risk** related to impaired skin integrity and suppressed inflammatory response

Expected Outcome. Client will remain free of infection.

Interventions	Rationales
Assess temperature, pulse rate, lung sounds, and characteristics of urine. Note the presence of a cough.	*Body temperature and pulse rate rise in response to infection. Pneumonia and urinary tract infections are common after surgery because of retained pulmonary secretions, urine stasis, or bacteria entering the urinary tract from the anus.*
Inspect the dressing and wound for evidence of purulent drainage.	*Impaired skin provides an entrance for microorganisms. Purulent drainage is characteristic of infection.*
Follow principles of asepsis when assessing the incision and changing the dressing.	*Asepsis reduces or eliminates pathogens.*
Administer prescribed antibiotics.	*They interfere with the growth and reproduction of pathogens.*

Evaluation of Expected Outcome

The surgical site remains free of infection; no other evidence of infection develops.

Nursing Analysis. **Thermal Injury Risk** related to hypothalamic dysfunction or infection

Expected Outcome. Client will maintain body temperature within normal range.

NURSING CARE PLAN 39-1 Care of the Client Undergoing Intracranial Surgery (*continued*)

Interventions	Rationales
Measure body temperature every 4 hours.	*Routine assessment of body temperature provides early indications of changes in client's thermoregulation.*
Help client maintain an adequate oral fluid intake.	*Perspiration assists with heat loss through evaporation.*
Remove heavy blankets if client develops a fever. Place client on an electrical cooling blanket to reduce fever.	*Blankets trap body heat and interfere with convection. A cooling blanket reduces body temperature through conduction.*
Administer a prescribed antipyretic when fever does not respond to heat reduction methods.	*Antipyretics lower the set point for body temperature in the hypothalamus.*

Evaluation of Expected Outcome

Temperature does not exceed 99.8°F.

Nursing Analysis. **Acute Confusion** related to cognitive deficits secondary to structural changes in brain tissue and physiology

Expected Outcomes. Client will be oriented to person, place, and time.

Interventions	Rationales
Orient client at frequent intervals.	*Until cognition and sensorium return to normal, client may not recall their location and the reasons for medical care.*
Provide environmental clues such as a calendar and clock with large numbers.	*An easy-to-read calendar and clock within client's vision helps reorient the client to time.*
Investigate contributing causes of disorientation and restlessness (e.g., full bladder, pain) and intervene as appropriate.	*Clients may sense that they are uncomfortable but be unable to identify specifics of their distress.*
Share current events, and turn on newsworthy TV or radio programs.	*Sensory stimulation and communication tend to elevate cognitive functions.*
Repeat explanations or answers to questions as needed.	*Repetition reinforces information and promotes storage of memory.*

Evaluation of Expected Outcome

Client is oriented to person, place, and time.

Nursing Analysis. **Injury** Risk related to confusion and poor judgment

Expected Outcome. Client will remain free of injuries.

Interventions	Rationales
Locate client near nursing station.	*Placing the client in an optimal site for nursing observation increases the nurses' ability to assist the client when necessary.*
Place a signal cord within the client's reach; remind client to use it when they need assistance.	*The signal cord can help prevent injuries if the client cannot make their needs known.*
Place a bed/chair alarm that sounds if the client attempts to get out of bed without assistance.	*Such an alarm calls attention to the need for assessment and assistance.*

Evaluation of Expected Outcome

No injuries occur.

(*continued*)

NURSING CARE PLAN 39-1 Care of the Client Undergoing Intracranial Surgery (*continued*)

Nursing Analysis. **Coping Impairment** related to multiple stressors involving physical losses, lengthy rehabilitation, and compromised finances

Expected Outcome. Client and family will cope with neurologic deficits, participate fully in rehabilitation, and seek assistance from social agencies.

Interventions	Rationales
Consult with the primary provider about the client's prognosis.	*Giving false reassurance is nontherapeutic; offering encouragement promotes motivation.*
Concur with primary provider's explanations if client or family raises questions.	*Giving consistent responses reinforces that the client has received the same information as other members of the health care team.*
Keep client and family informed of progress or changes as they occur.	*It is easier to cope with and adapt to small changes. Problem-solving is more effective when client and family are provided with facts.*
Accept client's and family's behavior under stress in a nonjudgmental manner.	*Responses to stress vary. Intolerance of a person's response interferes with a therapeutic alliance between the nurse, client, and family.*
Encourage problem-solving techniques and acknowledge positive outcomes.	*Unity and cohesiveness develop when client and family resolve problems collaboratively.*
Refer client and family to a social worker, discharge planner, or home health agency.	*Such providers can assist the client and family with the transition from the hospital to other options for care.*

Evaluation of Expected Outcomes

Client and family effectively cope with the stress of surgery and possibility of long-term disability.

Client and Family Teaching 39-1
Postintracranial Surgery

If the client is discharged directly home, the nurse must explain the purposes for prescribed medications (e.g., anticonvulsants, anti-inflammatory drugs, drugs to control gastric acidity), schedule for administration, and side effects to report. In addition, the nurse must provide the following verbal and written instructions:

- Watch for signs of intracranial bleeding and infection (expect swelling around the eye and below the incision).
- Expect sensory changes such as hearing a "clicking" sound around the bone flap, which will disappear as healing takes place. Understand that headaches are also common but notify the surgeon if a mild analgesic such as acetaminophen (Tylenol) fails to relieve them.
- Care for the surgical site as directed by the primary provider. Some recommendations include keeping the incision clean, avoiding scrubbing the incision, securing remaining hair away from the incision, resuming shampooing the hair when the staples or sutures are removed, and wearing a hat when outside to avoid sunburn until hair growth resumes.
- Maintain safety precautions at home including ambulating only with assistance and ensuring well-lit and clutter-free rooms. Do not drive until the risk of seizures has been eliminated.
- Engage in exercises that promote strength and endurance.
- Use techniques to ensure bowel and bladder elimination (see Chapter 40).
- Follow feeding and/or nutrition staff suggestions.
- Keep follow-up appointments for measuring anticonvulsant blood levels, electroencephalograms, and continued medical care and evaluation.

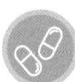

Pharmacologic Considerations

■ Fear of altering neurologic status prevents good postoperative pain management. Providers assume that opioids will affect neurologic findings, and this reluctance to medicate means pain is not well addressed. Acetaminophen is recommended if pain medicine is needed after a head injury (Concussion, 2020). Antileptics (e.g., gabapentin), corticosteroids, and morphine provided via client-controlled anesthesia all help reduce intracranial pain. The result is that clients assume movement and activity sooner, reducing hospital stays (Vadivelu, 2016).

››› *Stop, Think, and Respond 39-1*

You are caring for two clients with head injuries. Client A lost consciousness at the time of their head injury. They are alert and oriented on arrival in the ED, but 2 hours later, they do not respond even when you press on their nail beds. Client B has been hospitalized for 1 day. They have not been fully alert since admission and continue to be lethargic. They require more and more stimulation to obtain a response. Which client's condition is more serious? Explain your choice.

Skull Fractures

A skull fracture is a break in the continuity of the cranium. The most common types are simple, depressed, or comminuted fractures (Table 39-2).

Pathophysiology and Etiology

A skull fracture results from a blow to the head. It can be associated with an **open head injury**, in which the scalp, bony cranium, and dura mater (the outer meningeal layer) are exposed, or it may be a **closed head injury**, in which an intact layer of scalp covers the fractured skull.

Open head injuries create a potential for infection because they expose internal brain structures to the environment. They are less likely to produce rapid increased ICP because the opening gives the brain some room to expand as pressure increases.

Basilar skull fractures are located at the base of the skull. Trauma in this location is especially dangerous because it can cause edema of the brain near the origin of the spinal cord (*foramen magnum*), interfere with circulation of CSF, injure nerves that pass into the spinal cord, or create a pathway for infection between the brain and middle ear (Fig. 39-6), which can result in meningitis.

TABLE 39-2 Types of Skull Fractures

TYPE	DESCRIPTION
Simple	Linear crack without any displacement of the pieces
Depressed	Broken bone pushed inward toward the brain
Comminuted	Bone splintered into fragments

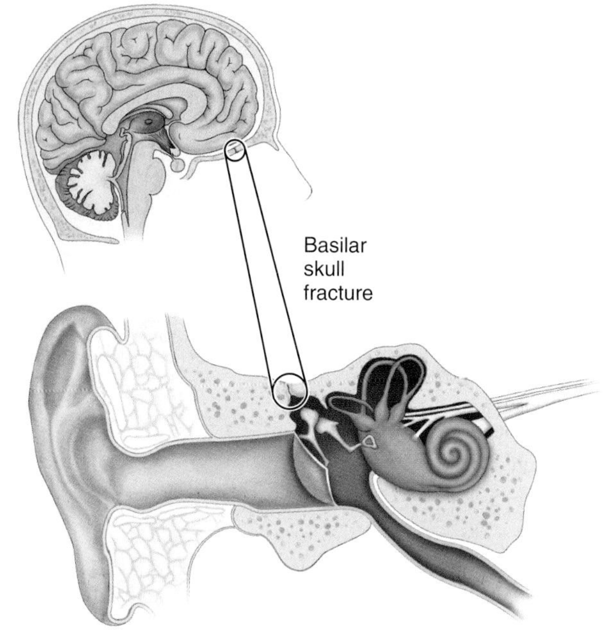

Figure 39-6 Basilar fractures allow cerebrospinal fluid to leak from the nose and ears. (Adapted from Hickey, J. V. (2008). *The clinical practice of neurological and neurosurgical nursing* (6th ed.). Wolters Kluwer Health/Lippincott Williams & Wilkins.)

Assessment Findings

Signs and Symptoms

Simple skull fractures produce few, if any, symptoms and heal without complications. The client may complain of a localized headache. A bump, bruise, or laceration may be visible on the scalp. Symptoms depend on the area of the brain that has been injured. For example, a large bone fragment that is pressing on the motor area can cause hemiparesis. In any type of skull fracture, shock can develop from injury to the skull or some other area of the body.

Because basilar skull fractures tend to tear the dura, **rhinorrhea**, leaking of CSF from the nose, or **otorrhea**, leakage of CSF from the ear, may occur. In some cases, **periorbital ecchymosis**, referred to as *raccoon eyes*, or bruising of the mastoid process behind the ear, called **Battle sign**, can be present (Fig. 39-7). Conjunctival hemorrhages can occur as well. Injury to the brain tissue may result in seizures. Epilepsy can develop as a sequela of head injury.

Diagnostic Findings

Skull radiographs, CT scan, or MRI show brain tissue injuries such as a fracture line or embedded skull fragments (compound skull fracture), cerebral edema, or a subdural or epidural hematoma.

Medical and Surgical Management

Simple skull fractures require bed rest and close observation for signs of increased ICP. If the scalp is lacerated, the wound is cleaned, debrided, and sutured. Depressed skull fractures require a craniotomy to remove bone fragments and control bleeding, elevation of the depressed fracture, and repair of damaged tissues. A piece of mesh is inserted to replace the bone fragments that are removed. Additional treatment

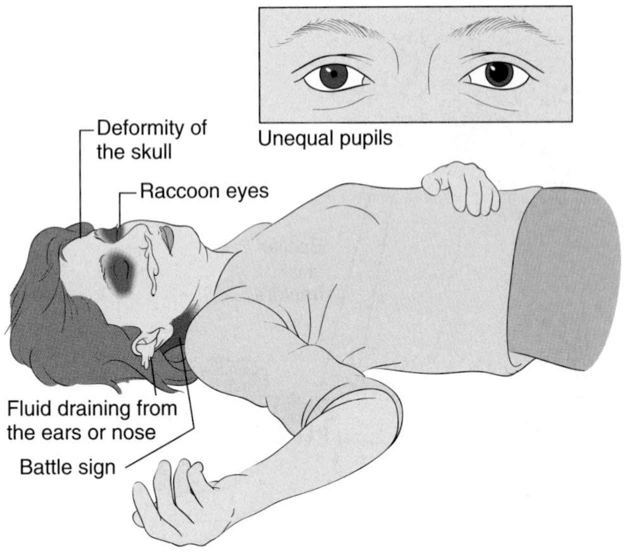

Figure 39-7 Signs of a skull fracture may include skull deformity, unequal pupils, periorbital ecchymosis (*raccoon eyes*), fluid from the ears or nose, and periauricular ecchymosis (*Battle sign*). (Source: LifeART image copyright (2022) Wolters Kluwer Health, Inc. Lippincott Williams & Wilkins. All rights reserved.)

includes antibiotics to control infection, an osmotic diuretic to prevent or treat cerebral edema, and an anticonvulsant to prevent or treat seizures. Use of corticosteroids following head injuries and neurosurgery is prescribed less and less because research studies are showing a higher incidence of deaths as compared with those not treated with corticosteroids (Cerebral Edema, 2020).

Nursing Management

Most clients are hospitalized for at least 24 hours after a significant head injury. The nurse examines the client to identify signs of head trauma and tests drainage from the nose or ear (Nursing Guidelines 39-1). To detect any CSF drainage, the nurse looks for a **halo sign**, which is a bloodstain surrounded by a clear or yellowish stain. If drainage is present, the nurse allows it to flow freely onto porous gauze and avoids tightly plugging the orifice.

The nurse performs neurologic assessments, which include an hourly evaluation of LOC and of pupil, motor, and sensory status, even if the injury appears mild. It is possible for a hematoma to accompany a skull fracture. The nurse obtains vital signs every 15 to 30 minutes and prepares for the possibility of seizures. For additional nursing care, see Chapter 37.

SPINAL CORD INJURIES

Spinal cord trauma is serious and sometimes fatal. The cervical and lumbar vertebrae are the most common sites of injury. Correct emergency management at the time of injury is crucial because moving the client incorrectly can permanently damage the spinal cord and the nerves that extend from it.

Pathophysiology and Etiology

Common causes of spinal cord injury include accidents and violence. Vehicular accidents, including those involving motorcycles, are the leading cause, followed by violence, falls, sports, and miscellaneous injuries.

NURSING GUIDELINES 39-1

Detecting Cerebrospinal Fluid in Drainage

Method #1

1. Wet a Dextrostix or Tes-Tape strip with drainage from the nose or ear.
2. Observe if the color change indicates the presence of glucose.
3. Use Method #2 if the test is positive because blood also contains glucose and can result in false results.

Method #2

1. Collect droplets of drainage on a white absorbent pad.
2. Observe the wet area after a few minutes for a halo sign.
3. Note if a pale yellow or clear ring encircles a central ring that is red: The red ring indicates blood; the pale yellow ring suggests CSF.

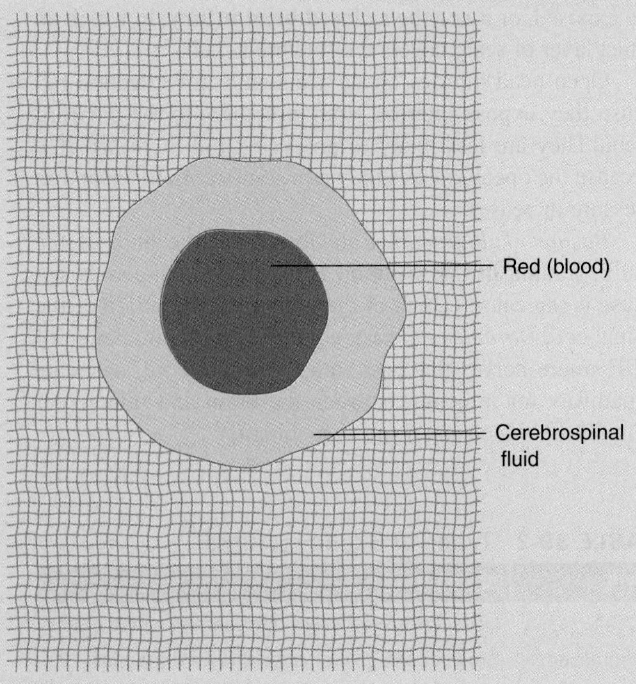

Halo sign

Trauma to the back can fracture or collapse one or more vertebrae, causing a portion of bone to injure the spinal cord and interfere with the transmission of nerve impulses (Fig. 39-8). Even without a fracture, edema may lead to cord compression, which may permanently damage the cord.

Spinal cord injury can also lead to bleeding within the cord. Because the blood has no place to drain, it forms a hematoma that occupies space and compresses the nerve roots. Injury to the cord can also completely or partially sever spinal cord nerve fibers. With such an injury, the client experiences various consequences of motor and sensory dysfunction below the site of the injury that affect functional abilities (Table 39-3).

Tetraplegia (a term that replaces *quadriplegia*) refers to weakness, paralysis, and sensory impairment of all extremities and the trunk when there is a spinal injury at or above the first thoracic (T1) vertebrae. **Paraplegia**, weakness or paralysis and compromised sensory functions of both legs and lower pelvis, occurs with spinal injuries below the T1 level. When the tracts of the spinal nerves are completely severed, no effective nerve regeneration occurs. Muscle spasms occur spontaneously, but they are not evidence that the client is regaining motor function. Many paraplegics return home, live independently, and, in some instances, resume work. Tetraplegics may return home but require extensive physical care.

Complications

Respiratory arrest and spinal shock are immediate complications of spinal cord injury. Long-term complications include autonomic dysreflexia, pressure ulcers, respiratory infections, urinary and fecal impairment, spasticity and contractures, weight gain or loss, calcium depletion, urinary calculi, sexual dysfunction, and pain.

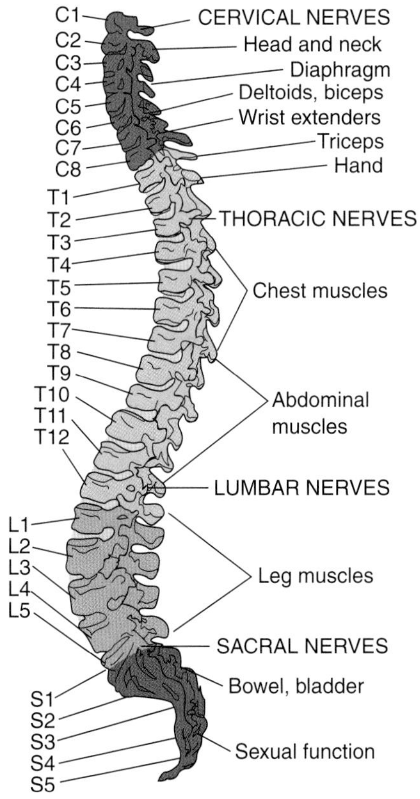

Figure 39-8 Structures affected by spinal nerves.

Spinal Shock (Areflexia)

Spinal shock is a loss of sympathetic reflex activity below the level of injury within 30 to 60 minutes of a spinal injury. It is characterized by immediate loss of all cord functions below the point of injury. In addition to paralysis, manifestations include pronounced hypotension, bradycardia, and warm, dry skin. If the level of injury is in the cervical or upper thoracic region, respiratory failure can occur. Bowel and bladder distention develop. The client does not perspire below the level of injury, which impairs temperature control. The client manifests **poikilothermia**, body temperature of the environment. Spinal shock may persist for 1 week to months until the body adjusts to the damage caused by the injury. Until then, vital functions require medical support.

Autonomic Dysreflexia (Hyperreflexia)

Autonomic dysreflexia is an exaggerated sympathetic nervous system response in people with spinal cord injuries above T6. It can occur suddenly at any time after spinal shock subsides. Box 39-1 lists factors that precipitate autonomic dysreflexia. Characteristics of this acute emergency are as follows:

- Severe hypertension
- Slow heart rate
- Pounding headache
- Nausea
- Blurred vision
- Flushed skin
- Sweating
- Goosebumps (erection of pilomotor muscles in the skin)
- Nasal stuffiness
- Anxiety

Uncontrolled autonomic dysreflexia can lead to seizures, stroke, and death. Prevention is the best treatment, but additional measures such as administering antihypertensive drug therapy with nifedipine (Procardia), nitroglycerin ointment, phentolamine (Regitine), hydralazine (Apresoline), or diazoxide (Hyperstat); raising the client's head; and relieving the precipitating cause are necessary once it develops.

Pressure Ulcers

One in three people with spinal cord injuries develop pressure ulcers in the first year following their injury, and many require three or more hospitalizations for the treatment of pressure ulcers during their lifetime (Pressure Ulcers, 2020). Risk factors include immobility, muscle atrophy, skin shear caused by spasticity and traumatic transfer techniques, skin contact with urine and feces, loss of sensation, and altered nutrition.

Respiratory Infections

Clients with spinal cord injuries may not be able to breathe normally and cough sufficiently to clear secretions. The spinal nerves that transmit impulses to the diaphragm, intercostal muscles, neck, and abdominal muscles may no longer function. Consequently, the risk of inadequate ventilation and pneumonia is high.

TABLE 39-3 Consequences of Spinal Cord Injuries

LEVEL OF INJURY	COMMON MOTOR EFFECTS	COMMON SENSORY EFFECTS	FUNCTIONAL ABILITIES
C1–C3	Paralysis below neck; impaired breathing; bowel and bladder incontinence; sexual dysfunction	No sensation below neck	Breathe with assistance of ventilator Swallow and speak Use a power wheelchair with movement of head and neck control Operate computer or appliances, such as TV or lights, using voice-activation device or mouth stick
C4–C5	Shoulder elevation possible; ventilation support required	No sensation below clavicle	Breathe with ventilator assistance or possibly independently Use a power wheelchair with sip-and-puff or hand control Drink independently using a long straw and bottle
C6–C8	Some elbow, upper arm, and wrist movement; can do diaphragmatic breathing	Some sensation in arms and thumb; sensation in chest impaired	Eat, groom, bathe, and attain bed mobility with assistive devices Transfer from bed to chair using a slide board Perform self-catheterization (men); more difficult for women Use manual wheelchair in flat environment Drive with hand controls
T1–T6	Paralysis below waist; control of hands; abdominal breathing	No sensation below midchest	Perform personal care and household activities independently Use manual wheelchair, including up and down curbs Stand between bars with leg splints
T7–T12	Varying degrees of trunk and abdominal control	Varying degrees of sensation below waist	Transfer from bed to wheelchair independently Propel wheelchair over uneven surfaces and rough terrain Care for bowel and bladder independently Perform light housekeeping and meal preparation Balance on legs Walk with splints or long leg braces
L1–L2	Hip adduction impaired	No sensation below lower abdomen; some sensation in inner thighs	Drive a car with hand controls
L3–L5	Knee and ankle movement impaired	No sensation below upper thighs	Walk with support of walker or crutches
S1–S5	Varying degrees of bowel/bladder control and sexual function	No sensation in perineum	Walk normally without assistive devices Control bladder, bowel, and sexual functions

C, cervical; L, lumbar; S, sacral; T, thoracic.

Urinary and Fecal Impairment

Although the kidneys continue to produce urine, the muscles of the bladder and urinary sphincter may no longer be controlled voluntarily. This may result either in reflexive emptying when the bladder fills with urine or failure to empty, which causes urine to reverse fill the ureters and renal pelvises as the bladder becomes overly distended. Bacteria are likely to colonize the bladder because clients may not completely empty it.

In addition, clients may have no urge to defecate and may be prone to fecal accumulation within the bowel. The connection between the spinal cord nerves and muscles needed for bowel elimination may be severed, or the rectal sphincter may not dilate to allow the passage of stool. In either case, there is a risk of fecal impaction.

BOX 39-1 Common Causes of Autonomic Dysreflexia

- Full bladder
- Abdominal distention
- Impacted feces
- Skin pressure or breakdown
- Overstretched muscles
- Sexual intercourse
- Labor and delivery
- Sunburn below the cord injury
- Infected ingrown toenail
- Exposure to hot or cold environmental temperature
- Taking over-the-counter decongestants

Spasticity and Contractures

Clients with spinal cord injuries experience **intermittent spasticity**, uncontrolled jerking movements, muscle stiffness, and rigidity. Spasticity occurs because nerve signals between the brain and nerves below the level of injury are interrupted. Instead of a coordinated effort, an unregulated spinal reflex may cause an overly active muscle response. Muscle spasms pull the joints into a shortened position, increasing the potential for skin impairment and contractures.

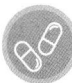

Pharmacologic Considerations

- In a study Botulinum Toxin A was used with clinical therapy and appeared to be highly effective at decreasing spasticity in the wrists, fingers, and elbows of persons with traumatic brain injury. Increased doses appeared to increase the length and intensity of response. Further studies are necessary to see the full effectiveness of this therapy (Injected Botulinum Toxin a Medication Appears to Reduce Severe Abnormal Excessive Muscle Tone, 2020).

Contractures result from the inability to move a joint freely because of an imbalance between opposing muscle groups; a stronger muscle overpowers a weaker one. After spinal cord injury, this may be a consequence of muscle spasticity. Contractures such as flexed elbows, wrists, hips, or knees; clenched fists; and thumb-in-palm may develop any time after the injury (Fig. 39-9).

Weight Change

After spinal cord injury, clients tend to lose weight initially but gain weight after weeks, months, and years of inactivity. Clients must be taught how to make healthy food choices by selecting foods that are relatively low in calories and nutritious.

Calcium Depletion

Following a spinal cord injury, clients experience demineralization of their bones because physical activity is one mechanism for maintaining bone density. The loss of muscle force contributes to bone demineralization. About 80% of those with spinal cord injuries have either osteopenia, lower than normal bone density, or osteoporosis, excessive loss of calcium from bones (Osteoporosis, 2020). This places clients at high risk for fractures from falls or even activities of daily living (ADLs) as well as the consequences of hypercalciuria such as renal and bladder stones (see discussion that follows). Preventive methods include administering calcium and vitamin D supplements and ossification agents such as bisphosphonates, calcitonin, and selective estrogen receptor modulators (see Chapter 63). Functional electrical stimulation, which is discussed later, may be helpful to increase bone density.

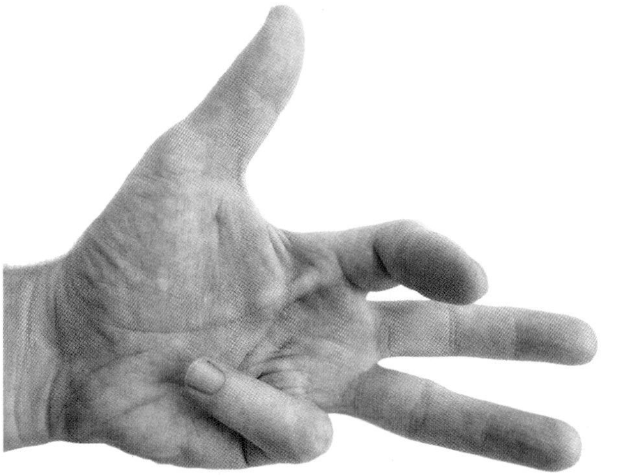

Figure 39-9 Contractures can occur when a joint is not exercised regularly. Use of the joint can be permanently lost. (Source: shutterstock.com/sokolenok)

Urinary Calculi

Clients with spinal cord injury are at risk for forming calculi (stones) in the kidneys or bladder at a higher rate than the general population. Following injury, hypercalciuria is two to four times that of persons without spinal cord injury who undergo prolonged bed rest (Weiss, 2015). The etiology of stone formation is discussed in Chapters 58 and 59. It is assumed that renal crystallization is associated with reabsorption of calcium by the kidneys, urinary retention, and immobility. Renal calculi can develop both soon after the injury and years later.

Sexual Dysfunction

Sexuality is affected differently in men and women who sustain spinal cord injuries. In most men whose S2 to S4 spinal nerves are undamaged, involuntary *reflex erections* may occur as a result of touching the penis or stimulating other erotically sensitive areas of the body such as the nipples, ears, or neck. *Psychogenic erections* occur depending on the level and extent of spinal cord injury when men experience an arousing thought, triggering nerve-stimulating impulses from the brain to the nerves of the spinal cord at the T10 to L2 levels. Drugs for erectile dysfunction such as tadalafil (Cialis) and others may help promote a reflex erection. Other alternatives for treatment of sexual dysfunction include penile injection therapy, application of a vacuum pump, or penile implant (see Chapter 55). Achieving an erection facilitates intercourse, but it may not ensure fertility. Men often have impaired ejaculation with decreased motility of sperm, reducing their ability to biologically father a child. Alternative fertility measures may facilitate pregnancy.

Women with spinal cord injuries can conceive and bear children. However, they experience decreased vaginal lubrication, impaired clitoral and vaginal sensations, and an inability to contract the pubococcygeal muscles of the pelvic floor. Although using a vibrator may help women with an injury below the T6 level achieve an orgasm, it may be unperceived or feel different than it did before the injury.

Pain

Eighty percent of clients with spinal cord injuries experience pain. Three types reported by clients are neuropathic, nociceptive (visceral), and musculoskeletal (Pain After Spinal Cord Injury, 2020) (see Chapter 11). Neuropathic pain is caused by an abnormal communication between spinal nerves and the brain. It is described with words such as sharp, shooting, burning, stinging, tearing, bursting, and stabbing. Some experience *allodynia*, pain from a stimulus that does not normally cause pain, and *hyperalgesia*, an increased response to a stimulus that is normally a little painful.

Neuropathic pain is long lasting and difficult to treat. Symptomatic pharmacotherapy is the mainstay of treatment. Currently, pain relief involves medications such as opioid and nonopioid analgesics, antidepressants such as duloxetine (Cymbalta) that are known to relieve pain, anticonvulsants such as pregabalin (Lyrica), muscle relaxants such as baclofen (Lioresal), antispasmodics such as tizanidine (Zanaflex), and topical lidocaine patch (Lidoderm). The results range from partially and transiently effective to totally ineffective, which has led to research for more efficacious treatment. One approach involves drugs that will target the glutamate release pathway (Nesic, n.d.) and another proposes a single spinal injection of fibronectin, a naturally produced glycoprotein that binds collagen, fibrin, and other proteins to cell membranes (Fibronectin, 2020). Drug therapy may be combined with psychologic treatments such as relaxation techniques, biofeedback, self-hypnosis, cognitive restructuring, and individual psychotherapy.

Assessment Findings

The degree and location of the spinal cord injury determines the immediate symptoms. There is pain in the affected area, difficulty breathing, numbness, and paralysis. If the injury is high in the cervical region, respiratory failure and death occur because the diaphragm is paralyzed. If the cord is completely severed, permanent loss of function below the level of the injury occurs. If damage to the cord is minimal, some function is maintained.

A neurologic examination reveals the level of spinal cord injury. Radiography, myelography, MRI, and CT scan show evidence of fracture or compression of one or more vertebrae, edema, or a hematoma.

Medical and Surgical Management

Initial Treatment

Initially, the head and back are immobilized mechanically with a cervical collar and back support. An IV line is inserted to provide access to a vein if shock develops. Vital signs are stabilized. Corticosteroids are given to reduce spinal cord edema, thereby decreasing potential damage to injured nerves. Riluzole (Rilutek), a neuroprotective drug that blocks the neurotoxic effects of glutamate, may be administered. Cethrin, a drug that promotes neuronal growth, has been granted "fast-tract" status by the U.S. Food and Drug Administration (FDA). It has shown evidence of promoting increased motor and neurologic recovery after acute spinal cord injury.

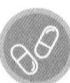

Pharmacologic Considerations

- Many agents are considered neuroprotective. These drugs range from tissue plasminogen activator (tPA) used during a stroke to riluzole (Rilutek) that protects nerves from glutamate buildup that hampers neural messages. For spinal cord injury and diseases such as amyotrophic lateral sclerosis (ALS), these agents maintain but do not increase function.

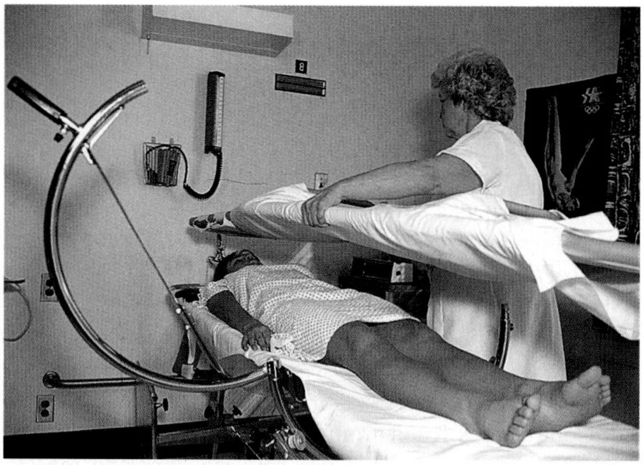

Figure 39-10 The nurse frequently turns a client on a mechanical turning frame to relieve pressure.

After the client is stabilized, the injured portion of the spine is further immobilized using a cast or brace or surgical intervention. Traction with weights and pulleys is applied to provide correct vertebral alignment and to increase the space between the vertebrae. Additional weight is added over the next few days to increase the space between the vertebrae and move them into correct alignment. A turning frame is used to change the client's position without altering the alignment of the spine (Fig. 39-10).

Depending on the extent of the injury, surgery may be necessary to remove bone fragments, repair dislocated vertebrae, and stabilize the spine. The vertebrae are fused with bone obtained from the iliac crest or stabilized with a steel rod. External immobilization with a brace or cast often is necessary.

Long-Term Management

After the initial period of therapeutic care, the focus of treatment turns to rehabilitative and restorative measures.

Functional Electrical Stimulation

While the client is undergoing physical and occupational therapy, **functional electrical stimulation** (FES) may be used to activate paralyzed muscles and prevent muscle atrophy. FES is used in a variety of ways. Surface or implanted electrodes attached to the quadriceps, hamstring, and gluteal muscles help paralyzed legs pedal a stationary bicycle, stand, or walk (Fig. 39-11). Electrodes attached to the forearm and flexors and extensors of the hand help the hand open and close to allow grasping of objects, reduce stiffness, maintain or increase range of motion, and increase circulation. FES is also being used to restore bladder continence by stimulating the sacral nerves, causing contraction of the detrusor muscle necessary for bladder emptying. In addition, FES improves breathing; when the electrodes are implanted in respiratory muscles, they reduce the need for mechanical ventilation.

Treadmill Training

Treadmill training, which is also known as weight-supported ambulation, is suitable only for those clients with an

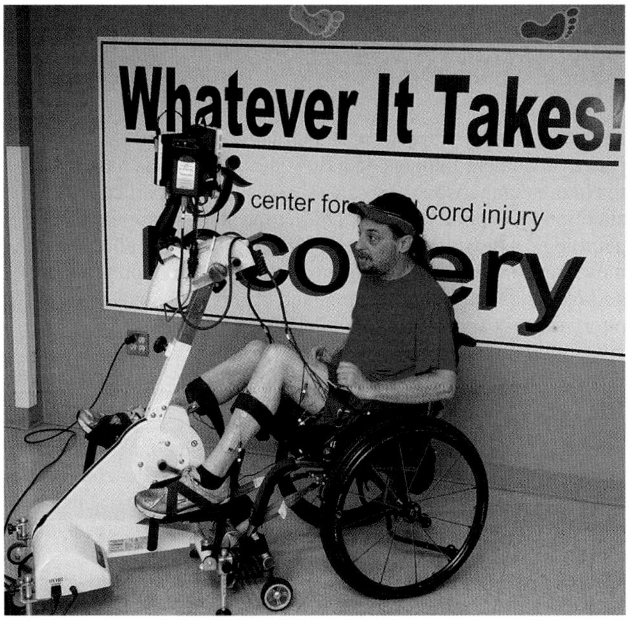

Figure 39-11 Functional electrical stimulation (FES) facilitates the movement of paralyzed muscles to pedal a modified bicycle. (Used with permission from Rehabilitation Institute of Michigan's Center for Spinal Cord Injury Recovery.)

incomplete spinal cord injury (i.e., some remaining connections between the spinal cord and brain). Treadmill training increases the function within the remaining connections. The client is suspended in a harness above the treadmill, and therapists move the person's legs in a walking fashion (Fig. 39-12).

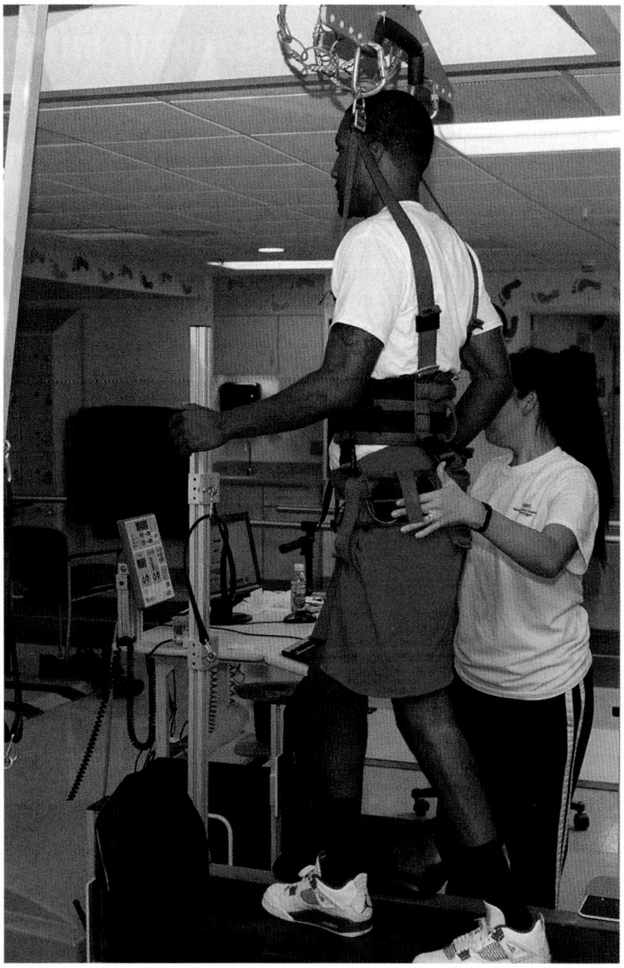

Figure 39-12 Walking is simulated by supporting body weight in a harness above a treadmill. (Used with permission from Rehabilitation Institute of Michigan's Center for Spinal Cord Injury Recovery.)

Tendon Transfer Surgery

Clients with injuries from vertebrae C5 through T1 have weak or nonfunctioning wrists and hands and may benefit from tendon transfer surgery. Tendon transfer is a surgical procedure that repositions tendons from a working muscle to a paralyzed one. The goal of the surgery is to restore a pinching motion with the thumb and flexion of the wrist. The presurgical preparation and postsurgical rehabilitation are both demanding for clients; strengthening and range-of-motion exercises and physical therapy are required.

Cell Transplantation

Nerve cells in the central nervous system, which includes the spinal cord, lose the ability to regenerate when injured. Consequently, there is a focus on finding cells that, when transplanted, can replace the nerve cells that have been damaged. Stem cells are *pluripotent*, that is, they can differentiate into a variety of cell types, including spinal nerves (see Chapter 18). However, use of embryonic stem cells is currently politically and ethically controversial. Autologous stem cells from bone marrow have been collected from clients and reimplanted in the area surrounding the injured spinal cord with promising results. (Other researchers are investigating the therapeutic effectiveness of using host stem-like Schwann cells and olfactory ensheathing cells harvested from the mucosa of nasal tissue for promoting nerve regeneration and growth of axons and restoring function when implanted into the injured spinal cord.)

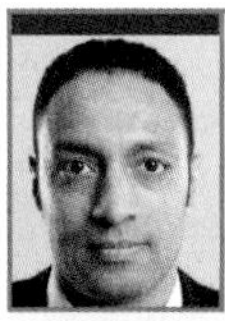

Clinical Scenario While riding a motorcycle, a 37-year-old client loses control on loose gravel and is thrown to the ground. They were wearing a helmet, but is unable to move their extremities. They call for help, and a nearby resident summons an ambulance. Upon arrival at the ED, the client is conscious and alert, but they tell the nurse that they cannot move or feel their arms or legs. **What nursing care is appropriate for managing this client's care? See the following Nursing Process section.**

NURSING PROCESS FOR THE INITIAL CARE OF THE CLIENT WITH SPINAL TRAUMA

The nurse provides immediate supportive care after the spinal cord injury and plans or administers rehabilitative measures to prevent long-term complications.

Assessment

On the client's arrival in the ED, obtain information about the injury and treatment given at the scene from family, witnesses, or those who transported the client to the hospital. After gathering such facts, perform a neurologic assessment, taking care to document findings on a flow sheet to provide a database for future comparison. Assess vital signs, paying particular attention to respiratory status. During the acute phase, repeat neurologic assessments frequently. Determine if the client has movement and sensation below the level of injury, look to see if neurologic damage is worsening, and observe for signs of respiratory distress and spinal shock.

Analysis, Planning, and Interventions

Keep the client's body and head aligned and limit all movement. If directed by the primary provider, insert a urinary retention catheter. Assist with immobilization of the injured spine (Fig. 39-13). Burr holes in the skull are required for inserting the pointed ends of traction tongs or the halo-vest traction apparatus. When applying traction, check that the weights hang free. Instruct others on the nursing team never to lift or remove the weights or increase or decrease the amount of prescribed weight. The use of external stabilizing devices such as the halo-vest facilitates early discharge from the acute care facility. Teach the client in a halo-vest measures to ensure their safety and prevent complications (Client and Family Teaching 39-2).

Besides monitoring for and intervening in cases of spinal shock and autonomic dysreflexia, the nurse's role may include the following:

Altered Breathing Pattern, Ineffective Airway Clearance, and Impaired Gas Exchange: Related to paralysis of respiratory, chest, and abdominal muscles

Expected Outcomes: (1) Client will breathe independently at a rate of 16 to 20 breaths/min. (2) The airway will be free of secretions. (3) The client's blood SpO_2 will be 90% or higher.

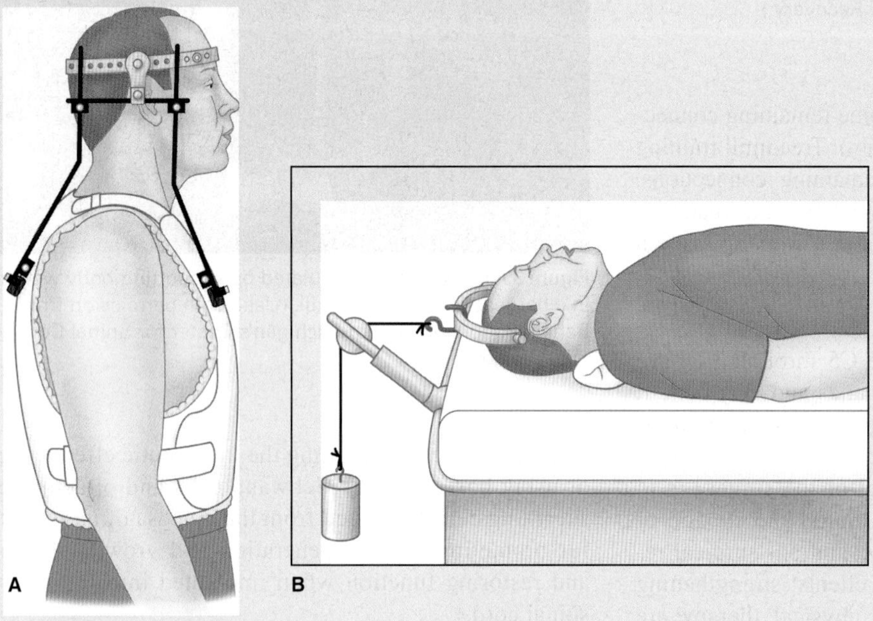

Figure 39-13 Cervical spine injuries are managed with immediate immobilization, early reduction, and stabilization of the vertebral column. Cervical traction with either **(A)** a halo-vest device or **(B)** cervical tongs accomplishes these goals.

- Maintain a patent airway. *A patent airway maximizes passage of air in and out of the lungs.*
- Be prepared for endotracheal intubation and mechanical ventilation if respiratory failure occurs. *An endotracheal tube provides an airway from the nose or mouth to an area above the mainstem bronchi. Mechanical ventilation provides a means to regulate respiratory rate, volume of air, and percentage of oxygen when a client cannot breathe independently.*
- Suction the airway to remove secretions. *A client with spinal trauma may not be able to cough effectively. An artificial airway increases the production of respiratory secretions. Suctioning helps ensure adequate ventilation and reduces the potential for pneumonia.*
- Administer oxygen as prescribed. *To prevent hypoxemia, the client may require more oxygen than available in room air.*
- Help the client use a spirometer as prescribed if the client is ventilator free. *This helps prevent atelectasis and pneumonia.*
- Encourage obtaining a pneumococcal pneumonia and yearly influenza immunization. *Prophylaxis of common community-acquired respiratory infections reduces the potential for pulmonary complications.*

Related complication of Neuropathic Pain: Related to irritated nerve root and soft tissue injury

Expected Outcome: The nurse will monitor to detect, manage, and minimize neuropathic pain.

- Administer analgesia by the prescribed route. *Pain management is a standard of care. An IV administration of an analgesic avoids administration of injections into tissues where absorption is compromised.*
- Assist the primary provider with nerve block procedures if analgesia is ineffective. *A nerve block is a form of regional anesthesia in which an anesthetic agent is injected close to the nerve that is transmitting pain impulses.*

NURSING PROCESS FOR THE INITIAL CARE OF THE CLIENT WITH SPINAL TRAUMA (continued)

Fall Risk and ADL deficit: Related to loss of motor function
Expected Outcomes: (1) Client's ability to be mobile will be maintained. (2) Client will use assistive devices to move and perform ADLs. (3) Client will not experience complications associated with inactivity and immobility.

- Position client to avoid joint contractures and foot drop. *Mobility depends on preventing permanent changes to the musculoskeletal system. Inactivity causes joints to assume a position of flexion.*
- Help client perform exercises identified by the physical therapist. *Active and passive exercises maintain joint flexibility and reduce muscle atrophy and atony. For exercises to be effective, clients must perform them several times a day.*
- Apply leg braces when ambulation is possible. *Braces support joints, allowing the client to ambulate independently or with a walker or crutches.*
- Maintain skin integrity and prevent pressure ulcers by changing client's position at least every 2 hours, using pressure-relieving devices, massaging bony prominences, using a mechanical lift for bed-to-chair transfers, and keeping skin clean and dry. *Position changes and pressure-relieving devices ensure that capillary pressure stays above 32 mm Hg, thus providing oxygenated blood to cells for their continued survival. Massage increases blood flow to temporarily deprived areas. Using a mechanical lift prevents injuries to the client as well as the nurse. Keeping skin clean and dry prevents maceration and decreases the potential for bacterial growth.*
- Facilitate urine elimination. Teach the client to perform intermittent catheterization every 3 to 4 hours if capable. If a leg bag is used, attach the catheter to the bag and empty and clean the device regularly. *Urinary retention and stasis may contribute to autonomic dysreflexia and formation of renal calculi.*
- Keep the bowel evacuated. If necessary, manually remove stool. *Infrequent bowel evacuation leads to constipation and impaction. A high-fiber diet and a bowel program using a suppository or enema every 3 days approximately 30 minutes after a meal normalize bowel movements.*
- Keep client hydrated. *Adequate hydration reduces potential for formation of thrombi and renal calculi.*
- Provide oral or enteral nutrition. *A well-balanced diet provides nutrients and elements necessary for energy and to sustain cellular growth and repair* (Nutrition Notes 39-1).

Acute Anxiety and Coping Impairment: Related to prognosis of neurologic deficits
Expected Outcomes: (1) Anxiety will be relieved. (2) Client will cope effectively with stressors.

- Discuss information about prognosis with the primary provider. *Communication facilitates mutual understanding of client's potential for recovery and rehabilitation.*
- Tell client and family that determining the severity of deficits immediately after a spinal cord injury is difficult. Explain that the outcome varies depending on the specific injury and client's response to rehabilitation. *Until the initial trauma and swelling have resolved, any assumptions about the client's outcome are premature. Successful rehabilitation depends on the level of the cord injury, development of complications, client's motivation and perseverance, and intervention of the health care team.*
- Be a good listener and offer encouragement as the client makes progress. *Such encouragement can contribute to the client's resolve to put forth continued effort.*

Evaluation of Expected Outcomes

Breathing is adequate to maintain oxygenation. Pain is relieved or reduced to a tolerable level. The client regains mobility using minimal assistive devices. Complications from inactivity are prevented or reduced. The client's level of anxiety is mild, and they begin to cope with the effects of the injury and the challenge of rehabilitation. The client and family demonstrate understanding of postdischarge home care.

Client and Family Teaching 39-2
Halo-Vest Management

The nurse teaches the client as follows:

- Turn your whole body rather than trying to turn your head; you will not be able to look down.
- Do not drive a car.
- Walk only on level surfaces until you become accustomed to the vest; avoid stairs, curbs, and uneven terrain unless assistance is available.
- Take care getting in and out of vehicles to avoid bumping the halo and loosening the pins.
- Use a mirror to inspect the pin sites and as a guide while cleaning them.
- Clean the pin sites two to three times a day with cotton-tipped applicators saturated with hydrogen peroxide; remove loose crusts.
- Use a clean applicator after making a full circle around the pin site.
- Clip the hair that grows around the pin sites.
- Report pain, redness, drainage from pin sites, fever, or neck tingling or pain to the primary provider.
- Never independently adjust the vest if it becomes tight or loose; consult the primary provider.
- Pad the vest if it causes pressure or friction.
- Take sponge baths to maintain hygiene; seek assistance for areas you cannot reach such as around the anus.
- Use a dry shampoo or consult primary provider on how to shampoo hair without wetting the vest.
- Use pillows for support and comfort when sleeping.
- Wear loose-fitting clothing with wide necklines for ease in dressing.
- Wear shoes with flat heels that are easy to slip on and off.

Nutrition Notes 39-1

The Client With a Spinal Cord Injury

- Clients have varying nutritional needs, depending on the nerves injured and the resulting complications.
- Tetraplegic and paraplegic clients have lower caloric requirements because their energy expenditure is reduced, and their caloric intake should be adjusted to avoid excessive weight gain. Nutrient needs, however, are stable or higher, depending on the complications. For example, prolonged immobility promotes nitrogen excretion, causing an increased protein requirement.
- Clients with skin breakdown have increased requirements for protein (meat, milk, supplements), vitamin C (citrus fruit and juices, strawberries, "greens," tomatoes), and zinc (meat, seafood, milk, egg yolks, legumes, whole grains), which are needed to promote healing.
- Extended immobility accelerates calcium loss from bone, leading to hypercalcemia and hypercalciuria. A high-fluid intake (up to 3 L/day) helps dilute urine, thus preventing the precipitation of calcium renal stones.

»> *Stop, Think, and Respond 39-2*

When providing hygiene to the client with a spinal cord injury, a red area that does not blanch is noted at the base of the coccyx. What actions are appropriate?

SPINAL NERVE ROOT COMPRESSION

There are two basic types of spinal nerve root compression: **intramedullary lesions** that involve the spinal cord and **extramedullary lesions** that involve the tissues surrounding the spinal cord. The most common site of nerve root compression is at the level of the three lower lumbar disks; however, nerve root compression also occurs in the cervical spine.

Pathophysiology and Etiology

Pressure on spinal nerve roots results from trauma, herniated (ruptured) intervertebral disks, and tumors of the spinal cord and surrounding structures (Fig. 39-14). Stress caused by poor body mechanics, age, or disease weakens an area in the vertebra, causing the spongy center of the vertebrae, the *nucleus pulposus*, to swell and herniate. This condition is commonly called a *slipped disk*; the displacement puts pressure on the nearby nerves.

Pain along the distribution of the nerve root is common. Actions that increase pressure intensify the pain. Weakness and changes in sensation occur. The symptoms intensify with increasing nerve root compression.

Assessment Findings

Symptoms vary depending on the cause of compression and level involved. They usually include weakness, paralysis, pain, and **paresthesia** (numbness, tingling). When a herniated disk in the lumbar region compresses the sciatic nerve, the client describes feeling pain down the buttocks and into the posterior thigh and leg. Physical examination reveals weakness or paralysis of the extremity innervated by the compressed nerve. If a nerve in the lumbar or sacral area is affected, the client experiences pain when lying supine and lifting the leg without bending the knee. The pain increases when straining, coughing, or lifting a heavy object. Walking and sitting become difficult. Spinal radiography, CT, MRI, myelography, and electromyography (EMG) show displacement or herniation of an intervertebral disk, tumor, or bleeding around the nerve root.

Medical Management

When a client has a herniated intervertebral disk, conservative therapy is tried first. Metastatic spinal cord tumors also are treated conservatively because removal is not feasible.

A herniated cervical disk is treated by immobilizing the cervical spine with a cervical collar or brace. Later, as inflammation subsides, the client wears the collar or brace intermittently when walking or sitting. Bed rest with a firm mattress and bed board is used for clients with a lumbar herniated disk.

Skin traction, which can be applied in the home, is used to decrease severe muscle spasm as well as increase the distance between adjacent vertebrae, keep the vertebrae

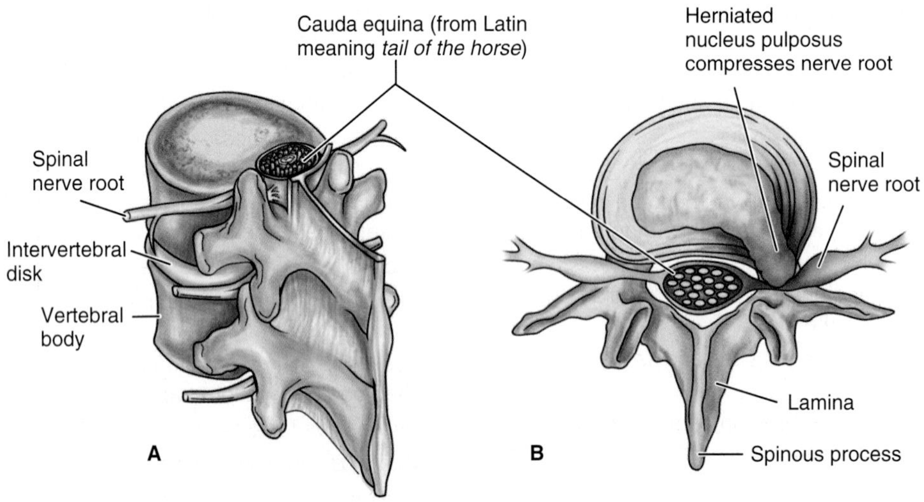

Figure 39-14 **(A)** Normal lumbar spine vertebrae, intervertebral disks, and spinal nerve root. **(B)** Ruptured vertebral disk.

correctly aligned, and, in many instances, relieve pain. Treatment relieves symptoms for an extended period.

Hot, moist packs are used to treat muscle spasm. Skeletal muscle relaxants, such as carisoprodol (Rela) and chlorzoxazone (Paraflex), help clients with a herniated intervertebral disk. Diazepam (Valium), a tranquilizer, is used for its twofold effect: to reduce anxiety associated with the pain of a herniated disk and to relax the skeletal muscle. Drugs such as aspirin and other nonsteroidal anti-inflammatory drugs (NSAIDs), phenylbutazone (Butazolidin), and corticosteroids are used to treat inflammation. Reducing inflammation and muscle spasm helps ease pain, but additional analgesics are given to control pain. Clients with an inoperable spinal cord tumor are given analgesics to maintain comfort.

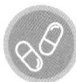

Pharmacologic Considerations

■ Clients taking a skeletal muscle relaxant or a sedative will experience drowsiness and dizziness. They may also experience relief of symptoms and decide to resume activities requiring mental alertness, yet lack judgment based on the drug effects. Caution clients regarding activities such as driving or operating equipment.

Surgical Management

If conservative therapy fails to relieve symptoms of a herniated disk with spinal nerve root compression, surgery is considered. Procedures for relieving spinal nerve root compression include the following:

- **Diskectomy**: removal of the ruptured disk
- **Laminectomy**: removal of the posterior arch of a vertebra to expose the spinal cord. The surgeon can remove whatever lesion is causing compression: a herniated disk, tumor, blood clot, bone spur, or broken bone fragment.
- **Diskectomy with spinal fusion**: removal of the ruptured disk followed by grafting a piece of bone taken from another area, such as the iliac crest, onto the vertebra to fuse the vertebral spinous process. Bone may also be obtained from a bone bank.
- **Chemonucleolysis**: injection of the enzyme chymopapain into the nucleus pulposus to shrink or dissolve the disk, which then relieves pressure on spinal nerve roots

Spinal fusion stabilizes the vertebrae weakened by degenerative joint changes, such as osteoarthritis, and by laminectomy. It results in a firm union; the client loses mobility and must become accustomed to a permanent area of stiffness. When a portion of the lumbar spine is fused, the client usually does not feel the stiffness after a short time because motion increases in the joints above the fusion. Motion is more limited when the area of fusion is in the cervical spine. Spinal fusion is also performed for spinal cord tumors, fractures and dislocations of the spine, and Pott disease (tuberculosis of the spine).

Nursing Management

The nurse performs a neurologic examination and notes any limitation of motion and the type of movement that

BOX 39-2 Maintaining Traction

For proper application and use of traction:

- The prescribed amount of weight must be used.
- Traction weights must hang above the floor.
- Ropes must move freely through the pulley grooves.
- The client's position must be in line with the pull of the traction apparatus.

NURSING GUIDELINES 39-2

Nursing Care After Specific Spinal Surgeries

Postcervical Diskectomy

- Keep a cervical collar in place at all times; do not remove without a primary provider's order.
- Instruct client to keep the neck straight in midline position until healing occurs.
- Support client's head, neck, and upper shoulders when moving from a lying to sitting to standing position or when getting into and out of a chair.
- Observe for Horner syndrome, a complication following anterior cervical diskectomy from cervical sympathetic nerve damage. Manifestations are lid ptosis (drooping), constricted pupil, regression of eye in the orbit, and lack of perspiration on one side of the face.

Postlumbar Laminectomy or Diskectomy With Spinal Fusion

- Logroll when turning client every 2 hours; maintain alignment at all times.
- Caution client to avoid turning self.
- Teach client to avoid twisting or jerking the back, sitting during the first week and prolonged sitting thereafter (client should use a straight-backed chair and not slump), and bending from the waist (client should bend from the knees and hips).

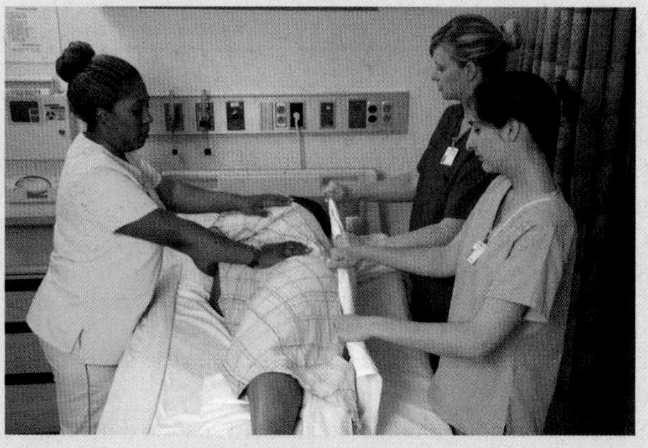

Roll client in a coordinated movement.

causes pain. Nursing Guidelines 39-2 outlines nursing responsibilities unique to various types of spinal surgery. For clients being treated conservatively, the nurse uses a firm mattress or applies a bed board because a firm surface supports the spine and promotes alignment. The nurse maintains the client on bed rest, placing them in semi-Fowler's position, with the knees and head slightly elevated to relieve lumbosacral pain. The nurse applies halo-vest traction. For intermittent pelvic or cervical skin traction, they attach the skin device to the client, supports the weights, and lowers them gently to avoid a sudden and strong pull (Box 39-2). The nurse reminds the client to roll from side to side without twisting the spine. When the client gets out of bed, the nurse reinforces the use of proper body mechanics. They advise clients with cervical nerve root compression to avoid extreme hyperextension of the neck and side-to-side rotation of the head. The nurse administers the prescribed muscle relaxants and analgesics. They apply moist heat for no longer than 20 minutes but repeats several times a day.

The nurse periodically evaluates the client's response to conservative therapy. It is important to note the activities and positions that increase pain and the gain or loss in motion or sensation since the previous observation. Comparison of current symptoms with those first exhibited provides an evaluation of response to therapy. It is important to note a change in symptoms when the client is removed from traction.

Nursing interventions after spinal surgery are as follows:

- Monitor vital signs.
- Assist client to perform hourly deep-breathing exercises while awake but avoid forced coughing because it increases pressure within the spinal canal.
- Examine the dressing for CSF leakage or bleeding.
- Assess neurovascular status (color, temperature, mobility, and sensation) in extremities below the area of surgery, which may result from edema or hemorrhage at the operative site.
- Report an inability to void or an output of less than 240 mL in 8 hours.
- Use a fracture bed pan.

KEY POINTS

- Concussion: is a result from a blow to the head that jars the brain.
  - Contusion: more serious than a concussion and leads to gross structural injury to the brain
  - Cerebral hematoma: bleeding within the skull
  - Skull fracture: a break in the continuity of the cranium
- Explain the cause and effects of CTE.
  - Epidural: Arterial blood collects between the skull and dura.
  - Subdural: Venous blood collects between the dura and subarachnoid layers.
  - Intracerebral hematomas: Blood collects within the brain.
- Skull fractures:
  - Open head injury: the scalp, bony cranium, and dura mater (the outer meningeal layer) are exposed.
  - Closed head injury: an intact layer of scalp covers the fractured skull.
- Spinal cord injuries:
  - Spinal cord trauma is serious and sometimes fatal. The cervical and lumbar vertebrae are the most common sites of injury
  - Spinal shock: a loss of sympathetic reflex activity below the level of injury within 30 to 60 minutes of a spinal injury.
  - Autonomic dysreflexia: an exaggerated sympathetic nervous system response in people with spinal cord injuries above T6
- Spinal nerve root compression:
  - Intramedullary lesions: that involve the spinal cord
  - Extramedullary lesions: that involve the tissues surrounding the spinal cord

CRITICAL THINKING EXERCISES

1. A client involved in a motor vehicle accident is brought to the ED. You are told that they were not wearing a seat belt and struck their head on the steering wheel. What neurologic assessments would you make? Why?
2. You are caring for a paraplegic client. What signs and symptoms suggest that the client is experiencing autonomic dysreflexia? What nursing measures are appropriate?
3. The family of a tetraplegic client in an extended care facility wants to assume home care of the client whose condition is stable. What recommendations would be appropriate at this time?
4. What health teaching is essential to provide a client who is recovering from back spasms associated with a herniated (ruptured) vertebral disk?

NCLEX-STYLE REVIEW QUESTIONS PrepU

1. When a nursing assessment of a 58-year-old client indicates that the client has symptoms of dementia, what information in the client's medical history suggests a potential etiology?
   1. The client has a brother who is schizophrenic.
   2. The client's mother drank alcohol when pregnant.
   3. The client played football while in college.
   4. The client had a recent motor vehicle accident.
2. A nurse on a medical flight crew is assessing an alert but lethargic client with a possible closed head injury. To what data is the nurse correct in giving priority attention as it relates to the client's neurologic status?
   1. Temperature and blood pressure
   2. Respiratory rate and breathing effort
   3. LOC and pupillary responses
   4. Peripheral vision and cranial nerve function

3. The nurse obtains a history from the wife of a client who has just arrived in the ED. What statement characterizes the progression of disease symptoms associated with an epidural hematoma?
1. "My husband had a headache all day. He rested in bed with the lights out."
2. "I noticed that he was confused and then collapsed in the kitchen. It happened so fast."
3. "I have noticed that he has become increasingly more forgetful over the past week."
4. "His coordination was poor this morning, but he still drove to the hospital."

4. What is the most important reason for the nurse to monitor a client's body temperature closely after intracranial surgery?
1. Hyperthermia increases the risk for paralysis.
2. Hyperthermia increases the risk for cerebral edema.
3. Hyperthermia increases the risk for immobility.
4. Hyperthermia increases the risk for brain damage.

5. In developing the plan of care, what is the priority for the nursing management of a client with a spinal cord injury at the lumbar level of the spine?
1. Total paralysis from the neck down
2. Symptoms of autonomic dysreflexia
3. Assistance needed with ambulation
4. Assistance needed with feeding

WANT TO KNOW MORE? There are a wide variety of online resources available on thePoint to enhance learning and understanding of this chapter.

Go to thePoint.lww.com/activate and use the activation code found in the front of this text to unlock these online resources.

40 Caring for Clients With Neurologic Deficits

Words To Know

Credé maneuver
cutaneous triggering
dysarthria
expressive aphasia
neurologic deficit
receptive aphasia
reflex incontinence

Learning Objectives

On completion of this chapter, you will be able to:

1. Define neurologic deficit.
2. Describe the three phases of a neurologic deficit.
3. Give the primary aims of medical treatment of a neurologic deficit.
4. Name six members of the health care team involved with the management of a client with a neurologic deficit.
5. Describe nursing management of a client with a neurologic deficit.

This chapter discusses the management of a client with a **neurologic deficit**, a condition in which one or more functions of the central and peripheral nervous systems are decreased, impaired, or absent. Examples include paralysis, muscle weakness, impaired speech, inability to recognize objects, abnormal gait or difficulty walking, impaired memory, impaired swallowing, or abnormal bowel and bladder elimination. The client with a neurologic deficit faces many problems. Often, the deficit affects more than one body system. The client may be unable to walk, talk, perform simple tasks such as feeding and bathing, or recognize family members.

Many members of the health care team are involved in the complex management of the client with a temporary or permanent neurologic deficit: the primary provider, nurse, nursing assistant, social worker, physical therapist, occupational therapist, speech therapist, prosthetist, psychotherapist, dietitian, pharmacist, and vocational counselor. With intensive therapy and a coordinated approach by all team members, many clients have the potential to regain normal or near-normal function or successful adaptation to functional changes.

PHASES OF A NEUROLOGIC DEFICIT

Neurologic deficits are divided into three phases: acute, recovery, and chronic. Not all clients with a neurologic deficit experience all three phases. Some clients have deficits that begin with an acute phase and move into a recovery phase or into a lifelong chronic phase.

Acute Phase

The acute phase follows a sudden neurologic event, such as a cerebrovascular accident (CVA) or a head or spinal cord injury. During the acute phase, the client is usually critically ill, with many signs and symptoms, such as altered level of consciousness (LOC), hypertension or hypotension, fever, difficulty breathing, or paralysis.

Gerontologic Considerations

- The slower response to stimuli that may accompany aging can lead to increased frustration, irritability, or depression. Teach caregivers and clients to allow extra time, if needed, to formulate answers to questions or perform activities. Encourage caregivers to use the family or community resources to prevent exhaustion.
- Older adults with a neurologic deficit may lack an adequate support system once they are discharged from the hospital. Involve social service and other agencies to assist these clients and their caregivers with rehabilitation and to prevent social isolation. For example, older adults without family may connect with others through past church or community involvement to schedule a brief phone conversation each morning or evening, or to obtain transportation to events of interest.
- A behavioral or cognitive change such as irritability may be the only sign of urinary retention in older adults with a neurologic deficit.
- Functional problems and diminished muscular strength that accompany aging may complicate recovery for a client with a neurologic deficit. For example, an age-related delay in the relaxation of the internal bladder sphincter can make bladder training more difficult.

Medical and Surgical Management

The focus of management during the acute phase is to stabilize the client and prevent further neurologic damage. The client with a CVA may require management of hypertension or hypotension through drug therapy. The client with a head or spinal cord injury may require respiratory support through mechanical ventilation or surgical intervention to stabilize the injured area or remove bone fragments, blood clots, or foreign objects. Sometimes, surgery is postponed until the client is stabilized and the acute phase has passed. In other instances, surgery is performed during the acute phase as a lifesaving measure.

Nursing Management

The nurse performs frequent and thorough neurologic assessments to evaluate the client's status, to check the need for additional medical or surgical interventions, and response to treatment. They use the Glasgow Coma Scale (see Chapter 36) or other neurologic assessment tools such as the Mini-Mental Status Examination (see Chapter 67). When significant changes occur, the nurse immediately reports them to the primary provider. The nurse assesses vital signs as often as necessary and maintains the blood pressure (BP) to ensure adequate cerebral oxygenation. They measure intake and output and observe for signs of electrolyte imbalances and dehydration. The nurse reports a urinary output of less than 500 mL/day or urinary or bowel incontinence.

Beginning basic rehabilitation during the acute phase is an important nursing function. Measures such as position changes and prevention of skin breakdown and contractures are essential aspects of care during the early phase of rehabilitation. The nursing goal is to prevent complications that may interfere with the client's potential to recover function. (For additional nursing management, see the Nursing Process section.)

Recovery Phase

The recovery phase begins when the client's condition is stabilized. It starts several days or weeks after the initial event and lasts weeks or months.

Medical and Surgical Management

Medical management during the recovery phase aims at keeping the client stable and preventing or treating complications, such as pneumonia, and further neurologic impairment.

Nursing Management

During recovery, the nurse works with team members to plan a rehabilitation program in several domains according to the client's abilities and limitations (Table 40-1). Various assessment tools can help identify a client's level of functioning and potential for improvement with a rehabilitation program, including

- The National Institutes of Health Stroke Scale (http://www.ninds.nih.gov/doctors/NIH_Stroke_Scale.pdf)
- The American Heart Association Stroke Outcome Classification (https://www.ahajournals.org/doi/full/10.1161/01.str.29.6.1274)
- The Barthel Index (Table 40-2)

Rehabilitation is designed to meet the client's immediate and long-term needs. Environmental changes may be necessary to help the client adapt to the disability and fully regain any remaining functions. Even though deficits can be temporary, a prolonged period and enrollment in a rehabilitation program are often necessary before recovery of partial or full function can occur. A successful rehabilitation program includes not only nurses and primary providers but also several other providers, such as physical therapists, occupational

TABLE 40-1 Domains of Neurologic Impairment

DOMAIN	DESCRIPTION
Motor	A single deficit or combination of deficits involving the face, arms, and legs, which affects speech, swallowing, muscle tone and strength, gait, coordination, and ability to use objects for their intended purpose
Sensory	Altered sensation (e.g., numbness, tingling, exaggerated sensation) or altered perception (e.g., inability to identify objects by touch, loss of writing ability)
Vision	Loss of vision in one eye or in the temporal or nasal fields; blindness
Language	Disturbances in comprehension, naming, repeating, clarity of speech, reading
Cognition	Changes in memory, attention, orientation, calculation, and construction
Affect	Altered mood, lability of mood

TABLE 40-2 Modified Barthel Index (MBI)

ITEM	UNABLE TO PERFORM TASK	SUBSTANTIAL HELP REQUIRED	MODERATE HELP REQUIRED	MINIMAL HELP REQUIRED	FULLY INDEPENDENT
Personal hygiene	0	1	3	4	5
Bathing self	0	1	3	4	5
Feeding	0	2	5	8	10
Toilet	0	2	5	8	10
Stair climbing	0	2	5	8	10
Dressing	0	2	5	8	10
Bowel control	0	2	5	8	10
Bladder control	0	2	5	8	10
Ambulation[a]	0	3	8	12	15
Wheelchair[a]	0	1	3	4	5
Chair/bed transfer	0	3	8	12	15

[a]Score only if client is unable to ambulate and is trained in wheelchair management.

DEPENDENCY NEEDS			
Categories	**MBI Total Scores**	**Dependency Level**	**Hours of Help Required per Week (Maximum)**
1	0–24	Total	27.0
2	25–49	Severe	23.5
3	50–74	Moderate	20.0
4	75–90	Mild	13.0
5	91–99	Minimal	<10.0

therapists, speech therapists, and enterostomal therapists, all of whom recommend devices or procedures to prevent complications and enhance the client's remaining abilities.

With continuous assessment and identification of the client's needs, the nurse plays an important role in rehabilitation. Devices that help a client walk, eat, groom, and perform other motor skills are recommended or devised to suit particular needs. Flotation pads for wheelchairs, walkers, padded ankle-foot boots to prevent foot drop, and range-of-motion (ROM) exercises are examples of the many appliances and procedures used in rehabilitation. (For additional nursing management, see the Nursing Process section.)

Chronic Phase

For some clients (e.g., those with amyotrophic lateral sclerosis [ALS], also known as Lou Gehrig disease, or Alzheimer disease), neurologic deficits result in a prolonged or lifelong chronic phase. In this phase, the client shows little or no improvement, remains stationary, or progressively worsens. Physical and psychologic rehabilitation continues in the chronic phase to prevent complications such as pressure ulcers and muscle contractures.

Medical and Surgical Management

Medical management continues throughout the chronic phase and uses a wide range of therapies and treatments, such as control of BP, physical therapy, dietary management, and treatment of complications related to disuse and immobility. In some cases, surgery is performed to correct deformities or problems that have developed. Examples include muscle and skin grafts to close a pressure ulcer, surgery to correct a contracture deformity, or removal of a kidney stone (a complication of prolonged immobility).

››› *Stop, Think, and Respond 40-1*

You have been caring for a client with a head injury who is being transferred to an extended care facility for rehabilitation. What information is important to include that will help nurses at the new facility plan the client's care?

Nursing Management

Clients in the chronic phase are often admitted to a hospital for treatment of complications. They are also transferred to a skilled nursing facility or long-term care facility when family members no longer can manage their care, or when the disease has progressively worsened so that skilled care is mandatory. Nursing management focuses on preventing physical and psychologic complications. Therapy in a rehabilitation center may include retraining in skills such as using the telephone, handling money, shopping, using public transportation, maintaining a household, and vocational training.

PSYCHOSOCIAL ISSUES AND HOME MANAGEMENT

Overview

It can be tremendously frightening to leave the inpatient setting, where the daily, intensive support of the health care team is readily available and return home with life-altering changes. The client and family need additional support to adapt to a new lifestyle. Although many clients recover sufficiently to assume responsibility for some aspects of their own care, others do not. The burden of care often falls on the spouse, who may have physical problems as well, or the adult children, who may not be available or willing to share this responsibility.

Financial resources are strained during a lengthy hospitalization and may continue after discharge. Adapting the home to accommodate a wheelchair or special bed can be costly. Wide doorways, ramps instead of stairs, and special fixtures in the bathroom for bathing and toileting are examples of changes that are often necessary. The client may have been the major wage earner. Some clients can enter training programs that allow them to find employment outside the home, whereas others can learn skills that enable them to be employed at home. Others, because of age or extreme physical disability, cannot be gainfully employed.

Nursing Management

The nurse listens and is alert to subtle hints about the client's and family's adaptation to the client's change in functional status. The nurse asks direct questions to identify problems and needs. They evaluate the client's ability to perform self-care, resume their role in the family, and call on a support system. The nurse takes appropriate steps to help the client and family attain and maintain a home life as near normal as possible. For example, the nurse assesses available facilities, the family support system, physical aids required (e.g., wheelchair, cane, walker), and the amount of assistance the client requires with activities of daily living. They encourage the family to help plan for the client's return home, to ask questions about care, and seek assistance from those agencies that can provide emotional, physical, and financial support.

Coping

The nurse addresses each client's status individually. They offer reassurance and emotional support and display empathetic understanding of the multiple problems that the client is facing. Many clients have difficulty coping with their disability. Crises such as being unable to move, having limited movement, being unable to attend to one's most basic needs, and having to totally depend on others for housing, clothing, mobility, and food generate strong emotional responses. Some clients eventually accept their disability, whereas others do not. The nurse provides encouragement and praise throughout rehabilitation and shows personal interest and pleasure in each accomplishment, no matter how small, to help clients accept what they cannot or never will be able to do.

The nurse gives clients time to talk about their problems, fears, and concerns. Once needs are identified, they encourage the client to set attainable goals, which may help maintain independence as long as possible. The nurse works with the client and family to develop solutions and possible alternatives. This helps the client and family meet each problem as it arises, understand the limitations, establish goals, and work toward a solution.

With rehabilitation comes the client's awareness of progress or lack thereof. At times, improvement is slow and barely noticeable. A client has often difficulty coping. Discouragement, depression, withdrawal, and anger are not unusual. The nurse suggests available support groups for those with neurologic deficits for emotional, physical, and social support.

Socialization

As soon as clients can respond to those around them, the nurse encourages socialization with others. However, communication difficulties may create barriers that some may interpret as a lack of intelligence. Clients with neurologic deficits may have any one or more of the following problems that affect communication: **expressive aphasia**, the inability to produce language, but may be able to write information; **receptive aphasia**, the inability to understand spoken or written language, but may retain the ability to understand very common words that are used most often; **dysarthria**, difficulty using the tongue, lips, palate, vocal cords, larynx, or breathing to produce speech. For interacting with clients with neurologic deficits, refer to Nursing Guidelines 40-1.

At first, socialization can be limited to health care team members and family. The nurse encourages the family to talk to the client, discuss current events, and motivate the client to respond.

Speech, occupational, and recreational therapies may be part of the rehabilitation program and require a team effort. In the beginning, speech and occupational therapies are designed to help strengthen muscles that are under voluntary control. Later, certain tasks are learned or relearned to help the client interact with others. Participation in these therapies increases socialization time and helps the client interact with others.

Family Processes

The nurse recognizes that the family faces many disruptions because of the permanent disability of a family member. Lifestyles are altered, financial resources are strained, conflicts arise, and people must accept new responsibilities. The nurse allows the family time to deal with and accept these changes. The nurse provides the family with opportunities to talk and openly express their anger, fears, guilt, and helplessness. Although no single perfect solution to any problem exists, the following suggestions may help the family adjust to present and future changes:

- Include the family in the client's rehabilitation.
- Give encouragement and praise when a family member is able to help with a part of home care or shows interest in becoming involved in the client's care.

NURSING GUIDELINES 40-1

Interacting With Clients With a Neurologic Deficit

Receptive Aphasia

Technique:

- Gain the person's attention
- Provide sensory aids such as glasses
- Limit environmental distractions, such as background noise or multiple people talking
- Use gestures, facial expressions, drawings, and pictures
- Speak in a normal tone of voice
- Use simple language on one topic at a time

Expressive Aphasia

Technique:

- Provide a list of words for the client's reference or use a communication board (refer to Chapter 7)
- Allow time for a response
- Guess the word the client has difficulty saying, and ask if it is correct
- Do not interrupt when the client speaks
- Admit that you do not understand
- Limit questions to "yes" or "no" answers

Dysarthria

Technique:

- Consult with a speech therapist
- Practice exercises recommended by speech therapist such as whistling; blowing bubbles, balls, or through straws
- Use a communication board or software
- Encourage changing the rate of speech
- Suggest pausing briefly between words
- Have the client write the word that is not understood
- Utilize prosthetics such as a dental retainer
- Enlist the aid of a speech generating device for creating a synthetic voice

- Explain the purpose of each segment of rehabilitation (e.g., ROM exercises, positioning).
- When the family expresses a desire to assume responsibility for certain procedures at home, teach each skill or task slowly and give the family time to practice under supervision.
- Prepare a list of public or private agencies that may assist with home care, transportation, and financial and emotional support.

Client and Family Teaching

The nurse develops a teaching plan for home care management that incorporates the therapies prescribed by the primary provider and other members of the team. The client and family have usually many questions. The nurse must begin teaching long before discharge so that the client and family have sufficient time to learn and understand home care management. The individualized teaching plan includes discussion of the topics presented in Client and Family Teaching 40-1.

Client and Family Teaching 40-1 Home Care for the Client With a Neurologic Deficit

The nurse addresses the following key areas and points when teaching the client and family.

Skin Care

- Know how to inspect and care for the skin. A pressure ulcer that is beginning to develop may not cause discomfort.
- Change position at least every 2 hours to relieve pressure on bony prominences.
- Contact a health care provider immediately if the skin is reddened and does not blanch upon a position change, warm, or disrupted.

Body Alignment

- Understand that good body alignment is important.
- Be able to demonstrate how to put joints through a full ROM. Perform ROM exercises several times per day or as ordered by the primary provider or physical therapist.
- Know how to use various devices, such as rolled blankets or pillows, to support or align areas of the body, such as the back, hips, and legs. Be able to explain the use of a footboard or other device to prevent foot drop.

Nutrition and Fluids

- Fluids should be consumed frequently. A high fluid intake is important to prevent urinary tract complications.
- A balanced diet is important in maintaining optimal health.
- It may be easier to tolerate small meals and between-meal snacks than three large meals.
- It is important to chew food and drink fluids carefully to avoid choking. Dietary liquids can be made semisolid with a thickening agent to facilitate swallowing if that is a problem.

Bowel and Bladder

- Continue a bowel and bladder training program.
- Include adequate dietary fiber to facilitate regular bowel elimination.
- Use a clean technique for irrigating, changing, or inserting catheters at home (as demonstrated by the nurse).
- Inspect the urine for cloudiness (which may indicate a urinary tract infection).
- Contact a primary provider if chills and fever occur or if the urine is bloody, cloudy, or has an offensive odor.

Client and Family Teaching 40-1 Home Care for the Client With a Neurologic Deficit (*continued*)

- Know how to perform skin care of the genitalia and perineum, including the special care that must be given to the anal area and the genitalia after defecation. (A client who is a man with an external urinary sheath should be able to demonstrate its application and know how to clean the penis daily to remove urine and dried secretions.)

Activity

- Make use of social contacts, hobbies, and changes in the daily routine to relieve boredom.
- Avoid fatigue and exposure to infection.
- Take deep breaths every 1 to 2 hours while awake and cough to raise secretions.

Therapies, Community Services, and Equipment

- Work with therapists and follow their advice about performance or practice of the therapies.
- When needed, use services available for home care.
- Contact agencies or retail stores from which home care equipment may be purchased, rented, or borrowed.
- If necessary, consult with a social service worker for information regarding financial assistance or the availability of loan closets that allow people who need certain types of equipment to borrow these materials.

Pharmacologic Considerations

- Clients with dysphagia often have difficulty taking pills or capsules. Liquid medications (in syrup form) can be an alternative; be aware that many of these contain sorbitol. This can cause diarrhea if multiple medications are given in syrup form.

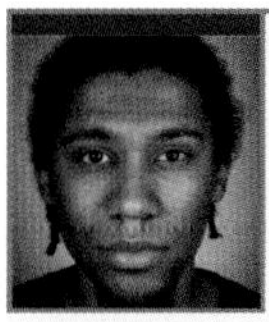

Clinical Scenario While seated unrestrained on the passenger side of a convertible, an 18-year-old man was thrown from the car when the driver swerved on a curve while traveling at high speed. When paramedics arrived, they noted that the client was conscious but had a loss of motor function and sensation below the C6 level of his spine. After he was transported to the hospital, the client's neck and spine were stabilized with traction, and later, a spinal fusion was performed. After 6 months of care, it was found that the client's paralysis is permanent. The consensus is that the client now requires supportive and rehabilitative care after his discharge. **What should the home care nurse include in this client's plan of care or in one for a client with a neurologic deficit caused by another type of neurologic disorder? See the following Nursing Process section.**

NURSING PROCESS FOR THE CLIENT WITH A NEUROLOGIC DEFICIT

Assessment

Obtain a thorough history (including drugs and allergies) from the client or family. Assess vital signs and level of comfort. Weigh the client for future comparisons. Perform a general neurologic assessment and use a standardized assessment tool (see Table 40-2) to note the extent of neurologic deficits related to swallowing, vision, weakness or paralysis of extremities, speech, and language comprehension. Evaluate airway, breathing, circulation, and LOC. Inspect the skin, auscultate the abdomen for bowel sounds, palpate the bladder for distension, and determine the client's ability to control bowel and bladder. Explore the client's emotional and rehabilitation needs. Determine if the client is at risk for falls (see Evidence-Based Practice 40-1).

Diagnosis, Planning, and Interventions

In addition to the diagnoses discussed in the following section, many nursing analysis may apply for the client and family facing a neurologic deficit (Box 40-1).

Altered Tissue Integrity Risk or Altered Skin Integrity Risk Altered Tissue Integrity Risk or Pressure Injury Risk: Related to immobility, incontinence, or other factors (specify)
Expected Outcome: Skin will remain intact and free from infection.

- Inspect all pressure points daily; keep skin clean and dry at all times. *Assessment enables identification of problems. Clean, dry skin reduces bacteria and the moisture that promotes their reproduction.*
- Massage bony prominences that blanch when pressure is relieved. *Massage increases circulation to the tissues, bringing oxygen and removing carbon dioxide and cellular wastes. Massage is contraindicated if the skin is already impaired, as evidenced by areas that remain reddened with relief of pressure.*
- Use a flotation mattress and other devices to relieve pressure when client is lying and sitting. *The integument becomes impaired when capillary pressure falls below 32 mm Hg* (Fig. 40-1).

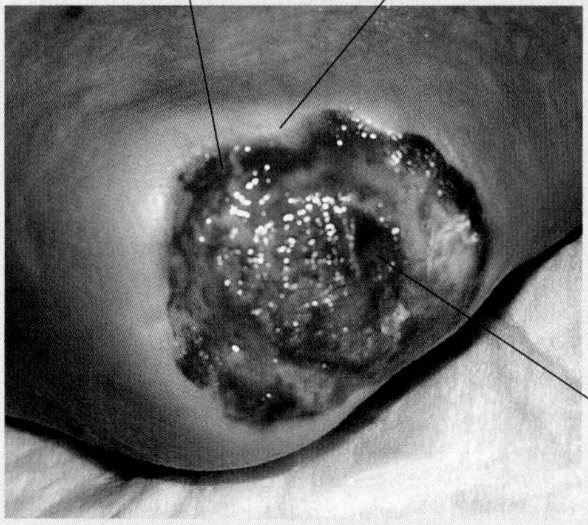

Figure 40-1 Pressure ulcer of the elbow in a client with a cerebrovascular accident (CVA) cared for at home. This client was admitted to the hospital for treatment of multiple pressure ulcers.

(continued)

NURSING PROCESS FOR THE CLIENT WITH A NEUROLOGIC DEFICIT (continued)

- Encourage adequate nutrition and provide supplements as ordered. *Protein, vitamin C, and zinc are important for healing/maintaining skin integrity. Supplements may be necessary to meet increased need for vitamin C and zinc.*
- Change client's position every 2 hours. *Doing so relieves pressure over bony prominences and maintains sufficient capillary pressure to keep integument intact.*

Constipation or Diarrhea (specify): Related to prolonged immobility, tube feedings, decreased fluid intake, effect of disease or injury on the spinal cord nerves
Expected Outcome: Client will have regular bowel movements at least every 3 days.

- Keep a daily record of all bowel movements. *A database helps identify problems.*
- Administer a prescribed stool softener daily. *Stool softeners moisturize the feces, which facilitates passage of stool without straining.*
- Increase client's daily fluid intake. *Oral fluids contribute to moisture in stool.*
- Institute a bowel training program (Nursing Guidelines 40-2). *Bowel training promotes bowel continence.*
- Perform a digital examination of the rectum if there is no bowel elimination in 3 days or if client passes liquid stools. *A digital examination helps determine if hard stool is in the rectum; passage of liquid stool may accompany fecal impaction.*
- Add high-fiber foods to the diet. *Fiber increases fecal bulk and pulls water into the feces, promoting regular bowel elimination.*
- Discuss persistent diarrhea with primary provider. *Bacterial growth in warm enteral formula, contamination of tube feeding equipment, and low-fiber formulas can cause enteritis and diarrhea.*

Reflex Urinary Incontinence or Urinary Retention: Related to effects of disease or injury to the nervous system or spinal cord nerves, loss of bladder tone
Expected Outcome: Client will void, the bladder will empty with no urinary retention, or both.

- Use an indwelling catheter or intermittent catheterization. *Some neurologic deficits are permanent; urinary elimination and continence may require a catheter.*
- Measure intake and output when client has an indwelling urethral catheter and takes fluids poorly and when first removing an indwelling urethral catheter. *Measuring intake and output helps identify whether fluid volume is within normal expectations.*
- Palpate the lower abdomen for bladder distention; notify the primary provider if client cannot void. *The bladder is not palpable unless it becomes distended. The urge to void occurs when the bladder contains 150 to 300 mL; urination needs to occur several times a day to avoid overdistension.*
- Ensure that client uses incontinence pads or absorbent underwear. *Disposable, porous pads and underwear wick urine away and keep bedding dry.*

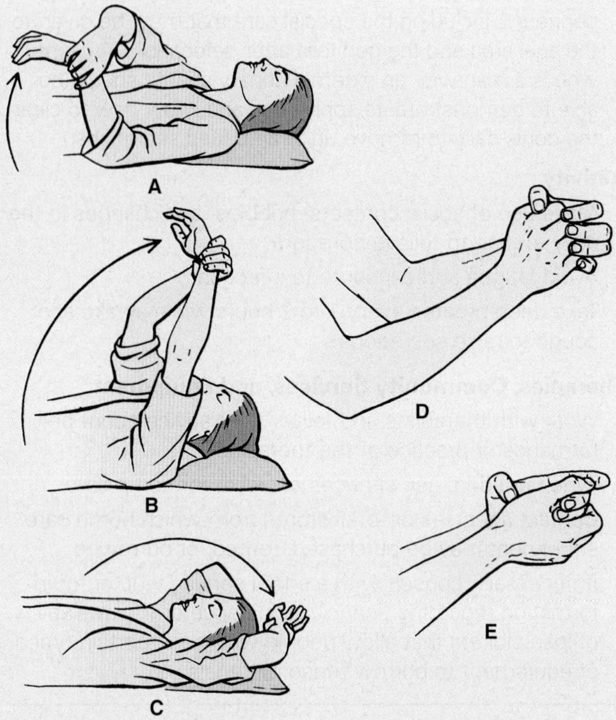

Figure 40-2 Range-of-motion exercises of the affected hand and arm that hemiplegic clients can learn to do themselves. **(A–C)** The client uses the unaffected hand to grasp the affected arm at the wrist and raise it over the head. **(D, E)** The client grasps the paralyzed hand and extends each affected finger slowly in turn.

- Institute a bladder training program as soon as possible (Nursing Guidelines 40-3). *Bladder training promotes urinary continence.*

Deconditioning: Related to muscle weakness and paralysis
Expected Outcome: Client will tolerate increased physical mobility as demonstrated by use of devices for mobility and remain free of contractures.

- Perform active or passive ROM exercises on the affected and unaffected extremities, or encourage client to perform ROM exercises independently (Fig. 40-2). *ROM exercises prevent contractures and muscle atrophy.*
- Regularly position clients with paraplegia or tetraplegia in an upright posture. *An upright posture helps the client take in the immediate environment and helps promote circulation through regulation of baroreceptors.*
- Apply an abdominal binder and elastic stockings before the client gets up. *An abdominal binder and elastic stockings decrease pooling of blood in distal areas, thereby preventing dizziness and faintness.*
- Implement fall precautions for clients with an unsteady gait or who are identified at risk using a fall risk assessment tool. *Clients with neurologic deficits are at higher risk for injuries associated with falls than most other clients.*
- Suggest using parallel bars or a walker (Fig. 40-3). *Before ambulating independently, clients can learn to support body weight and move forward with a variety of ambulatory aids.*

NURSING PROCESS FOR THE CLIENT WITH A NEUROLOGIC DEFICIT (continued)

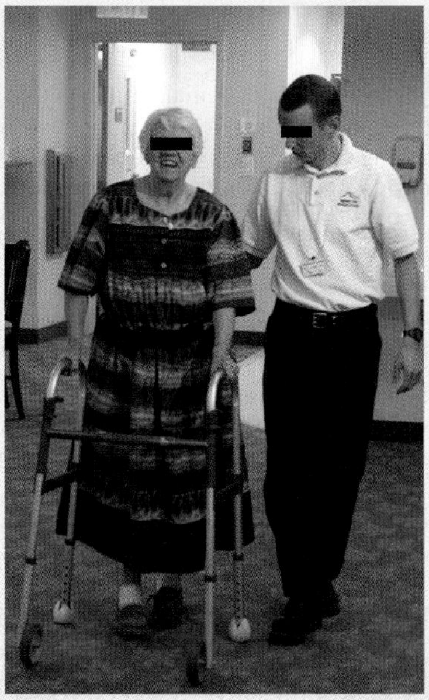

Figure 40-3 Ambulatory training in the physical therapy department starts as soon as the client can stand.

Psychosocial Needs: Related to disturbance or loss of nerve function to genitalia
Expected Outcome: Client will explore sexual alternatives.

- Be alert to subtle references to sexual dysfunction or problems. *Most clients are hesitant to discuss sexuality openly and frankly.*
- Allow client time to talk or ask questions. *Most clients refrain from sexual discussions if they sense the nurse is unreceptive or pressed for time.*
- Convey acceptance; recommend that the client and sexual partner speak with a primary provider or sexual therapist. *Medical and behavioral approaches may provide alternatives to former sexual activities.*
- Explain to paralyzed men that spontaneous erections may occur when the bladder is full. *Spontaneous erections are unpredictable and sometimes circumstantially inconvenient.*
- Offer information about penile implants (see Chapter 55). *A penile implant provides temporary or permanent penile erection, which facilitates vaginal penetration during intercourse.*
- Inform paralyzed men that ejaculation is rare and sperm motility is diminished, which reduces the potential for fathering children. *Clients with paraplegia or tetraplegia have the right to information about their potential for fertility.*
- Suggest that having intercourse on a water bed may facilitate sexual activity. *The buoyancy of a water bed promotes pelvic movement.*
- Share that some couples use mutual masturbation or electronic vibrators during sexual activity. *Orgasmic arousal can be achieved using alternatives.*
- Instruct clients who are women that they are still fertile and may need contraception if a pregnancy is undesired. *Motor paralysis does not affect ovulation.*

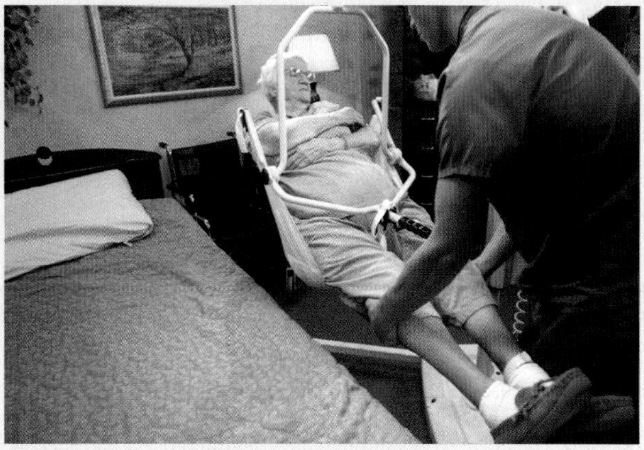

Figure 40-4 A mechanical lift may be used to transfer a client to and from the bed, wheelchair, or shower.

Injury Risk: Related to muscle weakness, paralysis, seizure disorder, loss of calcium from bone, other (specify)
Expected Outcome: Client remains free from injury.

- Use caution when moving and lifting a client who has been immobile. *Prolonged immobility results in calcium loss from bones and increased susceptibility to fractures.*
- Use a mechanical lift to safely transfer client (Fig. 40-4). *It uses principles of physics to raise, lift, and lower clients with minimal exertion on the part of caregivers.*
- Implement seizure precautions for clients with head injuries or brain tumors (see Chapter 37, Nursing Process for the Client With a Seizure Disorder, for specific interventions). *The client is at risk for injury during a seizure because they cannot implement self-protective interventions.*

Situational Low Self-Esteem: Related to effects of disability on perception of self-worth
Expected Outcome: Client will maintain positive self-regard, accept changes in body function, express feelings about the disability, and participate in rehabilitation.

- Assess for signs of negative responses, such as refusal to discuss loss, lack of participation in care, and increased isolation. *Nonverbal cues provide more reliable feedback about self-regard than do verbalizations.*
- Convey respect and hope; encourage verbalization of feelings. *Remaining nonjudgmental and giving the client an opportunity to express feelings help relieve stressors.*
- Help client identify their positive attributes and strengths from past experiences. *Focusing on successes rather than failures helps decrease feelings of helplessness and hopelessness.*
- Identify ways to support client's independence and role in the family. *Helping the client maintain their previous level of functioning maintains self-esteem.*

(continued)

NURSING PROCESS FOR THE CLIENT WITH A NEUROLOGIC DEFICIT (continued)

Grief: Related to loss of body function
Expected Outcome: Client will adaptively progress through various stages of grieving.

- Convey support and acceptance of client's feelings. *Grief is a normal response to loss; suppressing grief delays emotional healing.*
- Explain that grieving involves a sequence of emotions. *The grief process is a universal experience that begins with shock and progresses through denial, anger, depression, bargaining, and eventually acceptance.*
- Support grief work: explain denial, promote hope during depression, encourage adaptive outlets for anger, encourage decision-making in all aspects of self-care, and focus on present and future goals. *Grief work promotes acceptance of losses.*

Evaluation of Expected Outcomes

Expected outcomes vary, depending on the original goals and nursing diagnoses. The client has no evidence of skin breakdown. Complications associated with inactivity and immobility do not develop. The client works through the grieving process and accepts altered abilities. Defecation and urinary elimination are managed. The client is physically active, as demonstrated by use of trapeze, wheelchair, and other methods for mobility. The client continues sexual activities or learns about sexual alternatives. No injuries occur. The client participates in decision-making regarding daily activities, social outlets, vocational options, and applicable therapies.

Evidence-Based Practice 40-1

Risk for Falls and Neurologic Deficits

Clinical Question

What factors place a client with Parkinson Disease—neurologic deficits at risk for falls?

Evidence

In a study done in July 2020, reviewing clients diagnosed with Parkinson disease, it was noted that there was an increase in falls in the clients that had a decrease in gray matter volume in the brain. The study acknowledged that a diagnosis of Parkinson disease is associated with co-diagnoses of motor impairment and dementia. Parkinson disease and dementia clients exhibiting impaired motor function, lower gray matter volume in the brain, and notable cognitive deficits may have increased risk of falls (Parkinson disease, 2020).

Nursing Implications

Preventing falls is an important client safety goal for all health care facilities. Identifying clients who are at risk for falls early and implementing measures to prevent fall-related injuries are crucial to their care. The nurse can not only use the agency's fall risk assessment tool but also apply the principle that neurologic deficits put clients at a high risk for falls.

Reference
Cheng, K.-L., Lin, L.-H., Chen, P.-C., Chiang, P.-L., Chen, Y.-S., Chen, H.-L., Chen, M.-H., Chou, K.-H., Li, S.-H., Lu, C.-H., & Lin, W.-C. (2020). Reduced gray matter volume and risk of falls in Parkinson's disease with dementia patients: A voxel-based morphometry study. *International Journal of Environmental Research and Public Health, 17*, 5374. https://doi.org/10.3390/ijerph17155374.

BOX 40-1 Additional Nursing Diagnoses for the Client and Family Facing a Neurologic Deficit

Diagnoses for the Client

- **Knowledge deficiency** (specify) related to cognitive limitation, lack of recall, misinterpretation of information
- **Memory impairment** related to neurologic disturbances
- **Chronic confusion** related to cognitive changes
- **Situational low self-esteem** to feeling overwhelmed by prognosis
- **Coping impairment** related to chronic stress
- **Altered health maintenance** related to insufficient knowledge of tests, treatments, home care management, other (specify)
- **ADL deficit** related to inability to care for self, inadequacies such as housing, care, financial resources (specify)
- **Depression** related to inability to accept the physical changes, impaired cognition, aphasia, inability to control situation, dependence on others, and immobility
- **Grief** related to immobility, lack of transportation and loss of independence

Diagnoses for the Family

- **Caregiver fatigue** related to complexity or amount of care needed

NURSING GUIDELINES 40-2

Implementing a Bowel Training Program

Some clients can achieve self-controlled emptying of the bowel, provided they and those who care for them exert the persistent effort required. Bowel control typically is easier to achieve than bladder control.

For a bowel training program:

- Keep a record of bowel movements over several weeks. Doing so helps determine the time of day the client is most likely to have a bowel movement.

NURSING GUIDELINES 40-2 (*continued*)

- Encourage liquids throughout the day. Include foods that produce bulk, such as fresh fruits and vegetables, in the diet. Eliminate foods that cause loose stools.
- Assist client to the bathroom at a certain time each day. The physical activity involved in getting out of bed often increases peristalsis and encourages defecation.
- Administer a low-volume 1 oz. or less enema (mini enema such as Enemeez that contains liquid biscadoyl [Dulcolax] or docusate sodium [Colace]) or suppository each day at the same time to stimulate a bowel movement. Later, bowel function will become regulated so that the client can have a bowel movement at this time without these aids.

Steps for administering a suppository or enema:

1. Tape the paralyzed client's buttocks together to keep a suppository in place. Remove the tape at the time the suppository is expected to work.
2. Give enemas slowly, about 1 to 2 oz. or 5 mL of mini enema, followed by a 15- to 20-minute waiting period, to clients with tetraplegia or paraplegia who can retain sufficient enema solution.
3. Check the temperature of the enema solution immediately before administration. Insert the rectal tube gently, especially for clients who cannot feel, because they are vulnerable to trauma.
4. Allow the client privacy and about 30 minutes to have a bowel movement.
5. Digitally stimulate the rectum every 10 to 15 minutes until stool is expelled.

NURSING GUIDELINES 40-3

Implementing a Bladder Training Program

- Record the times the client voids over several weeks to help establish voiding patterns.
- Plan a voiding schedule that is similar to the assessed voiding patterns.
- Encourage increased fluid intake; clients who remain relatively immobile for the rest of their lives are subject to bladder infections and calculus (stone) formation in the urinary tract.
- Advise client to note any sensation (chilliness, lower abdominal discomfort, and restlessness) that precedes voiding. Doing so helps the client identify when they need to void.
- Encourage client to void every 30 minutes to 2 hours while awake. If the client can use the bedpan or urinal, keep these readily available and answer the call light promptly when the client requires assistance.
- Instruct client to bend at the waist or press inward and downward over the bladder, a technique referred to as **Credé maneuver**. It increases abdominal pressure and facilitates emptying the bladder.
- Use other measures to stimulate voiding, such as running water and placing a hand in a basin of water.
- Propose that paralyzed clients with **reflex incontinence**, which occurs spontaneously when the bladder is full, lightly massage or tap the skin above the pubic area, a method known as **cutaneous triggering** that stimulates relaxation of the urinary sphincter.

KEY POINTS

- Neurologic deficit: a condition in which one or more functions of the central and peripheral nervous systems are decreased, impaired, or absent, for example: paralysis, muscle weakness, impaired speech, inability to recognize objects, abnormal gait or difficulty walking, impaired memory, impaired swallowing, or abnormal bowel and bladder elimination
- Three phases of a neurologic deficit:
  - Acute phase: follows a sudden neurologic event, such as a CVA or a head or spinal cord injury; in the acute phase, the client is usually critically ill.
  - Recovery phase: begins when the client's condition is stabilized; it starts several days or weeks after the initial event and lasts weeks or months.
  - Chronic phase: neurologic deficits result in a prolonged or lifelong chronic phase; during this phase, the client shows little or no improvement, remains stationary, or progressively worsens.
- Goal of treatment for clients with neurological deficits:
  - improve function
  - reduce symptoms
  - improve the well-being of the client

CRITICAL THINKING EXERCISES

1. Discuss the methods to help clients achieve success in a bowel and bladder training program.
2. A client had a CVA 6 months ago and is paralyzed on his right side. He cannot speak and shows signs of mental changes. He now appears agitated and is

making motions with his left hand to various areas of his body, mainly his abdomen. What assessments could you make to determine the possible cause of his agitation?

3. A family is planning to care for a client who has had a CVA at home. Ideally, discharge planning begins at the time of admission. What equipment and supplies would you recommend that the family obtain?

4. A client had a spinal cord injury at T11 and is paraplegic. During a conference, team members mention his depression and withdrawal. What other members of the health care team and services may be helpful in this client's care?

NCLEX-STYLE REVIEW QUESTIONS PrepU

1. A client is in the skilled rehabilitation setting during the chronic phase of care. When developing the client's nursing plan of care, what long-term goal is most appropriate?
  1. The client will consume dietary carbohydrates for energy.
  2. The client will be free of skin breakdown or contractures.
  3. The client will be emotionally stable, with no signs of clinical depression.
  4. The client will regain use of all extremities.

2. When caring for a client with a neurologic deficit, what nursing intervention is most important for preventing the formation of a pressure ulcer?
  1. Promote a balanced nutritional intake.
  2. Massage reddened areas frequently.
  3. Relieve pressure over bony prominences.
  4. Cleanse the skin with antiseptic soap.

3. A home care nurse is helping a client and family cope with a recent neurologic deficit. What intervention is most important for the nurse to perform first?
  1. Identify solutions for the client and family's health problems.
  2. Encourage outside assistance from community agencies and resources.
  3. Assist the client and family to identify possible needs and solutions.
  4. Call the primary provider and ask for suggestions for meeting the client's needs.

4. The nurse initiates a teaching plan for the family and client with neurologic deficits because of Parkinson's disease. What nursing instruction is the highest priority?
  1. Encourage adequate sleep.
  2. Reduce home safety hazards.
  3. Use measures to improve self-esteem.
  4. Maintain social relationships.

5. When planning strategies for managing bowel elimination for the client with a neurologic deficit, what nursing intervention is most appropriate to include?
  1. Administer a tap water enema just before bedtime.
  2. Encourage a high-fiber diet to increase stool bulk.
  3. Change disposable absorbent undergarments when soiled.
  4. Pad the rim of the bedpan to prevent skin breakdown.

WANT TO KNOW MORE? There are a wide variety of online resources available on thePoint to enhance learning and understanding of this chapter.

Go to **thePoint.lww.com/activate** and use the activation code found in the front of this text to unlock these online resources.

UNIT 10 Caring for Clients With Sensory Disorders

41 Introduction to the Sensory System

Words To Know
accommodation
audiometry
caloric stimulation test
central vision
conductive hearing loss
conjunctivitis
decibels
electronystagmography
near point
nystagmus
ophthalmoscopy
otoscope
proptosis
ptosis
refraction
Rinne test
Romberg test
sensorineural hearing loss
tonometry
tuning fork
visual acuity
visual field examination
Weber test

Learning Objectives

On completion of this chapter, you will be able to:

1. Describe the anatomy and physiology of the eyes.
2. Discuss tests that are used for visual screening.
3. Identify questions to ask during an eye assessment.
4. Describe diagnostic studies for eye function.
5. Explain the anatomy and physiology of the ears.
6. Describe methods for assessing the ear and hearing acuity.
7. Describe specific diagnostic tests for ear function.

The special senses of vision and hearing allow humans to view their world, hear what is in their environment, communicate with others, and maintain their balance. Eye and ear disorders occur throughout the life cycle. Many of the disorders can result in changes in visual acuity or hearing loss as well as problems with balance and communication. Nurses can be instrumental in early identification of eye and ear problems, and they may play an important role in reducing the severity and/or long-term effects of eye and ear disorders. This chapter focuses on the structure and function of the eyes and ears and the diagnostic tests that are used to evaluate their function.

THE EYES

Anatomy and Physiology

The *eyeballs* are globes located in a protective bony cavity or *orbit* of the skull. The frontal, maxillary, zygomatic, sphenoid, ethmoid, lacrimal, and palatine bones form the walls of the orbit. Fat and muscle protect the posterior, superior, inferior, and lateral aspects of each eyeball.

The extraocular muscles that permit movement include the superior and inferior rectus (move eye up [*elevation*] and down [*depression*]), the medial and lateral rectus (move eye toward [*adduction*] and away from [*abduction*] the nose and the temple), and the superior and inferior oblique muscles (rotate around the optic axis [*intorsion* and *extorsion*]).

Gerontologic Considerations

- Teaching aids with black print at font size 22 or larger on ivory background minimizes glare and should be used for clients experiencing age-associated lens changes. Indirect lighting (over the shoulder) also minimizes glare.
- Color perception may be altered in older adults experiencing yellowing of the lens. Color identification should be considered when teaching older adults about medications by color of tablet or capsule because blue may be perceived as green.
- Older clients form drier cerumen and experience an increased incidence of impaction in the external acoustic meatus. Nonprescription preparations are available for softening hardened cerumen. Refer the client to a health care provider if hearing remains diminished.
- Careful documentation of conduction times assessed using the Rinne and Weber tests is important. This information enables early identification of hearing changes and may affect selection of assistive hearing devices (see Chapter 43).

A seventh muscle, called the *levator palpebrae superioris*, elevates the upper eyelid (Fig. 41-1). Three cranial nerves innervate the extraocular muscles: the trochlear nerve (*cranial nerve IV*) innervates the superior oblique muscle; the abducens nerve (*cranial nerve VI*) innervates the lateral rectus muscle; and the oculomotor nerve (*cranial nerve III*) innervates the remaining muscles (Porth, 2015).

Extraocular Structures

The eyelids, eyelashes, and tears protect the anterior or exposed surface of the eye. The upper and lower eyelids are folds of skin that meet at an angle referred to as the *canthus*. The outer or lateral canthus is the outer angle, and the inner or medial canthus is at the inner aspect of the eye. The line between the lateral and medial canthus usually is horizontal. Children with Down syndrome have a line that slants upward and outward. People of Asian origin have an *epicanthal fold*, which is a fold of skin that covers the inner canthus.

The eyelids protect against foreign bodies and adjust the amount of light that enters the eye. The eyelashes trap foreign debris. Periodic blinking clears dust and particles from the surface of the eyes. The eyelids also spread tears over the surface of the eye. The eyelids have multiple glands, including sebaceous, sweat, and accessory lacrimal glands. They are lined with a sensitive, transparent mucous membrane called *conjunctiva*. This membrane extends from the lid margins and meets the *cornea* (the transparent domelike structure that covers most of the anterior portion of the eyeball) at the *limbus*, which is the outermost edge of the iris. The lacrimal *caruncle* is a small, reddish elevation on the conjunctiva located at the inner canthus.

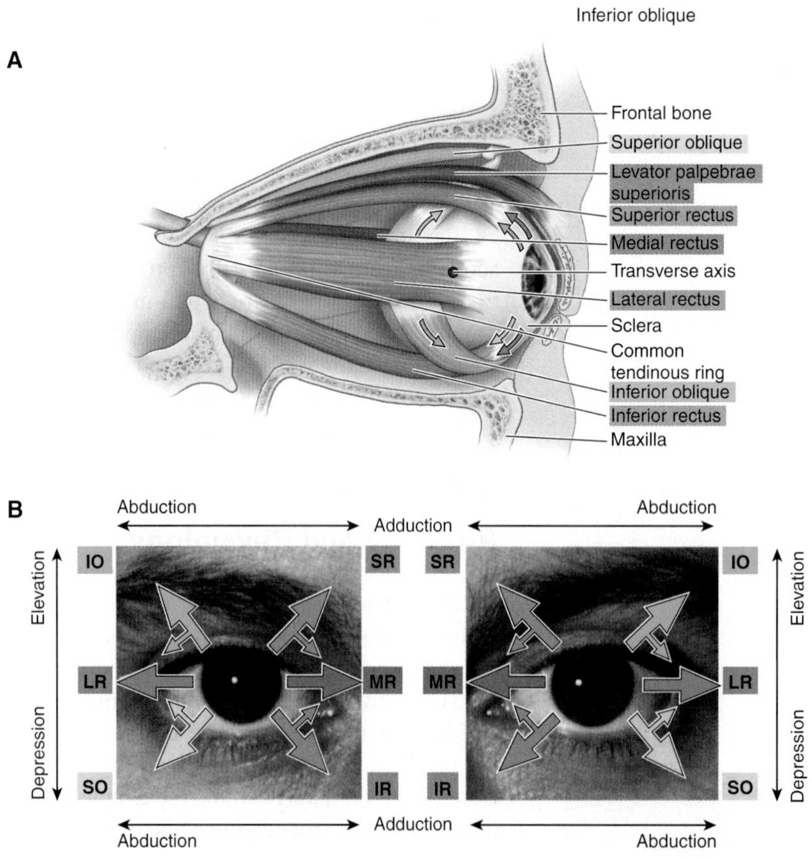

Figure 41-1 **(A)** Extraocular muscles. **(B)** The muscles used to move the eyes. (A and B reprinted with permission from Moore, K. L., Dalley, A. F., & Agur, A. M. R. (2014). *Clinically oriented anatomy* (7th ed.). Wolters Kluwer Health/Lippincott Williams & Wilkins.)

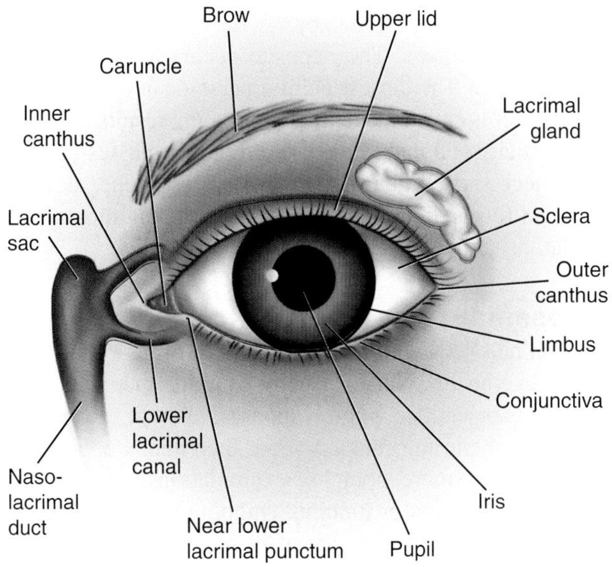

Figure 41-2 External structures of the eye and position of the lacrimal structures.

Tears, composed of water, sodium chloride, and lysozyme, an antibacterial enzyme, are produced by *lacrimal (tear) glands* found beneath the bony orbital ridge. The *lacrimal apparatus* includes the lacrimal glands, *punctum*, *lacrimal canals*, *lacrimal sac*, and *nasolacrimal ducts*. Tears flow across the eyes, continually bathing and lubricating the surface. The tears drain through the punctum into the lacrimal canals and lacrimal sac to the nasolacrimal ducts, tiny openings at the junction of the upper and lower lids, and then into the nose (Fig. 41-2).

Intraocular Structures

Three layers form the intraocular structures. The *first layer* is the *sclera*, commonly referred to as the "white of the eye." It is composed of tough connective tissue. The sclera protects structures in the eye. It connects directly to the cornea, anterior chamber, iris, and pupil.

The *middle layer* is the *uvea*, or vascular coat of the eye, located immediately under the sclera. The uvea includes the *choroid* (contains blood vessels and darkly pigmented cells that prevent light from scattering inside the eye) and the *iris* (the highly vascular, pigmented portion of the eye surrounding the pupil). The *pupil* is an opening that dilates and constricts in response to light. The choroid gives rise to the *ciliary body*, composed of *ciliary processes* and the *ciliary muscle*. The ciliary processes produce *aqueous humor*, a nutrient-rich liquid that nourishes eye structures. The ciliary muscle helps change the shape of the lens when adjusting to near or far vision. The *anterior chamber*, behind the cornea, is filled with clear aqueous humor, which provides nourishment to the cornea. The lens lies behind the pupil and iris.

The *posterior chamber* is a small space behind the lens. Aqueous fluid, produced in the posterior chamber by the ciliary processes, flows from the posterior chamber to the anterior chamber. It then drains into the *canal of Schlemm*.

Vitreous humor is thick, gelatinous material that maintains the spherical shape of the eyeball. It also maintains the placement of the retina (Fig. 41-3). The *retina*, the *innermost layer* of the eye, is composed of a pigmented outer layer and an inner neurosensory layer. Light stimulates this

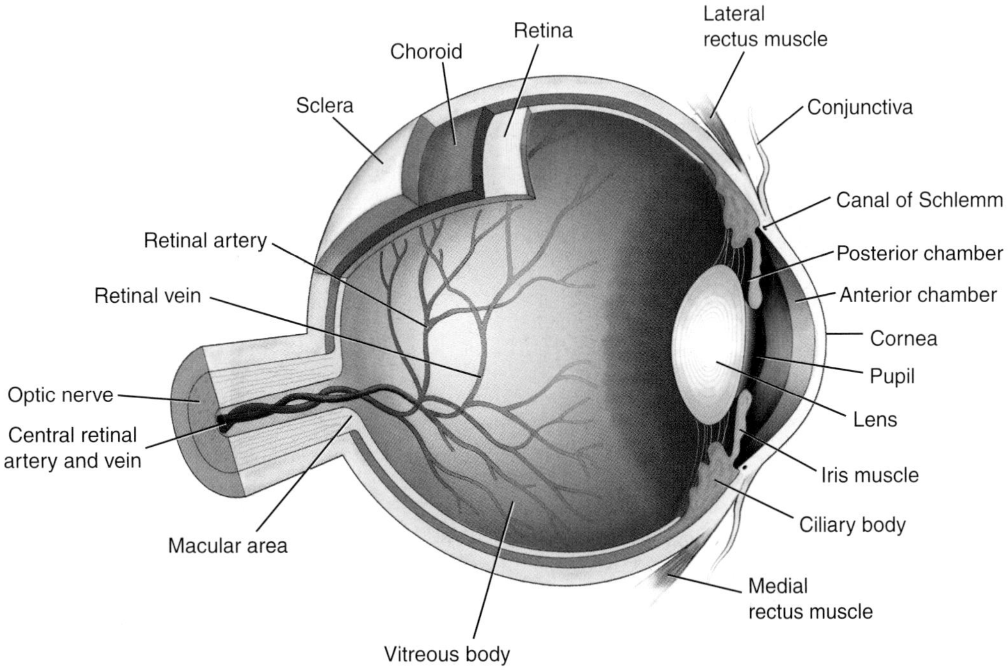

Figure 41-3 Three-dimensional cross-section of the eye.

neurosensory layer, which contains nerve cells called *rods* and *cones*. Rods function in night or dim light and assist in distinguishing black and white. Cones function in bright light and are sensitive to color. The nerve cells of the retina extend from the optic nerve.

The *macula lutea*, or the "yellow spot," is composed entirely of cones and allows for detailed vision. It lies in the center of the retina. The *fovea centralis* or *foveola* is at the center of the macula. The blood vessels are displaced from the fovea centralis, allowing light to pass to the cones. The density of the cones decreases away from the fovea centralis as the number of rods increases in the periphery of the retina. The *optic disk*, the anterior surface of the optic nerve, is easily distinguished from the macula because of the vasculature that radiates from the optic disk. No blood vessels radiate directly from the macula (Fig. 41-4). The macula is the area of the eye that provides **central vision**, the ability to discriminate letters, words, and the details of any image. If the macula degenerates or is damaged, only the ability to see movement and gross objects in the peripheral fields of vision remains.

Visual Function

The function of the eyeball is to convert light energy into nerve signals that are transmitted to and interpreted in the cerebral cortex. Every object reflects light. For a person to see it clearly, the reflected light must pass through the intraocular structures—the cornea, anterior chamber, pupil, lens, and vitreous humor. These structures cause **refraction**, which means that the light rays bend and change speed. The lens focuses the light into an upside-down and reversed image on the retina. The rods and cones in the retina send nerve impulses by way of the optic nerve and optic tract to the visual cortex of the occipital lobe. This is where the image is interpreted.

The lens is more convex on the posterior side and can change shape, a process known as **accommodation**. The ciliary muscles contract or relax to focus an image onto the retina, which allows the person to clearly see distant or near objects. For viewing distant objects, the ciliary muscles relax and the lens flattens. The opposite occurs to view objects that are closer. The closest point a person can clearly focus on an object is called the **near point**. Aging results in loss of lens elasticity and makes the use of reading glasses for near vision necessary. When the lens becomes opaque, as when a cataract forms, light is blocked from reaching the macula, and the visual image becomes blurred or cloudy.

Assessment

The ophthalmic assessment provides information about a client's eye health. Nurses usually examine the client's external eye appearance, pupil responses, and eye movements as well as obtain information about the client's ophthalmic condition. For more complex examinations, nurses need additional education or training. Ongoing eye examinations and treatment require the care of specialists. Box 41-1 provides a list of specialists and technicians who provide eye care and treatment.

Clients often ask nurses when to have an eye examination. The American Academy of Ophthalmology (2021) recommends that adults who do not have any signs of eye disease or risk of any eye disorders have a complete eye examination once in their 20s and twice in their 30s. A baseline comprehensive screening needs to be done at age 40 years because signs of disease and visual changes begin to occur at this time. Between ages 40 and 60 years, it is recommended that eye examinations occur every 2 years or as needed. After age 65 years, it is recommended that a complete eye exam ination occur every 1 to 2 years to check for age-related eye disorders. Adults with a personal or family history of eye disease, diabetes, or hypertension should see an ophthalmologist to determine how frequently they need an eye examination. Symptoms that require attention include bulging of the eyes; dark spot in the center of the client's field of vision; difficulty focusing; blurred, cloudy, double, or hazy

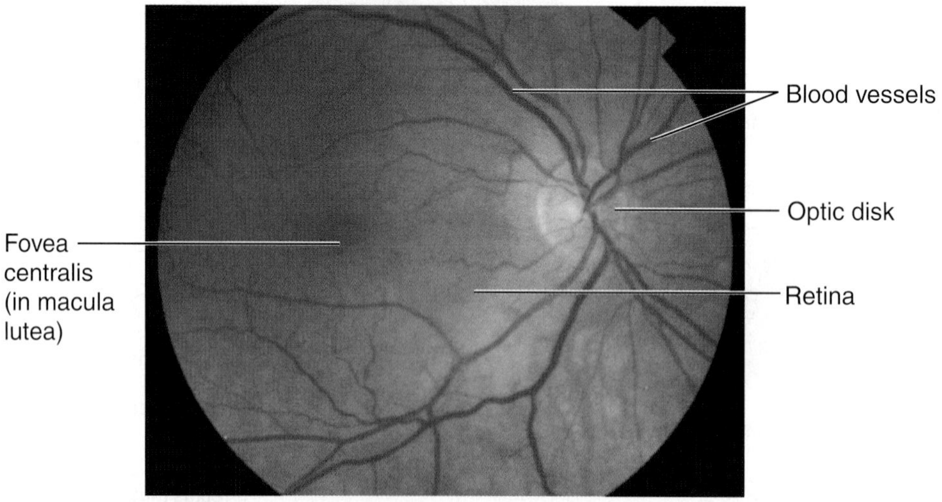

Figure 41-4 A normal ophthalmoscopic picture. The fundus or back of the eye as seen through an ophthalmoscope. The optic disc, with its radiating vasculature, is easily distinguished from the macula lutea. (Reprinted with permission from Moore, K. L., Dalley, A. F., & Agur, A. M. R. (2009). *Clinically oriented anatomy* (6th ed.). Wolters Kluwer Health/Lippincott Williams & Wilkins.)

BOX 41-1 Vision Specialists

Ophthalmologist: a primary provider (doctor of medicine [MD] or doctor of osteopathic medicine [DO]) who specializes in the medical and surgical treatment of eye diseases; licensed to diagnose and treat eye disorders, prescribe medications, perform surgery, and prescribe corrective lenses, including contact lenses.
Oculoplastic specialist: an ophthalmologist with advanced training in plastic and reconstructive surgery of the eye and surrounding structures.
Optometrist: a specialist who earns a doctor of optometry (OD) after undergraduate and graduate education. Optometrists test vision; examine eyes; prescribe corrective lenses and contact lenses; and in some states, treat limited eye diseases, including prescribing medications.
Optician: a specialist who makes eyeglass or contact lenses based on prescriptions from ophthalmologists and optometrists. The optician also ensures that corrective lenses fit properly.
Ophthalmic technician: assistants who are certified by The Joint Commission on Allied Health Personnel in Ophthalmology to assist in selected eye tests and procedures.

BOX 41-2 Questions to Ask During an Eye Assessment

- Are you having any problems with your eyes?
- Do you have any problems with your vision? Do you wear glasses or contact lenses?
- Have you experienced blurred, double, or distorted vision?
- Do you have any eye pain? Is it sharp or dull? Is it worse when you blink?
- Do you have any itching or feeling that something is in your eye?
- Is there any discharge? What does it look like (color, consistency, odor)?
- Are both eyes affected?
- How long have you had this problem?
- Has this happened before?
- What have you done to treat the problem?
- Does anything make the problem better or worse?
- What medications have you used to treat the eye problem?
- Do you have any other diseases or conditions?
- What medications are you taking?
- Have you ever had eye surgery? What? When?
- Do any family members have any eye conditions?

vision; loss of peripheral vision; or sudden loss of vision. Chapter 42 provides more information on eye disorders.

Nursing Assessment

The nurse obtains a history to identify any specific problems that the client is experiencing and possible causes. Box 41-2 lists questions that nurses may ask when taking an ocular history. The nurse gathers information related to eye problems: past and current ability to see; any discomfort, pain, or other symptoms; how long the client has experienced problems; any treatments and medications; and other illnesses that may affect eye health.

The nurse in the acute care, outpatient, or home setting performs a basic assessment of ocular health by obtaining the following:

- Client's description of vision changes, any visual or eye discomfort
- Use of glasses or contacts
- Use of prescription and nonprescription eye medication
- Previous eye trauma, ophthalmic and medical diseases, and surgery
- Family history of inherited eye diseases such as glaucoma
- Allergy history associated with seasonal **conjunctivitis** (inflammation of the conjunctiva) that often accompanies hay fever

After the interview, the nurse inspects the eyes for symmetry and also observes the lid margins for signs of inflammation, exudate, or loss of eyelashes. The nurse determines the pupil size and their change and response to light. Normal pupils are round, of equal size, and constrict simultaneously when stimulated (Fig. 41-5). The nurse checks the extraocular muscles by asking the client to keep their head still while following an object moved up, down, left, and right (Fig. 41-6). Other observations include looking for

- **Ptosis**: drooping upper eyelid
- **Proptosis**: an extended or protruded upper eyelid that delays closing or remains partially open
- **Nystagmus**: uncontrolled oscillating movement of the eyeball
- In addition, the nurse can examine the client for age-related changes in the eye. Table 41-1 reviews these changes.

Concept Mastery Alert

Cataract

A cataract interferes with focusing and causes increased glare, decreased vision, and changes in color perception. It does not affect central vision. Age-related macular degeneration affects central vision.

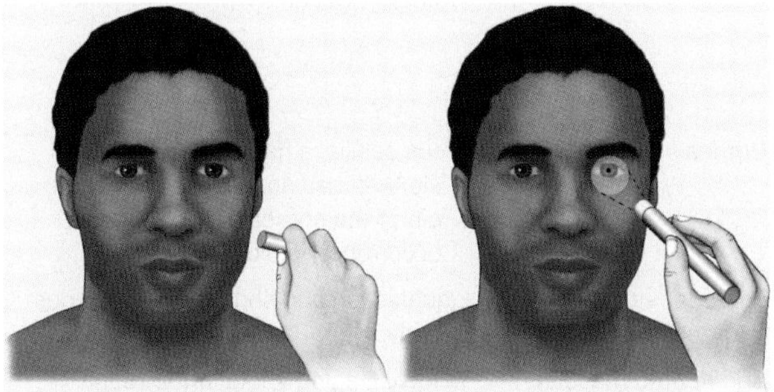

Figure 41-5 Assessing pupil response to light. Normal pupils constrict simultaneously when stimulated.

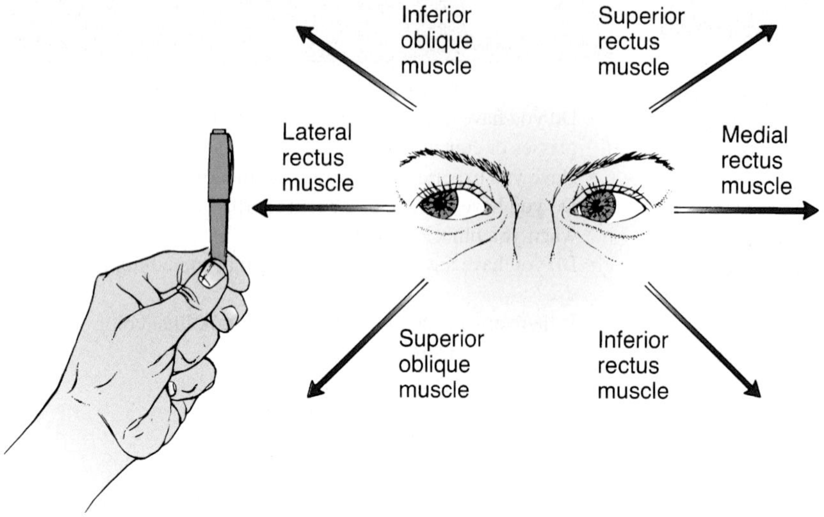

Figure 41-6 Assessing extraocular movements.

Visual Screening Tests

The *Snellen eye chart* (Fig. 41-7) is a simple screening tool for determining **visual acuity**, the ability to see far images clearly. With the chart 20 feet away, the examiner asks the client to cover one eye and identify letters of decreasing size. Results for each eye are expressed as a fraction that compares the client's vision with standard norms. If a client has 20/20 visual acuity (normal vision), it means that they see letters at 20 feet that others see clearly and accurately at 20 feet; a client with 20/40 vision sees letters at 20 feet that most others can read at 40 feet, and so on. For clients who cannot read or who do not read English, a tumbling E chart

TABLE 41-1 Age-Related Changes in the Eye

	STRUCTURAL CHANGE	FUNCTIONAL CHANGE	FINDINGS
Eyelids and lacrimal structures	Loss of skin elasticity and orbital fat; decreased muscle tone; development of wrinkles.	Turned-in lid margins (entropion) and turned-out lid margins (ectropion) cause irritation to cornea and conjunctiva or to the eyelids themselves.	Client reports burning and sensation of object in eye; increased tearing; inflammation; ulceration may occur.
Refractive changes; presbyopia	Lens cannot readily accommodate with aging (see Chapter 42).	Client holds reading materials at increasing distance to focus.	Client reports needing increased light; needs reading glasses or bifocals.
Cataract	Lens develops opacities.	Interference with focus of a sharp image on the retina.	Client reports increased glare, decreased vision, and changes in color perception.
Conjunctiva	The conjunctiva (white portion of the eye) becomes slack and more susceptible to chronic inflammations with age.	Part of the conjunctiva may become caught between the lids during blinking. Harmless degenerative plaques may appear on the conjunctiva; tear glands and the conjunctiva may lose the ability to lubricate the eye.	Client reports dry eyes and may have to use artificial tears.
Cornea	Arcus senilis, a harmless white circle that may appear on the margin of the cornea, is a common occurrence in older adults.	Composed of cholesterol and its derivatives; its presence does not necessarily indicate an overall increased cholesterol level.	No complaints.
Posterior vitreous detachment	Liquefaction and shrinkage of vitreous body.	May lead to retinal tears and detachment.	Client reports light flashes, cobwebs, and floaters.
Age-related macular degeneration	Yellowish aging spots in the retina (drusen) appear and coalesce in the macula.	Affects central vision (see Chapter 42).	Affects reading vision.

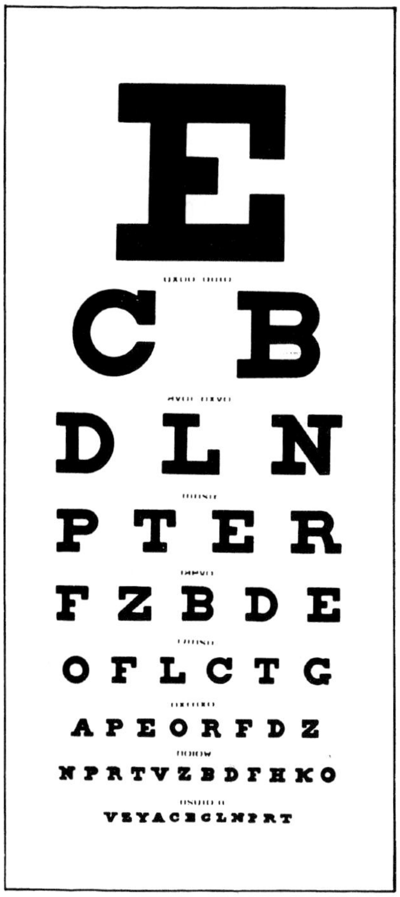

Figure 41-7 The Snellen chart is used to assess visual acuity, or far vision.

is used. It is set up like the standardized Snellen chart, but uses "E's" with the "fingers" pointing to one side or another or up or down. Clients are asked to indicate which way the "fingers" are pointing. If the client cannot identify even the largest letters or "E's" on the chart, the examiner asks them to count the number of fingers that the examiner holds up. If the finger count is inaccurate, the examiner tests the client's ability to distinguish light from dark. Visual acuity is also measured with a computerized refractor that records the strength and type of lenses necessary to correct the client's visual problem.

The *Jaeger chart* and *Rosenbaum Pocket Vision Screener* evaluate near vision. These charts contain words, numbers, and letters in various print sizes. The examiner instructs the client to cover one eye and then hold the chart approximately 14 inches away and read the smallest print that they can see comfortably. The size of the print the client reads indicates the quality of their near vision.

Color vision is assessed with *Ishihara polychromatic plates*. The client receives a series of cards on which the pattern of a number is embedded in a circle of colored dots. The numbers are in colors that color-blind individuals commonly cannot see. Clients with normal vision readily identify the numbers.

>>> ***Stop, Think, and Respond 41-1***

A client asks you what 20/200 visual acuity means. What is the best explanation?

Extraocular Muscle Function Tests

Corneal Light Reflex Test

The *corneal light reflex test* assesses the alignment of the eyes. The examiner holds a penlight approximately 12 inches from the client's face and asks the client to stare straight ahead. The reflection of light should be in the same spot on each eye, indicating parallel alignment. If the light reflex is uneven, it indicates deviated alignment of the eyes, possibly owing to muscle weakness or paralysis.

Cover–Uncover Test

The cover–uncover test assesses extraocular muscle function. The examiner asks the client to stare straight ahead and focus on an object in the distance while covering one eye with an opaque card. As the eye is covered, the examiner observes the uncovered eye for movement. The examiner then removes the card and observes the previously covered eye for movement. The test is repeated on the opposite eye. The client's uncovered eye should remain fixed on the object in the distance, as should the eye that is covered and then uncovered. If there is movement, it may indicate a deviation in alignment and muscle weakness.

Positions Test

The positions test or cardinal positions of gaze is done to assess eye muscle strength and cranial nerve function. The examiner asks the client to focus on an object that is approximately 12 inches away and moves this object through six cardinal positions in a clockwise direction. As the object is moved, the examiner observes the client's eye movements, which should be smooth and symmetrical in all six directions. If asymmetrical movements are noted, it indicates weakness in the extraocular muscles or dysfunction of the cranial nerve that innervates this muscle.

Diagnostic Studies

Ophthalmoscopy

Direct **ophthalmoscopy** is examination of the fundus or interior of the eye. This examination is done with a direct ophthalmoscope, an instrument that illuminates the internal surface of the eyes and allows the examiner to see the lens, retina, retinal blood vessels, and the optic disc under magnification (Fig. 41-8).

Indirect ophthalmoscopy involves the use of an instrument that produces a bright, intense light. The ophthalmologist uses this instrument in conjunction with an ophthalmoscope to see larger areas of the retina, although no magnification is involved.

Retinoscopy

Use of a *retinoscope* and trial lenses determines the focusing power of each eye. A retinoscope is a handheld instrument that produces a line of light. The light appears distorted in the eyes of clients with refractive errors. Trial lenses of

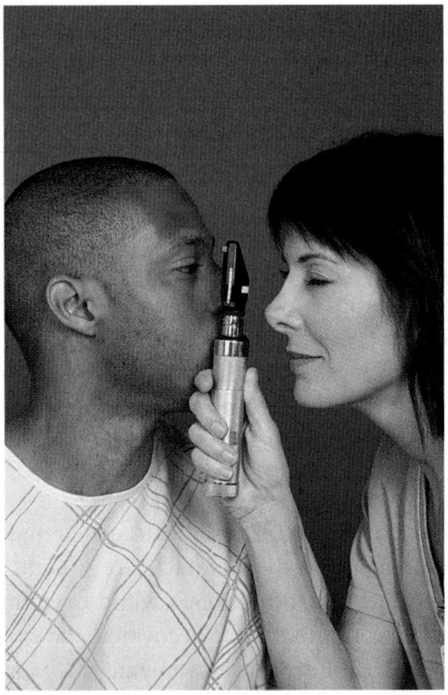

Figure 41-8 The examiner looks at the interior of the eye with a direct ophthalmoscope.

varying refractive powers are then placed in front of the eye until the light streak does not deviate in any direction.

Tonometry

Tonometry measures intraocular pressure (IOP) to screen for glaucoma. It is done by using a tonometer to indent or flatten (applanate) the surface of the eye. The principle is that a soft eye indents more easily than a hard eye. The force that produces indentation is measured and converted to a pressure reading. Normal IOP is 12 to 22 mm Hg. High readings indicate high IOP; low readings indicate low IOP.

There are various methods for performing tonometry. *Applanation tonometry* provides the greatest accuracy, but the *indentation* method may be used because it is smaller and more portable. Before either is used, a topical anesthetic solution is instilled in the lower conjunctival sac. Anesthesia begins almost immediately and lasts a few minutes. The client does not feel the tonometer while the eye is anesthetized. A *noncontact* tonometer, although less accurate, blows a puff of air against the cornea, and no local anesthetic is required.

Visual Field Examination

A **visual field examination** or perimetry test measures peripheral vision and detects gaps in the visual field. The client fixes their gaze on a stationary point straight ahead. A light or white object is moved from a point on the side, where it cannot be seen, toward the center. The client indicates the point at which they see the stimulus without directly looking at it. Certain disorders such as glaucoma, stroke, brain tumor, or retinal detachment are associated with changes in the visual field.

Color Vision Testing

Assessing a client's ability to differentiate color is essential for determining a person's ability to function within an environment dictated by color codes. For example, traffic lights or work equipment mandate that people be able to distinguish different colors. Ishihara polychromatic plates are the most common test for color vision. Different plates, bound in a book, have dots of primary colors embedded in a background of secondary colors. Clients must identify the hidden shape. Clients with diminished color vision are not able to do this successfully. For these clients, a quantitative color blind test may be used. These tests have trays with disks of various hues. The client is asked to arrange the disks in a continuum of the gradually changing hues. Quantitative color blindness tests help to distinguish the severity and type of color blindness.

Amsler Grid

Clients with macular problems are initially tested with an Amsler grid. It is made up of a geometric grid of identical squares with a central fixation point. The examiner instructs the client to stare at the central fixation point on the grid and report if they see any distortion of the squares. Clients with macular problems may say some of the squares are faded or wavy.

Slit-Lamp Examination

A *slit lamp* is a binocular microscope that magnifies the surface of the eye. A beam of light, narrowed to a slit, is directed at the cornea, facilitating an examination of structures and fluid in the anterior segment of the eye. This examination is used to identify disorders such as corneal abrasions, iritis, conjunctivitis, and cataracts.

Retinal Angiography

Retinal angiography or *fluorescein angiography* is used to detect vascular changes and blood flow through the retinal vessels. Sodium fluorescein, a water-soluble dye, is injected into a peripheral vein. The examiner uses a special camera to photograph the appearance and distribution of the dye in the retinal arteries, capillaries, and veins at 1-second intervals. The photographs provide a record of vascular filling and emptying defects. Many conditions affect retinal circulation, such as diabetes mellitus, hypertension, drug toxicity, tumors, and AIDS. In addition, lack of macular capillary perfusion or abnormal growth of new vessels around the macula (neovascularization as in macular degeneration) can be detected. Intravenous fluorescein causes skin to yellow slightly for 6 to 8 hours. The urine also turns bright yellow, but the color becomes less noticeable over the following 24 to 36 hours as the dye is excreted. Indocyanine green may be used instead for the contrast agent in order to visualize choroidal vasculature abnormalities with the use of digital video angiography.

Ultrasonography

Ultrasonography is used when pathologic changes such as an opaque lens, cloudy cornea, or bloody vitreous make it difficult to look directly at the posterior of the eye. Using sound waves, the contour and shape of contents in the eye are imaged and recorded. After instillation of anesthetic ophthalmic drops, an ultrasound probe is placed on the cornea, and a recording is made on an oscilloscope. This technique is helpful in detecting eye lesions and measuring for an intraocular lens implant before extracting a cataract.

Laser Scanning

An ophthalmologic screening tool uses a *retinal imaging* system to produce a high-resolution image of almost the entire retina without having to dilate the pupil. The Panoramic200 scanning laser ophthalmoscope (Optos, Dunfermline, Scotland) can detect retinal disorders such as diabetic retinopathy and provides an excellent baseline screening test.

Nursing Management

Although nurses may not be directly involved in caring for clients who are undergoing eye examinations and tests, it is essential that they engage in ensuring that clients receive eye care to preserve their eye function and/or prevent further visual loss. Careful assessment of the function and structure of the eyes provides the nurse with a baseline and assists with determining if further action is warranted. (See Evidence-Based Practice 41-1 regarding visual impairment and aging.)

Evidence-Based Practice 41-1

Visual Impairment, Aging, and Safety

Clinical Question

Does visual impairment increase with aging and become a safety factor?

Evidence

In today's world, the population increases with aging, people live longer, and there are more diseases that occur earlier, such as diabetes and high blood pressure. All of these factors increase the incidence of visual impairment and cause disabilities. A "homes-for-the-aged"-based population survey study was completed on about 1500 participants over age 60 years in India. The survey asked how visual impairment impacted their health status (Marmamula et al., 2021). The study concluded that people over 60 years of age had some visual impairment, but with prevention and scheduled eye examinations, planning ahead for clients and educating early would be helpful in achieving a goal of healthy lifestyle.

Nursing Implications

Nurses can use this evidence in their education and discharge teaching to make sure that older clients or clients with visual impairments are linked to necessary resources.

Reference

Marmamula, S., Barrenakala, N. R., Challa, R., Kumbham, T. R., Modepalli, S. B., Yellapragada, R., Bhakki, M., Khanna, R. C., & Friedman, D. S.. (2021). Prevalence and risk factors for visual impairment among elderly residents in "homes for the aged" in India: the Hyderabad Ocular Morbidity in Elderly Study (HOMES). *British Journal of Ophthalmology*, 105, 32–36. https://doi.org/10.1136/bjophthalmol-2019-315678

THE EARS

Anatomy and Physiology

Ears are sensory organs serving two primary functions: hearing and balance. Speech development and preservation are dependent on hearing, as is communication. The ability to have balance or equilibrium is also dependent on ear function; this includes having coordination, and ability to change positions and move safely.

The ear is divided into three areas: the outer, middle, and inner sections (Fig. 41-9). Sound is perceived because of a chain reaction involving all three areas of the ear. The inner ear also helps maintain balance. The outer ear and the middle ear transmit and amplify sound, referred to as *conductive hearing*. The inner ear's receptive organs are stimulated by the sound waves (hearing) and by head position or movement (balance). This is also referred to as *sensorineural hearing*. Sound is also conducted through skull bones to the inner ear. This pathway is not as effective as air conduction.

Outer Ear

The outer ear, or *auricle*, consists of the *pinna*, the fleshy external projection of the ear, and the *external acoustic meatus*, a 1-inch canal that extends to the *tympanic membrane*, or eardrum. The outer ear collects sound waves and directs them inward. The external acoustic meatus contains the glands that produce *cerumen*, a waxy substance that lubricates the ear canal, protects the eardrum, and helps prevent external-ear infections. Chewing and talking help to move cerumen to the outer area of the external acoustic meatus, where it is easily washed away. The outer ear transmits and amplifies sound as it travels down the ear canal, causing the tympanic membrane to vibrate.

Middle Ear

The middle ear is a small, air-filled cavity in the temporal bone. The *eustachian tube* extends from the floor of the middle ear to the pharynx and is lined with mucous membrane. It equalizes air pressure in the middle ear. A chain of three small bones, the *malleus*, the *incus*, and the *stapes* (collectively referred to as ossicles), stretches across the middle ear cavity from the tympanic membrane to the *oval window*. They move when struck by sound waves transmitted from the outer ear. When these bones are set in motion, the footplate of the stapes, which is very flexible, strikes the oval window, agitating the fluid in the inner ear.

Inner Ear

There are two sensory systems in the inner ear: the auditory (hearing) and vestibular (balance) systems. The inner ear, or *labyrinth*, consists of a series of cavities and canals that contain fluid. It contains the *cochlea*, which provides for hearing; the *semicircular canals*, which promote balance; and the *vestibulocochlear nerve* (*cranial nerve VIII*).

The fluid motion created by the vibrating stapes excites the nerve endings in the sensitive sound receptors of the *organ of Corti* located in the cochlea. The impulses are then converted to nerve impulses and transmitted along the cochlear nerve (or auditory or acoustic nerve) to the brain, where sound is perceived.

Nerve receptors for balance, motion, equilibrium, and spatial orientation are found in both the vestibule and semicircular canals (vestibular system). They transmit

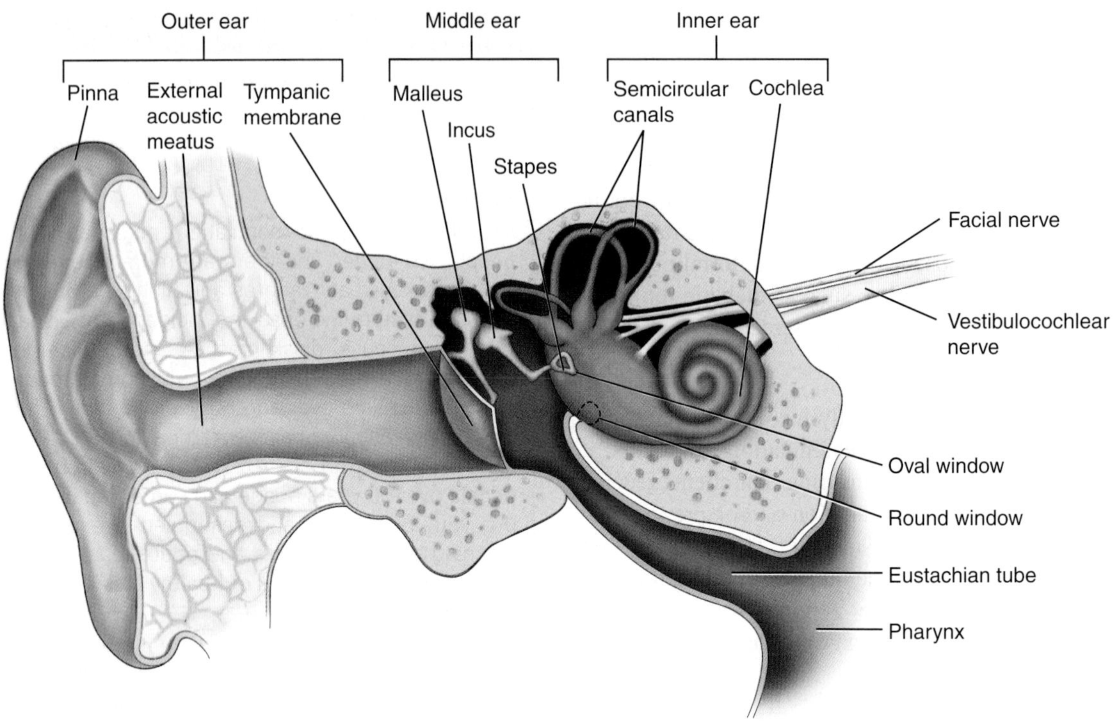

Figure 41-9 Anatomy of the ear. The outer, middle, and inner subdivisions are shown.

information about motion through the vestibular nerve, which joins with the cochlear nerve to form the eighth cranial nerve, the vestibulocochlear nerve. The sense of equilibrium is also reliant on vision and the stretch receptors in muscles and tendons, so that equilibrium is maintained or restored when head position changes or movement occurs. Response to body imbalance is fast and depends on reflexes: *vestibule-ocular reflexes* keep the eyes still while the head is moving and *vestibulospinal reflexes* permit the body to either maintain or regain equilibrium (Porth, 2015).

Assessment

The screening of hearing in adults is generally voluntary. General recommendations for asymptomatic adults include screening at least every decade through the age of 50 years and every 3 years thereafter. Although family practice primary providers assess and treat many ear disorders, they refer some clients to *otolaryngologists*, primary providers who specialize in the diagnosis and treatment of ear, nose, and throat disorders. An *audiologist* is a paraprofessional with special training in performing hearing tests, measuring hearing loss, and recommending methods for improving the perception of sound. Box 41-3 outlines the nursing assessment.

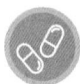

Pharmacologic Considerations

- Could impaired hearing, tinnitus, or vertigo be caused by a drug? Taking medications such as furosemide (diuretic), chemotherapy, salicylates (aspirin), and many antibiotics can have hearing-adverse effects. Medication reconciliation can discover if drugs are the cause of hearing loss.

Basic Auditory Acuity Tests

One general method is used to assess a client's gross auditory acuity. The method is referred to as the *whisper test*. For this test, the examiner covers the untested ear with their palm and stands 1 to 2 feet from the client's uncovered ear. They whisper a number or a phrase and ask the client to repeat it, providing several numbers to ensure valid test results. Another technique is to sit beside the client and bring a ticking watch toward the ear. The client should perceive the sound at the same time as the nurse, who is assumed to have normal hearing.

BOX 41-3 Nursing Assessment of the Ear and Basic Hearing Acuity

- Obtain client's appraisal of their hearing, including whether the client experiences tinnitus.
- Observe for actions that suggest a hearing problem such as leaning forward, turning the head, or cupping a hand to the ear to hear better.
- Document the use of a hearing aid.
- Ask client about allergies, a history of upper respiratory and middle-ear infections, high fevers, or exposure to loud sounds, because all these can cause hearing loss.
- Inspect external ear for signs of infection, such as swelling, redness, drainage, or evidence of trauma.
- Shine a penlight into the ear to grossly inspect the ear canal; straighten the ear canal by gently pulling the ear up and back for an adult and downward and backward for small children.
- Palpate the areas in front of and behind the ear lobe for tenderness and swelling.
- Perform a basic hearing acuity test.

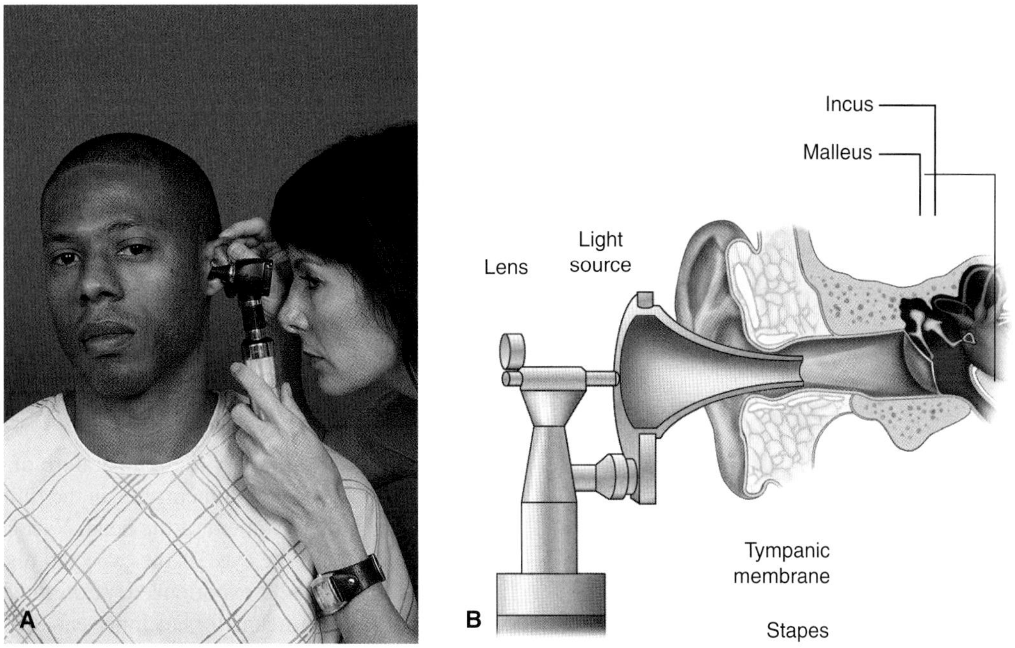

Figure 41-10 Technique for using the otoscope. **(A)** The examiner pulls the adult client's pinna up and back before inserting the otoscope. **(B)** Position of the otoscope in the ear.

Otoscopic Examination

An otoscopic examination involves inspecting the external acoustic canal and tympanic membrane using an **otoscope**, a handheld instrument with a light, lens, and optional speculum for inserting into the client's ear (Fig. 41-10). If normal, the canal appears smooth and empty. The normal tympanic membrane is intact, looks pearly gray, and transmits light. Excessive cerumen interferes with inspection.

Tuning Fork Tests

A **tuning fork** is an instrument that produces sound in the same range as human speech. It is used to screen for conductive or sensorineural hearing loss. A **conductive hearing loss** involves interference in the transmission of sound waves to the inner ear. **Sensorineural hearing loss** is the result of nerve impairment.

The Rinne test and Weber test identify types of hearing loss. For the **Rinne test** (Fig. 41-11), the tuning fork is struck, placed on the mastoid process behind the ear, and held there until the client indicates the sound is no longer heard. Immediately after that, the still-vibrating tuning fork is held beside the ear, and the client again says when the sound is no longer heard. Normally, air conduction beside the ear measures twice as long as by bone conduction through the mastoid.

The **Weber test** is performed by striking the tuning fork and placing its stem in the midline of the client's skull or center of the forehead (Fig. 41-12). A person with normal hearing perceives the sound equally well in both ears. If the sound seems lateralized to one ear, it suggests a conduction hearing loss in that ear or a sensorineural loss in the opposite ear.

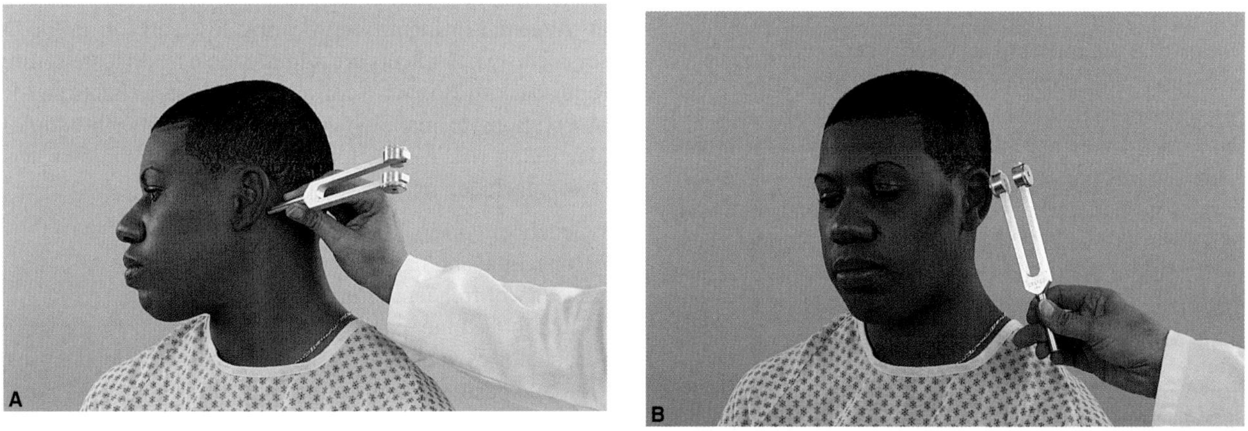

Figure 41-11 The Rinne test for both bone and air conduction of sound. **(A)** The tuning fork is first placed on the mastoid process behind the ear. **(B)** The tuning fork is then held beside the ear.

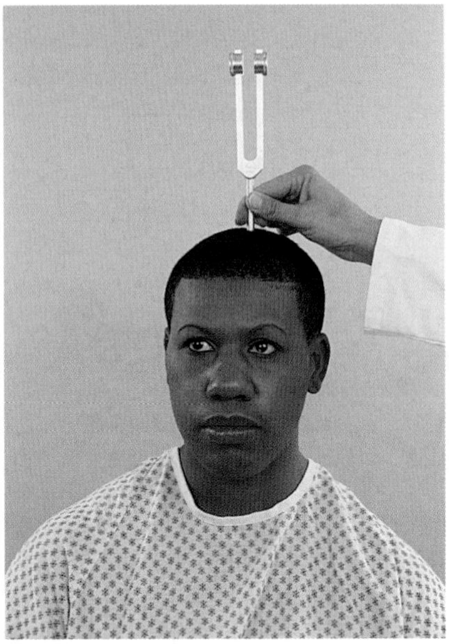

Figure 41-12 The Weber test for bone conduction of sound.

Romberg Test

The **Romberg test** is used to evaluate a person's ability to sustain balance. The client stands with feet together and both arms extended. The client closes their eyes. Swaying, losing balance, or arm drifting are abnormal responses. Because central nervous system lesions cause similar abnormal results, additional testing is needed to confirm an inner-ear dysfunction. For clients who are unsteady, this test may not be appropriate. For all clients, the examiner needs to be close by to prevent the client from completely losing their balance and falling.

Diagnostic Studies

Audiometry

Audiometry is done by an audiologist. Audiometric testing measures hearing acuity precisely. During the test, controlled intensities of sound, measured in **decibels** (dB), are projected to one ear at a time through a headset. The client indicates when the sound is heard. The lowest level of sound that normal individuals can first perceive is 20 dB; painful sounds occur at 120 dB. The sound of a jet engine would register around 180 dB. Hearing acuity is determined by measuring the intensity at which a person first perceives sound. Table 41-2 provides a description of hearing loss severity measured in decibels. There are two other aspects to audiometry—frequency and pitch. Frequency is the number of sound waves per second that come from a source—it is measured in Hertz (Hz)—or cycles per second. Frequency ranges from 20 to 20,000 Hz for humans. Normal speech range is 500 to 2000 Hz. Pitch refers to frequency; a tone of 100 Hz is low pitch and a tone of 10,000 Hz is high pitch (Hinkle & Cheever, 2014).

Caloric Stimulation Test

A **caloric stimulation test** assesses vestibular reflexes of the inner ear that control balance. Warm (40°C) or cool (25°C) water or air is instilled into the external meatus of each ear separately. The fluid alters the temperature of the temporal bone and creates convection currents in the fluid of the inner ear that simulate movement of the head. Nystagmus, a quivering movement of the eyes, is the expected response. Slight dizziness also may be experienced. A diminished response in one eye is significant for an inner-ear disorder such as Ménière disease (discussed in Chapter 43).

TABLE 41-2 Severity of Hearing Loss

LOSS IN DECIBELS	INTERPRETATION
0–15	Normal hearing
>15–25	Slight hearing loss
>25–40	Mild hearing loss
>40–55	Moderate hearing loss
>55–70	Moderate-to-severe hearing loss
>70–90	Severe hearing loss
>90	Profound hearing loss

Reprinted with permission from Hinkle, J. L., & Cheever, K. H. (2014). *Brunner & Suddarth's textbook of medical-surgical nursing* (13th ed., Table 64-2, p. 1886). Wolters Kluwer Health/Lippincott Williams & Wilkins.

Electronystagmography

Electronystagmography is a more precise method for evaluating vestibular function, the mechanisms that facilitate maintaining balance. It is performed in conjunction with caloric stimulation. When the fluid is instilled within the ear, a machine records the duration and velocity of the eye movements with electrodes attached superiorly, inferiorly, and laterally about the eyes.

>>> *Stop, Think, and Respond 41-2*

A client is having an assessment of balance. The primary provider tells you that the Romberg test is appropriate and will be performed. What is an important action for the nurse?

Nursing Management

Often, testing and care of ear function are done in outpatient settings. Assessment of ear structure and hearing function is done as screening in most health care settings, providing a foundation for further testing and referrals. Nurses can be instrumental in identifying hearing loss early in initial assessments when clients are admitted to a health care setting. Refer back to Box 41-3 for questions to ask clients and for observations to make when assessing clients. In addition, identifying risk factors for hearing loss is important. Risk factors include:

- Genetic predisposition
- Congenital anomalies
- History of frequent or prolonged otitis media
- Fluid in the inner ear
- Loud noises, including sustained exposure to loud noise or short exposure to sound greater than 110 dB
- Ototoxic medications
- Viral inner-ear infections
- Impacted cerumen

KEY POINTS

- Eyes:
  - Ptosis: drooping upper eyelid
  - Proptosis: an extended or protruded upper eyelid that delays closing or remains partially open
  - Nystagmus: uncontrolled oscillating movement of the eyeball
- Diagnostic tests:
  - Ophthalmoscopy: examination of the fundus or interior of the eye. Discuss tests that are used for visual screening.
  - Tonometry: measures intraocular pressure (IOP) to screen for glaucoma—normal IOP is 12 to 22 mm Hg.
  - Visual field examination (perimetry test): measures peripheral vision and detects gaps in the visual field.
  - Slit-lamp examination: magnifies the surface of the eye and is used to identify disorders such as corneal abrasions, iritis, conjunctivitis, and cataracts.
  - Retinal angiography (fluorescein angiography): used to detect vascular changes and blood flow through the retinal vessels.
- Ears:
  - Conductive hearing loss: involves interference in the transmission of sound waves to the inner ear.
  - Sensorineural hearing loss: is the result of nerve impairment.
- Basic auditory acuity tests:
  - Otoscopic examination: involves inspecting the external acoustic canal and tympanic membrane.
  - Tuning fork: an instrument that produces sound in the same range as human speech. It is used to screen for conductive or sensorineural hearing loss. Rinne test and Weber test
  - Romberg test: used to evaluate a person's ability to sustain balance
  - Audiometric testing: measures hearing acuity precisely.
  - Caloric stimulation test: assesses vestibular reflexes of the inner ear that control balance.
  - Electronystagmography: a more precise method for evaluating vestibular function, the mechanisms that facilitate maintaining balance

CRITICAL THINKING EXERCISES

1. If a client reports having difficulty seeing, what additional data are important to obtain?
2. A 60-year-old client tells you that he has not had his eyes examined in 5 years. What should you advise him?
3. What cues can a nurse observe in an older client with possible hearing loss?
4. A client tells you that her hearing has diminished over the years. She has seen an online advertisement for a hearing aid that gave the ordering information. What is your response?

NCLEX-STYLE REVIEW QUESTIONS PrepU

1. A 65-year-old client asks the nurse why his vision is not as sharp as it once was. What is the nurse's best response?
   1. "It is not unusual for older clients to have dry eyes."
   2. "Older adults are more prone to eye infections."
   3. "The lenses in an older adult's eyes accommodate more slowly."
   4. "Vision in older adults gradually worsens with age."
2. A nurse needs to test a client's ability to read small print and asks the client to hold a Jaeger chart. Which of the following instructions is the most appropriate?
   1. "Cover one eye while reading the smallest print with the other."
   2. "Hold the chart at arm's length while reading the chart with one eye."
   3. "Read the bottom line of the chart from right to left with both eyes."
   4. "Recite the smallest print on the chart that can easily be read with both eyes."
3. What advice would the nurse give to a client who has just undergone fluorescein angiography? Select all that apply.
   1. Expect hives or rashes within 4 hours.
   2. Expect mild headaches for 24 to 36 hours.
   3. Expect red and swollen eyes for 6 to 9 hours.
   4. Expect skin to appear slightly yellow for 6 to 8 hours.
   5. Expect urine to appear bright yellow for 24 to 36 hours.
4. A new nurse is receiving instruction on the best method for screening a client's hearing. Which statement by the new nurse indicates that more teaching is required?
   1. "I will cover one of the client's ears and whisper a number while standing 1 to 2 feet from the client's uncovered ear."
   2. "I will repeat the whisper test several times to make sure I have valid test results for each client."
   3. "I will say something in a normal voice with my back to the client and ask the client to repeat the statement."
   4. "I will sit beside the client and bring my ticking watch toward the client's ear and ask the client when they hear it."
5. A nurse is testing a client's hearing with a Weber test. Which statement by the client confirms the nurse's assessment that the client's hearing is normal?
   1. "I am able to hear the same sound in both ears."
   2. "I cannot hear any sound in either ear."
   3. "I can only hear the sound in my right ear."
   4. "I hear the sound better in my left ear."

WANT TO KNOW MORE? There are a wide variety of online resources available on thePoint to enhance learning and understanding of this chapter.

Go to **thePoint.lww.com/activate** and use the activation code found in the front of this text to unlock these online resources.

42 Caring for Clients With Eye Disorders

Words To Know

astigmatism
cataract
corneal transplantation
diplopia
emmetropia
endophthalmitis
enucleation
glaucoma
hordeolum
hyperopia
hypopyon
intraocular lens (IOL) implant
keratitis
keratoplasty
macular degeneration
myopia
photophobia
presbyopia
retinal detachment
uveitis
visually impaired

Learning Objectives

On completion of this chapter, you will be able to:

1. Explain the different types of refractive errors.
2. Differentiate the terms *blindness* and *visually impaired.*
3. Identify appropriate nursing interventions for a blind client.
4. Discuss the nursing management of clients with eye trauma.
5. Describe the technique for instilling ophthalmic medications.
6. Explain how different infectious and inflammatory eye disorders are acquired.
7. Specify the visual changes that result from delayed or unsuccessful treatment of macular degeneration.
8. Differentiate between open-angle and angle-closure glaucoma.
9. Distinguish categories and mechanisms of actions of medications used to control intraocular pressure.
10. Identify a category of drugs contraindicated in clients with glaucoma.
11. Name activities clients with glaucoma should avoid because they elevate intraocular pressure.
12. Describe methods for improving vision after a cataract is removed.
13. Discuss postoperative measures that help prevent complications after a cataract extraction.
14. Give classic symptoms associated with a retinal detachment.
15. Discuss the care and cleaning of an eye prosthesis.

One in three Americans has some form of vision-impairing eye disease by 65 years of age (Age related eyecare, 2020). More than 32 million people in the United States have some degree of visual impairment (Adults with Vision Loss, 2020). Legal blindness refers to a vision loss level that is defined in order to qualify individuals for specific benefits, such as social security disability benefits. Generally, this means that the client's better eye has a visual acuity of 20/200 or less with the best possible correction. This chapter discusses common disorders that can affect the eyes as well as the accompanying treatment and nursing care measures.

IMPAIRED VISION

Refractive Errors

Emmetropia, or normal vision, means that light rays are bent to focus images precisely on the retina. In refractive errors, vision is impaired because the eyeball is either shortened or elongated and, therefore, light rays cannot sharply focus on the retina. Refractive errors include myopia, hyperopia, presbyopia, and astigmatism.

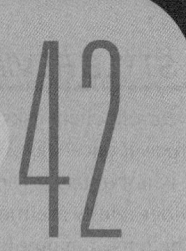

Gerontologic Considerations

■ Visual impairment curtails activities of older adults such as work, balancing financial statements, reading, watching television, and engaging in hobbies or other forms of recreation that are important aspects of personal identity. Nursing interventions include assessment of subtle specific changes and needs, referral to appropriate treatment, and referral to resources for visual assistive devices. Early identification and assistance with specific needs can help prevent depression, social isolation, and risk of falls.

■ Older adults should be encouraged to use the level and placement of lighting that best enables visibility for safety to navigate at night. Visual disturbances that occur concurrently with other comorbidities such as respiratory, renal, or cardiac concerns or pain increase the risk of falls. Objects, chairs, electrical cords, rugs, and foot stools are placed away from areas where the client walks, and assistance may be needed whenever the client is out of bed.

■ If an older adult has visual or arthritic changes or tremor, then the client should demonstrate self-administration of eye drops to ensure ability to place the drops into the eye in the appropriate amount.

Myopia is nearsightedness. People who are myopic hold things close to their eyes to see them well. **Hyperopia** is farsightedness. People who are hyperopic see objects that are far away better than objects that are close. **Presbyopia** is associated with aging and results in difficulty with near vision. People with presbyopia hold reading material or handwork at a distance to see it more clearly. **Astigmatism** is visual distortion caused by an irregularly shaped cornea. Many people have both astigmatism and myopia or hyperopia. Box 42-1 presents a summary of refractive errors.

BOX 42-1 Alterations in Refraction

- *Emmetropia (normal refraction)*: Parallel light rays are focused on the retina. Nearby vision requires contraction of ciliary muscle to bring object into focus. Vision defects are present if light rays converge in front of or behind the retina or if the eyeball is shaped abnormally.
- *Myopia (nearsightedness)*: Parallel light rays are focused in front of the retina as a result of increased anteroposterior diameter of the eyeball. Myopic persons cannot focus sharply on a distant object. As the individual moves closer to the object, the rays become more focused, and the focal point finally falls on the retina.
- *Hyperopia (farsightedness)*: The eyeball is abnormally short. Parallel light rays are focused beyond the retina. Focus on distant objects occurs through accommodation. As objects move closer to the eye, accommodation can no longer compensate, and images become blurred. The near point is abnormally distant.
- *Astigmatism (defect of the curvature of the cornea and lens producing refractive errors)*: Parallel rays are imperfectly focused on the retina. Light striking peripheral areas is bent at different angles and not focused on a single point on the retina.

Pathophysiology and Etiology

Refractive errors are inherited or occur as a result of surgical treatment of disorders of the cornea or lens. Myopia occurs in people with elongated eyeballs. Because of the excessive length of the eye, light rays focus on the vitreous body before they reach the retina. Hyperopia results when the eyeball is shorter than normal, causing the light rays to focus at a theoretical point behind the retina (Fig. 42-1). Presbyopia occurs because of degenerative changes. Presbyopia is caused by the gradual loss of elasticity of the lens, which leads to decreased ability to accommodate, or focus, for near vision. The loss of accommodation progresses gradually. Astigmatism results from unequal curvatures in the shape of the cornea.

Assessment Findings

People with refractive errors experience blurred vision. Some seek help for recurrent headaches caused by straining to see clearly. Refractive errors are detected with the Snellen and Jaeger charts. During retinoscopy, the vision of myopes (people who are myopic) improves when concave trial lenses correct the focusing power of the eyes. Hyperopes (people who are hyperopic) experience improvement when convex lenses are used. The amount of power needed to improve visual acuity indicates the degree of refractive error. The refractive error is not always the same in both eyes.

Medical Management

Refractive errors usually are corrected with eyeglasses or contact lenses. The lenses bend light rays to compensate for

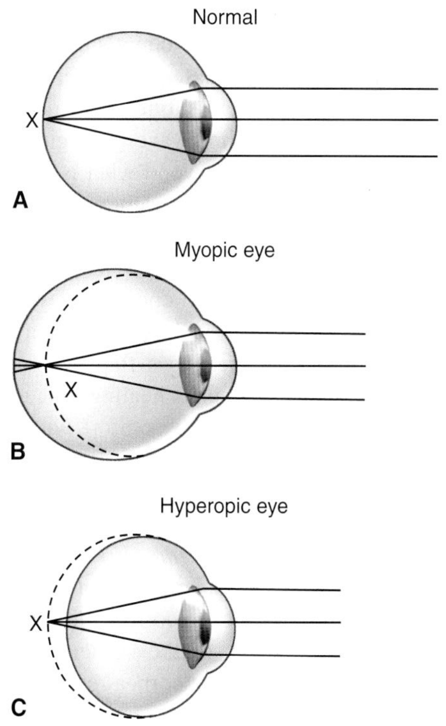

Figure 42-1 Eyeball shape affects visual acuity in some refractive errors. Ocular focusing of parallel light rays is shown in **(A)** normal, **(B)** myopic, and **(C)** hyperopic eyes.

the refractive error. Not everyone can wear contact lenses; people with a history of recurrent eye infections, low tear production, or severe allergic reactions are more likely to have trouble with them.

Surgical Management

A number of procedures are used to correct refractive errors. These include the following:

- *Incisional radial keratotomy (RK)*: Under local anesthesia, the eye surgeon reshapes the cornea by making incisions. It is made flatter for clients with myopia and more cone-shaped for clients with hyperopia, enabling light rays to converge directly at the back of the retina. This procedure is not always successful. Some clients report a worsening of their vision. When RK is successful, clients no longer need to wear corrective lenses.
- *Laser-assisted in situ keratomileusis (LASIK)*: This procedure is the most common surgery for refractive errors. The eye surgeon uses a laser called a femtosecond laser or a surgical blade (microkeratome) to create a thin corneal flap, which is gently folded back to expose the inner cornea. A cool-beam laser then resculpts the cornea; flattens the cornea for myopia; makes it more cone-shaped for hyperopia; and shapes the irregular corneal shape for clients with astigmatism. The flap is returned to its original position, and sutures are not required—it heals in place. Eye drops and/or ointments are used to promote healing. Vision generally is regained very quickly with little or no discomfort, but it can take 3 to 6 months for full stabilization of a client's vision.
- *Wave-front-guided LASIK*: This type of LASIK surgery uses computer imaging technology to create a three-dimensional "map" of the client's cornea, which is used to program the excimer laser for surgery. Wave-front technology can measure very subtle abnormalities in the surface of the cornea, enabling wave-front-guided LASIK to achieve vision correction beyond what is possible with glasses or conventional LASIK (American Academy of Ophthalmology, 2015).
- *Photorefractive keratectomy (PRK)*: This procedure uses an excimer laser to remove the epithelial layer (top surface) of the cornea. A laser sculpts the cornea to correct refractive errors without creating a flap. A bandage-type contact lens promotes epithelial healing and is used for about 4 days. There is some discomfort with PRK. Although LASIK is preferred because of more rapid recovery and lack of discomfort, PRK may still be used for clients with thin corneas.
- *Intrastromal corneal ring segments (ICRSs)*: The eye surgeon implants these semicircular pieces of plastic through a small incision in the cornea to correct mild myopia. The implant changes the shape of the cornea. If necessary, ICRS can be reversed, with the cornea resuming its original shape within a few weeks.
- *Phakic intraocular lenses (IOLs)*: Clients who do not have cataracts can have phakic IOLs surgically implanted in front of their natural lenses. Because this procedure involves a surgical incision into the eyeball, there is a higher risk of complications. This procedure is an option for clients who cannot safely have LASIK. It corrects more severe myopia or hyperopia but preserves the client's ability to focus for near vision.
- *Refractive lens exchange (RLE)*: This procedure is also referred to as clear lens extraction. An artificial lens is implanted in place of the client's lens (similar to cataract surgery). A multifocal lens can be implanted to correct all refractive errors. It does not have full U.S. Food and Drug Administration (FDA) approval. Currently, this procedure is generally done for clients with early-stage cataracts or severe hyperopia (American Academy of Ophthalmology, 2015).
- *Conductive keratoplasty (CK)*: This procedure, used only for clients with presbyopia, involves the application of heat (thermal refraction) to the periphery of the cornea to make it tighter and steeper. Clients generally experience immediate improvement without discomfort. Retreatment may be necessary as this is not a permanent correction.

Any procedure potentially provides complete correction of refractive error but can result in overcorrection or undercorrection. Other complications include decentered ablation, dry eye syndrome, epithelial abrasion, or infection. With RK, increased glare from microscarring of the cornea may occur. With LASIK, the most common procedure, complications include wrinkles in the flap, debris under the flap, a displaced flap, or infection or inflammation of the flap.

Nursing Management

Nurses, especially those in pediatric offices, industrial sites, community school systems, and public health clinics, perform screening examinations and refer clients to eye specialists. They are instrumental in teaching clients how to care for their corrective lenses and remove and clean contact lenses (Client and Family Teaching 42-1). In addition, nurses provide preoperative and postoperative care and teach clients about postoperative care at home. Client and Family Teaching 42-2 provides some postoperative teaching points for clients having LASIK or PRK.

Client and Family Teaching 42-1
Care of Eyeglasses and Soft Contact Lenses

The nurse emphasizes the following points in teaching the client and family:

For Eyeglasses

- Clean eyeglasses daily or more often if needed with warm water and soap or detergent or use a commercial glass cleaner.
- Rinse the glasses well and dry them with a microfiber cloth.
- Do not use paper tissues—the wood pulp from which they are made can scratch the lenses; soft T-shirt material is a better choice.

Client and Family Teaching 42-1 Care of Eyeglasses and Soft Contact Lenses (*continued*)

For Soft Contact Lenses

- Wear and replace contact lenses according to the prescribed schedule.
- Minimize contact with water, removing lenses before swimming or getting in a hot tub. Do not store or clean contact lenses with water.
- Wash and rinse hands well before touching lenses.
- Use a container that identifies the compartments for the right and left lenses.
- Remove a soft lens by sliding it onto the sclera and grasping it between thumb and forefinger.
- Use lens cleaner and eye drops recommended by your eye doctor. Follow directions for their use.
- Rub contact lenses with fingers, then rinse the lenses with solution before soaking them. The "rub and rinse" method is considered a superior cleaning method (American Academy of Ophthalmology, 2016).
- Rinse the empty lens case with fresh solution, not water. Let it air-dry. It is recommended that lens cases be replaced every 3 months. Do not use damaged or cracked lens cases.
- Take out the lenses and call the eye doctor right away if any of the following symptoms develop:
    - Significant vision changes
    - Red eyes
    - Eyes that hurt or feel itchy
    - Excessive tearing
- Do not use saliva to clean the lenses.
- Do not use solutions for cleaning lenses other than those that have been recommended.

Client and Family Teaching 42-2 Postoperative Instructions for Laser-Assisted In Situ Keratomileusis or Photorefractive Keratectomy

LASIK

- Understand that stitches are not needed—the corneal flap remains in place through natural eye pressure.
- Use antibiotic eye drops as ordered for up to 1 week to prevent infection.
- Resume normal activity within 3 days but avoid strenuous exercise for 1 week.
- Avoid rubbing eyes for about 1 week.
- Realize that healing occurs within 1 week but that it may take 3 to 6 months for vision to fully stabilize.
- Expect that discomfort may occur for 5 to 6 hours after the procedure. If necessary, use nonsteroidal anti-inflammatory drugs (NSAIDs) for relief.

PRK

- Use antibiotic and anti-inflammatory eye medications as ordered for 2 to 5 days after surgery.
- Understand that clear contact lenses are placed on each eye for 2 to 5 days to prevent infection.
- Understand that the epithelial layer begins to regenerate in 2 to 5 days but realize that complete healing takes 3 to 4 months.
- Avoid rubbing eyes for at least several weeks.
- Avoid strenuous exercise for 1 week.
- Use pain medication for 1 to 2 days after surgery if necessary. Pain fibers are located on the surface of the cornea.

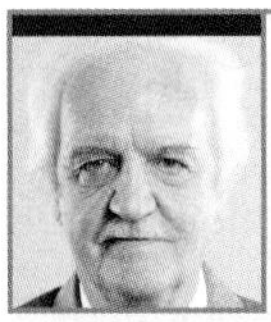

Clinical Scenario A 70-year-old client has recently had a significant loss of vision related to diabetic retinopathy. The client has been declared legally blind and will no longer be able to drive or engage in some activities independently. The client's 68-year-old wife is retired and in good health. They had hoped to pursue retirement plans, which included traveling and spending time with family. **What are important considerations for the care of this client to assist in their adaptation to diminished vision? See the following Nursing Process section.**

NURSING PROCESS FOR THE CLIENT WHO IS BLIND

Assessment

In addition to assessing the degree of the client's impairment, ask questions about how the client is coping with their visual problems. Grief is a normal response to being newly blind or having severely compromised vision. Anger and sadness are typical reactions as clients face their disability. Help and support clients during depression. It is therapeutic to acknowledge the grief rather than attempt to cheer clients. Another helpful approach is to express confidence that the client has the inner resources to deal with the adversity.

(*continued*)

NURSING PROCESS FOR THE CLIENT WHO IS BLIND (continued)

Diagnosis, Planning, and Interventions

One of the nurse's most important roles is to help the visually impaired client achieve independence. The following measures are appropriate:

- Introduce yourself each time you enter the room because many voices sound similar.
- Call the client by name during group conversations because the blind client cannot see to whom questions or comments are directed.
- Speak before touching the client.
- Tell the client when you are leaving the room.

In addition, the care of a client who is blind or whose vision is severely impaired includes, but is not limited to, the following:

Visual Impairment: Related to impaired vision
Expected Outcome: Client will independently complete activities of daily living (ADLs).

- Ask client's preference for where to store hygiene articles and other objects needed for self-care. *Involving the client promotes their control over the environment.*
- Keep personal care items in the same location at all times. *Doing so provides the client with the ability to locate toiletries easily.*
- Move food items from the tray to a larger surface area. *Doing so facilitates locating food and eating utensils without accidental spilling or dropping.*
- At mealtimes, describe where food is on the plate using the positions on the face of a clock. *This measure assists the client to identify the location of food.*
- Offer to open containers, butter bread, and so forth. *Allowing the client a choice facilitates independence.*

Injury Risk: Related to compromised vision
Expected Outcome: The client will remain free of trauma.

- Orient the client to the physical environment. *Orientation assists the client to remain familiar with the environment and to avoid injury.*
- Indicate the location of the signal cord for obtaining nursing assistance. *Doing so facilitates the client's ability to get help.*
- Keep doors fully open rather than ajar. *This measure helps maintain a safe environment.*
- Help the client to feel where the door to the bathroom is located. *This intervention promotes independence and prevents injury.*
- Remove chairs or objects that are in the client's walking pathway. *Doing so maintains a safe environment.*
- Instruct client to grasp your elbow and walk slightly behind and to the side when ambulating. *This positioning helps the client to feel secure and ensures safety.*

Activities of Daily Living Deficit: Related to decreased vision
Expected Outcome: The client will resume independent living.

- Discuss the client's network of support that can help with shopping, banking, and transportation. *This discussion assists the client to plan for meeting needs outside the home.*
- Offer a home health nursing referral for the purpose of assessing the client's needs for a home aide. *Home care nurses can assure the client has assistance with household tasks.*

Situational Low Self-Esteem: Related to impaired adjustment to the loss of vision
Expected Outcome: The client will redevelop a positive self-image.

- Call attention to tasks the client successfully performs without assistance if the client focuses on self-pity. *Encouragement promotes positive feelings about the ability to care for self.*
- Help the client clarify those activities that are essential and then develop a plan for mastering each one. *A plan reduces frustration and systematically helps client achieve short-term goals.*
- Review progress to nurture self-confidence, self-reliance, and improved self-image. *Reminding the client of progress promotes a positive self-image.*

Blindness

Definitions related to low vision refer to the *best corrected visual acuity* (BCVA). As indicated in Chapter 41, 20/20 is considered to be normal visual acuity. To pass a driving test, visual acuity of 20/40 in at least one eye is commonly required. *Low vision* is defined as a BCVA of 20/70 to 20/200. *Blindness* is a legal term for a BCVA of 20/200 or less even with corrective lenses. The term **visually impaired** is used to describe a BCVA between 20/70 and 20/200 in the better eye with the use of glasses. Many people who are considered blind perceive light and motion. People with severe loss of visual field are also referred to as *blind* and are not able to perceive light. The BCVA is defined as 20/400 to no light perception. Blindness can be congenital or caused by injury; a high fever that damages the optic nerve; or disorders such as cataracts, glaucoma, retinal detachment, macular degeneration, and tumors.

Medical Management

Vision is improved to its maximum extent with corrective lenses. Clients who are severely visually impaired or blind are referred to a rehabilitation center or other resource for supportive services. Blind or nearly blind clients are taught skills for independent living, how to use a cane for mobility, and how to read and write Braille, a system that uses raised dots to form letters of the alphabet and numbers. Some individuals use trained guide dogs. Also see Evidence-Based Practice 42-1, a discussion of teaching and earlier discovery of glaucoma.

Eye Trauma

Trauma or injury to the eye and surrounding structures can result in decreased or total loss of vision.

Pathophysiology and Etiology

Children and adults are subject to eye injuries from wind, sun, chemical sprays, direct blows to the eye, lacerations, and penetrating objects, such as fish hooks and bits of metal or wood. Cell and tissue injury causes an inflammatory response. Secondary infections may follow the initial injury. When trauma involves the cornea, scar tissue may affect the refraction of light. If the capsule that contains the lens is damaged, aqueous fluid and vitreous penetrate the lens, causing it to become an opaque cataract. Penetrating trauma can lead to **endophthalmitis**, a condition in which all three layers of the eye and the vitreous are inflamed; removal of the eye may be necessary. Orbital fractures are classified according to their location. Vision can be impaired and there can also be potential injury to the brain if the orbital roof is fractured.

Assessment Findings

Signs and Symptoms

The injured eye is painful or described as feeling "gritty." There is tearing, and the client usually tries to relieve the discomfort by squeezing the eyelids closed. The effort helps control eye movement and reduces the light entering the eye. Vision may be blurred. If the bony orbit is fractured, the eyes may appear asymmetrical, and the client has **diplopia** (double vision).

Blows to or near the eye usually result in swelling and bleeding into soft tissues with ultimate discoloration (black eye) of the area. On inspection, hemorrhage may be observed in the subconjunctival tissue. The eye may appear to recede into the orbit, and there may be a change in the normal size or shape of the iris or pupil. Adjacent lid structures may be lacerated, bloody, and swollen. Shining a penlight obliquely across the eye detects an obvious or obscured foreign body. Sometimes the upper lid must be everted to detect an object trapped beneath (Fig. 42-2). If treatment has been delayed, there may be purulent drainage in the conjunctival sac. A rust ring is seen in retained foreign bodies that contain iron.

Diagnostic Findings

Staining the surface with fluorescein dye identifies a minute foreign body or abrasion to the cornea. A slit-lamp examination provides magnification and light to visualize structures in the anterior and posterior segments. X-rays, computed tomography (CT), and possibly magnetic resonance imaging (MRI) help find a penetrating foreign body. An X-ray or CT confirms an orbital fracture.

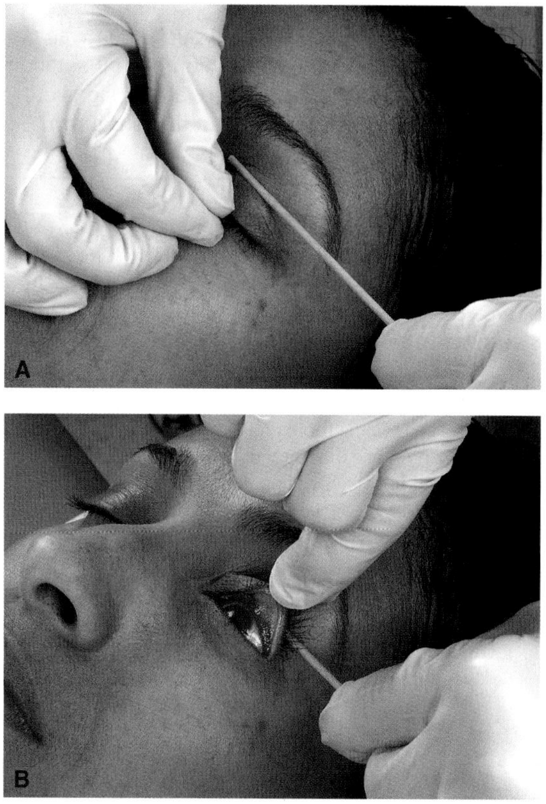

Figure 42-2 To evert the eyelid, **(A)** the examiner gently grasps the upper eyelashes and pulls downward, then places an applicator midway on the upper lid. **(B)** The examiner uses slight pressure to evert the lid over the applicator. The eyelid resumes its normal position when the client looks upward or the eyelash is pulled gently forward.

Medical and Surgical Management

Two types of ocular trauma require quick responses: chemical burns and foreign objects in the eye. Chemical burns require irrigation with tap water or normal saline. Foreign bodies should not be removed if they are penetrating. The eye should be protected from further jarring or movement of the object (American Academy of Ophthalmology, 2014). A metal eye shield, if available, or a stiff paper cup can be used to cover the eye following a traumatic injury until treatment is initiated by a qualified primary provider.

After emergency first aid is performed, the eye is anesthetized to ease examination. Antibiotic ointment or drops are instilled, and the eye may be patched, depending on the nature of the injury. Clients with blunt trauma are hospitalized to reduce the danger of intraocular complications. To repair a laceration of the eyelid, the primary provider injects a local anesthetic, and the lid margins are approximated with sutures. A cut on the eyeball, especially the cornea, is serious and requires immediate treatment. Surgery is performed if internal eye structures are damaged.

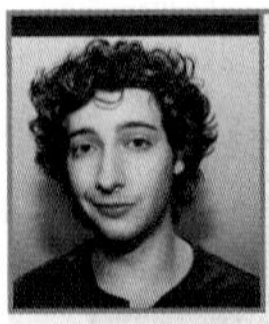

Clinical Scenario A young adult was mowing the lawn and had a small flying object strike their left eyeball. The client is seen in an outpatient setting for possible trauma to the eye. The client is holding their hand over their left eye. There are no signs of bleeding or an object protruding from the eye. **What actions by the nurse are important in this situation? See the following Nursing Process section.**

NURSING PROCESS FOR THE CLIENT WITH EYE TRAUMA

Assessment

Ask the client to remove their hand from their eye. Because the trauma does not appear to involve a penetrating injury, gently inspect the eye. Darken the room and direct a penlight at the eye to inspect for the presence of a foreign body. If none is visible, evert the lower lid and instruct the client to look up. Inspect the inferior conjunctival sac using direct vision or magnification. If this fails to locate a foreign body, evert the upper lid and direct the client to look down (see Fig. 42-2). If possible, perform a gross vision assessment. Prepare the client for examination with fluorescein dye to determine if a foreign object is still present and if the cornea is abraded.

Diagnosis, Planning, and Interventions

Obtain a brief history of the type or cause of injury from the client or a family member. If eye pain is severe, or the client cannot or is unwilling to permit an initial examination, loosely patch the eye and refer the client for immediate medical treatment. If a foreign body is present, avoid placing pressure on the eye that may push the object into the tissues of the eyeball. Provide instructions for home care and instilling eye medications if needed (Client and Family Teaching 42-3).

The care of a client with eye trauma includes, but is not limited to, the following:

Acute Pain: Related to trauma of the eye or surrounding structures
Expected Outcome: The client's eye discomfort will be reduced to a tolerable level.

- Implement emergency care, such as inspecting the eye for a foreign body, dimming bright lights, and protecting the affected eye. *These measures reduce pain from glare and movement.*
- Instill anesthetic eye drops under the direction or standing orders of a primary provider. *Anesthetic eye drops reduce pain. They must not be given repeatedly after corneal injury because of the risk for masking injury, delaying healing, and causing corneal scarring.*

Infection Risk: Related to disruption of corneal and conjunctival tissue
Expected Outcome: The client will not acquire a secondary ophthalmic infection.

- Wash hands before examining the eyes or performing any procedures about the face. *Hand hygiene prevents infection.*
- Use sterile solutions to irrigate the eye in nonemergency situations. *Sterile solutions reduce the introduction of microbes.*
- Instill antibiotic ointment or drops as prescribed. *Antibiotics prevent infection.*
- Do not use a container of ophthalmic medication for anyone other than the client. *This measure prevents cross-contamination.*
- Avoid contaminating the medication dropper or tube by holding the tip above the eye and adjacent tissue. *This position reduces the risk of infection and prevents trauma.*
- Change gauze eye dressings on a regular basis using aseptic technique. *Maintaining asepsis prevents the introduction and transmission of infection.*

Altered Health Care Maintenance: Related to client's desire to gain skill and knowledge to care for self at home
Expected Outcome: The client will demonstrate effective technique in the administration of eye medications and care of eye.

- Teach client to safely administer ordered antibiotic ointment. *Providing instructions for safe administration of antibiotic ointment gives the client the required information to carry out the procedure.*
- Inform the client to wash hands thoroughly before administering the eye medication. *Scrupulous hand hygiene prevents the introduction of infectious microbes.*
- Observe the client in the self-administration of antibiotic ointment to the eye. *This allows the nurse to assess the client's ability to self-administer eye medication and further teach the client if needed.*
- If the client needs a patch, instruct the client on changing the patch after the instillation of the antibiotic ointment. *A clean patch will promote asepsis and protect the eye from further trauma.*
- Inform the client to call the clinic if he or she experiences sudden pain or change in vision. *Such changes may indicate more trauma and will require examination and treatment.*
- Recommend the use of glasses with shatter-resistant lenses or safety goggles to prevent future eye trauma in situations where there is the potential for flying objects or substances that can injure the eyes. *Preventing injury promotes eye health and promotes the ability of the client to care for themselves.*

Evaluation of Expected Outcomes

Pain is reduced or eliminated. Trauma is minimized by immediate first aid measures. No signs of infection are noted. The client demonstrates effective management of the care required when discharged.

Client and Family Teaching 42-3
Instilling Eye Medications at Home

The nurse provides the following instructions for the client to instill eye medications at home:

- Wash hands thoroughly.
- Wipe the lids and lashes in a direction away from the nose with a moistened, soft gauze pad, paper tissue, or cotton ball. Use a separate item for each wipe.
- Pull the tissue near the cheek downward, forming a sac in the lower lid.
- Tilt the head slightly backward and toward the eye in which the medication is to be instilled.
- Do not allow the tip of the container to touch the eye.
- Instill the prescribed number of drops into the conjunctival pocket, or apply a thin ribbon of ointment directly into the conjunctival pocket beginning at the inner corner and moving outward.
- Close the eye gently.
- Wipe away excess medication that falls onto the skin.
- If there is a dressing, secure it to the face with tape and use an eye shield for additional protection, especially at night.
- Do not rub the eye, and visit an ophthalmologist or return to the emergency department if the eye is not completely comfortable within a short time.
- Keep all follow-up visits to check the condition of the eye and surrounding structures.

INFECTIOUS AND INFLAMMATORY EYE DISORDERS

Conjunctivitis

Conjunctivitis is an inflammation of the conjunctiva. It is commonly called *pinkeye* because of inflammation of the subconjunctival blood vessels (referred to as *hyperemia*) (see Fig. 42-3), which makes them more visible and causes the reddish or pink appearance. Some forms are highly contagious.

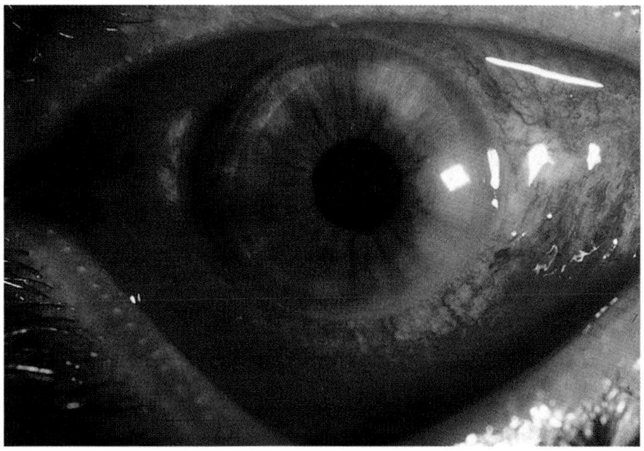

Figure 42-3 Conjunctival hyperemia in viral conjunctivitis. (Reprinted with permission from Hinkle, J. L., & Cheever, K. H. (2014). *Brunner & Suddarth's textbook of medical-surgical nursing* (13th ed.). Wolters Kluwer Health/Lippincott Williams & Wilkins.)

Pathophysiology and Etiology

Conjunctivitis results from a bacterial, viral, or rickettsial infection and can affect one or both eyes. The microorganisms most often are introduced by air transmission, direct contact with sources on the fingers, a contaminated face towel or washcloth, or transmission from infected lesions near the eye. Allergic reactions, trauma from chemicals, or foreign bodies in the eye also cause conjunctivitis. Allergic conjunctivitis affects both eyes. Exposure to allergens such as tree pollens causes production of the antibody immunoglobulin E (IgE) (see Chapter 33), which in turn causes the mast cells in the mucous membranes of the eyes and airways to produce histamines and other inflammatory substances. Untreated conjunctivitis, especially when caused by *Neisseria gonorrhoeae* and *Chlamydia trachomatis*, can lead to blindness (Mayo Clinic, 2015b).

Assessment Findings

Symptoms include redness, excessive tearing, swelling, pain, burning or itching, and, possibly, purulent drainage from one or both eyes. Clients may complain of **photophobia** (sensitivity to light). Infectious conjunctivitis generally starts in one eye but may spread to the other eye through hand contact. In infections with the herpes simplex virus, lesions appear on or near the lid margins. In severe cases, lymph nodes in the neck or throat area are enlarged.

Although a culture and sensitivity test can identify the causative microorganism, more often than not, the disorder is diagnosed by visual inspection and a history of exposure to someone with similar symptoms.

Medical Management

Treatment for bacterial conjunctivitis may include antibiotic ointment or drops, but often it will clear up without any treatment. There is no treatment for viral conjunctivitis, although an antiviral will most likely be prescribed for herpes simplex virus. Viral conjunctivitis generally runs its course in 1 to 2 weeks. Warm soaks or sterile saline irrigations are used to remove purulent drainage, reduce swelling, and relieve pain or itching. If an allergen causes the conjunctivitis, antihistamines and decongestants are prescribed.

Nursing Management

The nurse cleans the eye and instills or applies the prescribed medication. They provide health teaching so that the client can assume the necessary care independently. Because some forms of this condition are infectious, the nurse identifies methods for preventing its spread, including instructing the client to:

- Remain at home and apart from other people as much as possible while contagious.
- Use separate towels, linens, and other personal items.
- Wash hands often and thoroughly with soap and water.
- Use new tissue each time when wiping discharge from eye.
- Discard eye makeup items and do not use new makeup until conjunctivitis clears.

- Stop wearing contact lenses.
- For allergic conjunctivitis try to avoid the allergen(s) and wash clothes frequently.
- Return to the primary provider if discharge becomes thick and yellowish.

Uveitis

Uveitis is an inflammation of the uveal tract, which consists of the iris, ciliary body, and choroid.

Pathophysiology and Etiology

The cause of uveitis is not always identified, but one of the following may be the cause: eye injury or surgery, infections, or cancers such as lymphoma. Although the disorder occurs randomly, it is detected with some frequency among clients with juvenile rheumatoid arthritis, ankylosing spondylitis, tuberculosis, toxoplasmosis, histoplasmosis, and herpes zoster infection. Because some of these diseases are autoimmune disorders, uveitis may be an atypical antigen–antibody phenomenon (see Chapter 33). Complications such as glaucoma, cataracts, and retinal detachment are known to occur secondary to uveitis.

Assessment Findings

Symptoms include blurred vision and photophobia. Eye pain is experienced in varying degrees. The eye appears red and congested, and the pupil reacts poorly to light. In severe cases, a **hypopyon** can occur, which is an accumulation of pus in the anterior chamber behind the cornea. Uveitis is confirmed by its clinical appearance during slit-lamp examination. In severe cases, fluid from the eye may be extracted and examined. Angiography is used to determine retinal blood flow. Skin tests for primary disorders, such as tuberculosis, are performed to confirm or rule out this etiology.

Medical and Surgical Management

Treatment includes oral and topical corticosteroids (anti-inflammatory), mydriatic (dilating) eye drops such as atropine, and antibiotic eye drops. Analgesics are prescribed for pain. Sunglasses reduce the discomfort of photophobia. For the management of uveitis for some clients, a vitrectomy may be indicated to remove some of the vitreous. For conditions that are not resolving, a capsule is surgically implanted in the eye for the purpose of administering long-term, time-released corticosteroids. Clients may also be treated with long-term oral corticosteroids.

Nursing Management

The nurse instructs the client on the medication regimen and drug administration technique and emphasizes adherence to therapy. Failure to follow the medication regimen can result in serious complications. The nurse also emphasizes the importance of close follow-up during treatment. Other instructions are similar to those for conjunctivitis in the preceding section.

››› *Stop, Think, and Respond 42-1*

A 34-year-old client has had a cold for the last 5 days. Upon awaking, the client notes that the right eye is tearing a lot, is red, and feels like something is in it. The bright light in the bathroom causes the client to squint and cover the eye. The client visits the primary care primary provider's office. What instructions does the nurse need to include for this client?

Keratitis and Corneal Ulcer

Keratitis is an inflammation of the cornea. A corneal ulcer is an erosion in the corneal tissue.

Pathophysiology and Etiology

Trauma to the cornea (e.g., wearing hard contact lenses for an extended period or injury from an object that mars the integrity of the cornea), infectious agents (e.g., bacteria, fungi, viruses, parasites), or exposure to contaminated water can cause keratitis. Clients at risk include those who wear contact lenses and do not adhere to recommendations, those who are immunocompromised and/or are taking steroids, and those who live in a warm climate and are exposed to plant materials in their eyes. In addition, clients who have had prior corneal injuries are more vulnerable to developing keratitis. Secondary infections are common once the epithelium is damaged. Most clients experience severe pain because of the abundance of nerve endings in the cornea. Inflammation and disruption of the tissue interfere with the transparency and smoothness of the cornea, temporarily impairing vision. When and if scar tissue forms, visual impairment is permanent. The degree of visual change depends on the size and density of the corneal scar tissue.

Assessment Findings

Keratitis is associated with localized pain or the sensation that a foreign body is present. Blinking increases the discomfort. Photophobia, blurred vision, tearing, purulent discharge, and redness develop.

In addition to flashlight illumination and slit-lamp examination, fluorescein drops or strips provide evidence of corneal tissue erosion.

Medical and Surgical Management

Treatment is begun promptly to avoid permanent loss of vision. Keratitis is treated with topical anesthetics, mydriatics (drugs that dilate the pupil), and local and systemic antibiotics. Dark glasses are recommended to relieve photophobia. It is sometimes recommended that clients patch the affected eye. Treatment in the early stages of a corneal ulcer is the same as for keratitis. Once corneal scar tissue has formed, the only treatment is **corneal transplantation (keratoplasty)**.

Nursing Management

The nurse removes exudate that harbors microbes and instills antibiotic eye medication. They follow aseptic principles to avoid transferring microorganisms to the injured corneal tissues. The nurse advises the client who wears contact lenses to stop wearing them temporarily.

Blepharitis

Blepharitis is an inflammation of the lid margins, where eyelashes grow. It generally affects both eyes.

Pathophysiology and Etiology

One form of blepharitis is associated with hypersecretion from sebaceous glands, which causes greasy scales to form. This type often occurs in conjunction with dandruff of the scalp or seborrheic dermatitis found about the ears and eyebrows. Infectious agents such as staphylococci cause other cases. Some cases are combinations of both. Other causes can include rosacea, allergies, or lice or mites in the eyelashes. Blepharitis can coexist with conjunctivitis and lead to the development of hordeola and chalazia, which are discussed later.

Assessment Findings

The lid margins appear inflamed. Patchy flakes cling to the eyelashes and are readily visible about the lids. Eyelashes may be missing. Purulent drainage may be present. Clients may also experience watery red eyes, red swollen eyelids, photosensitivity, and frequent blinking.

The condition is definitively diagnosed by scraping or swabbing the lid margins and examining the scales microscopically, although that is usually not necessary.

Medical Management

Medications in topical form (drops or ointment) that treat the underlying infection are prescribed. Topical anti-inflammatories (drops or ointment) may be prescribed as well. Topical cyclosporine may be prescribed for blepharitis caused by seborrheic dermatitis, rosacea, or eczema (Mayo Clinic Staff, 2015a). The condition also improves with cleaning of the eyelids once or twice daily. Because seborrhea (excessive oiliness of the skin) of the face and scalp is associated with blepharitis, frequent washing of the face and hair is recommended. Baby shampoo is recommended because it does not cause burning of the eyes.

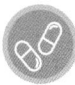

Pharmacologic Considerations

- Only preparations labeled as ophthalmic are instilled in the eye. Check the label of the preparation carefully for the name of the drug, the percentage of the preparation, and a statement indicating that the preparation is for ophthalmic use.

Nursing Management

The nurse reinforces the instructions for conscientious performance of hygiene measures. Many clients become discouraged because the condition takes some time to improve. Noncompliance contributes to the chronicity of the condition.

Hordeolum (Sty)

A **hordeolum** or sty is an inflammation and infection of the Zeis or Moll glands, types of oil glands at the edge of the eyelid.

Pathophysiology and Etiology

Staphylococcus aureus is the most common causative pathogen. The microorganisms multiply in the oil gland, which initiates an inflammatory response. A collection of purulent exudate accompanies the inflammation in the channel of the gland. As debris accumulates, it causes swelling and localized discomfort. Sties are common in clients with diabetes mellitus because their glucose-rich blood readily supports microbial growth.

Assessment Findings

A sty appears as a tender, swollen, red pustule in the internal or external tissue of the eyelid. A culture of the exudate, although seldom performed, identifies bacterial pathogens.

Medical and Surgical Management

Treatment of a sty includes warm soaks of the area and a topical antibiotic. Severe cases require incision and drainage.

Nursing Management

The nurse assures the client that treatment provides relief from pain and discomfort. The nurse explains how to avoid transferring microorganisms from the sty to areas of the body by cleaning the unaffected eye first and changing the washcloth, towel, and water after contact with the affected eye. The nurse also instructs the client to use separate fresh tissues, cotton balls, or gauze for each wiping stroke when cleaning exudate from the eye.

Chalazion

A *chalazion* is a cyst of one or more meibomian glands, a type of sebaceous gland in the inner surface of the eyelid at the junction of the conjunctiva and lid margin.

Pathophysiology and Etiology

A chalazion forms when the meibomian gland becomes obstructed and the release of sebaceous secretions is blocked. Consequently, the meibomian gland becomes inflamed and enlarged.

Assessment Findings

A chalazion appears similar to a sty, but the swelling in the upper or lower eyelid is not tender. As the chalazion matures, it feels hard. The enlargement within the eyelid causes clients to feel self-conscious about their appearance and affects their visual acuity. If a chalazion grows large enough to obscure the pupil or compress corneal tissue, the distortion of vision is similar to that caused by astigmatism.

Medical and Surgical Management

Treatment of a chalazion is not necessary if the cyst is small and does not interfere with vision. Warm soaks and massage of the surrounding area are prescribed to promote spontaneous drainage. If the cyst is firm, becomes infected, or interferes with the closure of the eyelid, it is surgically excised.

Nursing Management

The nurse prepares the client for examination and treatment by a primary provider and gives instructions on methods for carrying out the treatment measures. Some points to include when teaching clients with infectious and inflammatory eye disorders are as follows:

- Adhere to the full course of prescribed drugs to achieve satisfactory results.
- Wash hands thoroughly before cleaning the eyelids, instilling eye drops, or applying eye ointment.
- Do not rub the eyes; keep hands away from the eyes.
- Use a separate washcloth or towel if the disorder is infectious.
- Do not use nonprescription eye products during or after treatment unless approved by the primary provider.
- Eliminate the use of eye cosmetics or use hypoallergenic products and replace them frequently to avoid harboring microorganisms.
- Keep all follow-up appointments.

AGE-RELATED MACULAR DEGENERATION

Macular degeneration is the breakdown of or damage to the macula, the point on the retina where light rays converge for the most acute visual perception. The disorder usually occurs in both eyes, but the vision in one eye tends to deteriorate more rapidly.

Pathophysiology and Etiology

Age-related macular degeneration (AMD) tends to affect older adults. AMD is the leading cause of vision loss in clients older than 50 years of age (National Eye Institute, 2015a). Risk factors for developing AMD include race (it is more common in the White race), smoking, and family history. The National Eye Institute (2015a) states that genetic components have been identified, but as yet there is not a specific genetic test for AMD.

The two main types of AMD are referred to as the *dry type* (nonneovascular, nonexudative) and the *wet type* (neovascular, exudative). In the dry type, which is the most common, the outer layers of the retina break down over a long period of time, and characteristic small yellowish deposits (*drusen*) are apparent under the retina. When drusen form within the macula, the client gradually experiences a blurred vision. There are three stages defined for dry AMD:

- *Early dry AMD*: Clients either have small or very few drusen, and vision may not be affected.
- *Intermediate dry AMD*: The number of drusen is increased or there are a few large drusen; clients may have a blurred spot in their vision and need more light to do tasks that require close vision, such as reading.
- *Advanced dry AMD*: In addition to drusen, there is a breakdown of light-sensitive cells supporting tissue in the macula.

Dry AMD does not have any treatment or cure.

The wet type has two classifications. The first is called classic choroidal neovascularization. It has a more abrupt onset and is characterized by enlarged drusen. The underlying problem stems from an opening between one of the membranous layers of the retina and the choroid. Serous fluid seeps into the separation and elevates an area of the retina, like a blister. One or more blood vessels grow into the defect and produce a subretinal hemorrhage. After the bleed, scar tissue forms. The damage almost always is confined to the macular area, and vision loss can be severe. The second form of wet-type macular degeneration is termed occult choroidal neovascularization; it differs from the classic form in that the new vessel growth and leakage are less pronounced, resulting in vision loss that is less severe.

Assessment Findings

In dry macular degeneration, blurred vision is the first symptom of disease, which becomes more noticeable when clients try to read or do close work. In wet macular degeneration, clients experience distortion of vision, such as straight lines appearing wavy or letters in words looking broken. A client's perception of color may also be diminished. When the macula becomes irreparably damaged, clients compare their vision to a target in which the bull's-eye area of the image is absent (Fig. 42-4). The peripheral field, or side vision, is unaffected, but the client cannot see images by looking at them directly.

Fluorescein angiography shows pooling of the dye in the blister area. Optical coherence tomography uses fiberoptics to provide images of the ocular tissue structure. The Amsler grid (Fig. 42-5) is used to determine if the client has changes in central vision. AMD can cause lines on the grid to disappear or to appear wavy.

Medical Management

There are several treatment options for wet AMD:

- *Angiogenesis inhibitors*: used to inhibit the development and progression of abnormal blood vessel formation (angiogenesis); these medications are directly injected into the vitreous (intravitreal injection). Drugs include ranibizumab (Lucentis), pegaptanib (Macugen), bevacizumab (Avastin), and aflibercept (Eylea). These drugs are injected every 4 to 8 weeks. A transient loss of vision related to increased intraocular pressure (IOP), burning sensation, eye pain, and floaters may occur.
- *Photodynamic therapy*: uses an intravenous (IV) injection of a photosensitizing drug and a nonthermal laser application to reduce proliferation of abnormal blood vessels and eliminate the risk to the retina.
- *Laser photocoagulation*: seals the serous leak and destroys the encroachment of blood vessels in the area. It must be performed early to prevent the progression of the disorder.

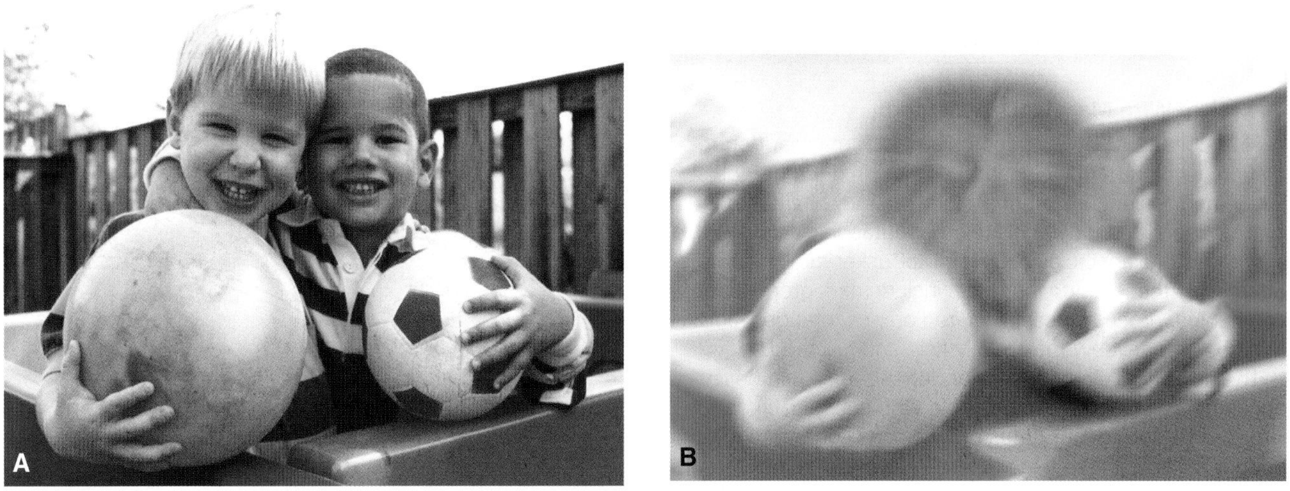

Figure 42-4 Visual loss associated with macular degeneration. **(A)** View with normal vision. **(B)** View with age-related macular degeneration. (Courtesy of the National Eye Institute, National Institutes of Health.)

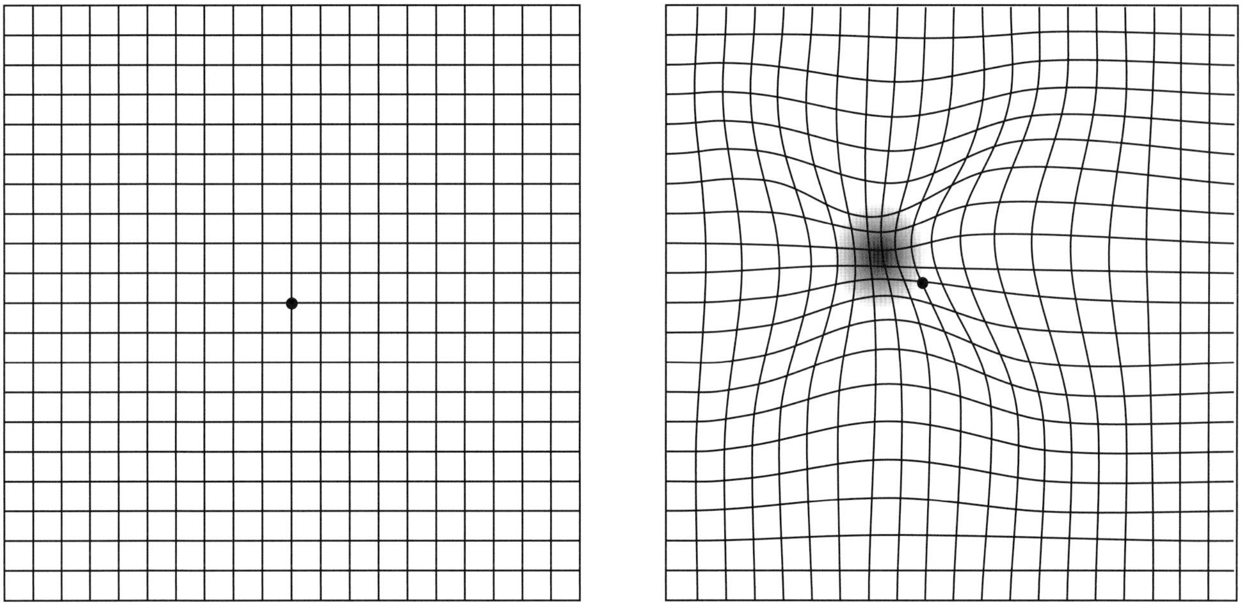

Figure 42-5 The Amsler grid is used to check central vision. **(A)** View with normal central vision. **(B)** What the grid may look like for someone with wet macular degeneration.

- *Macular translocation*: this is a surgical procedure for wet AMD. A **retinal detachment** is created, moving the retina to a healthier spot so that the macula is a slight distance from the area of choroidal neovascularization. Laser treatments can then be used without as much risk to the macula. Central vision is improved as a result.
- *Implantable miniature telescope (IMT)*: a tiny telescope inserted in one eye allows for central vision, whereas the other eye provides peripheral vision. Clients who have this procedure are at the end stage of wet AMD. They require some vision rehabilitation to adapt to the changes in sight.
- *Vitamin and mineral formulation*: a combination of vitamin C, vitamin E, beta-carotene (vitamin A), zinc oxide, and cupric oxide (copper) has been found to reduce the risk of developing advanced AMD and severe vision loss. Research has demonstrated that clients with intermediate AMD in one or both eyes or advanced AMD in one eye benefit from the vitamin and mineral formulation. Clients who are healthy or have early AMD do not benefit.
- *Diet*: clients with AMD are instructed to eat a healthy diet that includes two to three servings of cold-water fish (e.g., salmon) per week and daily servings of leafy green vegetables and a variety of fruits and other vegetables (Nutrition Notes 42-1).

Clients with AMD may be provided with suggestions for coping with visual impairment. Aids, such as magnifying glasses, may be of value, and high-intensity reading lamps have helped some people. The ophthalmologist may refer the client to a specialized center for evaluation and selection of assistive devices.

Nutrition Notes 42-1

The Client With Macular Degeneration

- Nutritional therapy to reduce the rate of macular degeneration development includes the inclusion of carotenoids (lutein and zeaxanthin), antioxidants (vitamin C, vitamin E, zinc, copper), and fatty acids (eicosapentaenoic acid [EPA] and docosahexaenoic acid [DHA]; McCusker et al., 2016). Sources of these phytochemicals include dark green leafy vegetables, broccoli, peas, kiwi, red grapes, oranges, corn, mangoes, honeydew melon, oily fish, and flaxseed.
- The risk of developing macular degeneration can be reduced by as much as half in people who eat spinach or collard greens two to four times per week as compared with people who eat these vegetables less than once per month.

Nursing Management

The nurse helps the client cope with loss of vision. For additional nursing management of the client with permanent visual impairment, review the information that accompanies the previous discussion of blindness.

GLAUCOMA

Glaucoma is a group of eye disorders caused by an imbalance between the production and drainage of aqueous fluid. When the drainage system is obstructed, the anterior chamber becomes congested with fluid and IOP rises. Optic nerve damage can occur as a result of the increased IOP. Although there is not a cure for glaucoma, the disease symptoms can be controlled, and optic nerve damage can be prevented.

Pathophysiology and Etiology

Glaucoma is the leading cause of blindness for people over 60 years old in the United States (Boyd, 2015). It is estimated that 3 million Americans have glaucoma, although as many as half are not diagnosed. Risk factors for being diagnosed with glaucoma include being over the age of 60; being of Black or Hispanic race; having a family history of glaucoma; and having conditions such as myopia (nearsightedness) and hypertension.

Normally aqueous humor fills the anterior and posterior chambers of the eye, flowing from the posterior chamber to the anterior chamber through the pupil (Fig. 42-6A). It flows through the trabecular mesh between the iris and the cornea, draining into the canal of Schlemm, a vein that circles around the iris, for return to the venous circulation. In normal eyes, the rate of secretion equals the rate of outflow and the IOP is between 10 and 21 mm Hg. IOP is a balance of several factors:

- Rate of aqueous humor production by the ciliary body
- The resistance to flow between the iris and ciliary body
- The rate of removal by the drainage system (trabecular meshwork and the canal of Schlemm; [Porth, 2015])

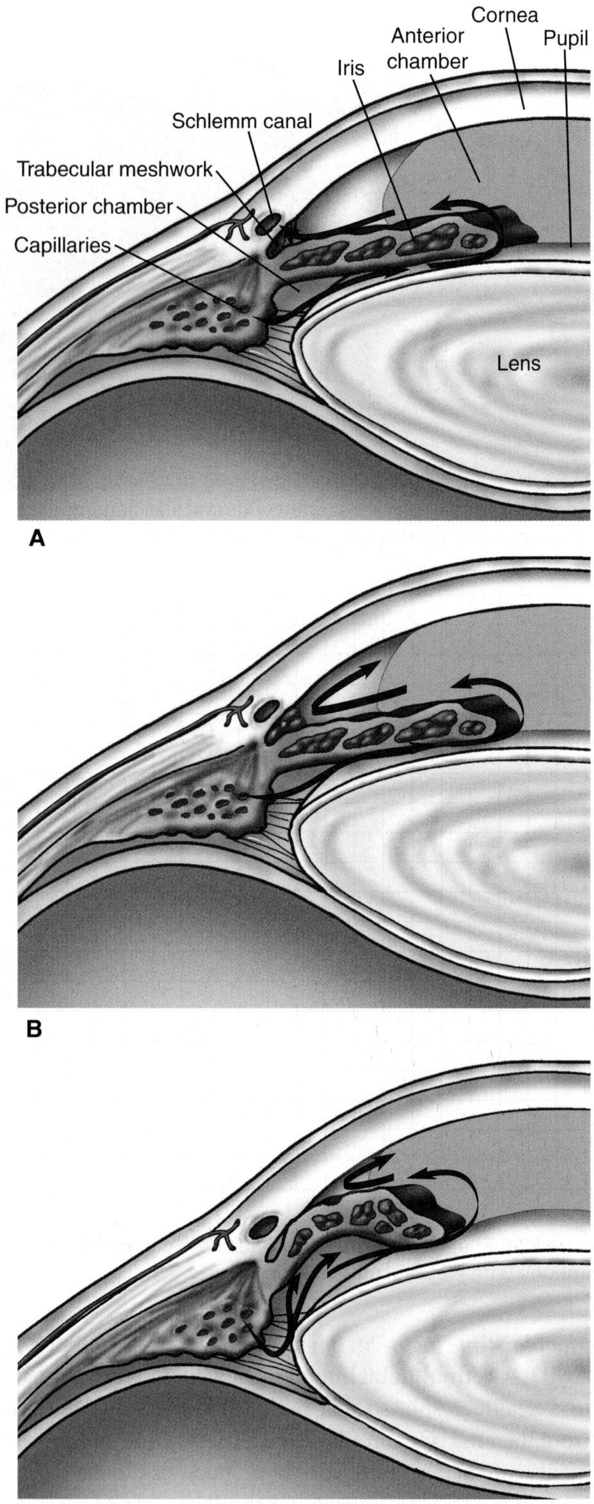

Figure 42-6 **(A)** In the normal eye, the pathway for aqueous humor to flow to the canal of Schlemm is wide and unobstructed. **(B)** In open-angle glaucoma, the flow is obstructed at the trabecular meshwork. **(C)** In angle-closure glaucoma, the movement of fluid is impaired because increased pressure in the posterior chamber produces a forward bowing of the iris, which narrows the approach to the canal of Schlemm.

For clients with glaucoma, the aqueous humor is impeded from flowing out properly. There are several types of glaucoma: open-angle or chronic glaucoma, angle-closure or acute glaucoma, normal-tension glaucoma, congenital glaucoma, or secondary glaucoma.

Open-Angle Glaucoma

Open-angle glaucoma is the most common form. Its onset is slow, and the client may not experience noticeable symptoms for several years. Open-angle glaucoma occurs when structures in the drainage system (i.e., trabecular meshwork and canal of Schlemm) degenerate and the exit channels for the aqueous fluid become blocked (Fig. 42-6B). As the IOP rises, it causes edema of the cornea, atrophy of nerve fibers in the peripheral areas of the retina, and degeneration of the optic nerve. This type of glaucoma develops painlessly, and visual changes occur slowly. When discovered, the ocular damage can already be severe.

Angle-Closure Glaucoma

Angle-closure glaucoma is less common, but the onset is very sudden, and immediate recognition and treatment are required to prevent blindness. It occurs in people who have an anatomically narrow angle at the junction where the iris meets the cornea (Fig. 42-6C). This deviation makes them vulnerable to angle closure when nearby structures protrude into the anterior chamber and occlude the drainage pathway. For example, an attack can be precipitated when the iris thickens in response to a mydriatic drug, by pupil dilation while sitting in the dark, or when the lens enlarges with age and bulges forward. This type of glaucoma is an emergency, and a delay in treatment may result in partial or total loss of vision in the affected eye.

Normal-Tension Glaucoma

Normal-tension glaucoma or low-tension glaucoma occurs in some individuals. IOPs are within normal range, but optic nerve damage and loss of vision still occur. *Congenital glaucoma* is seen early in life and is familial. *Secondary glaucoma* occurs following administration of some medications such as steroids, following ophthalmic infections, or as the result of systemic diseases or ocular trauma.

Assessment Findings

Signs and Symptoms

Clients with open-angle glaucoma may be asymptomatic, and the condition may not be discovered until the client has a routine ophthalmologic examination. When symptoms do occur, they are often ignored because they are not dramatic. Clients may complain of eye discomfort, occasional and temporary blurred vision, the appearance of halos around lights, reduced peripheral vision, and the feeling that their eyeglass prescription needs to be changed (Fig. 42-7).

In contrast, clients with acute angle-closure glaucoma become symptomatic quite suddenly. They experience severe headache and eye pain. The eyes become rock hard and sightless. Nausea and vomiting may occur. The conjunctiva is red; the cornea becomes cloudy and is commonly described as appearing "steamy." The attack is self-limiting, but with each subsequent attack, vision becomes more impaired.

Diagnostic Findings

The optic disc, when visualized directly with an ophthalmoscope or with retinal angiographic photographs, shows a cupping effect (widening and deepening). When the anterior chamber of the eye of a client with angle-closure glaucoma is inspected with a penlight or slit lamp, the angle between the iris and cornea is narrow. Tonometry reveals elevated IOP and reduced aqueous outflow. The visual field examination demonstrates a loss of peripheral vision; nasal and superior areas are usually impaired first.

Other tests used to monitor glaucoma, particularly the optic nerve and internal structures, include scanning laser polarimetry and optical coherence tomography. Ultrasound biomicroscopy evaluates how fluids flow through the eye angles. Pachymetry, using ultrasonography, measures corneal thickness, which affects IOP. A very thin cornea increases the risk of glaucoma. Gonioscopy uses special lenses to better visualize the eye structures, in particular, the drainage angle to determine the type of glaucoma. These methods not only establish a baseline but also determine whether glaucoma has progressed.

Medical Management

Treatment for glaucoma is aimed at achieving the greatest benefit at the least risk, cost, and inconvenience to the client. Although treatment cannot reverse optic nerve damage, further damage can be controlled. Treatment is most often begun with a topical medication at the lowest dose and then advanced to increase the dosage until the desired IOP level is reached and maintained. Clients with open-angle glaucoma use topical beta-blockers, such as timolol (Timoptic) (Drug Therapy Table 42-1). Beta-blockers decrease the flow rate of

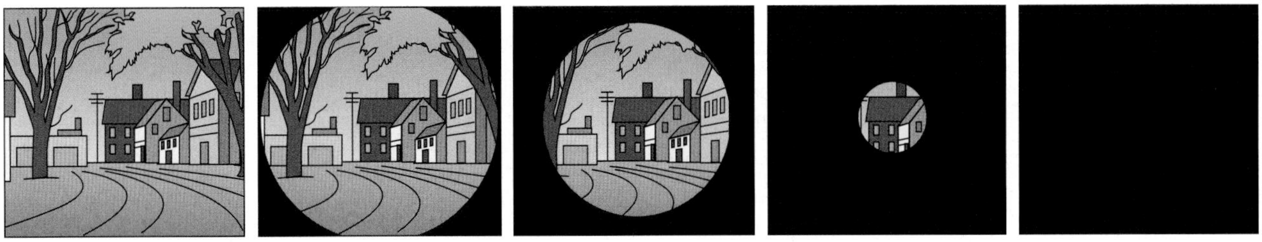

Figure 42-7 Gradual loss of vision from glaucoma.

aqueous humor into the eye. Prostaglandins such as latanoprost (Xalatan) and bimatoprost (Lumigan) that increase the outflow of the fluid in the eye and reduce IOP are also used to treat glaucoma. Other medications to control IOP may be given; as many as four topical medications may be used at a time. Miotics such as carbachol (Miostat) and pilocarpine (Pilocar) constrict the pupil. These medications pull the iris away from the drainage channels so that the aqueous fluid can escape. Other eye medications that are used for lowering IOP include echothiophate iodide (Phospholine Iodide), epinephrine, and dipivefrin (Propine). Acetazolamide (Diamox) and methazolamide (Neptazane), which are carbonic anhydrase inhibitors, slow the production of aqueous fluid. Oral medications, including carbonic anhydrase inhibitors such as acetazolamide (Diamox) and dichlorphenamide (Daranide), may be used to supplement or replace topical medications. However, side effects such as frequent urination, kidney stones, nausea, and depression are more problematic with oral preparations.

Surgical Management

When adherence to treatment is poor (e.g., client fails to instill eye drops as directed) or drug therapy no longer is effective (i.e., IOP fails to decrease sufficiently), or if the client develops severe adverse reactions to the medications, more aggressive treatment becomes necessary to preserve vision. There are a number of potential procedures that may be done to create accessory drainage channels, with the goal of promoting the drainage of aqueous humor and reducing IOP. Laser surgeries are used extensively in the treatment of glaucoma, depending on the type and severity of glaucoma. Table 42-1 describes some of the procedures currently available.

DRUG THERAPY TABLE 42-1 Drugs Used in Managing Glaucoma

Category and Common Generic (Brand) Drugs	Intended Use	Common Side Effects	Safety Warnings for Nurses
Alpha-2 Adrenergic Agonist			
Brimonidine (Alphagan-P)	Lowers IOP by decreasing aqueous humor production	Burning/stinging, discomfort, dry eyes	• Do not take with MAOI antidepressants • Confusion noted in frail elderly when used
Beta-Adrenergic Blocking Drugs			
Betaxolol (Betoptic) Carteolol (Ocupress) Timolol (Betimol)	Decreases the rate of production of aqueous humor and thereby lowers the IOP	Burning/stinging, discomfort, dry eyes, and eyelid erythema	• Use with caution when hypertensive beta-blocker drugs are used
Carbonic Anhydrase Inhibitors			
Brinzolamide (Azopt) Dorzolamide (Trusopt) Oral forms: acetazolamide and methazolamide	Inhibition of carbonic anhydrase in the eye decreases aqueous humor secretion, resulting in a decrease in IOP	Dry eyes, eyelid erythema	• Do not take if sulfa allergy
Prostaglandin Agonists			
Bimatoprost (Lumigan) Latanoprost (Xalatan) Travoprost (Travatan-Z)	These drugs act to lower IOP by increasing the outflow of aqueous humor through the trabecular meshwork	Darkening of the iris, conjunctival redness, stinging of the eyes, blurred vision	• Caution client about possible blurred vision
Combination Eye Drops Used to Treat Glaucoma			
Brimonidine/timolol (Combigan), dorzolamide/timolol (Cosopt)			
Less Frequently Used Drugs			
Miotics, direct acting, and cholinesterase inhibitors			
Carbachol (Carboptic) Pilocarpine (Pilopine HS)	IOP decreased by contracting the pupil of the eye (miosis), resulting in an increase in the space through which the aqueous humor flows	Periorbital pain, blurry vision	• Warning regarding difficulty with vision in evening or dark areas
Adrenergic Agonists			
Dipivefrin	Reduces production of aqueous humor and increases outflow	Eye redness and burning	• Systemic effects, including palpitations, elevated blood pressure, tremor, headaches, and anxiety

IOP, intraocular pressure; MAOI, monoamine oxidase inhibitor.

TABLE 42-1 Procedures to Treat Glaucoma

TYPE OF PROCEDURE	WHAT TYPE OF GLAUCOMA IS BEING TREATED	WHAT IS DONE
Selective laser trabeculoplasty (SLT)	Open-angle glaucoma	Uses low-level laser beams to selectively make openings in the trabecular meshwork that then open intratrabecular spaces. This procedure promotes drainage of aqueous humor. It may be safely repeated because much of the trabecular meshwork remains intact.
Argon laser trabeculoplasty (ALT)	Open-angle glaucoma	Uses laser beams to open the fluid channels of the eye, improving the drainage of aqueous humor. Generally, half of the fluid channels are treated first, in order to determine the effectiveness of the procedure, allowing for future procedures if required.
Micropulse laser trabeculoplasty (MLT)	Open-angle glaucoma	This newer laser procedure uses a specific diode laser delivered in short microbursts over a longer period of time to create the same effect as SLT and ALT but without as much tissue damage and residual postprocedure swelling.
Canaloplasty	Open-angle glaucoma	Canaloplasty places a microcatheter in the canal of Schlemm to enlarge the canal and promote improved drainage to reduce the IOP.
Trabectome surgery	Open-angle glaucoma	Trabectome surgery inserts the tip of the Trabectome (an electrocautery device), through the cornea to remove the trabecular meshwork. This increases the flow of aqueous humor into the drainage system.
Trabeculectomy	Open-angle glaucoma	Trabeculectomy involves making a small flap in the sclera and creating a filtration bleb or reservoir under the conjunctiva. The bleb looks like a blister on the cornea above the iris, but the upper eyelid usually covers it. The aqueous humor drains through the flap made in the sclera and collects in the bleb, where it is absorbed into blood vessels around the eye.
Aqueous shunt surgery	Open-angle glaucoma	An aqueous shunt or glaucoma drainage device is connected to a reservoir, which is placed on the outside of the eye beneath the conjunctiva through a tiny incision. Aqueous humor can now flow through the tube to the reservoir. The fluid is then absorbed into the blood vessels. When healed, the reservoir is not easily seen unless the eyelid is lifted and the client looks downward.
Laser Iridotomy	Angle-closure glaucoma	A laser creates a small opening in the iris to promote the drainage of aqueous humor to the drainage angle.
Peripheral iridectomy	Angle-closure glaucoma	This surgical procedure involves the removal of a small piece of the iris, providing access for the aqueous fluid access to the drainage angle (see image). The goal in treating closed-angle glaucoma with glaucoma medications and laser iridotomy is to avoid this procedure. It is not generally needed.

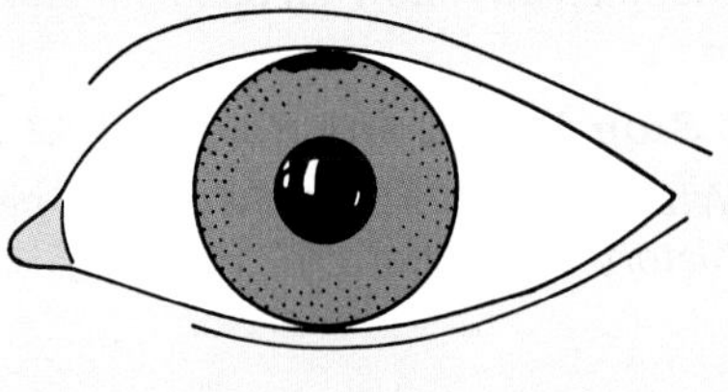

Appearance of the eye after peripheral iridectomy.

The particular laser surgery selected depends on the type of glaucoma and its severity. Lasers use a focused beam of light to create a very small burn or opening in the eye tissue, depending on the strength of the light beam. Laser surgeries are usually performed in an outpatient setting. During the laser surgery, the eye is numbed so that there is little or no pain. Procedures vary in length. Clients generally can resume normal activities within 24 hours.

The longevity of surgical results depends on the type of laser surgery, the type of glaucoma, age, race, and many other factors. Some people may need the surgery repeated to better control IOP. Medications are usually still needed to manage IOP, but possibly dosages can be reduced.

Nursing Management

The nurse determines the client's history of symptoms, the medications that have been prescribed, and whether the client is adhering to the prescribed medication schedule (or taking any other medications). It is also important to ask when the client was first diagnosed with glaucoma.

Acute angle-closure glaucoma is an emergency. The nurse refers the client for medical treatment immediately because vision can be permanently lost in 1 or 2 days. Severe pain requires analgesics. To promote the maximum effect from analgesic drug therapy, it is essential to limit sensory stimulation, such as loud noise, activity, and movement. The nurse informs the primary provider immediately if the client states that the pain has worsened despite treatment. While clients are incapacitated by their pain or if the disease results in loss of vision, the nurse assists with meeting basic needs. Mydriatics (drugs that dilate the pupil) must *never* be administered to clients with glaucoma. The nurse consults the primary provider if drugs with anticholinergic properties, such as atropine sulfate, are prescribed because the dilation of the pupil can further obstruct the drainage of aqueous fluid, raise IOP, and damage whatever vision remains.

Because glaucoma tends to run in families, the nurse advises adults to be examined regularly. Early diagnosis and treatment are essential for preventing loss of vision. Clients who are already diagnosed with glaucoma are encouraged to maintain close follow-up and comply with the medication regimen (Evidence-Based Practice 42-1). The nurse explains drug instillation techniques. Besides eye drops, some clients insert an ocular therapeutic system under the upper lid. An *ocular therapeutic system* is a small, thin film that contains eye medication. The film, which is replaced weekly, continuously releases the medication and eliminates the need for frequent eye drops instillation.

If a client has difficulty remembering when to take the medication, the nurse recommends a watch with a timer. For the client who does not understand the chronic and progressive nature of the disease, it is important to stress that glaucoma has no cure but can be controlled and that blindness caused by glaucoma is usually preventable. Self-care is important in managing the lifelong implications of glaucoma.

Other general instructions include the following:

- Obtain assistance from a family member, relative, or friend if you have trouble instilling eye drops.
- Avoid all drugs that contain atropine. Check with primary provider or pharmacist before using any nonprescription drug; preparations for cold or allergy symptoms may contain an atropine-like drug.
- Maintain regular bowel habits; straining at stool can raise IOP.
- Avoid heavy lifting and emotional upsets (especially crying) because they increase IOP.
- Limit activities that strain or tire the eyes.
- Keep an extra supply of prescribed drugs on hand for vacations, holidays, or in case some is lost or spilled.
- Seek medical attention immediately if pain or a visual disturbance occurs.
- Tell all primary providers that you have this disorder and the treatment prescribed by the ophthalmologist. Carry identification stating that you have glaucoma in case of illness or injury.
- Maintain all follow-up ophthalmology appointments.

Evidence-Based Practice 42-1

Teaching Clients About Glaucoma

Clinical Question

Does increasing awareness of glaucoma through teaching contribute to earlier diagnosis and treatment?

Evidence

Glaucoma is a disorder that is not detected or diagnosed until late in the process of the disorder, which means the eye could already have a large amount of damage. The symptoms of glaucoma are often not common knowledge or understood. A study was completed through a questionnaire, focusing on awareness of glaucoma and family history of glaucoma that might influence awareness in adult eye clients (Celebi, 2018). The results showed significant relationships between level of education and awareness of the disorder. The lower the educational level, the less likely adults were aware of the glaucoma disease and symptoms.

Nursing Implications

Nurses can use this evidence in their education when taking a history and assessment of clients over 40 years of age. Educating clients at the literacy level is important to make sure they have a clear understanding. Also, the nurse can enforce the importance of routine eye exams knowing the late detection may be after eye damage has occurred. A suggestion is that community education would be an effective and realistic public health plan to enhance knowledge and awareness of glaucoma, especially among individuals with a family history of the disease (Celebi, 2018).

Reference

Celebi A. (2018). Knowledge and awareness of glaucoma in subjects with glaucoma and their normal first-degree relatives. *Medical Hypothesis, Discovery & Innovation Ophthalmology Journal, 7*(1), 40–47. https://doi.org/10.4103/jhrr.JHRR_3_20

››› Stop, Think, and Respond 42-2

What is appropriate advice for a person with a family history of glaucoma?

CATARACTS

A **cataract** is a condition in which the lens of the eye becomes opaque. One or both eyes may be affected. If both are affected each eye may progress differently.

Pathophysiology and Etiology

Cataracts form on the lens, which is behind the iris and the pupil. The normal lens focuses light that passes into the eye, producing distinct and sharp images on the retina. With age and/or injury, the lens becomes less flexible and thicker, losing some of its transparency. A clear sharp image is impeded, and vision becomes more blurred.

Cataracts occur as a result of the aging process or are congenitally acquired, caused by injury to the lens, or secondary to other eye diseases. When cataracts occur in response to injury, they usually develop more quickly. Most cataracts result from degenerative changes associated with aging and develop slowly. A high incidence of cataracts occurs among people with diabetes and those with a family history. Prolonged exposure to ultraviolet rays (e.g., sunlight, tanning lamps), radiation, or certain drugs (e.g., corticosteroids) has been associated with cataract formation. In all cases, vision decreases because light no longer has a transparent pathway to the retina.

Assessment Findings

One of the earliest symptoms is seeing a halo around lights. Other symptoms include difficulty reading, changes in color vision (colors that look faded or yellow), glaring of objects in bright light, distortion of objects, blurred vision, poor night vision, and double vision in one eye. As the cataract worsens, visual acuity is so severely reduced that the client can only read the largest letter on a Snellen chart, count fingers, and distinguish movement. On inspection, a white or gray spot is visible behind the pupil (Fig. 42-8).

Under ophthalmoscopic and slit-lamp examination, the lens appears in varying stages of opacity. Some lenses are so cloudy that the examiner cannot see through the cataract to the posterior of the eye. Tonometry determines whether the cataract is increasing the IOP.

Surgical Management

Cataracts cannot be treated medically and are surgically removed. Surgery is generally done in outpatient settings with topical and intraocular anesthesia. Clients are awake and able to converse during the procedure. Clients who are highly anxious or agitated can receive IV sedation. For clients who have cataracts in both eyes, the surgery is done on one eye and the second one is done at least a few weeks later, and perhaps months later.

The most common surgical procedure is *phacoemulsification* (also referred to as *small incision cataract surgery*). With this method, a small portion of the anterior capsule is removed. A small probe is then inserted in the eye, and ultrasound waves are emitted through this device. Suction is used to extract the lens particles. When phacoemulsification is performed, most clients are able to return to full activity within a very short period of time. *Extracapsular extraction* is another method used to remove the lens. A longer incision is made, and the lens is extracted in one piece.

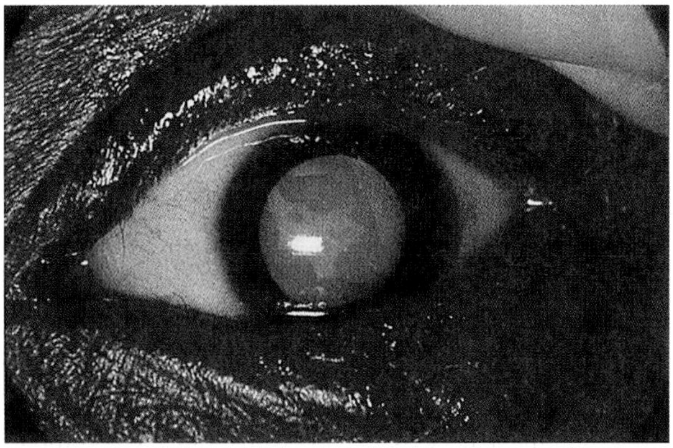

Figure 42-8 A cataract is a cloudy or opaque lens that appears gray or milky. (Reprinted with permission from Rubin, R., & Strayer, D. S., (Eds.). (2008). *Rubin's pathology: Clinicopathologic foundations of disease* (5th ed.). Wolters Kluwer Health/Lippincott Williams & Wilkins.)

After surgery, vision is restored with one of three methods: IOL implant (most common), corrective eyeglasses, or a contact lens. An **intraocular lens (IOL) implant** involves insertion of an IOL at the time of cataract surgery and is the most common method for improving vision. IOLs are inserted behind the iris. Ultrasonography is performed before surgery to determine the size and prescription of the IOL. A monofocal (single-vision) or multifocal lens is implanted and reduces the need for corrective glasses. When cataract eyeglasses are prescribed, the correcting lens for the *aphakic eye* (the eye without a lens) causes the client to see objects about one third larger than normal. These lenses also distort peripheral vision, and the client must learn to turn their head to see objects that are not in the center of vision. If only one lens is removed, the client must use one eye or the other to avoid seeing a distorted image. A coating is usually applied to the eyeglasses so that only the aphakic eye with a corrective lens is used.

A contact lens also can restore vision after cataract extraction. Advantages of the contact lens are that peripheral vision is not lost and objects appear about their actual size. A disadvantage is that the lens must be removed at night, cleaned, and reinserted daily, which can be difficult for an older client who has poor manual dexterity or a cataract in the other eye.

Clients may experience cloudy vision at some point after cataract surgery involving an IOL. The IOL is positioned on the posterior capsule or membrane, which is the back surface of the client's natural lens. This membrane may become cloudy, interfering with visual acuity. To restore the client's vision, a simple laser procedure is performed to open the membrane. Other complications of cataract surgery include infection, loss of vitreous, intraocular hemorrhage, retinal detachment, and displacement of the IOL implant. Loss of vitreous is serious because the vitreous body does not regenerate. Its loss, as well as hemorrhage, seriously damages the eye.

Nursing Management

Cataract surgery is usually performed in an outpatient setting. The client wears a protective eye shield for 24 hours after the procedure and then at night and during naps for about a week. Clients need to wear sunglasses when in bright light for at least 1 week. Eye drops, used several times a day, are prescribed for at least 1 week to prevent infection. There may be blurring for several days to weeks following cataract surgery. Clients may experience a small amount of eye discharge, especially when awaking. There could be some redness and a scratchy sensation for a few days. Clients need to notify the eye surgeon if they experience new floaters in their vision or increased redness, flashing lights, or change in vision. These are symptoms associated with retinal detachment, a complication of cataract surgery. Healing will be complete within about 8 weeks. However, clients with IOLs generally have functional vision soon after surgery.

The nurse is responsible for providing preoperative and postoperative care of the surgical client as well as discharge instructions, which include what the client must avoid for at least 1 week:

- Do not engage in strenuous activity and heavy lifting.
- Do not bend or stoop or do other exercises that potentially increase IOP.
- Do not immerse the eyes in water (clients may use a clean damp cloth to remove any eye discharge).
- Do not engage in any activity that potentially could cause dust or other particles to lodge in the eye.

Nutrition Notes 42-2 provides additional information.

Nutrition Notes 42-2

The Client With Cataracts

- Several studies have shown that vitamins C and E and beta-carotene can prevent or delay cataract formation. Five to 9 daily servings of richly colored fruits and vegetables are recommended for eye health.
- Recent research indicates that a low-sodium diet may help in preventing cataract development (Bae et al., 2015).
- Clients who have had cataract surgery should eat soft, easily chewable foods until healing is complete to avoid tearing from excessive facial movements.

RETINAL DETACHMENT

In retinal detachment, the sensory layer becomes separated from the pigmented layer of the retina (Fig. 42-9).

Pathophysiology and Etiology

In general, retinal separation is associated with a hole or tear in the retina caused by stretching or degenerative changes.

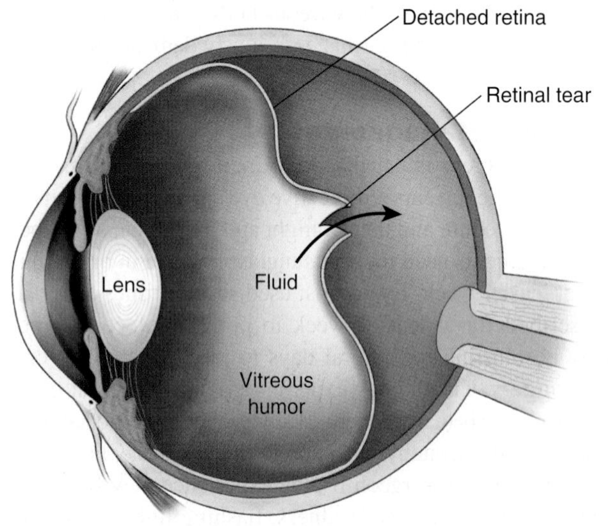

Figure 42-9 Retinal detachment.

Retinal detachment may follow a sudden blow, penetrating injury, or eye surgery. Tumors, hemorrhage in front of or behind the retina, and loss of vitreous fluid are particularly likely to lead to retinal detachment. This condition may also be a complication of other disorders, such as advanced diabetic changes in the retina. In many instances, the cause of retinal detachment is unknown. Retinal separation is more common after 40 years of age.

The separation of the two layers of the retina deprives the sensory layer of its blood supply. Vision is lost in the affected area because the sensory layer no longer can receive visual stimuli. Vitreous fluid moves between the separated layers of the retina, holding the layers apart and causing further separation.

Three types of retinal detachment have been identified:

- *Rhegmatogenous*: Fluid moves under the retina through a tear and separates it from the pigmented layer; this is the most common form.
- *Tractional*: Tension or a pulling force causes scar tissue to form on the retina's surface and eventually the retina separates from the pigmented layer.
- *Exudative*: Fluid moves under the retina secondary to inflammatory disorders or injury to the eye; there are no tears in the retina, macular degeneration, or uveitis.

Assessment Findings

Many clients notice definite gaps in their vision or blind spots. They describe the sensation of a curtain being drawn over their field of vision, and they often see flashes of light. Seeing spots, "cobwebs," or moving particles in one's field of vision, called *floaters*, is common. Complete loss of vision may occur in the affected eye. The condition is not painful, but clients are usually extremely apprehensive. When the retina is inspected with an ophthalmoscope, the tissue appears gray in the detached area.

Surgical Management

Surgical interventions for retinal reattachment include laser surgery, cryopexy, diathermy, retinopexy, and scleral buckling. The method chosen depends on the extent of detachment.

Several procedures are used for small tears or holes. *Laser surgery* (photocoagulation) involves making small burns around the tear to attach the retina back in place. The exudate that forms between the retina and choroid results in adhesion of the retina to the choroid. *Cryopexy* (freezing) involves the application of a supercooled probe to the tear, assisting the retina to reattach. *Diathermy* uses electric current to heat the tissue around the tear.

Pneumatic retinopexy is a less invasive method used to repair larger retinal tears. Methods described previously are used to seal the tear. A gas bubble is then injected within the vitreous to push the detached retina against the sclera. The gas bubble expands at first but then disappears within 2 to 6 weeks. A disadvantage of this procedure is that the client may have to position themselves in a facedown position for

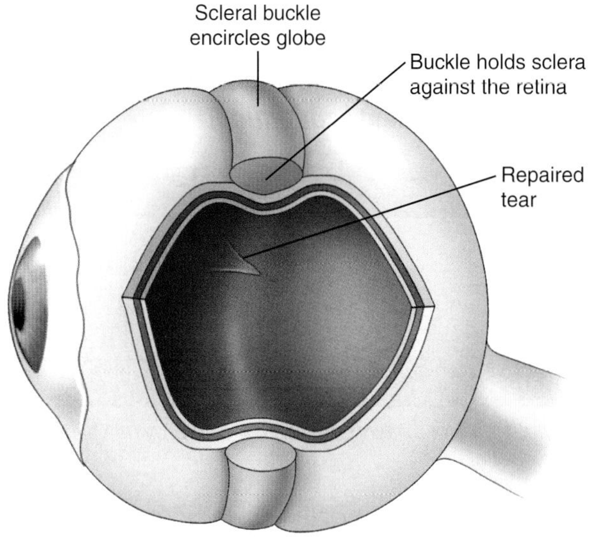

Figure 42-10 Scleral buckle.

a certain period of time each day for 7 to 10 days following the procedure. However, it is simpler and less expensive than other surgical procedures.

Scleral buckling (indenting of the surface of the eye) is a surgical procedure in which a tiny synthetic band is attached outside the eyeball to lightly push the wall of the eye against the detached retina (Fig. 42-10). Sometimes a vitrectomy, in which the vitreous is removed and replaced by gas to help reattach the retina, is also performed. As healing occurs, the eye produces fluid that fills the eye and takes the place of the gas. With both scleral buckling and vitrectomy, the use of laser or cryopexy "welds" the retina back in place.

Nursing Management

Anyone with a sudden loss of vision is referred immediately for examination by a primary provider. Clients are kept on bed rest and sometimes positioned on their side, with the affected eye in dependent position (e.g., if the tear is on the left side, the client will lie on their left side), until surgery is performed. Sedation may be ordered. The eyes are patched and covered with an eye shield. Mydriatic eye drops are instilled as ordered to dilate the pupil and facilitate further examination of the retina.

If surgery is performed, the client is kept on bed rest with position restrictions for several days. The head may be immobilized. The client is not turned or moved without orders. If an air bubble is instilled to promote contact between the retina and sclera, the client is positioned with the face parallel to the floor so that the bubble floats to the posterior of the eye. If floaters are still seen after the eye heals, the nurse can tell the client that they eventually become absorbed or settle to the inferior floor of the eye, out of the line of vision. For additional postoperative nursing management, see Nursing Care Plan 42-1.

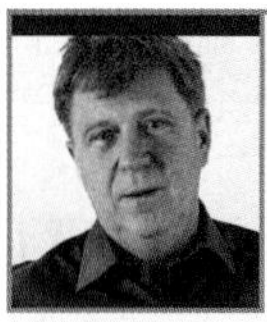

Clinical Scenario A 60-year-old client experienced flashing lights and a sensation that a curtain was drawn over their field of vision. The client is seen in the ophthalmologist's office and diagnosed with a retinal detachment. He has a scleral buckle procedure several hours later to repair the tear. **What are important considerations for this client's care in the postoperative period? See Nursing Care Plan 42-1.**

NURSING CARE PLAN 42-1 Postoperative Management of the Client Undergoing a Scleral Buckle Procedure for a Retinal Detachment

Assessment

Clients having any kind of eye surgery require the usual preoperative care. Frequently, they have surgery in ambulatory care settings, and so preoperative assessments may be done before the day of surgery. Preoperative vital signs provide a baseline for postoperative monitoring.

Because this client is having a scleral buckle procedure, it is important to ask about scheduled and other medications the client takes. Check to ensure that instructions (if applicable) about withholding any medications before surgery were followed. Examples include the following:

- Anticoagulation therapy withheld as ordered. For example, if the client takes warfarin (Coumadin), a prothrombin time of 1.5 is the desired level before surgery.
- Aspirin withheld for 5 to 7 days.
- NSAIDs withheld for 3 to 5 days.

In addition, check the postoperative orders and administer eye drops as ordered.

RC of Ophthalmic Hemorrhage or Increased Intraocular Pressure (IOP)

Expected Outcome. Bleeding and IOP will be managed and minimized.

Interventions	Rationales
Report sudden, intense, and persistent pain immediately.	*Pain may indicate hemorrhage or increased IOP, which may require emergency surgery.*
Instruct client to avoid coughing, vomiting, straining at stool, bending forward, or lifting anything heavier than 5 lb.	*Avoiding these activities prevents the IOP from rising.*

(*continued*)

NURSING CARE PLAN 42-1 Postoperative Management of the Client Undergoing a Scleral Buckle Procedure for a Retinal Detachment (*continued*)

Evaluation of Expected Outcome

Client experiences no complications.

Nursing Diagnosis. **Acute Pain** related to surgery

Expected Outcome. Client will experience little or no pain or discomfort.

Interventions	Rationales
Although postoperative discomfort is usually manageable, acknowledge the client's discomfort and administer prescribed analgesic that is appropriate for the level of pain.	*Acknowledging and treating the client's pain provide validation and pain relief.*
Keep room lights dim. Provide dark glasses if light causes discomfort.	*These measures reduce eye sensitivity to light.*
Use a clean cloth rinsed in very warm water (not scalding) as a gentle compress over the affected eye for mild discomfort.	*This measure promotes increased comfort.*

Evaluation of Expected Outcome

Client reports little or no pain.

Nursing Diagnosis. **Infection Risk** related to impaired tissue integrity

Expected Outcome. The incised tissue will heal without evidence of infection.

Interventions	Rationales
Perform conscientious hand washing before an eye assessment or treatment procedure.	*Consistent and meticulous hand washing remains the primary method to reduce or prevent the transmission of microorganisms.*
Follow principles of asepsis when cleaning the eye or reapplying a clean shield or warm compress.	*Asepsis prevents infection of the operative site.*
Keep the tips of all medication applicators clean.	*Doing so prevents contamination of equipment and prevents infection of the operative site.*
Report any yellow and/or foul-smelling drainage to surgeon.	*Some watery drainage and mucus are expected postoperatively, but yellow and/or foul-smelling drainage is indicative of an infection.*

Evaluation of Expected Outcome

The eye heals without evidence of redness, swelling, or unusual drainage.

Nursing Diagnosis. **Injury Risk** related to compromised vision and surgical procedure

Expected Outcome. Client's safety and vision will be maintained.

Interventions	Rationales
While client is in the postoperative unit, raise side rails and identify the location of the signal device.	*These measures provide client with security and orient the client as to how to get needed assistance.*
Encourage client to use a dim light or night light in the room after sundown.	*Total darkness presents safety challenges to the visually compromised client. Minimal light provides a light source and prevents injury.*
Apply a shield over the patched eye for at least 3 weeks at night.	*The shield provides additional protection and prevents client from rubbing or accidentally poking the eye or applying any pressure to the eye.*

NURSING CARE PLAN 42-1 Postoperative Management of the Client Undergoing a Scleral Buckle Procedure for a Retinal Detachment (*continued*)

Shower and wash hair carefully. Do not scrub vigorously and avoid getting soap in the eye. If shield is worn in the shower, replace it with a clean dry one after the shower.	*Being cautious with bathing protects the eye from water and chemical irritants and avoids injuring the eye.*
Position body according to instructions if needed to assist in holding the retina in place. This can be: • Facedown positioning—reclining: lie on stomach, hug soft pillows under chest and head, position head at an angle, direct eye gaze toward mattress. • Facedown positioning—seated: rest forehead on back of hand, position head parallel with floor, direct eye gaze toward floor. • Sitting up for meals and ambulating to bathroom is permitted as well as sitting for periods of time. • Do not lie on back. • Do not fly for at least 2 weeks until gas bubble is absorbed.	*Positioning assists in the healing process in that the gas bubble serves as a splint to hold the retina in place. Although specific positioning is required at all times, avoiding some positions is important to keeping the bubble in place until it is absorbed and the retina is more firmly attached.* *Gas is expandable at high altitudes, and thus flying needs to be avoided for at least 2 weeks until gas bubble is absorbed.*
Because vision will slowly improve following surgery, take care and do not drive or engage in activities that require visual acuity for a few weeks.	*Maintaining safety depends on activity restrictions that require visual acuity. It takes at least 6 weeks for vision to be restored fully, and often there are visual changes that will require corrective lenses.*
Maintain work restrictions for at least a month, especially if work requires straining or rapid activities.	*Heavy lifting, rapid activity, and straining increase IOP and cannot disrupt the surgical site.*

Evaluation of Expected Outcome

Client remains free of injury.

ENUCLEATION

Enucleation is the surgical removal of an eye. It is necessary when the eye is destroyed by injury or disease, when a malignant tumor develops (rare), or to relieve pain if the eye is severely damaged and sightless. Sometimes, only the contents of the eyeball are removed, and the sclera is left in place. Other times, the entire eyeball is removed as well as tissues in the bony orbit.

Medical and Surgical Management

When enucleation is performed, a metal or plastic ball is buried in the capsule of connective tissue from which the eyeball is removed. A pressure dressing is applied to control hemorrhage, a complication of enucleation. After the tissues have healed, a shell-shaped prosthesis is placed over the buried ball (Fig. 42-11). The shell is painted to match the client's remaining eye. The shell is the only portion that is removed for cleaning.

Nursing Management

The nurse observes the client after surgery for signs and symptoms of bleeding or infection. The client is usually allowed out of bed the day after surgery. When healing is complete, in about 2 to 4 weeks, the nurse teaches the client how to insert and remove the prosthetic shell. The prosthesis typically is removed before going to bed and inserted the next morning. The nurse instructs the client to hold the head over a soft surface, such as a bed or padded table, when removing or inserting the prosthesis to avoid damage if the prosthetic eye falls. The client should clean the shell after removal and keep it in a safe place where it will not become scratched or broken.

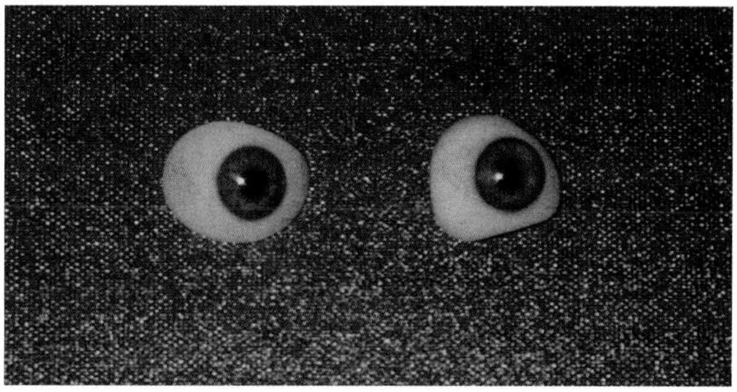

Figure 42-11 Eye prostheses. (*Left*) An ophthalmic ocular prosthesis. (*Right*) Scleral shell. (Reprinted with permission from Hinkle, J. L., & Cheever, K. H. (2014). *Brunner & Suddarth's textbook of medical-surgical nursing* (13th ed.). Wolters Kluwer Health/Lippincott Williams & Wilkins.)

KEY POINTS

- Vision:
  - Emmetropia or normal vision: means that light rays are bent to focus images precisely on the retina.
  - Myopia: nearsightedness
  - Hyperopia: farsightedness
  - Presbyopia: associated with aging and results in difficulty with near vision
  - Astigmatism: visual distortion caused by an irregularly shaped cornea
- Blindness: the inability to see; the condition of having severely impaired or absolutely no sense of sight
- Visually impaired or low vision: is a severe reduction in vision that cannot be corrected with standard glasses or contact lenses and reduces a person's ability to function at certain or all tasks; it is contagious.
- Uveitis: an inflammation of the uveal tract, which consists of the iris, ciliary body, and choroid
- Keratitis: an inflammation of the cornea
- Corneal ulcer: an erosion in the corneal tissue
- Blepharitis: an inflammation of the lid margins, where eyelashes grow. It generally affects both eyes.
- Hordeolum or sty: inflammation and infection of the Zeis or Moll glands, types of oil glands at the edge of the eyelid
- Chalazion: a cyst of one or more meibomian glands, a type of sebaceous gland in the inner surface of the eyelid at the junction of the conjunctiva and lid margin
- Macular degeneration: the breakdown of or damage to the macula, the point on the retina where light rays converge for the most acute visual perception
  - Dry type: the most common; the outer layers of the retina break down over a long period of time, and characteristic small yellowish deposits (*drusen*) are apparent under the retina.
    - Early dry AMD: Clients either have small or very few drusen, and vision may not be affected.
    - Intermediate dry AMD: The number of drusen is increased or there are a few large drusen; clients may have a blurred spot in their vision and need more light to do tasks that require close vision, such as reading.
    - Advanced dry AMD: In addition to drusen, there is a breakdown of light-sensitive cells supporting tissue in the macula.
  - Wet type: neovascular, exudative
    - Classic choroidal neovascularization: It has a more abrupt onset and is characterized by enlarged drusen. The underlying problem stems from an opening between one of the membranous layers of the retina and the choroid. Serous fluid seeps into the separation and elevates an area of the retina, like a blister. One or more blood vessels grow into the defect and produce a subretinal hemorrhage. After the bleed, scar tissue forms. The damage almost always is confined to the macular area, and vision loss can be severe.
    - Occult choroidal neovascularization: It differs from the classic form in that the new vessel growth and leakage are less pronounced, resulting in vision loss that is less severe.
- Glaucoma: a group of eye disorders caused by an imbalance between the production and drainage of aqueous fluid
  - Open-angle glaucoma: occurs when structures in the drainage system degenerate and the exit channels for aqueous fluid become blocked.
  - Angle-closure glaucoma: less common, but the onset is very sudden, and immediate recognition and treatment are required to prevent blindness. It occurs in people who have an anatomically narrow angle at the junction where the iris meets the cornea This deviation makes them vulnerable to angle closure when nearby structures protrude into the anterior chamber and occlude the drainage pathway.
  - Normal-tension glaucoma or low-tension glaucoma: occurs in some individuals. IOPs are within normal range but optic nerve damage and loss of vision still occur.
  - Congenital glaucoma: seen early in life and is familial
  - Secondary glaucoma: occurs following administration of some medications such as steroids, following ophthalmic infections, or as the result of systemic diseases or ocular trauma.
- Cataract: a condition in which the lens of the eye becomes opaque. One or both eyes may be affected.
- Retinal detachment: The sensory layer becomes separated from the pigmented layer of the retina. Three types of retinal detachment:
  - Rhegmatogenous: Fluid moves under the retina through a tear and separates it from the pigmented layer; this is the most common form.
  - Tractional: Tension or a pulling force causes scar tissue to form on the retina's surface and eventually the retina separates from the pigmented layer.
  - Exudative: Fluid moves under the retina secondary to inflammatory disorders or injury to the eye; there are no tears in the retina, macular degeneration, or uveitis.
- Enucleation: the surgical removal of an eye. It is necessary when the eye is destroyed by injury or disease, when a malignant tumor develops (rare), or to relieve pain if the eye is severely damaged and sightless. Degeneration.

CRITICAL THINKING EXERCISES

1. Discuss preventive measures for transmitting an infectious eye disorder.
2. Explain the preoperative and postoperative management for a client undergoing a cataract extraction.

3. A client has a family history of glaucoma and is concerned that they will suddenly go blind like their grandmother. What should you tell them would be reasons to seek immediate medical attention?

4. You are a new licensed practical nurse/vocational nurse (LPN/LVN) working in a primary provider's office that has a large percentage of older clients. Many of them use eye drops. After reviewing the procedure for administration of eye drops, outline what instructions you will provide to your clients.

NCLEX-STYLE REVIEW QUESTIONS PrepU

1. When caring for a client who is visually impaired, what are the best techniques for communication? Select all that apply.
   1. Avoid using words such as "see" or "look."
   2. Explain where items are on the diet tray.
   3. Provide a visual description of the room.
   4. Speak clearly and loudly to the client.
   5. Touch the client's arm when communicating.

2. A client arrives at an urgent care clinic and states that a chemical was inadvertently splashed in the right eye. What is the first action the nurse should initiate?
   1. Administer an analgesic as prescribed by the doctor.
   2. Ask the primary provider for an ophthalmic antibiotic.
   3. Examine the eyes for signs of redness and tearing.
   4. Flush the eye with normal saline solution.

3. A nurse is instructing a client about the eye drops prescribed for the new diagnosis of open-angle glaucoma. Which of the following statements indicates a need for further teaching?
   1. "I may experience difficulty seeing in the dark."
   2. "I should be careful about driving at night."
   3. "It is all right if I skip a dose every now and then."
   4. "My mouth may feel dry with this particular medication."

4. The nurse is assessing a client who reports a history of cataracts. Which of the following findings would indicate that the client is experiencing cataracts?
   1. The client's eyes are red and swollen.
   2. The client notices definite gaps in vision or blind spots.
   3. The client reports that the visual image is blurred or cloudy.
   4. The client states that tears flow incessantly.

5. The client with a detached retina undergoes a scleral buckling procedure. Postoperatively, which client problem should be the nurse's highest priority?
   1. Anxiety
   2. Boredom
   3. Pain
   4. Vomiting

WANT TO KNOW MORE? There are a wide variety of online resources available on thePoint to enhance learning and understanding of this chapter.

Go to thePoint.lww.com/activate and use the activation code found in the front of this text to unlock these online resources.

43

Caring for Clients With Ear Disorders

Words To Know

acoustic neuroma
American Sign Language
benign paroxysmal positional vertigo
cochlear implant
labyrinthitis
mastoidectomy
mastoiditis
Ménière disease
motion sickness
myringoplasty
myringotomy
otalgia
otitis externa
otitis media
otosclerosis
ototoxicity
presbycusis
speech reading
stapedectomy
tinnitus
tympanotomy
vertigo

Learning Objectives

On completion of this chapter, you will be able to:

1. List types of hearing impairment and the acuity levels for each.
2. Describe techniques used by clients with hearing impairment to communicate with others.
3. Give examples of support services available for the clients with hearing impairment.
4. Discuss the role of the nurse in caring for clients with a hearing loss.
5. Name conditions that involve the external ear.
6. Explain the technique for straightening the ear canal of adults to facilitate inspection and the administration of medication.
7. Discuss methods for preventing or treating disorders of the external ear.
8. Name conditions that affect the middle ear.
9. Describe nursing interventions appropriate for managing the care of a client with ear surgery.
10. Discuss the nursing management for clients experiencing vertigo.
11. Explain the symptoms clients have when diagnosed with Ménière disease.

Ear disorders occur throughout the life cycle. Many ear disorders result in hearing loss, a common sensory deficit among older adults. Hearing aids can compensate for some but not all forms of hearing loss. Nurses play a pivotal role in preventing hearing loss by reducing the severity and frequency of ear infections among children and advocating for measures that reduce exposure to loud noise. In addition to hearing loss, some ear disorders cause clients to have problems with balance. Depending on the nature of the disorder, there are various treatment options. Nurses are also key to assessing and evaluating clients with balance disorders and to promoting the safety of these clients.

Gerontologic Considerations

■ Unfamiliar environments may contribute to disorientation or confusion in the older adult with hearing impairment. Nursing interventions should include speaking clearly in a low tone of normal volume during frequent reorientations and teaching related to assistive hearing devices. Soft consonant sounds such as beginning and ending consonants should be clearly articulated, and the nurse should face the client if possible. The client's ability to care for the assistive device will influence selection of a hearing aid from various styles available.

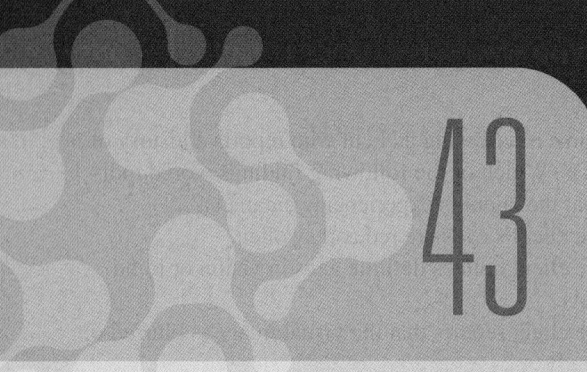

TABLE 43-1 Hearing Acuity

HEARING RANGE (DECIBELS NEEDED TO HEAR THE QUIETEST SOUNDS IN THE BETTER EAR)	DECIBELS (dB)	WITHOUT A HEARING AID	WITH A HEARING AID
Normal	0–25	Can hear faint to painful sounds	Unnecessary
Mild impairment	25–40	Cannot hear unvoiced consonants such as "s" and "f"; some difficulty keeping up with normal conversation, especially in noisy surroundings	Helpful but not necessarily worth the expense
Moderate impairment	40–70	Cannot hear conversational volume unless others talk loudly	Beneficial for restoring ability to hear normal conversations
Severe impairment	70–95	Misses most conversational content	Requires powerful hearing aids and often reads lips and perhaps uses sign language
Profound impairment	95–120	Depends heavily on speech reading	Helps hearing vowels, but amplified speech and background noise are painful
Total deafness	More than 120	Hears only painfully loud sounds or vibrations created by loud sounds	Not useful for understanding speech

HEARING IMPAIRMENT

Hearing is a sensory function that involves sound transmission, sensory receptors, and neural pathways. Hearing loss has many causes and implications for quality of life.

Pathophysiology and Etiology

Hearing impairment is described as mild, moderate, severe, or profound, depending on the intensity of sound required for a person to hear it (Table 43-1). Diminished hearing results from conductive loss, sensorineural loss, mixed hearing loss, or central hearing loss. *Conductive hearing loss* occurs from obstructions in the outer or middle ear, such as an accumulation of cerumen in the external acoustic meatus, or disease such as failure of the tiny ear bones to vibrate. *Sensorineural hearing loss* involves damage to the inner ear from conditions that affect the sensory hair cells or the nerves. Etiologies include atherosclerosis, tumors of the vestibulocochlear nerve, infections, and drug toxicity. A *mixed hearing loss* involves both conductive and sensorineural problems, involving damage within the outer or middle ear and in the inner ear or auditory nerve. *Central hearing loss* involves injury or damage to the nerves or the nuclei of the central nervous system.

Presbycusis is hearing impairment that is associated with old age. Clients with a hearing impairment often have **tinnitus**, in which the client hears buzzing, whistling, or ringing noises in one or both ears. Box 43-1 elaborates on causes of conductive and sensorineural hearing loss. Hearing loss also can result from repeated exposure to excessive noise, such as live concerts, high volumes from stereos or headphones, or a loud work environment (machinery or jackhammers). Risks for hearing loss include the following:

- Family history of sensorineural impairment
- Congenital malformations of the cranial structure (ear)
- Use of ototoxic medications (e.g., gentamycin, loop diuretics)
- Recurrent ear infections
- Bacterial meningitis
- Chronic exposure to loud noises
- Perforation of the tympanic membrane

BOX 43-1 Common Causes of Conductive and Sensorineural Hearing Loss

Conductive Hearing Loss
- External ear conditions
  - Impacted earwax or foreign body
  - Otitis externa
- Middle ear conditions
  - Trauma
  - Otitis media (acute and with effusion)
  - Otosclerosis
  - Tumors

Sensorineural Hearing Loss
- Trauma
  - Head injury
  - Noise
- Central nervous system infections (e.g., meningitis)
- Degenerative conditions
  - Presbycusis
- Vascular conditions
  - Atherosclerosis
  - Sudden deafness
- Ototoxic drugs (e.g., aminoglycosides, salicylates, loop diuretics)
- Tumors
  - Acoustic neuroma
  - Meningioma
  - Metastatic tumors
- Idiopathic
  - Ménière disease

Mixed Conductive and Sensorineural Hearing Loss
- Middle ear conditions
  - Otosclerosis
- Temporal bone fractures

Adapted from Grossman, S. C., & Porth, C. M. (2014). *Porth's pathophysiology: Concepts of altered health states* (9th ed., p. 624). Wolters Kluwer Health/Lippincott Williams & Wilkins.

Also see Evidence-Based Practice 43-1.

Hearing loss seriously impairs the ability to protect oneself and communicate with others. The age at which hearing loss occurs plus the severity of the impairment

Evidence-Based Practice 43-1

Client Experience With Tinnitus

Clinical Question

Why is tinnitus a problem, and what are the associated complaints?

Evidence

Tinnitus is often referred to as "ringing" in the ears or sometimes a hissing or roaring sound. When clients are assessed, this complaint may be made. It is sometimes hard to focus, balance, and complete tasks with this symptom. A retrospective analysis was completed to look at tinnitus and what common complaints it causes (Watts et al., 2018). A questionnaire was used to evaluate the study question. Eighteen domains of tinnitus-associated problems were identified. Reduced quality of life, tinnitus-related fear, and constant awareness were notably the most common problems described through the questionnaire (Watts et al., 2018).

Nursing Implications

Nurses can use this evidence in their education when taking a history and assessment of clients. The nurse will have an understanding that tinnitus is a symptom that is real and may affect how a client understands information, completes tasks, and is able to rest and relax when receiving care. This information is useful when planning care.

Reference
Watts, E. J., Fackrell, K., Smith, S., Sheldrake, J., Haider, H., & Hoare, D. J. (2018). Why is tinnitus a problem? A qualitative analysis of problems reported by tinnitus patients. *Trends in Hearing, 22.* https://doi.org/10.1177/2331216518812250

have extensive consequences. For example, hearing loss during the first 3 years of life, the most critical period for learning to make sounds, affects language acquisition at the word, phrase, and sentence levels. If uncorrected, hearing deficits can lead to depression and social isolation.

Approximately 15% of adults in the United States report some difficulty with hearing, with men more often than women reporting hearing issues. As people age from 45 years on, hearing impairment increases from 2% of adults to nearly 50% of adults age 75 years and over. The National Institute on Deafness and Other Communication Disorders (NIDCD, 2015a) estimates that nearly 15% of adults between the ages of 20 and 69 years experience high-frequency hearing loss because of exposure to noise during work or leisure activities.

Assessment Findings

Early detection of hearing loss can be beneficial to managing and treating what has caused the hearing loss and/or managing the consequences of the hearing impairment. Clients need an otoscopic examination to determine if there are underlying issues, such as impacted cerumen or injury to the tympanic membrane. Hearing tests will include audiometry and tuning fork tests. The client's history for exposure to occupational or other noise may be significant, as well as family history.

Medical Management

Besides treating the cause of the hearing loss, medical management includes a recommendation for a hearing aid, a battery-operated device that fits behind the ear, in the ear, or in the ear canal and amplifies sound. Clients with a conductive hearing loss benefit more from the use of a hearing aid because the structures that convert sound into energy and facilitate perception of sound in the brain continue to function. Hearing aids amplify sounds but do not improve a client's ability to distinguish words or speech. In addition, all sounds are amplified, including background noise (Hinkle & Cheever, 2018). Clients who use hearing aids are challenged with some related problems. Some experience a whistling noise because of a poor fit or improper function. Others may not have the appropriate hearing aid for their hearing loss. Hearing aids can also malfunction, in terms of the on/off switch, batteries, or other issues. It is important that clients seek assistance when they have hearing aid problems. Client and Family Teaching 43-1 provides tips for hearing aid care.

Client and Family Teaching 43-1
Tips for Hearing Aid Care and Maintenance

The nurse emphasizes the following points when teaching the client:

- Keep the hearing aid away from heat and moisture. Ear molds may be washed with soap and water after being removed from the hearing aid. They must be dried carefully with a small air dryer, such as those used to blow dust off keyboards. Carefully follow the manufacturer's directions for cleaning the hearing aid.
- Speak with the health care provider about having one of the staff keep the ears clean with ear lavage, as cerumen can cause damage to a hearing aid. The use of cotton swabs is not advisable, as they just push the cerumen deeper into the auditory canal. Many hearing aid companies provide a wax guard that fits over the hearing aid and prevents cerumen from getting in the hearing aid.
- Call health care provider (HCP) if ear drainage develops, as this can damage the hearing aid and may indicate an infection.
- Turn hearing aids off when not in use.
- Replace dead batteries as needed. Anticipate when the battery needs to be replaced, based on a personal record of usage and battery life. Make sure that the battery is placed correctly—if positioned backward, it will not function.
- Keep the hearing aid and batteries in a location that is not accessible to children or pets.
- Other issues that can occur include the following:
  - Ear discomfort related to a poorly fitting ear mold or hearing aid, jaw movement that impacts the hearing aid, improper placement of the ear mold or hearing aid. Contact the audiologist or technical specialist if the problem persists.
  - Acoustic feedback (or hearing aid squeal/whistling)—although this is a normal occurrence, if it interferes with hearing or is not usual, contact the audiologist or technical specialist for assistance.
  - Malfunction of the hearing aid requires assistance from the hearing or technical specialist.

Some clients with hearing deficits learn **American Sign Language** (ASL), a method for communication that uses a hand-spelled alphabet and word symbols (see Fig. 7-10). Clients also learn **speech reading**, also called *lip reading*.

Many technological devices have been developed to promote communication. The Federal Communications Commission (FCC) (2015) rules for television closed captioning assure that people with hearing impairment have full access to television programming. This entails accurate, synchronous, and complete display of words and sounds without impeding the visual content of the program.

Frequency modulation (FM) systems use radio frequency to amplify sounds. There is a transmitter microphone used by the speaker(s), such as in a classroom or church, and a receiver used by the person with hearing impairment. The receiver can be connected to a hearing aid device or be part of a headset. Many facilities such as schools, churches, and theaters provide FMs, but people can also get personal FMs. Other types of hearing-assistive technology systems (HATS) (American Speech-Language-Hearing Association [ASHA], n.d.) include the following:

- Infrared systems: Infrared light waves transmit sound from the television; can be used in homes, theaters, or classrooms.
- Induction loop systems: This system works with a client's hearing aid. An induction loop is installed in the ceiling or floor and connects with the speaker's microphone. The client turns the hearing aid to the "T" (telecoil/telephone) and the hearing aid telecoil receives the electromagnetic signal. The client can adjust the volume via the hearing aid.
- One-to-one communicators: In some situations, clients want to hear one person easily in a setting where there is extraneous noise. The client gives a person a microphone and the sound is amplified directly into the client's hearing aid. The client can adjust the volume.
- Other HATS:
  - Telephone-amplifying devices for all types of telephones
  - Text-based telecommunications devices for the deaf (TDD)
  - Amplified answering machines (text message telephones [teleprinter or teletypewriter])
  - Amplified telephones with different frequency responses
  - Specialized doorbells
  - Computers with specialized additions

Many other products allow people with hearing impairment to perceive (rather than hear) sound. For example, light-activated alarms in smoke detectors, alarm clocks, doorbells, and telephones flash when sound is produced. Hearing dogs, such as guide dogs for the blind, are specially trained to warn their owners when certain sounds occur.

Surgical Management

Sensorineural hearing loss is usually irreversible. For the client who is profoundly deaf or has severe hearing loss and for whom a hearing aid is ineffective, a **cochlear implant** may be beneficial. This device has an external microphone that captures incoming sounds as well as an external sound processor implanted behind the ear that captures the sound, converts it to digital signals, and sends them to an internal implant. This internal processor converts the signals into electrical energy and stimulates the auditory nerve. The brain then perceives this as sound (Fig. 43-1). A cochlear implant does not restore normal hearing, and what a person hears through a cochlear implant is not the same as the amplified sounds they hear through a hearing aid. However, the cochlear implant does provide a means for clients to learn or relearn sounds in the environment and to understand speech.

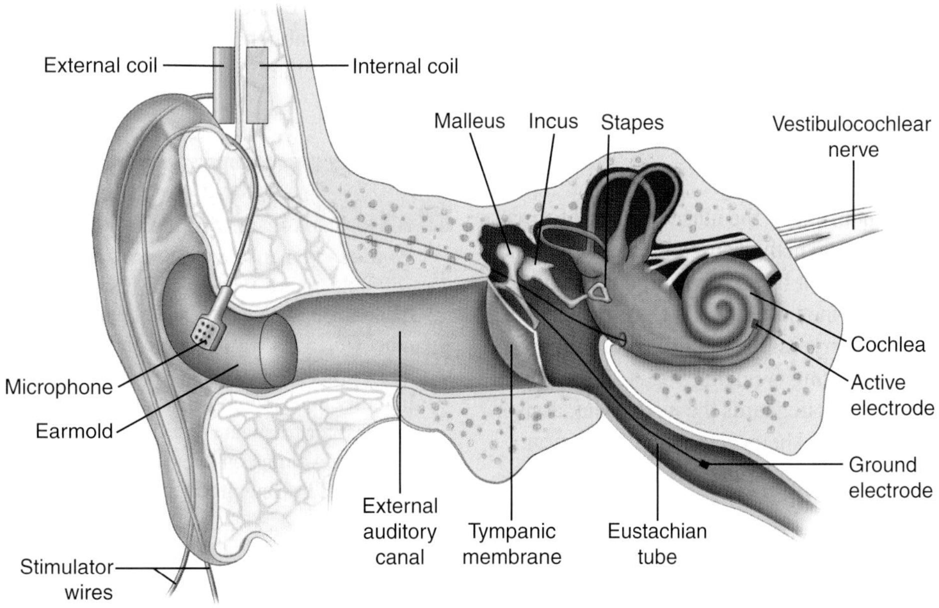

Figure 43-1 With a cochlear implant, sound is passed from the external transmitter to the inner coil by magnetic conduction and is then carried over an electrode to the cochlea.

Other implanted hearing devices may also be used. One type is a bone conduction device known as the bone-anchored hearing aid (BAHA). It is used as an alternative for clients who have mixed and conductive hearing loss or single-sided hearing loss. The device is implanted in a postauricular position under the skin into the skull. An external apparatus is then worn above the ear to transmit the sound through the skin. Although there are issues related to skin infections and loss of the implantable device as a result of trauma, there is a much improved sound quality for clients with hearing impairment. There is considerable innovation potential for other bone conduction devices with implanted transducers Bone conduction devices with implanted transducers (BCIs). One such device is middle ear implantation (MEI), in which the device is implanted in the middle ear cavity. Other devices in various stages of development are implanted through dental attachments.

Nursing Management

The nurse observes for signs of hearing impairment such as leaning forward, turning and cupping the ear to hear better, and asking that words be repeated (Box 43-2). They assess gross hearing using the techniques described in Chapter 41. The nurse also determines the clarity of the client's speech and may recommend a referral for the diagnosis and subsequent treatment of a hearing impairment as well as speech therapy. Many people reject the idea that their hearing is impaired. Some consider it a sign of aging and deterioration. If the client fears that wearing a hearing aid is a stigma, the nurse describes the various types of hearing aids that are available, some of which fit almost unnoticeably in the ear (Fig. 43-2). The nurse also stresses the importance of avoiding the purchase of a hearing aid from a mail-order catalog or a company salesperson.

Concept Mastery Alert

Suspiciousness

A nurse should be able to distinguish between suspiciousness and insecurity. For instance, if a client expresses fear that others are talking about them, it is a sign of suspiciousness and may indicate that the client may have a hearing impairment. Insecurity, on the other hand, is a lack of self-confidence.

If a hearing impairment exists, the nurse obtains information about its severity and the methods used to understand the speech of others. When a client hears poorly, the nurse determines the communication method the client prefers: speech reading, signing, writing, or typing. Suggestions for oral communication are listed in Nursing Guidelines 43-1. If the client uses a hearing aid, the nurse safeguards the instrument, assists the client with its insertion, and helps maintain its function.

To protect their self-esteem, some clients with a hearing impairment nod their heads as if they are following the conversation or laugh along with others to conceal the fact that they do not understand what has been said. The nurse encourages clients with a hearing loss to be forthright and inform others about the hearing deficit. In addition, they identify assistive hearing devices and aids for communication discussed earlier. The nurse advises clients to maintain previously established relationships because a physical impairment is unlikely to affect genuine friendships.

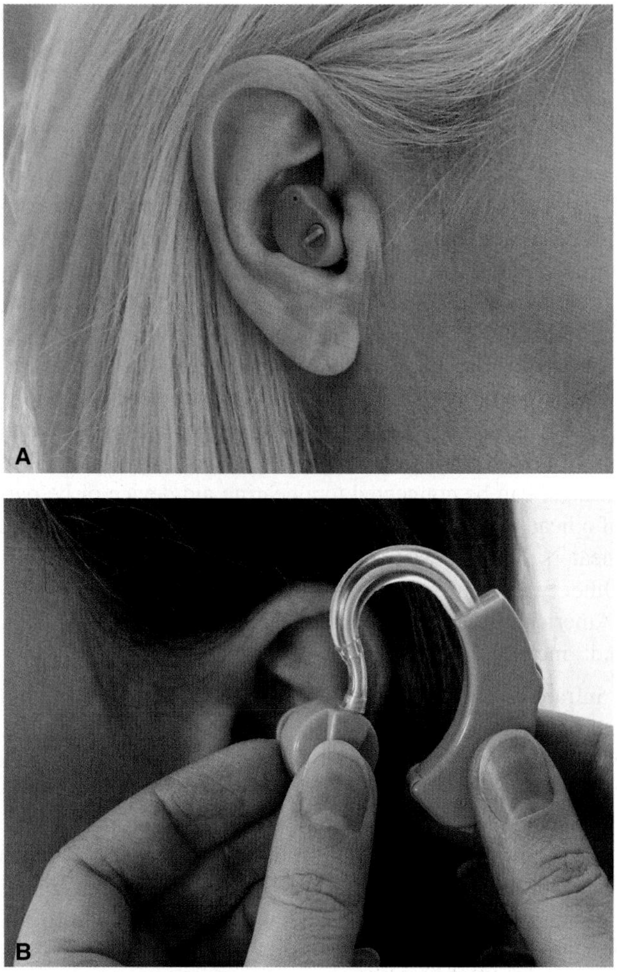

Figure 43-2 Examples of hearing aids: **(A)** In the ear. **(B)** Behind the ear. (Source **(A)**: shutterstock.com/Africa Studio, **(B)**: shutterstock.com/Andrey_Popov)

BOX 43-2 Client Symptoms of Hearing Loss

- Words and other sounds are muffled.
- Difficulty understanding conversations, especially if there is other noise, such as at a social gathering, public meeting, or other situations with background noise. Some clients avoid these situations, resulting in decreased socialization.
- Inability to hear complete words, particularly consonants.
- Request for frequent repetition during a conversation.
- Increased volume on televisions, radios, and other devices.
- Sense that hearing problems are interfering with normal activities.
- Friends and colleagues report that client's speech has deteriorated and the client is less understandable.

NURSING GUIDELINES 43-1

Hearing Loss

- Eliminate background noise as much as possible.
- Stand or sit on the side of the client's better ear.
- Ensure that there is adequate natural or artificial light.
- Get the client's attention.
- Face the client.
- Speak clearly and at a normal pace without exaggerating pronunciations.
- Do not shout, but avoid dropping conversational volume at the end of a sentence.
- Promote a clear image of your mouth; do not chew gum or cover your mouth.
- Use gestures and facial expressions to enhance what is being said orally.
- Rephrase whatever the client does not understand.
- Remain patient, positive, and relaxed.
- Provide paper and pencil if the client communicates by sign language or has speech that is difficult to understand.
- Use a support person who can communicate by signing.

The nurse uses illustrations, pamphlets, and written directions to aid teaching and includes a family member. They ask the client to repeat information and demonstrate technical skills. The nurse initiates a referral to a community agency to evaluate if and how well the client is performing self-care after discharge.

>>> ***Stop, Think, and Respond 43-1***

What recommendations can you make for someone to prevent injury to the ears or hearing loss?

DISORDERS OF THE EXTERNAL EAR

Various disorders such as impacted cerumen, injury from foreign objects, or otitis externa affect the external acoustic meatus. If these disorders are not treated carefully and adequately, they may spread to the middle ear.

Impacted Cerumen

Impacted cerumen is accumulated earwax that obstructs the external acoustic meatus.

Pathophysiology and Etiology

Impacted cerumen is more common among people who have excessive thick or dry cerumen. Both qualities interfere with drainage toward the proximal end of the meatus, where cerumen normally leaves the ear during regular shampooing and showering. The trapped cerumen interferes with the transmission of sounds carried on airwaves.

Assessment Findings

The client reports having a sense of fullness or pain in the ears, referred to as **otalgia**, and diminished hearing. The client asks that words be repeated, misinterprets questions, or raises the volume on the television or radio. Visual inspection with an otoscope shows an orange-brown accumulation of cerumen in the distal end of the external acoustic meatus. Audiometric, Rinne, and Weber tests reveal conductive hearing loss.

Medical Management

Dried cerumen is hydrated by instilling one or two drops of half-strength peroxide, warm glycerin, or mineral oil, or it is softened with commercial agents, such as carbamide peroxide (Debrox) and triethanolamine (Cerumenex). Cerumen is removed mechanically by irrigating the ear if the tympanic membrane is intact or using an instrument called a *cerumen spoon* or *curette*. A rubber-bulb syringe filled with warm water is sometimes used as well as microsuction devices by specially trained practitioners.

Nursing Management

The nurse inspects the ears and implements measures to remove excessive cerumen. Eardrops can be warmed by holding the container in the hand for a few moments or placing it in warm water. If irrigation or instillation of liquids is ordered, the nurse warms the liquid to body temperature. Cold or hot liquids cause dizziness, and the potential for injury exists if the liquid is hot. The nurse avoids inserting the irrigating syringe too deeply so as to close off the auditory canal. They direct the flow toward the roof of the canal rather than the tympanic membrane. It is important to teach clients not to clean the external auditory canal with objects such as cotton-tipped swabs or toothpicks because it is traumatic to the surface and can harm the tympanic membrane.

Foreign Objects

Pathophysiology and Etiology

Foreign objects find their way into the ear either by accident or by deliberate insertion. Sharp objects can scratch the skin or cause blunt penetration of the tympanic membrane. Insect stings cause local inflammation of the tissue.

Assessment Findings

The client describes discomfort, diminished hearing, feeling movement, or hearing a buzzing sound. On gross inspection, there is evidence of abrasion from trauma, or an insect or an object is seen. Inspection with a penlight or otoscope reveals swelling and redness in the auditory canal.

Medical Management

Mineral oil is instilled into the ear to smother an insect. Solid objects are removed with small forceps.

Nursing Management

The nurse instructs clients to clean the ears with a face cloth rather than inserting objects into the ears. A hat with earflaps or a scarf is recommended when venturing into the woods or other areas with a high insect population.

Otitis Externa

Otitis externa is an inflammation of the tissue in the external auditory canal.

Pathophysiology and Etiology

Inflammation is usually caused by an overgrowth of pathogens, such as *Staphylococcus aureus* or *Pseudomonas*, or a fungus such as *Aspergillus*. The microorganisms tend to follow trauma to the lining of the ear, or their growth is supported by retained moisture from swimming (swimmer's ear). Another possibility is that a hair follicle becomes infected, causing a furuncle or an abscess to develop. Skin conditions such as psoriasis or eczema can also lead to otitis externa. Seborrheic dermatitis or allergies to hair products that cause *dermatitis* (skin inflammation) can lead to otitis externa.

Assessment Findings

The tissue in the external ear looks red. Sometimes, it is difficult to see the tympanic membrane because of swelling. Clients describe discomfort that increases with manipulation during the examination. Hearing is reduced because of swelling. In severe infections, a fever develops and the lymph nodes behind the ear enlarge. Otoscopic examination reveals diffuse or confined inflammation, swelling, and pus. A culture of drainage identifies the specific pathogen.

Medical Management

Treatment includes warm soaks, analgesics, and antibiotic ear medication, often with corticosteroid medication, such as neomycin/polymyxin/hydrocortisone otic solution (Cortisporin, Otocort).

Nursing Management

The nurse instructs the client to carry out the medical treatment and provides health teaching to prevent recurrence. For example, they advise swimmers to wear soft plastic earplugs to prevent trapping water in the ear. If chewing produces or potentiates discomfort, the nurse encourages the client to temporarily eat soft foods or consume nourishing liquids. Above all, the nurse advises the client to avoid the use of nonprescription remedies unless they have been approved by the primary provider and to contact the primary provider if symptoms are not relieved in a few days (Box 43-3).

BOX 43-3 Preventing Recurrent Otitis Externa

- Do not use cotton swabs or other objects such as hairpins, matchsticks, or keys that can cause trauma to the external auditory canal.
- Avoid swimming in polluted water.
- Dry the outer ear and external auditory canal after the ears are immersed in water. A blow dryer on a low setting is usually effective.
- Washing ears with alkaline soap may leave a residue that interferes with the acidic pH of the ear canal, increasing the possibility of an infection.
- Instill eardrops with a 2:1 ratio of 70% isopropyl alcohol and acetic acid to dry the ears and restore the acidic pH of the auditory canal.
- Ear plugs may or may not be recommended (some HCPs feel they cause trauma to the external auditory canal). If used, they need to be cleansed with isopropyl alcohol.

DISORDERS OF THE MIDDLE EAR

Otitis Media

Otitis media is an acute inflammation or infection in the middle ear. Clients may have acute or chronic forms of either serous otitis media, also known as secretory or nonsuppurative otitis media, or the purulent or suppurative type. Although otitis media is more common among young children, adults can and do develop middle ear infections.

Pathophysiology and Etiology

Serous otitis media, a collection of pathogen-free fluid behind the tympanic membrane, results from irritation associated with respiratory allergies and enlarged adenoids. Purulent otitis media usually results from the spread of microorganisms from the eustachian tube to the middle ear during upper respiratory infections. Typical pathogens that cause otitis media include *Streptococcus pneumoniae* and *Haemophilus influenzae*.

Adults generally experience otitis media unilaterally (on one side). When fluid or pus collects in the middle ear, pressure increases and causes pain. This causes the tympanic membrane to bulge, with the potential of a spontaneous rupture in some cases. Rupture results in a jagged tear of tissue that heals slowly and sometimes incompletely. Scarring interferes with the vibration of the tympanic membrane, causing diminished hearing. Clients with perforated tympanic membranes are prone to repeated infections.

Other potentially serious complications can occur. Because the middle ear connects with the mastoid process, a part of the temporal bone, pathogens that are unresponsive to antibiotic therapy can spread, causing **mastoiditis**, or they can travel deeper in the inner ear, causing **labyrinthitis**. Infection also may extend to the meninges, causing meningitis, or brain abscess may result from its extension to the brain. If septicemia occurs, the infection can spread to the large veins at the base of the brain and cause lateral sinus thrombosis. Facial nerve damage and facial paralysis may result from the infection. With prompt and adequate treatment, complications are rare.

Assessment Findings

The client often describes a history of having had a recent upper respiratory infection or seasonal allergies. Signs and symptoms vary widely depending on the type and severity of the inflammation but may include a fever, tinnitus, malaise, severe earache, and diminished hearing. Tenderness behind the ear indicates mastoiditis. The tympanic membrane looks red and bulging. Pressure in the middle ear or dysfunction of inner ear structures can cause nausea, vomiting, and dizziness. If the tympanic membrane perforates, fluid drains into the external acoustic canal and pain is relieved.

The white blood cell count shows an elevated number of neutrophils and eosinophils. If the tympanic membrane has ruptured and drainage is present, the cultured drainage reveals a specific infectious microorganism.

Medical and Surgical Management

Prompt treatment usually prevents rupture of the tympanic membrane. In some cases, the fluid is aspirated by needle. Antibiotics are given to control the infection. The overuse of antibiotics, however, has created another problem: microorganisms are becoming resistant, and, for some infections, the available antibiotics are of limited benefit.

To reduce the consequences of spontaneous rupture of the tympanic membrane, subsequent scarring, and hearing loss, the primary provider performs a **myringotomy** or **tympanotomy**, an incisional opening of the tympanic membrane. The incised opening facilitates drainage of the purulent material, eases the pressure, and relieves the throbbing pain. The incision heals readily, with little scarring.

Plastic surgery (**myringoplasty**) is usually successful in repairing the perforated tympanic membrane. In one technique, the edges of the perforation are cauterized and a patch of blood-soaked absorbable gelatin sponge (Gelfoam) is used as scaffolding over which new tissue grows until it has filled in the defect. Chronic infections are prevented if the tympanic membrane is repaired. In the case of mastoiditis, a **mastoidectomy** is performed to remove the diseased tissue. With early and effective antibiotic therapy, mastoiditis is rare.

Nursing Management

After myringotomy, the discharge from the ear is bloody and then purulent. To remove the drainage, the nurse wipes the external ear repeatedly with a dry sterile cotton applicator. An alternative is to insert a loose (not tightly packed) cotton pledget in the external ear to collect drainage. The nurse changes the pledget when it becomes moist.

Otosclerosis

Otosclerosis is the result of a bony overgrowth of the stapes and a common cause of hearing impairment among adults. Fixation of the stapes occurs gradually over many years.

Pathophysiology and Etiology

The underlying cause of otosclerosis is unknown. The condition, which is more common in women than in men, usually becomes apparent in the second and third decades of life. It seems to be accelerated during pregnancy. Most clients have a family history of the disease, which indicates a possible hereditary relationship.

Otosclerosis interferes with the vibration of the stapes and the transmission of sound to the inner ear. Although hearing loss in otosclerosis is of the conductive type, when and if progression of the disease involving the cochlea of the inner ear occurs, a mixed type of hearing loss develops.

Assessment Findings

Signs and Symptoms

A progressive, bilateral loss of hearing is the most characteristic symptom. The client notices the hearing loss when it begins to interfere with the ability to follow conversation. There is particular difficulty hearing others when they speak in soft, low tones, but hearing is adequate when the sound is loud enough. Tinnitus appears as the loss of hearing progresses. It is especially noticeable at night, when surroundings are quiet, and can be quite distressing to the client.

The tympanic membrane appears pinkish-orange from structural changes in the middle ear. When the Rinne test is performed, the sound is heard best when the tuning fork is applied behind the ear. The sound lateralizes to the more affected ear when the Weber test is performed.

Diagnostic Findings

Audiometric tests reveal the type and severity of hearing loss. A computed tomography (CT) scan demonstrates the location and extent of excessive bone growth.

Medical and Surgical Management

Although otosclerosis has no cure, a hearing aid helps. The level of restored hearing depends greatly on the severity of the sensorineural involvement. The outcome is best when the hearing loss is purely conductive. If surgical treatment is selected, a **stapedectomy** is performed on the ear most affected. In this procedure, all or part of the stapes is removed, and a prosthesis is inserted that can vibrate the oval window (Fig. 43-3). Once the stapes is freed or replaced, the client experiences an immediate, dramatic improvement in hearing. Hearing temporarily diminishes after surgery because of swelling but eventually returns. Complications include dislodgment of the prosthesis and continued hearing loss, infection, dizziness, and facial nerve damage. Depending on the outcome of surgery, the procedure may be repeated for the opposite ear.

Nursing Management

The nurse uses selected alternatives for communicating with the client as identified earlier in Nursing Guidelines 43-1. It is important to give the preoperative client an explanation of what to expect in the immediate postoperative period. The nurse tells the client that activity is restricted for 24 hours or more after surgery and that hearing may be temporarily the same as or worse than before surgery.

After surgery, the nurse positions the client on the nonoperative side. They take care to prevent dislodgment of the prosthesis as a result of coughing, sneezing, or vomiting. Nausea and dizziness are common problems. The nurse assesses facial nerve function by checking symmetry when the client smiles or frowns.

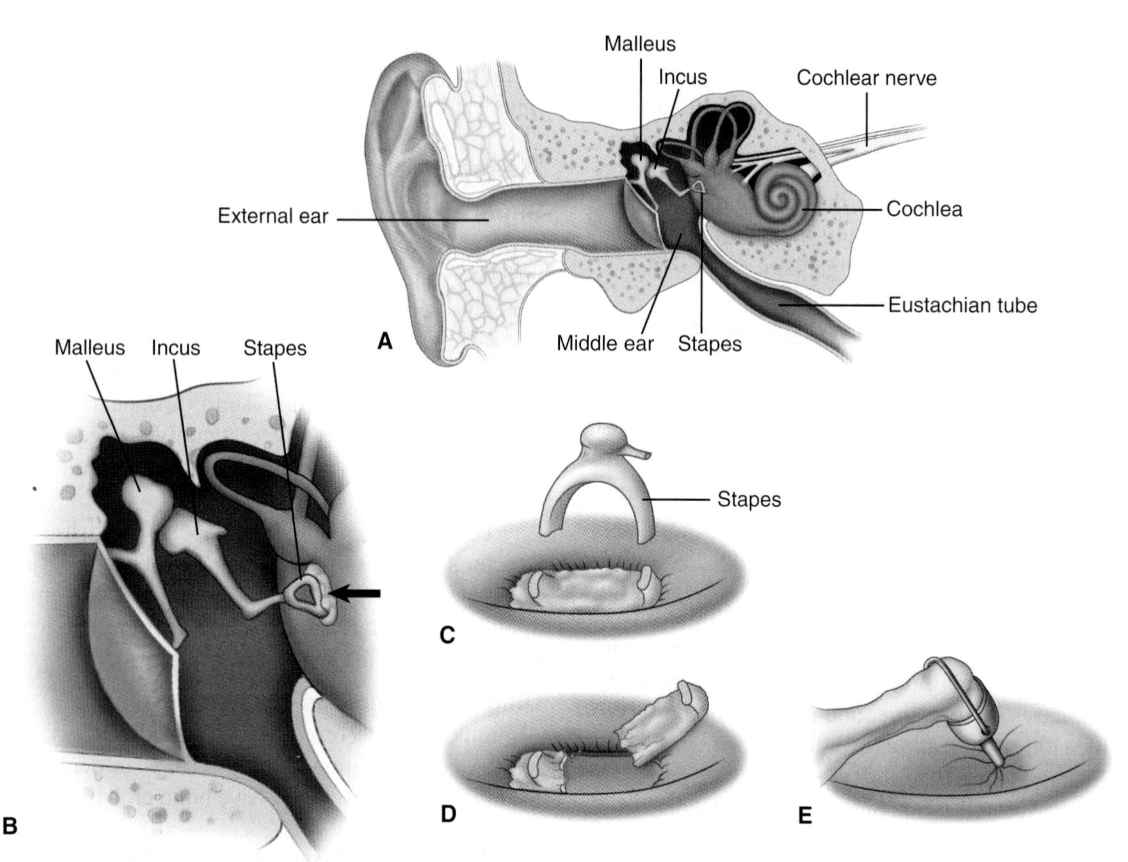

Figure 43-3 Stapedectomy for otosclerosis. **(A)** Normal anatomy. **(B)** Arrow points to sclerotic process at the foot of the stapes. **(C)** Stapes broken away surgically from its diseased base. The hole in the footplate provides an area where an instrument can grasp the plate. **(D)** The footplate is removed from its base. Some otosclerotic tissue may remain, and tissue is placed over it. **(E)** Robinson stainless steel prosthesis in position. (Reprinted with permission from Hinkle, J. L., & Cheever, K. H. (2014). *Brunner & Suddarth's textbook of medical-surgical nursing* (13th ed.). Wolters Kluwer Health/Lippincott Williams & Wilkins.)

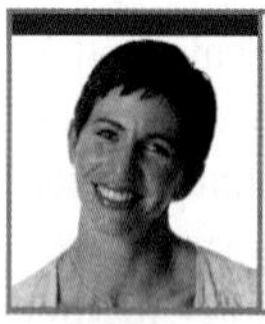

Clinical Scenario A client who is a woman of age 40 years has a stapedectomy and is transferred to a short-stay unit postoperatively. What are the major concerns for this client? See the following Nursing Process section.

NURSING PROCESS FOR THE CLIENT RECOVERING FROM STAPEDECTOMY

Assessment

After the client returns from surgery, take vital signs as well as monitor for complications, drainage from the affected ear, and level of discomfort. It is important to report any elevation in temperature.

Diagnosis, Planning, and Interventions

Impaired Comfort (pain, nausea, dizziness): Related to tissue disruption
Expected Outcome: Client will experience relief of discomfort to at least a tolerable level.

- Administer prescribed analgesic and assess again in 30 minutes. *Ongoing assessment determines effectiveness of pain medication. Response to pain and pain medication is unique for each client.*
- Give an antiemetic for nausea or vomiting. *Antiemetics promote relief of nausea.*
- Validate client's feelings of discomfort. *This measure promotes the nurse–client relationship and reassures the client that their needs are important.*
- Provide small, frequent sips of fluid or light food. *Doing so prevents nausea.*
- Limit head movement and avoid jarring the bed. *Movement aggravates dizziness. Limiting movement minimizes pain, dizziness, and nausea.*

NURSING PROCESS FOR THE CLIENT RECOVERING FROM STAPEDECTOMY (continued)

Infection Risk: Related to impaired tissue integrity secondary to the surgical incision
Expected Outcome: Client will remain free of a secondary infection.

- Adhere strictly to aseptic principles when changing a dressing or cleaning the ear. *Using aseptic technique reduces the introduction and transmission of microorganisms and protects the client from exposure to pathogens.*
- Administer prescribed antibiotics. *Appropriate and timely administration of antibiotics promotes a consistent blood level needed to treat or prevent infection.*
- Instruct client to keep their hands away from the dressing or packing. *Doing so maintains integrity of the dressings and prevents contamination from opportunistic infections.*
- Keep external ear and surrounding skin meticulously clean and free of purulent drainage. *This measure promotes healing and prevents infection through reduction of microorganisms.*

Injury Risk: Related to dizziness
Expected Outcome: Client will be free of injury.

- Encourage client to use the side rails and handrails for support when preparing to ambulate. *Side rails and handrails prevent client from falling or causing injury to the affected ear. Basic safety measures prevent injury.*
- Walk with the client who is dizzy. *Assistance promotes the client's safety and reduces the chance for injury.*

Evaluation of Expected Outcomes

The client remains comfortable, as evidenced by minimal complaints of pain and no complaints of nausea. They have no signs or symptoms of infection. The client experiences mild dizziness but maintains safety. The prescribed medical regimen and restrictions are discussed with the client or a family member. Client and Family Teaching 43-2 reviews other teaching points important to include in a discharge plan.

Client and Family Teaching 43-2
The Client With a Stapedectomy

The nurse teaches the client and family members to

- Refrain from blowing the nose because this action can dislodge the prosthesis.
- Avoid high altitudes or flying.
- Refrain from lifting heavy objects, straining when defecating, or bending over at the waist; these activities increase pressure in the middle ear.
- Prevent water from getting in the ear. Avoid swimming, showering, and washing the hair until approved by the primary provider.
- Follow the primary provider's instructions for keeping the ear clean.
- Stay away from people with respiratory infections. If a head cold occurs, contact the primary provider immediately.
- Notify the primary provider immediately if severe pain, excessive drainage, a sudden loss of hearing, or fever occurs.
- Adhere to the above restriction of activities recommended by the surgeon until told otherwise. Normal activities can usually be resumed within 2 to 4 weeks.

DISORDERS OF THE INNER EAR

Vertigo

Vertigo is the sensation of movement when there is none, or a sense of exaggerated motion when moving. The inner ear contains the semicircular canals and otolithic organs that sense the body's motion. Signals are quickly sent from the inner ear to muscles of the eyes, neck, trunk, and limbs so that stability can be maintained. When a disturbance occurs in the inner ear, vertigo occurs, along with problems with balance and stability. Vertigo is not a disease but a symptom of a disease.

There are two types of vertigo: objective vertigo, in which a person is stationary and the environment is moving (a sensation of things moving around oneself); and subjective vertigo, when a person feels motion but the surrounding environment is stationary (a spinning sensation) (Grossman & Porth, 2014). Syncopal episodes are usually indicative of cardiovascular disease and are not generally diagnosed as vertigo.

People experiencing vertigo are most likely to have a peripheral vestibular disorder, such as benign paroxysmal positional vertigo (BPPV) and Ménière disease (see related content in the sections that follow). Treatment of vertigo is based on the cause of the vertigo. Refer to Drug Therapy Table 43-1 for medications used to treat or manage symptoms related to vertigo. Nursing care focuses on the treatment of symptoms and maintenance of the client's safety.

Motion sickness is a form of physiologic vertigo. Repeated and constant motion causes this disturbance. Clients are most likely to experience motion sickness while in a car or plane, on a boat, or on carnival rides. Symptoms include nausea and vomiting, preceded by pallor and diaphoresis. Clients may use over-the-counter antihistamines, such as dimenhydrinate (Dramamine) or meclizine hydrochloride (Antivert) to prevent nausea and vomiting

DRUG THERAPY TABLE 43-1 Drugs Used to Treat Vertigo

Category and Common Generic (Brand) Drugs	Intended Use	Common Side Effects	Safety Warnings for Nurses
Antihistamines			
Meclizine (Antivert) Dimenhydrinate (Dramamine)	Reduces dizziness by suppressing receptors in vestibular (ear) system	Drowsiness, dry mouth, urinary hesitancy	• Possible allergy reaction with yellow dye #5 (tartrazine) • Monitor for urinary problems • Often taken at home, teach to refrain from driving or using dangerous equipment when drowsy
Benzodiazepines			
Clonazepam (Klonopin) Lorazepam (Ativan) Diazepam (Valium)	Enhance GABA action that depresses vestibular responses	Drowsiness, lightheadedness, headache, constipation, dry mouth	• Increased fall risk due to effects on balance • Dose must be titrated down when stopping drug
Antidepressants			
TCA Amitriptyline Nortriptyline (Pamelor) *SSRI* Citalopram (Celexa) Fluoxetine (Prozac) Paroxetine (Paxil) Sertraline (Zoloft)	Reducing anxiety associated with vestibular disorder	Anticholinergic effects (dry mouth, dry eyes, urinary retention) Nausea, dry mouth, sweating, insomnia, anorexia	• Screen for suicidal ideation • Monitor for cardiac symptoms with TCA • If taking SSRI monitor for serotonin syndrome • Dose must be titrated down when stopping drug • Taking the herbal supplement St. John's wort can increase risk of serotonin syndrome

GABA, γ-aminobutyric acid; TCA, tricyclic antidepressant; SSRI, selective serotonin reuptake inhibitors.
The drugs in column 1 indicate the drug that matches up with explanations in columns 2 through 4.

related to the motion sickness. Anticholinergic agents such as scopolamine patches are used to block the histamine response.

Benign paroxysmal positional vertigo involves brief periods of severe vertigo when clients move their heads, particularly if they move their head back and toward the affected ear. Many clients experience it when they roll over in bed onto their side. BPPV is the major cause of pathologic vertigo, affecting clients after the age of 40 years. Causes of this disorder are related to debris in the semicircular canals resulting from structural damage caused by infection, head trauma, or other events (Grossman & Porth, 2014). Meclizine may be used for a period of 1 to 2 weeks to treat the vertigo. If the vertigo persists, clients may engage in vestibular rehabilitation therapy (VRT), which is an intense physical therapy program designed to strengthen the vestibular sensory system and restore a client's balance.

Planning care for clients with vertigo requires careful assessment of symptoms, if the client has any chronic issues related to the vertigo, such as impaired fluid balance related to nausea and vomiting, or inability to manage activities of daily living because of the unpredictability of the vertigo, and fear of injury. Nursing care focuses on what type of vertigo the client has and/or the cause of the vertigo. In addition, treatment related to the vertigo and the client's ability to manage the issues caused by the vertigo are essential to providing appropriate care to the client.

Ménière Disease

Ménière disease, also referred to as endolymphatic hydrops, is a disorder characterized by fluctuations in the fluid volume and pressure in the endolymphatic sac of the inner ear. The disorder causes distention of the endolymphatic compartment, leading to a characteristic triad of symptoms, including hearing loss, vertigo, and tinnitus. Generally, Ménière disease affects only one ear, but it can affect both.

Pathophysiology and Etiology

Ménière disease most likely involves a primary lesion in the endolymphatic sac, where filtration and excretion of the fluids of the inner ear occur. The bony labyrinth protects the delicate membranous inner ear, and the membranous labyrinth is fluid filled. The pathology associated with this appears to include the following mechanisms:

- Increased production of endolymph
- Decreased production of perilymph
- Compensatory increase in the volume of the endolymphatic sac
- Decreased absorption of endolymph resulting from a malfunction of the endolymphatic sac or a blockage of the endolymphatic pathways (Grossman & Porth, 2014)

Clients with Ménière disease experience fluctuating periods of tinnitus, sensation of ear fullness, and severe vertigo. When a person moves their head, the endolymph also moves. Nerve receptors within the membranous labyrinth send signals to the brain about the movement.

In Ménière disease, an increase in endolymph causes the membranous labyrinth to dilate like a balloon, referred to as *endolymphatic hydrops*. The drainage system, or endolymphatic duct, becomes blocked. The blockage sometimes results from scar tissue or congenital narrowing of the duct. Eventually, hair cells in the inner ear are destroyed, which leads to functional deafness. In addition, the inner ear structures are disrupted and distorted, leading to chronic problems with imbalance and unsteadiness even when clients are not experiencing attacks.

Ménière disease typically is unilateral, appears during middle age, and occurs with equal frequency in men and women. When the fluid accumulates, it dilates the cochlear duct, which diminishes hearing. It also affects equilibrium as the vestibular system becomes damaged, and tinnitus occurs. At times, the client is symptom free except for permanent, residual hearing loss as the number of attacks increases. Occasionally, clients recover spontaneously. The cause of Ménière disease is not known. Generally, primary providers attribute the disease to viral infections of the inner ear, a head injury, hereditary factors, or allergic reactions. Approximately half of clients diagnosed with Ménière disease report a family history of the disease. More recent theories about its etiology center on autoimmune factors.

Assessment Findings

The onset of Ménière disease may be sudden, and symptoms may occur daily or infrequently. Vertigo is the most incapacitating symptom; clients report whirling dizziness and the need to lie down. Severe vertigo causes nausea and vomiting. Typically, clients also experience tinnitus and hearing loss that lasts for several hours as well as headaches and abdominal discomfort. Nystagmus of the eyes may result from an imbalance in vestibular control of eye movements. Generally, hearing returns between attacks but gradually becomes worse with repeated attacks.

An attack lasts from a few minutes to weeks. Because episodes can be unexpected, some clients are reluctant to leave their homes for fear they will have an attack in public. Continued employment becomes impossible for some clients.

In addition to a thorough medical history and physical examination, clients should have hearing and balance tests. Tests that measure inner ear function (Mayo Clinic Staff, 2015) include the following:

- *Videonystagmography (VNG)*: evaluates balance and eye movement by introducing warm and cool water and/or air into the auditory canal. Involuntary eye movements are measured in response to this stimulation through specialized video goggles. Sensors for balance in the inner ear send signals to the oculomotor muscles. Clients with Ménière disease cannot maintain focus on an object while having this stimuli. The eye movement demonstrates this phenomenon.
- *Rotary chair testing*: measures inner ear function. The client sits in a computer-controlled rotating chair and eye movement is measured.
- *Vestibular-evoked myogenic potentials (VEMP) testing*: determines if specific inner ear structures (the saccule, inferior vestibular nerve, and their central brain connections) are working normally. The saccule has slight sound sensitivity, which can be measured and recorded when sounds are presented to the ear.
- *Posturography*: determines issues of balance related to vision, inner ear function, or sensation from skin, muscles, tendons, or joints. The client, wearing a safety harness, stands barefoot on a platform and maintains (or tries to) balance while being exposed to various conditions.
- *Video head impulse test (vHIT)*: measures eye reactions to abrupt movements by having the client focus on a specific point while their head is turned abruptly. If the client cannot maintain focus, it is considered an abnormal response.
- *CT scan or magnetic resonance imaging (MRI)*: rules out other possible causes of the symptoms, such as a tumor that involves the vestibulocochlear nerve.
- *Audiometry*: identifies the type and magnitude of the hearing deficit.
- *Electrocochleography (ECoG)*: records the electrical activity of the inner ear in response to sound and helps to confirm the diagnosis.

Medical and Surgical Management

Treatment aims at reducing fluid production in the inner ear, facilitating its drainage, and treating the symptoms that accompany the attack. A low-sodium (1,000 to 1,500 mg/day or less) diet lessens edema. Smoking is contraindicated to prevent vasoconstriction, which interferes with fluid drainage. Treatment of the allergy or avoidance of the allergen is recommended. Bed rest may be necessary during acute attacks. Specific drug therapy may include the following:

- Meclizine (Antivert): an antihistamine often prescribed because it suppresses the vestibular system
- Diazepam (Valium) or other tranquilizers: may be ordered for acute episodes to help control vertigo; used only for short-term therapy because of the addictive potential
- Promethazine (Phenergan) or other antiemetics: ordered to help control nausea and vomiting; also has an antihistamine effect
- Hydrochlorothiazide or other diuretics: may decrease the fluid in the endolymphatic system and relieve symptoms

Dietary management is also advocated as an adjunct to other therapies. Clients on potassium-wasting diuretics are advised to eat foods that contain potassium, such as bananas, tomatoes, and citrus fruits. Other guidelines include the following:

- Limit foods high in salt and sugar. Be aware of hidden salts and sugars in foods.
- Eat meals and snacks and take fluids at regular intervals to maintain hydration.

- Drink sufficient fluids and select water, milk, and low-sugar juices. Limit coffee, tea, and soft drinks. Caffeine has a diuretic effect and as such is not recommended.
- Eat fresh fruits, vegetables, and whole grains, and avoid or limit intake of processed foods, especially those with high sodium content.
- Limit alcohol intake.
- Avoid monosodium glutamate (MSG), which can exacerbate symptoms.
- Avoid aspirin and aspirin products, which can increase tinnitus and vertigo. If clients become extremely incapacitated, surgery becomes an option. Surgeries range from decompression of the endolymphatic sac to insertion of intraotologic catheters to vestibular nerve section. Box 43-4 presents a brief description of specific surgical procedures.

Nursing Management

The nurse obtains a history of symptoms; their duration; and complete medical, drug, and allergy histories. They assess gross hearing and perform the Rinne and Weber tests. It is also important to determine the extent and effect of the client's disability.

The client with Ménière disease requires a great deal of emotional support because of the unpredictability of the attacks and the resulting impairments. During an attack, the nurse administers prescribed drugs, limits movement, and promotes the client's safety. They assist the client with activities of daily living because the least amount of motion can produce severe vertigo.

The nurse is available, empathic, and responsive to the client. Trust and confidence develop when the client does not feel abandoned or required to convince caregivers of the necessity for attention. Clients are comforted when the nurse acknowledges that dealing with temporary or permanent hearing loss is a challenge.

If a low-sodium diet is recommended, the dietitian provides a list of foods to avoid or a specific diet to follow. If an allergy is suspected as the cause of the disorder, the nurse advises the client to take the prescribed antihistamines as directed and to avoid known allergens. If a hearing aid is recommended, the nurse refers the client to an audiologist for instructions on its use and care.

BOX 43-4 Procedures to Reduce Severe Vertigo in Clients With Ménière Disease

- *Inner ear chemical infusions:* The process for infusion includes injecting the selected drug through the tympanic membrane. The medication passes into the inner ear. Dexamethasone (steroid) is the drug used most commonly. The mechanism of action is not fully understood, but its anti-inflammatory properties are considered to be the primary factor. Most clients get relief from the vertigo attacks and some also get improvement in their hearing. If this does not work, then gentamycin (antibiotic) is used as the second stage. It is generally used for clients who already have hearing loss because it is ototoxic and increases the possibility of further hearing loss.
- *Endolymphatic sac decompression*: This procedure involves opening the mastoid and decompressing the lymphatic sac and shaving some bone from the top of the sac. A shunt may be inserted to drain the inner ear. Hearing, although not improved, is preserved. The majority of clients experience relief from vertigo and also have a reduced sensation of fullness in the affected ear.
- *Vestibular neurectomy*: The vestibular nerve is cut, preventing the brain from receiving input from the semicircular canals. This procedure has a high success rate in relieving vertigo as well as preserving hearing. Some clients continue to experience imbalance issues.
- *Labyrinthectomy*: Clients with poor hearing in the affected ear may have this procedure done in order to relieve severe vertigo. The balance and hearing mechanisms are destroyed on one side by excising the labyrinth and resecting the vestibular nerve. Potential complications include facial nerve injury and total hearing loss.

››› *Stop, Think, and Respond 43-2*

A nurse admits a client with Ménière disease who is having an acute episode. After assessing the client, the nurse selects Risk for Deficient Fluid Volume as the best nursing diagnosis. Complete the diagnostic statement with expected outcomes.

Ototoxicity

Ototoxicity describes the detrimental effect of certain medications on the eighth cranial nerve or hearing structures. Signs and symptoms of ototoxicity include tinnitus and sensorineural hearing loss. Vestibular toxicity includes signs and symptoms of lightheadedness, vertigo, nausea, and vomiting. Drugs associated with ototoxicity include salicylates, loop diuretics, quinidine, quinine, and aminoglycosides. Box 43-5 lists selected ototoxic substances. It is important that nurses

BOX 43-5 Common Ototoxic Drugs

Alka-Seltzer (Acetylsalicylic acid)
Excedrin Extra Strength (Acetylsalicylic acid)
Prozac (Fluoxetine)
Benadryl (Diphenhydramine)
Depo-Provera (Medroxyprogesterone)
Ambien (Zolpidem)
Fentanyl DFC, PDR
Children's Tylenol (Acetaminophen) AC
Humira (Adalimumab)
Allegra (Fexofenadine)
OxyContin (Oxycodone)
Lithane (Lithium)
Marijuana (Cannabis sativa)
Codeine AHF, NTP
Advil (Ibuprofen)
Botox (Botulinum Toxin Type A)
Penicillamine CPS, PDR
Neosporin (Neomycin)

Adapted from Tinnitus. (2021). *Medications that can cause tinnitus.* https://www.tinnitus.net/medications-that-can-cause-tinnitus/

be knowledgeable about the ototoxic effects of certain medications. Nurses must carefully monitor the dosage and frequency of administration as well as assess the client for changes in hearing.

Acoustic Neuroma

An **acoustic neuroma**, also known as a vestibular schwannoma, is a benign Schwann cell tumor that progressively enlarges and adversely affects cranial nerve VIII (which consists of the vestibular and cochlear nerves). Most acoustic tumors arise in the auditory canal and extend into the cerebellar region, pressing on the brain stem. Acoustic neuromas are rare, occurring in 1 in 100,000 people. Men and women are affected equally, and diagnosis is usually made between 30 and 60 years of age. The cause of acoustic neuroma is unknown. The tumor is usually unilateral. Hearing loss occurs secondary to compression of the cochlear nerve or interference with the blood supply to the nerve and cochlea.

KEY POINTS

- Hearing impairment
  - Conductive hearing loss occurs from obstructions in the outer or middle ear, such as an accumulation of cerumen in the external acoustic meatus, or disease such as failure of the tiny ear bones to vibrate.
  - Sensorineural hearing loss involves damage to the inner ear from conditions that affect the sensory hair cells or the nerves. Etiologies include atherosclerosis, tumors of the vestibulocochlear nerve, infections, and drug toxicity.
  - Mixed hearing loss involves both conductive and sensorineural problems, involving damage within the outer or middle ear and in the inner ear or auditory nerve.
  - Central hearing loss involves injury or damage to the nerves or the nuclei of the central nervous system.
- Presbycusis: hearing impairment that is associated with old age. Clients with a hearing impairment often have
  - Tinnitus: the client hears buzzing, whistling, or ringing noises in one or both ears.
- Cochlear implant: has an external microphone that captures incoming sounds as well as an external sound processor implanted behind the ear that captures the sound, converts it to digital signals, and sends them to an internal implant.
- Middle ear disorders
  - Otitis media: an acute inflammation or infection in the middle ear
  - Otosclerosis: the result of a bony overgrowth of the stapes and a common cause of hearing impairment among adults
- Myringotomy or tympanotomy: an incisional opening of the tympanic membrane, the incised opening facilitates drainage of the purulent material
- Stapedectomy: in this procedure, all or part of the stapes is removed, and a prosthesis is inserted that can vibrate the oval window.
- Vertigo: the sensation of movement when there is none, or a sense of exaggerated motion when moving
- Ménière disease: a disorder characterized by fluctuations in the fluid volume and pressure in the endolymphatic sac of the inner ear; the disorder causes distention of the endolymphatic compartment, leading to a characteristic triad of symptoms including hearing loss, vertigo, and tinnitus.
- Ototoxicity: the damaging effect of certain medications on the eighth cranial nerve or hearing structures which produces tinnitus, sensorineural hearing loss, lightheadedness, vertigo, nausea, and vomiting. Drugs associated with ototoxicity include salicylates, loop diuretics, quinidine, quinine, and aminoglycosides.

CRITICAL THINKING EXERCISES

1. A client with a history of Ménière disease arrives at the clinic, complaining of severe vertigo and nausea. What precautions are important to take while the client is at the clinic?
2. A refugee from Somalia is scheduled for a mastoidectomy because of severe and untreated ear infections that affected the mastoid. Identify two goals for this client after they return from surgery.
3. A young client comes to the clinic complaining of severe pain in their left ear; it hurts to touch it. They say that they swim at least 3 days a week. They are diagnosed with otitis externa. The nurse practitioner prescribes analgesics and application of heat to the affected ear and also tells the client to avoid swimming for 2 weeks. Because this client swims regularly for exercise, what further instructions can the nurse provide to prevent future problems?
4. A client is diagnosed with an acoustic neuroma. The client asks the nurse why this is a problem because it is not cancerous.

NCLEX-STYLE REVIEW QUESTIONS PrepU

1. A nurse notes on the client's record that there is a history of moderate sensorineural hearing loss related to presbycusis. Which of the following strategies will best enhance the nurse's ability to interact with this client? Select all that apply.
   1. Exaggerate word pronunciations when speaking with the client.
   2. Face the client when communicating with them.
   3. Reduce background noise when conversing with the client.
   4. Rephrase whatever the client does not understand.
   5. Yell at the client to gain their attention.

2. What actions would the nurse perform while administering eardrops to remove excessive cerumen? Select all that apply.
1. Avoid inserting the irrigating syringe too deeply.
2. Boil the solution once.
3. Direct the flow of the eardrops toward the tympanic membrane.
4. Direct the flow of the eardrops toward the roof of the canal.
5. Shake the eardrops container vigorously.
6. Warm the eardrops by holding the container in the hand for a few minutes.

3. Which is the best evidence that the antibiotic the nurse is administering for the treatment of acute otitis media is having a therapeutic effect?
1. Ear discomfort is relieved.
2. Ear drainage is thin and watery.
3. Ringing sounds within the ear stop.
4. The ear feels less warm to the touch.

4. The nurse is assured that a client with chronic vertigo understands the safety measures needed to prevent injury by which of the following statements?
1. "I cannot drive within several hours of having a dizzy spell."
2. "I must learn to move my head slowly to prevent sudden dizziness."
3. "I need to remove clutter and throw rugs from my home."
4. "I should lie down in my bed whenever I am feeling dizzy."

5. A client tells the nurse of experiencing fluctuating issues with vertigo. What questions are important for the nurse to ask if Ménière disease is suspected? Select all that apply.
1. "Are you experiencing ringing in your ears?"
2. "Can you tell me about any impaired facial movements?"
3. "Do you have problems with your hearing?"
4. "Have you experienced a sense of fullness in your ears?"
5. "Is there any evidence of discharge from your ears?"

WANT TO KNOW MORE? There is a wide variety of online resources available on thePoint to enhance learning and understanding of this chapter.

Go to thePoint.lww.com/activate and use the activation code found in the front of this text to unlock these online resources.

UNIT 11

Caring for Clients With Gastrointestinal Disorders

44 Introduction to the Gastrointestinal System and Accessory Structures

Words To Know

barium enema
barium swallow
cholangiography
cholecystography
colonoscopy
enteroclysis
esophagogastroduodenoscopy
flexible sigmoidoscopy
gallbladder series
lower gastrointestinal series
panendoscopy
percutaneous liver biopsy
peristalsis
proctosigmoidoscopy
radionuclide imaging
ultrasonography
upper gastrointestinal series
virtual colonoscopy

Learning Objectives

On completion of this chapter, you will be able to:

1. Identify major organs and structures of the gastrointestinal system.
2. Discuss important information to ascertain about gastrointestinal health.
3. Identify facts in the client's history that provide pertinent data about the present illness.
4. Discuss physical assessments that are pertinent to gastrointestinal tract function.
5. Describe common diagnostic tests performed on clients with gastrointestinal disorders.
6. Describe nursing measures after liver biopsy.
7. Explain nursing management of clients undergoing diagnostic testing for a gastrointestinal disorder.

The gastrointestinal (GI) system (Fig. 44-1) may be considered as having three sections: the upper GI tract, the small intestine or middle portion of the GI tract, and the lower GI tract. The upper GI tract begins at the mouth and ends at the pyloric sphincter. The small intestine has three subdivisions: the duodenum, the jejunum, and the ileum. The lower GI tract begins at the cecum and ends at the anus. Accessory structures include the peritoneum, liver, gallbladder, and pancreas. The primary functions of the GI tract are digestion (Table 44-1) and distribution of food.

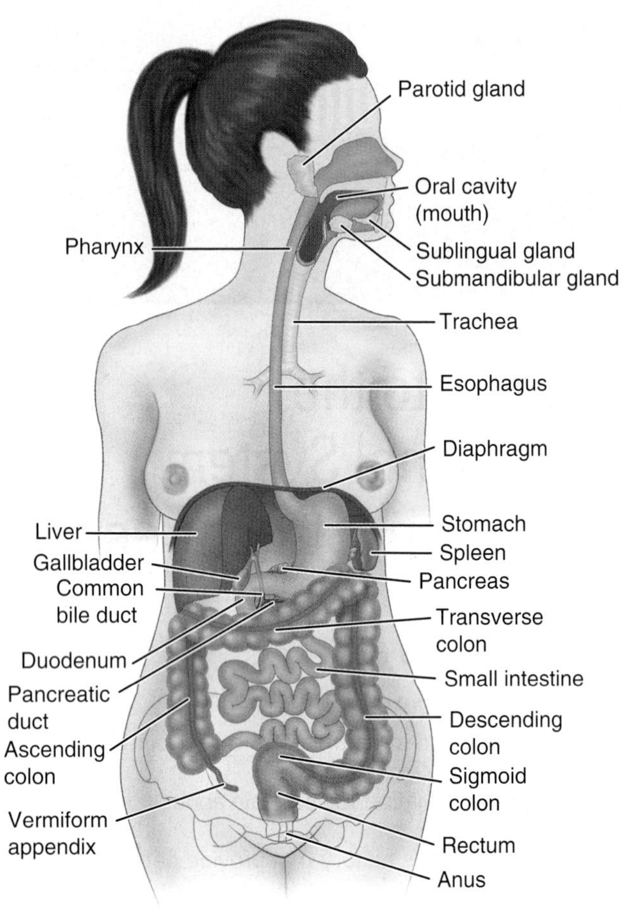

Figure 44-1 Organs of the gastrointestinal tract.

Gerontologic Considerations

- Assessment of older adults must include patterns of defecation. Changes in dietary intake or hydration, reduced abdominal or sphincter muscle tone, decreased awareness of the filling reflex or diminished control of the rectal sphincter due to changes in innervation can contribute to either constipation or incontinence.
- Dietary intake of fibrous fruits and vegetables, adequate fluid throughout the day, mobility or passive range-of-motion exercises, and scheduled times for defecation approximately 30 minutes after a meal can assist older adults with routine bowel evacuation.
- Before any diagnostic examination, provide a thorough explanation in terms the client can understand and answer any questions to help reduce anxiety. Anxiety regarding the diagnostic examination may be due to pain from positioning or being rushed.
- Fluid restrictions and the multiple enemas or laxatives required for GI tests may greatly impact fluid balance and electrolyte levels in the older adult. Older adults are at higher risk for dehydration than are younger people because they tend to have fewer physiologic reserves to compensate for fluid loss. A history of vomiting or diarrhea or diuretic therapy may compound the potential for fluid deficit. Additionally, any fluid deficit has potential for blood pressure decrease and associated risk of falls.
- After the diagnostic test, the older adult may experience dizziness or confusion secondary to prolonged time without food or fluids. Provide nourishment as soon as possible after the examination and give assistance with ambulation when necessary.
- Inform older clients and their families that diminished intestinal and sphincter muscle tone may contribute to constipation, diarrhea, or fecal incontinence following a diagnostic test; appropriate early nursing interventions should be implemented.

TABLE 44-1 Major Digestive Enzymes and Secretions

ENZYME/SECRETION	ENZYME SOURCE	DIGESTIVE ACTION
Action of Enzymes That Digest Carbohydrates		
Ptyalin (salivary amylase)	Salivary glands	Starch → dextrin, maltose, glucose
Amylase	Pancreas and intestinal mucosa	Starch → dextrin, maltose, glucose Dextrin → maltose, glucose
Maltase	Intestinal mucosa	Maltose → glucose
Sucrase	Intestinal mucosa	Sucrose → glucose, fructose
Lactase	Intestinal mucosa	Lactose → glucose, galactose
Action of Enzymes/Secretions That Digest Protein		
Pepsin	Gastric mucosa	Protein → polypeptides
Trypsin	Pancreas	Proteins and polypeptides → polypeptides, dipeptides, amino acids
Aminopeptidase	Intestinal mucosa	Polypeptides → dipeptides, amino acids
Dipeptidase	Intestinal mucosa	Dipeptides → amino acids
Hydrochloric acid	Gastric mucosa	Protein → polypeptides, amino acids
Action of Enzymes/Secretions That Digest Fat (Triglyceride)		
Pharyngeal lipase	Pharynx mucosa	Triglycerides → fatty acids, diglycerides, monoglycerides
Steapsin	Gastric mucosa	Triglycerides → fatty acids, diglycerides, monoglycerides
Pancreatic lipase	Pancreas	Triglycerides → fatty acids, diglycerides, monoglycerides
Bile	Liver and gallbladder	Fat emulsification

Note. →, converts to
From Hinkle, J. H., & Cheever, K. H. (2014). *Brunner & Suddarth's textbook of medical-surgical nursing* (13th ed., p. 1198). Wolters Kluwer Health/Lippincott Williams & Wilkins.

ANATOMY AND PHYSIOLOGY

Mouth

Food normally enters the GI system at the mouth, where it is chewed (masticated) before being swallowed. Food that contains starch undergoes partial digestion when it mixes with the enzyme *ptyalin (salivary amylase)*, which the *salivary glands* secrete. Table 44-2 outlines how oral structures participate in digestion.

Esophagus

The *esophagus* begins at the base of the pharynx behind the trachea and ends at the opening to the stomach. It is approximately 25 cm (10 inches) long. Layers of muscle tissue surround the esophagus. They consist of striated (banded or striped) muscle tissue in the proximal esophagus, striated and smooth muscle in the midesophagus, and smooth muscle in the lower esophagus. Coordinated movement of these muscle layers propels food from the pharynx into the stomach. These wavelike contractions are known as **peristalsis**. An *upper esophageal sphincter* or *pharyngoesophageal sphincter*, located at the upper end of the esophagus, prevents air from entering the esophagus and stomach during respiration. The *lower esophageal sphincter* or *gastroesophageal sphincter* is located where the esophagus joins the stomach. The lower sphincter remains contracted in order to prevent reflux of gastric contents into the esophagus. The esophagus passes through an opening in the diaphragm (*hiatus*) as it connects to the stomach.

Stomach

The stomach, which is located on the left side of the abdomen, temporarily holds ingested food and prepares it by mechanical and chemical action to pass in semiliquid form into the small intestine. The opening between the esophagus and stomach is called the *lower esophageal sphincter* or *cardiac sphincter* (so named because of its proximity to the heart). The opening between the stomach and duodenum is called the *pyloric sphincter*. Both sphincters are circular bands of muscle fibers. When contracted, these sphincters keep stomach contents enclosed (or confined). When the pyloric sphincter relaxes, stomach contents flow to the duodenum.

Gastric secretions that contain digestive enzymes are released continuously but increase when food is eaten. Gastric secretions are acidic because they contain hydrochloric acid (HCl). The contractions of the stomach mix the food with the gastric secretions and move the mixture of semiliquid food, called *chyme*, to the small intestine by peristalsis. The time required for the stomach to empty depends on the amount and composition of food. Fats, for example, delay stomach emptying.

Small Intestine

The small intestine or the middle portion of the GI tract is divided into three portions: duodenum, jejunum, and ileum. The *duodenum*, which is approximately 10 inches long, is the first region of the small intestine and contains the opening for the common bile duct and the primary pancreatic duct, which allow bile and pancreatic enzymes to enter. *Bile*, a fluid synthesized by the liver, breaks down fats (lipids). Pancreatic enzymes aid in the digestion of lipids, carbohydrates, and proteins. These secretions continue to promote the chemical breakdown of food and transform chyme to an alkaline state. Peristalsis mechanically propels the mixture, which is semiliquid at this point, into the jejunum and ileum, which have a combined length of approximately 23 feet.

The primary function of the small intestine is to absorb nutrients from the chyme. Absorption of different nutrients occurs at different sites in the small intestine (Table 44-3). When a part of the small intestine is diseased or removed surgically, absorption in that area is diminished or lost altogether.

The *ileocecal valve* lies at the distal end of the small intestine and the upper portion of the cecum and regulates the flow of intestinal contents, which are liquid at this point, into the large intestine. It also prevents the reflux of feces and bacteria from the large intestine, preserving the relative sterility of the small intestine.

Large Intestine

The large intestine, approximately 4 to 5 feet long and 2 inches in diameter, receives waste from the small intestine and propels waste toward the *anus*, the opening from the body for elimination. The large intestine absorbs water, some electrolytes, vitamin K, and bile acids. The cecum, colon, rectum, and anal canal make up the structures of the large intestine through which fecal material passes.

The *cecum* is a pouchlike structure at the beginning of the large intestine. The *appendix*, a narrow blind tube at the tip of the cecum, has no known function in humans.

The colon is divided into the *ascending*, *transverse*, *descending*, and *sigmoid* colons. The ascending colon starts at

TABLE 44-2 How Oral Structures Participate in Digestion

STRUCTURE	CONTRIBUTION TO THE DIGESTIVE PROCESS
Teeth	Reduce food to sizes appropriate for swallowing; break down dense particles
Tongue	Direct food toward the pharynx and esophagus mixes saliva to moisten and lubricate food
Salivary glands	Moisten and lubricate foods in the mouth; add ptyalin, amylase, and lipase enzymes for the initial digestion of starches and lipids
Muscles of mastication	Provide movement for the grinding of food into smaller particles; provide more surface area for the digestive enzymes to act

Adapted from Porth, C. M. (2015). *Essentials of pathophysiology: Concepts of altered health states* (4th ed.). Wolters Kluwer.

TABLE 44-3 Sites of and Requirements for Absorption of Dietary Constituents and Manifestations of Malabsorption

DIETARY CONSTITUENT	SITE OF ABSORPTION	REQUIREMENTS	MANIFESTATIONS OF MALABSORPTION
Water and electrolytes	Mainly small bowel	Osmotic gradient	Diarrhea Dehydration Cramps
Fat	Upper jejunum	Pancreatic lipase Bile salts Functioning lymphatic channels	Weight loss Steatorrhea Fat-soluble vitamin deficiency
Carbohydrates			
Starch	Small intestine	Amylase Maltase Isomaltase alpha-dextrins	Diarrhea Flatulence Abdominal discomfort
Sucrose	Small intestine	Sucrase	
Lactose	Small intestine	Lactase	
Maltose	Small intestine	Maltase	
Fructose	Small intestine		
Protein	Small intestine	Pancreatic enzymes (e.g., trypsin, chymotrypsin, elastin)	Loss of muscle mass Weakness Edema
Vitamins			
A	Upper jejunum	Bile salts	Night blindness Dry eyes Corneal irritation
Folic acid	Duodenum and jejunum	Absorptive; may be impaired by some drugs (i.e., anticonvulsants)	Cheilosis Glossitis Megaloblastic anemia
B_{12}	Ileum	Intrinsic factor	Glossitis Neuropathy Megaloblastic anemia
D	Upper jejunum	Bile salts	Bone pain Fractures Tetany
E	Upper jejunum	Bile salts	Uncertain
K	Upper jejunum; primarily the large intestine	Bile salts	Easy bruising and bleeding
Calcium	Duodenum	Vitamin D and parathyroid hormone	Bone pain Fractures Tetany
Iron	Duodenum and jejunum	Normal pH (hydrochloric acid secretion)	Iron deficiency anemia Glossitis

Adapted from Porth, C. M. (2015). *Essentials of pathophysiology: Concepts of altered health states* (4th ed., p. 718). Wolters Kluwer.

the cecum, traverses the underside of the liver, and turns at what is referred to as the *right hepatic flexure*. At this point, the transverse colon crosses the upper half of the abdomen from right to left and then it turns downward under the lower end of the spleen, to form the splenic flexure. The descending colon goes from this point to the rectum, which connects the sigmoid colon to the anus. In the colon, the unabsorbed material becomes fecal matter, which is composed of water, food residue, microorganisms, digestive secretions, and mucus. Water is reabsorbed by means of diffusion across the intestinal membrane as the mixture moves through the colon. By the time the mixture reaches the descending and sigmoid colon, it is a formed mass. The rectum holds and retains fecal matter through the contraction of the internal and external anal sphincters. As fecal mass accumulates, it distends the rectal wall, creating the urge to defecate. When the external anal sphincter relaxes, the fecal matter is expelled through the anus.

If any portion of the large intestine becomes diseased or is surgically removed, its absorptive function is diminished or lost. This may result in the passage of loose stools and potential fluid and electrolyte imbalance. Passage of liquid stool, which contains many bile salts, makes the client especially vulnerable to skin breakdown in the perianal area. If stool remains in the large intestine too long, constipation results. The client may then strain to evacuate hard, solid

TABLE 44-4 Age-Related Changes in the Gastrointestinal System

STRUCTURAL CHANGES	IMPLICATIONS
Oral Cavity	
• Injury/loss or decay of teeth • Atrophy of taste buds • ↓ Saliva production • Reduced ptyalin and amylase in saliva (enzymes in saliva that digest carbohydrates)	Difficulty chewing and swallowing
Esophagus	
• ↓ Motility and emptying • Weakened gag reflex • ↓ Resting pressure of lower esophageal sphincter	Reflux and heartburn
Stomach	
• Degeneration and atrophy of gastric mucosal surfaces with ↓ production of HCl • ↓ Secretion of gastric acids and most digestive enzymes • ↓ Gastric motility and emptying	Food intolerances, malabsorption, or decrease in vitamin B_{12} absorption
Small Intestine	
• Atrophy of muscle and mucosal surfaces • Thinning of villi and epithelial cells	↓ Motility and transit time, which lead to complaints of indigestion and constipation
Large Intestine	
• ↓ Mucus secretion • ↓ Elasticity of rectal wall • ↓ Tone of internal anal sphincter • Slower and duller nerve impulses in rectal area	↓ Motility and transit time, which lead to complaints of indigestion and constipation ↓ Absorption of nutrients (dextrose, fats, calcium, and iron) Fecal incontinence

Note. HCl, hydrochloric acid.
From Hinkle, J. H., & Cheever, K. H. (2014). *Brunner & Suddarth's textbook of medical-surgical nursing* (13th ed., p. 1200). Wolters Kluwer Health/Lippincott Williams & Wilkins.

stool, which can disrupt skin integrity. Table 44-4 describes the implications of age-related changes in the GI system.

Accessory Structures

The three accessory digestive organs are the liver, gallbladder, and pancreas. Although not an accessory structure itself, the peritoneum encloses the abdominal organs.

Peritoneum

The *peritoneum*, a membrane that lines the inner abdomen, encloses the viscera and the serous fluid that it secretes. It allows the abdominal organs to move about without creating friction. The walls of the digestive organs normally prevent the gastric and intestinal contents from escaping into the peritoneal cavity. Any perforation that allows material to seep out of the digestive tract is serious because the microorganisms and enzymes can cause a severe inflammation and infection of the surrounding tissue. This condition is known *as peritonitis*.

Liver

The *liver*, the largest glandular organ in the body, weighs between 1.0 and 1.5 kg (2 and 3 lb). It is located in the right upper abdomen just under the diaphragm, which separates the liver from the right lung. The liver is involved in many vital, complex metabolic activities. It forms and releases bile; processes vitamins, proteins, fats, and carbohydrates; stores glycogen; contributes to blood coagulation; metabolizes and biotransforms many chemicals (including drugs), bacteria, and foreign matter; and forms antibodies and immunizing substances (gamma globulin). See Chapter 47 for more information.

Gallbladder

The *gallbladder* is attached to the midportion of the undersurface of the liver. It normally has a thin wall and holds approximately 60 mL of bile. The liver forms approximately 1 L of bile each day. When the bile reaches the gallbladder from the common hepatic duct, water and minerals are absorbed from the bile to form a more concentrated product. Gallbladder contraction, triggered by ingested food (especially fats), causes bile to be released first through the cystic duct and then the common bile duct into the duodenum, where it aids in the absorption of fats, fat-soluble vitamins, iron, and calcium. Bile also activates the pancreas to release its digestive enzymes and an alkaline fluid that neutralizes stomach acids that reach the duodenum.

Pancreas

The *pancreas* is both an *exocrine gland*, one that releases secretions into a duct or channel, and an *endocrine gland*, one that releases substances directly into the bloodstream. As an endocrine organ, it produces the hormones insulin and glucagon (see Chapter 51). As an exocrine organ, it produces various protein-, fat-, and carbohydrate-digesting enzymes. At the appropriate time for digestion, the pancreatic enzymes are released in inactive forms and transported to the duodenum where they are activated.

ASSESSMENT

Many conditions can disrupt the normal function of the GI system. In addition to disorders of the GI tract and accessory organs, many disorders involving other organ systems can affect GI function. As a result, the client with a GI disorder may experience a wide variety of health problems that involve disturbances of ingestion, digestion, absorption, and elimination. Accurate recording of the client's health history and physical assessment findings helps the health care team to diagnose and treat GI disorders.

History

The objective of the history is to identify the client's specific problem and its possible cause. The history includes the chief complaint; a focused assessment of current nutritional, metabolic, and elimination patterns; and past history. The focus is on any abdominal pain, issues with digestion, nausea and/or vomiting, constipation or diarrhea, incontinence, or other complaints. It is also important to seek information about the client's dental hygiene and condition of the mouth, teeth, and gums and if the client wears dentures. The client's use of alcohol and tobacco (including smokeless chewing tobacco) is also important to ascertain. All of these factors can have an impact on GI health. Last, it is vital to ask the client about psychosocial or cultural influences that may be a factor in the client's overall health habits and issues. The nurse gathers as much data as possible about why the client has sought treatment and current symptoms. This includes how long the symptoms have been present and what appears to cause or be related to them. Pertinent information to elicit includes which types of food produce distress and when symptoms are most likely to occur. The nurse also determines what measures, if any, the client uses to relieve the symptoms and the effects of these measures. Again, it is important to determine if there are any psychosocial issues or cultural influences that are currently affecting/influencing the client.

During the GI assessment, the focus is on nutritional, metabolic, and elimination patterns, including quality of the client's appetite; problems associated with chewing or swallowing; what and how much the client eats each day; discomfort before, during, or after food consumption; nutritional supplements, if any, that the client uses (e.g., vitamins, herbs, home remedies); weight gain or loss; and bowel elimination patterns (usual consistency and color of stools, visible blood, stool frequency, effort or pain with passage of stool). After obtaining a current health history, the nurse obtains a history of all past medical and surgical disorders and their treatment. They compile a family history of illnesses and causes of death. A family history of digestive disorders is especially important because several diseases/disorders, such as colorectal cancer, have a hereditary link. The nurse also explores the client's work history to evaluate the possibility of exposure to environmental toxic wastes or radioactive materials.

The nurse obtains a complete allergy history, including adverse reactions to foods, because food allergies can cause various GI symptoms. The medication history includes prescription and nonprescription drugs, especially those affecting GI function. For each drug, the nurse lists the name, dose, frequency, and reason for taking.

››› *Stop, Think, and Respond 44-1*

A client says that they have been experiencing nausea and occasional vomiting for several days. What questions should you ask to gain more information?

Physical Examination

General Appearance

The nurse assesses the client's overall physical condition and measures weight, height, and vital signs. They evaluate general appearance with regard to age and body size, and assesses hygiene, energy, breathing pattern, emotional attitude, and mental status to the degree that they may affect the client's general appearance.

Skin

Using natural sunlight or bright artificial light, the nurse inspects the skin for any abnormal color, such as a yellowish tint indicating jaundice. In clients with very dark skin, the nurse inspects the hard palate, gums, conjunctiva, and surrounding tissues for discoloration. If the skin appears jaundiced, the nurse inspects the sclera to see if it is yellow. Inspection of the skin of the face and abdomen is necessary to look for other abnormalities, such as *spider angiomas* (superficial red discolorations consisting of blood vessels that assume a spider-shaped pattern), distended abdominal veins (*caput medusae*), and scars. The nurse also assesses for dryness of the oral mucosa and skin turgor. Mucous membranes may be dry, and skin turgor may be poor in clients who are dehydrated as a result of fluid losses from the GI tract.

Mouth

The nurse examines the lips for sores, cracks, lesions, or other abnormalities. Using a tongue blade and a flashlight, the nurse inspects the mouth for inflammation, sores, swellings, or discolorations. Assessment of the quality of oral care is essential and includes evaluating for missing teeth and partial plates, bridges, or dentures. If the client has dentures, the nurse asks if they fit well and whether the client can eat regular food. If the client can eat only soft foods, the nurse communicates this information to the primary provider and dietary department.

Abdomen

The nurse continues the physical assessment by having the client lie supine, with the knees flexed slightly, for the abdominal examination. (This position assists in relaxing the abdominal muscles.) Abdominal areas typically are described in quadrants (right upper, right lower, left upper, and left lower), with the umbilicus as the center point for both horizontal and vertical divisions (Fig. 44-2). The nurse then

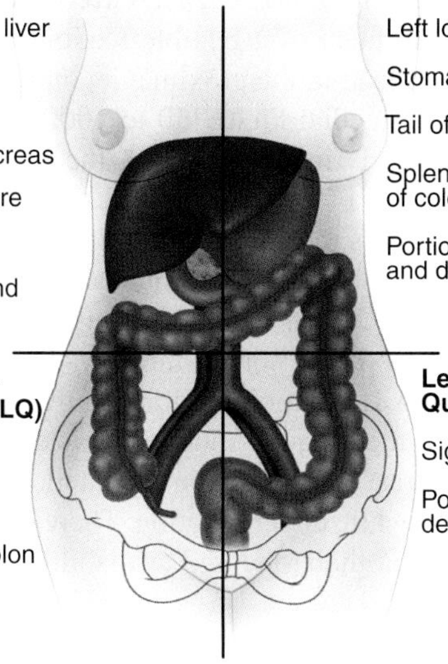

Figure 44-2 Abdominal quadrants.

observes the abdomen's contour, noting whether it is flat, round, concave, or distended as well as the effort associated with breathing. Distention may cause dyspnea as a result of upward pressure on the diaphragm (see Chapter 21).

Abdominal auscultation is done before palpation because palpation disrupts normal bowel sounds. Using a stethoscope, the nurse listens over each quadrant for bowel sounds, which sound like gurgles and normally occur every 5 to 20 seconds. The nurse describes the location, pitch quality, and frequency. Listening for a full 3 to 5 minutes over each quadrant is important to confirm absence of bowel sounds. Generally, bowel sounds are described as absent, normal, hypoactive (one or two sounds in 2 minutes), or hyperactive (five to six sounds in under 30 seconds). Measurement of abdominal girth is done at the widest point (usually at the umbilicus). Using a pen, the nurse marks the measurement location on the abdomen to ensure that additional examiners use the same reference point.

In the next part of the examination, the nurse percusses the abdomen to elicit changes in sounds from dullness over an area with a solid mass, such as the liver, to resonance over less dense structures or those filled with air.

The nurse next palpates the abdomen to determine whether it is soft or firm and to detect masses and areas of pain or tenderness. If the client reports tenderness, the nurse probes the lower liver margin. The nurse may feel an enlarged liver below the right lower rib cage. Pain or discomfort in this area may suggest a liver disorder, gallbladder or intestinal disease, or a pancreatic disorder.

Anus

The nurse examines the anal area for external hemorrhoids, skin tags, or fissures (small tears in the anal opening). They inspect the skin surrounding the anus for breaks, lesions, rash, inflammation, and drainage. If and when stool passes, the nurse examines its characteristics. The shape, color, and consistency of stool usually are helpful in the differential diagnosis of GI disorders. Foods and medications can alter the color of stool (Table 44-5).

Diagnostic Tests

Various studies, both radiographic and nonradiographic, are used to identify the location and structural appearance of organs or other space-occupying masses (air, fluid, tumors, foreign objects) in the abdomen, chest, or GI system. Radiographic studies involve the use of radiopaque contrast media. *Fluoroscopy* may be used to observe the shape and contour of empty organs and how these hollow structures fill with and evacuate radiopaque dye (contrast medium). Nonradiographic studies, such as magnetic resonance imaging (MRI), use forms of energy other than radiation to detect structural changes.

Upper Gastrointestinal Test

Sometimes referred to as a *barium swallow* or an *upper GI series*, this procedure involves a fluoroscopic study of the entire upper GI tract. Barium sulfate is a radiopaque solution used as a contrast agent. A thin barium solution such as diatrizoic acid (Hypaque) may be used instead. Both are sweetened and flavored but have a chalky taste. Clients are generally asked to drink 12 to 14 oz. As this contrast solution moves through the digestive tract, a fluoroscope is held over the part of the body being examined. Images of the esophagus, stomach, and part of the upper intestine are visualized on a video monitor. This test diagnoses structural abnormalities in the esophagus, such as tumors, strictures, varices, and hiatal hernia. Structural abnormalities below the esophagus include gastric tumors, peptic ulcers, and numerous gastric disorders (see Chapter 45).

Strictly speaking, a **barium swallow** (*esophagography*) is fluoroscopic observation of the client actually swallowing a flavored barium solution and its progress down the esophagus. Barium swallow facilitates the identification of structural abnormalities of the esophagus as well as swallowing

TABLE 44-5 Foods and Medications That Alter Stool Color

SUBSTANCE THAT AFFECTS NORMAL STOOL COLOR	VISIBLE COLOR
Meat protein and cocoa	Dark brown to dark red
Green leafy vegetables, purple or green food coloring, foods that contain chlorophyll, such as peas, asparagus, and leafy greens, as well as seaweed and whole-leaf green tea	Green
Carrots, beets, red gelatin, tomato juice, and red Kool-Aid	Red
Senna, carrots, sweet potato, yellow food coloring	Yellow
Bismuth, iron, licorice, and blueberries	Black
Barium and high amounts of fatty foods	Milky white to clay colored

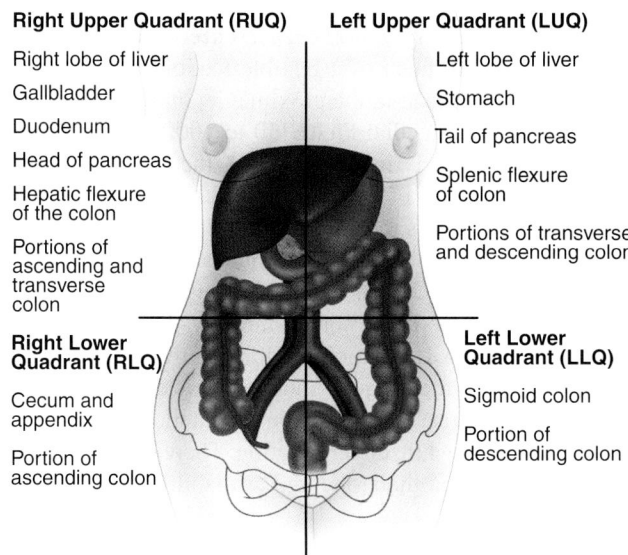

dysfunction and oral aspiration. An **upper gastrointestinal series** also includes radiographic observation of the barium moving into the stomach and the first part of the small intestine. If only a barium swallow is performed, the examination may take as little as 20 minutes. If stomach filling and emptying need to be observed, the test may take approximately 1 hour.

For 2 to 3 days before the procedure, the client is placed on a low-residue diet. Usually, they take nothing by mouth (NPO) for 8 to 12 hours before the test (Nutrition Notes). A laxative may be given to clean out the GI tract. Smoking stimulates gastric motility, so the client is asked not to smoke for 12 to 24 hours before the procedure. With rare exceptions (e.g., anticonvulsants, insulin), all medications are withheld on the day of the procedure.

Barium is very constipating. Once any test using barium is over, the nurse encourages the client to drink fluids liberally to dilute the barium and promote its elimination from the GI tract. They advise the client that stools will appear white, streaky, or clay colored from the barium. The nurse must wait to obtain stool specimens until the client has fully excreted the barium. In some cases, a laxative may help with evacuation. In all cases, failure to have a bowel movement within a reasonable time must be reported to the primary provider because the retained barium can cause a blockage.

Nutrition Notes

The Client Undergoing Diagnostic Gastrointestinal Testing

- Many GI tests require at least an 8-hour fast beforehand. Repeated or multiple tests performed over several days can compound potential or existing nutritional problems.
- Encourage adequate fluid intake to promote dilution and elimination of dyes and other test substances.
- Observe for subsequent signs and symptoms of intolerance in clients whose test requires ingesting a special solution, such as a carbohydrate solution. For instance, clients tested for lactose intolerance may experience cramping, abdominal distention, and diarrhea after ingestion of the substrate used for testing.

Lower Gastrointestinal Test or Small Bowel Series

A lower GI test or small bowel series is fluoroscopy of the small intestine after the ingestion of a contrast medium. It is used to identify tumors, inflammation, or obstruction in the jejunum or ileum. It is performed like an upper GI series, but the client must swallow more barium for the small intestine to be well visualized. If the health care provider suspects an obstruction or *fistula* (a leaking channel between two structures), a water-soluble contrast medium, such as methylglucamine diatrizoate (Gastrografin), is used instead of the barium. The test takes 5 to 6 hours, which is when the contrast medium reaches the lower portion of the small intestine. When a small bowel series fails to detect subtle small bowel disease, enteroclysis may be indicated.

Enteroclysis

Also known as a *small bowel enema*, **enteroclysis** requires nasal or oral placement of a flexible feeding tube, the tip of which is positioned in the proximal jejunum. This study uses two contrast media. First, 750 to 1000 mL of a thin barium suspension is infused through the tube, followed by 750 to 1000 mL of methylcellulose. The two contrast media fill in and pass through the intestinal loops. The examiner observes the intestine continuously by fluoroscopy and takes periodic X-rays of the various sections of the small intestine. Even with normal motility, this process can take up to 6 hours. If sedation is administered to ensure the client's comfort, they require monitoring accordingly. The risk that the contrast media may be aspirated is increased if the client vomits while under sedation. Therefore, positioning of the client on their side and availability of a suction apparatus are critical.

Barium Enema or Lower Gastrointestinal Series

A **barium enema** or **lower gastrointestinal series** is used to identify polyps, tumors, inflammation, strictures, and other abnormalities of the colon. It is performed in the radiology department. The radiographic technologist instills 1000 to 1500 mL of barium solution rectally. They observe the rectum, sigmoid colon, and descending colon fluoroscopically during filling. To facilitate this process, the examiner directs the client to make multiple position changes. The client must retain the barium during this test, which may take up to 30 minutes.

During the test, the client may experience abdominal cramping and a strong urge to defecate. The nurse reassures the client that most people can retain the instilled barium throughout the test. X-rays are taken again after the client expels the barium. In some cases, air is instilled to compress the barium residue against the wall of the lower intestine to aid in detecting mucosal defects. Stool specimens are not collected until the barium has been expelled completely.

To reduce the formation of stool and remove any residual stool, the client follows prescribed restrictions and procedures 24 to 48 hours before the barium enema:

- Low-residue diet 1 to 2 days before the test
- Clear liquid diet the evening before the test
- A laxative the evening before the test
- NPO after midnight
- Cleansing enemas the morning of the test (if not contraindicated by inflammation or active bleeding)

The amount of fluids is not restricted, and the client usually does not have to withhold oral medications. The client may have up to three cleansing enemas (or until the evacuated solution appears clear) before the procedure. After the examination is complete, the client may resume eating. The nurse encourages the client to rest and to drink fluids liberally. They also monitor the passage of stool and informs the client that feces will appear white until the barium is completely eliminated.

Oral Cholecystography or Gallbladder Series

Ultrasonography has mostly replaced oral cholecystography or **gallbladder series**. It is easier and quicker to perform and is as accurate as the other tests. It also has the benefit of not exposing clients to more radiation. In addition, ultrasound can be safely used for clients with liver disease and jaundice. However, if it is not available or ultrasound tests are not conclusive, **cholecystography** can be used to identify stones in the gallbladder or common bile duct and tumors or other obstructions. The test also determines the ability of the gallbladder to concentrate and store a dyelike, iodine-based, radiopaque contrast medium. After the dye is absorbed, it goes to the liver, is excreted into the bile, and passes into the gallbladder, making it radiographically visible. Radiography of the gallbladder should be performed before other GI examinations in which barium is used because residual barium tends to obscure the image of the gallbladder and its ducts.

Instructions before the procedure vary, but generally a client is asked to eat a fat-free meal the night before the test. It is important to ask the client whether they are allergic to iodine. Under the direction of a primary provider, the client swallows six iodine-containing contrast tablets—one every 5 minutes 10 to 12 hours before the procedure with a total of 250 mL of water or more. After the client ingests the contrast agent, they need to be NPO and may not eat or drink until after the test is complete. If the contrast dye causes nausea and vomiting, the client or nurse needs to notify the primary provider so that more tablets can be ordered or the test rescheduled. Once the initial X-rays are obtained, a fatty test meal or fatty synthetic substance may be given to stimulate gallbladder contraction and emptying. Additional X-rays are taken to determine the gallbladder's ability to empty.

Cholangiography

Performed in the radiology department or during surgery, **cholangiography** determines the patency of the ducts from the liver and gallbladder. It is used when the gallbladder is not distinctly visualized with an oral cholecystogram, vomiting interferes with the retention of the oral dye, or the status of the ductal system needs to be determined during or after surgery. There are four specific types of cholangiography:

- *Endoscopic retrograde cholangiopancreatography* (ERCP): With the use of endoscopy, dye is injected through a catheter into the common bile duct and the pancreatic duct. Direct visualization is accomplished with a flexible fiberoptic endoscope. It is inserted into the esophagus through the stomach into the descending duodenum (Fig. 44-3). The client is asked to change positions frequently in order to move the endoscope. In addition, fluoroscopy and multiple X-rays are required.
- *Intraoperative cholangiography*: The contrast agent is injected directly into the bile duct during gallbladder surgery.
- *Magnetic resonance cholangiopancreatography* (MRCP): This newer technique for visualizing the bile ducts, the pancreatic duct, and the gallbladder does not use contrast dye but rather MRI, thus obtaining computerized images. These images provide clear and detailed views.
- *Percutaneous transhepatic cholangiography* (PTC): Ultrasound is used to guide a needle into the bile ducts so that a water-soluble contrast agent can be directly injected into the biliary system. This procedure is safe for clients with liver disease and jaundice. It is used for clients with jaundice caused by liver disease, for clients with GI symptoms who do not have a gallbladder, to locate stones within the bile ducts, or to diagnose cancer within the biliary system. A flexible needle is inserted into the liver. Ultrasound assists the primary provider in guiding puncture of the bile duct.

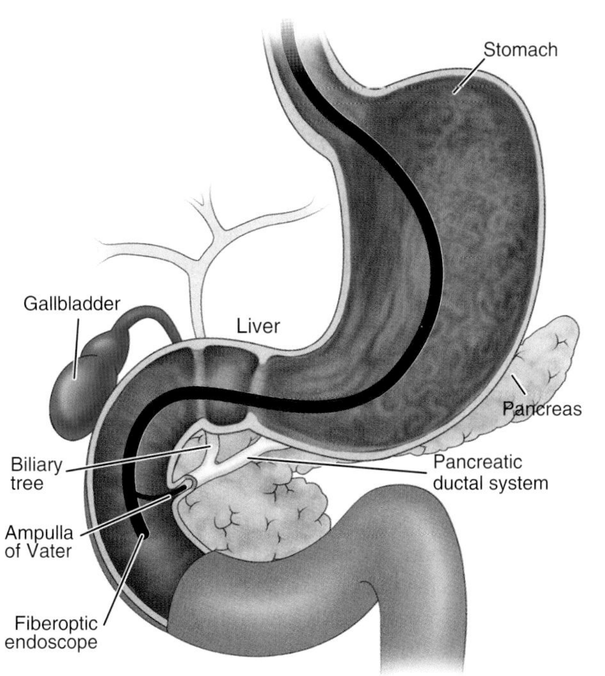

Figure 44-3 Endoscopic retrograde cholangiopancreatography (ERCP). A fiberoptic duodenoscope with side-viewing apparatus is inserted into the duodenum. The ampulla of Vater is catheterized, and the biliary tree is injected with contrast agent. The pancreatic ductal system is also assessed if indicated. This procedure is of special value in visualizing neoplasms of the ampulla area and extracting biopsy specimen.

If a contrast agent is used, no matter how it is introduced, it spreads into the biliary system. X-rays are then taken to show narrowing or blockages within the biliary system.

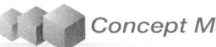

Concept Mastery Alert

Endoscopic Retrograde Cholangiopancreatography

When educating a client preparing to undergo an ERCP, the most important point for the nurse to emphasize is that the client's cooperation will be needed to change positions frequently throughout the procedure in order to prevent injuring the GI tract.

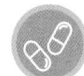

Pharmacologic Considerations

- Allergy to shellfish may signal risk for reaction to intravenous (IV) contrast. Study shows the link between shellfish and iodine allergy is no greater than other food allergies, yet it should always be investigated before a procedure (Long et al., 2019).

The client must sign a consent form. As part of this agreement, if the client is having an ERCP, the client must understand that their cooperation is essential in terms of frequent position changes and prevention of injury to the GI tract. If a contrast agent is going to be used, the nurse asks the client if they are allergic to iodine or shellfish. Clients having a PTC need to know they have to fast before the procedure and will have moderate sedation. Clients having a PTC are at risk for bleeding and infection. Therefore, coagulation studies and platelet counts are done. Clients also receive antibiotics during and after the procedure. Clients are repositioned frequently on the fluoroscopy table to enable multiple X-rays from different views.

Before the procedure, the nurse checks primary provider orders to determine if the client needs a cleansing enema. It may also be necessary to restrict food and fluids for several hours before the procedure. The nurse informs the client that they may experience a warm sensation and nausea when the contrast agent is instilled. After the procedure, the client may eat and drink. To promote dye excretion, the nurse encourages the client to drink liberally.

Radionuclide Imaging

Radionuclide imaging detects lesions of the liver or pancreas and assists in evaluating gastric emptying. A radionuclide is a radioactive natural or synthetic element, such as technetium. Once the radionuclide is injected intravenously or ingested orally, the radiologist may examine a body organ by passing the radionuclide imaging scanner over the structure. This test is helpful in demonstrating the size of the organ as well as defects or lesions such as tumors. Specialized radionuclide studies are done to identify sites of bleeding or inflammation in the GI tract. Radionuclides have rather short half-lives, lasting a few hours to days, during which they emit radiation, which is usually less than with diagnostic radiography.

Pretest measures include weighing the client to calculate the radionuclide dose and determining pregnancy and lactation. Breast milk may be pumped and discarded so that the nursing child remains safe from radioactivity. The test is contraindicated in pregnant women.

Computed Tomography

Computed tomography (CT) scanning may be performed to detect structural abnormalities of the GI tract. These tests help detect metastatic lesions that might not be apparent on regular GI X-rays. Oral barium sulfate or IV calcium phosphate may be given to provide contrast for the hollow GI organs examined by CT scan. The client is NPO for 6 to 8 hours before the CT test. Before the test, the bowel may be cleaned to reduce stool and gas. Drugs may be administered to decrease peristalsis or improve gastric motility.

Continuous motion (helical or spherical), three-dimensional CT scans enable examiners to have detailed pictures of GI organs and vessels. This procedure is referred to as *colonography*. Clients are prepared as they are for CT scanning. A small tube is inserted into the colon, air is introduced to inflate the colon, and computer images are produced.

Magnetic Resonance Imaging

MRI uses magnetic energy rather than radiation to visualize soft tissue structures. It is used to examine GI structures when CT scanning is inadequate. Oral contrast agents are used to enhance the evaluation of GI disorders, such as abscesses or bleeding.

The client is NPO for 6 to 8 hours before the MRI. They must remove any metal objects, credit cards, wristwatch, jewelry, and the like. Clients with pacemakers may need a cardiology consult before the MRI to determine if there are any risks or contraindications. IV fluids, if required, must be infused by gravity during MRI because the changes in electrical charges during the test can affect mechanical infusers or pumps. The nurse informs clients that the scanner, a narrow, tunnel-like machine that will enclose them during the test, makes loud repetitive noises while the test is in progress. Clients who are claustrophobic (fear enclosed spaces) may need sedation because it is imperative that they lie still and not panic during the test.

Magnetic Resonance Elastography

Magnetic resonance elastography (MRE) is a noninvasive methodology that combines MRI with low-frequency sound waves (referred to as *shear waves*). The resulting images enable primary providers to ascertain the firmness of the liver, thus allowing them to better predict clients who are at risk for developing fibrosis (scar tissue) and eventually cirrhosis (hardening of the liver). If detected early, treatment of the underlying cause can be initiated before the client develops cirrhosis, which is an irreversible and eventually fatal condition. Primary providers previously could only rely on palpation, which is inconclusive, or a liver biopsy, which is diagnostic for only a small portion of the liver, and very invasive, with risks of bleeding. MRE shows great promise for other parts of the body, such as breasts, muscles, and brain tissue.

Ultrasonography

In **ultrasonography** (also called *ultrasound*), high-frequency sound waves are directed through the body where they bounce off nearby structures such as the liver and pancreas. The returning sound waves are then interpreted and recorded electronically. Ultrasonography, which shows the size and location of organs and outlines structures and abnormalities, helps detect cholecystitis, cholelithiasis, pyloric stenosis, and some disorders of the biliary system. It may be useful in detecting changes caused by appendicitis. Although the client can drink water before ultrasonography, the nurse discourages drinking through a straw, smoking, or chewing gum. In these activities, the client may swallow air and thereby distort sound wave transmission.

Endoscopic ultrasonography uses a fiberoptic scope with a small high-frequency ultrasonic transducer to obtain direct images of specific areas along the GI tract. The images have higher resolution and help in staging tumors and evaluating changes in the intestinal walls.

Percutaneous Liver Biopsy

In a procedure called **percutaneous liver biopsy** (Fig. 44-4), the primary provider obtains a small core of liver tissue by

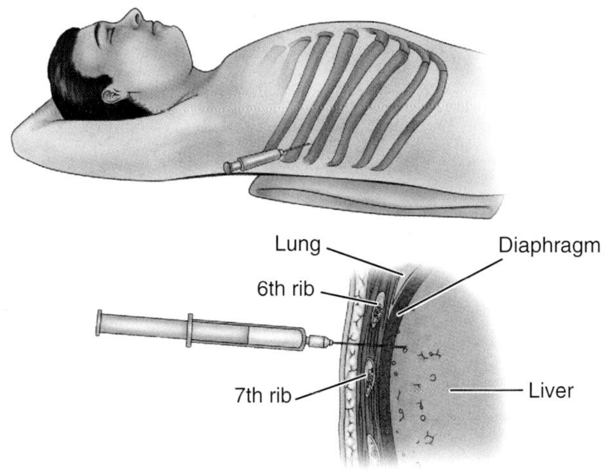

Figure 44-4 Percutaneous liver biopsy. (Reprinted with permission from Hinkle, J. L., & Cheever, K. H. (2014). *Brunner & Suddarth's textbook of medical-surgical nursing* (13th ed.). Wolters Kluwer Health/Lippincott Williams & Wilkins.)

placing a needle through the client's lateral abdominal wall directly into the liver. The tissue is then examined microscopically to detect abnormalities, which may include malignant changes, infectious or inflammatory processes, liver damage (cirrhosis), and signs of rejection in clients who have received a liver transplant.

Although the procedure is most often performed in the hospital operating room, it may be done in a primary provider's office or other outpatient site or in a radiology department. The client must have coagulation studies before the procedure because a major complication after a liver biopsy is bleeding. Ultrasound or CT scanning is performed before or during the biopsy to identify an appropriate site for placement of the biopsy needle. The client usually receives a sedative and anesthetic to promote comfort and cooperation.

When assisting with a percutaneous liver biopsy, the nurse ensures that the biopsy equipment is assembled and in order. They help the client assume a supine position with a rolled towel beneath the right lower ribs. Before the primary provider inserts the needle, the nurse instructs the client to take a deep breath and hold it to keep the liver as near to the abdominal wall as possible. After specimen cells are obtained, they are placed in a preservative. The nurse makes sure that the specimen container is labeled and delivered to the laboratory (Nursing Guidelines 44-1).

NURSING GUIDELINES 44-1

Assisting With a Percutaneous Liver Biopsy

- Explain that the purpose of the procedure is to obtain a small sample of liver tissue for a differential diagnosis of liver disease or to evaluate the extent of liver disease.
- Check the results of coagulation studies (aPTT, PT, INR, and platelet count).
- Check that the informed consent form has been signed.
- Instruct the client to lie supine with the right arm behind the head.
- Tell the client that the site will be cleansed and then draped with a sterile barrier.
- The primary provider will instruct the client to take a deep breath and hold it while the needle is introduced, sample obtained, and needle withdrawn; this takes only a few seconds.
- Monitor vital signs throughout the procedure.
- Place a pressure dressing over the biopsy site.
- Assist the client to lie on the right side after the procedure and place a small pillow under the costal margin.
- Instruct client to remain in this position for at least 2 hours to prevent the release of blood, bile, or both.
- Instruct the client that they should remain in bed for 8 to 12 hours, except to go to the bathroom. The client should avoid coughing or straining during this time.
- Continue to monitor vital signs according to agency policy. Changes in vital signs may indicate bleeding.
- Monitor the biopsy site frequently for bleeding, swelling, or hematoma.
- Assess breath sounds regularly. Report diminished breath sounds immediately.
- Assess the abdomen for distention or rigidity. Report if the client is experiencing abdominal pain.
- Instruct the client to avoid heavy lifting and strenuous activity for 5 to 7 days after the procedure.
- Instruct the client to follow primary provider orders for blood-thinning medications.
- Instruct the client to call if they experience the following symptoms:
  - Severe pain at the biopsy site
  - Shortness of breath
  - Chest pain
  - Bleeding from the biopsy site
  - Fever
  - Abdominal pain
  - Weakness or diaphoresis
  - Heart palpitations

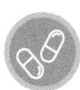

Pharmacologic Considerations

■ All anticoagulant medications (including nonsteroidal anti-inflammatory drugs [NSAIDs]) should be stopped 3 days to 1 week before liver biopsy. Clients with bleeding conditions, such as hemophilia, may be given an intramuscular (IM) injection of vitamin K before the procedure.

Gastrointestinal Endoscopy

GI endoscopy is the direct visual examination of the lumen of the GI tract. It facilitates evaluation of the appearance and integrity of the GI mucosa and detects lesions. It provides access for therapeutic procedures. GI endoscopy is performed using a flexible fiberoptic endoscope. Diagnostic uses include obtaining biopsies of the mucosa, obtaining samples of fluids found in the GI tract, and injecting dyes

BOX 44-1 Common Gastrointestinal Endoscopic Procedures

Esophagogastroduodenoscopy
Examination of the esophagus, stomach, and duodenum through an endoscope advanced orally to inspect, treat, or obtain specimens from any one or all of the upper GI structures.

Colonoscopy
Examination of the entire large intestine with a flexible fiberoptic colonoscope. Clients are sedated briefly (and monitored accordingly) with IV medication during the procedure. The colonoscope is advanced anally from the rectum to the cecum, allowing visualization of the rectum, sigmoid, and descending colon. The distal portion of the small intestine, the terminal ileum, may be inspected as well. Air may be instilled to promote visualization within the folds of the intestinal mucosa. Primary providers may remove polyps or perform biopsies as indicated.

Virtual Colonoscopy or CT Colonography
A noninvasive procedure requiring the same preparation as a colonoscopy. Sedation is not required. A small flexible rubber catheter is inserted in the rectum, and air or carbon dioxide is pumped through the tube to distend the colon. With the use of a CT scanner, images are taken with the client in a supine and prone position. Any other procedure cannot be done (e.g., removal of polyps and/or biopsies).

Although there are some concerns that the level of detail is not as great as with colonoscopy, it is a good diagnostic method. There is less risk of bowel perforation, and clients do not require sedation or pain relievers for this procedure. For clients on blood-thinning medications, virtual colonoscopy is a good alternative. Unfortunately, many insurance companies do not cover this procedure unless there are associated symptoms.

Proctosigmoidoscopy
Examination of the rectum and sigmoid colon using a rigid endoscope inserted anally about 10 inches. To facilitate examination, the client must lie in a knee–chest position. The test is brief and no sedation is needed.

Peritoneoscopy
Examination of GI structures through an endoscope inserted percutaneously through a small incision in the abdominal wall with the client receiving a local, spinal, or general anesthetic. Also called *laparoscopy*.

Small Bowel Enteroscopy
Endoscopic examination and visualization of the lumen of the small bowel.

Panendoscopy
Examination of both the upper and lower GI tracts.

for radiographic purposes. Therapeutic uses include inserting tubes and drains, electrocautery, and injecting medications. Among the variations of GI endoscopy (Box 44-1) are **proctosigmoidoscopy**, **esophagogastroduodenoscopy** (EGD) (Fig. 44-5), small bowel enteroscopy, peritoneoscopy, **colonoscopy** (Fig. 44-6), **virtual colonoscopy**, **flexible sigmoidoscopy**, and **panendoscopy**.

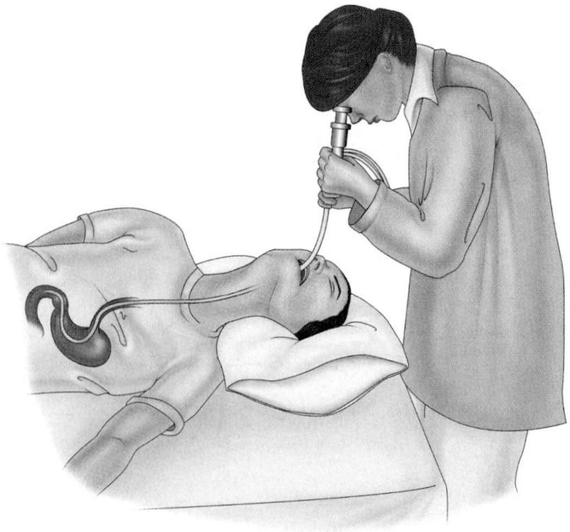

Figure 44-5 Esophagogastroduodenoscopy. (Reprinted with permission from Hinkle, J. L., & Cheever, K. H. (2014). *Brunner & Suddarth's textbook of medical-surgical nursing* (13th ed.). Wolters Kluwer Health/Lippincott Williams & Wilkins.)

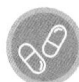

Pharmacologic Considerations

- Clear visualization of internal structures is important during endoscopic procedures. A clear liquid diet a number of hours before a procedure may suffice for viewing structures from the mouth to a portion of the small intestine. Viewing the lower bowel often requires cleansing, typically with laxatives. This is frequently done at home and may be taken orally as a pill or large-volume solutions.
- Emptying of the rectum may require enema solutions as well. The goal is to evacuate all intestinal contents. Instruct clients to call before the procedure if they feel evacuation of all contents was unsuccessful. The procedure may be rescheduled when visualization is better.

Before an endoscopic procedure, the client follows dietary and fluid restrictions and bowel preparation procedures if the examination involves the lower GI structures. For the client undergoing an EGD, it is necessary that they spray or gargle with a local anesthetic. For an EGD and a colonoscopy, the client receives an anxiolytic agent such as midazolam (Versed) before the procedure to provide sedation and relieve anxiety. Clients having these procedures must have someone drive them to and from the procedure site because they should not drive until the day after the procedure.

During an endoscopic procedure, the nurse monitors respirations and vital signs. Assessing the client's level of pain and discomfort during the procedure is important, as is medicating the client as indicated. After the test, the nurse assesses the client's vital signs, respiratory status, level of consciousness, and abdominal symptoms. The nurse monitors the client for complications, especially signs of perforation. These include fever, abdominal distention, abdominal or chest pain, vomiting blood, or bright red rectal bleeding. The nurse offers the client light food and fluids, unless the procedure was an EGD.

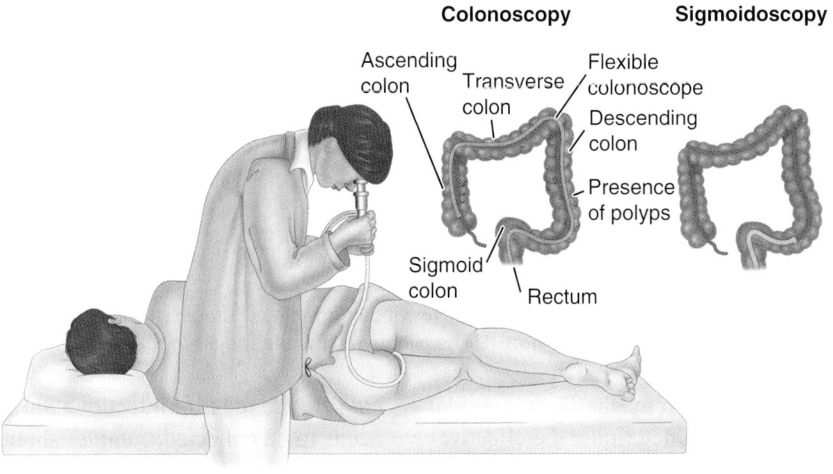

Figure 44-6 Colonoscopy and flexible fiberoptic sigmoidoscopy. For the colonoscopy, the flexible scope is passed through the rectum and sigmoid colon into the descending, transverse, and ascending colon. For the flexible fiberoptic sigmoidoscopy, the flexible scope is advanced past the proximal sigmoid and then into the descending colon. (Reprinted with permission from Hinkle, J. L., & Cheever, K. H. (2014). *Brunner & Suddarth's textbook of medical-surgical nursing* (13th ed.). Wolters Kluwer Health/Lippincott Williams & Wilkins.)

After an EGD, the client may not have food or fluids until the gag reflex returns. Once the gag reflex is present, the nurse may introduce clear fluids and advance the diet to regular foods and fluids according to the client's tolerance. Occasionally, the client may complain of a sore throat after EGD. If the client's gag reflex has returned, the nurse may offer saline gargles, ice chips, or cool drinks. Client and Family Teaching 44-1 outlines discharge instructions following a colonoscopy.

Laboratory Tests

Depending on the suspected or confirmed diagnosis, various blood and urine tests may be ordered. Laboratory tests may include a complete blood count, urinalysis, serum bilirubin, cholesterol, serum ammonia level, prothrombin time, protein electrophoresis, and enzymes such as amylase, lipase, aspartate aminotransferase, and lactic acid dehydrogenase. Common tumor marker blood studies include carcinoembryonic antigen and alpha fetoprotein. Tests specific to the GI system are described in the following sections.

Gastric Analysis

Analysis of gastric fluids assists in determining problems with the secretory activity of the gastric mucosa. It also helps evaluate gastric retention in clients who may have partial or complete pyloric or duodenal obstruction. For 8 to 12 hours before the test, the client is NPO. A small nasogastric tube is inserted into the stomach. Gastric contents are aspirated every 15 minutes for at least 1 hour and analyzed for acidity (pH), volume, and cytology if indicated.

Tests for *Helicobacter pylori*

Helicobacter pylori, a type of bacteria, are believed to be responsible for the majority of peptic ulcers. Gastric mucosal specimens, obtained during an endoscopy, are cultured for *H. pylori*. Blood tests are used to determine whether there are antibodies to *H. pylori* in the blood. Urea breath tests are also used to test for active infection from *H. pylori*. The client either drinks a urea solution or swallows a urea capsule. Breath tests are then conducted by having the client blow up a small balloon (Fig. 44-7) or by blowing bubbles in a small container of breath-collection liquid. If *H. pylori* bacteria are present, they break down the urea, releasing carbon. The blood carries the air to the lungs, where it is exhaled, and the

Client and Family Teaching 44-1 Discharge Instructions Following Colonoscopy

When the client is alert and managing fluids and small amounts of food, they may be discharged. The client must not drive the entire day following the procedure because they received sedative medication. The nurse provides the following instructions:

- Mild cramping and flatulence are expected; these symptoms will resolve within 24 hours.
- If you had a small growth or polyp removed, you may experience a slight amount of bleeding that resolves on its own.
- Avoid eating high-fat or high-fiber foods for at least 24 hours following the procedure.
- Biopsy results will be available in 5 to 7 days.
- Report the following problems that, if present, may indicate bowel perforation, hemorrhage, or infection:
  - Nausea
  - Vomiting
  - Fever
  - Excessive bleeding
  - Need to guard or protect abdomen
- Rebound abdominal tenderness
- Resume your usual medication regimen unless instructed otherwise.

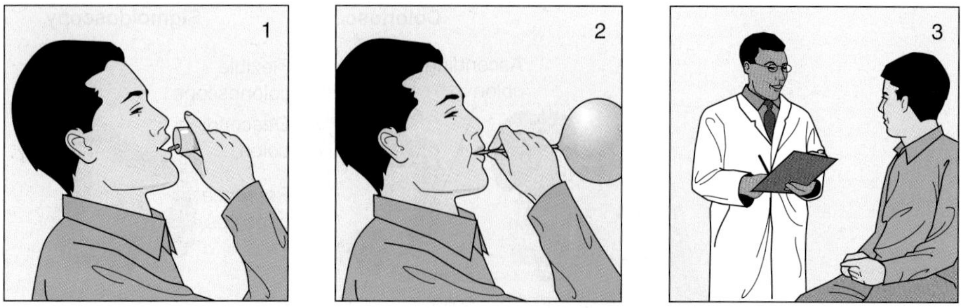

Figure 44-7 The breath test indicating *Helicobacter pylori* is performed in three easy steps: **(1)** The client takes a C-urea capsule and waits about 10 minutes. **(2)** The client blows up a balloon. **(3)** The client waits while the air in the balloon is analyzed for gastric urease.

air is analyzed. During and after therapy, the *H. pylori* stool antigen (HpSa) test can be done to determine the effectiveness of treatment.

Breath Hydrogen Test

This test involves collecting a breath sample before and at intervals after ingestion of a carbohydrate solution (used with glucose tolerance tests [GTT]). The two major gases in expired air are hydrogen and carbon dioxide. Elevated hydrogen levels in the expired breath sample indicate carbohydrate malabsorption. The type of solution used for the test depends on the suspected type of malabsorption. Lactose malabsorption (lactose intolerance) is the most common disorder investigated using this technique.

Stool Analysis

Stool specimens are collected to identify white blood cells (indicating inflammation), red blood cells (indicating GI blood loss), and fat (indicating malabsorption). They are also collected to identify infection. Only a small amount of stool needs to be collected; samples should always be placed in a covered container. To examine for microorganisms, specimens should be fresh and warm. Routine cultures may reveal bacterial infections (e.g., *Salmonella*, *Shigella*, *Campylobacter*). Placement of the specimen in a specific preservative to detect parasites and their ova allows diagnosis of parasitic infections (e.g., *Giardia*, *Cryptosporidium*).

A simple test that determines the presence of occult blood in the stool is the Hemoccult test. A positive result indicates that the client is bleeding or has recently bled from somewhere in the GI tract. Substances that may cause false positive results include red meat, iodine-containing antiseptic preparations, aspirin (greater than 325 mg/day) and other nonsteroidal anti-inflammatory agents, and excessive alcohol. Substances that may cause false negative results include ascorbic acid (vitamin C greater than 250 mg/day) and iron supplements.

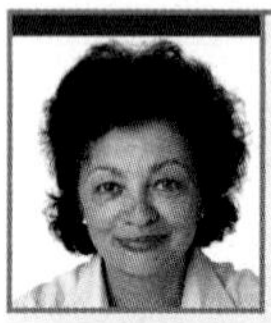

Clinical Scenario A client is seen by the primary care physician (PCP) for complaints of intermittent nausea, vague abdominal pain that is occasionally persistent, dyspepsia (indigestion), and some bouts of diarrhea. The client has been experiencing these symptoms for at least 6 months. The PCP schedules the client for several GI tests. **What nursing considerations are necessary for this client? See the following Nursing Process section.**

NURSING PROCESS FOR THE CLIENT UNDERGOING DIAGNOSTIC TESTING FOR A GASTROINTESTINAL DISORDER

Assessment

Interview the client to determine past familiarity with the test or similar procedure. Ask the client to discuss previous experiences or current expectations. If the client is responsible for self-preparation before the test, explain those preparations. Review the client's history and explore any data on prior hypersensitivity or allergy to test preparations. In particular, ask about reactions to radionuclide or iodine-based contrast medium (dye), possibly signaled by allergy to seafood. In some situations, label an allergic client's chart and apply a special band or tag to the client's identification bracelet.

Take vital signs and weigh the client if required before the procedure. Encourage the client to empty the bladder before some tests. It is important to record other essential baseline data for later comparison and identification of serious reportable changes or complications (e.g., rectal bleeding). In addition, record the client's informed consent.

Diagnosis, Planning, and Interventions

Acute Anxiety: Related to lack of knowledge of test procedure or possible test findings
Expected Outcomes: (1) Client will demonstrate knowledge of the test procedure. (2) Client will express feelings of relief from anxiety.

NURSING PROCESS FOR THE CLIENT UNDERGOING DIAGNOSTIC TESTING FOR A GASTROINTESTINAL DISORDER (continued)

- Explain the test's purpose and procedure and what to expect afterward. *Providing such information reassures the client about what will occur, thus relieving anxiety.*
- Review test preparations. *Such a review ensures that the client understands and carries out preparations as required.*
- Provide printed directions. *Printed directions reinforce verbal instructions.*
- Encourage client to express fears. *Expressing feelings assists in alleviating fear and clarifying misconceptions.*
- Discuss the client's perceptions and expectations of the test. *Having knowledge of the client's understanding provides an opportunity to reinforce the knowledge and to clarify expectations for the test.*
- Respect the client's individuality and remain nonjudgmental and supportive. *Respect makes the client more likely to ask questions without fear of ridicule.*

Acute Pain: Related to test procedure
Expected Outcome: Client will state no or minimal discomfort.

- Use pillows or blankets for positioning to relieve discomfort if the client has physical problems that cause pain (e.g., arthritis). *Supportive positioning alleviates and relieves pain.*
- Medicate the client with opioid analgesic or sedative if ordered before the procedure. *Analgesia or conscious sedation reduces pain and discomfort during the procedure.*
- Tell the client to inform test personnel if they experience pressure or cramping during the instillation of test fluids. *Test personnel can slow the instillation or take other measures to relieve discomfort.*
- Teach the client to expel gas and test fluids from the bowel when they experience the urge. *Ignoring the urge to expel bowel contents increases pain and discomfort.*

Hypovolemia: Related to fluid restriction or loss associated with diarrhea or vomiting
Expected Outcome: Client will maintain fluid volume balance as evidenced by normal findings on intake and output records.

- Weigh client and monitor the color and amount of urine. *These data provide a baseline for the client's response to tests, fluid loss related to diarrhea or vomiting, or both.*
- Monitor pulse rate and blood pressure. *Changes may indicate dehydration.*
- Report dizziness and confusion. *Such findings may indicate dehydration.*
- Administer oral fluids as soon as possible. *These fluids replace fluid loss.*
- When testing is complete, monitor intake and output and encourage liberal intake. *These measures ensure that client is taking in adequate fluids.*

Constipation Risk: Related to barium retention
Expected Outcome: Client achieves regular bowel elimination pattern within 2 to 3 days.

- Encourage client to drink at least 2000 mL of fluid per 24 hours after tests using barium. *This amount provides sufficient fluid to facilitate evacuation of stool.*
- Administer posttest laxative or enema if ordered. *A laxative or an enema promotes quicker evacuation of barium.*
- Monitor stool passage, observing the stool for barium. *Stools with barium appear light colored or white streaked.*
- Report diminished or hyperactive bowel sounds. *Such sounds may indicate barium retention.*

Evaluation of Expected Outcomes

The client reports minimal anxiety and pain, maintains adequate fluid balance, and evacuates all barium. Normal bowel elimination resumes as evidenced by statement from client.

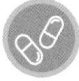

Pharmacologic Considerations

- Some, all, or none of the client's medications may be withheld before and during testing, depending on the test procedure, the client's medication regimen, and primary provider's orders.

KEY POINTS

- GI anatomy and physiology includes mouth, esophagus, stomach, small intestine, and large intestine.
- Accessory structures include peritoneum, liver, gallbladder, and pancreas.
- Assessment should include the following:
  - General appearance
  - Skin
  - Mouth
  - Abdomen
  - Anus
- Diagnostic tests are done for problems throughout the GI tract. These include barium swallow, upper GI series, small bowel series, enteroclysis (small bowel enema), barium enema, gallbladder series, ERCP, MRCP, CT, MRI, MRE, ultrasonography, percutaneous liver biopsy, and GI endoscopy.
- Laboratory tests include gastric analysis, *H. Pylori* testing, breath hydrogen test, and stool analysis.

CRITICAL THINKING EXERCISES

1. A client is preparing for an EGD. This includes withholding food and fluids for 6 to 12 hours and receiving a sedative before the test. In addition, the nurse will spray the client's throat with a local anesthetic or the client will gargle with the local anesthetic. What precautions does the nurse take before the client goes for the EGD?
2. When the client returns from the EGD, what is important for the nurse to assess?
3. A client is complaining of epigastric pain. What areas of the abdomen should be included in the nurse's assessment?
4. A client has a potential diagnosis of colon cancer. Which tests do you anticipate the primary provider will order for the client?

NCLEX-STYLE REVIEW QUESTIONS PrepU

1. The nurse, assessing a client's abdomen, does not hear any bowel sounds in the right lower quadrant (RLQ) for 5 minutes. What action is best for the nurse to do next?
   1. Ask the client if they have had a bowel movement.
   2. Auscultate in another quadrant for a minimum of 3 minutes.
   3. Document "bowel sounds absent" for this client.
   4. Listen for another 3 minutes over the RLQ.
2. The nurse needs to assess a client's abdomen. To best accomplish this, the nurse directs the client to lie in which of the following positions?
   1. In a semi-Fowler position
   2. On the right side with knees straight
   3. Prone with knees slightly bent
   4. Supine with knees flexed
3. A nurse is providing preprocedure instructions to a client scheduled for a barium enema. Which of the following statements indicates that the client understands the instructions?
   1. "I can eat whatever I want before the test."
   2. "I can only have clear liquids the day before the test."
   3. "I cannot eat any spicy foods for 7 days before the barium enema."
   4. "I have to abstain from all food and fluids for 24 hours before the test."
4. Before administering the contrast substance (oral tablets taken the evening before the procedure) to a client scheduled for an oral cholecystography, which question is essential for the nurse to ask?
   1. "Can the client tolerate holding still?"
   2. "Does the client want any anesthesia?"
   3. "How many X-rays has the client had?"
   4. "Is the client allergic to iodine?"
5. Which nursing action is most appropriate after a liver biopsy is done on a client with cirrhosis?
   1. Ambulating the client twice each shift
   2. Elevating the client's legs on two pillows
   3. Keeping the client in high Fowler position
   4. Positioning the client on the right side
6. A client has a colonoscopy. While recovering, the nurse assesses the client's abdomen. Which sign indicates a potential complication of the colonoscopy?
   1. Loose stools
   2. Mild cramping
   3. Nausea and vomiting
   4. Rebound tenderness

WANT TO KNOW MORE? There is a wide variety of online resources available on thePoint to enhance learning and understanding of this chapter.

Go to **thePoint.lww.com/activate** and use the activation code found in the front of this text to unlock these online resources.

45 Caring for Clients With Disorders of the Upper Gastrointestinal Tract

Words To Know

anorexia
bariatric surgery
diverticulum
dumping syndrome
dyspepsia
esophagitis
extreme obesity
fundoplication
gastrectomy
gastric decompression
gastritis
gastroesophageal reflux disease (GERD)
gastrostomy
hiatal or diaphragmatic hernia
jejunostomy
nasoenteric intubation
nasogastric intubation
odynophagia
orogastric intubation
peptic ulcer
percutaneous endoscopic gastrostomy
pyrosis

Learning Objectives

On completion of this chapter, you will be able to:

1. Discuss assessment findings and treatment of eating disorders, esophageal disorders, and gastric disorders.
2. Describe the nursing management of a client with a nasogastric or gastrointestinal tube or gastrostomy.
3. Identify strategies for relieving upper gastrointestinal discomfort.
4. Discuss the nursing management of clients undergoing gastric surgery.

Digestion begins in the mouth and continues in the stomach and small intestine, with food traveling through the esophagus in between. The nurse is responsible for managing the care of clients with disorders affecting the upper gastrointestinal (GI) tract (see Fig. 44-1, p. 746).

Gerontologic Considerations

- With age, the salivary glands become less active and the numbers of taste buds are reduced, contributing to anorexia in the older adult. Anorexia and weight loss in the older adult can also result from ill-fitting dentures or dysphagia or may be a manifestation of depression. Decreased appetite may result from diminished oxygenation to the appetite centers in the brain caused by atherosclerosis or decreased cardiac stroke volume.
- Severe and prolonged episodes of vomiting can be especially serious for older adults whose nutritional and fluid intake is marginal; more profound electrolyte imbalances and severe dehydration can result.
- Teach older adults about potential bradycardia, hypotension, or dizziness that accompany the Valsalva maneuver and the safety precaution of calling for assistance or remaining seated until the symptoms pass to decrease the risk of falling.
- Assess older adults for changes in type or dose of medications because side effects often include nausea or vomiting. Awareness of the anorexia/nausea/vomiting side effects of an increased level of medications such as digitalis is important to prevent toxicity.
- A diminished gag reflex that may occur with aging increases the risk for aspiration.

(continued)

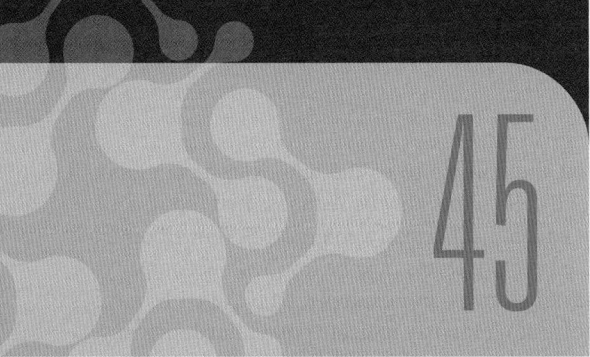

Gerontologic Considerations (*continued*)

- Changes in aging include thinning of the gastric mucosa, predisposing older adults to superficial gastritis and gastric ulcers.
- Common chronic conditions in older adults such as osteoarthritis, vascular, or cardiac problems may require medications such as aspirin, nonsteroidal anti-inflammatory drugs (NSAIDs), or anticoagulants, which increase the risk for gastritis, gastric bleeding, and gastric ulcers. These medications must be used with extreme caution in older adults who concurrently take prednisone, which also causes thinning of the gastric lining.
- Physical changes that occur with aging include degeneration of the gastric mucosa, resulting in a loss of parietal cells. The loss of parietal cells decreases the production of the intrinsic factor and hence decreases the absorption of vitamin B_{12}, leading to pernicious anemia.

DISORDERS THAT AFFECT EATING

Anorexia

Simple **anorexia**, or lack of appetite, is a common symptom of many diseases. (See Chapter 70 for information on *anorexia nervosa*, a complex psychological eating disorder.) Prolonged anorexia may lead to serious consequences such as malnutrition.

Pathophysiology and Etiology

The appetite center, which stimulates or suppresses the appetite, is located in the hypothalamus. Pleasant or noxious food odors, effects of drugs, emotional stress, fear, psychological problems, or illnesses may affect appetite.

Brief periods of anorexia are not life-threatening but can cause temporary malnutrition. During periods of reduced food consumption, most people have a sufficient reserve of stored glycogen, which provides energy through the process of *glycogenolysis*, the conversion of glycogen to glucose. Hormones such as glucagon, glucocorticoid hormones from the adrenal cortex, and thyroid hormones stimulate the liver to carry out *gluconeogenesis*, the synthesis of additional glucose by the liver from protein breakdown or lactate production. Selective reabsorption by the kidneys can temporarily maintain electrolyte balance.

Assessment Findings

Signs and Symptoms

Hunger usually is absent, and clients describe having no desire for food. Some clients state that they feel nauseous when they smell food or even think about eating. Some eat a small amount only because they feel they should or others coerce them to do so. Amounts of weight loss vary depending on how long the anorexia and reduced food intake have lasted. Eventually, the client may show signs of *hypovitaminosis* (vitamin deficiency). The body does not store any water-soluble vitamins (B vitamins, including folic acid and vitamin C) except for vitamin B_{12}. Therefore, deficiencies in these vitamins may be seen in more acute phases of illness. The body does store fat-soluble vitamins (A, D, E, and K) but requires fat absorption to do so. Chronic illnesses and those that directly affect fat absorption (e.g., cystic fibrosis, pancreatitis, liver disease) result in deficiency of the fat-soluble vitamins.

Diagnostic Findings

Depending on the chronicity of the anorexia, hemoglobin level and blood cell counts may be reduced. Red blood cells (RBCs) may become abnormally enlarged. Serum albumin, electrolyte, and protein levels may be low, with accompanying cardiac dysrhythmias. For example, an elevated U wave on the electrocardiogram may indicate potassium deficiency.

Medical and Surgical Management

Management depends on the cause. Short-term anorexia (less than 1 week) usually requires no medical intervention. Persistent anorexia may require various approaches, such as a high-calorie diet, high-calorie supplemental feedings, tube feedings, and total parenteral nutrition (TPN). Psychological support, psychiatric treatment, or both may be essential for the client whose anorexia is linked to *anorexia nervosa*, a psychiatric disorder, instead of a defined organic disease (see Chapter 70).

Nursing Management

To maintain sufficient nutrition and sustain normal body weight, the client must eat an adequate quantity of food. In assisting the client to meet this goal, the nurse monitors their weight daily. They also obtain a complete medical and allergy (drugs and food) history from the client or a family member and compiles a dietary history, including a description of the client's eating patterns and food preferences. For more information, see Nursing Guidelines 45-1.

Additional nursing measures depend on any consequences of anorexia. In the case of altered bowel patterns (diarrhea or constipation) from reduced bulk secondary to liquid supplements, potential interventions include the following:

- Keep a record of the client's bowel movements.
- If the client experiences diarrhea, consult with the primary provider and dietitian about changing the type of supplement.
- If the client is constipated, change the formula to one that contains fiber to add bulk to stools.
- Dilute the formula temporarily until the client adjusts to the concentrated contents.
- Assist the client and dietitian to increase dietary fiber.
- Administer a prescribed stool softener to promote ease and frequency of bowel elimination.

Nausea and Vomiting

Nausea and vomiting are common and often coexisting problems. If these symptoms are prolonged, weakness, weight loss, nutritional deficiency, dehydration, and electrolyte and acid–base imbalances may result.

Pathophysiology and Etiology

Some of the more common causes of nausea and vomiting include drugs, infections and inflammatory conditions of the GI tract, intestinal obstruction, systemic infections, lesions of the central nervous system, food poisoning, emotional stress, early pregnancy, and uremia. Nausea generally precedes vomiting and usually results from distention of the duodenum. Increased salivation and peripheral vasoconstriction, which causes cold, clammy skin, and tachycardia, accompany nausea. The vomiting center, located in the medulla, is particularly sensitive to parasympathetic neurotransmitters released in response to gastric irritation. The Valsalva maneuver, which

NURSING GUIDELINES 45-1

Managing the Care of Clients With Anorexia

- Provide foods that the client likes during meals.
- Offer nourishing beverages (eggnog, milk shakes, and commercial concentrates such as *Ensure* or *Instant Breakfast*) as between-meal snacks.
- If the client is hospitalized or in another health care facility, encourage family members to bring favorite foods that can be refrigerated or reheated.
- Conduct a daily caloric count if necessary to determine total proteins and carbohydrates in the client's diet.
- Keep serving sizes and containers small to avoid overwhelming the client.
- Serve and keep hot foods hot and cold foods cold.
- Encourage eating in the company of others.
- Formulate a nutritional plan with the client and dietitian that promotes weight gain (approximately 600 calories per meal).
- If necessary, arrange for supplementation based on documented deficiencies in the client's intake.
- Consult the primary provider and dietitian in cases of prolonged anorexia.

accompanies the forceful expulsion of stomach contents, causes dizziness, hypotension, and bradycardia.

Assessment Findings

Signs and Symptoms

The client describes an unpleasant feeling, identified as nausea, which usually is associated with loss of appetite and refusal to eat. When a client vomits, others may observe them retching while they evacuate the stomach contents. The process occurs once or several times in succession.

The client who experiences excessive fluid loss (dehydration) with vomiting may complain of excessive thirst and report decreased or no urine production. Eyes and oral mucosa appear dry or dull, and poor skin turgor reflects fluid loss (see Chapter 16).

The client's history may include ingestion of noxious substances, such as excessive amounts of alcohol, presumably contaminated food, or drugs that commonly cause GI side effects. Exposure to other people with similar symptoms suggests a bacterial or viral cause. When vomiting is secondary to intestinal obstruction, the abdomen is distended, tender, and firm to the touch. Bowel sounds may be absent or hypoactive.

Diagnostic Findings

Prolonged vomiting may lead to low levels of serum sodium and chloride. Bicarbonate levels may rise to compensate for the loss of chloride and accumulation of metabolic acids. The hematocrit value, if high, is secondary to the hemoconcentration that accompanies dehydration.

Medical and Surgical Management

Sometimes, nausea and vomiting are short-lived and do not require medical intervention. In some instances, intravenous (IV) fluids, electrolyte replacement, and drug therapy are necessary. Elimination of the cause necessitates various interventions, ranging from stopping a drug to surgical intervention for intestinal obstruction. Symptomatic relief may be achieved by administering an antiemetic agent (Drug Therapy Table 45-1), providing IV fluid and electrolyte replacement, and temporarily restricting food intake until the cause of vomiting is eliminated (Nutrition Notes).

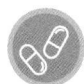

Pharmacologic Considerations

- Consult the primary provider for changes in drug orders if a client cannot retain a medication orally.

DRUG THERAPY TABLE 45-1 Antiemetic Medications

Category and Common Generic (Brand) Drugs	Intended Use	Common Side Effects	Safety Warnings for Nurses
Serotonin (5-HT3) Receptor antagonist Ondansetron (Zofran) Palonosetron (Aloxi) granisetron	Chemotherapy-induced nausea, post-op vomiting, hyperemesis in pregnancy; works by blocking neural receptors for 5HT3	Headache, dizziness (low blood pressure), myalgia (muscle aches and pains), malaise, fatigue, drowsiness	Do not use if the client has heart block or prolonged QT interval Increased sedation if used with opiates Emphasize prevention, must take consistently to prevent nausea and vomiting
Antidopaminergic Prochlorperazine	Control of nausea and vomiting, intractable hiccoughs by inhibiting the CTZ	Drowsiness, hypotension, dry mouth, nasal congestion	Dehydration greater when used in older adults Monitor for EPS
Cholinergic blocking drug Trimethobenzamide (Tigan)	Control of nausea and vomiting at CTZ	Hypotension (IM use), drowsiness, dizziness	Monitor for EPS, blurred vision
Antivertigo Dimenhydrinate (Dramamine)	Inhibits vestibular stimulation in the ear, thereby relieving motion sickness	Drowsiness, nervousness, restlessness, headache, dizziness	Must be started before travel to be effective Can cause difficulty in voiding for men with enlarged prostate

CTZ, chemoreceptor trigger zone; EPS, extrapyramidal symptoms; IM, intramuscular.

Nutrition Notes

The Client With Nausea

- The client should eat small meals and eat and drink slowly.
- Dry, salty foods, such as crackers and pretzels, may relieve nausea.
- Fried food, spicy food, and foods with strong odors should be avoided.
- Cold foods may be preferable to hot foods.

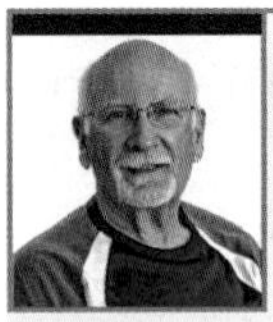

Clinical Scenario An older client seeks medical attention, complaining of nausea and vomiting that has persisted for more than 24 hours. The client states that family members had similar symptoms several days ago. **What issues are of concern for the nurse? See the following Nursing Process section.**

NURSING PROCESS FOR THE CLIENT WITH NAUSEA AND VOMITING

Assessment

Obtain a complete medical, dietary, drug, and allergy history. In addition, compile a list of symptoms that occurred before and along with nausea and vomiting; how long the problem has existed; and the frequency, color, and amount of vomited material. List the foods and where the client has eaten in the past 24 hours. In addition, assess the general appearance, weight, and vital signs. Documenting intake and output and monitoring for signs of fluid volume deficit are additional essential assessment requirements (see Chapter 16).

Diagnosis, Planning, and Interventions

Hypovolemia: Related to prolonged vomiting and decreased intake of oral fluids
Expected Outcome: Fluid balance will be restored as evidenced by intake of 1500 to 3000 mL/day with similar fluid loss.

- Offer clear fluids in small amounts. *Slow introduction of fluids allows the client to develop tolerance and determine if they can advance the diet.*
- Recommend commercial over-the-counter beverages such as Gatorade. *Gatorade replaces fluids and electrolytes.*
- Inform the primary provider if urine output is below 500 mL/day or serum electrolyte levels are abnormal. *Such findings indicate severe dehydration and the need for IV replacement fluids.*
- Monitor weight daily. *Daily monitoring helps to determine trends in weight loss or gain.*
- Assess skin turgor and mucous membranes. *Decreased skin turgor and dry mucous membranes indicate dehydration.*

Malnutrition Risk: Related to nausea and vomiting
Expected Outcome: The client's nutritional status will be adequate as evidenced by maintenance of weight and normal electrolyte and blood values.

- When the client tolerates clear fluids, advance diet to full liquids, then to soft, bland foods, such as creamed soups, crackers, or toast. *Advancing diet slowly helps the client develop tolerance for fluids and food.*
- Collaborate with the dietitian to provide nutritional foods. *The dietitian can help create a plan that assists the client to increase caloric intake with foods that they can tolerate.*
- Discourage caffeinated or carbonated beverages. *Such drinks may decrease appetite and lead to early satiety.*

Evaluation of Expected Outcomes

The client has an oral intake of 2500 mL and an output of 2600 mL. Weight is maintained or restored to preillness level. Serum electrolyte levels and other laboratory test results are within normal limits.

Cancer of the Oral Cavity and Pharynx

Cancer cells undergo changes in structure and appearance. They multiply, eventually forming a colony of abnormal and dysfunctional cells (see Chapter 18). When cancer affects the oral cavity, cells in the lips, mouth, or pharynx undergo malignant changes. When cancers of the oral cavity are detected early, the rate of cure is fairly good.

Pathophysiology and Etiology

Development of oral cancers is linked to smoking (includes cigarettes, cigars, and pipes), smokeless tobacco, drinking alcohol in excess, and human papillomavirus (HPV). Lip cancer is associated with pipe smoking and prolonged exposure to wind and sun. Tobacco, in particular, increases the risk of oral cancer, but clients who use both tobacco and alcohol have an extreme risk of developing oral cancer. It is hypothesized that tobacco and alcohol have a synergistic effect, in that they increase the others' carcinogenic effect. It is believed that alcohol dehydrates the cell walls on the oral mucosa, increasing the ability of tobacco carcinogens to permeate these cells. Research on this phenomenon is ongoing (The Oral Cancer Foundation, 2020).

As cancer cells in the oral cavity increase, the mass may distort a client's appearance; exert pressure on surrounding tissue, making it difficult to masticate (chew); cause local pain; or produce *dysphagia* (difficulty swallowing).

Although squamous cell carcinoma is the most common cause of oral cancers, HPV (specifically HPV 16) infection is the most common cause of oropharyngeal cancer, initially affecting the very back of the mouth. Other causes include repeated irritation from rough teeth, dentures, or fillings and poor oral and dental hygiene.

Malignant growths can be found anywhere in the oral cavity but usually occur on the lips, sides of the tongue, or floor of the mouth. Untreated, cancerous growths may extend into nearby tissue, such as the middle ear or nasal sinuses; infiltrate regional lymph nodes; or invade large blood vessels, such as the carotid arteries, that are near the oral cavity. Serious hemorrhage (carotid blowout) and death may result when cancer cells invade an artery that becomes ulcerated or when necrosis follows radiation therapy.

Assessment Findings

The early stage of oral cancer is characteristically asymptomatic. At first, the client may notice a lesion, lump, or other abnormality of the lips or mouth. Other changes such as pain, soreness, and bleeding follow. If a lesion is on the tongue, the client commonly experiences difficulty eating or tasting food. Pain and numbness also follow. Clients may also experience difficulty swallowing and/or persistent hoarseness. Dentists and oral hygienists may be the first to notice changes in mouth tissues, such as *leukoplakia*, a white patch on the tongue or inner cheek that may become cancerous. Other clients will have a red patch that does not heal. A biopsy of the lesion discloses malignant cells, which confirms the diagnosis of oral cancer.

Medical and Surgical Management

Prevention of oral cancers is the first goal. Eliminating high-risk behaviors such as smoking, using smokeless tobacco (chewing tobacco and snuff), and drinking large amounts of alcohol can prevent the development of cancer. Protecting lips against sun exposure with sunscreen designed for lips is also important, as is not smoking a pipe. Two HPV vaccines are available that protect against HPV strains that cause cervical cancer, and vaccination for girls between the ages of 11 and 26 years is recommended.

Treatment depends on the location and type of tumor, extent (or stage) of involvement, and the client's physical condition. In cases of hemorrhage, transfusions are given to replace lost blood. Ligation of the bleeding vessel usually is necessary. Drugs such as antianxiety agents are prescribed to relieve the client's apprehension.

Surgical treatment of most oral cancers includes tumor excision alone or with follow-up radiation therapy and chemotherapy. The radiation therapy may include a combination of external beam radiation and surgical implantation of radioactive interstitial implants. Surgical excision may result in complete cure, provided that it is performed early. A neck dissection is performed if the cancer has spread to the lymph nodes near the jaw or below the ears. Cancer of the tongue usually involves radical surgery to remove part or all of the tongue if radiation therapy and/or chemotherapy are not effective. Excision of the tumor from parts of the jaw or palate is disfiguring.

For clients with advanced disease, treatment is palliative only. Chemotherapy or radiation therapy is used to relieve pain and temporarily decrease tumor size. A tracheostomy and tube feedings are instituted to maintain an adequate airway and provide nourishment.

Nursing Management

General nursing management of the client with oral cancer is much the same as for any client with cancer (see Chapter 18). The focus of attention, however, is on maintaining a patent airway, promoting adequate fluid and food intake, and supporting communication that the tumor or treatment may have impaired. To review care of the client needing airway management, refer to Chapter 20 and the discussion of endotracheal intubation and tracheostomy care.

Nurses collaborate with speech pathologists to address communication problems. They must be patient when the client chooses to communicate by speaking and clarify or repeat what they say if speech is not understandable. Nurses may substitute written forms for communicating if speech is impaired. They also offer the client pencil and paper, a white dry-erase board, or an alphabet board, or they suggest that the client use hand signals.

When the client returns from the operating room after oral surgery, they should be positioned flat, either on the abdomen or side, with the head turned to the side to facilitate drainage from the mouth. After recovery from the anesthetic, the client is positioned with the head of the bed elevated, which makes it easier for the client to breathe deeply and cough up secretions. It also controls edema in the operative area.

After oral surgery, there should be equipment for suctioning, administration of oxygen, and tracheostomy at the client's bedside. If the client does not have a tracheostomy, a tracheostomy tray must be nearby for emergency use because respiratory distress or airway obstruction requires immediate attention. If the client has a tracheostomy, the nurse suctions secretions from the cannula and cleans it on a regular basis.

The nurse should not irrigate the client's mouth until the client is awake and alert. When and if mouth irrigation is carried out, the nurse should turn the client's head to the side to allow the solution to run in gently and flow out into an emesis basin. The nurse instills only a small amount of solution and then waits for the fluid to drain before administering more. In addition, they suction the mouth as necessary to remove secretions, blood, or irrigating solution.

The client must not receive oral liquids or foods until a written order exists. The nurse observes the client's ability to swallow small amounts of liquid. In cases of coughing or other difficulties, the nurse must suction the liquid from the mouth immediately.

The client may receive prescribed antiemetics if they experience nausea or vomiting. If the client has a gastric tube, the nurse checks it for patency. Clients should not use a straw because it causes the client to swallow air, which can distend the stomach.

The client's emotional response to radical oral surgery is a real and difficult problem. Extensive surgery of the mouth and adjacent structures is not only disfiguring but also incapacitating. It interferes with communication, eating, and control of saliva. Although health care providers explain the extent of surgery before the operation, many clients and families cannot grasp all the ensuing effects. The first time family members or clients see the effects of surgery, the experience usually is traumatic. The nurse needs to promote effective coping and therapeutic grieving at this time. Responses may range from crying or extreme sadness and avoiding contact with others to refusing to talk about the surgery or changes in appearance. Allowing the client time to mourn, accept, and adjust to losses is essential. To facilitate adaptation, the client needs opportunities to express feelings. Nurses must observe severely depressed clients closely. Clients who are suicidal need psychological evaluation and counseling. In addition, the nurse provides time for family members to express fears, ask questions, and grieve. It may help to refer clients and family members to support groups and counselors.

Nutritional management is a particular challenge when caring for clients with oral cancer. If the client can take oral nourishment, a nutritional consultation may be necessary to modify the diet according to the client's ability to chew and swallow. Because oral tissues are sensitive, the client should avoid hot and cold liquids and spicy foods. The nurse can consult with the primary provider about prescribing a topical anesthetic mouthwash containing lidocaine (Xylocaine), which numbs the tissues, or a systemic analgesic to relieve pain. Providing nourishment by a route other than the mouth may be necessary.

››› *Stop, Think, and Respond 45-1*

A client comes to the clinic complaining of difficulty chewing and swallowing. What questions should you ask?

Gastrointestinal Intubation for Feedings or Medications. At some time during the care of the client with oral cancer, as well as when caring for others with GI disorders, the nurse may have to perform GI intubation, which is the insertion and management of GI tubes. GI intubation is performed to:

- provide nutrition, medications, or both;
- carry out **gastric decompression**, which is removal of gas and fluids from the stomach; to lavage the stomach to remove ingested toxins;
- diagnose GI disorders, a process that may include aspiration of gastric contents for analysis;
- treat GI obstruction; or
- apply pressure to a GI bleed.

Determining placement of the tube, particularly for the client receiving feedings, is an important nursing role (Evidence-Based Practice 45-1). The goal is to prevent aspiration of the tube feeding. Although there are various methods used to determine placement, an X-ray is the most definitive. Once the placement is confirmed with an X-ray, then it is recommended that nurses aspirate stomach contents to further confirm placement. The aspirate is tested for pH. Research indicates that the pH level should be below 5.5.

Evidence-Based Practice 45-1

Ensuring Correct Feeding Tube Placement Clinical Question

What is the best method to use to ensure proper feeding tube placement?

Evidence

Researchers conducted a nationwide study of adult intensive care nurses to determine what clinical practices are used in the intensive care unit related to feeding tube placement and correct tube position confirmation. The results showed that various health care personnel perform feeding tube placements. Primary providers and registered nurses are responsible for most placements, followed, in order of frequency, by advanced practice registered nurses, physician assistants, and licensed practical nurses. The most common practice related to initial feeding tube placement confirmation was radiographic confirmation with the entire length of the tube visualized. The most frequently used method to confirm placement before and during feedings was auscultation, followed by measurement of the external length of the tube, and assessment of the appearance of the aspirate. The researchers point out that current guidelines and standards of practice recommend against using auscultation because evidence from other studies has shown that auscultation is not a valid way to confirm tube placement. Also, there is no consistent recommendation in the guidelines about using the appearance of the aspirate to confirm correct placement. Overall, the researchers recommend a higher reliance on measuring the external length of the tube, which is easy to do and considered reliable if the tube is accurately marked after correct initial placement is confirmed with radiographic assessment.

Nursing Implications

The current study makes the following recommendations related to tube placement confirmation: (1) use various bedside methods to confirm placement, including capnography if available, observing for respiratory distress, and measuring the pH of feeding tube aspirates; (2) auscultation should not be used to determine location; (3) radiographic confirmation should always be done before the tube is used for feedings or medication administration; (4) ultrasonography for select client population group; (5) mark the tube exit site right after radiographic confirmation and then use the marker to ensure that the correct location is maintained during use; and (6) monitor the aspirate for a sudden change in amount.

Reference

Mak, M., & Tam, G. (2020). Ultrasonography for nasogastric tube placement verification: an additional reference. *British Journal of Community Nursing, 25*(7), 328–334. https://doi-org.americansentinel.idm.oclc.org/10.12968/bjcn.2020.25.7.328

TABLE 45-1 Nasogastric, Nasoenteric, and Feeding Tubes

TUBE TYPE	LENGTH	SIZE (FRENCH)	LUMEN	OTHER CHARACTERISTICS
Nasogastric Tubes				
Levin (plastic or rubber)	125 cm	14–18	Single	Circular markings serve as guidelines for insertion.
Gastric sump or Salem (plastic)	120 cm	12–18	Double	Smaller lumen acts as a vent.
Moss	90 cm	12–16	Triple	Tube contains both a gastric decompression lumen and a duodenal lumen for postoperative feedings.
Sengstaken–Blakemore (rubber)	100 cm	12–16	Triple	Two lumens are used to inflate the gastric and esophageal balloons; one lumen attached to suction to aspirate gastric contents or for drainage of gastric contents.
Minnesota	100 cm	12–16	Quadruple	As above, but fourth lumen is attached to suction esophageal contents to prevent aspiration.
Nasoenteric Decompression Tubes				
Miller–Abbott (rubber)	3 m	16	Double	Used for decompression for a small bowel obstruction or ileus. One lumen is Tungsten weighted; the other is used as a vent.
Nasoenteric Feeding Tubes				
Dobbhoff or Enteraflo (polyurethane or silicone rubber)	160–175 cm	8–12	Single	Tungsten-weighted tip; radiopaque stylet.

GI tubes are advanced to the upper GI tract by way of the mouth or nose or introduced directly into the stomach or small intestine through the abdominal wall. The nasal route is the preferred route for passing a tube when the client's nose is intact and free from injury. Examples of different types of GI intubation include **nasogastric intubation** (tube passes through the nose into the stomach via esophagus), **orogastric intubation** (tube passes through the mouth into the stomach), **nasoenteric intubation** (tube passes through the nose, esophagus, and stomach to the small intestine), **gastrostomy** (tube enters the stomach through a surgically created opening into the abdominal wall), and **jejunostomy** (tube enters jejunum or small intestine through a surgically created opening into the abdominal wall). A gastric tube lies in the stomach; an intestinal tube extends past the pylorus. See Table 45-1.

The type of tube selected depends on the reason for placing the tube. In general, smaller (narrower), more flexible tubes are used for feeding because they tend to be more easily tolerated by clients; larger tubes are used for decompression because they allow for the evacuation of large pieces of debris or blood clots from the upper GI tract. Tubes used for feeding are longer and end in the upper, small intestine; instilling the feeding formula below the pylorus reduces the potential for vomiting and aspiration. The disadvantage of the long tubes is that the distal location is difficult to assess without a chest or abdominal X-ray. Nurses may be involved with inserting feeding tubes and/or nasogastric tubes for gastric decompression.

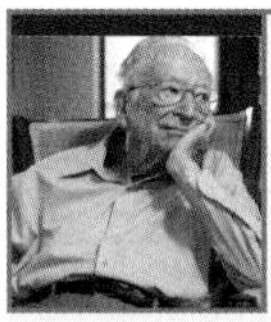

Clinical Scenario A client with chronic difficulty swallowing has agreed to have a feeding tube placed. What are the important nursing approaches for managing the care of a client receiving a tube feeding? See the following Nursing Process section.

NURSING PROCESS FOR THE CLIENT RECEIVING ENTERAL TUBE FEEDINGS

Assessment

Before beginning a tube feeding, determine why the client requires it—such as to improve nutritional and hydration status for chronic illness. It is essential to evaluate renal function and check for any digestive issues, just as it is important to assess previous stool patterns, present weight, and any vomiting.

Diagnosis, Planning, and Interventions

When a client is receiving tube feedings, medications, or both (Table 45-2), ensure that the lungs remain free of liquid substances, infection does not develop, and intake and output are appropriate for the client's age and size. Additional objectives include providing adequate nutrition, promoting appropriate stool patterns (amount, consistency, and frequency), and preserving intact skin and nasal mucosa. Keep mucous membranes moist because they tend to dry from mouth breathing and restricted oral fluids. Provide frequent mouth care to relieve discomfort from dryness and unpleasant tastes and odors. Ice chips and analgesic throat lozenges,

(continued)

NURSING PROCESS FOR THE CLIENT RECEIVING ENTERAL TUBE FEEDINGS (continued)

gargles, or sprays may help if the client's mouth and throat become sore. Provide mouth care after removal of the tube and inform the client that a sore throat (an aftereffect of intubation) may persist for several days.

The client is at risk not only for dry mouth but also fluid volume deficit resulting from insufficient fluid intake. Be aware of the client's normal fluid needs and whether the formula alone can meet them. Observe for signs and symptoms of dehydration. For example, if urine output is less than 500 mL/day, administer formula and additional water as ordered.

While ensuring adequate hydration, protect the client from infections that stem from microbes in the tube-feeding formula. Signs and symptoms of infection include diarrhea, fever, or abnormal white blood cell count. To prevent infection, wash hands before handling equipment; keep the feeding formula refrigerated or unopened until it is ready for use; warm the bolus, intermittent, or cyclic feeding formula (Box 45-1) to room temperature just before administering; hang continuous formula-feeding containers with only the volume necessary for 4 to 6 hours; flush the tubing with water before adding more formula and after giving a bolus or intermittent feeding or medications; discard any premixed formula after 24 hours; thoroughly clean and dry all equipment used for bolus feedings (i.e., syringe, feeding adapters, tubing, containers) after each use; and replace the infusion container and tubing used for a continuous tube feeding every 24 hours or as directed by agency policy.

The plan of care contains the following diagnoses, outcomes, and interventions:

Malnutrition Risk: Related to inadequate dietary intake
Expected Outcome: Nutrition will be adequate as evidenced by stable body weight.

- Maintain feeding schedule, drip rate, and amount administered by gravity drip, bolus feeding, or continuous controlled pump. *Feeding at set rate and amount ensures that the client will receive the appropriate amount, calories, and nutrients and assists the client to digest the feeding without discomfort.*
- Aspirate and measure residual content before each intermittent feeding or every 4 to 8 hours for continuous feedings. Delay feeding if residual content measures more than 100 mL or 10% to 20% of the hourly amount of a continuous feeding. Readminister the residual amount. *Measuring the residual content ensures that the client digests feedings and will not be overfed. Readministering residual amounts ensures that the client does not lose nutrients and digestive enzymes.*
- Maintain tube function by
- Administering 15 to 30 mL of water before and after medications and feedings (every 4 to 6 hours with continuous feedings). *This measure ensures tube patency and decreases the risk of bacterial infection and crusting or blockage of the tube.*
- Changing tube-feeding container and tubing per agency policy. *Regular changes prevent blockage and infection.*
- Monitor weight daily. *Daily monitoring checks for trends in weight loss or gain.*
- Consult with primary provider and dietitian if the client experiences any problems with tube feeding, such as nausea, bloating, diarrhea, or cramping. *Such problems may indicate poor tolerance of feeding, wrong formula for the client, or other issues.*

Aspiration Risk: Related to the presence of feeding tube, enteral feedings, potential increase in gastric residual, potential depressed gag reflex
Expected Outcome: The nurse will manage tube feedings to reduce the risk aspiration during feedings or vomiting episodes.

- Check tube placement and gastric residual before feedings. *Checking prevents improper infusion and assists in preventing vomiting.*
- Place the client in semi-Fowler position during and 30 to 60 minutes after an intermittent feeding and at all times for a continuous feeding. *Proper positioning prevents regurgitation.*
- Stop feeding if client vomits or aspiration is suspected. *In these cases, cessation prevents further problems and allows for treatment of the immediate problem.*

Diarrhea: Related to hypertonic feeding solutions, lack of dietary fiber, high carbohydrate and electrolyte content, or other factors (e.g., gastroenteritis, deficient fluid volume)
Expected Outcome: Client will have normal bowel patterns with formed stool.

- Consult with a primary provider about decreasing the infusion rate. *A decreased infusion rate provides time for carbohydrates and electrolytes to be diluted, preventing increased fluid from the vascular system going to the jejunum.*
- Administer feedings at room temperature. *Cold or warm feedings stimulate peristalsis.*
- If possible, administer feedings continuously. *Bolus or intermittent feedings cause sudden distention of the small intestine.*
- Instruct client to remain in semi-Fowler position during and after feedings (as discussed previously). *This position slows the movement of feeding into the intestine.*
- Consult with primary provider and dietitian if diarrhea persists. *Client may require a different formula if all other possible causes for diarrhea are ruled out.*

Evaluation of Expected Outcomes

The client maintains their weight. Lungs are clear to auscultation, and the client has not vomited. Bowel patterns are normal with formed stool.

BOX 45-1 Tube-Feeding Methods

Liquid nourishment is administered by bolus, intermittent, cyclic, or continuous methods. Intermittent cyclic and bolus tube feedings are physiologically preferable to continuous feedings for long-term use because they resemble a more normal pattern of intake, allowing hormone and enzyme levels to rise and fall rather than being constantly stimulated. Continuous feedings, however, may be preferred to decrease the risk of aspiration.

Depending on institutional policy and individual feeding orders, the feeding tube is flushed with water at various intervals to ensure patency. Many tube-feeding formulas are available to suit a client's different nutritional needs. Nursing observation of tolerance of the feeding is essential to determine which tube and formula are best suited for the client.

Bolus Tube Feedings
- Allow introduction of 250 to 400 mL formula through the tube in a short period (usually 15 to 30 minutes).
- Administered by syringe or gravity flow system attached to the distal end of the feeding tube.
- Usually administered 3 to 4 times daily.

Intermittent Tube Feedings
- Allow delivery of between 250 and 400 mL formula over 30 to 60 minutes.
- Delivered by gravity flow system or an electronic feeding pump.

Continuous Tube Feedings
- Allow formula to be administered at lower rates—usually 1.5 mL/min over a longer time (usually 12 to 24 hours).
- Delivered by gravity flow system or an electronic feeding pump.

Cyclic Tube Feedings
- Allow formula to be administered continuously for 8 to 12 hours during sleep followed by a 12- to 16-hour pause.
- Ensure adequate nutrition during weaning from tube to oral feeding.
- Alternate with oral food intake until the client can take most nutrition orally.

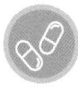

Pharmacologic Considerations

■ Although liquid medications are preferred for enteral administration, they can cause GI distress. Sorbitol, an inactive ingredient, is used as a sweetener for oral liquid medications. In large amounts, such as multiple medications administered via enteral tube, sorbitol acts as an osmotic laxative. Tablets crushed and mixed with water may reduce diarrhea should this occur.

Gastrointestinal Intubation for Decompression. The larger GI tube is used to relieve abdominal distention caused by problems after surgery, episodes of acute upper GI bleeding, or symptoms associated with intestinal obstruction, or for diagnostic purposes. It is inserted by following the same procedure as is used for the insertion of a feeding tube (Fig. 45-1).

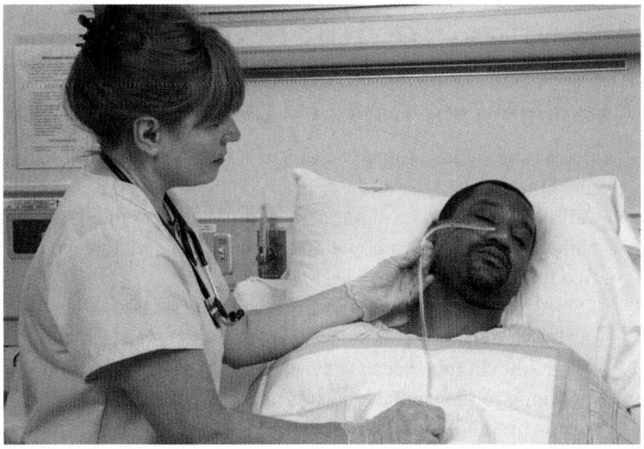

Figure 45-1 The nurse determines the length of nasogastric tubing for a client by measuring from the tip of the nose to the tip of the earlobe and then to the tip of the xiphoid process.

Some tubes, such as a gastric sump tube, have a double lumen (two-channeled), one of which serves as a vent, allowing a small amount of air to be drawn in when the tube is connected to suction. Sump tubes decrease the possibility of the stomach wall adhering to and obstructing the tube openings during gastric decompression. A common problem associated with vented tubes is leakage from the vent lumen. The nurse may prevent this by keeping the vent above the level of the client's stomach. Newer gastric sump tubes have a one-way antireflux valve that allows air to enter but prevents gastric contents from escaping. In many cases, decompression tubes are connected to a source of suction (Nursing Guidelines 45-2).

Gastrostomy Tubes for Long-Term Feeding. A client with a gastrostomy has a transabdominal opening into the stomach that provides long-term access for administering fluids and liquid nourishment. Creating a gastrostomy is a relatively minor procedure that can be performed surgically or endoscopically.

General Considerations. Surgical placement of a gastrostomy involves laparotomy and surgical creation of an external stoma through which a gastrostomy tube is placed. When a **percutaneous endoscopic gastrostomy** (PEG) is performed, an endoscope is introduced orally and advanced into the stomach so that the primary provider can see the correct location for the tube. This location also is identified on the external abdominal surface before an incision is made. Two primary providers or one primary provider and a specially trained nurse usually perform the PEG, which can be done either in the endoscopy suite or at the bedside with the client needing minimal sedation (Fig. 45-2). Because of the reduced risks, endoscopic placement is preferred to surgical laparotomy unless the client has ascites, is morbidly obese, or has had previous gastric surgery. If the client's condition eventually improves, the gastrostomy tube is removed and the opening closes over time. On rare occasions, the gastrostomy opening may require surgical closure.

Gastric feedings are administered by bolus, intermittent, cyclic, or continuous feeding methods using the same

NURSING GUIDELINES 45-2

Managing the Care of a Client Needing Gastrointestinal Suction and Decompression

- Locate the suction source, usually a wall outlet or portable machine.
- Adjust the suction level on the wall outlet or portable machine to provide the amount and frequency of suction specified by the primary provider.
- Select intermittent high, low, or continuous suction when using a Salem sump tube; select low intermittent suction when using a Levin tube because the single lumen may adhere to the lining of the stomach during continuous suction. (If the tube is used only to obtain specimens for diagnostic purposes, manual suction may be achieved by attaching a syringe to the end of the tube and drawing back on the plunger.)
- Insert the gastric decompression tube in accordance with accepted standards and connect it to the suction.

Maintain Safe Suction

- Observe the amount and quality of the gastric contents being suctioned and the client's response.
- Monitor the procedure frequently because abdominal or gastric distention caused by suction failure may have serious consequences such as strain on surgical sutures or vomiting around the tube.
- Check equipment frequently to make sure it is operating properly. If the suction is not operating satisfactorily, obtain another suction machine.

Maintain Tube Patency

- If the decompression tube is occluded, irrigate or replace it.
- First, review the client's medical record. The primary provider may order irrigation on an as-needed basis.
- When irrigating the tube, use normal saline solution to prevent disturbance of electrolyte balance. Also, use a large syringe to instill the irrigant into the distal end of the tube.
- After the fluid is instilled, remove it by gently pulling back on the plunger.
- Document the amount of solution used and the amount of fluid returned on the client's intake and output.

Ensure Client Comfort

- Provide ice chips sparingly because water pulls electrolytes into the gastric secretions, which are then removed by suction, increasing the risk an electrolyte disturbance.

techniques described previously. Bolus feedings are not given through tubes inserted below the pylorus because such placement causes abdominal cramping and diarrhea. Intermittent, cyclic, or continuous feedings simulate the normal passage of food into the small intestine and usually are well tolerated.

Gastrostomy feeding devices may be skin-level devices (known as *buttons*) or tubes. Some tubes have a double lumen to allow infusion of two different fluids at once, such as administration of medications and delivery of feeding formula without interruption. For stabilization, most gastrostomy tubes have an external bumper and a firm internal bumper or an inflatable balloon. The advantage of the firm internal bumper is that it is difficult to dislodge accidentally; the disadvantage is that it may be difficult or painful to remove when replacement is desired. The advantage of the balloon-style internal bumper is that it is relatively painless and easy to replace; disadvantages include relative ease of accidental dislodgment and gradual loss of fluid from the inflated balloon, resulting in leakage. The volume of fluid placed in the balloon is measured regularly and replaced as necessary. Box 45-2 provides further information about preventing complications for clients with a PEG tube.

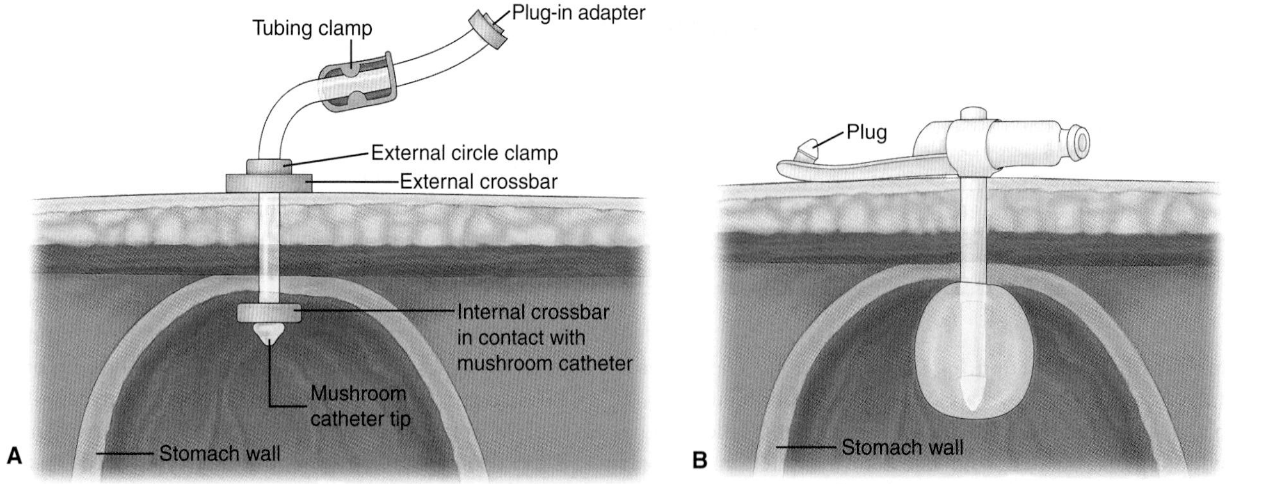

Figure 45-2 (A) A detail of the abdomen and the percutaneous endoscopic gastrostomy tube showing catheter fixation with internal bumper. **(B)** A detail of the abdomen and the gastrostomy device showing balloon fixation. (Reprinted with permission from Hinkle, J. L., & Cheever, K. H. (2018). *Brunner & Suddarth's textbook of medical-surgical nursing* (14th ed.). Wolters Kluwer.)

BOX 45-2 Prevention of Complications Related to Percutaneous Endoscopic Gastrostomy Tubes

- PEG tubes are most often stabilized with internal and external bumpers. The internal bumper prevents the tube from being dislodged from the stomach or intestine. The external bumper secures the tube to the abdominal wall and prevents the tube from migrating.
- Bumpers that are too tight may cause
- Pressure ulcer on the abdomen
- "Buried bumper syndrome," in which the internal bumper becomes buried in the abdominal wall, possibly leading to gastrointestinal bleeding, perforation, or peritonitis
- Bumpers that are too loose may cause
- Free movement of the tube, leading to irritation, ulceration of the tract, or granulation tissue (granuloma) forming
- Dislodgment
- A new PEG tube insertion site may have a slight amount of bleeding, mucus, or both; report any prolonged drainage or other problems.
- The tube insertion site should be inspected for signs of irritation, infection, drainage, or gastric leakage.
- Sites should be cleaned with water and soft cloth, dressing, or gauze only needed for any drainage or client comfort.
- New PEG tubes are usually taped or sutured until the tract heals.
- Once the tract heals, there is less risk for trauma to the abdominal wall. The PEG tube is more easily replaced in a healed tract.

Reference
Thompson, R. (2017). Troubleshooting PEG feeding tubes in the community setting. *Journal of Community Nursing, 31*(2), 61–66. https://doi.org/10.3748/wjg.v20.i26.8505

Nursing Management. Before insertion of a PEG tube, the nurse weighs the client, assesses vital signs, auscultates bowel sounds, and offers an opportunity to empty the bladder. Other activities include determining the client's perception of the procedure, clarifying information, and checking that proper consent forms are signed and in order. The nurse prepares the client's skin and conducts other ordered preprocedural activities, such as inserting an IV line and administering sedatives.

The nurse monitors vital signs (i.e., respiratory rate, oxygen saturation, heart rate and rhythm) throughout the procedure according to institutional protocol. They monitor and document the client's tolerance of the procedure. Monitoring of vital signs and response to the procedure continues in the postprocedural period. The nurse observes the stoma and surrounding skin for signs of infection and checks dressings frequently for evidence of bleeding and drainage.

The nurse must examine the appearance and volume of the drainage from the gastrostomy tube during the first 24 hours when the tube may be temporarily attached to gravity drainage. They auscultate bowel sounds and palpate the abdomen lightly for signs of distention and tenderness. They inspect the oral mucosa for excessive dryness. In addition, the nurse notes the client's tolerance of the instilled formula when tube feeding is initiated, promptly reporting abdominal distention, vomiting, fever, and severe pain to the primary provider. Another important nursing intervention is to monitor the characteristics and pattern of bowel elimination and trends in daily weight.

Accidental removal of the gastrostomy device necessitates immediate replacement. Clients who have recently placed gastrostomy devices (less than 2 weeks) do not have a well-established tract and are at high risk for inadvertent replacement into the peritoneum instead of the stomach. If fluids are administered into this device, the resulting peritonitis may be life-threatening. For this reason, the nurse notifies the primary provider immediately and takes steps to ensure proper placement of the replacement device. For clients with well-established tracts, the nurse can maintain patency of the tract by inserting a clean catheter (i.e., Foley) and inflating the balloon to hold the catheter in place. The diameter of the replacement device should be the same as that of the device that was removed. The nurse notifies the primary provider so a new feeding device can be inserted. It is safe to administer gastric feedings through a catheter until it is replaced.

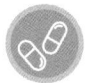

Pharmacologic Considerations

- Never crush and administer an enteric-coated drug through any type of enteral feeding tube (nasogastric, nasoenteric, or gastrostomy).

DISORDERS OF THE ESOPHAGUS

Various disorders can affect the esophagus. Examples include gastroesophageal reflux disease (GERD), esophageal diverticulum, hiatal hernia, and cancer. Esophageal varices, which result from hypertension in the portal venous system, are discussed in Chapter 47.

Gastroesophageal Reflux Disease

Gastroesophageal reflux disease (GERD) is a common disorder that develops when gastric contents flow upward into the esophagus. All adults and children normally have some degree of reflux, especially after eating. Gastroesophageal reflux is considered a disease process only when it is excessive or causes undesirable symptoms such as pain or respiratory distress.

Pathophysiology and Etiology

GERD results from an inability of the lower esophageal sphincter (LES; also called the *cardiac sphincter*) to close fully, allowing the stomach contents to flow freely into the esophagus. Obesity and pregnancy increase susceptibility to GERD because of the upward pressure that increased abdominal girth associated with these conditions places on the diaphragm.

Assessment Findings

Signs and Symptoms

The most common symptoms associated with GERD are epigastric pain or discomfort (**dyspepsia**), burning sensation in the esophagus (**pyrosis**), and regurgitation. Other symptoms include difficulty swallowing (dysphagia), painful swallowing (**odynophagia**), inflammation of the lining of the esophagus (**esophagitis**), aspiration pneumonia, and respiratory distress. Clients with esophagitis related to GERD may experience bleeding from the lining of the esophagus, manifested by vomited blood (*hematemesis*) or tarry stools (*melena*). Sometimes, *occult* (hidden) *bleeding* for long periods produces iron-deficiency anemia. Because the esophagus is anatomically close to the heart, clients with epigastric pain may think they are having a heart attack. Until a myocardial infarction (MI) is ruled out as a cause for the discomfort, it is considered a potential diagnosis. Prolonged or severe esophagitis can lead to scarring and stricture formation. In these events, the client may report a sensation of feeling food "stick" in the esophagus for varying periods. Chronic GERD can be a risk factor for developing Barrett esophagus, a known precursor of cancer of the esophagus. Barrett esophagus, in which the esophageal lining becomes more like the intestinal mucosa, occurs in a small percentage of clients who have chronic GERD.

Diagnostic Findings

Upper endoscopy with biopsy confirms esophagitis. Tests of stool may show positive findings of blood. Ambulatory 12- to 36-hour esophageal pH monitoring uses a wireless disposable capsule (eventually is passed through the digestive system) that is inserted endoscopically into the esophagus about 2 inches above the LES. This capsule transmits pH levels to a receiver that is worn around the client's waist. It records the frequency of reflux episodes and their associated symptoms. A barium swallow may be done to determine whether there is inflammation or stricture formation from chronic esophagitis.

Bronchoscopy with analysis of fluids found in the lungs and nuclear medicine scans may be used to test for aspiration. Esophageal motility testing is used to evaluate the muscles of the esophagus by assessing pressures with a catheter and sensor. It is usually performed in clients who do not respond to treatment for GERD to determine what surgery might be needed. A gastric emptying study may also be done to evaluate the effectiveness of the stomach to empty its contents into the duodenum. Ineffective gastric emptying may lead to gastroesophageal reflux and aspiration. The gastric emptying study may help determine what medications and/or surgery are needed.

Medical and Surgical Management

Treating GERD begins with conservative measures first, depending on the symptoms and presence of erosive esophagitis. Education and lifestyle changes may include weight loss, maintaining an upright position following meals, elevating the head of the bed when sleeping, avoiding food and fluids 2 to 3 hours before bedtime, and avoiding foods that intensify symptoms.

TABLE 45-2 Medication Administration by Way of Feeding Tube

FORM OF MEDICATION	HOW TO ADMINISTER
Liquid	Administer in its liquid form
Basic compressed tablets	Crush and dissolve the tablet in water
Buccal or sublingual tablets	Administer according to the prescribed route
Soft gelatin capsules filled with liquid	Puncture the capsule with a sterile needle and squeeze the contents into a medicine cup
Enteric-coated tablets	Do not administer through a feeding tube—contact the pharmacist to change the form of the medication
Timed-release tablets	Do not crush timed-release tablets. This can result in an overdose because the client will receive too much of the medication over a very short period of time. Contact the pharmacist to change the form of the medication.

Medications may also be effective. Antacids, whether aluminum, magnesium, or calcium-based, continue to be a primary treatment because they neutralize stomach acids. A newer foam antacid tablet, composed of alginic acid and sodium bicarbonate, is used with other drugs. The tablet disintegrates as it reaches the stomach and turns into a foam that forms a barrier to the reflux of liquid. It reduces the number of reflux incidents and is particularly useful after the client has eaten a meal and when they are lying down. Other medications used to control esophageal reflux are discussed in Drug Therapy Table 45-2. Generally, histamine type 2 (H_2)-receptor antagonists (reduce acid production), proton pump inhibitors (PPIs) (such as Prilosec or Nexium, which blocks acid production), or both are used for 2 to 3 months if GI bleeding or other symptoms are present. Some studies suggest that there is an increased risk of MI with the use of PPIs. However, the research also suggests that for clients with chronic GERD, the benefits of PPIs may outweigh the risk of MI. H_2-receptor antagonists, such as ranitidine, cimetidine, or famotidine, are used for the short-term treatment of duodenal and gastric ulcers for managing GERD. Prokinetic or promotility drugs may be used for mild-to-moderate GERD caused by incompetence of the LES or delayed gastric emptying. Drugs such as metoclopramide (Reglan) increase LES pressure and promote the movement of food through the stomach.

The most common surgical procedure performed for GERD is Nissen **fundoplication**, a procedure that tightens the LES by wrapping the gastric fundus around the lower esophagus and suturing it into place. Fundoplication may be performed using laparoscopic technique, endoscopic technique, or open laparotomy. Esophageal strictures may be managed by endoscopic dilatation. Recurrent strictures may require repeat dilatation. In some cases, clients are taught

DRUG THERAPY TABLE 45-2 Medications Used to Treat Problems in the Upper Gastrointestinal Tract

Category and Common Generic (Brand) Drugs	Intended Use	Common Side Effects	Safety Warnings for Nurses
Acid Neutralizers			
Antacids Aluminum hydroxide (AlternaGEL) Calcium carbonate (Tums) magnesia (magnesium hydroxide or oxide) Sodium bicarbonate	Neutralizes gastric acid to relieve heartburn and sour stomach	Constipation Diarrhea, electrolyte imbalance with chronic use	Do not give oral drugs within 1–2 hours Consider cardiac status and sodium restrictions when using sodium bicarbonate
Acid Reducers			
Histamine H_2 Antagonists Cimetidine (Tagamet) Famotidine (Pepcid) Nizatidine (Axid)	Gastric/duodenal ulcers, GERD, gastric hypersecretory conditions, GI bleeding, heartburn by inhibiting H_2 receptor in the stomach	Headache, somnolence, diarrhea	Should not take maximum dose for more than 2 weeks without medical consultation
Proton Pump Inhibitors Esomeprazole (Nexium) Lansoprazole (Prevacid) Omeprazole (Prilosec)	Erosive esophagitis, GERD, *H. pylori* eradication, NSAID-associated gastric ulcers by suppressing gastric acid secretion	Headache, nausea, diarrhea	Rapid IV administration can cause cardiac arrhythmia Long-term use may be associated with bone fractures
Miscellaneous Acid Reducers Sucralfate (Carafate)	Short-term duodenal ulcer treatment	Constipation	Best option for pregnant women with GERD symptoms
Gastrointestinal Motility Agents Metoclopramide (Reglan)	Diabetic gastroparesis, GERD, prevention of nausea and vomiting by rapid transit out of stomach	Restlessness, dizziness, fatigue	Monitor for EPS and tardive dyskinesia
Agents Used to Eradicate Helicobacter pylori of Duodenal Ulcers			
Bismuth, metronidazole, tetracycline (Pylera)	*H. pylori* eradication in clients with duodenal ulcer	Nausea, diarrhea, abdominal pain	Metronidazole is carcinogenic in mice, avoid if possible Capsules must be swallowed whole with a full glass of water

EPS, extrapyramidal symptoms; GERD, gastroesophageal reflux disease; GI, gastrointestinal; IV, intravenous; NSAID, nonsteroidal anti-inflammatory drug.

self-dilatation using a tapered flexible dilator in the home setting. Newer devices to treat GERD are listed as follows:

- *Transoral incisionless fundoplication (TIF)* uses a device called an EsophyX. It is inserted surgically through the mouth into the stomach that folds tissue at the base of the stomach to create a replacement for the sphincter valve, preventing reflux.
- The *Stretta system* uses electrodes to create tiny lesions on the LES. As the lesions heal, the tissue tightens, increasing the muscle mass of the LES and preventing reflux.
- The *LINX device* is a series of titanium beads connected with titanium wires to form a ring; it is surgically implanted around the LES to prevent reflux. The magnetic attraction of the beads is strong enough to prevent acid reflux but allows for the passage of food (Mayo Clinic Staff, 2014).

These minimally invasive procedures take approximately 45 minutes and may be performed using conscious sedation. Recovery time for clients is short—generally 1 to 2 days. Because these procedures are still relatively new, long-term effects are unknown.

Nursing Management

The nurse educates the client with GERD about diet and lifestyle changes needed to reduce reflux symptoms. Dietary management consists of eating smaller meals and avoiding foods and beverages that increase gastric acidity (e.g., black and red pepper, regular and decaffeinated coffee, alcohol) and avoiding items that lower pressure in the LES (e.g., alcohol, chocolate, peppermint, licorice, citrus fruits, caffeine, high-fat foods). Additional measures include losing weight, avoiding tight-fitting garments, elevating the head of the bed, stopping smoking, and avoiding food and drink for several hours before bedtime. Nurses must advise pregnant clients that symptoms of GERD usually resolve after delivery. The nurse teaches the client how to self-administer medications to control reflux. They emphasize strict compliance with drug therapy to reduce symptoms. The nurse also teaches the client about the importance of controlling severe GERD to prevent possible complications, such as esophageal stricture formation and esophageal cancer. They closely observe the client having fundoplication for postoperative abdominal distention and nausea because many clients cannot belch or vomit after undergoing this procedure.

>>> ***Stop, Think, and Respond 45-2***

You are assigned to care for a client with GERD. After lunch, the client tells you that they need to take a nap. What should you advise?

Esophageal Diverticulum

A **diverticulum** is a sac or pouch in one or more layers of the wall of an organ or structure. Esophageal diverticula (plural) are found at the junction of the pharynx and the esophagus or in the middle or lower portion of the esophagus.

Pathophysiology and Etiology

The most common esophageal diverticulum, known as *Zenker diverticulum* (Fig. 45-3), occurs at the pharyngeal–esophageal juncture. Men are more likely than women to have this condition. Diverticula result from a congenital or an acquired weakness of the esophageal wall. They trap food and secretions, which then narrow the lumen; interfere with the passage of food into the stomach; and exert pressure on the trachea. The trapped food decomposes in the esophagus, causing esophagitis or mucosal ulceration.

Assessment Findings

The client has foul breath (*halitosis*) and experiences difficulty or pain when swallowing, belching, regurgitating, or coughing. Auscultation of the middle to upper chest may reveal gurgling sounds. A barium swallow determines the structural abnormalities in the esophagus. Esophagoscopy usually is contraindicated secondary to the risk of esophageal perforation.

Medical and Surgical Management

For mild symptoms, treatment usually includes a bland, soft, semisoft, or liquid diet to facilitate the passage of food. Eating four to six small meals a day is recommended. If symptoms are more severe, surgical excision of the diverticulum may be done. The goals are to relieve any obstruction and repair the weakened esophageal wall. Several types of surgical procedures can be used to excise diverticula depending on their size and location. Although open surgical methods are still used, surgeons are also able to do minimally invasive methods through laparoscopy, which promotes earlier recovery.

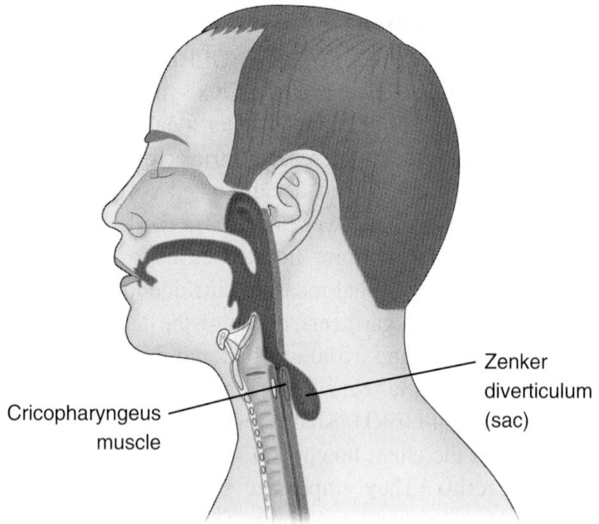

Figure 45-3 Zenker diverticulum. (Reprinted with permission from Hinkle, J. L., & Cheever, K. H. (2014). *Brunner & Suddarth's textbook of medical-surgical nursing* (13th ed.). Wolters Kluwer Health/Lippincott Williams & Wilkins.)

Nursing Management

The nurse explains that oral hygiene will not alleviate the foul breath. They provide instructions for dietary modifications or arrange a consultation with a dietitian. (See the section on Nursing Management of hiatal hernia and Nursing Care Plan 45-1 as well.)

Concept Mastery Alert

Zenker Diverticulum

In severe cases of Zenker diverticulum, the standard treatment is the surgical removal of the diverticulum. In mild cases, bland, soft, semisoft, or liquid diets are recommended.

Hiatal Hernia

A **hiatal or diaphragmatic hernia** is a protrusion of part of the stomach into the lower portion of the thorax. There are two types of hiatal hernias:

- *Axial or sliding*: The junction of the stomach and esophagus and part of the stomach slide in and out through the weakened portion of the diaphragm (Fig. 45-4A). This is the most common type of hiatal hernia.
- *Paraesophageal*: The fundus is displaced upward, with the greater curvature of the stomach going through the diaphragm next to the gastroesophageal (GE) junction (Fig. 45-4B).

Pathophysiology and Etiology

A hiatal hernia results from a defect in the diaphragm at the point where the esophagus passes through it. It is particularly common in women. There is congenital muscle weakness or weakness resulting from trauma. Factors that increase intra-abdominal pressure also contribute to the potential for hiatal hernia and include multiple pregnancies, obesity, and loss of muscle strength and tone that occurs with aging. Smoking, as well as aging, is a factor in developing a hiatal hernia. Hiatal hernia develops in approximately 60% of people older than 70 years. When the upper portion of the stomach slips from its usual position and becomes trapped, gastroesophageal reflux occurs.

Assessment Findings

The client describes having heartburn, belching, nausea, and a feeling of substernal or epigastric pressure or pain after eating and when lying down. They may report increased symptoms when bending at the waist. If scars form, swallowing becomes difficult. As food distends the

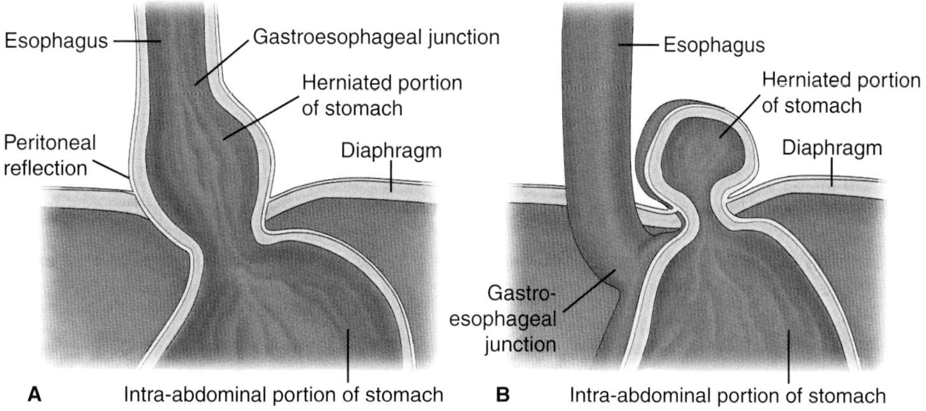

Figure 45-4 **(A)** Sliding hiatal hernia. **(B)** Paraesophageal hiatal hernia.

esophagus, the client may vomit. Reflux does not usually accompany GI hernias because the GI sphincter remains intact. Sliding hernias, however, are often associated with reflux. A barium swallow confirms the diagnosis by outlining the abnormal positioning of the stomach. An esophagoscopy shows the extent of irritation and scarring in the esophagus.

Medical and Surgical Management

Medical management of hiatal hernia is the same as that of GERD. The narrowed esophagus is stretched endoscopically, but the procedure may need to be repeated often. Clients who do not respond to a rigid medical regimen are treated surgically, which involves restoring the stomach to its proper position and repairing the diaphragmatic defect.

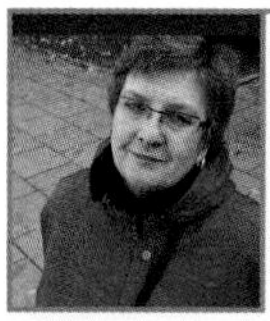

Clinical Scenario A client is diagnosed with a sliding hiatal hernia. The treatment for this client will not require surgery. What are the important elements when planning care for this client? See the following Nursing Process section.

NURSING PROCESS FOR THE CLIENT WITH AN ESOPHAGEAL DISORDER

Assessment

Ask the client about their appetite, particularly changes, difficulty swallowing, and problems after meals, such as discomfort, bloating, regurgitation, and belching. If the client indicates that they have pain after meals, ask if the pain follows every meal or certain foods, if other things (e.g., a particular position) seem to aggravate it, and if the pain is a burning sensation or associated with stomach fullness or pressure. In addition, determine if the client has experienced any weight loss. It is important to ask the client if they have tried antacids or other over-the-counter medications to relieve symptoms. Weigh the client and check for signs of malnutrition and dehydration. When completing the history, ask about past infections, exposure to irritants, and alcohol and tobacco use.

Diagnosis, Planning, and Interventions

For clients who undergo thoracic surgery to repair a hiatal hernia, nursing care is the same as for clients who have chest surgery (see Chapter 20). Regardless of the surgical approach, postoperative care will most likely involve intubation for gastric decompression to prevent stomach distention and avoid pressure on the surgical repair (see Nursing Guidelines 45-2).

Malnutrition Risk: Related to difficulty swallowing
Expected Outcome: Client will consume adequate nutrients to gain or maintain weight.

- Encourage the client to eat frequent, small, well-balanced meals. *This meal plan provides adequate nutrition without overloading the upper GI system.*
- Instruct client to eat slowly and to chew food thoroughly. *Slow eating and thorough chewing promote easy passage of food to the stomach through the esophagus.*
- Suggest that the client avoid foods and beverages that cause discomfort. *Clients with GERD should avoid foods and beverages that are irritating and decrease LES pressure and stimulate gastric acid secretion (e.g., caffeine, chocolate).*
- Record daily weights. A *daily record reveals trends in weight gain or loss.*
- Instruct client to avoid alcohol or tobacco products. *They may suppress the appetite and can irritate the digestive tract.*

Acute Pain: Related to pressure, reflux of gastric secretions, and/or difficulty swallowing
Expected Outcome: Client will experience relief from epigastric discomfort.

(*continued*)

NURSING PROCESS FOR THE CLIENT WITH AN ESOPHAGEAL DISORDER (continued)

- Tell the client to avoid very hot or cold fluids or spicy foods. *These foods stimulate esophageal spasms and the secretion of hydrochloric acid in the stomach.*
- Inform client to remain upright for at least 2 hours after meals. *An upright position helps prevent reflux.*
- Discourage the client from eating before bedtime. Raise the head of the bed on blocks 4 to 8 inches. *These measures help to prevent reflux.*
- Tell the client to avoid activities that may involve the Valsalva maneuver (e.g., lifting heavy objects, straining for bowel movements). *The Valsalva maneuver increases intra-abdominal pressure and may cause the stomach to wedge above the diaphragm.*
- Instruct the client to take medications as prescribed. *Excessive antacids may cause rebound stomach acidity. Prescribed medications reduce acidity effectively, prevent esophageal irritation, and relieve pain.*

Evaluation of Expected Outcomes

The client consumes adequate nutrients as evidenced by maintenance of weight and adherence to small, frequent meals. The state relief from epigastric pain.

Cancer of the Esophagus

Esophageal cancer is a serious condition. Clients usually do not experience symptoms until the disease has progressed to interfere with swallowing and passage of food, leading to weight loss.

Pathophysiology and Etiology

Esophageal cancer affects men more often than women. Clients usually are diagnosed in the fifth or sixth decade of life. There are two types of esophageal cancer. The most common is squamous cell carcinoma, which begins in the cells lining the esophagus. It generally occurs in the middle to upper part of the esophagus. The other type is adenocarcinoma, which begins in the glandular tissue of the lower part of the esophagus. As the cancer advances, the mass occupies space and interferes with swallowing. If the tumor grows unchecked, it may obstruct the passage of food into the stomach, promoting the possibility of aspiration, or the tumor may ulcerate, leading to occult or frank blood loss.

In general, the major cause of esophageal cancer is chronic irritation of the esophagus from any source. Esophageal cancer is strongly correlated with alcohol abuse and cigarette smoking. Clients with GERD are at higher risk of adenocarcinoma of the esophagus. Other risk factors include habitual ingestion of hot liquids or foods, chewing tobacco, poor or inadequate oral hygiene, poor intake of fruits and vegetables, obesity, and a history of radiation therapy to the upper abdomen or chest.

Assessment Findings

Symptoms usually develop slowly. Beginning symptoms are mild, with vague discomfort and difficulty swallowing some foods. Weight loss accompanies progressive dysphagia. As the disease continues, solid foods become almost impossible to swallow, and the client resorts to consuming liquids only. They may experience regurgitation of food and liquids. The tumor also may hemorrhage, resulting in hemoptysis. By the time swallowing difficulty is pronounced, cancer may have invaded surrounding tissues and lymphatics. Expansion of the tumor causes back pain and respiratory distress. Pain is a late symptom. The client also exhibits weight loss and weakness.

A barium swallow demonstrates a filling defect caused by a space-occupying mass. A biopsy of tissue removed during esophagoscopy or an esophagogastroduodenoscopy (EGD) reveals malignant cells. A bronchoscopy may determine whether the cancer cells have affected the trachea. An endoscopic ultrasound or mediastinoscopy may evaluate for cancer in the surrounding lymph nodes or other mediastinal structures. Computed tomography (CT) of the chest and abdomen and positron emission tomography (PET) also determine whether metastasis has occurred.

Medical and Surgical Management

If esophageal cancer is diagnosed in early stages, treatment is directed at a cure and includes surgery, chemotherapy, and/or radiation. If the tumor is very small and has not extended beyond the superficial layers of the esophagus, the tumor and surrounding margin of healthy tissue can be removed with an endoscopic procedure. If the cancer is more extensive, a complete resection of the esophagus (esophagectomy) will be done, which involves removing the tumor and a wide margin of tumor-free tissue as well as surrounding lymph nodes. If the tumor is in the upper two thirds of the esophagus, the surgeon removes the affected area and replaces that portion of the esophagus with a section of the jejunum or colon. This surgery is particularly risky because of pulmonary complications and problems with the anastomosis and the transplant to replace the cancerous esophageal tissue (American Cancer Society, 2020). If the tumor is in the lower one third of the esophagus, the surgeon removes the affected area and attaches the remaining esophagus to the stomach. In cases where the cancer is more extensive, the surgeon removes part of the esophagus, surrounding lymph nodes, and the upper part of the stomach (esophagogastrectomy).

Clients who are not candidates for surgery are treated with palliative measures and, possibly, endoscopic laser surgery to destroy some of the tumor. Esophageal dilatation may be used to enlarge the obstructed area. A prosthesis (stent placement) may be inserted at the tumor site to widen the narrowed area or when a fistula forms at the tumor site. Radiation, chemotherapy, laser therapy, and/or photodynamic therapy may also be used as palliative measures. Laser therapy may be used to destroy the cancerous tissue and relieve obstruction when surgery is not effective or cannot be used. Photodynamic therapy combines chemotherapy with a special light to eliminate cancer cells and relieve symptoms such as difficulty swallowing.

Nursing Management

The nurse must consult with the dietitian before instituting measures for weight reduction or gain as ordered. A major nursing goal is adequate or improved nutrition and, eventually, stable weight. The nurse encourages small, frequent meals. If the client has difficulty swallowing, the nurse ensures that the client receives soft foods or high-calorie, high-protein, semiliquid foods. The client needs to refrain from consuming foods that contain significant air or gas, such as carbonated drinks. To reduce bloating, the client should avoid drinking from straws or narrow-necked bottles to reduce the volume of air trapped in the esophagus or stomach. The client should receive liquid supplements between meals.

The nutritional needs of the client with inoperable cancer of the esophagus are met with nasogastric or gastrostomy tube feedings or TPN. In such cases, essential nursing management involves caring for the skin at the tube insertion site, preventing infection, administering nourishment, maintaining tube patency, and preparing the client or family for self-care or home care after discharge. (See the earlier sections on GI intubation and gastrostomy.)

Clients who return from esophageal or gastric surgery need to be turned and to perform deep breathing and coughing every 2 hours. They must also know how to support the surgical incision for coughing and deep breathing. The nurse may use an incentive spirometer to motivate the client and provide immediate feedback on respiratory efficiency. The client must ambulate to mobilize secretions, increase the depth of respiration, and promote expulsion of intestinal gas.

To avoid gastric distention, the client should not have oral nourishment until bowel sounds resume and are active. The nurse provides oral liquids, when allowed, to thin secretions. To minimize dyspnea, the nurse gives frequent, small meals and does not allow the client to lie down immediately after eating.

The nurse explains the rationale underlying the prescribed treatment and instructs the client and family to adhere to the therapeutic regimen, follow the necessary dietary modifications, and attend medical follow-up appointments regularly. They emphasize that the client should inform the primary provider immediately of worsening symptoms, steady weight loss, difficulty swallowing soft foods, abnormal bleeding, or other new problems.

GASTRIC DISORDERS

Gastritis

Gastritis is inflammation of the stomach lining (gastric mucosa). It may be acute or chronic.

Pathophysiology and Etiology

The causes of gastritis include dietary indiscretions; reflux of duodenal contents; use of aspirin, steroids, NSAIDs, alcohol, or caffeine; cigarette smoking; ingestion of poisons or corrosive substances; food allergies; infection; and gastric ischemia secondary to vasoconstriction caused by a stress response. The bacterium *Helicobacter pylori* may contribute to chronic gastritis. Autoimmune gastritis occurs when the client's own body attacks the lining of the stomach and erodes the protective layer. This can be associated with other autoimmune disorders and vitamin B_{12} deficiency.

Gastric secretions are highly acidic. *Parietal cells* in the stomach increase acid production (hydrochloric acid) in response to seeing, smelling, and eating food. The parasympathetic vagus nerve releases histamine and acetylcholine, chemicals that also stimulate the parietal cells. An increasing level of acid triggers the conversion of pepsinogen to pepsin, creating a chemical mixture strong enough to digest the stomach wall. However, because mucus protectively coats the stomach lining, pepsin normally has little effect on the stomach wall.

Prostaglandin E, a lipid compound secreted in the stomach, apparently promotes the production of mucus, which contains buffering substances and mechanically bars penetration by stomach acids. The submucosal layers of the stomach can become inflamed, however, when irritating substances reduce or penetrate the mucous layer. Consequently, the client experiences epigastric discomfort often described as *heartburn*. The mucus-producing cells usually heal and regenerate in 3 to 5 days. Chronic irritation leads to ulceration.

Assessment Findings

Usually, the client complains of epigastric fullness, pressure, pain, anorexia, nausea, and vomiting. When a bacterial or viral infection causes gastritis, the client may experience vomiting, diarrhea, fever, and abdominal pain. Drugs, poisons, toxic substances, and corrosives can cause gastric bleeding. Clients may describe seeing blood in emesis or note a darkening of their stool color. Chronic gastritis may give rise to no symptoms or symptoms similar to mild indigestion.

A complete blood count may reveal anemia from chronic blood loss. Stool testing for occult blood often detects RBCs. In difficult cases, gastroscopy may be performed to visualize the mucosa and obtain specimens, which are examined for pathogens or cellular abnormalities. Clients may also be tested for *H. pylori*.

Medical and Surgical Management

Treatment depends on the cause and symptoms. Ingestion of poisons requires emergency treatment. In acute cases, eating is restricted and IV fluids are given to correct dehydration and electrolyte imbalances, particularly if vomiting is severe. Antiemetics are prescribed to control nausea and vomiting, and antibiotics may be prescribed to inhibit or destroy the infection.

The usual treatment of chronic gastritis is the avoidance of irritating substances, such as alcohol and NSAIDs. Some clients may wish to avoid spicy foods, high-fat foods, and caffeine, depending on the degree to which these items aggravate their symptoms. Various drugs such as antacids, H_2-receptor antagonists, and PPIs may be prescribed. A combination of drugs may be used to treat *H. pylori.* (See the section on Medical and Surgical Management of peptic ulcer disease [PUD].)

Nursing Management

The nurse monitors the client's symptoms. Evaluating the client's response to dietary modifications and prescribed medications is important. The nurse observes the color and characteristics of any vomitus or stool that the client passes. In addition, they teach about diet, drug therapy, and the need for continued medical follow-up. For complications such as ulcer formation, refer to the section on Nursing Management of PUD.

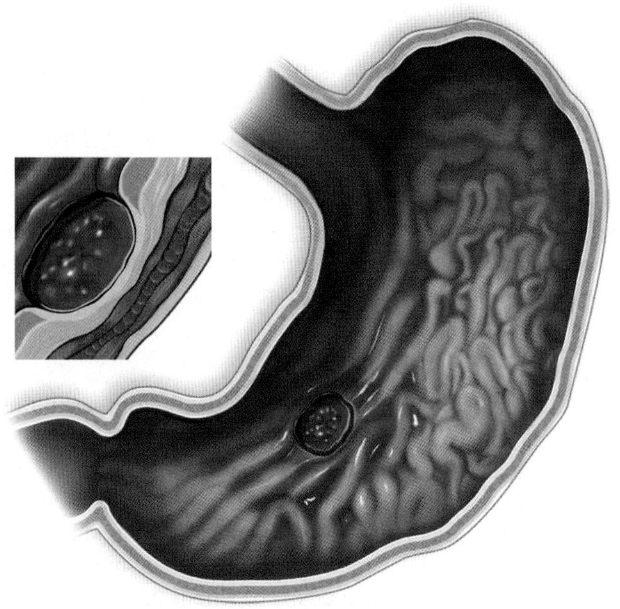

Figure 45-5 Peptic ulcer disease. (Reprinted with permission from Kyle, T., & Carman, S. (2020). *Essentials of pediatric nursing* (4th ed.). Wolters Kluwer.)

Peptic Ulcer Disease

A **peptic ulcer** is a circumscribed loss of tissue in an area of the GI tract that is in contact with hydrochloric acid and pepsin. Most peptic ulcers occur in the duodenum; however, they may develop at the lower end of the esophagus, in the stomach, or in the jejunum after the client has had surgery at the spot where the stomach and the jejunum were sutured. Gastric ulcers are more likely to recur and have the highest incidence of undergoing malignant changes. Men are affected more frequently by PUD than women are. The highest incidence occurs during middle life, but the condition can occur at any age.

Pathophysiology and Etiology

PUD occurs when the normal balance between factors that promote mucosal injury (gastric acid, pepsin, bile acid, ingested substances) and factors that protect the mucosa (intact epithelium, mucus, and bicarbonate secretion) is disrupted. The single greatest risk factor for the development of PUD is infection with the Gram-negative bacterium *H. pylori.* Transmission of the bacterium is thought to be by fecal–oral or oral–oral pathways. *H. pylori* are present in the gastric or duodenal mucosa of 80% to 90% of clients with PUD. The bacteria, which shelter themselves in the bicarbonate-rich mucus, are a factor in chronic gastritis and PUD. The mechanism by which this microorganism makes the mucosa more susceptible to erosion is not yet completely understood. It appears that *H. pylori* secrete an enzyme that theoretically depletes gastric mucus, making it more vulnerable to injury.

Family history is thought to be an additional risk factor for the development of PUD. A genetic component may exist, as demonstrated by the high incidence among first-degree relatives. Another explanation is the clustering of infection with *H. pylori* in families. Other risk factors include chronic use of NSAIDs, cigarette smoking, and physiologic stress. PUD resulting from physiologic stress is seen most often in the intensive care unit and may accompany increased intracranial pressure (Curling ulcer), burns (Cushing ulcer), and sepsis.

Ulcers develop when there is prolonged hyperacidity or chronic reduction in mucus. Once gastric acid has penetrated the mucosal layer, the acid begins to digest the stomach wall (Fig. 45-5). Histamine, released from the injured cells, aggravates the condition by triggering hypersecretion of more hydrochloric acid and pepsin. The body responds with the inflammatory process. Capillary permeability is increased; the mucosa swells and bleeds easily.

Because food dilutes stomach acid, clients with PUD experience more discomfort when the stomach is empty than after eating food. Unless the process is controlled, the erosion can lead to obstruction from scar formation or penetrate the entire thickness of the stomach wall, spilling gastric contents into the peritoneal cavity, a process that may be accompanied by hemorrhage.

Aging and chronic stomach inflammation, such as in recurrent gastric ulcers, cancer of the stomach, or a long history of alcoholism, lead to atrophy of the glandular epithelium of the stomach. The chronic gastric inflammation causes the parietal cells to secrete less hydrochloric acid, resulting in hypochlorhydria (reduced gastric acidity) or achlorhydria (absence of hydrochloric acid). In addition, the gastric mucosa produces intrinsic factor, which the body requires for the absorption of vitamin B_{12}. Chronic gastric inflammation inhibits the production of intrinsic factor, leading to poor absorption of this essential nutrient. As a result, the client is at high risk of pernicious anemia.

Assessment Findings

Signs and Symptoms

Most clients with PUD have abdominal pain, which usually is confined to the epigastrium and does not radiate. Clients most often describe it as having a "burning" quality. They usually complain of pain that occurs 1 to several hours after meals and disturbs sleep. Eating food may relieve the pain. Back pain suggests that the ulcer is irritating the pancreas. Approximately 20% of clients may have bleeding as the first sign of the ulcer. Hemorrhage, hematemesis, or melena may occur. Protracted vomiting secondary to scarring and resultant obstruction also are seen among those who have ignored earlier symptoms. Some clients also have unexplained weight loss.

Diagnostic Findings

The diagnosis is suggested by the history and confirmed by results of an upper GI series or EGD. To differentiate between benign and malignant ulcers, a gastric washing or biopsy for cytologic analysis may be performed. Typically, the hemoglobin level and RBC count are low from chronic blood loss. Vomiting alters electrolyte levels. In addition, tests for *H. pylori* are performed.

Medical and Surgical Management

Most clients with PUD have *H. pylori*. Thus, the goals of treatment are to (1) eradicate the bacteria and (2) reduce the acid levels in the digestive system to relieve pain and promote healing. Use of only one antibiotic is inadequate to kill the bacterium; eradication therapy includes a combination of antibiotics for at least 2 weeks. Drugs are also prescribed to reduce acid, relieve pain, and promote healing, including H_2-receptor antagonists, antacids, PPIs, and cytoprotective agents. These drugs may be prescribed for longer than 2 weeks. The following list provides examples of drugs used to treat PUD:

- *Antibiotics*: Commonly prescribed antibiotics are amoxicillin (Amoxil), clarithromycin (Biaxin), and tetracycline, which exert bactericidal effects to eradicate *H. pylori*.
- *Amebicides*: Metronidazole (Flagyl) assists in the eradication of *H. pylori*.
- *H_2-receptor antagonists*: Cimetidine (Tagamet), famotidine (Pepcid), and nizatidine (Axid) block H_2 receptors and decrease hydrochloric acid secretion in the stomach, relieving pain and promoting healing.
- *Antacids*: These drugs initially are used to neutralize existing stomach acid and provide quick pain relief. They are not absorbed from the GI tract and therefore do not produce alkalosis, even when given in large doses.
- *PPIs*: Omeprazole (Prilosec), lansoprazole (Prevacid), esomeprazole (Nexium), rabeprazole (AcipHex), and pantoprazole (Protonix) block the final step in acid production at the surface of parietal cells. These medications also promote healing and appear to inhibit the growth of *H. pylori*.
- *Cytoprotective agents*: Sucralfate (Carafate) forms a seal over the ulcer, protecting it from irritation. Misoprostol (Cytotec), a synthetic prostaglandin, is used to sustain the mucosal layer especially among clients who require large doses or long-term treatment with aspirin or NSAIDs. Bismuth salts such as bismuth subsalicylate (Pepto-Bismol) suppress *H. pylori*, assist in healing mucosal lesions, and protect the lining of the stomach and intestines.
- *Combination drugs*: Some drug companies provide medication combinations for the treatment of PUD, which include two antibiotics with an H_2-receptor antagonist or cytoprotective agent. Examples include Prevpac and Helidac.

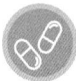

Pharmacologic Considerations

- Sucralfate is administered 2 hours after an H_2-receptor antagonist to ensure the absorption of the H_2-receptor antagonist. It may be given for 4 to 6 weeks.

Clients with PUD may experience obstruction resulting from edema and inflammation. Gastric intubation is necessary, along with treatment for the ulcer. Treatment of hemorrhage includes complete rest for the GI tract, blood transfusions, and gastric lavage with saline solution. IV fluids are administered until the bleeding has stopped. If more conservative measures are unsuccessful, endoscopic laser therapy or endoscopic injections of epinephrine or anhydrous alcohol into the ulcer bed may be used to control bleeding.

Ulcers that persist (referred to as *refractory ulcers*) despite medical interventions, repeatedly recur, cause severe hemorrhage, create unrelieved obstruction, cause perforation, or are predisposed to malignant changes justify surgical interventions as described in Table 45-3. If a total **gastrectomy** (removal of the stomach) is performed, the client receives vitamin B_{12} injections or intranasal vitamin B_{12} for life because, without the stomach, the intrinsic factor necessary for the absorption of vitamin B_{12} is no longer produced. Vitamin B_{12} therapy usually is not necessary for 1 or 2 years after surgery because the body uses very small amounts of this vitamin and body reserves usually are sufficient for several years.

Clients with a gastrojejunostomy are at risk of developing dumping syndrome when they begin to take solid food. **Dumping syndrome**, which produces weakness, dizziness, sweating, palpitations, abdominal cramps, and diarrhea, results from the rapid emptying (dumping) of large amounts of hypertonic chyme (a liquid mass of partly digested food) into the jejunum. This concentrated solution in the gut draws fluid from the circulating blood into the intestine, causing hypovolemia. The drop in blood pressure (BP) can produce syncope. As the syndrome progresses, the sudden appearance of carbohydrates in the jejunum stimulates the pancreas to secrete excessive amounts of insulin, which, in turn, causes hypoglycemia.

Nursing Management

The nurse must explore each symptom of PUD in depth. For example, if pain occurs, the nurse determines its type, onset

TABLE 45-3 Surgical Procedures to Treat Peptic Ulcer Disease

PROCEDURE	DESCRIPTION	ILLUSTRATION
Vagotomy	A branch of the vagus nerve is cut to reduce gastric acid secretion.	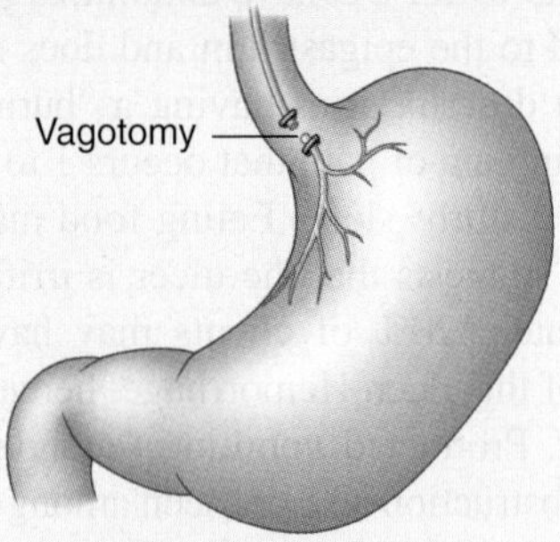
Pyloroplasty	The pylorus is repaired or reconstructed to expand the stomach outlet narrowed by scarring or improve gastric motility and emptying.	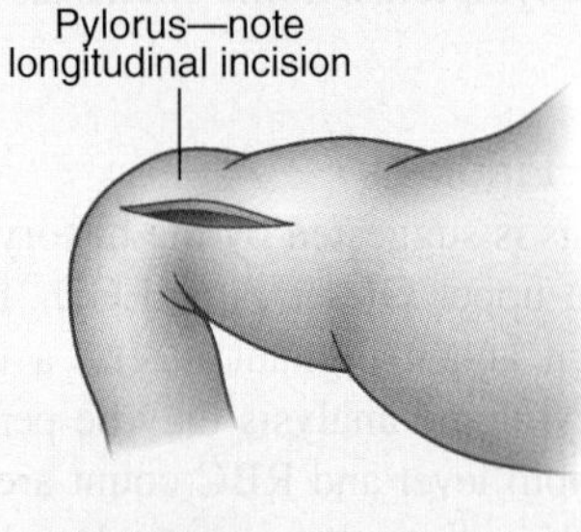 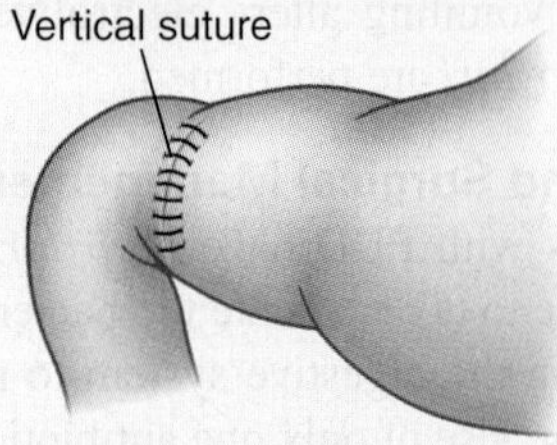
Antrectomy	The antrum (lower portion of the stomach, including the pylorus) is removed to eliminate a benign ulcer in the lesser curvature of the stomach if the ulcer has not healed after 12 weeks of medical treatment or is recurring.	
Gastroduodenostomy (Billroth I)	Part of the stomach is removed, while the remaining portion is connected to the duodenum. Usually, a vagotomy also is performed. This procedure is done to remove an ulcerated area in the stomach that is prone to hemorrhage, perforation, and obstruction.	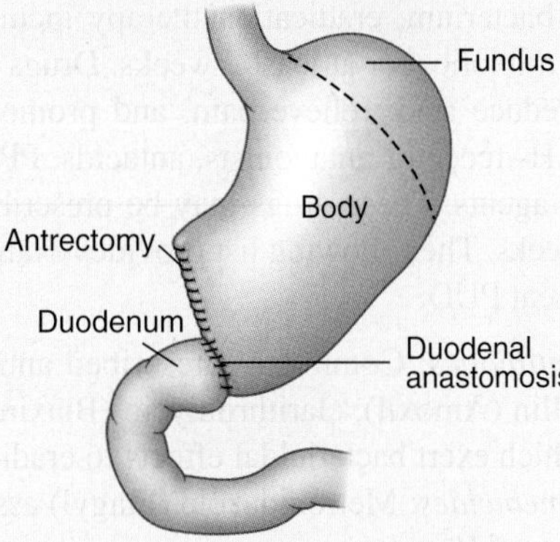
Gastrojejunostomy (Billroth II)	Same as Billroth I, except that the remaining portion is connected to the jejunum in cases of extensive duodenal inflammation or perforation.	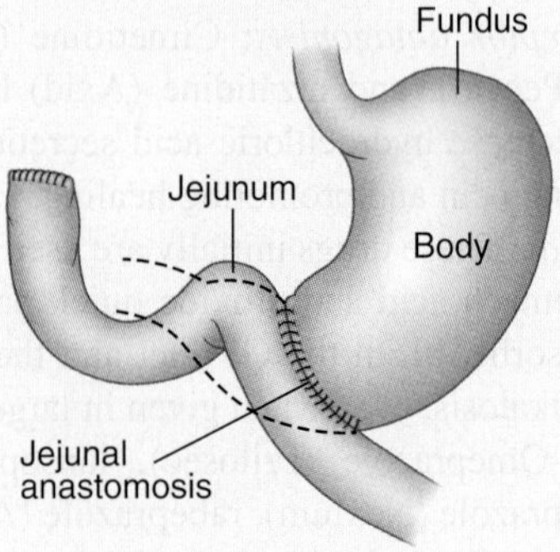
Total Gastrectomy	The entire stomach is removed and the esophagus is joined to the jejunum to remove an ulcer high in the stomach near the gastroesophageal junction. It is performed to treat a gastric malignancy.	

in relation to eating food, location, and duration. A dietary history must include relevant questions pertaining to foods that cause distress, the amount of food eaten at each meal, and whether eating food relieves pain.

For a client to continue eating, it may be necessary to modify ingredients, temperature, or consistency of foods as well as to use smaller portions on smaller plates. Clients need nutritional supplements. If the client is receiving tube feedings, reinstilling the gastric residual is necessary because it contains partially digested nutrients and essential electrolytes.

In addition, the nurse notes the client's bowel patterns and stool characteristics. They also evaluate the client's emotional status and response to activity. The nurse monitors the nonsurgical client closely for medical complications, which includes assessing vital signs and fluid status. Nursing Guidelines 45-3 describe the assessment of gastric pH. For a discussion of appropriate nursing management of a surgical client, refer to the Nursing Management section that accompanies the discussion of cancer of the stomach.

NURSING GUIDELINES 45-3

Assessing the pH of Aspirated Fluid

Purpose: To evaluate the effectiveness of antacid or H_2-receptor antagonist therapy in PUD by aspirating stomach fluid and testing gastric pH. Desired pH range is 4.0 to 6.0.

- Obtain a pH test kit.
- Put on gloves.
- Verify that the distal tip of the client's nasogastric tube is in the stomach and has not migrated to the intestine.
- Use a separate syringe for withdrawing the test specimen because antacid residue or irrigating solution in the nasogastric tube will falsely raise the gastric pH.
- Connect the syringe to the tube.
- Instill a small amount of air to clear fluid from the gastric tube just before aspirating.
- Aspirate a small amount of fluid.
- Drop a sample of the gastric fluid onto a pH color indicator strip.
- Compare the color on the test strip with the color guide supplied in the test kit.
- Record the findings.

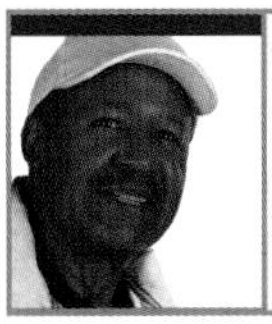

Clinical Scenario A client just diagnosed with PUD has experienced the following signs and symptoms: burning epigastric pain, poor appetite, occasional vomiting of dark red contents, stools that appear darker, and weight loss. The client is being seen for a complete GI workup and treatment. **What are the important foci of care for the nurse assigned to this client? See the following Nursing Process section.**

NURSING PROCESS FOR THE CLIENT WITH A GASTRIC DISORDER

Assessment

Ask about current symptoms, looking for specific information about such symptoms as indigestion, fullness, heartburn, nausea, and vomiting. How long has the client had these symptoms? When do they occur? For example, does the client experience problems before or after eating or with certain foods? Do situations such as stress make the problems worse? Does anything relieve the problem? Having the client provide a record of dietary intake for the last 72 hours may be useful. Also, ask about previous gastric problems and treatments/surgery. Assess for signs of abdominal discomfort/pain, malnutrition, and dehydration.

Diagnosis, Planning, and Interventions

Acute Pain: Related to the effects of gastric acid on damaged mucosal tissue
Expected Outcome: Client states that pain is relieved.

- Administer medications as prescribed. *Administering medications as ordered can destroy bacteria causing the ulcer, block acid production and promote healing, neutralize stomach acid, and protect the lining of the stomach and small intestine, thus alleviating pain.*
- Instruct the client to avoid aspirin and caffeine as well as alcohol and nicotine. *Avoiding these substances minimizes increased acid production and irritation to the GI mucosa, thus relieving pain.*
- Eat a healthy diet at regular times. *Pacing meals and choosing nutritionally adequate foods promote healing and reduce pain.*

Hypovolemia: Related to vomiting, diarrhea, and/or bleeding
Expected Outcome: Client will maintain adequate fluid balance.

- Assist client to set a goal for minimum oral liquid intake during waking hours. *Involving the client in planning helps meet their needs.*
- Provide fluids with calories and electrolytes hourly. Offer different choices. *Frequent fluid intake maintains fluid balance. Various choices prevent monotony.*
- Monitor fluid intake and output. *This record helps indicate trends in fluid balance and early signs of dehydration.*

(continued)

NURSING PROCESS FOR THE CLIENT WITH A GASTRIC DISORDER (continued)

Knowledge Deficiency: About dietary management and gastric disorder
Expected Outcome: Client will demonstrate knowledge of dietary management as evidenced by appropriate choices of foods and fluids.

- Review client's fluid and nutritional needs. *Understanding of fluid and nutritional needs promotes better compliance and intake.*
- Provide a list of foods and substances to avoid. *Doing so may help prevent gastric irritation.*
- Review medications with the client, including reasons for medications, schedule, and side effects and their management. *Such review promotes better compliance and outcomes.*

Evaluation of Expected Outcomes

Client states that pain is relieved. Fluid intake is 2000 mL/24 hours, with a urine output of 1850 mL/24 hours. Nutritional intake is adequate as evidenced by maintenance of preillness weight. The client adheres to medical regimen as evidenced by appropriate choice of foods and fluids and compliance with medication schedule.

Cancer of the Stomach

Pathophysiology and Etiology

Cancer of the stomach is a malignancy characterized by either an enlarged mass or ulcerating lesion that expands or penetrates several tissue layers. Stomach malignancies are most common among Asian and Pacific Islanders as well as in African Americans and Latinos. Although a single etiology has not been identified, factors that are linked to stomach cancer include (1) heredity; (2) chronic inflammation; (3) *achlorhydria* (absence of free hydrochloric acid in the stomach), which may promote bacterial growth; (4) chronic ingestion of highly salted, smoked, or pickled foods; (5) nitrates and nitrites, nitrogen-based chemical additives in cured meats, which combine with other nitrogen-containing substances in the stomach to produce nitrosamines—known carcinogens; (6) a diet low in fresh fruits and vegetables; (7) infection with *H. pylori*; (8) tobacco and alcohol use; and (9) stomach polyps. The most common type of stomach cancer is adenocarcinoma, which arises from the glandular cells in the inner layer of the stomach. Stomach cancer often spreads to the lymph nodes and metastasizes to the liver, pancreas, esophagus, or duodenum.

Assessment Findings

Early symptoms are vague. As the tumor enlarges, symptoms include a prolonged feeling of fullness after eating, indigestion, heartburn, nausea, vomiting, anorexia, weight loss, fatigue, and anemia. Stool usually contains occult blood. Pain is a late symptom. Endoscopy, a barium swallow or CT scan, and a tissue biopsy obtained by gastroscopy or open laparotomy help confirm the diagnosis. Gastric analysis may disclose no free hydrochloric acid. CT or PET scanning, ultrasonography, or magnetic resonance imaging (MRI) helps determine the depth of the cancer.

Medical and Surgical Management

Small cancers limited to the inside lining of the stomach can be removed with endoscopic mucosal resection. A subtotal (partial) or total gastrectomy is used for more extensive tumors and is the only curative approach. The type and extent of surgery usually depend on tumor location, symptoms, and any metastasis. A subtotal gastrectomy preserves more normal digestion. Even though surgery may not achieve a complete cure, it still may be performed to control bleeding or relieve obstruction at the cardiac or pyloric junction.

Chemotherapy with drugs such as 5-fluorouracil (5-FU) or doxorubicin (Adriamycin) and palliative radiation therapy also may be used. For some clients with a specific genetic mutation in their cancer cells, a drug called imatinib mesylate (Gleevec), used in the treatment of leukemia, may be taken orally every day in capsule form. A newer medication, sunitinib (Sutent), is showing better promise for clients who cannot take imatinib. Imatinib targets the specific mutation, preventing cell growth without harming healthy tissue. Sunitinib is an antineoplastic that interferes with the growth of cancer cells. Surgery remains the treatment of choice.

Nursing Management

The nurse's role in the management of gastric cancer includes teaching the public, especially susceptible ethnic groups or clients with a family history of stomach cancer, how to change their dietary habits to reduce the predisposition for this disease. The nurse may also instruct high-risk groups, such as those who have undergone vagotomy or must take medications to reduce hydrochloric acid formation, on the early warning signs of cancer and the value of frequent health assessments. Nursing roles in managing clients undergoing surgery for gastric cancer are extensive. (See Nursing Care Plan 45-1 and Client and Family Teaching 45-1.)

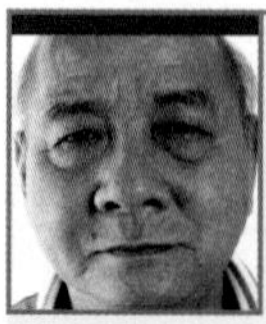

Clinical Scenario A client is scheduled for GI surgery related to esophageal cancer. What are the general considerations for a client undergoing surgery of the upper GI tract? See Nursing Care Plan 45-1.

NURSING CARE PLAN 45-1 The Client Undergoing Gastrointestinal Surgery

Preoperative Assessment

In addition to performing assessments for the client with a GI disorder:

- Obtain a complete health, drug, tobacco, and allergy history.
- Ask approximately how long symptoms have lasted, whether eating is normal, and how much weight, if any, the client has lost.
- Assess bowel sounds for presence and quality.
- Ask about food intolerance and current dietary management.
- Determine bowel elimination patterns and stool characteristics.
- Assess understanding of diagnostic tests, scheduled surgery, and preparations for surgery.

Nursing Diagnosis. **Acute Anxiety** related to test results, diagnosis, and surgical procedure

Expected Outcome. Anxiety will be mild as evidenced by a calm demeanor, appropriate questions, and expressions of fear.

Interventions	Rationales
Provide time for client to verbalize fears and express needs related to diagnosis and surgery.	*Being present and supportive encourages communication.*
Allow client to express their personal reaction to the threat to well-being.	*Expressing feelings without being judged can help reduce fears.*
Explain tests, procedures, and surgery using nonmedical speech and allowing time for questions.	*Education helps to increase coping skills.*
Keep client informed of progress and explain delays or changes in plans.	*Adequate explanations make clients feel more secure and less anxious.*
If surgery is emergent (such as in GI hemorrhage), provide explanations to family members and anticipate questions and concerns that client will have after surgery.	*Family members will have decreased anxiety and be less anxious and better able to provide support when seeing client after surgery.*

Evaluation of Expected Outcome

Client is less anxious, expressing fears and questions about diagnosis and surgery.

Nursing Diagnosis. **Knowledge Deficiency** related to preoperative preparation

Expected Outcome. Client will demonstrate exercises satisfactorily and acknowledge the purpose of equipment and procedures that may be used after surgery.

Interventions	Rationales
Using nonmedical language, instruct client about common postoperative equipment: IV line, infusion pump, nasogastric suction, oxygen, urinary catheter, wound drain, cardiac monitor, and pulse oximeter.	*Providing understandable explanations helps client learn information effectively.*
Prepare client by explaining reasons for postoperative treatments and procedures, such as frequent assessment of vital signs and performance of breathing exercises.	*Such explanation promotes postoperative compliance with needed treatments and procedures.*
Explain postoperative administration of analgesics to reduce and manage pain.	*Client fears pain—understanding that pain will be managed reduces fear.*
Evaluate client's learning through return demonstrations of deep breathing, coughing, moving legs, and turning as well as verbalization of instructions.	*Having client provide explanations and demonstrations reinforces instructions and helps the nurse determine if client needs further teaching.*

Evaluation of Expected Outcome

Client can discuss the surgical procedure and demonstrate how to turn, deep breathe, cough, and splint incision.

Postoperative Assessment

Refer to standards of postoperative care in Chapter 14. When the client returns from surgery:

- Assess vital signs.
- Review the record about the type of surgery performed and the client's progress during surgery and in the postanesthesia recovery unit.
- Inspect the surgical dressing for drainage and tubes or catheters for placement, patency, and type of drainage.
- Carefully observe nasogastric tube drainage for evidence of bleeding. Although the nasogastric tube may contain a small amount of dark blood when the client first returns from the operating room, the drainage should promptly return to the yellow-green of normal gastric secretions.
- Inspect the IV site and note the current rate and progress of fluid infusion.
- Document fluid intake and output as well as the level of consciousness and comfort.
- Closely monitor the client for change in vital signs, especially fluctuations in BP (BP may increase initially in response to shock), increased pulse rate, and elevated temperature; extreme

(continued)

NURSING CARE PLAN 45-1 The Client Undergoing Gastrointestinal Surgery (*continued*)

restlessness; difficulty breathing (increased respiratory rate, cyanosis); severe pain, especially after an analgesic has been given or in an area other than the operative site; abdominal distention or rigidity; excessive or absent nasogastric output; urinary output less than 35 mL/hour if catheterized or failure to void within 8 hours of surgery; failure to pass flatus or stool more than 48 hours after surgery; profuse diaphoresis; excessive bloody drainage from the nasogastric tube, surgical drains, or surgical dressing; separation of the surgical wound edges; and unusual color or odor of drainage.

Nursing Diagnosis. **Malnutrition Risk** related to poor nutritional intake before surgery and changed GI system after surgery

Expected Outcome. Client will achieve optimal caloric intake to maintain weight.

Interventions	Rationales
Assess client for changes in physiologic status that will interfere with nutrition.	*Malnutrition contributes to poor recovery from surgery.*
Administer TPN as ordered (see Chapter 13).	*TPN provides adequate calories, nutrition, and fluid replacement and supports metabolic needs.*
Administer nasogastric feedings as ordered (see section Gastrointestinal Intubation for Feedings or Medications).	*Nasogastric feedings provide adequate calories, nutrition, and fluid replacement and support metabolic needs.*
When bowel sounds return, advance oral diet as ordered and tolerated. Encourage small, frequent meals.	*An advanced diet provides opportunity for client to eat and adjust. Small, frequent meals prevent fullness and nausea.*
Monitor food intake.	*Such monitoring helps identify trends in client's nutritional status.*
Weigh client twice a week.	*Weighing determines weight loss, gain, or maintenance.*
Report laboratory values such as low blood cell and hemoglobin counts and decreased iron, serum protein, transferrin, or ferritin level.	*Such findings may indicate malnutrition.*

Evaluation of Expected Outcome

Client attains optimal nutrition as evidenced by reasonable weight and tolerance of six small meals of soft foods and liquids.

Client and Family Teaching 45-1 Discharge Instructions for the Client With Stomach Cancer

The type and extent of teaching depends on the surgery that is performed. If tube or gastrostomy feedings, tracheostomy care, and suction techniques will continue after discharge, the nurse involves the client and a family member in practicing these procedures while the client is still hospitalized. They identify where medical supplies can be purchased and offer a referral for home care from a local community agency. Other points to instruct the client and family about in the discharge teaching plan include the following:

- Adhere to the diet (e.g., foods to eat or avoid) recommended by the primary provider.
- Also adhere to the dietary, fluid, and positional modifications to avoid the dumping syndrome.
- Take medications exactly as prescribed. Follow the directions on the label, paying particular attention to when you should take the drug (e.g., before, after, or with food or meals).
- Monitor weight weekly. Report any significant weight loss to the primary provider.
- Keep appointments for periodic medical follow-up.

Extreme Obesity

Extreme obesity is defined as a body mass index (BMI) of 40 or higher (Box 45-3) or a body weight of more than 20% of the ideal.

Pathophysiology and Etiology

Obesity has now reached epidemic levels in the United States, with more than one third of the population categorized as obese (having a BMI of 30 or higher; Centers for Disease Control and Prevention [CDC], 2020). The etiology of obesity involves several factors. Genetic predisposition to obesity is a factor, but it is sometimes difficult to separate hereditary factors from learned diet and lifestyle habits. It is clear that obesity results from excessive caloric intake, ready access to an abundance of food, and a sedentary lifestyle. A low resting metabolic rate may also be a factor. Pregnancy and lack of sleep can be factors that contribute to obesity. Some medications such as antidepressants, diabetes medications, steroids, beta-blockers, antiseizure medications, and antipsychotic medications may contribute to obesity, although it is sometimes difficult to ascertain if inactivity and overeating while taking these medications are also factors. Clients with extreme obesity are at greater risk of diabetes, heart disease, hypertension, stroke, osteoarthritis, gallbladder disease, and some forms of cancer, including colorectal and kidney cancer.

BOX 45-3 Calculating Body Mass Index (BMI)

To calculate BMI, multiply weight in pounds by 703 and then divide that by height in inches squared.

Example: A client weighs 160 lb and is 5 feet 6 inches tall. The weight of 160 is multiplied by 703, which equals 112,480. The height is 66 inches—when squared, it equals 4356. Divide 112,480 by 4356, which equals a BMI of 25.8, which identifies this client as overweight.

To calculate BMI using the metric, divide the client's weight in kilograms by height in meters squared.

Using the above example, the client weighs 72.7 kg and is 167.6 cm or 1.676 m. Divide 72.7 by 1.676^2 (2.81), which equals a BMI of 25.8.

$$\text{BMI} = \frac{\text{Weight (pounds)}}{[\text{Height (inches)}]^2} \times 703$$

The Centers for Disease Control and Prevention (2016) classifies weight as follows:

- BMI < 18.5 = Underweight
- BMI 18.5 to < 25 = Normal weight
- BMI 25 to 30 = Overweight
- BMI higher than 30 = Obesity

Obesity is sometimes classified into three categories:

Class 1—BMI of 30 to < 35

Class 2—BMI of 35 to < 40

Class 3—BMI of 40 or higher. Class 3 obesity is sometimes categorized as "extreme" or "severe" obesity.

Assessment Findings

Clients with extreme obesity often weigh 100 lb more than their ideal body weight. They may already have hypertension, heart disease, and type 2 diabetes. Many clients are unable to engage in physical activity without getting severely short of breath, and they cannot participate easily in normal activities of daily living such as bathing and other self-care activities. In addition, they may have poor self-esteem and suffer from depression. A health history reveals dietary habits, weight loss efforts, and exercise routines. Measuring weight, BMI, and waist circumference are important measures. Women with a waist circumference of more than 35 inches and men with circumference of more than 40 inches tend to have more health issues related to obesity.

Medical and Surgical Management

Treatment centers on weight loss, dietary changes, increase in exercise and activity, and behavior modifications. Several prescription medications are currently approved for the treatment of obesity. Orlistat (Xenical, Alli) works to bind to gastric and pancreatic lipase to prevent the digestion of 30% of ingested fat, thereby decreasing caloric intake. Undigested fat is excreted in the stool. Clients with gallbladder problems or those with chronic problems related to absorption of food cannot take orlistat. Clients taking this medication may experience an increased number of bowel movements, increased flatus and oily discharge from the rectum, and decreased absorption of fat-soluble vitamins. To compensate for this problem, clients are advised to take a multivitamin. Lorcaserin (Belviq) is used to decrease the appetite and promote a sensation of fullness by activating brain receptors for *serotonin*, a neurotransmitter that triggers feelings of satiety and satisfaction (see Chapter 70). If there is no significant weight loss within 12 weeks, the medication is discontinued. Another drug being used for weight control is phentermine/topiramate (Qsymia). It is known to promote appetite suppression and the sensation of satiety in a way similar to that of amphetamines, but its precise action is not understood. Side effects include increased heart rate, insomnia, and dizziness. Bupropion and naltrexone (Contrave) combine an antidepressant (which also depresses appetite) and a drug that curbs appetite and food cravings. Saxenda, a drug used for diabetes, is now approved for weight loss treatment.

Bariatric Surgical Procedures

Bariatric surgery, weight loss surgery, or gastric bypass surgery are procedures designed to help clients reduce their weight through surgical changes to the upper GI digestive system. Surgery is performed only after other methods for weight reduction have failed. Selected clients should be extremely obese and motivated to lose weight, and they should accept the surgery-related risks and the lifestyle changes necessary for weight management. In addition, they can have no associated physiologic reasons for obesity, such as endocrine problems, or any psychopathology that interferes with understanding of the risks involved, such as bipolar disorder or schizophrenia (Mayo Clinic Staff, 2020).

There are several types of bariatric surgery:

- *Standard Roux-en-Y gastric bypass (RYGB)*: This procedure creates a small stomach pouch by stapling the stomach and then dividing the upper jejunum, rerouting the upper half (called the *Roux limb*), and attaching it to the stomach pouch. The other end of the jejunum is attached to the Roux limb at a lower point. The end effect is that food moves through the esophagus into the small gastric pouch, passes through the pouch into the Roux limb, and then passes into the remaining small intestine, bypassing the lower stomach and duodenum. The RYBG procedure can be performed laparoscopically.
- *Modified RYGB*: This surgical procedure is used on severely obese clients. In this procedure, the bypassed segment of the intestine that contains the digestive juices is attached to the intestine that carries food closer to the large intestine in order to restrict more nutrient and calorie absorption.
- *Biliopancreatic diversion with duodenal switch*: This procedure is similar to the RYBG procedure, but it keeps some stomach function intact while bypassing the small intestine.
- *Laparoscopic gastric banding (LAGB)*: This procedure restricts food intake into the stomach by creating a small pouch from the top of the stomach and narrowing the passage into the lower part of the stomach through the use of an inflatable band. It reduces the amount of food the stomach can hold and slows passage of food through the stomach. The two types widely used for restrictive purposes are called vertical banded gastroplasty (VBG) and LAGB (Lap-Band).
- *Sleeve gastrectomy*: This procedure involves surgical removal of the left half of the stomach, thus reducing the size of the stomach.

As with any surgical procedure, there are risks. Postoperative bleeding, blood clots, bowel obstruction, and infection may occur. Other problems may involve nausea and/or distention in the stomach pouch related to overeating or poor chewing of food, dumping syndrome, diarrhea or constipation, and nutritional deficiencies. Long-term goals for this surgery are resolution of chronic health problems, such as type 2 diabetes, hypertension, increased cholesterol and triglycerides, and obstructive sleep apnea. It is hoped that clients will gain increased mobility and greater quality of life.

Nursing Management

The nurse manages the care of clients having bariatric surgery as they would for clients having any other type of gastric surgery. However, clients have greater risk of complications related to their extreme obesity. For example, obstructive sleep apnea may be a problem. The client may require continuous positive airway pressure (CPAP) or bilevel positive airway pressure (BiPAP) (see Chapter 20). Obesity can also contribute to poor wound healing, infection, and wound dehiscence. Pain is another possible complication, and effective management is needed so that clients better comply with breathing and mobility exercises.

Discharge teaching must emphasize the preoperative instruction related to lifestyle changes and the need for medical follow-up. During the first 3 to 6 months following this surgery, clients may experience flu-like symptoms such as body aches, fatigue, chills, as well as dry skin, thinning and/or hair loss, and mood changes. Postoperative dietary guidelines for clients having an RYGB are presented in Client and Family Teaching 45-2.

Client and Family Teaching 45-2 Dietary Guidelines After Roux-En-Y Gastric Bypass (RYGB) Surgery

Postoperatively, clients who have had RYGB surgery have a stomach about the size of an egg. Although it will stretch some, it will never be more than the size of a cup. As time passes, some dietary restrictions will ease. When teaching the client about avoiding discomfort and complications, the nurse emphasizes the following points:

- Gradually progress to five or six small meals daily, with each feeding providing protein, fat, and complex carbohydrate. Restrict the total amount to less than one cup.
- Plan to take an hour to eat, chewing food slowly and thoroughly.
- Do not drink fluids with meals. Withhold fluids for 15 minutes before eating to 90 minutes after eating. Take fluids in sips. Drink adequate amounts of water. Avoid liquid calories, such as juice and sodas.
- Choose breads, cereals, and grains that provide less than 2 g of fiber per serving.
- Avoid commonly problematic foods such as tough, fibrous, or overcooked meats; doughy breads, pasta, rice, skins and seeds of fruits and vegetables, nuts, and popcorn.
- Avoid all sweets.
- Avoid any foods that cause discomfort. Maintain a food diary to track what causes discomfort.
- Stop eating when you feel full.

KEY POINTS

- Disorders that affect eating:
  - Anorexia—lack of appetite
  - Nausea and vomiting
  - Cancer of oral cavity and pharynx—may necessitate need for GI intubation for feedings and/or medications
- Disorders of the esophagus:
  - GERD—reflux
  - Esophageal diverticulum—pouch in the wall of esophagus
  - Hiatal hernia—can be sliding or paraesophageal
  - Cancer of the esophagus
- Gastric disorders:
  - Gastritis—inflammation of the stomach lining
  - Peptic ulcer disease
  - Cancer of the stomach
  - Extreme obesity

CRITICAL THINKING EXERCISES

1. An older adult is admitted to a health care facility because of unexplained weight loss. What assessments are appropriate?
2. A client is diagnosed with a peptic ulcer. They tell you that they had an ulcer many years ago and that they watched their diet carefully and used antacids, and eventually, the symptoms subsided. They ask if they should start doing this again. What should you advise?
3. Clients having upper abdominal surgery are more prone to pulmonary complications. What are some reasons for this?
4. A few days after a client had a gastrectomy, they ate a small meal of rice with cooked vegetables, bread, vanilla pudding, and 8 oz of juice. Shortly afterward, they complained of feeling weak, dizzy, sweaty, and very crampy. The nurse suspects dumping syndrome. What actions should the nurse take?

NCLEX-STYLE REVIEW QUESTIONS PrepU

1. The nurse is assisting a client following an episode of severe vomiting and dehydration. The client is now tolerating fluids. What food choice suggestion by the nurse is most appropriate as the client progresses with the diet?
   1. Dry toast
   2. Grilled cheese
   3. Poached egg
   4. Tomato soup

2. Which of the following actions by the nurse promotes safety for a client receiving bolus tube feedings via a nasogastric tube? Select all that apply.
   1. Administer the tube feeding within 10 minutes.
   2. After feeding, aspirate gastric contents and test the pH of the aspirate.
   3. Assess tube placement according to agency policy.
   4. Check the residual volume prior to the bolus feeding.
   5. Irrigate the nasogastric tube with 30 mL water following the bolus.

3. During a routine home visit, a client describes what the nurse believes may be symptoms related to a hiatal hernia. Which modification to the client's bed is most appropriate to recommend at this time?
   1. Consider sleeping in a waterbed temporarily.
   2. Elevate the legs on pillows when retiring at night.
   3. Place a bed board between the mattress and springs.
   4. Raise the head of the bed on 4-inch blocks.

4. The nurse implements the teaching plan on dumping syndrome for the client who has recently undergone a gastrojejunostomy. After the nurse provides information about restricting carbohydrates, which additional information should the nurse plan to teach this client to help reduce the potential for experiencing the symptoms of dumping syndrome?
   1. Lie down for a short time after eating.
   2. Meditate or relax just prior to eating.
   3. Sleep with the head of the bed elevated.
   4. Walk several times a day between meals.

5. The nurse reviews the results of diagnostic tests for a client experiencing persistent indigestion, feeling of gastric fullness, and unexplained weight loss. Which finding best suggests that the client's symptoms are related to cancer of the stomach?
   1. An elevated level of gastrin is found in the blood.
   2. Gastric irritation is noted during a gastroscopy.
   3. Gastric analysis shows the absence of hydrochloric acid.
   4. Hemoglobin and hematocrit are decreased.

WANT TO KNOW MORE? There are a wide variety of online resources available on thePoint to enhance learning and understanding of this chapter.

Go to thePoint.lww.com/activate and use the activation code found in the front of this text to unlock these online resources.

46 Caring for Clients With Disorders of the Lower Gastrointestinal Tract

Words To Know

abdominoperineal resection
appendectomy
appendicitis
colectomy
Crohn disease
diverticula
diverticulitis
diverticulosis
encopresis
fissure
fistula
fistulectomy
fistulotomy
fulminant colitis
hemorrhoidectomy
hemorrhoids
hernia
hernioplasty
herniorrhaphy
inflammatory bowel disease
intussusception
irritable bowel syndrome
melena
pancolitis
paralytic ileus
peritonitis
pilonidal sinus
segmental resection
short bowel syndrome
skip lesions
tenesmus
toxic megacolon
ulcerative colitis
ulcerative proctitis
volvulus

Learning Objectives

On completion of this chapter, you will be able to:

1. List factors that contribute to constipation and diarrhea and describe nursing management for clients with these problems.
2. Explain the symptoms of irritable bowel syndrome.
3. Contrast Crohn disease and ulcerative colitis.
4. Describe the features of appendicitis and peritonitis.
5. Describe nursing management for a client with acute abdominal inflammatory disorders.
6. Describe the nurse's role as related to care measures for the client with intestinal obstruction.
7. Differentiate diverticulosis and diverticulitis.
8. Identify factors that contribute to the formation of an abdominal hernia.
9. Discuss nursing management for a client requiring surgical repair of a hernia.
10. Describe warning signs of colorectal cancer.
11. List common problems that accompany anorectal disorders.

The lower gastrointestinal (GI) tract includes the small and large intestines from the duodenum to anus (see Fig. 44-1, p. 746). The material that moves down the lower GI tract consists of food residues, microorganisms, digestive secretions, and mucus. The mixture of these substances composes feces. Disorders of the lower GI tract usually affect the movement of feces toward the anus, absorption of water and electrolytes, and elimination of dietary wastes.

Gerontologic Considerations

■ Constipation is a common problem in older adults and often results from inadequate intake of dietary fiber, lack of exercise, and decreased fluid intake. The risk of constipation is also increased by an age-related decrease in the peristaltic action of the GI tract. Constipation can also occur in older adults who feel rushed when defecating or cannot get to the toilet in time, or as a common side effect of many medications, especially narcotic pain relievers.

■ Older adults with appendicitis may not display the type of acute pain that younger adults with the condition experience. Severe pain may be absent, minimal, or referred in the older adult, causing a delay in diagnosis and a greater incidence of complications. Additionally, the temperature may not be elevated in older adults with an infection.

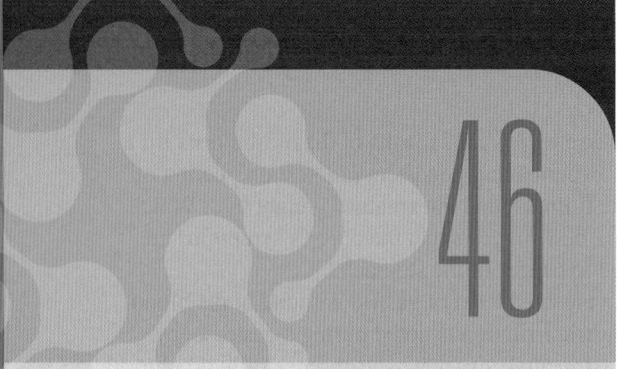

Gerontologic Considerations (*continued*)

- Regular health examination and screenings for colorectal cancer should be encouraged because of increased incidence of cancer in older adults.
- Older adults who have limited fluid or fiber intake, or who take medications with constipation as a side effect, are at higher risk of development of hemorrhoids. Careful screening for this risk includes physical assessment and assessment of knowledge.
- Older adults may take anticoagulant medication for commonly experienced chronic vascular conditions or if they are at risk of pulmonary embolism. Assessment of risk for constipation is important to prevent the development of hemorrhoids and the accompanying risk of bleeding.

ALTERED BOWEL ELIMINATION

People differ greatly in their bowel habits. Normal bowel patterns range from three bowel movements per day to three bowel movements per week. In differentiating normal from abnormal, the consistency of stools and the comfort with which a person passes them are more reliable indicators than is the frequency of bowel elimination. The type and amount of food a person consumes greatly affect stool consistency. High-fiber diets, such as those containing whole grains, fresh fruits, and uncooked vegetables, form an increased residual of cellulose, an insoluble, indigestible product, in the bowel. Cellulose absorbs water. The combination of cellulose and water increases and softens fecal volume, which speeds the passage of feces through the lower GI tract.

Diseases or disorders of the lower GI system usually manifest themselves as changes in bowel elimination. The most common problems are constipation and diarrhea. Irritable bowel syndrome (IBS) is a motility problem in which constipation and diarrhea are alternately present.

Constipation

Pathophysiology and Etiology

Constipation is a condition in which stool becomes dry, compact, and difficult and painful to pass. Fewer than three bowel movements a week for several weeks is often the defining factor for a diagnosis of chronic constipation. Normally, fecal matter collects in the rectum and presses on the internal anal sphincter, creating an urge to defecate (eliminate stool). Peristalsis and distention of the colon facilitate the signal to release stool. The gastrocolic reflex facilitates stool passage by accelerating peristalsis. This reflex is most active after eating, particularly after the first meal of the day.

A diet low in fiber predisposes people to constipation because the stools produced are small in volume and dry. The lower GI tract propels low-volume stools more slowly. Whenever stool remains stationary in the large intestine, moisture continues to be absorbed from the residue. Consequently, retention of stool, for any number of reasons, causes stool to become dry and hard.

Constipation may result from insufficient dietary fiber and water, ignoring or resisting the urge to defecate, emotional stress, use of drugs that tend to slow intestinal motility, or inactivity. It may stem from several disorders, either in the GI tract or systemically. Anatomic disorders of the colon, rectum, and anus, which predispose a person to constipation, include strictures (e.g., secondary to disease or intestinal resection), anal stenosis, and anterior displacement of the anus.

For clients with chronic constipation, the underlying cause(s) include the following:

- A partial or complete blockage in the colon or rectum
- Neurologic factors related to neuropathy or a neurologic disorder such as multiple sclerosis
- Muscular disorders that interfere with normal contraction and relaxation of the muscles in and around the pelvis
- Hormonal conditions such as diabetes may lead to constipation

To elaborate, impaired GI motility can lead to chronic constipation. Motility may be impaired in the absence of other disorders (intestinal pseudo-obstruction) or as a result of visceral myopathies, musculoskeletal disorders, neuropathy, or spinal cord lesions. Systemic disorders that predispose clients to constipation include hypothyroidism, diabetes, pheochromocytoma, porphyria, and hypercalcemia (resulting from hyperparathyroidism and excessive production of vitamin D). Constipation may also result from chronic use of laxatives ("cathartic colon") because such use can cause a loss of normal colonic motility and intestinal tone. Laxatives also dull the gastrocolic reflex. Chronic lead poisoning or concurrent medications such as opioids, tranquilizers, antidepressants, and antihypertensives may also result in constipation. Older adults are more prone to constipation because they take more drugs that can interfere with bowel elimination, have more chronic illnesses, and many have decreased mobility.

Assessment Findings

Signs and Symptoms

Bowel elimination is infrequent or irregular. Clients describe feeling bloated. The abdomen may be tympanic or distended, and bowel sounds may be hypoactive. The client experiences rectal fullness, pressure, and pain when attempting to eliminate stool. What they pass usually is hard and dry. Rectal bleeding may result as the tissue stretches and tears while the person tries to pass the hard, dry stool. When a nurse inserts a gloved and lubricated finger in the rectum, the stool may feel like small rocks, a condition referred to as *scybala*.

Sometimes, if the constipation has lasted for a long time, the client may begin passing liquid stool around an obstructive stool mass (**encopresis**), a phenomenon sometimes misinterpreted as diarrhea. The liquid stool results from dry stool stimulating nerve endings in the lower colon and rectum, which increases peristalsis. The increased peristalsis sends watery feces from higher in the bowel than the retained stool. This symptom is most common in residents of nursing homes and school-aged children who have a long-standing history of constipation, stool-withholding behavior, or both. It may be necessary to check for a fecal impaction.

Diagnostic Findings

A thorough history and physical examination are necessary to determine the underlying cause and need for further diagnostic testing. Frequently, treatment is based on findings of the history and physical examination, precluding the need for a more aggressive approach. Abdominal radiography helps determine the extent of constipation. A barium enema is performed if a structural abnormality is suspected. In *defecography*, a thick barium paste is inserted into the rectum. X-rays are taken as the client expels the barium to determine whether there are any anatomic abnormalities or problems with the muscles surrounding the anal sphincter. Anorectal motility and/or colonic motility studies may be performed to confirm a motility disorder. These studies use flexible catheters with sensors that measure the pressure of muscle contractions.

Colonic transit or marker studies are used to determine how long it takes for food to travel through the intestines. For one or more days, clients swallow capsules that contain radiographically visible plastic particles. After 5 to 7 days, X-rays are taken to determine whether any particles are left and if so, where they are. The location of the particles can help determine whether there is colonic inertia related to muscle and/or nerve impairment or pelvic floor dysfunction. Sigmoidoscopy or colonoscopy may be ordered to examine the sigmoid colon or the entire colon to determine if there are any issues.

Medical and Surgical Management

Treating the cause provides the best relief. For quick symptomatic relief, the primary provider prescribes an enema or a laxative in oral or suppository form, followed by prophylactic administration of a stool softener. Drug Therapy Table 46-1 provides information about types of laxatives that may be used to treat constipation. Fiber supplements, stimulants such as bisacodyl (Dulcolax) or senna (Senokot), lubricants, or stool softeners may be ordered. Dietary management also is promoted.

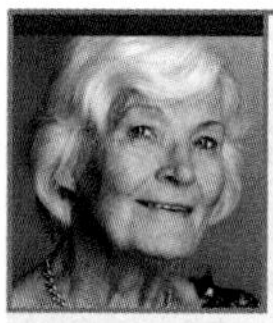

Clinical Scenario An older client is experiencing constipation. **What does the nurse need to consider when caring for this client? See the following Nursing Process section.**

NURSING PROCESS FOR THE CLIENT WITH CONSTIPATION

Assessment

Complete the assessments performed on any client with a GI disorder (see Chapter 44). Obtain a complete history as well as a drug history, including the frequency with which the client uses laxatives or enemas. In discussing bowel elimination, determine the client's definition of constipation. Some clients are unaware that a daily bowel movement is not necessarily a rigid standard for proper bowel function.

Obtain a description of the bowel elimination pattern, asking about frequency, overall appearance and consistency of stool, blood in the stool, pain, and effort necessary to pass stool.

Keep a record of the client's bowel elimination. In addition, assess dietary habits, fluid intake, and activity level. Physical examination includes the anal area, looking for fissures, redness, and hemorrhoids. Auscultate the abdomen for bowel sounds and palpate for distention and masses. Finally, inspect the stool or gently insert a lubricated, gloved finger in the anal canal to assess the characteristics of the unpassed stool.

Diagnosis, Planning, and Interventions

Major goals of nursing management are restoring normal bowel function, relieving rectal discomfort and anxiety, and helping the client understand how to maintain normal bowel function. To make these goals measurable, the nurse must add specific criteria.

When constipation is related to dietary habits, decreased fluid intake, stress, lack of exercise, or other factors, suggest a high-fiber diet that includes plenty of raw fruits and vegetables, whole-grain bread, and coarse brans and cereals (Nutrition Notes). Teach clients to drink eight or more full glasses of water and fruit juice daily to promote regularity, because fructose is a natural laxative. In addition, urge the client to schedule a time to exercise each day because such activity promotes intestinal motility.

The client must respond quickly to the urge to defecate and allow sufficient time to evacuate the bowel. Encourage the client to use the toilet at regular intervals even without the urge to defecate, particularly after meals, when the gastrocolic reflex is most active. Help the client and family understand the need for privacy during bathroom times. Instruct the client to avoid excessive straining to have a bowel movement.

Discourage self-treatment with daily or frequent enemas or laxatives. Chronic use of such products causes natural bowel function to be sluggish. In addition, laxatives containing stimulants can be habit forming, requiring continued use in increasing doses. Teach the client about the use of fiber supplements, such as those containing psyllium. Agents considered "natural" sometimes contain ingredients that lead to chronic laxative dependence. The client must discuss any medication they use for control of chronic constipation with the primary provider or nurse practitioner. If long-term treatment with stool softeners is indicated, the nurse provides a list of safe medications, such as those containing mineral oil, magnesium, or nonabsorbable sugar (i.e., sorbitol, lactulose).

NURSING PROCESS FOR THE CLIENT WITH CONSTIPATION (continued)

Constipation: Related to immobility or inadequate fluid intake as evidenced by infrequent passage of stool and abdominal distention
Expected Outcomes: Client attains a normal pattern of elimination, and stools are soft and easily passed.

- Review usual pattern of elimination. *Constipation has many possible reasons; assessing usual pattern is the first step in identifying the cause.*
- Review current medications. *Many medications affect bowel elimination.*
- Encourage client to slowly increase dietary fiber intake to 25 g/day. Bran cereals, fresh fruits and vegetables, and beans are excellent sources of insoluble fiber, which promotes normal bowel function. Remind client to add these foods gradually. *Fiber absorbs water in the colon and forms a gel, adding bulk and easing defecation. Adding fiber gradually helps to avoid bloating, gas, and diarrhea.*
- Instruct client to increase fluids to six to eight glasses per day. *This intake prevents hard, dry stools.*
- Encourage client to be out of bed, increase activity, or develop a regular exercise program. *Activity increases peristalsis and promotes bowel elimination.*
- Administer laxatives, suppositories, and enemas as ordered. *Treatments should be used only as ordered to avoid cathartic bowel.*

Acute Pain: Related to rectal distention, difficulty passing stool, or anal tears
Expected Outcome: Client will state reduced or no rectal discomfort.

- Apply lubricant in rectum and around the anus with a glove. *Lubricant provides emollient action for the passage of stool and healing of anal tears.*
- Assist client to soak rectal area in a tub of warm water. *Soaking in a warm tub relieves pain, helps to heal anal tears, and soothes rectal distention.*

Evaluation of Expected Outcomes

The client has soft, formed stool every 2 days. They report feeling more comfortable after warm soaks and application of lubricant. Refer to Nursing Guidelines 46-1 for ways to promote healthy defecation and prevent constipation.

DRUG THERAPY TABLE 46-1 Agents Used to Treat Constipation

Category and Common Generic (Brand) Drugs	Intended Use	Common Side Effects	Safety Warnings for Nurses
Bulk-Producing Laxatives			
Methylcellulose (Citrucel) Psyllium (Metamucil)	Relief of constipation, irritable bowel syndrome, severe watery diarrhea by holding fluid in stool	Diarrhea, nausea, vomiting, bloating, flatulence, cramping, perianal irritation, fainting	
Emollients			
Mineral oil	Relief of constipation, fecal impaction	Perianal discomfort and itching due to anal seepage	• Respiratory aspiration • Anal seepage
Stool Softeners/Surfactants			
Docusate (Colace)	Relief of constipation, prevention of straining during bowel movement by forming slippery coating	Diarrhea, nausea, vomiting, bloating, flatulence, cramping, perianal irritation, fainting	• Do not give if using mineral oil • Report rectal bleeding immediately
Hyperosmotic Agents			
Lactulose (Cephulac) Lubiprostone (Amitiza)	Relief of constipation, hepatic encephalopathy Chronic idiopathic constipation	Headache, nausea, diarrhea	• Syrups contain sugars, caution with diabetics

(continued)

DRUG THERAPY TABLE 46-1 Agents Used to Treat Constipation (*continued*)

Category and Common Generic (Brand) Drugs	Intended Use	Common Side Effects	Safety Warnings for Nurses
Irritant or Stimulant Laxatives			
Sennosides (Senokot) Bisacodyl (Dulcolax)	Acts directly on intestinal mucosa and alters water/electrolytes	Diarrhea, nausea, vomiting, bloating, flatulence, cramping, perianal irritation	• Chronic use may lead to dependence
Saline Laxatives and Bowel evacuants			
Milk of magnesia magnesium citrate (Fleets) Polyethylene glycol (PEG) solution (MiraLAX, Golytely)	Evacuate colon for endoscopy, relieve constipation by increasing fluid in colon	Nausea, abdominal bloating	• Not to be combined with other laxatives • Call primary provider if hives and rash emerge
Methylnaltrexone (Relistor)	Opioid-induced constipation reduced by direct inhibition of pain receptors in gut	Gastric distress, nausea, vomiting, diarrhea	• Given as daily subcutaneous injection

Nutrition Notes

The Client With Constipation

■ A *high-fiber diet* is a vague term that does not quantify or qualify fiber content. Individual tolerance and "need" for fiber vary. To achieve a high-fiber intake, most daily grain choices should be whole grains (e.g., 100% whole wheat bread, whole wheat or bran cereal, oats, brown rice, whole-wheat pasta). Clients should look for whole-grain breads that provide at least 2 g of fiber per serving and whole-grain cereals that provide at least 5 g fiber per serving. An adequate fluid intake is essential. In addition, encourage clients to

■ Consume approximately one-half cup of dried peas or beans (legumes) daily. These vegetable proteins are low-fat, high-fiber alternatives to meat. Legumes include split peas; black-eyed peas; pinto, kidney, and navy beans; and red and yellow lentils.

■ Consume plenty of fruits and vegetables daily; actual amounts recommended vary with total calories consumed. Because the skin and seeds of the fruit are especially rich in insoluble fiber, whole fruits are recommended over canned fruit or fruit juice. Likewise, minimal peeling and scraping of vegetables are encouraged. Most fruits and vegetables provide 1 to 3 g of fiber per serving.

■ Consider slowly adding coarse, unprocessed wheat bran, a natural laxative, to the diet. Start with 1 teaspoon daily and work up to 2 to 3 tablespoons daily to decrease the likelihood of flatus, distention, cramping, and diarrhea. Mix wheat bran with juice or milk; add it to muffins, quick bread, or casseroles; or sprinkle it over cereal, applesauce, or other foods.

■ Seeds and nuts (sesame, sunflower, and poppy seeds; crunchy peanut butter; popcorn) are also sources of fiber.

NURSING GUIDELINES 46-1

Strategies to Prevent Constipation

- Eat a diet that includes fruits, vegetables, and grains.
- Limit high-fat meats and dairy products.
- Limit sweets, which also can be high in fat.
- Drink fluids, especially water, and fluids that are sugar-free.
- Engage in regular physical activity, including exercises that involve toning abdominal muscles.
- Do not ignore the urge to defecate.
- Try to establish a regular time for a bowel movement; generally best within 30 minutes of a meal.

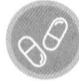

Pharmacologic Considerations

■ Opiates (pain medications) bind to nerve receptors in the bowel to decrease motility and delay transit of bowel contents. Methylnaltrexone is a drug that blocks receptors and reduces constipation due to opioid use.

Diarrhea

Pathophysiology and Etiology

Diarrhea is the frequent passage of larger-than-normal amounts of liquid or semiliquid stool (more than three bowel movements per day and over 200 g/day). It results from increased peristalsis, which moves fecal matter through the GI tract much more rapidly than normal. The swift velocity causes intestinal cramping and decreases the time available for water to be absorbed from stool in the large intestine. Consequently, the stool is either very soft or liquid.

Diarrhea can be acute or chronic. Acute episodes generally are short-lived, lasting at most 7 to 14 days. Chronic diarrhea occurs for more than 2 or 3 weeks and can persist with periods of no diarrhea and then resumption of symptoms can occur.

Three major problems associated with severe or prolonged diarrhea include dehydration, electrolyte imbalances, and vitamin deficiencies. When diarrhea results from a disease that causes malabsorption, the client is at risk of a nutritional deficiency. The sudden onset of acute abdominal pain or a rise in temperature may indicate perforation of the bowel.

Diarrhea may be related to bacterial or viral infections affecting the intestine; lactose intolerance; fructose intolerance; food allergies or intolerance; artificial sweeteners, such as sorbitol or mannitol (found in chewing gum and other artificially sweetened products); uremia; intestinal disease such as diverticulitis, ulcerative colitis, malabsorption, or intestinal obstruction; rapid addition of fiber to the diet; consumption of highly spiced or seasoned food; food poisoning, overuse of laxatives; and adverse effects of drugs, especially antibiotics or concentrated tube-feeding formulas. The most common cause is infection by bacterial, parasitic, or viral agents. The client may give a history of contacts with people who are ill in their household, foreign travel, or use of water from an impure source (e.g., lakes, streams). The client also may mention long-standing abdominal pain or diarrhea or a family history of metabolic or inflammatory disorders.

Diarrhea also may result from several metabolic disorders and diseases such as cystic fibrosis, pancreatic insufficiency, or inflammatory bowel disease (IBD). It may be caused by surgical resection of large portions of the small bowel (**short bowel syndrome**). Other causes include immunoglobulin A deficiency, overeating, concurrent medication (especially antibiotics), and IBS.

Assessment Findings

Signs and Symptoms

Stools are watery and frequent. In severe cases, blood and mucus pass with the stool. The client usually experiences urgency (**tenesmus**) and abdominal discomfort. Bowel sounds are hyperactive. Skin around the anus may become excoriated from contact with fecal matter and products of the digestive process (e.g., gastric acid, bile salts). Fever may be present. Infectious diarrhea typically has a sudden onset, with accompanying generalized malaise.

Diagnostic Findings

Routine stool cultures are obtained to identify bacterial infections as the cause for infectious diarrhea. Identifying parasites involves placing stool specimens in special preservatives for analysis of parasites and their ova by the microbiology department. Several samples may be needed because parasites are not typically shed with each stool. Routine ova and parasite analysis may identify amebic infections; however, such infections may require serologic (blood) tests.

A complete blood count (CBC) and blood chemistries may be done, depending on symptoms and if a cause of the diarrhea is not evident. A urinalysis may be done as well. Blood in the stool may be common with certain infections and disease processes. Nurses typically test stool specimens, collecting a specimen from the client (e.g., fecal occult blood test [FOBT] or guaiac smear test [gFBOT]). A proctosigmoidoscopy or colonoscopy may be performed to identify chronic inflammation or alteration in the mucosal layer of the large intestine. These studies often are carried out to identify the cause of chronic inflammation. An upper GI series with small bowel follow-through allows for radiologic examination of the small bowel and identification of inflammation. Upper GI endoscopy allows for the identification of malabsorptive disorders such as celiac disease.

Medical and Surgical Management

Treatment of diarrhea that is mild or of short duration, such as that caused by dietary changes or acute illness, involves resting the bowel by limiting intake to clear liquids for one or two meals and gradually advancing to a regular diet. When diarrhea persists and stools are frequent and large, or if the person is very young, an older adult, or debilitated, medical treatment may include one or more of the following measures:

- Administration of an antidiarrheal agent, such as diphenoxylate hydrochloride with atropine sulfate (Lomotil), loperamide hydrochloride (Imodium), or a combination product such as kaolin and pectin (Kaopectate)
- Fluid and electrolyte replacement by either the oral or intravenous (IV) route
- Dietary adjustments, which may involve eliminating foods that cause diarrhea
- Total parenteral nutrition (TPN) if diarrhea is severe and prolonged and if the introduction of oral fluid and food results in another episode of diarrhea

Chronic diarrhea depletes the bowel of helpful organisms and allows yeasts and fungi to thrive unchecked. To recolonize the bowel, capsules or granules containing *Lactobacillus acidophilus* (Bacid or Lactinex) are prescribed. These agents are referred to as *probiotics*.

Irritable Bowel Syndrome

Irritable bowel syndrome, also known as spastic bowel, is a functional motility disorder primarily affecting the colon. It refers to a cluster of symptoms that occur despite the absence of an identifiable disease process. The intestinal mucosa does not exhibit any changes. People with IBS experience abdominal pain and cramping, bloating and flatus, as well as diarrhea and/or constipation, with or without the presence of mucus. Often, either diarrhea or constipation predominates. IBS does not cause inflammation of the bowel or changes in bowel tissue, and it does not increase the risk of colorectal cancer.

It is estimated that 10% to 15% of people in the United States have IBS (International Foundation for Functional Gastrointestinal Disorders [IFFGD], 2020). Women are affected more often than men, which suggests a hormonal influence. People younger than 45 years are more likely to be diagnosed with IBS. In addition, a family history of IBS places clients at an increased risk of developing IBS.

Pathophysiology and Etiology

Fluctuating intestinal motility tends to be an underlying factor that causes symptoms. Clients with IBS have stronger and longer intestinal contractions that can cause diarrhea, or they experience just the opposite, with weaker contractions to propel digested food through the gastrointestinal tract, causing dry, hard stools and infrequent defecation.

The cause of IBS is not understood. Affected clients appear to be overly sensitive to changes in the bowel, such as the presence of food, gas, or stool. There may also be an imbalance or alteration of bacteria that are necessary for normal digestion. Other factors may also be involved, such as certain foods (different for each client), stress and anxiety, hormonal changes for women, infection or irritation, as well as disturbances in the vasculature of the bowel or metabolism.

Assessment Findings

Signs and Symptoms

Many clients experience various degrees of abdominal pain that defecation relieves. Most clients with IBS describe having chronic constipation with sporadic bouts of diarrhea. Some report the opposite pattern, although less commonly. Many clients suffer from belching and flatulence (intestinal gas). In general, symptoms do not awaken people from sleep. Some clients with IBS report anxiety, insecurity, depression, or anger.

Weight usually remains stable, indicating that when diarrhea occurs, malabsorption of nutrients does not accompany it. There often is white or yellow mucus in the stools and clients may report that they do not feel like their bowels completely empty with a bowel movement. They may also experience urgency. Blood usually is not found in the stool because the bowel is not locally inflamed.

Diagnostic Findings

There are two international sets of criteria used to diagnose IBS because diagnosis often is made by ruling out other intestinal disorders. The first is the Rome set of criteria, which includes abdominal pain for at least 3 days a month for at least 3 months, accompanied by two of the following: relief of pain with defecation, alteration in frequency of stools, and/or a change in the consistency of the stool—either harder or softer. The Manning criteria are similar. They focus on relief of pain with defecation, incomplete emptying of the bowel with each movement, the presence of mucus in the stools, and changes in stool consistency (Mayo Clinic Staff, 2020). The likelihood of IBS increases with an increase of these signs and symptoms.

Radiographic and endoscopic tests rule out other disorders with similar symptoms, such as peptic ulcer disease, colorectal cancer, diverticulitis, or IBD. Specifically, a barium enema and colonoscopy may show the spasms, distention, and mucus accumulations associated with IBS (Fig. 46-1).

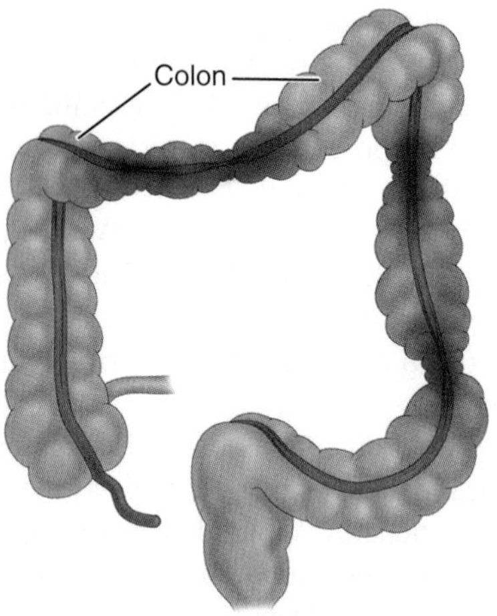

Figure 46-1 In irritable bowel syndrome, the spastic contractions of the bowel are visible in X-ray contrast studies.

Medical and Surgical Management

Dietary changes reduce flatulence and abdominal discomfort. By trial and error, the client eliminates common food sources that cause discomfort or intestinal gas, such as beans or cabbage. At the same time, a high-fiber diet (30 to 40 g/day) or a bulk-forming agent, such as products containing psyllium (e.g., Metamucil), is prescribed to regulate bowel elimination. The fiber draws water into constipated stool and adds bulk to watery stool. An anticholinergic, such as dicyclomine (Bentyl), has an antispasmodic effect if taken before meals. Either a prescription or nonprescription antidiarrheal is used for temporary relief from diarrhea. Antidepressant medications may be prescribed not only to help with depression but also to inhibit neuron activity that impacts intestinal motility.

Nursing Management

Most clients with IBS are not hospitalized. Nurses become involved in their care during diagnostic testing, follow-up visits, or hospitalization for a concurrent problem. During these encounters, the nurse gathers a comprehensive database of symptoms, helps manage the problems associated with constipation and diarrhea, explains treatments, evaluates the client's understanding of the regimen for self-care, and monitors the response to therapy. By keeping a diary where they record daily food consumption and symptoms, clients can determine what foods cause problems. Avoiding problem foods helps alleviate symptoms. Eating at regular intervals helps many clients. For clients with diarrhea, eating frequent small meals may be effective. Clients with IBS may also have the following recommendations:

- Eliminate alcohol
- Stop smoking
- Participate in stress management strategies, such as regular exercise and/or relaxation techniques
- Engage in counseling if depression or anxiety worsens

For more specific nursing interventions, refer to the preceding discussions of clients with constipation and diarrhea.

>>> *Stop, Think, and Respond 46-1*

A neighbor confides that they have IBS. They wonder if you can provide them with any tips about managing their condition. What is your best response?

INFLAMMATORY BOWEL DISEASE

Inflammatory bowel disease is a chronic illness characterized by exacerbations and remissions. The term *IBD* refers to several chronic digestive disorders believed to result from the immune system attacking the bowel. In general, IBD causes severe diarrhea with pain, weight loss, and chronic fatigue. Crohn disease and ulcerative colitis are the most common inflammatory diseases that include IBD. These two distinct disorders are grouped together because of their similar symptoms and treatments (Table 46-1). Because of the similarity in presenting symptoms and results of diagnostic procedures, differential diagnosis may be difficult. Unlike IBS, IBD does not resolve without medical intervention.

TABLE 46-1 Comparison of Crohn Disease and Ulcerative Colitis

FACTOR	CROHN DISEASE	ULCERATIVE COLITIS
Course	Prolonged, variable	Exacerbations, remissions
Pathology		
Early	Transmural thickening	Mucosal ulceration
Late	Deep, penetrating granulomas	Minute mucosal ulcerations
Clinical manifestations		
Location	Ileum, right colon (usually)	Rectum, left colon
Bleeding	Usually not, but may occur	Common—severe
Perianal involvement	Common	Rare—mild
Fistulae	Common	Rare
Rectal involvement	About 20%	Almost 100%
Diarrhea	Less severe	Severe
Diagnostic study findings		
Barium studies, video capsule endoscopy and double-balloon endoscopy, CT scan, MRI, small bowel imaging	Regional, discontinuous skip lesions ("cobblestone" appearance) Narrowing of colon Thickening of bowel wall Mucosal edema Stenosis, fistulae	Diffuse involvement No narrowing of colon No mucosal edema Stenosis is rare Shortening of colon
Flexible sigmoidoscopy	May be unremarkable unless accompanied by perianal fistulae	Abnormal inflamed mucosa
Colonoscopy	Distinct ulcerations separated by relatively normal mucosa in ascending colon	Friable mucosa with pseudopolyps or ulcers in descending colon
Therapeutic management	Corticosteroids, aminosalicylates (sulfasalazine [Azulfidine]) Antibiotics Parenteral nutrition Partial or complete colectomy, with ileostomy or anastomosis Rectum can be preserved in some clients Recurrence is common	Corticosteroids, aminosalicylates (sulfasalazine) useful in preventing recurrence Bulk hydrophilic agents Antibiotics Proctocolectomy, with ileostomy Rectum can be preserved in only a few clients "cured" by colectomy
Systemic complications	Small bowel obstruction Right-sided hydronephrosis Nephrolithiasis Cholelithiasis Arthritis Retinitis, iritis Erythema nodosum	Toxic megacolon Perforation Hemorrhage Malignant neoplasms Pyelonephritis Nephrolithiasis Cholangiocarcinoma Arthritis Retinitis, iritis Erythema nodosum

Crohn Disease

Crohn disease is also called *regional enteritis*. This chronic inflammatory condition can occur in any portion of the GI tract but predominantly affects the bowel in the terminal portion of the ileum. In general, this disease begins in adolescence or young adulthood, although it can occur in adults aged 50 or 60 years. Clients who are more prone to this disorder include those who are of Eastern European, including Jewish, descent, and those who smoke.

Pathophysiology and Etiology

Crohn disease can impact any portion of the GI tract, but it most commonly occurs in the distal ileum and less commonly in the ascending colon. The mucosa initially thickens and is edematous, with ulcers forming in the inflamed areas. The chronic inflammation in Crohn disease extends transmurally through all the layers of the bowel, but the submucosal layer is most involved. Hyperemia (increased blood supply), edema, and ulcerations characterize affected areas. Endoscopic examination shows inflamed areas alternating with healthy tissue. The inflamed areas occur randomly, a phenomenon described as **skip lesions**. The bowel is described as having a "cobblestone" appearance because of the deep ulcerations that form amid the edematous tissue in a longitudinal and transverse manner (Fig. 46-2).

Because Crohn disease is a transmural inflammatory process, inflammation can extend beyond the lining of the bowel. As a result, inflammatory channels containing blood, mucus, pus, or stool may develop. Such an inflammatory channel is called a **fistula**; two or more are referred to as *fistulae*. Fistulae may form a channel between the bowel and the skin surface (enterocutaneous fistulae). Common sites for enterocutaneous fistulae are perianal and perilabial sites. Inflammation also may extend between the bowel and other pelvic organs (e.g., vagina), between the bowel and bladder, or between loops of bowel (enterovaginal, enterovesical, and enteroenteric fistulae, respectively). Fistulae also may form between the rectum and vagina in women as evidenced by passage of stool from the vagina. Chronic inflammation in Crohn disease also may lead to scarring and stricture formation and eventual obstruction of the lumen. Transportation of the digestive products is impeded, leading to abdominal pain.

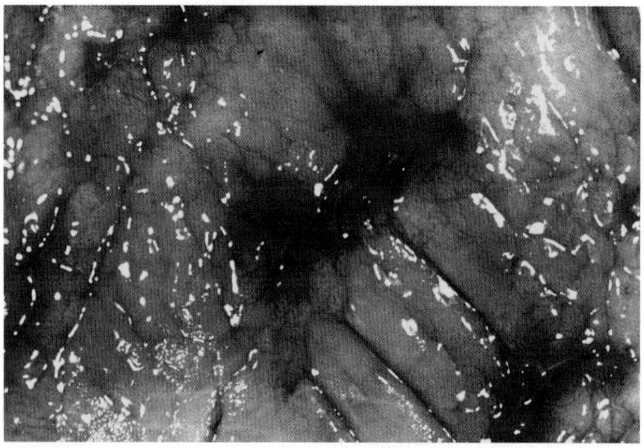

Figure 46-2 Crohn disease. Gross features include the presence of small irregular ulcers which may result from deep but discrete ulcers of the gastrointestinal mucosa. The ulcers can be longitudinal or transverse, giving the mucosa a characteristic cobblestone appearance. (Reprinted with permission from Riddell, R., & Jain, D. (2014). *Lewin, Weinstein and Riddell's gastrointestinal pathology and its clinical implications* (2nd ed.). Wolters Kluwer Health.)

The cause of Crohn disease is unknown. Because incidence is increased among family members, a genetic predisposition is presumed. Other possible contributing factors include allergic and autoimmune responses triggered by diet or infectious microbial antigens. Recurrent attacks on the tissue are believed to result from an exaggerated immune response, which explains the chronic nature of the disease. The role of stress in the development of symptoms and subsequent exacerbations is believed to be a contributing factor but not a cause of Crohn disease. As with any chronic illness, stress may influence the client's ability to cope with symptoms. This issue is certainly confused by the fact that many clients with IBD may also have IBS. Diarrhea as a response to anxiety may be confused with exacerbation of the disease.

Assessment Findings

Signs and Symptoms

Crohn disease is known for periods of remission and exacerbation. Usually, the onset is insidious, and the course of the disease varies. Most clients have abdominal pain, distention, and tenderness in the lower abdominal quadrants, especially on the right side. Pain may be associated with eating. As such, clients stop eating and fail to ingest required nutrition, resulting in weight loss. The client may have a history of chronic diarrhea and fatigue. Growth failure is a common early symptom in children and adolescents. Fever may be present. As Crohn disease progresses, anorexia, more weight loss, dehydration, and signs of nutritional deficiencies occur. Symptoms gradually increase in some clients, whereas acute exacerbations alternate with remissions in other clients. The symptoms may go into remission spontaneously.

The systemic nature of this disease is evidenced by symptoms outside the GI tract, referred to as *extraintestinal manifestations of IBD*. They include arthritis, arthralgias, skin lesions (erythema nodosum and pyoderma gangrenosum), inflammation in the eyes (uveitis, conjunctivitis, and iritis), and disorders of the liver and gallbladder. Usually, extraintestinal manifestations become quiescent when the bowel disease is under control.

During the physical examination, palpation may reveal an abdominal mass. Inspection of the perineum and perianal areas may reveal scars from previous fissures, skin tags, or evidence of fistulae or perianal abscesses.

Diagnostic Findings

An examination of stool specimens reveals *steatorrhea* or excessive fat and occult blood and white blood cells (WBCs). Stool cultures fail to disclose an etiologic microorganism or parasite. Results of blood studies indicate anemia from chronic blood loss and nutritional deficiencies. The WBC count and erythrocyte sedimentation rate may be elevated, confirming an inflammatory disorder. Serum protein and albumin levels may be low because of malnutrition. Low serum levels of the fat-soluble vitamins also reflect the client's malnourished state.

All these laboratory findings do not confirm IBD because they can be associated with several other disorders, especially acute infections. Abnormal serum electrolyte levels and a disturbed acid–base balance may accompany severe diarrhea. Serologic tests for IBD may be helpful in some cases. These tests allow for the identification of certain antibodies common to those with Crohn disease (anti-*Saccharomyces* antibodies [ASCAs]) and those with ulcerative colitis (antineutrophil cytoplasmic antibodies [ANCAs]). These tests do not confirm IBD because clients with IBD may not test positive for the antibodies, and some clients who do not have IBD may test positive. These tests may, however, serve as an important adjunct to other diagnostic tests.

Barium enema findings may show inflammation in the large intestine, but confirmation of the diagnosis requires endoscopic examination (colonoscopy or sigmoidoscopy). Endoscopic evaluation allows for identification of mucosal abnormalities (e.g., skip lesions, ulcerations, cobblestone appearance, bowel wall thickening, and presence of fistula tracts). Biopsies taken during colonoscopy or sigmoidoscopy are examined under the microscope for evidence of chronic inflammation and possible granuloma. A granuloma is an aggregate of inflammatory cells and, when identified on biopsy, confirms the diagnosis of Crohn disease. The absence of a granuloma does not rule out the diagnosis of Crohn disease.

Clients with Crohn disease are vulnerable to intestinal perforation during barium enema and endoscopy because of poor integrity of the bowel wall. They are monitored accordingly. Esophagogastroduodenoscopy (EGD) with biopsy is indicated when inflammation is suspected in the upper GI tract. A barium study of the upper GI tract is the most definitive for radiographic examination of the small intestine and identification of inflammation that endoscopy cannot evaluate. Video capsule endoscopy may be the preferred mode for examining the small bowel and reducing the risk of perforation. If further examination is needed, a double-balloon endoscopy may be performed, using a longer scope for examination of the small intestine. In addition, computed tomography (CT) scans and CT enterography (special CT scanning for the small bowel) will be done.

Medical Management

Treatment is supportive. The dietary approach varies. A high-fiber diet may be indicated when it is desirable to add bulk to loose stools. A low-fiber diet may be indicated in cases of severe inflammation or stricture. A high-calorie and high-protein diet helps replace nutritional losses from chronic diarrhea. The client may need nutritional supplements, depending on the area of the bowel affected. When the small intestine is inflamed, some clients experience lactose intolerance, requiring avoidance of lactose-rich foods.

Some clients need an elemental diet formula, such as Tolerex, Vivonex, or Peptamen, that reduces proteins, fats, and carbohydrates to an easily absorbed form. Elemental diets effectively induce remission in Crohn disease without medications. Unfortunately, clients are not allowed to eat or drink normally while on the elemental diet, making this treatment modality unacceptable for many. In addition, elemental formulas are not very palatable. Some may need to be administered through a nasogastric tube. Success with elemental diet therapy requires extensive education and client motivation. Newly introduced polymeric diets (Modulen) may provide the benefit of inducing remission and are more palatable. TPN may become necessary to provide intestinal rest. IV fluids, electrolytes, and whole blood are given to correct anemia and restore fluid and electrolyte balance.

Drug therapy involves supplementary vitamins, iron, antidiarrheal and antiperistaltic drugs to reduce peristalsis and rest the bowel, anti-inflammatory corticosteroids and 5-aminosalicylic acid (5-ASA) medications, immune-modulating agents, and antibiotics (Drug Therapy Table 46-2). Vitamin and iron supplements are used for known deficiencies and malabsorption. Antidiarrheal agents, such as diphenoxylate (Lomotil) and loperamide (Imodium), usually are used sparingly and only when clients do not have an infection. Decreasing motility in cases of infection predisposes clients with IBD to toxic megacolon, a complication that is discussed in the section on Ulcerative Colitis.

Considered first-line treatment for IBD, 5-ASA drugs contain salicylate, which is bonded to a carrying agent that allows the drug to be absorbed in the intestine. These drugs work by decreasing the inflammatory response. The 5-ASA medications include sulfasalazine (Azulfidine), olsalazine (Dipentum), and mesalamine (Asacol, Pentasa). Mesalamine also is available in enema or suppository form (Rowasa) and may be used to treat distal disease. Folic acid usually is recommended for clients taking sulfasalazine, which interferes with the absorption of this nutrient. Corticosteroids (prednisone) are used during acute exacerbations of symptoms and when 5-ASA drugs cannot control the symptoms. Hydrocortisone is available in enema form (Cortenema) and is effective in controlling distal disease without posing a high risk of systemic side effects. Long-term corticosteroid use is undesirable because of the potentially severe side effects; the dose usually is tapered and discontinued when the symptoms are in remission.

Failure to maintain remission necessitates the use of immune-modulating agents such as 6-mercaptopurine (6-MP) or azathioprine (Imuran). These agents often allow clients to discontinue corticosteroids without exacerbating symptoms. Other immune modulators are cyclosporine (Sandimmune), tacrolimus (Prograf), and methotrexate (MTX). Antibiotics such as metronidazole (Flagyl) and ciprofloxacin (Cipro) are effective adjuncts to treating Crohn disease, especially related fistulae.

Treatment of moderate to severely active and fistulizing Crohn disease includes infliximab (Remicade), which has proved safe and effective in achieving and maintaining

DRUG THERAPY TABLE 46-2 Agents for Disorders of the Lower Gastrointestinal (GI) Tract

Category and Common Generic (Brand) Drugs	Intended Use	Common Side Effects	Safety Warnings for Nurses
Antidiarrheals			
Bismuth (Pepto-Bismol)	Coats the wall of the GI tract and absorbing substances	Dry skin and mucous membranes, nausea, constipation	• Do not take bismuth if hypersensitive to aspirin
Loperamide (Imodium) Diphenoxylate w/ atropine (Lomotil) Difenoxin w/ atropine (Motofen)	Slows GI motility	Dry skin and mucous membranes, constipation	• Products containing atropine are opiate-based • Do not drive if product is opiate-based
Crofelemer (Fulyzaq)	HIV/AIDS-related diarrhea	Bronchitis	
Laxatives, Cathartics, and Bulk-Forming Agents (see Drug Therapy Table 46-1)			
Drugs Used to Treat Inflammatory Bowel Disease			
Aminosalicylates (5-ASA) Balsalazide (Colazal) Mesalamine (Pentasa) Olsalazine (Dipentum) Sulfasalazine (Azulfidine)	Ulcerative colitis by topical inhibition of inflammation of intestinal mucosa	Headache, abdominal pain, nausea	• Do not take if hypersensitive to aspirin • Monitor blood urea nitrogen (BUN) and creatinine if preexisting kidney disease • Staining of clothes and flooring when using mesalamine rectally
Anti-inflammatory Corticosteroids Prednisone, methylprednisolone (Medrol)	Ulcerative colitis by inhibiting inflammatory immune response	Acne, water retention, weight gain, hair loss, increased appetite	• With food to decrease gastric irritation • Monitor for higher blood glucose in clients with diabetes • Abrupt withdrawal may precipitate Addison disease crisis
Immune-Modulating Agents Mercaptopurine azathioprine (Imuran) Lesser-used agents, reserved when disease is unresponsive: methotrexate, cyclosporine	Ulcerative colitis by inhibiting inflammatory immune response	Increased vulnerability to infection, rash, nausea, vomiting, diarrhea	• Immune suppression makes more susceptible to infections • Frequent lab work for immune suppression • Use barrier method birth control
Biologic Agents Adalimumab (Humira) Certolizumab (Cimzia) Infliximab (Remicade) Natalizumab (Tysabri)	Ulcerative colitis, Crohn disease, rheumatoid arthritis by neutralizing immune proteins reducing inflammation	Fever, chills, headache, muscle aches, diarrhea	• Immune suppression makes more susceptible to infections • Frequent lab work for immune suppression • Owing to pancytopenia risks, special permission must be obtained for natalizumab therapy
Miscellaneous Drugs for Bowel Disorders			
Alosetron (Lotronex)	Second-line treatment of irritable bowel syndrome with severe diarrhea in women	Gastric distress, hemorrhoids, constipation	• Owing to ischemic bowel risk, special permission must be obtained for therapy
Eluxadoline (Viberzi)	Irritable bowel syndrome with diarrhea	Constipation, nausea	• Gallbladder or alcohol problems are a contraindication for use • Do not take with opiates • Monitor for acute abdominal pain, may indicate pancreatitis
Linaclotide (Linzess)	Chronic idiopathic constipation, irritable bowel syndrome with constipation	Diarrhea	• Do not use under 17 years of age • Monitor for dehydration

remission in many clients with Crohn disease. Infliximab is an antibody that interferes with the inflammatory process early in the immune response by inhibiting tumor necrosis factor (TNF). Adalimumab (Humira) is a similar medication used in clients for whom infliximab has not been effective. Clients learn to self-administer adalimumab by subcutaneous injection every other week. The potentially serious risk of infection, including tuberculosis, is associated with its use. Certolizumab pegol (Cimzia) also inhibits TNF. Injections are given every other week initially and then monthly if the medication is effective. Certolizumab poses a risk of infection because of its effect on the immune system.

Surgical Management

Surgical treatment is reserved for complications such as intestinal obstruction, perforation, or fistula formation. The need for surgical intervention is common in Crohn disease. In fact, more than 75% of clients with Crohn disease require surgery within 20 years of the onset of symptoms, and 90% require surgery within 30 years. Unlike surgical treatment for ulcerative colitis, removing the inflamed portion of the intestine does not alter disease progression or recurrence. Many clients who undergo surgery for Crohn disease require additional surgery within a few years. An intestinal transplant, a new approach to surgical intervention for clients with severe Crohn disease, may be performed on clients who have lost intestinal function. The procedure does not provide a cure but does improve the client's quality of life.

Surgical removal of a large amount of intestine results in the loss of absorptive surface, called short bowel syndrome. Massive bowel resection results in dependence on TPN, possibly for life. Removal of the colon requires a permanent ileostomy because the disease tends to recur in any rectal pouch. Ileostomy is discussed in Chapter 48.

Nursing Management

A health history assists in determining the onset, duration, and nature of the client's GI problems. Medical, drug, allergy, and diet histories also are important. Nursing care focuses on monitoring the client for complications, managing fluid and nutrition replacement, supporting the client emotionally, and teaching about diet and medications.

The nurse determines the average number of stools the client passes each day and their appearance. Providing regular skin care to avoid breakdown is essential. In addition, the nurse asks the client about weight loss and whether any foods increase the frequency of bowel movements or cause discomfort. The client requires assistance to maintain adequate nutritional intake. The nurse monitors the client's intake and collaborates with the dietitian to replace uneaten food with something more acceptable.

Physical examination includes auscultating and lightly palpating the abdomen and inspecting the rectal area. The nurse takes vital signs, weighs the client, and measures and documents intake and output. Advising the client to report whenever a bowel movement occurs is important so it can be inspected and a sample sent to the laboratory for occult blood and other analyses.

ULCERATIVE COLITIS

In **ulcerative colitis**, the chronic inflammation usually is limited to the mucosal and submucosal layers of the colon and rectum. The inflammation causes small ulcers to form that produce mucus and pus and result in bleeding (Fig. 46-3). The disease is most common in young and middle-aged adults but can occur at any age. Some clients experience prolonged remission, whereas others experience mild-to-severe (and potentially life-threatening) exacerbations of symptoms.

Pathophysiology and Etiology

Although the exact cause is unknown, some believe that multiple factors trigger ulcerative colitis, including genetic predisposition, infection, allergy, and abnormal immune response. The connection between the disease and a malfunction of the immune system is supported by the fact that clients with ulcerative colitis often have other coexisting immune-related disorders such as ankylosing spondylitis and other extraintestinal manifestations.

Inflammation usually begins in the rectum and extends proximally and continuously. As a rule, no healthy tissue appears between inflamed areas, as in Crohn disease. When inflammation remains confined to the most distal area of the large intestine, the client has **ulcerative proctitis**. When inflammation extends beyond the sigmoid colon, the client has ulcerative colitis. **Pancolitis** occurs when a client's entire colon is affected with ulcerative colitis, and they experience severe bouts of bloody diarrhea, pain, cramps, fatigue, and

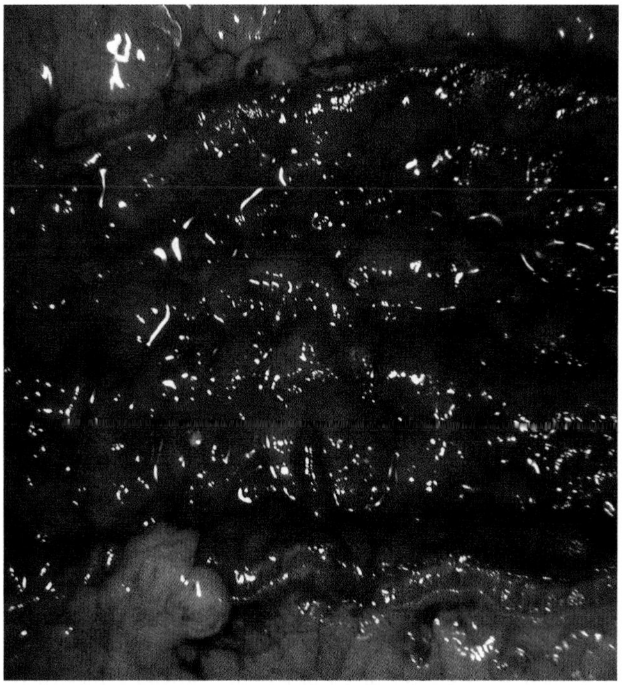

Figure 46-3 Ulcerative colitis. Longitudinal furrows of denuded mucosa alternate with islands of heaped-up mucosa, demonstrating how loss of mucosal integrity contributes to fluid and electrolyte depletion. (Reprinted with permission from Corman, M. L. (2013). *Corman's colon and rectal surgery* (6th ed.). Wolters Kluwer Health/Lippincott Williams & Wilkins.)

weight loss. **Fulminant colitis**, also affecting the entire colon, is a progression of severity of the ulcerations, with severe pain, copious diarrhea, and potential dehydration and shock.

The lining of the colon tends to bleed easily in ulcerative colitis. Ulceration may extend to the muscular layer of the bowel wall. Superficial abscesses form in depressions in the mucosa. Poor integrity of the bowel wall may lead to **toxic megacolon**, a complication in which the colon dilates and becomes atonic (lacks motility). The thin bowel wall is vulnerable to perforation under these conditions, leading to peritonitis, septicemia, and the need for emergency surgical repair.

Assessment Findings

Signs and Symptoms

The onset of the disease usually is abrupt. Clients experience severe diarrhea and expel blood, pus, and mucus along with fecal matter. Cramps and abdominal pain in the left lower quadrant (LLQ) accompany diarrhea. Eating precipitates cramping and diarrhea, resulting in anorexia, dehydration, and fatigue. Clients usually experience weight loss. The urge to defecate may come so suddenly and with such urgency that the client is incontinent. Some clients experience such incontinence during sleep. Despite intense tenesmus, clients may expel very little stool, or they may have 10 to 20 stools/day. This disease is usually marked by exacerbations and remissions.

Diagnostic Findings

Laboratory findings are similar to those described in the section on Crohn Disease. Barium enema reveals evidence of inflammation. Definitive diagnosis requires proctosigmoidoscopy or colonoscopy with biopsy. Endoscopic examination and biopsy of the lining of the colon reveal characteristic inflammatory lesions. Biopsies of the intestinal mucosa reveal evidence of chronic inflammation. These diagnostic studies usually are withheld in cases of toxic megacolon because of the high risk of perforation. Typical preparation for these procedures often is modified because clients cannot tolerate cathartics, which can lead to exacerbation of ulcerative colitis. Instead, clients have a clear liquid diet before the procedure and a gentle tap water enema on the day of the examination.

Medical and Surgical Management

Medical treatment aims toward achieving and maintaining remission. The diet is kept as normal as possible but modified to increase caloric and nutritional content. The client is instructed temporarily to refrain from eating foods associated with discomfort. If all foods cause discomfort, the symptoms are likely from the disease itself and not food. The client may be given TPN and intermittent lipid infusions to rest the bowel completely. The use of an elemental diet, as described with Crohn disease, has not proved effective in ulcerative colitis.

Blood transfusions and iron are given to correct anemia. The client also may need parenteral fluids and electrolytes. Because frequent bowel movements interfere with the absorption of nutrients, supplementary vitamins are prescribed.

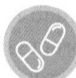

Pharmacologic Considerations

- Prevent accidental parenteral administration by always using oral syringes to prepare an enteral medication.

Medications used to treat Crohn disease also are used to treat ulcerative colitis (see section on Crohn Disease and Drug Therapy Table 46-2). Corticosteroids, given orally, intravenously, or rectally, are used if the disease does not respond to other measures. Because of unacceptable side effects associated with long-term use of corticosteroids, the dose is tapered and discontinued according to the client's response. When tapering corticosteroids without exacerbating the disease becomes impossible, immunomodulating agents (azathioprine, 6-MP) are used to decrease the immune response and allow tapering. The goals of therapy are to induce and retain remission, allowing the client to be as healthy as possible when contemplating elective surgery, or both.

Surgery is necessary when the disease does not respond to medical treatment or with complications such as dysplastic tissue (a precancerous condition), perforated colon, or hemorrhage. Removal of the colon under elective, nonemergent circumstances offers the client the best possible outcome and is the definitive cure. The current standard treatment is ileoanal pull-through and anastomosis (see Chapter 48). This procedure typically is performed in two stages, several weeks apart. In the first stage, the colon is removed, and a rectal "pouch" is created from a section of the ileum. The rectal mucosa is removed to create a temporary ileostomy. In the second stage, the surgeon closes the ileostomy and connects the intestine to the rectum, allowing the client to defecate normally. When an emergency **colectomy** is performed (i.e., partial or complete surgical removal of the colon for toxic megacolon or perforation), an anastomosis (rejoining of the bowel) may be impossible, necessitating creation of a permanent ileostomy.

Nursing Management

The nurse obtains a health history to identify the nature of the abdominal pain, number and frequency of stools, anorexia, and weight loss. They ask the client about dietary patterns, including daily amounts of alcohol and caffeine. The nurse auscultates the abdomen for bowel sounds and their characteristics and palpates the abdomen to determine any pain or tenderness.

The nurse compiles a comprehensive database and conducts frequent focused assessments to identify early changes in the symptoms, which may herald rapidly progressing complications. Until the disease is confirmed, preparing clients for diagnostic tests is necessary. The nurse needs to question radiographic and endoscopic protocols for harsh laxatives and cleansing enemas when the client is experiencing severe diarrhea because bowel irritation and stimulation tend to aggravate the client's symptoms.

Client and Family Teaching 46-1 Inflammatory Bowel Disease

The nurse should include the following topics when teaching the client and family about IBD:

- Comply with special dietary modifications and understand that compliance with these is important.
- Know the name, purpose, dosage, and adverse effects of prescribed drugs.
- Use medications to control symptoms rather than cure the disease.
- Keep all follow-up primary provider and laboratory appointments so that potentially dangerous complications of the disease and side effects of medications can be monitored.
- Use proper techniques for rectal hygiene and skin care.
- Know signs to report immediately to the primary provider such as more frequent bowel movements, extreme fatigue, severe abdominal pain, visible blood in the stool, adverse drug effects, or weight loss.
- Have regular medical checkups, even when symptoms subside, because clients with ulcerative colitis have an increased risk for the development of colon cancer.

Once the diagnosis is confirmed, the primary provider orders drug and fluid therapy. If antispasmodics and opiates are prescribed, the nurse must exercise great caution when administering them because they may trigger the development of toxic megacolon. The nurse reports any sudden onset of abdominal distention, severe pain, or fever in a client with acute ulcerative colitis. In addition, they observe the client receiving steroids for subtle changes because these drugs mask inflammatory symptoms accompanying complications. The dosage and frequency of steroids gradually are tapered when clients no longer need them. As soon as the client is well enough to learn, the nurse provides information about the disease and teaches measures for self-care (Client and Family Teaching 46-1).

Clients who are discharged and need high levels of care, such as enteral feedings or TPN, require extensive teaching specific to their home care needs. Central venous catheter care and maintenance of TPN are a few examples of these special learning needs. The nurse thoroughly covers all technical procedures for the client or significant other to perform and allows time for the client or caregiver to perform them with nursing supervision before discharge. The nurse makes a referral to a home care agency to provide continuity of care and to ease the transition from acute care to home care.

ACUTE ABDOMINAL INFLAMMATORY DISORDERS

Appendicitis and peritonitis are among disorders known as *acute abdominal inflammatory disorders*.

Appendicitis

Appendicitis is inflammation of a narrow, blind protrusion called the *vermiform appendix* located at the tip of the cecum just below the ileocecal valve in the right lower quadrant (RLQ) of the abdomen. Appendicitis can occur at any age but is most common in adolescents and young adults. It is difficult to diagnose at its onset because the initial symptoms resemble a host of other disorders such as gastroenteritis, Crohn disease, ovarian cyst, tubal pregnancy, and inflammation of the kidney or ureter.

Pathophysiology and Etiology

Like other parts of the bowel, the appendix fills with food and empties digested material regularly. Its location and shape contribute to the inefficiency of this process. The inflammation begins when the opening of the appendix narrows or becomes obstructed (Fig. 46-4). The obstruction may result from a hard mass of feces, called a *fecalith*; a foreign body; local edema; or a tumor. The blockage interferes

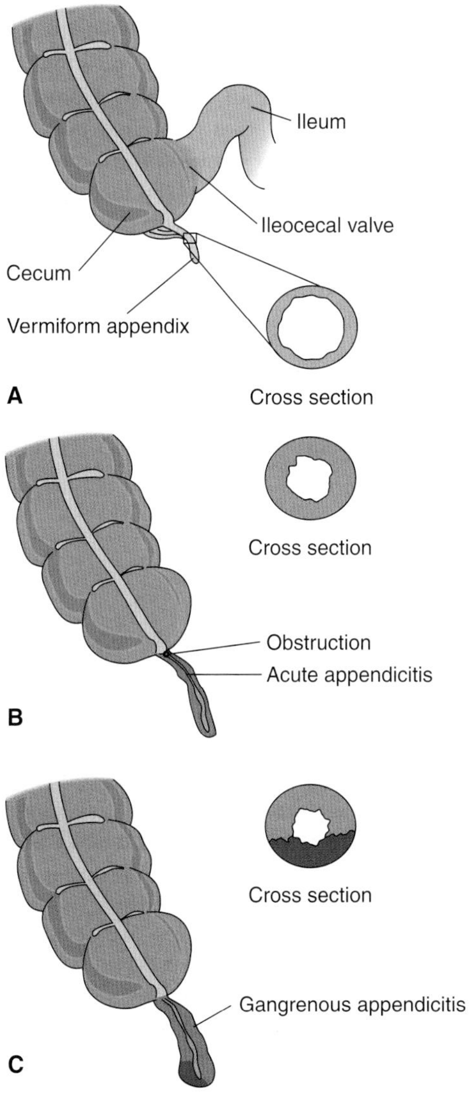

Figure 46-4 **(A)** Normal appendix. **(B)** Acute appendicitis resulting from obstruction (note the narrowing in the cross-section). **(C)** Appendicitis and gangrene.

with the drainage of secretions from the appendix, and they accumulate in the confined space. The appendix enlarges and distends, and the swelling compresses surrounding blood vessels. The locally damaged cells are then easily infected with bacteria from within the intestinal lumen. Unless the inflammation resolves, the appendix can become gangrenous or it ruptures, spilling bacteria throughout the peritoneal cavity.

Assessment Findings

An attack of abdominal pain is the most frequent symptom. At first, the pain is generalized throughout the abdomen or around the umbilicus. Later, the pain localizes in the RLQ at McBurney point, an area midway between the umbilicus and the right iliac crest. Often, the pain is worse when manual pressure near the region is suddenly released, a condition called *rebound tenderness*. When an examiner deeply palpates the left lower abdominal quadrant and the client feels pain in the RLQ, this is referred to as a *positive Rovsing sign* and suggests acute appendicitis. Low-grade fever, nausea, and vomiting may be present. The abdomen is tense, and the client usually flexes the right hip to relieve the discomfort. The position of the appendix influences the type of pain. For example, clients may have pain with defecation if the appendix is against the rectum. If the appendix circles toward the cecum, clients may complain of lumbar pain and tenderness. Clients can have pain with urination if the tip is pressing near the bladder or a ureter. Box 46-1 describes precautions to follow when a client may have appendicitis.

If the appendix perforates, clients experience more diffuse abdominal pain. The abdomen appears distended secondary to a **paralytic ileus** (intestine lacks peristalsis). Perforation generally occurs 24 hours following the onset of abdominal pain. Clients have a fever of 37.7°C (100°F) or higher and are very ill.

Concept Mastery Alert

Rovsing Sign

When assessing a client with appendicitis, the nurse should palpate the LLQ to elicit a Rovsing sign. This causes pain to be felt in the RLQ.

BOX 46-1 Precautions When Assessing a Client for Appendicitis

- Avoid multiple or frequent palpation of the abdomen—there is danger of causing the appendix to rupture.
- Perform the test for rebound tenderness at the end of the examination. A positive response causes pain and muscle spasm and makes it difficult to complete the rest of the assessment.
- Do not administer laxatives or enemas to a client who is experiencing fever, nausea, and abdominal pain, even though the client may complain of feeling constipated. Laxatives and cathartics may cause the appendix to rupture.

A WBC count can be elevated, revealing moderate leukocytosis. When a differential count of leukocytes is performed, it shows an ever-increasing number of immature neutrophils, indicating a progressive worsening of the inflammatory condition. A CT scan or abdominal ultrasound shows enlargement at the cecum.

Medical and Surgical Management

Antibiotics are given, and the client is restricted from eating or drinking while a decision is made about surgery. IV fluids are prescribed to meet the client's fluid needs. Analgesics may be withheld initially to avoid masking symptoms that may affect the diagnosis. If symptoms worsen, the surgeon performs an **appendectomy**, either via several small laparoscopic incisions or as an open incision procedure to remove the appendix before it spontaneously ruptures. The appendix has no known function in the body. Its removal results in cure with no physiologic changes. If the appendix perforates or ruptures, an abscess or peritonitis can develop. Open appendectomy will then be performed to allow for a thorough cleaning of the abdominal cavity. Some complications may occur, which can include wound infection or abscess formation at the site where the appendix was removed or at the site of the surgical incision(s). Rarely are there any issues with an ileus or peritonitis (see next section), but with any abdominal surgery this is a potential risk.

Nursing Management

The nurse assesses vital signs and the client's pain to detect early changes in the symptoms. If ordered, the nurse administers IV fluid therapy and observes the client's response to antibiotics. When analgesics are withheld, the nurse is empathetic and facilitates comfort with positioning, imagery, and distraction.

When surgery is indicated, preparing the client quickly is important to avoid delay that may cause surgical complications. Soon after surgery, if no complications occur, the client ambulates and tries light nourishment. Convalescence may be rapid, although postoperative progress depends on the client's age, general physical condition, and extent of complications. A healthy young adult usually can return to normal activities soon. Clients need to avoid heavy lifting or unusual exertion, however, for several months. For more specific nursing interventions when caring for a client undergoing surgery, see Chapter 14.

>>> *Stop, Think, and Respond 46-2*

An older adult client presents with vague symptoms of lower abdominal pain, nausea, and one episode of vomiting. In the initial assessment, what is an important question to ask?

Peritonitis

Pathophysiology and Etiology

In **peritonitis**, the peritoneum, a serous sac lining the abdominal cavity, becomes inflamed. Peritonitis may be caused

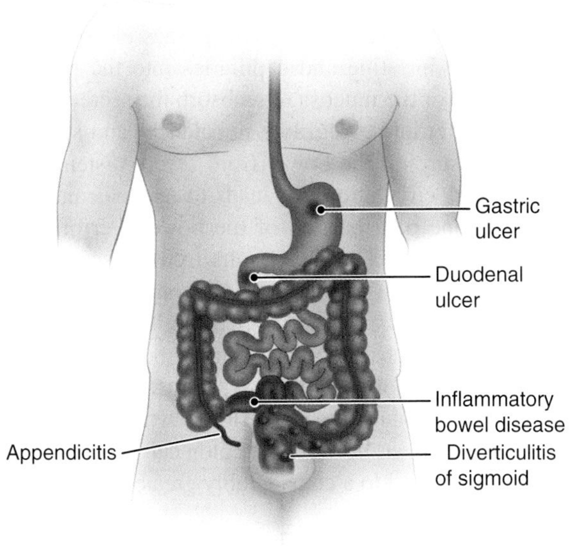

Figure 46-5 Common causes of peritonitis.

by perforation of a peptic ulcer, the bowel, or the appendix; abdominal trauma, such as gunshot or knife wounds; IBD; ruptured ectopic pregnancy; or infection introduced during peritoneal dialysis, a procedure used to treat kidney failure. Figure 46-5 illustrates common causes of peritonitis.

Spillage of chemical contents and bacteria inflames the peritoneum, which leads to localized abscess formation or generalized inflammation. The intestinal tract initially responds with hypermotility, but eventually *paralytic ileus* ensues, with air and fluid trapped in the bowel. The proliferation of bacteria leads to tissue edema and leakage of fluid. Fluid in the abdominal cavity has increasing amounts of bacteria, protein, blood, cellular debris, and WBCs. As generalized peritonitis occurs, vascular fluid shifts to the abdomen, lowering blood pressure (BP) and producing hypovolemic shock or septic shock. If the condition is not treated promptly or adequately, death may follow.

Assessment Findings

Signs and Symptoms

Symptoms include severe abdominal pain, distention, tenderness, nausea and vomiting, anorexia, and diarrhea initially, followed by inability to pass stool or gas. Fever may be absent initially, but the temperature rises as infection becomes established. The client avoids moving the abdomen when breathing because movement increases pain. They may draw the knees up toward the abdomen to lessen the pain. Lack of bowel motility typically accompanies peritonitis. The abdomen feels rigid and boardlike as it distends with gas and intestinal contents. Bowel sounds typically are absent. The pulse rate is elevated, and respirations are rapid and shallow. If the peritonitis is unresolved, severe weakness, hypotension, and a drop in body temperature occur as the client nears death.

Diagnostic Findings

The results of a WBC count show marked leukocytosis. Abdominal X-rays reveal free air and fluid in the peritoneum. A CT scan or ultrasonography identifies structural changes in abdominal organs. Cultures of peritoneal fluid and blood usually reveal bacteria such as *Escherichia coli*, *Klebsiella*, *Proteus*, and *Pseudomonas*. If untreated, clients develop sepsis and septic shock, which, if untreated, can lead to death.

Medical and Surgical Management

A nasogastric tube is used to relieve abdominal distention by suctioning the accumulated gas and stagnant upper GI fluids. IV fluids and electrolytes replace substances relocated in the peritoneal cavity and lost through vomiting and drainage from gastric intubation. Large doses of antibiotics are prescribed to combat infection. Analgesics such as fentanyl or IV morphine sulfate are ordered to relieve pain and promote rest. Antiemetics are prescribed for nausea and vomiting. The perforation is surgically closed so that intestinal contents can no longer escape.

Nursing Management

The nurse monitors the acutely ill client while completing preparations for diagnostic tests or surgery. They administer analgesics and infuses IV fluids with secondary administrations of antibiotics. If ordered, a nurse passes a nasogastric tube and connects it to suction (see Chapter 45). The client may need a urinary retention catheter. The nurse assesses the circulatory status by taking vital signs frequently and monitoring central venous and pulmonary artery pressures.

For the client who has had surgery, the nurse assesses the client's vital signs, fluid balance, incision, dressing, and drains. Assessing the client's pain level is important, as is medicating according to the medical orders. For clients who have prolonged recovery time, TPN may be initiated.

Clients are fearful of the emergent nature of the peritonitis and subsequent surgery. The nurse provides frequent explanations and emotional support. Clients also need monitoring for continued abdominal infection. If the client experiences abdominal distention, fever, changes in level of consciousness, or deviations in vital signs, the nurse must notify the primary provider quickly. Refer to Chapter 14 for further management of the postoperative client.

INTESTINAL OBSTRUCTION

Intestinal obstruction occurs when a blockage interferes with the normal progression of intestinal contents through the intestinal tract. Obstruction is more common in the small intestine than in other parts of the tract. Obstruction in the large intestine generally occurs in the sigmoid colon. The causes are classified as mechanical or functional (adynamic or lacking peristalsis; also called *paralytic ileus* or *pseudo-obstruction*) and as partial or complete. The severity depends on the region of the bowel affected, degree to which the lumen is obstructed, and degree to which blood circulation to the intestine is impeded. An intestinal obstruction is extremely dangerous and may be fatal if not treated promptly.

Pathophysiology and Etiology

Mechanical obstructions result from a narrowing of the bowel lumen with or without a space-occupying mass. A mass may include a tumor, *adhesions* (fibrous bands that constrict tissue), incarcerated or strangulated hernias, **volvulus** (kinking of a portion of intestine), **intussusception** (telescoping of one part of the intestine into an adjacent part), or impacted feces or barium (Table 46-2).

In functional obstruction, the intestine can become adynamic from an absence of normal nerve stimulation to intestinal muscle fibers. Paralytic ileus is common 12 to 36 hours after abdominal surgery. It also can result from inflammatory conditions (e.g., peritonitis), electrolyte disturbances (e.g., hypokalemia), or adverse drug effects (e.g., narcotics, cholinergic blockers). Even a vascular embolus or low blood flow during shock can interfere with the neuromuscular function of the bowel.

When the intestinal contents cannot move freely, the portion above the obstruction distends, whereas the portion below the obstruction is empty. If the obstruction is complete, no gases or feces are expelled rectally. Both forward and reverse peristalses become forceful in an attempt to clear the obstruction. Stasis of the accumulating volume and the violent muscular peristaltic contractions potentiate the risk of intestinal rupture.

Locally, the increased pressure pushes electrolyte-rich fluid from the intestine and capillaries into the peritoneal cavity. Failure of the mucosa to reabsorb the secretions contributes to water and electrolyte imbalances and shock. Increasing pressure on the bowel from severe distention and edema impairs circulation and leads to necrosis and, eventually, gangrene of a portion of the bowel. Perforation of the gangrenous bowel, which results from pressure against weakened tissue, causes the intestinal contents to seep into the peritoneal cavity, resulting in peritonitis.

Small bowel obstruction and large bowel obstruction are similar in terms of development and resulting pathophysiology. Dehydration occurs more slowly with large intestine obstruction, however, because the colon can absorb the fluid contents and distend to a considerably greater size.

Assessment Findings

Signs and Symptoms

Nausea and abdominal distention are common. When an obstruction occurs high in the GI tract, the client usually vomits whatever contents are in the stomach and small intestine. The

TABLE 46-2 Mechanical Causes of Obstruction

CAUSE AND COURSE OF EVENTS	APPEARANCE
Adhesions: Loops of intestine adhere to areas that heal slowly or scar after abdominal surgery. The adhesions cause the intestinal loop to kink 3–4 days later.	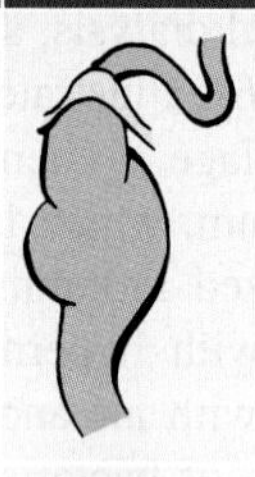
Intussusception: One part of the intestine slips into another lower part (like a telescope shortening). The intestinal lumen narrows.	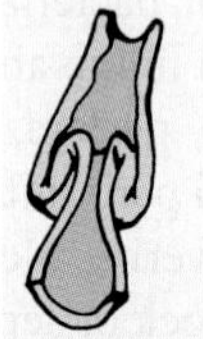
Volvulus: The bowel twists and turns on itself, obstructing the intestinal lumen. Gas and fluid accumulate in the trapped bowel.	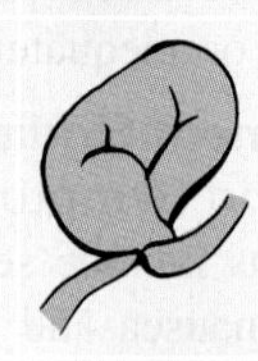
Hernia: The intestine protrudes through a weakened area in the abdominal muscle or wall. Intestinal flow and blood flow to the area may be completely obstructed.	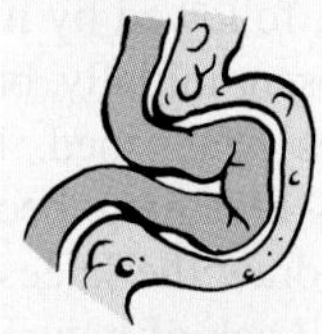
Tumor: A tumor in the intestinal wall extends into the intestinal lumen; or a tumor outside the intestine causes pressure on the intestinal wall. The lumen becomes partially obstructed; if the tumor is not removed, complete obstruction results.	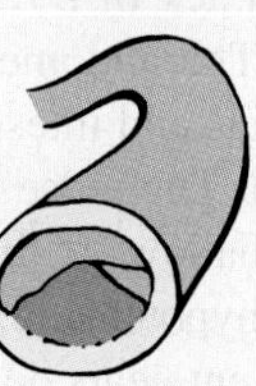

emesis appears to contain bile or fecal material. If the obstruction is lower in the GI tract, vomiting may occur later or not at all. The client may have one or two bowel movements soon after the intestine has been obstructed because they are expelling material already past the obstruction. The client may experience severe intermittent abdominal cramps. Sudden, sustained pain; abdominal distention; and fever are symptoms of perforation.

In a functional obstruction, peristalsis is absent; therefore, bowel sounds are not heard. In a mechanical obstruction, the bowel sounds usually are high-pitched above the obstructed area. Pulse and respiratory rates are elevated. BP falls, and urine output decreases if shock develops.

Clinical symptoms associated with large bowel obstruction occur more slowly. Constipation may be the only symptom for many days. Eventually, the client experiences abdominal distention. It is possible to see loops of bowel outlined through the abdominal wall, and the client complains of lower abdominal cramps and pain. Fecal vomiting also may occur. The client can have symptoms of shock.

Diagnostic Findings

A radiographic study of the abdomen shows air and fluid collecting in a segment of the intestine. A barium enema (used when the risk of perforation is low) pinpoints the location of the obstruction. CT scans are done to better visualize the obstruction. Tests of serum electrolytes may indicate low levels of sodium, potassium, and chloride. Metabolic alkalosis is evidenced by arterial blood gas results. CBC shows an increased WBC count in instances of infection. The hematocrit level is elevated if dehydration develops.

Medical and Surgical Management

While diagnostic tests are performed to determine the cause and appropriate treatment for the client's obstruction, the client receives medical support. The client receives nothing by mouth (NPO). IV fluids with electrolytes are administered to correct fluid and electrolyte imbalances, and antibiotics are ordered to treat the infection.

To relieve intestinal distention, cramping, and vomiting and to reduce the potential for intestinal rupture with peritonitis, intestinal decompression is begun. Intestinal decompression is accomplished by suctioning large amounts of accumulated secretions and gas through a nasogastric tube or longer intestinal tube, which may or may not be weighted. Nasogastric tubes are used when the obstruction is partial or located high in the small intestine.

Before surgery, decompression alone may be sufficient to relieve a functional obstruction or symptoms in clients who are undergoing surgery for mechanical obstruction. In some cases, mechanical obstructions are treated during colonoscopy by removing obstructing polyps or destroying benign tumors with laser therapy or electrocautery. Most mechanical obstructions, however, require surgery. Usually, a section of the obstructed bowel is removed and then the proximal and distal sections are reconnected (bowel resection and anastomosis). In some cases, a temporary or permanent ostomy (see Chapter 48) may be performed.

Nursing Management

In addition to the assessments performed on the client with a GI disorder, the nurse obtains complete medical, drug, and allergy histories; assesses fluid intake and output; and takes vital signs. Documenting all symptoms and obtaining detailed information about each is important. For example, if vomiting has occurred, the nurse gathers information regarding its onset, amount, and color. If an intestinal tube has been inserted, the nurse monitors its progress (Nursing Guidelines 46-2).

The care of a client with an intestinal obstruction involves managing pain, maintaining fluid balance to prevent deficits related to fluid shifts and losses from vomiting, and helping the client deal with fear related to severe, possibly life-threatening symptoms and an unstable condition. The nurse also manages pain by maintaining the patency of the decompression tube and administering a prescribed narcotic analgesic as long as BP and respiratory rate indicate that doing so is safe. The nurse maintains uninterrupted infusion of IV fluids and shortens the siege of vomiting by maintaining intestinal decompression, even though intestinal fluid is lost in the suctioning. It is crucial to monitor urinary output hourly and to report output below 50 mL per hour, a finding that may indicate that the client is going into shock.

DIVERTICULAR DISORDERS

Diverticula are sacs or pouches caused by herniation of the mucosa through a weakened portion of the muscular coat of the intestine or other structure (Fig. 46-6). They can appear anywhere in the GI tract, but they appear most commonly in the colon, especially the sigmoid area, in people older than 50 years.

Diverticulosis and Diverticulitis

Asymptomatic diverticula are called **diverticulosis**. When the diverticula become inflamed, the term **diverticulitis** is used.

Pathophysiology and Etiology

The incidence of diverticula is higher in people who have a low intake of dietary fiber. There also may be a congenital predisposition. It is thought that most diverticula result from weakness in the muscular coat associated with aging. Other factors that contribute to the formation of diverticula include obesity, lack of exercise, smoking, and certain medications such as steroids, opiates, and nonsteroidal anti-inflammatories.

Diverticula become inflamed when fecal material is trapped in one or more blind pouches. The inflammation causes swelling of the tissue in the area. If the localized swelling involves several diverticula in one area, the edema may be severe enough to cause an intestinal obstruction. Abscesses form when the inflamed tissue becomes infected with intestinal bacteria present in the bowel. The swollen tissue has the potential to rupture into the peritoneal cavity or form a fistular connection with an adjacent organ such as the bladder.

NURSING GUIDELINES 46-2

Managing the Care of Client With an Intestinal Tube

Preparations

- Auscultate and examine the abdomen for bowel sounds, distention, and tenderness.
- To provide a baseline for reference, measure abdominal girth, placing a measuring tape about the largest diameter of the abdomen.
- Mark the measuring location on the skin (with an indelible marker) to facilitate consistency when obtaining future comparison measurements.
- Assemble all the equipment the primary provider will need. If a weighted double-lumen tube is selected, label the tip of the adapter leading to the lumen through which tungsten gel is instilled to avoid confusing which lumen to use for suction.

Tube Advancement

- After the primary provider inserts the tube, ambulate the client, if possible, to facilitate tube passage through the pylorus. When a radiographic image indicates that the tube has advanced beyond the stomach, position the client as follows:
- On the right side for 2 hours, then
- On the back in a Fowler position for 2 hours, then
- On the left side for 2 hours.
- Observe the lines or numbers on the tube periodically to evaluate the tube's progressive movement and approximate anatomic location.
- Advance the tube several inches at specified intervals as directed to avoid tension as it descends into the intestine.
- Stabilize or tape the tube to the nose after a radiographic image verifies that the tube has reached the obstruction. Coil the excess length, securing it to the client's hospital gown.
- Attach the proximal end to suction.
- Prepare for radiography to be performed daily to evaluate progress toward relieving the obstruction.

Removal

- Remove the tube once the obstruction is relieved or another treatment replaces intubation.
- Disconnect the tube from suction.
- If removing a weighted tube, withdraw the tungsten gel by aspirating it with a 10-mL syringe. Remove the tungsten gel in the other types of tubes after the tube is withdrawn.
- Withdraw 6 to 10 inches of the tube between 10-minute pauses. When the tube is in the esophagus, as determined by 18 inches of length remaining in the client, flush the tube with a small amount of air to remove debris.
- Clamp the tube to prevent secretions from being deposited in the client's upper airway and instruct the client to hold the breath while the tube exits the esophagus.
- If removing a Cantor-like or Harris-like tube, grasp the bag of tungsten gel with forceps and withdraw it from the client's mouth when it reaches the oropharynx.
- Once the tungsten gel is removed from the bag, remove the tube from the client's nose. Provide nasal and oral hygiene immediately afterward.

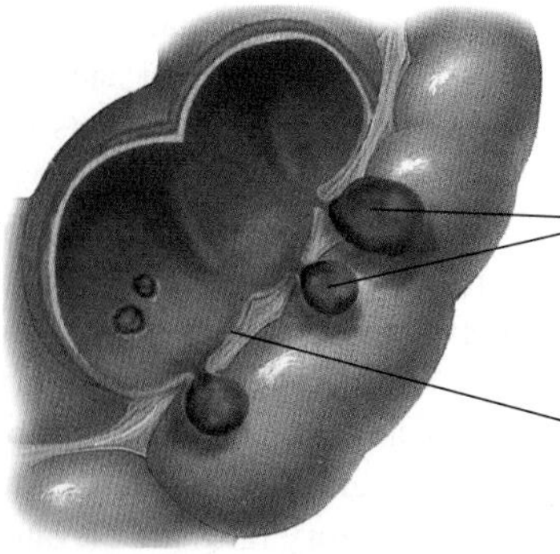

Figure 46-6 Intestinal diverticula, particularly common in the sigmoid colon of older adults, usually do not cause symptoms except for occasional rectal bleeding. They may become inflamed and infected from fecal matter that becomes lodged in the pouchlike herniations. (From Anatomical Chart Company (2006). *Atlas of pathophysiology* (2nd ed.). Lippincott Williams & Wilkins.)

Assessment Findings

Constipation alternating with diarrhea, flatulence, pain and tenderness in the LLQ, fever, and rectal bleeding may occur. A palpable mass may be felt in the lower abdomen. When the diverticula bleed, the stools appear maroon and are sometimes described as resembling "currant jelly."

A barium enema shows an irregular mucosal wall. A colonoscopy helps visualize the areas of inflammation. A CT scan generally is used first as an alternative to a barium enema or colonoscopy because both require an aggressive bowel preparation that may be contraindicated when the large intestine is acutely inflamed. Risk of perforation is increased. A CBC shows leukocytosis. A stool specimen may reveal occult blood.

Medical and Surgical Management

Diverticula noted during routine examination require no treatment if they do not cause symptoms. A high-fiber diet supplemented with bran or prescription of a bulk-forming agent (e.g., Metamucil) helps avoid constipation. The goal is for clients to consume 20 to 35 g of fiber daily.

When symptoms occur, the diet is temporarily adjusted to low-residue foods. If the inflammation is severe and accompanied by pain and local tenderness, the client is maintained on IV fluids for several days with no oral intake. As the inflammation subsides with antibiotic therapy, oral fluids and food are reintroduced.

If diverticulitis does not respond to medical treatment, or if complications such as perforation, intestinal obstruction, or severe bleeding occur, surgery becomes necessary. The portion of colon that contains the diverticula is removed, and the continuity of the bowel is reestablished by joining the remaining portions of the colon. Depending on the location and extent of the disease and whether there is intestinal obstruction, a temporary colostomy may be necessary (see Chapter 48). The continuity of the bowel is restored, and the colostomy is closed 3 to 6 weeks later.

Nursing Management

In addition to the assessments performed on the client with a GI disorder, the nurse obtains a history of symptoms, diet, drug use, and allergies and asks questions regarding pain, bowel elimination, and diet habits. They take vital signs to establish a baseline and to determine if the client is febrile. The nurse examines the abdomen for pain, tenderness, and masses.

Explaining the underlying pathology and rationale for treatment is important. Because dietary compliance reduces the potential for recurrences, consulting the dietitian for teaching is useful. If surgery becomes necessary, the nurse prepares the client before surgery and manages the postoperative care. A dietary consult or a list of foods to eat or avoid is necessary. The nurse also includes the following points in the teaching plan:

- Follow the diet recommended by the primary provider, which will probably reduce pain and discomfort.
- Bran adds bulk to the diet. Unprocessed bran can be sprinkled over cereal or added to fruit juice. Add other high-fiber foods such as fresh fruits and vegetables and other whole grains.
- Avoid the use of laxatives or enemas except when recommended by the primary provider.
- Avoid constipation. Do not suppress the urge to defecate.
- Drink at least 8 to 10 large glasses of fluid each day.
- Take prescribed medications as directed, even if symptoms improve.
- Exercise regularly if the current lifestyle is somewhat inactive.
- If severe pain or blood in the stool occurs, see a primary provider immediately.

ABDOMINAL HERNIA

Although **hernia** refers to the protrusion of any organ from the cavity that normally confines it, the term most commonly is used to describe the protrusion of the intestine through a defect in the abdominal wall. Certain areas in the abdominal wall are weaker than other areas and more vulnerable to the development of a hernia. These areas include the inguinal ring, the point on the abdominal wall where the inguinal canal begins; the femoral ring at the abdominal opening of the femoral canal; and the umbilicus.

If the protruding structures can be replaced in the abdominal cavity, it is a *reducible hernia*. Placing the client in a supine position and applying manual pressure over the area may reduce the hernia. An *irreducible* or *incarcerated hernia* is one in which the intestine cannot be replaced in the abdominal cavity because of edema of the protruding segment and constriction of the muscle opening through which it has emerged. If the process continues without treatment, the blood supply to the trapped segment of the bowel can be cut off, leading to gangrene. This development is referred to as a *strangulated hernia*.

Pathophysiology and Etiology

The most common abdominal hernias are *inguinal*, *umbilical*, *femoral*, and *incisional* (Box 46-2), with inguinal hernias the most common type. Inguinal hernias are more prevalent in men than in women. Umbilical and femoral hernias are more frequent in women than in men.

A hernia develops when intra-abdominal pressure increases, such as while straining to lift something heavy, having a bowel movement, or coughing or sneezing forcefully. When abdominal pressure increases, a segment of the intestine moves through a weak area of abdominal muscle. In the areas that are naturally predisposed to weakness, the abdominal wall may be thin or stretched from an inadequate amount of collagen. Such a condition may be present at birth or develop as a result of aging, abdominal surgery, or obesity.

At first, the defect in the abdominal wall is small. As the hernia persists and the organs continue to protrude, the defect grows larger. Eventually, the bowel becomes trapped

BOX 46-2 Types of Hernias

Inguinal: Protrusion of the hernial sac contains the intestine at the inguinal opening.

- *Direct*: Hernia extends through inguinal ring; it follows spermatic cord in men and the round ligament in women.
- *Indirect*: Protrusion follows the posterior inguinal wall; it often descends into the scrotum in men.

Umbilical: Hernia occurs in the umbilical region, through which the hernial sac protrudes. This type occurs in children when the umbilical orifice fails to close shortly after birth. It may occur in obese adults who have prolonged abdominal distention.

Femoral: Intestines descend through the femoral ring where the femoral artery passes into the femoral canal below the inguinal ligament. Incidence of strangulation is high.

Incisional: This type occurs through the scar of a surgical incision when healing is impaired. Careful surgical technique, particularly prevention of wound infection, can prevent incisional hernias. Obese, older, or malnourished clients are prone to the development of incisional hernias.

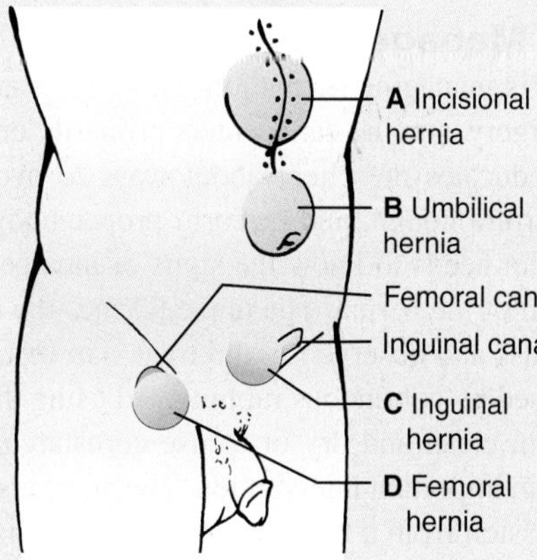

in the weakened pouch. If blood supply to the bowel is compromised, it becomes gangrenous.

Assessment Findings

A hernia initially causes swelling in the abdomen with no other symptoms. When the client coughs or bears down, the protrusion is more obvious. Sometimes, the swelling is painful, but the pain subsides when the hernia is reduced. Incarcerated hernias cause severe pain and, if not treated, may become strangulated. In this case, the client suffers extreme abdominal pain. The severe pressure on the loop of the intestine protruding outside the abdominal cavity causes intestinal obstruction.

Medical and Surgical Management

When a hernia forms, it tends to enlarge, leading to serious complications. Surgery is the only method of eliminating a hernia. Some clients, either because they are unwilling to have or are not candidates for surgery, may wear a truss, an apparatus that presses over the hernia and prevents protrusion of the bowel. The client also may lie supine while manual pressure is applied over the protruding area to reduce the hernia periodically. Some clients learn to do this procedure themselves.

A **herniorrhaphy**, the surgical repair of a hernia, is the recommended treatment. When a herniorrhaphy is performed, the protruding intestine is repositioned in the abdominal cavity and the defect in the abdominal wall is repaired. Herniorrhaphy is performed under local, spinal, or general anesthesia. Some types of hernias can be treated using a laparoscopic approach. When a hernia is neglected for many years, the tissues in the area weaken, and postoperative healing may be impaired. Obese people who have put off surgical repair for a prolonged period are especially prone to recurrence of the hernia despite surgical repair. For these cases, the surgeon also may perform a **hernioplasty**. The weakened area is reinforced with wire, fascia, or mesh. The obese client usually is advised to lose weight before the surgery to lessen the possibility of recurrence.

Strangulation is an acute emergency. Unless surgery is performed promptly, blood flow to the intestine is impaired. If necrosis occurs, the gangrenous part of the intestine must be excised and portions of the intestine reconnected.

Nursing Management

If the client is managing herniation with a truss and not undergoing surgery, nursing care centers primarily on teaching. The nurse educates the client about ways to avoid constipation, control a cough, and perform proper body mechanics. The client needs to know the signs of incarceration and strangulation of the hernia. The nurse teaches the client how to wear a truss and observe for and treat skin irritation from friction caused by continuous rubbing. Advising the client to keep the skin clean and dry or to use cornstarch to absorb moisture is an important intervention. The nurse also explains that compression from a truss may produce localized edema from interference with lymphatic and venous blood flow.

When surgery is scheduled, the nurse prepares the client and manages postoperative care (see Chapter 14). The assessment of clients undergoing surgery includes obtaining a complete medical and drug history because malnutrition, diabetes, or concurrent use of corticosteroids or antimetabolite cancer drugs can affect wound healing. The nurse also obtains the client's allergy history, especially to seasonal inhalants (i.e., ragweed pollen), and smoking history because sneezing and coughing can increase intra-abdominal pressure after surgery and place the client at risk of weakening the surgical repair.

Before surgery, the nurse takes vital signs, auscultates the lungs to identify infectious or respiratory risk factors, and documents the client's weight and duration of the hernia. These factors influence the potential for postoperative healing complications. The client's previous surgical experience may affect how the client feels about this surgery. The nurse also assesses the client's urinary and bowel patterns to determine if the client has any preexisting problems affecting elimination. After surgery, the nurse inspects the scrotum of men clients because it is common for edema to follow surgical repair.

Hernia repairs are performed mainly on an outpatient basis. Therefore, the nurse teaches measures to the client and significant others who will provide care after discharge. The nurse needs to reinforce verbal instructions with written instructions about signs and symptoms of possible complications (i.e., bleeding, infection) and the need to report these symptoms to the primary provider. The instructions include techniques for avoiding constipation and straining to have a bowel movement. The nurse also includes instructions to avoid strenuous exertion and heavy lifting until the primary provider determines that the client can safely undertake such activities. For clients who perform heavy physical labor, it is essential to explore how they may modify the manner in which they perform their jobs, take an extended sick leave, or apply for a temporary leave of absence. The nurse explains to those whose work is sedentary or light that they usually can return to full employment with few activity restrictions within a few weeks.

CANCERS OF THE COLON AND RECTUM

Intestinal malignancies may develop anywhere in the lower GI tract. Colorectal cancer ranks as the third most common cancer among men and women in the United States. The death rate from colon cancer has decreased over the last few decades, in part owing to increased screening and removal of precancerous or cancerous polyps that are small, making treatment easier and more effective. In addition, overall treatment for colorectal cancers has improved (American Cancer Society, 2020). The incidence of the disease increases with age. For colorectal screening, fecal occult blood testing is recommended every 1 to 2 years and colonoscopy every 5 to 10 years in clients older than 50 years. This screening may be performed in younger clients with risk factors, such as a family history of colorectal cancer or ulcerative colitis.

Pathophysiology and Etiology

Most malignant colorectal tumors develop from benign adenomas in the mucosal and submucosal intestinal layers (American

Cancer Society, 2020). A benign polyp may become malignant and then invade the surrounding tissues and structures. Cancer cells break away and spread to other body parts, most commonly the liver and the lungs. It is believed that genetic, environmental, and lifestyle factors spark the transformation from a benign to a cancerous state. Catalysts seem to include chronic bowel inflammation, as in ulcerative colitis, and a lifetime pattern of eating low-fiber, high-fat foods.

Having a blood relative with this disease is a high-risk factor. Genetic testing may be done to identify some types of familial colon cancer. At some point, the normal cells undergo mutation, which affects their proliferation and growth pattern. It is theorized that an *oncogene*, a genetic messenger that stimulates tumor growth, is not adequately suppressed. Without growth inhibition, the neoplastic cells reproduce rapidly and later proceed to invade the muscle wall. Other research suggests that a gene mutation interferes with the ability of colon cells to copy their DNA molecule correctly. It is also hypothesized that *tumor suppressor genes*, which normally control cell division and/or cause appropriate cell death, are impacted by gene mutations and do not function properly, leading to cellular proliferation of the tumor.

Although the primary malignant growth may remain in situ (confined to its site of origin), it can change the shape of the stool, compressing it or making it appear pencil-like as it passes by the protruding mass. Untreated, the cancer extends to other organs by way of the mesentery lymph nodes or portal vein leading to the liver.

Assessment Findings

The chief characteristic of cancer of the colon is a change in bowel habits, such as alternating constipation and diarrhea, and a narrowing of the stool. These changes last more than a few days. Occult or frank blood may be present in the stool. There may be a sense of urgency to defecate, but a bowel movement does not remove that sensation. Sometimes, a client may feel dull, vague abdominal discomfort. Pain is a late sign of cancer. On physical assessment, the abdomen feels distended, and a mass may be palpated in the abdomen or rectum.

Except for changes in bowel habits, clients' complaints may not be as specific. Cancers that start in the ascending colon often grow to a large size before causing symptoms because this part of the colon has a larger circumference and more flexibility. Eventually, clients complain of vague abdominal pain. Stools will appear black or tarry (**melena**) because of blood loss from the surrounding tissue. As a result, there can be iron-deficiency anemia and fatigue. Tumors in the descending colon, which has a narrower circumference, are more likely to cause obstruction—partial or total. Clients often complain of pain and cramping, constipation or diarrhea, abdominal distention, narrowing of stools, and bright red blood in the stools. Tumors in the rectum also cause bloody stools, as well as rectal pain, *tenesmus* (defecation is incomplete and painful), and constipation or diarrhea.

A number of diagnostic tests are performed for colorectal cancer, including FOBT, sigmoidoscopy, double contrast barium enema, colonoscopy, and digital rectal examination. Other imaging tests such as CT, ultrasound, positron-emission tomography (PET), and magnetic resonance imaging (MRI) may be done to examine suspicious areas or to determine if there is metastasis.

Newer diagnostic tests include virtual colonoscopy and (see Chapter 44) CT colonography, and DNA testing of stools, which involves looking for cellular genetic changes that can be a sign of cancer. Genetic screening may detect chromosomal markers for particular types of colon cancer. An elevated carcinoembryonic antigen (CEA) test or carbohydrate antigen 19-9 (CA 19-9) tumor marker test result suggests a tumor. Unfortunately, these tests are not effective in identifying colorectal cancer in its earliest, most treatable stages. Unless malignant growths are elevated from the mucosal wall, a barium enema may not provide conclusive evidence either. A tissue sample taken during a proctosigmoidoscopy or colonoscopy may detect malignant cells in the area of the biopsy. A CBC may show a low erythrocyte count from chronic blood loss. Liver enzymes may be checked to determine if liver function is impaired by metastasis to the liver.

Medical and Surgical Management

When polyps are discovered during endoscopic examination, they are removed (*polypectomy*) and examined. Even if the polyps are benign, the client continues to undergo periodic radiographic and endoscopic examinations to identify recurrent polyps for early malignant changes. The primary treatment of colorectal cancer is surgical, but sometimes treatment involves a combination of surgery, radiation therapy, chemotherapy, and targeted therapy (e.g., drugs that interfere with angiogenesis, such as bevacizumab [Avastin]).

An encapsulated colorectal tumor may be removed without taking away surrounding healthy tissue. This type of tumor, however, may call for partial or complete surgical removal of the colon (colectomy). Occasionally, the tumor causes a partial or complete bowel obstruction. If the tumor is in the colon and upper-third of the rectum, a **segmental resection** is performed. In this procedure, the surgeon removes the cancerous portion of the colon and rejoins the remaining portions of the GI tract to restore normal intestinal continuity.

Cancers in the lower-third of the rectum are treated with an **abdominoperineal resection**—wide excision of the rectum and creation of a sigmoid colostomy. The surgical procedures used to treat cancers in the middle-third of the rectum vary. A low resection with a temporary colostomy usually is attempted to preserve the anal sphincter. Radiation therapy is indicated in many cases of colon cancer, whereas chemotherapy usually is reserved for those with evidence of lymphatic infiltration or metastasis. If the cancer metastasizes, a colostomy may be performed to relieve an intestinal obstruction. In some cases, the obstruction is relieved or bleeding is controlled with laser surgery.

Nursing Management

The nurse advises and prepares clients for routine colorectal screening. They follow standard guidelines for collecting

Client and Family Teaching 46-2
Fecal Occult Blood Testing (FOBT)

The nurse should include the following points when instructing a client about the procedure for FOBT, which the client may perform at home:

Seven to 10 Days Before and Throughout the Test

- Do not drink alcohol or take aspirin, NSAIDs, vitamin C, or iron preparations.
- Check with the primary provider if anticoagulants, steroids, colchicines (used to treat gout), or cimetidine (for peptic ulcer treatment) have been prescribed.

Two Days Before and Throughout the Test

- Consume a high-fiber diet and avoid red meat, substituting with poultry and fish.
- Avoid turnips, cauliflower, broccoli, cantaloupe, horseradish, and parsnips.

During the Test

- Collect stool within a toilet liner or bedpan.
- Use an applicator stick and remove a sample from the center of the stool.
- Apply a thin smear of stool onto the test area supplied with the screening kit.
- Take care to cover the entire space.
- Place two drops of developer solution onto the test area.
- Wait precisely 60 seconds.
- Observe for a blue color, indicating a positive reaction (for more valid results, test samples from several stools over 3 to 6 days).

stool specimens and sending them to the laboratory for analysis. The nurse instructs the client how to collect specimens at home, if applicable (Client and Family Teaching 46-2). The nurse advises anyone who is asymptomatic but whose stool test results are positive for blood to undergo a colonoscopy, the next step in cancer detection. Nursing management of the client with a colostomy is discussed in Chapter 48.

ANORECTAL DISORDERS

Clients with anorectal disorders usually experience localized pain and bleeding, and thus seek medical attention. They may also have problems with perianal itching, tenderness, and swelling. They may delay defecation secondary to pain and other discomfort.

Hemorrhoids

Hemorrhoids are dilated veins outside or inside the anal sphincter (Fig. 46-7). Thrombosed hemorrhoids are veins that contain clots.

Pathophysiology and Etiology

Chronic straining to have a bowel movement or frequent defecation with chronic diarrhea likely weakens the tissue supporting the veins. Clients whose work requires prolonged sitting are at increased risk for the development of

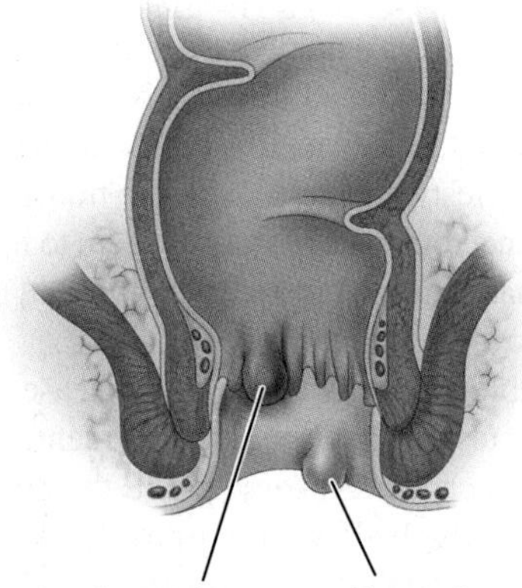

Figure 46-7 Internal and external hemorrhoids.

hemorrhoids. Pregnancy, prolonged labor, portal hypertension, or other intra-abdominal conditions that interfere with venous blood return can cause or aggravate the condition. The veins near the anal sphincter probably are displaced downward from their natural location as the result of a loss of supporting tissue. Without adequate connective tissue and smooth muscle support, the veins dilate and fill with blood. Dry stool passes by the engorged hemorrhoids, which stretches and irritates the mucosa, giving rise to the local symptoms of burning, itching, and pain. Passing dry, hard stool causes the hemorrhoids to bleed.

Assessment Findings

External hemorrhoids may cause few symptoms, or they can produce pain, itching, and soreness of the anal area. They appear as small, reddish-blue lumps at the edge of the anus. Thrombosed external hemorrhoids are painful but seldom cause bleeding.

Internal hemorrhoids cause bleeding but are less likely to cause pain unless they protrude through the anus. The amount of bleeding varies from an occasional drop or two of blood on toilet tissue or underwear to chronic loss of blood, leading to anemia. Internal hemorrhoids usually protrude each time the client defecates but retract after defecation. As the masses enlarge, they remain outside the sphincter.

An anoscope, an instrument for examining the anal canal, or a proctosigmoidoscope, allows visualization of internal hemorrhoids. A colonoscopy rules out colorectal cancer, which has similar symptoms.

Medical Management

Small external hemorrhoids may disappear without treatment, or the client may obtain relief through symptomatic treatment. The primary provider may recommend warm soaks, an ointment that contains a local anesthetic for the relief of pain and itching, topical astringent pads to relieve swelling, a diet that corrects or prevents constipation, and a stool softener. In some cases, the hemorrhoid is ligated (tied off) with a rubber band. Coagulation techniques use infrared light, laser, or heat to coagulate the hemorrhoids so that the protein and water in hemorrhoidal tissue are destroyed as an alternative to traditional surgery. Sclerotherapy is an injection of a hardening chemical directly into the hemorrhoid to shrink it.

Surgical Management

A **hemorrhoidectomy**, the surgical removal of hemorrhoids, may be necessary in chronic and severe cases. The procedure is performed using conventional surgery or laser surgery; the client receives a local anesthetic or regional nerve block. Internal packing of lubricated gauze, external gauze dressing, or a perineal pad is applied to absorb blood. A T-binder holds the absorbent material in place. Hemorrhoid stapling (stapled hemorrhoidopexy) is a procedure that interrupts blood flow to the hemorrhoid. Although it is less painful than a hemorrhoidectomy and has a shorter recovery period, there is a higher chance of recurrence and rectal prolapse.

Nursing Management

The nurse gathers a complete history, including drug and allergy histories. Because bleeding accompanies many colorectal disorders, it is important to ask the client to describe the bleeding as well as other related symptoms. The nurse determines if there is a history of constipation or alternating diarrhea and constipation and if the client uses any prescription or nonprescription drugs. In addition, the nurse obtains a diet history, paying particular attention to the type of foods (especially fiber) included in the diet. The physical examination involves putting on gloves, draping the client, and inspecting the anus.

Health teaching is focused on self-management. The nurse reviews the primary provider's home care instructions, demonstrates wound care to the client or responsible caregiver and provides an opportunity for returning the demonstration, provides dietary recommendations and offers a list of high-fiber foods, instructs about stool softeners as indicated, emphasizes the importance of an active lifestyle and increased fluid intake, and cautions against the prolonged use of laxatives.

Anorectal Abscess

An anorectal abscess is an infection with a collection of pus in an area between the internal and external sphincters.

Pathophysiology and Etiology

The original source of the infection may be microorganisms harbored in the intestine itself. An anorectal abscess is common in clients with Crohn disease. Anorectal infections, however, also are transmitted from others through anal intercourse or insertion of foreign bodies into the rectum.

Usually, infectious microorganisms invade anal crypts, small tubular cavities in the anal skin and rectal mucosa. A purulent exudate collects, and the pressure causes pain and swelling. The abscess eventually may develop into a fistulous tract (channel).

Assessment Findings

Clients with an anorectal abscess experience pain that is aggravated by walking and sitting or other activities that increase intra-abdominal pressure such as coughing, sneezing, and straining to have a bowel movement. A swollen mass is evident in the anus. Fever and abdominal pain develop if the abscess has extended into deeper tissues. Foul-smelling drainage may leak from the anus if the abscess spontaneously ruptures. A culture of anal drainage reveals the infectious microorganism.

Medical and Surgical Management

Analgesics and sitz baths are prescribed to relieve symptoms. Antibiotic therapy is used to treat gonorrheal, staphylococcal, streptococcal, or other drug-sensitive bacteria. An incision and drainage to remove the infected material may be necessary. If a fistula has formed, deeper excision and removal of the fistulous tract are necessary. Because fistula formation frequently is associated with Crohn disease, additional diagnostic testing may be necessary to determine the presence of this condition.

Nursing Management

To limit the spread of infectious microorganisms, the nurse instructs the client to practice scrupulous hand washing after each bowel movement, to use separate hygiene articles, to cleanse the bathtub after each use, and to use a condom if having anal intercourse. Refer to the nursing management of a client with an anorectal disorder for specific nursing interventions.

Anal Fissure

An anal **fissure** (*fissure in ano*) is a linear tear in the anal canal tissue.

Pathophysiology and Etiology

Constipation is the leading cause of anal fissures. Other factors that may lead to the formation of a slit-like tear include eversion of the anus during vaginal delivery and trauma to the anus, such as during anal intercourse or through the insertion of foreign bodies or medical instruments. When the anal canal is excessively stretched, the skin rips apart, exposing the underlying tissue.

Assessment Findings

Severe pain and bleeding on defecation are common. If constipation was not an original problem, it becomes one. Most clients with an anal fissure are reluctant to defecate because of the associated pain. The torn area may be visible when the anus is visually inspected, and the irregular surface of the fissure may be felt during a digital examination. Anoscopy provides evidence of the altered integrity of the anal mucosa.

Medical and Surgical Management

Treatment includes applying anesthetic creams, ointments, or suppositories; taking sitz baths and analgesics; and preventing constipation. Surgical excision of the area may be necessary.

Nursing Management

The nurse includes the following in the plan of care:

- Teach the client how to insert a suppository.

- Instruct the client in how to take a sitz bath.
- Discuss strategies to relieve constipation.

Refer to Nursing Care Plan 46-1 for more information.

Anal Fistula

An anal fistula (*fistula in ano*) is a tract that forms in the anal canal.

Pathophysiology and Etiology

When healing of an anorectal abscess is inadequate, an inflamed tunnel develops, connecting the area of the original abscess with perianal skin (Fig. 46-8). Purulent material drains from the opening.

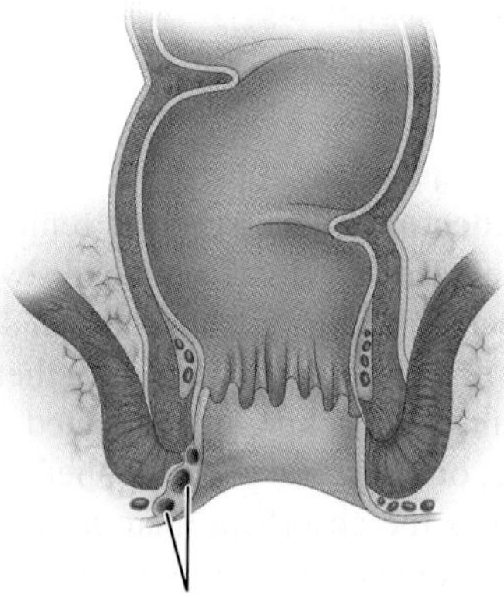

Figure 46-8 Anal fistula.

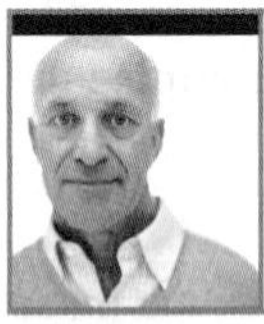

Clinical Scenario A client is seen at a local clinic with complaints of rectal pain that gets worse with activities that increase pressure on that area. The client has had bleeding when defecating and complains of constipation. **What is the major focus for the nurse when gathering data and planning care for this client? See Nursing Care Plan 46-1.**

NURSING CARE PLAN 46-1 The Client With an Anorectal Condition

Assessment

Include the following questions in the health history:

- Do you have any burning, itching, or pain in the anorectal area? If so, when do these symptoms occur—with defecation? How long do they last? Do you have any other discomfort, such as abdominal cramps?
- Is there any blood in the stool or on the toilet tissue when you wipe the rectum? How much? Is the blood bright or dark red?
- Is there mucus or pus from the rectal area?
- What is your stool pattern?
- Do you use laxatives? If so, how often?
- What is your typical diet?
- Do you exercise regularly? If so, what is the exercise?
- Do you sit or stand for long periods?

Nursing Diagnosis. Constipation Risk related to fear of painful elimination

Expected Outcome. Client identifies measures that prevent or treat constipation.

Interventions	Rationales
Instruct client, unless contraindicated, to increase intake of water to 2 L/day.	*Such fluid intake prevents hard, dry stools and eases defecation.*
Provide a list of high-fiber foods.	*A high-fiber diet promotes bulk of stool and prevents constipation.*
Instruct client in the use of laxatives or stool softeners as ordered.	*Prolonged use of these measures is not encouraged; they should be used only as indicated.*
Teach the client to heed the urge to have a bowel movement.	*This measure prevents constipation.*

Evaluation of Expected Outcome

Client practices measures that prevent constipation as evidenced by increased fluid and fiber intake and the passage of soft, formed stools.

Nursing Diagnosis. Acute Pain related to surgical procedure

Expected Outcome. Client will report that pain management regimen relieves their pain.

Interventions	Rationales
Administer pain medications as ordered.	*Medications promote ongoing pain relief.*
Encourage client to rest in a comfortable position that removes pressure from the surgical site, or to use a flotation device.	*These measures relieve pressure and decrease pain at the surgical site.*

NURSING CARE PLAN 46-1 The Client With an Anorectal Condition (*continued*)

Apply ice and analgesic ointments as indicated.	*These measures promote pain relief.*
Use warm compresses or sitz baths three to four times daily as indicated.	*Warmth through compresses or baths relaxes the rectal sphincter spasm and soothes irritated tissues.*

Evaluation of Expected Outcome

Client states that positioning and use of sitz baths relieve pain.

Nursing Diagnosis. **Knowledge Deficiency** related to unknown needed care

Expected Outcome. Client will demonstrate an ability to manage therapeutic regimens.

Interventions	Rationales
Instruct client to cleanse perianal area with warm water and to dry with cotton wipes.	*These measures prevent infection and irritation.*
Teach client how to do sitz baths at home using warm water three to four times each day.	*Sitz baths promote healing, decrease skin irritation, and relieve rectal spasms.*
Instruct client to take a sitz bath after each bowel movement.	*Sitz baths also help keep the perianal area clean.*
Encourage client to follow diet and medication instructions.	*Encouragement promotes compliance with therapeutic regimen and prevents complications.*
Encourage moderate exercise.	*Activity promotes healing and normal stool patterns.*

Evaluation of Expected Outcomes

(1) Incision heals without complications. (2) Client has no signs of infection and eats a diet high in fiber. (3) Vital signs are normal. (4) Stools are soft formed and regular.

Assessment Findings

The client reports pain on defecation. The opening of the fistula appears red, and pus leaks from the external opening of the fistula or can be expressed if the area is compressed. If the fistula is superficial, it feels cordlike on palpation. A proctosigmoidoscopy or colonoscopy may identify Crohn disease, which predisposes the client to an anorectal abscess or anal fistula.

Medical and Surgical Management

Antibiotics are prescribed to treat infection. Treatment of underlying Crohn disease often allows for resolution of the fistula without surgical intervention. Most simple low-lying fistulae can be managed by **fistulotomy**. This procedure involves incising the fistula along with partial sphincter division and is reserved for those fistulae that arise from relatively normal surrounding tissue. Another surgical procedure, referred to as **fistulectomy**, involves an excision of the fistulous tract. This type usually is the recommended surgery.

If a sphincter division compromises fecal continence, a noncutting seton may be placed into the fistula to allow for drainage of the fistula and to minimize the risk of future abscesses. A *seton* is a nonabsorbable suture or drain that is passed from the cutaneous opening of the fistula into the lumen of the anal canal and then back out onto the skin, where it is tied to itself. The seton can be gradually tightened to cut through the sphincter or left in place as a drain.

Nursing Management

The nurse teaches the client to self-administer medications, keep the anal region clean, and avoid transferring microorganisms to other hygiene articles that they share with family members (e.g., bar soap). (See Nursing Care Plan 46-1 for additional nursing management.)

Pilonidal Sinus

Pilonidal means "a nest of hair." A **pilonidal sinus** is an infection in the hair follicles in the sacrococcygeal area above the anus (Fig. 46-9). Other local infections, such as osteomyelitis and furuncles of the skin, also have common presenting signs and symptoms and must be ruled out. The terms *pilonidal sinus* and *pilonidal cyst* are both used to describe the condition.

Pathophysiology and Etiology

The condition typically occurs after puberty. People who have a deep intergluteal cleft and those who have abundant hair in the perianal and lower back regions are predisposed to the condition. Inadequate personal hygiene, obesity, and trauma to the area also contribute to its development.

A sinus or cyst begins to form when the skin deep in the cleft softens as a result of being chronically moist. Stiff hairs then irritate and pierce the soft, macerated skin, becoming embedded in it. The irritation inflames the tissues. Infection readily follows because the break in the skin allows microorganisms to enter. Several channels may lead from the sinus to the skin.

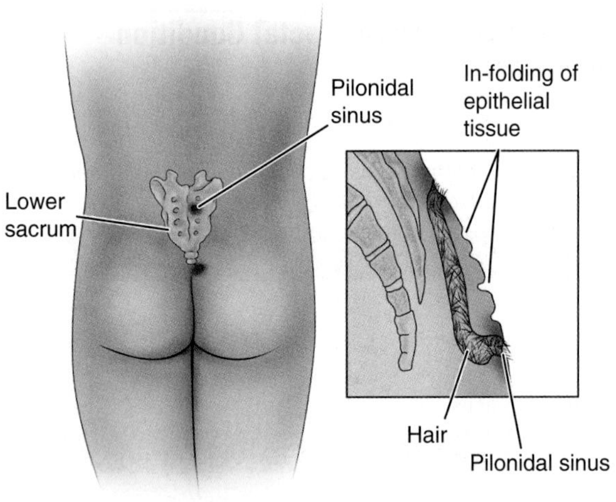

Figure 46-9 Pilonidal sinus on lower sacrum about 5 cm (2 inches) above the anus in the intergluteal cleft. Hair particles emerge from the sinus tract, and localized indentations (pits) can appear on the skin near the sinus openings.

Assessment Findings

Pain and swelling at the base of the spine and purulent drainage occur. On inspection, the sinus opening may be located in the gluteal fold. Dilated pits of the hair follicles in the sinus are a unique characteristic.

Medical and Surgical Management

The abscess is drained, and the tissue is incised. The sinus and all its connecting channels are laid open, and purulent material and hair are removed. Packing is inserted into the cavity, and the wound heals by secondary intention. In some cases, the wound edges are approximated. Healing by primary intention, however, sometimes allows the purulent material to reform and collect, causing another abscess. Because the infection is localized, systemic antibiotics usually are not prescribed.

Nursing Management

The nurse teaches the client how to minimize discomfort and facilitates postoperative bowel elimination. As appropriate, the nurse instructs a family member in the procedures of removing the packing, cleaning the incised tissue, and redressing the area. (See Nursing Care Plan 46-1 for additional nursing management.)

KEY POINTS

- Altered bowel elimination includes the following:
  - Constipation
  - Diarrhea
  - Irritable bowel syndrome
- Inflammatory bowel disease—several types, has episodes of exacerbations and remissions
  - Crohn disease
- Ulcerative colitis—chronic inflammation
- Acute abdominal inflammatory disorders
  - Appendicitis—inflammation of the appendix
  - Peritonitis—peritoneum is inflamed
- Intestinal obstruction—blockage interferes with progression of intestinal contents
- Diverticular disorder
  - Diverticulosis—pouches in intestinal wall
  - Diverticulitis—pouches (diverticula) becomes inflamed
- Abdominal hernia—protrusion of organ from its normal cavity
  - Incisional, umbilical, inguinal, femoral
- Cancers of colon and rectum
- Anorectal disorders
  - Hemorrhoids—dilated veins at the anal sphincter
  - Anorectal abscess
  - Anal fissure—linear tear in the anal canal tissue
  - Anal fistula—tract that forms in the anal canal
  - Pilonidal sinus—infection in the hair follicle in the sacrococcygeal area

CRITICAL THINKING EXERCISES

1. The admitting department notifies the nursing unit to expect a client with ulcerative colitis. Based on the characteristics of the disease process, what assessments are essential to obtain at the time of admission?
2. As you assist an older adult with using a bedpan, you notice blood on the toilet tissue. What other data are appropriate to gather at this time?
3. A 65-year-old client recently diagnosed with diverticulosis tells you that they are very concerned about having acute problems with diverticulitis like their mother. What information could you provide that can most help them prevent diverticulitis?
4. A 45-year-old friend tells you that their primary provider has scheduled them for a colonoscopy. The friend asks you why they need to have one since they feel fine and are not having any bowel problems. What is most important to ask?

NCLEX-STYLE REVIEW QUESTIONS PrepU

1. Which of the following outcomes demonstrates the client's understanding of methods to relieve constipation?
   1. The client exercises regularly four to six times a week.
   2. The client has two servings of fruits or vegetables per day.
   3. The client limits water intake to 24 oz/day.
   4. The client states that whole grains are not part of the daily diet.
2. A nurse is preparing a client with a long history of ulcerative colitis for first-stage surgery to remove the colon. Which of the client's statements indicates that the client requires more preoperative education?
   1. "I eventually will be able to eat regular food."
   2. "I will have an ileostomy for the rest of my life."
   3. "My stools will be more liquid than they are normally."
   4. "The surgeon said that the second stage will be done in a few weeks."

3. What does the nurse recognize as important assessments on a 24-year-old client seen in the emergency room with complaints of abdominal pain? The diagnosis is "rule out appendicitis." Select all that apply.
1. Abdominal pain currently localized in RLQ
2. Generalized abdominal pain for 24 hours
3. Indigestion after eating meals
4. Stools with high-fat content
5. WBC of 16,500 cells/mm^3

4. Which of the following signs would the nurse expect when assessing a client with suspected peritonitis? Select all that apply.
1. Abdomen feels rigid.
2. Pulse rate is elevated.
3. Rectal bleeding is present.
4. Respirations are slow and labored.
5. Stools appear maroon.

5. A client is admitted with a diagnosis of diverticulitis. The client has nausea, vomiting, and dehydration. Which sign requires immediate attention by the nurse?
1. Abdominal distention
2. Boardlike abdomen
3. Low-grade fever
4. Pain in LLQ

WANT TO KNOW MORE? There are a wide variety of online resources available on thePoint to enhance learning and understanding of this chapter.

Go to thePoint.lww.com/activate and use the activation code found in the front of this text to unlock these online resources.

47 Caring for Clients With Disorders of the Liver, Gallbladder, or Pancreas

Words To Know

alpha-fetoprotein
ascites
balloon tamponade
biliary colic
caput medusae
cholecystitis
choledocholithiasis
cholelithiasis
cholestasis
cirrhosis
esophageal varices
fetor hepaticus
hepatic encephalopathy
hepatic lobectomy
hepatitis
hepatorenal syndrome
injection sclerotherapy
laparoscopic cholecystectomy
lithotripsy
open cholecystectomy
pancreatitis
pancreatoduodenectomy (Whipple procedure)
partial or total pancreatectomy
portal hypertension
steatorrhea
T-tube

Learning Objectives

On completion of this chapter, you will be able to:

1. Explain possible causes of jaundice.
2. List common findings manifested by clients with cirrhosis.
3. Discuss common complications of cirrhosis.
4. Identify the modes of transmission of viral hepatitis.
5. Discuss nursing management for clients with a medically or surgically treated liver disorder.
6. Identify factors that contribute to signs and symptoms of and medical treatments for cholecystitis.
7. Name techniques for gallbladder removal.
8. Summarize the nursing management of clients undergoing medical or surgical treatment of a gallbladder disorder.
9. Describe the treatment and nursing management of pancreatitis.
10. Describe the treatment of pancreatic carcinoma.
11. Explain the nursing management of clients undergoing pancreatic surgery.

The liver, gallbladder, and pancreas play important roles in digestion. They are also responsible for many other physiologic activities (see Chapter 44). Their poor function impairs the digestive process and the client's overall nutritional status.

Gerontologic Considerations

- Changes in the liver that accompany the aging process include decreases in organ weight, blood flow, and size and number of hepatocytes; increase in fibrous tissue; and changes in metabolism of medications. However, liver function is not significantly affected unless disease is present.
- Assessment of liver function can be important for determining side effects owing to alterations in medication metabolism and excretion.
- Although hepatitis A commonly is found in younger people, older adults may contract hepatitis through contact with younger people who have the disease, such as grandchildren, wait staff, or supermarket or nursing home employees.

Gerontologic Considerations (continued)

■ Although recurrent severe pain is the predominant symptom of chronic hepatitis in young to middle-aged adults, older adults report the pain with chronic hepatitis as being mild or absent.
■ The incidence of gallstones is common in older adults. Older adults may recover more slowly from surgery of the gallbladder. If changes owing to aging, respiratory, or vascular disease are present, individuals are more prone to develop postoperative complications, such as pneumonia and thrombophlebitis.
■ Teaching for self-care or appropriate supportive nursing care must include adequate movement in bed, performance of deep-breathing exercises, and ambulation shortly after surgery.

DISORDERS OF THE LIVER

The liver has four lobes. Each lobe is surrounded by connective tissue that extends in the lobe itself and divides the liver into smaller units referred to as *lobules*. The liver is supported by intra-abdominal pressure and various attachments called *mesenteries*, which connect the liver to the adjacent intestines, abdominal wall, and diaphragm. Unless it is abnormally enlarged, the liver usually is not palpable. Figure 47-1 illustrates the liver and the surrounding structures.

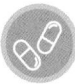

Pharmacologic Considerations

■ Drug availability is controlled by the liver's first pass effect. When a drug is absorbed by the small intestine, it travels to the liver where a portion of the drug is metabolized. As a result, less active drug is circulated to the tissues.

BOX 47-1 Functions of the Liver

- Metabolizes glucose
- Regulates blood glucose concentration
- Converts glucose to glycogen to glucose to maintain normal glucose levels
- Synthesizes amino acids from the breakdown of protein or from lactate that muscles produce during exercise to form glucose (*gluconeogenesis*)
- Converts ammonia (by-product of gluconeogenesis) into urea
- Metabolizes proteins and fats
- Stores vitamins A, B_{12}, D, and some B-complex vitamins as well as iron and copper
- Metabolizes drugs, chemicals, bacteria, and other foreign elements
- Forms and excretes bile
- Excretes bilirubin
- Synthesizes factors needed for blood coagulation (e.g., prothrombin, fibrinogen)

The liver has various functions (Box 47-1) and a rich blood supply. It receives arterial blood from the hepatic artery, an indirect branch of the aorta. This blood, which provides approximately 20% of the blood supply to the liver, is rich in oxygen. The portal vein transports blood from the intestinal tract to the liver and provides about 80% of the liver's blood supply. It is low in oxygen but high in nutrients. After blood has traversed vascular pathways inside the liver, the hepatic veins collect the blood and transport it to the inferior vena cava and then back to the heart (Fig. 47-2).

Microscopically, the liver's internal structure includes smaller branches of the hepatic artery, the hepatic and portal veins, the lymphatics, and the bile ducts. The cellular

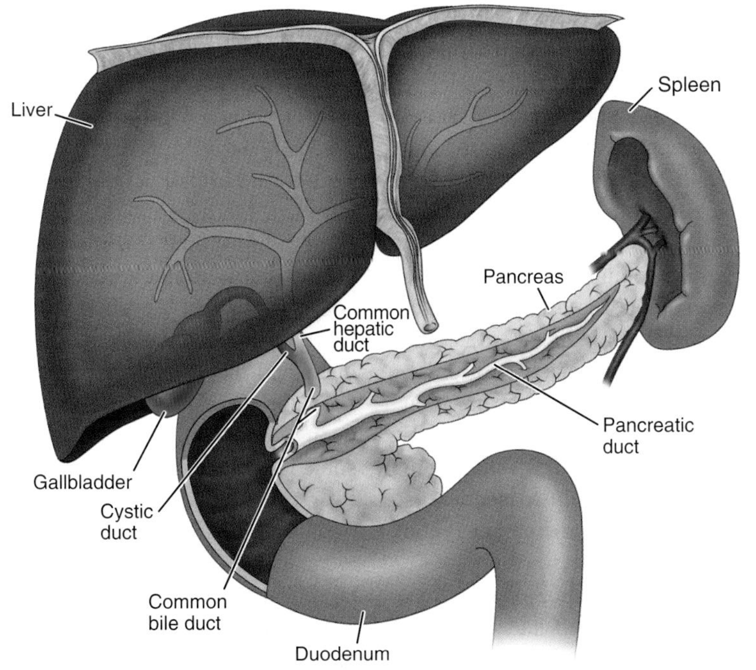

Figure 47-1 The liver and biliary system.

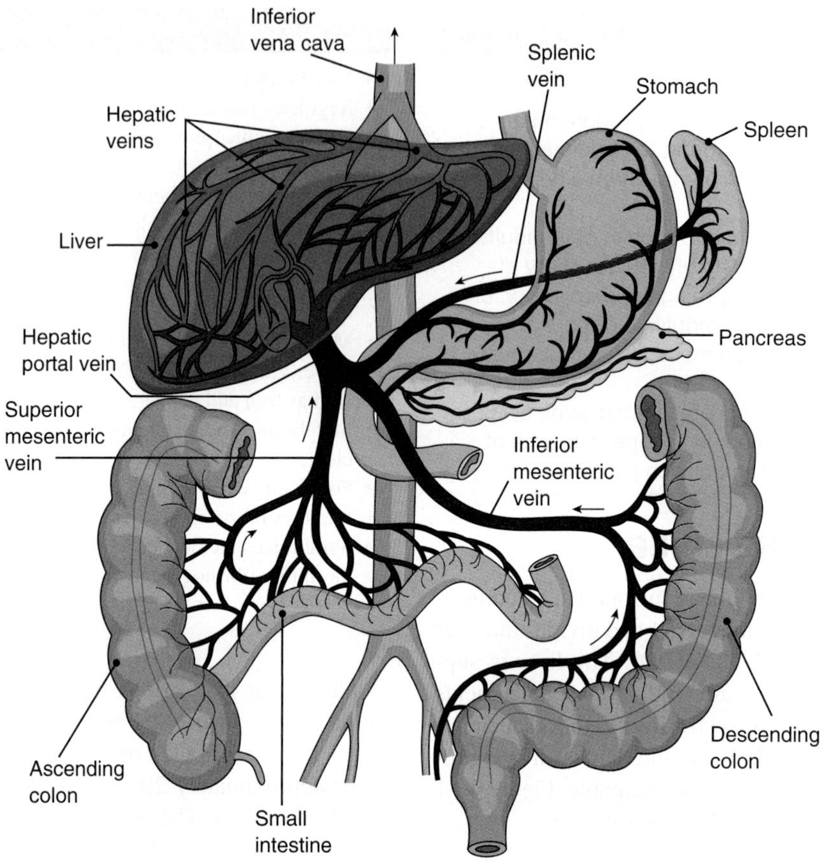

Figure 47-2 Hepatic portal system. Veins from the abdominal organs carry blood to the hepatic portal vein leading to the liver. After blood travels through vascular pathways inside the liver, the hepatic veins carry it to the inferior vena cava and back to the heart.

constituents of the liver are the hepatic parenchymal cells (hepatocytes), which perform most of the liver's metabolic functions, and the Kupffer cells, which engage in the liver's immunologic, detoxifying, and blood-filtering actions. The smallest bile ducts, *canaliculi*, are between the lobules of the liver. They receive secretions from the hepatocytes, carrying them to larger bile ducts and, eventually, to the hepatic duct. This duct joins with the cystic duct from the gallbladder to form the common bile duct, which empties into the small intestine. The sphincter of Oddi controls the amount of bile that enters the duodenum from the common bile duct.

Jaundice

Jaundice is a greenish-yellow discoloration of tissue. It is a sign of disease, but it is not itself a unique disease. Jaundice accompanies many diseases that directly or indirectly affect the liver and is probably the most common sign of a liver disorder.

Jaundice results from an abnormally high concentration of the pigment *bilirubin* in the blood. Normally, total bilirubin concentration ranges from 0.2 to 1.3 mg/dL. If the serum bilirubin level exceeds 2.5 mg/dL (43 fmol/L), jaundice is visible, notably on the skin, oral mucous membranes, and (especially) sclera.

To understand the scope and significance of jaundice, it is important to know how bile is formed and excreted. Bilirubin is produced in the liver, spleen, and bone marrow. It also results from hemoglobin metabolism and is a by-product of hemolysis (red blood cell [RBC] destruction). The reticuloendothelial system also produces bilirubin. The liver removes bilirubin from the body, excreting it in *bile*, of which bilirubin is the major pigment. Thus, serum contains a normal amount of bilirubin. Serum bilirubin levels increase when (1) there is excessive destruction of RBCs or (2) the liver cannot excrete bilirubin normally.

There are two forms of bilirubin. *Indirect* or *unconjugated bilirubin* binds with protein as it circulates in the blood. This form normally circulates in the blood; when its level is elevated, the usual cause is increased hemolysis. The other form of bilirubin is *direct* or *conjugated bilirubin*, which circulates freely in the blood until reaching the liver. The liver conjugates direct bilirubin with glucuronide. The conjugated bilirubin is excreted in the bile. As the bile enters the bile ducts and moves into the intestine, bacterial enzymes transform the direct bilirubin into *urobilinogen*. Some urobilinogen is changed into *urobilin*, the brown pigment of stool; some is excreted in the urine; and some is carried back to the liver by the bloodstream for reexcretion in the bile (Fig. 47-3).

There is no direct test for indirect bilirubin levels. They are calculated by subtracting direct bilirubin levels from total bilirubin levels. For example, if the total bilirubin level is 1.0 mg/dL and the conjugated bilirubin level is 0.1 mg/dL, then the indirect bilirubin level is 0.9 mg/dL.

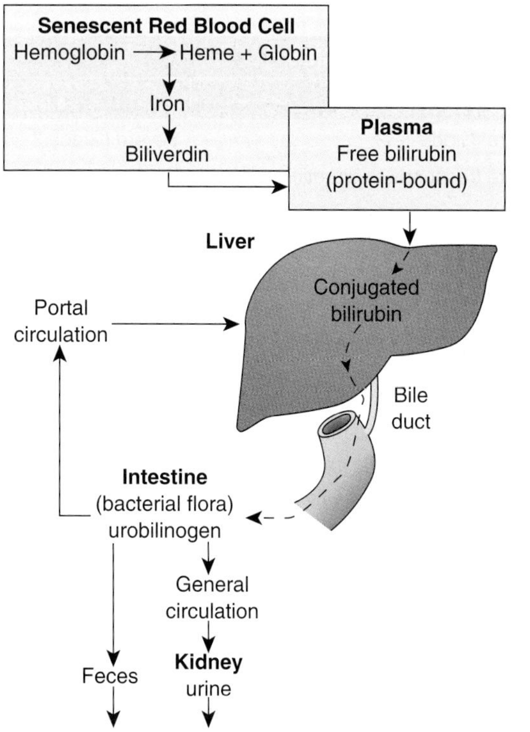

Figure 47-3 Formation, circulation, and elimination of bilirubin.

There are three forms of jaundice: (1) *hemolytic jaundice*, caused by excess destruction of RBCs (see Chapter 31); (2) *hepatocellular jaundice*, caused by liver disease (damaged liver cells cannot clear normal amounts of bilirubin from the blood); and (3) *obstructive jaundice*, caused by a block in the passage of bile between the liver and intestinal tract (Table 47-1). Because unconjugated and conjugated bilirubin are distinct and can be differentiated, they are important in the differential diagnosis of diseases that produce jaundice.

Cirrhosis

Cirrhosis is a chronic, degenerative liver disorder caused by generalized cellular damage.

Pathophysiology and Etiology

Once liver cells are irreversibly damaged, nonfunctional fibrous connective scar tissue replaces them, which leads to considerable anatomic distortion and partial or complete occlusion of blood channels in the liver. The liver becomes increasingly unable to carry out its many functions. This leads to disturbances in digestion and metabolism, defects in blood coagulation, fluid and electrolyte imbalances, and impaired ability to metabolize hormones and detoxify chemicals. Because bile begins to drain into the intestine, the client experiences fat malabsorption and an inability to absorb fat-soluble vitamins (A, D, E, and K). Portal hypertension, esophageal varices, ascites, and hepatic encephalopathy are complications of advanced cirrhosis (see later discussion).

There are several types of cirrhosis: alcoholic, postnecrotic, biliary, and nonalcoholic steatohepatitis. *Alcoholic cirrhosis*, the most common type, results from chronic alcohol intake and is frequently associated with poor nutrition. It can also follow chronic poisoning with certain chemicals (e.g., carbon tetrachloride, a cleaning agent) or ingestion of hepatotoxic drugs (e.g., acetaminophen). Alcoholic cirrhosis is characterized by necrotic liver cells, which gradually are replaced by scar tissue. Eventually, the amount of scar tissue exceeds functional liver tissue. The liver takes on a characteristic "hobnail" appearance, in which there are islands of normal tissue, regenerating tissue, and scar tissue. The disease develops over a long period of 30 years or more.

Postnecrotic cirrhosis results from destruction of liver cells secondary to infection (e.g., hepatitis), metabolic liver disease, or exposure to hepatotoxins or industrial chemicals. Broad bands of scar tissue form within the liver as a result of the cellular destruction. Cirrhosis caused by chronic hepatitis C is the second leading cause of cirrhosis (American Liver Foundation, 2020).

In *biliary cirrhosis*, scarring occurs around the bile ducts in the liver. The cause usually is related to chronic biliary obstruction and infection. Primary biliary cirrhosis refers to a progressive autoimmune disease of the liver. Chronic inflammation causes destruction to the small intrahepatic biliary ducts, preventing the flow of bile into the small intestine. Eventually, cirrhosis and liver failure result.

Another cause of cirrhosis is referred to as *nonalcoholic steatohepatitis* (NASH). This type involves the building up of fat. Most likely NASH is a result of other diseases, such as diabetes, elevated cholesterol, and/or coronary artery disease.

The prognosis for clients with cirrhosis is based on bilirubin and albumin levels, presence of **ascites** (accumulation of serous fluid in the peritoneal cavity), neurologic involvement, and nutritional status. Table 47-2 provides information on classification of severity of cirrhosis.

TABLE 47-1 Types of Jaundice

TYPE	DESCRIPTION	CHANGES IN BILIRUBIN LEVELS
Hemolytic	Hemolytic processes (e.g., multiple blood transfusions, pernicious anemia, sickle cell anemia) cause an overproduction of bilirubin.	Elevated unconjugated bilirubin levels
Hepatocellular	Liver cells damaged by viral infections, medications, or chemical toxicity cannot clear bilirubin from the blood.	Elevated conjugated and unconjugated bilirubin levels
Obstructive	Gallstones, inflammation, or tumors obstruct the bile duct, causing reabsorption of bile into the blood.	Elevated conjugated bilirubin levels

TABLE 47-2 Child–Turcotte–Pugh Classification for Severity of Cirrhosis

	POINTS ASSIGNED[a]		
PARAMETER	**1**	**2**	**3**
Encephalopathy	None	Mild to moderate (Grade 1–2)	Severe (Grade 3–4)
Ascites	Absent	Mild to moderate (responds to diuretics	Severe
Bilirubin (mg/dL)	≤2	2–3	>3
Albumin (g/dL)	>3.5	2.8–3.5	<2.8
International normalized ratio (INR)	<1.7	1.7–2.3	>2.3

[a]Total score of 5–6, grade A; 7–9, grade B; 10–15, grade C.
U.S. Department of Veterans Affairs. (2018). *Child-Turcotte-Pugh Calculator.* http://www.hepatitis.va.gov/provider/tools/child-pugh-calculator.asp

Assessment Findings

Signs and Symptoms

Signs and symptoms of cirrhosis increase in severity as the disease progresses and are categorized as compensated or decompensated (Box 47-2). *Compensated cirrhosis* is less severe, and signs and symptoms are vague. As the disease progresses, it is referred to as *decompensated cirrhosis.* Signs and symptoms of decompensated cirrhosis are very pronounced and indicate liver failure.

The client's history often correlates with factors that predispose to cirrhosis, such as chronic alcohol use, hepatitis, or exposure to toxins. The client typically experiences chronic fatigue, anorexia, dyspepsia, nausea, vomiting, and diarrhea or constipation, with accompanying weight loss. Many clients report passing clay-colored or whitish stools as a result of no bile in the gastrointestinal (GI) tract. They may also report dark or "tea-colored" urine from increased concentrations of urobilin. Abdominal discomfort and shortness of breath are common complaints as a result of organ compression from the enlarged liver. Many clients mention nosebleeds, bleeding from the gums, or easy bruising. Skin may itch (pruritus) from accumulated bile salts.

A client with cirrhosis has an enlarged liver and sometimes an enlarged spleen, causing the abdomen to appear distended. Ascites occur late in the disease as a result of liver dysfunction and portal obstruction. Some clients will have peritonitis because of intestinal flora that migrates to the peritoneum. The skin, sclera, or oral mucous membranes are jaundiced. Edema may be present in the legs and feet. Vessels over the abdomen may be dilated (**caput medusae**). Gastric varices occur because blood flow through the liver is obstructed, leading to distended blood vessels throughout the entire GI tract, but most frequently in the upper GI tract. These vessels are not intended for high pressures and thus are prone to rupture and bleeding.

Because the dysfunctional liver cannot fully metabolize estrogen, men may present with *gynecomastia* (enlarged breasts) and testicular atrophy. *Palmar erythema* (bright pink palms) and *cutaneous spider angiomata* (tiny, spider-like blood vessels) may be visible. These findings are also related to an inability to inactivate estrogen. Vitamin deficiencies and anemia occur secondary to impaired GI function, poor dietary intake, and the body's inability to use or store vitamins, especially vitamins A, C, and K. For clients with bleeding disorders, the lack of vitamin K prevents effective clotting.

BOX 47-2 Clinical Manifestations of Cirrhosis

Compensated
- Intermittent mild fever
- Vascular spiders
- Palmar erythema (reddened palms)
- Unexplained epistaxis
- Ankle edema
- Vague morning indigestion
- Flatulent dyspepsia
- Abdominal pain
- Firm, enlarged liver
- Splenomegaly

Decompensated
- Ascites
- Jaundice
- Weakness
- Muscle wasting
- Weight loss
- Continuous mild fever
- Clubbing of fingers
- Purpura (owing to decreased platelet count)
- Spontaneous bruising
- Epistaxis
- Hypotension
- Sparse body hair
- White nails
- Gonadal atrophy

Diagnostic Findings

A liver biopsy, which reveals hepatic fibrosis, is the most conclusive diagnostic procedure. The biopsy is obtained percutaneously with mild sedation (see Nursing Guidelines 44-1, p. 755) or through a surgical incision. It can also be performed in the radiology department with ultrasound or computed tomography (CT) to identify appropriate placement of the trochar or biopsy needle.

Certain blood tests provide information about liver function (Box 47-3). Prolonged prothrombin time (PT) and low platelet count place the client at high risk for hemorrhage.

BOX 47-3 Common Blood Test Findings in Cirrhosis

Blood studies of clients with cirrhosis are likely to show the following:

- Increased unconjugated and conjugated bilirubin levels
- Consistently increased liver enzyme levels of AST, ALT, ALP, and GGT (elevated levels indicate liver and/or bile duct damage)
- Low RBC count—cells appear large
- Decreased leukocytes and thrombocytes
- Low fibrinogen level
- Prolonged PT
- Decreased platelet count
- Low serum albumin level
- Increased globulin level
- Hypokalemia

ALP, alkaline phosphatase; ALT, alanine aminotransferase; AST, aspartate transaminase; GGT, gamma-glutamyl transferase; RBC, red blood cell; PT, prothrombin time.

The client may receive intravenous (IV) administration of vitamin K or infusions of platelets before liver biopsy to reduce the risk of bleeding. Ultrasound scanning may be done to distinguish the density of scar tissue and parenchymal cells. Other tests used to examine the liver include CT, magnetic resonance imaging (MRI), and radioisotope liver scan, all of which may demonstrate the liver's enlarged size, nodular configuration, and distorted blood flow.

Medical and Surgical Management

No specific cure for cirrhosis exists. The principal aim of therapy is to prevent further deterioration by abolishing underlying causes and preserving what liver function remains. Various approaches are used to relieve associated symptoms. An optimal diet and vitamin and nutritional supplements promote healing of liver cells (Nutrition Notes 47-1). Improved nutritional status helps the client feel better. Malnutrition may be treated with enteral or parenteral feedings. Because absorption of the fat-soluble vitamins is impaired, special attention is given to their supplementation (see Table 44-1, p. 746). Vitamin K also is used to correct coagulopathy, which results from prolonged PT and partial thromboplastin time (PTT). Vitamin B complex, vitamin C, and iron also may be prescribed. IV albumin may be given if hypoproteinemia is severe. The client *must not* consume alcohol.

Altered ammonia metabolism may be responsible for precipitating hepatic encephalopathy (see Complications of Cirrhosis). Lactulose is administered to detoxify ammonium and to act as an osmotic agent, drawing water into the bowel, which causes diarrhea in some clients. Antacids or histamine type 2 (H_2)-receptor antagonists may be used to reduce gastric disturbances and to decrease the potential for GI bleeding. Potassium-sparing antidiuretics such as spironolactone are used to treat ascites (see Complications of Cirrhosis).

Transfusions of platelets may be necessary to correct thrombocytopenia (low platelet count). Packed RBCs may be administered in cases of anemia or blood loss.

Nutrition Notes 47-1

The Client With Cirrhosis

- Nutrition therapy for clients with cirrhosis is individualized according to symptoms and tolerance.
- Dietary restrictions are used only when they can be expected to improve symptoms. Fat is restricted for clients with fat malabsorption (steatorrhea). Medium-chain triglyceride oil may be given for calories when fat intake is limited. Sodium is restricted to 2 g/day when ascites is present. Fluid restriction is imposed in clients with hyponatremia.
- A high-calorie diet is recommended for clients with malnutrition, weight loss, or infection. Adequate calories are essential to ensure protein sparing. A high-protein diet is used to prevent muscle wasting. A protein-restricted diet is no longer recommended for most people with hepatic encephalopathy because it may worsen malnutrition and muscle wasting, and protein intolerance is much less common than previously thought.
- A carbohydrate-controlled diet is used for clients with diabetes or insulin resistance.
- Small, frequent meals and the use of nutritional supplements may help boost intake in clients who have nausea, vomiting, or fatigue.

Cholestyramine may be prescribed to bind bile salts and relieve pruritus. Additional measures to relieve pruritus include skin care and routine cleansing with a nondrying agent. Skin is patted dry, and moisturizing lotion is applied immediately after bathing. Ursodeoxycholic acid (Actigall) may be used to promote bile flow from the liver. Sodium intake is carefully regulated and often restricted because of the potential for water retention, which can lead to edema, circulatory congestion, and heart failure. Fluid intake also may be restricted. Liver transplantation is an option for treating liver failure as well as chronic liver disease (Box 47-4).

Nursing Management

If the client has active alcoholism, the nurse monitors vital signs closely. A rise in blood pressure (BP), pulse, and temperature correlates with alcohol withdrawal; the nurse must recognize and treat these appropriately along with the other presenting symptoms (see Chapter 71).

The nurse weighs the client daily and keeps an accurate record of intake and output. If the abdomen appears enlarged, the nurse measures it according to a set routine (Fig. 47-4). Because of the anorexia that accompanies severe cirrhosis, the client may better tolerate frequent, small, semisolid, or liquid meals rather than three full meals a day.

Careful evaluation of the client's response to drug therapy is important because the liver cannot metabolize many substances. The nurse reports any change in mental status or signs of GI bleeding immediately because they indicate secondary complications.

The nurse provides educational information specific to the liver disorder. They can refer the client to the American Liver Foundation (or a similar organization) for information

BOX 47-4 Liver Transplants and Organ Donation

The United Network for Organ Sharing (UNOS) is a private, nonprofit organization that manages the nation's organ transplant system under contract with the federal government. Through this network, the organization adds clients who need transplants to a national waiting list and generates a list of potential recipients when a donor organ becomes available. The UNOS bases its list of potential recipients on such factors as genetic similarity, organ size, medical urgency, and time on the waiting list. Only medical and logistical factors are used in organ matching. Personal or social characteristics such as celebrity status, income, or insurance coverage play no role in transplant priority.

Many transplanted livers are from cadaver donors. Some centers, however, now have "living related donor" programs, in which portions of livers for transplantation come from living donors. In either type of transplant, recipients need lifelong immunosuppressant therapy to suppress the immune system and prevent rejection of the transplanted organ.

The organs available are nowhere close to the number needed. Many potential recipients succumb to liver failure while waiting for donor organs. Transplantation costs are high, and the condition of potential recipients is fragile, jeopardizing the chances for successful transplantation. The decision to do a liver transplantation is based on careful scrutiny and assessment of the client, with consideration of the potential for success and improved quality of life.

From United Network for Organ Sharing. (2021). https://www.unos.org/

about available support groups. The nurse emphasizes the need for abstinence from alcohol and all nonprescription drugs unless approved by the primary provider. In addition, they contact social services about referrals to alcohol or drug cessation programs. Additional teaching depends on the type and cause of the disorder and the primary provider's prescribed or recommended home care (Client and Family Teaching 47-1). See Nursing Care Plan 47-1 later in this chapter for a description of additional nursing management.

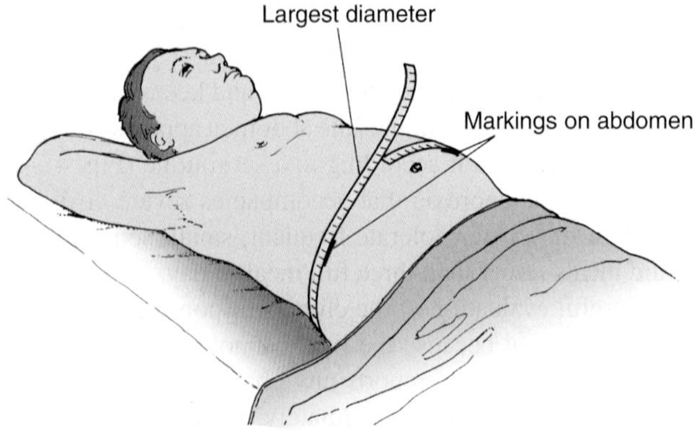

Figure 47-4 To measure abdominal girth, place a tape measure around the largest diameter of the abdomen. Make guide marks on the skin so that future measurements are obtained from the same site.

Client and Family Teaching 47-1
Cirrhosis

The following topics are appropriate for a teaching plan:

- Follow the diet recommended by the primary provider.
- Consult a dietitian if you require a special diet (e.g., a low-sodium diet to prevent edema and ascites). Many metabolic liver disorders require highly specialized diets and necessitate extensive teaching from nursing and nutritional staff. Some diets require routine monitoring and home care.
- Avoid situations that could further damage the liver, such as drinking alcohol, taking tranquilizers, or inhaling chemicals such as benzene or vinyl chloride, which are toxic.
- Rest frequently, especially if activity causes fatigue.
- Avoid exposure to people with known infections.
- Continue skin care.
- Avoid nonprescription drugs (especially aspirin and products that contain it because they contribute to bleeding problems) unless approved by the primary provider.
- Be prepared for rejection as a blood donor because of liver disease.
- Contact the primary provider immediately about vomiting of blood, tarry stools, extreme fatigue, yellow skin, light-colored stools, or dark urine.

Complications of Cirrhosis

Portal Hypertension

The portal system consists of gastric veins from the stomach, the mesenteric vein from the intestines, the splenic vein from the spleen and pancreas, and the portal vein. All these veins drain into and through the liver and out the hepatic veins into the inferior vena cava.

In the scarred cirrhotic liver, intrahepatic veins may be compressed. Consequently, blood backs up into the portal system, which is the venous pathway through the liver. This congestion and increased fluid pressure in the portal system are called **portal hypertension**. As the normal pathway for blood is obstructed, the collateral veins become distended and engorged with blood (Fig. 47-5). These distended collateral vessels develop primarily in the esophagus (esophageal varices) and rectum (hemorrhoids) and on the abdominal surface (caput medusae). Clients with portal hypertension can experience the following signs and symptoms:

- GI bleeding as evidenced by vomiting of blood, or black, tarry stools or bloody stools
- Ascites
- Encephalopathy
- Decreased platelets

Methods of treating portal hypertension aim to reduce fluid accumulation and venous pressure. Administration of a beta-adrenergic blocker, such as propranolol (Inderal), reduces BP and lowers pressure in the portal system. Sodium is restricted. A diuretic, usually an aldosterone antagonist such as spironolactone (Aldactone), is prescribed (Drug

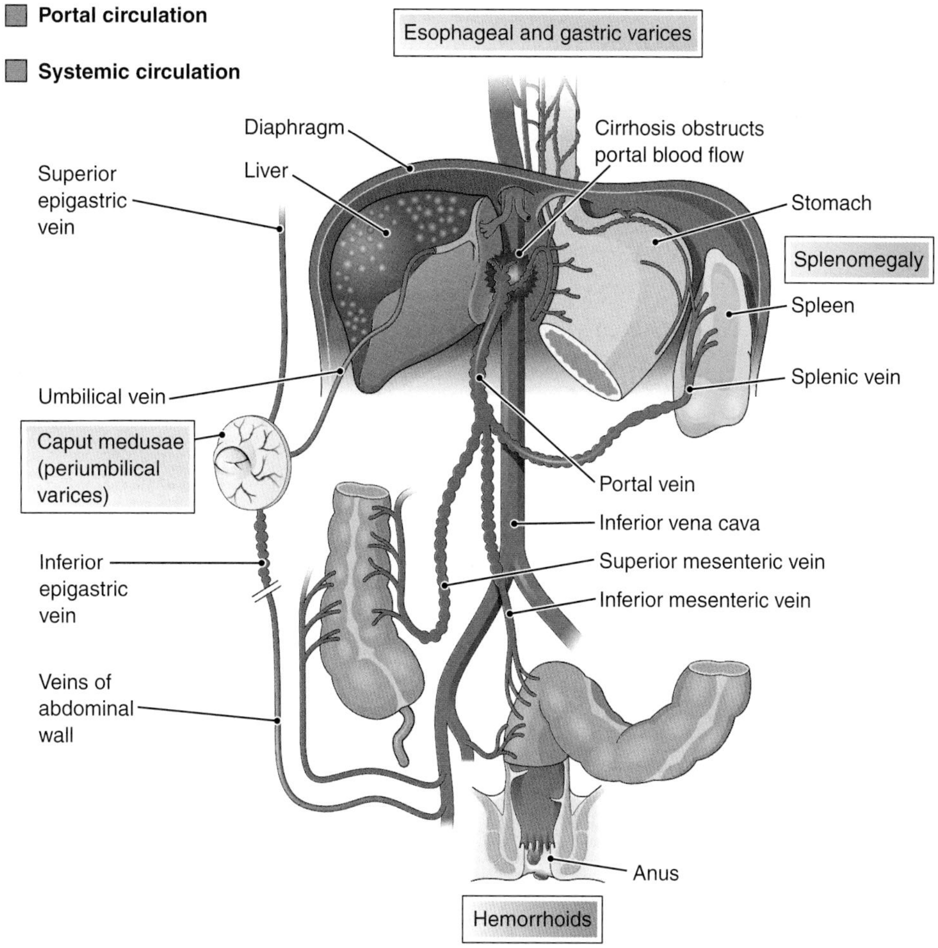

Figure 47-5 Portal hypertension results from obstruction of blood in the portal circulation in cirrhosis and other disorders. With the increased pressure, collateral vessels become distended, primarily in the esophagus, rectum, and abdominal surface.

Therapy Table 47-1). Diuretics such as furosemide (Lasix) also may be given to promote urinary excretion of excess fluids. These diuretics must be administered with caution, however, because long-term use can cause sodium depletion.

A *surgical shunt* may be created. This procedure uses a graft to decompress the portal system by diverting blood flow into the systemic circulation. It is not frequently performed, however, because of the high incidence of complications and shunt failure. An alternative, nonsurgical method of shunt placement is a *transjugular intrahepatic portosystemic shunt* (TIPS). This invasive radiologic procedure involves the creation of a tract from the hepatic to the portal vein. In TIPS, a cannula with an expandable stent is inserted into the portovenous system through the jugular vein. The stent serves as the intrahepatic shunt between the hepatic vein and portal circulation to relieve portal hypertension. TIPS may be carried out using conscious sedation or anesthesia (see Chapter 14).

Esophageal Varices

Dilated, bulging esophageal veins are referred to as **esophageal varices**. A single dilated, bulging esophageal vein is called a *varix*. Esophageal varices overfill as a result of portal hypertension. They are especially vulnerable to bleeding because they lie superficially in the mucosa, contain little protective elastic tissue, and are easily traumatized by rough food or chemical irritation. Figure 47-6 depicts the pathogenesis of esophageal varices.

Esophageal bleeding is a cardinal sign of esophageal varices. It may be slight but chronic, or massive and rapid. Massive bleeding from esophageal varices is a life-threatening medical emergency requiring immediate intervention. Once bleeding begins, clotting disorders common to liver damage occur. Barium swallow or esophagoscopy confirm the diagnosis of esophageal varices. A CT scan and/or MRI may also be done to further delineate esophageal varices.

Measures to treat portal hypertension reduce the potential for bleeding varices. In addition, a soft diet and elimination of alcohol, aspirin, and other locally irritating substances may prevent varices. Antitussives and stool softeners are prescribed when the client is symptomatic to reduce coughing or straining, which increases vascular pressure.

Esophageal varices also are treated with injection sclerotherapy or variceal banding. In **injection sclerotherapy** (also referred to as *endoscopic sclerotherapy*), the primary provider passes an endoscope orally to locate the varix.

DRUG THERAPY TABLE 47-1 Selected Medications Used for Liver and Pancreatic Disorders

Category and Common Generic (Brand) Drugs	Intended Use	Common Side Effects	Safety Warnings for Nurses
Liver Disorders			
Palliative treatment of cirrhosis			
Antibiotic/ammonia reduction kanamycin (Kantrex)	Hepatic encephalopathy, destroys GI ammonia forming bacteria	Nausea, vomiting, diarrhea	Can be nephrotoxic
Laxative/ammonia reduction *Hyperosmotic agents* lactulose (Cephulac) lubiprostone (Amitiza)	Hepatic encephalopathy, binds with ammonia to remove from blood	Headache, nausea, diarrhea	Syrups contain sugars, caution with diabetics
Diuretic spironolactone (Aldactone)	Blocks aldosterone which reduces 3rd space fluids (ascites)	Hyperkalemia	Monitor serum potassium and renal function at day 3, week 1, monthly × 3, 4 × yearly while taking drug Gynecomastia in men
Vitamins K (Mephyton) B complex C	Promotes blood coagulation in bleeding conditions resulting from liver disease Enhances neurotransmission Tissue building		Bleeding assessed by prothrombin time Avoid IV/IM owing to anaphylaxis
Octreotide (Sandostatin)	Bleeding esophageal varices by reducing blood pressure in portal veins, reducing blood flow	Headache, dizziness	Monitor cardiac status for dysrhythmias Possible biliary/gallstone formation
Agents used to treat hepatitis C infections			
Boceprevir (Victrelis) Daclatasvir (Daklinza) Simeprevir (Olysio) Sofosbuvir (Sovaldi)	Prevents replication of hepatitis C virus	Flu-like symptoms	Monitor for liver failure
Combinations Ribavirin/interferon (Copegus) Ledipasvir/sofosbuvir (Harvoni) Ombitasvir/paritaprevir/ritonavir (Technivie) Ombitasvir/paritaprevir/ritonavir/dasabuvlr (Viekira Pak)			Monitor for liver failure Women must use two forms of nonhormonal birth control up to 6 months following treatment
Pancreatic Disorders—Enzyme Replacement			
Pancrelipase (Creon, Pancreaze, Creon, Zenpep, Ultresa, Viokace Pertzye)	Lipase, protease, and amylase supplement for pancreatic insufficiency	Nausea, diarrhea	If given to infants, do not mix with breast milk Products not interchangeable

The drugs in column 1 indicate the drug that matches up with explanations in columns 2 through 4.

They then pass a thin needle through the endoscope into the varix and then directly inject a sclerosing agent (sodium tetradecyl, sodium morrhuate). The sclerosing agent solidifies and stops circulation to the varix.

In *variceal banding* (*variceal band ligation*), another endoscopic procedure, the primary provider uses a device with small rubber bands at the end of the endoscope. After locating the varix, the primary provider places a rubber band over it. The band restricts blood flow to the varix, which sloughs off after a few days. Persistent portal hypertension allows varices to form again, making it necessary to repeat sclerotherapy or banding procedures regularly.

Another procedure involves placing a distal splenorenal shunt (DSRS). The splenic vein is detached from the portal vein and reattached to the left renal vein. This procedure helps reduce pressure in the varices and controls bleeding.

Acute hemorrhage from esophageal varices is life-threatening. Resuscitative measures include administration of IV fluids and blood products. IV octreotide (Sandostatin) is started as soon as possible. Octreotide reduces pressure in

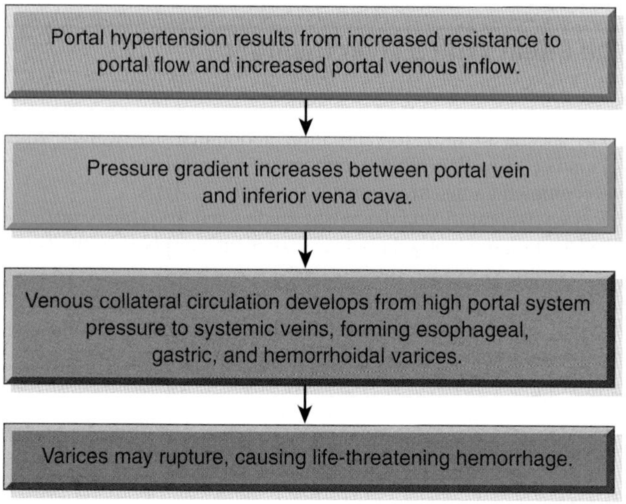

Figure 47-6 Pathogenesis of esophageal varices.

the portal venous system and is preferred to the previously used agents, vasopressin or terlipressin. Urgent endoscopy is indicated to allow for treatment with sclerotherapy or banding. If a skilled endoscopist is not available, or bleeding is too rapid to permit endoscopy, **balloon tamponade** with a Sengstaken–Blakemore tube may be useful in compressing the varices and stemming the flow of blood (Fig. 47-7). Unfortunately, this method usually allows only temporary relief from hemorrhage, necessitating endoscopy with sclerotherapy or banding after the client's condition is stabilized.

Ascites

Ascites is the collection of fluid in the peritoneal cavity. Undoubtedly, portal hypertension is a major underlying factor in the development of ascites. It leads to a cascade of events, referred to as the **hepatorenal syndrome**, which ultimately alters fluid distribution and interferes with fluid excretion.

Increased pressure in the portal system forces serum proteins into the peritoneal cavity. The proteins draw plasma from the circulating blood by osmosis. The kidneys respond to decreases in blood volume and renal BP by initiating the renin–angiotensin–aldosterone system (see Chapter 27). In response, the body conserves sodium ions, which further contributes to fluid retention. Low renal blood volume also may suppress antidiuretic hormone, causing water to be reabsorbed rather than eliminated as urine. These combined factors promote fluid accumulation in the abdomen. Ascites is visible as extensive and massive abdominal swelling.

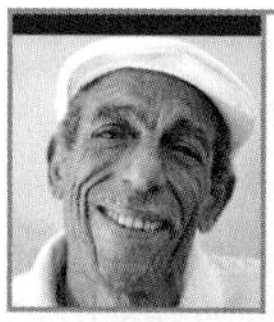

Clinical Scenario A 64-year-old client is hospitalized with cirrhosis of the liver related to a long history of alcoholism and substance abuse. The client presents with jaundice. He complains of feeling weak and reports a steady loss of weight for several weeks. The muscles appear wasted. What are important foci when caring for a client with multiple symptoms related to liver disease? See Nursing Care Plan 47-1.

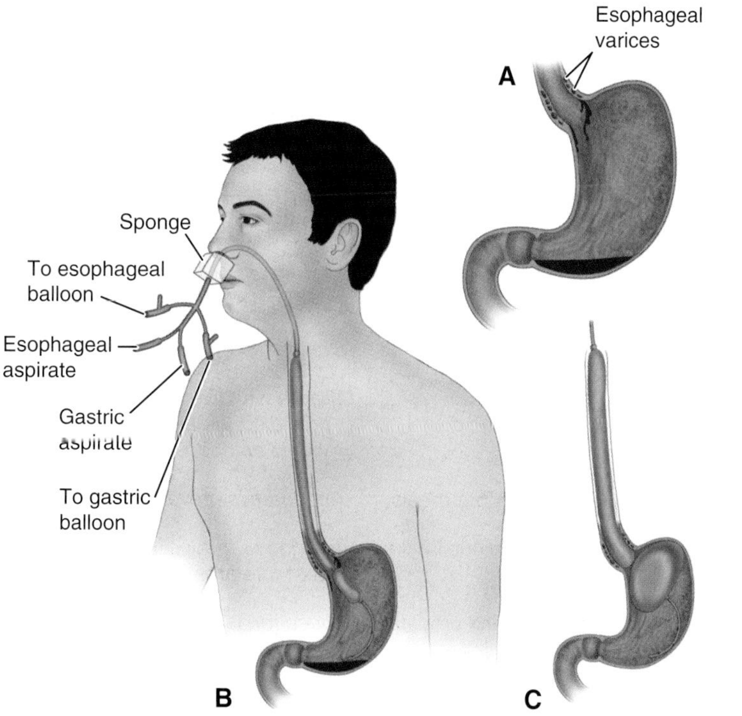

Figure 47-7 Balloon tamponade to treat esophageal varices. **(A)** Dilated, bleeding esophageal veins (varices). **(B)** A Sengstaken–Blakemore tube in place with uninflated balloons in the esophagus and stomach. The tube has four separate openings: Two are used to inflate the two balloons, and two allow for aspiration of esophageal and gastric secretions. **(C)** Inflated balloons compress bleeding esophageal varices.

NURSING CARE PLAN 47-1 The Client With a Liver Disorder

Assessment

- Obtain complete diet, drug, and allergy histories and a history of symptoms from client or family. Depending on the circumstances, in-depth questioning may be necessary. Contributing factors may include exposure to toxic chemicals, history of hepatitis, or long-term alcohol abuse.
- Pay special attention to ventilation, abdominal size, weight, and jaundice as well as other symptoms of liver disease.
- Recommend a nutrition consult for intake analysis.
- Review laboratory and diagnostic studies and the primary provider's progress notes daily to assess client's response to therapy.

Nursing Diagnosis. **Activity Intolerance** related to fatigue and malaise

Expected Outcome. Client will engage in ways to conserve energy and will report improved energy levels.

Interventions	Rationales
Assess client's ability to perform activities of daily living and pattern of fatigue.	*Data provide a baseline for comparison and help nurse and client to target ways to conserve energy.*
Assist client to set small, short-term goals that will be easy to achieve.	*Such goals help the client accomplish tasks without being overwhelmed or exhausted.*
Encourage client to separate essential and nonessential tasks and to delegate.	*Doing so creates a realistic picture of what must be done and who should do it.*
Encourage the client to limit demands on their time.	*Doing so helps the client set priorities and balance demands with available energy.*
Teach strategies for energy conservation such as sitting instead of standing in the shower, storing items within easy reach, and breaking large tasks into smaller ones.	*These strategies enhance energy and give a client more control over activities.*
Offer a high-protein (if client does not have severe liver disease) and high-calorie diet.	*Inadequate nutrition contributes to fatigue.*
Encourage client to rest frequently.	*Inadequate sleep contributes to fatigue.*

Evaluation of Expected Outcome

Client begins to participate in appropriate activities, gradually increases activities, and reports feeling stronger and more energetic.

Nursing Diagnosis. Malnutrition Risk. related to loss of appetite, nausea, and vomiting

Expected Outcome. Client will identify nutritional requirements and consume adequate nutrition.

Interventions	Rationales
Encourage client to eat six small meals a day.	*Small, frequent meals reduce the sensation of fullness and the stimulus for vomiting.*
Consult the dietitian for ways to provide nutritional meals that complement the prescribed diet.	*Such meals will provide foods that the client is likely to eat within dietary restrictions.*
Provide high-carbohydrate snacks or supplements to meals.	*Doing so provides additional calories.*
Offer highest-calorie meal when the client's appetite is greatest.	*Clients with liver disease usually are hungriest at breakfast, so providing the highest-calorie meal at the beginning of the day would be most logical.*
If vomiting is a problem, administer antiemetics before meals.	*Antiemetics prevent nausea and vomiting.*
Monitor food intake and ask dietitian to calculate caloric intake.	*Tracking nutritional intake provides a record of foods the client best tolerates at different times of the day.*
Ask family members to assist with meal planning and preparation, adapting to the client's cultural preferences.	*These measures enhance the client's ability to eat preferred foods and meet nutritional requirements within dietary restrictions.*

Evaluation of Expected Outcome

Client reports improved appetite, identifies appropriate foods that meet dietary requirements, and demonstrates appropriate weight gain.

NURSING CARE PLAN 47-1 The Client With a Liver Disorder (*continued*)

Nursing Diagnosis. **Altered Breathing Pattern** related to ascites and liver enlargement

Expected Outcome. Client will breathe without effort.

Interventions	Rationales
Assess respiratory pattern, noting what causes and relieves dyspnea.	*Assessing the cause of dyspnea helps the nurse provide relief measures and improves client's ventilatory efforts.*
Elevate head of bed at least 30 degrees.	*Elevating the head reduces abdominal pressure on the diaphragm and facilitates lung expansion.*
Schedule rest periods after activity.	*Rest reduces metabolic and oxygen requirements.*
Provide supplemental oxygen if client becomes short of breath.	*Oxygen therapy decreases dyspnea by reducing the central drive mediated by chemoreceptors in the carotid bodies.*

Evaluation of Expected Outcome

Client reports decreased shortness of breath and improved comfort with breathing.

Nursing Diagnosis. **Fluid Overload Risk** related to peripheral edema, ascites, and sodium retention

Expected Outcome. Client will maintain fluid balance.

Interventions	Rationales
Assess location and extent of edema. Measure and record abdominal girth daily.	*These measures help locate changes in peripheral edema and ascites.*
Monitor weight daily.	*Abdominal girth and weight reflect changes in body fluid volume.*
Restrict sodium and fluid intake as ordered.	*Such restrictions reduce peripheral edema and ascites.*
Administer prescribed diuretics and potassium.	*These measures promote fluid excretion through the kidneys to maintain fluid and electrolyte balance.*
Monitor serum albumin levels. Administer protein supplements as ordered.	*Low albumin levels can cause severe peripheral edema because they lead to impaired movement of fluid from interstitial spaces to intravascular spaces.*
Maintain IV infusion rates carefully.	*Doing so prevents inadvertent infusion of excess fluid volumes.*
Encourage client to turn at least every 2 hours when in bed.	*Edematous tissue is vulnerable to ischemia and pressure ulcers.*

Evaluation of Expected Outcome

Client maintains fluid balance as evidenced by stable BP, adequate urine output, and decreased peripheral edema and ascites.

Nursing Diagnosis. **Bleeding Risk and/or Infection Risk** related to risk for impaired blood coagulation, bleeding from portal hypertension, and infection

Expected Outcome. Client will have no evidence of new bleeding or infection.

Interventions	Rationales
Carefully monitor vital signs.	*Changes may indicate the onset of bleeding or infection.*
Notify primary provider promptly when client has signs of infection: fever, chills, or drainage.	*Prompt treatment reduces the risk of morbidity and mortality.*
Monitor bleeding times, clotting studies, and platelet counts.	*Abnormal results indicate increased risk for bleeding.*
Teach client to avoid aspirin or nonsteroidal anti-inflammatory drugs and to use electric razors and toothbrushes.	*These drugs can cause GI bleeding, and aspirin interferes with platelet function. Electric razors and soft toothbrushes can minimize unnecessary trauma.*

(*continued*)

NURSING CARE PLAN 47-1 The Client With a Liver Disorder (*continued*)

Practice aseptic measures and teach family members to do so.	*Asepsis reduces the risk of infection.*
Observe stools for color and consistency.	*Tests detect blood in stool and may indicate issues with GI bleeding.*
Test stool for occult blood.	
Note any complaints of anxiety, epigastric fullness, weakness, and restlessness.	*These findings may indicate bleeding and early shock.*
Monitor for ecchymosis, epistaxis, petechiae, and bleeding from gums.	*These findings indicate altered clotting mechanisms.*
Monitor client carefully during blood transfusions.	*Doing so can help detect a transfusion reaction.*
Administer vitamin K as ordered.	*Vitamin K promotes clotting.*

Evaluation of Expected Outcome

Client does not exhibit any new signs of bleeding or infection. Vital signs are stable, and laboratory values are normal.

Nursing Diagnosis. Altered Skin Integrity related to pruritus, jaundice, bleeding tendencies, and edema

Expected Outcome. Skin will remain intact.

Interventions	Rationales
Provide frequent skin care, avoid drying soaps and alcohol-based lotions.	*Skin care removes waste products deposited in skin and prevents drying.*
Encourage client to keep fingernails short and smooth.	*Doing so prevents excoriation and infection from scratches.*
Turn client at least every 2 hours, massaging bony prominences with emollients.	*Turning and massage mobilize edema and improve circulation.*
Use nonallergenic bed linens; instruct family to avoid harsh detergents.	*These measures decrease skin irritation.*

Evaluation of Expected Outcome

Skin remains intact with no evidence of pressure ulcers.

Nursing Diagnosis. Chronic Pain related to liver enlargement and ascites

Expected Outcome. Client will report increased level of comfort.

Interventions	Rationales
Encourage client to remain on bed rest when experiencing abdominal discomfort, changing position frequently.	*These measures relieve pressure and promote comfort.*
Administer prescribed analgesics.	*These drugs relieve chronic pain.*
Explain the pain management regimen.	*Adequate explanations help the client understand implementation of the pain-control plan.*
For client receiving opioids, monitor sedation and respiratory status when dose is increased.	*Usually, clients receiving long-term opioids develop a tolerance to the respiratory depressant effects. They still require monitoring for sedation and respiratory problems.*
Instruct client in nonpharmacologic techniques to relieve pain.	*Other interventions supplement pain medications and improve comfort level.*

Evaluation of Expected Outcome

Client reports that pain medication is effective and that comfort is improved.

NURSING CARE PLAN 47-1 The Client With a Liver Disorder (*continued*)

RC of Hepatic Encephalopathy

Expected Outcome. The nurse will minimize and manage problems associated with hepatic encephalopathy.

Interventions	Rationales
Assess cognitive and neurologic status at least every 8 hours.	*Baseline data provide a means by which to determine change.*
Restrict dietary protein as ordered.	*Protein is a source of ammonia, which contributes to encephalopathy.*
Give small and frequent feedings high in carbohydrates.	*Carbohydrates provide energy and space protein breakdown.*
Restrict medications that increase encephalopathy.	*Sedatives, hypnotics, and opioids may precipitate hepatic encephalopathy and increase confusion.*
Monitor laboratory results, especially ammonia levels.	*Increased ammonia levels indicate hepatic encephalopathy, which can lead to coma.*
Administer medications that reduce serum ammonia levels, such as lactulose.	*Reduced serum ammonia levels are a key goal.*
Identify potentially dangerous items and modify the environment.	*Doing so promotes the client's safety.*
Report any new or sudden increase in mental confusion.	*Confusion indicates increased hepatic encephalopathy and possible coma. It requires immediate medical intervention.*
Orient client to name, place, time, and date as needed.	*Doing so reinforces reality and provides the client with cues about the world.*
If hepatic coma develops, monitor respiratory status and initiate measures to prevent complications.	*Clients in hepatic coma are at increased risk for pneumonia and infection.*
Implement measures to prevent skin breakdown and pressure.	*These clients are at increased risk for skin breakdown and pressure ulcers.*

Evaluation of Expected Outcome

Client remains free from injury.

Abdominal paracentesis may be performed to remove ascitic fluid. Abdominal fluid is rapidly removed by careful introduction of a needle through the abdominal wall, allowing the fluid to drain. This usually eases severe discomfort caused by distension and relieves breathing difficulty secondary to a high volume of abdominal fluid pressing on the diaphragm and lungs. Up to 5 to 6 L of fluid may be removed over 60 to 90 minutes. IV albumin is simultaneously infused to pull fluid back into the vascular space. Monitoring of BP and urine output is crucial to evaluate the effects of the fluid shifts. Diuretic therapy is prescribed if the circulatory volume becomes excessive.

Additional treatment includes maintenance diuretic therapy and a sodium-restricted diet. The potassium-sparing diuretic spironolactone (Aldactone) may be chosen because it specifically antagonizes the hormone aldosterone. Reversing the effects of aldosterone causes the excretion of sodium and water, retention of potassium, and reduction of ascitic fluid.

If ascites repeatedly develop despite conservative treatment, the primary provider may surgically insert an internal catheter to redirect the ascitic fluid back into the vascular space. (See the section on Portal Hypertension under Complications of Cirrhosis for more information.)

Hepatic Encephalopathy

Hepatic encephalopathy, or portosystemic encephalopathy, is a central nervous system (CNS) manifestation of liver failure that often leads to coma and death. This neurologic complication is related to an increased serum ammonia level but not singularly. Ammonia forms in the intestine by bacterial action on ingested proteins. The liver normally detoxifies ammonia by converting it to urea, which the kidneys then excrete in urine. A failing liver, as in advanced cirrhosis, can no longer break down ammonia, causing it to accumulate in the blood. Ammonia can cross the blood–brain barrier and enter brain cells, where it interferes with brain metabolism, cell membrane pump mechanisms, and neurotransmission.

Indications of CNS effects include disorientation, drowsiness, confusion, personality changes, mood swings, agitation, memory loss, a flapping tremor called *asterixis*, a positive Babinski reflex, slightly sulfurous (fecal) breath odor (referred to as **fetor hepaticus**), and lethargy to deep coma. Symptoms usually worsen after the client eats a high-protein meal or has active GI bleeding, because both dietary protein and digested blood cells increase ammonia volume in the intestine. In addition to an elevated serum ammonia level, electroencephalography may show abnormal waveforms.

Treatment includes eliminating dietary protein; removing residual protein (such as blood if the client had a recent GI hemorrhage); and depleting intestinal microorganisms with drugs, laxatives, and enema therapy. Antibiotics, such as neomycin or kanamycin (Kantrex), which are poorly absorbed from the GI tract, are prescribed to destroy intestinal microorganisms and thereby decrease ammonia production. The administration of lactulose (Cephulac) reduces the serum ammonia concentration. In the colon, lactulose splits into lactic acid and acetic acid, attracts ammonia from the blood, and forms a compound that can be eliminated in the feces. Levodopa (L-dopa) is a precursor of dopamine that restores normal neurotransmission in the brain. Supportive measures include administering IV fluids containing electrolytes and multivitamins or total parenteral nutrition (TPN).

The prognosis for clients with hepatic encephalopathy is grim. Only a few survive without a liver transplant. Clients who do survive face a prolonged rehabilitation.

Hepatitis

Hepatitis is inflammation of the liver. The disease may be acute or chronic.

Pathophysiology and Etiology

The liver may become inflamed shortly after exposure to hepatotoxic chemicals or drugs, after lengthy alcohol abuse, or by invasion with an infectious microorganism. The most common cause of hepatitis is a viral infection, which is the focus of this discussion. The letters A, B, C, D, E, and G identify the viruses that infect the liver (Table 47-3). The modes of transmission and incubation periods differentiate

TABLE 47-3 Forms of Viral Hepatitis

TYPE	CAUSE	MODE OF TRANSMISSION	INCUBATION	SIGNS AND SYMPTOMS	OUTCOME
Hepatitis A (previously called *infectious hepatitis*)	Hepatitis A virus (HAV)	Oral route from feces and saliva of persons who are infected; water, food, and equipment contaminated with HAV	3–5 weeks	May occur with or without symptoms; flu-like illness Preicteric phase: headache, malaise, fatigue, anorexia, fever Icteric phase: dark urine, jaundice, tender liver	Usually mild with full recovery; fatality rate <1%; no carrier state or increased risk of chronic hepatitis, cirrhosis, or hepatic cancer
Hepatitis B (previously called *serum hepatitis*)	Hepatitis B virus (HBV)	Infected blood or plasma; needles, syringes, surgical or dental equipment contaminated with infected blood; also sexually transmitted through vaginal secretions and semen of carriers or those actively infected	2–5 months	Arthralgias, rash; anorexia, dyspepsia, abdominal pain; generalized malaise, weakness, and aching; jaundice may be present and accompanied by clay-colored stools and dark urine; may occur without symptoms	May be severe; fatality rate 1%–10%; carrier state possible; increased risk of chronic hepatitis, cirrhosis, and hepatic cancer; some people who are infected become carriers
Hepatitis C (previously called *non-A, non-B hepatitis—NANB*)	Hepatitis C virus (HCV); may be more than one virus	Infected blood or blood products; sexual contact	2–20 weeks	Similar to HBV, although less severe and without jaundice	Frequent occurrence of chronic carrier state and chronic liver disease; increased risk of hepatic cancer
Hepatitis D (also called *delta hepatitis*)	Hepatitis D virus (HDV)	Same as HBV; cannot infect alone; occurs as dual infection with HBV	2–5 months	Similar to HBV	Similar to HBV with greater likelihood of carrier state, chronic active hepatitis, and cirrhosis
Hepatitis E	Hepatitis E virus (HEV)	Fecal–oral routes; low risk of person–person contact; found more in countries with poor sanitation and water quality	2–9 weeks	Similar to HAV—very severe in pregnant women	Similar to HAV—very severe in pregnant women
Hepatitis G	Hepatitis G virus (HGV, GB virus C, or GBV-C)	Infected blood or blood products	14–145 days	Similar to HCV	Causes persistent infection; does not affect clinical course or cause chronic liver disease

BOX 47-5 Risk Factors for Acquiring Blood-Borne Hepatitis

- History of illicit IV drug use
- Occupational exposure through sharps injuries (needlesticks)
- Perinatal exposure (child born to woman who has hepatitis)
- Blood transfusion
- Organ transplant
- Exposure to contaminated equipment that penetrates the skin (includes tattoos and body piercings)
- Sexual contact with a person who is infected
- Hemodialysis
- Impaired immune response

each virus. Box 47-5 lists risk factors for the spread of hepatitis through infected blood.

Once the virus invades the *hepatocytes* (liver cells), it alters their structure. An immune reaction ensues, in which the infected cells become inflamed and dysfunctional. The active disease process affects the uptake, conjugation, and excretion of bilirubin.

Most people recover from acute infection, but a few suffer from chronic active hepatitis and subsequent liver damage. In chronic persistent hepatitis (most common with hepatitis B, C, and D), liver damage does not worsen, but it does not improve, and the liver remains enlarged. Some clients may develop cirrhosis. Others deteriorate rapidly with liver failure and die unless liver transplantation is performed. Invasion of the transplanted liver by the virus is common, but it usually takes years before the newly transplanted liver develops cirrhosis.

Transmission of Hepatitis

Hepatitis A virus (HAV) and hepatitis E virus are usually transmitted via the oral–fecal route (eating or drinking something contaminated by the feces of a person who is infected). If food or drinking water is contaminated because of inadequate hand washing or poor sanitation, the virus can spread rapidly. Hepatitis A can also occur as a result of eating raw or undercooked shellfish from water contaminated by sewage. Occasionally, hepatitis A is transmitted via blood transfusions. Hepatitis A rarely leads to chronic illness, but clients may need to be hospitalized. Hepatitis E is not as common. It is self-limited, and there is no chronic form of the disease.

Hepatitis B and C are transmitted through the blood or sexual contact. Hepatitis B and C commonly are associated with hepatocellular carcinoma. Therefore, routine monitoring (e.g., blood test for alpha-fetoprotein and ultrasound) should be carried out for clients with chronic forms of these diseases. Hepatitis D occurs in some people infected with hepatitis B. It is similar to hepatitis B in terms of how infection occurs and how it is treated. Anti-delta antibodies are present when blood tests are done—this confirms the diagnosis.

Hepatitis G is considered to be non-A, non-B, and non-C disease. It occurs 14 to 145 days after a blood transfusion. It cannot be identified as can the other types, and thus it is designated type G. Hepatitis G is similar to hepatitis C.

Other types of hepatitis include the following:

- *Autoimmune hepatitis*: results from an abnormal immune system response. Treatment of this uncommon form consists of the administration of corticosteroids and immune-modulating agents (azathioprine or 6-mercaptopurine; see Drug Therapy Table 46-1). Without treatment, many of these clients will die or require a liver transplant.
- *Toxic hepatitis*: develops when certain chemicals toxic to the liver (e.g., chloroform, phosphorus, carbon tetrachloride) cause liver necrosis. Treatment includes removing the toxin and treating symptoms. If liver damage is severe and prolonged, the prognosis is not good without a liver transplant.
- *Drug-induced hepatitis*: occurs when a drug reaction damages the liver. This form of hepatitis can be severe and fatal. Examples of drugs that may cause a severe reaction are anesthetic agents, antidepressants, or anticonvulsants. High-dose corticosteroids are administered to treat the reaction. Liver transplantation may be necessary.

Pharmacologic Considerations

- Clients should know that more than 3000 mg of acetaminophen in a day can damage the liver. This over-the-counter pain reliever is also found in many cough and cold remedies. When taken together for cold and flu symptoms, the accumulative amount of acetaminophen can potentially harm a person's liver.

Assessment Findings

Signs and Symptoms

The signs and symptoms of the various forms of hepatitis sometimes are indistinguishable. The phases of all forms of hepatitis are as follows:

1. *Incubation phase*: the virus replicates within the liver; the client is asymptomatic. Late in this phase, the virus can be found in blood, bile, and stools (for hepatitis A). At this point, the client is considered infectious.
2. *Preicteric or prodromal phase*: nausea; vomiting; anorexia; fever; malaise; arthralgia; headache; right upper quadrant (RUQ) discomfort; enlargement of the spleen, liver, and lymph nodes; weight loss; rash; and urticaria.
3. *Icteric phase*: jaundice, pruritus, clay-colored or light stools, dark urine, fatigue, anorexia, and RUQ discomfort; symptoms of the preicteric phase may continue.
4. *Posticteric phase*: liver enlargement, malaise, and fatigue; other symptoms subside; liver function tests begin to return to normal.

Not all clients with hepatitis experience all the listed symptoms, and the severity of any one symptom may vary. Even though the symptoms are categorized, not all clients with hepatitis necessarily develop jaundice.

Diagnostic Findings

Serologic analysis can detect specific viral antibodies. RNA testing may be performed to identify the virus itself. Test results may take up to 1 week. The white blood cell (WBC) count may be elevated. Evidence of **cholestasis** (ineffective bile drainage) is seen with elevated bilirubin levels. Hepatic aminotransferase (alanine aminotransferase [ALT] and aspartate aminotransferase [AST]) levels rise during the incubation period and begin to fall once symptoms appear. Chronic disease may result in persistent elevation of the transaminases. A prolonged PT or PTT reflects poor synthetic liver function. Additional indicators of poor synthetic function include low blood glucose and serum albumin levels. Liver biopsy and histologic examination of the specimen allow for evaluation of the severity of the disease by identifying inflammation, fibrosis, and cirrhosis. Table 47-4 presents terms and abbreviations related to hepatitis and specific tests for types of hepatitis.

Medical and Surgical Management

Treatment is symptomatic and includes bed rest, a balanced diet of small feedings at intervals, and IV fluid administration if the client is extremely ill or has a low oral fluid intake. Supplementation of vitamins, especially the fat-soluble vitamins, is necessary regardless of oral intake because these vitamins are poorly absorbed. In some cases, antiemetics are given to relieve vomiting, but usually drug therapy is avoided until the liver recovers.

Recombinant interferon alfa-2b (Intron A) may be given to clients with chronic hepatitis B, C, and D to force the virus into remission. It frequently is administered in combination with ribavirin (Rebetol), a synthetic antiviral also used to treat respiratory syncytial virus infection. The combination therapy increases the likelihood of a sustained virus-free response (more than 6 months). Ribavirin may cause birth defects, so clients of childbearing age need to be counseled about using strict birth control methods while taking this drug.

For clients with chronic disease who do not respond to medical treatment, a liver transplantation may be performed (see Box 47-4). This involves total removal of the diseased liver and transplantation of a healthy liver in the same location. Immunosuppression must be done for transplantation to succeed. Immunosuppressant agents include cyclosporine, tacrolimus, sirolimus, corticosteroids, and azathioprine. The goal is to find immunosuppressive agents that effectively reduce rejection of transplanted organs and cause the fewest side effects.

Nursing Management

The nurse practices preventive techniques to control the spread of hepatitis viruses and teaches the family and general public how to reduce the risk of infection (Box 47-6). Nursing care in the early stages focuses on maintaining physical rest, supporting nutritional intake (Nutrition Notes 47-2), and preventing complications. Before discharge, the nurse teaches self-care measures to promote health and avoid transmitting the infection to others. The client must avoid alcohol and drugs that can further damage the liver. For clients who develop chronic active or persistent hepatitis and require liver transplants, see Nursing Process for the Client Having Surgery for a Liver Disorder.

TABLE 47-4 Hepatitis Terms and Abbreviations

Hepatitis A	
HAV	Hepatitis A virus
Anti-HAV	Antibody to HAV; appears in serum soon after onset of symptoms; disappears after 3–12 months
IgM anti-HAV	IgM antibody to HAV; indicates recent infection with HAV; positive up to 6 months after infection
Hepatitis B	
HBV	Hepatitis B virus; etiologic agent of hepatitis B
HBsAg	Hepatitis B surface antigen; indicates acute or chronic hepatitis B or carrier state; indicates infectious state
Anti-HBs	Antibody to HBsAg; indicates prior exposure and immunity to hepatitis; may indicate passive antibody from HBIG or immune response from hepatitis B vaccine
HBeAg	Hepatitis B e antigen; present in serum early in course; indicates highly infectious stage of hepatitis B; persistence in serum indicates progression to chronic hepatitis
Anti-HBe	Antibody to HBeAg; suggests low titer of HBV
HBcAg	Hepatitis B core antigen; found in liver cells; not easily detected in serum
Anti-HBc	Antibody to HBcAg; most sensitive indicator of HBV; appears late in the acute phase; indicates infection of HBV at some time in the past
IgM anti-HBc	IgM antibody to HBcAg; present for up to 6 months after infection
Hepatitis C	
HCV	Hepatitis C virus
Hepatitis D	
HDV	Hepatitis D virus; etiologic agent to hepatitis D; HBV required for replication
HDAg	Hepatitis delta antigen; detectable in early acute HDV infection
Anti-HDV	Antibody to HDV; indicates past or present infection with HDV
Hepatitis E	
HEV	Hepatitis E virus; etiologic agent of hepatitis E
Hepatitis G	
HGV	Hepatitis G virus

HBIG, hepatitis B immune globulin; IgM, immunoglobulin M.
Adapted from Hinkle, J. L., & Cheever, K. H. (2018). *Brunner & Suddarth's textbook of medical-surgical nursing* (14th ed., p. 1362). Wolters Kluwer.

>>> Stop, Think, and Respond 47-1

You are assigned to a client who is recovering from abdominal surgery. She tells you that the client in the next room has chronic hepatitis and that she is afraid she will catch it. Which answer would best help this client?

- *"Don't worry. That kind of hepatitis can only be transmitted sexually."*
- *"There are many kinds of hepatitis—do you know which kind she has?"*
- *"Hospital staff always use precautions to prevent any possibility of transmission of infectious diseases to other clients."*
- *"There is no problem—that client is not a carrier of the disease."*

BOX 47-6 Measures for Preventing Viral Hepatitis Transmission

Preventing Hepatitis A[a]

- Receive hepatitis A virus (HAV) vaccine, especially when considered at high risk (health care workers, day care workers, food preparers, foreign travel).
- Obtain immune globulin (IG) injection if exposed (in household or sexual contacts with infected individuals) to hepatitis without previous immunization.
- Observe standard precautions. Wear gloves if hands come into contact with body fluids; wear gown and face shield if body fluids may be splashed.
- Require child care staff to wear gloves during diaper changes and to perform adequate hand washing.
- Perform conscientious hand washing, even after removing gloves.
- Screen food handlers.
- Avoid eating from public salad bars and buffets that do not have sneeze guards or other hygienic devices and practices to prevent food contamination.
- Use liquid soap dispensers and hand dryers in public restrooms rather than bar soap and cloth towels.
- Avoid placing fingers and handheld objects in mouth.
- Do not share cigarettes, eating utensils, or beverage containers.
- Avoid eating raw seafood or seafood harvested from possibly polluted water.
- Use a pocket mask when giving pulmonary resuscitation.
- Drink bottled water in developing countries. Avoid ice unless it was made from bottled water.

Preventing Hepatitis B[b]

- Receive hepatitis B virus (HBV) vaccine, especially if in a high-risk category (dialysis, blood dyscrasias, IV drug abuser, homosexual, health care worker, school teacher).[c]
- Adhere to American Academy of Pediatrics guidelines for immunization.
- Obtain hepatitis B immune globulin (HBIG) if exposed to HBV and not previously vaccinated within 24 hours but no later than 7 days after blood contact.
- Observe standard precautions (wear gloves if hands may come into contact with body fluids; wear gown and face shield if body fluids may be splashed).
- Do not recap needles.
- Dispose of needles and other sharp objects in a puncture-resistant container.
- Use a condom when engaging in sexual intercourse.
- Do not share razors, fingernail tools, toothbrushes, or any personal care item that may come into contact with blood or body fluids.
- If contemplating surgery, investigate the possibility of donating and storing your own blood for later use.
- Wear a mouth shield when giving mouth-to-mouth resuscitation.

[a]Prevention of hepatitis A also prevents hepatitis E; no vaccine or postexposure treatment is available for hepatitis E.
[b]Prevention of hepatitis B also prevents hepatitis C, D, and G; no vaccine or postexposure treatment is available for hepatitis C, D, or G.
[c]Hepatitis B vaccination is not routinely given to older adults. In general, older adults should receive the vaccine only if they are traveling to areas where they may be exposed to the disease. Immunogenicity is somewhat reduced in older adults.

Nutrition Notes 47-2

The Client With Hepatitis

- Nutrition therapy for clients with hepatitis is based on symptoms and tolerance. Some clients may not require any nutrition intervention; others may need a high-calorie, high-protein diet to replenish losses and small, frequent meals to maximize intake.
- A high-protein diet of 1.5 to 2.0 g/kg is used to promote liver cell regeneration in clients with hepatitis.

Tumors of the Liver

A tumor of the liver is an abnormal mass of cells in the liver. Liver tumors may be benign or malignant (see Chapter 18). If malignant, the tumor may be a primary lesion (classified as a *hepatoma*) or a metastasis.

Pathophysiology and Etiology

Primary malignancies (hepatomas) are rare but appear to have an increased incidence in people with previous hepatitis B or D virus infections or cirrhosis, especially those with the postnecrotic form. The most common liver malignancy is a metastatic lesion from the breast, lung, or GI tract. Causes of benign liver tumors are tuberculosis and fungal and parasitic infections. Oral contraceptives and anabolic steroids also have been implicated in the development of benign hepatic lesions.

Tumor cells grow at an accelerated rate. They function in a disorganized manner and eventually impair the liver's physiologic activities. They may obstruct bile flow, leading to jaundice, liver failure, portal hypertension, and ascites.

Assessment Findings

Symptoms can be vague and confused with those of cirrhosis. Jaundice is common. Once the tumor is sufficiently large, the client may report pain in the RUQ. Weight loss and debilitation are common. The client usually experiences bleeding tendencies. Eventually, the abdomen becomes distended from liver enlargement and related ascites.

Alpha-fetoprotein, a serum protein normally produced during fetal development, is a marker that, if elevated, can indicate a primary malignant liver tumor. Total bilirubin and serum enzyme (ALT, AST, alkaline phosphatase) levels are elevated. A liver scan, ultrasonography, MRI, or CT scan identifies the tumor and its location. A biopsy, performed to identify the specific type of tumor cells, also can define and disclose damage to adjacent liver tissue. (See Evidence-Based Practice 47-1.)

Medical and Surgical Management

If the tumor is confined to a single lobe of the liver, a **hepatic lobectomy** (removal of a lobe of the liver) may be

Evidence Based Practice 47-1

Alpha-Fetoprotein Levels and Liver Cancer

Clinical Question

What does the diagnostic lab alpha-fetoprotein screen indicate in liver cancer?

Evidence

Adult liver cancer incidence is increasing. This could be linked to the increasing spread of hepatitis C virus. Alpha-fetoprotein (AFP) levels can be used as part of the diagnostic screening. The test can be elevated in the intrahepatic cancer and is sometimes indicated when there is also spreading from the colon. If the client has a possible tumor and the AFP level is high, it does not necessarily indicate liver cancer but it could be used to show that the tumor has reoccurred after diagnosis (National Institute of Health National Cancer Institute, n.d.).

Nursing Implications

Nurses should be educated in the types of diagnostic tests, procedures, and screening that may be needed in clients with liver cancer. This is important in educating the client on the procedure and supporting the client with any questions before and after the screenings or procedures are completed.

Reference

National Institute of Health National Cancer Institute (NIH). (n.d.). *Adult primary liver cancer treatment (PDQ®)–health professional version.* http://www.cancer.gov/types/liver/hp/adult-liver-treatment-pdq#link/_3_toc

attempted to remove primary malignant or benign tumors. Metastatic tumors usually are considered inoperable because they often are scattered throughout the liver. The frequency of metastasis and poor survival rate usually eliminate liver transplantation as a therapeutic option. Sometimes, biliary ducts obstructed by disease are bypassed with percutaneous biliary or transhepatic drainage. This is referred to as *percutaneous biliary drainage*. A catheter is inserted under fluoroscopy through the abdominal wall, past the obstruction, into the duodenum. This procedure relieves the pressure and pain caused by bile buildup and decreases jaundice and pruritus.

In some cases, *cryosurgery* or *cryoablation* is used. This technique uses liquid nitrogen at −196°C to destroy tumors. It is injected directly into the tumor through a cryoprobe. Two or three freeze-and-thaw cycles are administered through probes inserted with open laparotomy. Another procedure called *radiofrequency ablation* may be used to destroy cancer cells. This technique uses electric current to heat and destroy the cells. Ultrasound or CT scanning is required to guide the one or more needles used to pass the electric current. In addition, alcohol is sometimes used to kill cancer cells; pure alcohol is injected directly into the liver tumor (American Cancer Society, 2019).

For malignant tumors, short-term improvement may be achieved using IV chemotherapy or infusions directly into the hepatic artery or in the peritoneum. Doxorubicin hydrochloride (Adriamycin) and 5-fluorouracil (5-FU) are common choices for drug therapy. Unfortunately, results from chemotherapy tend to be transient. Radiation therapy may be administered to reduce pain and discomfort.

Nursing Management

In the terminal stages of the disease, the nurse keeps the client as comfortable as possible by administering analgesics, supporting ventilation compromised by ascites, and reducing discomfort from pruritus. When the liver fails and coma develops, the nurse institutes safety measures and continues performing total care. While the client is alert, the nurse provides support for the client and family as both begin grieving their potential losses. As appropriate, they make referrals for hospice care. Additional nursing management depends on symptoms and treatment. Client and Family Teaching 47-2 provides information regarding tumors of the liver.

Client and Family Teaching 47-2
Tumors of the Liver

The nurse emphasizes the following points when teaching the client and family:

- Follow diet recommended by primary provider.
- Plan rest periods during the day.
- Avoid heavy lifting.
- Take medications exactly as prescribed. Follow directions on the label, particularly with regard to taking the drug before, after, or with food or meals.
- Record weight weekly or as recommended by the primary provider. Report any significant weight gain or loss to the primary provider.
- Contact primary provider about significant increase in abdominal size, fever, nausea, vomiting, vomiting of blood (bright red, coffee grounds), tarry stools, difficulty with concentration or changes in level of consciousness, jaundice, or swelling of the ankles.
- Make and keep appointments for periodic follow-up office visits.

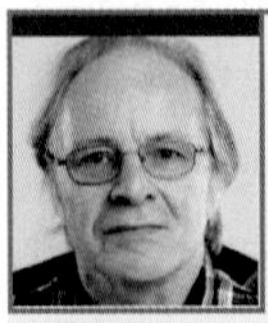

Clinical Scenario A client is diagnosed with a primary liver tumor in one lobe of the liver with no evidence of the tumor in the remainder of the liver. The client is admitted to the postsurgical unit following a hepatic lobectomy. **What are important nursing considerations when caring for this client? See the following Nursing Process section.**

NURSING PROCESS FOR THE CLIENT HAVING SURGERY FOR A LIVER DISORDER

Assessment

Determine whether the client will be undergoing a lobectomy or a liver transplantation (see Chapter 14 for perioperative nursing management). Postoperative assessments include checking vital signs and the function of drains and tubes. Observe carefully for potential complications (hemorrhage, shock, infection, rejection in cases of transplant, electrolyte imbalances, and hepatic coma). In addition, observe the client with cirrhosis for signs of alcohol withdrawal. Standard postsurgical assessments include evaluating breathing pattern, airway patency, and pain.

Diagnosis, Planning, and Interventions

Hypovolemia: Related to hemorrhage from surgical site and fluid loss from drainage, tubes, or both
Expected Outcome: Client will maintain fluid balance as evidenced by adequate urine output and normal BP and pulse.

- Monitor intake and output at least every 8 hours. *Urine output less than 30 mL is inadequate for renal function and indicates hypovolemia.*
- Monitor vital signs at least every 4 hours; do so more frequently if client is hypovolemic. *Hypovolemia causes hypotension and decreased oxygenation.*
- Monitor IV infusion replacement solutions and rates. *Fluids replace intravascular volume and promote kidney function.*
- Monitor serum and urine osmolality, serum sodium, blood urea nitrogen (BUN), creatinine, and hematocrit levels. *Decreased intravascular volume will elevate these fluid volume levels.*

Thermal Injury Risk: Related to infection
Expected Outcome: Body temperature will be below 101°F.

- Monitor temperature frequently. Report elevation above 101°F immediately. *This finding may indicate wound infection and require cultures.*
- If the client is diaphoretic, assist with bathing and changing into dry clothes. *These measures increase comfort and minimize shivering caused by water evaporation from the skin.*
- If the client is shivering, cover with light blanket. If the client is not shivering, cover with a sheet only. *Shivering increases body temperature. A light blanket will prevent shivering. A sheet should be sufficient to keep a client who is not shivering covered but not too warm.*
- Administer antipyretics as ordered. *They help reduce fever, which enhances the immune response.*
- Notify primary provider if client's mental status changes. *This finding can indicate septic shock.*
- Place client on hypothermia blanket as ordered. *Cooling blankets are used if temperature rises to 105°F to control fever.*

Malnutrition Risk: Related to anorexia; impaired use of proteins and carbohydrates; and nausea, vomiting, and sluggish peristalsis
Expected Outcome: Weight will remain stable, and the client will tolerate oral feedings.

- Initially administer nutrition by IV access. *Client will not tolerate oral liquids until bowel sounds resume and they pass flatus or stool.*
- After removal of the IV line or nasogastric tube, give small sips of clear liquids. *Small sips prevent nausea and vomiting.*
- Progress diet to full liquids and then soft foods. *Advancing the diet as tolerated prevents nausea, vomiting, or gastric discomfort.*

Evaluation of Expected Outcomes

Fluid balance is adequate as evidenced by moist mucous membranes, good skin turgor, intake of 2400 mL and output of 2300 mL, BP of 136/88 mm Hg, and pulse rate of 84 beats/min. Body temperature remains below 101°F. The client tolerates food, nourishment meets metabolic needs, and the client's weight stabilizes.

DISORDERS OF THE GALLBLADDER

Several disorders affect the *biliary system*, which refers to the *gallbladder* and *bile ducts*, which carry bile (Fig. 47-8). These disorders impair the drainage of bile into the duodenum. Box 47-7 defines terms related to the biliary system.

Cholelithiasis and Cholecystitis

Cholelithiasis refers to stones that form in the gallbladder. Gallstone formation represents the most common abnormality of the biliary system. If the stones are located in the common bile duct, the condition is referred to as **choledocholithiasis**. The formation of stones often leads to **cholecystitis**, an inflammation or infection of the gallbladder. Cholecystitis may be chronic or acute.

Pathophysiology and Etiology

Cholelithiasis and cholecystitis are intimately related and almost always coexist. Their incidence increases progressively with age. Gallstones are more frequent in women than in men, particularly women who are middle-aged or have a history of multiple pregnancies, diabetes, and obesity or frequent weight changes. The cause of cholelithiasis remains unestablished, but bile stasis, dietary factors, and infection

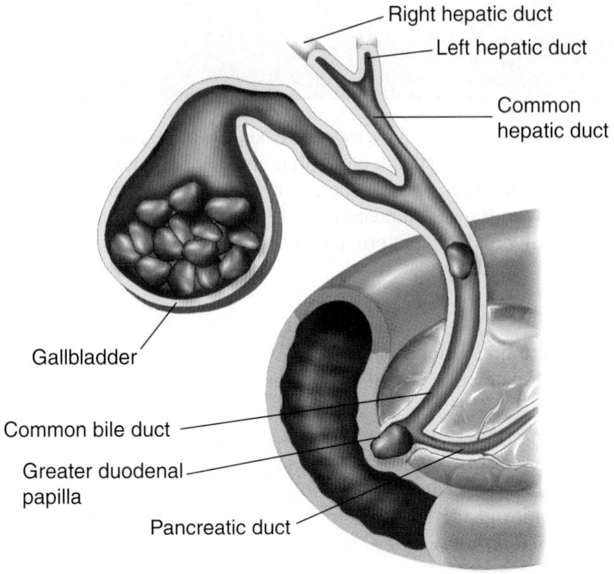

Figure 47-8 Gallstones may form in many locations within the biliary tree.

are suspected. It is also possible to have a tumor that blocks the cystic duct. The bile duct can also become scarred or kinked, leading to blockage and subsequent cholecystitis. The formation of pigmented stones is associated with hemolytic anemia, which increases free bilirubin (see Chapter 31). Cholesterol-type stones are linked to a high-fat diet or predisposition to hypercholesterolemia. Box 47-8 lists risk factors for cholelithiasis.

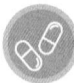

Pharmacologic Considerations

- Orlistat (for obesity) and ursodiol (bile acid) are drugs which may reduce bile acid during weight loss and decrease the risk of gallstone formation.

BOX 47-7 Terms Related to the Biliary System

Cholecystitis: inflammation of the gallbladder
Cholelithiasis: the presence of calculi in the gallbladder
Cholecystectomy: removal of the gallbladder
Cholecystostomy: opening and drainage of the gallbladder
Choledochotomy: opening into the common duct
Choledocholithiasis: stones in the common duct
Choledocholithotomy: incision of common bile duct for removal of stones
Choledochoduodenostomy: anastomosis of common duct to duodenum
Choledochojejunostomy: anastomosis of common duct to jejunum
Lithotripsy: disintegration of gallstones by shock waves
Laparoscopic cholecystectomy: removal of gallbladder through endoscopic procedure
Laser cholecystectomy: removal of gallbladder using laser rather than scalpel and traditional surgical instruments

BOX 47-8 Risk Factors for Cholelithiasis

- Obesity
- Women, especially those who have had multiple pregnancies or who are of Native American or Hispanic of Mexican descent
- Frequent changes in weight
- Rapid weight loss (leads to rapid development of gallstones and high risk of symptomatic disease)
- Treatment with high-dose estrogen (e.g., in prostate cancer)
- Low-dose estrogen therapy—a small increase in the risk of gallstones
- Ileal resection or disease
- Cystic fibrosis
- Diabetes mellitus

Reprinted with permission from Hinkle, J. L., & Cheever, K. H. (2018). *Brunner & Suddarth's textbook of medical-surgical nursing* (14th ed., p. 1392). Wolters Kluwer.

Symptoms tend to develop when one or more gallstones partially or totally impair the passage of bile, causing the gallbladder to become inflamed, swollen, and distended with bile. Each time the person eats fatty foods, *cholecystokinin*, a hormone secreted by the small intestine, stimulates the gallbladder to send bile for its digestion. The gallbladder responds by contracting forcefully. Discomfort results from a combination of the inflammation and contractile spasms. Digestion problems result from the reduced or absent bile. If the swelling and distended volume remain unrelieved, the gallbladder can become necrotic or rupture, leading to peritonitis.

Assessment Findings

Signs and Symptoms

Initially, clients experience belching, nausea and/or vomiting, and RUQ discomfort, with pain or cramps after high-fat meals. Symptoms become acute when a stone blocks bile flow from the gallbladder. With acute cholecystitis, clients usually are very sick with fever, vomiting, abdominal tenderness over the liver, and severe RUQ pain called **biliary colic**. The pain may radiate to the back and right shoulder. The gallbladder may be so swollen that it becomes palpable. Slight jaundice may be noted. The urine appears dark brown; the stools may be light-colored.

Diagnostic Findings

Various tests are performed to rule out other disorders with similar symptoms. Eventually, the stones and structural changes in the gallbladder are imaged by means of *cholecystography* (gallbladder imaging), ultrasonography, CT scan, or radionuclide imaging—cholescintigraphy. This last procedure may be used if ultrasonography is inconclusive. Percutaneous transhepatic cholangiography distinguishes jaundice caused by liver disease from jaundice caused by gallbladder disease. A hepatobiliary iminodiacetic acid (HIDA) scan uses radioactive dye that binds to bile-producing cells. The scan then tracks the flow of bile from the liver to the small intestine, showing obstructions in the flow. Endoscopic retrograde cholangiopancreatography (ERCP) locates stones that have collected in the common bile duct. Magnetic resonance cholangiopancreatography is a noninvasive technique that uses MRI to detect gallstones and gallbladder disorders.

Clients with jaundice have elevated bilirubin levels. Leukocytosis findings correlate with inflammation. In addition, serum liver enzymes may be elevated. The PT may be prolonged as a result of interference with absorption of vitamin K.

Medical and Surgical Management

When the gallbladder is acutely inflamed, the client takes nothing by mouth. Instead, a nasogastric tube is inserted, and antibiotics and parenteral fluids are prescribed until the inflammation subsides. Treatment of mild or chronic cholecystitis involves a low-fat diet. To relieve pain and discomfort, analgesics, anticholinergics, and even nitroglycerin are prescribed. Fat-soluble vitamins may be ordered to compensate for their reduced absorption. A bile-binding resin, such as cholestyramine (Questran), is prescribed to relieve pruritus.

Clients who are at surgical risk and whose gallstones appear radiolucent on diagnostic studies receive oral bile acids, either chenodeoxycholic acid (CDCA; chenodiol [Chenix]) or ursodeoxycholic acid (UDCA; ursodiol [Actigall]), in an attempt to dissolve the gallstones. These drugs, which may take at least 6 to 12 months to be effective, are only moderately successful. The success rate is greatest when the stones are small, but the rate of recurrence within 5 years is high.

Lithotripsy techniques may be performed. These include:

- *Extracorporeal shock wave therapy*: Also referred to as **lithotripsy** or ESWL. This is a nonsurgical procedure that uses shock waves, generated by a machine called a *lithotripter*, to break up some types of gallstones. The shock waves are directed at the gallbladder while the anesthetized client lies in a specially designed water tank. After the shock waves fragment the gallstones, endoscopy or direct contact dissolution removes the fragments. In some instances, the client may pass the fragments naturally.
- *Extracorporeal lithotripsy*: One type of extracorporeal lithotripsy uses laser pulses to create a mechanical shock wave to fragment some types of gallstones. Fluoroscopy is used in tandem to guide the devices. Another type uses an electrohydraulic probe with two electrodes that deliver electric sparks in rapid pulses to fragment the stones. The process may use direct visualization with an endoscope or a percutaneous balloon or basket system.

Stones in the common bile duct can be removed by performing a *sphincterotomy* (opening of the sphincter of Oddi where the common bile duct joins the duodenum) using an endoscope. The stone is snared or retrieved using a basket-like attachment on the endoscope. Other nonsurgical techniques for removing gallstones are depicted in Figure 47-9.

Laparoscopic cholecystectomy is the preferred surgical procedure for gallbladder removal. It is the treatment of choice for about 80% of clients with gallbladder disease. The procedure requires general anesthesia, but the surgery is performed

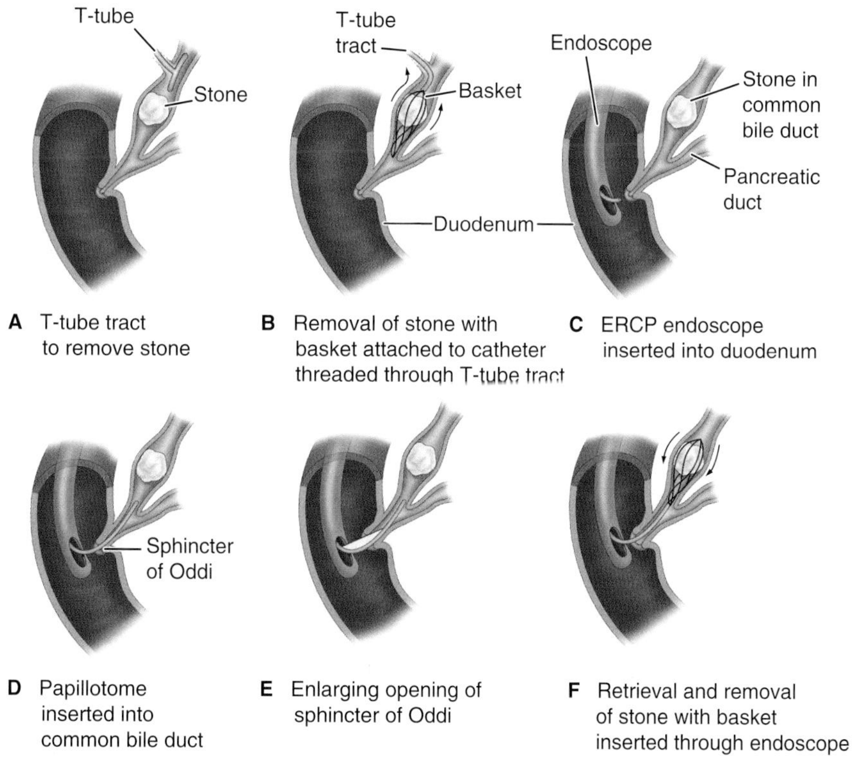

Figure 47-9 Nonsurgical techniques for removing gallstones. ERCP, endoscopic retrograde cholangiopancreatography.

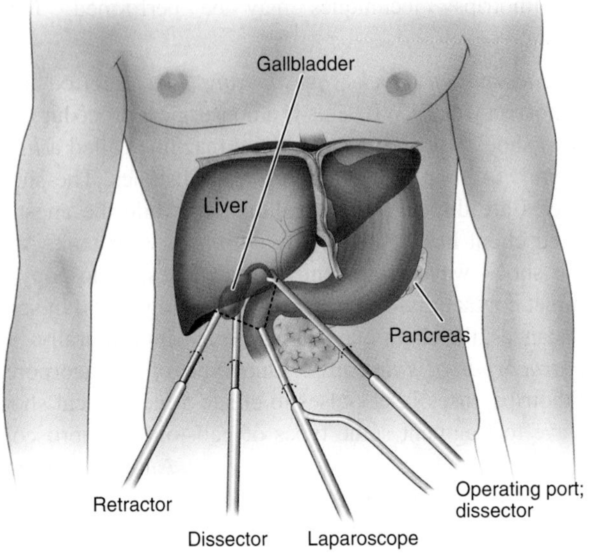

Figure 47-10 In laparoscopic cholecystectomy, the abdominal organs are viewed on a television monitor while the gallbladder is removed.

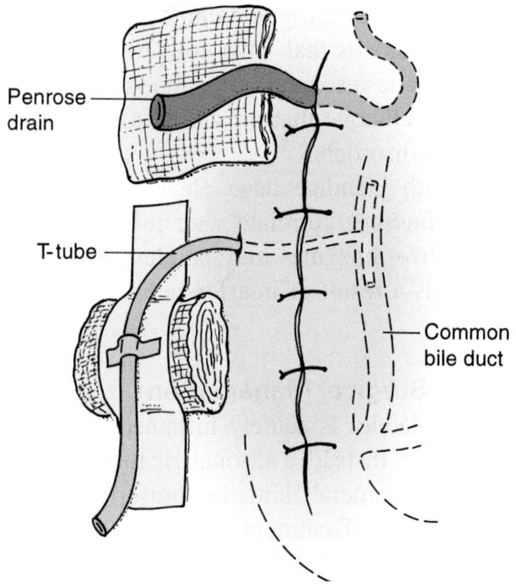

Figure 47-11 After an open cholecystectomy, a wound drain removes exudates from the area formerly occupied by the gallbladder, and a T-tube diverts bile, which the liver is still forming.

with an endoscope inserted in one of three or four small puncture sites in the abdomen (Fig. 47-10). After inflating the abdomen with carbon dioxide to displace abdominal structures and provide a better view, the surgeon drains the gallbladder, dissects the vessels and ducts, and then grasps and removes the gallbladder. Next, the surgeon staples the puncture sites closed and covers the incisions with a light dressing.

Most clients return home in the evening or the morning after the procedure. Although a nasogastric tube may have been inserted during surgery, it is removed before the client is awake and alert. Mild analgesics are administered to relieve minor discomfort. The client may eat food once the effects of the anesthetic subside. A prolonged recovery period usually is unnecessary. Most clients resume normal activities within 1 week.

For some clients, laparoscopic removal is inappropriate. When the gallbladder is extremely distended and fragile from inflammation and infection or contains unusually large or multiple stones, its removal through a small abdominal opening may be impossible or dangerous. In these cases, the surgeon performs an **open cholecystectomy**. This procedure involves a laparotomy (abdominal incision). A *Penrose drain*, a wide, flat rubber tube, or a *vacuum drain*, a plastic tube connected to a bulb or other collecting device, is inserted in the wound to remove serosanguinous fluid. After surgery, clients experience a lengthy period of gastric decompression and acute postoperative pain. Hospitalization lasts about 1 week, and a 6-week recovery period follows discharge.

During cholecystectomy, a *choledochotomy*, surgical opening and exploration of the common bile duct, may be performed. A **T-tube** (a tube used to drain bile) usually is inserted while the surgical wound heals (Fig. 47-11). The T-tube is brought through the abdomen near the incision and connected to gravity drainage.

Nursing Management

During an attack of biliary colic, the nurse ensures that the client rests, monitors the client's tolerance to eating, and administers prescribed antispasmodics or analgesics. Nutrition Notes 47-3 outlines other dietary considerations. If gastric decompression is required, the nurse inserts a nasogastric tube and connects it to suction (see Chapter 45). If lithotripsy or another procedure is initiated to remove the stones, close observation of the client after the procedure for increased pain, shock, or signs of internal bleeding is important.

Same-Day Surgery

When outpatient or laparoscopic surgery is scheduled, the nurse instructs the client about presurgical procedures, laboratory testing, and the consent form. On the day of surgery, the nurse completes preoperative skin preparation, inserts an IV line, and administers sedation. After the client recovers from anesthesia and before discharge, the nurse provides intensive instruction to the client and the accompanying caregiver regarding self-care. Giving written instructions for reference is useful. In accordance with agency policy, the nurse performs follow-up measures, such as telephoning the client the day after surgery to inquire about recovery progress.

Nutrition Notes 47-3

The Client With Gallbladder Disease

- A low-fat diet is commonly recommended prior to gallbladder surgery, even though its efficacy has not been established.
- After gallbladder surgery, there is no need for a fat-restricted diet. A regular diet is resumed.

Cholecystectomy

The nurse asks the client to describe symptoms experienced before admission such as the type and location of pain or discomfort. They ask whether any foods cause pain or discomfort and discuss other problems, such as nausea, vomiting, or abdominal cramping. The nurse inspects the skin and sclera for jaundice and palpates the abdomen for tenderness. Routine presurgical and postsurgical assessments are necessary when the client returns from surgery (Nursing Care Plan 47-2). If a T-tube is in place after an open cholecystectomy, the nurse monitors and records the drainage and maintains tube patency by keeping the collector below the level of the incision. This prevents bile from flowing back into the duct. A primary provider's order is necessary to clamp a T-tube. As healing occurs, the primary provider may direct that the T-tube be clamped temporarily before a meal and reopened later after eating.

The nurse measures bile drainage every 8 hours or according to agency policy. If more than 500 mL of bile drains within 24 hours or if drainage is significantly reduced, the nurse notifies the primary provider. Preventing tension on the tubing is important because it may become dislodged internally. A return of normal color to stool and urine indicates that bile is being deposited normally in the GI tract. Client and Family Teaching 47-3 provides more information related to teaching a postoperative cholecystectomy client about their care.

Client and Family Teaching 47-3 Postoperative Teaching Following a Cholecystectomy

The nurse emphasizes the following points when teaching the client and family:

- Meet with a dietitian to review foods that should be avoided.
- Read labels on food products to determine their fat content.
- If applicable, explain the purpose of drug therapy, the schedule to follow for administration, and the potential side effects.
- Continue taking medication as long as prescribed, even if symptoms disappear.
- Understand that frequent monitoring of the effect of drug therapy may be necessary.
- Notify the primary provider immediately of severe pain, jaundice, fever, or if the color of the stools or urine changes.

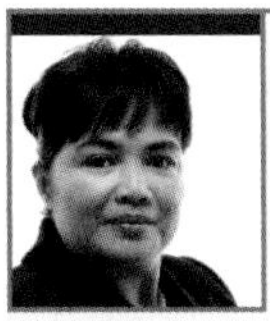

Clinical Scenario A 45-year-old woman was admitted early in the morning for a cholecystectomy. The surgery went well, and the client was admitted to an inpatient surgical unit. The nurse assigned to care for this client needs to focus on several issues for this client. What are the priorities for this client's care? See Nursing Care Plan 47-2.

NURSING CARE PLAN 47-2 The Client Having Gallbladder Surgery

Postoperative Assessment

See Chapter 14 for perioperative management. When the client returns from surgery:

- Assess vital signs.
- Review chart for type of surgery and client's progress during surgery and in the postanesthesia recovery unit.
- Inspect surgical dressing for drainage and tubes or catheters for placement, patency, and type of drainage.
- Carefully observe nasogastric tube for type and amount of drainage. If there is a T-tube, monitor drainage for amount. If there is a Penrose drain, observe and change dressing as needed.
- Inspect IV site; note current rate and progress of fluid infusion.
- Document fluid intake and output as well as level of consciousness and comfort.
- Closely monitor for the following complications:
  - Change in vital signs, especially BP fluctuations, increased pulse rate, and elevated temperature
  - Change in respiratory status, including difficulty breathing and increased respiratory rate
  - Abdominal discomfort
  - Urine output less than 35 mL/hour if catheterized, or failure to void within 8 hours of surgery
  - Jaundice

Nursing Diagnosis. **Acute Pain** related to surgical incision

Expected Outcome. Client will report that analgesics relieve pain.

Interventions	Rationales
Administer analgesics as ordered.	*Timely administration provides maximum and effective pain control.*
Teach client to splint incision when moving or coughing.	*Splinting reduces pain and discomfort.*
Maintain patency of nasogastric and T-tubes if present.	*Doing so maintains drainage flow, preventing pressure of accumulated fluids and reducing pain.*

Evaluation of Expected Outcome

Client reports decreased abdominal pain and demonstrates good splinting technique when moving or coughing.

(continued)

NURSING CARE PLAN 47-2 The Client Having Gallbladder Surgery (*continued*)

Nursing Diagnosis. **Altered Breathing Pattern** related to proximity of incision to lungs, inhibiting deep breathing

Expected Outcome. Client will report comfort with breathing and exhibit unlabored breathing and effective respirations.

Interventions	Rationales
Place client in upright or semi-Fowler position.	*These positions facilitate lung expansion.*
Encourage client to deep breathe, cough, and splint incision at least every 2 hours.	*These measures provide for lung expansion and mobilize secretions.*
If client has shallow breaths, instruct them to use incentive spirometer.	*It promotes deeper breathing and more lung expansion.*
Ambulate client as soon as possible at least four times a day, increasing distance each time. Encourage client to sit at least twice a day.	*Ambulation and sitting prevent pulmonary complications and promote lung expansion.*
Auscultate lung sounds at least every 8 hours.	*Auscultation detects retained secretions and atelectasis early, helping prevent respiratory complications.*

Evaluation of Expected Outcome

Client demonstrates adequate lung function as evidenced by ability to take deep breaths and cough and no signs of respiratory complications.

Nursing Diagnosis. **Altered Skin Integrity** related to altered biliary drainage after surgery and insertion of T-tube, Penrose drain, or both

Expected Outcome. Incision and skin around T-tube and drain will remain intact and not be irritated.

Interventions	Rationales
Inspect all drainage tubes to ensure that they are connected to drainage bags, appropriately covered with sterile dressings, and fastened to client's clothing to prevent dislodgment or kinking.	*Doing so prevents bile from leaking onto skin.*
Keep drainage collector for T-tube below incision and maintain connection to gravity drainage.	*These measures promote drainage of bile through T-tube.*
Change dressings frequently as needed. Apply protectants such as zinc oxide or petrolatum to skin around drainage tubes.	*These measures prevent skin irritation.*
Observe sclerae for jaundice. Report abdominal pain, nausea, vomiting, bile drainage around T-tube, or clay-colored stools.	*These findings may indicate obstruction of bile drainage.*

Evaluation of Expected Outcome

Skin around drainage tubes remains intact and free of irritation.

Nursing Diagnosis. **Malnutrition Risk** related to high metabolic needs and decreased ability to digest fatty foods

Expected Outcome. Client will maintain weight and optimal nutritional status.

Interventions	Rationales
Offer a diet low in fats and high in carbohydrates and proteins. Instruct client that fats are restricted for 4–6 weeks after surgery.	*Initially, bile is drained and unavailable for fat digestion. As the biliary ducts dilate to accommodate the bile volume once held by the gallbladder, sufficient bile will be released into the GI tract to emulsify fats and allow for digestion.*
Administer vitamins A, D, E, and K as indicated.	*These fat-soluble vitamins are needed for adequate nutritional intake.*
Consult with dietitian if client is having difficulty meeting nutritional needs.	*Doing so provides client with a resource for nutritional information and alternatives to dietary restrictions.*

NURSING CARE PLAN 47-2 The Client Having Gallbladder Surgery (*continued*)

Instruct client to weigh themselves weekly.	*This provides a record of weight maintenance, loss, or gain.*
Encourage client to increase activity.	*Increased activity promotes appetite.*
Instruct client to maintain a record of nutritional intake and any problems with GI symptoms during or after meals.	*This method helps client to track and avoid foods that cause GI symptoms.*

Evaluation of Expected Outcome

Client reports that weight remains stable and that they are tolerating the diet very well.

Nursing Diagnosis. Altered Health Maintenance related to insufficient knowledge for self-care

Expected Outcome. Client will demonstrate knowledge of discharge instructions as evidenced by adequate wound care and repetition of dietary and medication instructions.

Interventions	Rationales
Reinforce diet instructions described in Nursing Diagnosis Imbalanced Nutrition, with rationales as to why client must restrict fat.	*Knowledge improves understanding of and compliance with dietary restrictions.*
Provide verbal and written information that the client can understand about any prescriptions.	*Clients learn in various ways. Presenting understandable information promotes learning.*
Demonstrate and have client or family member return demonstration of wound care, dressing changes, and care of T-tube and drainage collector.	*Return demonstrations allow the nurse to determine the client or family member's ability and knowledge, reinforce instructions, and correct misconceptions.*
Instruct client or family member to notify the primary provider if the wound appears red or swollen or has purulent drainage, or if T-tube output increases.	*Such findings indicate infection or obstruction below the T-tube, which needs intervention.*
Explain that initially, stools may be loose and frequent.	*Bile will initially trickle continuously into the digestive system because the gallbladder no longer stores bile.*
Instruct client to notify primary provider of clay-colored stools, dark brown urine, or jaundice.	*These findings indicate obstruction and require early intervention.*
Recommend that the client avoid lifting anything over 5 lb for at least 1 month.	*This will prevent incisional hernia formation.*

Evaluation of Expected Outcome

Client manages self-care at home as evidenced by proper wound healing, compliance with dietary and medication regimen, and no complications.

DISORDERS OF THE PANCREAS

The pancreas is in the upper abdomen. Disorders of the pancreas can affect both exocrine and endocrine functions.

Acute Pancreatitis

Pancreatitis, inflammation of the pancreas, may be acute or chronic with a long history of relapse and recurrences. Acute pancreatitis ranges from mild to severe and can be fatal. Characteristics of the mild form are inflammation and edema of the pancreas. Although the client is very ill, pancreatic function usually returns to normal within 6 months. In the severe form, more generalized and complete enzymatic digestion of the pancreas occurs. The tissue becomes necrotic, and the client develops many local and systemic complications. Mortality rates in the United States are about 10% of clients diagnosed with acute pancreatitis (The National Pancreas Foundation, 2014).

Pathophysiology and Etiology

Primarily, the pancreas becomes inflamed when the organ's own enzymes—especially trypsin—cause the pancreas to digest itself (*autodigestion*). Autodigestion develops when there is reflux of bile and duodenal contents into the pancreatic duct, which activates the exocrine enzymes that the pancreas produces. Swelling of the opening to the pancreatic duct impairs or even obstructs the release of bicarbonate, which neutralizes chyme as it enters the small intestine.

It also obstructs the release of the enzymes trypsin, which digests proteins; amylase, which digests carbohydrates; and lipase, which digests fats. As the enzymes accumulate in the gland, they begin to digest the pancreatic tissue itself. Eventually, destruction of the pancreas leads to impairment of endocrine functions.

The causes of acute pancreatitis vary widely. Known causes include structural abnormalities, abdominal trauma, infections, metabolic disorders (e.g., hyperlipidemia, hypercalcemia), vascular abnormalities, inflammatory bowel disease, hereditary factors, ingestion of alcohol or certain other drugs, or refeeding after prolonged fasting or anorexia. Sometimes, however, acute pancreatitis develops without any of these predisposing factors or other identifiable causes.

Complications from severe acute pancreatitis are serious and sometimes fatal. Hyperglycemia results from an imbalance of glucagon, insulin, and somatostatin. Necrosis and hemorrhage of the gland, peritonitis, severe fluid and electrolyte imbalance, shock, pleural effusion, acute respiratory distress syndrome, and blood coagulation problems ensue. When lipase digests the fatty tissue around the pancreas, calcium binds with the released fatty acids. In rare cases, this reduces the level of circulating calcium to a dangerous degree, resulting in tetany and convulsions. Pancreatic cysts and abscesses also can develop.

Assessment Findings

Signs and Symptoms

The most common complaint of clients with pancreatitis is severe mid-abdominal to upper abdominal pain, radiating to both sides and straight to the back. Clients relate that it is worse following eating. Nausea, vomiting, and flatulence usually are present. The client may describe the stools as being frothy and foul-smelling, a sign of **steatorrhea**, increased fat in the stool, from poor fat digestion. The symptoms, which worsen after the client eats fatty foods or drinks alcohol, are relieved when the client sits up and leans forward or curls into a fetal position.

Physical examination may reveal jaundice. Bowel sounds are diminished or absent with accompanying distension, and the abdomen is tender to palpation. The client may be hypotensive, indicating hypovolemia and shock caused by the release of large amounts of protein-rich fluid into the tissues and peritoneal cavity. The client may be feverish and tachycardic. Breathing is shallow from severe pain. Severe pancreatitis may result in bruising around the umbilicus or on the flanks.

Diagnostic Findings

Elevated serum and urine amylase, lipase, and liver enzyme levels accompany significant pancreatitis. If the common bile duct is obstructed, the bilirubin level is above normal. Blood glucose levels and WBC counts can be elevated. Serum electrolyte levels (calcium, potassium, and magnesium) are low. Pancreatic edema and necrosis appear on CT scan with vascular enhancement. Abdominal ultrasound reveals pancreatic inflammation. Various endoscopic examinations may be performed to assist the differential diagnosis and to determine the presence of pancreatic cysts, abscesses, and pseudocysts (fibrous capsules filled with fluid, blood, enzymes, pus, and tissue debris). An MRI may be ordered to see if there are abnormalities in the gallbladder, pancreas, and ducts. Stools may be tested for fat content—this indicates inadequate absorption of nutrients.

Medical and Surgical Management

Medical treatment concentrates on relieving pain; reducing pancreatic secretions; restoring fluid and electrolyte losses; and preventing or treating systemic complications such as respiratory distress syndrome, acute (renal) tubular necrosis, and bleeding abnormalities. The client usually receives nothing by mouth, and a nasogastric tube may be inserted and connected to suction if the client is experiencing problems with nausea and vomiting. This relieves nausea, distension, and vomiting.

Along with general fluid therapy for hydration purposes, IV albumin may be given to pull fluid trapped in the peritoneum back into the circulation. Parenteral nutrition may be administered if the client is weak and debilitated to reduce the metabolic stress associated with acute pancreatitis and cannot tolerate enteral feedings. Otherwise, enteral feedings are started early to provide nutritional support. Diuretics are given if circulating fluid is excessive. Pain management is important to meet the client's comfort needs, but also to keep the client calm. Pancreatic secretions can increase secondary to a client's discomfort and/or restlessness, increasing a client's pain. Opioids are generally prescribed and administered parenterally. Morphine, fentanyl, and hydromorphone are generally the medications ordered. H_2-receptor antagonists such as famotidine (Pepcid) or proton pump inhibitors such as omeprazole (Prilosec) may be administered to suppress gastric acid and decrease pancreatic activity. IV antibiotic therapy is prescribed to prevent localized abscesses or to treat systemic sepsis. If pseudocysts develop, they may be located by CT scan and drained by percutaneous needle aspiration. Improvement, if it is forthcoming, usually occurs in about 1 week. A clear liquid diet is prescribed initially, with a slow progression to a low-fat diet. Alcohol, caffeine, and pepper, which are digestive stimulants, are withheld. If pancreatic exocrine function is impaired, pancreatic enzyme replacement therapy is administered with meals to promote digestion (Nutrition Notes 47-4).

Nutrition Notes 47-4

The Client With Pancreatic Disease

- If motility and absorption are not impaired, malnourished clients may be given nasojejunal feedings of an elemental formula during an acute attack of pancreatitis; their extremely low fat content causes only minimal pancreatic stimulation.
- TPN is used cautiously; some clients with pancreatitis cannot tolerate a high-glucose concentration even with insulin coverage.
- IV lipids are used sparingly when pancreatitis is related to hyperlipidemia.

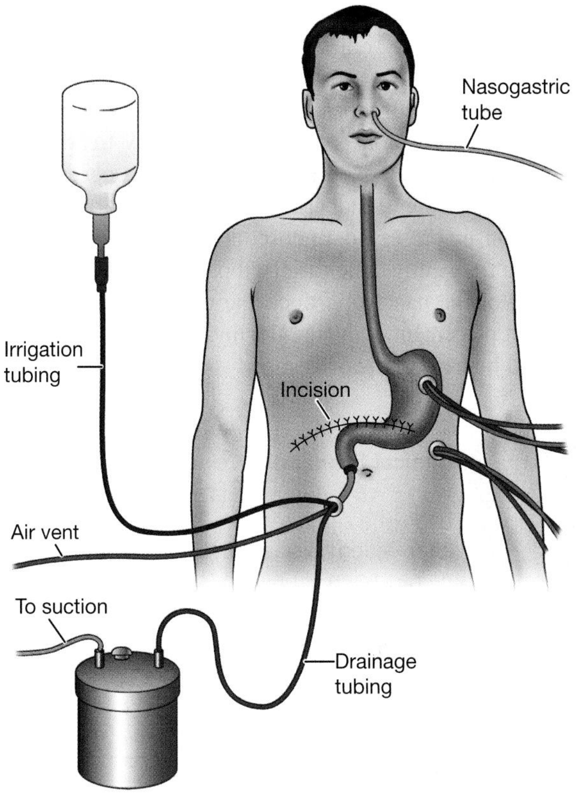

Figure 47-12 Multiple sump tubes are used after pancreatic surgery. Triple-lumen tubes consist of ports that provide tubing for irrigation, air venting, and drainage.

In severe cases, surgical management involves opening the abdomen to debride necrotic tissue. Every 2 to 3 days, the process is repeated to prevent the spread of infection. Multiple sump drains, inserted into the cavity to remove debris, are attached to continuous irrigation (Fig. 47-12). If acute cholecystitis or obstruction of the common duct is thought to be a coincidental or inciting factor, drainage and simple stone removal may be necessary. Sphincterotomy may be done to enlarge the bile duct or pancreatic duct opening. This procedure is done with an endoscope and small wire. Additionally, stents may be placed in the ducts to keep them open.

Nursing Management

Nursing management involves monitoring the client for life-threatening changes and alcohol withdrawal if substance abuse is part of the client history. It also entails performing the prescribed treatment measures. The nurse is responsible for inserting a nasogastric tube, maintaining its patency, and infusing IV fluids. If gastric decompression is prolonged, the client can receive nasojejunal feedings of a low-fat formula or TPN. The nurse must monitor blood glucose levels closely. Clients with acute pancreatitis require frequent administrations of analgesics. Most clients with acute pancreatitis are severely ill. The nurse must continuously monitor intake and output, especially urine volume. If the primary provider inserts a pulmonary artery or central venous catheter, the nurse monitors pressure measurements. Cardiac monitoring is continuous because electrolyte imbalances can produce dysrhythmias. The nurse continues to perform other assessments, including vital signs, lung sounds, serum electrolyte values, and observes for bleeding tendencies. If the client develops severe respiratory problems, they may require intubation and mechanical ventilation. The nurse must report any sudden change in the client's general condition or symptoms (i.e., pain or abdominal distension) to the primary provider immediately.

When surgery is performed, the nurse infuses irrigation solution and ensures that suction is functioning effectively. They also provide skin care if pancreatic drainage leaks from the sump drain sites.

Chronic Pancreatitis

Pathophysiology and Etiology

Chronic pancreatitis is prolonged and progressive inflammation of the pancreas, with gradual destruction of the pancreatic tissue. Fibrous tissue causes increased pressure within the pancreas, eventually leading to obstruction of the pancreatic and biliary ducts. In most cases, alcohol consumption is the cause of chronic pancreatitis. It leads to edema of the duodenum and decreases the tone of the sphincter of Oddi. Consequently, duodenal contents can move into the pancreatic duct. Other causes include hereditary predisposition, hyperparathyroidism, hypertriglyceridemia, autoimmune pancreatitis, trauma, and anatomic abnormalities. In about 20% of cases, no particular cause is identifiable. With chronicity, the gland undergoes fibrotic scarring from the recurring inflammation. The pancreas hardens, and exocrine and endocrine functions are partly or completely lost as pancreatic tissue is destroyed.

Assessment Findings

Signs and Symptoms

In chronic pancreatitis, the client has severe-to-persistent pain; weight loss; and digestive disturbances such as flatulence, vomiting, and diarrhea. If pseudocysts form, they contribute to the severity of the symptoms by putting pressure on adjacent organs or by rupturing. If secondary diabetes develops, the client may experience increased appetite, thirst, and urination. A firm mass may be palpated in the upper left quadrant. The urine may be dark; the stools may be light-colored and foul-smelling. Fatty streaks appear in the stool. With the loss of plasma proteins from the blood, peripheral edema and ascites develop.

Diagnostic Findings

Abnormal laboratory findings are the same for chronic pancreatitis as for acute disease. CT scans, MRI, ultrasound, and ERCP studies of the pancreas show diagnostic results similar to those in clients with acute pancreatitis. Results of a glucose tolerance test show an impaired ability to metabolize carbohydrates because of malfunctioning endocrine cells in the islets of Langerhans.

Medical and Surgical Management

Treatment depends on the cause and whether the pancreatic duct is obstructed. If the duct is not obstructed, treatment consists of abstinence from alcohol; a clear liquid to bland, fat-free diet; and correction of associated biliary tract disease or hyperparathyroidism. The client who adheres to treatment may have good results.

Abdominal pain for clients with chronic pancreatitis may initially be relieved by abstinence from alcohol in order to slow the disease process and decrease pain. Pain management strategies for clients with chronic pancreatitis begin with nonopioid oral analgesics such as NSAIDs or acetaminophen. If clients continue to have persistent pain then oral mild opioids, such as acetaminophen with codeine, may be used. If more potent analgesia is needed, clients may have morphine, fentanyl, or hydromorphone through pumps or with the use of patches.

Treatment for insulin and digestive enzyme deficiencies includes diet, insulin, and pancreatic enzyme products (PEP). Because items sold as enzyme supplements contain variable amounts of enzyme, the FDA began to regulate PEPs in 1991. PEPs are used to improve food digestion and contain the active ingredient pancrelipase with a mixture of other digestive enzymes—amylase, lipase, and protease.

When surgery is part of treatment, some or all of the pancreas (**partial or total pancreatectomy**) may be removed. If there is scarring, with stricture and stenosis of portions of the pancreatic duct, various surgical measures can be performed to attempt reconstitution of the duct. A pancreaticojejunostomy (joining of the pancreatic duct to the jejunum) can relieve ductal obstruction. Pancreatic autotransplantation is a recent surgical development. It involves excision and relocation of the pancreas. During this procedure, innervation is severed, effectively treating pain symptoms. Although exocrine function is lost, necessitating enzyme replacement, endocrine function, and normal insulin production are preserved. Endoscopic or laparoscopic procedures are frequently done for distal pancreatectomy, decompression of the pancreatic duct, the denervation of nerves, and stent placement, reducing the invasiveness of the procedure and improving the outcomes.

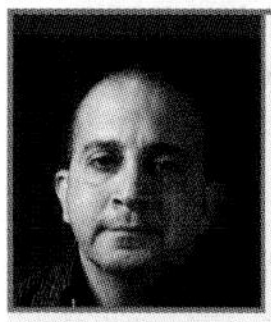

Clinical Scenario A client is admitted with severe abdominal pain radiating to the back. The client reports that it is even worse after eating. His appetite is diminished, and he has been experiencing nausea and vomiting. The client also has a temperature of 38.8°C, and he is slightly agitated. A diagnosis of acute pancreatitis is made. **What does the nurse need to include in the client's plan of care? See the following Nursing Process section.**

NURSING PROCESS FOR THE CLIENT WITH PANCREATITIS

Assessment

Initial assessment includes a history of symptoms the client experienced before admission as well as a complete medical history. Ask about the frequency and amount of alcohol ingestion and determine when the client had their last drink as a method of evaluating if or how soon withdrawal symptoms may occur. For reliability, involve family members in compiling assessment data (if possible), especially if the client's condition is serious. During the interview, obtain a description of pain with respect to location, type, severity, and circumstances that aggravate or relieve it. The physical examination includes gentle palpation of the abdomen, especially the epigastric area, for pain, tenderness, distension, or rigidity.

Include an immediate evaluation of vital signs, because shock often is an outstanding symptom of acute pancreatitis. A description of the client's general appearance is important. Periodic weights provide a comparison for when more serious symptoms occur. Instruct the client to save stool for inspection or laboratory testing. Initiate blood glucose testing as indicated.

Diagnosis, Planning, and Interventions

Administer prescribed analgesics. The client may exhibit or develop tolerance as a result of cross-addiction to alcohol or chronic use of analgesics. Monitor for signs of alcohol withdrawal, which may develop within the first 24 hours of admission. Implement measures to manage nutrition and blood glucose levels and administer insulin as indicated. The client requires therapeutic skin care to prevent breakdown from frequent, loose stools. If surgery is planned, manage preoperative and postoperative care. Diabetic and diet teaching begin before the client is discharged from the hospital (Client and Family Teaching 47-4). Provide referrals to a community substance abuse rehabilitation program if appropriate.

Other care can include the following nursing diagnoses, expected outcomes, and interventions:

Chronic Pain: Related to distension, edema, and irritation of the inflamed pancreas
Expected Outcome: Client will report reduced pain.

- Administer analgesics as ordered. *Prompt administration of analgesics provides a therapeutic level of analgesia and promotes pain relief.*
- Withhold oral feedings. *Doing so limits the reflux of bile and duodenal contents into the pancreatic duct, preventing activation of the exocrine enzymes produced by the pancreas.*
- Instruct client to remain on bed rest. *Bed rest reduces metabolic rate and thus decreases secretion of pancreatic and gastric enzymes.*
- Report unrelieved pain or sudden increased intensity of pain. *Increased pain stimulates secretion of pancreatic enzymes. Sudden increased pain may indicate pancreatic rupture.*
- Administer anticholinergic medications as ordered. *They reduce gastric and pancreatic secretions.*
- Maintain continuous nasogastric drainage. *Drainage removes gastric contents and prevents gastric secretions from entering the duodenum.*

NURSING PROCESS FOR THE CLIENT WITH PANCREATITIS (continued)

Altered Breathing Pattern: Related to severe pain and pancreatic distension, edema, and inflammation
Expected Outcome: Client will maintain adequate lung function as evidenced by improved breathing patterns and clear lungs.

- Position client with head of bed elevated or in semi-Fowler position. *These measures reduce pressure on the diaphragm from abdominal distension and promote lung expansion.*
- Reposition client at least every 2 hours. *Repositioning prevents atelectasis and pooling of respiratory secretions.*
- Monitor pulse oximetry. Report episodes of desaturation to primary provider. *Pulse oximetry helps show changes in respiratory status and promotes early interventions.*
- Encourage client to deep breathe and cough every 2 hours. *Deep breathing and coughing clear the airway and reduce atelectasis.*

Hypovolemia: Related to vomiting, decreased fluid intake, fever, diaphoresis, and fluid shifts
Expected Outcome: Client will be adequately hydrated as evidenced by sufficient urine output and normal BP and skin turgor.

- Monitor intake and output at least every 8 hours. *This record can show if fluid loss is excessive.*
- Monitor serum electrolytes and BUN levels. *Findings might indicate a need for fluid and electrolyte replacements.*
- Administer IV fluids and electrolytes as ordered. *Replacing fluids and electrolytes restores fluid balance.*
- Administer plasma, albumin, and blood products as ordered. *Clients with severe pancreatitis lose large amounts of blood and plasma, which decreases effective circulating blood volume.*

Diarrhea: Related to impaired fat and protein digestion
Expected Outcome: Client experiences decreased diarrhea.

- Monitor number and characteristics of stools. *Such monitoring provides a baseline for determining fluid and electrolyte loss from stools.*
- Maintain low-fat diet if client is allowed food. *Decreased fat intake reduces the amount that the client cannot properly digest.*
- Administer antidiarrheal medications if ordered. *They assist in decreasing diarrhea and, in turn, reduce fluid and electrolyte losses.*

Injury Risk: Related to alcohol withdrawal
Expected Outcome: Client remains uninjured with stable vital signs and no seizures.

- Monitor client for signs of CNS stimulation, such as agitation or belligerence. Observe for signs of hand tremors and emotional lability. *Such findings may indicate that the depressant effects of alcohol are wearing off.*
- Report if client's heart rate is over 100 beats/min, diastolic BP is greater than 100 mm Hg, or temperature is above 100°F (36.6°C). *Such findings may indicate signs of alcohol withdrawal and the need for medical intervention.*
- Minimize environmental stimuli. *Extraneous lights and noise can increase agitation and possibly cause confusion.*
- Administer prescribed sedatives. *They provide appropriate sedation as the client withdraws from the effects of alcohol.*
- Provide a safe environment for the client if they are extremely agitated or at risk for seizures. Place client near nurses' station if they require close observation. *Anticipating safety needs prevents harm to the client. If the client is near the nurses' station, the nurses can more closely monitor their activities.*
- Pad side rails and keep oral suction available. *If the client has a seizure or becomes extremely agitated, padded side rails, other safety measures, and immediate availability of suction can prevent further injury.*
- If a seizure occurs, initiate seizure precautions by protecting, but not restraining, the client. Observe the client throughout the seizure. After the seizure, ensure that the airway is clear and administer oxygen briefly according to agency policy. *Restraining a client during a seizure can cause more injury. Staying with the client during and after the seizure provides protection for the client and ensures that their airway is patent.*

Evaluation of Expected Outcomes

The client reports relief of pain, with an increased ability to sleep and rest more comfortably. They breathe deeply at a rate of 12 to 20 breaths/min and maintain adequate pulmonary ventilation as evidenced by clear lungs and 95% saturation by pulse oximetry. Fluid intake and output are balanced as evidenced by urine output of at least 50 mL/hour and normal BP and skin turgor. The client reports fewer stools and that stools have more form. Alcohol withdrawal occurs without hypertension or seizures.

Client and Family Teaching 47-4
Pancreatitis

Most clients with pancreatitis require a prolonged recovery period. The following instructions are usual:

- Follow the written instructions for a bland, low-fat, calorie-controlled diet.
- Eat four or more small meals daily.
- Take prescribed medications, including enzyme replacements, as directed.
- If alcohol abuse is known to cause acute or chronic pancreatitis, avoid all alcoholic beverages. Strongly consider self-referral to Alcoholics Anonymous or a medical treatment center. Urge the family to attend Al-Anon meetings. (If insulin administration is necessary because of diabetes mellitus, see Chapter 51.)

Carcinoma of the Pancreas

Pancreatic cancers account for 3% of all cancers and 7% of cancer deaths in the United States (American Cancer Society, 2021). Carcinoma of the pancreas may occur in the gland's head, body, or tail. Some tumors are primary lesions, whereas others are metastases from other locations. Because tumors of the head of the pancreas tend to cause obstructive jaundice, they usually are diagnosed earlier. Nevertheless, most are discovered late in the disease and invariably have a lethal prognosis.

Pathophysiology and Etiology

When sufficient malignant cells accumulate, they block the pancreatic duct, producing symptoms similar to chronic pancreatitis. There is some question as to whether the pancreatitis is a precursor or consequence of tumor development. Tumors in the body or tail of the pancreas can press on the portal vein and lead to the formation of varices and bleeding. Once a tumor develops, it tends to grow rapidly. By the time symptoms are serious enough for the client to seek medical assistance, the tumor may have spread to adjacent structures, such as the liver or spleen.

Besides pancreatitis, factors that correlate with pancreatic cancer include diabetes mellitus, a high-fat diet, and chronic exposure to carcinogenic substances (i.e., petrochemicals). Although data are inconclusive, a relationship may exist between cigarette smoking and high coffee consumption (especially decaffeinated coffee) and the development of pancreatic carcinoma. Other factors that may contribute to pancreatic cancer are: excess body weight and family history of pancreatic cancer.

Assessment Findings

Signs and Symptoms

Symptoms may not appear until the disease is far advanced. The most common symptoms are left upper abdominal pain that may be referred to the back, jaundice, anorexia, and weight loss. The client may describe light-colored stools but dark urine, typical symptoms of obstructive jaundice. Pruritus may accompany jaundice.

A mass may be palpated in the left upper quadrant. The mass may be a tumor or an enlarged gallbladder, which tends to expand as a result of obstructed passage of bile. Ascites may be present in late stages of the disease. Some clients develop thrombophlebitis from pancreatic tumor products, which increase the blood's coagulability.

Diagnostic Findings

Abdominal ultrasonography or CT scan demonstrates pancreatic enlargement. Spiral or helical CT scans give a more accurate view of organs and is very useful in diagnosing and staging pancreatic tumors. An endoscopic ultrasound (EUS) is done to take images of the pancreas from inside the abdomen. The scope is inserted down the esophagus and into the stomach to get the images. An ERCP is done to obtain a biopsy or percutaneous needle aspiration to provide evidence of malignant cells. Magnetic resonance cholangiopancreatography (MRCP) provides a noninvasive way to examine the pancreatic and bile ducts. Unlike ERCP, contrast dye is not required. Biopsy samples cannot be obtained with this procedure. Elevated serum amylase, alkaline phosphatase, and bilirubin levels support the evidence that the pancreas is diseased, but they do not confirm carcinoma. The level of carcinoembryonic antigen is elevated, but this elevation is a less specific tumor marker than is CA 19-9.

Medical and Surgical Management

Treating pancreatic cancer remains challenging. Often the prognosis is poor. Ablative procedures, using heat or cold, may be done to prevent the spread of the cancer. Embolization of arteries or veins is done to block the flow of blood to the cancer cells. Chemotherapy, targeted therapy, and radiation therapy are done to alleviate symptoms and destroy cancer cells.

Surgery can be curative if the cancer can be totally resected. Palliative surgery is done to remove as much of the cancer as possible and to alleviate symptoms and/or prevent complications such as intestinal or bile duct obstruction. The most common surgical procedure is a **pancreatoduodenectomy (Whipple procedure)** (Fig. 47-13). This surgical procedure involves removing the head and perhaps the body of the pancreas, resecting the duodenum and stomach, and redirecting the flow of secretions from the stomach, gallbladder, and pancreas into the jejunum. The tumor may be irradiated during surgery, or radioactive seeds may be implanted. Because metastasis to the spleen is so common, some surgeons also may perform a splenectomy. Rather than do an extensive resection, others are inclined to do a total pancreatectomy. This radical surgery then creates a malabsorption syndrome and historically brittle diabetes, which must be treated after surgery. A distal pancreatectomy involves the resection of the tail and part of the body of the pancreas, and usually the spleen.

A cholecystojejunostomy, a rerouting of pancreatic and biliary drainage, may be done to relieve obstructive jaundice. This measure is considered palliative only. For inoperable tumors, radiation therapy or chemotherapy with gemcitabine and/or other agents may be tried. These treatments do not cure the disease. Despite surgery, chemotherapy, or radiation

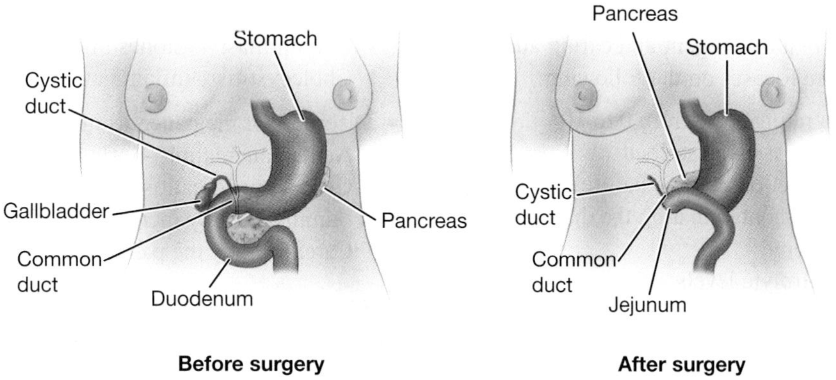

Figure 47-13 Radical pancreatoduodenectomy (Whipple procedure). The head of the pancreas is removed as well as the gallbladder. The common duct is sutured to the end of the jejunum, and the remaining portion of the pancreas and the end of the stomach are sutured to the side of the jejunum.

therapy, many clients die within 3 to 12 months after the onset of symptoms.

- The complexity of these surgical procedures raises the potential for complications, which may include the following: Bleeding tendencies related to vitamin K deficiency
- Liver and/or kidney failure
- Infection
- Leaks from the many anastomoses required
- Digestive issues related to inadequate stomach emptying, ineffective digestion (may require pancreatic enzymes), and anorexia
- Weight loss
- Diabetes
- Changes in bowel habits

Nursing Management

Nursing management for those treated medically is the same as for any client with a terminal malignant disorder (see Chapter 18). Clients undergoing palliative surgery require care similar to that of clients having general abdominal surgery. If clients have severe anorexia and weight loss, they are poor risks for immediate surgery. These clients may receive preoperative IV fluids, TPN, or a special diet to improve nutritional status and correct any fluid or electrolyte imbalances. Most surgical clients have a nasogastric tube inserted. Once the biliary obstruction is relieved, the color of the skin, stools, and urine returns to near normal. Clients undergoing the Whipple procedure or one of its variations require more intensive nursing management because of the profoundly invasive nature of the procedure.

Initially, the nurse evaluates the client's general physical condition and obtains a history of all symptoms present before admission. They ask about the onset of symptoms, weight loss, bleeding tendencies, and the type of pain or abdominal discomfort. Physical examination includes inspection for jaundice, a visual examination of stools and urine, and palpation of the abdomen for tenderness and distension. Laboratory tests include blood or urine samples for analysis and detection of glucose. The nurse records vital signs and weight and assesses nutritional status.

The nurse observes the client after surgery for complications such as shock, pancreatic abscess formation, and hemorrhage. See Chapter 14 for postoperative nursing management measures for pain control, anxiety, and impaired skin integrity. Immediate postoperative assessments include vital signs and a review of the chart for the type and extent of surgery. The nurse also checks the surgical dressing and all drains and tubes for patency as well as noting the amount and color of drainage throughout the entire postoperative course.

Close observation for signs of bleeding, such as easy bruising, blood in the urine or stool, or bleeding from the incision, drains, or tubes, is important. The nurse also monitors for signs of infection (elevated temperature, increased pain, abdominal distension, abdominal tenderness, and purulent drainage from the incisional site).

››› *Stop, Think, and Respond 47-2*

A friend calls and tells you that his abdominal pain is so severe that he cannot find a position to be comfortable. You advise him to seek medical attention. What suggestions could you make to prepare for the appointment?

The surgery for carcinoma of the pancreas is very serious, with potentially major complications and poor outcomes. Nursing diagnoses can include the following.

- **Acute Pain** related to surgical procedure
- **Hypovolemia** related to hemorrhage and loss of fluids
- **Altered Breathing Pattern** related to abdominal discomfort and drainage tubes
- **Infection Risk** related to invasive procedure and poor physical condition
- **Malnutrition Risk** related to high metabolic requirements and decreased ability to digest food
- **Injury Risk** related to failure to consume adequate calories or get enough insulin
- **Death Anxiety** related to shortened lifespan and poor prognosis

Clients who have surgery for pancreatic carcinoma and their significant others require diligent and caring attention. The nurse providing care focuses on the following:

- Assessing pain with a rating scale from 0 to 10
- Administering medications as prescribed
- Emptying drainage collection devices before they become full, taking care to avoid contaminating the drainage port
- Replacing fluids as ordered
- Monitoring serum electrolyte levels
- Auscultating lung sounds
- Instructing client to splint abdomen when turning or moving
- Encouraging client to deep breathe and cough at least every 2 hours
- Using aseptic technique to change or reinforce dressings when they become moist
- Following agency policy for changing IV sites, tubing, and infusing solutions
- Reassigning staff with potentially infectious symptoms to assignments that do not require direct client care or advising them to take sick leave
- Discouraging family or friends who may be ill from visiting until they are well
- Monitoring blood glucose levels several times each day
- Administering IV solutions, TPN, or both per orders
- Monitoring oral and IV caloric intake
- Teaching client about pancreatic enzyme replacement and a low-fat diet
- Providing support to client and family members as they begin to cope with the prognosis
- Helping client and family gain access to support services, hospice, and other organizations for palliative care and support

Care for clients with pancreatic tumors also must consider the psychological and emotional outcomes. If the client is discharged home, they and their family members require extensive teaching and home health services. The teaching plan should address schedules and techniques for administering prescribed medications, how to check the blood glucose level, recommended diet, importance of drinking fluids and eating, skin care (particularly around the incision), and the future schedule for follow-up visits, radiation therapy, or chemotherapy. The nurse also must review with the client and family symptoms to report to the primary provider: jaundice, dark urine, bleeding tendencies, vomiting, tarry stools, increased pain, swelling of the extremities, abdominal enlargement, decreased urine output, weight loss, and calf pain.

KEY POINTS

- Disorders of the liver include
  - Jaundice: yellowing of the skin
  - Cirrhosis: Chronic degenerative liver disorder
    - Complications: portal hypertension, esophageal varices, ascites, hepatic encephalopathy
  - Hepatitis: inflammation of the liver, multiple types
  - Tumors of the liver: abnormal cell mass
- Disorders of the gallbladder include
  - Cholelithiasis—stones in gallbladder
  - Cholecystitis—inflammation or infection of gallbladder
- Disorders of the pancreas include
  - Acute pancreatitis—inflammation of the pancreas
  - Chronic pancreatitis—prolonged and progressive inflammation of pancreas
  - Carcinoma of the pancreas—cancer

CRITICAL THINKING EXERCISES

1. A client has jaundice. What questions can you ask to help determine the cause?
2. How would you reassure someone who is interested in becoming a nurse yet has reservations because of potentially acquiring a blood-borne disease, such as hepatitis B?
3. A clinic nurse hears a client who is a man with hepatitis telling the medical assistant that he is taking cough syrup for his bad cold and cough. Does the nurse need to follow up?
4. A client with acute pancreatitis is admitted to the medical-surgical unit. They have poor skin turgor and tachycardia, and they complain of nausea and have dry heaves. In addition, they rate their abdominal pain as 8 on a 0-to-10 scale. An IV line is running, and the client is taking nothing by mouth. After about 2 hours, the client is more comfortable. The client asks for something to drink by signaling with the call light. How do you respond?

NCLEX-STYLE REVIEW QUESTIONS PrepU

1. The nurse notes that the client's total bilirubin is 1.0 mg/dL. Which action by the nurse is correct?
   1. Assess the client's sclerae for evidence of jaundice.
   2. Check the client's stool for presence of occult blood.
   3. Record the results as normal.
   4. Test the client's urine for blood.
2. After a liver biopsy on the client with cirrhosis, which nursing intervention is most appropriate to add to the plan of care?
   1. Ambulate the client twice each shift.
   2. Elevate the client's legs on two pillows.
   3. Keep the client in high Fowler position.
   4. Position the client on their right side.
3. Which action by the nurse best reduces the risk of transmitting the virus for a client diagnosed with HAV?
   1. The nurse puts on a mask and gown when providing direct care.
   2. The nurse maintains the client in a private room at all times.
   3. The nurse performs vigorous hand washing after leaving the room.
   4. The nurse wears gloves when entering the client's room.

4. A nurse inspects a breakfast tray for a client with pancreatitis who has not had any food for several days, and had a nasogastric tube removed. The client is now on a bland, low-fat diet. Which food item, if found on the client's breakfast tray, should be removed?
1. Whole wheat toast
2. Scrambled eggs
3. Skim milk
4. Stewed prunes

5. What nursing interventions should the nurse consider for a client who had surgery for pancreatic carcinoma? Select all that apply.
1. Advise the client to avoid splinting the abdomen when turning.
2. Discourage visitors who are ill from visiting until they are well.
3. Empty drainage collection devices regularly.
4. Instruct the client to avoid deep breathing and coughing.
5. Monitor blood glucose levels several times each day.

48 Caring for Clients With Ostomies

Words To Know

abdominoperineal resection
anastomosis
appliance
colostomy
continent ileostomy (abdominal pouch)
double-barrel colostomy
effluent
enterostomal therapist
ileoanal reservoir
ileostomy
loop transverse colostomy
ostomate
ostomy
segmental resection
single-barrel colostomy
standard or Brooke ileostomy
stoma
wound, ostomy, and continence nurse (WOCN)

Learning Objectives

On completion of this chapter, you will be able to:

1. Differentiate between ileostomy and colostomy.
2. Explain how stool is excreted from three types of ileostomies.
3. Describe the two-part procedure needed to create an ileoanal reservoir.
4. Discuss various types of colostomies.
5. Explain ways that clients with descending or sigmoid colostomies may regulate bowel elimination.
6. Discuss preoperative nursing care of a client undergoing ostomy surgery.
7. List complications associated with ostomy surgery.
8. Discuss postoperative nursing management of a client with an ileostomy and colostomy.
9. Describe the components used to apply and collect stool from an intestinal ostomy.
10. Cite reasons for changing an ostomy appliance.
11. Summarize how to change an ostomy appliance.

The term **ostomy** refers to a surgical opening between an internal body structure and the skin. The most common intestinal ostomies are the ileostomy, an opening from the distal small intestine, and the colostomy, an opening from the colon. Table 48-1 provides a summary of the common ostomy procedures. Fecal material exits through a **stoma**, an opening on the exterior abdominal surface. Most ostomies are created in response to an inflammatory bowel disorder that fails to respond to medical treatment or complications such as rupture of a portion of intestine, irreversible obstruction, compromised blood supply to the intestine, or cancerous tumor. Whether an ostomy is temporary or permanent, each client requires an individually adapted plan of care that incorporates preparation for surgery, recovery from surgery, and knowledge required for ongoing self-care.

Gerontologic Considerations

■ Older adults with ostomies who also experience chronic disorders such as poor vision and arthritis may encounter difficulty in changing the appliance, performing skin care, irrigating the colostomy stoma, and caring for the permanent appliance. Consult with a wound, ostomy, and continence nurse about which equipment may best meet the client's needs.

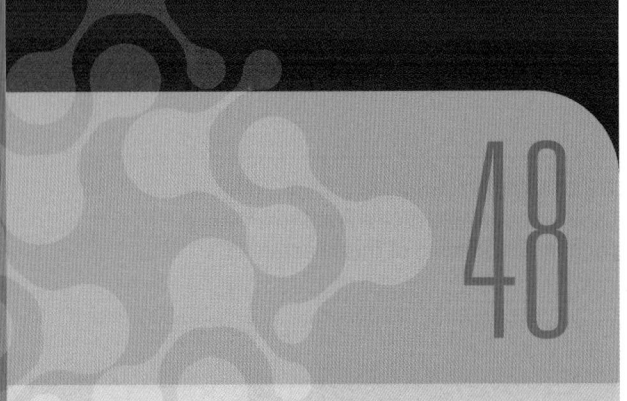

Gerontologic Considerations (continued)

■ Health care providers must assess the older adult's ability to provide long-term self-care for the ostomy, or identify available resources such as a family member, visiting nurse, or home health care nurse. In some instances, a skilled nursing facility or nursing home may be necessary.

ILEOSTOMY

Ileostomies are most frequently done for clients who have inflammatory bowel disease or cancer. They can be permanent or temporary, depending on why it needed to be done. A permanent **ileostomy** can involve removing the entire colon, rectum, and anus or bypassing these structures. A temporary ileostomy entails removing all or a portion of the colon, but the rectum (at least part of it), and the anus remain intact.

There are three types of ileostomies: **standard or Brooke ileostomy** (may be referred to as a conventional ileostomy), continent ileostomy or abdominal pouch, and ileoanal reservoir, or J-pouch or pelvic pouch.

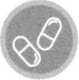

Pharmacologic Considerations

■ Clients with an ileostomy may need fat-soluble vitamin supplementation and approximately 25% eventually develop vitamin B_{12} deficiency requiring regular supplementation.

Standard or Brooke Ileostomy

In the usual surgical procedure for a standard ileostomy, the entire colon and rectum are removed (total colectomy) or are temporarily bypassed. The terminal end of the ileum is brought out through a separate area on the right lower quadrant of the abdomen slightly below the umbilicus, near the

TABLE 48-1 Intestinal Ostomies

OSTOMY	DESCRIPTION	FECAL CONSISTENCY	FECAL CONTROL
Ileostomy	The ileum (the third part of the small intestine) is brought to the surface through an opening in the right side of the abdomen following removal or bypass of the colon and rectum. An ileostomy can be permanent or temporary.	Liquid, semi-liquid, mushy, or pasty	
	Types:		
	Standard or Brooke ileostomy—most frequently done; a stoma is formed to drain fecal contents into a pouch.	Liquid to pasty	Continuous output—pouch needs to be emptied 6–10 times per day
	Continent or abdominal ileostomy—a modification of the standard ileostomy; a reservoir is created with a nipple valve to drain fecal contents. A pouch is not needed—the client inserts a catheter to drain the reservoir.	Liquid	By siphoning 5–8 times per day
	Ileoanal reservoir or J-pouch or pelvic pouch (or ileoanal anastomosis)—an internal pouch created from the ileum. The colon and rectum are removed and the reservoir/pouch is connected to the anus. This procedure often follows a temporary ileostomy. Once the ileum heals it is then connected to the pouch and the ileostomy is closed. Anal sphincter control and continence are preserved, and an external pouch is not required for defecation.	Liquid, mushy, or pasty	Once healing occurs, 7–10 movements per day
Colostomy	A stoma is created through an opening in the abdomen from a portion of the colon; location is dependent upon which portion of the colon is used to create the stoma. A colostomy can be permanent or temporary.	Liquid to formed	
	Types:		
	Ascending colostomy—stoma is placed in the right abdomen; only a small portion of the colon is preserved. Fecal contents contain digestive enzymes and acids. This procedure is the least common.	Liquid to pasty; similar to ileostomy	Continuous output—pouch needs to be emptied 5–8 times per day
	Transverse colostomy—Two types:		
	1. *Loop transverse colostomy*—One stoma is created in the mid-abdomen—stoma has two openings: the proximal opening expels stool; the distal or resting colon opening expels mucus. The stool contains digestive enzymes and acids.	Semi-liquid to soft	Pouch must be worn at all times; emptying times vary from 4–8 times per day.
	2. *Double-barrel transverse colostomy*—Similar to the loop colostomy, but the colon is completely separated into two stomas: one for expelling stool and one for mucus (referred to as the mucus fistula).	Semi-liquid to soft	As above
	Descending colostomy—Located in the lower left abdomen, there is more functional colon remaining.	Soft	Continence can sometimes be achieved. Pouch may be worn.
	Sigmoid colostomy—Located lower in the left abdomen than the descending colostomy. The most functional colon remains. This is the most common type of colostomy.	Soft to formed.	Continence can often be achieved. Pouch may be worn.

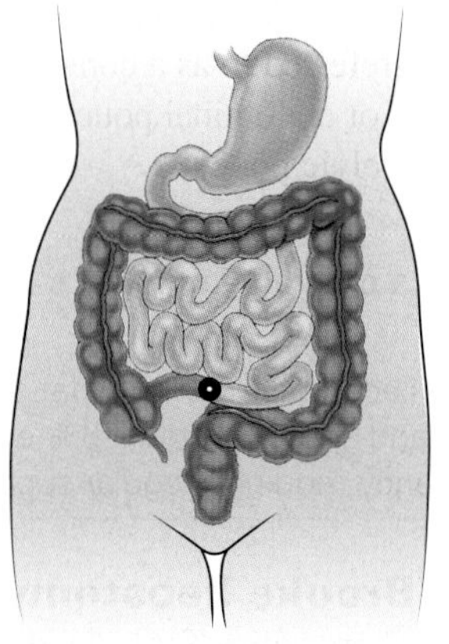

Figure 48-1 Total colectomy is removal of the entire colon and rectum. The terminal end of the ileum is brought out through the abdomen to form an ileostomy. (Blue color represents the section that has been removed.)

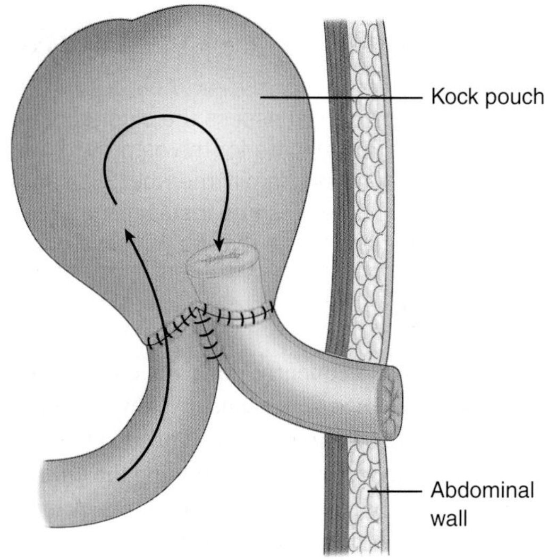

Figure 48-2 Continent ileostomy.

outer border of the rectus muscle (Fig. 48-1). The cut end is everted and sutured to the skin, a process referred to as creating a *matured* stoma. When an ileostomy is performed, the stoma continually releases stool and gas. The fecal material discharged from an ileostomy is liquid, mushy, or pasty, and it contains digestive enzymes and acids.

Continent Ileostomy or Abdominal Pouch

A **continent ileostomy (abdominal pouch)** is similar to the standard ileostomy but involves the creation of an internal reservoir for the storage of GI **effluent** (discharged fecal material or liquid feces). The reservoir stores this effluent for several hours until the client removes it with a catheter. Doing so eliminates the need for an external appliance. After removing the diseased portion of the ileum, the surgeon forms a reservoir with a portion of the terminal ileum and creates a nipple valve by telescoping (*intussusception*) the distal ileal segment into the reservoir. The surgeon then forms an external stoma and anchors it to the abdominal wall (Fig. 48-2).

During the operation, the surgeon inserts a temporary catheter through the nipple valve and sutures the catheter in place so that its end protrudes from the external stoma. Then the surgeon packs the perineal area from which the lower intestine was removed with gauze. The packing remains in place for about 1 week.

Ileoanal Reservoir or J-Pouch or Pelvic Pouch

The **ileoanal reservoir**, also called an ileoanal **anastomosis** (a surgical connection between two structures; Fig. 48-3), is a procedure that maintains bowel continence. It is performed on selected clients who have chronic ulcerative colitis or whose disease does not affect the anorectal sphincter. Besides allowing the client to control bowel elimination, this procedure, as opposed to a standard ileostomy with total colectomy, preserves innervation to the male genitalia. Subsequently, clients who are men are unlikely to experience bladder dysfunction, erectile dysfunction, or infertility.

An ileoanal anastomosis is performed in two stages. In the first stage, the surgeon creates a temporary ileostomy, removes a large length of diseased colon down to the terminal section of the rectum above the anal sphincter, joins several distal loops of healthy ileum to form a pouch for holding stool, and connects the ileal reservoir to the anal cuff. After the first stage of surgery, clients experience an almost continuous discharge of mucus from the anus and a frequent discharge of fecal material from the ileostomy. Initially, clients cannot control the frequent watery discharge.

The second stage is performed 2 or 3 months later. At this time, the surgeon closes the temporary ileostomy and

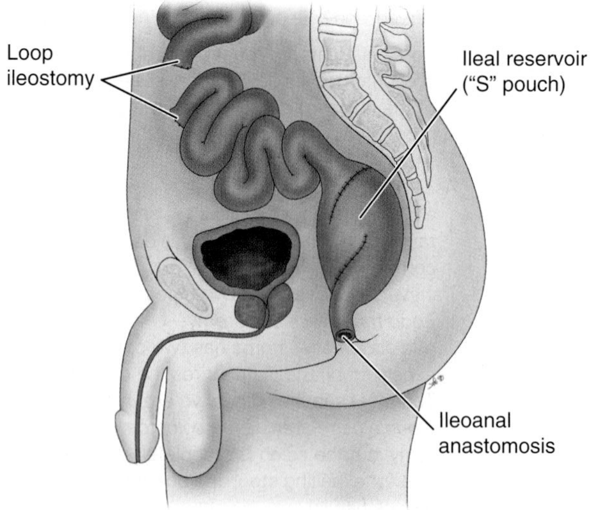

Figure 48-3 An ileoanal anastomosis joins a section of ileum to create an ileal reservoir. The distal end of the ileum is sutured above the anus. Intestinal effluent is temporarily discharged through the proximal stoma of a loop ileostomy until the second stage of surgery is performed.

reunites the two sections of ileum. The area where the two sections of bowel are joined is called an *anastomosis*. The anastomosis establishes a normal flow of fecal material through the ileum to the reservoir. The fecal material, which is stored in the ileal reservoir, is then expelled from the anus. Control is achieved as edema subsides and the anal sphincter becomes stronger.

Preoperative Period

Surgical Management for Ileostomy Surgery

Before surgery, the primary provider explains the purpose for the surgical procedure along with its benefits and risks. They describe the appearance and function of the stoma, where it will be placed, and its required care. The primary provider carefully marks the site to ensure that it is away from bony prominences, skin creases, and scars; is within the rectus abdominis muscle; is unobstructed; and is visible to the client. Clients benefit from preoperative interactions with a specially certified nurse, referred to as an *enterostomal therapy nurse*, **enterostomal therapist**, or **wound, ostomy, and continence nurse (WOCN)**. This nurse assists with marking placement of the stoma and collaborates with the surgeon regarding placement and the client's educational needs.

The surgeon identifies potential risks from the total colectomy, such as possible bladder and sexual dysfunction secondary to parasympathetic nerve injury. Sexual dysfunction in men after a total colectomy is unusual but sometimes occurs. If such dysfunction persists after a colectomy, operative and nonoperative options are available to facilitate erection. Clients who are young men may wish to collect and store sperm for later use if they plan to have children. A colectomy may slightly diminish fertility in women; however, this procedure does not preclude the ability to achieve a full-term pregnancy with a normal vaginal delivery.

Cleansing of the bowel before surgery is carried out using dietary restrictions in combination with laxative or lavage agents (e.g., GoLYTELY, Miralax, Dulcolax), depending on the client's condition (i.e., presence or absence of obstruction) and according to the surgeon's preference. Opinions vary regarding the need for antibiotic prophylaxis. Many surgeons order a combination of intravenous (IV) antibiotics (i.e., a third-generation cephalosporin and metronidazole) before surgery and continue administration after surgery.

Whenever possible, prednisone should be tapered and discontinued before surgery to avoid negative effects of the drug on tissue healing. A preoperative "stress dose" of IV steroid (i.e., hydrocortisone) is given to clients who have been on prednisone within the previous 6 months to prevent adrenal crisis. Adrenal crisis is potentially life-threatening and can result from the abrupt withdrawal of corticosteroids or significant stress after the client has been treated with corticosteroids. See Chapter 50 for additional information on adrenal crisis.

Immunosuppressive agents such as azathioprine, 6-mercaptopurine, and cyclosporine should be discontinued 3 to 4 weeks before surgery to prevent negative effects on tissue healing. Aspirin-containing compounds are discontinued at least 1 week before surgery to minimize the risk of bleeding. Blood samples are taken before surgery, and the client's blood is typed and crossmatched for replacement of losses that occur during surgery.

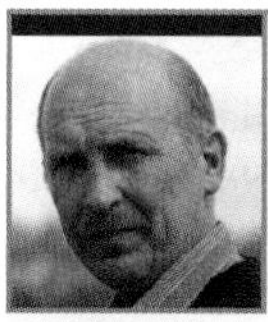

Clinical Scenario A 50-year-old man with chronic ulcerative colitis is admitted for a total colectomy with ileostomy. Knowing that this client faces major changes postoperatively, **what are important aspects of the client's care that the nurse must consider preoperatively? See the following Nursing Process section.**

NURSING PROCESS FOR THE CLIENT BEFORE ILEOSTOMY SURGERY

Assessment

Obtain complete medical, allergy, diet, and drug histories. Ask the client if they have been taking corticosteroids. If so, monitor the client closely for signs and symptoms of adrenal insufficiency such as weakness, lethargy, hypotension, nausea, and vomiting as the dosage is tapered. Perform a physical assessment, paying particular attention to inspecting the skin over the abdomen, auscultating bowel sounds, and obtaining the client's vital signs and weight. In addition, check the preoperative laboratory test results to determine if blood cell counts and serum electrolyte levels are within normal ranges. Obtain a description of preoperative measures the client may have been asked to take, such as dietary modifications and antibiotic therapy. Implement medical orders for cleansing the bowel, inserting a nasogastric tube, and preparing the client for surgery.

Referral to community and professional resources before surgery may positively affect the client's postoperative quality of life. Resources for education and support include the medical and surgical teams and the lay public (e.g., Crohn's & Colitis Foundation of America, United Ostomy Associations of America).

Health care teams hold several views about beginning ostomy instructions before surgery. Some believe that such teaching helps clients to accept the ostomy. Others believe that this type of teaching creates premature stress and anxiety. Often, a WOC nurse provides ostomy instruction, whether before or after surgery. They are certified to care for ostomates and manage their unique problems. This nurse is also an excellent resource for nurses providing direct care to ostomates. If the client expresses a readiness to learn or asks questions about ostomy care, provide information about ostomy equipment and general principles of ostomy management. Also, if the client so desires, arrange a preoperative visit with the WOC nurse.

(continued)

NURSING PROCESS FOR THE CLIENT BEFORE ILEOSTOMY SURGERY (continued)

Diagnosis, Planning, and Interventions

Knowledge Deficiency: About the surgical procedure and the creation of an ileostomy
Expected Outcome: Client demonstrates knowledge of preoperative expectations, the surgical procedure, and initial understanding of an ileostomy.

- Ask the client what they have been told about their surgery. *Clarifying what the client knows is helpful in order to supplement or provide information or correct any misconceptions.*
- Provide illustrations and/or written materials depending on the client's level of understanding and desire for information. *Teaching at the client's level and needs is important so that the client is not unnecessarily alarmed.*
- Discuss preoperative medications (antibiotics) and preparations (bowel cleansing) that will be given. *Client's understanding of the need for preoperative antibiotics and bowel cleansing alleviates anxiety.*

Acute Anxiety: Related to change in health status and fear of the unknown
Expected Outcome: Client will experience reduced anxiety.

- Provide an overview of preoperative procedures, using explanations the client understands. *Explanations enable the client to know what to expect.*
- Allow time for the client to ask questions and express fears. *Adequate time and support promote communication and assist the client to verbalize anxiety.*
- Assess previous positive coping skills and assist client to access them again. *Past successful coping methods are likely to be effective now.*

Altered Body Image: Related to the stoma and altered bowel elimination
Expected Outcome: Client verbalizes what the changes will be and the benefits to future health.

- Encourage the client to discuss feelings about the stoma. *Such discussion enables the client to express concerns and fears about the fecal diversion.*
- Inform the client that an assigned staff nurse will be there when the client first views and touches the stoma. *Such information gives reassurance that a familiar nurse will be available to answer questions and give support.*
- If the client expresses interest, provide a list of appropriate community resources. *Knowing that others have experienced the same surgery and can share their experience and offer advice and support may help the client.*

Evaluation of Expected Outcomes

The client is able to discuss what will occur preoperatively and is able to describe the surgical procedure. The client verbalizes fears and demonstrates positive coping skills. They discuss what physical changes to expect.

Postoperative Period

Nursing Management

Standard or Brooke Ileostomy

The nurse monitors the anus for drainage that may come from the rectum which is packed with gauze during surgery to absorb drainage and promote gradual healing. The rectal pack usually is removed in 5 to 7 days. Afterward, irrigations may be ordered to promote healing. A nasogastric tube is used for gastrointestinal (GI) decompression until normal bowel motility resumes. Fluid, electrolyte, and nutritional balances are maintained with IV fluids until oral nourishment is possible. Within several days, the nasogastric tube is removed and oral feedings begin. Antibiotic therapy continues. Analgesics are prescribed for pain relief. Wound healing is monitored, and complications that develop are managed.

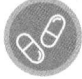

> **Pharmacologic Considerations**
>
> ■ Clients with an ileostomy should avoid medications that are slowly absorbed in the GI tract. This includes enteric-coated and sustained-release drugs. Gelatin capsules and liquid forms of drugs dissolve the best. Any laxatives may cause severe dehydration and should not be taken.

The nurse observes the client for possible postoperative complications, which include intestinal obstruction; bleeding; and impaired blood supply to, stenosis of, or prolapse or excessive protrusion of the stoma. Intestinal obstruction, a serious complication, may result from a twisted, strangulated, or incarcerated segment of the remaining intestine or a bolus of poorly chewed or inadequately digested food. When a collection of food causes obstruction, the primary provider may irrigate the stoma in an attempt to correct the problem. If the bowel is twisted or strangulated, surgical intervention is necessary.

Prolapse or protrusion of the ileostomy is fairly common. If it is moderate (1 or 2 inches), no treatment is required. A severe prolapse of the stoma is a serious complication, however. If edema occurs, it may cause an obstruction and restrict stomal blood supply. Stomal necrosis results if the prolapse is not promptly and skillfully managed. Once the stoma prolapses, recurrence is likely.

Continent Ileostomy

The nurse reinforces the perineal packing, as needed, during the postoperative period. In addition, the nurse checks the abdominal dressing for drainage and connects the stomal catheter, if ordered, to low intermittent suction that empties the reservoir continuously, thereby preventing tension on healing suture lines. They check the ileal catheter frequently for the following signs of obstruction: lack of fecal drainage, the client's complaint of feeling full in the area of the ileal pouch, or leakage of liquid stool around the catheter. The nurse notes the color and amount of drainage, observes the size and color of the stoma, and administers either routine or as-needed irrigations of the ileal catheter, using small amounts of normal saline solution if the catheter appears to be obstructed, according to primary provider's orders. They keep the skin clean around the stoma, change the gauze dressing over the stoma when it becomes wet with mucus or serosanguineous drainage, and change the dressing every 6 to 8 hours as drainage decreases.

The nurse also monitors ileal output carefully during the entire postoperative period. As GI function resumes, the initial amount of ileal drainage is usually high. If excessive fluids and electrolytes are lost, parenteral fluid and electrolyte replacement is necessary. When ileal drainage stabilizes, about 10 to 14 days after surgery, the primary provider removes the ileal catheter. The reservoir then holds the accumulating effluent until the nurse or client siphons it. Initially, the reservoir is emptied every 2 to 4 hours. As the capacity of the reservoir increases, usually in about 6 months, the client or caregiver performs the procedure three or four times daily.

The nurse includes the information presented in Client and Family Teaching 48-1 in their teaching plan. For additional nursing management, refer to the discussion that addresses similar problems experienced by a client with ileoanal reservoir.

Ileoanal Reservoir

The postoperative assessment after the first stage of ileoanal reservoir surgery includes making the same observations and assessments as those for an ileostomy. In addition, the nurse inspects the anal area for drainage and checks the drain or drainage tube in the presacral area if there is one. After the second stage, when the ileostomy is closed and the ileum is connected to the anal reservoir, the nurse inspects the anal area and the operative sites for drainage.

The postoperative plan of nursing care involves measures pertaining to general surgery and related client problems, such as risk for fluid volume deficit, risk for bowel incontinence, and impaired perianal skin integrity to reduce the risk for bowel incontinence, the nurse instructs the client to perform perineal exercises to reestablish anal sphincter control and enlarge the ileoanal reservoir. These exercises involve tightening the anus as if trying to prevent a bowel movement and holding the contraction for a count of 10 before relaxing. The nurse should urge the client to do 10 repetitions of this exercise four to six times a day.

Keeping the perianal area clean is especially important. After first-stage ileoanal surgery, the nurse teaches the client to use a squirt bottle to clean the perianal area and avoid skin irritation. After the second-stage repair, the nurse instructs the client to cleanse the anus with warm, soapy water to remove mucus, stool, or both. The client also must dry the area well. Refer to Client and Family Teaching 48-2 for information that the nurse teaches the client and family.

Client and Family Teaching 48-1
Care of the Stoma and Catheter After a Continent Ileostomy

The nurse emphasizes the following points when teaching the client:

- Assemble a clean catheter, lubricant, basin, tissues, irrigating syringe and solution, and gauze dressing.
- Sit on or beside the toilet or on the side of the bed.
- Warm the catheter to body temperature and lubricate the tip. Insert it about 2 inches into the stomal opening.
- Expect resistance when the catheter reaches the nipple valve (about 2 inches), which controls the retention of waste matter. Gently push the catheter a little further into the ileal pouch. At the same time, exhale, cough, or bear down as if to pass stool until fecal material begins to drain.
- Direct the external end of the catheter into a basin or the toilet about 12 inches below the stoma.
- If the catheter is obstructed, try the following measures:
  - Bear down as if to have a bowel movement.
  - Rotate the catheter tip inside the stoma.
  - Milk the catheter.
  - If these are not successful, remove the catheter, rinse it, and try again.
  - Notify the primary provider if efforts to unblock the catheter do not result in any drainage.
  - Never wait longer than 6 hours without obtaining drainage.
- Allow 5 to 10 minutes for drainage to cease; then remove the catheter, clean it with soapy water, and store it in a sealable plastic bag until needed again.
- Wash the area around the stoma and pat the skin dry.
- Place an absorbent pad or dressing over the stoma.

Client and Family Teaching 48-2 Postoperative Ileoanal Reservoir Care

The nurse discusses the following issues with the client and their family:

- Continue performing perineal strengthening exercises daily.
- Apply protective ointments or creams as recommended by the primary provider.
- Inspect the anal area daily using a handheld mirror.
- Contact primary provider if the anal area becomes sore or skin changes (e.g., ulceration, bleeding) are apparent.
- Use a thin sanitary shield or disposable, lined underwear to absorb fecal drainage until anal sphincter control is achieved.

The Ostomy Appliance

The matured stoma promotes healing and provides a smooth peristomal area that permits the immediate postoperative application of an **appliance**, the collection device worn over a stoma. Clients with an ileostomy always wear an appliance, which requires frequent emptying. Ostomy suppliers provide various appliances to meet the individual needs of the **ostomate** (client with an ostomy). Appliances consist of one-piece or two-piece devices with a pouch for collecting feces an a faceplate, or disk, which is attached to the abdomen with an opening through which the stoma protrudes (Fig. 48-4). The faceplate adheres to the skin either with self-adhesive backing or another bonding substance such as an adhesive powder, paste, or wafer. Clients are taught to protect the skin around the stoma with a skin barrier. Some products have the skin barrier built in to the adherent surface.

A disposable, or temporary, appliance is preferred in the immediate postoperative phase because the size of the stoma changes over time as a result of swelling from the procedure itself. The size of the stoma may change rapidly and differ from one appliance change to the next. After the stoma heals and reaches its final size and shape (approximately 3 months), a permanent (reusable) appliance is fitted.

Reusable equipment consists of a sturdier pouch with a custom-sized faceplate and "O" ring. The pouch is designed to fasten into position when pressed over the ring, much like snapping a lid on a plastic margarine tub. The pouch has a clamp at the bottom, which can be released when the pouch needs to be emptied. The pouch may be fastened to a belt for more security. The belt supports the weight of the liquid fecal material and prevents the faceplate from being pulled away from the abdominal skin. Foam rubber, gauze, or flannel padding is placed under a belt if the belt cuts into the flesh. The client requires two sets of permanent appliances so that one can be cleaned periodically. Disposable equipment may be appropriate for some clients. Disposable bags, faceplates, and attachment rings are replaced with new ones with each change of the ostomy appliance (usually daily with bathing).

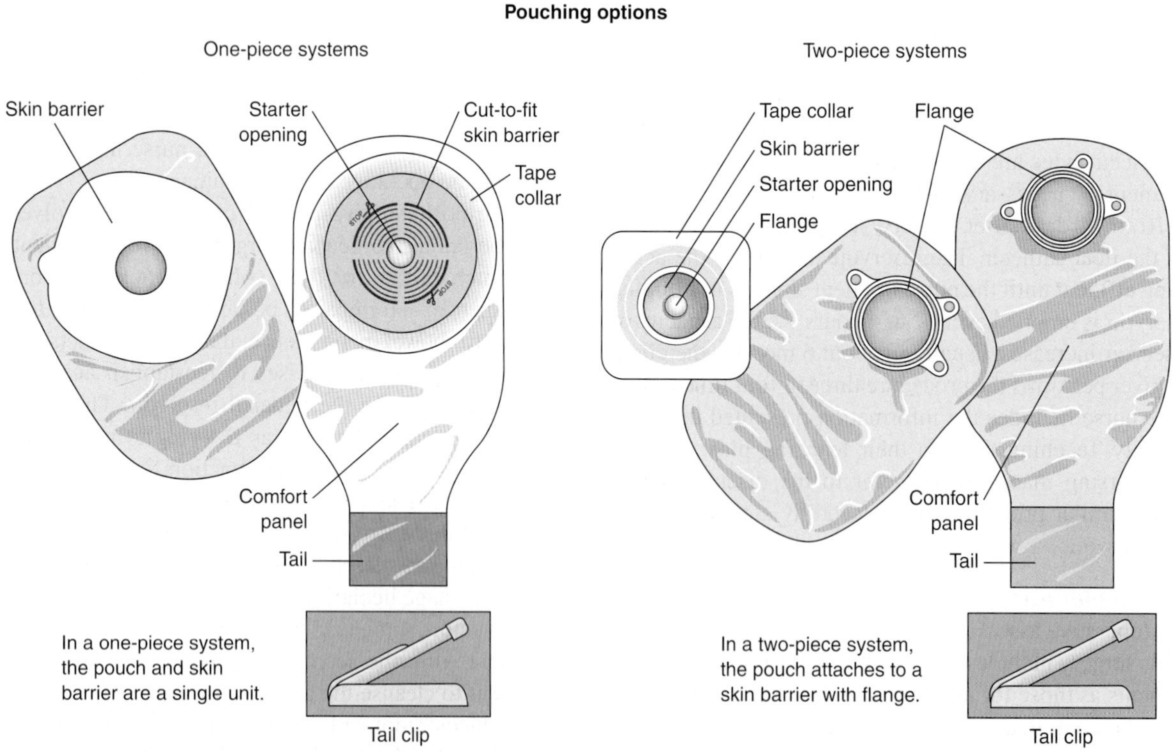

Figure 48-4 Ostomy appliance. (Reprinted with permission from Hinkle, J. L., & Cheever, K. H. (2014). *Brunner & Suddarth's textbook of medical-surgical nursing* (13th ed.). Wolters Kluwer Health/Lippincott Williams & Wilkins.)

Pharmacologic Considerations

- Some medications, especially vitamins, cause particularly strong odors that cling to the appliance. Talk to the health care provider regarding alternatives.

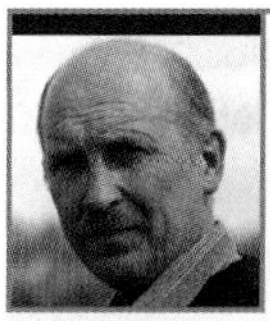

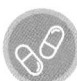

Clinical Scenario The 50-year-old client has the total colectomy and ileostomy and an uneventful stay in the postanesthesia care unit. He is transferred to the postsurgical unit. **What does the nurse need to include in this client's care? See the following Nursing Process section.**

NURSING PROCESS FOR THE CLIENT RECOVERING FROM ILEOSTOMY SURGERY

Assessment

Review the medical record for information regarding the type of surgery and any problems during or immediately after surgery. Obtain vital signs; inspect the dressing and stoma for bleeding and signs of infection (Table 48-2); monitor the rate and progress of fluid and blood infusions; check the function of the gastric suction; measure intake and output; and inspect the collection appliance, special drains, packing, or tubes. Record all immediate postoperative findings to provide a database.

Diagnosis, Planning, and Interventions

Nursing Guidelines 48-1 provides instructions for replacing an ostomy appliance. In logical steps and at a pace that promotes comprehension, teach the client and another family member about managing the ostomy, adopting dietary modifications, recognizing how drug therapy affects bowel elimination, and adjusting to various surgery-related changes, such as possible sexual dysfunction. Client and Family Teaching 48-3 lists additional topics to include in the teaching plan.

In addition to the measures discussed in the following pages, postoperative care includes standard pain management (see Chapter 11) and postoperative interventions (see Chapter 14).

Altered Skin Integrity Risk: Related to effects of fecal material and adhesives on the skin
Expected Outcome: Client will maintain intact peristomal skin.

- Demonstrate safe, gentle removal of the pouch. *This type of removal prevents skin irritation.*
- Gently cleanse the peristomal area with warm water and mild soap. *Gentle cleansing minimizes skin irritation and abrasions.*
- Teach the client to apply a skin barrier, such as a wafer, gel, paste, or powder. *The skin barrier protects the peristomal skin from digestive enzymes and bacteria.*

Infection Risk: Related to fecal contamination of the surgical wound
Expected Outcome: Client's wound is free from infection.

- Apply dressing securely, covering the surgical wound completely. *The dressing protects the incision from contact with fecal material.*
- Change the ostomy pouch when it is loose and leaking. *Changing at the appropriate time minimizes the risk of fecal drainage entering the incision.*
- When drainage leaks near the incision, wipe it away from the incision and change the dressing if soiled at all. *These measures keep fecal drainage away from incision, ensuring that the dressing always is clean.*
- Observe for signs of wound infection: wound drainage, abdominal pain, and elevated temperature. *These signs indicate possible wound infection.*

Bowel Incontinence: Related to loss of sphincter control and change in intestinal motility
Expected Outcome: Client will have no or minimal leaking from the appliance or soiling with fecal material.

- Instruct the client how to prepare the drainage pouch for a secure fit around the stoma, leaving an extra 1/8 inch in the appliance opening. (Use a gauge for measuring, provided by the manufacturer.) *Accurate preparation provides room for stoma clearance and potential swelling.*
- Press the adhesive faceplate around the stoma for about 30 seconds. *This measure ensures secure attachment of the pouch to the peristomal skin.*
- Demonstrate frequent emptying of the pouch. *Frequent emptying prevents tension on the pouch and skin from the weight of the drainage.*
- Use the following measures to prevent leakage:
  - Press the adhesive faceplate from the stomal edge outward. *This technique prevents the formation of wrinkles.*
  - Ask the client to remain inactive for 5 minutes. *This period allows time for body heat to strengthen the adhesive bond.*
  - Allow a small amount of air to be trapped in the pouch. *Liquid feces will then drain to the bottom of the pouch, placing less tension on it.*
  - Make several pinhole-sized punctures at the upper edge of the pouch. *Punctures allow excess gas to escape and decrease tension on the pouch.*

(continued)

NURSING PROCESS FOR THE CLIENT RECOVERING FROM ILEOSTOMY SURGERY (continued)

Dehydration or Hypovolemia: Related to decreased appetite, vomiting, or increased loss of fluids and electrolytes from ileostomy
Expected Outcome: Client maintains adequate fluid and electrolyte balance.

- Assess fluid balance. *This evaluation determines any deficits.*
- Examine serum and urine test results for sodium and potassium levels. *Review may indicate imbalances and other potential problems (e.g., acidosis, cardiac dysrhythmias).*
- Observe skin turgor and appearance of the tongue. *Poor skin turgor and dry tongue indicate fluid deficits.*

Altered Body Image Perception: Related to altered body image and risk for sexual dysfunction
Expected Outcome: Client will plan modifications for maintaining sexual fulfillment.

- Encourage the client and partner to verbalize fears and concerns about intimacy. *Discussion allows client and partner to express feelings and explore needs.*
- Reassure the client who is not experiencing sexual dysfunction that intercourse will not harm the healed ostomy. *Fear can interfere with sexual relations; reassurance assists clients to reestablish sexual relationships.*
- Recommend alternative sexual positions and modifications (Client and Family Teaching 48-4). *Different positions and other modifications may enable the client to avoid embarrassment about the stomal appearance until they are more comfortable.*
- Refer clients who experience sexual dysfunction to a sexual therapist, enterostomal therapist, or advanced practice nurse. *Clients and partners may need assistance to determine problems and solutions, including alternative methods to achieve sexual satisfaction.*

Coping Impairment: Related to disturbed body image and altered bowel function
Expected Outcome: Client will cope effectively with body changes.

- Ensure privacy when teaching and providing ileostomy care. *Privacy allows client to get used to changes without fear of embarrassment in front of others.*
- Help the client to set realistic goals and identify personal skills and knowledge. *Participation in the care plan allows the client to make decisions and move toward independence.*
- Use empathetic communication, allowing time for client to express fears and concerns. *A supportive environment promotes coping.*
- Refer the client to support networks, such as ostomy groups or other ostomates. *Resources help client to problem solve and increase coping skills.*

Evaluation of Expected Outcomes

Peristomal skin is not reddened, there is no evidence of edema or drainage, and the client does not complain of burning sensations. The incision heals without infection. Stool is contained in the ostomy pouch. The client maintains adequate fluid balance as evidenced by balanced intake and output, good skin turgor, moist tongue and mucous membranes, and normal serum and urine sodium and potassium levels. The client reports that they have attained satisfactory sexual performance. They also demonstrate coping skills as evidenced by interest in self-care, ability to seek assistance, and ability to maintain relationships.

TABLE 48-2 Characteristics of Healthy and Unhealthy Stomas

CHARACTERISTICS	HEALTHY STOMA	UNHEALTHY STOMA
Color	Bright pink or red	Dusky blue or black
Size	Comparable in diameter with the intestine from which it has been formed; may be somewhat large after surgery because of edema	Larger or smaller in comparison to size after resolution of postoperative edema
Opening	Patent, unobstructed	Tight or narrow
Surface	Moist, shiny with an overlying layer of mucus; may bleed slightly when being cleansed	Dull, dry; excessive bleeding
Length	Protrudes from or is just flush with the skin	Protrudes beyond 2 inches from the skin or retracts beneath it
Sensation	Painless	Peristomal burning
Function	Regular passage of feces	Sparse or absent elimination of feces

NURSING GUIDELINES 48-1

Changing an Ostomy Appliance

Assemble clean gloves; scissors; ostomy belt; stoma gauge; faceplate; pouch; adhesive or skin barrier or protectant; and cleaning materials such as gauze pads, water, or adhesive solvent.

- Wash hands and put on gloves.
- Empty pouch when it is one-third full.
- Change the faceplate only when needed, that is, if it becomes loose or tight or if client experiences discomfort. If the faceplate is changed too frequently, skin around stoma may become raw and excoriated secondary to removal of protective layers of epithelium with the faceplate.
- If the ostomy appliance is being replaced routinely, schedule the change when the gastrocolic reflex is less active. For many clients, this time is early in the morning, before eating, or 2 or 3 hours after mealtime.
- Gently ease the faceplate from the skin. If the faceplate was applied with adhesive, roll the adhesive from the skin and appliance. If it does not roll off, use a small amount of solvent, which chemically loosens the adhesive bond. Because some solvents irritate the skin, apply solvent sparingly between the body and faceplate using a sprayer, medicine dropper, or gauze pad. Avoid rubbing, which may further irritate skin. Clean the area with soap and water and pat dry after a solvent has been used.
- Inform the client that the most common causes of discomfort are reactions to the adhesive or solvent used to remove it or irritation from leaking fecal drainage. In such cases, the client may experience stinging, tingling, or itching immediately after an appliance change. These sensations should quickly subside. If a sensation is prolonged or intensified, remove the appliance regardless of whether it has been on for 1 hour or several days. When using a new adhesive product, remember to patch test it first on nonirritated skin at the inner aspect of the client's forearm.
- After removing the faceplate and pouch, protect the peristomal area from drainage by placing a tissue cuff around the stoma or using a receptacle such as a small paper cup to collect the drainage. Use a soapy washcloth to clean the skin around the stoma and wipe the soap from the skin. Pat the area or allow it to air dry.
- Inspect the stoma and skin carefully. If excoriation is observed, use a temporary appliance or hydrocolloid dressing, such as Duoderm or Tegaderm, to cover the excoriated skin to promote moist healing. If there is yeast growth, nystatin (Mycostatin) powder may be ordered. Triamcinolone acetonide (Kenalog) spray (topical corticosteroid) may be used.
- Create an even surface for reapplying the pouch by filling irregular hollows in the peristomal skin with hydrocolloid paste, such as Karaya paste, before replacing the faceplate.
- Measure the circumference of the stoma and cut a comparable hole in the faceplate, allowing 18-inch margin to account for potential swelling in a new stoma.
- Secure the pouch to the faceplate. Be sure to smooth out ridges or openings in the closure. Also, be sure to seal the pouch.
- Peel the backing from the faceplate.
- Affix the faceplate to the skin.

Client and Family Teaching 48-3
Postoperative Ileostomy Care

The nurse discusses the following issues with the client and their family:

- Restrict oral intake only with medical supervision.
- Eat slowly and chew food well with the mouth closed to help lessen the development of gas.
- Avoid foods that cause discomfort, excessive gas, or loose stools.
- Drink extra fluids, especially in warm weather.
- Dilate the stoma if the volume of stool decreases for some unexplained reason. To do this, cut the nail on the index or little finger, cover the finger with a finger cot, lubricate it thoroughly, and then insert the finger gently into the stoma for a few minutes.
- Clean the pouch thoroughly to prevent odors.
- Use an internal odor-absorbing substance or one that can be added to the pouch to control lingering or stubborn odors.
- Use an old or disposable pouch when medications or offending foods that cause disagreeable odors are excreted.
- Slip a plastic cover over the pouch to act as a second barrier against escaping odors.
- Check with a primary provider before self-administering any drug, especially a laxative or antidiarrheal agent.

Client and Family Teaching 48-4
Sexual Modifications for Ostomates

The nurse offers the following suggestions to clients with ostomies:

- Always practice good hygiene. Bathe and apply a fresh pouch before having sex.
- Disguise the pouch by enclosing it within a purse-string cloth cover.
- When anticipating sexual activity, avoid eating or drinking substances that activate the bowel or create a lot of gas.
- Fashion a cummerbund with a pocket or fold into which the pouch can be held.
- Remove the belt and temporarily secure the pouch to the skin with tape.
- If accidents happen, cultivate a sense of humor, which may relieve the anxiety of the sexual partner as well.
- Consult with members of a local ostomy group who also may provide support and counseling regarding sexual matters.

COLOSTOMY

A **colostomy** is an opening in the large bowel created by bringing a section of the large intestine out to the abdomen and fashioning a stoma. A cancerous lesion, an ulcerative inflammatory process, multiple polyposis (condition of numerous polyps), and traumatic injury to the bowel are indications for a colostomy.

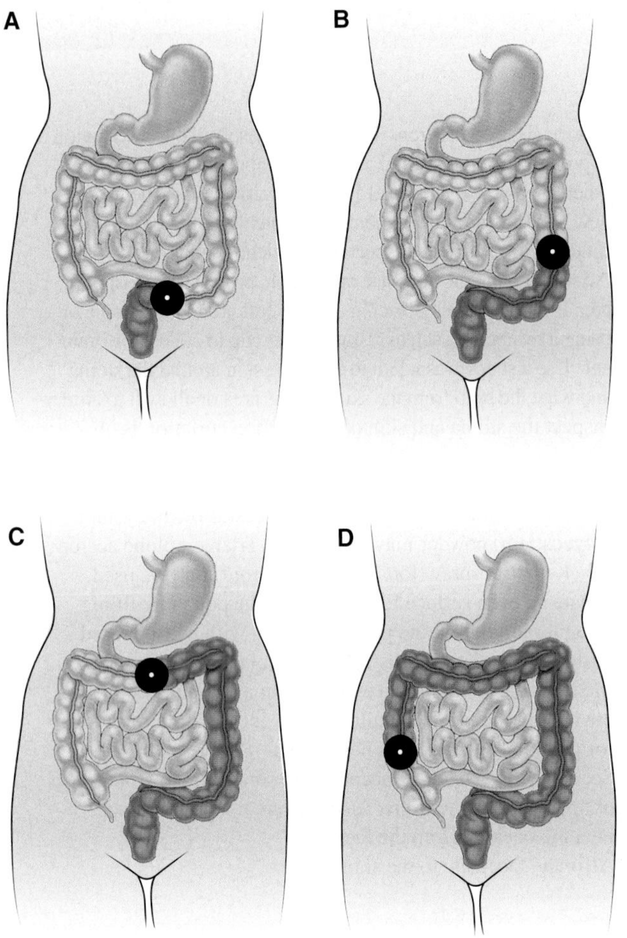

Figure 48-5 Placement of colostomies, with shaded areas representing the sections of the bowel that have been removed or are currently inactive: **(A)** Sigmoid colostomy—feces are solid. **(B)** Descending colostomy—feces are semi-mushy. **(C)** Transverse colostomy—feces are mushy. **(D)** Ascending colostomy—feces are fluid.

Types of colostomies are described according to their placement. A temporary or permanent colostomy may be created in the sigmoid, descending, transverse, or ascending areas of the colon (Fig. 48-5). The consistency of the fecal material ranges from semiliquid to formed depending on the intestinal area from which the colostomy is formed (see Table 48-1). Regular irrigations may control a sigmoid colostomy, and sometimes a descending colostomy, thus eliminating the need for the client to constantly wear an appliance (Nursing Guidelines 48-2).

The stoma may be found anywhere from the lower right, center, to middle, or lower left positions on the abdomen. The terms *single barrel*, *double barrel*, and *loop* are used to describe the appearance of the colostomy.

Surgical Management

Single-Barrel Colostomy

The term **single-barrel colostomy** indicates that the ostomy has a single stoma through which fecal matter passes. The colon is cut above the diseased area, and the healthy end is brought through the abdominal wall to form the matured stoma. The diseased portion of the bowel is removed, with the remaining distal end closed for later reconnection (**segmental resection**). For tumors in the lower third of the sigmoid, that portion, the rectum, and anus may be surgically removed through a perineal incision in a procedure referred to as an **abdominoperineal resection**. After performing an abdominoperineal resection, the surgeon leaves a drain or pack in the perineal area for about 1 week, after which it is removed, and irrigations of the perineal wound may be ordered.

Double-Barrel Colostomy

A **double-barrel colostomy**, which is performed most often in the transverse section of the large intestine, contains both a proximal and distal stoma. Each stoma is everted and sutured in place. The proximal stoma expels the fecal material. The distal stoma leads from the lower portion of the cut bowel to the anus. Because fecal drainage has been diverted, the distal

NURSING GUIDELINES 48-2

Performing Colostomy Irrigation

Irrigation for Single-Barrel Colostomy

Colostomy irrigation begins on the fourth or fifth postoperative day. Standard irrigation is a scheduled irrigation using 500 to 1500 mL tepid water. Check primary provider's orders. Try to use colostomy irrigation equipment that the client will use at home.

- Ask client to sit on a toilet seat or chair near the toilet.
- Prepare the irrigation, purging air from the tubing.
- Place the irrigation sheath over the stoma, directing the sheath into the toilet.
- Lubricate the distal end of the catheter.
- Hang the container of irrigant so that the bottom of the solution bag is about 12 inches above the stoma.
- Gently insert the catheter tip into the stoma and advance it 2 to 3 inches (Fig. A).
- If there is resistance, remove the catheter, release the tubing clamp, and gently reinsert the catheter while the solution is flowing.
- Allow the irrigant to flow slowly and gradually into the stoma (Fig. B).
- If the client complains of cramping, clamp the tubing and ask the client to take a few deep breaths.
- Once the cramping subsides, continue the irrigation.
- If water escapes from the stoma during the irrigation, clamp the tubing until it stops. If a catheter tip is used instead of a cone, introduce the catheter further into the stoma but no more than 6 inches.
- When the prescribed amount of solution is instilled, remove the catheter. The client may remain sitting or walk around

NURSING GUIDELINES 48-2 (*continued*)

(clamp the distal end of the irrigation sheath). Complete drainage usually takes 30 minutes.
- If the irrigant fails to return properly, gently massage the lower abdomen or have the client take several deep breaths and relax or reposition their body. Notify the primary provider if these measures do not work.
- Document the procedure, including the amount of irrigant used, appearance of returns, and client's response.

Irrigation for Double-Barrel Colostomy

If the client has a double-barrel colostomy, irrigate the proximal stoma in the same manner as a single-barrel colostomy. To irrigate the distal stoma, try the following:
- Have the client sit on a toilet or a bedpan, because the irrigation fluid and a small amount of mucus will leave by way of the anus. During the immediate postoperative period, necrotic tissue also may be expelled.
- Use a bulb syringe (Fig. C), short catheter, container of solution, plastic sheath or apron, and an emesis basin as another technique for irrigation. This method calls for several instillations of 250 to 500 mL solution at a time, sometimes twice a day. Some clients have found this method effective for controlling spillage for 24 hours or more. It may be used as an alternate choice when the standard method cannot be used.

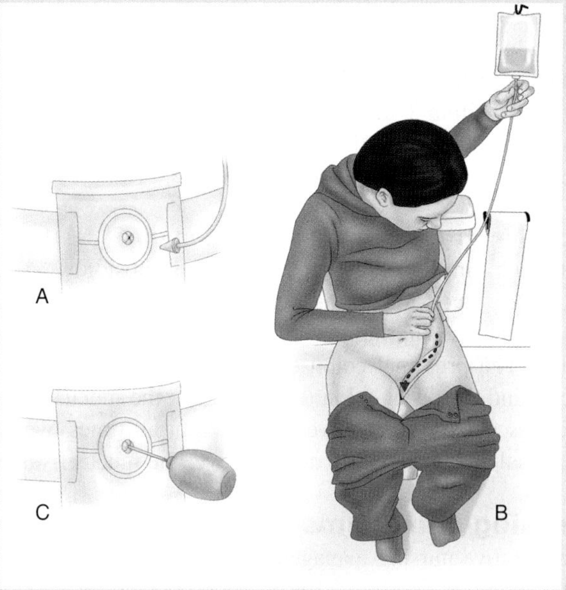

(A) Irrigating catheter has a cone attachment to prevent injury to stomal tissue. **(B)** Irrigating fluid is instilled with sleeve in place; drainage empties into toilet. **(C)** A bulb syringe method may be used to stimulate fecal drainage.

portion of the bowel does not pass feces. The distal stoma and the anus may expel mucus. When a double-barrel colostomy has been performed, the primary provider is asked to identify the distal and proximal stomas. A diagram is provided in the medical record, and the nurse may duplicate it on the nursing care plan. This information is essential when assessing bowel function and whether irrigations are required. Irrigation may be ordered for both the proximal and distal portions of the bowel or for the proximal portion only.

A double-barrel colostomy often is temporary and usually performed to rest a portion of the bowel to treat a disorder such as acute diverticulitis, chronic constipation, or inflammatory bowel disease. The interval before reestablishing the continuity of the bowel may be 16 months or longer. When the diseased portion of the bowel is removed or healed, the bowel is reconnected and functions normally. In the meantime, the stoma may need irrigation or alternative methods for regulating bowel elimination (Box 48-1).

››› *Stop, Think, and Respond 48-1*

A client calls the primary provider's office 4 months after a double-barrel colostomy. He tells the triage nurse that the stool is more liquid than usual and that he is emptying the pouch every 4 hours. What questions does the triage nurse need to ask?

Transverse Colostomy

A transverse colostomy is usually a temporary colostomy located in the transverse colon. They are most often done for clients experiencing cancer, diverticulitis, inflammatory bowel disease, or obstruction. There are two types: loop transverse colostomy and double-barrel transverse colostomy.

Loop Transverse Colostomy

A **loop transverse colostomy** involves lifting a loop of bowel through an opening in the upper abdomen. The loop

BOX 48-1 Regulating Bowel Elimination Without Irrigating

Some ostomates learn to regulate bowel elimination without irrigating frequently. The following tips may be encouraging to new ostomates, who may be able to establish regular elimination patterns:
- Insert a suppository, such as glycerin or bisacodyl (Dulcolax), into the stoma. The suppository should be recommended by the primary provider. Up to 7 days or more of daily use may be needed before a regular elimination pattern is established. Initially, movements may occur three or four times daily, but each day, movements should decrease until only one or two movements occur daily.

Other methods to stimulate bowel elimination and a regular schedule include the following:
- Drinking prune or fruit juice
- Eating fiber-rich foods and dried fruits and performing mild exercise
- Using a stool softener, mineral oil, or milk of magnesia if recommended by the primary provider

is supported in place by a plastic rod or bridge. An opening may be created at the time of surgery, or 24 to 72 hours following the procedure. When opened there are actually two openings—one for the proximal end of the colon, which excretes loose to soft feces, and the other for the distal end, which excretes mucus. The plastic rod or bridge is generally removed within 1 to 2 weeks. A client wears a pouch for stool collection at all times. In most cases reanastamosis of the colon occurs within 2 to 3 months.

Double-Barrel Transverse Colostomy

Although similar to a loop transverse colostomy, in this procedure two stomas (as opposed to openings) are created, totally separating the colon into a proximal and distal colon. The proximal colon excretes liquid to semi-formed feces, and the distal colon (referred to as the mucus fistula) excretes mucus. Clients wear a pouch at all times over the proximal end and a gauze dressing over the mucus fistula.

Nursing Management

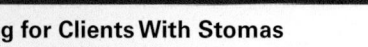

Preoperative nursing management is similar to that for clients having an ileostomy. Because a colostomy may be performed for cancer of the colon or rectum, however, the client may be more anxious about the procedure. Postoperative cancer treatment options also may serve to increase the client's anxiety. Nurses and/or dieticians will review postoperative dietary restrictions and expectations (Nutrition Notes). Also see Evidence-Based Practice 48-1.

Evidence-Based Practice 48-1

Caring for Clients With Stomas

Clinical Question

How can community nurses have an impact on clients with stomas?

Evidence

Using literature review, data analysis, and consumer surveys Schluter and Sinasac (2020) determined that clients with a stoma would benefit from a community-based stoma nurse. Many clients are sent home prior to feeling completely comfortable with their appliance, with some only acquiring the skill to empty appliance.

When a stoma is created in a client, it affects that client in many ways. Body image is affected and sometimes certain activities or hobbies are affected. The community nurse can make an impact by educating the client on cleaning, removal, applying, and problem solving for activities. The review concluded that providing support can help identify those with peristomal skin complication (Schluter & Sinasac, 2020).

Nursing Implications

Nurses should be educated in the types of stomas, appliances, and care methods. A community-based stomal nurse should have initial contact with a new client within 2 to 7 days post discharge from a facility and for the life of the stoma (Schluter & Sinasac, 2020).

Reference

Schluter, J. E., & Sinasac, P. A. (2020). Community stomal therapy services: a needs analysis and development of an evidence based model of care. *Journal of Stomal Therapy Australia, 40*(1), 8–13. https://10.33235/jsta.40.1.8-13

Nutrition Notes

The Client With an Ostomy

For Both Colostomy and Ileostomy Clients:

- Fiber is restricted after ostomy surgery to prevent irritation and slow transit time until healing is complete. Thereafter, small amounts of foods containing fiber are added individually to the diet so that the client's tolerance can be evaluated. Foods not tolerated initially may be reintroduced weeks or months later. Most clients resume a normal diet within 6 weeks after surgery.
- The primary nutrition concerns are fluids and electrolytes. Eight to 10 cups of fluid are recommended daily. Reassure the client that extra fluids do not contribute to watery stools but are excreted as urine. Fluid restriction should not be used to control liquid feces. Sodium and potassium requirements may increase because of increased losses.
- Eating small, frequent meals at regular times is recommended. Eating a large meal in the middle of the day instead of in the evening may help decrease stool output at night.
- Clients should take small bites of food and chew food thoroughly.
- Foods that may help decrease odor include buttermilk, parsley, yogurt, kefir, and cranberry juice. Odor-causing foods include dried peas and beans, fish, eggs, onion, garlic, vegetables from the cabbage family, asparagus, beer, and other alcoholic beverages.
- Banana flakes, applesauce, pasta, potatoes, smooth peanut butter, and cheese may help thicken stools. Because they may cause obstruction, nuts, corn, cabbage, coconut, dried fruit, unpeeled apples, and grapes should be avoided.

For Colostomy Clients:

- Eventually, a high-fiber diet may improve stool consistency and regularity in clients with a colostomy. Increase fiber gradually.

For Clients With an Ileostomy:

- Lactose intolerance may occur.
- Limit liquids with meals if output is high.
- Oral rehydration formulas, such as Gatorade, may help maintain fluid and electrolyte balance.
- Depending on the placement of the ileostomy, there is a potential for nutrient malabsorption. Recent research indicates that over a period of 2 years following resection, the remaining large intestine undergoes adaptation to increase its absorptive capacity. However, clients are prone to deficiency of vitamins, minerals, and essential fatty acids. Serum levels should be monitored periodically and supplements provided as indicated (Matarese, 2013).
- Diet should include complex carbohydrates, and simple sugars should be avoided.

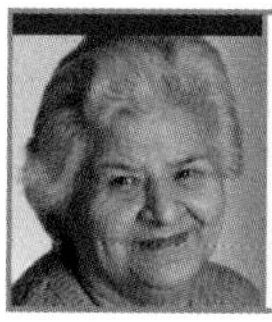

Clinical Scenario A 70-year-old client diagnosed with colon cancer has colostomy surgery. What do the nurses need to focus on when providing postoperative care to this client? See the following Nursing Process section.

NURSING PROCESS FOR THE CLIENT FOLLOWING COLOSTOMY SURGERY

Assessment

After the client returns from surgery, assessments include taking vital signs, checking dressings, and monitoring nasogastric tubes and IV infusions. Review the client's chart for the type of colostomy and the location of the stoma(s). If an abdominoperineal resection was performed, check the drain or packing in the perineal area and note the characteristics of the drainage.

Monitor vital signs every 4 hours or as ordered. Take the client's temperature by a route other than rectal. Report a sudden elevation in temperature over 101°F (38.3°C) or an increase in pain and abdominal tenderness or distension to the primary provider immediately. Also, check the surgical dressing frequently in the early postoperative period and observe the characteristics of the stoma. Monitor urine output and the volume of suctioned gastric secretions. If urine output is markedly decreased or less than 500 mL/day, inform the primary provider immediately.

Diagnosis, Planning, and Interventions

Perform standard postsurgical measures to maintain the airway and relieve pain and anxiety. Also, perform nasogastric decompression (see Chapter 45), if ordered, and monitor fluid and electrolyte status. It may be necessary to measure fluids lost through decompression and replace them with additional IV fluids. An indwelling catheter may be used to relieve abdominal pressure and prevent urine retention during the first few days after surgery.

Teach the client how to care for the colostomy by demonstrating the irrigating procedure and, if possible, outlining nonirrigation methods for keeping the ostomy patent and establishing a regular pattern of bowel elimination. The time between the use of these methods and eventual regularity is unique to each client. Natural methods are the least predictable for regulating the bowel, but many clients learn to recognize subtle clues that the bowel will be moving. They then have sufficient time to reach a bathroom and eliminate in private.

In addition, demonstrate skin and stoma care and appliance application and removal. To provide ample learning time, divide material that the client must learn into small units. After demonstrating one aspect of care, have the client return the demonstration. When the client feels self-confident, add additional material. Reinforce verbal information and demonstrated skills with printed material that may be available from ostomy associations or the WOC nurse. Finally, arrange a dietary consultation to discuss nutrition and food modifications. Client and Family Teaching 48-5 outlines important teaching for the client with a colostomy.

Bowel Incontinence: Related to unpredictable bowel elimination pattern
Expected Outcome: Client will not experience accidental soiling.

- Instruct the client how to keep the ostomy appliance intact. Proper application prevents accidental soiling.
- Schedule colostomy irrigation or suppository insertion for a descending or sigmoid colostomy. These measures assist with maintaining predictable bowel elimination.

Diarrhea or Constipation: Related to changes in bowel motility
Expected Outcome: Client will maintain expected consistency of feces according to location of the colostomy.

Diarrhea

- Instruct client to keep a record of food intake, noting time of problems with loose stools or diarrhea. *A food record helps identify specific foods that irritate the GI tract.*
- Inform client about the need to reduce or eliminate offending foods. *Such information helps prevent diarrhea.*
- Teach client to report prolonged problems with increased stool volume, watery stool consistency, nausea, vomiting, or abdominal pain to the primary provider. *Ostomates can experience gastroenteritis.*

Constipation

- Gently dilate the stoma with a lubricated, gloved finger. *Dilation stimulates the colon and assists with expelling stool.*
- Advise client to increase fluid intake. *Increased intake will add fluid to stool, making it easier to pass.*
- Encourage client to eat regular meals. *Dieting or fasting can decrease stool volume and slow elimination.*
- Provide high-fiber, nonirritating foods. *Such foods increase stool bulk and moisture.*
- Offer foods such as coffee or stewed prunes. These foods promote elimination.
- Consult with primary provider if preceding measures fail. *Client may benefit from irrigation, suppository, or laxative.*

Evaluation of Expected Outcomes

The client reports a predictable stool pattern and no problems with soiling. Stool consistency is as expected, and the client has not had constipation or diarrhea.

Client and Family Teaching 48-5 Postoperative Colostomy Care

The nurse emphasizes the following points when teaching the client and their family:

- Inspect the stoma for changes in appearance. Changes in the size and color of the stoma vary with activity and emotional status. Anger or extreme annoyance may cause the stoma to turn red or purple. Small beads of blood may ooze from the surface. Fright may cause the stoma to blanch. These reactions are normal and insignificant as long as the tissues revert to their normal state when the cause is alleviated.
- Eat a regular diet, but avoid gas-forming foods to control intestinal gas.
- If experiencing problems with constipation, increase fiber in the diet and drink extra water—these measures generally correct the problem.
- Eliminate food items that result in diarrhea. This may help to control the problem because diarrhea may be related to diet. Characteristics of diarrhea include both increased stool output and liquid nature of the stool. One or two loose stools per day do not necessarily indicate a problem. If diarrhea persists for more than 2 days, contact the primary provider.
- Eat slowly with the mouth closed and chew food well to decrease gas that results chiefly from swallowing air rather than from digestion.
- With the exception of tight clothing, do not alter preferences in clothing. If you require firm support (e.g., wear girdles or braces, have back problems), find a stoma shield that is helpful in preventing irritation or undue pressure on the stoma.
- Check body weight weekly. Contact primary provider if there is a sudden weight loss or gain.
- Perform irrigations at approximately the same time each day. The best time to irrigate is after a meal because food in the digestive tract stimulates peristalsis and defecation.
- The primary provider may recommend that the schedule for irrigations gradually progress to every other day, every third day, or even twice a week. If constipation occurs, contact primary provider regarding a change in the irrigation schedule.
- Do not restrict travel or activities outside the home. Changes in stool pattern may be normal when daily routines change. Preassembled kits that contain all materials needed for irrigation and changes of the colostomy appliance are available. If traveling by air, take ostomy supplies in carry-on luggage to prevent their loss if luggage is misdirected or lost. Necessary items also may be assembled individually and placed in waterproof containers.

KEY POINTS

- Ileostomy
  - Standard or Brooke: entire colon and rectum are removed or bypassed
  - Continent ileostomy: abdominal pouch created for internal reservoir
  - Ileoanal reservoir: performed in two stages, allows control of bowel elimination when complete
  - Ostomy appliances are used, requires correct placement and proper care
- Colostomy
  - Single-barrel: single stoma
  - Double-barrel: has both proximal and distal stomas, usually temporary with plan for reversal
  - Transverse: temporary and located in the transverse colon

CRITICAL THINKING EXERCISES

1. In what ways does the care of a 20-year-old client with an ileostomy differ from that of a 60-year-old client with a colostomy?
2. A client with an ileostomy is disturbed by having to empty liquid stool from their appliance frequently. They intend to reduce their intake of fluids. What information is important to give this client?
3. What recommendations are appropriate for the client with a colostomy who has been experiencing an unusual amount of intestinal gas?
4. Discharge is planned for a client with a new colostomy. They tell the nurse that when they get home, they will just drink liquids and avoid solid food until the colostomy is working more normally. What should the nurse teach this client?

NCLEX-STYLE REVIEW QUESTIONS PrepU

1. The nurse is caring for a client scheduled for an ileostomy. Which of the following statements by the client indicates that they require more education about the surgery?
   1. "Eventually, I will have more control over bowel movements."
   2. "I need to drink extra fluids to prevent dehydration."
   3. "I will be able to have a sexual relationship when I heal."
   4. "I will need to wear an appliance/collection bag all the time."

2. Which of the following nursing interventions will be most effective in helping the client to cope with body changes?
   1. Involve family members when providing ileostomy teaching.
   2. Provide detailed written instructions about ileostomy care.
   3. Reassure the client that the changes are common and temporary.
   4. Set realistic goals with the client to approach the ileostomy.

3. A nurse is caring for a client who is 24 hours postoperative for a resection of the colon. When auscultating the client's abdomen, the nurse does not hear any bowel sounds. What is the next best action by the nurse?
   1. Ambulate the client.
   2. Ask the client about fullness or bloating.
   3. Check vital signs and call the doctor.
   4. Record this anticipated finding.

4. A client is scheduled for a sigmoid colostomy. As part of the client teaching, the nurse asks the client about the surgery and to indicate on the diagram where the stoma will be located. Where should the client mark the diagram? ____________________

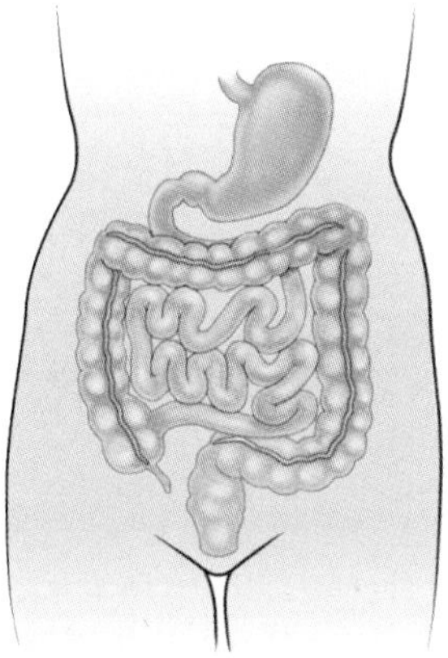

5. During a conversation concerning the client's feelings about a colostomy, the client says to the nurse, "How will I ever adjust to this colostomy?" Which nursing response is most appropriate at this time?
   1. Encourage the client to express concerns.
   2. Reassure the client that adjustment will come with time.
   3. Recommend that the client seek assistance from home care aides.
   4. Say nothing, but quote the statement in the chart.

WANT TO KNOW MORE? There are a wide variety of online resources available on thePoint to enhance learning and understanding of this chapter.

Go to **thePoint.lww.com/activate** and use the activation code found in the front of this text to unlock these online resources.

UNIT 12
Caring for Clients With Endocrine Disorders

49 Introduction to the Endocrine System

Words To Know

adenohypophysis
adrenal cortex
adrenal glands
adrenal medulla
adrenocorticotropic hormone
corticosteroids
corticotrophin-releasing hormone
estrogen
feedback loop
follicle-stimulating hormone
glucagon
glycogenolysis
gonadotropin-releasing hormone
growth hormone–releasing hormone
hormones
hypophysis
hypothalamic dopamine
hypothalamus
insulin
islets of Langerhans
luteinizing hormone (LH)
melatonin
neurohormones
neurohypophysis
ovaries
pancreas
pancreatic polypeptide
parathormone
parathyroid glands
pars intermedia
pineal gland
pituitary gland
progesterone
prolactin
radioimmunoassay
radionuclide
somatostatin
somatotropin
testes

Learning Objectives

On completion of this chapter, you will be able to:

1. Identify the chief function of the endocrine glands.
2. Describe the general function of hormones.
3. Explain the relationship between the hypothalamus and the pituitary gland.
4. Discuss the regulation of levels of hormones.
5. List endocrine glands and the hormones they secrete.
6. Name other organs that are not classified as endocrine glands but secrete hormones.
7. Outline information to include when taking the health history of a client with an endocrine disorder.
8. Describe physical assessment findings that suggest an endocrine disorder.
9. List examples of laboratory and diagnostic tests that identify endocrine disorders.
10. Discuss the nursing management of clients undergoing diagnostic tests to detect endocrine dysfunction.

The endocrine glands (Fig. 49-1) secrete **hormones**, chemicals that accelerate or slow physiologic processes, directly into the bloodstream. This characteristic distinguishes endocrine glands from exocrine glands, which release secretions into a duct. Hormones circulate in the blood until they reach receptors in target cells or other endocrine glands. They play a vital role in regulating homeostatic processes such as

- Metabolism
- Growth
- Fluid and electrolyte balance
- Reproductive processes
- Sleep and wake cycles

Words To Know (*continued*)
testosterone
tetraiodothyronine
thymopoietin
thymosin
thymus gland
thyroid gland
thyroid-stimulating hormone
triiodothyronine

Gerontologic Considerations

- Obtaining a drug history is essential before a diagnostic examination of an older adult because side effects or interactions may contribute to changes in endocrine function. If the older adult is cognitively impaired, a family member or the caregiver should provide information regarding the onset and course of the cognitive changes, medications, and dosage history.
- Effective teaching strategies for diagnostic tests include verbal and written instructions, including rationale for actions if possible. If the older adult has cognitive changes, a family member or caregiver should be included in the instructions and allowed to remain with the client as much as possible.

Table 49-1 presents an overview of the hormones involved in the endocrine system.

››› Stop, Think, and Respond 49-1

Give examples of hormones that affect metabolism, growth, fluid and electrolyte balance, reproductive processes, and sleep and wake cycles.

ANATOMY AND PHYSIOLOGY

Pituitary Gland

Many endocrine glands respond to stimulation from the **pituitary gland** (or **hypophysis**), which is connected by a stalk to the hypothalamus in the brain. The pituitary is divided into three lobes: the anterior lobe (**adenohypophysis**), intermediate lobe (**pars intermedia**), and posterior lobe (**neurohypophysis**). The pituitary gland is called the *master gland* because it regulates the function of other endocrine glands. The term is somewhat misleading, however, because the hypothalamus influences the pituitary gland.

Hypothalamus

The **hypothalamus**, a portion of the brain between the cerebrum and the brain stem, projects down toward the pituitary gland. This creates a pathway for **neurohormones**, also known as releasing hormones or factors, that stimulate and inhibit secretions from the anterior and posterior lobes of the pituitary gland. Under the influence of the hypothalamus, the lobes of the pituitary gland secrete various hormones (Fig. 49-2).

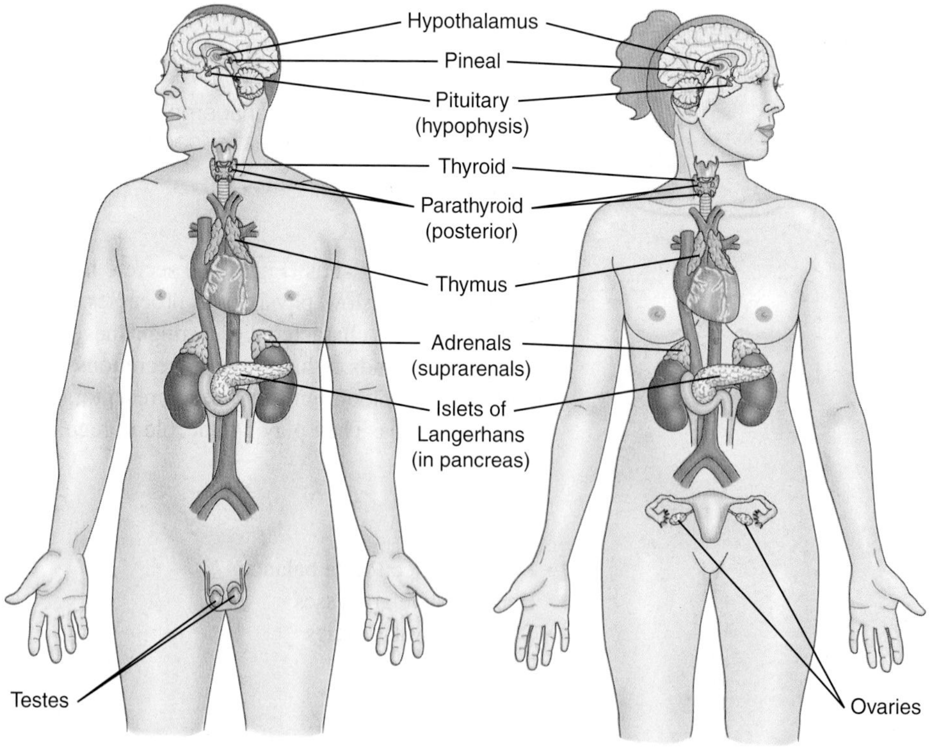

Figure 49-1 The glands of the endocrine system.

TABLE 49-1 Endocrine Hormones

GLAND	HORMONE RELEASED	HORMONE FUNCTION	HORMONE REGULATOR
Posterior pituitary	Antidiuretic hormone (ADH)	Increases water absorption from kidneys; raises blood pressure	Hypothalamic secretions, blood osmolarity
	Oxytocin	Stimulates contraction of pregnant uterus and release of breast milk after childbirth	Hypothalamic secretions, uterine stretch, suckling
Anterior pituitary	Somatotropin (growth hormone)	Stimulates bone and muscle growth; promotes protein synthesis and fat mobilization	Hypothalamic secretions
	Prolactin	Promotes production and secretion of milk after childbirth	Hypothalamic hormones
	Thyroid-stimulating hormone (TSH)	Stimulates production and secretion of thyroid hormones	Blood thyroxine levels; hypothalamic secretions
	Adrenocorticotropic hormone (ACTH)	Stimulates adrenal cortex to secrete cortisol and other steroids	Corticotropin-releasing hormone (CRH) from the hypothalamus; blood cortisol levels
	Luteinizing hormone (LH) in women and interstitial cell–stimulating hormone (ICSH) in men	Initiates ovulation and the secretion of sex hormones in both genders	Hypothalamic secretions, estrogen and testosterone levels
	Follicle-stimulating hormone (FSH)	Stimulates development of ovum in ovaries and sperm in testes	Hypothalamic secretions, progesterone
Thyroid	Tetraiodothyronine (thyroxine or T_4) and triiodothyronine or T_3	Increases oxygen consumption and heat production; stimulates, increases, and maintains metabolic processes	TSH regulated by thyrotropin-releasing hormone (TRH) from the hypothalamus
	Calcitonin	Inhibits calcium release from bone, thus lowering blood calcium levels	Blood calcium concentrations
Parathyroids	Parathyroid hormone (PTH)	Increases blood calcium by stimulating calcium release from bone; decreases blood phosphate level	Calcium concentrations in blood
Thymus	Several thymosin and thymopoietin hormones; thymic humoral factor; thymostimulin; factor thymic serum	Stimulate T-cell development in thymus and maintenance in other lymph tissue; involved in some B cells developing into antibody-producing plasma cells	Not known
Pineal gland	Melatonin	Involved in circadian rhythms; antigonadotropic effect induces sleep	Exposure to light–dark cycles; darkness stimulates release and light diminishes release
Adrenal medulla	Epinephrine (adrenaline)	Constricts blood vessels in skin, kidneys, and gut, which increases blood supply to heart, brain, and skeletal muscles, leading to increased heart rate and blood pressure; stimulates smooth muscle contraction; raises blood glucose levels	Sympathetic nervous system
	Norepinephrine	Constricts blood vessels; increases heart rate and contraction of cardiac muscles; increases metabolic rate	Sympathetic nervous system
Adrenal cortex	Corticosteroids:		
	Glucocorticoids	Regulate blood glucose by affecting carbohydrate metabolism; affect growth; decrease effects of stress and anti-inflammatory agents	ACTH; stress and serum electrolyte concentrations
	Mineralocorticoids (mainly aldosterone)	Regulate sodium, water, and potassium excretion by the kidneys	Renin and angiotensin
	Gonadocorticoids (mainly androgens—male sex hormones)	Contribute to secondary sex characteristics (greater androgenic effect in women after menopause)	ACTH
Pancreas (islets of Langerhans)	Insulin	Lowers blood sugar; increases glycogen storage in liver; stimulates protein synthesis	Blood glucose concentrations
	Glucagon	Stimulates glycogen breakdown in liver; increases blood sugar (glucose) concentration	Blood glucose and amino acid concentration

(continued)

TABLE 49-1 Endocrine Hormones (*continued*)

GLAND	HORMONE RELEASED	HORMONE FUNCTION	HORMONE REGULATOR
Ovary follicle	Estrogens	Develop and maintain female sex organs and characteristics; initiate building of uterine lining	FSH and LH
Ovary (corpus luteum)	Progesterone and estrogens	Influence breast development and menstrual cycles; promote growth and differentiation of uterine lining; maintain pregnancy	FSH
Testes	Androgens (mainly testosterone)	Develop and maintain male sex organs and characteristics; aid sperm production	FSH and ICSH

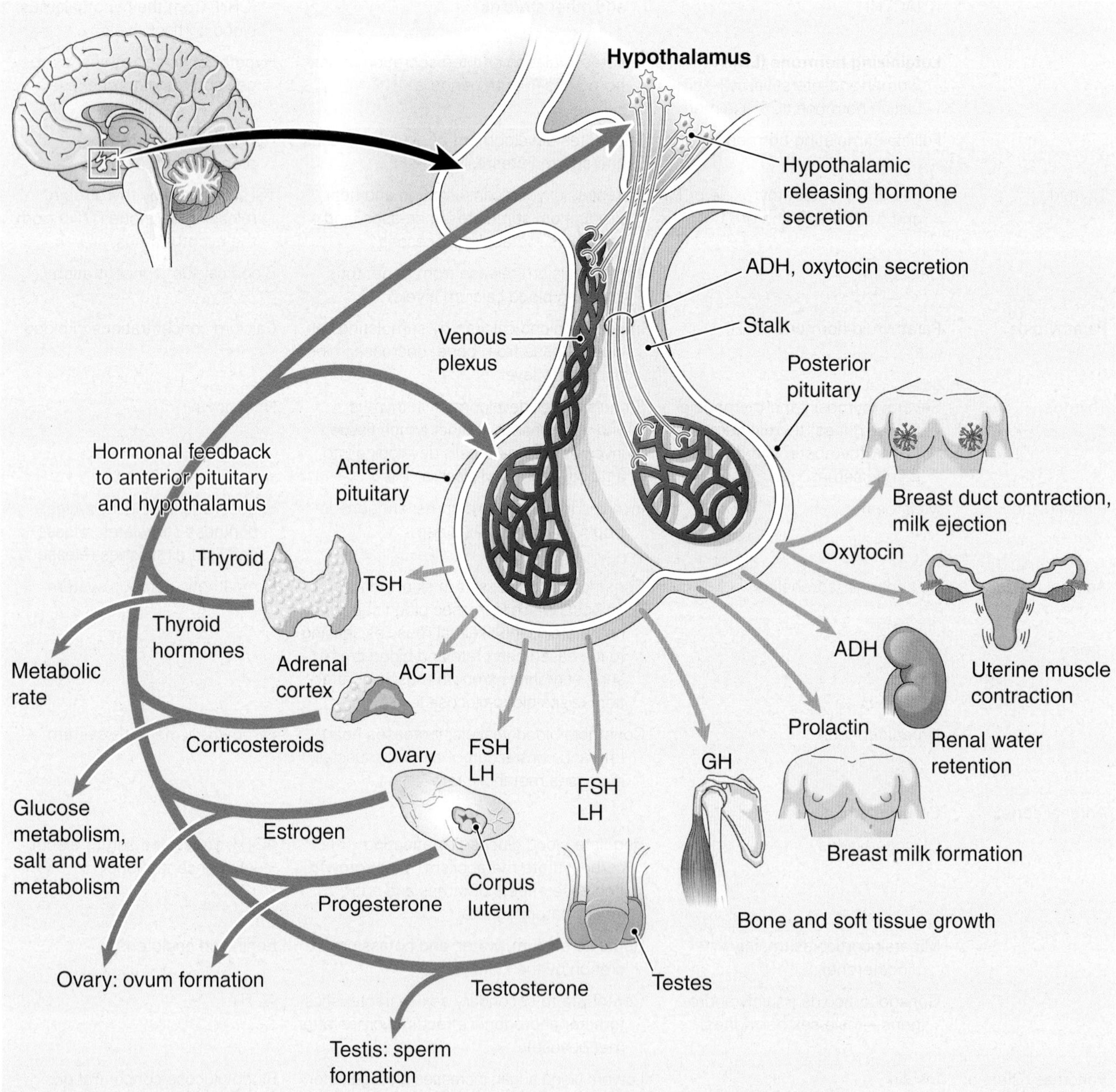

Figure 49-2 The relationship of the hypothalamus to the pituitary gland and the hormones secreted by the anterior and posterior lobes of the pituitary gland. ACTH, adrenocorticotropic hormone; ADH, antidiuretic hormone; FSH, follicle-stimulating hormone; GH, growth hormone; LH, luteinizing hormone; TSH, thyroid-stimulating hormone.

There are six hypothalamic neurohormones:

- **Thyrotropin-releasing hormone**, which stimulates the release of **thyroid-stimulating hormone** (TSH) from the anterior pituitary gland
- **Corticotrophin-releasing hormone** (CRH), which causes the anterior pituitary gland to secrete **adrenocorticotropic hormone**
- **Gonadotropin-releasing hormone**, which triggers sexual development at the onset of puberty and continues to cause the anterior pituitary gland to secrete **luteinizing hormone** and **follicle-stimulating hormone**
- **Growth hormone–releasing hormone** (GHRH), which results in the release of **somatotropin** (growth hormone) from the anterior pituitary gland. GHRH secretion is controlled by another hypothalamic hormone, somatostatin, which is also secreted by other tissues outside the hypothalamus such as the pancreas.
- **Somatostatin**, which inhibits GHRH and TSH and also blocks the secretion of several gastrointestinal hormones, including gastrin, cholecystokinin, and secretin; lowers the blood flow within the intestine; suppresses the release of insulin and glucagon from the pancreas; and suppresses the release of exocrine enzymes from the pancreas.
- **Hypothalamic dopamine**, which inhibits the release of prolactin from the anterior pituitary gland (Dopamine, of which there are five variants, is produced in several structures within the brain, one of which is the hypothalamus.)

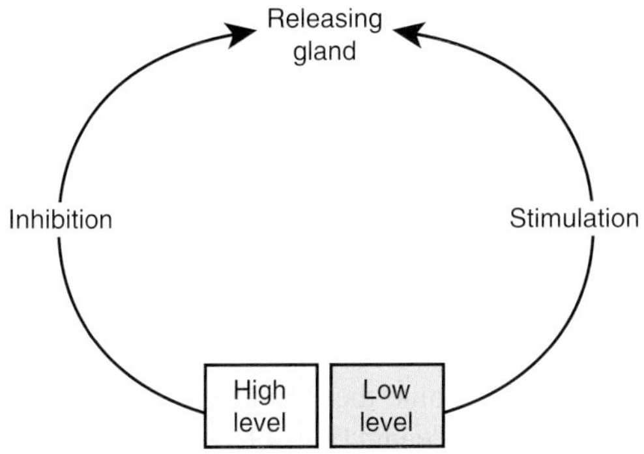

Figure 49-3 A feedback loop regulates hormone levels.

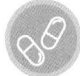

Pharmacologic Considerations

■ Octreotide (Sandostatin), a drug that mimics the actions of somatostatin, may be used as an urgent measure to reduce bleeding esophageal varices in clients with erectile dysfunction (Carale & Azar, 2015).

Hormone Regulation

A feedback loop controls hormone levels. A **feedback loop** is a mechanism that turns hormone production off and on to keep concentrations of hormones within a stable range at all times (Fig. 49-3). Feedback can be either negative or positive. Most hormones are secreted in response to negative feedback, a decrease in levels stimulates the releasing gland; in positive feedback, the opposite occurs. Most endocrine disorders result from overproduction or underproduction of specific hormones.

Thyroid Gland

The **thyroid gland** is located in the lower neck anterior to the trachea (Fig. 49-4). It is divided into two lateral lobes joined by a band of tissue called the *isthmus*. The thyroid concentrates iodine from food and uses it to synthesize **tetraiodothyronine** (thyroxine or T_4) and **triiodothyronine** (T_3). These

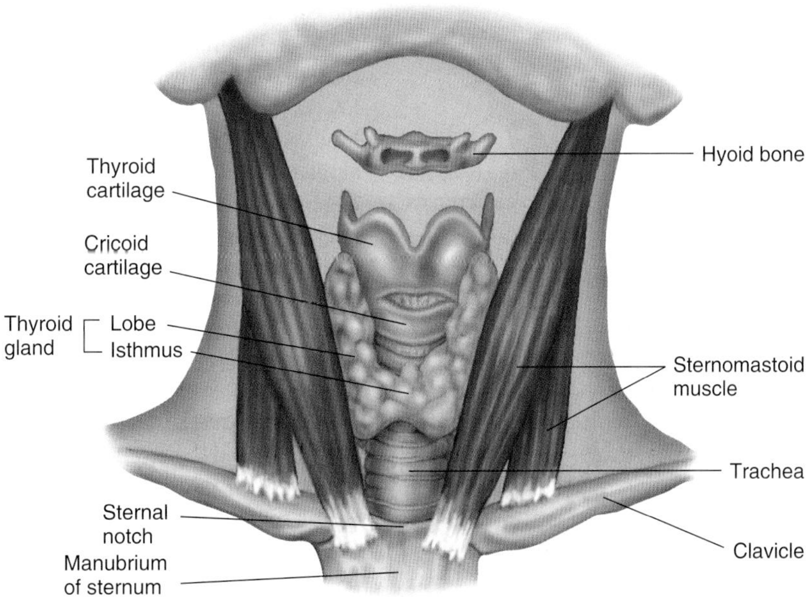

Figure 49-4 The thyroid gland and surrounding structures.

two hormones regulate the body's metabolic rate. **Calcitonin**, another thyroid hormone, inhibits the release of calcium from bone into the extracellular fluid. A rise in the serum calcium level stimulates the release of calcitonin from the thyroid gland.

Parathyroid Glands

There are four (some people have more than four) **parathyroid glands**: small, bean-shaped bodies, each surrounded by a capsule of connective tissue and embedded within the lateral lobes of the thyroid (Fig. 49-5). The upper parathyroids are found posteriorly at the junction of the upper and middle thirds of the thyroid. The lower parathyroids typically lie among the branches of the inferior thyroid artery. They secrete **parathormone**, which increases the level of calcium in the blood when there is a decrease in the serum level. Parathormone does so by (1) causing calcium and phosphorus to be released from bones; (2) interfering with the urinary excretion of calcium but promoting the urinary excretion of phosphorus; and (3) activating vitamin D, which causes an increase in calcium absorption within the intestine.

Thymus Gland

The **thymus gland** is located in the upper part of the chest above or near the heart (refer Fig. 49-1). It secretes **thymosin** and **thymopoietin**, which aid in developing T lymphocytes, a type of white blood cell involved in immunity (see Chapter 33). The thymus gland is large during childhood but usually shrinks by adulthood. Despite its reduced size, the thymus gland continues to support the production of T lymphocytes, but the rate of production decreases with age. Functional disorders of the gland are rare.

Pineal Gland

The **pineal gland** is attached to the thalamus in the brain (see Fig. 49-1). It secretes **melatonin**, which aids in regulating sleep cycles and mood (see Chapter 69). Melatonin is believed to play a role in hypothalamic–pituitary interaction.

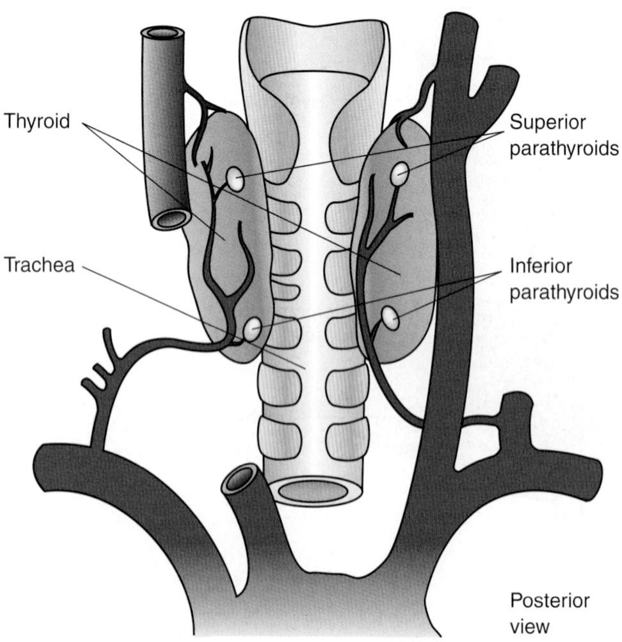

Figure 49-5 Posterior view of the thyroid gland with the embedded parathyroid glands.

Adrenal Glands

The **adrenal glands** are located above the kidneys (Fig. 49-6). The outer portion is called the *cortex*, and the inner portion is called the *medulla*.

The **adrenal cortex** manufactures and secretes glucocorticoids, mineralocorticoids, and small amounts of androgenic sex hormones. Collectively, these hormones are called **corticosteroids**. Glucocorticoids and mineralocorticoids are essential to life and influence many organs and structures of the body. Glucocorticoids, such as cortisol, affect body metabolism, suppress inflammation, and help the body withstand stress. Mineralocorticoids, primarily aldosterone, maintain water and electrolyte (sodium, potassium, chloride) balances (see Chapter 16). The androgenic hormones convert to testosterone and estrogens. Anabolic steroids, derivatives of adrenal androgens, promote the development of muscle mass and other masculinizing characteristics.

The **adrenal medulla** secretes epinephrine and norepinephrine. These two hormones are released in response to stress or threat to life. They facilitate what is referred to as the *physiologic stress response*, also known as the *fight-or-flight response* (see Chapter 67). Many organs respond to the release of epinephrine and norepinephrine. Responses include increased blood pressure and pulse rate, dilation of the pupils, constriction of blood vessels, bronchodilation, and decreased peristalsis.

Pancreas

The **pancreas** lies behind the stomach, with the head of the gland close to the duodenum (Fig. 49-7). It is both an exocrine and an endocrine gland. The exocrine portion secretes digestive enzymes that the common bile duct carries to the small intestine. The hormone-secreting cells of the pancreas, called the **islets of Langerhans**, release hormones from alpha, beta, delta, and gamma islets, clusters of cells each being distinct from the others. **Insulin**, a hormone released by beta islet cells, lowers the level of blood glucose when it rises beyond normal limits (see Chapter 51). **Glucagon**, a hormone released by alpha islet cells, raises blood sugar levels by stimulating **glycogenolysis**, the breakdown of glycogen into glucose, in the liver. **Somatostatin**, a hormone secreted by delta islet cells as well as the hypothalamus, helps maintain a relatively constant level of blood sugar by inhibiting the release of insulin and glucagons. **Pancreatic polypeptide** from gamma islet cells controls exocrine secretions from the pancreas.

Ovaries and Testes

The sex glands, the female **ovaries** and the male **testes**, are important in the development of secondary sex characteristics, manufacture of hormones, and development of the ovum (female) and sperm (male).

The ovaries produce **estrogen** and **progesterone**. The testes are the major source of the hormone **testosterone**, which is involved in the development and maintenance of male secondary sex characteristics, such as facial hair and a deep voice. The functions and roles of these hormones are discussed in Chapters 52, 53, and 55.

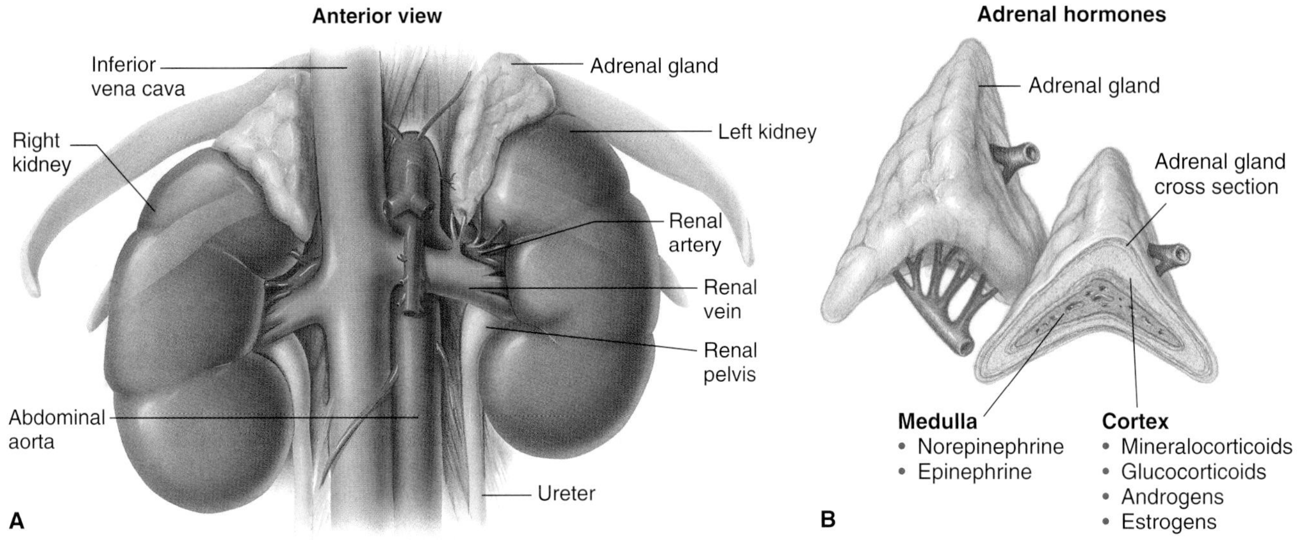

Figure 49-6 **(A)** The adrenal glands sit on top of each kidney. **(B)** Cross-section of one adrenal gland; each gland is composed of the outer cortex and the inner medulla, both of which secrete specific hormones.

Additional Hormone-Releasing Organs

Other organs are not typically considered endocrine glands, yet they secrete one or more hormones among the other major functions that they perform. For example, the atria of the heart secrete *atrial natriuretic peptide*, a hormone that helps reduce blood volume by promoting urinary excretion of sodium (see Chapter 16). Conversely, the kidneys release *renin*, a hormone that initiates the production of angiotensin and aldosterone to increase blood pressure and blood volume. The kidneys also secrete *erythropoietin*, a substance that promotes the maturation of red blood cells.

During pregnancy, the placenta not only provides maternal circulation to the developing fetus but also secretes hormones such as estrogen; progesterone; CRH, which determines the length of gestation and the onset of labor; and human chorionic gonadotropin (Marieb & Hoehn, 2018). When exposed to sunlight, epidermal skin cells form a precursor of vitamin D; the liver continues the conversion, and the kidneys complete the activation process. And lastly, hormone-secreting cells within the gastrointestinal tract aid in the regulation of digestion. For example, gastrin is released within the stomach to increase the production of hydrochloric acid. Cholecystokinin released from

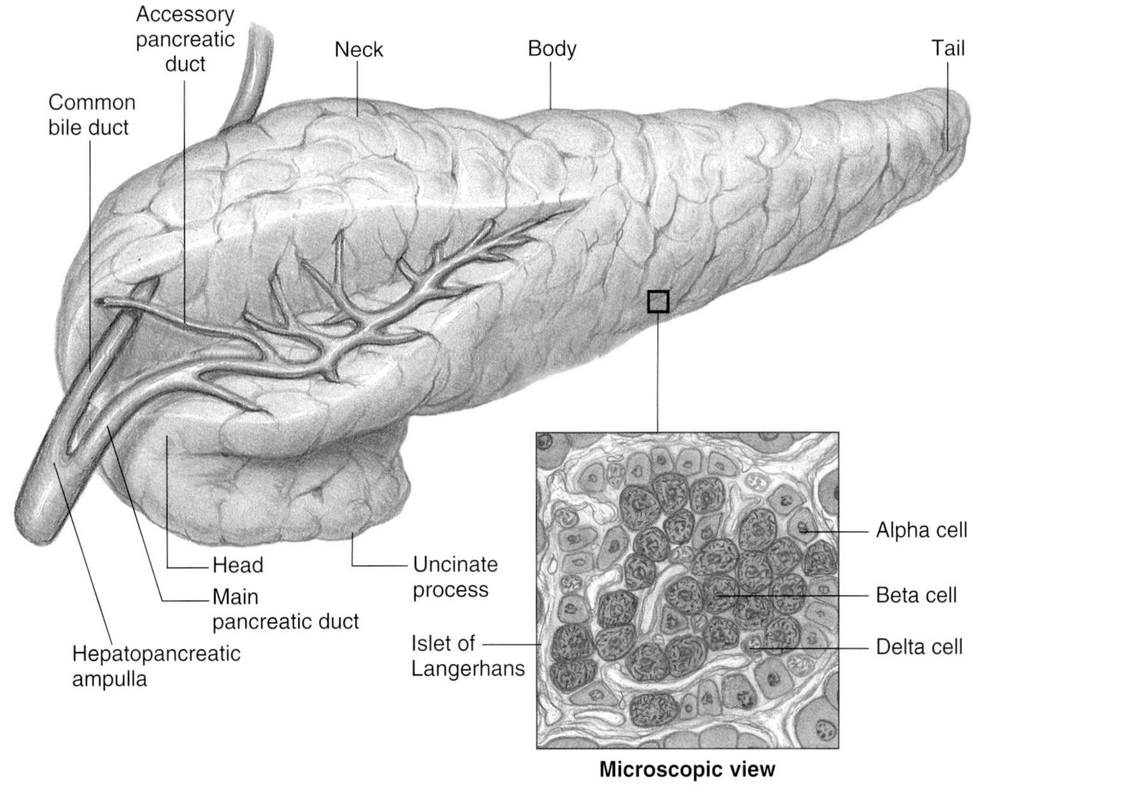

Figure 49-7 The pancreas secretes endocrine hormones from the islets of Langerhans. Exocrine digestive enzymes are released from the pancreas through the common bile duct.

cells in the small intestine stimulates contraction of the gallbladder to release bile when dietary fat is ingested.

ASSESSMENT

History

The health history becomes especially significant in the diagnosis of many endocrine disorders. Some endocrine disorders are inherited or have a tendency to occur in families; therefore, a complete family history is essential. The nurse also obtains diet and drug histories.

The nurse documents an allergy to iodine, a component of contrast dyes, or shellfish and informs the primary provider. They also report whether the client has had a diagnostic test that used iodine (e.g., intravenous pyelography, gallbladder series) within the past 3 months. This information is essential before initiating a thyroid test. The nurse identifies the current symptoms. Sometimes, the symptoms of endocrine disorders are vague or resemble other physical or mental disorders. Examples are fatigue, personality changes, inability to sleep, and frequent urination. At other times, symptoms are dramatic, such as a change in mental acuity or sudden weight loss.

Physical Examination

The nurse obtains the client's height, weight, and vital signs and notes their general physical appearance. The nurse examines body structures to detect evidence of hypersecretion or hyposecretion of hormones (see Chapters 50 and 51 for assessment findings unique to specific endocrine glands). They inspect the skin for excessive oiliness or dryness, excessive or absent areas of pigmentation, excessive hair growth or loss, and skin breaks that heal poorly. The nurse examines the shape and color of the nails and determines whether they are thin, thick, or brittle. They examine the eyes for *exophthalmos*, abnormal bulging or protrusion of the eyes (Fig. 49-8), and periorbital swelling. The nurse observes the client's facial expression and general features. They visually inspect the neck for thyroid enlargement and gently palpates the thyroid gland (Fig. 49-9). Repeated or forceful palpation of the thyroid in the case of thyroid hyperactivity can result in a sudden release of a large amount of thyroid hormones, which can have serious implications. The nurse notes the pulse rate and rhythm. They examine the extremities for edema and changes in pigmentation, auscultates the lungs for abnormal sounds, and examines outstretched hands for tremors. The nurse also determines if the client has experienced any loss of motor function or decreased sensitivity to pain or touch in the extremities.

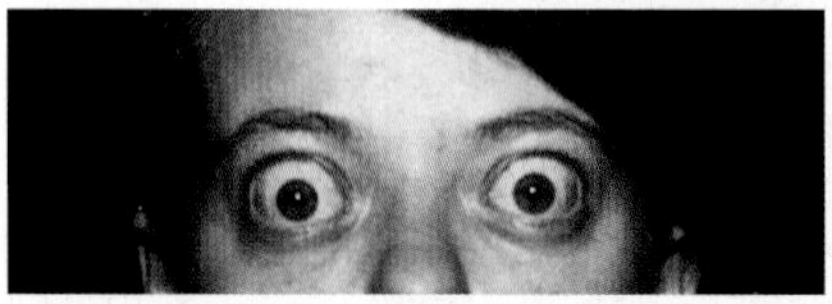

Figure 49-8 Exophthalmos in a person with hyperthyroidism. (Reprinted with permission from Rubin, E., and Strayer, D. S., (Eds.). (2014). *Rubin's pathology: Clinicopathologic foundations of medicine* (7th ed.). Wolters Kluwer.)

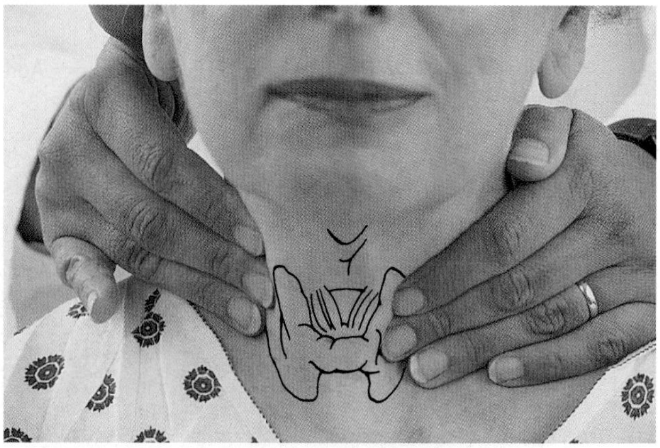

Figure 49-9 With the client's head slightly tilted to the side, the examiner displaces the thyroid laterally with their fingers and palpates the thyroid as the client swallows. The examination is repeated on the opposite side. (Photo by B. Proud.).

The nurse assesses the client's mental and emotional status and evaluates their demeanor (e.g., dull, apathetic, extremely nervous). They determine the client's ability to process information and respond to questions.

Diagnostic Tests

The type and extent of laboratory and diagnostic testing depend on the tentative medical diagnosis (see Chapters 50 and 51). Because the physical symptoms may be vague, multiple and varied laboratory tests may be necessary to ultimately determine the etiology of the client's symptoms. A complete blood count and chemistry profile are performed to determine the client's general status and to rule out disorders.

Hormone Levels

Measuring blood or urine and sometimes salivary hormone levels helps evaluate the functioning of some endocrine glands. These tests include cortisol levels (morning and evening) to determine adrenal hyperfunction or hypofunction, antidiuretic hormone (ADH) levels to determine the presence or absence of ADH, estrogen and testosterone to detect reproductive hormone levels, and a thyroid panel that measures TSH, T_3, and T_4 levels to identify diseases associated with increased or decreased thyroid hormones.

Radiography, Computed Tomography, and Magnetic Resonance Imaging

Radiographs of the chest or abdomen are taken to detect tumors as well as to determine organ size and placement. A computed tomography (CT) or magnetic resonance imaging (MRI) scan is performed to detect a suspected pituitary tumor or to identify calcifications or tumors of the parathyroid glands.

Radionuclide Studies

A **radionuclide** is an atom with an unstable nucleus that emits electromagnetic radiation as alpha, beta, or gamma particles. A radioactive iodine (RAI) uptake test (^{131}I uptake, ^{123}I uptake) and TSH test are radionuclide studies performed to determine thyroid function.

Pharmacologic Considerations

- Thyroid test results can be altered by the following medications:
  - *TSH decrease:* dopamine, levodopa, bromocriptine, glucocorticoids, octreotide, amphetamines
  - *TSH increase*: metoclopramide, amiodarone, contrast medium for radiographs
  - *T_4 decrease*: phenytoin, carbamazepine
  - *T_4 increase*: furosemide, heparin, amiodarone, contrast medium for radiographs

A **radioimmunoassay** determines the concentration of a substance in plasma. Venous blood samples are required for radioimmunoassay tests. A radioactively labeled substance (e.g., hormone, protein, antibodies, antigens) is combined in the laboratory with a blood sample to determine the quantity of the substance to be identified. For example, a T_3 determination by radioimmunoassay evaluates thyroid function.

A nuclear scan uses a radioactive substance that is taken orally or injected intravenously. The dose of the radioactive substance is larger than the dose used for radionuclide studies. Certain endocrine organs are visualized or their activity is determined by means of special equipment. Examples of scans include thyroid scan, adrenergic tumor scan, and parathyroid scan.

NURSING MANAGEMENT

The nurse prepares the client for laboratory and diagnostic testing. They explain the general purpose of the test, type of test, and how it will be performed. The nurse encourages the client and family to ask questions and discuss the results with the primary provider.

Nurses must consult the institution's procedure manual and the primary provider's orders for the required preparation for each diagnostic procedure. Some tests, such as a CT scan, require no special preparation other than a general explanation. Some tests require fasting; others require a temporary elimination of certain foods from the diet.

The nurse explains to the client how to participate in the test. For example, some tests require the client to save all voided urine during a particular time frame or to return for additional testing.

If a client is anxious about the use of radioactive materials for tests, the nurse offers assurance that these substances are safe and ordinarily pose no danger to the client or others. Also see Evidence-Based Practice 49-1.

Evidence-Based Practice 49-1

Complications From Thyroidectomy

Clinical Question

In clients receiving a thyroidectomy, how does traditional thyroidectomy compare to robotic-assisted thyroidectomy in relation to postoperative complications?

Evidence

Traditionally, thyroidectomies have been performed by making an incision across the front of the neck (anterior approach), often leaving a visible scar that leaves clients feeling self-conscious. In addition, using an anterior incision can leave clients with localized pain; sensations of numbness and tingling (paresthesia); sensations of burning, itching, or pins and needles (dysesthesia); and sunken-in scars or keloids (overgrowth of skin where the incision is made) (Ryu et al., 2020).

New technology in robotic-assisted surgery allows surgeons to make all three incisions in the armpit (transaxillary approach), using a robotic-assisted endoscope with a gas insufflation to access the thyroid gland (Ryu et al., 2020). Other approaches include a single long axillary incision, or incisions in the axilla, breast, and chest (Tae et al., 2019). Although these new approaches offer some benefits, they are not free from complications. In addition to the typical complications that can happen with traditional thyroid surgery (bleeding, infection, localized pain) another complication that must be monitored is the potential for nerve damage (Ryu et al., 2020; Tae et al., 2019). Different approaches lend themselves to different complications. For example, when a transaxillary approach and robotic-assisted endoscopes are used, some clients have suffered partial upper arm or lower arm paralysis because of the way the body is positioned during surgery (Ryu et al., 2020). Another documented complication with robotic-assisted endoscopic thyroid surgery is temporary vocal cord paralysis, which typically goes away within 3 months after having the surgery (Ryu et al., 2020).

Nursing Implications

When caring for a client after a thyroidectomy, it is important for the nurse to know whether a traditional anterior incision or robotic-assisted surgery was performed. Knowing which surgical approach was used helps the nurse determine the types of complications to look for. The nurse must assess for nerve damage (paralysis, paresthesia, or dysesthesia) and carefully document and report assessment findings. Clients should be closely monitored postoperatively to see if the condition is transient (goes away) or permanent. During this time, the nurse must be mindful of the effects nerve damage may have on the client's safety and ability to perform typical activities of daily living, such as the ability to self-feed and swallow (depending on the location of the potential nerve damage). Client safety concerns must be assessed if nerve damage is suspected. Support and assistance should be offered when needed. If indications of nerve damage continue, the nurse should discuss with the provider regarding consultations with physical therapy, occupational therapy, and/or speech and language pathology, depending on the functions that are affected. In addition, the nurse should support the client's emotional well-being by keeping lines of communication between the client and staff open, lending physical and emotional support as needed, and making the client aware of actions being taken.

References

Ryu, C. H., Seok, J., Jung, Y. S., & Ryu, J. (2020). Novel robot-assisted thyroidectomy by a transaxillary gas-insufflation approach (TAGA): A preliminary report. *Gland Surgery, 9*(5), 1267–1277. https://doi.org/10.21037/gs-20-450

Tae, K., Ji, Y. B., Song, C. M., & Ryu, J. (2019). Robotic and endoscopic thyroid surgery: Evolution and advances. *Clinical and Experimental Otorhinolaryngology, 12*(1), 1–11. https://doi.org/10.21053/ceo.2018.00766

Concept Mastery Alert

Nuclear Scan Anxiety

If a client scheduled for a nuclear scan expresses anxiety about the safety of intravenous radioactive substances, the nurse should offer assurance that radioactive substances are safe and ordinarily pose no danger to the client or others.

KEY POINTS

- Anatomy and physiology:
  - Pituitary gland
  - Hypothalamus
  - Thyroid gland
  - Parathyroid glands
  - Thymus gland
  - Pineal gland
  - Adrenal glands
  - Pancreas
  - Ovaries and testes
- Assessment:
  - History
  - Physical examination
  - Diagnostic tests to include the following:
    - Hormone levels
    - Radiography
    - CT
    - MRI
    - Radionuclide studies

CRITICAL THINKING EXERCISES

1. Explain why the pituitary gland is considered the master gland. Give some examples that support the terminology.
2. Discuss the meaning and purpose of a feedback loop.
3. Based on the principle of the feedback loop, if a client's T_3 and T_4 hormone levels are low, what hormone level(s) is/are most likely elevated?
4. When examining a client, the nurse notes that the client's eyes bulge and protrude from the bony orbits. What is the term for this condition, and what hormonal disorder may be the cause? What diagnostic test would be ordered to confirm or rule out a hormonal cause for the condition?

NCLEX-STYLE REVIEW QUESTIONS PrepU

1. A client diagnosed with parathormone deficiency is admitted to the hospital. As the nurse initiates the care plan, what body system should be the focus of care?
   1. Skeletal
   2. Urinary
   3. Respiratory
   4. Integumentary
2. The nurse takes vital signs for a client scheduled for open-heart surgery in the next few minutes and notes that the client's pulse, respiration, and blood pressure are slightly elevated. The nurse explains to the client that the elevations are a normal response to stress and anxiety and are because of the release of what hormone?
   1. Insulin
   2. Epinephrine
   3. Thyroxine
   4. Aldosterone
3. Match the pancreas, ovary, adrenal gland, pituitary, thymus, and thyroid gland with numbers 1 through 6 in the following figure.

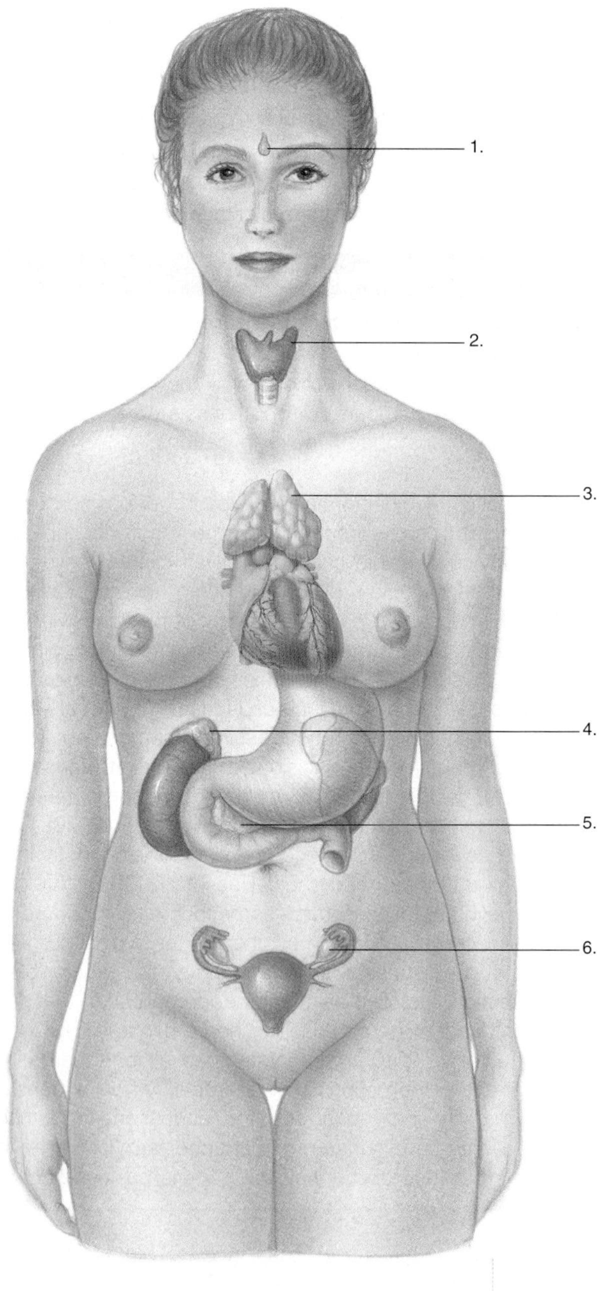

4. The nurse gently palpates the neck of a client diagnosed with a thyroid disorder. The client asks why the nurse's touch is so gentle. What response by the nurse is most appropriate?
   1. "Forceful palpation can result in excessive release of thyroid hormone from the gland."
   2. "This type of palpation is the way my instructor in nursing school taught me to do it."
   3. "Gentle palpation prevents closing off the trachea, which would cause you to gasp for air."
   4. "Forceful palpation causes pain in an area that is already enlarged and tender to touch."

5. When assessing a client with a suspected thyroid disorder prior to a nuclear scan, what type of allergy is most important for the nurse to report?
   1. Peanuts
   2. Shellfish
   3. Eggs
   4. Wheat

WANT TO KNOW MORE? There are a wide variety of online resources available on thePoint to enhance learning and understanding of this chapter.

Go to **thePoint.lww.com/activate** and use the activation code found in the front of this text to unlock these online resources.

50 Caring for Clients With Disorders of the Endocrine System

Words To Know

acromegaly
Addisonian crisis
adrenalectomy
adrenal insufficiency
carpopedal spasm
cushingoid syndrome
Cushing syndrome
diabetes insipidus
goiter
hyperaldosteronism
hyperparathyroidism
hyperplasia
hyperthyroidism
hypertrophy
hypoparathyroidism
hypophysectomy
hypothyroidism
myxedema
pheochromocytoma
Simmonds disease
syndrome of inappropriate antidiuretic hormone secretion
tetany
thyroidectomy
thyroiditis
thyrotoxic crisis

Learning Objectives

On completion of this chapter, you will be able to:

1. Describe the physiologic effects of hyposecretion and hypersecretion of the pituitary, thyroid, parathyroid, and adrenal glands.
2. Describe the nursing management of clients with pituitary gland disorders.
3. Describe thyroid disorders and nursing management of clients with these disorders.
4. Compare the differences in physiologic effects, assessment findings, and management of disorders affecting the parathyroid glands.
5. Identify disorders of the adrenal glands and describe nursing management of clients with these disorders.
6. Identify symptoms of emergency conditions resulting from endocrine disorders.

A disorder of any endocrine gland can profoundly affect the other endocrine glands as well as many major body systems. This chapter discusses the care of clients with various endocrine disorders and considers the ways in which these disorders affect systemic physiology. The chapter focuses on disorders affecting the pituitary, thyroid, parathyroid, and adrenal glands. Diabetes mellitus is presented separately in Chapter 51. Disorders of the ovaries and testes are discussed in Chapters 53 and 55, respectively.

Gerontologic Considerations

- Older adults have an increased incidence of nodules and small goiters on the thyroid gland.
- Symptoms of thyroid disease in older adults often are atypical or minor and easily attributed to normal aging or other chronic conditions. For example, older adults may not experience restlessness or hyperactivity and may not appear nervous. Symptoms seen most often in older adults include anorexia, weight loss, palpitations, angina, and atrial fibrillation.
- A component of health assessment includes determination of the client's and caregiver's awareness of symptoms that should be reported to the health care provider.

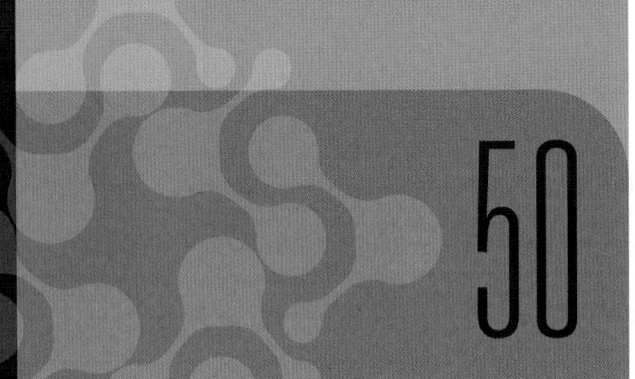

Gerontologic Considerations (*continued*)

- Specific teaching regarding reporting subtle symptoms such as those listed previously is critical for early identification of disease processes.
- Changes in thyroid hormone levels may accompany atrophy of the thyroid gland due to aging, thyroidectomy, iodine deficiency or excess, medications, radiation (American Thyroid Association, 2017), lifetime exposure to organic pollutants (Grova et al., 2019), or diseases that affect the thyroid.
- Hypothyroidism is difficult to identify in older adults because symptoms closely resemble normal aging—for example, anorexia, constipation, weight loss, muscular weakness and pain, joint stiffness, apathy, and depression. Older adults should be encouraged to seek further evaluation for any of these symptoms to determine if diagnostic examinations are needed to identify potential underlying disorders.
- Dosages of thyroid replacement drugs are lower in older adults, and drug therapy is initiated slowly and increased cautiously.
- Older adults receiving thyroid replacement therapy are at increased risk of adverse reactions associated with cardiac function.
- Untreated hypothyroidism becomes a risk factor for coronary artery disease, indicating a need for cardiac stress testing and lipid level monitoring.
- Metabolic changes of hypothyroidism can be corrected with proper treatment.
- Older adults and family members should be advised that T_4 replacement with levothyroxine sodium must be maintained for life, with at least annual follow-up visits.
- Comorbid thyroid disorders and congestive heart failure may warrant adjustment in medications (American Thyroid Association, 2017).

DISORDERS OF THE PITUITARY GLAND

Pituitary gland disorders usually result from excessive or deficient production and secretion of specific hormones. When oversecretion of growth hormone (GH) occurs before puberty (when the ends [epiphyses] of the long bones are not yet fully united), *gigantism* results. When secretion of GH during childhood is insufficient, *dwarfism* occurs. Refer to a pediatric text for further discussion of gigantism and dwarfism. Oversecretion of GH during adulthood results in *acromegaly*. Conversely, an absence of pituitary hormonal activity causes panhypopituitarism or *Simmonds disease*.

Acromegaly (Hyperpituitarism)

Pathophysiology and Etiology

Acromegaly results when GH is oversecreted after the epiphyses of the long bones have sealed. GH is overproduced when the pituitary gland is insensitive to feedback-inhibiting hormones such as *somatostatin*, a hypothalamic hormone, and *insulin-like growth factor 1* (IGF-1). IGF-1, a hormone released by the liver, stimulates the growth of bones and tissue (National Institute of Diabetes and Digestive and Kidney Diseases [NIDDK], 2020). Unchecked GH allows sustained production of IGF-1, a hormone synthesized and secreted by the liver, which supports cellular division and growth but is less potent than insulin. The sustained production of IGF-1 leads to lengthening and widening of bones, organ enlargement, and hyperlipidemia (Utiger, n.d.). Hypersecretion causes **hypertrophy** (increase in cell size) and **hyperplasia** (increased numbers of cells), which results in an *adenoma*, a benign tumor. As with other cranial tumors, a benign pituitary tumor becomes a space-occupying lesion and can affect other cerebral structures (see Chapter 37).

Assessment Findings

Signs and Symptoms

A client with acromegaly has coarse features, a huge lower jaw, thick lips, a thickened tongue, a bulging forehead, a bulbous nose, and large hands and feet (Fig. 50-1). When the

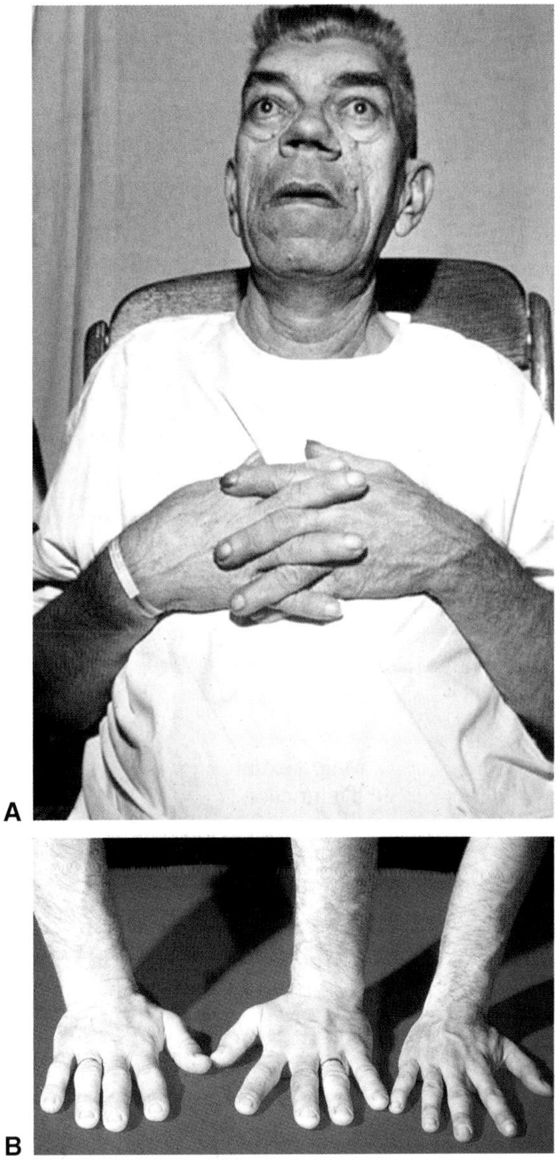

Figure 50-1 Acromegaly is characterized by **(A)** enlarged coarse facial features and **(B)** large hands. Note single, normal-sized hand on right. (Reprinted with permission from McConnell, T. H. (2007). *The nature of disease: Pathology for the health professions.* Wolters Kluwer Health/Lippincott Williams & Wilkins.)

overgrowth is from a tumor, headaches caused by pressure on the sella turcica, a bony depression in which the pituitary gland rests, are common. Partial blindness may result from pressure on the optic nerve. The heart, liver, and spleen may be enlarged. Despite enlarged tissues, muscle weakness is common, and hypertrophied joints become painful and stiff. Osteoporosis of the spine and joint pain develop. Many men experience erectile dysfunction, and women may have amenorrhea (absence of menstruation), increased facial hair, and deepened voices that result from compression of areas of the pituitary gland responsible for producing sex-related hormones (Fig. 50-2). Some people develop diabetes mellitus.

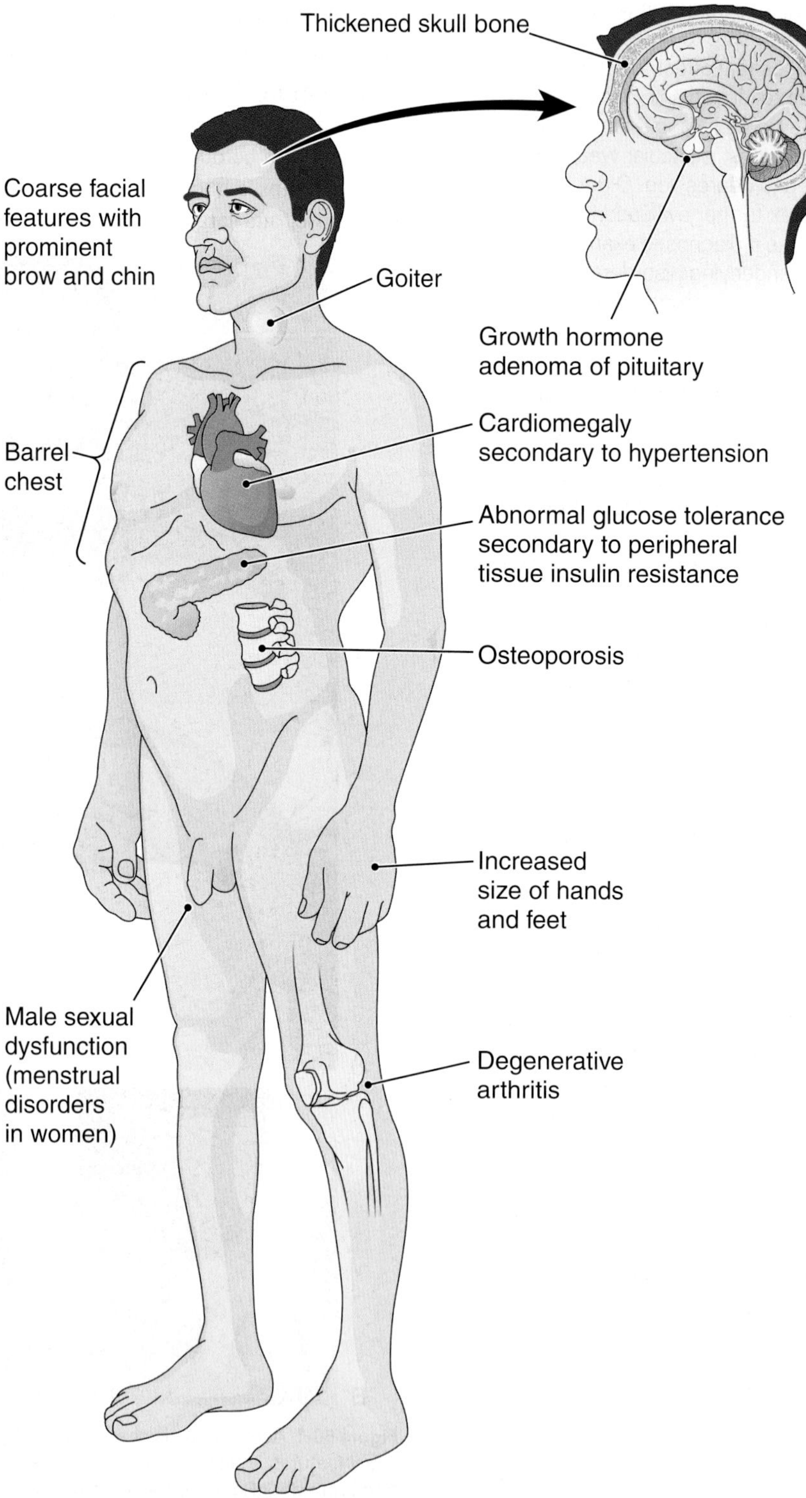

Figure 50-2 Clinical manifestations of acromegaly. (Reprinted with permission from McConnell, T. H. (2007). *The nature of disease: Pathology for the health professions.* Wolters Kluwer Health/Lippincott Williams & Wilkins.)

Diagnostic Findings

Skull radiography, magnetic resonance imaging (MRI), and computed tomography (CT) reveal pituitary gland enlargement. Bone radiographs show thickened long bones and skull bones. A glucose tolerance test in combination with a GH measurement is the most reliable method of confirming acromegaly. Ingestion of a bolus of glucose should lower GH levels, but GH levels remain elevated in persons with acromegaly (NIDDK, 2020). Increased blood levels of IGF-1, which supports cellular division and growth, can also indicate acromegaly in nonpregnant women; they typically have IGF-1 levels two to three times higher than normal in pregnant women.

Medical and Surgical Management

The treatment of choice is **hypophysectomy**, surgical removal of the pituitary gland, which lies within the sella turcica, a saddle-shaped depression in the sphenoid bone. The gland is removed by piercing the sphenoid with either a *sublabial* (under the upper lip) approach or, more recently, with a minimally invasive endoscopic *endonasal* (through the nose) method (Fig. 50-3), which reduces surgical trauma, leaves no residual scar, and results in a recovery time of 2 days. However, because the pituitary gland is surrounded by the optic nerves and carotid arteries, many primary providers who use the endoscopic technique request assistance from a neurosurgeon, an otolaryngologist, neuro-ophthalmologist, or interventional radiologist (Petersenn, 2019).

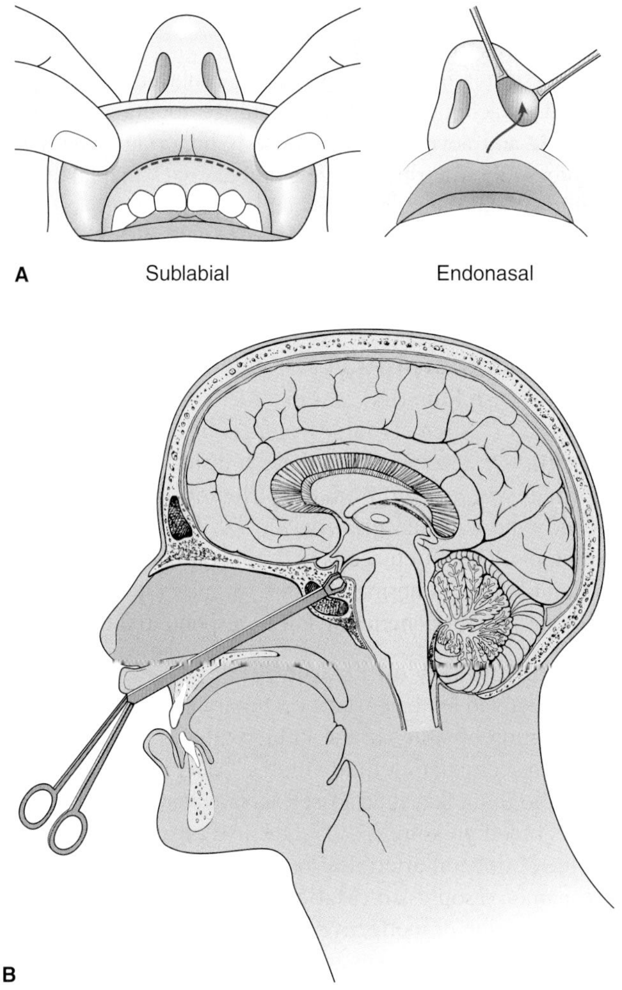

Figure 50-3 **(A)** External views of the sublabial and endonasal approaches to remove the pituitary gland. **(B)** A sublabial transsphenoidal hypophysectomy is performed to remove the pituitary gland.

The client who is a surgical risk may undergo a primary method of treatment that includes a series of radiation treatments over 4 to 6 weeks. Clients undergo frequent monitoring for evidence of tumor recurrence. Even if the disease is arrested successfully, physical changes are irreversible. If surgery or radiation therapy removes or destroys normal pituitary tissue, replacement therapy with thyroid hormone, corticosteroids, antidiuretic hormone (ADH), and sex hormones is necessary.

Medical treatment includes oral administrations of bromocriptine mesylate (Parlodel), an oral antiparkinsonism drug that inhibits the release of GH in clients with acromegaly, or cabergoline (Dostinex), or parenteral injections of octreotide (Sandostatin), lanreotide (Somatuline), or pegvisomant (Somavert).

Bromocriptine and cabergoline are used alone or in conjunction with pituitary gland irradiation or surgery to reduce the serum GH level. Octreotide, a synthetic form of somatostatin, stops the production of GH and IGF-1 and effectively relieves symptoms for a short time. One form of octreotide is injected subcutaneously every 8 hours; a longer acting form, Sandostatin LAR Depot, is injected intramuscularly every month. Both forms may cause gastrointestinal (GI) side effects, gallstones, and diabetes. Pegvisomant, a GH receptor antagonist, is the newest and most effective drug for treating acromegaly. Injected subcutaneously once a day, it normalizes the IGF-1 level by blocking the GH stimulation of IGF-1 produced by the liver (Ilie et al., 2019). Pegvisomant may be combined with octreotide or lanreotide (Corica et al., 2020). Clients who take pegvisomant must be monitored for liver damage.

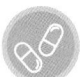

Pharmacologic Considerations

- Parenteral Somavert (pegvisomant) must be administered within 6 hours of reconstitution. The internet provides client instruction materials to assist in successful teach-back sessions for self-administration, empowering clients in managing their disease.

Nursing Management

Until the client has surgery or receives radiation treatment, nursing priorities include helping the client cope with changes in physical appearance, pacing activities to accommodate the client's fatigue, and relieving discomfort from headaches, abdominal distention resulting from organ enlargement, and skeletal pain. The nurse evaluates the client's pain, discerning type and location; gives analgesics as prescribed; and notes whether the client reports relief from pain. The nurse encourages self-care and activities when the client's strength and endurance permit.

The client may experience severe psychological stress because of the prominent physical changes, sexual dysfunction, and decreased libido. The nurse discusses such issues to help the client cope with changes. If the client expresses concern over sexual dysfunction, the nurse brings it to the primary provider's attention. Referral to a sex therapist could be indicated.

Postoperatively, the client undergoes frequent neurologic assessments to detect signs of increased intracranial pressure and meningitis (see Chapter 36). If the client has nasal packing, the nurse monitors drainage from the nose and postnasal drainage for the presence of cerebrospinal fluid. The nurse modifies oral and facial hygiene to promote cleanliness without contributing to trauma near the operative site. The nurse also reminds the client to avoid drinking from a straw, sneezing, coughing, and bending over to prevent dislodging the graft that seals the operative area between the cranium and nose.

Panhypopituitarism (Simmonds Disease)

Pathophysiology and Etiology

Simmonds disease is a rare disorder caused by destruction of the pituitary gland followed by cessation of pituitary hormonal activity. Events such as postpartum emboli or hemorrhage, surgery, tumor, and tuberculosis can destroy pituitary function. This disease affects all hormones of the anterior pituitary gland (Fig. 50-4).

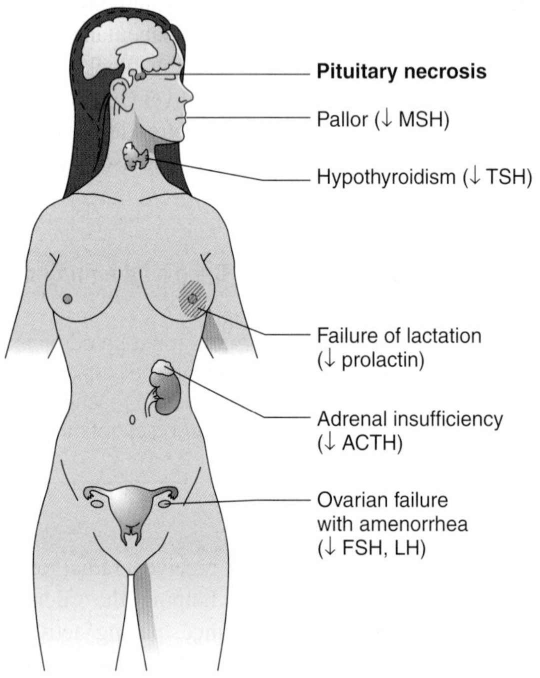

Figure 50-4 Major clinical manifestations of panhypopituitarism. ACTH, adrenocorticotropic hormone; FSH, follicle-stimulating hormone; LH, luteinizing hormone; MSH, melanocyte-stimulating hormone; TSH, thyroid-stimulating hormone. (Reprinted with permission from Rubin, E., & Strayer, D. S., (Eds.). (2014). *Rubin's pathology: Clinicopathologic foundations of medicine* (7th ed.). Wolters Kluwer.)

Assessment Findings

The gonads and genitalia atrophy. Because of the impaired pituitary stimulus, the thyroid and adrenals fail to secrete adequate hormones. Signs and symptoms of hypothyroidism, hypoglycemia, and adrenal insufficiency (Addison disease—see later discussion) are apparent. The client ages prematurely and becomes extremely cachectic (showing physical wasting). The skin becomes pale because of a decrease in melanocyte-stimulating hormone (MSH), which is under the control of adrenocorticotropic hormone (ACTH). Results of laboratory tests show decreased hormone levels (e.g., thyroid, corticosteroid, reproductive hormones).

Medical Management

Treatment includes administration of replacement hormones for the glands that depend on the pituitary gland for stimulation. If untreated, the disease is fatal. GH replacement is necessary only for children. Deficiency of thyroid-stimulating hormone (TSH) requires replacement with levothyroxine (Synthroid) or liothyronine (Cytomel) for the client's lifetime. Clients who are men receive testosterone, and clients who are women receive estrogen; both sexes receive follicle-stimulating hormone (FSH) and luteinizing hormone (LH).

Nursing Management

The nurse administers all hormone replacements as prescribed. Teaching the client to adhere to the medication schedule and never to omit a dose is important. The nurse monitors blood hormone levels and assesses mental status, emotional state, energy level, and appetite. They are alert to any alterations in nutrition. Most clients with Simmonds disease tolerate four to six small meals per day better than three regular meals.

Diabetes Insipidus

Diabetes insipidus (DI) is a disorder characterized by the excretion of extremely large volumes of urine. *Neurogenic* or *central DI* develops when there is insufficient ADH (also known as *vasopressin*) from the posterior pituitary gland. A second type is called *nephrogenic DI*. Both have identical symptoms. The difference is that in nephrogenic DI, the secretion of ADH is normal, but the receptors in the renal tubules partially or completely fail to respond to the hormone.

Pathophysiology and Etiology

ADH, secreted by the posterior pituitary gland, regulates the reabsorption of water in the kidney tubules. Its function is to increase circulating fluid volume. ADH is released in response to thirst and fluid losses such as hemorrhage, which lowers blood pressure (BP). ADH also raises BP by signaling the peripheral arterioles to constrict; hence, its alternative name, vasopressin (Marieb & Hoehn, 2018). Lack of ADH secretion or ineffective response to it causes the client to produce large volumes of dilute urine. If the client fails to drink a compensatory volume of fluid, dehydration with concentrated levels of electrolytes occurs.

Neurogenic DI can result from head trauma that damages the pituitary gland or from primary or metastatic brain tumors. In some congenital incidences, symptoms occur shortly after birth. Neurogenic DI also can occur after *hypophysectomy*, surgical removal of the pituitary gland.

Nephrogenic DI is less common than neurogenic DI. The client generally acquires nephrogenic DI as a side effect from drugs such as lithium (Eskalith), a drug used for managing bipolar disorder, which is usually reversible after discontinuing the drug (see Chapter 69); demeclocycline (Declomycin), an antibiotic in the tetracycline family; and amphotericin B (Amphocin), an antifungal antibiotic (Priya et al., 2021). Nephrogenic DI also is associated with elevated levels of prostaglandin E_2, which has been shown to interfere with the action of vasopressin.

Assessment Findings

Signs and Symptoms

Urine output may be as high as 20 L/24 hours. Urine is dilute, with a specific gravity of 1.002 or less. Limiting fluid intake does not control urine excretion. Thirst is excessive and constant. Activities are limited by the frequent need to drink and void. Weakness, dehydration, and weight loss develop.

Diagnostic Findings

A fluid deprivation test can diagnose DI and differentiate neurogenic DI from nephrogenic DI. The protocol for a fluid deprivation test involves withholding fluid from the client for 5 to 6 hours while concurrently measuring their urine volume, urine specific gravity, and serum osmolality (osmotic pressure of the serum compared with water). In both types of DI, the excreted urine volume continues to be excessive, with a low specific gravity almost equal to that of water; the serum osmolality is high because of the client's dehydration from the water restriction. At the completion of the fasting phase of the test, the client receives an infusion of desmopressin acetate (DDAVP), a synthetic analogue of vasopressin. If the urine becomes more concentrated following the infusion, the symptoms are attributed to insufficient ADH (i.e., neurogenic DI). If the urine continues to be dilute, with low specific gravity, the symptoms are the result of a failure of the renal tubules to respond to ADH, and the diagnosis is nephrogenic DI.

Medical Management

DDAVP nasal solution and lypressin (Diapid) nasal spray are synthetic drugs with ADH activity that reduce urine output to 2 to 3 L/24 hours (Client and Family Teaching 50-1). If the client cannot take oral fluids to meet the excessive fluid volume loss, intravenous (IV) fluids are necessary.

The management of nephrogenic DI is different. Besides ensuring that the client has a sufficient intake of fluid, the primary provider also needs to reduce the client's urine output by reducing the amount of sodium excreted by the renal tubules. Therefore, the primary provider restricts the client's use of dietary sodium. The primary provider prescribes a thiazide diuretic, such as hydrochlorothiazide (HydroDIURIL). The thiazide acts at the proximal convoluted tubule, leaving less fluid for excretion in the distal convoluted tubules, the portion affected by nephrogenic DI. Consequently, the client excretes water, but the total volume is less than in an untreated state. Sometimes the primary provider prescribes the thiazide diuretic combined with spironolactone (Aldactone) or amiloride (Midamor), potassium-sparing diuretics to help prevent hypokalemia. In addition, the primary provider prescribes indomethacin (Indocin), an anti-inflammatory drug that acts as a prostaglandin inhibitor, to reduce the level of prostaglandin E_2 (Priya et al., 2021). Lastly, the primary provider restricts the client's intake of dietary protein to reduce the work of the kidney to excrete protein nitrogenous wastes.

Client and Family Teaching 50-1
Self-Administration of Lypressin Nasal Spray

The nurse teaches the client the following administration steps:

1. Hold container upright.
2. Place nozzle in nostril while in sitting position.
3. Spray prescribed number of times in each nostril.
4. Avoid exceeding the number of sprays per self-administration; the excess is not absorbed and therefore wastes the volume of the prescribed drug.
5. Do not inhale medication.
6. Report nasal irritation to the primary provider.
7. Monitor urine output and level of thirst.

Nursing Management

Nursing measures include correcting fluid volume deficit. The nurse closely monitors the rate of IV infusions to ensure that the prescribed amount is given over the required period and measures fluid intake and output. If the client is acutely ill, extremely dehydrated, fails to take oral fluids, or is beginning to receive medical treatment, the nurse measures urine output every 30 minutes while administering prescribed fluid and drug therapy. They weigh the client daily to identify weight gain or loss and observes for signs of fluid excess or deficit. The nurse notifies the primary provider of sudden or steady weight gain or loss.

The nurse teaches the client to consume sufficient fluid to control thirst and to compensate for urine loss. In addition, the nurse explains other methods for reducing fluid loss, such as remaining in air-conditioned areas during hot and humid weather and avoiding strenuous physical activity. The nurse stresses adherence to drug (and diet) therapy and reassures the client that treatment can control symptoms.

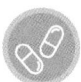

Pharmacologic Considerations

- A person with DI who is in an accident may be unable to take their routine medication. To alert Emergency Medical Services (EMS) of a possible severe fluid deficit, encourage clients to wear medical alert identification.

Syndrome of Inappropriate Antidiuretic Hormone Secretion

The **syndrome of inappropriate antidiuretic hormone secretion (SIADH)** is characterized by renal reabsorption of water rather than its normal excretion.

Pathophysiology and Etiology

Causes of SIADH include lung tumors; central nervous system (CNS) disorders; brain tumors; cerebrovascular accident; head trauma; and drugs such as vasopressin, general anesthetic agents, oral hypoglycemics, and tricyclic antidepressants. The continued release of ADH increases fluid volume and causes *hyponatremia* (decreased serum sodium level).

Assessment Findings

Water retention, headache, muscle cramps, and anorexia develop. As the condition worsens, the client experiences nausea, vomiting, muscle twitching, and changes in the level of consciousness (LOC). Diagnosis is based on symptoms and a history of a disorder associated with SIADH. Serum sodium levels and serum osmolarity (solute concentration) are decreased. Urine sodium levels and osmolarity are high.

Medical Management

When possible, treatment aims at eliminating the underlying cause. Osmotic diuretics, such as mannitol (Osmitrol), and loop diuretics, including furosemide (Lasix), help correct water retention. Severe hyponatremia is treated with IV administration of a 3% hypertonic sodium chloride solution.

Nursing Management

The nurse closely monitors fluid intake and output and vital signs. They carefully assess LOC and immediately reports any changes to the primary provider. The nurse checks closely for signs of fluid overload (confusion, dyspnea, pulmonary congestion, hypertension) and hyponatremia (weakness, muscle cramps, anorexia, nausea, diarrhea, irritability, headache, weight gain without edema).

The nurse gives the client and family extensive information about the medication schedule and adverse effects of drug therapy, especially if several medications are prescribed. They stress the importance of adhering to the medication schedule and not omitting a dose.

DISORDERS OF THE THYROID GLAND

Under the direction of thyroid-releasing hormone from the hypothalamus and the anterior pituitary gland's release of TSH, the thyroid gland, which depends on serum iodine, produces two hormones that are responsible for regulating body metabolism (Fig. 50-5). One hormone is *thyroxine*, also called T_4 because it contains four iodine molecules, and the second is *triiodothyronine*, called T_3 for a similar reason. T_4 is more abundant than T_3, but it is less potent. T_4 exists in two forms: the form bound to protein is not metabolically active; the unbound form is referred to as *free* T_4 (FT_4). It is considered a prohormone or precursor of T_3 because it can become T_3, a more powerful regulator of body metabolism, by eliminating one of its iodine molecules. If there is sufficient T_3, any unused FT_4 is converted to *reverse* T_3 (RT_3),

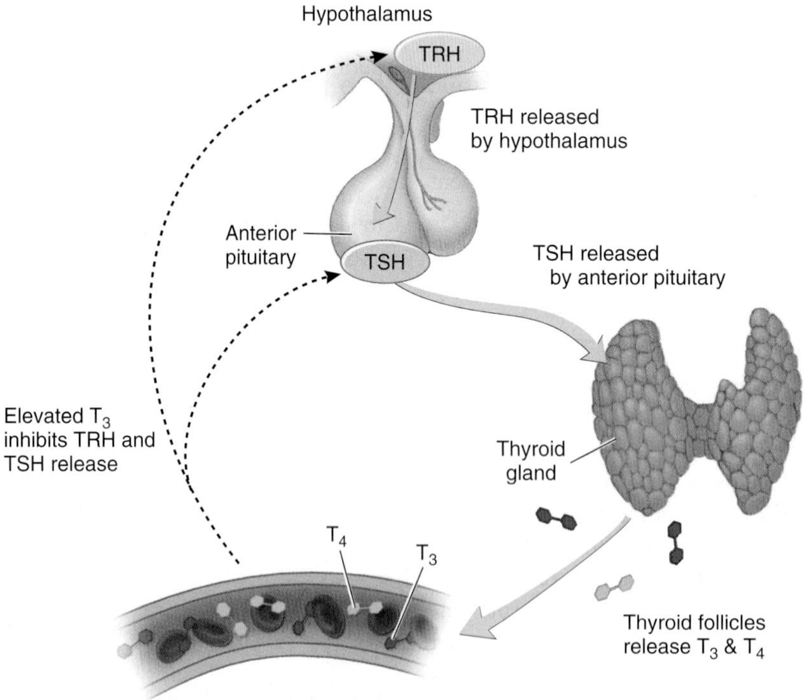

Figure 50-5 Cycle of thyroid stimulation and inhibition. T_3, triiodothyronine; T_4, thyroxine; TRH, thyrotropin-releasing hormone; TSH, thyroid-stimulating hormone. (Reprinted with permission from Premkumar, K. (2012). *Anatomy and physiology: The massage connection* (3rd ed.). Wolters Kluwer Health/Lippincott Williams & Wilkins.)

an inactive state, by the liver and kidneys (American Thyroid Association, 2019). Calcitonin is another hormone produced by separate cells in the thyroid gland; its function is discussed later under "Disorders of the Parathyroid Glands."

Thyroid disorders due to hyperfunction or hypofunction of thyroid hormones are difficult to detect because symptoms are vague until the disease progresses. Treatment often is long-term, and the client requires periodic follow-up to monitor response. Thyroid disorders include hyperthyroidism, thyrotoxic crisis, hypothyroidism, thyroid tumors, and endemic and multinodular goiters.

Hyperthyroidism

Hyperthyroidism also is called *Graves disease*, *Basedow disease*, *thyrotoxicosis*, or *exophthalmic goiter*.

Pathophysiology and Etiology

There is no single etiology for hyperthyroidism. Researchers have suggested that it may be autoimmune or inherited. Hypersecretion of thyroid hormones accompanies thyroid tumors, pituitary tumors, and hypothalamic malignancies. It also may result from stress or infection. The metabolic rate increases because of the oversecretion of the thyroid hormones thyroxine (T_4) and triiodothyronine (T_3). Both T_4 and T_3 increase the metabolic rate. Hyperthyroidism is more common in women than in men.

Assessment Findings

Signs and Symptoms

Symptoms vary from mild to severe. Clients with hyperthyroidism characteristically are restless despite feeling fatigued and weak, highly excitable, and constantly agitated. Fine tremors of the hands occur, causing unusual clumsiness (Fig. 50-6). Clients cannot tolerate heat and have an increased appetite but lose weight. Diarrhea also occurs. Visual changes, such as blurred or double vision, can develop. *Exophthalmos*, seen in clients with severe hyperthyroidism, results from enlarged muscle and fatty tissue surrounding the rear and sides of the eyeball (see Fig. 49-8). Neck swelling caused by the enlarged thyroid gland often is visible. Table 50-1 compares the signs and symptoms of hyperthyroidism and hypothyroidism.

> *Concept Mastery Alert*
>
> **Hyperthyroidism**
>
> Clients with hyperthyroidism are characteristically sensitive to heat and often perspire unusually freely. They are highly excitable and have an increased appetite, but they lose weight because their metabolism burns excessive calories.

Diagnostic Findings

The protein-bound iodine; free thyroxine (FT_4)—T_4 that is not bound to protein; thyroglobulin; and serum T_3 and T_4 levels are elevated. The TSH level is decreased. Thyroid ultrasonography shows an enlarged thyroid gland. A thyroid scan indicates an increased uptake of radioactive iodine (RAI; ^{131}I and ^{123}I) throughout the gland or confined to a single nodule.

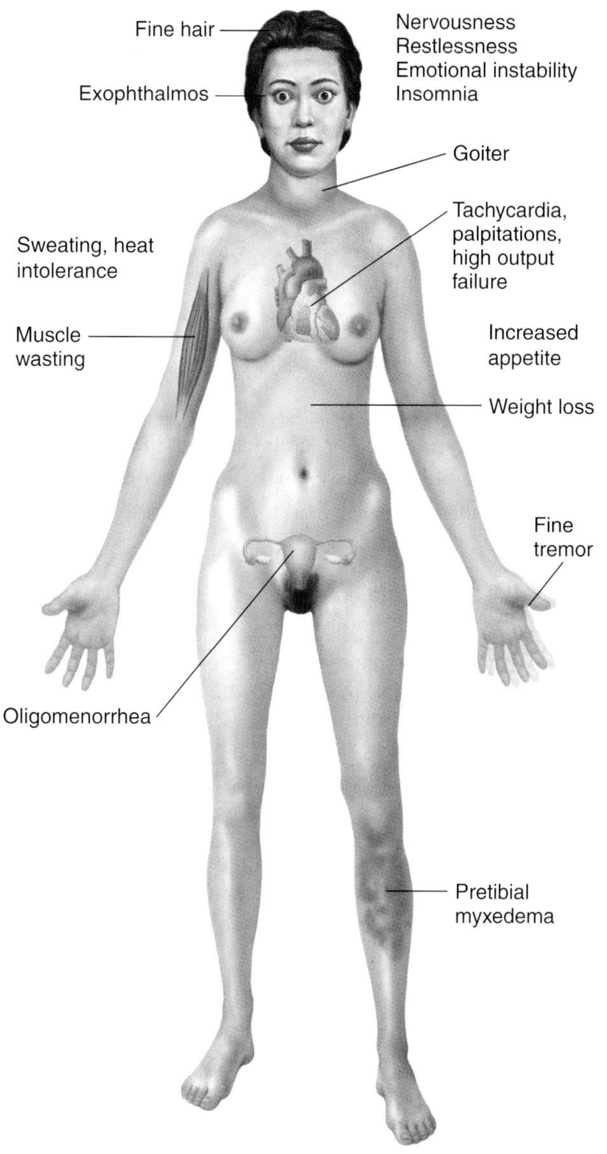

Figure 50-6 Clinical manifestations of hyperthyroidism. (Reprinted with permission from Grossman, S. C., & Porth, C. M. (2014). *Porth's pathophysiology: Concepts of altered health states* (9th ed.). Wolters Kluwer Health/Lippincott Williams & Wilkins.)

Medical and Surgical Management

Antithyroid drugs, such as propylthiouracil (PTU; Propyl Thyracil) and methimazole (Tapazole), are given to block the production of thyroid hormone preoperatively or for long-term treatment for clients who are not candidates for surgery or radiation treatment. If clients receive antithyroid drugs as the only treatment and do not comply with prescription therapy early in its management, the disorder may reactivate. About 40% to 70% of those who comply with antithyroid drug therapy for 1 to 2 years experience remission, but they need to continue with follow-up care to detect any sign of recurrence (Stoppler, 2019).

Antithyroid drugs can curb thyroid activity before surgery to reduce the postoperative potential for bleeding and thyrotoxicosis (discussed later). Antithyroid medications, however, are avoided during pregnancy because they can

TABLE 50-1 Symptoms of Thyroid Dysfunction

BODY SYSTEM OR FUNCTION	HYPERTHYROIDISM	HYPOTHYROIDISM
Metabolism	Increased, with symptoms of increased appetite, intolerance to heat, elevated body temperature, weight loss despite increased appetite	Decreased, with symptoms of anorexia, intolerance to cold, low body temperature, weight gain despite anorexia
Cardiovascular system	Tachycardia, moderate hypertension	Bradycardia, moderate hypotension
Central nervous system	Nervousness, anxiety, insomnia, tremors	Lethargy, sleepiness
Skin and skin structures	Flushed, warm, moist	Pale, cool, dry; face appears puffy, hair is coarse; nails are thick and hard
Ovarian function	Irregular or scant menses	Heavy menses, may be unable to conceive, loss of fetus is also possible
Testicular function		Low sperm count

induce hypothyroidism, or cretinism, in the fetus. Drug Therapy Table 50-1 discusses these and other drugs used to treat thyroid disorders.

Pharmacologic Considerations

- When treating pregnant women who have hyperthyroidism, it is recommended to use PTU during the first trimester, then switch to methimazole (Tapazole) for the remainder of the pregnancy, then switch back to PTU should the mother elect to breastfeed the infant (Ross, 2021).

^{131}I is used to destroy hyperplastic thyroid tissue by radiation. The thyroid is quick to remove iodine, including RAI, from the bloodstream. Antithyroid drugs are given for 6 months or more before administration of ^{131}I. If symptoms do not improve, a second and perhaps a third dose of ^{131}I is given. About 6 to 8 weeks after the initial dose of ^{131}I, most clients notice some remission of symptoms. The extended time lag before relief of symptoms is a disadvantage of this treatment method. A more common and unfortunate result of treatment is hypothyroidism because accurately determining the precise amount of thyroid tissue that radiation will destroy is very difficult. This complication may not develop until long after the administration of ^{131}I, and clients must remain under medical supervision for many years.

Thyroidectomy is the removal of part or all of the thyroid gland. *Subtotal thyroidectomy* (partial removal of the thyroid gland) or a *partial thyroid lobectomy* (removal of the upper or lower portion of one lobe) is an effective treatment for a confined area or nodule within the thyroid that is increasing

DRUG THERAPY TABLE 50-1 Agents to Treat Thyroid Disorders

Category and Common Generic (Brand) Drugs	Intended Use	Common Side Effects	Safety Warnings for Nurses
Thyroid Hormones			
Levothyroxine—T_4 (Levothroid, Levoxyl, Synthroid, Unithroid) Liothyronine—T_3 (Cytomel, Triostat) Liotrix—T_3/T_4 (Thyrolar) Thyroid, desiccated (Armour)	Hypothyroidism, thyroid-stimulating hormone suppression, thyroid diagnostic testing	Palpitations, headache, nervousness, insomnia, weight loss, fatigue, sweating, flushing	• One drug cannot be substituted for another • Severe tachycardia, fever, diarrhea, vomiting, change in mental status can indicate thyrotoxicity
Antithyroid Preparations			
Methimazole (Tapazole) Propylthiouracil (PTU)	Hyperthyroidism, thyrotoxicosis	Numbness, headache, loss of hair, skin rash, nausea, vomiting	• Monitor labs for agranulocytosis
Iodine Products			
Sodium iodide (^{131}I)	Eradicate hyperthyroidism, selected cases of thyroid cancer	Nausea, vomiting, tachycardia, gland tenderness	• Have client use separate toilet facilities 2–4 days after dosing or flush 2–3 times after each use • Stay away from children and pregnant women 2–4 days after dosing
Ancillary Agents			
Beta-adrenergic blocker Propranolol (Inderal)	Symptom management of hyperthyroidism	Nausea, dizziness, bradycardia	• Monitor for cardiac symptoms • Symptoms can worsen when medication stopped suddenly

production of thyroid hormones. Occasionally, an entire lobe with or without the isthmus is removed. *Total thyroidectomy* (removal of the entire thyroid gland) is performed if a cancerous tumor is present or if the hyperthyroidism is in an advanced stage and involves all of the glandular tissue.

Those who have a small thyroid nodule or a thyroid volume less than 30 mL may be candidates for minimally invasive surgery with an incision that measures 0.5 to 1 inch, as compared with a traditional thyroidectomy incision of 2 to 4 inches. As with most minimally invasive techniques, the advantages are less blood loss, less pain, shorter recovery time, and an almost imperceptible scar.

Clients commonly receive antithyroid drug therapy for several weeks before surgery to prevent a dramatic release of thyroid hormones into the bloodstream during surgery. Complications of thyroidectomy include the following:

- Accidental removal of or alteration in the blood supply to the parathyroid glands, which are embedded in thyroid tissue, resulting in hypocalcemia. One or more parathyroid glands may be reimplanted into nearby muscular tissue where they will eventually attach, grow, and function normally.
- Hemorrhage caused by the vascularity of the thyroid and surrounding tissue
- Thyrotoxicosis (or thyroid storm) as a result of excessive secretion of thyroid hormones during surgical excision
- Damage to the recurrent laryngeal nerve, which affects the function of the vocal cords. If the recurrent laryngeal nerve is damaged either temporarily or partially, breathing may be impaired because the vocal cords cannot open properly during inspiration; the voice may sound weak, hoarse, or breathy; and aspiration and pneumonia may occur if the vocal cords do not close completely during swallowing.

Nursing Management

The nurse monitors respirations, heart rate, and BP regularly. Evidence of bleeding that may be present on the anterior dressing or that which may drain behind the neck is assessed frequently. Manifestation of hypocalcemia is determined using Chvostek and Trousseau signs (refer to Chapter 16) and involuntary muscle spasms in the event the parathyroid glands have been accidentally removed. They record the client's sleep pattern and daily weights. The nurse promotes rest and helps the client avoid excess physical stimulation.

Nutrition Notes 50-1

The Client With Hyperthyroidism

- Calorie needs increase between 10% and 50% above normal to replenish glycogen stores and correct weight loss. A high-protein intake helps replenish losses from muscle catabolism.
- Clients experiencing steady weight loss despite eating large amounts of food often are frustrated and discouraged. Encourage frequent meals and the intake of nutritionally dense foods (fortified milkshakes, foods fortified with skim milk powder, eggs, cheese, butter, or milk).
- After treatment restores normal metabolism, calories are adjusted downward to avoid excess weight gain.

Increased caloric intake can compensate for increased metabolism (Nutrition Notes 50-1).

The nurse informs the client that the effects of antithyroid therapy usually are not apparent until the thyroid gland ceases to secrete the excess thyroid hormone into the bloodstream. This process may take several weeks or more. If RAI is used to destroy thyroid tissue, the nurse tells the client that it does not seriously affect other tissues. Possible transient effects after use of ^{131}I are nausea, vomiting, malaise, fever, and gland tenderness.

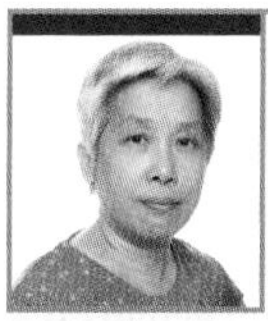

Clinical Scenario A 49-year-old woman has been experiencing heart palpitations, difficulty sleeping, irritability, and heat intolerance, which she attributes to menopause. She has come to her primary provider's office to confirm her self-diagnosis. She tells the nurse that she has been losing weight and feels like her mind is "racing." The nurse notes that the client has fine hand tremors and her eyes seem to bulge from the surrounding bony orbits. Her pulse rate is 130 beats/min, and BP is 160/92 mm Hg. Upon gently palpating her neck, the nurse notes fullness in the area of the thyroid gland. After test results ordered by the primary provider indicate she has hyperthyroidism and options for treatment are explained, the client chooses to have her thyroid surgically removed. **What should be included in this client's plan of care? See Nursing Care Plan 50-1.**

NURSING CARE PLAN 50-1 The Client Undergoing Thyroid Surgery

Assessment

- Obtain complete medical, drug, and allergy histories.
- Check and compare present weight with preillness weight.
- Measure vital signs each shift and more often if findings are abnormal.
- Perform a physical examination but avoid palpating the thyroid gland (manipulation releases excess thyroid hormones).
- Determine client's preoperative compliance with antithyroid drug therapy.
- Explore client's knowledge of the operative procedure and perioperative care.

Nursing Diagnosis. **Acute Anxiety** related to the perception of pending surgery

Expected Outcome. Anxiety will be reduced to a tolerable level as evidenced by a rating below 5 on a scale from 0 to 10, uninterrupted sleep, no restlessness or purposeless activity, and moderate emotional responses.

(continued)

NURSING CARE PLAN 50-1 The Client Undergoing Thyroid Surgery (*continued*)

Interventions	Rationale
Be calm and confident during interactions with client.	*A nurse who conveys expertise helps reduce anxiety and builds a sense of security.*
Interact with client frequently and respond promptly to requests for assistance.	*Trust develops when a client obtains attention and support in a reasonable amount of time.*
Give client opportunities to talk and ask questions about the surgery and subsequent health management issues.	*If a nurse is receptive to questions, the client is more likely to verbalize concerns about the impending procedure.*
Encourage the presence of those who give the client emotional support.	*Significant others with whom the client has emotional bonds potentiate security.*

Evaluation of Expected Outcome

Client reports decreased anxiety.

Nursing Diagnosis. **Knowledge Deficiency** related to unfamiliarity with perioperative measures that reduce potential postoperative complications

Expected Outcome. Client will demonstrate deep breathing and leg exercises and the technique for postoperative head support.

Interventions	Rationale
Provide routine instructions for deep breathing and leg exercises (see Chapter 14).	*These measures decrease the potential for pneumonia, thrombi, and other complications.*
Show client how to support the neck with the hands when rising to sit (see Fig. 50-7).	*Supporting the head avoids straining neck muscles or the surgical incision.*

Evaluation of Expected Outcome

Client performs exercises and supports the head as taught before surgery.

Nursing Diagnosis. **Altered Breathing Pattern** related to compression of the trachea from edema of the glottis, accumulated blood in the operative area, recurrent laryngeal nerve damage, or retained secretions

Expected Outcome. Breathing will be regular, noiseless, and effortless with oxygen saturation (SpO_2) of at least 90%.

Interventions	Rationale
Elevate the head of the bed 30 degrees or more.	*Head elevation reduces edema.*
Apply an ice bag to the neck if prescribed.	*Cold promotes vasoconstriction, thereby reducing edema and bleeding.*
Place a tracheostomy set in the client's room.	*Having a means for establishing a patent airway is an emergency lifesaving measure.*
Assemble oral/pharyngeal suction equipment at client's bedside and suction client if they cannot raise respiratory secretions.	*Suctioning clears the airway of substances that compromise the movement of gases into and out of the lungs.*
Observe for dyspnea and restlessness.	*Increased breathing effort is evidence of a compromised airway.*
Report signs of respiratory distress to the nurse in charge and the primary provider.	*Sharing information aids in collaborative efforts to prevent complications.*

Evaluation of Expected Outcome

Client maintains normal ventilation with no airway obstruction.

Nursing Diagnosis. **Bleeding Risk** related to surgical incisions, wounds, and tissue trauma

Expected Outcome. The nurse monitors to detect, manage, and minimize signs of hemorrhage.

Interventions	Rationale
Monitor vital signs every 1–4 hours.	*Tachycardia and hypotension suggest cellular hypoxia and fluid volume deficit secondary to bleeding.*
Inspect the surgical dressing frequently for bleeding.	*Gauze dressing material wicks blood from the surgical incision.*

NURSING CARE PLAN 50-1 The Client Undergoing Thyroid Surgery (*continued*)

Check the back of the neck for bloody drainage.	*Gravity causes blood to drain posteriorly, which interferes with its visibility on the surface of the surgical dressing.*
Attend to client's complaints of fullness in or around the surgical incision.	*Blood may accumulate beneath the sutured incision rather than drain externally.*
Place suture or staple removal equipment in client's room or stock equipment in a clean utility room.	*The incision may need to be opened to remove clotted blood or ligate blood vessels that continue to bleed.*

Evaluation of Expected Outcome

There is no evidence of excessive bleeding in or around the operative site.

Nursing Diagnosis. **Impaired Verbal Communication** related to hoarseness secondary to recurrent laryngeal nerve damage

Expected Outcome. Client will regain normal volume and quality of speech.

Interventions	Rationale
Minimize unnecessary vocalizations for client.	*Resting the voice reduces strain on the vocal cords.*
Deliver bedside humidification.	*Inhalation of moist air helps relieve hoarseness.*
Provide an alternate means (pad of paper, magic slate, alphabet board) for the client to ask questions or make needs known.	*Written communication provides a substitute for verbal interactions.*
Ensure that client has access to a signal cord or bell with which to summon a caregiver.	*A light or bell signals a need for assistance and is essential when a client cannot call for help.*
Assess the quality of client's voice periodically every 2–4 waking hours for the first 2 postoperative days.	*The nurse must report a weakening of the voice or loss of the ability to project sounds.*

Evaluation of Expected Outcome

Speech is at the presurgical volume.

Nursing Diagnosis. **Aspiration Risk** related to recurrent laryngeal nerve damage

Expected Outcome. Lungs will be free of food or liquids.

Interventions	Rationale
Prepare oral/pharyngeal suction equipment.	*Suctioning provides a way to clear the airway.*
Have client sit upright.	*An upright position promotes the mechanics of swallowing and a more forceful cough if substances enter the airway.*
Provide thickened substances initially.	*Watery food and beverages are more difficult to swallow.*
Encourage client to place a very small amount in their mouth at any one time.	*Controlling ingested substances increases the potential success for swallowing the mass.*

Evaluation of Expected Outcome

Client does not experience respiratory distress, and lungs are clear on auscultation.

Nursing Diagnosis. **Acute Pain** related to tissue trauma secondary to operative procedure

Expected Outcome. Client will report an increased comfort level within 30 minutes of a pain relieving intervention.

Interventions	Rationale
Administer analgesics as prescribed.	*They interfere with pain transmission and perception.*
Place pillows under the head, neck, and shoulders.	*Pillows support the operative area, preventing excessive muscular pulling and possible separation of the incision.*
Maintain head support when client's position is changed.	*Head support reduces muscle contraction and tension on the surgical incision.*

Evaluation of Expected Outcome

Client is comfortable or pain-free.

RC of Tetany. Related to accidental removal of parathyroid glands

Expected Outcome. The nurse will monitor to detect, manage, and minimize tetany.

(*continued*)

NURSING CARE PLAN 50-1 The Client Undergoing Thyroid Surgery (*continued*)

Interventions	Rationale
Observe for spontaneous spasm of the fingers or toes, mouth twitching, or jaw tightening when you tap the cheek anterior to the earlobe (Chvostek sign), and spasm of the fingers toward the wrist when you inflate a BP cuff midway between systolic and diastolic pressures for 3 minutes (Trousseau sign) (see Chapter 16).	*Tetany develops when the parathyroid glands, which regulate blood calcium levels, are accidentally removed during a thyroidectomy. Hypocalcemia results in neuromuscular hyperexcitability.*
Note crowing respirations and dyspnea.	*Manifestations of hypocalcemia include symptoms caused by laryngeal spasm.*
Be prepared to implement seizure precautions.	*Seizures may occur when the blood calcium level falls below normal.*
Have calcium gluconate for IV administration available if prescribed by the primary provider.	*Calcium replacement controls symptoms of tetany.*

Evaluation of Expected Outcomes

No complications develop.

RC of Thyrotoxic Crisis. Related to excessive level of thyroid hormones

Expected Outcome. The nurse will monitor to detect, manage, and minimize thyrotoxic crisis.

Interventions	Rationale
Assess for hyperthermia, tachycardia, chest pain, cardiac arrhythmias, and altered LOC.	*Excess levels of thyroid hormones raise body temperature and accelerate cardiac activity by increasing the rate of metabolism.*
Notify the primary provider if symptoms of thyrotoxic crisis develop.	*Collaborative measures are necessary to control symptoms and their consequences.*
Implement measures to reduce body temperature such as administering antipyretics or placing the client on an aquathermia pad.	*Measures to reduce body temperature help prevent complications such as seizures and brain damage.*
Follow medical orders for measures to reduce heart rate and arrhythmias.	*Tachycardia increases myocardial demands for oxygen: Unless managed, it can lead to myocardial infarction, acute heart failure, or cardiac arrest.*

Evaluation of Expected Outcome

No complications develop.

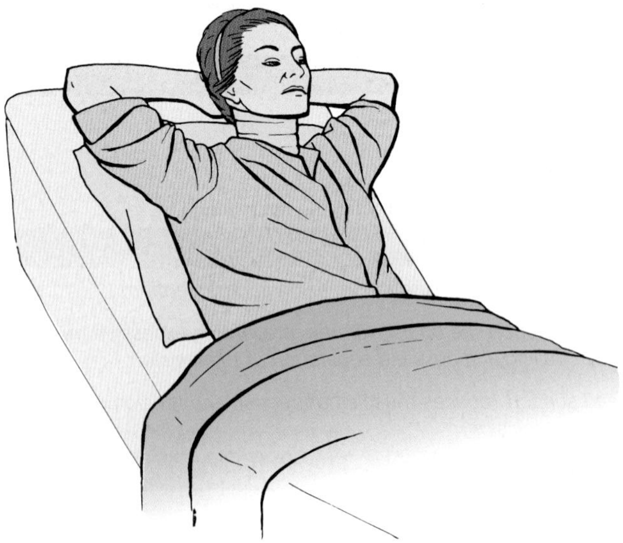

Figure 50-7 After a thyroidectomy, the client uses the hands to support the head while rising to a sitting position. This type of support helps avoid strain to the neck muscles and surgical incision.

Thyrotoxic Crisis

Pathophysiology and Etiology

Thyrotoxic crisis (also known as thyroid storm and thyrotoxicosis), an abrupt and life-threatening form of hyperthyroidism, is thought to be triggered by extreme stress, infection, diabetic ketoacidosis, trauma, toxemia of pregnancy, or manipulation of a hyperactive thyroid gland during surgery or physical examination. Although rare, this condition may occur in clients with undiagnosed or inadequately treated hyperthyroidism.

The oversecretion of T_3 and T_4 is followed by a release of epinephrine. Metabolism is markedly increased. The adrenal glands produce excess corticosteroids in response to the stress created by the hypermetabolic state.

Assessment Findings

The temperature may be as high as 106°F (41°C). The pulse rate is rapid, and cardiac arrhythmias are common. The client may experience persistent vomiting, extreme restlessness with delirium, chest pain, and dyspnea.

The diagnosis is based on the symptoms and a recent medical history that indicates symptoms of severe hyperthyroidism. Laboratory tests, such as a thyroid panel with measurements of TSH, serum T_3, and T_4, may be used to confirm the diagnosis. In thyrotoxic crisis, serum T_3 and T_4 laboratory values are markedly elevated.

Medical Management

Immediate treatment is necessary. Antithyroid drugs (e.g., PTU, methimazole) are used to block the synthesis of thyroid hormones. An IV corticosteroid may be given to replace depletion that results from overstimulation of the adrenals during the hypermetabolic state. IV sodium iodide prevents the thyroid gland from releasing additional thyroid hormones. Propranolol (Inderal), a beta-blocker, reduces the effect of thyroid hormones on the cardiovascular system. Supportive therapy includes IV fluids, antipyretic measures, and oxygen therapy.

Nursing Management

The client with thyrotoxic crisis is acutely ill. The nurse monitors vital signs, especially the temperature, frequently. Failure to respond to an antipyretic drug requires other measures such as a cooling blanket or ice application. A cool room also may help reduce body temperature. The nurse gives all therapeutic treatment measures as ordered because the situation must be corrected as soon as possible.

Hypothyroidism

Hypothyroidism occurs when the thyroid gland fails to secrete adequate thyroid hormones.

Pathophysiology and Etiology

This condition may originate in the thyroid (primary hypothyroidism) or in the pituitary gland, in which case insufficient TSH is secreted. Regardless of the cause, inadequate thyroid hormone secretion results in a slowing of all metabolic processes (see Table 50-1). Severe hypothyroidism is called **myxedema**. Advanced, untreated myxedema can progress to myxedemic crisis or what some call myxedemic coma. Signs of this life-threatening event are hypothermia, hypotension, and hypoventilation. A client with hypothyroidism experiencing infection, trauma, or excessive chills, or taking narcotics, sedatives, or tranquilizers, may develop myxedemic crisis.

Assessment Findings

Signs and Symptoms

Signs and symptoms are opposite those of hyperthyroidism in many respects (Fig. 50-8). Metabolic rate and physical and mental activity slow down. The client is lethargic, lacks energy, dozes frequently during the day, is forgetful, and has chronic headaches. The face takes on a masklike, unemotional expression, yet the client often is irritable. The tongue may be enlarged and the lips swollen, and there may be edema of the eyelids. Temperature and pulse rate are decreased; the client is intolerant to cold. Weight increases despite a low-calorie intake. The skin is dry, and hair characteristically is coarse and sparse and tends to fall out. Menstrual disorders are common. Constipation may be severe. The voice is low pitched and hoarse, and speech is slow. Hearing may be impaired. The client may experience numbness or tingling in the arms or legs that is unrelieved by position change.

Hypothyroidism may lead to an enlarged heart caused by pericardial effusion and an increased tendency toward atherosclerosis and excessive effort by the heart to pump blood. Anemia also may be present. Early recognition of hypothyroidism is difficult because many of the symptoms are nonspecific and may not be sufficiently dramatic to bring the client to the primary provider. This condition can go untreated for years.

Diagnostic Findings

In primary hypothyroidism, levels of TSH are increased because of the negative feedback to the pituitary gland; that is, the low levels of thyroid hormones cause the pituitary gland to increase secretion of TSH (see Chapter 49). The level of FT_4 is decreased. The RAI uptake may be decreased. The T_3 and T_4 levels show no response in primary untreated hypothyroidism but may show a response if hypothyroidism results from failure of the pituitary gland to secrete TSH.

Medical Management

Hypothyroidism is treated with thyroid replacement therapy (see Drug Therapy Table 50-1). Thyroid hormone in the form of desiccated thyroid extract, or with one of the synthetic products, such as levothyroxine sodium (Synthroid) or liothyronine sodium (Cytomel), are oral thyroid preparations. A low dose of thyroid hormone is given initially and then increased or decreased until the optimal dose is achieved.

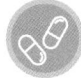

Pharmacologic Considerations

- Thyroid hormones should not be used as a means of weight loss. When combined with other weight loss agents, life-threatening toxicity can occur.

Symptoms associated with hyperthyroidism and hypothyroidism often affect learning and retention ability. The nurse carefully explains the treatment regimen, including the dose of the medications and possible adverse effects. If a special diet has been recommended, the nurse obtains a dietary consultation and reviews sample diets with the client. A teaching plan includes the following:

- Weigh self weekly; keep a record of symptoms and weight in case the medication dose needs adjustment.
- Avoid stressful situations.
- Maintain good nutrition (Nutrition Notes 50-2).
- Notify the primary provider if symptoms worsen or adverse drug effects occur.

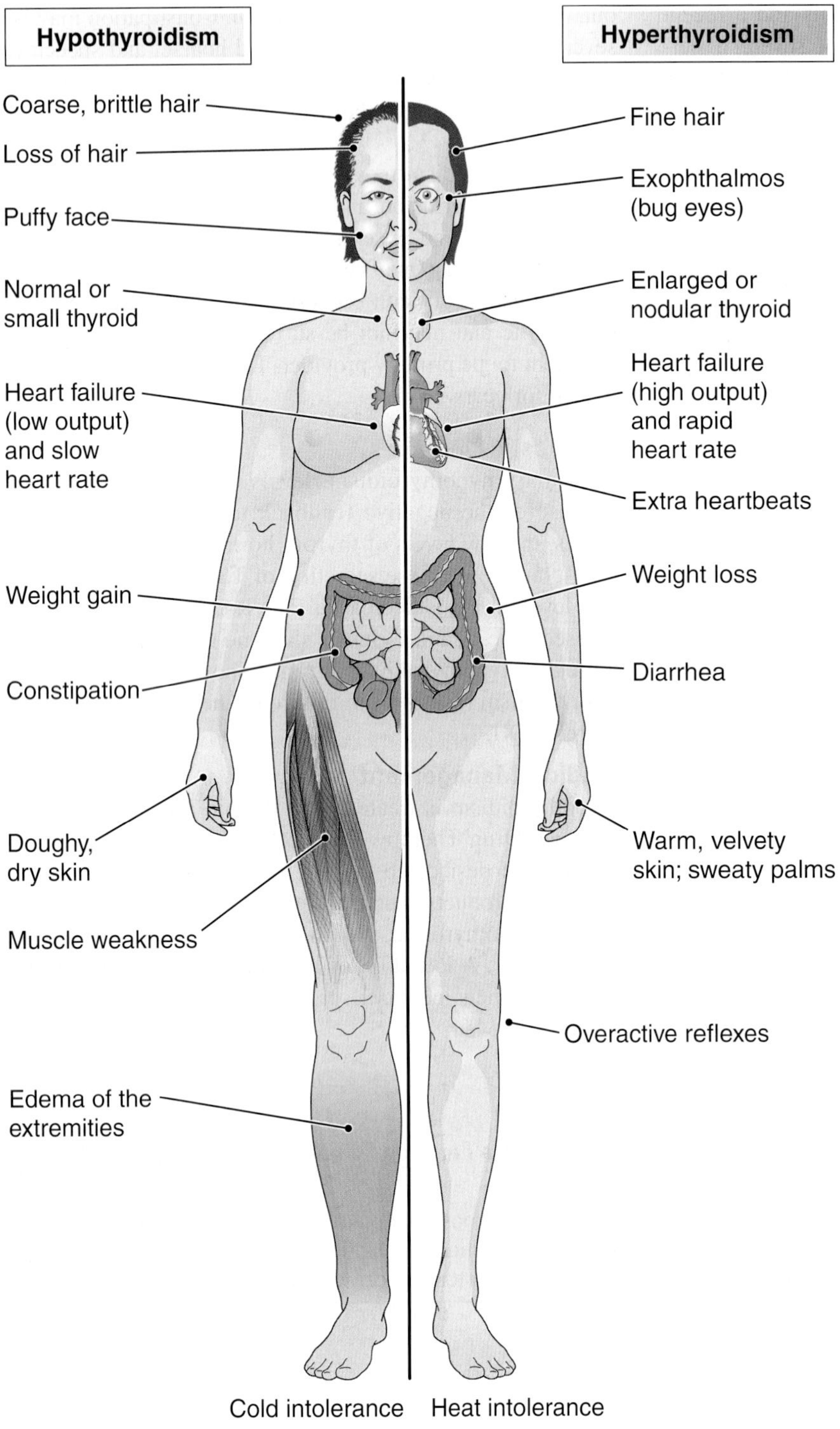

Figure 50-8 Comparison of hypothyroidism and hyperthyroidism. (Reprinted with permission from McConnell, T. H. (2007). *The nature of disease: Pathology for the health professions.* Wolters Kluwer Health/Lippincott Williams & Wilkins.)

Nutrition Notes 50-2

The Client With Hypothyroidism

- Until normal metabolism is restored, clients experience weight gain even if calorie intake is low.
- After hormone replacement therapy begins, the client may still need to follow a low-calorie diet to attain or maintain a normal weight. A high-fiber diet promotes satiety and bowel regularity.
- Additional modifications, such as low-fat, low-cholesterol, and low-sodium diets, are necessary if the client has cardiovascular complications.

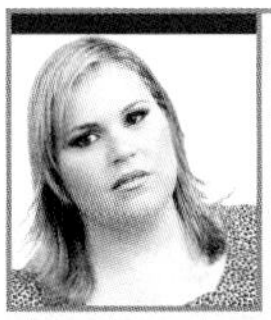

Clinical Scenario A 38-year-old woman has been experiencing progressive fatigue, weight loss, dizziness, nausea, and vomiting. During the nursing assessment, the nurse notes that the client's skin tents when assessing its turgor, indicating dehydration. The client's skin appears bronzed, but she denies any unusual exposure to the sun or use of a tanning service. The client's BP is 104/64 mm Hg when lying down and falls to 72/56 mm Hg when sitting. Her nonfasting capillary blood sugar measures 60 mg/dL with a glucometer. The nurse consults the client's primary provider, who suspects that the client has Addison disease. **What is important to include in this client's nursing care? See the following Nursing Process section.**

NURSING PROCESS FOR THE CLIENT WITH ADDISON DISEASE

Assessment

Obtain a complete health history that includes presence or absence of weight loss, salt craving, nausea and vomiting, abdominal cramps, diarrhea, muscle weakness, and decreased stress tolerance. Take vital signs frequently. Monitor blood sugar levels; hypoglycemia may occur in clients with primary adrenal insufficiency. These clients must never receive insulin by error because insulin lowers the blood glucose to a critically low level that could result in brain damage, coma, or death.

Diagnosis, Planning, and Interventions

Nursing management of the client with primary adrenal insufficiency is essentially the same as that of the client with secondary adrenal insufficiency because the major problem in both types is a lack of adrenal cortical hormones. The client with secondary adrenal insufficiency because of surgery (bilateral adrenalectomy, surgical removal of the pituitary gland) has a controlled deficiency that hormone replacement therapy corrects.

Hypovolemia: This is related to inadequate fluid intake, vomiting, and fluid loss secondary to inadequate adrenal hormone secretion.
Expected Outcome: Fluid intake will be 1500 to 3000 mL/day.

- Keep careful records of fluid intake and urine output. *Data collection is necessary to determine if a problem is developing.*
- Weigh the client daily on the same scale, at a similar time, with similar clothing. *Consistency in data collection helps the nurse accurately compare assessment findings.*
- Notify the primary provider if dehydration, signs of hyponatremia, or progressive weight loss occurs. *The primary provider and nurse collaborate to manage a client's problem.*
- Encourage the client to drink fluids and eat the prescribed diet to maintain fluid and electrolyte balance (Nutrition Notes 50-4). *Fluid and nutritional needs are easier to meet orally than parenterally.*
- If serum sodium levels are decreased, instruct the client to add salt to food. If excessive perspiration occurs, increase fluid and salt intake. *Salt is sodium chloride. Sodium is an electrolyte that attracts water and reduces its excretion. Increasing oral fluid intake compensates for the unusual loss of body fluid.*

RC of Hypoglycemia: Related to adrenocortical insufficiency
Expected Outcome: The nurse will monitor to detect, manage, and minimize episodes of low blood glucose.

- Minimize any reason for fasting, such as before a diagnostic test. *Eating carbohydrates regularly maintains the blood glucose level.*
- Observe for symptoms of hypoglycemia: hunger, headache, sweating, weakness, trembling, emotional instability, visual disturbances, and, finally, disorientation and loss of consciousness. *Physiologic and emotional changes accompany a low blood glucose level.*
- Check the client's blood glucose level with a glucometer 30 minutes before each meal, at bedtime, and whenever the client is symptomatic. *Checking capillary blood glucose provides a numeric assessment of the blood glucose level.*
- Follow agency protocol for raising the client's blood glucose level, which may include offering the client the equivalent of 15 g of carbohydrate such as 1/2 cup of grape juice or administering three to four glucose tablets if the level is below 70 mg/dL and rechecking the level in 15 minutes. If the blood glucose level continues to be low, repeat the method for increasing blood sugar. *Glucose, a monosaccharide found in various carbohydrate food sources and commercially available in glucose tablets that contain 4 or 5 g of glucose per tablet, should raise the blood glucose level within 15 minutes of consumption.*
- Give the client milk and graham crackers or provide the next meal when the blood glucose level recovers to a level above 70 mg/dL. *Milk and graham crackers contain forms of carbohydrates that take longer to absorb and tend to maintain the blood glucose level for an extended period.*
- Contact the primary provider if the client continues to be symptomatic and the blood glucose level is below 80 mg/dL. *Regulation of blood glucose level may require parenteral administration of glucose, which the nurse cannot implement independently.*
- Instruct the client to remain in bed. *Dizziness and fainting may accompany the low blood glucose level; maintaining bed rest protects the client from injuries from a fall.*
- Offer five or six small meals per day rather than three regular meals to control hypoglycemic episodes; if client is eating three meals per day, give between-meal snacks of milk and crackers. *Frequent and regular eating of carbohydrates helps stabilize blood glucose levels within a normal range.*

(continued)

NURSING PROCESS FOR THE CLIENT WITH ADDISON DISEASE (continued)

Fatigue: Related to fluid, electrolyte, and glucose imbalances
Expected Outcome: Client will demonstrate endurance to meet self-care needs independently.

- Assist with bathing and grooming as needed. *The nurse helps the client until the client can resume total self-care.*
- Provide rest between activities. *Rest replenishes energy.*
- Control environmental stimuli to promote rest. *Stimulation interferes with client's ability to relax physically and become refreshed.*

Injury Risk: Related to hypotension and muscle weakness
Expected Outcome: Client will experience no injuries or falls.

- Tell the client to lie down if they become dizzy when rising or changing position. *Blood tends to pool temporarily in dependent areas, causing a deficit in the brain when assuming an upright position.*
- Take the client's BP if symptoms such as weakness and fainting occur. *Measuring BP provides objective data for assessing hemodynamic changes.*
- Keep side rails raised. *They remind the client that they should not ambulate independently.*
- Instruct the client to ask for assistance getting out of bed. *Assistance can support and reposition the client if syncope develops.*
- Emphasize the importance of getting out of bed slowly. *Moving quickly aggravates symptoms of hypotension and potentiates the risk of fainting and falling.*

Evaluation of Expected Outcomes

Fluid intake approximates output; electrolytes remain within normal limits. The client has sufficient energy for ADLs. No injuries occur.

Thyroid Tumors

Tumors of the thyroid can cause hyperthyroidism. They are more commonly benign, but all nodules must be evaluated.

Pathophysiology and Etiology

A *follicular adenoma* is the most common benign thyroid lesion. A thyroid nodule is most likely this type in adult women, but as it enlarges, surgical excision and pathologic examination are necessary to be certain. *Papillary carcinoma* is the most common malignant lesion; it usually occurs in clients who have received radiation treatments to the head or neck region in the past. It tends to spread only to nearby lymph nodes and rarely to other parts of the body. The cure rate of thyroid cancer depends on the type of tumor.

Assessment Findings

Symptoms are vague, and the client may be unaware of the lesion. Often, a routine physical examination reveals a nodular thyroid. As the tumor enlarges, the client often notices a swelling in the neck. Benign tumors cause symptoms of hyperthyroidism in some clients. Malignant tumors can cause voice changes, hoarseness, and difficulty swallowing. Biopsy of the lesion confirms the diagnosis. Thyroid cancer is suspected when the gland is firm and palpable and when results of RAI studies show poor concentration in the suspected area.

Medical and Surgical Management

If there are no symptoms of hyperthyroidism with a benign nodule, treatment usually is not needed. The nodule is examined yearly. If the enlargement causes symptoms, such as difficulty swallowing and noticeable neck swelling, surgical removal of the lesion is considered. Although treatment of malignant lesions varies, a thyroidectomy (total or subtotal) typically is performed. A modified radical neck dissection is indicated if there is metastasis. After a thyroidectomy, thyroid hormone replacement therapy is given to restore thyroid function and suppress pituitary TSH so that it no longer stimulates the growth of residual thyroid tissue. ^{131}I is administered to destroy remaining thyroid tissue as well as to treat lymph node metastasis if present.

Nursing Management

If the thyroid tumor is malignant, the primary provider explains the planned treatment and expected outcome. The nurse provides emotional support, especially if the tumor has metastasized and radical surgery is necessary. When RAI is used after surgery, the client is isolated and placed on radiation precautions (see Chapter 18). The nurse handles body fluids carefully to prevent radioactive contamination.

Endemic and Multinodular Goiters

The word **goiter** refers to an enlarged thyroid gland.

Pathophysiology and Etiology

An *endemic goiter* is caused by a deficiency of iodine in the diet, by the inability of the thyroid to use iodine, or by relative iodine deficiency caused by increasing body demands for thyroid hormones. *Nontoxic goiter* (also called *simple*

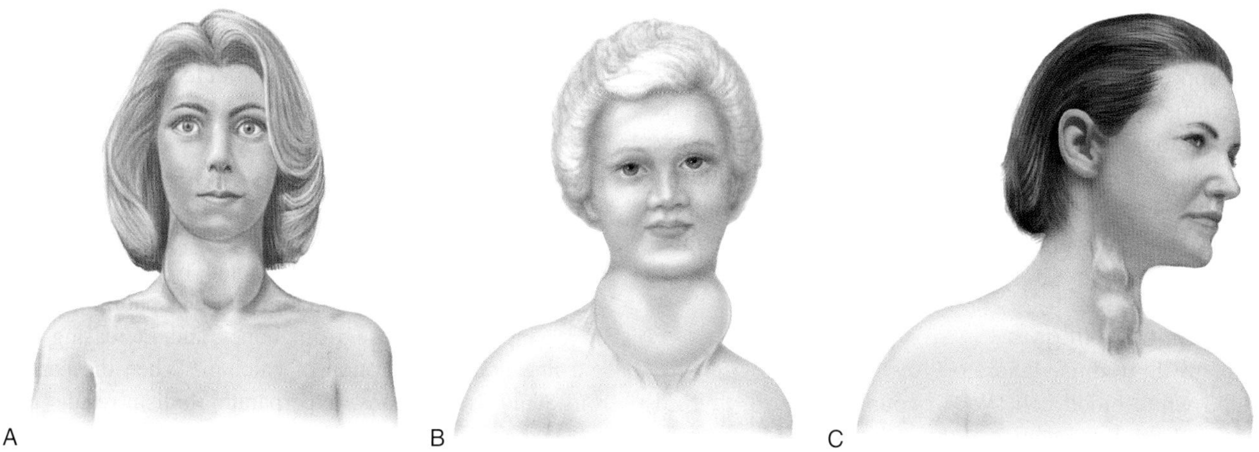

Figure 50-9 Thyroid abnormalities. **(A)** Toxic goiter (Graves disease) with exophthalmos. **(B)** Nontoxic goiter. **(C)** Nodular goiter. (Provided by Anatomical Chart Co.)

or *colloid goiter*) is an enlarged thyroid, usually with no symptoms of thyroid dysfunction. The gland may enlarge as a result of consuming excessive goitrogenic foods such as gluten, soy products, and cruciferous vegetables such as broccoli and brussels sprouts (Pick, 2016), peanuts, pine nuts, and flaxseed (or taking certain drugs such as lithium that may cause hyperplasia of the gland). *Nodular goiters* contain one or more areas of hyperplasia. This type of goiter appears to develop for essentially the same reasons as an endemic goiter (Fig. 50-9).

Assessment Findings

The thyroid gland enlarges. The client has a sense of fullness in the neck area. Continued gland enlargement eventually results in difficulty swallowing and breathing as the thyroid presses on the trachea and esophagus. When the gland has enlarged, it is visible as a swelling in the neck. Nodular goiters also produce enlargement, but the gland has an irregular surface on palpation. A thyroid scan shows an enlarged gland and a decreased uptake of ^{131}I. Tests of thyroid function are performed, but results may or may not be abnormal and thus may be inconclusive.

Medical Management

Treatment depends on the cause. If the diet is deficient in iodine, foods high in iodine, such as seafood or iodized salt, are recommended. Potassium iodide to supplement iodine intake may be given. In some instances, a thyroidectomy is recommended, especially when the gland is grossly enlarged.

Nursing Management

If the client has respiratory distress because of the enlarged thyroid, the nurse closely observes respiratory status and elevates the head of the bed to relieve respiratory symptoms. They provide a diet high in iodine and iodized salt. Natural iodine content is highest in seafood/shellfish; it is also found in varying amounts in bread, milk, eggs, meat, and spinach. Fish, lentils, and yogurt are nongoitrogenic alternatives to soy protein (McLaughlin, 2015). A soft diet may be necessary if the client has difficulty swallowing.

Thyroiditis

Thyroiditis, inflammation of the thyroid gland, can be acute, subacute, or chronic.

Pathophysiology and Etiology

There are multiple etiologies and, consequently, subtypes of thyroiditis that involve inflammation of the gland, release of higher than normal levels of hormone, and changes in thyroid function from hyperactivity to hypoactivity. Inflammation causes the gland to enlarge and become tender in some cases. Excess thyroid hormone released from stores within the thyroid gland rather than from stimulation from the pituitary gland produces a hypermetabolic state. As the stores of thyroid hormone deplete, a hypometabolic state ensues. In some cases, the thyroid gland recovers; in other cases, hypothyroidism becomes permanent.

Acute thyroiditis, most common in children, appears to result from bacterial infection of the gland. Acute thyroiditis is fairly rare due to the efficacy of antibiotic therapy. One type of *subacute thyroiditis* can follow an upper respiratory viral infection. The most common type is *Hashimoto thyroiditis*, a chronic form of thyroiditis, believed to be an autoimmune disorder that develops in the postpartum period.

Assessment Findings

Signs and Symptoms

Signs and symptoms of acute thyroiditis include high fever, malaise, and tenderness and swelling of the thyroid gland. Subacute thyroiditis produces symptoms of a swollen and painful or painless gland. Chills, fever, and malaise approximately 2 weeks after infection accompany thyroiditis of a viral etiology. When signs of hyperthyroidism develop, the client experiences tachycardia, tremors, intolerance of heat, weight loss, and emotional irritability. Once the gland is destroyed, symptoms of hypothyroidism such as lethargy, weight gain, weakness, constipation, and dry hair develop.

Diagnostic Findings

In acute thyroiditis, laboratory test results show an elevated white blood cell (WBC) count. During a thyroid scan, inflamed and damaged thyroid cells fail to concentrate RAI. During the hypermetabolic phase of the disease, thyroid function tests elevate. In Hashimoto thyroiditis, high titers of antimicrosomal and antithyroglobulin antibodies are evident, reflecting the autoimmune nature of the disease.

Medical and Surgical Management

Acute thyroiditis requires administration of appropriate antibiotics. The treatment of subacute thyroiditis is symptomatic and includes analgesics for pain and discomfort. Corticosteroids also may be prescribed to reduce inflammation. The treatment of Hashimoto thyroiditis includes thyroid hormone replacement therapy. Surgery is required if the gland becomes excessively large.

Nursing Management

Management depends on the type of thyroiditis and severity of symptoms. The nurse gives antipyretics for fever. They elevate the head of the bed if the client has difficulty breathing. The nurse offers a soft diet if the gland is markedly enlarged and the client has difficulty swallowing.

If a client has undergone surgery (Nursing Care Plan 50-1), the nurse instructs the client before discharge about the care of the surgical wound and to avoid excessive strain on the wound until it is healed. Because the incision is made in a neck crease, the healed scar is barely visible. If a client appears concerned about scarring, the nurse may suggest that the client wear clothing that covers the neck until the scar is almost invisible.

The nurse discusses the symptoms of hypothyroidism, hyperthyroidism, and hypoparathyroidism (see later discussion), with instructions to notify the primary provider immediately if they occur. If medication is prescribed, the nurse reviews the dosage, schedule for self-administration, and adverse effects of each drug. A teaching plan includes techniques for wound care, the need to take thyroid replacement medication in the morning at the same time each day to avoid insomnia and CNS stimulation, and side effects that require notification of the primary provider (chest pain, tachycardia, and dyspnea).

››› *Stop, Think, and Respond 50-1*

When reviewing a client's medical record, you read that the primary provider has detected an enlarged thyroid gland. What are some possible causes?

DISORDERS OF THE PARATHYROID GLANDS

Parathormone, the hormone secreted by the parathyroid glands, maintains serum calcium and phosphorus levels by increasing their release from bones and increasing renal and intestinal reabsorption of calcium. When the parathyroid gland dysfunctions, hyperparathyroidism results in an elevated level of serum calcium; hypoparathyroidism results in a low serum calcium level. Phosphorus levels become elevated because of kidney reabsorption.

Calcitonin, a thyroid hormone, functions in opposition to parathormone to maintain a balance of serum calcium. Calcitonin suppresses osteoclasts, cells that break down bone, so calcium remains within the osteocytes (bone cells) of the skeletal system. In doing so, it prevents an elevation of calcium in the blood. Maintaining the density of bones explains the rationale for using calcitonin when managing osteoporosis (see Chapter 63).

Hyperparathyroidism

Hyperparathyroidism, an excess of parathormone, can be a primary or secondary condition.

Pathophysiology and Etiology

The most common cause of *primary hyperparathyroidism* is an adenoma (benign tumor) of one of the parathyroid glands. In primary hyperparathyroidism, excessive secretion of parathyroid hormone (parathormone) removes calcium from the bones. The bones become demineralized as the calcium leaves and enters the bloodstream. Renal stones may develop when calcium becomes concentrated in the urine.

In *secondary hyperparathyroidism*, the parathyroid glands secrete excessive parathormone in response to hypocalcemia (low serum calcium level), which may result from vitamin D deficiency, chronic renal failure, large doses of thiazide diuretics, and excessive use of laxatives and calcium supplements.

Assessment Findings

Signs and Symptoms

Excessive calcium in the blood depresses the responsiveness of the peripheral nerves, accounting for fatigue and muscle weakness. The muscles become hypotonic (loss of or decrease in muscle tone). Cardiac arrhythmias may develop. Because the bones have lost calcium, there is skeletal tenderness and pain on bearing weight; the bones may become so demineralized that they break with little or no trauma (pathologic fractures). Other possible effects include nausea, vomiting, and constipation. Large amounts of calcium and phosphorus passing through the kidneys predispose the client to the formation of stones in the urinary tract, pyelonephritis, and uremia (see Chapter 58).

Diagnostic Findings

The diagnosis is based on elevated serum calcium and decreased serum phosphorus levels (the latter of which is excreted and not reabsorbed by the kidneys) when other causes of hypercalcemia are excluded. The results of a 24-hour urine test show increased urine calcium levels. Skeletal radiographs show calcium loss from bones. An MRI or CT scan identifies a parathyroid adenoma if it is present. As noted earlier, parathormone levels are elevated in hyperparathyroidism.

Medical and Surgical Management

Secondary hyperparathyroidism is managed by correcting the cause (e.g., vitamin D therapy for a vitamin D deficiency, correction of renal failure, calcium-restricted diet). Sodium and phosphorus replacements often are ordered. Hormone replacement with synthetic calcitonin (Calcimar) is avoided because it is associated with allergic reactions and drug resistance. The latter is caused by antibodies that neutralize the hormone.

The only treatment for primary hyperparathyroidism is the surgical removal of hypertrophied glandular tissue or an individual tumor of one of the parathyroid glands. Before surgery, the primary provider determines the number of the four glands to be removed based on the cause of hyperparathyroidism and laboratory and diagnostic test results. One or more of the parathyroids is left in place for maintaining calcium and phosphorus metabolism.

Nursing Management

The nurse closely measures the client's intake and output. They observe for signs of urinary calculi from hypercalcemia, flank pain, and decreasing urine output (see Chapter 58). The nurse encourages a large volume of fluid to keep the urine dilute (Nutrition Notes 50-3). They assess the client's ability to perform self-care, provide a safe environment to prevent falls and other injuries, encourage frequent rest periods, and monitor fatigue level.

The primary nursing responsibility is teaching the client about the effects of the disease, the planned medical management, and the importance of following the prescribed treatment. If the client undergoes surgery, the nursing management is similar to that for thyroid surgery. In addition, the nurse observes the client for symptoms of hypoparathyroidism.

Nutrition Notes 50-3

Clients With a Parathyroid Disorder

- Clients with hyperparathyroidism should use a low-calcium diet (fewer dairy products) and drink at least 3 to 4 L of fluid daily to dilute the urine and prevent renal stones from forming. It is especially important that they drink fluids before going to bed and periodically throughout the night to avoid concentrated urine.
- Clients with hypoparathyroidism need more calcium and vitamin D than can be provided through food alone, yet they should be encouraged to eat foods rich in calcium, such as milk, yogurt, green leafy vegetables, and fortified orange juice. Carbonated beverages should be avoided because they are high in phosphorus (phosphoric acid). It is critical to stress the importance of these two aspects of treatment. Consultation with a dietitian may be necessary to provide a list of foods to include or to avoid in the prescribed diet.

Hypoparathyroidism

Hypoparathyroidism is a deficiency of parathormone that results in hypocalcemia.

Pathophysiology and Etiology

Hypocalcemia affects neuromuscular functions. It causes hyperexcitability, resulting in spastic muscle contractions and *paresthesias* (abnormal sensations). The most common causes of hypoparathyroidism are trauma to the glands and inadvertent removal of all or nearly all these structures during thyroidectomy or parathyroidectomy. The idiopathic form of this disorder is rare but may be autoimmune in origin or caused by the congenital absence of the parathyroids.

Assessment Findings

Signs and Symptoms

The main symptom of acute and sudden hypoparathyroidism is **tetany**. The client may report numbness and tingling in the fingers or toes or around the lips. A voluntary movement may be followed by an involuntary, jerking spasm. Muscle cramping may be present. Tonic (continuous contraction) flexion of an arm or a finger may occur. If a nurse taps the client's facial nerve (which lies under the tissue in front of the ear), the client's mouth twitches and the jaw tightens. The response is identified as a positive Chvostek sign (see Chapter 16). The nurse may elicit a positive Trousseau sign by placing a BP cuff on the upper arm, inflating it between the systolic and diastolic BP, and waiting 3 minutes. The nurse observes the client for spasm of the hand (**carpopedal spasm**), which is evidenced by the hand flexing inward (see Chapter 16).

Laryngeal spasm can occur, causing dyspnea with long, crowing respirations as air passes around the constriction. Cyanosis may be present, and the client is in danger of asphyxia and cardiac arrhythmias. Nausea, vomiting, abdominal pain, and seizures can develop.

In chronic hypoparathyroidism, the client experiences neuromuscular irritability, constipation or diarrhea, numbness and tingling of the arms and legs, loss of tooth enamel, and muscle pain. Positive Chvostek and Trousseau signs may or may not be elicited, depending on the degree of hypocalcemia.

Diagnostic Findings

The serum calcium level is decreased, the serum phosphorus level is increased, and the urine levels of both are decreased.

In chronic hypoparathyroidism, radiographs show increased bone density.

Medical Management

Tetany and severe hypoparathyroidism are treated immediately by the administration of an IV calcium salt, such as calcium gluconate. Endotracheal intubation and mechanical ventilation may be necessary if acute respiratory distress occurs. Bronchodilators also are used.

Long-term treatment after trauma or inadvertent removal of the parathyroids includes administration of oral calcium, vitamin D, or vitamin D_2 (calciferol), which increases the serum calcium level. The dose is related to the degree of hypocalcemia, which is determined by frequent monitoring of serum and urine calcium levels. Parathyroid replacement therapy with recombinant human parathormone (rhPTH) has been approved to normalize serum calcium and reduce the need for calcium supplements and vitamin D (Mannstadt et al., 2019). It is administered by daily injections but is only available via a restricted distribution program due to the increased risk of osteosarcoma (Drugs.com, 2019). A diet high in calcium and low in phosphorus usually is recommended (see Nutrition Notes 50-3).

Nursing Management

The nurse is alert for signs of tetany and assesses for Chvostek and Trousseau signs. They monitor the client with chronic hypoparathyroidism for increasing severity of symptoms. The nurse is prepared to administer IV calcium salt and observes the client during such administration for adverse effects, such as flushing, cardiac arrhythmia (usually bradycardia), tingling in the arms and legs, and a metallic taste. Local tissue necrosis may occur if the IV medication escapes into surrounding tissues. The nurse monitors serum calcium levels to determine the effectiveness of therapy.

If the client has chronic hypoparathyroidism, the nurse obtains complete medical, drug, and allergy histories. They examine the client for symptoms of the disorder, primarily for the effect of hypocalcemia on the CNS. The nurse assesses the arms and legs for evidence of muscle spasm. They auscultate the lungs because the client may have dyspnea or other respiratory difficulties. During the assessment of vital signs, attention to heart rate and rhythm is particularly important.

The nurse prophylactically keeps an emergency tracheostomy tray, mechanical ventilation equipment, artificial airway, and endotracheal intubation equipment at the client's bedside following a thyroidectomy or if hypocalcemia is severe. They insert an IV line for the emergency administration of calcium. The nurse observes frequently for respiratory distress and notifies the primary provider immediately if this problem occurs.

Until hypocalcemia is corrected, the nurse must assist the client with activities of daily living (ADLs). Movement, noise, and other environmental disturbances can trigger muscle contractions or convulsions. Thus, minimizing all forms of stress is essential until serum calcium levels approach normal and symptoms are relieved.

Clients who require lifetime treatment of the disorder need a careful review of the prescribed treatment. The nurse must emphasize the importance of drug and diet therapy to normalize calcium levels. The nurse gives the client a list of the symptoms of hypercalcemia and hypocalcemia, either of which can occur if the dose of the prescribed supplement is too high or too low or if the supplement is omitted. They emphasize the need to contact the primary provider immediately about any symptoms. The nurse reminds the client that the primary provider may need periodically to adjust the dose of the supplement; therefore, recognizing the symptoms associated with hypercalcemia and hypocalcemia is essential. Client and Family Teaching 50-2 outlines more teaching points.

Client and Family Teaching 50-2
Hypoparathyroidism

The nurse develops a teaching plan that includes the following points:

- Take supplements at the doses and intervals prescribed.
- Never increase, decrease, or omit supplement doses unless advised by the primary provider. Increasing the dose can cause symptoms of hypercalcemia; decreasing or omitting the dose can cause the original symptoms to return.
- If nausea, vomiting, or severe diarrhea develops, contact the primary provider.
- Read food labels carefully so that you include foods that are part of the diet and avoid those that are not. Adherence to the recommended diet is necessary.

DISORDERS OF THE ADRENAL GLANDS

Adrenal dysfunction includes pathology of the outer portion of the adrenal gland, the *cortex*, which synthesizes and secretes the hormones known as *corticosteroids*, mineralocorticoids, glucocorticoids, and gonadocorticoids, or sex hormones, sometimes referred to as *androgens*. The sex hormones are secreted in small amounts by the adrenal glands in comparison with that secreted by the testes and ovaries. Androgenic gonadocorticoids, one source of testosterone, cause masculinizing effects in women after menopause when ovarian estrogen levels decline. Disorders of the adrenal glands also involve the *medulla*, the inner portion, which secretes the catecholamines norepinephrine (noradrenaline) and epinephrine (adrenaline). Proper secretion of these hormones is essential to life.

Adrenal Insufficiency (Addison Disease)

Adrenal insufficiency, inadequate production of steroid hormones, is classified as either primary or secondary.

Pathophysiology and Etiology

Primary adrenal insufficiency (Addison disease) results from the destruction of the adrenal cortex by diseases such as tuberculosis. It also may be an autoimmune disorder, in which antibodies formed by the client's immune system destroy adrenal tissue. In many instances, the cause is unknown.

The consequences of decreased adrenal cortical function include decreased available glucose and hypoglycemia. The glomerular filtration rate of the kidneys slows dramatically, causing decreased urea nitrogen excretion.

Secondary adrenal insufficiency is the result of surgical removal of both adrenal glands (*bilateral adrenalectomy*), hemorrhagic infarction of the glands, hypopituitarism (caused by pituitary failure or surgical removal of the pituitary gland), or suppression of adrenal function by the administration of corticosteroids. Clients with secondary adrenal insufficiency after bilateral **adrenalectomy** or surgical removal of the pituitary gland do not experience true adrenal insufficiency because corticosteroids are administered to replace the hormones no longer secreted by the adrenals.

Assessment Findings

Signs and Symptoms

Decreased or absent adrenocortical hormones lead to symptoms of adrenal insufficiency (Fig. 50-10), which are the same in primary and secondary adrenal insufficiency (Box 50-1). Clients with primary adrenal insufficiency usually experience symptoms gradually. Clients with secondary adrenal insufficiency develop symptoms suddenly or over several days to weeks. Although many believed President John Kennedy's tanned appearance was due to his outdoor activities like sailing and playing touch football, it more than likely was due to Addison disease.

Diagnostic Findings

A dose of synthetic ACTH, cosyntropin (Cortrosyn), is administered intramuscularly as a screening test for adrenal function. In primary adrenal insufficiency, an absent or a low cortisol response indicates adrenal insufficiency. In secondary insufficiency, the decrease in serum cortisol levels is less significant.

The serum cortisol level is decreased. Serum sodium and fasting blood glucose levels are low, and serum potassium, calcium, and blood urea nitrogen levels are increased. The WBC count often is elevated. A glucose tolerance test shows evidence of hypoglycemia. In Addison disease, the glucose level in the bloodstream does not rise as high as normal and returns to its fasting level more quickly than it would under normal conditions. The fasting blood glucose level may be low. Radiographs of the adrenals show calcification. An abdominal CT scan reveals atrophy of the adrenal glands.

Medical Management

Clients with primary adrenal insufficiency require daily corticosteroid replacement therapy for the rest of their lives. Fludrocortisone (Florinef), a synthetic corticosteroid preparation that possesses mineralocorticoid and some

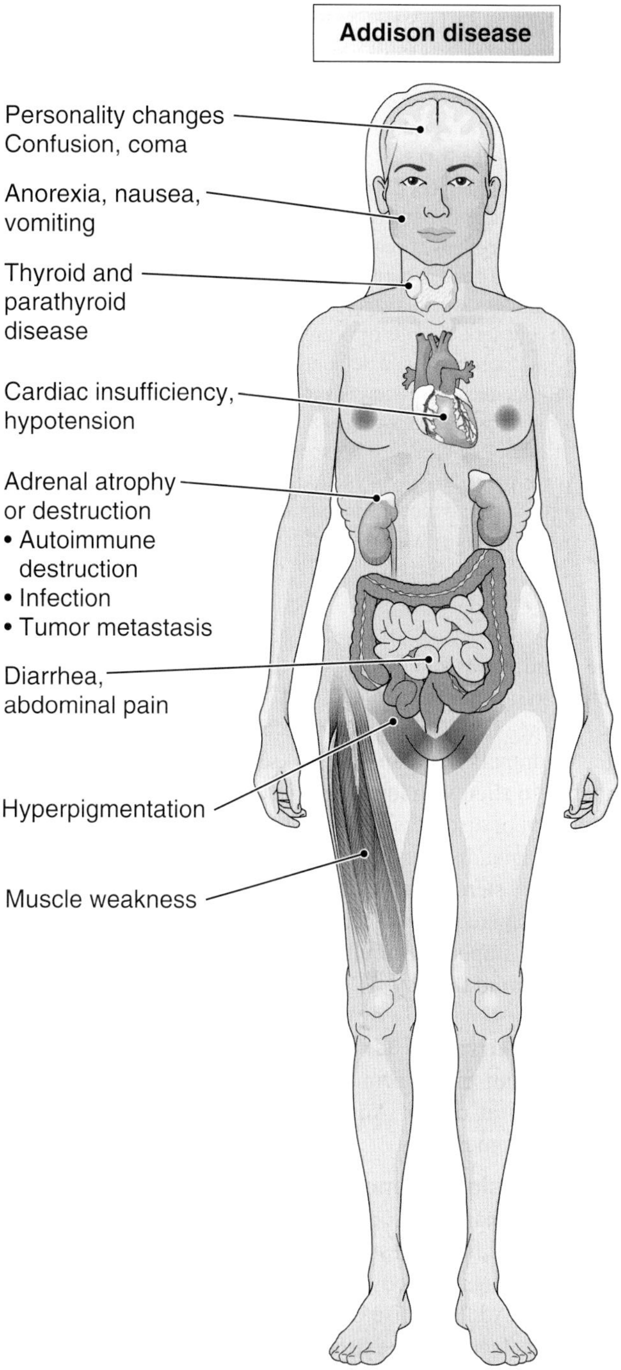

Figure 50-10 Clinical manifestations of Addison disease. (Reprinted with permission from McConnell, T. H. (2007). *The nature of disease: Pathology for the health professions.* Wolters Kluwer Health/Lippincott Williams & Wilkins.)

glucocorticoid properties, frequently is selected for replacement therapy. An additional glucocorticoid may be necessary depending on the client's response to therapy.

Treatment for secondary adrenal insufficiency caused by bilateral adrenalectomy or pituitary failure is the same as treatment for primary adrenal insufficiency. Treatment of secondary adrenal insufficiency resulting from discontinuation of corticosteroid therapy or hemorrhagic infarction of

BOX 50-1 Signs and Symptoms of Adrenal Insufficiency

- Increased urinary excretion of sodium and retention of potassium followed by dehydration and reduced blood plasma volume
- Weakness, fatigue, dizziness, hypotension, postural hypotension, hypothermia
- Vascular collapse because of poor myocardial tone, decreased cardiac output, weak and irregular pulse
- Weight loss, anemia, anorexia, gastrointestinal symptoms
- Nervousness, periods of depression
- Hypoglycemia from a deficiency of the hormones that facilitate the conversion of protein into glucose; episodes of hypoglycemia may occur 5 to 6 hours after eating—the period before breakfast is especially dangerous.
- Abnormally dark pigmentation, especially of exposed areas of the skin and mucous membranes, and decreased hair growth (primary adrenal insufficiency)

Client and Family Teaching 50-3 Corticosteroid Therapy for Adrenal Insufficiency

The nurse explains adrenal insufficiency and the importance of lifetime corticosteroid replacement. A teaching plan includes the following points:

- Never omit, increase, or decrease a dose. Lifetime corticosteroid replacement therapy is necessary. If the prescribed drug is not taken, adrenal insufficiency, which is life-threatening, will occur.
- Seek medical attention for dosage readjustment whenever there is stress. The body has limited ability to handle stress of any kind. Examples of stress include an infection, a motor vehicle accident (even if not noticeably hurt), a family crisis, and a heavy workload.
- Avoid exposure to infections and excessive fatigue.
- If an infection (e.g., sore throat, upper respiratory tract infection) or any other type of illness occurs, contact the primary provider immediately. An increased medication dose may be necessary.
- Seek immediate medical attention if vomiting, diarrhea, or any other condition prevents the medication from being taken orally or interferes with proper drug absorption. Parenteral administration will be necessary. (The primary provider instructs the client on the procedures to follow if the medication cannot be taken orally.)
- Wear identification, such as a MedicAlert tag or bracelet, stating that the wearer has adrenal insufficiency. If an accident or any other problem occurs, medical personnel must be made aware of the need for corticosteroids.
- Follow the diet recommended by the primary provider.

the gland varies and depends on the ability of the adrenals to return to normal function.

If the client is not given or does not take the medication, acute adrenal crisis can develop (see next section). This also applies to clients on long-term corticosteroid therapy for the treatment of disorders such as allergies, rheumatoid arthritis, and collagen diseases who abruptly discontinue taking their prescribed steroid. If the drug is to be discontinued, the dose must be tapered over time. Client and Family Teaching 50-3 discusses important information to teach clients receiving corticosteroid therapy.

Acute Adrenal Crisis (Addisonian Crisis)

Clients with either primary or secondary adrenal insufficiency are at risk of **Addisonian crisis**, a life-threatening endocrine emergency.

Pathophysiology and Etiology

Acute adrenal crisis occurs when the adrenal glands fail. Because the hormones of the adrenal cortex are prominent in facilitating the body's adaptive reactions to stress, clients with Addison disease may develop acute adrenal crisis when faced with extreme stress. Even uncomplicated surgery requires more physiologic adaptive ability than a client with Addison disease usually possesses. Salt deprivation, infection, trauma, exposure to cold, overexertion, or any abnormal stress can cause adrenal crisis. Acute adrenal crisis also can occur when corticosteroid therapy is suddenly discontinued. If the condition is untreated, coma and death result.

Assessment Findings

Adrenal crisis may be sudden or gradual. It may begin with anorexia, nausea, vomiting, diarrhea, abdominal pain, profound weakness, headache, intensification of hypotension, restlessness, or fever. Unless the corticosteroid dose is increased or restored to meet the demand, the client progresses to acute adrenal crisis. The BP markedly decreases and shock develops.

Diagnosis is based on symptoms and history. Case findings can show an omission of daily corticosteroid therapy. (See section on diagnostic findings for adrenal insufficiency in this chapter.)

Medical Management

Adrenal crisis is an emergency; death may occur from hypotension and vasomotor collapse. Corticosteroids are given intravenously in solutions of normal saline and glucose. Antibiotics are administered because of extremely low resistance to infection.

Nursing Management

Two important nursing tasks are the recognition of signs and symptoms of adrenal crisis and the accurate administration of corticosteroid drugs. A client with a diagnosis of adrenal insufficiency is a candidate for acute adrenal crisis; therefore, the nurse constantly observes such clients for this problem. They administer the correct dose of corticosteroid therapy at the correct time. Doses must never be omitted or

Nutrition Notes 50-4

The Client With Addison Disease

- A high-protein, moderate-carbohydrate diet that is low in refined carbohydrates is recommended to reduce the risk of hypoglycemia from excess insulin secretion. The risk of hypoglycemia is also lessened by consuming frequent meals and snacks, especially a substantial bedtime snack.
- A high-sodium intake is necessary unless fludrocortisone (Florinef), a sodium-retaining hormone, is used.
- Unless otherwise contraindicated, 2–3 L of fluid per day are recommended.
- Potassium requirements are determined on an individual basis.

abruptly discontinued because this can result in an adrenal crisis. Once the condition is recognized, the nurse takes vital signs frequently, paying special attention to heart rate and rhythm. They observe for signs of hyponatremia and hyperkalemia. The nurse keeps the client warm and as quiet as possible until treatment is initiated and the condition is stabilized. Client teaching includes instructing clients never to discontinue taking prescribed corticosteroids abruptly. Gradually decreasing the prescribed dosage under the direction of a primary provider is preferred to promote endogenous secretion of glucocorticoid production by the adrenal cortex.

Pheochromocytoma

Pheochromocytoma is a tumor of the adrenal medulla that causes hyperfunction.

Pathophysiology and Etiology

A pheochromocytoma usually is a benign tumor. Hyperfunction causes the adrenal medulla to secrete excessively the catecholamines epinephrine and norepinephrine. Exercise, emotional distress, trauma such as surgery, manipulation of the tumor, and postural changes can trigger episodic symptoms. Excessive secretion of epinephrine leads to hypertension and increases the potential for cerebrovascular accident, palpitations, and tachycardia. People who should be assessed for pheochromocytoma include those who (1) have hypertension that is difficult to control, (2) take more than four medications to control their BP, or (3) develop hypertension before 35 years of age.

Assessment Findings

Symptoms include elevated BP (intermittent or, more frequently, persistent), tremors, nervousness, sweating, headache, nausea, vomiting, hyperglycemia, polyuria, and vertigo. The level of vanillylmandelic acid in a 24-hour urine specimen is markedly increased. Urinary catecholamine determination on the same or a different specimen may be elevated. CT, MRI, ultrasonography, aortography, and retrograde pyelography reveal the tumor. A drop in BP after a test injection of the alpha-adrenergic blocker phentolamine (Regitine) supports the presence of a pheochromocytoma; when compared with baseline measurements, the systolic BP falls more than 35 mm Hg and the diastolic BP falls more than 25 mm Hg.

Medical and Surgical Management

Treatment involves surgical or minimally invasive laparoscopic removal of the tumor by means of *unilateral adrenalectomy* (removal of one adrenal gland). Phentolamine is given before and during surgery to control hypertension. Alpha-adrenergic blockers, such as phenoxybenzamine (Dibenzyline), are used to control hypertension before surgery or when surgery is contraindicated, or to treat a malignant pheochromocytoma. Medical treatment includes metyrosine (Demser), an enzyme inhibitor that reduces the synthesis of catecholamines to decrease hypertensive attacks.

Nursing Management

The nurse monitors the BP closely when initiating drug therapy or during dose changes. They notify the primary provider of a sudden decrease in BP. If the client undergoes adrenalectomy, the nurse assesses for signs and symptoms of acute adrenal insufficiency (see earlier discussion).

Cushing Syndrome (Adrenocortical Hyperfunction)

Cushing syndrome is an endocrine disorder that results from excessive secretion of hormones by the adrenal cortex.

Pathophysiology and Etiology

An overproduction of adrenocortical hormones results from the following: (1) overproduction of ACTH by the pituitary gland, with resultant hyperplasia of the adrenal cortex and excessive production and secretion of glucocorticoids, mineralocorticoids, and gonadocorticoids; (2) benign or malignant tumors of the pituitary gland or adrenal cortex; or (3) prolonged administration of high doses of corticosteroids. Those clients who take corticosteroids are advised to continue taking them and avoid discontinuing their administration abruptly to avoid adrenal (Addisonian) crisis. When these types of medications are no longer necessary, they are discontinued gradually (see the section on adrenalectomy later in this chapter).

Hyperadrenalism affects most body systems and causes many changes in appearance and physiology. The term **cushingoid syndrome** refers to the physical changes that accompany this disorder (Fig. 50-11). Examples of physiologic alterations include suppression of the inflammatory response, hyperglycemia, hypokalemia, hypernatremia with subsequent weight gain and elevated BP, peptic ulcer, demineralization of bones, and muscle weakness. Increased levels of androgenic gonadocorticoid hormone cause women to acquire secondary sex characteristics of men. People of both sexes experience decreased sexual drive. Many clients suffer from depression, and the endocrine imbalance may cause psychosis.

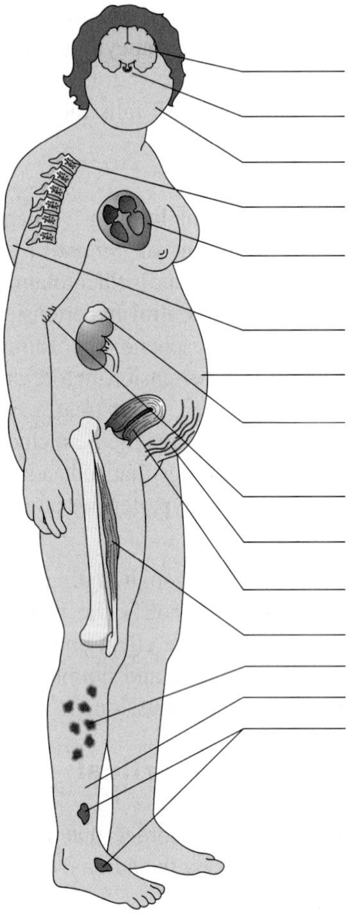

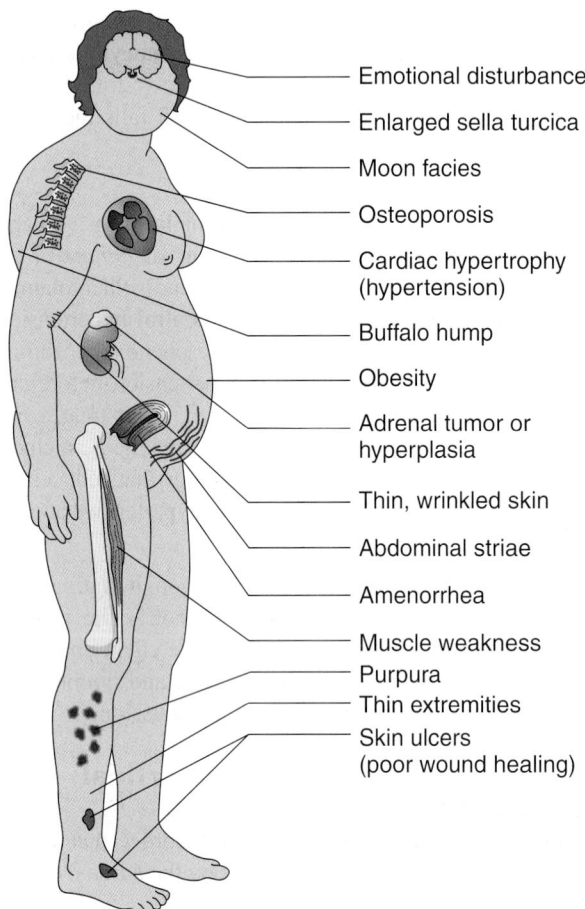

Figure 50-11 Clinical manifestations of Cushing syndrome. (Reprinted with permission from Rubin, E., Strayer, D. S., (Eds.). (2014). *Rubin's pathology: Clinicopathologic foundations of medicine* (7th ed.). Wolters Kluwer.)

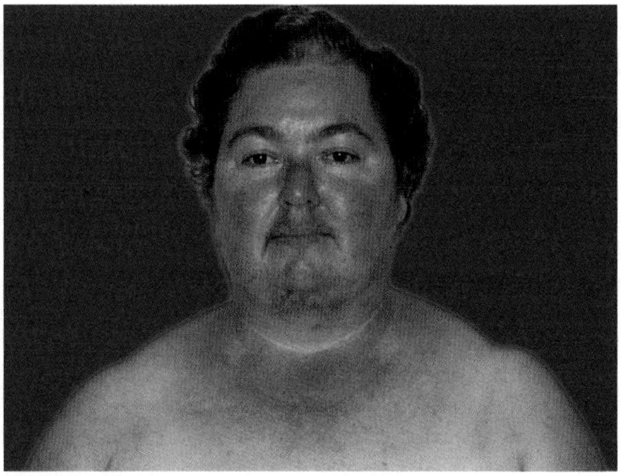

Figure 50-12 This woman with Cushing syndrome exhibits a moon face, buffalo hump, increased facial hair, and thinning of the scalp hair. (Reprinted with permission from Rubin, R., & Strayer, D. S., (Eds.). (2008). *Rubin's pathology: Clinicopathologic foundations of disease* (5th ed.). Wolters Kluwer Health/Lippincott Williams & Wilkins.)

Assessment Findings

Signs and Symptoms

Physical examination reveals muscle wasting and weakness resulting from extensive protein depletion. Carbohydrate tolerance is lowered, and signs and symptoms of diabetes mellitus develop (see Chapter 51). Fat is redistributed, leading to facial fullness and the characteristic moon face and buffalo hump. The skin is thin, and the face is ruddy. The client has increased susceptibility to wounds, and healing is prolonged; however, the immunosuppressive effects of the disorder usually mask symptoms of infection.

Because the blood vessels are fragile, the client bruises easily, and striae often form over extensive skin areas. The bones become so demineralized that the client may have backache, kyphosis, and collapse of the vertebrae. They retain sodium and water, and peripheral edema and hypertension develop. The client reports mood changes and difficulty coping with stressors that were manageable in the past. The family may report serious mental changes. In women, Cushing syndrome produces masculinization with hirsutism and amenorrhea. These sexual changes and alterations in appearance are reversible when adrenocortical hormone levels return to normal (Fig. 50-12).

See Evidence-Based Practice 50-1 for research on Cushing syndrome and weight loss.

Diagnostic Findings

Diagnosis is tentatively based on the physical changes. Urine levels of 17-hydroxycorticosteroids (17-OHCS) and 17-ketosteroids (17-KS) usually are increased. Plasma and urine cortisol levels are elevated. An overnight dexamethasone suppression test is used as an initial screening. The client takes 1 mg oral dexamethasone; the next morning, plasma cortisol levels are obtained. If these results are above normal (5 mg/dL), 0.5 mg dexamethasone is given every 6 hours, and 24-hour urine collections are tested for 2 consecutive days. Clients without the disorder have decreased 17-OHCS and 17-KS levels; these levels remain elevated in those with Cushing syndrome.

To determine whether the symptoms of Cushing syndrome are the result of pituitary stimulation, plasma ACTH is measured in conjunction with the administration of dexamethasone. If ACTH levels subsequently are found to be low or normal and the cortisol level is elevated, it suggests that the adrenal gland alone is hyperfunctioning. If both the ACTH and cortisol levels are elevated, a pituitary or hypothalamic etiology is more likely.

Laboratory blood test results also reveal increased serum sodium, decreased serum potassium, and increased blood glucose levels. Abdominal radiographs, CT, or MRI may show adrenal enlargement, and an IV pyelogram may show changes in the renal shadow caused by an abnormally large adrenal gland.

Evidence-Based Practice 50-1

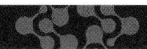

Cushing Syndrome and Weight Loss

Clinical Question

Does weight loss occur with the treatment of mifepristone for Cushing syndrome?

Evidence

Clients with Cushing syndrome struggle with obesity and weight issues. This can occur even after surgery. Mifepristone, which is classified as a glucocorticoid receptor antagonist, was trialed in a study by Fein, Vaughan, Kushner, Cram, and Nguyen (2015). The study had clients with Cushing syndrome undergo a 24-week trial with mifepristone. The study concluded that a substantial weight loss occurred during the 24-week trial and for up to 2 years after for clients who continued treatment with mifepristone (Fein et al., 2015). Chang et al. (2021) were able to see the effectiveness of mifepristone medication therapy for clients that were presurgical and preradiation. Effects of weight loss, BP control, and improvements in glycemic statuses were noted.

Nursing Implications

Nurses need knowledge of new treatments and medications for Cushing syndrome. The nurse should take a thorough history of nutrition, weight loss, and medications. The nurse may also do a baseline weight to track the client over the treatment period.

Reference

Chang, A. Y., Mirfakhraee, S., King, E. E., Mercado, J. U., Donegan, D. M., & Yuen, K. C. (2021). Mifepristone as bridge or adjunct therapy in the management of challenging Cushing disease cases. *Clinical Medicine Insights: Endocrinology and Diabetes.* https://doi.org/10.1177/1179551421994102

Fein, H. G., Vaughan III, T. B., Kushner, H., Cram, D., & Dat, N. (2015). Sustained weight loss in clients treated with mifepristone for Cushing's syndrome: A follow-up analysis of the SEISMIC study and long-term extension. *BMC Endocrine Disorders, 15,* 63. https://doi.org/10.1186/s12902-015-0059-5

Medical and Surgical Management

Treatment depends on whether a tumor or adrenal hyperplasia causes the disorder. It is directed toward removing the cause and lowering plasma cortisol levels. Radiation therapy or removal of the pituitary gland may be used for adrenal hyperplasia. Bilateral adrenalectomy may be preferred if both adrenals are involved.

Drug therapy includes diuretics for edema as well as an antihypertensive agent. A diet low in sodium and carbohydrates controls edema and blood glucose level. Antibiotics are used to treat infection.

If cushingoid syndrome results from exogenous administration of a corticosteroid preparation, the drug is slowly withdrawn by tapering the dose over days or weeks. In some instances, as in the treatment of a disorder such as leukemia, or to prevent rejection of transplanted organs, the syndrome is allowed to persist.

Hyperaldosteronism

Hyperaldosteronism is due to the excessive secretion of aldosterone leading to extreme electrolyte imbalances. Aldosterone, a mineralocorticoid, is regulated by serum levels of potassium and sodium, the renin-angiotensin system, and ACTH.

Pathophysiology and Etiology

The cause of primary hyperaldosteronism may be a benign aldosterone-secreting adenoma of one of the adrenals, an adrenal malignant tumor, or unknown. Pregnancy, heart failure, narrowing of the renal artery, and cirrhosis can cause secondary hyperaldosteronism.

Excessive secretion of aldosterone results in increased reabsorption of sodium and water and excretion

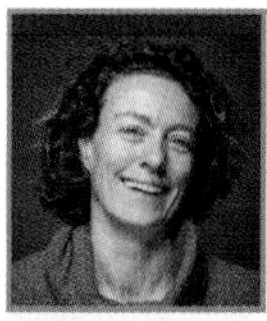

Clinical Scenario A 52-year-old woman has returned to her primary provider's office because her recent laboratory blood work indicated an elevation of blood sugar. The nurse interviews and examines the client prior to being seen by her primary provider. The nurse notes the following: round, moon face and growth of facial hair; fatty deposit over her upper back; evidence of bruising and striae on the client's skin; and a pendulous abdomen yet thin arms and legs. The client's BP is 172/96 mm Hg while resting. Based on the client's basic physical assessment, Cushing syndrome is suspected. **What nursing actions are appropriate during the management of the client's care? See the following Nursing Process section.**

NURSING PROCESS FOR THE CLIENT WITH CUSHING SYNDROME

Assessment

Obtain thorough medical, drug, and allergy histories and observe for symptoms of an adrenal disorder: altered skin pigmentation and integrity; decreased energy level; mental changes; sexual dysfunction; and changes in mood, appetite, weight, and bowel patterns. Monitor vital signs every 4 hours and test the blood or urine (or both) for glucose three or four times per day. If the urine tests positive for glucose or the blood glucose level is elevated, report the information to the primary provider.

Because the client is at risk of the development of peptic ulcers, observe the color of each stool and test the stool for occult blood. If the client reports epigastric pain or discomfort or the stool has a black appearance or tests positive for blood, make the primary provider aware of the assessment findings.

(continued)

NURSING PROCESS FOR THE CLIENT WITH CUSHING SYNDROME (continued)

Diagnosis, Planning, and Interventions

If corticosteroid therapy has caused a cushingoid appearance and the dose is to be tapered over time, give the client and family a detailed explanation of the tapering schedule. Review the directions printed on the prescription container and emphasize the importance of strictly following the tapering schedule. The client may find it helpful to use a calendar to enter the dosage for each day. Another option to ensure compliance is to write the entire tapering schedule on a card and instruct the client to cross off each day.

Depending on many factors such as age and severity of the disorder, clients with Cushing syndrome may or may not be scheduled for adrenalectomy or irradiation of the pituitary gland. Until further treatment is scheduled, emphasize the importance of continued medical supervision. Highlight important points such as avoiding trauma to the skin; contacting the primary provider if sores or cuts do not heal or become infected, if easy bruising occurs, or if stools are dark or black; following the recommended diet; reading food labels carefully; avoiding exposure to infection; avoiding nonprescription drugs (unless approved by the primary provider); weighing self weekly; and reporting marked weight gain or edema to the primary provider. Diagnoses, expected outcomes, and interventions include, but are not limited to, the following:

Fluid Overload Risk: Related to sodium and water retention
Expected Outcome: Fluid volume will be normal as evidenced by equivalent fluid intake and output volumes, reduced or no dependent edema, consistent daily weights, and BP measurements within normal limits.

- Examine extremities for increased or decreased edema. *Fluid retention is manifested by swelling in dependent areas, pitting when pressure is applied to the skin over a bone, tight-fitting shoes or rings, the appearance of lines in the skin from stockings, and seams in the shoes or areas where they lace.*
- Measure intake and output daily, weekly, or as ordered. *Acutely ill clients require more frequent assessment. A gain of 2 lb in 24 hours suggests 1 L of water retention.*
- Assess vital signs each shift; report systolic BP that exceeds 139 mm Hg or diastolic BP that exceeds 89 mm Hg. *Hypertension is defined as a consistently elevated BP above 139/89 mm Hg (see* Chapter 27*). One factor that contributes to hypertension is excess circulatory volume.*
- Administer prescribed diuretics. *They promote the excretion of sodium and water.*
- Provide a sodium-restricted diet at the level prescribed by the primary provider. *Limiting sodium reduces the potential for fluid retention.*

Altered Skin Integrity Risk: Related to thinning of skin and edema
Expected Outcome: Skin will remain intact.

- Inspect the skin daily, especially over bony prominences, for open lesions or ulcers. *The skin is thin, fragile, and prone to breaking down with minimal trauma.*
- Encourage the client to change positions frequently. *Relieving pressure on capillaries helps maintain a supply of oxygenated blood to cells and tissues. Cells deprived of oxygenated blood are prone to cellular death.*
- Handle the client gently; use interventions that relieve pressure on the skin. *Gentleness reduces the potential for skin abrasions, and interventions that cushion the weight and force of gravity against body surfaces help prevent the development of pressure ulcers.*
- Exercise care when performing tasks that may damage the skin, such as removing tape when discontinuing an IV infusion. *The skin's fragility increases its potential for injury.*

Fatigue: Related to muscle wasting and protein depletion
Expected Outcome: Client will demonstrate energy to complete ADLs.

- Provide frequent rest periods between activities. *Rest restores energy and improves endurance.*
- Assist the client with activities when muscle wasting or pain secondary to osteoporosis is severe. *The nurse relieves client of responsibilities until the client can safely and comfortably manage self-care.*

Infection Risk: Related to suppressed inflammatory response and immune function
Expected Outcome: Client will be free of infection.

- Observe for signs and symptoms that indicate an infection: a skin injury that does not heal, increased temperature, sore throat, or cough. *Signs of infection or inflammation are less dramatic in these clients than in others. What may appear to be a minor problem could be masking a more serious problem.*
- Make every effort to prevent exposing the client to infectious microorganisms. *Microorganisms are spread by direct and indirect contact. A client with suppressed defenses is more likely to succumb to an infection.*
- Immediately notify the primary provider if an infection is suspected. *The nurse collaborates with the primary provider on medical interventions.*

Injury Risk: Related to demineralization of bones
Expected Outcome: Client will be safe and free from injury such as a bone fracture.

NURSING PROCESS FOR THE CLIENT WITH CUSHING SYNDROME (continued)

- Protect the client from falls by applying supportive slippers and keeping the environment free of clutter and water spills. *The force of a fall is more likely to cause a fracture when the bones are porous. Environmental safety reduces the potential for injury.*
- Instruct the client to seek assistance when getting out of bed. *Assistance reduces the incidence and consequences of a fall.*

Suicide Attempt Risk: Related to mood changes and depression
Expected Outcome: Client will reveal the absence of suicidal ideation; the client's mood will be stable with no significant depressive symptoms.

- Assess mental status, including suicidal ideation, regularly. *A depressed client is likely to appear sad, be tearful, have difficulty sleeping or sleep more than expected, neglect hygiene, have a poor appetite and reduced energy, and lack interest in the future. Clients who entertain thoughts of suicide usually admit to their despair when openly questioned.*
- Explain that a depressed mood is a common symptom of the disorder or side effect of corticosteroid therapy. *Depressed clients may blame themselves for their inability to cope with stressors. Providing information about the cause of the depressed mood may help the client to persevere with the treatment regimen.*
- Maintain safety by removing items that could be used for suicide, checking on the client frequently, transferring the client to a room close to the nursing station, and offering to stay with the client when they are feeling self-destructive. *Eliminating the opportunity or methods by which the client can harm themselves may prevent a suicide attempt.*
- Collaborate with the primary provider about a referral to a mental health practitioner or agency if suicidal thoughts occur or depression is ongoing. *Counseling, drug therapy, and psychotherapy after discharge provide long-term measures for keeping a client safe from self-harm.*

Altered Body Image Perception: Related to changes in physical appearance
Expected Outcome: Client will express a positive self-image.

- Offer the client opportunities to express feelings over physical changes. *Verbalizing feelings with a supportive person increases the client's ability to cope with stress.*
- Explain that when the cause of the disorder is eliminated, some physical changes gradually improve, but others, such as striae and kyphosis, are permanent. *Being honest and sharing accurate information promotes the client's trust and confidence.*
- Offer suggestions such as wearing loose clothing, a hat, or cap to help disguise physical changes that the client finds difficult to tolerate. *Although the client's perception of physical changes probably is more exaggerated than that of others, they may feel more confident in social situations with techniques that minimize changes in appearance.*

Evaluation of Expected Outcomes

Fluid volume is normal, with no evidence of edema, hypertension, or weight gain. The client meets self-care needs without fatigue. Temperature and WBC count are within normal limits. Skin is intact. The client is free from injury, such as pathologic fractures. They demonstrate normal range of moods and deny suicidal ideation. The client copes effectively with physical changes.

of potassium by the kidneys. Figure 50-13 presents an overview of the renin-angiotensin-aldosterone system.

Assessment Findings

Headache, muscle weakness, increased urine output, fatigue, hypertension, and a potential for cardiac arrhythmias are a cluster of signs and symptoms that develop. Serum potassium levels are decreased, and serum sodium levels are increased in the absence of other causes, such as diuretic therapy or diarrhea. The serum bicarbonate, serum aldosterone, and plasma renin levels are increased. CT or MRI may rule out or locate an adrenal tumor. Adrenal venography may identify small tumors that CT scanning fails to reveal.

Medical and Surgical Management

If the cause is an adrenal tumor, unilateral adrenalectomy may be performed. Medical management may include administration of spironolactone, a potassium-sparing diuretic, and an antihypertensive agent to control BP. A sodium-restricted diet may be necessary.

Nursing Management

The nurse monitors vital signs every 4 hours or as ordered. They report marked elevations to the primary provider. The nurse measures fluid intake and output and weighs the client every 2 to 7 days. Daily examination of the extremities for edema is essential. The nurse observes for signs of hypokalemia and hypernatremia (see Chapter 16).

Adrenalectomy

An adrenalectomy may be performed laparoscopically through several keyhole-size incisions or by open adrenalectomy through a large flank or subcostal incision following

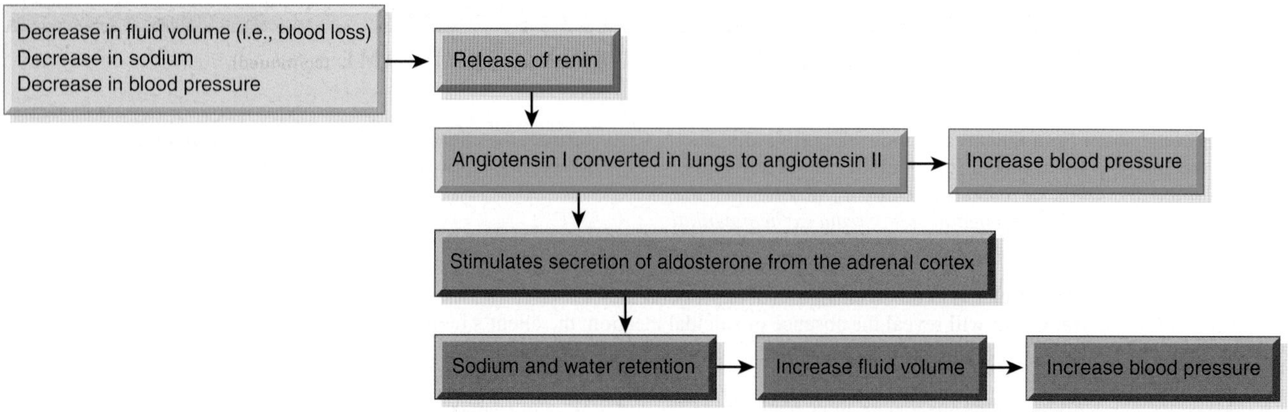

Figure 50-13 The renin-angiotensin-aldosterone system.

the position of the 12th rib. Surgeons prefer an open adrenalectomy to a laparoscopic approach when malignancy is present or the gland is 4 inches or more in diameter. In some instances, removal of the ovaries, testes, and both adrenal glands (which secrete male and female hormones) is considered to control cancers of the breast and prostate, which depend on hormones for growth. When an open adrenalectomy is performed, the client is at increased risk of deep vein thrombosis secondary to decreased mobility, and pneumonia secondary to impaired respiratory effort due to pain at the operative site (Miles, 2016).

Nursing Management

Preoperative Period

Major goals include reduced anxiety and an understanding of preparations for surgery and possible postoperative events. The nurse keeps the client on bed rest and minimizes anxiety. The client who requires surgery to halt the progression of a metastatic disease may be anxious as well as depressed and needs time to discuss the surgery and anticipated results. If the client has a pheochromocytoma, the nurse monitors BP frequently before surgery. When bilateral adrenalectomy is scheduled, the nurse may start IV administration of a solution containing a corticosteroid preparation the morning of surgery. Some surgeons prefer to initiate corticosteroid administration during the removal of the adrenals. Additional preparations are the same as for the client having general surgery (see Chapter 14).

Postoperative Period

When the client returns from surgery, the nurse reviews the surgical record because postoperative observations and management depend on whether one or both adrenal glands were removed. In addition to the complications associated with general anesthesia, the nurse observes for problems such as hemorrhage, atelectasis, and pneumothorax because the adrenals are located close to the diaphragm and inferior vena cava. They monitor vital signs frequently and closely observes for signs of adrenal insufficiency (adrenal [Addisonian] crisis), which may occur when the following happen:

- The prescribed dose of a corticosteroid preparation is inadequate to meet the client's needs (bilateral adrenalectomy).
- The remaining adrenal gland does not produce sufficient hormone to meet the client's needs (unilateral adrenalectomy).
- The prescribed dose of a corticosteroid preparation is not given.

If symptoms of adrenal insufficiency occur, the nurse notifies the primary provider immediately. They should never omit administering a prescribed corticosteroid because corticosteroid replacement is essential to life. Acute adrenal insufficiency is managed with infusions of IV solutions, glucose, and cortisol. Client and Family Teaching 50-4 provides detailed instructions for postdischarge management of the client who has undergone bilateral adrenalectomy.

Client and Family Teaching 50-4
Discharge Instructions After Adrenalectomy

The nurse emphasizes the following points when teaching the client:

- The functions of the adrenal glands include providing a physiologic response to stress, suppressing inflammation, raising blood sugar levels, conserving sodium to maintain blood volume and BP, and contributing hormones that affect sexual characteristics.
- Follow the prescribed treatment regimen.
- Care for the surgical wound as directed until it has healed.
- Adhere to the prescribed medication schedule.
- Obtain sufficient sleep and rest to prevent fatigue and support ADLs.
- Eat a well-balanced diet.
- Keep appointments for scheduled blood tests and health care appointments.
- Avoid infections and stressful situations.
- Carry identification indicating that the adrenal glands have been surgically removed.
- Seek immediate medical help if it is not possible to take the prescribed corticosteroid drug or if symptoms of adrenal insufficiency and adrenal crisis develop.

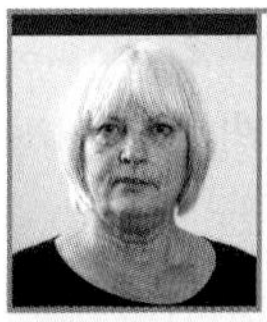

Clinical Scenario A 56-year-old woman has had persistent hypertension that has not responded to prescribed antihypertensives. Her elevated BP has been accompanied by headaches. Subsequent laboratory tests revealed low serum potassium levels. An abdominal CT scan revealed a unilateral adrenal mass. The client is scheduled to undergo an open adrenalectomy because there is a possibility that the mass is malignant. **How might the nurse plan for the client's immediate postoperative care? See the following Nursing Process section.**

NURSING PROCESS FOR THE CLIENT UNDERGOING AN ADRENALECTOMY

Assessment

Check vital signs as soon as the client returns to the unit to establish a baseline. Conduct other routine postoperative assessments such as examining the dressing over the incision and the patency and characteristics of fluid from incisional drains, noting LOC, checking infusion of IV fluids, auscultating the lungs and abdomen, observing breathing patterns, identifying the level of pain, measuring intake and output, and monitoring whether the client is performing leg exercises. Closely observe for acute adrenal crisis evidenced by hypotension and shock, nausea, vomiting, dehydration, muscle weakness, and hypoglycemia. Monitor blood studies for electrolyte imbalances and assess closely for any signs of infection. Throughout the postoperative period, continue to monitor pulse, BP, temperature, breath sounds, blood glucose levels, and urinary output.

Diagnosis, Planning, and Interventions

Acute Pain: Related to tissue trauma
Expected Outcome: Pain will be eliminated or reduced to a tolerable level within 30 minutes of nursing intervention.

- Assess pain whenever assessing vital signs. *Pain assessment is the fifth vital sign; assess pain whenever you take vital signs and more often if indicated.*
- Give an analgesic promptly before pain increases. *Giving an analgesic before pain becomes intolerable more easily relieves and controls pain.*
- Assess and note the client's response to the analgesic. *The nurse is obligated to manage the client's pain; the client may require additional measures if the analgesic is ineffective.*
- Offer comfort measures such as massage, skin care, and emotional support. *Nonpharmacologic approaches complement and supplement pain-relieving medications.*

Ineffective Airway Clearance: Related to inadequate coughing secondary to incisional pain
Expected Outcome: The airway will be clear as evidenced by normal breath sounds and respiratory rate and effort.

- Support the incision firmly when turning or changing the client's position. *Movement of the skin and tissue underlying the incision stimulates nociceptors that transmit pain impulses to the CNS. Limiting pain facilitates movement, circulation, and breathing.*
- Apply firm support over the incision when the client deep breathes and coughs. *Pressing on the incision with a pillow or folded bath blanket promotes fuller lung expansion and more effort when coughing, both of which help to maintain a patent airway.*
- Change the client's position every 2 hours. *Movement helps prevent stasis of respiratory secretions.*
- Encourage deep breathing and coughing every 2 hours. *Deep breathing and coughing open and clear respiratory passages.*
- Encourage adequate (2000 mL) intake of oral fluids. *When oral fluids are absorbed, they contribute to the volume in all fluid compartments. Adequate oral intake thins mucus.*
- Consult with the primary provider about the need for suctioning or aerosolized respiratory treatments if the lungs sound congested or if sputum is thick and difficult to raise. *Suctioning is a mechanical means to remove retained secretions; it is useful if the client's natural cough is ineffective. Respiratory treatments provide medications that dilate the bronchi and thin mucoid secretions so that they are more easily expelled.*

Infection Risk: Related to decreased cortisol secretion or immunosuppression secondary to steroid therapy replacement
Expected Outcome: The wound is clean and dry with no signs of infection.

- Observe strict aseptic technique for all procedures, such as changing the dressing on the surgical wound. *Medical asepsis reduces microorganisms; surgical asepsis uses techniques in which microorganisms are absent or destroyed before contact with a susceptible host.*
- Notify the primary provider if vital signs change, purulent drainage is found on the dressing, or analgesics do not control pain. *The nurse reports findings that may require medical interventions.*
- Inspect the wound during each dressing change. Notify the primary provider about excessive redness, swelling of the suture line, or purulent drainage. *Impaired skin from an incision increases the potential for infection. Nurses must report abnormal wound characteristics immediately.*

(continued)

NURSING PROCESS FOR THE CLIENT UNDERGOING AN ADRENALECTOMY (continued)

Injury Risk: Related to postural hypotension and weakness secondary to adrenal insufficiency
Expected Outcome: Client will be free from injury.

- Assist with ambulatory activities and observe for weakness and dizziness. *Until the client's condition is stable and BP is normal, they require assistance.*
- Notify the primary provider of continued hypotension or weakness. *Persistent symptoms may represent an impending adrenal crisis, which requires more definitive medical treatment.*

Evaluation of Expected Outcomes

Client reports pain relief and improved comfort. Lungs are clear to auscultation; client coughs and breathes effectively. There is no evidence of infection. Safety is maintained; the client is injury-free.

KEY POINTS

- Disorders of the pituitary gland
  - Acromegaly (hyperpituitarism): oversecretion of GH after the epiphyses of the long bones have sealed
  - Panhypopituitarism (Simmonds disease): destruction of the pituitary gland followed by cessation of pituitary hormonal activity
  - Diabetes insipidus: excretion of an extremely large volume of urine
  - Syndrome of inappropriate antidiuretic hormone secretion (SIADH): renal reabsorption of water rather than normal excretion
- Disorders of the thyroid gland
  - Hyperthyroidism (Graves disease): oversecretion of thyroid hormones
  - Thyrotoxic crisis (thyroid storm): life-threatening episode of hyperthyroidism
  - Hypothyroidism: secretion of inadequate amounts of thyroid hormone
  - Thyroid tumors: generally benign but must be evaluated, cause excess secretion of thyroid hormones
  - Endemic and multinodular goiters (enlarged thyroid gland): can be caused by deficiency of iodine (endemic), enlarged with no thyroid dysfunction symptoms (nontoxic), or may contain one or more areas of hyperplasia (nodular)
  - Thyroiditis: inflammation of the thyroid gland
- Disorders of the parathyroid glands
  - Hyperparathyroidism: excess amount of parathormone
  - Hypoparathyroidism: deficiency of parathormone levels that result in hypocalcemia
- Disorders of the adrenal glands
  - Adrenal insufficiency: inadequate production of steroid hormones, can be primary or secondary
  - Acute adrenal crisis (Addisonian crisis): life-threatening endocrine emergency
  - Pheochromocytoma: tumor of the adrenal medulla that caused hyperfunction
  - Cushing syndrome (adrenocortical hyperfunction): excessive secretion of hormones by the adrenal cortex
  - Hyperaldosteronism: excessive secretion of aldosterone, leading to extreme electrolyte imbalance

CRITICAL THINKING EXERCISES

1. When caring for a client receiving fludrocortisone (Florinef) orally after bilateral adrenalectomy, nurses have a team conference to review the client's potential for acute adrenal insufficiency. What information is appropriate to discuss?
2. A nurse is assigned to a client recently admitted because of unexplained weight loss, insomnia, and fullness in the throat. The attending primary provider, several medical students, and a primary provider's assistant subsequently palpate this enlargement. Later, the client becomes restless and disoriented. The heart rate increases to 165 beats/min, respirations are rapid, and the temperature is recorded at 103.8°F (39.8°C). What is a possible explanation for the changes in the client's condition and what methods would be used to manage them?
3. A client had a thyroidectomy this morning. It is now 8 p.m., and the client complains of difficulty swallowing clear liquids and pressure in the area of the throat incision. The BP is normal, but the pulse rate is elevated. You see no drainage on the surface of the dressing. What actions would you take at this time?
4. How do the clustered terms "sugar, salt, and sex" relate to hormones produced by the adrenal cortex?

NCLEX-STYLE REVIEW QUESTIONS PrepU

1. What nursing assessment indicates that a client with DI is experiencing a therapeutic response to treatment?
   1. The client's coarse facial features are more normal.
   2. Sexual dysfunction is no longer occurring.
   3. The client has a significant weight loss.
   4. The client's urine output is a normal amount.

2. What items should the nurse have available when a client recovers after a thyroidectomy? Select all that apply.
   1. Pulse oximeter
   2. Oral airway
   3. Tracheostomy tray
   4. Ice bag
   5. Tourniquet
   6. Calcium gluconate

3. A nurse assesses a client immediately following a thyroidectomy and documents that the dressing over the incision is dry and intact. In what other location should the nurse check for signs of bleeding and hemorrhage?
   1. Within the pharynx with a tongue blade
   2. Inside the oral cavity with a flashlight
   3. At the back of the neck with a gloved hand
   4. Over the sternum using light palpation

4. Prior to discharge from the hospital, the nurse instructs the client who will be taking thyroid replacement medication to report any side effects of the drug, such as chest pain, insomnia, and hyperactivity. What is the best explanation for the nurse's instruction?
   1. The side effects indicate that the dosage is too low and needs to be increased.
   2. The side effects determine whether the medication should be discontinued.
   3. The side effects of thyroid replacement often mimic those of hyperthyroidism.
   4. The side effects indicate that a tranquilizer or sedative may be needed.

5. A client who has been on long-term corticosteroid therapy is unhappy with the accompanying weight gain and changes in physical appearance, and confides to the nurse that they intend to stop taking the prescribed medication. What is the best nursing response to the client's statement?
   1. Discontinuing this medication should be done under the direction of the primary provider.
   2. Unwanted side effects of this medication can be controlled with other drugs.
   3. Report the results that occur to the primary provider after discontinuing the medication.
   4. Discuss how to control side effects with the pharmacist who fills your prescription.

WANT TO KNOW MORE? There are a wide variety of online resources available on thePoint to enhance learning and understanding of this chapter.

Go to thePoint.lww.com/activate and use the activation code found in the front of this text to unlock these online resources.

51

Caring for Clients With Diabetes Mellitus

Words To Know

bariatric surgery
diabetes mellitus
diabetic ketoacidosis
diabetic nephropathy
diabetic retinopathy
fasting blood glucose
gangrene
glucometer
glycemic index
glycosuria
glycosylated hemoglobin
hyperglycemia
hyperosmolar hyperglycemic nonketotic syndrome
hypoglycemia
insulin independence
insulin resistance
ketoacidosis
ketonemia
ketones
ketonuria
Kussmaul sign
lipoatrophy
lipohypertrophy
lipolysis
metabolic syndrome
microalbuminuria
oral glucose tolerance test
polydipsia
polyphagia
polyuria
postprandial glucose
prediabetes
random blood glucose
renal threshold
rule of 15
tight glucose control

Learning Objectives

On completion of this chapter, you will be able to:

1. Define and distinguish the two types of diabetes mellitus.
2. Identify the three classic symptoms of diabetes mellitus.
3. Name three laboratory methods used to diagnose diabetes mellitus.
4. Describe the methods used to treat diabetes mellitus.
5. Identify categories of medications used to manage diabetes mellitus and their mechanism of action.
6. Discuss the nursing management of the client with diabetes mellitus.
7. Explain the source of ketones and the cause of diabetic ketoacidosis.
8. List three main goals in the treatment of diabetic ketoacidosis.
9. Identify two physiologic signs of hyperosmolar hyperglycemic nonketotic syndrome.
10. Describe the treatment of hyperosmolar hyperglycemic nonketotic syndrome.
11. Explain the cause and treatment of hypoglycemia.
12. Differentiate between the symptoms of hypoglycemia and hyperglycemia.
13. Describe common chronic complications of diabetes mellitus.

Diabetes mellitus, a metabolic disorder of the pancreas, affects carbohydrate, fat, and protein metabolism. This disease is reaching epidemic proportions in the United States. Some experts believe that diabetes in adults is one consequence of **metabolic syndrome**, which includes obesity, especially in the abdominal area; high blood pressure (BP); elevated triglyceride, low-density lipoprotein, blood glucose levels; and a low high-density lipoprotein level (see Chapter 25).

No age group is exempt from diabetes. The American Diabetes Association (2018) estimates that there are 34.2 million Americans with diabetes, of whom 7.3 million are yet undiagnosed. Incidence is highest among persons over 65 years of age, Native Americans, and Alaska Natives followed by non-Hispanic Blacks. At present, diabetes is the seventh leading cause of death in the United States (Centers for Disease Control and Prevention [CDC], 2020d). Because of the chronic nature of diabetes, affected people experience many debilitating and life-threatening complications before death. Older aged diabetics experience higher mortality, reduced functional status, and increased risk for institutionalization (Sesti et al., 2018). Research is providing exciting discoveries, however, that may eventually cure this disease.

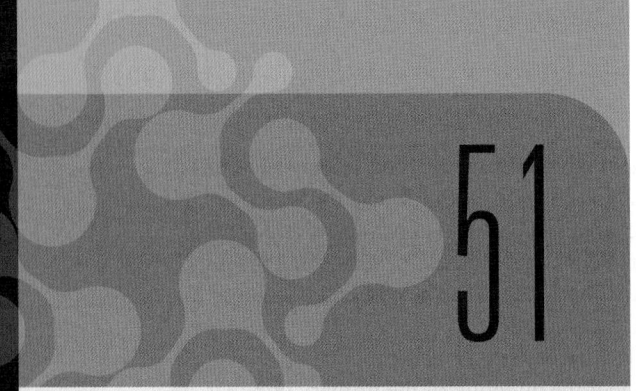

Gerontologic Considerations

- Diabetes is associated with an increased risk for developing dementia. Hypoglycemia risk, a side effect of diabetic medications, is higher in older adults and is more likely to occur simultaneously with cognitive impairment. Additionally, older adults may be more vulnerable to hypoglycemia because of diabetes duration, cognitive changes, renal dysfunction, risk for frailty (Sesti et al., 2018), and impaired functional balance abilities (Tsai et al., 2016).
- Older adults may experience complex challenges to diabetes self-care. Comorbidities may affect cognitive or functional ability to monitor and accurately administer medications.
- Family or caregivers should be included in teaching about monitoring and treatment. Interventions can be determined to meet individual needs, potentially preventing progressive decline or readmissions. For example, newer devices that can monitor blood sugar and interface with mobile electronic devices allow remote caregivers to track results (Bradway et al., 2018).
- Client abilities, preferences, comorbidities, and stress levels influence potential complications.
- Changes in taste sensation (sweet and salty) that accompany aging may contribute to older adults' unintentional consumption of foods higher in sugar content, resulting in the risk for hyperglycemia. Teaching plans should emphasize blood glucose testing prior to insulin administration.
- Some older clients experience difficulty in administering insulin because of problems such as decreased visual acuity or arthritis. Assess the client's ability and resources for self-administration of insulin before developing a teaching program. Appropriate aids, such as a magnifier that fits over the syringe, prefilled syringe, or insulin pens, are available.
- Older adults may take several medications for chronic comorbidities. Prescription and nonprescription drugs and any other complementary or alternative therapy should be assessed for interactions with oral antidiabetic agents.
- The eating and sleeping habits of older adults often differ from those of young or middle-aged persons. This should be taken into consideration when planning meals and scheduling the dosage of insulin or an oral hypoglycemic agent.
- Good foot care is especially important in older adults because other diseases are common in this population, such as peripheral vascular disease and osteoarthritis.

DIABETES MELLITUS

The Centers for Disease Control and Prevention (CDC, 2020d) has identified and described the two major forms of diabetes mellitus:

- *Type 1*, formerly called insulin-dependent diabetes mellitus, is characterized by an absence of insulin production by the beta cells in the islets of Langerhans of the pancreas (Fig. 51-1). The onset of type 1 diabetes is more likely in people younger than 20 years of age. Type 1 diabetes accounts for approximately 1.6 million of all diagnosed cases of diabetes, with 200,000 being below the age of 20 (Juvenile Diabetes Research Foundation, 2021).

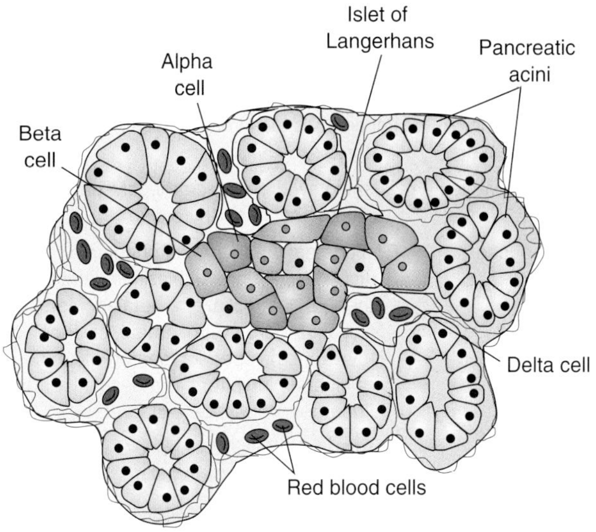

Figure 51-1 Islet of Langerhans in the pancreas. (Reprinted from Guyton, A. C., & Hall, J. E. (2011). *Guyton and Hall Textbook of medical physiology* (12th ed.). W. B. Saunders. Copyright ©2011 Elsevier. With permission.)

- *Type 2*, formerly known as non–insulin-dependent diabetes mellitus (NIDDM), is characterized by **insulin resistance** or insufficient insulin production that may or may not result in the eventual need for insulin therapy. Type 2 diabetes is more common in aging adults. In 2018, adults aged 45 to 64 years were the highest among newly diagnosed age groups for type 2 diabetes (CDC, 2020b). Type 2 diabetes also is being detected in obese children.

Prediabetes Mellitus

The American Diabetes Association (2021d) has developed criteria that identify people with **prediabetes**, which can lead to type 2 diabetes, heart disease, and stroke. People with prediabetes are overweight or obese, have risk factors for diabetes, and may have one or more abnormal blood glucose level tests such as *hemoglobin A1c (HbA1c)*, *fasting blood glucose*, or *oral glucose tolerance* or all three. A person with an HbA1c of 5.7% to 6.4%, a **fasting blood glucose** level of 100 to 125 mg/dL after an overnight fast, or an **oral glucose tolerance test** level of 140 to 199 mg/dL after a glucose tolerance test lasting 2 hours is considered prediabetic (American Diabetes Association, 2021f). Estimates in 2020 indicated 88 million Americans were prediabetic (CDC, 2020d). A significant number of those with prediabetes will develop the disease; however, many can delay or avoid type 2 diabetes with weight loss and increased physical activity.

Hyperglycemia

Hyperglycemia, an elevated blood glucose level, is associated with other disorders or their management (Table 51-1). For example, pancreatitis (see Chapter 47) causes both exocrine and endocrine disturbances. When the production of adrenocortical hormones is excessive, as in Cushing syndrome (see Chapter 50), or with the administration of glucocorticoid drugs for immunosuppressive purposes, secondary diabetes develops. Impaired glucose metabolism and hyperglycemia also are associated with drugs such as loop and

TABLE 51-1 Nondiabetic Conditions Associated With Hyperglycemia

DISORDER	EXAMPLES
Exocrine pancreatic disease	Pancreatitis, pancreatic cancer, cystic fibrosis
Endocrinopathies	Cushing syndrome, acromegaly, pheochromocytoma, hyperthyroidism
Drug induced	Corticosteroids, thiazides, phenytoin, nicotinic acid, phenothiazines, lithium, theophylline, diltiazem, beta-agonists, alpha interferon, furosemide, calcitonin, thyroxine, haloperidol, pentamidine, calcineurin inhibitors, protease inhibitors, fluoroquinolones, beta-blockers
Viral induced	Congenital rubella, Coxsackie B virus, cytomegalovirus, adenovirus, mumps
Genetic disorders	Down syndrome, Klinefelter syndrome, Turner syndrome, Prader–Willi syndrome
Pregnancy	Gestational hyperglycemia
Nutritional support	Total parenteral nutrition (TPN)

Adapted from Solis-Herrera, C., Triplitt, C., Reasner, C., DeFronzo, R.A., & Cersosimo, E. (2018). Classification of diabetes mellitus. *MDText.com, Inc.* Retrieved February 24, 2018, from https://www.ncbi.nlm.nih.gov/books/NBK279119/

thiazide diuretics, antipsychotics, levodopa, and oral contraceptives and with the administration of total parenteral nutrition (TPN). Insulin may be used in the management of these disorders, but that does not indicate that the client has diabetes mellitus. A normal blood glucose level is restored once these diabetogenic regimens are discontinued.

Pathophysiology and Etiology

Type 1 Diabetes Mellitus

Insulin has three functions: (1) It carries glucose into body cells as their preferred source of energy, (2) it promotes the liver's storage of glucose as glycogen, and (3) it inhibits the breakdown of glycogen back into glucose. In type 1 diabetes, the islet cells, or endocrine portion of the pancreas, cease to produce insulin. Without insulin, the blood glucose level rises beyond its normal range—sometimes to 300 to 1000 mg/dL, and the body breaks down fat and protein as alternative sources of cellular energy (Norris, 2018). The breakdown of fat, known as **lipolysis**, results in the accumulation of fatty acids and ketones, metabolic by-products of fat metabolism. When ketones accumulate in the blood, clients with diabetes are prone to developing a form of metabolic acidosis known as **ketoacidosis**. In type 1 diabetes, ketoacidosis develops quite suddenly because of the total cessation of insulin production.

Type 1 diabetes is considered an autoimmune disorder. Several researchers have shown that killer (CD8) T-cell lymphocytes attack and destroy the insulin-producing islet cells (Sun et al., 2020; Roep et al., 2021). The hypothesis is that people with type 1 diabetes lack a protein marker known as major histocompatibility complex, or MHC, that helps the T cells identify natural cells as "self." Consequently, the T cells misidentify islet cells as unnatural and subsequently destroy them. This same research has now found a way to destroy the islet-attacking T cells using tumor necrosis factor-alpha and stimulate the growth of new islet cells with the bacillus Calmette–Guérin (BCG) vaccine, which heretofore has been used as a vaccine against tuberculosis. The first clinical trial using the BCG vaccine showed a successful, but transient, effect on research participants, which may mean that lifelong, repeated administration of BCG vaccine may be required. Clinical trials continue currently to test the role of the BCG vaccine (Massachusetts General Hospital, 2018). If successful, the outcome of this research may eventually mean that type 1 diabetes can be controlled and perhaps cured without daily injections of insulin (Kühtreiber et al., 2018).

Type 2 Diabetes Mellitus

Diabetes mellitus, especially type 2, runs in families, although a specific gene for diabetes has not been isolated. The consensus is that type 2 diabetes mellitus is an inherited disease, and that obesity, especially intraabdominal obesity, is likely a cofactor that triggers its onset. Scientists possibly have found the link between obesity and type 2 diabetes (Essers et al., 2014). Their findings show that chronic low-grade inflammation results in insulin resistance, a decreased sensitivity to insulin at the tissue level, as well as type 2 diabetes. The belief is that anti-inflammatory therapies could play a role in the prevention and treatment of type 2 diabetes that then causes changes in liver function accompanied by hyperglycemia and insulin resistance.

Concept Mastery Alert

Type 2 Diabetes Mellitus

A major concern with type 2 diabetes mellitus is insulin resistance. Obesity is a contributing factor to insulin resistance.

When type 2 diabetes is manifested, the beta cells of the islets of Langerhans secrete increased levels of insulin into the bloodstream to offset hyperglycemia, but the blood glucose level remains higher than normal because there is a deficiency of *transmembrane glucose transporters* on the surface of cells. Transmembrane glucose transporters form channels that facilitate diffusion of glucose into cells (Fig. 51-2), and they may function only at 20% efficiency in people with type 2 diabetes. This contributes to hyperglycemia. Exercise increases transmembrane glucose transporter levels in skeletal muscles, which explains how exercise helps reduce blood sugar (Vargas et al., 2020). Eventually, the overstimulated beta cells become exhausted, resulting in a decline in insulin production, and the client with type 2 diabetes may also become insulin deficient, like those with type 1 diabetes. The correlation of obesity, sedentary lifestyle, and insulin resistance helps explain how dieting, exercise, and weight loss control type 2 diabetes and delay, reduce, or eliminate the need for medication to treat the disease.

An excessive level of glucose in the blood leads to **glycosuria**, glucose in the urine, and urinary excretion. Glycosuria

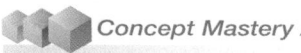

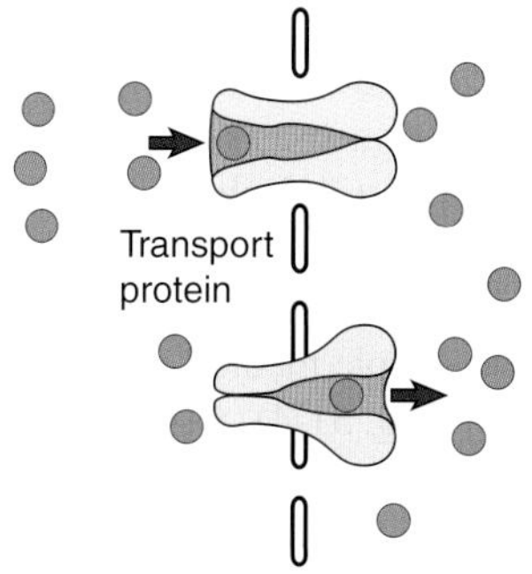

Figure 51-2 Glucose transporters called GLUT4 that are responsible for facilitated diffusion bind to glucose outside the cell membrane then change their conformation to allow glucose inside the cell. In type 2 diabetes, glucose transporters are less efficient resulting in elevated levels of glucose in the blood. (Reprinted with permission from Timby, B. K. (2016). *Fundamental nursing skills and concepts* (11th ed.). Wolters Kluwer.)

appears when the blood glucose level rises above 180 mg/dL. At this level, the kidneys' **renal threshold**, the ability to reabsorb glucose and return it to the bloodstream, is impaired. The hypertonicity from concentrated amounts of glucose in the blood pulls fluid into the vascular system, resulting in **polyuria**, excessive urine production. The client experiences urinary frequency accompanied by increased excreted urine. Because so much water is lost, **polydipsia**, excessive thirst, develops.

While the needed glucose is being wasted, the body's requirement for fuel continues. The person with diabetes feels hungry and eats more (**polyphagia**). Despite eating more, they lose weight as the body uses fat and protein to substitute for glucose. **Ketones**, chemical intermediate products in fat metabolism, such as beta-hydroxybutyric acid, acetoacetic acid, and acetone, cause ketoacidosis when they accumulate.

The bicarbonate buffer system attempts to neutralize the ketones. Thus, **ketonemia** (increased ketones in the blood) causes a decreased alkali (base) reserve, leading to acidosis. **Kussmaul sign** (fast, deep, labored breathing) are common in ketoacidosis (Fig. 51-3). Acetone, which is volatile, can be detected on the breath by its characteristic fruity odor. If treatment is not initiated, the outcome of ketoacidosis is circulatory collapse, renal shutdown, and death. Ketoacidosis is more common in people with diabetes who no longer produce insulin, such as those with type 1 diabetes. People with type 2 diabetes are more likely to develop **hyperosmolar hyperglycemic nonketotic syndrome** (HHNKS; see later discussion), because with limited insulin, they can use enough glucose to prevent ketosis but not enough to maintain a normal blood glucose level.

Infection and stress invite ketosis because they increase the demand for insulin, which the pancreas cannot accommodate in diabetes. In addition, people with diabetes mellitus are at increased risk for vascular disorders such as atherosclerosis, cerebrovascular accidents, myocardial infarction, peripheral vascular disease with decreased ability to heal, renal failure, blindness, and neuropathy. Women are prone to complications during pregnancy; men are prone to erectile dysfunction (see Chapter 55).

››› *Stop, Think, and Respond 51-1*

Identify some differences between type 1 and type 2 diabetes mellitus.

Assessment Findings

Signs and Symptoms

The three classic symptoms of both types of diabetes mellitus are polyuria, polydipsia, and polyphagia. Additional symptoms include weight loss, weakness, thirst, fatigue, and dehydration. These signs and symptoms have an abrupt onset in clients with type 1 diabetes. Clients with type 2 diabetes have a gradual onset of symptoms. Some develop skin, urinary tract, and vaginal infections, possibly because the elevated level of blood glucose supports bacterial growth. There may be changes in visual acuity manifested by blurred vision because the hypertonicity of body fluid affects the cells in the lens and retina (Norris, 2018).

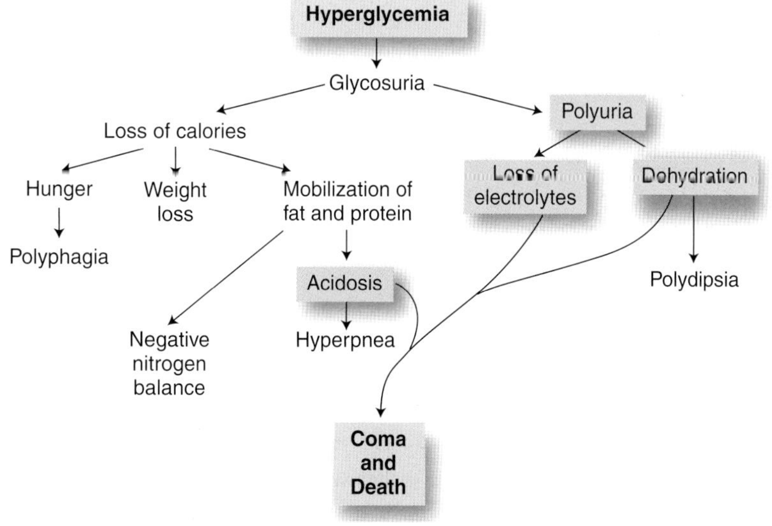

Figure 51-3 Signs and symptoms of uncontrolled hyperglycemia in diabetes mellitus. (Reprinted with permission from Rubin, E., Strayer, D. S., (Eds.). (2014). *Rubin's pathology: Clinicopathologic foundations of medicine* (7th ed.). Wolters Kluwer.)

NURSING GUIDELINES 51-1

Performing Urine Testing for Glucose and Ketones

Method: Tes-Tape and Diastix

- Have the client empty their bladder to eliminate glucose and ketones that have been stored in the bladder for hours; save this specimen in case the client cannot void later.
- Encourage the client to drink water; ask the client to void in 30 minutes.
- For the client with an indwelling catheter, clamp the catheter for 30 minutes and take the specimen directly from the catheter, not the drainage bag.
- Test the second voided specimen to detect current concentration of glucose and ketones.
- Dip the testing strip into the urine and wait for the recommended time.
- Observe the color change and document the results.

Diagnostic Findings

Although diabetes mellitus is a highly complex disease, screening for its detection in blood and urine is relatively simple. Normally, urine contains no detectable glucose or ketones; in diabetes, one or both may be present. Because the body fails to use glucose adequately, it excretes glucose in the urine. If the body metabolizes fats faster than it can use the ketones, ketones also appear in the urine. The relative ease of these urinary tests facilitates early detection of diabetes (Nursing Guidelines 51-1).

Blood Sugar Testing. Because glycosuria (glucose in urine) and **ketonuria** (substances in urine from the breakdown of fat metabolism) may not become evident until glucose exceeds the renal threshold, blood tests are helpful in establishing the diagnosis. Blood tests such as random blood sugar, fasting blood glucose, **postprandial glucose**, and the oral glucose tolerance test are based on measuring glucose intolerance (Table 51-2).

One quick and simple method of blood sugar testing involves a glucometer (Fig. 51-4). A **glucometer** measures capillary blood glucose from blood sampled from a finger stick. Primary providers now recommend self-monitoring of blood glucose levels with a glucometer for clients taking insulin, clients with unstable diabetes, or clients with frequent hypoglycemic episodes. Self-monitoring with a glucometer is helpful for those taking an oral hypoglycemic agent to determine the effects of diet, exercise, and medications. Ideally, with finger testing, the blood sugar should measure 90 to 130 mg/dL before meals and less than 180 mg/dL 1 to 2 hours after meals.

A glucometer can also be used to obtain blood sugar levels from alternate sites such as the upper arm, forearm, thigh, or calf. These tests are described as less painful or even painless because the fingertips have a higher number of nerve endings. However, alternate sites are regarded as lagging test sites because they actually provide a measurement of blood glucose as it was 20 to 35 minutes prior to the test (U.S. Food and Drug Administration [FDA], 2019). Consequently, alternate sites are only an option for people whose glucose levels are relatively stable and are not an option for people who require tight glucose control. **Tight glucose control** involves maintaining near-normal blood glucose levels by taking short-acting insulin throughout the day and intermediate-acting insulin at bedtime. Controlling blood glucose levels can delay the onset of complications associated with diabetes.

TABLE 51-2 Diagnostic Tests for Detecting Glucose Intolerance

TEST	IMPLEMENTATION	DIAGNOSTIC RESULT
Random blood glucose	Blood specimen is drawn without preplanning	In nondiabetics, 79–140 mg/dL; ≥200 mg/dL in the presence of symptoms is suggestive of diabetes mellitus
Fasting blood glucose	Blood specimen is obtained after 8 hours of fasting	In clients who are nondiabetic, the glucose level will be <100 mg/dL. In clients who are diabetic, glucose is ≥126 mg/dL
Postprandial glucose	Blood sample is taken 2 hours after a high-carbohydrate meal	In clients who are nondiabetic, the glucose level will be between 80 and 160 mg/dL. In clients who are diabetic, the result is ≥180 mg/dL
Oral glucose tolerance test	Diet high in carbohydrates is eaten for 3 days. Client then fasts for 8 hours. A baseline blood sample is drawn, and a urine specimen is collected An oral glucose solution is given, and time of ingestion is recorded Blood is drawn at 30 minutes and 1, 2, and 3 hours after the ingestion of glucose solution. Urine is collected simultaneously. Drinking water is encouraged to promote urine excretion	In clients who are nondiabetic, the glucose returns to <140 mg/dL in 2 hours, and urine is negative for glucose. In clients who are diabetic, blood glucose level will be ≥ 200 mg/dL in 2 hours; urine is positive for glucose
Glycosylated hemoglobin or hemoglobin A1c	Single sample of venous blood is withdrawn	The amount of glucose stored by the hemoglobin is elevated above 7.0% in the newly diagnosed client with diabetes mellitus, in one who is noncompliant, or in one who is inadequately treated

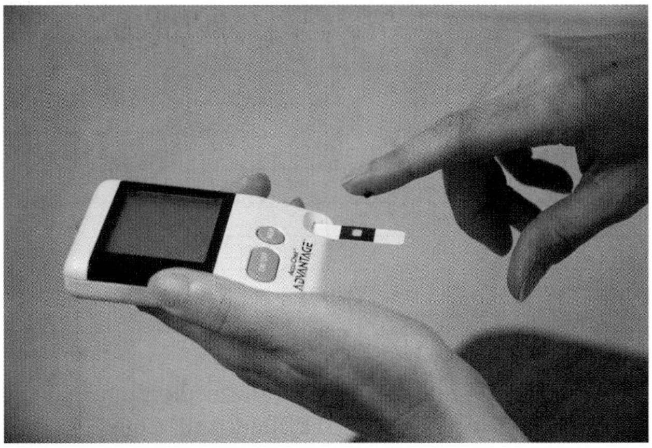

Figure 51-4 Example of a blood glucose monitor that uses blood sampled from a finger stick.

Glycosylated Hemoglobin. Once a client with diabetes receives a treatment regimen to follow, the primary provider can assess the effectiveness of treatment and the client's adherence to that treatment by obtaining a **glycosylated hemoglobin**, also called an HbA1c test. The results of this test reflect the amount of glucose that is stored in the hemoglobin molecule during its lifespan of 120 days. The level of glycosylated hemoglobin among diabetics should be less than 7%. According to the American Diabetes Association (2015a), an HbA1c of 7% is the equivalent of an average blood glucose level of 154 mg/dL. Amounts of 8% or greater indicate that control of the client's blood glucose level has been inadequate during the previous 2 to 3 months.

Medical Management

Treatment depends on many factors, such as the type of diabetes and the ability of the pancreas to manufacture insulin, and involves combinations of the following:

- Diet and weight loss
- Exercise
- Insulin
- Oral antidiabetic agents
- Pancreas transplantation
- Islet cell transplantation

Diet and Weight Loss

Diet is a major component of treatment for every person with diabetes. Formulation of a diabetic diet depends on the client's sex, age, height and weight, activity level, occupation, state of health, former dietary habits, and cultural background (Nutrition Notes).

Nutrition Notes

The Client With Diabetes Mellitus

Carbohydrate counting is a flexible alternative to using the exchange system. This method of dietary management involves an individualized meal pattern that specifies the number of carbohydrate "choices" (one choice = 15 g carbohydrate) for each meal and snack. Most adults are allowed three to five carbohydrate choices per meal and one to two for each snack, depending on their caloric needs. Carbohydrate choice lists can help clients with identifying sources of carbohydrates and the appropriate portion sizes. Clients also need to know how to read the Nutrition Facts label in order to count carbohydrates accurately.

For some clients, dietary modifications alone can control type 2 diabetes. These clients have a mild form of diabetes, with the pancreas producing some insulin. The client with diabetes who is overweight is placed on a weight reduction diet because diabetes is less easily controlled in the presence of obesity. Even a moderate weight loss improves the body's use of insulin.

Clients may also use the **glycemic index**, a measure of how fast a carbohydrate food is likely to raise blood sugar, to help maintain normal blood sugar levels. The glycemic index assigns a number to various foods relative to glucose, which is given an arbitrary value of 100. Glycemic index values are generally divided into three categories:

- Low glycemic index: 1 to 55
- Medium glycemic index: 56 to 69
- High glycemic index: 70 and higher

Foods with glycemic indices greater than 70, such as a waffle (76), raise low blood sugar quickly and are designed to cover brief periods of intense exercise. Foods with indices less than 55, such as low-fat yogurt (14), slowly help prevent **hypoglycemia** (low blood glucose level) during the night or when a person exercises for long periods. However, the glycemic index does not indicate the amount of the recommended food to consume (Mayo Clinic Staff, 2020).

When dietary allowances (calories, percentages of carbohydrates, fats, and proteins) are prescribed, the client is given a diet prescription and a list of substitutions and choices to vary the diet. For example, the primary provider determines that the client with diabetes may have 1500 calories/day. The calories are then distributed according to the percentage of carbohydrates, fats, and proteins that equal the total prescribed caloric amount. A dietitian provides the client with a list of foods in six different categories—starch/bread, protein (animal and plant based), vegetable, fruit, milk, and fat—and indicates how many items from each category the client can consume for breakfast, lunch, dinner, and snacks (Fig. 51-5). The dietitian gives the client a list of foods in each category and their equivalent amounts. The client can then substitute one food in the list for another in the specified amount for variety (Box 51-1).

Exercise

Exercise helps metabolize carbohydrates and control blood glucose levels because glucose-transporting receptors within skeletal muscles allow the muscles to take in glucose from the blood *independent* of insulin. This provides energy during exercise and lowers blood sugar. Exercise, therefore, reduces the need for insulin because blood sugar can be lowered without it, an advantage for those with diabetes. It also explains why hypoglycemia can accompany exercise.

Exercise also improves the circulation of blood, which is compromised in the client with diabetes. Exercise also

	1 STARCH/BREAD	2 MEAT	3 VEGETABLE	4 FRUIT	5 MILK	6 FAT
BREAKFAST	2			1	1	1
SNACK TIME						
LUNCH	2	1	1	1		1
SNACK TIME				1		
DINNER	2	2	1	1		2
SNACK TIME	1			1	1	

Figure 51-5 A sample diabetic meal plan for 1500 calories.

lowers cholesterol and triglyceride levels and improves muscle tone. An exercise program for the client with diabetes specifies the type of exercise and the length of time to perform it. The American Diabetes Association (2021e) recommends that adults with diabetes perform at least 150 minutes a week of moderate-intensity aerobic physical exercise spread over at least 3 days a week with no more than 2 consecutive days without exercise. Sporadic periods of exercise are discouraged because wide fluctuations in blood glucose levels can occur. It is necessary to regulate food and insulin requirements during times of increased activities.

Insulin

All clients with type 1 diabetes must rely on insulin therapy. The goal of pancreas and islet cell transplantation (see later discussion), which is performed only for clients with type 1 diabetes, is that the client will acquire **insulin independence**—that is, the client's own naturally produced insulin will regulate blood glucose levels within consistently normal ranges. Better yet, the use of techniques to reverse autoimmunity or to stimulate islet cell regeneration with gene therapy (discussed earlier) may eventually cure clients with type 1 diabetes. Additional possibilities for eliminating the need for exogenous insulin include transplantation of stem cells. Until then, clients with type 1 diabetes continue to require daily, multiple, or continuous injections of insulin. Clients with type 2 diabetes eventually may become dependent on insulin therapy when the beta cells cease to function and antidiabetic agents are no longer effective.

BOX 51-1 Sample Starch/Bread Choices for Substitution and Equivalent Amounts

Starches contain 15 grams of carbohydrate and 80 calories per serving. One serving equals:

MEASUREMENT	INGREDIENT
1 slice	Bread (white, pumpernickel, whole wheat, rye)
2 slices	Reduced-calorie or "lite" bread
1/4 (1 oz)	Bagel (varies)
1/2	English muffin
1/2	Hamburger bun
3/4 C	Cold cereal
1/3 C	Rice, brown or white, cooked
1/3 C	Barley or couscous, cooked
1/3 C	Legumes (dried beans, peas or lentils), cooked
1/2 C	Pasta, cooked
1/2 C	Bulgar, cooked
1/2 C	Corn, sweet potato, or green peas
3 oz	Baked sweet or white potato
3/4 oz	Pretzels
3 C	Popcorn, hot air popped or microwave (80% light)

Food Exchange Lists. https://www.nhlbi.nih.gov/health/educational/lose_wt/eat/fd_exch.htm

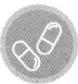

Pharmacologic Considerations

- Three important properties of insulin are as follows:
1. onset, when the insulin first begins to act in the body;
2. peak, the time when insulin is exerting maximum action;
3. duration, the time the insulin remains in effect.

These properties determine which insulin or analogue will be used as the long-acting, intermediate, rapid, or short-acting dose.

Table 51-3 includes commonly used insulin preparations, which are divided into four categories: rapid acting, short acting, intermediate acting, and long acting. Some clients with type 2 diabetes maintain glycemic control with a once-daily injection of an intermediate-acting insulin, combination of intermediate-acting and short-acting insulin in a 70:30 or 50:50 proportion, or long-acting insulin. Clients with type 1 diabetes may self-administer three to four injections or more throughout the day unless they use an insulin pump (discussed later).

Human Insulin. Human forms of insulin are gradually replacing purified insulin extracts from beef and pork pancreas. Beef and pork insulins are essentially "foreign" substances, and the human immune system produces antibodies that blunt their effect, requiring higher doses of insulin (Kimball, 2019). Human insulin also appears to cause fewer allergic reactions

TABLE 51-3 Insulin/Insulin Analogue Preparations and Activity

INSULIN TYPE	ONSET	PEAK	DURATION
Rapid-acting insulins			
Insulin analogues			
Aspart (NovoLog)	5–15 min	1–3 hr	3–5 hr
Glulisine (Apidra)	15–30 min	30–60 min	4 hr
Lispro (Humalog)	5–10 min	30 min–1.5 hr	3–5 hr
Human insulin rDNA—inhaled Regular (Afreeza)	12–15 min	1 hr	2 hr
Short-acting insulins			
Human insulin rDNA			
Regular (Humulin R, Novolin R)	30–60 min	2–4 hr	5–8 hr
Intermediate-acting insulin			
Isophane insulin suspension (NPH; Humulin N, Novolin N)	1.5 hr	4–10 hr	14 hr
Long-acting insulins (all insulin analogues)			
Degludec (Tresiba)	1 hr	9 hr	25 hr
Detemir (Levemir)	3–4 hr	6–8 hr	24 hr
Glargine (Lantus, Toujeo [300 u/mL])	1 hr	Steady, no peak	24 hr
Combined insulins (all insulin analogues)			
70% Aspart protamine/30% aspart (Novolog 70/30)	10–20 min	1–1.5 hr	18–24 hr
70% Degludec/30% aspart (Ryzodeg 70/30)	15 min	72 min	24 hr
70% NPH/30% regular (Humulin 70/30, Novolin 70/30)	30–60 min, then 1–2 hr	2–4 hr, then 6–12 hr	6–8 hr, then 18–24 hr

Note. These are ordered according to the American Association of Clinical Endocrinologists (AACE) 2016 guidelines for use.

than insulin obtained from animal sources; however, clients who switch from animal to synthesized human insulin must be monitored for low blood glucose levels initially because the human form of insulin is used more effectively.

Several methods are used to produce human insulin through genetic engineering. First, the conversion of pork insulin to human insulin results from changing one amino acid. Second, insertion of the human gene for insulin into strains of the bacteria *Escherichia coli* produces Humulin insulin; use of yeast organisms instead of *E. coli* yields Novolin insulin detemir (Levemir), and degludec (Tresiba). Third, further modification of human insulin to work faster than Humulin has led to the development of lispro (Humalog) and aspart (NovoLog); conversely, glargine insulin (Lantus and others) is human insulin that has been modified to work more slowly than other human insulins.

Gastrointestinal (GI) enzymes inactivate insulin; therefore, insulin cannot be administered in forms that move through the GI tract. Most insulins are injected subcutaneously; some may be administered intravenously. In the United States, Afreeza, an oral inhaled form of human insulin, is sometimes referred to as an ultrarapid-acting insulin. Afreeza must be used in conjunction with a long-acting insulin and is contraindicated in those with chronic lung disease.

Recently, a transdermal insulin patch system has been developed. The transdermal system uses ultrasonic waves to enlarge the diameter of skin pores to enable the insulin to permeate and enter the dermis through sweat pores and eventually enter the bloodstream. Although the transdermal technology sounds promising, it requires further human clinical trials before becoming available (Dansinger, 2019a).

››› *Stop, Think, and Respond 51-2*

Identify which of the following insulins is rapid acting, short acting, intermediate acting, and long acting: glargine (Lantus), Lente, lispro (Humalog), Novolin R.

Administration of Insulin. Insulin is prescribed in units. U100 means that 1 mL contains 100 units of insulin; inhaled insulin is supplied in 4-, 8-, and 12-unit single-use cartridges. The primary provider specifies both the dosage and the type of insulin to be used. When combining two types of injectable insulin in the same syringe, the short-acting insulin is withdrawn into the syringe *first* and the intermediate-acting insulin is added next, a practice referred to as "clear to cloudy" because short-acting insulin is clear and intermediate-acting insulin contains an additive that makes it cloudy. The mixture is administered within 15 minutes to ensure that the onset, peak, and duration of each separate insulin remain intact. Glargine (Lantus) insulin and detemir (Levemir) cannot be mixed with other types of insulin in the same syringe. Combination mixtures of insulin, such as Humulin 70/30, Novolin 70/30, and Humulin 50/50, eliminate the need for mixing insulins from two separate vials.

Rapid-acting and short-acting insulin can be administered IV and subcutaneously. The IV route is used to (1) treat severe hyperglycemia or (2) prevent or control elevated blood sugar by adding it to a TPN solution that contains a high concentration of glucose. The subcutaneous route is used most commonly for administering insulin (Fig. 51-6); insulin is absorbed more rapidly when injected in the abdomen than in the arms or thighs. Clients with diabetes are taught to use the abdomen for self-administration of insulin. Subcutaneous

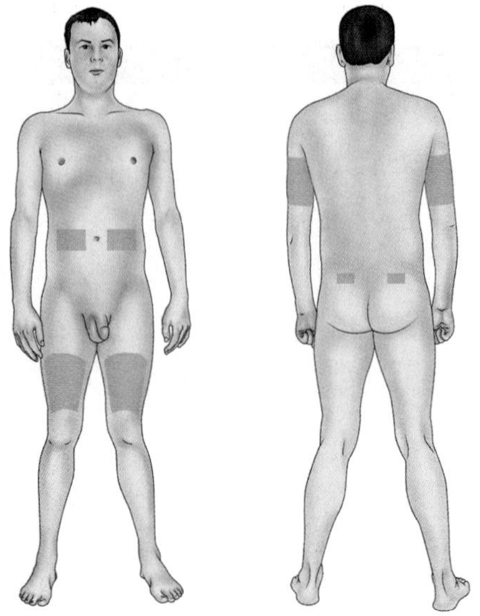

Figure 51-6 Subcutaneous injection sites used for administering insulin.

injection sites require rotation to avoid **lipoatrophy**, breakdown of subcutaneous fat at the site of repeated injections, and **lipohypertrophy**, buildup of subcutaneous fat at the site of repeated injections, either of which eventually interferes with insulin absorption in the tissue. Because insulin is an anabolic hormone, it also causes weight gain.

Other techniques for injecting insulin subcutaneously include an insulin pen, jet injector, or insulin pump. See Evidence-Based Practice 51-1 for research on insulin administration.

Insulin Pen. An insulin pen is a device in which a cartridge containing 150 to 300 units of insulin is loaded into an injecting pen and a disposable needle attached. Each time the insulin is injected, a new needle is attached. Once the device is loaded, the client (1) selects the number of units for injection by dialing in the dose in 1- to 2-unit increments, (2) cleans and pierces the skin, and (3) injects the programmed amount (Fig. 51-7).

Jet Injector. A jet injector uses high pressure and rapid speed, rather than a needle, to instill insulin through the skin. The pressure transforms the liquid into a fine mist that is distributed over a wide area of tissue, resulting in faster absorption (Fig. 51-8). Although a jet injector offers several advantages, such as reducing pain at the site and eliminating the use of needles and their appropriate disposal, the cost tends to make this form of administration less practical.

Insulin Pump. An insulin pump provides a means for delivering insulin by continuous infusion. The device has three components: pump, tubing, and needle (Fig. 51-9).

Evidence-Based Practice 51-1

Insulin Administration

Clinical Question

In clients receiving insulin, how does needle length compared to injection technique affect hypoglycemic episodes?

Evidence

Proper insulin administration is an important part of good blood sugar control and diabetes management. In the stable client, insulin is meant to be injected into the subcutaneous layer of tissue. Evidence supports that injection techniques should be adjusted depending on the thickness of the subcutaneous tissue at the injection site and the length of the needle being used. When injection techniques are not adjusted, insulin can mistakenly be injected into muscle tissue, speeding up the rate at which it is absorbed into the body, causing what can be life-threatening episodes of hypoglycemia (or low blood sugar; Al Hayek & Al Dawish, 2020; Pozzuoli et al., 2018; Thewjitcharoen et al., 2020).

Insulin needles come in various sizes, ranging from 4, 5, and 6 mm (standard sizes of needles in most insulin pens) to 8 mm (5/16 inch) and 12.7 mm (1/2 inch) (found in most insulin syringes). Injection sites should be rotated including those within the abdomen (Thewjitcharoen et al., 2020). Al Hayek and Al Dawish (2020) found that the longer the needle and the less fatty tissue over the injection site, the greater the chance of injecting insulin into the muscle when using an 8-mm needle (straight into the skin).

Nursing Implications

It is important for the nurse to consider needle length and the thickness of the subcutaneous layer at the injection site when deciding whether to inject insulin at a 90-degree angle (straight into the tissue) or at a 45-degree angle (at a slant). When using needles that are 12.7 or 8 mm, inserting the needle into the skin at a slant can help lessen the chance that the insulin is accidentally injected into the muscle. Evidence also supports folding up the skin (sometimes referred to as pinching up the skin) at the injection site to lower further the chance of injecting the insulin into the muscle (Diggle, 2015). Using shorter needle lengths (4, 5, or 6 mm needles, which are now standard on most insulin pens) whenever possible can lessen the chance of accidental injection into the muscle regardless of how thin or obese the client is. Using assessment and critical thinking skills to evaluate the length of the needle on the insulin pen or syringe and assessing the injection site will help the nurse make good decisions about whether to inject the insulin at a 90-degree angle (straight into the skin) or at a 45-degree angle (at a slant). This will help increase the chance of injecting the insulin into the subcutaneous tissue and not the muscle, giving clients the best results.

References

Al Hayek, A. A., & Al Dawish, M. (2020). Evaluating the user preference and level of insulin self-administration adherence in young patients with type 1 diabetes: Experience with two insulin pen needle lengths. *Cureus, 12*(6), e8673. https://doi.org/10.7759/cureus.8673

Pozzuoli, G. M., Laudato, M., Barone, M. M, Crisci, F., & Pozzuoli, B. (2018). Errors in insulin treatment management and risk of lipohypertrophy. *Acta Diabetol, 55*, 67–73. https://doi.org/10.1007/s00592-017-1066-y

Thewjitcharoen, Y., Prasartkaew, H., Tongsumrit, P., Wongjom, S., Boonchoo, C., Butadej, S., Nakasatien, S., Karndumri, K., Veerasomboonsin, V., Krittiyawong, S., & Himathongkam, T. (2020). Prevalence, risk factors, and clinical characteristics of lipodystrophy in insulin-treated patients with diabetes: An old problem in a new era of modern insulin. *Diabetes, Metabolic Syndrome and Obesity: Targets and Therapy, 13*, 4609–4620. https://doi.org/10.2147/DMSO.S282926

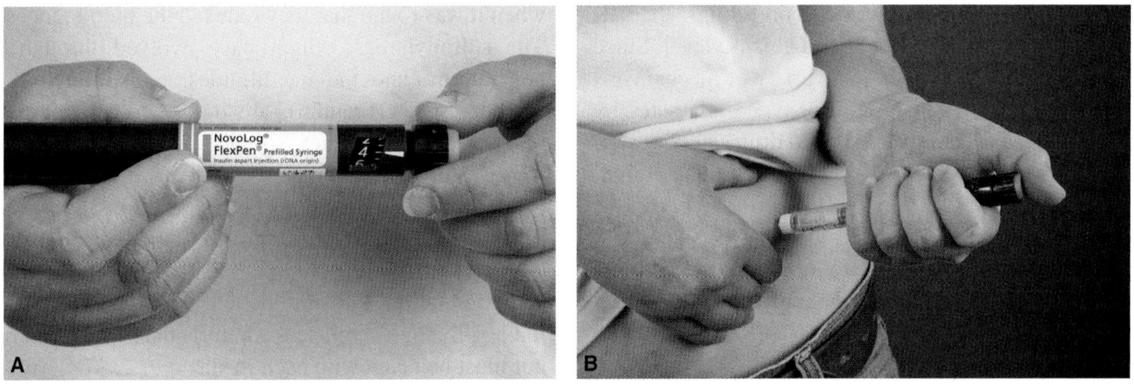

Figure 51-7 To use an insulin pen, the person **(A)** dials in the dose and **(B)** injects the needle into the cleaned site, pressing the button to deliver insulin.

Pharmacologic Considerations

■ Insulin pens are client-specific. They are designed for one client to use multiple times. A separate needle is used in these devices, yet can still be contaminated by the client's blood and should never be shared by more than one client.

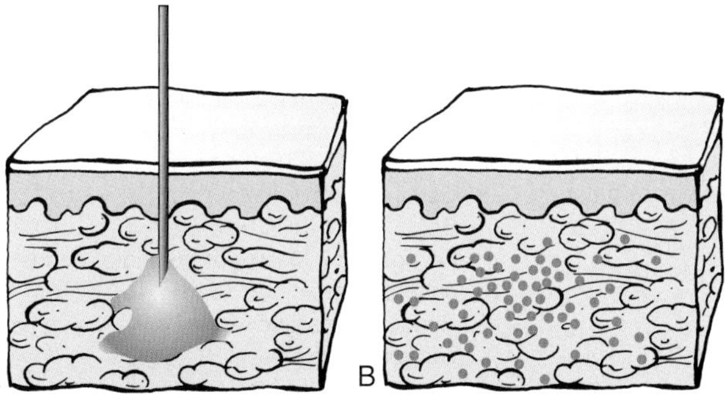

Figure 51-8 **(A)** Needle produces a pool of insulin beneath the skin, which is slowly absorbed. **(B)** Jet injector produces an insulin mist beneath the skin, which is absorbed more quickly.

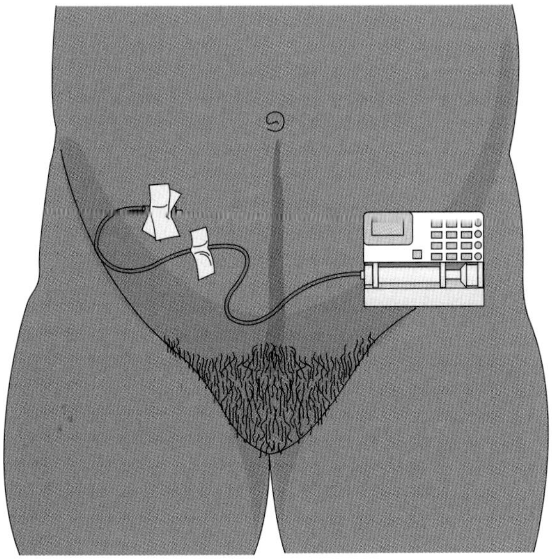

Figure 51-9 An insulin pump contains a syringe preloaded with insulin that is delivered to a client through tubing and needle in the abdomen. (Reprinted with permission from Pillitteri, A. (2014). *Maternal and child health nursing* (7th ed.). Wolters Kluwer Health/Lippincott Williams & Wilkins.)

The pump itself contains a reservoir for rapid-acting or short-acting insulin, a battery-operated infuser, and a computer chip that enables a person to regulate basal (continuous) and premeal bolus doses in 0.05- to 0.10-unit increments. The pump, which is worn in a pouch or belt holder, is attached to tubing with a needle. The needle is inserted in the subcutaneous tissue of the abdomen and can remain in the same site for up to 3 days. Clients who are interested in controlling their diabetes with an insulin pump need to consider both its advantages and disadvantages (Box 51-2).

Oral Antidiabetic Agents

Oral antidiabetic drugs also known as hypoglycemic agents are prescribed for clients with type 2 diabetes who meet the following criteria:

- Fasting blood glucose level less than 200 mg/dL
- Insulin requirement of less than 40 units/day
- No ketoacidosis
- No renal or hepatic disease

BOX 51-2 Insulin Pump Considerations

Advantages

- Resembles the normal pancreatic release of insulin
- Decreases the necessity for multiple daily injections in different sites
- Helps maintain consistent blood sugar levels; reduces the potential for episodes of hyperglycemia and ketoacidosis
- Provides more flexibility for eating food at varying times during the day
- Facilitates the instillation of smaller doses than those of insulin syringes

Disadvantages

- Requires high motivation to control diabetes by frequently checking blood glucose levels and adjusting the infusion
- Creates a potential for hyperglycemia if the pump fails, the tubing becomes kinked or obstructed, or the needle is displaced
- Interferes or creates a nuisance factor when participating in active sports, sexual intercourse, or bathing; the pump can be temporarily disconnected without removing the needle, but doing so stops the delivery of insulin until it is reconnected

Before 1995, only one category of oral drugs, the sulfonylureas, was used to lower the blood glucose level. Since then, many new drugs that work in a variety of mechanisms have been developed that help control type 2 diabetes by various mechanisms. Recently developed drug categories include biguanides, alpha-glucosidase inhibitors, thiazolidinediones (TZDs), meglitinides, dipeptidyl peptidase-4 (DPP-4) inhibitors, also known as gliptins, glucagon-like peptide 1 (GLP-1) receptor agonists, and sodium-glucose cotransporter 2 (SGLT2) inhibitors. Drug Therapy Table 51-1 lists examples of oral hypoglycemic drugs.

Sulfonylureas and Meglitinides. Sulfonylureas such as glyburide (DiaBeta, Glynase, Micronase) and glipizide (Glucotrol) were modified from sulfa-containing antibiotics when it was found that they reduced the blood glucose level. The sulfonylureas, which have evolved through several generations, and the meglitinides, nonsulfonylureas such as repaglinide (Prandin), are described as being "insulin releasers" because they stimulate the pancreas to secrete more insulin. Although they are effective drugs, they tend to cause weight gain, hypoglycemic reactions, and *secondary failure*, a phenomenon in which the pancreas cannot continue making sufficient insulin, perhaps as a result of the gland's overstimulation. Repaglinide has a short duration of action, making hypoglycemia less common than with sulfonylureas, but must be taken with each meal.

Biguanides and TZDs. Metformin (Glucophage) is the only biguanide approved for use together with the TZDs, which

DRUG THERAPY TABLE 51.1 Antidiabetic Agents (Other Than Insulins)

Category and Common Generic (Brand) Drugs	Intended Use	Common Side Effects	Safety Warnings for Nurses
Biguanide			
Metformin (Fortamet, Glucophage, Riomet)	Prediabetes, type 2 diabetes mono-/combotherapy; sensitizes the liver, reduces glucose absorption, reduces liver production of glucose	Nausea, vomiting, flatulence, diarrhea	• Monitor kidney function, reduction makes greater risk for lactic acidosis • Do not take for 48 hours following radiographs using contrast medium
Glucagon-like peptide 1 (GLP-1) agonists			
Albiglutide* (Tanzeum) Dulaglutide* (Trulicity) Exenatide* (Byetta) Liraglutide* (Saxenda)	Type 2 diabetes mono-/combotherapy; supplements GLP-1 hormone to stimulate insulin release	Injection site irritation	• Used in chronic weight control over 27 BMI • Do not use if history of thyroid or endocrine cancers • Reduces effectiveness of oral contraceptives
Sodium glucose cotransporter 2 (SGLT-2)			
Canagliflozin (Invokana) Dapagliflozin (Farxiga) Empagliflozin (Jardiance)	Type 2 diabetes mono-/combotherapy; allows kidney to release more glucose in the urine	Hypoglycemia, genital/urinary yeast infections	• Monitor kidney function especially if compromised before therapy initiated • Monitor for *hypo*tension and *hyper*kalemia
Dipeptidyl peptidase-4 inhibitors (Gliptins)			
Alogliptin (Nesina) Sitagliptin (Januvia) Linagliptin (Tradjenta) Saxagliptin (Onglyza)	Type 2 diabetes mono-/combotherapy; enhances incretin hormone to stimulate insulin release	Headache, nasopharyngitis, upper respiratory infection	• Not to be used for Type 1 diabetes
Thiazolidinediones (TZD)			
Pioglitazone (Actos) Rosiglitazone (Avandia)	Type 2 diabetes mono-/combotherapy; improve peripheral cell insulin sensitivity	Headache, muscle pain, respiratory symptoms, weight gain, swelling of face and extremities, chest pain, irregular heart rate	• Monitor liver enzymes • Do not use when symptomatic heart failure is evident • Use effective barrier birth control • Anovulatory women may start ovulation; use effective birth control
Alpha-glucosidase inhibitors			
Acarbose (Precose) Miglitol (Glyset)	Type 2 diabetes mono-/combotherapy; prevents postprandial blood glucose surge	Flatulence, bloating, diarrhea, abdominal pain	• Do not give with digestive enzymes
Amylinomimetic			
Pramlintide* (Symlin)	Type 2 diabetes, Type 1 adjunct, supplements amylin hormone	Headache, nausea, anorexia	• Monitor for severe hypoglycemia • Do not mix with insulin

DRUG THERAPY TABLE 51.1 Antidiabetic Agents (Other Than Insulins) (*continued*)

Category and Common Generic (Brand) Drugs	Intended Use	Common Side Effects	Safety Warnings for Nurses
Sulfonylureas			
Third generation— glimepiride (Amaryl)	Type 2 diabetes mono-/combotherapy, stimulates pancreas beta cells to release insulin	Nausea, weight gain, headache, epigastric discomfort, heartburn	• Monitor for hypoglycemia • Produces weight gain
Second generation— glipizide (Glucotrol) glyburide (DiaBeta, Glynase) *First generation—* chlorpropamide (Diabinese)	Type 2 diabetes monotherapy		
Meglitinides			
Nateglinide (Starlix) Repaglinide (Prandin)	Type 2 diabetes mono-/combotherapy; stimulates pancreas beta cells to release insulin	Respiratory tract infection, headache	• Monitor for hypoglycemia in debilitated or older clients
Antidiabetic combination drugs used for type 2 diabetes			
Metformin based Metformin/canagliflozin (Invokamet) Metformin/dapagliflozin (Xiqduo XR) Metformin/empagliflozin (Synjardy) Metformin/linagliptin (Jentadueto) Metformin/saxagliptin (Kombiglyze) Metformin/sitagliptin (Janumet) Metformin/alogiptin (Kazano) Metformin/glyburide (Glucovance) Metformin/glipizide Metformin/rosiglitazone (Avandamet) Metformin/pioglitazone (Actoplus) Metformin/repaglinide (Prandimet) Alogliptin/pioglitazone (Oseni) Lingliptin/empagliflozin (Glyxambi) Pioglitazone/glimepiride (Duetact) Rosiglitazone/glimepiride (Avandaryl) Sitagliptin/metformin (Janumet)			

*Parenteral drug, comes in the form of a single injection pen
BMI, body mass index.
The drugs in column 1 indicate the drug that matches up with explanations in columns 2 through 4.

include rosiglitazone (Avandia) and pioglitazone (Actos), and are categorized as "insulin sensitizers"—they help tissues use available insulin more efficiently. Metformin does not promote weight gain like the sulfonylureas, and it does not trigger low blood glucose levels. It may, however, cause upset stomach, flatulence, and diarrhea, and it is associated with a small risk of lactic acidosis. TZDs, on the other hand, are known to cause weight gain, edema, and liver damage; heart failure; heart attacks; and bladder cancer; anyone taking a TZD should have liver function tests performed every 2 months during the first year of treatment. Troglitazone (Rezulin), the first developed TZD, was withdrawn from the market after its initial approval because several deaths were related to its use.

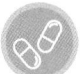

Pharmacologic Considerations

■ Oral hypoglycemic drugs may be used in conjunction with insulin therapy in some clients with insulin-dependent diabetes; this reduces the insulin requirements and decreases the incidence of hypoglycemic reactions.

Mitochondrial Target of TZD Modulators. A new class of insulin sensitizers known as mitochondrial target of TZDs (mTOTs) is not available yet. This class of drugs is intended to be an alternative to TZDs such as Actos and the now restricted-use drug, Avandia, both of which carry black box warnings. Developers of mTOTs report that the drugs have less serious side effects than TZDs because they target a different molecular mechanism for lowering plasma glucose and have less potential for causing peripheral edema and heart failure like other TZDs. The results of research with mTOTs indicate that the normal metabolism of carbohydrates is reestablished, insulin resistance is reduced, the production of calorie-burning brown fat is increased, the function of pancreatic beta cells is preserved, and, possibly, neurons in the brain are protected (Chen et al., 2017).

Alpha-Glucosidase Inhibitors. Alpha-glucosidase inhibitors include drugs such as miglitol (Glyset) and acarbose (Precose). Alpha-glucosidase is an intestinal enzyme that breaks down complex carbohydrates into glucose, a simple sugar. When this enzyme is inhibited, the process of forming glucose is slowed and glucose is absorbed more slowly from the small intestine. Consequently, blood glucose is balanced with the body's available insulin. Drugs in this category must be taken 15 minutes before each meal. They are most effective in reducing postprandial (after a meal) hyperglycemia. Occasionally, clients with type 1 diabetes take both insulin and an alpha-glucosidase inhibitor because this category of drug tends to equalize blood glucose levels and prevents swings between hyperglycemia and hypoglycemia.

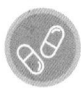

Pharmacologic Considerations

- Risk for lactic acidosis, a subtype of metabolic acidosis from an accumulation of lactate, has occurred among those taking a biguanide such as metformin (Glucophage). The risk is greater with decreased kidney function. Symptoms include malaise, abdominal or muscular pain, short or rapid breathing.

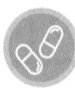

Pharmacologic Considerations

- Women specifically are at an increased risk for upper limb bone fractures when taking rosiglitazone or pioglitazone (TZDs). This risk falls dramatically when the medications are stopped (Mohn et al., 2018).

Unfortunately, a person who develops hypoglycemia while taking an alpha-glucosidase inhibitor cannot respond to one of the first lines of treatment, which is drinking fruit juice, because the drug interferes with the conversion of fructose in the juice to glucose. In this case, the better treatment is to give glucose either in tablets or by injection because glucose requires no further breakdown for absorption.

GLP-1 Receptor Agonists. Pramlintide (Symlin) and exenatide (Byetta) are GLP-1 agonists known as *secretagogues*, hormones that stimulate the secretion of another substance, in this case, insulin. They are used along with traditional drugs for managing diabetes. Pramlintide is similar to *amylin*, a hormone that is secreted by the beta cells of the pancreas. Amylin lowers blood sugar after meals and causes a sense of satiety that controls overeating. Exenatide mimics *incretin*, a hormone released from cells that line the ileum and colon. Incretin promotes the secretion of insulin and improves the metabolism of carbohydrates. When combined with other diabetic agents, both pramlintide and exenatide regulate blood sugar more effectively and result in weight loss, an advantage over medications that affect only insulin levels. Until 2012, the disadvantage of these adjuvant drugs was that they required multiple daily injections. A new long-acting injection now has been developed. Bydureon, an extended-release injectable suspension of exenatide, allows type 2 diabetics to achieve glycemic control with just one dose per week.

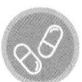

Pharmacologic Considerations

- Injectable incretin hormones increase insulin production, slow gastric emptying, and inhibit glucagon release. These hormones should not be confused with insulin products nor be mixed with insulin or any other drug in a syringe for injection.

DPP-4 Inhibitors (Gliptins). DPP-4 is an enzyme that destroys incretin, a hormone released after eating that promotes the secretion of insulin. By inhibiting DPP-4 with drugs known as gliptins such as sitagliptin (Januvia) and saxagliptin (Onglyza), they sustain insulin levels subsequently lowering blood sugar. These drugs also reduce glucagon, delay gastric emptying, and promote satiety (feeling of fullness). DPP-4 inhibitors are used as monotherapy or combined with metformin. Side and adverse effects include headache, hypoglycemia, dizziness, cough, peripheral edema, hypertension, acute pancreatitis, and urticaria. The U.S. FDA (2015a) issued a warning that this group of drugs may cause severe and disabling joint pain and required the information added to the drug label.

SGLT2 Inhibitors. The newest category of drugs used to manage type 2 diabetes is SGLT2 inhibitors which include canagliflozin (Invokana), dapagliflozin (Farxiga), and empagliflozin (Jardiance). SGLT2 is responsible for reabsorbing glucose from the urine back into the blood. Inhibiting SGLT2 causes increased excretion of glucose, thereby lowering blood glucose levels. Unfortunately, glycosuria can lead to urinary tract and genital infections in both men and women. Other possible side effects include elevated serum potassium, cholesterol, hypoglycemia, and postural hypotension. Recently, the U.S. FDA (2015b) has warned that taking this drug may lead to ketoacidosis.

>>> *Stop, Think, and Respond 51-3*

Name at least one oral antidiabetic agent in each of the following categories: (1) promotes release of insulin, (2) enhances response to insulin (insulin sensitizer), and (3) slows the breakdown of complex carbohydrates.

Bariatric Surgery

Bariatric surgery, operative procedures on the stomach and small intestine for the purpose of achieving weight loss (see Chapter 70), is an option for some clients with type 2 diabetes. National Institute of Diabetes and Digestive and Kidney Diseases (NIDDK, 2020) recommends that it should only be considered by individuals who are severely obese with a body mass index >35 kg/m^2 with uncontrolled hyperglycemia despite medical treatment, and cardiovascular risks such as dyslipidemia, sleep apnea, and joint problems. Successful outcomes include complete resolution of type 2 diabetes or an improvement in glycemic control. Disadvantages of bariatric surgery include vitamin and mineral deficiencies, osteoporosis, and dumping syndrome. Those considering bariatric surgery are encouraged to select surgeons and institutions that perform this type of surgery on a high-volume basis. A surgeon, cardiologist, endocrinologist, psychiatrist, and nutritionist make up a comprehensive team involved in the preoperative and postoperative care of a client undergoing bariatric surgery.

Pancreas Transplantation

Replacing the pancreas involves a whole or partial organ transplant (Fig. 51-10). The usual candidate is a client with type 1 diabetes who has renal failure and will benefit from a combined kidney and pancreas transplant. Clients with type 2 diabetes are not offered the option of a pancreas transplant because usually their problem is insulin resistance, which does not improve with a transplant.

Because the pancreas is both an exocrine and endocrine gland, transplanting it requires a means for exocrine enzymatic drainage and venous absorption of insulin. Exocrine drainage is accomplished by establishing a duodenal or urinary bladder connection with the transplanted pancreas. Insulin is released into the portal vein, which carries blood to the liver. Although bladder connections have a lower incidence of organ rejection, they also tend to cause urologic complications and are used less often than originally.

As with any transplant, lifelong immunosuppressive drug therapy is required because without it, the new organ is destroyed. Because type 1 diabetes can be managed with insulin, many experts believe that the risks involved with immunosuppression outweigh the benefit that can be achieved with a pancreas transplant, unless a kidney transplant also is necessary.

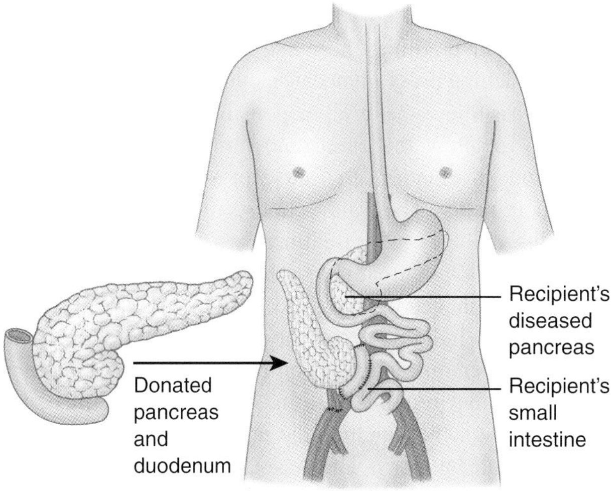

Figure 51-10 The donated pancreas is inserted in the abdomen and connected to local blood vessels. The nonfunctioning pancreas is left in place. The portion of donor duodenum is attached to the recipient's intestine or bladder to facilitate a pathway for pancreatic digestive enzymes.

Islet Cell Transplantation

Some clients with type 1 diabetes are recipients of islet cell transplants, the insulin-producing components of the pancreas, rather than a transplant of the entire organ or part of the organ (Fig. 51-11). One human organ donor pancreas, but more often two, or a portion of the pancreas from a living donor is necessary to obtain sufficient numbers of islet cells for transplantation. The fragile islet cells must be transplanted soon after removal (NIDDK, 2018).

After the pancreas is harvested, the islet cells are separated from the tissue and injected through the abdominal wall into the client's portal vein, where they migrate to the liver and begin to release insulin. The bone marrow, spleen, and the liver are being used as alternate transplant sites (Addison et al., 2020).

Presently, islet cell transplantation surgeons use a combination of tacrolimus (Prograf), sirolimus (Rapamune), and daclizumab (Zenapax) to prevent rejection. The current practice is to avoid using a steroid with other immunosuppressive drugs because steroids raise the blood glucose to levels that the new islet cells have difficulty overcoming. However, progress is being made to prevent rejection and avoid lifelong immunosuppression by encapsulating the islet cells in a subcutaneously implanted chamber that acts as an immunobarrier (Gamble et al., 2018).

Transplanted islet cells tend to lose their ability to function over time, and approximately 70% of recipients resume insulin administration within 2 years. However, the amount of insulin and the frequency of its administration are reduced because of improved control of blood glucose levels.

Nursing Management

The nurse obtains a complete medical, drug, and allergy history, including a list of all symptoms and their duration. They determine when the client was diagnosed with diabetes and if others in the family also are diabetic. If the client is a diagnosed diabetic, the nurse asks the client to identify their prescribed treatment regimen and when they last consumed food and self-administered medications. The nurse weighs the client and performs a complete head-to-toe physical examination because diabetes affects many systems. The nurse looks for physical changes associated with diabetes:

- Changes in the skin over insulin injection sites, impaired skin areas that appear to be healing poorly, ulcerations or evidence of skin or soft-tissue infection
- Vital signs, peripheral pulses, temperature of the extremities, inspection of the extremities for edema or changes in color

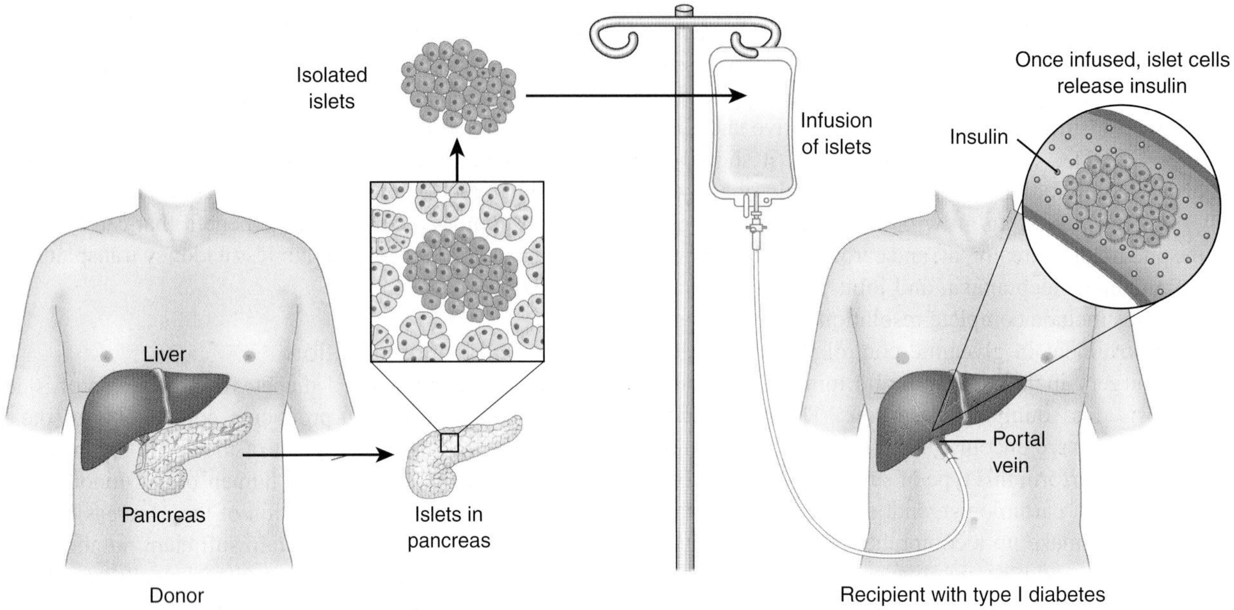

Figure 51-11 Pancreatic cells are extracted from the donor organ. The islet cells are isolated and injected into the portal vein of the recipient, where they begin to secrete insulin.

- Decreased visual acuity and visual changes such as blurred vision
- Muscle atrophy, weakness, or loss of sensation

The nurse monitors the client's blood glucose level before meals and at bedtime. It is also necessary to monitor postprandial blood sugar for the client on tight glucose control. The nurse tests the urine for ketones if the blood glucose level is high. They administer prescribed medications and evaluates the client's response to their effects. If hypoglycemia develops, the nurse uses the **rule of 15**: give 15 g of rapidly absorbed carbohydrate (Box 51-3), wait 15 minutes, recheck the blood sugar, and administer another 15 g of glucose if the blood sugar is not above 70 mg/dL. See Nursing Care Plan 51-1 for information about managing a client with diabetes mellitus.

The nurse initiates or reinforces information the client must know to manage their condition independently. They refer the client to a diabetic educator if one is available; consultation with a dietitian may be appropriate. The extent of the teaching program depends on whether the client has been diabetic for some time or is newly diagnosed; even those who have had the disorder for years may have inaccurate ideas about their disorder and treatment regimen. Before teaching begins, the nurse confers with the primary provider regarding the following:

- Type of diet for the client to follow
- Medication regimen (insulin, oral antidiabetic agents, adjuvant medications, or some combination)
- Materials for insulin administration, such as needle and syringe, insulin pen, insulin jet injector, or insulin pump
- Technique for monitoring blood glucose levels, self-testing devices (glucometer), and the suggested brand to use
- Materials for and frequency of urine testing
- Additional information such as skin care, signs of diabetic ketoacidosis (DKA), HHNKS, and hypoglycemia (discussed later)

Whenever possible, the nurse includes the family in a diabetic teaching program because one or more family members may assume some or all responsibility for the treatment regimen. To allow the client and family member time to understand information, the nurse presents the material in small increments. They may choose to begin teaching by explaining diabetes, why treatments are necessary, and the various methods of treatment. The nurse uses audiovisual materials to enhance learning. Because the treatment of diabetes is highly individualized, they emphasize that the treatment of one person cannot be compared with that of another.

If the client requires insulin, the nurse identifies sites for injections, which include the upper arms, upper thighs, abdomen, and buttocks. The Association of Diabetes Care & Education Specialists (2020) advocates rotating insulin injections in an anatomic injection site—not site to site—to ensure consistent rates of absorption. Abdominal injections are absorbed most quickly followed by the arms, thighs, and buttocks and have the least rate variability.

BOX 51-3 Examples of 15 g of Rapidly Absorbed Carbohydrate

3 to 4 glucose tablets
1 small tube of glucose gel
½ cup fruit juice or regular soft drink
1 tbsp honey or syrup
1 tbsp of sugar or 5 small sugar cubes
2 tbsp raisins
6 to 8 LifeSavers candies
8 oz of skim or 1% milk

If the primary provider has recommended the use of a glucometer to monitor blood glucose levels, the nurse allows time for the client to use the glucometer and monitor their own blood glucose levels. Additional teaching topics include the following:

- Signs and symptoms of hyperglycemia and hypoglycemia
- The importance of weight reduction, if necessary
- Methods of terminating hypoglycemia with a rapidly absorbed carbohydrate, such as food or beverage sources, glucose tablets, or glucose gel
- Problems that require contacting the primary provider, such as skin infection, pain in the extremities, visual problems, change in color or temperature of the skin of the extremities, frequent episodes of hypoglycemia, prolonged nausea and vomiting, and illness
- The importance of following an exercise regimen suggested by the primary provider. The nurse stresses that during exercise, the client needs to have some food or other primary provider-approved form of glucose if symptoms of hypoglycemia occur. This is especially important for clients taking insulin or those subject to episodes of hypoglycemia while taking an oral antidiabetic agent.
- How to integrate the dietary exchange list throughout the day
- The information that is printed on food labels to promote compliance with the prescribed diet
- The definitions of products labeled as "low calorie" and "dietetic," and that these terms are not synonymous with "no sugar." They may contain sugar.
- The importance of drinking adequate water, especially in warm weather, when exercising and when perspiring
- Foot care
- The necessity for regular appointments with an ophthalmologist for comprehensive eye examinations
- The need to consult the primary provider regarding dosage adjustments for insulin or oral antidiabetic agent if the client becomes ill or cannot eat

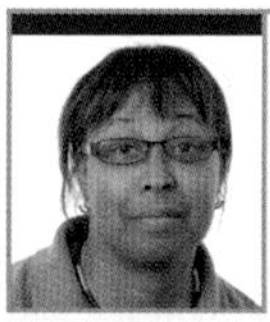

Clinical Scenario Prior to a routine physical examination, laboratory blood work indicated that a 48-year-old woman had an elevated fasting blood sugar. She indicated to the primary provider that she has been losing weight despite eating more food, has been thirsty, and has been urinating more frequently. An oral glucose tolerance test confirms that the client has type 2 diabetes. **What problems should the nurse identify and manage as priorities in this client's care? Refer Nursing Care Plan 51-1 for examples.**

NURSING CARE PLAN 51-1 The Client With Diabetes Mellitus

Assessment

Determine the following:

- Evidence of polyuria, polydipsia, and polyphagia
- Current weight; recent weight changes
- Vital signs, especially BP in lying, sitting, and standing positions
- Blood glucose level before each meal and at bedtime
- Any ketones or albumin in the urine
- Serum electrolyte, cholesterol, lipid, triglyceride, blood urea nitrogen, and creatinine levels
- Condition of the skin and feet
- Any abnormal sensations such as pain, tingling, burning, and numbness
- Visual acuity and last date of ophthalmic examination
- Knowledge of therapeutic management

Nursing Diagnosis. **Malnutrition Risk** related to the body's need for an alternate nutrient for energy, altered satiety, decreased activity, and habituation of preillness eating habits

Expected Outcome. Client will adhere to a prescribed calorie-controlled diet.

Interventions	Rationales
Provide three meals and snacks within prescribed caloric limits.	*Restriction of calories promotes weight loss and balances glucose with naturally produced or parenterally administered insulin.*
Suggest free foods such as up to 1 cup of raw vegetables like salad greens and sugar-free gelatin, unlimited sugar-free drinks, or low-sodium bouillon if the client becomes hungry between meals or snacks.	*Free foods contain fewer than 20 calories/serving; their consumption provides negligible calories.*
Encourage client to drink 8 oz of water before eating a meal.	*Water is calorie-free, distends the stomach, and provides a feeling of fullness.*
Advise client to eat slowly and wait 15 seconds between chewing thoroughly, swallowing, and taking the next bite.	*Slowed eating prolongs the pleasure of eating and allows time for the brain to sense satiation.*

Evaluation of Expected Outcome

Client follows and eats the prescribed diet and verbalizes understanding of restrictions and allowances.

(continued)

NURSING CARE PLAN 51-1 The Client With Diabetes Mellitus (*continued*)

Nursing Diagnosis. **Hypoglycemia Risk** related to inadequate monitoring of blood glucose levels, increased insulin administration, overcalculating carbohydrate intake

Expected Outcome. The nurse will monitor for, manage, and minimize hypoglycemia.

Interventions	Rationales
Test capillary blood glucose level with a glucometer 30 minutes before each meal and at bedtime.	*Hypoglycemia is more likely before the client consumes food.*
Monitor for signs of hypoglycemia such as shakiness, diaphoresis, hunger, and disturbed cognition.	*Low blood glucose level causes physiologic stimulation and diminishes the ability to think clearly.*
Follow agency policy for administering a quick-acting source of simple carbohydrate to lower the limit of blood glucose level	*Simple carbohydrates are absorbed quickly and tend to raise the blood glucose level within 15 minutes to eliminate the symptoms of hypoglycemia.*
Recheck the capillary blood glucose level 15 minutes after treating a hypoglycemic episode.	*Rechecking the level helps determine the client's response to the nursing intervention.*
Repeat the administration of simple carbohydrate if the client continues to be symptomatic; reassess capillary blood glucose level.	*The client may need additional simple carbohydrate to successfully raise blood glucose.*
Notify the primary provider if the client's symptoms continue after two attempts to raise the blood sugar with oral substances.	*Parenteral interventions to raise the blood glucose level are medically prescribed.*
Offer client complex carbohydrates when hypoglycemia is controlled.	*Complex carbohydrates are digested and absorbed more slowly than simple carbohydrates, which reduces the potential for another hypoglycemic episode.*
Withhold insulin when the client must fast before laboratory or diagnostic procedures.	*Eating and administration of insulin are timed according to insulin's onset, peak, and duration of action.*
Ask a second nurse to double-check the vial of insulin and the number of units in the syringe before administering the injection.	*Double-checking helps avoid errors in insulin administration. Giving more than the prescribed amount or mistaking rapid-acting or short-acting insulin for intermediate- or long-acting insulin can cause hypoglycemia.*

Evaluation of Expected Outcome

Client's blood sugar is at least 70 mg/dL.

Nursing Diagnosis. **Hypoglycemia Risk** related to inadequate monitoring of blood glucose levels, increased insulin administration, undercalculating carbohydrate intake

Expected Outcome. The nurse will monitor for, manage, and minimize hyperglycemia.

Interventions	Rationales
Monitor capillary blood glucose levels before each meal and at bedtime; check urine for ketones if glucose levels are elevated.	*Elevated blood glucose level before a client eats suggests that they are not compliant with the diet and may require a higher dose of an oral antidiabetic agent or coverage with rapid-acting or short-acting insulin. Ketonuria increases the potential for DKA.*
Assess for clinical signs and symptoms of hyperglycemia such as thirst, increased urination, and sleepiness.	*Hyperglycemia has a gradual onset with symptoms similar to the undiagnosed state; hyperglycemia can progress to DKA or HHNKS.*
Administer insulin or oral antidiabetic agents as prescribed.	*Insufficient insulin results in elevated blood glucose level.*
Implement medical orders for insulin administration according to a sliding scale established by the primary provider.	*Insulin lowers blood glucose level.*
Notify the primary provider if the client with hyperglycemia is noninsulin-dependent.	*Modifications in the diet or changes in antidiabetic medications are medically prescribed.*
Reinforce the importance of compliance with the prescribed diet, exercise, and medication regimen.	*These measures manage hyperglycemia.*

NURSING CARE PLAN 51-1 The Client With Diabetes Mellitus (*continued*)

Evaluation of Expected Outcome

Blood glucose levels are within 80–120 mg/dL in a nonfasting state.

Nursing Diagnosis. **Hypovolemia** related to hyperglycemia and polyuria

Expected Outcome. Client will maintain proper fluid balance.

Interventions	Rationales
Monitor intake and output.	*A deficit in fluid intake or excess urine output suggests a deficit in fluid volume.*
Provide at least 1500–3000 mL of fluid/day.	*The average fluid requirement/24 hours is 1500–3000 mL.*

Evaluation of Expected Outcome

Client is well hydrated as evidenced by a fluid intake of between 1500 and 3000 mL with similar urine output.

Nursing Diagnosis. **Injury Risk** related to orthostatic hypotension and impaired vision secondary to neuropathy and retinopathy

Expected Outcome. Client will be free from injury.

Interventions	Rationales
Assist client when rising from a sitting or lying position.	*Autonomic neuropathy causes orthostatic hypotension and the potential for fainting and falling.*
Have the client dangle on the side of the bed before ambulating.	*Dangling allows a period during which blood flow is restored to the brain.*
Keep the floor dry and the environment free of clutter.	*Retinopathy may interfere with the client's ability to see potential safety hazards.*

Evaluation of Expected Outcome

There is no evidence of trauma.

Nursing Diagnosis. **Altered Skin Integrity Risk** related to loss of sensation in feet and impaired blood circulation

Expected Outcome. Skin will remain intact.

Interventions	Rationales
Examine skin and feet daily.	*Client may be insensitive to injuries and slow to heal because of peripheral neuropathy and vascular disturbances.*
Assess skin for signs of breakdown, poor healing, change in color or temperature, or infection.	*Impaired blood supply compromises the integrity of the integument.*
Dry client's skin well after bathing, especially in areas of the body that are dark and moist.	*Fungal infections are common in creases and folds of skin.*
Rotate insulin injection sites; give each injection ½ to 1 inch away from the previous injection.	*Rotating injection sites prevents lipoatrophy and lipohypertrophy.*
Inspect inside the client's shoes for foreign objects or disrepair.	*Friction or pressure can impair the integrity of the feet.*
Provide foot care with daily hygiene.	*Care of the feet prevents injury and skin breakdown.*

Evaluation of Expected Outcome

Skin is warm, dry, and intact, with no evidence of tissue breakdown in the feet.

Nursing Diagnosis. **Altered Health Maintenance** related to complexity of therapeutic regimen

Expected Outcome. Client will verbalize and demonstrate knowledge of diabetes and self-management techniques.

(*continued*)

NURSING CARE PLAN 51-1 The Client With Diabetes Mellitus (*continued*)

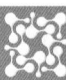

Interventions	Rationales
Assess client's ability and willingness to learn about diabetes and self-management.	*Teaching is more effective when the learner is capable and motivated to acquire information.*
Teach client about oral medications and/or insulin, and how to self-administer using proper technique.	*Clients learn in various ways: verbal explanations, reading information, seeing a demonstration, or using a hands-on application.*
Allow client opportunities to practice administering insulin.	*Practice promotes self-confidence and develops expertise.*
Show client how to monitor blood glucose using a glucometer.	*Using the same method as the client will use after discharge increases knowledgeable self-management.*
Arrange for the dietitian to teach client about their nutrition therapy.	*Dietitians are experts in nutrition therapy.*
Review the importance of exercise and methods for daily activity.	*Exercise reduces blood glucose level, helps with weight loss, and improves circulation.*

Evaluation of Expected Outcome

Client demonstrates knowledge and skills to independently manage their disease.

ACUTE COMPLICATIONS OF DIABETES MELLITUS

Some clients, despite careful control of their disease, develop one or more serious complications over time. Some complications can be controlled when detected in the early stages.

Diabetic Ketoacidosis

Diabetic ketoacidosis (DKA), a type of potentially life-threatening metabolic acidosis, occurs when there is an accumulation of ketones, a product of fat metabolism when cells cannot utilize glucose for energy. It occurs as a consequence of an acute insulin deficiency or an inability to use whatever insulin the pancreas secretes. DKA is sometimes the event that leads to an initial diagnosis of diabetes.

Pathophysiology and Etiology

DKA can develop despite the client's adherence to the prescribed treatment regimen. Clients who develop DKA often have a severe, hard-to-control form of the disease (brittle or unstable diabetes). Occasionally, a client admitted to the hospital in DKA has undiagnosed diabetes. Other causes of this serious event are infection and nonadherence to the treatment regimen. (See the discussion of ketoacidosis under Pathophysiology and Etiology of diabetes mellitus.)

When the amount of glucose transported across cell membranes decreases, the liver increases its production of glucose. The blood glucose level becomes extremely elevated. The kidneys attempt to excrete the glucose, which is well beyond the renal threshold. In the process, excessive amounts of water, sodium, and potassium are excreted as well. The client becomes dehydrated; the skin is warm, dry, and flushed. Stored fat is broken down, causing ketones to accumulate in the blood and urine. As ketones mount, the pH of the blood becomes acidic. The client begins breathing rapidly and deeply in an attempt to eliminate carbon dioxide and prevent it from forming carbonic acid, which would contribute even more to the acidotic state. If the condition is severe and prolonged, the client becomes comatose. Death results from untreated or ineffective treatment of DKA.

Assessment Findings

Early symptoms are vague and become more definite and serious as increasing ketones accumulate in the bloodstream. Weakness, thirst, anorexia, vomiting, drowsiness, and abdominal pain develop. The cheeks are flushed, and the skin and mouth are dry. The breath has an odor of acetone. Kussmaul sign often is evident. The pulse is rapid and weak. The BP is low. The client may become unresponsive but restless. Blood glucose levels are elevated to 300 to 1000 mg/dL or more. Urine contains glucose and ketones. The blood pH ranges from 6.8 to 7.3. The serum bicarbonate level is decreased to levels from 0 to 15 mEq/L. The compensatory breathing pattern can lower the partial pressure of carbon dioxide in arterial blood ($PaCO_2$) which is normally 35 to 45 mm Hg to levels of 10 to 30 mm Hg. Serum sodium and potassium levels reflect the degree of dehydration (i.e., they may be elevated because they are concentrated in a low volume of body fluid); however, intracellular levels are low, but they are unmeasurable.

Medical Management

Treatment depends on the severity of DKA. The main goals of treatment are to (1) reduce the elevated blood glucose, (2) correct fluid and electrolyte imbalances, and (3) clear the urine and blood of ketones. To accomplish these goals, insulin is given IV. Insulin reduces the production of ketones by making glucose available for oxidation by the tissues and by restoring the liver's supply of glycogen. Regular insulin is added to an IV solution and infused continuously. The amount of insulin and the rate of infusion depend on the blood glucose levels, but the rate may be in the range of 5 units/hour. Isotonic fluid is instilled at a high volume, for example, 250 to 500 mL/hour for several hours. The rate is adjusted once the client becomes rehydrated and diuresis is less acute. As insulin begins to lower the blood glucose level, the IV solution is changed to include one with glucose. This helps to avoid the potential for hypoglycemia. Potassium replacements are given despite elevated serum levels to raise intracellular stores. Periodic monitoring of serum electrolytes and blood glucose levels is necessary. The urine is tested for glucose and ketones.

Nursing Management

The nurse monitors IV infusions closely and takes vital signs frequently. Older adults and those with cardiopulmonary or renal disorders are prone to fluid overload. The nurse inserts an indwelling urinary catheter and monitors urine output to ensure that replaced potassium has a means for excretion. Besides checking serum electrolyte findings, the nurse attaches cardiac leads and observes the client's heart conduction pattern to detect evidence of hyperkalemia such as peaked T waves and bradycardia. Blood glucose level is measured frequently; the urine is similarly checked for the presence of ketones. They keep the primary provider informed of the client's response, or lack of response, to therapy. See Nursing Care Plan 51-1 for additional nursing care.

Hyperosmolar Hyperglycemic Nonketotic Syndrome

HHNKS, an acute complication of diabetes, is characterized by hyperglycemia without ketosis. It is not unusual to find the blood glucose level well over 500 mg/dL, but the pH of the blood remains within the normal range of 7.35 to 7.45. Fluid and electrolyte imbalances accompany HHNKS.

Pathophysiology and Etiology

HHNKS often results from a serious illness during which metabolic needs exceed the limits of available insulin. Because of persistent hyperglycemia, fluid moves from the intracellular compartment to the extracellular compartment. Diuresis occurs with a subsequent loss of sodium and potassium. Because the client still is secreting some insulin, which can transport glucose in the cells, fat metabolism is minimal or unaffected; hence, ketosis does not develop. HHNKS is more common in undiagnosed or older clients with type 2 diabetes. It also occurs among clients who do not have diabetes who receive drugs that elevate blood glucose, or who require kidney dialysis or TPN.

Assessment Findings

Hypotension, mental changes, extreme thirst, dehydration, tachycardia, and fever develop. Neurologic signs include paralysis, lethargy, coma, and seizures. Symptoms of hypokalemia and hyponatremia usually are present. Physical examination reveals dry mucous membranes and poor skin turgor. Blood glucose levels are exceedingly high, and serum potassium and sodium levels are low. The serum osmolarity is increased.

Medical Management

Treatment includes the administration of insulin and correction of fluid and electrolyte imbalances. A central catheter may be used to monitor the client's hemodynamic response to fluid replacement.

Nursing Management

The nurse measures the client's blood glucose level and assesses for electrolyte imbalances and dehydration. They implement medical orders for insulin, fluids, and electrolyte replacement and closely monitors the client's response to treatment. The nurse's priority areas for evaluation include hydration status, intake and output, skin turgor, vital signs, and electrolyte studies. The nurse observes the client's neurologic and cognitive symptoms; cognition may be significantly impaired in the early stages of care. The nurse protects the client's safety if cognition is impaired and judgment is poor. Additional management depends on symptoms (see Nursing Care Plan 51-1).

Hypoglycemia

Hypoglycemia, a low blood glucose level, is always a potential adverse reaction when administering medications for diabetes.

Pathophysiology and Etiology

When too much insulin is in the bloodstream relative to the amount of available glucose, hypoglycemia occurs. The blood glucose level falls below 70 mg/dL. Because glucose is the primary source of cellular energy, especially for the brain, hypoglycemia tends to manifest in neurologic changes such as confusion, difficulty processing information, anxious feelings, emotional irritability, and headache. The client feels hungry, a homeostatic mechanism to stimulate eating. If the condition is untreated, seizures, permanent brain damage, or death can rapidly occur.

Hypoglycemia occurs when a client with diabetes is (1) not eating at all and continues to take insulin or oral antidiabetic medications, (2) not eating sufficient calories to compensate for glucose-lowering medications, or (3) exercising more than usual, which lowers available blood glucose. Alcohol consumption also interferes with the liver's ability to synthesize glucose from noncarbohydrates, placing clients with diabetes who drink at higher risk for hypoglycemia; the effect may persist for up to 24 hours (American Diabetes Association, 2021a).

Assessment Findings

Signs and Symptoms

The pattern of symptoms varies somewhat depending on the degree of hypoglycemia, the individual reaction, and the type of insulin taken. Initial symptoms include tachycardia, weakness, headache, nausea, drowsiness, nervousness, hunger, tremors, malaise, and excessive perspiration. Some clients have characteristic personality or behavioral changes. Confusion and dizziness can occur. If hypoglycemia is not

TABLE 51-4 Characteristics of Hyperglycemia and Hypoglycemia

CHARACTERISTIC	HYPERGLYCEMIA	HYPOGLYCEMIA
Predisposing factors	Insufficient or omitted insulin	Excessive insulin
	Concurrent infection	Unusual exercise
	Dietary indiscretion	Too little food
Onset	Slow; hours to days	Sudden; minutes
Mental status	Drowsy	Disoriented; eventually becomes comatose
Skin	Flushed, dry, hot	Pale, moist, cool
Blood pressure	Low	Normal
Pulse	Rapid, weak	Normal or slow, bounding
Respiration	Air hunger	Normal to rapid, shallow
Hunger	Absent	Often present
Thirst	Present	Absent
Vomiting	Present	Maybe absent
Urine glucose	Present in large amounts	Absent in second voided specimen
Response to treatment	Slow	Rapid

corrected, symptoms can progress to difficulty with coordination. The client may complain of double vision. If left untreated, unconsciousness and seizures can develop.

Although symptoms vary, each client tends to have a uniquely repetitious pattern when hypoglycemia develops. The manifestation of hypoglycemic symptoms usually is quite rapid, with unconsciousness or seizures occurring shortly after onset.

When a client with diabetes is found unconscious, DKA or hypoglycemia needs to be ruled out. These conditions are direct opposites: In ketoacidosis, the blood glucose level is high; in hypoglycemia, it is low. The nurse and client must be familiar with the symptoms of hypoglycemia and hyperglycemia to recognize and differentiate the complication as it is developing and treat it appropriately (Table 51-4).

Diagnostic Findings

Diagnosis is based on symptoms, client history, and blood glucose levels. The history is important in differentiating between DKA and hypoglycemia. If the client had insulin or oral antidiabetic drugs, especially those that are insulin releasers like the sulfonylureas, and has not eaten, it is most likely that hypoglycemia is present. If the client has eaten and has not taken or received insulin, DKA is more likely. Recognition of hypoglycemia must be immediate; therefore, a bedside glucometer test and sharp assessment skills are important.

Medical Management

The medical treatment for a hypoglycemic reaction is the administration of 15 g of simple carbohydrates as soon as possible. If the client is unconscious, glucose gel can be applied to the buccal cavity of the mouth. If the client does not respond after two administrations of rapidly absorbed carbohydrate, the primary provider may order glucagon, a hormone that stimulates the liver to release glycogen, or 20 to 50 mL of 50% glucose is prescribed for IV administration. Once the hypoglycemic symptoms are relieved, the client with diabetes is given complex carbohydrates such as graham crackers and milk to sustain and prolong an adequate level of blood glucose.

Nursing Management

If the client is conscious and can swallow, the nurse gives an oral form of rapidly absorbed carbohydrate. Whenever a client with diabetes mellitus is in a hospital unit, glucose tablets and quick-acting carbohydrates are stocked and available. In a severe reaction, the nurse may provide more than an initial offering of carbohydrates after monitoring the client's blood glucose level to evaluate the effect. If the symptoms do not abate and the blood glucose level remains low, the nurse collaborates with the primary provider concerning additional medical measures. The nurse implements medical orders for parenteral medications such as IV glucose or parenteral glucagon.

Above all, the nurse stays with the hypoglycemic client until the pronounced symptoms are corrected. When an episode of hypoglycemia occurs, the regulation of glucose metabolism may be tenuous for about 24 hours. The nurse observes the client at frequent intervals for further episodes of hypoglycemia.

The nurse can prevent hypoglycemia by:

- Ensuring that the meal is served within 15 minutes of administering rapid-acting insulin and within 30 minutes of giving short-acting insulin
- Ensuring that the client eats the prescribed diet and between-meal snacks
- Informing the primary provider immediately if nausea, vomiting, or diarrhea occur, or if the client refuses to eat
- Administering the correct type and dose of insulin at the prescribed times
- Asking a colleague to check the label on the insulin vial and the number of units in the insulin syringe against that which is ordered before administering insulin to avoid a medication error

Additional nursing management of hypoglycemia depends on the symptoms presented (see Nursing Care Plan 51-1).

CHRONIC COMPLICATIONS OF DIABETES MELLITUS

Although clients with diabetes can develop many complications, extremely common ones include peripheral neuropathy, nephropathy, retinopathy, and vascular changes.

Peripheral Neuropathy

Neuropathy is a general term that refers to pathologic changes in nerves. Neuropathies in clients with diabetes can affect motor, sensory, and autonomic nerves. Neuropathies develop 10 or more years after the onset of diabetes, but the incidence increases with the duration. Because their onset is gradual, the client usually is oblivious to the development in the early stages.

Pathophysiology and Etiology

Neuropathy results from poor glucose control and decreased blood circulation to nerve tissue. Manifestations of peripheral neuropathies are more common among clients with diabetes who smoke and whose blood glucose level is poorly controlled. Because nitric acid dilates blood vessels, some believe that consistently elevated blood glucose levels lower nitric acid levels, impair circulation, and subsequently damage peripheral nerves. This may explain the development of erectile dysfunction in men with diabetes (see Chapter 55).

Motor Neuropathy

When motor nerves are affected, the muscles weaken and atrophy. Joint support is diminished. The feet widen. Eventually, bone structure is affected, resulting in skeletal deformities, usually in the feet and ankles, with subsequent changes in gait. Areas of skin and soft tissue that are subjected to friction and pressure are prone to ulcerate (Fig. 51-12). If there is infection or impaired healing, portions of the affected extremity may require amputation (see Chapter 61).

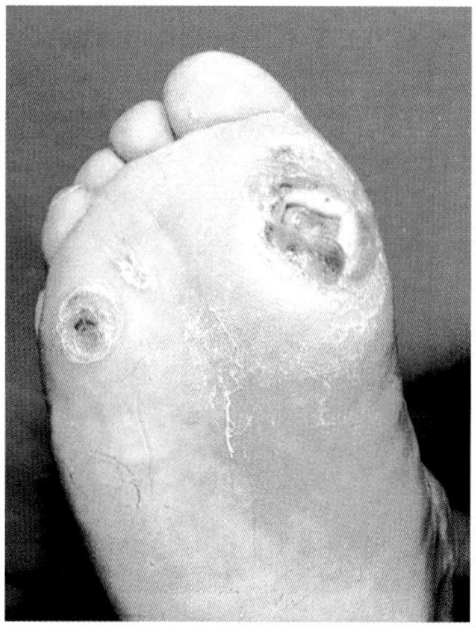

Figure 51-12 Neuropathic ulcers occur on pressure points in areas with diminished sensation in diabetic polyneuropathy. Pain is absent (and therefore, the ulcer may go unnoticed). (Reprinted with permission from Hinkle, J. L., & Cheever, K. H. (2014). *Brunner & Suddarth's textbook of medical-surgical nursing* (13th ed.). Wolters Kluwer Health/Lippincott Williams & Wilkins; Originally from Bates, B. B. (1995). *A guide to physical examination and history taking* (6th ed.). J.B. Lippincott.)

Sensory Neuropathy

Neuropathy involving sensory nerves leads to *paresthesias*, abnormal sensations such as prickling, tingling, burning, or needle-like pain in the feet, legs, and sometimes hands. In severe cases, feeling is totally lost. This lack of sensitivity increases the potential for soft tissue injury without the client's awareness.

Autonomic Neuropathy

Neuropathy of autonomic nerves that affect organ functioning has several consequences. *Gastroparesis*, atony of the stomach, retards the movement of food from the stomach. If nerves that innervate the bladder are affected, the client does not sense the urge to void, and retained urine supports bacterial growth, causing frequent urinary tract infections. Incontinence also may occur when the bladder is overfilled. As many as 50% of men with diabetes develop erectile dysfunction when nerves that promote erection become impaired (Dansinger, 2019b). When autonomic nerves that affect cardiovascular function fail to function effectively, episodes of orthostatic hypotension occur. Clients with diabetes often do not sense the chest pain of angina as acutely as those without diabetes, which delays or interferes with prompt assessment and treatment of coronary artery disease and myocardial infarction.

Assessment Findings

Signs and Symptoms

Pain is one of the leading symptoms that accompany motor and sensory nerve changes. Skeletal muscles in the extremities become smaller. The feet swell and become insensitive to temperature or other tactile stimuli. Disturbing sensations develop that often are intensified by maintaining a position for an extended period, such as occupational tasks that require standing in place, holding the steering wheel while driving, or performing a repetitive motion such as knitting. The client may report digestive, urinary, and sexual dysfunction and dizziness when rising.

Diagnostic Findings

A neurologic examination validates that when a tuning fork is in contact with the skin of the extremities, the client has diminished vibratory sense. Loss of protective sensation, the ability to sense and differentiate hot and cold, sharp and dull, and soft and rough stimuli, occurs. This is demonstrated with a screening test in which areas of the feet are touched with a nylon monofilament that delivers 10 g of force without the client's perception (Fig. 51-13). Electromyography studies demonstrate a slowed conduction of electrical stimulation along nerves (see Chapter 36).

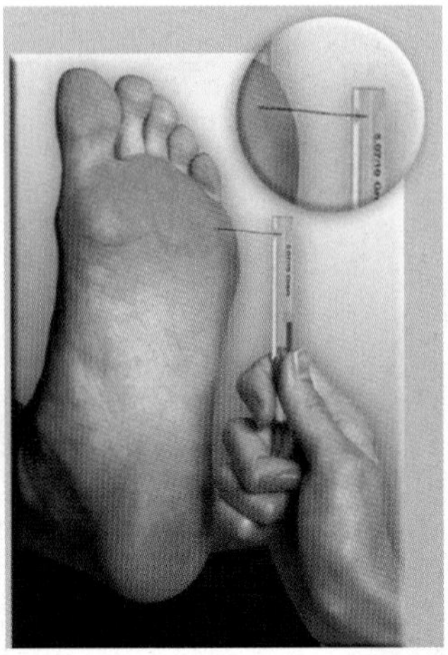

Figure 51-13 A strand of monofilament line is used to assess sensation in clients with diabetes. (Adapted with permission from Cameron, B. L. (2002). Making diabetes management routine: How Often do you and your patients screen for complications? *American Journal of Nursing, 102*(2), 26–32.)

Medical Management

Diet, exercise, and medication control blood glucose levels. Several medications can reduce pain, such as non-narcotic analgesics or a tricyclic antidepressant such as imipramine (Tofranil). Anticonvulsants such as pregabalin (Lyrica), gabapentin (Neurontin), or carbamazepine (Tegretol) also provide pain relief. Nonpharmacologic pain relief can be facilitated with transcutaneous electrical nerve stimulation. Elastic compression stockings; increasing dietary sodium; or using fludrocortisone (Florinef), which increases fluid volume, or an antihypotensive agent such as midodrine (Pro-Amatine) help reduce orthostatic hypotension. Small, frequent meals or administration of metoclopramide (Reglan) is recommended for the relief of symptoms associated with gastroparesis. Antibiotic therapy, increased oral fluid intake, and urinating every 3 hours help eliminate urinary tract infections. Various options are available for men who are concerned about erectile dysfunction (see Chapter 55).

Several pharmaceutical companies are developing drugs that might reverse diabetic neuropathies. Clinical trials include aldose reductase inhibitors (ARIs), which reduce the conversion of high blood glucose to sorbitol, known to damage nerve and renal cells, and insulin-like growth factor-1, a protein that promotes neural conduction and regrowth of nerve axons. Ranirestat, an ARI, has been shown to relieve diabetic sensory neuropathy, and it is considered a promising agent for the treatment of complications of diabetes, especially neuropathy (Asano et al., 2019). Anticonvulsants like pregabalin (Lyrica) and gabapentin (Neurontin) are also used to provide relief from pain associated with diabetic neuropathy affecting the feet.

Nursing Management

The nurse implements a teaching plan for the management of diabetes and its potential complications. If possible, the primary care nurse refers the client for classes with a diabetes educator. The nurse stresses foot care (Client and Family Teaching 51-1) and advises the client with peripheral autonomic neuropathy to rise slowly from a lying or sitting position, to drink generous fluids, and to wear knee-high or thigh-high elastic stockings during waking hours. The nurse emphasizes compliance with prescribed medications and warns the client to avoid taking more than the recommended doses of analgesics. For digestive problems, they explain that consuming a large volume of food at any one sitting and eating fatty foods delays stomach emptying. The nurse refers clients with erectile dysfunction to a urologist.

Client and Family Teaching 51-1 Foot Care in Diabetes

The nurse instructs the client and family as follows:

- Inspect the feet daily for blisters, corns, calluses, long or ingrown nails, or any reddened areas; use a mirror if necessary to visualize all aspects of the foot.
- Wash the feet daily in warm (not hot) water.
- Dry the feet thoroughly, being careful to dry between the toes.
- Keep toenails short and cut straight across.
- Apply a moisturizer to feet daily.
- Do not use razor, abrasive, or commercial products to remove corns or calluses.
- Use lamb's wool between toes that overlap.
- Wear well-fitting shoes that fit comfortably when first worn; do not wear rubber, plastic, or vinyl shoes that cause the feet to perspire. Consult primary provider about wearing sneakers or canvas shoes.
- Never go barefoot.
- Visit a podiatrist regularly for foot care.
- Wash, dry, and cover any injuries with sterile gauze and call health care provider immediately for evaluation.
- Notify the primary provider about a blister, abrasion, or foot injury.

Diabetic Nephropathy

Diabetic nephropathy refers to the progressive decrease in renal function that occurs with diabetes mellitus. Clients with type 1 diabetes are more likely to develop diabetic nephropathy, but clients with type 2 diabetes also are affected.

Pathophysiology and Etiology

Nephropathy is a consequence of glomerular deterioration resulting in impaired filtration of blood during urine formation (see Chapter 57). There are five stages of nephropathy, each characterized by a successive progression of renal dysfunction (Table 51-5). Essentially, the glomeruli excrete serum proteins, especially albumin, and lose their ability to excrete nitrogen waste products.

Poor glucose control contributes to the onset of nephropathy. Although hypertension is an eventual consequence of diabetic nephropathy, when it occurs in the prediabetic or prenephropathic state, it accelerates the onset and progression of renal damage. Nephropathy is associated with retinopathy and systemic vascular changes (discussed later).

TABLE 51-5 Stages of Diabetic Nephropathy

STAGE	CHARACTERISTICS	EFFECTS	AVERAGE ONSET AFTER DIAGNOSIS OF DIABETES (YEARS)
Stage I	Hyperfiltration	Blood flow through kidneys is increased	10
	Glomerular hypertrophy	Kidneys are enlarged	
Stage II	**Microalbuminuria**	Albumin, a blood protein, is excreted in small amounts	
Stage III	Gross albuminuria	Large amount of albumin is excreted; urine consistently tests positive for its presence. Blood pressure becomes elevated. Excretion of nitrogen wastes is impaired	15
Stage IV	Advanced dysfunction	Severe impairment of glomerular filtration is evidenced by excessive proteinuria, hypertension, and rise in blood urea nitrogen and creatinine levels	15–20
Stage V	End-stage renal failure	Kidney functions are severely impaired; dialysis or renal transplantation is necessary	20–25

Assessment Findings

In the early stages, the client does not manifest any obvious signs and symptoms. Eventually, they notice swelling of the feet and hands, most likely from the loss of albumin, a colloid that pulls water into the vascular system. The BP increases gradually. The client feels tired and weak. A routine urinalysis or dip with a chemical strip detects albumin in the urine. The blood urea nitrogen and serum creatinine become elevated. The renal creatinine clearance is decreased.

Medical Management

Controlling both blood glucose levels and hypertension can prevent or delay the development of diabetic nephropathy. The American Diabetes Association (2021c) recommends that clients with diabetes maintain their BP at or below 140 mm Hg systolic and diastolic pressure less than 90 mm Hg. Angiotensin-converting enzyme (ACE) inhibitors such as captopril (Capoten) and angiotensin II receptor antagonists such as losartan (Cozaar) slow the progressive nature of nephropathy. A moderate reduction in dietary protein is beneficial. Smoking cessation is strongly recommended.

Nursing Management

The nurse monitors the client's blood glucose and HbA1c results. They check the urine with a test strip to detect evidence of albuminuria. The nurse provides additional teaching if the client's blood glucose level is not controlled. They refer the client to programs that assist with smoking cessation or discuss the possibility of nicotine patches or gum to control further habituation. The nurse explains the therapeutic regimen associated with prescribed antihypertensive drugs and dietary measures for lowering BP and complications from vascular disease (see Chapter 27). Because nephropathy is progressive, the nurse encourages the client to keep appointments for regular medical follow-up.

Diabetic Retinopathy

Diabetic retinopathy refers to pathologic changes in the retina that are experienced by persons with diabetes. On average, it develops 10 or more years after the onset of diabetes. The earlier retinopathy develops, the more likely it is that vision will rapidly deteriorate.

Pathophysiology and Etiology

Diabetic retinopathy is a consequence of inadequately controlled blood glucose levels, which cause vascular changes in the retina (Fig. 51-14).

There are two types: (1) nonproliferative retinopathy is the milder manifestation and (2) proliferative retinopathy, the more severe form, can lead to blindness. In nonproliferative

A

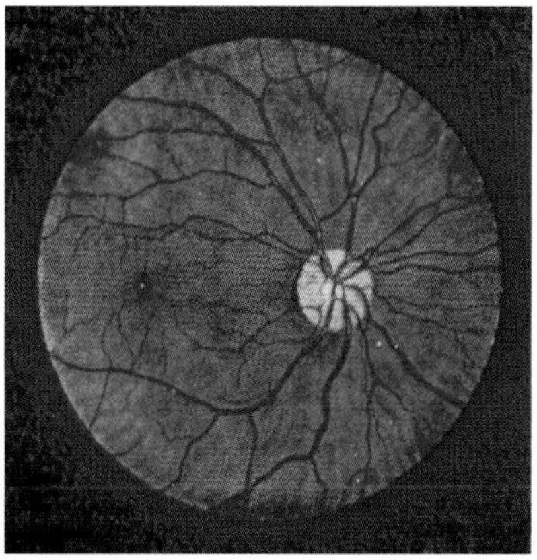

B

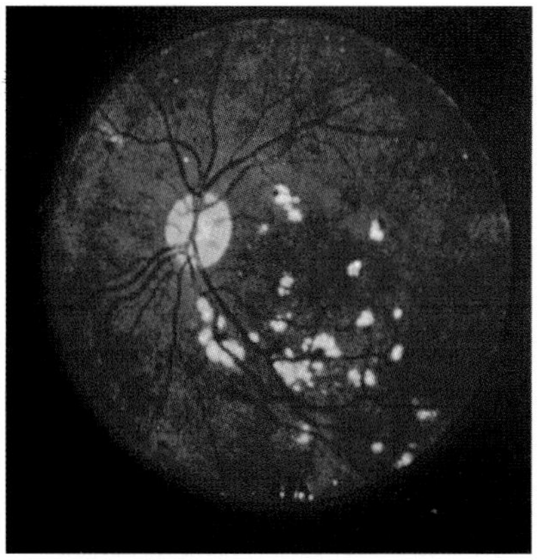

Figure 51-14 **(A)** In the normal eye, the light circular area over which several blood vessels converge is the optic disc, where the optic nerve meets the back of the eye. **(B)** In diabetic retinopathy, the fundus photograph shows characteristic waxy-looking lesions, microaneurysms, and hemorrhages.

retinopathy, *microaneurysms*, outpouchings in retinal capillaries, develop from high vascular pressure and compromised circulation. The stasis of blood flow interferes with transferring substances between the retina and blood vessels. The deprived retinal cells swell.

In the more advanced, proliferative form, damaged blood vessels are replaced with new ones that grow along the surface of the retina. The newer blood vessels, however, are more fragile. They tend to rupture and leak blood into the vitreous, the gel-like fluid that fills the posterior portion of the eye. Inelastic scar tissue forms, which alters the shape of the retina, causes distorted vision, and pulls at the retina, increasing the potential for retinal detachment.

Assessment Findings

Clients with nonproliferative and proliferative retinopathy may not experience any visual changes for some time. When symptoms do occur, the client reports blurred vision, no vision in spotty areas, or seeing debris floating about the visual field.

Visual acuity is diminished. Ophthalmic examination reveals swelling near the macula of the eye, an area lateral to the optic nerve that provides acute central vision. Fluorescein angiography documents changes in retinal blood vessels photographically (see Chapter 42).

Medical Management

The client with diabetes is referred for an ophthalmic evaluation within 3 to 5 years after diagnosis. If there is no evidence of retinopathy for one or more eye exams, they may be repeated every 2 years (American Diabetes Association, 2021b). If there is evidence of retinal vessel changes, an ACE inhibitor such as lisinopril (Prinivil) is prescribed to dilate the retinal blood vessels and improve blood flow. If vitreous hemorrhage already has occurred, some primary providers prefer to let the condition resolve on its own, which may take up to 18 months. A more expeditious technique is to seal leaking or newly forming blood vessels with laser photocoagulation. A vitrectomy, removal of bloodied vitreous, also improves the clarity of vision. Ovine hyaluronidase (Vitrase), a genetically engineered form of angiopoietin, a vascular growth factor that stimulates the repair of leaky retinal blood vessels, has been shown to clear the bloodied vitreous after intraocular injection in approximately 1 month.

Nursing Management

The nurse encourages clients with diabetes to follow their therapeutic regimen to facilitate tight glucose control. They teach clients about complications associated with diabetes and encourages recommended ophthalmic examinations. When medications are prescribed, the nurse explains their purpose, techniques for self-administration, side effects, and symptoms that are important to report to the prescribing primary provider.

Vascular Disturbances

Vascular disturbances affect many tissues and organs, as described in previous discussions of peripheral neuropathy, diabetic nephropathy, and retinopathy. In clients with diabetes, however, all the arteries and arterioles are more susceptible to accelerated atherosclerotic and arteriosclerotic changes than in clients without diabetes.

Pathophysiology and Etiology

A consistent finding among clients with diabetes is thickening of the arterial walls. The incidence of coronary artery disease also is increased. One possible explanation for obesity in clients with diabetes is that the brain may be insensitive to leptin, a chemical that signals satiation. A lack of response to leptin promotes overeating, which contributes to hyperlipidemia.

Assessment Findings

Peripheral vascular changes are one of the most common complications associated with diabetes (see Chapter 25). Because of a decreased blood supply, the extremities are pale and cool. Leg cramps can occur. **Gangrene** (death of tissue) develops if blood supply to the extremities is markedly diminished. Uncontrolled infection leads to skin ulcers. Clients with diabetes are likely to develop chest discomfort when the coronary arteries are affected. Myocardial infarctions occur at a much earlier age than among the nondiabetic population. Hyperlipidemia and elevated triglyceride levels correlate with the predisposition to atherosclerosis. Angiography and Doppler ultrasonic flow studies indicate peripheral vascular disease.

Medical and Surgical Management

Atherosclerosis is managed with lipid-lowering measures such as a low-fat diet, exercise, and medications. Vasodilators are prescribed to combat the effects of arteriosclerosis. Drugs that reduce platelet aggregation (e.g., aspirin) are prescribed prophylactically. Smoking cessation is advised. Impaired skin is managed with aggressive measures to promote healing (see Chapter 25). Uncontrolled gangrene of the extremities can result in amputation. The lower extremities are involved most often. Any type of surgery or hospitalization is an enormous stressor. The glucose levels of the client with diabetes increase, with a concomitant increased demand for insulin. The health care team closely monitors the client's blood glucose levels. Either higher doses of insulin or antidiabetic drugs are prescribed or elevated blood glucose levels are covered by administering rapid-acting or short-acting insulin before meals and at bedtime.

Nursing Management

Nursing management is geared toward the type of vascular disturbance and the signs and symptoms the client experiences.

KEY POINTS

- Diabetes mellitus
  - Prediabetes: HbA1c of 5.7% to 6.4%, fasting blood glucose of 100 to 125 or an oral glucose tolerance test of 140 to 199
  - Hyperglycemia: elevated blood glucose level
  - Type 1 DM: absence of insulin production by the beta cells in the islets of Langerhans, must have insulin therapy
  - Type 2 DM: insulin resistance or insufficient insulin production, many times can be controlled by diet, exercise, weight loss, and/or oral medication prior to insulin therapy

- Medical management
  - Insulin: rapid acting, short acting, intermediate acting, long acting, and combined
  - Generally administered subcutaneously, but can be given IV (rapid and short acting only), can be done by an insulin syringe, insulin pen, or an insulin pump
  - Multiple types of oral medications can be used for type 2 DM
  - Alternative therapies include bariatric surgery and islet cell transplantation
- Acute complications of DM
  - DKA: life-threatening acidosis
  - HHNKS: severe hyperglycemia without ketosis
  - Hypoglycemia: low blood glucose
- Chronic complications of DM
  - Peripheral neuropathy: changes to the nerves of the motor, sensory, and autonomic systems
  - Diabetic nephropathy: progressive decrease in renal function for clients with DM
  - Diabetic retinopathy: pathologic changes in the retina
  - Vascular disturbances: affects many tissues and organs

CRITICAL THINKING EXERCISES

1. A client with diabetes mellitus has not followed the diet prescribed by the primary provider. What information would you include in a teaching plan for this client? What approach would you take to reinforce the importance of diet in the management of diabetes?
2. Explain the differences between the signs and symptoms of hyperglycemia and hypoglycemia.
3. A client's fasting blood sugar is 128 mg/dL and the HbA1c is 8.8%. How would you explain the results of the laboratory tests to the client?
4. A client with diabetes says, "Nurse, I have diabetes, so why are you examining my feet?" What is an appropriate response from the nurse?

NCLEX-STYLE REVIEW QUESTIONS PrepU

1. The prescribed treatment for a client with diabetes involves the self-administration of a combination of two insulins, short-acting insulin (Humulin R) and intermediate-acting insulin (Humulin N). What action indicates that the client needs more practice?
   1. The client instills air into the short-acting and intermediate-acting insulin vials.
   2. The client withdraws the intermediate-acting insulin first and then the short-acting insulin.
   3. The client rolls the vial of intermediate-acting insulin to mix it with its additive.
   4. The client inverts each vial prior to withdrawing the specified amount of insulin.
2. In addition to insulin, the primary provider has prescribed pramlintide (Symlin) 120 mcg subcutaneously before each meal. Pramlintide is supplied in 5-mL vials with a supply dosage of 600 mcg/mL. Fill in the blank with the volume the nurse should administer to the client. Round the answer to one decimal place.

   ____
3. In what location should the nurse recommend injecting a bedtime injection of glargine (Lantus) insulin?
   1. Upper arm
   2. Upper thigh
   3. Abdomen
   4. Buttocks
4. What signs will the nurse detect if a client with diabetes mellitus develops hypoglycemia? Select all that apply.
   1. Flushed, warm skin
   2. Confusion
   3. Drowsiness
   4. Hunger
   5. Thirst
   6. Tremors
5. When a client with long-standing diabetes comes to the clinic for a routine visit, what statement best indicates that the nurse is assessing for a complication related to the disease?
   1. "What does your blood pressure usually run?"
   2. "Have you had any heart palpitations?"
   3. "What is the color of your urine?"
   4. "Have you had your eyes checked recently?"

WANT TO KNOW MORE? There are a wide variety of online resources available on thePoint to enhance learning and understanding of this chapter.

Go to thePoint.lww.com/activate and use the activation code found in the front of this text to unlock these online resources.

UNIT 13
Caring for Clients With Breast and Reproductive Disorders

52 Introduction to the Female and Male Reproductive Systems

Words To Know

breast self-examination
clinical breast examination
conization
digital rectal examination
dilatation and curettage
ejaculation
emission
erection
fertilization
gynecologic examination
implantation
lactation
mammography
menarche
menopause
menstruation
oocytes
ovulation
ovum
Papanicolaou test
procreate
prostate-specific antigen
puberty
spermatocytes
spermatogenesis
spermatozoon
transillumination
tumor markers
vulva
zygote

Learning Objectives

On completion of this chapter, you will be able to:

1. Name the major external structures of the female reproductive system.
2. Name four internal female reproductive structures and their functions.
3. Discuss the process of ovulation.
4. Explain the physiologic changes that lead to menstruation.
5. List at least five types of reproductive data that are obtained when taking a woman's health history.
6. Discuss the purpose of the cytologic test known as a Papanicolaou test.
7. Review the instructions a nurse provides for a client who is scheduling a gynecologic examination and Papanicolaou test.
8. Name diagnostic tests used for diagnosing disorders of the female reproductive system.
9. Describe the anatomy and physiology of the breast.
10. Explain the differences between a clinical breast examination and a breast self-examination.
11. Discuss the advantage of a mammographic examination.
12. Name three techniques for performing a breast biopsy.
13. Identify the major external structures of the male reproductive system.
14. Name the chief internal male reproductive structures and their functions.
15. List three accessory structures of the male reproductive system.
16. Explain the terms: erection, emission, and ejaculation.
17. List at least five types of reproductive data that are obtained while taking a male's health history.
18. Name the techniques for physically assessing male reproductive structures.
19. List methods that are used to diagnose prostate cancer.
20. Name two tests for determining infertility problems in men.

The reproductive systems of females and males form during embryonic development, and the external structures are evident at birth. However, the reproductive system does not become active and functional until **puberty** (the onset of sexual maturation). As the reproductive structures mature during adolescence, they facilitate the development of gender-specific physical characteristics and the ability to **procreate** (reproduce).

In both males and females, the reproductive system consists of external and internal structures involved in reproduction. The breasts are included as part of the woman's reproductive system because they are important for nourishing infants. This chapter reviews the anatomy and physiology unique to each gender and the assessment techniques used to determine normal and abnormal function. Subsequent chapters in this unit address common disorders of the reproductive system that occur among women and men and the nurse's role in managing the care of clients who develop these disorders.

Gerontologic Considerations

- The female genitalia change during the aging process. Changes include thinning of pubic hair; decrease in the size of the labia majora and minora; shortening and narrowing of the vagina; and atrophy of Bartholin glands, which results in less lubrication. The cervix, uterus, fallopian tubes, and vulva atrophy, causing a loss of vascularity and elasticity, which may contribute to irritation or excoriation of the tissue.
- As women age, reproductive hormones produced by the pituitary gland and ovaries begin to decrease years before menses cease. Menopause on average occurs around age 50 years in most women (see Chapter 53).
- Loss of estrogen leads to atrophy of mammary tissue and increased fat tissue, resulting in pendulous breasts.
- Loss of muscular tone with age causes the scrotum to become more pendulous. As the scrotum drops, there is an increased risk of trauma and injury to this area.
- Older men experience individual differences in the decrease in testosterone and sperm production (termed andropause). Although production of viable sperm decreases, an older man may continue to be able to reproduce.
- The prostate gland enlarges with age as fibrotic tissue replaces the glandular tissue. Prostate enlargement can compromise urination because it compresses the urethra.

THE FEMALE REPRODUCTIVE SYSTEM

Anatomy and Physiology

External Structures

The major external structures of the female reproductive system include the *mons pubis*, vaginal orifice (opening), *labia majora*, *labia minora*, and *clitoris* (Fig. 52-1). These structures are also referred to as the **vulva** (collective term for external genitalia).

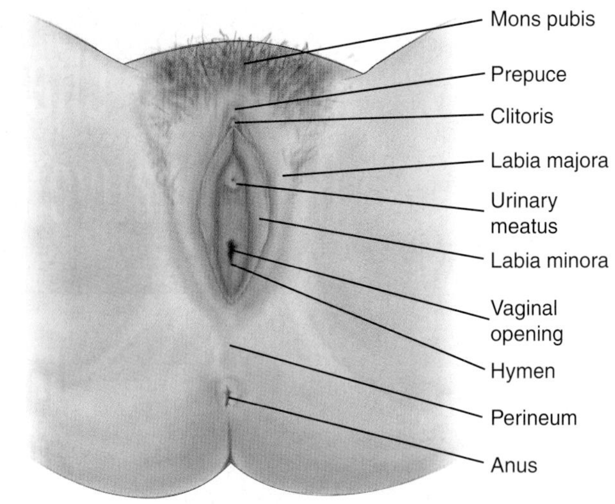

Figure 52-1 Female external genitalia.

The *mons pubis* is a pad of fat located centrally in the lower pelvis. Once reproductive hormones are produced at puberty, the *mons pubis* develops a covering of hair. The *labia majora* and *labia minora* are the large and small hairless skinfolds that, when separated, reveal the urethral and vaginal openings.

At the superior junction of the labia, there is a fleshy protrusion of tissue known as the *clitoris*. The clitoris is erectile tissue that enlarges and becomes extremely sensitive when stimulated by the penis or touching that accompanies sexual foreplay. On either side of the vaginal opening are mucus-secreting glands, called *Bartholin glands* or bulbourethral glands, that lubricate the vaginal opening during sexual arousal and facilitate the ease of penile penetration of the vagina during intercourse. The *fourchette* is the area beneath the vaginal opening at the base of the labia majora. Significant trauma to this tissue is often used as forensic evidence in rape trials.

The *hymen* (a mucosal membrane) is located at the vaginal opening. The hymen's absence does not necessarily confirm the loss of virginity. The hymen may rupture at the time of the first sexual intercourse, but it can be perforated by physical activity, insertion of a tampon, or pelvic examination.

Internal Structures

The internal female reproductive structures (Fig. 52-2) consist of the *vagina*, the *uterus*, two *fallopian tubes*, and two *ovaries*. The *vagina*, an expandable, tube-shaped structure, extends from the opening between the labia to the uterus. The vagina (1) provides a pathway for menstrual blood, (2) receives the penis and sperm during intercourse, and (3) serves as the structure through which an infant descends during the birth process. *Döderlein bacilli*, nonpathogenic bacteria residing in the vagina, use vaginal glycogen, a type of carbohydrate, to produce lactic acid. Routine douching of the vagina is discouraged because douching reduces the acidic medium, predisposing to the growth of infectious bacteria.

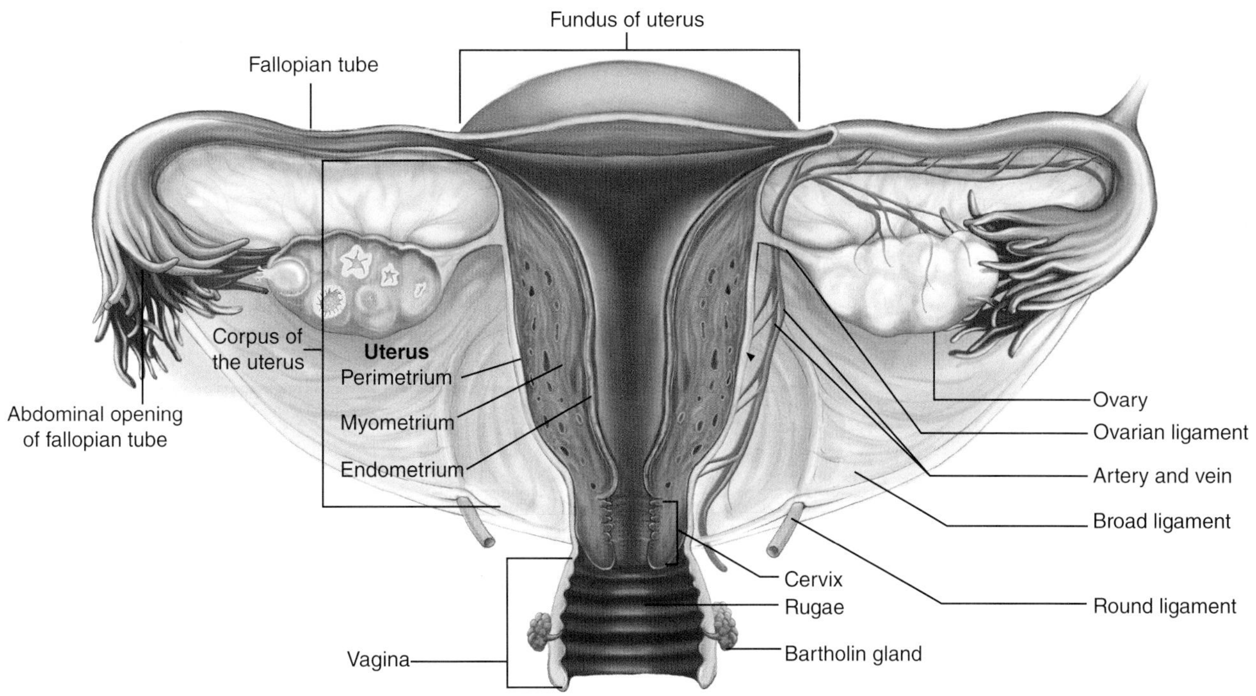

Figure 52-2 Internal female reproductive structures. The uterus, vagina, and a portion of the fallopian tube are shown in cross-section.

The *uterus*, the largest of the internal female reproductive structures, is approximately the size of a pear in the nonpregnant state. Various ligaments and muscles within the pelvis support and suspend the uterus, which is subdivided into the *corpus* (body), or major central portion; the *fundus*, or upper area; and a narrow neck, called the *cervix*. The cervix is lined with cells that secrete mucus, which is very thick except at the time of ovulation (discussed later). Thick mucus repels bacteria; thinner cervical mucus facilitates the movement of sperm (male sex cells) toward the **ovum** (pl., *ova*; matured female reproductive cell, or egg).

The uterine wall is composed of three layers: the *perimetrium*, the outer serous membrane; the *myometrium*, a smooth muscle layer that contracts to expel an infant during labor; and the mucosal *endometrium*, the innermost layer that sheds monthly during the menstrual cycle.

One or the other *fallopian tube* receives an extruded ovum every month and serves as the place where the ovum is most commonly fertilized. The sweeping motion of the *fimbriae*, which resemble fringes at the distal end of the fallopian tube, directs the released ovum into the fallopian tube.

The two ovaries (female gonads) lie behind and slightly below the ends of the fallopian tubes. Various ligaments hold the ovaries in place. In follicles of the cortex (outer layer) of each ovary, approximately one-half million **oocytes** (developing egg cells) are present in a woman at birth. The ovaries also secrete two hormones: estrogen, which is responsible for secondary sexual characteristics such as breast development and the preparation of the uterus for conception, and progesterone (discussed later).

After puberty and until **menopause** (the termination of female fertility; see Chapter 53), three processes occur: ovulation, pregnancy, and menstruation.

››› *Stop, Think, and Respond 52-1*

What health teaching is appropriate when a client says she self-administers a douche every week for the purpose of routine feminine hygiene?

Ovulation

The roles of the internal structures are to release and transport the ovum and to support the development of a fertilized ovum. **Ovulation** is the expulsion of an ovum from an ovary. The cyclical release of the ovum is influenced by pituitary hormones. The anterior pituitary hormone, known as follicle-stimulating hormone (FSH), initiates ovulation monthly. FSH triggers the maturation of a follicle in one of the ovaries and an increased production of ovarian estrogen. A second pituitary hormone, luteinizing hormone (LH), causes the mature follicle to rupture, thereby releasing an ovum from the ovary (Fig. 52-3).

After the ovum is released, movement of the fimbriae at the end of the fallopian tube and the muscular contractions of the tube itself draw the ovum into the tube toward the uterus. The cells surrounding the ruptured follicle transform into the *corpus luteum* (yellow body), which secretes progesterone and estrogen. The endometrium, the inner lining of the uterus, becomes thick and vascular in response to the hormonal secretions.

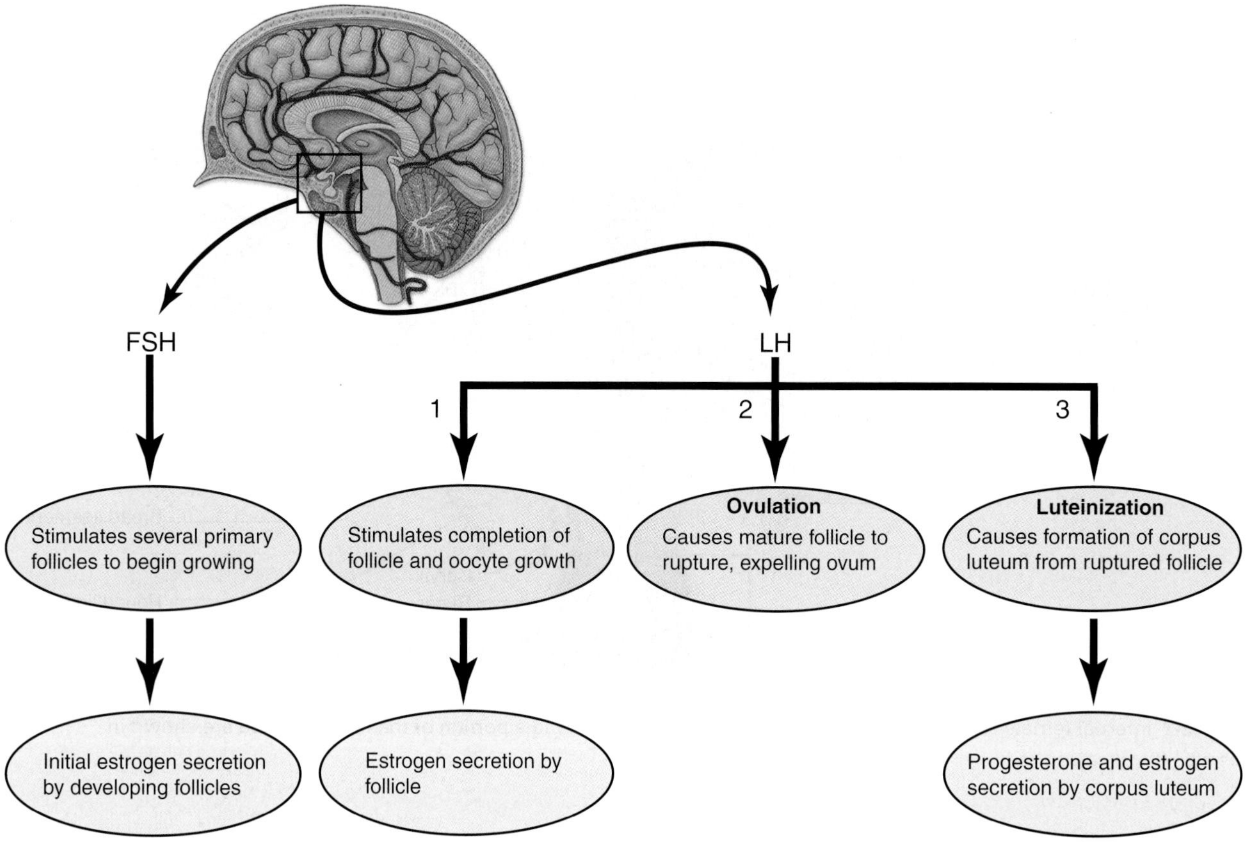

Figure 52-3 The effects of gonadotropins on the ovaries. FSH, follicle-stimulating hormone; LH, luteinizing hormone.

Pregnancy

Pregnancy occurs as a result of fertilization and implantation. **Fertilization**, the union of an ovum and a **spermatozoon** (pl., *spermatozoa*, the male reproductive cell), normally occurs in the fallopian tube (Fig. 52-4). At the moment a sperm penetrates the ovum, the number of chromosomes is complete, making it possible for an embryo to develop. The fertilized ovum, or **zygote**, then proceeds down the uterus and attaches itself in the endometrium (**implantation**). Once fertilization and implantation occur, the pituitary production of FSH is inhibited so that ovulation temporarily stops.

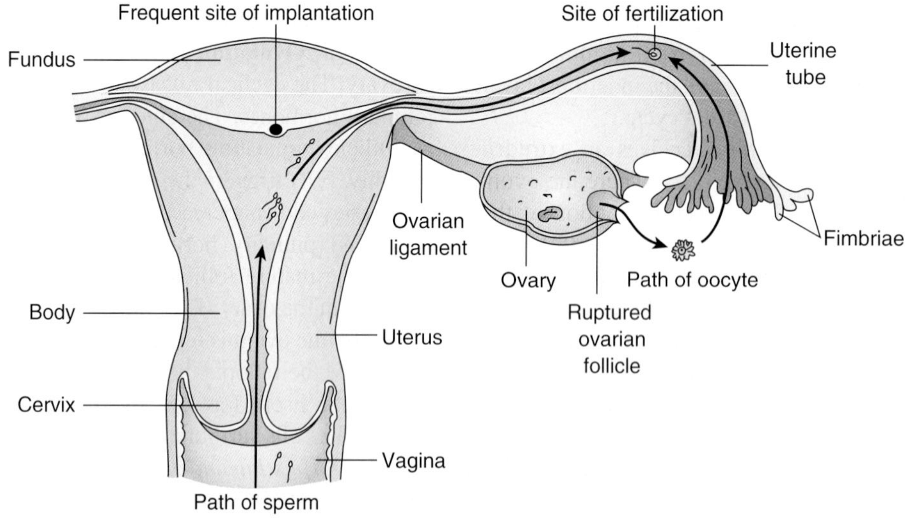

Figure 52-4 Schematic drawing of female reproductive organs, showing path of ovum from ovary into the fallopian tube, path of spermatozoa, and the usual sites of fertilization and implantation.

Menstruation

If the ovum is not fertilized, the production of progesterone by the corpus luteum begins to decrease until it changes from a yellow to a white spot on the ovary (corpus albicans). Without a high level of progesterone, the endometrium degenerates and sheds, a process referred to as **menstruation**, which begins about 2 weeks after ovulation (Fig. 52-5). Menstrual flow usually lasts 4 to 5 days, with a normal loss of 30 to 60 mL of blood. Women who have heavy menses, or menstrual flow, lose more blood. After menstruation, the endometrium becomes thicker and more vascular again in preparation for a possible pregnancy.

Because of these hormone-dependent changes, the microscopic characteristics of the uterus are in a cyclical state of transition. Thus, it is important that each gynecologic specimen sent to the laboratory be marked with the beginning date of the client's last menstrual period (LMP).

Pharmacologic Considerations

- Drugs containing estrogen and/or progestin are used to manipulate the processes of female fertility. As a result, pregnancy can be prevented, regulation of flow may be controlled, or severe menstrual symptoms can be relieved.

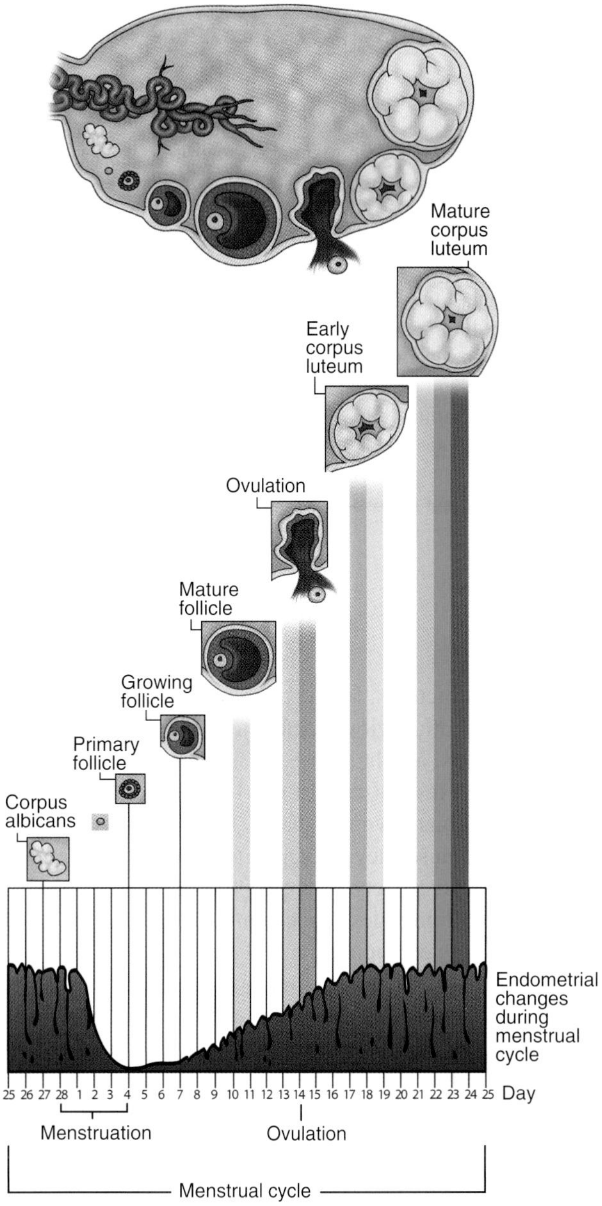

Figure 52-5 One menstrual cycle and the corresponding endometrial changes.

Assessment

Health History

To ensure a thorough baseline history, the nurse obtains the following information:

- General health and family history
- Age of **menarche**, the first menstruation
- Date of client's LMP, description of the menstrual pattern and flow, and other symptoms associated with menstruation
- Risks for sexually transmitted infections (STIs) (see Chapter 56)
- Pregnancy history: number of pregnancies, live births, stillborn births; type of fetal abnormalities
- Abortion history
- Contraceptive practices
- Age of menopause, associated symptoms, and use of hormone replacement therapy (HRT)
- Date of last gynecologic and breast examination, including mammograms and Papanicolaou tests
- Prior treatments or surgery for a gynecologic disorder
- Drug, allergy, substance abuse, and smoking history
- Symptoms of present disorder, such as painful intercourse or characteristics of vaginal discharge, and duration

See Nutrition Notes for nutrition factors that may influence reproductive health.

Nutrition Notes

Nutrition and Reproductive Health

- A severe reduction in body fat caused by extreme caloric restriction or excessive exercise can cause female reproductive abnormalities such as delayed or cessation of menstruation, small breasts, and impaired potential for implantation of a fertilized ovum (Polotsky, 2010). In men, the same factors can cause the genitals to appear or remain juvenile.
- Obese women may experience problems with subfertility or infertility. A cause of infertility in women is polycystic ovarian syndrome, a multiendocrine disorder linked to insulin resistance.

Gynecologic Examination (Pelvic Examination)

A primary provider, clinical nurse specialist, primary provider's assistant, or nurse practitioner performs the **gynecologic examination**, an inspection and palpation of pelvic

NURSING GUIDELINES 52-1

Assisting the Client Undergoing a Pelvic Examination

- Have the client void before the examination.
- Ask the client open-ended questions to promote verbalizing anxiety.
- Provide information on what to expect during the examination and when results from tissue samples will be available.
- Answer questions and use the opportunity to educate the client on health maintenance and health promotion activities.
- Have a drape available.
- Assist the client to assume a lithotomy position immediately before the examination.
- Put pleasing posters on the walls or ceiling to help distract the client.
- Guide the client to breathe deeply during the examination.

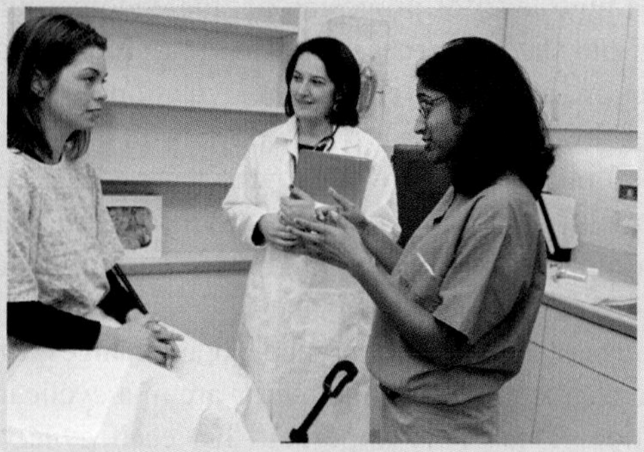

reproductive structures. In preparation for the test, the nurse obtains examination gloves, lubricant, several sizes of bivalve speculums, a light source, and materials for obtaining a Papanicolaou test (discussed next). The nurse is sensitive to the fact that many women dislike having gynecologic examinations because they anticipate discomfort, are embarrassed, and have anxiety over possible diagnoses. Nursing Guidelines 52-1 provides suggestions on assisting the client undergoing a gynecologic examination.

Inspection of the external genitalia and adjacent structures occurs first, followed by the inspection of the vaginal wall and cervix using a bivalve speculum (Fig. 52-6). Next, one or two fingers of a lubricated, gloved hand are placed into the vagina. By vaginal–abdominal palpation, the structures beyond the vaginal orifice are examined, and the position, size, and contour of the uterus, ovaries, and other pelvic structures are assessed (Fig. 52-7). At the end of the examination, a gloved finger may be inserted into the rectum to palpate the posterior surface of the uterus.

Diagnostic Tests

Cytologic Test for Cervical Cancer (Papanicolaou Test)

A **Papanicolaou test** (Pap test), an important cervical cancer screening tool, involves obtaining a sample of exfoliated cells (dead cells that are shed). The specimens, which are best obtained 2 weeks after the first day of the LMP, are removed by scraping and brushing tissue during the pelvic examination (Fig. 52-8). The test is used mainly to detect early cancer of the cervix and secondarily to determine estrogen activity as it relates to menopause or endocrine abnormalities. Box 52-1 presents the classification system used to describe Pap test results.

According to the American Cancer Society (ACS, 2020), the recommendations for human papillomavirus (HPV) and Pap testing have made significant changes from the 2012

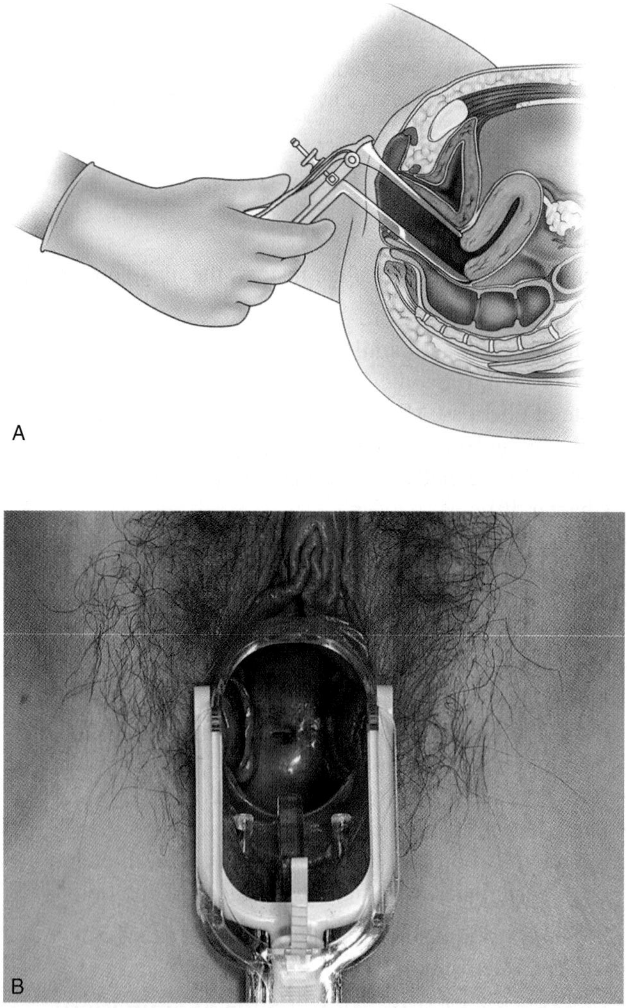

Figure 52-6 Technique for speculum examination of the vagina and cervix. **(A)** After the examiner spreads the woman's labia and inserts the speculum in the vagina, the blades are spread apart **(B)** to reveal the cervical os opening. (Photo by B. Proud.)

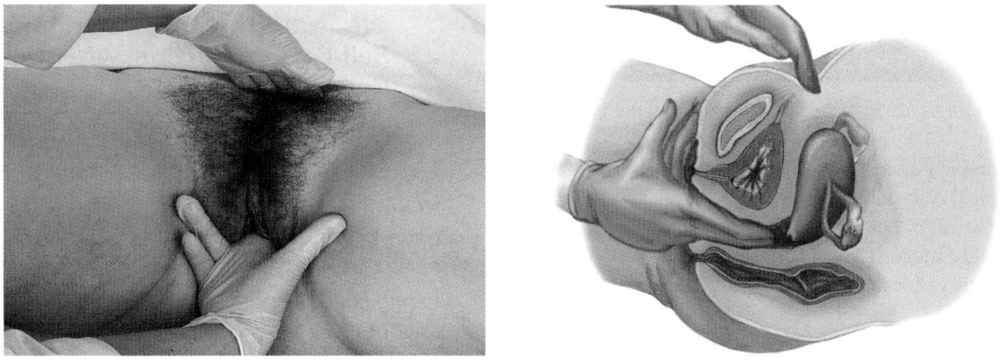

Figure 52-7 Bimanual examination of pelvic structures.

testing recommendations. Women aged 21 to 24 years have no recommended testings/screenings. Women between the ages of 25 and 29 years have the recommendation for HPV testing to be every 5 years (preferred), the HPV/Pap co-test every 5 years (acceptable), or the Pap test every 3 years (acceptable). Women between the ages of 30 and 65 years are recommended for HPV testing to be every 5 years (preferred), the HPV/Pap co-test every 5 years (acceptable), or the Pap test every 3 years (acceptable). Screenings can be discontinued for women older than age 65 who have had a series of previous screenings with normal results for 10 years and no history of cervical changes in the last 25 years. Once screenings have been stopped, they are not recommended to start again. Those who have been diagnosed with cervical precancerous changes or who have been infected with HIV, are immunosuppressed, or were exposed to diethylstilbestrol (DES) before birth should continue to be screened beyond age 65 based on their provider's recommendations (ACS, 2020).

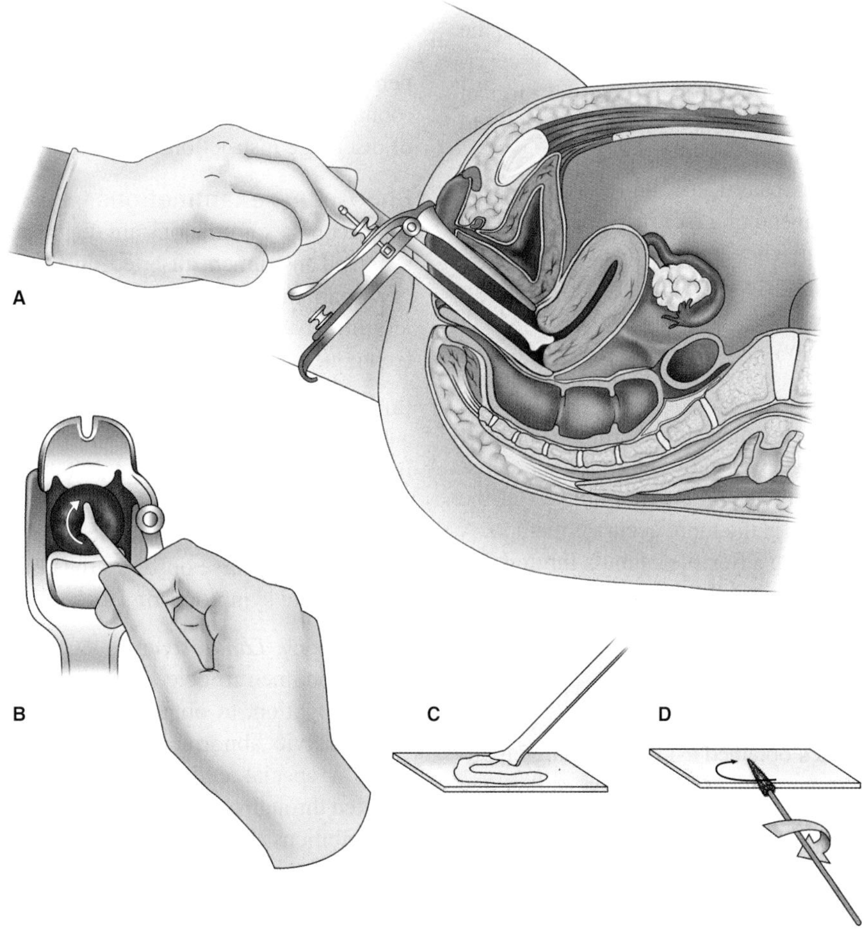

Figure 52-8 Specimen collection for Pap test. **(A)** With the speculum in place, the examiner uses a spatula to obtain cervical secretions. **(B)** They place the spatula tip in the cervical os and rotates the spatula 360 degrees. **(C)** Examiner smears material that clings to the spatula smoothly on a glass slide and promptly places in a solution. **(D)** They rotate the cytobrush in the cervical os and rolls it onto a glass slide.

BOX 52-1 Papanicolaou Classification System

Papanicolaou findings are described using the following numerical system:

- *Class 1*: No atypical or abnormal cells
- *Class 2*: Atypical cells but no evidence of malignancy
- *Class 3*: Suggestive of but not conclusive for malignancy
- *Class 4*: Strongly suggestive of malignancy
- *Class 5*: Conclusive for malignancy

The nurse advises the client to schedule an appointment at a time other than during menstruation and prior to the examination: (1) avoid intercourse and the use of tampons for 2 days; (2) refrain from douching for 48 hours; and (3) cease the use of vaginal creams, sprays, powders, or medications for at least 48 hours (Centers for Disease Control and Prevention [CDC], 2019). When assisting with the examination, the nurse obtains the required materials, prepares the client, and labels and preserves the specimens.

Cervical Biopsy

A cervical biopsy is performed when results from a Pap test are positive or questionable. Tissue is obtained by punching out multiple small samples or by performing **conization**, the process of removing a larger, cone-shaped section of cervical tissue (cone biopsy). Conization is an invasive surgical procedure performed on an outpatient basis; it is also used to treat early-stage cervical cancer.

If the client is premenopausal, the nurse schedules the biopsy for 1 week after the end of a menstrual period, when the cervix is least vascular. They tell the client that cramps and slight spotting may occur afterward. The nurse recommends a mild analgesic for discomfort and advises the client to report severe pain or heavy bleeding.

Endometrial Smears and Biopsy

Diagnosing cancer of the endometrium, the inner lining of the uterus, is accomplished by aspirating endometrial tissue specimens or performing an endometrial biopsy. Of the two, the endometrial biopsy is the more accurate method. A smear is obtained by inserting a flexible cannula through the cervix and into the uterine cavity. The cannula is attached to a syringe used to aspirate secretions. This procedure usually is performed without anesthesia.

To obtain a biopsy specimen, a dilating instrument called a *uterine sound* is inserted through the cervical opening. A tissue sample is then obtained using a scraping instrument called a *curette* or by aspiration. This procedure can be performed without anesthesia in the primary provider's office.

Dilatation and Curettage

Dilatation and curettage (D&C) is a surgical procedure in which the cervix is stretched (dilatation) and the endometrium is scraped (curettage). A D&C is performed to diagnose or treat various gynecologic problems (e.g., abnormal uterine bleeding) and to remove fetal and placental tissue. Samples of endometrial scrapings are obtained when the client is under general or light intravenous (IV) anesthesia. A vaginal and cervical pack is usually left in place, and a sterile perineal pad is applied before the client leaves the operating room. Client and Family Teaching 52-1 provides examples of discharge instructions.

Client and Family Teaching 52-1
Self-Care Instructions After Dilatation and Curettage

Following a D&C, the nurse instructs the client as follows:

- Expect slight cramping and a dark, bloody discharge for a few days to several weeks.
- Report bright red bleeding, foul vaginal discharge, a fever, or pain that is intolerable despite mild analgesia.
- Change soiled perineal pads frequently and avoid tampons.
- Take showers rather than tub baths for 3 or 4 days.
- Refrain from strenuous exercises and heavy household cleaning for 4 to 5 days, after which full activity may be resumed.
- Wipe from front to back after bowel elimination to avoid introducing microorganisms into the vaginal canal or urethra.
- Delay intercourse and douching for 1 to 2 weeks or until the primary provider indicates that they may be resumed.

Endoscopic Examinations

Endoscopic examinations are diagnostic procedures that use a lighted instrument inserted into the body for the purpose of visualizing structures not otherwise accessible. They are less invasive and more economical than the use of surgical techniques.

Culdoscopy. *Culdoscopy*, performed under local or general anesthesia, allows visualization of the uterus, broad ligaments, and fallopian tubes by inserting an endoscope through an incision made in the posterior vaginal wall. Ectopic pregnancy and pelvic masses can be visualized. Afterward, the nurse observes the client for signs of internal bleeding and symptoms of shock.

Laparoscopy. *Laparoscopy* is an examination of the interior of the abdomen to detect an ectopic pregnancy, to perform a tubal ligation, to obtain ovarian tissue for biopsy, and to detect pelvic abnormalities. The procedure is performed using a special endoscope called a *laparoscope* that is inserted through a small incision located one-half inch below the umbilicus (Fig. 52-9). About 2 or 3 L of carbon dioxide or nitrous oxide gas are introduced into the peritoneal cavity, creating a pneumoperitoneum to separate the intestines from the pelvic organs and to facilitate visualization.

The nurse can tell the client undergoing laparoscopy that she will experience discomfort in the shoulder as a result of the instillation of gas. Afterward, the nurse checks incisional

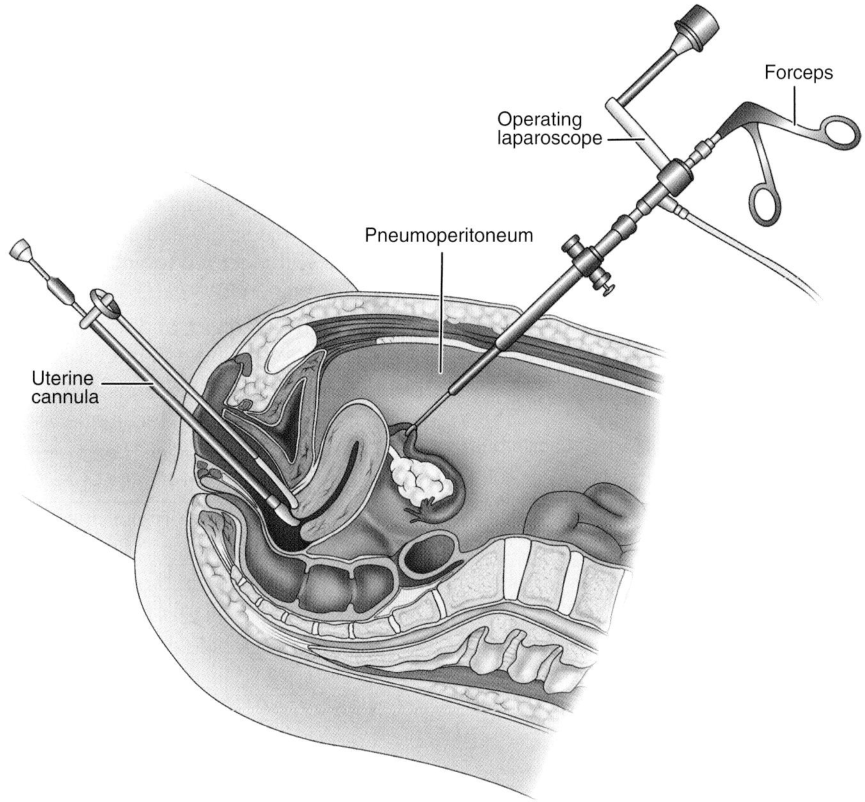

Figure 52-9 Laparoscopy is used to visualize the interior of the abdomen.

sites for bleeding and relieves discomfort by administering a prescribed analgesic.

Colposcopy. A *colposcopy* is a procedure used to visualize the cervix and vagina. A speculum is inserted into the vagina, and the surface areas are examined with a light and magnifying lens (colposcope). A cervical biopsy and Pap test can be taken at this time.

Hysterosalpingogram

A *hysterosalpingogram* is a radiographic examination that visualizes the uterus and fallopian tubes. It is used to detect deviations such as adhesions and to determine fallopian tube patency, other tubal abnormalities, or congenital malformations of these structures. Bowel preparation usually is necessary to clear the intestine of gas and fecal material that interfere with proper visualization of the uterus and fallopian tubes. A cannula is inserted into the cervix, and contrast media is injected. For clients who indicate an allergy to iodinated contrast media, a reaction may be minimized or prevented by administering an IV steroid the day before the examination along with diphenhydramine (Benadryl) prior to administering the contrast media. Fluoroscopic or radiographic films are taken after contrast media is administered.

Abdominal Ultrasonography (Sonogram)

Ultrasonography aids in visualizing soft tissue by recording the reflection of sound waves. An abdominal ultrasound detects pelvic abnormalities such as tumors and the size and location of fetal and placental tissue. The nurse instructs the client to drink at least 1 quart of water 45 minutes to 1 hour before the test and not to void until after the test is completed. A full bladder facilitates the transmission of the ultrasound waves and elevates the bowel away from the other pelvic organs. The client should restrict solid food for 6 to 8 hours to avoid having images obscured with gas and intestinal contents.

Laboratory Tests

Various laboratory tests, such as a complete blood cell count, hemoglobin, and serum electrolytes, are ordered to obtain a baseline of the client's health status. Culture and sensitivity tests are also ordered if an infection is suspected. Ovarian hormone activity is evaluated by total urine estrogen and urine pregnanediol tests.

THE BREASTS

Anatomy and Physiology

The breasts are modified sweat glands known as mammary glands that contain 15 to 20 lobes surrounded by fatty tissue. Each breast has a central nipple that is bordered by darker pigmented skin called the *areola*. Smooth muscle in the nipples contract, causing the nipples to become erect when cold, touched, or sexually stimulated. The nipples are connected to an internal system of ducts where several lobules (subdivisions of a lobe) converge (Fig. 52-10). Although men and

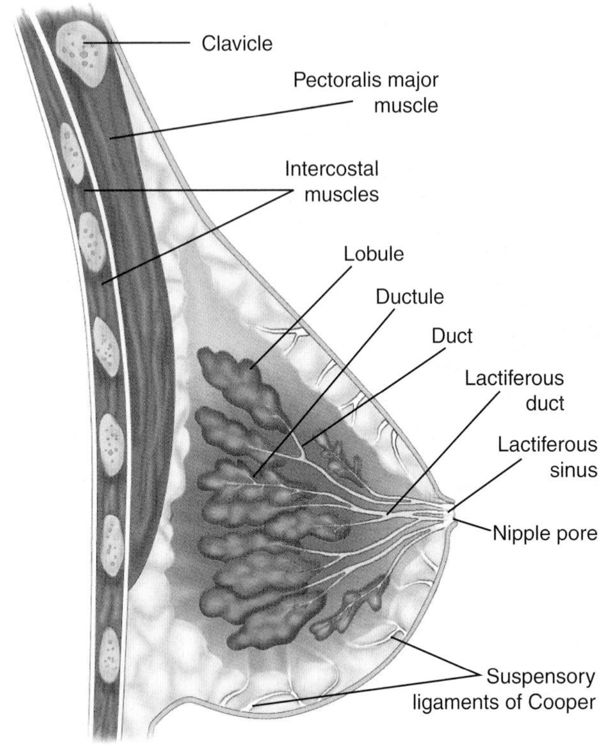

Figure 52-10 Anatomy of the female breast (lateral view).

women have breasts, a primary function of the female breast is to produce milk, a process called **lactation**.

Estrogen secreted by the ovaries at the onset of puberty causes the growth and development of the female mammary system. The amount of fatty tissue determines the size of the breast. Further growth and development that occurs during pregnancy is hormone-dependent. Prolactin promotes the production of milk from elements in the blood. Progesterone, secreted by the placenta, stimulates the development of alveoli, which secrete the milk. Estrogen, also secreted by the placenta, stimulates increased production of tubules and ducts to transport milk to the lactiferous ducts, which drain at the nipple.

The breasts have an abundant supply of blood vessels and lymphatics. The axillary lymph nodes and the internal mammary lymph nodes drain venous blood from the breasts. It is through these blood vessels and lymphatics that cancer in the ducts of the breast spreads to distant areas of the body.

Assessment

Breast Examination

Clinical breast examination is a manual palpation of the breast performed by a primary provider, nurse, or primary provider's assistant. During a clinical breast examination, the examiner notes breast size, symmetry, and any unusual changes in the skin of the breasts and nipples. With the client lying down and arm raised over the client's head, the examiner checks for masses, dimpling, flattening, rashes, ulceration, or discharge from the nipple. Using the flat part of the fingertips, the examiner palpates the breasts and axillae for masses and tenderness and examines the lymph nodes for other abnormalities.

Client and Family Teaching 52-2
Breast Self-Examination

The nurse instructs the client as follows:

- Examine your breasts 3 days after the end of menstruation or anytime if you no longer menstruate.
- Begin the examination in the shower when the breasts are wet and soapy and again after the shower when lying down with a folded towel under the shoulder on the side being examined (A).
- Use light, medium, and firm pressure applied with the pads of three fingers when checking each breast (B).
- Move your fingers in circles, spokes of a wheel, or rows, but follow the same technique with each BSE.
- Feel every part of each breast, including the nipple area and the armpit to the collarbone.
- Raise your arms over your head and look at the breasts in a mirror.
- Look for changes in breast shape, size, and contour; puckering (dimpling) of the skin; or areas that appear red.
- Squeeze each nipple and look for liquid drainage.

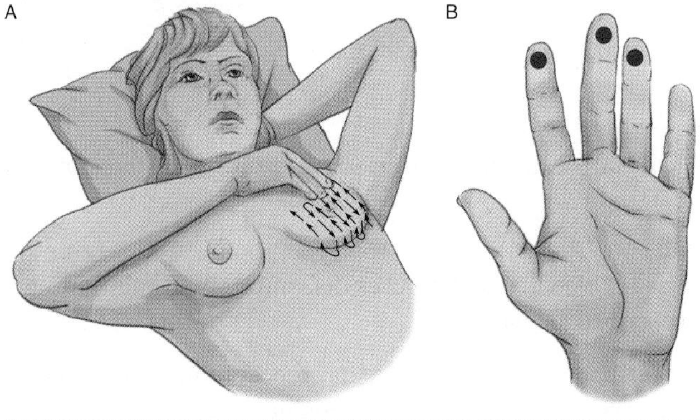

Breast self-examination (BSE), described and illustrated in Client and Family Teaching 52-2, is one way women may discover early breast changes. The ACS (2020) now states that clinical breast examinations by a health care provider and BSEs are no longer recommended because there is no clear evidence that the practice plays a role, or one that is very small, in detecting breast cancer. BSE, when done occasionally, is still appropriate for learning how the breasts feel and look and reporting any changes to a primary provider. Because breast cancer can also occur in men, examination of the male breasts and axillae may be included in the annual physical examination.

Mammography

Mammography (mammogram) is a radiographic technique considered the "gold standard" for detecting cysts or tumors of the breast, some of which may be too small to palpate. Conventional mammography is used as a screening tool to detect breast cancer (Fig. 52-11). Most mammograms are done digitally, either in the standard two-dimensional (2D) or in three-dimensional (3D) images.

The ACS (2020) recommends the ages and frequency at which mammography should be performed, although this is currently being updated (Box 52-2). The National Cancer

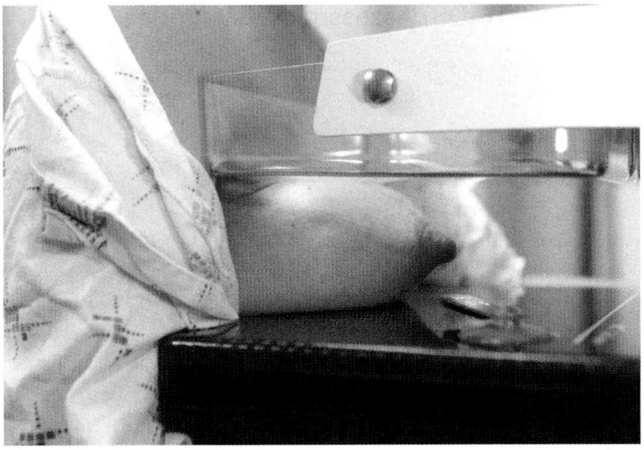

Figure 52-11 A client undergoing mammography.

Institute (2020), on the other hand, has not issued guidelines for mammography. Rather, it advises that women discuss the benefits and risks of mammography, when to start them, and how frequently they should be done. See Evidence-Based Practice 52-1 for information about culture and communication regarding mammography.

When a mammogram is scheduled, the nurse explains the radiographic procedure and instructs the client to omit using a deodorant with aluminum hydroxide or body talc on the day of the test to avoid artifacts on the X-ray film. If the client forgets or fails to receive this information, the nurse provides a premoistened wipe to cleanse the axillae just before the test. The nurse determines if and how often the client performs BSEs and may ask her to demonstrate or describe the technique. For women who are unfamiliar with BSE yet want to learn how it should be done, the nurse provides instructions and a demonstration using an anatomic teaching model. The nurse ensures privacy throughout the examination, advises clients to have their mammograms at the same health agency, or arranges for records to be transferred so that previous mammogram results can be compared.

One of the reasons why women avoid or postpone mammographic examination is the discomfort that they experience with breast compression. Some mammography testing centers are now using a radiolucent (allowing X-rays to penetrate tissue with a minimum of absorption) cushioning pad to reduce discomfort. Use of the pad does not compromise the quality of the mammographic image.

BOX 52-2 Guidelines for Mammography

The U.S. Preventive Services Task Force provides the following recommendations for screening in women at average risk for breast cancer:

- **Women aged 40 to 49 years:** The decision to start screening should be an individual one.
- **Women aged 50 to 74 years:** Screen every 2 years.
- **Women aged 75 years and older:** No recommendation.

From U.S. Preventive Services Task Force. (2016). Final recommendation statement—Breast cancer: Screening. *Annals of Internal Medicine, 164*(4), 279–297. https://www.uspreventiveservicestaskforce.org/Page/Document/RecommendationStatementFinal/breast-cancer-screening1.

Evidence-Based Practice 52-1

Cultural Sensitivity, Communication, and Breast Cancer Screenings

Clinical Question

How is client communication with Latina clients important in mammogram screenings?

Evidence

The incidence of actual breast cancer in the United States in Latina women is low; however, they are at the greatest risk due to decreased follow-up after receiving abnormal results (Molina et al., 2014). A qualitative study was done to explore the communication barriers to Latina and non-Latina White women in the United States. The results found that ethnic and cultural differences surrounding communication and previous experience with health care providers may influence follow-up care (Molina, Hohl, Ko, Rodriguez, Thompson, & Beresford, 2014).

Nursing Implications

Nurses must be familiar with cultural differences among clients. How clients comprehend test results and follow-up care may differ in different cultures. The communication and approach by the nurse may also be perceived differently in different cultures. The nurse should refer to culture-related resources when needed. With the development of the National Breast and Cervical Cancer Early Detection Program (NBCCEDP), the CDC assists low-income, uninsured, and underinsured women to obtain access to screening, diagnostic testing, and treatment for breast and cervical cancer (CDC, 2020).

References

Centers for Disease Control and Prevention (CDC). (2020). *National Breast and Cervical Cancer Early Detection Program (NBCCEDP).* https://www.cdc.gov/cancer/nbccedp/about.htm

Molina, Y., Hohl, S. D., Ko, L. K., Rodriguez, E. A., Thompson, B., & Beresford, S. A. (2014). Understanding the patient-provider communication needs and experiences of Latina and non-Latina white women following an abnormal mammogram. *Journal of Cancer Education, 29*(4), 781–789. https://doi.org/10.1007/s13187-014-0654-6

Regardless of which mammography technique (2D or 3D) is used, the American College of Radiology has established a uniform method for reporting the results of the examination. It is referred to as the *Breast Imaging Reporting and Database System* or BI-RADS for short (Table 52-1).

Ultrasonography

Ultrasonography (ultrasound) is often used with a mammogram to differentiate fluid-filled cysts from other types of breast lesions. The process involves the use of high-frequency sound waves to produce a visual picture. Ultrasonography has been useful for women with very dense breasts, especially younger women and those on HRT.

>>> Stop, Think, and Respond 52-2

A 52-year-old woman tells you she has never had a mammogram and has heard they are painful. How would you respond to her?

TABLE 52-1 Breast Imaging Reporting and Database System (BI-RADS) Assessment Categories

Category 0	**Mammography**: Incomplete—need additional imaging evaluation and/or prior mammograms for comparison **Ultrasound and MRI**: Incomplete—need additional imaging evaluation		
Category 1	Negative		
Category 2	Benign		
Category 3	Probably benign		
Category 4	Suspicious	Mammography and ultrasound	Category 4A: Low suspicion for malignancy Category 4B: Moderate suspicion for malignancy Category 4C: High suspicion for malignancy
Category 5	Highly suggestive of malignancy		
Category 6	Known biopsy-proven malignancy		

MRI, magnetic resonance imaging.
Reprinted with permission from American College of Radiology BI-RADS® poster. https://www.acr.org/-/media/ACR/Files/RADS/BI-RADS/BIRADS-Poster.pdf.

Breast Biopsy

A breast biopsy is performed to determine if a breast lesion is malignant. A specimen of tissue from the breast may be obtained through incisional biopsy, excisional biopsy, or aspiration biopsy.

Incisional Biopsy

Incisional biopsy is performed in the operating room, where one or more sections of tissue are removed. The specimen is frozen quickly and then examined microscopically by a pathologist while the client remains anesthetized. If the tissue is negative (i.e., benign), the remainder of the benign tissue is removed (if it has not been completely removed for biopsy), the incision is closed, and the client is sent to the recovery room. If the removed specimen is malignant, the surgeon may then perform the surgical procedure that offers the best chance of cure. The decision to operate immediately when there is a malignancy is thoroughly discussed with the client before surgery.

Excisional Biopsy

Some surgeons prefer an excisional biopsy, which is removal of the entire lesion. A pathologist examines the excised specimen later and more comprehensively. Clients may be discharged from the hospital before the results of the biopsy are obtained, or they may remain hospitalized. If the lesion is malignant, the biopsy results and the proposed treatment are discussed with the client.

Aspiration Biopsy

Aspiration biopsy, a procedure usually performed on an outpatient basis, uses a needle and syringe to obtain a sample of the suspect tissue. A local anesthetic is first injected around the area, and a sample of tissue is removed. A pathologist examines the tissue sample. Sometimes this procedure is done in the hospital under mammographic guidance to ensure an accurate sample of suspect tissue.

Nursing Management

The nurse allows the client time to ask questions and listens to concerns before the breast biopsy is performed. The client may have concerns about not only the procedure but also the results of the biopsy and possible diagnosis of cancer.

An aspiration biopsy usually causes minimal discomfort after the procedure, but there may be redness and soreness in the area. The nurse instructs the client to notify the primary provider if either drainage or bleeding from the biopsy site is more than slight or if increased redness, pain, or fever occurs. Incisional and excisional biopsies require sutures, but pain usually is minimal and relieved with a mild analgesic.

The nurse provides instructions regarding caring for the wound, using a mild analgesic, wearing a supportive brassiere, and timing of a follow-up appointment. They review the signs and symptoms that suggest wound infection.

THE MALE REPRODUCTIVE SYSTEM

Anatomy and Physiology

The anatomic structures and physiologic functions of the male reproductive system include the development of gender-specific sexual characteristics and the manufacture and transportation of sperm and seminal fluid. The lower urinary tract and reproductive system structures are shared and closely associated with each other.

External Structures

The external male genitalia consist of the penis and scrotum. The *penis*, a cylindrical structure, contains the urethra through which both urine and sperm are released. The penis contains nerves very sensitive to sexual stimulation. The tip of the penis is the *glans*. In an uncircumcised man, the *prepuce*, sometimes referred to as the foreskin, covers the glans. Three columns of erectile tissue run throughout the internal body, or shaft, of the penis. The pair on the dorsum is the *corpora cavernosa* (sing., corpus cavernosum), and the *corpus spongiosum* is on the ventral surface of the penis (Fig. 52-12).

The *scrotum* is the divided sac of skin that contains the right and left *testes* (male gonads), also called testicles. Since the testes cannot produce viable sperm when temperatures are at or above body temperature, their location within the scrotal sac ensures optimum conditions for sperm production. To maintain the temperature of the testes 3-degrees cooler than body temperature, smooth and skeletal muscles in the scrotum

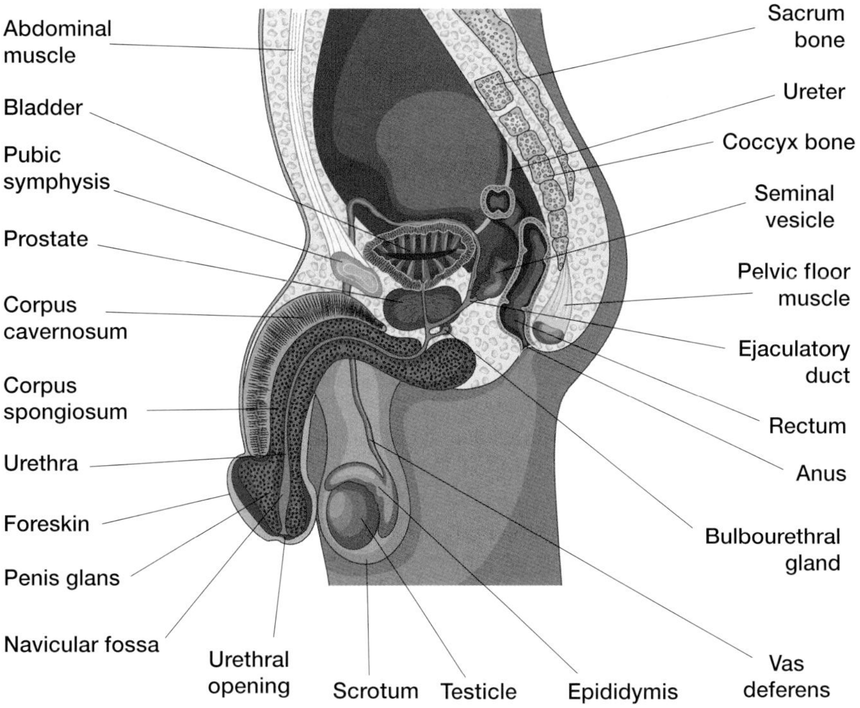

Figure 52-12 Anatomy of the male reproductive system. (Source: shutterstock.com/Vecton)

pull the tissue toward the body when external temperatures are cold. On the other hand, the smooth muscles relax, causing the scrotum to become loose and hang away from the body, when environmental temperatures are hot (Marieb & Hoehn, 2018).

Internal Structures

The chief internal structures of the male reproductive system include the *testes*, *seminiferous tubules*, *epididymis*, *ductus deferens*, and the *spermatic cord*. The testes (sing., *testis*) lie within the scrotum and are responsible for **spermatogenesis**, or sperm production, and secretion of testosterone. Testosterone, the male sex hormone, affects the development and maintenance of secondary male sex characteristics.

The testes are subdivided into lobules containing coiled seminiferous tubules. **Spermatocytes** (immature spermatozoa) form within the seminiferous tubules. Adult men produce approximately 400 million spermatocytes per day (Marieb & Hoehn, 2018).

Spermatogenesis is a result of both testosterone and the secretion of FSH, which is released by the anterior pituitary gland. Leydig cells in the spaces between the seminiferous tubules secrete testosterone. The secretion of testosterone is controlled by LH released by the anterior pituitary gland.

The *epididymis* collects the spermatocytes from the seminiferous tubules. The spermatocytes are nourished in the epididymis until they become motile. Mature spermatozoa (i.e., sperm) contain a head with a nucleus and 23 chromosomes, a midpiece that stores adenosine triphosphate (ATP) to supply energy during propulsion, and a tail that enables them to move toward the ovum.

The *vas deferens*, also called the *ductus deferens*, is connected to the epididymis. The vas deferens is joined with a network of blood vessels and nerves collectively referred to as the *spermatic cord*. The spermatic cord loops through the inguinal canal and into the pelvic cavity before it descends to the prostate gland. The wall of the vas deferens contains smooth muscle that moves sperm along the ductal pathway.

Accessory Structures

There are various accessory structures that support the transport and survival of sperm. They include the *seminal vesicles*, which join with the vas deferens to become the ejaculatory duct; the *prostate gland*; and the *bulbourethral glands*.

The *seminal vesicles* are a pair of glands that produce fluid with various substances that function to (1) nourish sperm, (2) enhance sperm motility by enzymatically liquefying ejaculated semen, (3) stimulate contraction of the uterus to help the sperm reach the ovum, and (4) resist sperm destruction by female antibodies (Marieb & Hoehn, 2018). Because seminal fluid fluoresces under ultraviolet light, criminologists are able to support charges of sexual assault when examining clothing or other fibers on which seminal fluid is present (Marieb & Hoehn, 2018).

The ejaculatory duct extends into the *prostate gland*, which encircles and empties into the urethra. The prostate gland contains secretory cells that produce alkaline fluid. The prostatic fluid mixes with sperm and fluid from the seminal vesicles during ejaculation (see later discussion). The alkalinity of the prostatic fluid neutralizes the acidic metabolic wastes released by sperm and counteracts the acid pH within the vagina to ensure mass survival of sperm.

Lastly, *bulbourethral glands*, also known as *Cowper glands*, lie within the external urethral sphincter. Their function is similar to the Bartholin glands of the woman: They secrete a mucous fluid that serves to facilitate penetration of the vagina by lubricating the head of the penis.

Erection, Emission, and Ejaculation

Erection refers to a state in which the penis becomes elongated and rigid, facilitating its insertion into the vagina. Erection takes place as a result of parasympathetic nerve activity. The parasympathetic nerves that innervate the penis cause the release of nitric oxide, a chemical with vasodilating properties. Dilation of the penile arteries compresses the veins within the penis, causing engorgement of blood within the tissue. Drugs used for erectile dysfunction work to mimic the body's natural method of achieving an erection. For example, sildenafil (Viagra) and other similar drugs act to increase smooth muscle relaxation and inflow of blood. This allows for an improved and more sustained erection.

The movement of sperm and their mixture with fluid from the seminal vesicles and prostate gland into the urethra is called **emission**, a process mediated via the sympathetic nervous system.

Ejaculation is the discharge of semen, or fluid that contains sperm, from the penis. The process of ejaculation results from rhythmic contraction of the muscles of the vas deferens and the penis during orgasm and sexual climax. The normal volume of ejaculate is 2 to 6 mL, which contains an average of 60 to 100 million spermatozoa/mL. Infertility occurs when there are less than 20 million spermatozoa/mL.

Following ejaculation, the sympathetic nervous system causes the arteries to constrict, allowing the accumulated blood to drain into the venous system. The penis then resumes its pre-erection state. Because a man's sexual response is regulated via nervous system intervention, an absolute refractory period follows. This means that there is an interim period of time, ranging from a few minutes to several hours, which must elapse before a man can achieve a subsequent erection and ejaculation.

Assessment

History

The nurse obtains a general health and family history (see Chapter 4) and a detailed sexual history. A sexual history includes questions that elicit information about

- Risks for STIs
- Contraceptive practices
- Ability to achieve or sustain an erection
- Pain during sexual intercourse
- Premature ejaculation or other concerns of a sexual nature
- Inability of a sex partner to conceive
- Prior treatment (including drug therapy, diagnostic tests, or surgery) relative to the genitourinary system

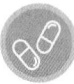

Pharmacologic Considerations

■ Some types of medications, such as certain antihypertensives, can reduce a man's ability to achieve or sustain an erection.

Physical Examination

The nurse inspects the external genitalia, looking for abnormalities such as skin lesions and urethral discharge. They palpate the testes for tumors and examines the scrotum. **Transillumination**, shining a light through the scrotum, provides clues about the density of scrotal tissue. A **digital rectal examination** (DRE) is performed to assess the prostate for size as well as evidence of tumor (Fig. 52-13). Yearly DREs are recommended for men older than 40 to 50 years.

Diagnostic Tests

Several diagnostic tests are commonly performed to evaluate the male genitourinary tract. Table 52-2 describes appropriate nursing care for clients undergoing specific tests.

Transrectal Ultrasonography

Transrectal ultrasonography (TRUS) is a test in which a lubricated probe is inserted into the rectum to obtain a view of the prostate gland from various angles. The test is indicated in cases in which the prostate gland is enlarged or the blood level of prostate-specific antigen (PSA) (see later discussion) is elevated.

Cystoscopy

In a cystoscopy, an illuminated optical instrument called a *cystoscope* is inserted into the urinary meatus to inspect the bladder, prostate, and urethra. This aids in evaluating the degree of encroachment by the prostate on the urethra.

Tissue Biopsy

A biopsy of tissue from various reproductive structures may be removed for diagnostic purposes. A needle biopsy of prostatic tissue is obtained to diagnose a definitive cancer of the prostate when other assessment findings like DRE and PSA appear suspiciously abnormal. The biopsy of the prostate is obtained via the perineal or rectal approach and is generally performed as a medical office procedure.

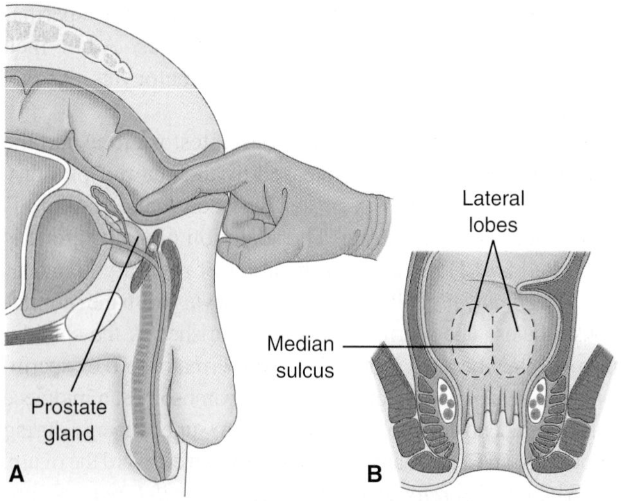

Figure 52-13 (A) Palpation of the prostate gland during digital rectal examination (DRE). **(B)** The prostate is round, with a palpable median sulcus or groove that separates the two lobes.

TABLE 52-2 Nursing Management of the Client Undergoing Genitourinary Diagnostic Testing

TEST	PREPROCEDURE CARE	POSTPROCEDURE CARE
All tests	Explain the procedure and answer questions in a calm and reassuring manner. Use techniques of therapeutic communication to provide an opportunity for the client to express concerns. Talk with client and inform them of each step as the test proceeds.	Assist client to resume a comfortable position and remove gels or lubricants. Answer questions about when test results will be available and when normal activity can resume. Provide written posttest instructions, if applicable.
Transrectal ultrasonography (ultrasound of prostate)	Assure client that test is not painful; administer or have client self-administer an enema; encourage client to focus on breathing slowly to reduce anxiety.	Assist client in removing excess lubricant. Explain that client may resume normal activities.
Cystoscopy	Inform client that he will experience bladder fullness and a strong desire to void. Inform client that an anesthetic lubricant will be instilled into the urethra to minimize discomfort and facilitate passage of cystoscope.	Instruct client to monitor voiding pattern and to report any bleeding or difficulty urinating. Inform client that prophylactic antibiotics will be given and stress that medication be taken as ordered.
Prostatic biopsy	Inform client that a local anesthetic may be used to minimize discomfort; administer or have client self-administer an enema if a rectal approach is used.	Provide information about site care. Instruct client that sitz baths and a mild analgesic will reduce discomfort. Tell client that a prophylactic antibiotic will be given and stress that medication be taken as ordered.
Testicular biopsy	Inform client that a local anesthetic will be administered.	In the case of an incisional rather than a needle biopsy, instruct the client to refrain from tub baths until the sutures are removed.

A testicular biopsy, requiring a specimen from one or both testes, evaluates spermatozoa production for diagnosing infertility problems or testicular malignancy. Although this procedure can be done in the primary provider's office, it may also be performed in a hospital's ambulatory surgery department.

Culture and Sensitivity Tests

Culture and sensitivity tests are obtained from urethral secretions, skin lesions, or urine. Prostatic fluid can be expressed during a DRE and also sent for culture.

Fertility Tests

Fertility studies include a semen analysis to determine sperm count, sperm motility, and abnormal sperm. Other laboratory tests may include measuring the level of plasma LH, which is necessary for the release of testosterone from the testes. A decrease in the blood level of LH may be responsible for decreased testosterone production and infertility.

Tumor Markers

Tumor markers are substances synthesized by abnormal tissue that are released into the circulation in excessive amounts. The **prostate-specific antigen** (PSA) assay is a blood test that, when elevated above 4 ng/mL, may correspond with prostate cancer. However, an elevated PSA does not always indicate a malignancy; it may indicate benign disease or other factors such as an enlarged prostate gland, older age, prostatitis, recent ejaculation, and other innocuous causes.

PSA screening at levels between 4 and 10 ng/mL is considered to be the "borderline range" with a 1 in 4 chance of developing prostate cancer, and a PSA level of more than 10 ng/mL increasing to a 50% chance of developing prostate cancer (ACS, 2021). The ACS (2020) recommends that clients make an informed decision regarding prostate screening exams, after discussion with their health care provider. Other blood test findings that suggest prostate cancer are elevated levels of alpha-fetoprotein, beta-human chorionic gonadotropin (bHCG), and total urine estrogens. Alkaline and acid phosphatase blood tests determine if prostatic cancer has spread to the bone.

>>> *Stop, Think, and Respond 52-3*

What health teaching is important for men to ensure early diagnosis and treatment of disorders that affect the male reproductive system?

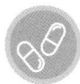

Pharmacologic Considerations

■ Women and men who are athletes may self-administer anabolic steroids similar to testosterone to increase muscle mass and to facilitate physical endurance. However, such regimens have consequences for the reproductive system and general health. Men experience reduced and abnormal sperm production, atrophy of the testes, erectile dysfunction, breast enlargement, increased aggressiveness, depression, and suicidal tendencies. Women using steroids experience development of facial hair, breast reduction, cessation of menstruation, and hypertrophy of the clitoris. Both experience acne, risk of liver damage, and hypercholesterolemia.

KEY POINTS

- Female reproductive system
  - External structures: mons pubis, vaginal orifice, labia majora, labia minora, clitoris
  - Internal structures: vagina, uterus, fallopian tubes, uterus
  - Cycles consist of ovulation, pregnancy, and menstruation.
- Breasts: mammary glands of lobes surrounded by fatty tissue; primary function: lactation
- Male reproductive system
  - External structures: penis and scrotum
  - Internal structures: testes, seminiferous tubules, epididymis, ductus deferens, spermatic cord
  - Accessory structures: seminal vesicles, prostate gland, bulbourethral glands

CRITICAL THINKING EXERCISES

1. When a client says she has "female problems," what information is important to ask?
2. What nursing activities are appropriate when a woman has a pelvic examination during which a sample will be obtained for a Pap test?
3. A 50-year-old man is offered a PSA test but refuses following his primary provider's explanation concerning its advantages and disadvantages. Explain the rationale for this man's decision.
4. A couple is experiencing infertility, and the man agrees to have his sperm examined. The man's volume of the semen specimen is 4 mL and contains a total of 300 million sperm. Explain the results of the test as it relates to the couple's fertility.

NCLEX-STYLE REVIEW QUESTIONS PrepU

1. What is the best action a nurse can take when a client says she douched just prior to coming for a gynecologic examination that will include a Pap test?
   1. Note the information on the specimen form.
   2. Proceed with the examination as usual.
   3. Explain that the test results may be invalid.
   4. Reschedule the Pap test after no prior douching.
2. Discharge instructions from the nurse following a D&C should include notifying the primary provider if what sign or symptom develops?
   1. Slight cramping
   2. Dark, bloody discharge
   3. Elevated temperature
   4. Mild abdominal pain
3. What instructions are essential by the nurse when preparing a client for a mammogram? Select all that apply.
   1. Wear a supportive bra.
   2. Omit applying deodorant.
   3. Schedule the test within a week after menstruation.
   4. Perform a breast self-examination prior to the test.
   5. Avoid body powder containing talc.
   6. Bathe or shower with an antiseptic soap.
4. During physical examination of the male reproductive system, what method is best for providing the nurse with information about the density of the client's scrotal tissue?
   1. Performing digital rectal examination
   2. Using transillumination
   3. Inspecting the size of the scrotum
   4. Using a scrotal radiography
5. Following a prostatic biopsy, what suggestion can the nurse provide to help relieve the client's discomfort?
   1. Take a sitz bath.
   2. Void frequently.
   3. Apply a scrotal support.
   4. Sit on several pillows.

WANT TO KNOW MORE? There are a wide variety of online resources available on thePoint to enhance learning and understanding of this chapter.

Go to **thePoint.lww.com/activate** and use the activation code found in the front of this text to unlock these online resources.

53 Caring for Clients With Disorders of the Female Reproductive System

Words To Know

amenorrhea
bioidentical hormones
carcinoma in situ
cervicitis
conization
cystocele
dilation and curettage
dysmenorrhea
dyspareunia
endometrial ablation
endometriosis
enterocele
fibroid tumors
fistula
hormone replacement therapy
hysterectomy
infertility
libido
menopause
menorrhagia
menstrual diary
metrorrhagia
myomectomy
oligomenorrhea
oophorocystectomy
oophorectomy
panhysterectomy
pelvic inflammatory disease
pessary
polycystic ovarian syndrome
premature ovarian failure
premenstrual syndrome
rectocele
salpingo-oophorectomy
toxic shock syndrome
uterine fibroid embolization
uterovaginal prolapse
vaginitis

Learning Objectives

On completion of this chapter, you will be able to:

1. Describe at least four conditions that deviate from normal menstrual patterns.
2. Describe the purpose of a menstrual diary and how to maintain it.
3. Give two examples of disorders characterized by amenorrhea and oligomenorrhea.
4. Discuss therapeutic techniques and nursing management for menstrual disorders.
5. List several physiologic consequences of menopause.
6. Give reasons for and against hormone replacement therapy.
7. Name four infectious and inflammatory conditions common in women and one cause for each.
8. Describe the signs and symptoms that differentiate three types of vaginal infections.
9. Discuss methods that may help prevent vaginal infections or their recurrence.
10. Describe the technique for inserting vaginal medications.
11. Name at least four aspects of nursing care for clients with pelvic inflammatory disease.
12. Give at least two suggestions that can help women avoid toxic shock syndrome.
13. List four structural abnormalities of the female reproductive system and their effects on fertility or sexuality.
14. Discuss methods the nurse can use to help a client select an appropriate treatment for endometriosis.
15. List three problems experienced by women who develop vaginal fistulas, and related nursing management.
16. Give examples of appropriate information when teaching a client to use a pessary.
17. Explain the term *carcinoma in situ* and how it applies to the prognosis of women with gynecologic malignancies.
18. Identify the most common reproductive cancers and methods for early diagnosis.
19. Discuss nursing diagnoses and potential complications among clients who undergo a hysterectomy and nursing interventions important to include in their care.
20. Give two reasons that explain the high lethality associated with ovarian cancer.
21. Name three possible causes of vaginal cancer.
22. Discuss the nursing management of and appropriate discharge instructions for a client who has a radical vulvectomy for vulvar cancer.

Diseases or disorders of pelvic reproductive structures can profoundly affect a woman's health and sexuality. This chapter discusses some common problems for which adult women seek health care, including disturbances in menstruation, infectious and inflammatory disorders, structural abnormalities, disorders affecting fertility, and benign and malignant tumors of the reproductive system. Menopause, although it is a normal physiologic process and not a disorder, is also discussed in this chapter because it often requires symptomatic management.

Gerontologic Considerations

- Vaginal flora change with age, causing the environment to become more alkaline predisposing older women to vaginitis.
- Older women may develop perineal pruritus. To discover the cause, ask questions about diet, type of clothing worn, vaginal discharge, or other contributing factors. The client may be tested for glucose in the blood and urine, and a pelvic examination may be performed to rule out other abnormalities, such as cervicitis, cystocele, rectocele, or cancer of the vulva, cervix, or uterus, which are discussed later.
- Older women who experience uterine prolapse must carefully consider risks and benefits of various types of surgery, especially if the surgery may have an impact on other chronic conditions.

DISORDERS OF MENSTRUATION

Premenstrual Syndrome

Premenstrual syndrome (PMS) or its more severe form, known as *premenstrual dysphoric disorder* (PMDD), is a group of physical and emotional symptoms that occur in some women 7 to 10 days before menstruation. Its cause is unknown; however, it has been proposed that PMS results from excess estrogen, deficient progesterone, or both; hypothalamic–pituitary dysregulation; or the effect of reproductive hormones on brain chemicals such as endorphins, melatonin, and serotonin.

Women experience several symptoms, including weight gain; headache; nervousness; irritability; personality changes; depression; abdominal bloating; pain or tenderness of the breasts; breast enlargement; craving for sweets; swelling of the ankles, feet, and hands; anxiety; or increased physical activity. Diagnosis is based on data from a **menstrual diary** in which the client keeps daily recordings of her symptoms for at least 2 months. The classic finding is that the client is symptom-free during the period between the onset of menstruation and ovulation.

Treatment of PMS depends on the severity and type of symptoms experienced. Hormonal drug therapy aims at manipulating the cyclic fluctuation in estrogen and progesterone. This is accomplished with oral contraceptives, progesterone, synthetic androgens, or gonadotropin-releasing hormone (GnRH) analogues such as histrelin (Supprelin) and nafarelin (Synarel) for 6 months. In some instances, short-term therapy with tranquilizers or antidepressants such as fluoxetine (Prozac), which has been particularly beneficial, is indicated. Nonopioid analgesics, such as mefenamic acid (Ponstel), ibuprofen (Motrin), and naproxen (Anaprox), are given for discomfort. Some vitamins and mineral supplements may also relieve PMS symptoms (see Nutrition Notes).

To supplement medical treatment, the nurse encourages the client to make healthful lifestyle changes, such as the following:

- Eating six small meals per day
- Including complex carbohydrates and foods high in calcium while reducing sugar and salt
- Reducing or eliminating caffeine to relieve irritability and ease breast tenderness
- Eliminating alcohol prior to menstruation to avoid depression or mood swings
- Exercising aerobically 30 minutes most days of the week
- Getting sufficient sleep each night
- Managing stress more effectively by performing progressive muscle relaxation, deep-breathing exercises, or practicing yoga (Mayo Clinic Staff, 2020)

The nurse explains how to maintain an accurate menstrual diary. The nurse also explains drug therapy using oral contraceptives. Because estrogen levels are pharmacologically suppressed, the client who takes a GnRH analogue may experience vaginal dryness that can make intercourse uncomfortable and a loss of bone density similar to osteoporosis (refer to the Nursing Management section that accompanies the discussion of menopause for additional interventions). If the client takes nonsteroidal anti-inflammatory drugs (NSAIDs) to relieve pain, the nurse stresses the importance of taking the NSAIDs with food or after meals to avoid gastric distress.

Dysmenorrhea

Dysmenorrhea is painful menstruation; it may be primary or secondary. Primary dysmenorrhea usually is idiopathic, and no abnormality is found. Secondary dysmenorrhea is a result of other disorders such as endometriosis, displacement of the uterus, or fibroid uterine tumors that are discussed later. Symptoms are lower abdominal pain and cramping, which may become more severe with fatigue, cold, and tension. Dysmenorrhea is treated with mild nonnarcotic analgesics and by treating the underlying cause if one is identified. Taking one of the various forms of hormonal contraceptives for several months usually reduces the symptoms of dysmenorrhea (Smith & Kaunitz, 2019).

For symptomatic relief of pain and discomfort, suggest local applications of heat, such as a warm shower, moist heating pad, or water bottle. Demonstrate how to assume a knee–chest position (Fig. 53-1) to relieve discomfort caused by retroversion (backward tilt) of the uterus. Encourage the client to obtain adequate rest, nutrition, and relief from stress to facilitate coping with periodic discomfort.

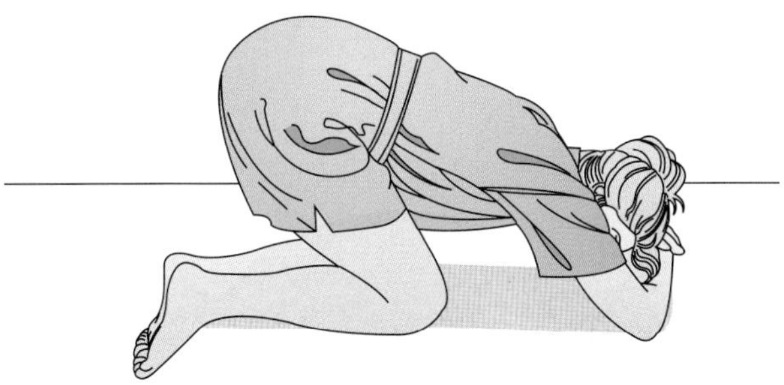

Figure 53-1 Knee–chest position. (Reprinted with permission from Pillitteri, A. (2014). *Maternal and child health nursing* (7th ed.). Wolters Kluwer Health/Lippincott Williams & Wilkins.)

Nutrition Notes

The Client With PMS

- Several vitamins and minerals taken on a daily basis may relieve symptoms associated with PMS, such as 100 mg vitamin B_6 to reduce irritability, fatigue, and depression; 400 International Units of vitamin E to reduce breast tenderness; 1200 mg calcium in divided doses three times a day to relieve bloating and body aches; and 400 mg magnesium to relieve pain, water retention, and dysphoria (Thielen, 2018).
- Some studies suggest that megadoses of vitamin B_6 relieve PMS symptoms, but large doses (i.e., 500 mg) can cause sensory neuropathy, which disappears after supplement use stops. Until the relationship between nutrients and PMS is more clearly defined, discourage self-medicating with megadoses of vitamins and minerals.

Amenorrhea and Oligomenorrhea

Amenorrhea is the absence of menstrual flow. *Primary amenorrhea* is the term used when a woman of reproductive age has never menstruated. If menstruation stops after menstrual cycles have occurred, it is called *secondary amenorrhea*. Secondary amenorrhea occurs normally during pregnancy, after menopause, sometimes throughout lactation, and when the ovaries or uterus is surgically removed. **Oligomenorrhea** is infrequent menses. It is perfectly normal for adolescent women to experience oligomenorrhea for 1 year or more before they establish regular menses.

Oligomenorrhea and amenorrhea are usually caused by endocrine imbalances resulting from pituitary disorders or hypothyroidism, the stress response, or severely lean body mass. Women who are athletes, women with anorexia nervosa, or women with debilitating diseases can have such low levels of estrogen that menstruation ceases. Treatment focuses on the correction of the underlying cause. Two reproductive system disorders that can cause oligomenorrhea and amenorrhea are premature ovarian failure (POF) and polycystic ovarian syndrome (PCOS).

Premature Ovarian Failure

Premature ovarian failure (POF) is a disorder in which the ovaries cease to function in women younger than 40 years of age, some even early in their teens. It is characterized by irregular menses and symptoms that resemble natural menopause.

Although most women are born with approximately 2 million ovarian follicles with the potential to respond to stimulation by follicle-stimulating hormone (FSH), those with POF may not because their ovarian follicles are depleted or their follicles are unresponsive to FSH. In some women, the condition may result from an autoimmune attack that destroys the ovarian follicles. For most others, the follicle that is programmed to mature with stimulation of FSH lacks the support of other less mature follicles to help its development. The dominant follicle becomes luteinized, but it does not release an ovum (Mayo Clinic Staff, 2019).

POF is diagnosed by determining the level of FSH in a sample of blood. A higher-than-normal level of FSH combined with the history of irregular menses or premature cessation of menstruation suggests POF.

Polycystic Ovarian Syndrome

Polycystic ovarian syndrome (PCOS), a condition characterized by a cluster of signs and symptoms that include amenorrhea and oligomenorrhea, affects women between 20 and 40 years of age (Evidence-Based Practice 53-1). Affected women generally consult a primary care provider because of infrequent and irregular menses and a failure to become pregnant.

During a gynecologic examination, the primary care provider palpates the ovaries that are enlarged from multiple

Evidence-Based Practice 53-1

Polycystic Ovarian Syndrome

Clinical Question

What is the support for probable anxiety, depression, and problematic eating in PCOS?

Evidence

PCOS is a disorder of the endocrine system that affects approximately 4% to 8% of women in the reproductive phase (Correa et al., 2015). In this disorder, the woman has an imbalance of hormones that may cause the following: obesity, a resistance to insulin, and possible infertility. The woman may also experience side effects from the imbalanced hormones and this could cause issues with the state of her mental health (Correa, Sperry, & Darkes, 2015).

Nursing Implications

Nurses should encourage clients to make lifestyle changes that include diet, exercises, and coping strategies. The nurse can make educational resources obtainable for the client. If a referral is made, the nurse can encourage follow-up appointments. The changes mentioned can have an impact on the client's mental health state and provide a positive outlook.

Reference

Correa, J., Sperry, S., & Darkes, J. (2015). A case report demonstrating the efficacy of a comprehensive cognitive-behavioral therapy approach for treating anxiety, depression, and problematic eating in polycystic ovarian syndrome. *Archives of Women's Mental Health, 18*(4), 649–654. https://doi.org/10.1007/s00737-015-0506-3

fluid-filled cysts that form in the ovarian follicles. Vaginal ultrasonography and blood tests to measure hormone levels confirm the findings of the physical examination. The affected follicles neither secrete progesterone that suppresses menstruation nor release an ovum.

PCOS is associated with multiple endocrine abnormalities such as overproduction and inefficient use of insulin and high testosterone levels. Women with this disorder tend to have problems including interference with menstruation and ovulation, weight gain, excessive growth of body hair, acne, thinning hair or baldness, abnormal lipid levels, and hypertension.

Treatment includes prescribing an oral contraceptive to offset the excess of testosterone and to regulate the menstrual cycle. For those women who want to conceive, the primary care provider may prescribe an oral hypoglycemic agent such as metformin (Glucophage) and progestin-containing medications. Primary care providers prescribe lipid-lowering agents and antihypertensives to women who also manifest hyperlipidemia and high blood pressure (BP).

››› *Stop, Think, and Respond 53-1*

What are the similarities and differences among primary and secondary amenorrhea, POF, and PCOS?

Menorrhagia

Menorrhagia is excessive bleeding at the time of normal menstruation. It may be quantified as a menstrual flow that lasts more than 7 days, that requires the use of an additional two pads per day, or that extends 3 or more days longer than usual. Menorrhagia can be caused by endocrine, coagulation, or systemic disorders.

Symptomatic relief is accomplished with NSAIDs, progestins, and hormonal contraceptives with combinations of estrogen and progestin. NSAIDs reduce prostaglandins, biologic chemicals that exist in endometrial tissue, where they exert a stimulating effect on the uterus. Progestins, natural and synthetic forms of progesterone, transform the proliferative endometrium into a secretory endometrium that simulates a pregnant state. When combination hormonal contraceptives are administered, they produce a "pill period," which is characterized by light menstrual bleeding.

Dilation and curettage (D&C) is performed for symptomatic relief; however, effectiveness sometimes lasts only 1 to 2 months. **Endometrial ablation** (detachment of the lining of the uterus) by photodynamic therapy or uterine balloon therapy is a potential nonsurgical alternative (American Colleges of Obstetricians and Gynecologists [ACOG], 2020). When photodynamic therapy is used, a light-sensitive substance is applied to endometrial tissue, after which a laser probe is inserted through the cervix. The absorption of laser light by the tissue causes the endometrium to slough, in contrast to being removed with a surgical curette. Uterine balloon therapy produces the same effect by introducing a balloon into the uterus, filling the balloon with isotonic saline solution, and heating the solution to 87° for 8 minutes (Fig. 53-2). Both procedures are gaining popularity because they are cost-effective. The posttreatment course is similar to that after a D&C (see Client and Family Teaching 52-1 for education guidelines).

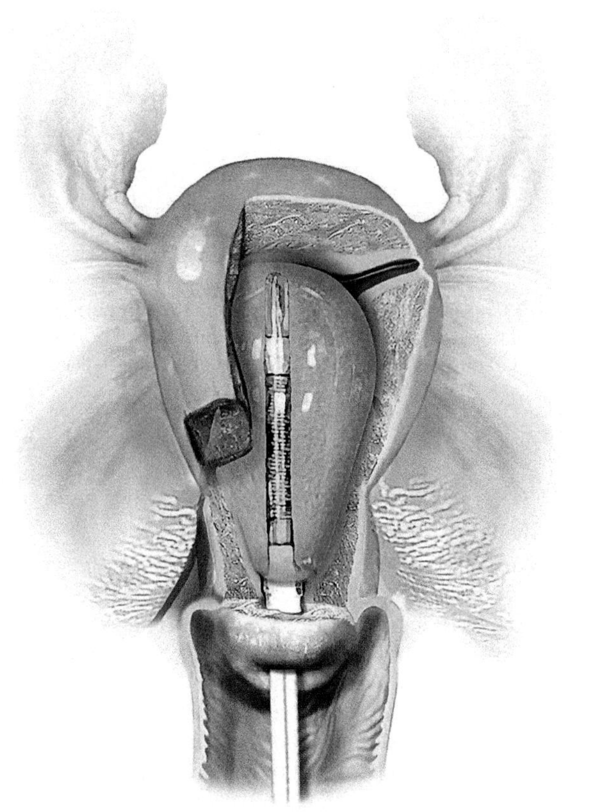

Figure 53-2 Uterine balloon therapy. This cutaway of the uterus shows a heating coil within a saline-filled balloon. (Reprinted with permission from Baggish, M. S., Guedj, H., & Valle, R. F. (2007). *Hysteroscopy: Visual perspectives of uterine anatomy, physiology and pathology* (3rd ed.). Wolters Kluwer Health/ Lippincott Williams & Wilkins.)

Metrorrhagia

Metrorrhagia is vaginal bleeding at a time other than a menstrual period. The amount of blood is not important; the fact that it occurs unexpectedly is significant. Irregular bleeding often results from an erratic stimulation of or response to pituitary or ovarian hormones, especially in adolescent girls and perimenopausal women. Some women "spot" for a day or two midway between menstrual periods. This functional bleeding is attributed to ovulation and is not considered abnormal. However, other causes for atypical bleeding include uterine malignancies, cervical irritation, or breakthrough bleeding that occurs with hormone replacement therapy (HRT) or low-dose hormonal contraceptives. Intermenstrual or postcoital (after intercourse) bleeding needs to be evaluated promptly. Treatment depends on the underlying cause.

The nurse advises the client with unexplained bleeding to see a primary care provider. For metrorrhagia or any menstrual disorder, the role of the nurse is the same: gather appropriate information, assist with gynecologic examinations, offer suggestions for relieving discomfort, instruct clients about their drug therapy, prepare clients for surgical interventions, care for them during recovery, and provide specific health teaching instructions.

MENOPAUSE

Menopause ("change of life") is the cessation of the menstrual cycle. The climacteric or perimenopausal period refers to the time during which ovarian activity gradually ceases; the postmenopausal period begins 1 year after menstruation ceases. Menopause normally occurs as a natural physiologic process between 45 and 55 years of age. Surgical menopause that occurs when the ovaries are removed can occur at any age.

The changes in hormone levels that accompany menopause cause a variety of reproductive and systemic effects. Some women have symptoms so mild and transitory that they go unnoticed; other women experience severe symptoms. Some women seek health care for symptomatic relief or to reduce the risk of osteoporosis and cardiovascular disease that occur when estrogen production decreases.

Physiology

Menopause occurs when ovarian function diminishes. Levels of estrogen and progesterone are reduced, ovulation gradually ceases, menstruation becomes irregular until it stops, and natural reproductive capacity ends. As the levels of estrogen and progesterone drop, the hypothalamus attempts to raise them by releasing GnRH, which stimulates the anterior pituitary gland to release FSH and luteinizing hormone (LH). The surge of hypothalamic–pituitary stimulation is thought to be responsible for alterations in temperature regulation, sleep disturbances, and disequilibrium in mood. Estrogen deficiency causes thinning of the vaginal walls, breast and uterine atrophy, and loss of bone density. The risks of heart disease and stroke increase with estrogen reduction. Depression, should it occur, is thought to be related more to an individual's perception of the social or psychological implications of menopause rather than to biologic factors. Depression and menopause share many of the same symptoms, indicating the need for further evaluation to determine if a mood disorder is present (Maki et al., 2019).

Assessment Findings

Changing menstrual patterns, including irregular periods and scanty or sometimes unusually copious menstrual flow, signal the onset of menopause. During the perimenopausal period (the transitional period surrounding menopause), women may experience vasomotor disturbances such as hot flashes accompanied by sweating, sleep disturbance, irritability or depression, vaginal dryness, diminished **libido** (interest or desire for sex), or **dyspareunia** (discomfort during intercourse). These common symptoms often are the ones for which women seek treatment. A cytologic examination of vaginal and cervical smears (Papanicolaou test [Pap test]) shows a decrease in estrogen production.

Medical Management

The decision to administer **hormone replacement therapy** (HRT), estrogen combined with progestin, or estrogen replacement therapy (ERT), estrogen alone, is made for each client on an individual basis (Table 53-1). The Women's Health Initiative study, a 15-year clinical trial involving HRT and ERT among postmenopausal women, ended 3 years prematurely in 2002 because of an increase in breast cancer, heart disease, blood clots, and stroke among participants. Subsequently, there have been additional studies to confirm or refute the previous recommendation to avoid HRT and ERT. The National Cancer Institute (2018) confirms that women should discuss with their health care provider the risks and benefits of HRT on an individual basis, based on their medical status (National Cancer Institute, 2018).

If HRT or ERT is indicated, it is prescribed in the lowest appropriate dose for the shortest time necessary. It is believed that estrogen in small doses can help prevent osteoporosis and relieve menopausal symptoms such as hot flashes, night sweats, and vaginal dryness. The risks of endometrial or breast cancer and the seriousness of future myocardial infarction and stroke may outweigh the potential benefit of preventing hip fractures and kyphosis that are secondary to osteoporosis.

TABLE 53-1 Risks and Benefits of Menopausal Hormone Replacement Therapy (HRT)

THERAPY	RISKS	BENEFITS
Estrogen alonea	Increased risk of fatal and nonfatal strokes	See below
	Increased risk of endometrial cancer in women with a uterus	
Estrogen with or without progestin[a]	Increased risk of strokes and blood clots	Decreased potential for osteoporosis
	Increased risk of dementia in women 65 years or older	Relief from hot flashes, night sweats, and vaginal dryness
	Increased risk for gallbladder disease	
Estrogen with progestin[a]	Increased risk for breast cancer and heart attacks (but not with estrogen alone)	Decreased risk for colorectal cancer

[a]Estrogen and progestin are prescribed for women with a uterus; estrogen alone is prescribed for women with no uterus.

References
National Institutes of Health. (2008). *Women's Health Initiative (WHI) follow-up study confirms the health risk of long-term combination therapy outweighs benefits for postmenopausal women.* http://public.nhlbi.nih.gov/newsroom/home/GetPressRelease.aspx?id2554
Todd, N. (2020). Hormone Replacement Therapy (HRT): Benefits and Risks. *WebMD.* https://www.webmd.com/menopause/hrt-risks-benefits

It may be necessary to treat some of the symptoms associated with menopause. Vaginal itching and drying is prevented or reduced by drugs such as an estrogen or cortisone cream or ointment. Low-dose androgens are added to the hormone replacement regimen to restore interest in sexual activity. Antidepressants or minor tranquilizers are prescribed for women experiencing emotional problems that are separate or related to hormonal fluctuations. Drugs such as bisphosphonates or selective estrogen receptor modulators (SERMs) (see Chapter 63) are available to reduce the potential for osteoporosis rather than prescribing HRT. **Bioidentical hormones**, U.S. Food and Drug Administration (FDA)–approved prescription substances made from soy and yams, are indistinguishable and similarly effective as those from naturally occurring estrogen and progesterone (see Chapter 9). Diets rich in phytoestrogens, such as isoflavones in soy products and lignans in flaxseed, may reduce menopausal symptoms, especially hot flashes (Watson, 2019).

See Drug Therapy Table 53-1 for specific drug treatment during menopause.

DRUG THERAPY TABLE 53-1 Drug Therapy During Menopause

Category and Common Generic (Brand) drugs	Intended Use	Common Side Effects	Safety Warnings for Nurses
Estrogen Replacement Therapy (ERT)			
Estrogens • Oral conjugated (Premarin, Menest) • Topical (Divigel) • Transdermal (EstroGel) • Vaginal (ESTRING, Femring) *Estradiols* • Oral (Femtrace) • Topical (Estrasorb) • Transdermal (Climara, Estraderm) • Injectable Delestrogen) • Vaginal (Vagifem) *Synthetic conjugated Estrogens* (Cenestin, Enjuvia)	Vasomotor symptoms associated with menopause, atrophic vaginitis, osteoporosis	Headache, dizziness, melasma, venous thromboembolism, nausea, vomiting, abdominal bloating and cramps, breakthrough bleeding/spotting, vaginal changes, rhinitis, changes in libido, breast enlargement and tenderness, weight changes, generalized pain	• Monitor for emboli in extremities or lungs • Monitor for certain cancers, stroke symptoms, and heart disease • Low-sodium diet and diuretics may help fluid/weight gain
Hormone Replacement Therapy (HRT)			
Estrogen/progestin Combined (Activella, Angeliq, Climara Pro, CombiPatch, Femhrt, Prempro, YAZ*)	Treatment of moderate to severe vasomotor symptoms associated with menopause, treatment of vulval and vaginal atrophy, osteoporosis	Same as for ERT	Same as for ERT
Bone Resorption Inhibitors			
Bisphosphonates • Alendronate (Fosamax) • Etidronate (Didronel) • Ibandronate (Boniva) • Pamidronate (Aredia) • Risedronate (Actonel) • Zoledronic acid (Zometa)	Reduce bone loss caused by resorption, reversing osteoporosis	Nausea, dyspepsia, diarrhea, headache	• Do not use if delayed esophageal emptying
Selective estrogen receptor modulators (SERM) Denosumab (Prolia) Raloxifene (Evista) Teriparatide (Forteo)	Osteoporosis prevention and treatment; increases bone mineral density by decreasing bone resorption	Hot flashes, flu-like symptoms, arthralgia, rhinitis, increased cough, leg cramping	• Dental check and repair before starting to reduce risk for osteonecrosis of jaw bone Increased fracture risk
Estrogen/bazedoxifene (Duavee) combined estrogen and SERM see above			

*The U.S. Food and Drug Administration (FDA) completed its review of recent observational (epidemiologic) studies regarding the risk of blood clots in women taking drospirenone-containing birth control pills. Drospirenone is a synthetic version of the female hormone, progesterone, also referred to as a progestin. Based on this review, FDA has concluded that drospirenone-containing birth control pills may be associated with a higher risk for blood clots than other progestin-containing pills. FDA is adding information about the studies to the labels of drospirenone-containing birth control pills such as YAZ. From the Food and Drug Administration (2018). *FDA Drug Safety Communication: Updated information about the risk of blood clots in women taking birth control pills containing drospirenone.* https://www.fda.gov/drugs/drug-safety-and-availability/fda-drug-safety-communication-updated-information-about-risk-blood-clots-women-taking-birth-control

The drugs in column 1 indicate the drug that matches up with explanations in columns 2 through 4

Concept Mastery Alert

Soy milk can be recommended to a client with hypertension who is seeking herbal remedies to treat hot flashes. The natural estrogens in soy milk may help reduce perimenopausal symptoms, especially hot flashes.

Nursing Management

The nurse collects a database that includes a menstrual, reproductive, sexual, and psychosocial history. They prepare and support the client during physical and diagnostic examinations. Health teaching addresses topics such as normal developmental changes during middle adulthood, coping strategies, health promotion techniques, methods to achieve symptomatic relief, and treatment-related information.

Because normal and abnormal structural changes are easily confused, the nurse recommends regular gynecologic and breast examinations during and after menopause. The nurse also gives the following suggestions:

- Use bland skin creams or lotions to reduce skin dryness.
- Use a water-based lubricant prior to intercourse for vaginal lubrication.
- Plan an exercise program to prevent weight gain and loss of calcium from the bones.
- Increase calcium intake by eating calcium-rich foods or by taking a calcium supplement containing vitamin D_3.
- Discuss with the prescriber the benefits, risks, and alternatives for HRT or ERT.
- Discuss a schedule for routine gynecologic and breast examinations.
- Contact the primary care provider if breakthrough vaginal bleeding or other symptoms occur while taking hormonal replacements. Changing the dosage, using a different combination of hormones, or substituting alternative medications may eliminate undesirable effects.
- Cultivate new interests and hobbies or resume those that have been abandoned because of other responsibilities.

INFECTIOUS AND INFLAMMATORY DISORDERS

Vaginitis

Vaginitis is a condition in which the vagina is inflamed.

Pathophysiology and Etiology

Vaginal inflammation is caused by chemical or mechanical irritants such as feminine hygiene products, allergic reactions, age-related tissue changes (atrophic vaginitis with menopause), and the most common etiology, infections. The pathogenic microorganisms frequently associated with vaginitis are the bacterium *Gardnerella vaginalis*, the protozoan *Trichomonas vaginalis*, and the yeastlike fungus *Candida albicans* (see Chapter 56).

Although the vagina is self-protected by mucus-secreting cells and an acidic environment (pH of 3.5 to 4.5), the tissue still may become disrupted. Some situations predispose to vaginitis because they alter protective mechanisms. For example, antibiotics or frequent douching eliminate the bacilli that promote an acidic vaginal environment. Decreased estrogen at menopause reduces the thick, moist consistency of vaginal tissue. Pregnant women, those with unregulated diabetes, and those who take hormonal contraceptives containing estrogen have an excess of glycogen in vaginal mucus, which supports the growth of microorganisms.

Assessment Findings

An abnormal vaginal discharge is the primary symptom of vaginal infection, and the characteristics of the discharge often are indicative of the infecting organism (Table 53-2). The discharge often is accompanied by itching, burning, redness, and swelling of surrounding tissues. Diagnosis is confirmed by visual and microscopic examination of secretions.

Medical Management

Infectious vaginitis is remedied by using drugs to which the microorganism is particularly sensitive. They include antifungal, antiprotozoal, and antibiotic agents (Drug Therapy Table 53-2). In some cases, the sexual partner also is infected, and vaginitis recurs if both are not treated simultaneously.

Atrophic vaginitis is relieved with estrogen replacement administered as a topical cream. If the client has diabetes mellitus, regulating blood glucose is an important aspect of treatment.

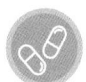

Pharmacologic Considerations

- A panty liner may be worn after vaginal insertion of the drug to prevent staining of clothing and bed linen.

Nursing Management

The nurse informs the client not to douche before the physical examination because washing away the secretions removes the characteristics of the vaginal discharge and interferes with obtaining an adequate diagnostic smear. After

TABLE 53-2 Characteristics of Vaginal Infections

MICROORGANISM	COLOR OF DISCHARGE	CONSISTENCY	ODOR	OTHER SYMPTOMS
Candida albicans	Curdy white	Thick	Strong	Burning with urination
Trichomonas vaginalis	Yellow white	Foamy	Foul	Severe itching
Gardnerella vaginalis	Grayish white	Watery	Fishy	More discharge after intercourse

DRUG THERAPY TABLE 53-2 Agents to Treat Vaginitis

Category and Common Generic (Brand) drugs	Intended Use	Common Side Effects	Safety Warnings for Nurses
Antifungal Clotrimazole (Gyne-Lotrimin) Miconazole (Monistat) Terconazole (Terazol) Tioconazole (Vagistat-1)	Treatment of candidiasis fungal infection	Cramping, nausea, urinary frequency, erythema, stinging	Instruct partner to use condom to prevent reinfection.
Antiprotozoal Metronidazole (Flagyl)	Treatment of *trichomoniasis vaginalis*	Unpleasant metallic taste, anorexia, nausea, diarrhea, darkening of urine	• Do not use in first trimester of pregnancy. • Sexual partner may need to be treated.
Antibiotic Sulfisoxazole (Gantrisin)	Treat bacterial vaginitis (*Gardnerella vaginalis)*	Headache, nausea	• Photosensitivity, instruct to wear sun protection • Discontinue immediately if hypersensitivity reaction occurs.

diagnosis, the nurse may insert the first dose of vaginal medication while teaching the client how to repeat the technique. Nonprescription drugs for the treatment of yeast/fungal infections are available. The nurse informs clients that although these drugs usually are effective, the initial diagnosis of vaginitis is best made by a primary care provider. The nurse emphasizes the importance of completing the course of therapy.

The nurse also informs the client to avoid routine douching. Taking *Lactobacillus acidophilus* in capsule form or eating yogurt containing active cultures of lactobacilli can replenish normal vaginal microorganisms. Sitz baths are recommended to relieve itching, burning, and swelling of the vulva and perineum. Skin protectants containing zinc oxide promote healing. The nurse offers additional suggestions for preventing a recurrence of vaginal infections, as presented in (Client and Family Teaching 53-1).

Client and Family Teaching 53-1
Preventing Vaginal Infections

The nurse teaches the client to do the following:

- Bathe daily with particular attention to perineal hygiene.
- Wipe from front to back after bowel movements.
- Avoid feminine hygiene products and douching more than once per week.
- Wear cotton undergarments and change them daily.
- Refrain from wearing layers of clothing, such as underwear plus pantyhose plus slacks, which increase warmth and interfere with air circulation around the genital area.
- Change from a wet swimsuit as soon as possible.
- Wash hands and devices that are inserted into the vagina, such as medication applicators, douche tips, and diaphragms, and store them in clean containers.
- Change sanitary pads before they become saturated; substitute a sanitary pad for a tampon at night.
- Use a condom or avoid intercourse if either client or her sex partner(s) has genitourinary symptoms.

Cervicitis

Cervicitis is an inflammation of the cervix.

Pathophysiology and Etiology

Cervical inflammation results from infectious microorganisms, decreased estrogen levels during menopause, or trauma during gynecologic procedures, or occurs as a consequence of inserting tampons or vaginal medication applicators. Streptococcal, staphylococcal, gonorrheal, and chlamydial (see Chapter 56) infections are the most common etiologies. The potential is greater during pregnancy and after childbirth, when the microorganisms can enter cervical tissue through small lacerations. The infection can travel upward through uterine and tubal structures, leading to pelvic inflammatory disease (PID) (see later discussion). Inflammation and subsequent formation of scar tissue increase the potential for ectopic pregnancy or difficulty conceiving. Chronic cervicitis decreases the amount and quality of cervical mucus and alters the pH, both of which are underlying causes of infertility.

Assessment Findings

Early cervicitis may be asymptomatic. The client eventually spots or bleeds intermenstrually or develops a vaginal discharge. Dyspareunia (painful intercourse) or slight bleeding after sexual intercourse may occur. Severe cervicitis sometimes causes a sensation of weight in the pelvis.

Diagnosis is made by visual examination of the cervix. Microscopic examination of cervical smears identifies the causative microorganism.

Medical Management

Douches and local or systemic antibiotics are the treatment of choice for acute cervicitis. Chronic cervicitis is treated with electrocautery, a heat-generating device. Frank bleeding requires cervical or vaginal packing or electric coagulation of the bleeding vessel. Healing often takes 6 to 8 weeks. Severe chronic cervicitis is treated by **conization** (removal of the diseased portion of the cervical mucosa). This outpatient procedure uses an instrument that simultaneously cuts tissue and coagulates the bleeding area. Dilatation is done if there is cervical stenosis. Successful treatment eliminates the inflammation, relieves the symptoms, and aids fertility.

Nursing Management

The nurse schedules treatment procedures 5 to 8 days after the end of the menstrual period to reduce the potential for bleeding. The nurse positions the client for a gynecologic examination and explains that a momentary cramping sensation may be felt during the electrocautery procedure. After electrocautery, the nurse instructs the client to do the following:

- Rest more than usual for 1 to 2 days.
- Avoid straining or heavy lifting.
- Rest in bed and report if slight bleeding does occur; frank bleeding requires a return visit to the primary care provider.
- Expect a grayish-green, malodorous discharge for about 3 weeks after cautery.
- Anticipate slight bleeding about the 11th day.
- Return for a follow-up visit to the primary care provider in 2 to 4 weeks.
- Abstain from sexual relations until tissues are healed.
- Expect that healing may take 6 to 8 weeks.

Pelvic Inflammatory Disease

Pelvic inflammatory disease (PID) is an infection of the pelvic organs other than the uterus, including the ovaries (oophoritis), fallopian tubes (salpingitis), pelvic vascular system, and pelvic supporting structures.

Pathophysiology and Etiology

Microorganisms enter pelvic structures through the cervix from the vagina (Fig. 53-3). The cause usually is bacterial, with gonococci and *Chlamydia trachomatis* being the most common pathogens. The infection travels up the uterus to the fallopian tubes (salpingitis) and ovaries (oophoritis) and can result in a pelvic abscess or peritonitis as pus from the infected tubes leaks into the abdomen.

Assessment Findings

Signs and symptoms include an infectious malodorous discharge, backache, severe or aching abdominal and pelvic pain, a bearing-down feeling, fever, dyspareunia, nausea and vomiting, menorrhagia, and dysmenorrhea. Some women experience milder symptoms such as pain during a pelvic examination. Severe infection may cause urinary symptoms.

Diagnosis is based on symptoms as well as a gynecologic examination. A culture and sensitivity test of the vaginal discharge is obtained to identify the causative microorganism. Ultrasonography, magnetic resonance imaging (MRI), or computed tomography (CT) may disclose a pelvic abscess.

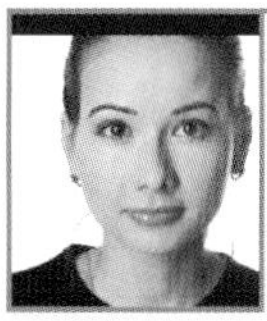

Clinical Scenario A 20-year-old college student is brought to the emergency department by her roommate. The client tells the nurse who obtains her history that she has had a purulent vaginal discharge for a week or more. She admits to being sexually active but consistently takes an oral hormonal contraceptive to avoid pregnancy. The client currently has a fever of 102.2°F by the oral route. While being prepared for a gynecologic examination, the client winces with pain, identifying it as being in her lower abdomen. **What nursing actions should take precedence at this time? Refer to the Nursing Process section that follows for examples.**

Medical Management

Hospitalization with complete bed rest often is necessary. Parenteral or oral antibiotics are administered as soon as culture and sensitivity tests are obtained. Intravenous (IV) fluids are ordered if the client is dehydrated, and antipyretics are used if the temperature is elevated. A ruptured pelvic abscess requires emergency surgery.

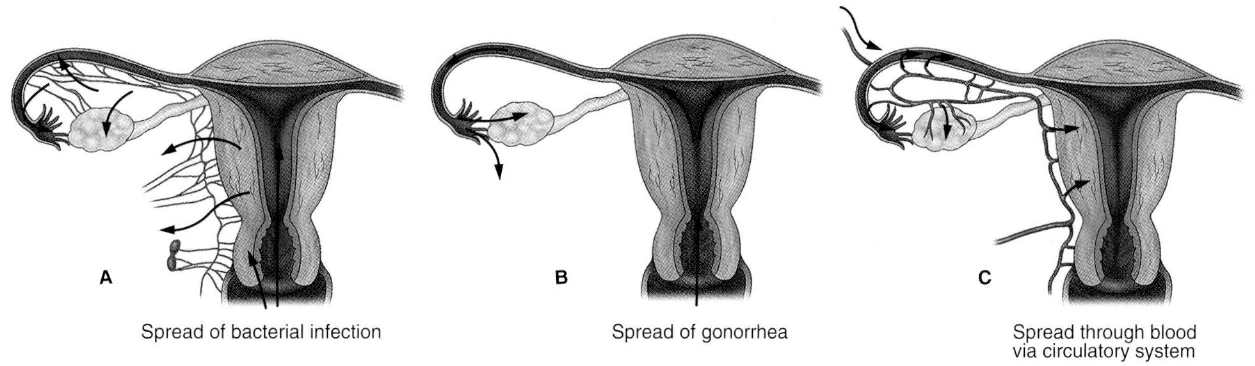

Figure 53-3 **(A)** Bacteria spread from the vagina and uterus through the lymphatics. **(B)** Gonorrhea spreads from the vagina and uterus through the tubes and ovaries. **(C)** Bacteria can also reach the reproductive organs through the bloodstream.

NURSING PROCESS FOR THE CLIENT WITH PELVIC INFLAMMATORY DISEASE

Assessment

Obtain a complete medical, drug, and allergy history, and ask the client to describe all symptoms. A vaginal smear may be necessary. If the client is an outpatient, instruct the client to refrain from douching for 48 hours before being examined. If the client is admitted to the hospital and a vaginal smear is ordered, inquire whether the client has douched within the last 48 hours.

Diagnosis, Planning, and Interventions

The nurse's role in caring for a client with PID includes, but is not limited to, the following:

Thermal Injury Risk: Related to infectious illness
Expected Outcome: The client's body temperature will return to the normal range.

- Assess body temperature every 4 hours using a temporal or tympanic thermometer. *The pattern and trend in body temperature indicate the efficacy of nursing measures. A temporal or tympanic thermometer is best for determining core body temperature.*
- Assist client to put on light clothing and cover with minimum bed linen. *Exposing skin to ambient air promotes heat loss by radiation.*
- Circulate room air using a portable fan. *Reduces temperature by convection as cooler air blows across the body's surface.*
- Administer a tepid sponge bath if body temperature exceeds 103°F; discontinue if shivering develops. *Heat loss can be facilitated by conduction and evaporation. Shivering increases body heat via muscular contraction.*
- Provide oral fluids of at least 100 mL/hour. *Oral intake replaces fluid losses caused by perspiration and increased metabolism.*
- Limit activity to bathroom only. *Reduced activity lowers metabolic demands and heat production.*
- Administer an antipyretic as prescribed for fever over 101°F. *Antipyretics inhibit heat-producing chemicals such as prostaglandin E_2 that affect thermoregulation by the hypothalamus.*
- Administer prescribed oral or parenteral antibiotic as directed. *Antibiotics inhibit microbial reproduction, which relieves bacterial infection.*

Infection Risk: Related to systemic spread of pathogenic microorganisms
Expected Outcome: The nurse will monitor to detect, manage, and minimize sepsis if it occurs.

- Monitor vital signs and results of white blood cell (WBC) counts. *Increased temperature, pulse rate, and leukocytosis indicate an infectious process.*
- Maintain IV site and administer parenteral fluids and antibiotic therapy as scheduled. *The nurse implements prescribed medical therapy for treating an infectious process.*
- Keep the client in a semi-sitting position. *Keeping the upper body elevated facilitates pelvic drainage and minimizes upward extension of infection.*

Infection Risk: Related to direct or indirect contact with infectious microorganisms and their transmission
Expected Outcome: No nosocomial infections will occur among other clients or staff that can be traced to the client with the primary infection.

- Provide the client with a private room with a toilet and sink. *Separating the client from others confines the source of transmission to one location.*
- Follow contact isolation precautions. *Contact isolation is a category of transmission-based precautions for controlling the spread of infectious microorganisms found in wound drainage and other body fluids.*
- Wrap and dispose of soiled perineal pads in a lined biohazard container. *Confining objects that are heavily contaminated with infectious microorganisms reduces the potential for transmitting them to other susceptible people.*
- Bag soiled linen according to infection control policies of the institution. *Linen that has been in contact with a person with infectious body fluids is contained in specially marked bags to avoid transmitting pathogens to personnel who handle laundry.*
- Leave a disposable stethoscope and thermometers in the room for assessments. *Instruments used for frequent assessments are restricted to the infectious client and then destroyed.*
- Perform hand hygiene after removing gloves. *Hand hygiene reduces the number of pathogens on the skin, which tend to grow and multiply in the warmth of latex or vinyl gloves.*
- Clean the cover on the BP cuff with a disinfectant when the client is discharged. *A disinfectant destroys microorganisms on the surface of objects in the environment.*
- Instruct housekeeping personnel to damp mop the client's room after cleaning other clients' rooms and change the mop head when finished. *A principle of medical asepsis is to always clean the most heavily soiled area last. Changing the mop head prevents spreading microorganisms to other areas.*

Acute Pain: Related to inflamed tissue and pelvic congestion
Expected Outcome: Client's comfort will be maintained within a level of tolerance.

NURSING PROCESS FOR THE CLIENT WITH PELVIC INFLAMMATORY DISEASE (continued)

- Administer prescribed analgesic. *Analgesics relieve pain by various biochemical mechanisms.*
- Provide diversional activities to distract client from pain. *Distraction reduces pain perception by providing alternative stimuli to the brain.*
- Position for comfort and limit unnecessary activity. *An uncomfortable position and movement tend to increase pain intensity.*

Altered Skin Integrity Risk: Related to excoriating potential of vaginal drainage
Expected Outcome: Vulvar and perineal tissue will be intact.

- Wash the perineum well with soap and water every 4 hours. *Removing drainage from contact with the skin promotes skin integrity.*
- Pat or blot the skin dry. *Touching the skin gently rather than vigorously reduces trauma to the skin. Keeping the skin dry reduces the potential for maceration.*
- Change perineal pads frequently. *Changing perineal pads frequently increases the potential for absorbing and wicking drainage from the skin surface.*

Evaluation of Expected Outcomes

Expected outcomes are that vital signs and WBC count are normal. Infection control measures are effective. The client's pain or discomfort is relieved or eliminated. The genital tissue is free of redness and excoriation.

After discharge from the hospital, tell the client to temporarily abstain from sexual intercourse to prevent extending the infection and infecting the partner. In addition, explain that subsequent episodes of PID can be prevented by seeking medical attention when symptoms of infection, such as a feeling of pressure in the pelvic area, burning on urination, or vaginal drainage, first appear. Early treatment prevents the infection from moving up the reproductive tract, resulting in complications such as peritonitis, abscess formation, and obstruction of the fallopian tubes. When early treatment of acute PID is delayed or inadequate, the infection may become chronic.

Toxic Shock Syndrome

Toxic shock syndrome (TSS), a type of septic shock (see Chapter 17), is a life-threatening systemic reaction to the toxin produced by several kinds of bacteria. Some causative microorganisms include *Staphylococcus aureus*, *Streptococcus pyogenes*, and *Clostridium sordellii*. TSS also occurs in men and nonmenstruating women with soft tissue and postoperative infections.

Pathophysiology and Etiology

TSS is associated with the use of superabsorbent tampons that are not changed frequently and internal contraceptive devices that remain in place longer than necessary. The syndrome occurs when virulent bacteria reproduce suddenly and abundantly in the body and remain unchecked by normal physiologic defense mechanisms. The bacteria produce chemicals that cause blood vessels to dilate, which keeps the major portion of the blood volume in the periphery, reduces cardiac output, and causes severe hypotension (shock). The toxin also seems to inhibit the ability of affected cells to use oxygen (Norris, 2019).

Assessment Findings

Signs and Symptoms

A sudden onset of high fever, chills, tenderness or pain in the muscles, nausea, vomiting, diarrhea, hypotension, hyperemia (increased redness and congestion) of vaginal mucous membranes, disorientation, and headache occurs. The skin is warm despite the client being in shock. A rash that first appears on the palms of the hands or the body a few hours after the infection later results in shedding of the superficial layer of the skin (desquamation). The pulse is rapid and thready.

Diagnostic Findings

The infecting microorganism is found in cultures of specimens from the vagina, blood, urine, or other sites. The blood urea nitrogen, serum creatinine, and serum bilirubin levels are increased. The serum enzymes aspartate aminotransferase (AST) and alanine aminotransferase (ALT) are elevated. The platelet count may be decreased.

Medical Management

Circulation is supported with IV fluids while combating the infection with IV antibiotic therapy. Some drugs that are used include oxacillin (Prostaphlin), nafcillin (Nafcil), and methicillin (Staphcillin). Potent adrenergic drugs such as dopamine (Intropin) or dobutamine (Dobutrex) are given to counteract peripheral vasodilation and maintain renal perfusion. Oxygen is given to promote aerobic metabolism at the cellular level.

Nursing Management

The nurse frequently assesses vital signs. They administer the first dose of antibiotics immediately and as ordered thereafter. The nurse applies pressure to venipuncture or injection sites to control bleeding and oozing if the platelet count is low. They carefully measure intake and output and report any sudden decrease in the urinary output or a urinary output of less than 500 mL/day to the primary care provider.

Before discharge, the nurse teaches preventive measures such as using perineal pads rather than tampons or changing tampons frequently. They tell clients who use a diaphragm, vaginal sponge, or cervical cap for birth control to remove the device within 24 hours after use. The nurse emphasizes hand hygiene and keeping vaginal devices clean.

Concept Mastery Alert

Endometriosis occurs when tissue similar to the endometrium is found outside the uterus. Heavy bleeding and cramping are symptoms of endometriosis, but endometriosis is not caused by a thicker than usual uterine lining.

STRUCTURAL ABNORMALITIES

Endometriosis

Endometriosis is a condition in which tissue with a cellular structure and function resembling that of the endometrium is found outside the uterus. The atypical locations for endometrial tissue include the ovaries, the pelvic cavity, and occasionally the abdominal cavity.

Pathophysiology and Etiology

The cause of endometriosis is not clearly understood. It may result from remnants of embryonic tissue that remain in the abdominal cavity. Another possible cause is retrograde menstruation, in which the fallopian tubes expel fragments of endometrial tissue that eventually become implanted outside the uterus.

The ectopic tissue responds to stimulation by estrogen and, perhaps, to progesterone. The tissue bleeds when the endometrium of the uterus is shed, but unfortunately, there is no outlet for the extrauterine bleeding. The trapped blood causes pain and ultimately adhesions in the peritoneal cavity. If the fallopian tubes are affected, they may become occluded and result in **infertility**, an inability to conceive. If endometrial tissue is enclosed in an ovary, a chocolate cyst (named because it collects dark blood) develops. Occasionally, this cyst ruptures, spilling old blood and endometrial cells into the pelvic or abdominal cavity. The condition is relieved naturally when endometrial tissue atrophies after menopause or regresses during pregnancy.

Assessment Findings

Severe dysmenorrhea and copious menstrual bleeding are typical symptoms of endometriosis. The client may experience dyspareunia and pain on defecation. Rupture of a chocolate cyst results in severe abdominal pain that can mimic other abdominal pathologies such as appendicitis or bowel obstruction.

A pelvic examination reveals fixed, tender areas in the lower pelvis. Restricted mobility of the uterus from adhesions may be noted. A laparoscopy confirms the diagnosis.

Medical and Surgical Management

Endometriosis is cured by natural or surgical menopause. To preserve the potential for having children, many women are managed medically as long as possible. Estrogen–progestin contraceptives are administered to keep the client in a nonbleeding phase of her menstrual cycle for about 9 months. The goal is to control the ectopic tissue so that the client is symptom-free for several years. The progestin norethindrone (Norlutin) and the synthetic androgen danazol (Danocrine) are effective in causing atrophy of endometrial tissue.

Without destroying the possibility for childbearing, surgery is performed to remove the cysts, as much of the ectopic tissue as possible, and lyse adhesions caused by bleeding. Laparoscopy is used to remove small areas of endometrial tissue as well as relieve adhesions. Endometriosis that is widespread throughout the pelvic organs, however, may necessitate a **panhysterectomy**, removal of the uterus, both fallopian tubes, and ovaries.

A newer drug, elagolix (Orilissa) which is a GnRH receptor antagonist, is designed to suppress estrogen just enough to relieve the pain of endometriosis without the harsh side effects of drugs that reduce estrogen to such low levels that hot flashes, bone loss, and mood swings result. This drug was FDA approved in 2018 to help control moderate to severe endometriosis pain (MedlinePlus, 2018).

Nursing Management

The nurse obtains a complete reproductive history, asking the client to describe all symptoms, including their duration, type, and location of pain; number of days of menses; amount of menstrual flow; and regularity or irregularity of the menstrual cycle. They offer information on methods for relieving menstrual pain (see discussion of dysmenorrhea) and assists the client through the decision-making process as it applies to family planning and medical or surgical treatment of endometriosis before natural menopause. Some techniques for resolving decisional conflict include the following:

- Reinforce or clarify explanations of treatment options and the consequences of each option.
- Emphasize that the condition does not require an immediate decision and avoid giving advice or influencing the client's opinions.
- Suggest that the client include her significant other in the discussion of options.
- Offer the option of seeking a second medical opinion.
- Suggest the client list the pros and cons of each option to help determine which choice is most compatible with her values and goals.

The nurse emphasizes the importance of adhering to the prescribed medication schedule, if that is the client's choice, and the importance of regular gynecologic evaluations. They instruct the client to seek care if pain increases, the menstrual flow is extremely heavy, or pregnancy occurs. Refer to the information on nursing management of clients undergoing a hysterectomy (removal of the uterus) (later in this chapter) for those who choose that treatment option.

Vaginal Fistulas

A **fistula** is an unnatural opening between two structures. The opening may be between a ureter and the vagina (ureterovaginal fistula), between the bladder and the vagina (vesicovaginal fistula), or between the rectum and the vagina (rectovaginal fistula; Fig. 53-4).

Pathophysiology and Etiology

Vaginal fistulas are caused by cancer, radiation treatment, surgical or obstetric injury, congenital anomaly, or a complication of Crohn disease (see Chapter 46). They result in the continuous drainage of urine or feces from the vagina. The vaginal wall and the external genitalia become excoriated and often infected. The client may not void through the urethra because urine does not accumulate in the bladder.

Assessment Findings

The client reports that urine or stool leaks from the vagina. Diagnosis is made by physical examination of the vaginal wall. A sterile probe is inserted if the fistula is easily seen or a dye (usually methylene blue) is used to detect the exact location of the fistula. When a vesicovaginal fistula is suspected, the colored dye is instilled into the bladder through a urethral catheter. A ureterovaginal fistula requires IV administration of the dye. An IV pyelogram (IVP) detects the flow of radiopaque dye through the lower genitourinary tract. A rectovaginal fistula is located by looking for fecal drainage on the posterior vaginal wall.

Medical and Surgical Management

Surgery is performed after inflammation and edema have disappeared. This may require months of treatment. Sometimes, the tissues are in such poor condition that surgical repair is not possible. In the meantime, or if the fistula cannot be repaired, symptomatic treatment to reduce the risk for infection and manage skin excoriation is provided.

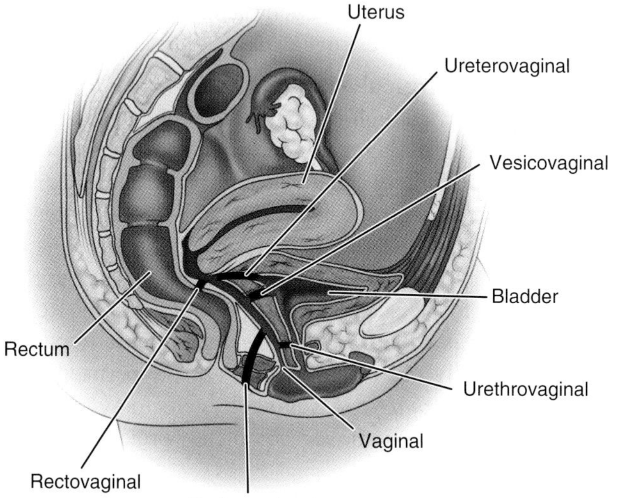

Figure 53-4 Types of vaginal fistulae.

Nursing Management

Before repair of a rectovaginal fistula, administer neomycin (Mycifradin), kanamycin (Kantrex), or any other prescribed antibiotic to clean the bowel of microorganisms. Provide a light, low-residue diet to keep stool soft; give an enema and a cleansing vaginal irrigation the morning of surgery; and insert an indwelling catheter to keep the bladder empty.

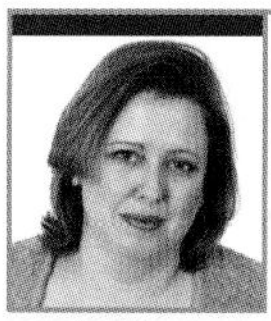

Clinical Scenario A 45-year-old woman arrives for an appointment with her gynecologist. When the nurse obtains the client's health history, she reports having continuous vaginal drainage of urine following a laparoscopically assisted vaginal hysterectomy a few months earlier. She says her underwear is constantly wet and she and her environment smell of urine, which prevents having friends and family visit and interferes with a sexual relationship with her husband. **How can the nurse help this client manage the problems she has identified?**

After surgery, serosanguineous vaginal drainage on the perineal pad is normal. No urine or feces from the vagina indicates healing of the repaired fistula. Prevent pelvic pressure and stress on the suture line by monitoring catheter drainage closely. The pressure of a full bladder from an obstructed catheter may break down the surgical repair and cause the fistula to reappear. Prevent and relieve pressure on perineal structures. Warm perineal irrigations and heat lamp treatments are effective in promoting healing and lessening discomfort. Douches used during the postoperative period remove drainage, keep the suture area clean, and lessen chances of infection. About the third or fourth postoperative day, a rectal suppository or a stool softener may be ordered to prevent straining during a bowel movement.

Pelvic Organ Prolapse

The term *prolapse* indicates a structural protrusion. Women experience any number of problems of this nature in the vagina. They include cystocele, rectocele, enterocele, and uterine prolapse (Fig. 53-5).

A **cystocele** is the bulging of the bladder into the vagina. A **rectocele** is a herniation of the rectum into the vagina. An **enterocele** is a protrusion of the intestinal wall into the vagina. A **uterovaginal prolapse** is the downward displacement of the cervix anywhere from low in the vagina to outside the vagina.

Pathophysiology and Etiology

Pelvic organ prolapse is a consequence of congenital or acquired weaknesses in the muscles and fascia that are needed to support pelvic structures. Common causes include unrepaired postpartum tears; stretching during pregnancy and

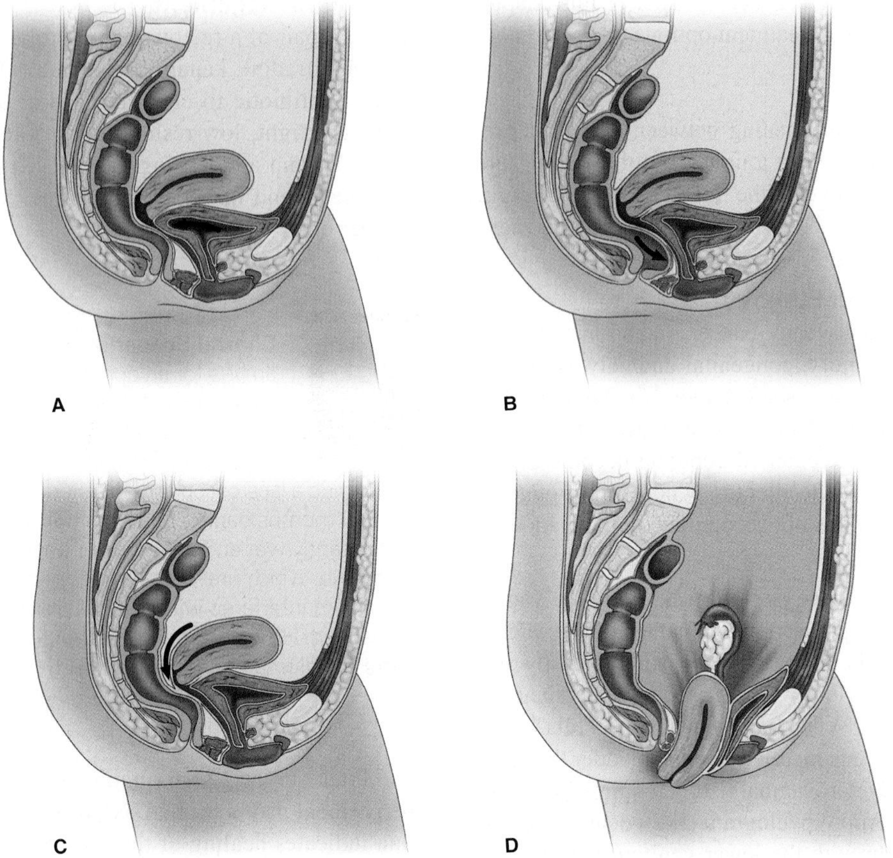

Figure 53-5 Types of pelvic organ prolapse. **(A)** Cystocele. **(B)** Rectocele. **(C)** Enterocele. **(D)** Uterine prolapse.

childbirth or with tumorous masses, ascites, and obesity; and postmenopausal atrophy. As the pelvic floor relaxes, the uterus, rectum, intestine, and bladder, alone or in combination, herniate downward. Structural displacement of the bladder and bowel leads to alterations in urinary and bowel elimination. Uterine tissue that protrudes below the vaginal orifice is subject to irritation from clothing or rubbing against the thighs while walking; ulceration and infection frequently follow. Clients with severe uterovaginal prolapse are at greater risk for cervical cancer.

The functional consequences of pelvic organ prolapse can be disruptive. The client often experiences difficulty standing for long periods, walking with ease, lifting, and other activities that are hard to avoid.

Assessment Findings

Signs and Symptoms

Clients with a cystocele may experience stress incontinence—a little urine seeps every time the woman coughs, sneezes, laughs, bears down, or strains. Cystitis (inflammation of the bladder; see Chapter 59) results from the stagnation of urine in the bladder. With a rectocele, constipation often is a problem. In some instances, the client has to put her finger into the vagina and apply pressure to the posterior vaginal wall to reduce the herniation before being able to evacuate stool. Symptoms of a uterovaginal prolapse include backache, pelvic pain, fatigue, and a feeling that "something is dropping out," especially when lifting a heavy object, coughing, or standing for prolonged periods.

Diagnostic Findings

Diagnosis is confirmed during a pelvic examination and visual inspection of the vagina. Urinary tests are performed to reproduce stress incontinence or to determine the volume at which a client senses an urgent need to void. A Pap test determines the client's estrogen status.

Medical and Surgical Management

A **pessary**, a firm, doughnut-shaped or ring device, may be inserted in the upper vagina to reposition and give support to the uterus when surgery cannot be done or the client declines surgery. Pelvic floor strengthening exercises (see Chapter 59) are recommended when there is stress incontinence.

Surgical repairs are done transvaginally. The surgical repair of a cystocele is called *anterior colporrhaphy*. Repair of a rectocele is called *posterior colporrhaphy*. Repair of the tears (usually old obstetric tears) of the perineal floor is called *perineorrhaphy*. A vaginal hysterectomy (see later discussion) is done to remove a completely prolapsed uterus.

Nursing Management

The nurse obtains a comprehensive medical history, including the chief complaint and symptoms; inserts a catheter for diagnostic testing; assists with the pelvic examination and collection of specimens; and provides appropriate health teaching based on the primary care provider's plan for treatment. They show the client how to remove, clean, and reinsert a pessary, including the following information:

- Remove the pessary and thoroughly wash it with warm, soapy water, followed by rinsing and drying.
- Inspect the pessary to be sure that all secretions have been removed.
- Apply a sterile lubricant to the pessary before it is reinserted. Discomfort may indicate that it has been inserted incorrectly, the pessary has moved, or that it is causing irritation. Contact the primary care provider if these problems occur.
- See the primary care provider immediately if a white or yellow discharge from the vagina develops. It may indicate an infection.
- Assume the knee–chest position for a few minutes once or twice a day to keep the pelvic organs and the pessary in good position.
- Avoid heavy lifting and straining when having a bowel movement.

The nurse tells clients not wishing to manage their own pessary to see their primary care provider at least every 2 months, or sooner if vaginal discharge or changes in voiding develop.

After an anterior colporrhaphy, some women have temporary difficulty voiding or emptying the bladder completely. Therefore, clients are discharged with a retention catheter in place or are taught to perform clean intermittent catheterization (see Chapter 59) for 7 to 10 days until they can void sufficiently to empty the bladder. The client learns pelvic floor strengthening exercises after surgical repairs.

Uterine Displacement

In some women, the uterus, which normally is flexed about 45 degrees anteriorly with the cervix positioned posteriorly, is displaced. *Retroversion*, the most common displacement, describes a uterus that tilts posteriorly with a cervix that tilts anteriorly. *Retroflexion* refers to a uterus that bends backward. *Anteversion* describes a uterus that bends forward as a whole unit (the opposite of retroversion). *Anteflexion* describes a uterus that is bent forward on itself (the opposite of retroflexion; Fig. 53-6).

Pathophysiology and Etiology

Displacement usually is congenital; sometimes, backward displacement is from childbearing or scar tissue that forms in clients who have endometriosis or PID. Positional displacement may not cause any noticeable problems, or it may be the underlying reason for discomfort during menstruation and intercourse. Some cases of infertility are caused by retrodisplacement of the uterus.

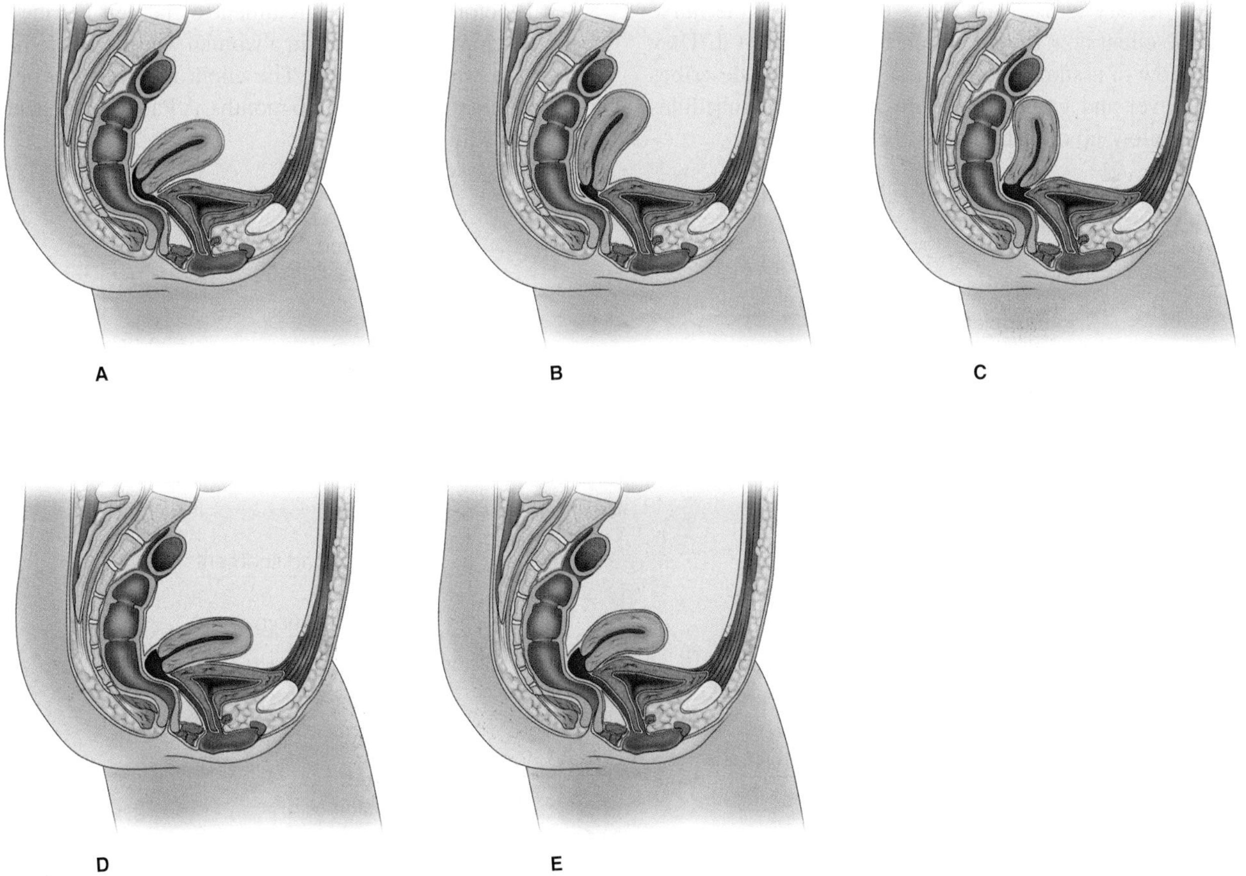

Figure 53-6 Variations in uterine position. **(A)** Normal. **(B)** Retroversion. **(C)** Retroflexion. **(D)** Anteversion. **(E)** Anteflexion.

Assessment Findings

Clients with a malpositioned uterus describe having backache, dysmenorrhea, or dyspareunia. Sometimes, the client seeks a medical examination to investigate the reason pregnancy has not occurred. A bimanual pelvic examination locates the abnormal position of the uterus.

Medical and Surgical Management

If the displacement causes severe discomfort, or if infertility can be corrected, abdominal surgery is performed to relocate and suture the uterus to a more natural position. Age or complicating diseases sometimes make surgery too great a risk. Under such circumstances, the displacement is reduced by inserting a pessary, which repositions the uterus, and having the client assume the knee–chest position several times a day.

››› *Stop, Think, and Respond 53-2*

Give examples of conditions that are associated with dysmenorrhea.

Nursing Management

The nurse performs an initial interview, collects pertinent data, and assists with the gynecologic examination. If surgery is performed, the nurse assesses the client for complications, manages wound drains, maintains patency of the indwelling catheter, inspects vaginal packing, and notes the condition of dressings. They include deep breathing, pain management, and early ambulation in postoperative management.

If a pessary is used to correct the prolapse, the nurse shows the client how to remove, clean, and reinsert it. They explain how to assume a knee–chest position and describes activity level and hygiene measures. The nurse schedules medical follow-up or instructs the client to do so.

TUMORS OF THE FEMALE REPRODUCTIVE SYSTEM

Uterine Leiomyoma

A *leiomyoma*, sometimes shortened to *myoma*, is a benign uterine growth principally consisting of smooth muscle and fibrous connective tissue. Myomas, the most common tumors in a woman's pelvis, often are referred to as **fibroid tumors** or fibromyomas.

Pathophysiology and Etiology

Estrogen is believed to stimulate the development of fibroids. Tumors may be small or large, single or multiple. Growth usually is slow except during pregnancy. They shrink during and after menopause. Fibroids can occur in various locations in the uterus: subserosal (on the outside of the uterus and below the serous membrane), intramural (within the wall), and submucosal (below the mucous membrane; Fig. 53-7). The latter are associated most frequently with excessive menstrual bleeding.

Assessment Findings

When symptoms exist, menorrhagia is most common. There can be a feeling of pressure in the pelvic region, dysmenorrhea, anemia (from loss of blood), and malaise.

Benign uterine tumors may be detected during a pelvic examination. A Pap test is done to rule out a malignancy. A sonogram reveals uterine and fibroid size. Microscopic examination of the excised tumor confirms the diagnosis.

Medical and Surgical Management

Several factors govern the treatment of benign uterine tumors. A symptomatic tumor in a woman who wishes to have children is watched closely. The client receives a gynecologic examination every 3 to 6 months. A Pap test is repeated every 6 to 12 months.

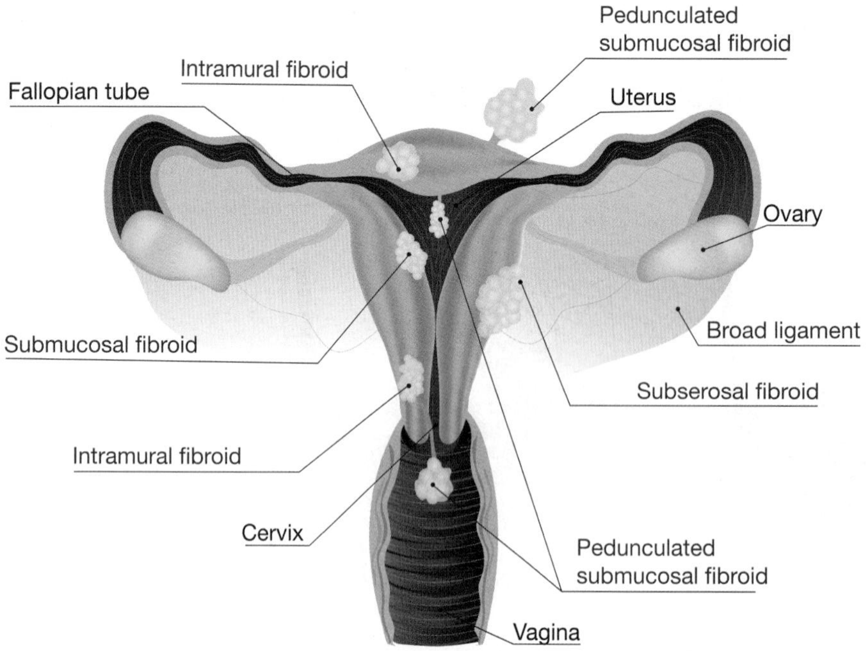

Figure 53-7 Submucosal, intramural, and subserosal leiomyomas (fibroids). (Source: shutterstock.com/Annakek)

When the client has abnormal bleeding, a **dilation and curettage** (D&C)—surgical procedure that removes tissue from inside the uterus—is performed to determine the cause of or to control the bleeding. Although a D&C does not remove the tumor, it may make more extensive surgery unnecessary. A **myomectomy** (surgical removal of a fibromyoma tumor only) through an abdominal incision or with a laparoscope inserted through the cervical canal preserves the uterus if a woman of childbearing years wishes to become pregnant in the future. Another option is to perform **uterine fibroid embolization,** a minimally invasive procedure using fluoroscopic imaging during which embolic agents are instilled to block arteries supplying the fibroids causing them to shrink (Society of Interventional Radiology, 2019). Drug therapy with leuprolide (Lupron), a GnRH agonist that decreases estrogen, may be administered for 2 to 3 months to temporarily reduce blood loss and shrink fibromyomas prior to surgery. If surgery is delayed or does not take place, fibromyomas will reoccur after leuprolide is discontinued. A **hysterectomy**, surgical removal of the uterus, is performed when symptoms are severe and incapacitating, if the client is past childbearing years, or future pregnancy is not desired.

Nursing Management

The nurse assists with the gynecologic examination, reinforces medical explanations, and provides preoperative instructions. During the postoperative period, the nurse assists in the safe recovery of the client who undergoes surgery similar to that discussed for cervical and endometrial cancer.

Cervical and Endometrial Cancer

Cervical cancer, which affects the lowest portion of the uterus, is the second most common malignancy of the female reproductive system (breast cancer is first), but ranks 20th in frequency among types of cancer (National Institutes of Health, 2020). The decrease in the incidence of cervical cancer is attributed to performing the Pap test and administering the human papillomavirus (HPV) vaccine to preteens and teens (Centers for Disease Control and Prevention [CDC], 2019).

Cancer of the endometrium affects the lining of the uterus, usually in the area of the fundus or corpus, and is more common in postmenopausal women.

Pathophysiology and Etiology

Cancer of the cervix has its peak incidence among women between 35 and 50 years of age and is associated with the following risk factors:

- Being born to mothers treated with diethylstilbestrol (DES) while pregnant
- Becoming sexually active at an early age
- Having multiple sexual partners or having intercourse with a high-risk man (one who has had multiple partners or penile condyloma [warts])
- Acquiring genital infections caused by HPV
- Having chronic cervicitis secondary to uterine prolapse
- Having a history of cigarette smoking
- Having had pelvic radiation

The risk of endometrial cancer increases after 50 years of age, especially in those women taking estrogens without the addition of progesterone for 5 or more years during and after menopause. Other risk factors include early menarche, late menopause, never having been pregnant (nulliparity), and obesity.

Cervical and endometrial cancers probably begin as premalignant lesions that later undergo malignant changes. The localized malignancy is referred to as **carcinoma in situ**. Untreated, it subsequently invades other areas of the uterus and adjacent tissue.

Assessment Findings

Signs and Symptoms

Bleeding is the earliest and most common symptom of both endometrial and cervical cancer. In early cervical cancer, spotting occurs first, especially after slight trauma such as douching or intercourse. The bleeding from endometrial cancer can be mistaken for menorrhagia in premenopausal women. Late symptoms for both include pain, symptoms of pressure on the bladder or bowel, and the generalized wasting associated with advanced cancer.

Diagnostic Findings

All vaginal bleeding is investigated, first by a gynecologic examination, then by diagnostic tests. Cervical cancer is detected with Pap tests and biopsies of suspect tissue. Cells obtained by endocervical aspiration or endometrial biopsy during a hysteroscopy identify abnormal cells higher in the uterus. Radiography, MRI, or CT scanning is used to determine if there is metastasis; a barium study or IVP is ordered to determine bowel or bladder metastasis. Both types of cancer are classified according to the stage (Table 53-3).

Medical and Surgical Management

Treatment of cervical and endometrial cancer depends on the stage of the tumor. Prognosis depends on how early the cancer is diagnosed. Methods for treating cervical and endometrial cancer include one of various types of hysterectomy (Box 53-1), external or internal radiation therapy (Fig. 53-8), and chemotherapy (see Chapter 18).

The uterus is removed using an abdominal or vaginal approach—the choice usually depends on the pathology and the client's condition. An abdominal approach is always used for a radical hysterectomy or when there is a risk for excessive bleeding during the operative procedure. The vaginal approach has fewer complications, reduced recovery time, and lower cost. Laparoscopically assisted vaginal hysterectomy, a combination of surgical and endoscopic techniques, is being used to perform vaginal hysterectomies that otherwise would have been performed abdominally.

Nursing Management

A major role of the nurse is to make women aware that a vaccine against several strains of HPV that predispose them to cervical cancer is available for women who are not yet

TABLE 53-3 Stages of Uterine Cancers

TYPE	STAGE	DESCRIPTION
Cervical	I	Limited to the cervix, but deeper tissues, not just surface tissues
	II	Extends beyond the cervix to the upper two thirds of the vagina, extends beyond the cervix and uterus
	III	Involves the lower third of the vagina and is fixed to the pelvic wall, may block ureters
	IV	Involves the rectum, bladder, or extends beyond the true pelvis
Endometrial	I	Growing in uterus, may affect part of cervix
	II	Involves the corpus and cervix, into the supportive connecting tissue of cervix
	III	Extends outside the uterus, but not the true pelvis, bladder, or rectum
	IV	Involves the rectum, bladder, or extends outside the true pelvis

From American Cancer Society. (2019). *Endometrial cancer stages.* https://www.cancer.org/cancer/endometrial-cancer/detection-diagnosis-staging/staging.html; American Cancer Society. (2020). *Cervical cancer stages.* https://www.cancer.org/cancer/cervical-cancer/detection-diagnosis-staging/staged.html

BOX 53-1 Types of Hysterectomies

Total hysterectomy: Removal of the entire uterus and cervix

Subtotal hysterectomy: Removal of the uterus only, with a stump of the cervix left intact

Panhysterectomy: Removal of the uterus, fallopian tubes, and ovaries

Radical hysterectomy: Removal of the uterus, cervix, ovaries, and fallopian tubes; part of the upper vagina and some pelvic lymph nodes also may be removed at this time.

Pelvic exenteration: Removal of all reproductive organs, rectum, colon, bladder, distal ureters, iliac blood vessels, and pelvic lymph nodes and peritoneum

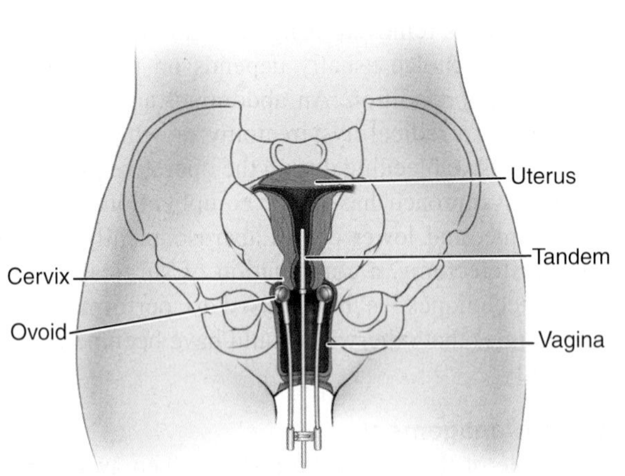

Figure 53-8 Placement of tandem and ovoids, devices containing sources for internal radiation therapy.

BOX 53-2 Cervical Cancer Vaccine

- Gardasil is a vaccine that protects against four types of HPV, which cause 70% of cervical cancers and 90% of cervical warts (see Chapter 56).
- The recommended age for administering the vaccine is 11 to 26 years of age (i.e., prior to becoming sexually active and possibly infected with HPV).
- The vaccine does not protect against types of HPV with which the person has already been infected.
- The vaccine consists of three injections over the course of 6 months.
- Side effects include injection site reactions, fever, nausea and vomiting, dizziness, and fainting.
- Routine cervical cancer screening is recommended regardless of vaccine use, because cervical cancer can develop from other causes, other strains of HPV not included in the vaccine, and from a prevaccination infection with one or more of the HPV vaccine strains.

sexually active between the ages of 11 and 26. The vaccine is also recommended for boys of similar ages who have not already received a full series of the immunization (Box 53-2) (see Chapter 56).

All women should also have regular gynecologic examinations and Pap tests. Theoretically, all uterine cancers begin in situ (*in situ* means the cancerous cells remain in the place where they first formed, that is, in this case, the uterus). Therefore, regular cytologic (cell) examinations increase the potential for an early diagnosis before invasion occurs. Specific nursing management depends on the selected treatment. In the interim between diagnosis and treatment, the nurse offers emotional support and information about the various options for treatment. See Chapter 18 for a discussion of radiation therapy and chemotherapy and nursing management.

Preoperative and Postoperative Care

Preoperative preparations vary depending on the surgeon's preference and the planned surgical approach (abdominal or vaginal). A douche is given before a vaginal hysterectomy, and an enema is given before either surgery. The nurse inserts an indwelling catheter before surgery and administers an antibiotic, usually one of the cephalosporins, during or after surgery to prevent infection. For general postoperative care, refer to perioperative standards of care discussed in Chapter 14.

Ovarian Cysts and Benign Ovarian Tumors

A cyst is a membranous sac filled with fluid, cells, or both. Ovarian cysts, which are benign, are filled with fluid. Benign ovarian tumors are noncancerous growths of solid tissue.

Pathophysiology and Etiology

The exact etiologic mechanism for the variety of ovarian cysts and tumors is essentially unknown, but endocrine dysfunction has been implicated in some types. Follicular

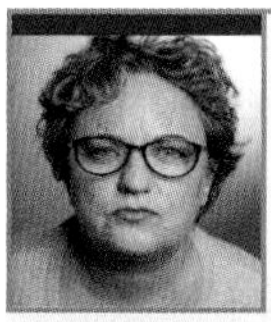

Clinical Scenario A 49-year-old woman who has been experiencing heavy menses lasting 10 days comes to the gynecologist's office to determine the cause of her symptoms and receive subsequent treatment. The nurse, who prepares the client, gathers data prior to the consultation with the primary care provider. The nurse notes that the client's abdomen is enlarged similar to that of a midtrimester pregnancy. The client indicates she is tired most of the time, which the nurse attributes to chronic blood loss. The primary care provider determines that the client has a very large leiomyoma that is best removed by performing an abdominal, rather than vaginal, hysterectomy because of its size. The client's ovaries and fallopian tubes will be left intact. **What problems and nursing interventions can the nurse caring for this client postoperatively include in her care? Review the example in Nursing Care Plan 53-1.**

cysts are thought to develop when a ripening ovum fails to be released. Another type forms when the corpus luteum fails to regress after ovulation and continues to produce progesterone. Chocolate cysts are secondary to endometriosis. Ovarian cysts and benign tumors tend to affect menstruation and fertility, depending on the specific type. Some benign tumors have a potential to become malignant (Norris, 2019).

Assessment Findings

The client may experience pressure in the lower abdomen, backache, menstrual irregularities, and pain, which can be mistaken for appendicitis, ureteral stone, or other abdominal disorders. Clients with tumors associated with or influenced by hypothalamic, pituitary, or adrenal hormones can develop hirsutism (growth of facial hair), atrophy of the breasts, and sterility.

Tumors and cysts may be detected during a pelvic examination. Ultrasonography and laparoscopy are used to determine tumor size. Surgery is the only means for confirming a diagnosis of a benign tumor or cyst.

NURSING CARE PLAN 53-1 The Client With a Total Abdominal Hysterectomy

Assessment

- Assess vital signs and level of consciousness.
- Evaluate pain intensity.
- Monitor condition of the dressing, location of drains (nasogastric, wound), and patency of urinary catheter.
- Check the type, volume, and rate of IV fluid and the location and appearance of the IV site regularly.
- Note the presence of antiembolic stockings.

Nursing Diagnosis. **Acute Pain** related to tissue trauma

Expected Outcome. Pain will be reduced to a tolerable level within 30 minutes of a nursing intervention.

Interventions	Rationales
Assess the type of pain, intensity, and location each time vital signs are assessed and as needed.	*Pain assessment is the fifth vital sign.*
Administer analgesics as ordered.	*They reduce pain perception.*
Implement nonpharmacologic interventions, such as distraction, imagery, and repositioning, to augment analgesia.	*Substituting alternative stimuli to the brain decreases pain perception.*

Evaluation of Expected Outcome

Client reports decreased discomfort; pain is adequately controlled.

Nursing Diagnosis. **Bleeding Risk** Related to vaginal hemorrhage

Expected Outcome. The nurse will monitor to detect, manage, and minimize hemorrhage.

Interventions	Rationale
Record the number of perineal pads used.	*Counting perineal pads facilitates the assessment of blood loss.*
Assess blood pressure and pulse every 15 minutes if bleeding seems severe.	*Blood pressure falls and pulse rate increases in relation to loss of circulating blood volume.*
Record the color of bloody drainage.	*Bright red bleeding correlates with arterial bleeding; dark red blood is more likely venous.*
Report excessive bleeding or passage of blood clots to the primary care provider.	*A blood transfusion or an increased rate of IV fluid may be necessary to maintain blood volume to prevent shock.*

(*continued*)

NURSING CARE PLAN 53-1 The Client With a Total Abdominal Hysterectomy (*continued*)

Evaluation of Expected Outcome

Client has normal postoperative vaginal drainage; vital signs are within normal range.

RC of Abdominal Distention, Paralytic Ileus. Related to decrease in GI motility Venous Thromboembolism Risk: Related to decrease in peripheral blood circulation, surgical trauma, and a decrease in mobility

Urinary Retention. Related to surgical procedure, decrease in fluid intake, and effects of anesthetic medications

Expected Outcome. The nurse will monitor to detect, manage, and minimize abdominal distention.

Interventions	Rationale
Palpate the abdomen every 4 hours for signs of rigidity.	*The abdomen loses its soft quality as it distends with gas.*
Encourage ambulation.	*Movement promotes intestinal peristalsis, which moves gas toward the rectum.*
Report abdominal discomfort, nausea, abdominal distention, or diminished or faint bowel sounds to the primary care provider.	*Elimination of intestinal gas may be facilitated by using a rectal tube, which must be medically ordered.*

Evaluation of Expected Outcome

Abdomen is soft; bowel sounds are active; client passes flatus rectally.

Nursing Diagnosis. **Venous Thromboembolism Risk**

Expected Outcome. The nurse will monitor to detect, manage, and minimize thrombophlebitis.

Interventions	Rationale
Remove and reapply antiembolic stockings every 8 hours.	*Antiembolic stockings support valves in veins and reduce venous stasis.*
Encourage active leg exercises every 2–4 hours.	*Skeletal muscle contraction propels venous blood toward the heart.*
Assess for calf swelling and tenderness bilaterally every shift.	*Calf tenderness and swelling are suggestive of a thrombus in the lower extremities.*
Do not place pillows beneath the knees or raise the knees with the electric bed.	*Bending the knees interferes with venous circulation and promotes venous stasis and clot formation.*
Ambulate as much as possible.	*Walking requires skeletal muscle contraction, which promotes venous circulation.*

Evaluation of Expected Outcome

No evidence of thrombus formation.

Nursing Diagnosis. **Urinary Retention**

Expected Outcome. The nurse will monitor to detect, manage, and minimize urinary retention after indwelling catheter is removed.

Interventions	Rationale
Measure intake and output every shift.	*Intake and output facilitate assessment of fluid status.*
Palpate the lower abdomen for distention.	*The bladder is palpable when distended with urine.*
Measure the volume of each voiding.	*Voiding small amounts can indicate urinary retention with overflow.*
Encourage liberal fluid intake.	*Urinary elimination is related to fluid intake.*

NURSING CARE PLAN 53-1 The Client With a Total Abdominal Hysterectomy (*continued*)

Report bladder distention in the absence of voiding to the primary care provider.	*Medically prescribed interventions such as inserting a straight or indwelling catheter require an order from the primary care provider.*

Evaluation of Expected Outcome

Client voids in sufficient quantity.

Nursing Diagnosis. **Altered Body Image Perception** related to misconceptions about physical and sexual consequences of hysterectomy

Expected Outcome. Client will maintain an accurate body image after surgery.

Interventions	Rationale
Give client an opportunity to verbalize perceptions and fears.	*Clients are less apt to discuss personal problems or fears if they sense that the nurse does not have time to engage in a discussion.*
Clarify that a hysterectomy does not physically compromise libido or ability to achieve orgasm or cause premature aging, depression, or masculinization.	*Many women accept common myths and misperceptions as fact.*

Evaluation of Expected Outcome

Client has a realistic understanding of the physical outcomes of surgery.

Client and Family Teaching 53-1 Preventing Vaginal Infections

Depending on the client's treatment, the teaching plan includes some or all of the following:

- Take any prescribed medication as ordered. Seek care if adverse drug effects occur.
- Avoid heavy lifting, sexual intercourse, vigorous physical exercise, and douching until permitted by the primary care provider.
- Ambulate at intervals and avoid sitting in one position for a prolonged period.
- Clean the incision as directed.
- Seek medical care if any of the following signs and symptoms occurs: fever; redness, swelling, pain, or drainage of the incision; vaginal discharge that has a foul odor; vaginal bleeding; pain in the chest, abdomen, or legs.
- Avoid constipation and straining to have a bowel movement. Drink plenty of fluids. If constipation occurs, contact the primary care provider.

Medical and Surgical Management

Some ovarian cysts and benign tumors require no treatment or are treated with oral contraceptives to provide symptomatic relief. If the cyst ruptures, surgery, which can entail complete **oophorectomy** (removal of the ovary), **oophorocystectomy** (removal of the cystic tissue) only, or a **salpingo-oophorectomy** (removal of the ovary and fallopian tube), is required.

Nursing Management

The nurse explains measures for relieving menstrual discomfort and provides referrals to support groups that are devoted to infertile women. The preoperative preparation and postoperative management are the same as for any client having abdominal surgery and a general anesthetic (see Chapter 14). After surgery, some women develop abdominal distention, which is relieved by ambulating, inserting a rectal tube, or applying an abdominal binder. The nurse informs the client who has had surgery but not a hysterectomy to continue having regular gynecologic examinations and Pap tests because she is still at risk for uterine cancer.

Cancer of the Ovary

Although other types of female reproductive system cancers occur with greater incidence, ovarian tumors are the leading cause of death from gynecologic malignancies (CDC, 2020). Tumors of the ovary have been lethal largely because they present with nonspecific symptoms; there is no effective screening test, and therefore tumors frequently are far advanced and inoperable by the time they are diagnosed.

Pathophysiology and Etiology

It is believed that some ovarian tumors have a hereditary link and that others arise from ovarian cysts. Recent research has shown that the more times a woman ovulates during her lifetime, the greater the risk of ovarian cancer. Women who are nulliparous, those with a family history of ovarian cancer, and those who have been diagnosed with other types of cancer such as endometrial, colon, or breast cancer tend to develop ovarian cancer more often than others.

Malignant tumors of the ovary are classified according to the type of cell from which they originate. Most are epithelial, followed by germ cell (an ovum) tumors. Other types are very rare.

Assessment Findings

In the beginning, clients experience vague lower abdominal discomfort. As the tumor grows larger, urinary frequency and urgency may develop because of pressure on the bladder. Later, ascites, weight loss, severe pain, and gastrointestinal symptoms occur. A mass may be felt during a pelvic examination. Many primary care providers believe that ovarian enlargement found on pelvic examination requires surgical exploration.

The CDC and the American Cancer Society indicate that there is no evidence that supports any benefit from routine screening for ovarian cancer among asymptomatic, healthy women (CDC, 2019; American Cancer Society, 2020). However, that opinion does not apply to using diagnostic tests such as transvaginal and transabdominal ultrasound scans and the tumor marker blood test, CA 125, for women who are at high risk because they carry a genetic mutation for ovarian cancer or have a family history of the disease.

Laboratory studies measuring tumor marker antigens, such as alpha-fetoprotein, a carcinoembryonic antigen, and CA 125, may be ordered. An ultrasound and Doppler imaging of ovarian vessels are used in an effort to detect early-stage ovarian cancer. A breakthrough in detecting early-stage ovarian cancer occurred in 2002 with the development of proteomic technology, the ability to study proteins inside cells. Proteomic technology uses computer software to identify patterns of proteins. These methods are being used to detect patterns indicating ovarian cancer in serum blood samples. An abdominal CT scan, proctoscopy, barium study, chest X-ray, and IVP are performed to detect metastasis to other areas. A positive diagnosis is made by microscopic examination.

Medical and Surgical Management

Preventive measures recommended to at-risk populations include having at least two full-term pregnancies followed by breastfeeding and using oral contraceptives for more than 5 years. In addition, prophylactic bilateral oophorectomy is recommended for women at risk for hereditary ovarian cancer syndrome after they reach 35 years of age or after childbearing is completed. After diagnosis of a malignant tumor, the diseased ovary is removed. A total hysterectomy may or may not be performed. If both ovaries are removed, HRT may be prescribed.

Surgical treatment, which reduces the tumor load, is followed by chemotherapy. The current antineoplastic drug regimen of choice is a combination of carboplatin (Paraplatin), paclitaxel (Taxol), and docetaxel (Taxotere; American Cancer Society, 2018). The use of radiation therapy rather than chemotherapy is controversial at this time but may be used as an adjunct treatment.

Nursing Management

Only a small percentage of clients with malignant tumors of the ovary survive 5 years or more despite intensive treatment. The emotional effects of the diagnosis require support and understanding on the part of the nurse and other members of the health team. Many of these clients are young, the treatment is difficult, and the prognosis is poor for those diagnosed with late-stage ovarian cancer. Women who are diagnosed in the early stage of the disease, when the cancer is still confined to the ovary, have a much better prognosis.

Preoperative and postoperative nursing care is similar to that of other clients who undergo abdominal surgery (see "Preoperative and Postoperative Care" in the nursing management discussion of the client with cervical and endometrial cancer). See Nursing Care Plan 53-1 for nursing diagnoses and interventions for the client undergoing a total abdominal hysterectomy.

Cancer of the Vagina

Cancer of the vagina is rare and usually seen in women older than 40 years.

Pathophysiology and Etiology

The incidence of vaginal cancer is higher among women infected with HPV, a sexually transmitted microorganism (see Chapter 56), and among those who use a pessary but neglect to remove and clean it. Studies have shown a relationship between the development of vaginal carcinoma in (young) adult women offspring whose mothers were administered DES early in their pregnancy. DES is no longer used to treat problems associated with pregnancy.

The upper posterior third of the vagina is the most common site of vaginal cancer. Metastatic lesions may occur in the cervix or adjacent areas such as the vulva, uterus, or rectum.

Assessment Findings

Abnormal vaginal bleeding usually is the predominant symptom. Dyspareunia also may occur. Visual examination of the vaginal canal discloses the lesion. A biopsy then confirms the diagnosis.

Medical and Surgical Management

Cancer of the vagina is treated according to the extent of the tumor. Most clients undergo laser photovaporization treatments, although a partial or total vaginectomy is a possibility. Radiation therapy also is used. Complications, such as fistulas and bleeding, arise from the tumor itself and from radiation therapy. These complications are difficult to correct and control.

Nursing Management

The poor prognosis and complications associated with vaginal cancer and its treatment present a nursing challenge. The nurse keeps the client as comfortable as possible and changes bedding and clothing frequently. Urine or fecal drainage from fistulas makes odors difficult to control, but a room deodorizer and frequent gown and linen changes help.

The nurse encourages all women who took DES during pregnancy to tell their daughters and advise them to have complete gynecologic examinations regularly. After treatment, clients may profit from techniques to reduce the discomfort during sexual intercourse caused by narrowing of the vagina. Some suggestions include using a water-based lubricant or prolonged foreplay to lubricate the vagina, having one's sex partner dilate the vagina with fingers before penetration with the penis, and taking a slower pace during sexual activities.

Cancer of the Vulva

Cancer of the vulva, the external female genitalia, is relatively rare. It usually occurs in women older than 60 years, but cases among younger women have arisen recently. Vulvar cancer is highly curable when diagnosed at an early stage.

Pathophysiology and Etiology

Infections with carcinogenic agents such as HPV and herpes simplex virus type 2 increase the risk of vulvar cancer (see Chapter 56). These infections are treatable but not curable, which explains the lifelong threat of genital cancer.

Atypical cells, which appear as white or pigmented raised patches, most commonly involve the labia majora. Cancer also occurs in the labia minora, clitoris, and Bartholin glands. Because of the widespread presence of the viruses in the vulvar epithelium and their potential for carcinogenesis, multiple cancerous sites may coexist or occur again after treatment. Although the cancer is slow growing, it can and does spread to the vagina, urethra, and anus through regional lymph nodes.

Assessment Findings

Pruritus and genital burning are the most frequent early symptoms. Later, a bloody discharge, enlarged lymph nodes, ulceration and swelling of the vulva, and a visible mass develop. Eventually, the client experiences severe pain. As the cancer ulcerates, a bloody and sometimes purulent discharge from the vulva occurs.

The lesions are first noted during inspection of the genitalia. Application of acetic acid tends to accentuate the abnormal tissue. Biopsy confirms the diagnosis.

››› *Stop, Think, and Respond 53-3*

Which type of pelvic reproductive cancer has the highest incidence? Which reproductive cancer has the highest mortality rate?

Medical and Surgical Management

Vulvectomy (removal of the vulva) with or without the removal of lymph nodes (radical vulvectomy) is the standard for treatment. Laser photo vaporization is being used as an alternative, however, to preserve the cosmetic appearance of the genitalia, especially if the lesions do not exceed a depth of 3 mm. The efficacy of preoperative chemotherapy plus radiation before surgery for advanced disease is being investigated.

When cancer of the vulva is inoperable, wet dressings and perineal irrigations with a deodorizing solution help control the odor and the infection that usually occur in the ulcerating neoplasm. Narcotic analgesics usually are necessary in the terminal stage of the disease.

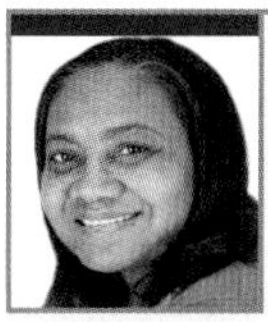

Clinical Scenario A 67-year-old woman has delayed consulting her primary care provider about persistent itching in her labial region. The itching has continued and she has found no relief from hygiene and home remedies she has tried. When she examined her vulva earlier this month, she found a lesion on her labia minora that had a different appearance than the surrounding tissue. The primary care provider performed several diagnostic tests, including a Pap test and biopsy of the lesion. The biopsy identified cancer of the vulva that included the labia and a portion of the perineum. The client was referred to a gynecologist who will perform a wide excision of the tissue and adjacent lymph nodes followed by radiation therapy. **While awaiting surgery and during the client's postoperative recovery, how can the nurse manage the client's care? Refer to the following Nursing Process section.**

NURSING PROCESS FOR THE CLIENT WITH CANCER OF THE VULVA UNDERGOING SURGERY

Assessment

Determine the location and level of discomfort or pain. Check the status of peripheral circulation and integrity of the skin. Discuss the client's perception of body image and explore concerns she may have about sexual function.

Diagnosis, Planning, and Interventions

Offer emotional support in relation to the results of the biopsy. Provide appropriate preoperative and postoperative care.

Before surgery, instruct the client to begin initial skin preparation by washing the lower abdomen, genitalia, perineum, and upper thighs with antibacterial soap for several days before surgery. On the day of surgery, insert a Foley catheter and provide standard teaching for deep-breathing and leg exercises. Antibiotic therapy may begin before the operative procedure.

(continued)

NURSING PROCESS FOR THE CLIENT WITH CANCER OF THE VULVA UNDERGOING SURGERY (continued)

Plan measures to prevent postoperative complications, manage pain, relieve edema in the lower extremities, prevent wound infection, and preserve and restore skin integrity. In addition, intervene therapeutically to assist the client in maintaining an acceptable body image, preparing for the resumption of sexual function, and performing self-care activities after discharge. Refer to perioperative standards of care in Chapter 14.

Other nursing measures include, but are not limited to, the following diagnoses, expected outcomes, and interventions:

Acute Pain: Related to tissue trauma and swelling
Expected Outcome: Pain will be relieved to a tolerable level within 30 minutes of a nursing intervention.

- Administer prescribed analgesics liberally. *Pain is best relieved by administering analgesia before it becomes severe.*
- Place an air or egg crate mattress on the bed. *These mattresses promote comfort by distributing pressure more evenly.*
- Place client in a semi-recumbent position. *It relieves pressure on the sutures.*
- Change the client's position at least every 2 hours. *Any position becomes uncomfortable if maintained for a prolonged period.*
- Use as many pillows as necessary to promote comfort. *Pillows support, elevate, and relieve pressure.*
- When in a lateral position, bend and support the upper leg on pillows. *Bending and supporting the upper leg in a lateral position prevents tension in the operative area.*

Venous Thromboembolism Risk: Related to decrease in peripheral blood circulation, surgical trauma, and a decrease in mobility
Expected Outcome: The nurse will monitor to detect, manage, and minimize risk for the development of thrombophlebitis.

- Assess for and report calf pain, swelling, or tenderness. *Calf pain, swelling, or tenderness indicates the possible development of a blood clot.*
- Remove and reapply antithrombotic stockings or pneumatic leg compression devices at regular intervals each day. *Compression of valves in the veins prevents venous stasis.*
- Ensure that the client performs leg exercises while in bed and ambulates as tolerated. *Skeletal muscle contraction promotes venous circulation.*
- Administer prescribed anticoagulants; monitor laboratory tests for therapeutic levels. *Anticoagulants interfere with blood clotting; dosages of anticoagulants are based on assessments of the partial thromboplastin time, prothrombin time, or international normalized ratio.*

Altered Tissue Perfusion: Related to compromised lymphatic and venous circulation secondary to excision of lymph nodes and ligation of blood vessels
Expected Outcome: Dependent edema will be absent by discharge.

- Elevate the lower extremities whenever possible. *Gravity promotes venous and lymphatic circulation.*
- Dangle the client's legs the evening of surgery and assist to ambulate daily. *Skeletal muscle movement that is required for ambulation promotes venous circulation.*

Infection Risk: Related to compromised skin integrity in close proximity to the rectum
Expected Outcome: Client will remain free of infection.

- Perform conscientious hand hygiene and put on gloves before caring for the wound. *Hand hygiene is the best method for preventing the transmission of microorganisms; gloves are one type of universal precautions that act as a barrier to prevent contact with blood and infectious microorganisms.*
- Inspect and change perineal dressing following principles of asepsis. *Using aseptic principles and universal precautions reduces the potential for transmitting pathogens.*
- Cleanse the anus after putting on gloves with moistened antiseptic wipes after bowel elimination. *Stool contains pathogens that can be introduced into the wound.*
- Empty surgical drains and catheter drainage bag aseptically. *A drain or catheter provides a portal through which microorganisms can enter the client's body.*
- Observe and record the appearance and amount of drainage. *Evidence of purulent drainage suggests infection.*

Altered Skin Integrity: Related to unresolved tissue healing
Expected Outcome: The wound will become approximated.

- Irrigate the wound with sterile saline, hydrogen peroxide, or a medically prescribed antiseptic solution at least three times daily. *Removing wound debris facilitates healing.*
- Dry the wound with a heat lamp or hair dryer. *Pressure or friction increases pain and can disrupt healing.*
- Give warm sitz baths after sutures have been removed. *Sitz baths increase circulation to the area and promote healing.*
- Cover intact skin with a transparent or air- and water-occlusive dressing. *Intact skin is protected from contact with moist drainage.*
- Support surgical drain during periods of ambulation. *An unsupported drain may be displaced from internal areas of the wound.*
- Explore the need to refer the client for home health nursing. *Home health nursing services are necessary if family or a significant member is unavailable for postdischarge wound care.*

NURSING PROCESS FOR THE CLIENT WITH CANCER OF THE VULVA UNDERGOING SURGERY (continued)

Altered Body Image Perception: Related to emotional distress secondary to amputated genitalia
Expected Outcome: Client will maintain a positive self-image.

- Ensure privacy when assessing the wound or carrying out treatment measures. *Privacy demonstrates respect for the client's dignity.*
- Keep the client clean, odor-free, and well groomed. *Attention to personal appearance promotes feeling attractive.*
- Listen when the client expresses emotions regarding her changed appearance. *Verbalizing feelings relieves stress.*
- Encourage significant others to be genuinely attentive and to express acceptance through hand holding, sitting close, or other actions. *Touching is a nonverbal method for expressing continued regard for one another.*

Coping Impairment: Related to potential sexual dysfunction due to anatomic changes in external genitalia
Expected Outcome: Client will find satisfactory techniques for experiencing sexual intimacy.

- Act as a liaison for information between the client and her surgeon as to the physical consequences of surgery. *Clients sometimes are reluctant to discuss sexual issues.*
- Role-play or encourage discussions regarding sexual issues between the client and significant other. *Role-playing can help client communicate about sensitive topics.*
- Explore the idea of using a vaginal dilator, liberal lubrication, and a side-lying position for intercourse once healing is complete. *Alternative sexual practices promote comfort and pleasure during sexual activities.*
- Suggest that the client seek a referral from her primary care provider to a sexual counselor if sexual issues are unresolved. *Sexual counselors have expertise in helping clients resolve problems with sexuality.*

Evaluation of Expected Outcomes

Expected outcomes are that pain is reduced or eliminated. The calves are of normal size and not tender. There is no dependent edema. Temperature is normal, with no wound tenderness or purulent drainage; WBC count is normal. The wound heals and the skin becomes intact. The client interacts with others and resumes previous lifestyle activities. The client can experience sexual intimacy.

Before discharge, instruct the client on the following measures for self-care:

- Expect that wound healing may take as long as 6 months.
- Elevate the legs and wear antiembolic stockings to reduce dependent edema in the lower extremities.
- Eat a high-protein diet with sources of vitamin C to promote healing.
- Try to stand and straddle the toilet when attempting to void after the catheter is removed in 7 to 10 days so that urine is directed into the toilet rather than down the leg or perineum.
- After urination, cleanse the periurethral area with water or normal saline in a plastic container with a spout.
- Continue to take the prescribed stool softener after discharge.
- Take a sitz bath using a portable basin after each bowel movement.
- Report any unusual odor, fever, fresh bleeding, separation of the wound margin, inability to void or constipation, and perineal pain.

KEY POINTS

- Disorders of menstruation include PMS, dysmenorrhea, amenorrhea, POF, PCOS, and menopause
- Infectious and inflammatory disorders:
  - Vaginitis: inflammation of the vagina
  - Cervicitis: inflammation of the cervix
  - PID: infection of the pelvic organs other than the uterus
  - TSS: type of septic shock
- Structural abnormalities
  - Endometriosis: endometrial tissue outside the uterus
  - Vaginal fistulas: unnatural opening between pelvic structures
  - Pelvic organ prolapse: structural protrusion
  - Uterine displacement: uterus positioned abnormally in the pelvis
- Tumors of the female reproductive system
  - Uterine leiomyoma: benign uterine growth
  - Cervical and endometrial cancer: cancer of the cervix and the uterus lining
  - Ovarian cysts and benign ovarian tumors
  - Cancer of the ovary
  - Cancer of the vagina
  - Cancer of the vulva

CRITICAL THINKING EXERCISES

1. What suggestions are useful to help a young adult woman maintain reproductive health?
2. A client reports that she becomes very moody every month and wonders if she has PMS. What additional information should the nurse obtain?

3. The parent of an adolescent woman asks why the cervical cancer vaccine is recommended for women from 9 through 26 years of age. What information can the nurse provide?
4. A woman who experiences severe dysmenorrhea has been diagnosed with endometriosis. What questions would you anticipate that this client might ask?

NCLEX-STYLE REVIEW QUESTIONS PrepU

1. A client believes that she experiences PMS. When the nurse interviews the client, which statement is most suggestive of this condition?
   1. The client has severe abdominal cramping during her menses.
   2. The client's breasts feel tender during her mid-menstrual cycle.
   3. The client feels temporarily depressed when menstruation ceases.
   4. The client's symptoms begin 2 weeks before menstruation.
2. When a 50-year-old menopausal client seeks a nurse's advice regarding prevention of chronic conditions like heart disease and osteoporosis with HRT, what is the most accurate information?
   1. Hormonal therapy is no longer recommended for this purpose.
   2. Low-dose, short-term HRT may help.
   3. Estrogen replacement alone is better than when combined with progestin.
   4. It is best to use bioidentical hormone therapy as prophylaxis.
3. A client who experiences infectious vaginitis on a frequent basis consults the nurse in the local health clinic about how to reduce or eliminate these infections. When the nurse gathers information from the client, what is a possible etiologic cause?
   1. The client says her sexual partner uses latex condoms.
   2. The client uses tampons during menstruation.
   3. The client says she douches after each period.
   4. The client has a sensitivity to dietary gluten.
4. The primary care provider orders doxycycline 0.3 g p.o. bid. Calculate the number of capsules to administer when the supplied dose is 150 mg/capsule. Record your answer in a whole number.
5. Internal radiation therapy with an applicator containing a radioactive substance is inserted within a client's vagina and cervix to treat cancer. What nursing order is most appropriate to add to the client's plan of care?
   1. Elevate the head of the bed to 90 degrees.
   2. Maintain strict continuous bed rest.
   3. Check vaginal drainage daily.
   4. Weigh daily before breakfast.

WANT TO KNOW MORE? There are a wide variety of online resources available on thePoint to enhance learning and understanding of this chapter.

Go to thePoint.lww.com/activate and use the activation code found in the front of this text to unlock these online resources.

54 Caring for Clients With Breast Disorders

Words To Know

adjuvant therapy
breast abscess
breast augmentation
breast cancer
breast reconstruction
fibroadenoma
fibrocystic breast disease
HER2 positive
in situ
lumpectomy
mammoplasty
mastalgia
mastectomy
mastitis
mastopexy
metastasis
modified radical mastectomy
neoadjuvant therapy
partial or segmental mastectomy
radical mastectomy
reduction mammoplasty
sentinel lymph node mapping
simple or total mastectomy
subcutaneous mastectomy
tomosynthesis

Learning Objectives

On completion of this chapter, you will be able to:

1. List four signs and symptoms common in breast disorders.
2. Name two infectious and inflammatory breast disorders and explain how they are acquired.
3. Discuss health teaching that may help prevent or eliminate infectious and inflammatory breast disorders.
4. Compare and contrast two benign breast disorders.
5. Name groups at high risk for developing breast cancer.
6. List common signs and symptoms of breast cancer.
7. Describe four methods for treating breast cancer, including six surgical techniques used to remove a malignant breast tumor.
8. Give two criteria that are used when selecting a mastectomy procedure.
9. Name a serious complication of breast cancer treatment.
10. Discuss the nursing management of clients who undergo surgical treatment for breast cancer.
11. List four sites to which breast cancer commonly metastasizes.
12. Describe three elective cosmetic breast procedures for clients with a mastectomy.
13. Describe three cosmetic breast procedures that women with nondiseased breasts may elect.

Female breasts are part of the female reproductive system, and they respond to the hormonal cycle associated with ovulation, menstruation, and pregnancy. Their primary function is the production of milk, a process referred to as *lactation*. This chapter discusses common disorders that affect breast tissue such as infectious and inflammatory disorders and benign and malignant breast lesions, which generally manifest with one or more of the following symptoms: breast tenderness or pain, breast mass, nipple discharge, and change in breast appearance. Also discussed are cosmetic breast procedures.

Gerontologic Considerations

- With age, the breast tissue atrophies and may become more fibrotic. The fibrotic tissue may be palpable or may cause some retraction of the nipple in older women, but may not be a sign of cancer. Occasionally, preexisting breast tumors become more evident with age.

INFECTIOUS AND INFLAMMATORY BREAST DISORDERS

Mastitis

Mastitis, an inflammation of breast tissue, can occur in one or both breasts. It is most common in women who are breastfeeding. Although mastitis can occur at any time, it is most common during the second or third postpartum week.

Pathophysiology and Etiology

Breast inflammation is caused or contributed to by one or more plugged lactiferous ducts or an infectious agent that enters through cracked or fissured nipples. Ducts become plugged as a consequence of infrequent nursing, failure to alternate breasts at each feeding, or an infant nursing weakly.

Lactating breasts have an elaborate blood supply and ductal system that easily supports microbial growth. If an infection develops, the most common causative microorganism is *Staphylococcus aureus*, which often is resistant to antibiotic therapy. The infectious process results from inadequate maternal hand washing, an infant infected by microorganisms at the hands of nursery personnel, or by organisms on the mother's skin.

Assessment Findings

Fever and malaise accompany breast tenderness, pain, and redness. The breast later becomes swollen, firm, and hard. A crack in the nipple or areola develops, and the axillary lymph nodes enlarge. Rarely, a breast abscess will develop. A culture and sensitivity test on expressed breast milk identifies the infectious agent.

Medical Management

Drug therapy generally involves 10 days of an antibiotic from the penicillin group based on culture and sensitivity tests. For those clients who are allergic to penicillin, the primary provider may substitute erythromycin (E-mycin, Ilosone, Erythrocin). For organisms that are penicillin resistant, oxacillin (Prostaphlin); cephalosporins such as cefazolin (Kefzol), which are safe for women to take while breastfeeding; or vancomycin (Vancocin) are given. Analgesics are prescribed for pain. Local heat also can be applied. To prevent engorgement and to maintain lactation, the breasts are emptied using a breast pump. The client may be referred to a lactation consultant or to health care providers, such as nurses with special training and experience in helping breastfeeding mothers, for additional teaching and support (Mayo Clinic Staff, 2020).

Nursing Management

The nurse obtains a health history (which includes identifying allergies to antibiotics), prepares the client for a physical examination, and collects the specimen of breast milk using standard precautions and aseptic principles. Client teaching includes information for self-administering antibiotic medications, principles of medical asepsis, and techniques to promote comfort and temporary alternatives to breastfeeding. Specific instructions to the client include the following:

- Take antibiotics as prescribed for the entire treatment period. The American Academy of Pediatrics says that in general, if an antibiotic can be administered directly to a premature infant or a neonate, then it is safe for the mother to take during breastfeeding (Wisner, 2020).
- Report side effects from the medication such as rash, gastrointestinal upset, and opportunistic infections in the mouth or vagina.
- Perform scrupulous hand hygiene before touching the breast.
- Bathe or shower regularly and apply a medical-grade lanolin ointment such as Lansinoh to dry or cracked nipples.
- Wear a supportive brassiere.
- Avoid wearing breast shields, which trap breast milk and moisture around the nipple.
- Apply warm soaks to the breast or let warm water from a shower flow over the breast.

See Evidence-Based Practice 54-1 for research on breast massage compared with alternative positioning of the baby for breastfeeding.

Evidence-Based Practice 54-1

Mastitis

Clinical Question

In lactating mothers, how does breast massage compare with alternative positioning of an infant when nursing affects mastitis resolution?

Evidence

In lactating mothers, mastitis happens when the breast is not adequately drained, breast engorgement (overfilling of the breast) is not managed well, and/or there is an oversupply of milk. Other causes include a sudden, significant change in feeding schedules (e.g., separation of mother and baby, as in the case of premature birth requiring a neonatal ICU stay, or when the mother returns to work) or weaning (Pevzner & Dahan, 2020). Although antibiotics may treat the infection in case of infectious mastitis, addressing its underlying cause is necessary to prevent recurrence, and effective milk removal is a must (Wilson et al., 2020). Preventative measures such as good breastfeeding management and avoidance of situations that cause sore nipples or engorgement (or overfilling of the milk ducts) can be very effective. Treatments for mastitis include rest, frequent breastfeeding using alternate positioning, breast massage, medications to treat pain and inflammation, and warm compresses. Antibiotics may be necessary (if infection occurs), but the underlying cause must be addressed. Although some sources encourage mothers to discontinue breastfeeding on the affected side, evidence supports encouraging continuation of breastfeeding, as the infant's suckling is the most effective form of milk removal (Pevzner & Dahan, 2020).

Nursing Implications

Prevention, early identification, and treatment of mastitis are key. Good breastfeeding management is the first line of defense for prevention of mastitis. This entails encouraging new mothers who choose to breastfeed to do so often, ideally 8 to 12 times per day during the first few days of the infant's life. Education will help prevent

Evidence-Based Practice 54-1 (*continued*)

mastitis and should include the importance of nursing on both sides each time, alternative holds such as the clutch (or football) hold, side-by-side, and the leaning-over position to maximize draining milk from all parts of the breast, as well as considerations of good breast care. If mastitis symptoms occur, good assessment skills will help identify the difference between uncomplicated breast pain due to conditions such as breast engorgement (overfilling) and actual mastitis. If mastitis is suspected, conservative treatment measures such as those described in this chapter should be initiated, but if symptoms do not improve within 12 to 24 hours or worsen quickly, then evaluation by a medical provider is necessary. Emotional support and encouragement are also important roles for the nurse, because mastitis is not only painful but can also leave the new mother feeling inadequate, frustrated, and confused. Support and encouragement from the nurse can help her move past those feelings, empower her to work with the baby to resolve the condition, and help her make decisions that she feels are best for her and her new baby.

References

Pevzner, M., & Dahan, A. (2020). Mastitis while breastfeeding: Prevention, the importance of proper treatment, and potential complications. *Journal of Clinical Medicine, 9*(8), 2328. https://doi.org/10.3390/jcm9082328

Wilson, E., Woodd, S.L., & Benova, L. (2020). Incidence of and risk factors for lactational mastitis: A systematic review. *Journal of Human Lactation, 36*(4), 673–686. https://doi.org/10.1177/0890334420907898

Breast Abscess

A **breast abscess** is a localized collection of pus in breast tissue.

Pathophysiology and Etiology

An abscess occurring in the breast is most frequently a complication of postpartum mastitis. Purulent exudate accumulates in a confined, local area of breast tissue. *S. aureus* again is the most common cause.

Assessment Findings

The client experiences the signs and symptoms of mastitis; in the case of an abscess, however, pus may drain from the nipple. A physical examination of the breast determines diagnosis. A culture and sensitivity test of nipple drainage identifies the infecting microorganism and indicates to which antibiotics it is sensitive.

Medical and Surgical Management

The client usually is hospitalized and placed on contact isolation precautions because the soiled dressings are highly infectious. The client is started on intravenous (IV) antibiotic therapy. The abscess may be incised, drained, and packed.

Nursing Management

The nurse removes and reapplies dressings following aseptic principles. To avoid irritating the skin from frequent removal of tape, the nurse uses a binder to hold the dressing in place. They apply zinc oxide to the surrounding skin to avoid maceration from irritating drainage or wound compresses. To reduce swelling, the nurse supports the arm and shoulder with pillows. They instruct the client not to shave axillary hair on the side with the abscess until healing is complete.

The mother who is temporarily separated from her newborn needs emotional support. The nurse helps the client to pump the breasts to remove milk and prevent engorgement. If the mother decides to terminate breastfeeding, the nurse applies a tight-fitting brassiere.

BENIGN BREAST LESIONS

Fibrocystic Breast Disease

Fibrocystic breast disease, also called *mammary dysplasia* (abnormal development of breast tissue) or *chronic cystic mastitis*, is a benign breast condition that affects women primarily between the ages of 30 and 50 years.

Pathophysiology and Etiology

Fibrocystic disease results from hormonal changes during the menstrual cycle. The use of caffeine may aggravate the condition.

When fibrocystic disease develops, single or multiple breast cysts appear in one or both breasts (Fig. 54-1). The cysts grow in size and become increasingly tender in proportion to the secretion of estrogen during each menstrual cycle. Cyst formation tends to continue throughout the reproductive years. Some cysts disappear, although others can remain permanently. The condition resolves with menopause.

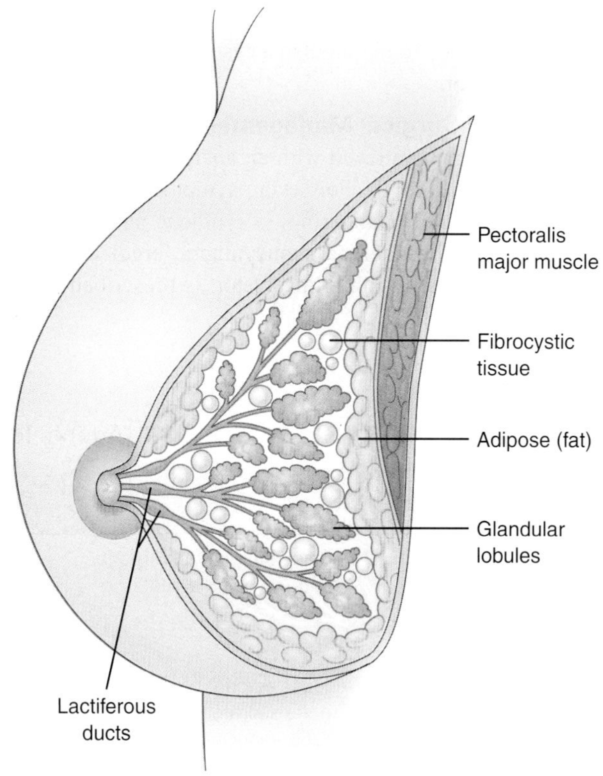

Figure 54-1 Breast with multiple cysts.

Although a correlation between fibrocystic disease and breast cancer was reported years ago, current studies have indicated no cause-and-effect relationship between these two conditions. Women with fibrocystic disease, however, may mistake a cancerous mass for a fibrocystic mass and delay medical diagnosis; if breast self-examination (BSE) is performed, it may be less vigorous because of breast tenderness, or the client may fail to palpate a malignant mass disguised by scar tissue from a previous incisional biopsy.

Assessment Findings

Signs and Symptoms

Fibrocystic disease of the breast may produce no symptoms. However, many women report having tender or painful breasts and feeling one or more, often multiple, lumps within the breast tissue. The fibrous tissue feels rubbery; moveable nodules are not fixed to any particular site within the breast (Anderson, 2015). Some report their symptoms are reduced or relieved by avoiding substances containing caffeine. The fibrous cysts are most noticeable just before menstruation and usually abate during menstruation. The size of the cysts often changes with the menstrual cycle, becoming larger before menstruation. Straining the pectoralis major muscle with activities such as weight training, boat rowing, or shoveling can cause or increase **mastalgia** (breast pain).

Diagnostic Findings

A preliminary diagnosis is made by examination of the breasts. The characteristic breast mass of fibrocystic disease is soft to firm, movable, and unlikely to cause nipple retraction. Fluid from the cysts is aspirated for cytologic examination, or an incisional biopsy is performed. If the results are questionable, mammography and ultrasonography are performed to distinguish a cystic lesion from a solid malignant tumor.

Medical and Surgical Management

Mild discomfort is relieved with an analgesic such as aspirin or ibuprofen (Advil). For severe symptoms, oral contraceptives or danazol (Danocrine), a synthetic androgen, and bromocriptine (Parlodel), a semisynthetic ergot derivative that mimics prolactin-inhibiting factor, is prescribed (Drug Therapy Table 54-1).

Pharmacologic Considerations

■ Tamoxifen (a drug typically used for breast cancer) may be used "off label" for fibrocystic breast pain. Stroke, pulmonary emboli, and uterine malignancies are also associated with its use. Therefore, this drug is reserved for cases when severe breast pain is unrelieved with conventional treatment.

Occasionally, one or more cysts are removed surgically. Widespread disease that causes severe discomfort is treated with **partial,** also called **segmental, mastectomy** (surgical procedure to remove part of the breast, but not the entire breast itself). Care is taken to preserve the areola to provide a cosmetic appearance to the breast after surgery.

Nursing Management

The nurse obtains a health history and asks focused questions about the characteristics and timing of symptoms in relation to the menstrual cycle. During diagnostic examinations, the nurse prepares and supports the client, labels tissue or fluid specimens, and arranges for laboratory analysis. The nurse teaches the client with fibrocystic disease to do the following:

- Use the same technique each time if BSE is performed to become familiar with the feel and location of cystic masses.
- Schedule a breast examination with a primary provider every 6 months, or whenever a new or unusual lump develops.
- Follow the guidelines of the American Cancer Society (ACS) concerning mammography (see Chapter 52). Wear a well-fitting, supportive brassiere day and night.
- Take mild analgesics or prescription medications according to label directions.
- Apply cold compresses to the breasts when symptomatic.
- Avoid coffee, tea, chocolate, and caffeinated soft drinks for several months to determine if it helps symptoms subside.
- Restrict activities that may cause trauma to the breasts such as playing soccer or other sports in which the breasts are unprotected.
- Consult with the primary provider about taking vitamin E supplement or oil of evening primrose (a herbal preparation), which some clients have found helpful.

DRUG THERAPY TABLE 54-1 Agents for Severe Fibrocystic Disease

Category and Common Generic (Brand) Drugs	Intended Use	Common Side Effects	Safety Warnings for Nurses
Synthetic Androgen Danazol (Danocrine)	Reduces amount of hormone made by ovaries, reducing breast pain	Acne, deepened voice, weight gain, flushing, sweating	• Women need to use effective barrier method birth control • Amenorrhea may occur • Monitor liver function
Ergot Derivative Bromocriptine (Parlodel, Cycloset)	Reduces amount of prolactin hormone secreted from pituitary gland, reducing breast pain from menstrual cycle variations	Lightheadedness, dizziness, insomnia, confusion, nausea, constipation, dry mouth, orthostatic hypotension	• Do not give with MAOI (monoamine oxidase inhibitor) antidepressants • Do not use with type 1 diabetes

Fibroadenoma

A **fibroadenoma** is a solid, benign breast mass composed of connective and glandular tissue. This type of breast lesion usually occurs in women during late adolescence and early adulthood, but is occasionally found in older women.

Pathophysiology and Etiology

The cause of fibroadenomas is unknown. There may be a hormonal influence, however, because the mass grows during pregnancy and shrinks after menopause. Classically, the benign tumor is a single nodule that grows slowly in non-pregnant women until it reaches a fixed, stable size. It usually does not enlarge and regress with each menstrual cycle, like those in fibrocystic disease, and it, too, is not considered precancerous.

Assessment Findings

A fibroadenoma presents as a painless, nontender lump in the breast. The lesion usually is encapsulated, mobile, and firm when palpated. If the size of the mass is large, the breasts may appear asymmetric.

Ultrasound, digital mammography, and breast **tomosynthesis** (three-dimensional [3D] mammography) that puts multiple images together into a 3D image can reveal physical characteristics unique to a fibroadenoma versus a malignant mass with a higher degree of accuracy than standard mammography (Mayo Clinic Staff, 2020). In the case of very young women—an atypical age for breast cancer—an excisional biopsy is performed only if the mass changes or becomes larger. If the mass is detected in a woman with a higher risk for developing breast cancer, such as one with a family history or of an older age, a biopsy is performed to confirm that the tissue is indeed benign.

Medical and Surgical Management

Based on the diagnostic findings, the client and her primary provider either to continue to observe the mass or excise it. Surgery involves removal of the benign tumor but not a **mastectomy** (excision of the breast). The client is discharged a few hours after recovery from anesthesia.

Nursing Management

The nurse provides emotional support while the diagnosis is tentative, because finding a mass in the breast conjures up fears that it may be malignant. The nurse teaches the client as follows:

- Continue BSE if it is performed, and follow recommendations for mammography.
- Consult a primary provider if the characteristics of the mass change or if a pregnancy occurs.
- If surgery is performed, following instructions to:
- Keep the wound clean and covered until the incision heals.
- Wear a firm, supportive brassiere to reduce incisional discomfort.
- Follow label directions for taking a mild nonnarcotic analgesic to relieve minor pain that may last 1 to 3 days.
- Contact the surgeon to schedule a postoperative evaluation or call immediately if there is exceptional incisional pain, or if swelling, wound drainage, or a fever develops.

MALIGNANT BREAST DISORDERS

Cancer of the Breast

The incidence of **breast cancer**, a mass of abnormal cells, began to decline after the results of the Women's Health Initiative study linked the use of hormone replacement therapy (HRT) to an increased incidence of breast cancer and heart disease. Since then, the incidence of breast cancer has stabilized, affecting one woman in eight (ACS, 2021). The risk for breast cancer in women increases with age. Although breast cancer does occur in men, the risk for men is 1:833 compared to 1:8 for women (Susan G. Komen Organization, 2021). In terms of cancer-related deaths in women in the United States, breast cancer is second only to lung cancer. When the disease is localized and treated early, the 5-year survival rate is at least 99%, but decreases to 85% when regionalized with a limited spread beyond its site of origin, and 26% if there is distant **metastasis**, spread to other parts of the body (Susan G. Komen Organization, 2021).

Pathology and Pathophysiology

Certain factors appear to increase the risk of breast cancer. Being female, being older than 50 years of age, and having a family history of breast cancer are the most common risk factors. Relatives of women with breast cancer who inherited a mutated gene (*BRCA1* or *BRCA2*) are very likely to develop breast cancer. Additional factors include exposure to ionizing radiation in childhood or adolescence, previous breast cancer, a history of colon or endometrial cancer, chronic alcohol consumption, early menarche, late menopause, obesity, having no children, or having children after 30 years of age. White women are at higher risk for breast cancer than African American women, but African American women are more likely to die of it. Most of the women diagnosed with breast cancer have none of the identified risk factors except being female or being older than 50 years of age (Mayo Clinic Staff, 2020).

Each normal breast contains 15 to 20 lobes connected by ducts to smaller lobules (refer to Fig. 52-10). The most common malignancy is invasive ductal carcinoma (70% to 80%); followed by invasive lobular carcinoma (5% to 10%); inflammatory breast cancer (1% to 5%), the rarest but most aggressive form of breast cancer; with medullary carcinoma, mucinous carcinoma, and invasive papillary carcinoma making up the rest (Susan G. Komen Organization, 2020). Some malignant breast tumors are hormone dependent, meaning that estrogen or progesterone enhances tumor growth. Regardless of the type or its etiology, untreated breast cancer spreads elsewhere through the axillary lymph nodes to distant areas such as the lungs and brain.

Assessment Findings

Signs and Symptoms

The primary sign of breast cancer is a painless mass in the breast, most often in the upper outer quadrant (Fig. 54-2). The tumor may have been developing **in situ**, in a localized area without invading the surrounding tissue, for as long as 2 years before becoming palpable. Other signs of breast

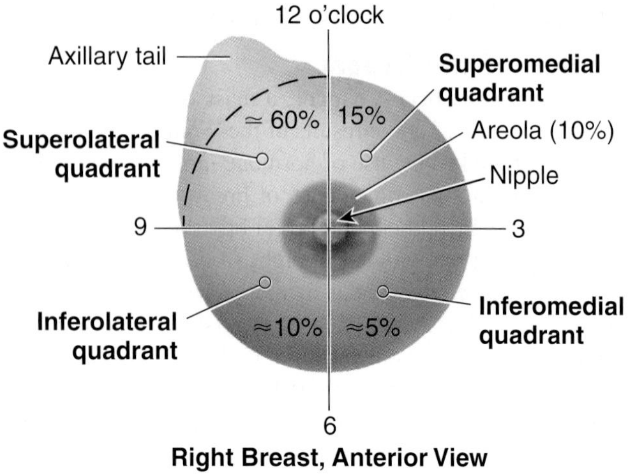

Figure 54-2 Locations of primary malignant breast tumors. (Reprinted with permission from Agur, A. M. R., & Dalley, A. F. (2016). *Grant's atlas of anatomy* (14th ed.). Wolters Kluwer.)

cancer include a bloody discharge from the nipple, a dimpling of the skin over the lesion, retraction of the nipple, peau d'orange (orange peel) appearance of the skin overlying the tumor, and a difference in size between the breasts (Fig. 54-3). The lesion may be fixed or movable, and axillary lymph nodes may be enlarged. Many of these signs depend on several factors, such as the type, location, and duration of the tumor.

Diagnostic Findings

Mammography, especially digital mammography and tomosynthesis (3D mammography), detects breast lesions earlier than they can be palpated; it is advocated particularly for women with dense breast tissue. The radiologist often can differentiate a benign tumor from a malignant one on a radiograph. Even in women who are 55 years of age or older,

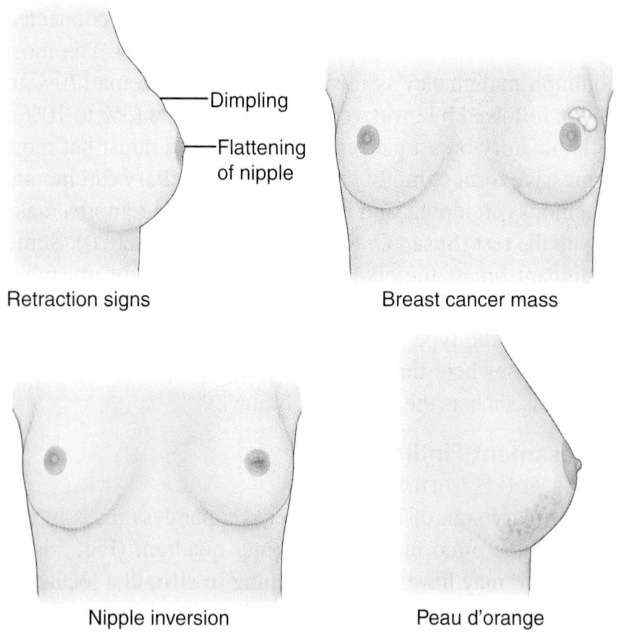

Figure 54-3 Signs and symptoms of breast cancer.

mammograms performed every 2 years, or yearly if they wish, ensure an early diagnosis and a decreased mortality rate from breast cancer. In addition to an annual mammography, breast magnetic resonance imaging (MRI) is recommended for women at high risk for breast cancer, such as those with a strong family history and/or a mutation in genes such as *BRCA1* or *BRCA2* (Susan G. Komen Organization, 2020). Biopsy and microscopic cell examination confirm the diagnosis.

Medical and Surgical Management

Treatment depends on the stage and type of breast tumor (Fig. 54-4). It includes surgery, which may be combined with chemotherapy (including hormone therapy) and radiation therapy. The use of immunotherapy has been added to the options for treatment and clinical trials of vaccines are in progress (see discussion later in the chapter).

Surgery

Surgery is performed immediately after obtaining the results of the biopsy or after completion of radiation and chemotherapy, depending on the type and stage of the cancer. The type of surgery recommended depends on the stage of the tumor and the client's informed decision about treatment options (Table 54-1). The current trend is to perform the least disfiguring procedure necessary to obtain a favorable prognosis. Compared with more extensive types of mastectomy procedures, breast-conserving surgeries such as **lumpectomy**, partial mastectomy, and segmental mastectomy followed by radiation have demonstrated equivalent outcomes in terms of survival rate for treatment of early-stage breast cancer (Breastcancer.org, 2020).

Sentinel lymph node mapping determines whether complete removal of axillary lymph nodes is necessary. Sentinel lymph node mapping involves identifying the first (sentinel) lymph nodes through which the breast cancer cells would spread to regional lymph nodes in the axilla (Fig. 54-5). The sentinel lymph nodes are located by injecting a nuclear isotope around the breast tumor followed by the instillation of blue dye. After the breast tumor is excised, a Geiger counter is passed over the perimammary tissue to find the area of most intense radioactivity. A small incision is made, and the blue dye is tracked to the sentinel lymph nodes. The sentinel lymph nodes are removed with a minimum of surrounding tissue and examined for cancer cells. An absence of cancer cells in the sentinel lymph nodes suggests that all lymph nodes are free of cancer cells. Validating the lack of lymph node metastasis allows the surgeon to preserve more breast, axillary tissue, and chest muscle. Leaving many normal lymph nodes intact reduces the potential for complications, such as lymphedema, delayed wound healing, and altered skin sensation caused by the extensive disruption of lymphatic circulation.

Lymphedema, soft-tissue swelling from accumulated lymphatic fluid (see Chapter 32), occurs in some women after they have undergone breast cancer surgery. The condition, a consequence of removing or irradiating the axillary lymph nodes, is evidenced by temporary or permanent

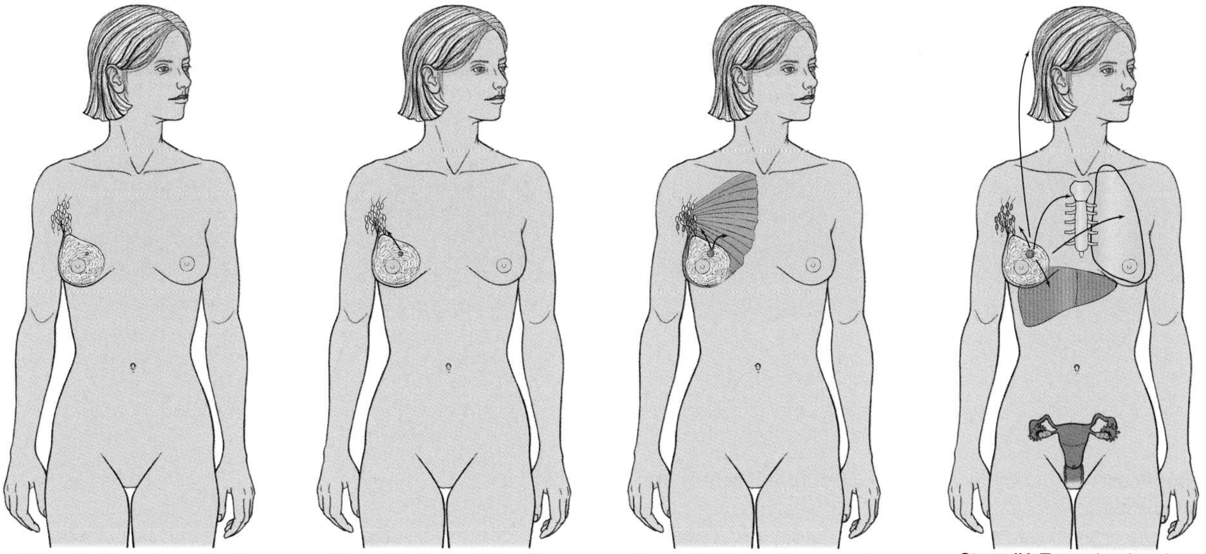

Stage 0: Tumor is confined to the milk duct or lobule.

Stage I: Tumor is less than 2 cm in diameter and confined to the breast.

Stage IIA: Tumor is less than 5 cm, or tumor is smaller with 1, 2, or 3 axillary lymph node involvement.

Stage IIB: Tumor is greater than 5 cm. Up to 3 axillary lymph nodes may be involved.

Stage IIIA: Tumor is greater than 5 cm and is confined to 4 to 10 lymph nodes.

Stage IIIB: Tumor, regardless of size, has spread to the chest wall or skin.

Stage IIIC: Tumor of any size with involvement of 10 or more lymph nodes, but no distant metastases.

Stage IV: Tumor involves lymph nodes, and there are distant metastases.

Figure 54-4 Breast cancer stages.

TABLE 54-1 Surgical Procedures for Breast Cancer

PROCEDURE	DESCRIPTION	ILLUSTRATION
Lumpectomy	Only the tumor is removed; some axillary lymph nodes may be excised at the same time for microscopic examination.	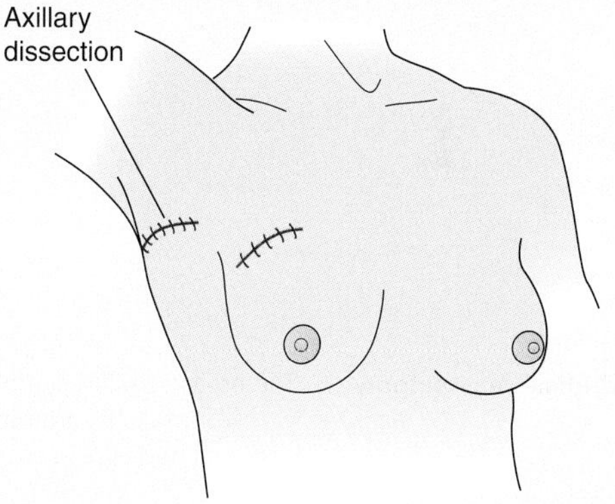
Partial or segmental mastectomy	The tumor, some breast tissue, and some lymph nodes are removed.	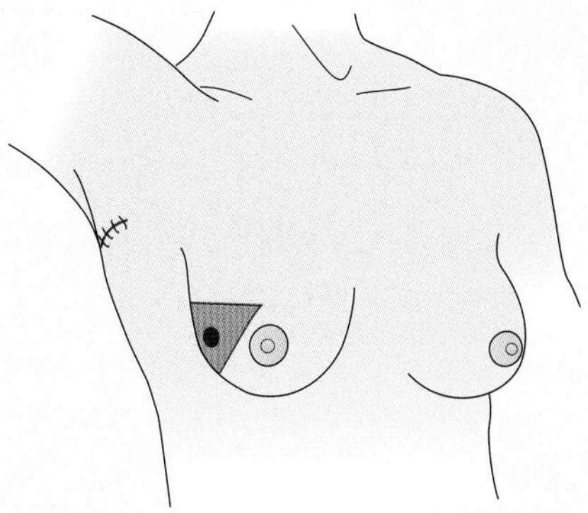

(continued)

TABLE 54-1 Surgical Procedures for Breast Cancer (*continued*)

PROCEDURE	DESCRIPTION	ILLUSTRATION
Simple or total mastectomy	All breast tissue is removed. No lymph node dissection is performed.	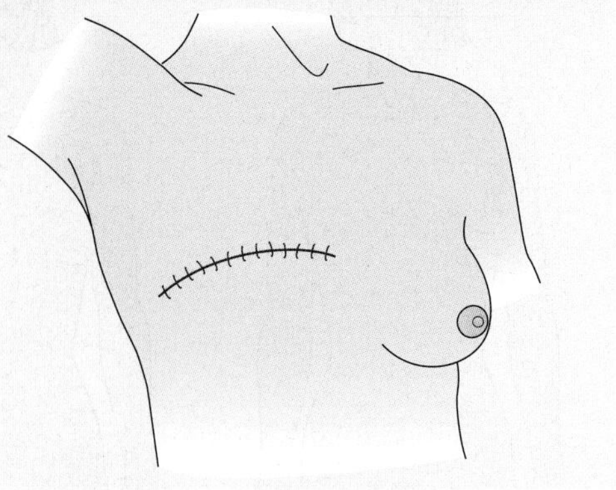
Subcutaneous mastectomy	All breast tissue is removed, but the skin and nipple are left intact.	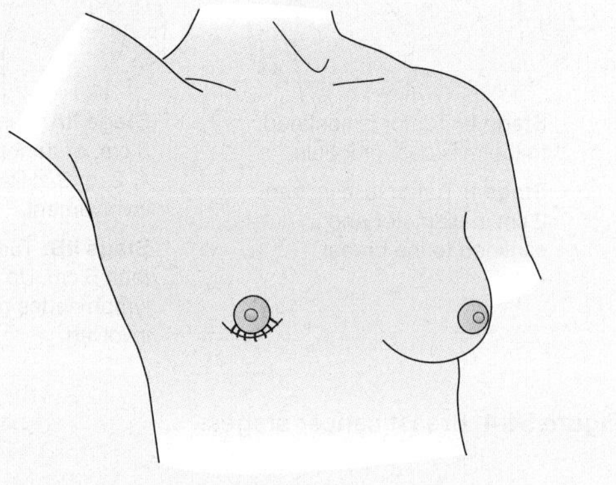
Modified radical mastectomy	The breast, some lymph nodes, the lining over the chest muscles, and the pectoralis minor muscle are removed.	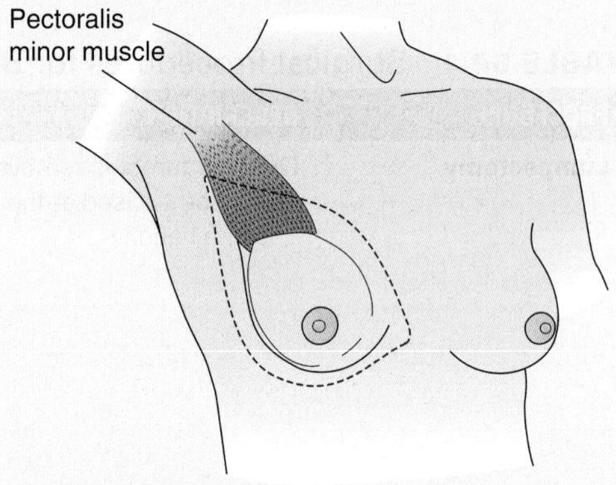
Radical mastectomy	The breast, axillary lymph nodes, and pectoralis major and minor muscles are removed. In some instances, sternal lymph nodes also are removed.	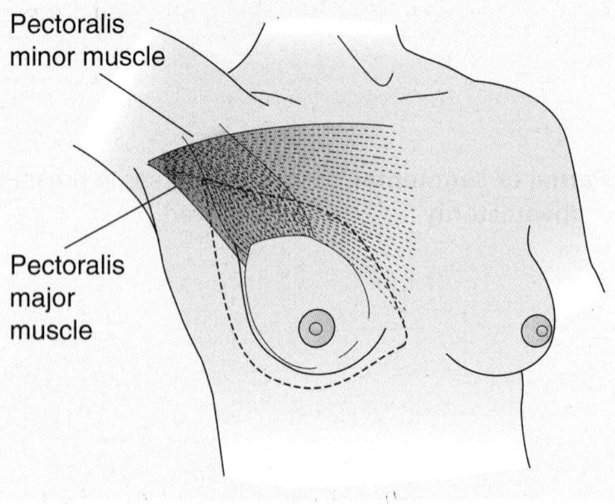

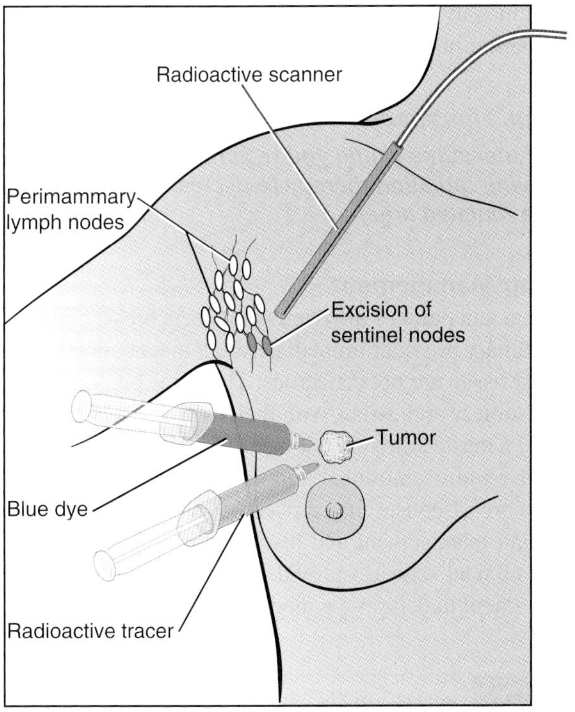

Figure 54-5 Sentinel lymph node mapping and excision to detect the spread of breast cancer to regional lymph nodes. The absence of cancer cells in sentinel lymph nodes suggests that the cancer is confined to breast tissue only.

enlargement of the arm and hand on the side of the amputated breast. Impaired lymphatic circulation predisposes to disfigurement, reduced range of motion, heaviness of the limb, skin changes, infection, and, in severe cases, tissue necrosis that may require amputation of the limb.

Depending on circumstances, chemotherapy and chemotherapy plus for adjunctive treatment and radiation therapy are common surgical adjuncts. The choice depends on factors, such as the type of cancer, sensitivity to estrogen, stage of the tumor, presence of metastasis, and client's age. Bone marrow transplantation may be used if the breast cancer resists other forms of treatment.

Chemotherapy

The goal of chemotherapy is to destroy any cancer cells that may have escaped surgical removal. Recent drug research has affected chemotherapy recommendations and proposals for candidates who may benefit from them. Most women with stage I breast cancer who choose surgery alone have an excellent prognosis. However, clinical trials suggest that clients with estrogen-sensitive tumors may benefit from one of two categories of drugs: tamoxifen or an aromatase inhibitor (AI) such as letrozole (Femara) for 5 years or more following mastectomy. Tamoxifen blocks estrogen receptors on breast cancer cells; AIs prevent prehormones from becoming estrogen but are not very effective in premenopausal women, because the ovaries produce more estrogen as a result of a negative feedback loop (see Chapter 49). AIs either after or instead of tamoxifen have been found to be superior to tamoxifen alone for preventing breast cancer recurrence and metastatic disease.

One or more of the following drugs have extended survival and prevented disease recurrence when used as **neoadjuvant therapy** (treatment prior to surgery) or **adjuvant therapy** (treatment after surgery):

- An antiestrogen drug, such as tamoxifen, for postmenopausal women whose tumors are hormone dependent. Although tamoxifen has been the mainstay of drug therapy for breast cancer, many women develop resistance to the drug; some primary providers may prefer to give an AI initially or after 5 years of tamoxifen.
- Trastuzumab (Herceptin), a monoclonal antibody, binds and selectively inhibits breast cancer cells that express a genetic protein called **H**uman **E**pidermal growth factor **R**eceptor 2 (HER2) that causes breast cancer cells to reproduce uncontrollably. Trastuzumab can be used alone or in combination with antineoplastic drugs to treat tumors that are HER2-positive (see later discussion in Immunotherapy).
- An antiprogestin drug, mifepristone (RU486), which blocks progesterone-dependent breast cancers as determined by progesterone receptor assay on excised tissue
- Androgen therapy for advanced breast cancer in postmenopausal women using testolactone (Teslac)
- Single or combined antineoplastic agents, such as doxorubicin (Adriamycin), cyclophosphamide (Cytoxan), paclitaxel (Taxol), docetaxel (Taxotere), or carboplatin (Paraplatin); antineoplastic drugs also are combined with drugs mentioned earlier that influence hormonal physiology.

Radiation Therapy

Radiation therapy can be given before or after surgery. If the surgeon finds that the axillary nodes contain cancer cells, that there is chest wall involvement, or that the tumor is larger than 5 cm, a series of radiation treatments usually is ordered prophylactically, even after a modified radical mastectomy. Side effects of radiation therapy include fatigue, skin redness similar to bad sunburn, rash, minor discomfort, or pain (see Chapter 18). Some clients develop pneumonitis, rib fractures, and breast fibrosis.

Immunotherapy and Cancer Vaccines

Immunotherapy is the basis for various drugs and therapeutic cancer vaccines. Rather than prevent breast cancer, it stimulates the immune system's ability to attack and rid the body of cancer cells. Currently, monoclonal antibodies (mABs) such as trastuzumab (Herceptin) and others are being administered to clients with **HER2-positive** breast cancer. HER2 is a protein that promotes the growth of cancer cells in about 1 of every 5 cases of breast cancer. The mABs facilitate the immune system's ability to attack the HER2-positive cancer cells (Susan G. Komen Organization, 2021).

Immunotherapy drugs have several advantages when compared with traditional chemotherapy drugs:

- They have fewer side effects than traditional chemotherapy drugs.
- They can be administered for a longer time.
- They can be combined with other drugs without added toxicity.
- There is a lower potential for developing resistance to the mABs (Breastcancer.org, 2020).

Pharmacologic Considerations

■ Preventive vaccines are used prophylactically to inhibit a disease in healthy people. Therapeutic vaccines may be used in the future to treat various diseases in diagnosed people, but none is currently available outside of clinical trials. Those being developed for breast cancer treat by helping the immune system to recognize, respond, and kill cancer cells.

Breast cancer vaccines are also being developed. The nelipepimut-S vaccine (NeuVax), is currently in phase III clinical trials. The vaccine stimulates CD8 and cytotoxic T lymphocytes to recognize and destroy HER2 cancer cells and surrounding micrometastatic cells. Experimental work on other breast cancer vaccines is ongoing. A second vaccine known as the HER2 DNA vaccine also facilitates the immune system's ability to recognize the HER2 cells, destroy them, and prevent them from spreading. In addition, researchers are working on a breast cancer vaccine that stimulates the immune system to attack a protein called mammaglobin-A, which is found in 80% of primary and metastatic breast cancer tumors. Lastly, researchers in the United States are testing a vaccine that involves the injection of telomerase peptide, an antigen found in 90% of breast tumors, to stimulate an immune response to the tumor. Currently, there are no vaccines available for breast cancer other than to those participating in research projects.

>>> *Stop, Think, and Respond 54-1*

What measures would you recommend to your client receiving radiation therapy to decrease skin irritation to the radiated area?

Nursing Management

The nurse encourages anyone who detects breast changes to see a primary provider immediately, but in fact, most changes in breast tissue are not cancerous. The nurse prepares the client for surgery and assists with their safe recovery. Men who undergo a mastectomy do not face extreme physical changes, but still require emotional support because of the diagnosis. For breast-conserving procedures, nursing care focuses on wound management and discharge instructions. The following clinical scenario provides more specific information about a client undergoing a modified radical mastectomy.

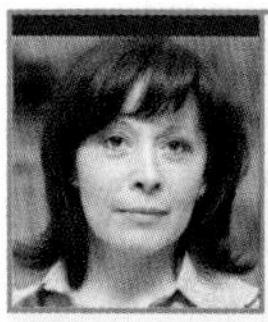

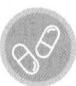

Clinical Scenario A 48-year-old woman noticed a change in the appearance of her left breast as compared with the right breast. Upon self-examination, she could feel a thick, hard mass in the upper outer quadrant of her left breast. Prior to the clinical breast examination, she had told the nurse that she had a family history of breast cancer. A subsequent mammogram and MRI revealed a fixed mass that could very likely be cancerous. A biopsy confirmed a diagnosis of ductal carcinoma. After completing neoadjuvant chemotherapy, the client will undergo a modified radical mastectomy and subsequent postoperative radiation. What problems might she encounter? How can the nurse proactively manage them? Consider the examples in Nursing Care Plan 54-1.

NURSING CARE PLAN 54-1 The Client Undergoing a Modified Radical Mastectomy

Assessment

- Discuss the client's medical, drug, allergy, and family history.
- Take vital signs and weight.
- Determine the location of the breast lesion.
- Establish what diagnostic tests were performed before admission (if any).
- Discuss information the primary provider has given the client about the type and extent of surgery.

Nursing Diagnoses. **Acute Anxiety** and **Fear** related to undergoing an unfamiliar experience and the potential consequences of the disease and its treatment

Expected Outcome. Client will indicate increased emotional comfort.

Interventions	Rationale
Provide an opportunity for the client to express feelings and discuss concerns.	*Verbalizing helps the client deal openly with feelings.*
Answer all questions; consult with other team members about matters that involve their expertise.	*Presenting facts provides the client with reality-based information and reduces exaggerated perceptions.*

NURSING CARE PLAN 54-1 The Client Undergoing a Modified Radical Mastectomy (*continued*)

Collaborate with primary provider on arranging for a visit from a Reach to Recovery or I Can Cope volunteer sponsored by the American Cancer Society.	*People who have recovered from a similar diagnosis and surgery can serve as role models and answer questions from their own personal experiences.*
Do not stifle crying; stay with client when emotions are overwhelming.	*Crying relieves tension when a person can find no other coping strategy.*
Encourage client's significant other or whomever the client turns to for support to remain with client as much and as long as possible.	*The presence of others who provide emotional support reduces anxiety.*
Keep client informed of the routine that will be followed in preparation for surgery and postoperative care.	*Dealing with unexpected events heightens anxiety; knowledge facilitates a sense of control.*

Evaluation of Expected Outcome

Anxiety is reduced.

Nursing Diagnosis. **Knowledge Deficiency** related to surgical routines

Expected Outcome. Client will be able to paraphrase the preoperative and postoperative routines.

Interventions	Rationale
Explain that the arm on the surgical side may be elevated, and movement away from the body (abduction) may be temporarily restricted.	*Elevation reduces edema. Abduction is temporarily restricted until healing progresses.*

Evaluation of Expected Outcomes

Client demonstrates an understanding of the type of surgery and potential postsurgical treatment modalities; preoperative preparations; and postoperative management, including coughing, deep breathing, and leg exercises.
Client openly discusses and asks questions about surgery.

Nursing Diagnosis. **Hypovolemia and Bleeding Risk** Related to tissue excision

Expected Outcome. The nurse will monitor to detect, manage, and minimize hemorrhage and shock.

Interventions	Rationale
Obtain vital signs according to agency routines. Do not take blood pressure on the arm on the side of the mastectomy.	*The circulation of blood and lymph can be further compromised if the arm on the side of the mastectomy is used to measure blood pressure, to take blood specimens, or for IV infusions or injections.*
Check color and amount of blood loss from the wound and drain, if one is present.	*An increase in the volume or change to bright red color suggests excessive or arterial blood loss.*
Feel underneath client's side or back for obscured bleeding.	*Gravity can cause blood to drain posteriorly.*
Administer IV fluids or blood transfusions at the rate prescribed.	*Fluid replacement offsets fluid losses.*

Evaluation of Expected Outcome

Bleeding is controlled; shock does not occur.

Nursing Diagnoses. **Altered Breathing Pattern** and **Ineffective Airway Clearance Risk** related to pain, weak cough, and bulky dressing

Expected Outcome. Client will breathe effortlessly and be well oxygenated.

Interventions	Rationale
Instruct client to deep breathe and cough every 2 hours during waking hours or use an incentive spirometer.	*Deep breathing expands alveoli and promotes increased gas diffusion.*

(*continued*)

NURSING CARE PLAN 54-1 The Client Undergoing a Modified Radical Mastectomy (*continued*)

Splint incision to reduce discomfort.	*Pain or fear of pain interferes with deep breathing.*
Administer oxygen as prescribed.	*Supplemental oxygen provides a higher concentration than found in room air.*
Instruct client to self-administer analgesia before deep breathing and coughing if a patient-controlled analgesia (PCA) pump is available.	*Pain is more adequately controlled when an analgesic is given before severe pain develops.*

Evaluation of Expected Outcome

Gas exchange is adequate as evidenced by oxygen saturation (SpO_2) of 90% or greater and clear lung sounds.

Nursing Diagnosis. **Acute Pain** related to tissue trauma

Expected Outcome. Discomfort will be controlled within a tolerable level.

Interventions	Rationale
Administer pain medication liberally according to prescribed dose and frequency.	*Clients have the right to pain relief.*
Avoid giving injections in the arm on the same side as the surgery.	*Circulation of blood and lymph is impaired, which can affect the absorption of parenteral medication and increase the potential for infection.*
Monitor response to analgesia 30 minutes after administration or more frequently if PCA is in use.	*The nurse is obligated to use additional measures to reduce the client's pain until it is at their tolerable level.*
Pin the tubing of the drain or the drain collection chamber to the client's gown.	*Stabilizing the drain helps prevent it from pulling at the insertion site and increasing discomfort.*
Implement nursing techniques such as changing positions, relaxation, distraction, and guided imagery (see Chapter 11).	*Nonpharmacologic measures supplement or complement analgesia.*
Collaborate with the primary provider if pain control is inadequate.	*The nurse consults with the primary provider to determine possible changes in the type of analgesic, its dose, or frequency.*

Evaluation of Expected Outcome

Pain is controlled.

Nursing Diagnoses. **Altered Skin Integrity** and **Infection Risk** secondary to surgical wound

Expected Outcome. The incision will heal; no infection will develop.

Interventions	Rationale
Limit movement, especially abduction, of the arm on the side of surgery until the wound edges are intact.	*Activity can disrupt the approximation of the incision.*
Inspect the wound for swelling, unusual drainage, odor, redness, or separation of the suture line.	*Wound infections are accompanied by signs of inflammation and a delay in healing.*
Empty and reestablish negative pressure in closed wound drains at least once per shift.	*Negative pressure (suction) pulls fluid from the incisional area, which facilitates healing.*
Administer antibiotic therapy as prescribed.	*Antibiotics destroy or inhibit the growth of microorganisms.*
Monitor the trend in temperature and white blood cell counts.	*A fever and leukocytosis suggest that an infection is developing.*
Allow the client to shower after the sutures and drains are removed.	*Hygiene reduces the number of microorganisms on the skin.*

Evaluation of Expected Outcome

Incision heals without complications.

NURSING CARE PLAN 54-1 The Client Undergoing a Modified Radical Mastectomy (*continued*)

Nursing Diagnosis. **Altered Tissue Perfusion** (lymphedema) related to compromised flow of lymphatic fluid

Expected Outcome. Soft tissue in the arm on the side of surgery will be comparable with the opposite arm in color, size, and temperature.

Interventions	Rationale
Do not take blood pressure, give injections, administer IV infusions, or have blood drawn from the arm on the side of the mastectomy.	*Procedures that affect the circulation in the affected arm can contribute to ineffective tissue perfusion.*
Support and elevate the arm on the side of the mastectomy with pillows such that it is kept higher than the heart.	*Elevation promotes gravity drainage of fluid trapped in the soft tissue.*
Place the arm in a sling when the client ambulates initially; eventually, the arm can be positioned at the client's side.	*A sling prevents stasis of fluid in distal areas of the arm.*
Show the client how to squeeze and release a soft rubber ball or a rolled pair of cotton socks several times a day.	*Venous blood and lymph circulate with contraction of skeletal muscles.*
Remove and reapply an elastic roller bandage from the fingers to the axilla twice a day, or insert the affected arm into a pneumatic sleeve, an air-filled device that mechanically pumps the arm, for a half hour or the prescribed amount of time twice a day.	*An elastic roller bandage or pneumatic sleeve compresses the valves in veins to promote circulation.*
Assess the hand for swelling, dusky color, delayed nail blanching, coldness, and tingling; report abnormal findings.	*The nurse is responsible for reporting abnormal findings to reduce the potential for complications.*

Evaluation of Expected Outcome

The circulation is maintained in the operative arm; both arms are of comparable size.

Nursing Diagnosis. **Dressing ADL deficit** related to alteration in pectoral chest muscles

Expected Outcome. Client will achieve full range of arm motion.

Interventions	Rationale
Start active exercises of the affected arm on the first or second postoperative day, or later if the primary provider indicates a need to postpone them. (Skin grafts may need additional time to heal.)	*Active exercise reduces the potential for contractures.*
Begin with flexing and extending the fingers, wrist, and elbow. Later, encourage the client to use the affected arm to perform oral hygiene, hair combing, and face washing.	*Exercise gradually restores the ability to flex, extend, and abduct the arm.*
Show the client how to face and "finger walk" up a wall in the room (see Client and Family Teaching 54-1). Mark the client's progress with masking tape so that the height can be exceeded with subsequent efforts.	*Finger walking increases the ability to raise the arm. Marking progress provides an incentive to meet or exceed heights during previous exercises.*
Loop a rope or cord around a shower rod and raise and lower each arm in pulley fashion.	*Modification in the technique for performing arm exercises facilitates rehabilitation.*
Tie a string or rope to a doorknob and have the client turn the rope in a circular fashion.	*Turning a rope promotes circumduction.*

Evaluation of Expected Outcomes

Client improves the use of the arm and hand of operative side. The client performs postmastectomy exercises.

Nursing Diagnosis. **Injury Risk** related to change in center of gravity secondary to extensive removal of chest tissue

Expected Outcome. The client will not fall.

(*continued*)

NURSING CARE PLAN 54-1 The Client Undergoing a Modified Radical Mastectomy (*continued*)

Interventions	Rationale
Assist the client during periods of ambulation.	*The nurse supports the client when or if client loses balance.*
Walk on the client's unaffected side.	*The client is more likely to drift toward the heavier side of the body.*
Instruct the client to keep the shoulders level and the muscles relaxed when walking.	*Clients tend to accommodate for the change in the center of gravity by leaning to the side.*

Evaluation of Expected Outcome

The client remains injury-free.

Nursing Diagnosis. **Grief** related to loss of breast

Expected Outcome. Client will express grief and deal with losses in an appropriate amount of time.

Interventions	Rationale
Avoid trying to diminish the significance of the loss.	*Grief work involves dealing with the reality of a significant loss.*
Acknowledge client's grief and reinforce that feeling angry or sad is normal and expected.	*Validating client's feelings gives permission for them to experience true emotions.*
Stay with client and ensure privacy during emotional periods.	*The nurse's presence provides support.* *Ensuring privacy demonstrates respect for the client's dignity.*
Avoid administering prescribed sedatives or tranquilizers as a substitute for spending time with the client.	*Numbing the mind interferes with grieving.*
Encourage sharing with those who can be empathic, such as another breast cancer survivor.	*Sharing the significance of a loss with a person who has survived a similar experience provides a bond for healing.*

Nursing Diagnoses. **Altered Body Image Perception and Coping Impairment** related to perceived loss of physical attractiveness and sexual desirability

Expected Outcomes. Client will accept body changes, use positive coping strategies, and experience satisfactory sexual activity.

Interventions	Rationale
Suggest that client pad a brassiere with one or two cotton socks until a prosthesis is fitted in 6 to 8 weeks.	*Padding a brassiere gives the outward appearance that the client has both breasts. Purchasing a prosthetic brassiere is delayed until the tissue heals.*
Inform client that cosmetic breast reconstruction is an option to discuss with the surgeon.	*Cosmetic breast reconstruction provides an alternative for simulating natural breast tissue.*
Advocate that client and sexual partner openly express to each other how the surgery has affected them emotionally.	*Open communication facilitates mutual understanding and acceptance of body change.*
Discuss methods for dealing with the removed breast during sexual activities such as using no or low lighting during intercourse or wearing the upper portion of lingerie.	*Modifying sexual activities reduces self-consciousness.*

Evaluation of Expected Outcome

Client adjusts to the loss of the breast.

The nurse prepares the client for common side effects of neoadjuvant or adjuvant chemotherapy, such as nausea, vomiting, changes in taste, alopecia (hair loss), mucositis, dermatitis, fatigue, weight gain, and bone marrow suppression. Some clients also experience mild short-term memory loss and difficulty with thought processes, known as "chemo brain." It is not known whether this results from chemotherapy or the depression that frequently accompanies a cancer diagnosis. Administering antiemetics and anxiolytic medications before a chemotherapy treatment helps lessen the potential for vomiting. The nurse provides instructions regarding when and how the client should take medications at home to alleviate nausea and mouth sores and to boost the white blood cell or red blood cell production. If alopecia is likely, the nurse offers the client a list of wig suppliers (usually provided through the ACS). Catalogs from which the client can purchase scarves, turbans, or hats to camouflage hair loss are available through the ACS.

Most clients are not hospitalized long after mastectomy. Therefore, providing early discharge instructions and making arrangements for home care are important interventions. Information that nurses commonly must address with the client includes the following:

- Explain wound and drain care or arrange for home health nursing.
- Assess the availability of family assistance at home.
- Look for and report any signs of infection or impaired wound healing such as drainage or significant pale or dusky appearance to the skin around the incision.
- Provide instructions for performing arm exercises and stress their continuation (Client and Family Teaching 54-1).

Client and Family Teaching 54-1
Performing Arm Exercises Following Surgery for Breast Cancer

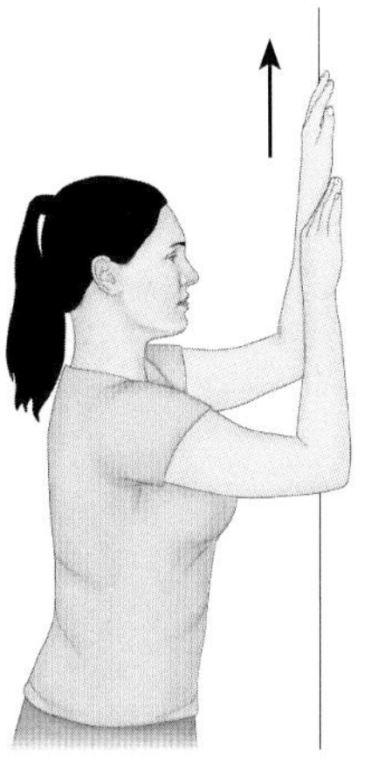

1. *Wall hand climbing.* Stand facing the wall with feet apart and toes as close to the wall as possible. With elbows slightly bent, place the palms of the hand on the wall at shoulder level. By flexing the fingers, work the hands up the wall until arms are fully extended. Then reverse the process, working the hands down to the starting point.

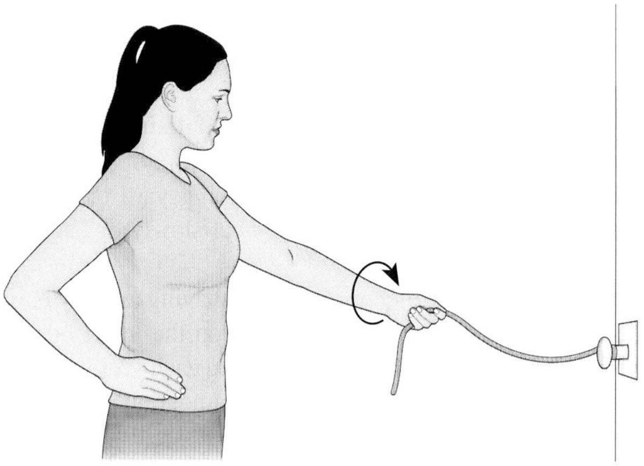

2. *Rope turning.* Tie a light rope to a doorknob. Stand facing the door. Take the free end of the rope in the hand on the side of the surgery. Place the other hand on the hip. With the rope-holding arm extended and held away from the body (nearly parallel with the floor), turn the rope, making as wide swings as possible. Begin slowly at first; speed up later.

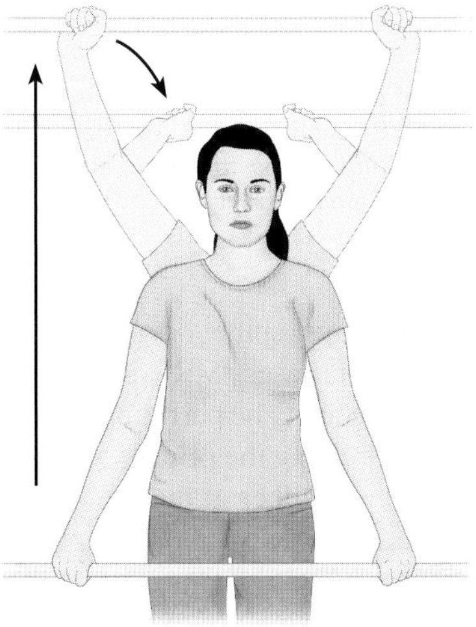

3. *Rod or broomstick lifting.* Grasp a rod with both hands, held about 2 feet apart. Keep the arms straight and raise the rod over the head. Bend elbows to lower the rod behind the head. Reverse maneuver, raising the rod above the head, then return to the starting position.

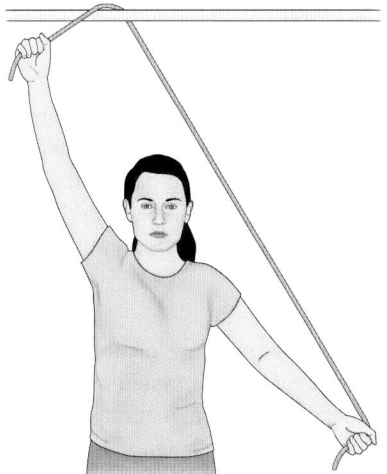

4. *Pulley tugging.* Toss a light rope over a shower curtain rod or doorway curtain rod. Stand as much under the rope as possible. Grasp an end in each hand. Extend the arms straight and away from the body. Pull the left arm up by tugging down with the right arm, then the right arm up and the left down in a seesawing motion.

- Arrange for follow-up examinations by the surgeon.
- Instruct on the self-administration of prescribed drug therapy.
- Inform that some residual numbness or tingling on the chest wall and the inner side of the arm from the axilla to the elbow may occur and take as long as 1 year to resolve.
- Suggest the application of cream or lotion to the arm if the skin tends to be dry.
- Explain that in the selection of a prosthesis, one filled with fluid assumes natural contours like the other breast, feels like normal breast tissue, and even radiates body warmth.
- Advise against lifting or carrying objects that weigh more than 15 lb and making vigorous repetitive movements with the affected arm.
- Discourage sleeping on the affected arm or wearing constrictive clothing that impairs circulation.
- Reinforce that blood pressure measurements, injections, blood donations, and IV infusions are contraindicated lifelong in the arm on the side of the mastectomy.
- Recommend wearing gloves while doing yard or housework to prevent injuries that may heal slowly or become infected.
- Advise the use of an electric razor for shaving axillary hair.
- Encourage the client to perform BSE on the intact breast, have the intact breast clinically examined each year by a primary provider, and obtain a yearly mammogram and MRI.

>>> *Stop, Think, and Respond 54-2*

A client has had a modified radical mastectomy (a surgical procedure to remove the breast, some lymph nodes, the lining over the chest muscles, and the pectoralis minor muscle). While trying to teach her how to care for the incision, she avoids looking at the wound. How can you help her cope with the change in body image?

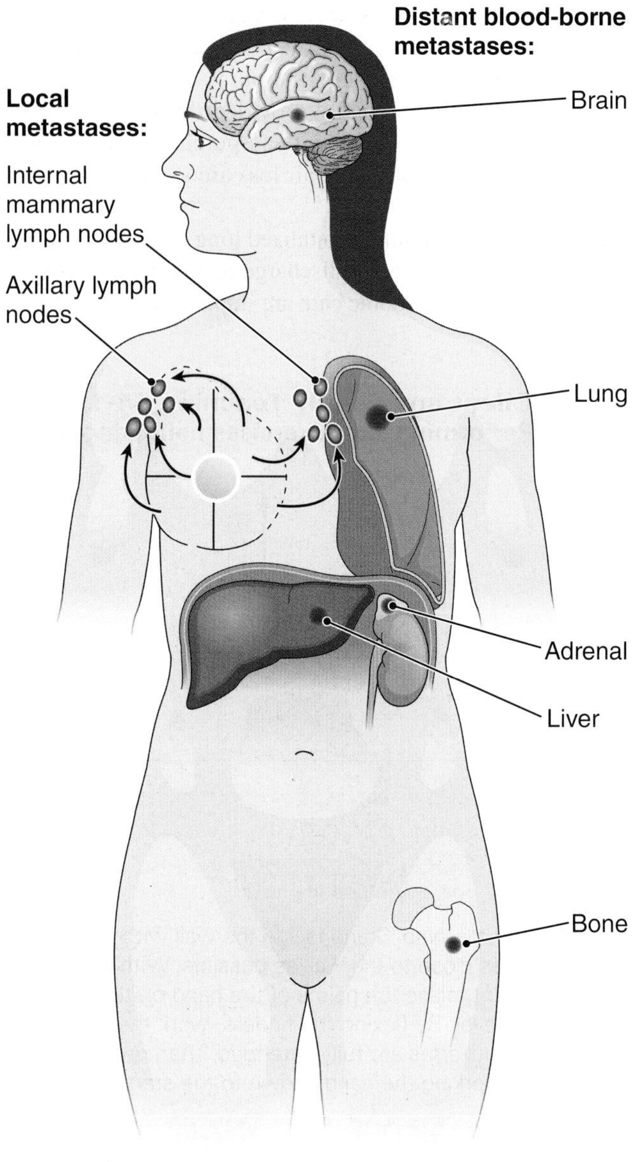

Figure 54-6 Sites of breast cancer metastasis. (Reprinted with permission from McConnell, T. H. (2014). *The nature of disease: Pathology for the health professions* (2nd ed.). Wolters Kluwer Health/Lippincott Williams & Wilkins.)

Metastatic Breast Cancer

Despite treatment even in the early stages of breast cancer, some women develop metastatic disease. Metastasis is the migration of cancer cells from one part of the body to another (Fig. 54-6). Malignant cells spread by direct extension, through the lymphatic system, bloodstream, and cerebrospinal fluid.

Pathophysiology

Lymph nodes most commonly are involved in metastasis, and the skeletal and pulmonary systems may also be involved (in that order). In addition, metastases may be found in the brain, adrenals, and liver. Once metastasis occurs, the prognosis is less favorable. Some metastases progress slowly, but others progress more rapidly.

Assessment Findings

Signs and Symptoms

Metastases often cause pain in the new site. When bone becomes involved, pathologic fractures (a fracture after slight or no trauma) are possible.

Diagnostic Findings

Radiographs of the lungs, spine, or other areas of the body are used to detect metastases. MRI or computed tomography (CT) scanning also may be performed. These studies are done before or after treating the primary tumor. Lymph node dissection is performed either at the time of breast surgery or later to evaluate metastasis to the lymph nodes draining the breasts.

Medical Management

Treatment aims at providing the greatest period of palliation (relieving symptoms without curing the disease) for the client. It varies with the primary provider and the specific type of metastasis. Research has shown that in women with estrogen receptor–positive breast cancer, the rate of recurrence can be reduced by administering tamoxifen, a selective estrogen receptor modulator, or an AI such as letrozole (Femara), one of a group of drugs that stops the conversion of androgen into estrogen, for 10 years following diagnosis (Susan G. Komen Organization, 2021).

Large doses of estrogen or testosterone sometimes alleviate the pain, weight loss, and malaise of metastatic cancer. Intramuscular androgen (testosterone) therapy is used especially when metastases are to bone. All forms of treatment carry the possibility of unpleasant side effects and complications. For palliative purposes, radiation therapy may be used to treat regional or distant metastases (especially to bone) or local tumor recurrence of the chest wall. Sometimes, surgery, chemotherapy, radiation, immunotherapy, or a therapeutic vaccine is used to manage metastasis.

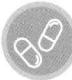

Pharmacologic Considerations

- Metastases of breast cancer to soft tissue and bone may respond to antineoplastic drugs. These drugs may cause bone marrow depression, granulocytopenia, anemia, nausea, vomiting, hypotension, dermatitis, malaise, diarrhea, and stomatitis.
- In treating clients with breast cancer metastases, pain management is important. The opioid analgesics morphine and fentanyl (Duragesic) are most often used for relief of cancer pain.

Nursing Management

For nursing care of the client undergoing chemotherapy or radiation and caring for the terminally ill client with cancer, see Chapters 10 and 18.

Breast Cancer Prevention

Three options are available to women with increased risk of developing breast cancer: (1) long-term follow-up, (2) bilateral prophylactic mastectomy, and (3) chemoprevention with tamoxifen, or letrozole (Femara). Those who choose long-term follow-up receive an annual mammogram and MRI, with a clinical breast examination and perform monthly BSE. Prophylactic bilateral mastectomy is the most invasive of the three options. Clients considering this option are informed that removing the breasts reduces the risk of breast cancer but does not eliminate it.

A breast cancer preventive study determined that tamoxifen reduced the occurrence of estrogen receptor-positive tumors, but did not affect the occurrence of estrogen receptor-negative tumors. Besides reducing the risk of breast cancer, tamoxifen preserves bone mineral density, thus preventing osteoporosis. It also lowers the low density lipoprotein (LDL) cholesterol levels. On the other hand, tamoxifen can have detrimental effects. It increases the incidences of endometrial cancer, deep vein thrombosis, pulmonary embolism, and cataracts. Other side effects include increased hot flashes, cold sweats, vaginal discharge, genital itching, and pain with intercourse. AIs cause fewer side effects than tamoxifen, but are associated with joint pain, joint stiffness, bone loss, and fractures. There may be damage to a developing embryo; therefore, they are contraindicated for women who are pregnant or wish to become pregnant. A nonhormonal form of birth control is best until an AI is discontinued (Breastcancer.org, 2020).

The U.S. Preventive Services Task Force (2019) indicated that women who are at increased risk for breast cancer and low risk for adverse medications may be offered raloxifene (Evista), a drug used to prevent osteoporosis, to reduce the risk of estrogen receptor-positive breast cancer. As with tamoxifen, no reduction in estrogen receptor-negative breast cancers was evident. However, the risk of thromboembolic disease increased, because raloxifene is a selective estrogen receptor modifier (SERM; Nelson et al., 2019).

There is some evidence that the risk for breast cancer is reduced among women who take aspirin and nonsteroidal anti-inflammatory drugs (NSAIDs), which block prostaglandins that are elevated in cancer cells, increase the risk for metastasis, and reduce survival. However, aspirin, if used for cancer protection, should be taken 3 or more times per week, even as a low-dose (81 mg) regimen (Bertrand et al., 2020; Clark et al., 2017). The role of diet (see Nutrition Notes), maintaining an ideal body weight, and avoiding alcohol are all factors that affect the development or prevention of breast cancer.

Nutrition Notes

The Client at Risk for Breast Cancer

- There is suggestive evidence that a diet high in fats, sugars, red meats, and processed meats increases the risk of both premenopausal and postmenopausal breast cancer. The use of the Mediterranean diet, which is low in fats, red and processed meats, and limited use of low-fat dairy products shows a slight decrease in the risk of breast cancer in the postmenopausal client (Laudisiol et al., 2019). However, there is convincing evidence that increased body fat raises the risk of postmenopausal breast cancer, and abdominal obesity and adult weight gain are identified as probable risks. Being overweight and weight gain are epidemiologic evidence consistently demonstrating that a high body mass index (BMI; above 28 kg/m^2) increases the occurrence of breast cancer after menopause.
- Adult weight gain has been associated with postmenopausal breast cancer in several studies.
- The strongest link between diet and breast cancer is with alcohol, it is not the type of alcohol but the amount of alcohol consumed that increases cancer risk (ACS, 2020).
- It is possible that the greatest effect of nutrition on breast cancer occurs during puberty or adolescence, when breasts are still forming.

American Cancer Society. (2020). Diet and physical activity: What's the cancer connection? https://www.cancer.org/cancer/cancer-causes/diet-physical-activity/diet-and-physical-activity.html.

Laudisiol, D., Barreal, L., Muscogiuril, G., Annunziata, G., Colaol, A., & Savastanol, S. (2019). Breast cancer prevention in premenopausal women: Role of the Mediterranean diet and its components. *Nutrition Research Reviews, 33*(1), 1–14. https://doi.org/10.1017/S0954422419000167

COSMETIC BREAST PROCEDURES

Some women undergo various cosmetic breast procedures, collectively referred to as **mammoplasty**, for several reasons but primarily to improve their appearance.

Breast Reconstruction

Breast reconstruction is a surgical procedure in which the area of a mastectomy is refashioned to simulate the contour of a breast and optionally to create a nipple and areola. This is accomplished by using either autogenous (self) tissue or an artificial implant filled with saline or silicone gel. Reconstruction can begin at the time of mastectomy if sufficient skin is spared, or it can be performed later.

Autogenous Tissue

When reconstructing the breast with autogenous tissue, the surgeon harvests tissue in a manner similar to a "tummy tuck" (abdominoplasty) from the rectus abdominis muscle along with its adjoining skin and fat or the latissimus dorsi muscle (Fig. 54-7). Removing donor tissue tends to leave a physical deformity, with some defects being more obvious than others.

If a woman desires a nipple, it is reconstructed from tissue from the opposite nipple, the ear, or toe. Tissue for the areola is selected from a site with a similar color, like the inner thigh or vaginal labia. It also may be created by pigmented tattoo.

Artificial Implants

Artificial implants are either filled with saline or silicone gel, both of which are enclosed within a silicone shell. It was previously believed that the silicone gel filling posed a health risk if it ruptured. After years of data collection, the U.S. Food and Drug Administration (FDA, 2020) has determined that silicone gel–filled as well as saline-filled implants are safe despite the fact that local complications and adverse outcomes may occur. Created out of a highly cohesive silicone gel implant, "gummy bear" implants are more stable, soft when squeezed, cannot leak, and go back to their original shape when released. However, some find them too firm and require a larger incision when implanted. When a client desires breast reconstruction or breast augmentation (discussed later), the pros and cons of each type should be considered (Table 54-2; Fig. 54-8).

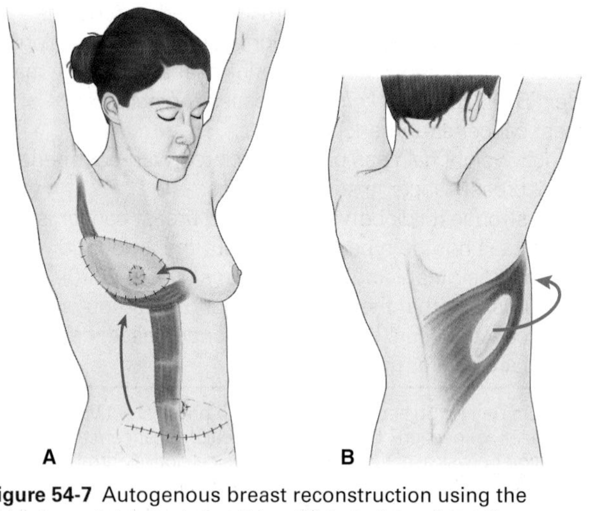

Figure 54-7 Autogenous breast reconstruction using the **(A)** rectus abdominal muscle or **(B)** latissimus dorsi flap. A breast mound is created by tunneling skin, fat, and muscle to the mastectomy site.

Before an implant for breast reconstruction can produce an optimum cosmetic appearance, the skin and tissue on the chest wall are expanded to provide a large enough space to fill and approximate the size of the remaining breast. Tissue expansion is achieved by stretching the chest wall over several months with an inflatable or saline-filled pocket (Fig. 54-9).

The FDA states that (1) breast implants are not expected to last a lifetime and one or more additional surgeries may be necessary; (2) changes in the breast are irreversible; (3) an initial MRI screening is recommended 3 years after receiving a silicone-gel implant to detect a rupture, followed by regular screenings every 2 years thereafter; and (4) either type of implant requires surgical removal if it ruptures. Manufacturers of silicone gel implants collect data about the long-term type and rates of complications, which allows the FDA to track device failures and to have procedures in place to notify recipients of potential hazards.

Breast Augmentation

Women who wish to enlarge their natural, malignancy-free breasts may choose **breast augmentation**, which is similar to breast reconstruction using an artificial implant. This generally involves same day or overnight surgery with discharge following recovery. Before leaving the surgical facility, the nurse provides instructions that include the following:

- Take a mild aspirin-free analgesic for discomfort and prescribed antibiotic according to the primary provider's directions.
- Apply a bag of crushed ice or bag of frozen vegetables to the breasts if they feel tight and swollen; maximum swelling occurs in about 3 to 5 days and resolves gradually thereafter.
- It is normal to hear squishing or sloshing sounds around the breast from trapped air and fluid until they disappear approximately a week after surgery.
- Shower after 24 hours; discard the initial dressing, but leave the Steri-Strips in place until advised by the surgeon to remove them.
- Restrict arm movements for 3 days, and then resume nonstrenuous activities.
- Avoid activities, such as vigorous sports, that may result in injury to the breasts until healing is complete.
- Wear a sports or supportive (wireless) brassiere day and night for several weeks.
- Sleep in whatever position is comfortable; most prefer sleeping on their side or back.
- Report excessive drainage, excessive pain, and fever to the primary provider immediately.
- Continue regularly scheduled mammograms at a facility with expertise in imaging the breasts of clients with implants.

TABLE 54-2 Comparison of Breast Implants

ADVANTAGES	DISADVANTAGES
Silicone Gel–Filled	
• Currently considered safe • Softer, lighter, and more natural feel, especially in thin clients with little breast tissue • Lasts longer • All U.S. manufacturers offer a lifetime implant replacement warranty	• More expensive • Requires larger incision because they are prefilled • Fixed prefilled volume • Capsules subject to scar tissue formation with hardening over time • Less potential for rippling • Must be at least 22 years of age • Rupture silently (rupture is harder to detect) • Must be inserted with inframammary, periareolar, or transaxillary incision, which leaves a visible scar (see Fig. 54-9) • Replacement is more involved • Periodic MRI monitoring is most likely not covered by insurers.
Highly Cohesive Silicone	
• Teardrop shape for natural appearance • Firmer • Stays in place • Will not leak • No danger if rupture occurs • No wrinkling, rippling, or folding • Adjustable volume facilitates symmetrical appearance	• Feels less natural due to firmness • Larger incision required; discreet armpit incision is nearly impossible • Can rotate and cause breast distortion • More expensive than others • More data needed on long-term complications
Saline-Filled	
• Safe • Less expensive • Smaller incision (See Fig. 54-9) • No danger if rupture occurs • Adjustable volume facilitates symmetrical appearance • No age restriction • Can be inserted using a transumbilical incision (through the umbilicus), which leaves no visible scar, or through any other surgical site options used with silicone gel–filled implants • Easily replaced by removing outer shell	• Firmer, heavier, and can ripple • Breast becomes immediately smaller if a rupture occurs

MRI, magnetic resonance imaging.

Reduction Mammoplasty

A **reduction mammoplasty** is an overnight surgical procedure in which glandular breast tissue, fat, and skin are removed bilaterally to decrease the size of large, pendulous breasts. Most candidates for a reduction mammoplasty wear a size D cup or larger brassiere and experience discomfort in the shoulders or back, skin irritation beneath the breasts, difficulty in finding suitable clothing, self-consciousness, or low self-esteem.

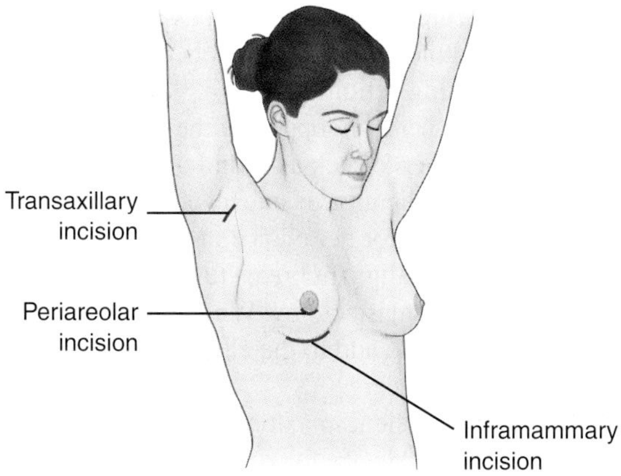

Figure 54-8 Incisional sites for placement of implants.

To reduce the size of the breasts, an incision is made around the nipple through which tissue is removed. The loose skin is tightened to reposition the areola and nipple. The client is discharged with a bulky chest dressing and sometimes a small wound drain.

Opposite Breast Reduction

The size of a reconstructed breast is limited by the amount of tissue that remains; thus, there may be potential asymmetry. Opposite breast reduction is a surgical procedure that is performed to reduce the volume of a healthy breast so that it more closely resembles the size of a reconstructed breast. The procedure, although done for different reasons, is the same as a reduction mammoplasty.

Breast Lift

Ptosis, or drooping, of the breast(s) is corrected with a breast lift or, more technically, **mastopexy**. The sagging skin and low nipple placement that accompany weight loss or aging are corrected in a procedure similar to reduction mammoplasty, although the incision and scar line are smaller and the recovery time is shorter. In some cases, the size or contour of the breast is enhanced with breast augmentation techniques.

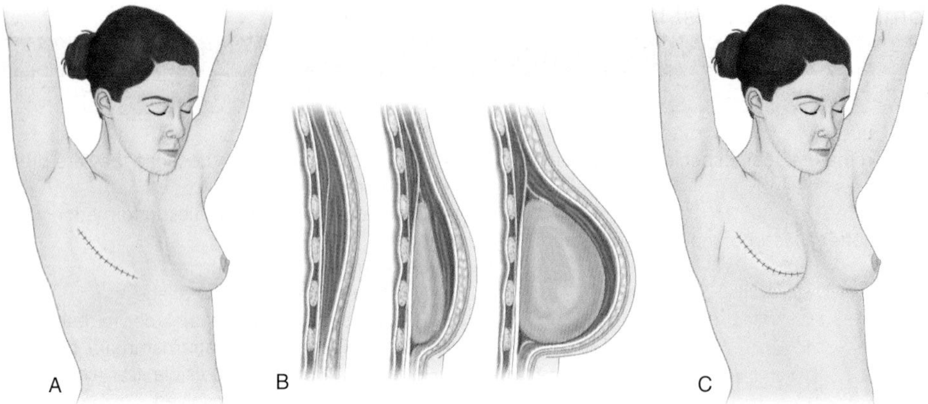

Figure 54-9 Breast reconstruction with tissue expander and artificial breast implant. **(A)** Mastectomy incision line before tissue expansion. **(B)** The expander is placed under the pectoralis muscle and is gradually filled with saline solution to stretch the skin. **(C)** The breast mound is restored. (The nipple and areola may be reconstructed later.) (Images used with permission from the American Society of Plastic Surgeons (plasticsurgery.org).)

KEY POINTS

- Infectious and inflammatory breast disorders:
  - Mastitis: inflammation of breast tissue
  - Breast abscess: localized collection of pus in breast tissue
- Benign breast lesions
  - Fibrocystic breast disease: benign, results from hormonal changes
  - Fibroadenoma: solid but benign breast mass
- Malignant breast disorders
  - Cancer of the breast
  - Treatments include: surgery, chemotherapy, radiation therapy
  - Surgery types: lumpectomy, partial or segmental mastectomy, simple or total mastectomy, subcutaneous mastectomy, modified radical mastectomy, radical mastectomy
  - Metastatic breast cancer: migration of cancer cells to other parts of the body
  - Breast cancer prevention
- Cosmetic breast procedures
  - Breast reconstruction: area of mastectomy refashioned to simulate breast, can be with autogenous tissue or implants
  - Breast augmentation: enlargement of natural, malignancy-free breasts
  - Reduction mammoplasty: reducing the size of large breast
  - Opposite breast reduction: reduces size of one breast to resemble size of the other
  - Breast lift: adjusts sagging of breast

CRITICAL THINKING EXERCISES

1. How might the signs and symptoms differ among women with fibrocystic breast disease, a fibroadenoma, and malignant breast tumor?
2. What advice is appropriate for preventing breast cancer?
3. How does sentinel lymph node mapping contribute to breast conservation?
4. What information is appropriate for a client considering breast augmentation with silicone gel implants?

NCLEX-STYLE REVIEW QUESTIONS PrepU

1. What nursing information is a correct explanation about when fibrocystic lesions usually become larger and more tender?
   1. Nearer to beginning menopause
   2. Just before menstruation
   3. After the menstrual cycle
   4. Following sexual intercourse
2. What groups of clients are at higher risk for developing breast cancer? Select all that apply.
   1. Women with a family history of breast cancer
   2. Women who are obese
   3. Women with multiple sex partners
   4. Women who consume a high-fat diet
   5. Women having had no pregnancies
   6. Women who are beyond menopause
3. A client tells the nurse that she would prefer to postpone the modified radical mastectomy recommended by her primary provider until she has more information about her treatment options. What is the most appropriate initial nursing action?
   1. Discourage her from opposing the primary provider.
   2. Encourage her to seek a second opinion.
   3. Suggest the client have an excisional biopsy.
   4. Help advocate for her choice of treatment.
4. A client with a malignant breast tumor undergoes a left modified radical mastectomy. What nursing order is most appropriate to add to the client's immediate postoperative plan for care?
   1. Maintain the client in a dorsal recumbent position.
   2. Limit oral fluid intake to no more than 2000 mL/day.
   3. Use the right arm when assessing blood pressures.
   4. Inspect the incision at least once each shift.

5. What are the current options for women at high risk for breast cancer? Select all that apply.
   1. Long-term follow-up
   2. Bilateral prophylactic mastectomy
   3. Breast cancer vaccine
   4. Chemoprotection with tamoxifen
   5. Screenings with MRI of the breast
   6. Bilateral oophorectomy to reduce estrogen

WANT TO KNOW MORE? There are a wide variety of online resources available on thePoint to enhance learning and understanding of this chapter.

Go to **thePoint.lww.com/activate** and use the activation code found in the front of this text to unlock these online resources.

55 Caring for Clients With Disorders of the Male Reproductive System

Words To Know

azoospermia
benign prostatic hyperplasia
benign prostatic hypertrophy
brachytherapy
cryotherapy
cryptorchidism
digital rectal examination
epididymitis
erectile dysfunction
hydrocele
impotence
orchiectomy
orchiopexy
orchitis
paraphimosis
phimosis
priapism
prostatectomy
prostatitis
retrograde ejaculation
spermatocele
therapeutic vaccine
torsion of the spermatic cord
varicocele
vasectomy
vasoepididymostomy
vasovasostomy

Learning Objectives

On completion of this chapter, you will be able to:

1. Give four examples of structural disorders that affect the male reproductive system.
2. Explain the technique and purpose for performing testicular self-examination.
3. List three infectious or inflammatory conditions of the male reproductive system and how they are acquired.
4. Discuss two erectile disorders and explain their effects on fertility and sexuality.
5. Identify two methods for treating erectile dysfunction.
6. Describe nursing care for a client being treated for erectile dysfunction.
7. Explain how prostatic hyperplasia compromises urinary elimination, and the symptoms it produces.
8. Discuss the nursing management of a client undergoing a prostatectomy.
9. Compare and contrast three male reproductive cancers in terms of age of onset, incidence, and treatment outcomes.
10. List homecare instructions after a vasectomy.

A variety of conditions are threats to male reproductive health. This chapter provides information about genitourinary conditions that are specific to male clients, such as congenital or acquired structural abnormalities, infectious and inflammatory conditions, erectile disorders, benign prostatic enlargement, and cancer.

Gerontologic Considerations

- Pressure from a urologic tumor may precipitate congestion of blood in the scrotum in older men with new-onset varicoceles.
- Although impotence is not a normal part of aging, its incidence increases as men age. More than half of all men 75 years of age or older are chronically impotent. Impotence may have many causes, and contributing factors should be identified. Assessment for pain, chronic comorbidities (diabetes, coronary artery disease, peripheral vascular disease, respiratory issues, arthritis, etc.), or possible side effects of medications should be a part of evaluation.

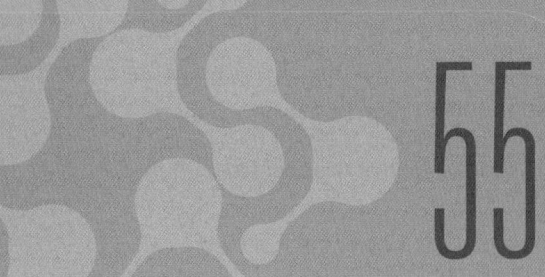

STRUCTURAL ABNORMALITIES

Structural abnormalities of the male reproductive system may be congenital or acquired. These various abnormalities, including cryptorchidism, torsion of the spermatic cord, disorders of the foreskin, and benign scrotal swelling, often require surgical repair. Nursing management after surgeries in these cases is similar.

Cryptorchidism

Cryptorchidism is a condition due to which one or both testes fail to descend into the scrotum. The undescended testis (singular) or testes (plural) may lie in the inguinal canal, in the abdominal cavity, or, rarely, in the perineum or femoral canal. The scrotum essentially is empty, but the client is asymptomatic otherwise. During childhood or at puberty, undescended testes occasionally find their way into the scrotum without treatment. At least one testis must be in the scrotum to ensure production of sperm.

The cause of undescended testes is unknown. The longer the testis remains undescended during childhood, the greater is the potential for fertility to be compromised. If the condition is not corrected by 2 years of age, the seminiferous tubules atrophy and fibrose. Treatment generally consists of surgery to secure the testis in the scrotum; the procedure is called **orchiopexy** and performed preferably between 1 and 2 years of age. If the problem remains uncorrected, the risk of testicular cancer is greater than 20% to 40% (see later discussion). When one or both testicles are permanently absent, a saline testicular prosthesis may be implanted within the scrotum to provide a normal anatomic appearance.

Nurses teach men who are at high risk for developing testicular cancer, such as those who have had cryptorchidism, to perform testicular self-examination monthly, preferably when warm, such as in the shower, to detect any abnormal mass in the scrotum (Client and Family Teaching 55-1). The American Academy of Family Physicians does not recommend routine testicular self-examinations in asymptomatic clients because the incidence of testicular cancer is rare, and there is a high survival rate even when detected at symptomatic stages (Baird et al., 2018). Men are advised to consult a primary provider if they detect a consistent, changing mass in a testis.

Client and Family Teaching 55-1
Performing Testicular Self-Examination

The nurse provides the following instructions:

1. Use both hands to palpate the testis. The normal testicle is smooth and uniform in consistency.
2. With the index and middle fingers under the testis and the thumb on top, roll the testis gently in a horizontal plane between the thumb and fingers (A).
3. Feel for any evidence of a small lump or abnormality.
4. Follow the same procedure and palpate upward along the testis (B).
5. Locate and palpate the epididymis (C), a cordlike structure on the top and back of the testicle that stores and transports sperm. Also, locate and palpate the spermatic cord.
6. Repeat the examination for the other testis, epididymis, and spermatic cord. It is normal to find that one testis is larger than the other.

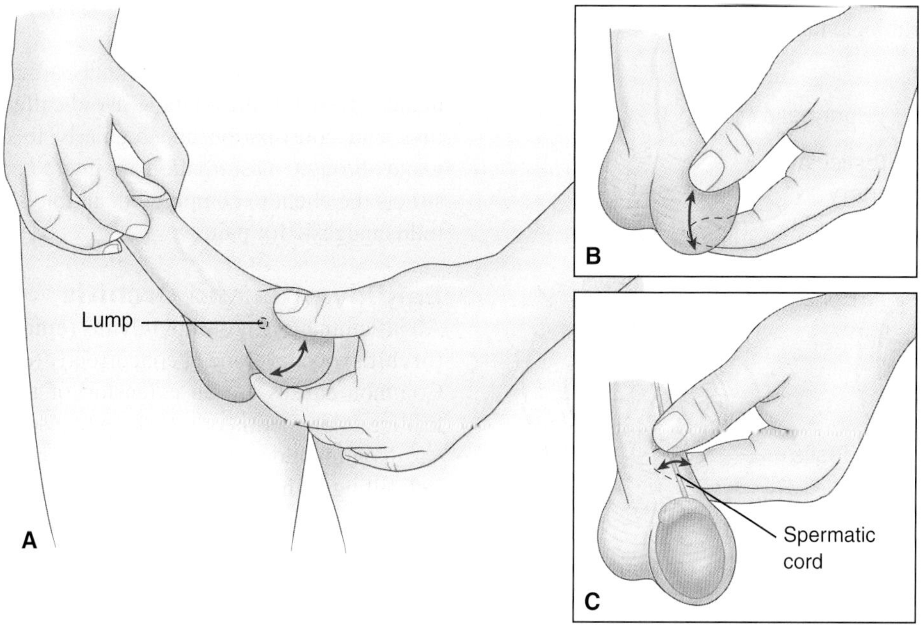

Torsion of the Spermatic Cord

Torsion means to twist. In this case, **torsion of the spermatic cord** involves rotation of the testicle that twists the spermatic cord around the testicular artery compromising blood flow to the testicle (Fig. 55-1). The condition occurs in prepubescent boys and in men whose spermatic cords are congenitally unsupported in the tunica vaginalis, the membrane surrounding the testes. Clients report a sudden, sharp testicular pain, with visible local swelling. The pain may be so severe that nausea, vomiting, chills, and fever occur. Torsion may follow intense exercise, but it also may occur during sleep or after a simple maneuver such as crossing the legs. Physical examination reveals an extremely tender testis. Elevation of the scrotum intensifies the pain by increasing the degree of twist.

Immediate surgery is necessary to prevent atrophy of the spermatic cord and preserve fertility. The torsion is reduced, excess tunica vaginalis is excised, and the testis is anchored with sutures in the scrotum. A prophylactic procedure may be performed on the opposite side.

Preoperatively, the nurse administers prescribed analgesia to relieve pain. After surgery, they apply a commercial scrotal suspensory, sometimes referred to as a jockstrap, especially when the client is out of bed. The nurse inspects the dressing for signs of drainage and gives antibiotics if medically ordered. They report any sudden onset of pain to the primary provider.

Phimosis and Paraphimosis

Phimosis and paraphimosis are conditions that occur among uncircumcised male clients, when the opening of the foreskin is constricted. **Phimosis** refers to an inability to retract the foreskin (prepuce); **paraphimosis** is a strangulation of the glans penis from an inability to replace the retracted foreskin. These phimotic conditions often are caused by a congenitally small foreskin; however, chronic inflammation at the glans penis and prepuce secondary to poor hygiene or infection are also etiologic factors.

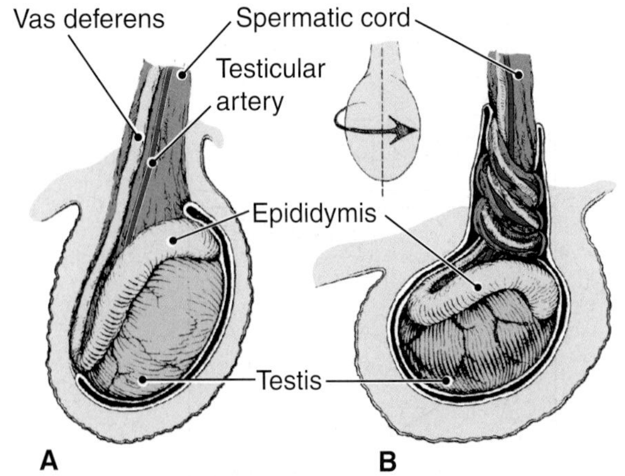

Figure 55-1 Torsion of the spermatic cord. **(A)** Normal. **(B)** Torsion. (Reprinted with permission from Cohen, B. J., & Hull, K. L. (2015). *Memmler's the human body in health and disease* (13th ed.). Wolters Kluwer.)

Clients with phimosis report pain with erection and intercourse and difficulty cleaning under the foreskin. Clients with paraphimosis experience painful swelling of the glans. If the condition continues, severe edema and urinary retention may occur. Circumcision—surgical removal of the foreskin—is recommended to relieve these conditions permanently; if surgery is not indicated, the client is instructed to wash under the foreskin daily and seek care if he cannot retract the tissue.

Hydrocele, Spermatocele, and Varicocele

The suffix *cele* means swelling. **Hydrocele**, **spermatocele**, and **varicocele** all present as a swelling of the scrotum (Fig. 55-2), but in each case the conditions are somewhat different. Often, hydrocele and spermatocele are not clinically significant and do not require treatment; however, varicoceles are thought to be an underlying cause of infertility in men and may be surgically repaired (Table 55-1).

INFECTIOUS AND INFLAMMATORY CONDITIONS

Prostatitis

Prostatitis is an inflammation of the prostate gland and is most often caused by microorganisms that reach the prostate by way of the urethra. *Escherichia coli* and microbes that cause sexually transmitted infections often are responsible (see Chapter 56), but in some instances no evidence of bacterial infection is found. Occasionally, a psychosexual problem may be the suspected cause of the client's symptoms. In any case, inflammation causes glandular swelling and tenderness. Because the prostate surrounds the urethra, a combination of genitourinary problems develops. Clients experience perineal pain or discomfort, an unusual sensation preceding or following ejaculation, low back pain, fever, chills, dysuria, and urethral discharge. Treatment consists of up to 30 days of antibiotic therapy, mild analgesics, and sitz baths.

The nurse stresses that sexual partners also need to be treated. They tell the client to avoid caffeine, prolonged sitting, and constipation and regularly to drain the prostate gland through masturbation or intercourse. The nurse instructs the client to comply with antibiotic therapy and use a mild analgesic for pain.

Epididymitis and Orchitis

An inflammation of the epididymis (**epididymitis**) and testis (**orchitis**) occurs alone or concurrently (epididymo-orchitis). Common causes are an extension of the infectious agent, leading to prostatitis or an infection elsewhere in the body.

Noninfectious epididymitis may result from long-term indwelling catheter use or genitourinary procedures such as cystoscopy or **prostatectomy** (surgical removal of the prostate). Orchitis without epididymal involvement is associated with a viral mumps infection that occurs after puberty and may result in testicular atrophy and sterility. Bilateral epididymitis frequently leads to permanent **azoospermia** (absence

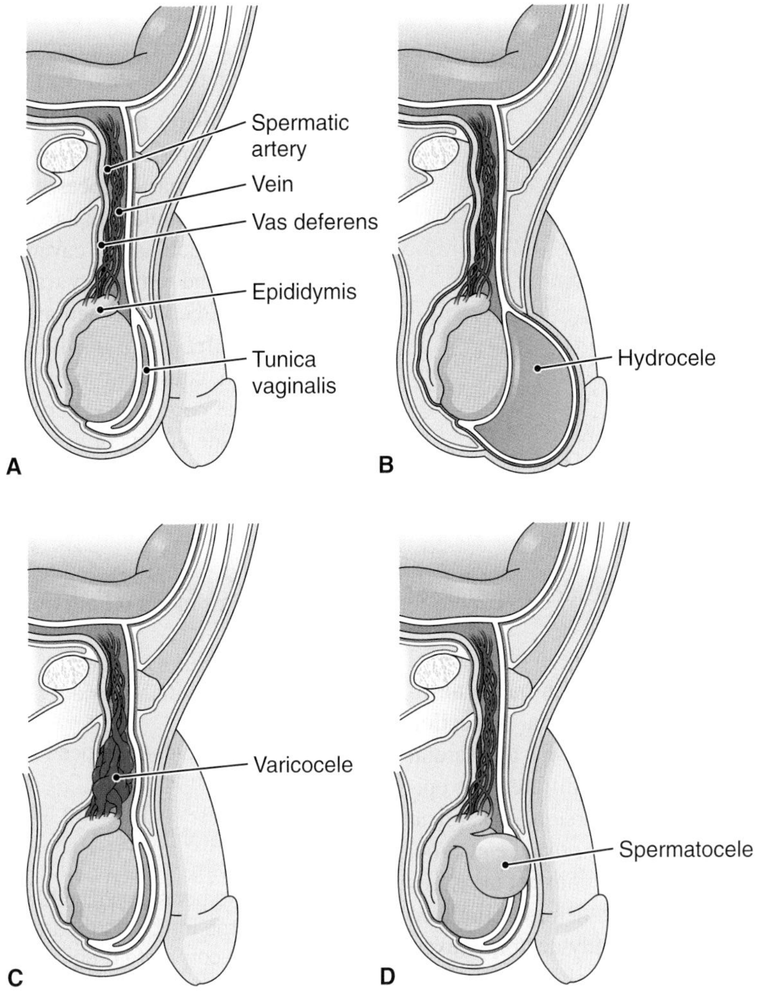

Figure 55-2 **(A)** Normal anatomy. **(B-D)** Causes of scrotal swelling: **(B)** Hydrocele is an accumulation of fluid around the testicle. **(C)** Varicocele is characterized by dilation of the veins of the spermatic cord. **(D)** Spermatocele is a self-contained cystic mass on the epididymis. (Reprinted with permission from Cohen, B. J. (2003). *Medical terminology* (4th ed.). Lippincott Williams & Wilkins.)

TABLE 55-1 Comparison of Hydrocele, Spermatocele, and Varicocele

CONDITION AND ETIOLOGY	DESCRIPTION	SIGNS AND SYMPTOMS	DIAGNOSTIC AIDS	MEDICAL AND SURGICAL MANAGEMENT
Hydrocele				
Congenital defect, injury, infection, lymph obstruction, tumor, side effect of radiation, or unknown cause	Accumulation of as much as 100 mL of lymphatic fluid between the testis and tunica vaginalis	Swollen testicle, heaviness in scrotum or lower back; may be asymptomatic; pain if testicular blood flow is impaired	Palpation, transillumination	No treatment if asymptomatic; aspiration of fluid as a temporary measure; surgical excision of fluid-filled sac; treatment of primary condition (i.e., infection)
Spermatocele				
Unknown cause	Epididymal; sperm-containing cyst	Small, freely movable mass; usually asymptomatic; may be painful if large	Palpation, transillumination	No treatment unless cyst is large and causes pain
Varicocele				
Incompetent valves in the spermatic veins	Venous dilation with damage to elastic fibers and hypertrophy of vein walls	Feeling of heaviness in scrotum; may be asymptomatic or have pain and swelling	Palpation, auscultation of venous rush, ultrasound, blood flow studies	No treatment, surgical ligation, or sclerosing

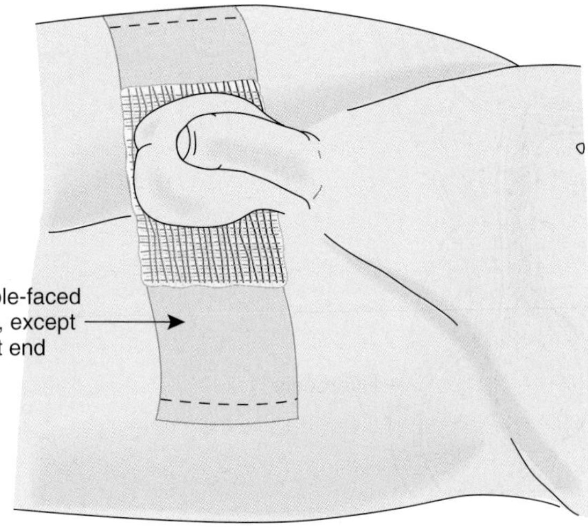

Figure 55-3 Technique of scrotal elevation.

of sperm), especially when the infection recurs frequently or becomes chronic.

The chief complaint is pain and swelling in the inguinal area and scrotum. Fever and chills occur with bacterial infections, and the urine contains pus and bacteria. Inspection reveals a markedly swollen testis and epididymis and scrotal skin that is red and tense. It is important to differentiate epididymitis from testicular torsion because torsion is a surgical emergency. Treatment consists of bed rest, scrotal elevation, analgesics, anti-inflammatory agents, and comfort measures such as local cold applications. Antibiotic therapy is initiated to eliminate the infectious agent. An epididymectomy (excision of the epididymis) is performed on clients who have recurrent, chronic, or intractable infections, but this results in sterility if it is performed bilaterally.

To relieve pain by lessening the weight of the testes, the nurse elevates the scrotum with a commercial scrotal suspensory or improvises with a folded towel, a four-tail bandage, or adhesive tape across the upper thighs (Fig. 55-3). They place an ice bag under the tender scrotum, not on top of it or leaning against it. The nurse avoids keeping the cold bag constantly next to the skin because it may damage tissue. They may use a routine such as on for 60 minutes and off for 30 minutes. As with any infection, the nurse encourages copious fluid intake.

Homecare includes instructions to continue taking prescribed antibiotics, take sitz baths, apply local heat after scrotal swelling subsides, and avoid lifting and sexual intercourse until symptoms are relieved. Nurses also advocate for infant and childhood immunizations against infectious diseases, such as mumps, to reduce potential adult complications such as orchitis.

ERECTION DISORDERS

Erectile Dysfunction

Erectile dysfunction (ED), also known as **impotence**, is (1) the inability to achieve an erection, (2) the inability to achieve an erection that is sufficiently rigid for sexual activity, or (3) the inability to sustain erection for a satisfactory period of time. There must be multiple or persistent incidences of failed erection for the disorder to be considered pathologic.

Pathophysiology and Etiology

ED may have physical and psychological origins. Erection depends on three basic processes (see Chapter 52): appropriate neurologic stimulation; adequate arterial blood flow into blood vessels such as the cavernous artery, which expands penile tissue; and temporary trapping of venous blood so as to sustain an erection. When any one or more of these processes are ineffective or insufficient, ED occurs.

Common causes of ED include neurologic disorder such as spinal cord injury, perineal trauma, testosterone insufficiency, side effects of drug therapy, atherosclerosis, hypertension, and complications of diabetes mellitus. ED may also be related to anxiety or depression.

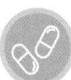

Pharmacologic Considerations

ED can be caused by a number of medications:

- Antidepressants/antianxiety agents
- Antihistamines
- Antihypertensives/diuretics
- Anti-Parkinson agents
- Cancer agents for prostate treatment
- Anticholesterol drugs
- Antiretrovirals
- Opioids and nonsteroidal anti-inflammatory pain relievers
- Proton pump inhibitors (heartburn agents)

Conduct a complete drug reconciliation when ED is mentioned, be sure to include over-the-counter and herbal supplements.

Assessment Findings

Signs and Symptoms

When discussing a sexual health history, the client reports difficulty in achieving or maintaining an erection. If an erection occurs, the client may reveal that there is insufficient rigidity for penetrating the vagina or that intercourse is less than satisfactory because penetration cannot be sustained.

Diagnostic Findings

Men typically have three to five erections while sleeping. A nocturnal penile tumescence and rigidity test can determine if the client is experiencing any spontaneous erections during sleep. The test involves applying sensors at the base and tip of the penis at bedtime for one, two, or three nights. The sensors detect the tumescence (enlargement) and firmness of the penis (Fig. 55-4). No spontaneous erections during sleep suggest a physiologic etiology for ED. Evidence of spontaneous erections during sleep but ED in a waking state suggests a psychological etiology. Test results may prove invalid, however, if the tester does not apply the sensors well or if the client sleeps restlessly.

For men who do not achieve erections using phosphodiesterase type 5 (PDE5) inhibitors like sildenafil (Viagra)

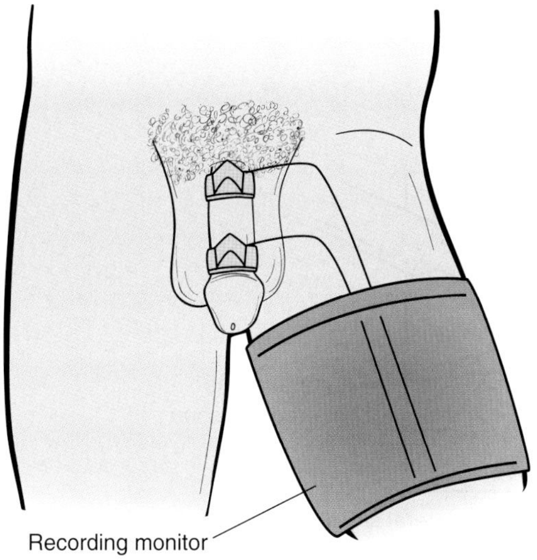

Figure 55-4 Nocturnal penile tumescence test. Sensing rings are located at the tip and base of the penis at night. The rings are attached to a monitor on the leg that records the force and duration of erections that occur during sleep.

or tadalafil (Cialis; see later discussion), vascular ultrasound studies using a Doppler may be performed. During a penile Doppler sonography, a pharmacostimulant such as alprostadil (Caverject) intracavernosal injection is given. When an erection occurs, the cavernosal artery is visualized with an ultrasonic scanner to quantify the perfusion of the penis with arterial blood. An insufficient response indicates that the ED is likely due to arterial insufficiency or a related mixed ED (Jung et al., 2018).

Medical and Surgical Management

Several approaches exist to help restore sexual function. Substituting other drugs for those that cause impotence or treating the contributing cause may restore potency (erectile ability). The American Urologic Association (2018) recommends oral PDE5 inhibitors as first-line therapy; if PDE5 therapy is unsuccessful, clients receive information about other available options for managing ED in progressive order based on invasiveness (Table 55-2).

The PDE5 inhibitors, such as sildenafil (Viagra), tadalafil (Cialis), vardenafil (Levitra, Staxyn), or avanafil

TABLE 55-2 Treatment Options for Erectile Dysfunction

TREATMENT	EFFECT	ADVANTAGES	DISADVANTAGES
Oral agents, PDE5 inhibitors avanafil (Stendra), sildenafil (Viagra, Revatio) Tadalafil (Cialis, Adcirca) Vardenafil (Levitra, Staxyn—immediate release)	Inhibition of PDE5 dilates arterial vessels in the corpus cavernosum, producing an erection	Easy to use Relatively short half-life	• Taken prior to sexual activity, unless (Cialis) daily dose is taken. • Contraindicated if taking nitrates because the combination increases the potential for hypotension. • May cause prolonged erection, hypotension, headache, flushing, dyspepsia, nasal congestion, hearing loss, sensitivity to light, altered color perception, and blurred vision.
Urethral suppository of alprostadil (Muse)	Relaxes penile muscles, promoting vascular filling	Produces an erection within 15 minutes	Less effective than penile injection route. May cause urethral burning and irritation. Hypotension and dizziness may develop during initial therapy.
Self-injection with prostaglandin E1, alprostadil (Caverject), papaverine HCl (Pavatine), or phentolamine (Regitine)	Relaxes arterial blood vessels, resulting in increased blood flow into penis	Produces an erection in 5–20 minutes Erection is sustained up to 1 1/2 hours	Discomfort at injection site. No more than 10 injections per month at equal intervals. Painful, sustained erections lasting ≥4 hours are more likely to occur with papaverine and phentolamine.
Vacuum constriction devices	Draws blood into the penis, producing an erection that is sustained with a tension band	Least expensive of treatment options Sustains erection for as long as 30 minutes Can be used daily	Some find the device cumbersome. May cause pain and decreased sensation. Obstructs ejaculation.
Surgical implantation of semirigid or inflatable penile prosthesis	Provides penile rigidity sufficient for vaginal penetration	Permanent outcome; failure rate is 2.5%	Produces less penile enlargement compared with normal erections. Requires 6 weeks to recover from surgery before sexual activity. Besides the expense of surgery, there may be surgical complications such as infection, urethral or corporal perforation, prolonged pain, and damage or malfunction, which may require additional surgery.

PDE5, phosphodiesterase type 5.

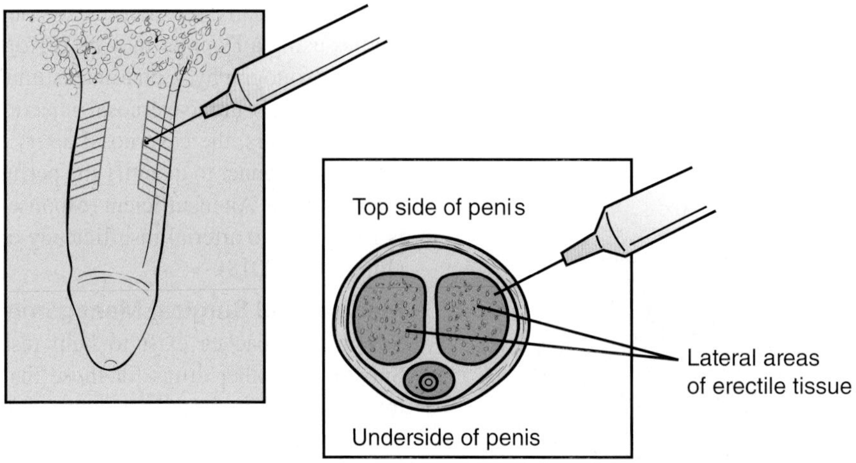

Figure 55-5 Penile injection technique. An injection site is selected on either of the lateral sides of the penis. The prescribed drug is injected into the erectile tissue at a 90-degree angle.

(Stendra), facilitate penile erection by producing smooth muscle relaxation in the corpora cavernosa, facilitating an inflow of blood. These drugs have no erectile effect without sexual stimulation. Depending on the drug, most are taken "on demand" 15 minutes, 30 minutes, or 1 hour before sexual activity. Daily dosing has been introduced in an effort to provide an alternative for on-demand nonresponders. Daily dosing is well tolerated with minimal side effects, but there is some question of whether the cost justifies its use, considering the frequency or infrequency of sexual intercourse.

Apomorphine (Uprima), a dopamine agonist, an older drug used in the treatment of Parkinson disease (see Chapter 37), is a possible alternative to phosphodiesterase inhibitors for the treatment of ED. This drug, which is administered as a nasal spray, has some advantages over sildenafil: (1) It acts within 15 to 25 minutes of administration and (2) it is safer for men with coronary artery disease.

Some clients elect to facilitate penile engorgement by self-administering a urethral suppository of alprostadil or self-injecting drugs, such as papaverine HCl (Pavatine) with phentolamine (Regitine) or alprostadil (Caverject) into the corpora cavernosa to achieve an erection (Fig. 55-5). As an alternative, they may prefer to attach a vacuum device to the penis (Fig. 55-6).

Although vascular surgery is an option for some clients, many choose a surgically implanted penile prosthesis (Fig. 55-7). One type contains a saline reservoir that is pumped to fill the implant, when sexual activity is desired; the other type maintains the penis in a semi-erect state at all times. The nurse informs the client before surgery that when a pump-type implant is inserted, the erect penis tends to be shorter than experienced in preillness erections because the cylinders do not fill the glans portion of the penis.

Nursing Management

If the client prefers to self-inject a vasodilator, the nurse provides instruction on technique, suggested frequency of injections, and side effects. If the client undergoes a penile implant, the nurse assesses for pain, swelling, bleeding, and surgical complications such as infection. The nurse

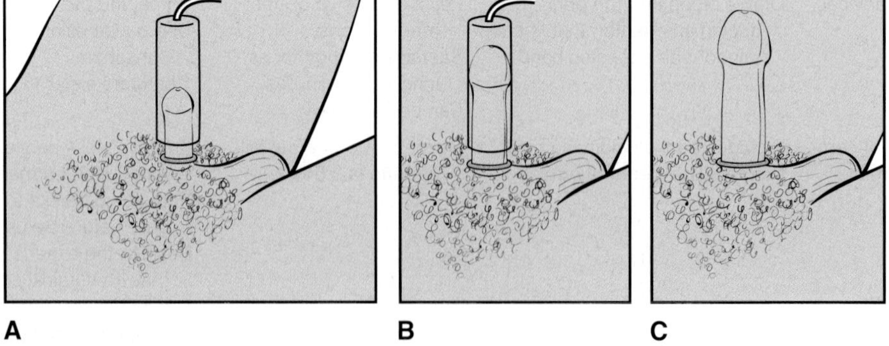

Figure 55-6 An erection is produced by **(A)** placing a vacuum device around the penis with a constricting attachment to the base of the penis. **(B)** The vacuum engorges the penis with blood. **(C)** When the vacuum device is removed, the constricting attachment prohibits the outflow of blood to sustain the erection.

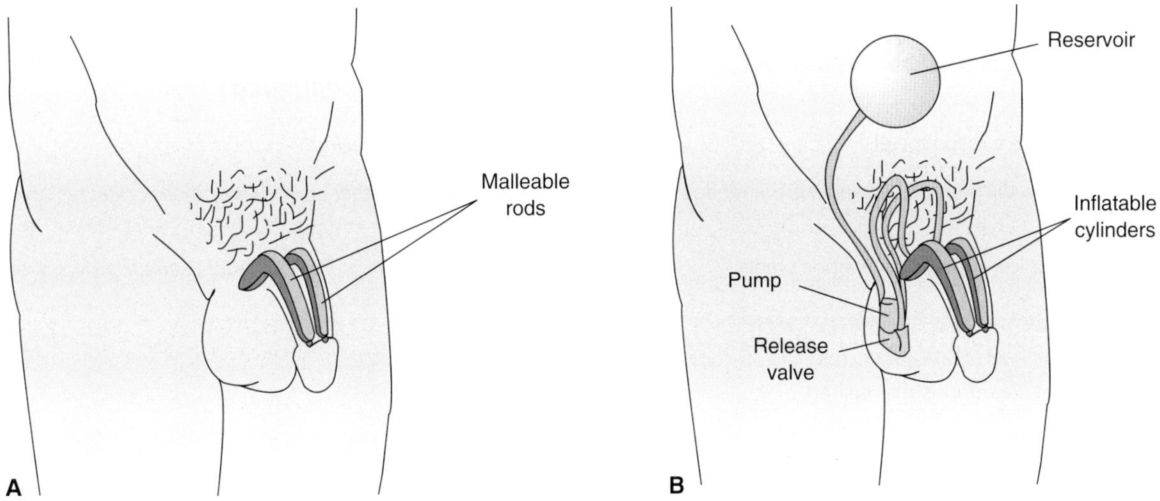

Figure 55-7 Examples of penile implants. **(A)** Semirigid. **(B)** Inflatable.

reinforces the information the primary provider identifies as possible complications after discharge, such as

- Erosion of penile or urethral tissue from a midsized implant, pressure, and friction of the implanted cylinders, which is evidenced by seeing the implant through the skin.
- Erosion of scrotal, bowel, or bladder tissue if an implant with a fluid reservoir is used, which is detected by changes in scrotal skin texture and elimination.
- Migration of the cylinders, pump, or reservoir from their intended location, which is accompanied by pain, tenderness, and dysfunction of components that are part of the device.
- Malfunction of the device characterized by underinflation, bulging of the cylinders during inflation, and loss of fluid from the implant, which can occur with migration, accidental trauma such as a fall, or aggressive or improper use of the device.

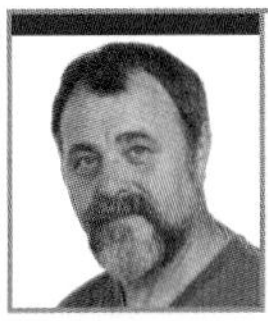

Clinical Scenario A 62-year-old man reports that he has gradual difficulty achieving an erection over the last year. The client has been a type 2 diabetic for the last 10 years and currently takes a long-acting insulin each evening. He reports that for the most part, his blood sugar levels are within near-normal ranges. The client has been on sildenafil for 6 months at gradually increasing doses, but he still feels that he is sexually inadequate, when he and his wife attempt intercourse. This has led to stress and disharmony in his marriage. The client refuses to use penile injections or a vacuum device as an alternative; he prefers to have a penile implant. **What measures should the nurse implement to ensure a safe postoperative recovery? Refer to Nursing Care Plan 55-1.**

NURSING CARE PLAN 55-1 Postoperative Management of the Client With a Penile Implant

Assessment

- Determine the level of consciousness and vital signs.
- Check the condition of dressing and incision.
- Assess the client's level of pain.
- Evaluate the amount of penile and scrotal swelling.
- Check the status of the IV infusion (type of solution, drip rate, location of IV site).
- Note the urinary catheter and volume of urine elimination.
- Assess the client's knowledge of postoperative care and discharge instructions.

Nursing Diagnosis. **Acute Pain** related to tissue injury and swelling

Expected Outcome. Pain will be eliminated or reduced to the client's level of tolerance.

Interventions	Rationales
Assess level of discomfort as needed and whenever assessing vital signs.	*An assessment of pain level is the fifth vital sign.*
Administer analgesia as prescribed.	*Clients have the right to pain relief.*

(continued)

NURSING CARE PLAN 55-1 Postoperative Management of the Client With a Penile Implant (*continued*)

Elevate genitalia with a rolled towel.	*Elevation reduces swelling.*
Apply an ice pack to the incision and replace as needed.	*Facilitating vasoconstriction with an ice pack reduces swelling and pain.*
Suspend linen over lower pelvis with a bed cradle.	*A cradle prevents pressure on painful tissue from the weight of bed linen.*

Evaluation of Expected Outcome

Pain is relieved, and comfort is maintained.

Nursing Diagnosis. **Bleeding Risk** related to inadequate hemostasis

Expected Outcome. The nurse will monitor for, manage, and minimize incisional bleeding.

Interventions	Rationales
Assess for frank bleeding or an enlarging hematoma around the incision, usually at the base of the penis where it joins the scrotum.	*A large amount of obvious blood or its collection in the skin and underlying tissue indicates significant blood loss.*
Ensure that the implant is semirigid.	*Implant rigidity provides localized pressure that reduces bleeding.*

Evaluation of Expected Outcome

Blood loss is minimal, and swelling of the genitalia remains within acceptable limits.

Nursing Diagnosis. **Urinary Retention** related to urethral compression

Expected Outcome. Client will void without difficulty and empty his bladder with each voiding.

Interventions	Rationales
Monitor frequency and amount of each voiding.	*Urinary retention is evidenced by the absence of voiding or voiding small, frequent amounts.*
Palpate the lower abdomen.	*The bladder is palpable when it is distended with urine.*
Report an inability to void or lack of sufficient quantity per voiding.	*Catheterization may be required to empty the bladder, or the primary provider may choose to order a medication to induce voiding.*

Evaluation of Expected Outcome

Client voids in sufficient quantities; the bladder remains nonpalpable.

Nursing Diagnosis. **Altered Skin Integrity Risk** related to dermal deterioration secondary to a tight prosthesis

Expected Outcome. Skin in the operative area will remain supple and intact.

Interventions	Rationales
Look for pale, thin skin near the glans penis.	*The prosthesis occupies space, stretches the skin, and reduces the diameter of blood vessels.*
Report signs of inadequate capillary perfusion and skin erosion.	*Prolonged interruption of blood flow causes tissue necrosis.*

Evaluation of Expected Outcome

Skin in the operative area remains supple and intact.

Nursing Diagnosis. **Situational Low Self-Esteem** related to possible spectator curiosity concerning the outcome of the surgical procedure

Expected Outcome. Client retains positive self-esteem.

NURSING CARE PLAN 55-1 Postoperative Management of the Client With a Penile Implant (*continued*)

Interventions	Rationales
Explain the purpose for genital inspection.	*Genital inspection is performed for the purpose of assessing local tissue response rather than satisfying curiosity.*
Provide privacy and draping during genital assessments.	*The client has the right to privacy and to be treated with dignity.*
Avoid unprofessional comments about the client's reasons for or outcome of surgery.	*The client's decision for elective surgery is private and personal.*
Provide opportunities for the client to privately share his feelings about his changed appearance.	*Clients are more likely to openly discuss their feelings, when they feel secure that others will not overhear the conversation.*
Describe techniques for concealing the semi-erect appearance of the penis, such as wearing untucked shirts and pleated trousers or pants with an elastic waist.	*Disguising the state of semi-erection decreases self-consciousness in social situations.*

Evaluation of Expected Outcome

Client's self-esteem is undisturbed.

Nursing Diagnosis. **Knowledge Deficiency** related to desire to obtain information about the postoperative course after discharge

Expected Outcome. Client will relate techniques that promote healing and prevent complications during the recovery process.

Interventions	Rationales
Explain that the penis should be taped against the skin in a straight position for 1 week or longer, but can be untaped for voiding.	*Taping acts as a splint to keep the penis from moving about while healing takes place.*
Identify the period for sexual abstinence (usually 3 to 6 weeks).	*Sexual intercourse is safe once healing is complete.*
Instruct on how to inflate and deflate an inflatable prosthesis.	*An erect penis facilitates vaginal penetration; the client empties the penile implant after intercourse.*
Inform client to avoid tight-fitting underwear.	*Pressure and friction can cause tissue erosion and curvature of the penis.*
Advise client to avoid contact sports.	*The force of physical contact may alter the position or integrity of the penile implant.*
Explain that the client must avoid heavy lifting for at least 3 weeks.	*Straining can disrupt internal sutures and reconstructed tissue.*
Emphasize the need to report persistent pain and swelling.	*Pain and swelling are common signs of infection, erosion, and migration.*

Evaluation of Expected Outcome

Client can verbalize discharge instructions and receives written information to which he can refer for self-care at home.

Priapism

Priapism is a condition in which the penis becomes engorged and remains persistently erect without any sexual stimulation. The underlying etiology is usually a vascular problem, a medical condition that causes blood to thicken, or a side effect of medications, including those prescribed to treat ED. The engorged penis produces significant discomfort and interferes with arterial blood flow and, in some cases, urinary elimination. If the erection lasts longer than 6 hours, the tissue may be sufficiently damaged to result in impotence.

Treatment options include administering vasoconstrictive medications such as terbutaline (Brethine) or phenylephrine (Neo-Synephrine) or draining the trapped blood with a needle placed in the side of the penis. If these interventions fail, emergency surgery is performed to shunt blood temporarily out of the corpora cavernosa. Health care providers must extend respect for the client's feelings and understandable embarrassment throughout interactions.

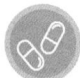

Pharmacologic Considerations

- Pseudoephedrine immediate release (Sudafed) 120 mg orally is the antidote for erections lasting more than 2 hours. Men should be instructed to have this medication on hand while using drugs for ED. Health care providers should be contacted when an erection lasts for 3 hours or the pseudoephedrine does not work after 1 hour.

BENIGN PROSTATIC HYPERPLASIA

When the number of cells in a structure increases, the condition is referred to as *hyperplasia*. If the cells are nonmalignant, it is called *benign hyperplasia*. Thus, **benign prostatic hyperplasia** (BPH) indicates that the prostate gland contains more than the usual number of normal cells. When the gland enlarges, the condition is known as **benign prostatic hypertrophy**.

Pathophysiology and Etiology

BPH occurs as men age. The outward expansion of the gland is of no clinical importance. Inward encroachment, however, diminishes the diameter of the prostatic section of the urethra and interferes with emptying the bladder (Fig. 55-8).

Assessment Findings

Signs and Symptoms

The symptoms of BPH appear gradually. At first, the client notices that it takes more effort to void. Eventually, the urinary stream narrows and has decreased force. The bladder empties incompletely. Because residual urine accumulates, the client has an urge to void more often and nocturia occurs. Because residual urine is a good culture medium for bacteria, symptoms of cystitis (inflammation of the bladder) may develop (see Chapter 59).

Diagnostic Findings

A **digital rectal examination** (DRE), the palpation of the prostate gland through the rectum, reveals an enlarged and elastic gland (Fig. 55-9). Cystoscopy exposes the extent of the infringement on the urethra and the effects on the bladder. Intravenous (IV) and retrograde pyelograms and blood chemistry tests give information about possible damage to the upper urinary tract from urinary retention. Measurement of a significant quantity of residual urine adds to the data that confirm the diagnosis. The prostate-specific antigen (PSA) test results may be slightly elevated. Transrectal ultrasonography indicates prostatic size and helps rule out the possibility that a malignancy is causing the enlargement.

Medical and Surgical Management

In the early stages of BPH, the progression of prostatic enlargement is monitored with periodic DREs. Drug therapy is the second line of treatment (Drug Therapy Table 55-1).

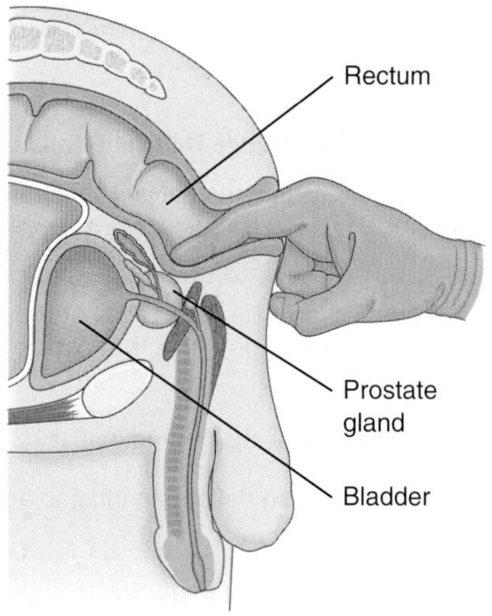

Figure 55-9 A digital rectal examination is a method for assessing the size and texture of the prostate gland. Normally, the prostate gland feels smooth and the size of a walnut. Prostate enlargement, hardness, irregular contour, and tenderness indicate a need for further assessment.

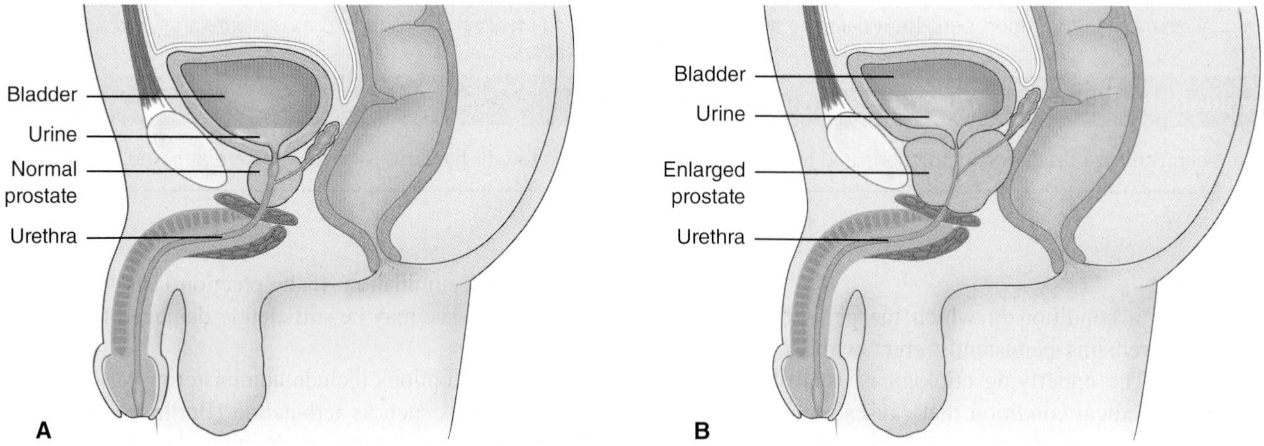

Figure 55-8 Comparison of normal prostate and enlarged prostate. **(A)** Normal prostate gland allows free flow of urine from the bladder to the urethra. **(B)** An enlarged prostate gland compresses the urethra, forcing urine to be retained in the bladder.

DRUG THERAPY TABLE 55-1 Agents for BPH

Category and Common Generic (Brand) Drugs	Intended Use	Common Side Effects	Safety Warnings for Nurses
Alpha-Adrenergic Blockers (Peripherally Acting Anti-Adrenergics)			
Alfuzosin (Uroxatral) Doxazosin (Cardura) Silodosin (Rapaflo) Tamsulosin (Flomax) Terazosin (Hytrin)	Reduces the tone of smooth muscle in the bladder neck and prostatic urethra, used for hypertensive therapy also	Headache, dizziness, ejaculatory dysfunction, diarrhea, and rhinitis	• Reduce orthostatic hypotension by taking at bedtime • Symptoms worsen when medication stopped suddenly
Androgen Hormone Inhibitors			
Dutasteride (Avodart) Finasteride (Propecia, Proscar)	Inhibits the conversion of testosterone into androgen, causing the prostate gland to shrink	Impotence, decreased libido, asthenia, dizziness, and postural hypotension	Teratogenic, may pass in blood, men should not donate blood for 6 months after discontinuing drug Teratogenic, pills should not be handled by women without gloves
Miscellaneous Agents			
Dutasteride/tamsulosin (Jalyn)	See separate drug class categories above		
Tadalafil (Cialis only)	Tadalafil increases the level of cyclic guanosine monophosphate, which relaxes smooth muscle in the bladder and prostate as well as increasing blood flow to the penis. Orally, 5 mg daily is used to treat both ED and BPH.		

The drugs in column 1 indicate the drug that matches up with explanations in columns 2 through 4.
BPH, benign prostatic hyperplasia; ED, erectile dysfunction.

Terazosin (Hytrin) or other alpha-adrenergic blockers help relax the muscles in the prostate and relieve urinary symptoms. Finasteride (Proscar, Propecia) and similar drugs that are androgen hormone inhibitors (also classified as 5-alpha reductase inhibitors) can be used to decrease symptoms and also appear to arrest the progression of prostate enlargement in some clients. Combination therapy with an alpha-adrenergic blocker, such as doxazosin and finasteride, is another option. Side effects with both drugs can occur (see Drug Therapy Table 55-1).

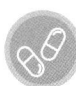

Pharmacologic Considerations

■ Dutasteride (Avodart) may pass in the blood; therefore, clients should not donate blood while taking and up to 6 months after discontinuing the drug. This is to prevent the possibility of a pregnant woman receiving the drug in a transfusion and harming the fetus.

Some men have found that taking *saw palmetto*, an herbal substance from the fruit of the palm tree, or *Pygeum africanum*, an herb extracted from the bark of an African evergreen, relieves the symptoms of BPH. Saw palmetto interferes with the enzyme that converts testosterone to dihydrotestosterone. When dihydrotestosterone is inhibited, the stimulus for growth of the prostate gland is reduced. This herb may also inhibit cyclooxygenase, an enzyme that plays a role in inflammation, which may explain the manner in which the symptoms of prostatitis are relieved (Saper, 2016). *P. africanum* probably reduces inflammation and removes cholesterol deposits within the prostate gland (Deters, 2015). Before self-administering any substance that is considered alternative therapy, clients should discuss the matter with their primary provider.

Other forms of treatment are used when glandular enlargement results in pronounced symptoms. The aim of all surgical prostatectomy procedures for BPH is to enlarge the bladder outlet by removing a portion or all of the prostate gland using an open, laparoscopic, or robotic-assisted approach (Table 55-3). Surgeries performed through the urethra include transcystoscopic urethroplasty, transurethral resection of the prostate (TURP), transurethral incision of the prostate (TUIP), transurethral laser incision of the prostate (TULIP), and transurethral needle ablation (TUNA). Operations performed through an external incision include suprapubic, retroperitoneal, or perineal prostatectomy (Fig. 55-10). In almost all cases, a continuous bladder irrigation is ordered after TURP to remove blood clots and residual tissue.

After a TURP, between 66% and 75% of clients experience **retrograde ejaculation**, a condition in which the semen is deposited in the bladder rather than discharging through the urethra at the time of orgasm, rendering the

TABLE 55-3 Procedures for Prostatic Enlargement

PROCEDURE	DESCRIPTION
Transurethral Approaches	
Transcystoscopic urethroplasty	The balloon tip of a catheter is inflated for 10–20 minutes to stretch the prostatic urethra.
Urethral stent or coils	A flexible tube is permanently placed in the urethra to dilate the lumen.
Thermotherapy	A heated instrument inserted in a urethral catheter destroys prostatic tissue but preserves the urethra.
TURP	Part of the prostate is removed with a cutting instrument inserted through an endoscope.
TUIP	No tissue is removed; the bladder outlet is enlarged by making an incision in the prostate, which relieves pressure on the urethra.
TULIP	A laser is used to incise and destroy prostate tissue.
TUNA	Needles within the prostate deliver low-level radiofrequency energy to remove excess tissue.
Open Surgical Approaches	
Suprapubic prostatectomy	The prostate gland is removed by making a midline abdominal incision into the bladder. A suprapubic catheter and a Foley catheter are inserted.
Retropubic prostatectomy	The prostate gland is removed through an abdominal incision, but the bladder is not entered.
Open radical prostatectomy	The prostate gland is removed through a long incision made either in the abdomen or between the scrotum and anus. The prostate gland and its capsule, seminal vesicles, and lymph nodes are removed. This procedure is reserved for clients with prostatic cancer.
Laparoscopic radical prostatectomy	A minimally invasive procedure in which the surgeon uses magnified visualization of the prostate gland and surrounding structures through small abdominal incisions. Poses technical difficulty for the surgeon.
Robotic-assisted laparoscopic radical prostatectomy	A minimally invasive procedure in which the surgeon remains distant from the operative field and removes the prostate gland using 10 times the magnification on a video monitor and robotic arms inserted through small keyhole-size incisions in the abdomen.

TUIP, transurethral incision of the prostate; TULIP, transurethral laser incision of the prostate; TUNA, transurethral needle ablation; TURP, transurethral resection of the prostate.

client sterile. After a TURP and open prostatectomies, clients may have temporary or permanent urinary incontinence, depending on the procedure used and the surgeon's technical skill. Perineal surgical approaches often result in permanent ED, although some nerve-sparing techniques are being performed.

Nursing Management

For the client who is not yet a candidate for surgery, the nurse teaches how to maintain optimal bladder emptying (Client and Family Teaching 55-2).

The surgical client requires support and information to allay anxiety and promote a postoperative period that is free of complications. The nurse teaches deep-breathing and leg exercises and explains that the client will have continuous bladder irrigation for at least 24 hours after surgery.

Urethral catheterization before surgery is necessary for clients with sudden or acute retention. If difficulty is encountered while inserting a urethral catheter, a coude catheter, which has a curved tip, and instillable anesthetic lubricant are used to facilitate the procedure. If the catheter cannot be passed urethrally, a temporary suprapubic catheter, also called a cystostomy tube, is required to relieve bladder distention. See Nursing Care Plan 55-2 for caring for a client undergoing a prostatectomy and Nursing Guidelines 55-1 for the care of a client with a suprapubic catheter.

Client and Family Teaching 55-2
Maintaining Optimal Bladder Function

The nurse instructs the client as follows:

- Void often and assist bladder emptying by leaning forward on toilet and "bearing down" (Valsalva maneuver), or pressing down on the bladder while seated on the toilet (Credé maneuver).
- Drink frequent small volumes of oral fluids so that the bladder does not become extremely full at any one time.
- Limit alcohol and caffeine, which increase the urgency to urinate.
- Limit the use of cough, cold, or allergy medications containing decongestants, which can interfere with urination.
- Note any signs and symptoms of acute urinary obstruction and urinary infection such as distended bladder, lower abdominal discomfort, inability to urinate, small and frequent urination, fever and chills, and flank pain that indicate a need for medical attention.

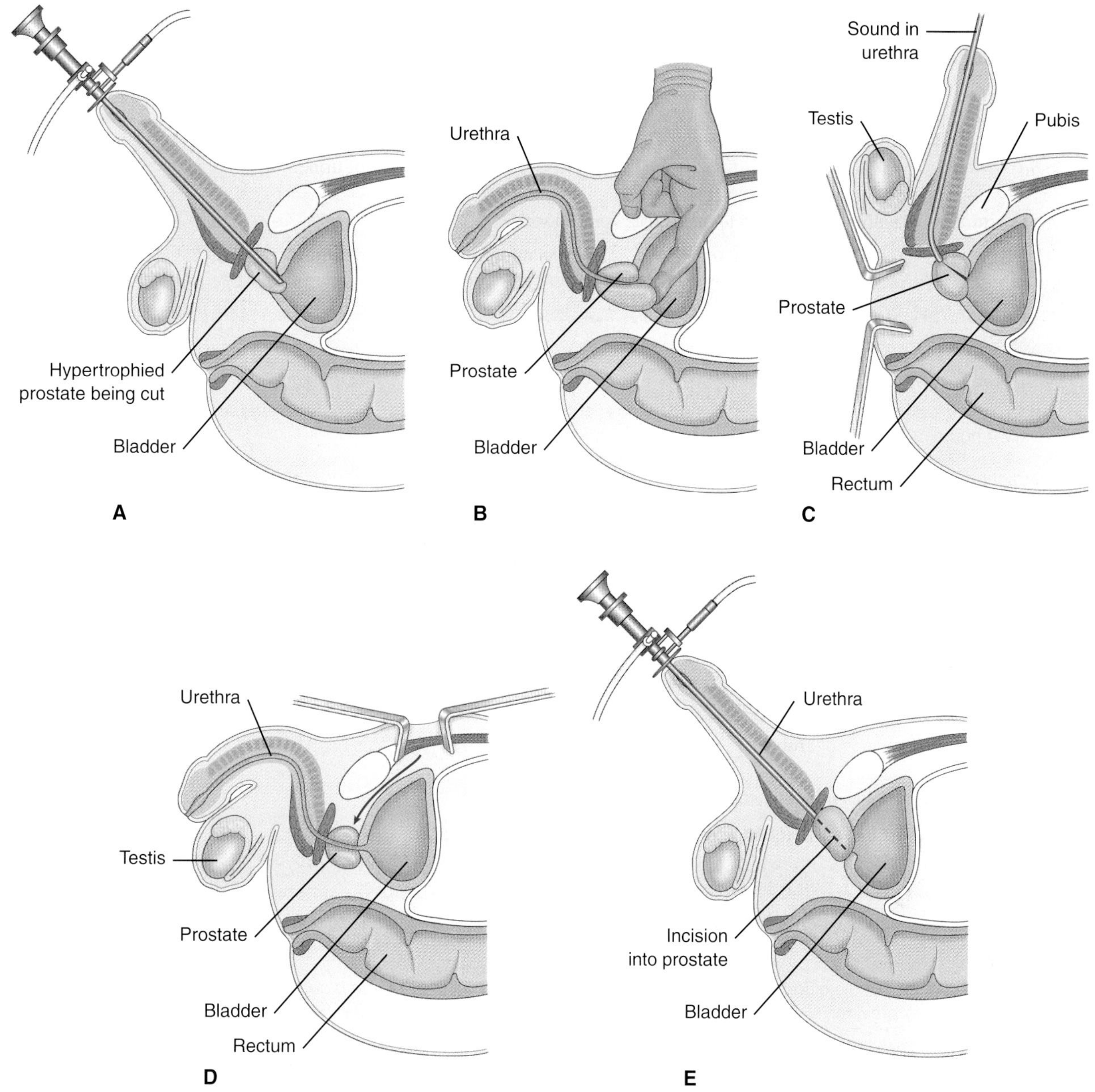

Figure 55-10 Examples of prostate surgery techniques. **(A)** Transurethral resection of the prostate (TURP). **(B)** Suprapubic prostatectomy. **(C)** Perineal prostatectomy. **(D)** Retropubic prostatectomy. **(E)** Transurethral incision of the prostate (TUIP).

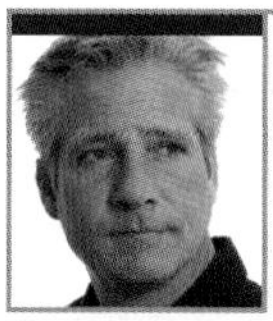

Clinical Scenario A 62-year-old man has been undergoing medical treatment with an androgen inhibitor for an enlarged prostate gland, but he has had a poor response. He is unhappy that the drug has caused occasional impotence. He continues to feel that his bladder is full, which leads to frequent efforts to urinate. During attempts to void, he has difficulty initiating urination without straining and pushing on his lower abdomen. After discussing other methods for reducing the size of his prostate with his primary provider, the client will have his prostate gland surgically removed. When the client returns from surgery, what nursing actions are appropriate when managing his care? See Nursing Care Plan.

NURSING CARE PLAN 55-2 The Client Undergoing a Prostatectomy

Assessment

Determine the following after surgery:

- Level of consciousness
- Vital signs
- Level of discomfort
- Location of urinary catheter(s)
- Volume and color of urine

Nursing Diagnosis. **Bleeding Risk** related to inadequate hemostasis

Expected Outcome. The nurse will monitor to detect, manage, and minimize excessive bleeding.

Interventions	Rationales
Monitor vital signs every 15 minutes until stable and then every 4 hours.	*Hypotension and tachycardia suggest a loss of blood volume.*
Assess color of urine and status of dressing, if there is one, at least every 4 hours.	*A change from burgundy to bright red, like catsup, suggests fresh bleeding.*
Maintain traction on the urinary catheter for at least 6 hours after surgery.	*Traction provides pressure on blood vessels, which facilitates hemostasis.*
Discourage straining to have a bowel movement, attempts to void with the catheter in place, and lifting heavy objects.	*Bearing down increases blood pressure, which can trigger fresh bleeding.*
Report signs of hypovolemic shock to the primary provider.	*The primary provider determines the medical measures such as administering blood transfusions and medications for stabilizing the client's condition.*

Evaluation of Expected Outcome

Client's urine is light pink, clear, or amber.

Nursing Diagnosis. **Hypovolemia** related to postoperative bleeding

Expected Outcome. The nurse will monitor to detect, manage, and minimize anemia.

Interventions	Rationales
Monitor laboratory test results when a complete blood count is performed.	*Low erythrocyte, hemoglobin, and hematocrit results indicate that the client may require the replacement of blood.*
Assist with administering whole blood or packed cells as prescribed by the primary provider.	*Transfusions of whole blood or packed cells replace depleted cells and intravascular fluid volume faster than the bone marrow can reproduce erythrocytes.*

Evaluation of Expected Outcome

Client's hemoglobin is at least 10 g/dL.

Nursing Diagnosis. **Urinary Retention** related to obstruction of urinary catheter with tissue debris and blood clots or urethral stricture

Expected Outcome. Catheter will remain patent.

Interventions	Rationales
Instill bladder irrigation solution at a rate to maintain light pink or clear urine (Fig. 55-11).	*Irrigating solution dilutes blood cells and tissue debris and facilitates removal from the bladder by gravity drainage.*
Encourage client to drink about one glass of water every hour while awake.	*A generous fluid intake keeps the urine dilute and the catheter patent.*
Palpate bladder and assess true urine volume every 4 hours whenever client complains of pain or if urine leaks around catheter.	*The bladder is not palpable unless distended.* *Interference with gravity drainage results in urine accumulation in the bladder.*
Avoid dependent loops and kinks in urinary catheter, never clamp urinary catheter, and do not allow client to lie on the drainage tubing.	*True urine volume is assessed by subtracting the volume of irrigating solution from the total urinary output. Pain and leaking fluid suggest accumulated urine with no appropriate outlet.*

NURSING CARE PLAN 55-2 The Client Undergoing a Prostatectomy (*continued*)

Keep drainage bag below the level of the bladder.	*Fluid (urine in this case) flows by gravity from higher to lower locations. If the urinary drainage bag is above the bladder, urine flows backward into the bladder.*

Evaluation and Expected Outcome

Urine drains freely from the catheter or with spontaneous voiding.

Nursing Diagnosis. **Electrolyte Imbalance Risk** related to absorption of bladder irrigation solution

Expected Outcome. The nurse will monitor to detect, manage, and minimize hyponatremia.

Interventions	Rationales
Analyze if there is a realistic relationship between the amount of instilled irrigation solution and the drainage volume.	*A deficit in irrigation volume suggests systemic absorption of a portion of the full amount.*
Monitor and report if client develops weakness, muscle cramps, nausea, vomiting, confusion, seizures, or elevated blood pressure.	*Hyponatremia is manifested in physical signs and symptoms, and serum sodium <135 mEq/L.*
Slow or interrupt the bladder irrigation if you suspect hyponatremia or fluid excess; report assessment data to the primary provider.	*The nurse collaborates with the primary provider when the management of the client's problems involves medical interventions.*

Evaluation of Expected Outcome

Client's serum sodium level is 135–145 mEq/L.

Nursing Diagnosis. **Acute Pain** related to tissue injury or bladder spasms

Expected Outcome. Pain will be controlled within the client's level of tolerance.

Interventions	Rationales
Check that catheter is patent and draining before administering medication.	*Obstruction in the flow of urine contributes to pain.*
Administer a prescribed antispasmodic, such as a belladonna and opium suppository, or prescribed medications such as oxybutynin (Ditropan) or propantheline (Pro-Banthine), or an analgesic for incisional pain.	*Anticholinergics relieve bladder spasms. Analgesics interfere with the perception of pain.*
Explain that the large balloon holding the catheter in place, traction on the catheter, and the volume of instilling irrigant tend to produce the urge to void, but an effort to do so contributes to discomfort.	*Offering the client an explanation helps alleviate the anxiety concerning the cause of discomfort.*
Use nursing measures such as placing a rolled towel beneath the scrotum, assisting with the application of an athletic support, suggesting the use of a recliner rather than sitting on a hard surface, changing position, and diversional activities.	*Alternative measures enhance the response to drug therapy.*

Evaluation of Expected Outcome

Pain and discomfort are tolerable.

Nursing Diagnosis. **Infection Risk** related to impaired tissue and potential contamination of catheters and incisional drains

Expected Outcome. Client will be free of infection as evidenced by progressive wound healing, no fever, no purulent drainage, expected white blood cell count, and urine free of bacteria.

Interventions	Rationales
Practice conscientious hand hygiene before providing nursing care.	*Hand hygiene is the single most important method to reduce the potential for spreading microorganisms.*

(continued)

NURSING CARE PLAN 55-2 The Client Undergoing a Prostatectomy (*continued*)

Keep ports used for emptying drainage clean.	*A contaminated port provides a portal for microorganisms that can ascend to other structures in the urinary tract.*
Reinforce or change moist dressings using surgical asepsis.	*Moisture on a dressing wicks microorganisms into the wound.*
Keep perineum clean after a bowel movement for clients with a perineal prostatectomy.	*Stool contains many bacteria that can easily enter a perineal wound because of its close proximity to the anus.*
Report tenderness, unusual drainage, foul odor, and fever.	*An infection produces a cluster of common signs and symptoms.*

Evaluation of Expected Outcome

There is no evidence of infection; vital signs are normal.

Nursing Diagnosis. **Altered Skin Integrity Risk** related to leaking urine from suprapubic catheter

Expected Outcome. Skin will remain free of redness and excoriation around the catheter site.

Interventions	Rationales
Clean skin around suprapubic catheter with mild soap and water; dry skin thoroughly (Nursing Guidelines 55-1).	*Wet skin causes maceration of tissue. Strong soaps can irritate the skin.*
Apply and change drain gauze around suprapubic catheter because it becomes moist.	*A drain gauze absorbs moisture.*
Enclose the suprapubic catheter in an ostomy appliance.	*Ostomy equipment can be used as a means to collect urine and prevent contact between the skin and the urine.*
Consult an enterostomal therapist on substances such as karaya that can be applied to the skin.	*Karaya provides a moisture-resistant barrier and protects the skin.*

Evaluation of Expected Outcome

Skin remains intact or the wound heals normally.

Nursing Diagnosis. **Reflex Urinary Incontinence** related to altered urinary sphincter or nerve damage secondary to surgical procedure if nerves have not been spared

Expected Outcome. Client will learn methods to disguise incontinence or regain continence.

Interventions	Rationales
Suggest wearing absorbent pads or underwear.	*Absorbing urine reduces embarrassment associated with incontinence.*
Teach pelvic floor–strengthening exercises (Client and Family Teaching 55-3).	*Pelvic floor exercises strengthen the muscles that promote urinary continence.*
Suggest using a penile clamp, which is molded to comfortably fit around the shaft of the penis.	*A penile clamp compresses the urethra externally, preventing incontinence.*

Evaluation of Expected Outcome

Continence problems are controlled.

Nursing Diagnosis. **Sexual Dysfunction** related to structural changes secondary to surgical procedure

Expected Outcome. Sexual activity will be satisfactory.

Interventions	Rationales
Provide information on support groups.	*Others who have experienced sexual dysfunction after prostatectomy may be both supportive and influential in solving sexual problems.*
Clarify information concerning potential sexual consequences of the specific surgical procedure.	*Sexual problems may be temporary or permanent depending on the type of prostatectomy that is performed.*

NURSING CARE PLAN 55-2 The Client Undergoing a Prostatectomy (*continued*)

Evaluation of Expected Outcome

Client resumes sexual activity, when appropriate, or adapts to sexual changes.

Nursing Diagnosis. Altered Health Maintenance related to lack of knowledge about care after discharge

Expected Outcome. Client will refer to written instructions that correlate with drug teaching, wound and catheter care, and medical follow-up.

Interventions	Rationales
Emphasize ongoing medical care.	*Medical follow-up ensures progressive recovery and monitoring for developing complications.*
Advise client to avoid self-administering aspirin.	*Aspirin interferes with platelet aggregation, which promotes bleeding.*
Explain drug action, frequency of drug administration, and side effects of medications that will be taken after discharge.	*Knowledge about discharge medications promotes compliance and safe use of prescribed drugs.*
Demonstrate and have client return demonstration for catheter and wound care.	*Appropriate catheter and wound care reduce the potential for infection.*
Identify when client can resume activity, including sexual intercourse.	*Physical exertion increases the potential for bleeding.*
Suggest consuming 10–12 glasses of oral fluid each day, increasing dietary fiber, or using a mild laxative or stool softener.	*Preventing constipation decreases the potential for bleeding if effort is required to eliminate stool.*
Instruct client to immediately report pain in the pelvis or perineum, cloudy or bloody urine that persists despite drinking fluids, or fever or chills.	*Unusual signs and symptoms indicate the possibility of a developing complication.*

Evaluation of Expected Outcome

Client demonstrates an understanding of perineal exercises, medication schedule, activities to avoid, when to contact primary provider, and wound care.

NURSING GUIDELINES 55-1

Managing the Care of a Client With a Suprapubic Catheter*

Purpose: To drain urine from the bladder through a catheter that is inserted through the anterior abdominal wall and anchored with external skin sutures. The client may or may not have a urethral (Foley) catheter as well.

- Stabilize the catheter by taping it to the skin of the abdomen.
- Keep the catheter connected to a sterile drainage system.
- Keep the drainage system below the level of the insertion site.
- Empty the urine from the bag periodically to reduce tension on the catheter and skin.
- Record the urine output from the suprapubic catheter separate from voided urine output or output from another catheter.
- Keep the skin clean and dry at the insertion site to avoid skin irritation and compromised skin integrity.
- For "trial voiding":
  - Clamp the catheter for 4 hours.
  - Have the client void naturally.
  - Unclamp the suprapubic catheter.
  - Measure the residual urine.
- Collaborate with the primary provider on removing the suprapubic catheter, when the residual urine is repeatedly <100 mL.
- To remove the catheter:
  - Offer an analgesic 30 minutes before proceeding.
  - Wash hands and put on gloves.
  - Empty the urinary drainage container and record amount.
  - Position the client on his back.
  - Free the tape from the skin.
  - Remove gloves and rewash hands.
  - Open a suture removal kit.
  - Put on sterile gloves.
  - Remove the skin sutures.
  - Pull gently on the catheter until it is free.
  - Place a sterile dressing over the insertion site.
  - Remove gloves and wash hands.
- Change the dressing when it becomes moist until the site heals in approximately 2 days.

*A suprapubic catheter may also be called a *cystostomy tube*.

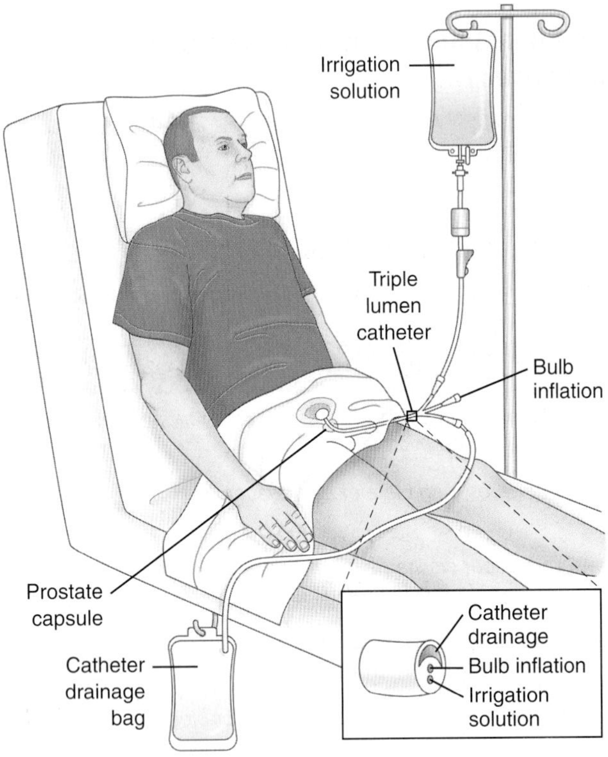

Figure 55-11 A three-way system for bladder irrigation.

Client and Family Teaching 55-3 Performing Pelvic Floor–Strengthening Exercises

The nurse emphasizes the following points when teaching the client:

- Squeeze the pelvic floor muscles (those used to stop urination and hold back a bowel movement) for up to 10 seconds—longer is not better.
- Relax completely for 10 seconds—less is not better.
- Repeat sequence as many times as possible in 5 minutes or a cycle of 15 contractions followed by relaxation.
- Interrupt exercises when muscles can no longer be contracted tightly.
- Perform exercises in the morning and evening.
- Perform shorter pelvic floor exercises four or five times during the day:
- Squeeze pelvic floor muscles and hold for 1 second.
- Relax for 1 second.
- Repeat five times in succession within 2 minutes.
- Continue long and short exercises for 3 to 4 months or until continent.

MALIGNANCIES OF THE MALE REPRODUCTIVE SYSTEM

Cancer of the Prostate

Prostate cancer is second to skin cancer in frequency among American men. It ranks second after lung cancer as the cause of deaths from cancer for men. The incidence is higher in African Americans and men with a father or brother diagnosed with the disease at a young age. About 1 in 8 American men will be diagnosed with prostate cancer, and 1 in 41 will die of the disease. The cancer grows slowly, however, and has a high survival rate. The survival rate 5 years after diagnosis is nearly 100%; after 10 years, it is 98%; and after 15 years, it is 95% (American Cancer Society, 2021a).

Pathophysiology and Etiology

The cause of prostatic cancer is unknown, but there seems to be a relationship with increased testosterone levels and a diet that is high in fat. A man with blood relatives who have prostate cancer has an increased risk of developing the disease. Most prostatic carcinomas occur in the periphery of the gland. As it enlarges, it causes genitourinary symptoms similar to a variety of other conditions (e.g., BPH and cystitis). If untreated, tumor cells spread by way of the bloodstream and lymphatics to the pelvic lymph nodes and bone, particularly the lumbar vertebrae, pelvis, and hips.

Assessment Findings

Signs and Symptoms

At first, no symptoms occur, and none may develop for years. When the tumor grows large enough, it compromises urinary flow and causes frequency, nocturia, and dysuria (difficult or painful urination); hematuria (blood in the urine); hemospermia (blood in semen); and ED. The first symptoms of metastases may be back pain or pain down the leg from nerve sheath involvement. When pain develops, the disease often is in an advanced stage.

Diagnostic Findings

DRE detects a prostatic nodule. A PSA greater than 4 ng/mL is the basis for performing more definitive diagnostic procedures, and a PSA greater than 10 ng/mL indicates a prostatic malignancy. A PSA greater than 80 ng/mL indicates advanced metastatic disease. However, some men with normal PSA levels have prostatic cancer, whereas others with elevated PSA levels are cancer free.

Screening measurements of PSA are controversial. The U.S. Preventive Services Task Force (USPSTF, 2018) believes that there is insufficient evidence for routine PSA screening. In men aged 55 to 69 years, the decision for a PSA screening should be an individual one. In men aged 70 years or older, the USPSTF recommends no PSA-based screening. The rationale for the recommendation is that some prostatic cancers grow slowly, and the benefits of treatment may be minimal. In fact, there are potential quality-of-life consequences for treating prostate cancer in men who would never have developed cancer-related symptoms during their lifetime. According to the USPSTF, there is inadequate evidence that PSA screening actually improves health outcomes; treatment results after clinical detection with DRE are comparable (see Chapter 52).

On the other hand, the American Cancer Society (2020) recommends that screening for prostatic cancer using PSA and DRE should be offered to men beginning at age 40 years who have more than one first-degree relative who developed prostate cancer at an early age; at 45 years of age for African Americans and men at high risk with a father, brother, and son diagnosed with prostate cancer when younger than age 65 years; or at 50 years of age for those who are at average risk for prostate cancer and have at least a 10-year life expectancy. The American Urological Association (AUA, 2018) recommends against routine screening for men under age 54 at average risk for prostate cancer and men over age 70 with a less than 10- to 15-year life expectancy. The AUA indicates that the greatest benefit of screening is among men in the age range of 55 to 69 years, but it should be a shared decision after weighing the benefits of screening and potential harm from treatment.

Transrectal ultrasound confirms the presence of a mass. Definitive diagnosis is made by biopsy and microscopic examination of tissue. Sometimes, the malignancy is detected after microscopic examination of tissue removed during a TURP or open prostatectomy for BPH.

Pelvic or spinal radiographs, bone scan, and magnetic resonance imaging (MRI) or computed tomography (CT) scanning detect metastases to bones. An elevated serum acid phosphatase is associated with bone metastasis. An IV pyelogram (IVP) and other renal function studies detect kidney damage caused by long-standing urethral obstruction and urinary retention (if present).

Medical and Surgical Management

The tumor size, microscopic characteristics (sometimes referred to as the *Gleason score*), and any metastases are used to establish the stage, which in turn determines treatment (Table 55-4). The client's age, general health status, potential life expectancy, and the possible negative effects of treatments, such as incontinence and impotence, are also considered when planning treatment. Common treatment regimens include active surveillance to monitor the cancer closely as often as every 6 months; observation, which is sometimes called "watchful waiting," using fewer tests in lieu of relying on changes in symptoms; surgery; cryotherapy, which freezes and kills prostate cancer cells; external or internal radiation (**brachytherapy**); hormone therapy; immunotherapy; or a combination of these.

Surgery

If the nodule is localized, an open suprapubic prostatectomy is the treatment of choice. A radical prostatectomy, performed through a perineal or retropubic approach, is the surgical preference if the tumor is large enough to be palpated or if it has spread to adjacent tissue.

When a radical prostatectomy is performed, the entire prostate, its capsule, and the seminal vesicles are removed. The bladder neck is sutured to the membranous urethra over an indwelling urethral catheter, which is left in place for 10 to 14 days. Potential complications of this surgery include a 25% to 50% chance of impotence, difficulty with urinary control, and genital and lower extremity edema. A TURP may be performed if the client has urethral obstruction and his physical status is not amenable to treatment. Occasionally, permanent suprapubic urinary drainage may need to be established.

The removal of a cancerous prostate can also be performed laparoscopically. Although this procedure is technically more difficult, it has the same advantages as other similar, minimally invasive procedures: less pain, less blood loss, shorter recovery period, and quicker resumption of previous lifestyle. The American Cancer Society (2019a)

TABLE 55-4 Staging and Treatment of Prostatic Cancer

STAGE	DESCRIPTION	TREATMENT
Stage I	Cancer is small, grows slowly, and may never cause symptoms or other health problems.	Observation or external radiation, or brachytherapy (sealed source radiation) for asymptomatic men or older men with other serious health problems; for younger and healthier men, options include observation, radical prostatectomy, external radiation, or brachytherapy.
Stage II	Tumor is larger than stage I yet confined to the prostate gland; if left untreated, the cancer is more likely to spread beyond the prostate and cause symptoms.	For asymptomatic men or those who have other serious health problems, same treatment as for stage I or radical prostatectomy and radiation. For younger and otherwise healthy men, radical prostatectomy with removal of pelvic lymph nodes, followed by external radiation if the cancer has spread at the time of surgery or the PSA level is still detectable several weeks after surgery. If there is a greater chance for reoccurrence based on pathologic examination of the tissue and PSA scores, external or internal radiation (or both), several months of hormone therapy, and participating in a clinical treatment trial.
Stage III	Tumor has spread beyond the prostate but has not reached the bladder, rectum, lymph nodes, or other organs; likely to recur after treatment.	Observation for asymptomatic older men or those with other more serious illness; for others, hormone therapy alone or combined with external radiation, radical prostatectomy, followed by radiation and participation in a clinical treatment trial.
Stage IV	Tumor has spread to the bladder, rectum, lymph nodes, or distant organs such as the bones; not considered curable.	Same as stage III; in addition, TURP to relieve symptoms, chemotherapy to manage a tumor that continues to grow and spread, and adjuvant treatment to relieve bone pain or other symptoms; immunotherapy once FDA approved.

FDA, U.S. Food and Drug Administration; PSA, prostate-specific antigen; TURP, transurethral resection of the prostate.

indicates that laparoscopic and robotic-assisted laparoscopic radical prostatectomies are as effective as open radical prostatectomy; the long-term results have not been determined at this time. A bilateral **orchiectomy** (surgical removal of the testes) may be performed to eliminate the production of testosterone in men with advanced prostatic carcinoma (stage IV). Permanent side effects are impotence, loss of libido, hot flashes, and possible psychological disturbances. Many men do not accept surgical castration, and lower levels of testosterone can be achieved with hormone therapy.

Cryotherapy

Cryotherapy is an outpatient treatment modality that destroys the prostate gland using a gas cooled to −40°F passing through as many as 30 hollow probes inserted through the perineum. The tubes, which are observed with transrectal ultrasound, freeze and decimate the prostate gland within 3 minutes. The procedure is more effective if used before any type of radiation treatment. Clients can be discharged with a retention catheter on the same day as the treatment or after a brief stay in the hospital. Hematuria may be observed for a few days during the few weeks that the catheter is in place. There may be temporary discomfort in the location, where the probes were placed. ED is common as well as short-term swelling of the penis or scrotum. The PSA levels are monitored regularly to detect a recurrence of the cancer (American Cancer Society, 2019b).

Radiation Therapy

Radiation therapy (see Chapter 18) may be used alone or in conjunction with other treatment modalities, especially when there is local metastasis. Possible side effects include impotence, diarrhea, and urinary frequency and urgency.

Hormone Therapy

Men with stages III or IV carcinoma of the prostate are candidates for hormone therapy (Drug Therapy Table 55-2). With the use of luteinizing hormone-releasing hormone (LHRH) agonists and antagonists, a CYP17 inhibitor that blocks an enzyme that fuels cancer growth, and antiandrogenic (male) hormones or estrogenic hormones, the progression of the malignancy may be retarded and there may be a

DRUG THERAPY TABLE 55-2 Hormonal Therapy for Prostate Cancer

Category and Common Generic (Brand) Drugs	Intended Use	Common Side Effects	Safety Warnings for Nurses
LHRH Antagonist			
Degarelix (Firmagon)	Blocks release of gonadotropin, which reduces testosterone; reversible	Hot flashes, injection site pain, and weight gain	• Monitor hepatic function
LHRH Analogs			
Goserelin (Zoladex) Histrelin (Vantas) Leuprolide (Eligard, Lupron) Triptorelin (Trelstar)	Inhibit pituitary gonadotropin secretion, which reduces testosterone to same as castration levels	Hot flashes, headache, emotional lability, depression, sweating, acne, sexual dysfunction, pain, and edema	• Provide arm care instructions following implant • Monitor blood glucose for changes in clients with diabetes mellitus
Antiandrogens			
CYP17 Inhibitor Abiraterone (Zytiga)	Enzyme blocking slows cancer growth	Hot flashes, nocturia, urinary frequency, peripheral edema, general pain, and upper respiratory infection	• Must be taken with prednisone, be sure ample supply is given • Teratogenic, pills should not be handled by women without gloves
Bicalutamide (Casodex) Enzalutamide (Xtandi) Flutamide (Eulexin) Nilutamide (Nilandron)	Competes with androgen for receptor sites, used with an LHRH analog	Hot flashes, dizziness, diarrhea, peripheral edema, general pain, and asthenia	• Monitor blood glucose for changes in clients with diabetes mellitus • Monitor hepatic function
Miscellaneous Agents			
Adrenal Steroid Inhibitor Aminoglutethimide (Cytadren)	Blocks adrenal gland release of hormones	Drowsiness, skin rash, nausea, and vomiting	• Monitor thyroid function
Estrogen Estramustine (Emcyt)	Palliative use, to block estrogen receptors	Breast tenderness and enlargement, nausea, diarrhea, and edema	• Dietary calcium interferes with absorption

The drugs in column 1 indicate the drug that matches up with explanations in columns 2 through 4.
LHRH, luteinizing hormone-releasing hormone.

prolonged period of palliation (comfort). Estramustine (Emcyt) is a combination of estrogen and an antineoplastic drug that is also used for palliative treatment.

Feminizing side effects occur with hormone therapy. The client's voice may become higher, hair and fat distribution may change, and breasts may become tender and enlarged. Libido and potency are also diminished. When estrogens are used in lower doses, the client may not experience these problems.

Immunotherapy

The U.S. Food and Drug Administration (FDA) has approved sipuleucel-T (Provenge), a therapeutic vaccine for prostate cancer. A **therapeutic vaccine** is one that treats an existing disease as opposed to a vaccine that prevents disease. The Provenge vaccine is made from the client's harvested white cells that are stimulated in a laboratory with a prostatic acid phosphatase antigen present in about 95% of prostate cancer cells. The stimulated cells are returned to the client intravenously every 2 weeks for three treatments. The vaccine is palliative rather than curative; it extends the client's life by approximately 4 months. Vaccine side effects seem to be minor and short-lived and include chills, fever, headache, fatigue, shortness of breath, vomiting, and mild tremor. Pembrolizumab (Keytruda) was approved by the FDA in 2017 for immunotherapy against solid tumors. Other treatments must have been attempted and ruled out prior to use with pembrolizumab (Prostate Cancer Foundation, 2021). Additional clinical trials of yet approved therapeutic vaccines are being developed.

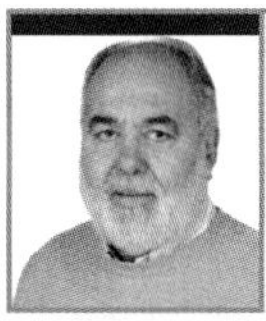

Clinical Scenario During a routine physical that included a DRE, the primary provider noted that the 68-year-old man had an enlarged nodular prostate gland. A PSA test was subsequently ordered. The test results measured a PSA of 38 ng/mL. The client was referred to a urologist for a needle biopsy of the prostate gland. The biopsy revealed cancerous cells. The client was given several options for treating prostate cancer. He will undergo an open radical prostatectomy. What nursing interventions are appropriate when managing this client's care? Refer to the nursing process discussion that follows.

NURSING PROCESS FOR THE CLIENT WITH PROSTATIC CANCER

Assessment

Obtain a health history from the client and focus on identifying information such as changes in patterns of urinary elimination (frequency, urgency, and nocturia), hematuria, low back pain, and a family history of prostatic cancer. After extensive surgical treatment for prostatic cancer, assess the client for signs of infection, urinary incontinence, and sexual dysfunction and reinforce health teaching that aids in the detection of metastasis.

Diagnosis, Planning, and Interventions

Refer to Chapter 14 for general preoperative and postoperative standards of care. Radical prostatectomy is similar to other prostatectomy procedures and the same immediate postoperative nursing diagnoses and interventions apply. Sexual consequences vary depending on whether the surgery involved nerve-sparing techniques. Diagnoses, expected outcomes, and interventions for clients with prostatic cancer include, but are not limited to, the following:

Infection Risk: Related to homecare of Foley catheter
Expected Outcome: Client will be free of a urinary tract infection as evidenced by clear urine without bacteria or white blood cells.

- Tell the client to use soap and water to clean around the urethral meatus and several inches of the catheter at least twice a day. *Medical asepsis decreases the growth of microorganisms that can ascend upward into the urinary tract.*
- Demonstrate and have the client return the demonstration for keeping the connection between the catheter and leg bag clean when changing and replacing leg bags for routine cleaning. *Keeping connections and equipment clean reduces the portals for microbial entry into the urinary tract.*
- Tell the client or caregiver to clean the leg bag by using soap and water and then rinsing it with a 1:7 solution of vinegar and water. *Vinegar is a weak acid (acetic acid) that chemically interferes with the growth of microorganisms.*

Reflex Urinary Incontinence: Related to surgical compromises to internal and external urinary sphincter muscles
Expected Outcome: Urinary control will be reestablished within 3 months after surgery or client will use equipment to collect urine.

- Teach pelvic floor–retraining exercises (see Client and Family Teaching 55-3) if incontinence is not permanent. *Pelvic floor–retraining exercises improve sphincter tone and bladder control.*
- For permanent incontinence, show the client how to apply a penile clamp or an external catheter connected to a leg bag. *Devising a method for mechanically controlling urinary incontinence or collecting urine unobtrusively decreases social embarrassment.*

Sexual Dysfunction: Related to temporary impotence, when the pudendal nerve (responsible for erection and orgasm) is spared
Expected Outcome: Client will use alternatives other than intercourse for sexual pleasure until potency resumes.

(continued)

NURSING PROCESS FOR THE CLIENT WITH PROSTATIC CANCER (continued)

- Explain to the client and sexual partner that it may take from 3 to 12 months for sexual potency to return. *Providing a timeline helps the client and his sexual partner cope with temporary sexual dysfunction.*
- See interventions for impotence for additional suggestions. *Various alternatives to sexual intercourse may be useful for managing sexual dysfunction.*

RC of Impotence: Related to pudendal nerve damage secondary to non–nerve-sparing radical perineal prostatectomy
Expected Outcome: The nurse will assist the client and sexual partner to manage ED.

- Recommend demonstrating sexual feelings in ways other than intercourse. *Intimacy is communicated in many different ways. Becoming asexual is counterproductive.*
- Discuss the use of manual stimulation or a mechanical vibrator if it does not compromise the sex partner's values. *Stimulating the clitoris of a woman manually or with a vibrator is an alternative method to sexual penetration for promoting orgasm in women.*

RC of Metastasis: Related to dissemination of cancerous cells beyond the prostate gland
Expected Outcome: The nurse will assist the client to manage and minimize the possibility of a recurrence of the primary cancer or metastasis.

- Explain that the PSA level will decrease after prostatectomy; a subsequent rise may indicate the cancer has reoccurred. *Having regular PSA levels after treatment aids in the early detection of cancer recurrence or metastasis. A phenomenon called a PSA "bounce," a rise in the PSA levels within 2 years of radiation therapy, is not pathologic; it may be caused by the release of PSA from dead and damaged cancer cells.*
- Clarify that repeat lymph node biopsies may be part of the surgical follow-up. *One method, by which cancer cells are spread, is the lymphatic system.*
- Inform the client that blood tests for measuring serum acid phosphatase are used to monitor evidence of bone metastasis. *A rise in acid phosphatase is a tumor marker for a client who has been treated for cancer of the prostate.*

Evaluation of Expected Outcomes

Expected outcomes for the client who is treated for cancer of the prostate are urinary continence and no evidence of infection. The client finds acceptable techniques for sexual expression, when impotence is permanent. He identifies techniques that assist in monitoring for a recurrence of the primary cancer or its metastatic spread.

As the client recovers, promote increased self-care and provide instructions for home management. The discharge plan of care includes, but is not limited to, the following:

- Maintain medical follow-up.
- Take medications as prescribed.
- Decrease dietary fat and increase fiber.
- Exercise regularly to increase lean body mass and decrease insulin levels, which is a catabolic hormone that promotes weight gain.
- Join a support group to learn more about the disease process and clinical research trials.

Consult with the family primary provider or oncologist before self-treating with herbal supplements.

Concept Mastery Alert

Prostatectomy

Some prostatectomies include the risk of damage to the pudendal nerve. Therefore, postoperatively, the nurse should assess for impotence. The pudendal nerve innervates the penis and the perineum. It can be damaged during prostate surgery, leading to the complication of impotence. It is not always a permanent condition.

Cancer of the Testes

Cancer of the testes is the most common cancer in American men between the ages of 15 and 35; the average age at diagnosis is 33 (American Cancer Society, 2021b; Mayo Clinic, 2020). The incidence has increased in the last 50 years, but is currently slowing. Despite the numbers of men who develop testicular cancer, it is one of the most treatable cancers even if it has metastasized; the overall survival rate at 5 years is 95%. Significant advancement in treatment in recent years has resulted in a 99% cure rate if the cancer has not spread beyond the testicles (American Cancer Society, 2021c; Evidence-Based Practice 55-1).

Pathophysiology and Etiology

The incidence of testicular cancer is higher in non-Hispanic White men and men with a history of cryptorchidism regardless of whether an orchiopexy was performed. Other clients who are at increased risk for testicular cancer include those with a family history of the disease, those who are human immunodeficiency virus (HIV) positive or have developed AIDS, and those who already have had cancer in one testicle. In most cases, only one testicle is affected, but the other may become cancerous at a later time.

The exact etiology is unknown, but one possible explanation is that the cells in the undescended testis or testes degenerate earlier than occurs with natural aging. The degenerative process then leads to abnormal cellular changes.

Evidence-Based Practice 55-1

Breast Cancer in Men

Clinical Question

Are men at risk for breast cancer?

Evidence

Although breast cancer is 100 times more common in women, 1990 new cases of breast cancer in men are diagnosed each year (Kraft, 2017). The average age is in the late 60s and increases with each year of age. Similar to women, men that have a family history of a blood relative with breast cancer also increases their risk. The following are risks for men and breast cancer: inherited Breast Cancer2 (*BRCA2*) gene mutation; Klinefelter syndrome, a disorder in which a man is born with one or more extra X chromosomes; being exposed to radiation; use of alcohol; liver disease; hormone treatment for prostate cancer; overweight; testicular abnormalities; and environmental exposure (American Cancer Society, 2018).

Nursing Implications

Nurses should obtain a thorough history when assessing clients who are men. Nurses can educate men on signs and symptoms of breast cancer, how to perform breast self-examinations, resources for treatment, and referrals. Clients should be encouraged to discuss concerns with the health care provider.

Reference

American Cancer Society. (2018). *Risk factors for breast cancer in men*. https://www.cancer.org/cancer/breast-cancer-in-men/causes-risks-prevention/risk-factors.html

Nearly all testicular tumors involve the sperm-forming germ cells. Those that consist of immature germ cells are called *seminomas*; *nonseminomas* develop among more mature, specialized germ cells. Nonseminomas grow more rapidly and tend to metastasize at a faster rate; therefore, treatment is more aggressive. Testicular cancers tend to spread to the lymph nodes near the kidneys, liver, lungs, bone, and rarely to the brain (Eggener & Campbell, 2016).

Assessment Findings

Gradual or sudden swelling of the scrotum or a lump felt on palpation always deserves prompt medical attention. The tumor usually presents as a hard, nontender nodule of the testis with additional coexisting symptoms (Box 55-1). Ultrasound of the testis may follow. Unless discovered early through testicular self-examination, the first symptoms such as unrelenting back pain or shortness of breath may be those of tumor metastasis.

BOX 55-1 Signs and Symptoms of Testicular Cancer

- Testicular lump that is hard or granular
- Increase in the size of one testicle
- Heavy or dragging feeling in the scrotum
- Dull ache in the groin or above the pubis
- Diminished sensitivity to testicular pressure

Tumor markers include repeated blood elevations of alpha-fetoprotein and hCG. An IVP may show lymph node enlargement that displaces the ureters. Lymphangiography is also used to detect lymph node involvement. For detection of metastases, CT is preferred over MRI. Because biopsy risks spreading the highly malignant tumor cells, surgery is recommended immediately.

Medical and Surgical Management

Treatment of testicular tumors depends on the stage of the disease (Table 55-5) and includes surgery, chemotherapy, and radiation. Before medical or surgical treatment, however, the topic of sperm banking should be discussed to ensure future paternity. Locating a sperm bank and then collecting two or three semen samples may delay and jeopardize the outcome of treatment.

Surgery

A radical inguinal orchiectomy and the removal of the spermatic cord are performed through an inguinal incision. The scrotal sac on the operative side looks and feels empty. It is possible to implant a testicular prosthesis filled with silicone gel at a later date.

Clients with nonseminomas usually undergo a radical, nerve-sparing procedure known as retroperitoneal lymph node dissection (RPLND) within 6 weeks of an orchiectomy as well. RPLND decreases potential metastasis from the testis and the need for chemotherapy. If only one testis is removed, sexual activity, libido, and fertility are usually unaffected. After a radical lymph node dissection, libido and erections are preserved, but unless the nerve-sparing procedure is performed, the surgery results in retrograde ejaculation.

Chemotherapy

A multiple antineoplastic drug regimen with combinations of bleomycin (Blenoxane), etoposide (Vespid), and cisplatin (Platinol), or others may be given depending on the type of tumor, stage of cancer, and surgery that was performed. Chemotherapy, which usually is aggressive initially, is modified as the tumor markers show a response. An autologous (self-donated) bone marrow transplantation may be recommended for recurrent disease or for clients who are resistant to drug therapy.

TABLE 55-5 Staging and Treatment of Germ Cell Tumors of the Testis

STAGE	DESCRIPTION	TREATMENT
Stage I	Tumor confined to the testis	Orchiectomy and RPLND
Stage II	Involvement of testis plus retroperitoneal nodes	Orchiectomy, RPLND, and possible chemotherapy
Stage III	Distant metastasis	Orchiectomy, RPLND, four cycles of chemotherapy, and surgery to resect residual masses

RPLND, retroperitoneal lymph node dissection.

Sperm tends to be destroyed or mutated when exposed to toxic cancer drugs, but spermatogenesis may eventually resume months or within 2 years after chemotherapy. Men with low sperm counts prior to chemotherapy and those who receive very high doses of chemotherapy are less likely to recover sperm counts that are adequate for impregnation (Cancer Research UK, 2017). Those with normal sperm counts before treatment, although they are the minority, may develop normal sperm counts afterwards; up to 70% have been known to father children naturally or with cryopreserved semen (National Cancer Institute, 2021).

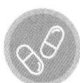

Pharmacologic Considerations

■ When many drugs are used with the same side effects, they can intensify. Many of the chemotherapeutic drugs used to treat testicular cancer affect the nervous system. Monitor and instruct clients to report signs and symptoms of neuropathy immediately.

Radiation

Seminomas are sensitive to radiation, and most clients receive radiation to the retroperitoneal lymph nodes. Shielding of the remaining testis minimizes impairment of sperm production. For clients with nonseminomas, radiation is considered an adjunct to lymphadenectomy and chemotherapy.

Nursing Management

Preoperative Period

One of nursing's chief concerns is responding to the client's emotional distress over having a life-threatening diagnosis, being unfamiliar with the surgical experience, and confronting alterations in body image and sexuality. Most clients are understandably concerned over the potential change in their sexual image and fertility; however, it may be of even greater concern to men in the age group most often affected. The nurse provides private opportunities for the client to ask questions and uses therapeutic communication techniques to encourage the client to verbalize his feelings.

Postoperative Period

Refer to Chapter 14 for postoperative standards of care. After an orchiectomy, the nurse applies a scrotal support. If drains have been inserted, they are connected to closed (Jackson–Pratt) or open (machine) suction. The nurse gives prophylactic antibiotics to prevent infection. They manage pain, which may be severe after a radical lymph node dissection, with narcotic analgesics. If pain is not relieved and nursing measures to augment the effect of analgesics are inadequate, the nurse collaborates with the primary provider to modify drug therapy.

As the client's comfort improves, the nurse may discuss the effects of the diagnosis and treatment and again provide opportunities for the safe expression of anxiety, fear, and grief. The nurse provides the client with names of local support groups and encourages him to contact them for emotional support after discharge.

A teaching plan includes the following instructions for homecare:

- Drink plenty of fluids and eat a well-balanced diet to avoid constipation.
- Obtain adequate rest; avoid fatigue and heavy lifting.
- Wash the incision with soap and warm water. Report any redness, drainage, pain, or swelling of the incision or scrotum.
- Take any prescribed medication exactly as directed.
- Perform self-examination of the remaining testicle every month and immediately report any changes.
- Seek care if any of the following occur: fever, chills, adverse drug effects, weight loss, or anorexia.

For clients who are concerned about future reproduction, the nurse discusses issues as appropriate for the client's particular situation. If a client has banked sperm, the nurse informs him that normal pregnancies have occurred with sperm stored until they are 55 years of age (Cancer Research UK, 2020). For clients for whom treatment has proceeded without collecting and storing sperm, the nurse identifies other options, such as donor insemination or adoption. They may suggest contacting the Department of Social Services to become a foster parent, volunteering as a Big Brother, or leading a scout troop or youth group.

Cancer of the Penis

Penile cancer is rare and occurs more often in men who are uncircumcised. The cause is unknown, but it is thought that chronic irritation leads to a precancerous skin lesion that eventually undergoes malignant changes. Medical attention is sought when the lesion, which typically has been present for years, becomes infected. Biopsy confirms the existence of malignant cells, and lymphangiography identifies if the lymph nodes are involved. The tumor is staged using MRI and CT scanning.

Treatment includes tumor excision, chemotherapy, external or interstitial radiation therapy, or all three. In some cases, the penis is partially or completely amputated and the scrotum and testes excised. Full amputation of the penis requires the insertion of a permanent drainage tube in the perineal tissue to empty the bladder. The 5-year survival rate for cancer of the penis is 65% (American Cancer Society, 2021d).

ELECTIVE STERILIZATION

A **vasectomy** is a minor surgical procedure done in a primary provider's office or clinic. It involves the ligation of the vas deferens and results in permanent sterilization by interrupting the pathway that transports sperm (Fig. 55-12). On occasion, the client may complain of impotence, although the procedure has no effect on erection or ejaculation. It may take several weeks or more after surgery before the ejaculatory fluid is free of sperm, and the client is informed to use

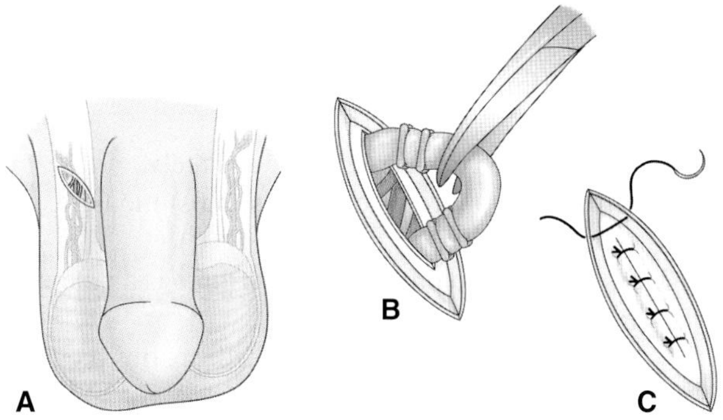

Figure 55-12 Vasectomy procedure. **(A)** An incision is made to expose the vas deferens. **(B)** The vas deferens is isolated and severed. **(C)** The severed ends are occluded with sutures or sealed with electrocautery, and the incision is closed.

a reliable method of contraception until sperm no longer are present. The client may wish to consider banking sperm before undergoing the procedure. Some men feel ambivalent about having this procedure, and the nurse provides the client with an opportunity to express these feelings.

The nurse reinforces the following important information for homecare after a vasectomy:

- Expect some bruising and incisional soreness after the local anesthetic wears off.
- Apply ice packs to the scrotum to reduce swelling; remove the cold application after 20 minutes and replace again after the tissue rewarms.
- Take a mild analgesic, such as aspirin or acetaminophen, for discomfort.
- Wear an athletic support for several days for comfort.
- Resume usual activities in 2 to 3 days, but avoid strenuous exercise for up to 5 days.
- Resume sexual activity when comfort allows, usually in 1 week.
- Use a reliable method of contraception until the primary provider indicates that sperm no longer are present, which may be determined after 10 or more ejaculations.
- Report severe pain, fever, or swelling at the top of the testes.

A **vasovasostomy** is a surgical attempt to reverse a vasectomy by restoring patency and continuity to the vas deferens; a **vasoepididymostomy** connects the stump of the vas deferens directly to the epididymis. It may take from 3 to 6 months after reversal procedures before sperm counts and motility are normal. Lack of success usually is the result of either scar formation or sperm leakage from the surgical connection.

KEY POINTS

- Structural abnormalities:
  - Cryptorchidism: one or both testes fail to descend into scrotum
  - Torsion of the spermatic cord: rotation of the testicle that twists the spermatic cord around the testicular artery, affecting blood flow to the testicle
  - Phimosis: inability to retract foreskin
  - Paraphimosis: strangulation of the glans penis due to the inability to replace retracted foreskin
- Infectious and inflammatory conditions:
  - Prostatitis: inflammation of the prostate gland
  - Epididymitis: inflammation of the epididymis
  - Orchitis: inflammation of the testis
- Erection disorders:
  - Erectile dysfunction (ED): inability to achieve or maintain an erection. May be caused by physical or psychological reasons
  - Priapism: condition when penis becomes engorged and persistently erect without sexual stimulation
- Benign prostatic hyperplasia: enlarged prostate gland due to the increase of cells
- Malignancies of the male reproductive system
  - Cancer of the prostate: second most common cancer in men, second most common cause of death due to cancer in men
  - Cancer of the testes: most common cause of cancer in men between ages of 15 and 35, one of the most treatable types of cancer
  - Cancer of the penis: rare, occurs more often in men who are uncircumcised
- Elective sterilization: vasectomy—minor surgical procedure done in the provider's office

CRITICAL THINKING EXERCISES

1. Assume you are attending a team conference to plan the care of a client who is having a suprapubic prostatectomy. What nursing interventions are appropriate?
2. Describe the typical client who acquires benign prostatic hypertrophy versus one who develops testicular cancer.
3. What information can the nurse provide to a man who is experiencing ED?
4. A man is considering a vasectomy but is worried that the procedure will affect his sexuality. How would the nurse respond?

NCLEX-STYLE REVIEW QUESTIONS PrepU

1. What factor is most likely responsible for a young adult client's development of orchitis?
   1. The client was never immunized for mumps.
   2. The client is an active homosexual.
   3. The client has multiple sexual partners.
   4. The client is a military veteran.

2. What is the best reason for the nurse to advise a client who has been prescribed sildenafil (Viagra) for ED to avoid taking a nitrate such as sublingual nitroglycerin (Nitrostat)?
   1. The combination interferes with an erection.
   2. Sildenafil counteracts vasodilation by nitroglycerin.
   3. The client is likely to experience hypotension.
   4. Priapism is likely to occur when used together.

3. A client describes experiencing nocturia. To gather more information about symptoms associated with benign prostatic hypertrophy, what question is most important for the nurse to ask next?
   1. "Have you noticed any changes in sexual function?"
   2. "Have you felt any lumps in your scrotum recently?"
   3. "Do you have difficulty starting to void?"
   4. "Do you have problems controlling urination?"

4. Following a suprapubic prostatectomy, the client has a catheter in the urethra and another in an abdominal incision. When documenting the urinary output in the medical record, what is the most accurate nursing documentation?
   1. Record only the output from the urethral catheter.
   2. Record only the output from the wound catheter.
   3. Record the output from each catheter separately.
   4. Record the combined output from both catheters.

5. Following a vasectomy, a client questions how soon he can be sure that his sexual partner will not become pregnant. What nursing response is most accurate?
   1. You are considered sterile immediately.
   2. After 10 or more ejaculations, most men are sterile.
   3. As long as you produce semen, there is a potential for pregnancy.
   4. Once scrotal swelling diminished, sperms are no longer produced.

WANT TO KNOW MORE? There are a wide variety of online resources available on thePoint to enhance learning and understanding of this chapter.

Go to **thePoint.lww.com/activate** and use the activation code found in the front of this text to unlock these online resources.

56 Caring for Clients With Sexually Transmitted Infections

Words To Know

autoinoculation
chancre
chancroid
Charcot joints
chlamydia
condylomata
dental dam
genital herpes
genital warts
gonorrhea
gummas
herpes simplex virus type 2
human papillomavirus (HPV) infection
microcephaly
neuropathic joint disease
nucleic acid amplification testing
sexually transmitted infections
syphilis
tabes dorsalis
venereal diseases
Zika virus

Learning Objectives

On completion of this chapter, you will be able to:

1. Name five common sexually transmitted infections (STIs) and identify those that are curable.
2. List five STIs that, by law, must be reported.
3. Give two reasons why statistics on reportable STIs are not totally accurate.
4. Discuss several factors contributing to the transmission of STIs.
5. Give two reasons why women acquire STIs more often than men.
6. Name the most common and fastest spreading STI.
7. Explain two ways STIs are spread.
8. Discuss methods that are helpful in preventing STIs.
9. Discuss information that is important to teach clients about using condoms.
10. Name the type of infectious microorganism that causes each of the common STIs.
11. Identify complications that are common among clients who acquire each of the most common STIs.
12. Name drugs used to treat common STIs.

Sexually transmitted infections (STIs), also known as *sexually transmitted diseases* (STDs) or **venereal diseases**, are a diverse group of infections spread through sexual activity with a person who is infected. The term *STI* is increasingly used to emphasize that a person can be infected without experiencing symptoms of the disease. STIs are a significant public health problem. Some, such as HIV/AIDS (see Chapter 35), hepatitis (see Chapter 47), and skin infestations with lice and mites (see Chapter 65), are spread by additional routes as well. The pathogens that cause STIs include bacteria, fungi, parasites, protozoans, and viruses.

The STIs that require national reporting to the Centers for Disease Control and Prevention (CDC) include chlamydia, gonorrhea, hepatitis B, HIV, syphilis, and chancroid, and Zika virus (CDC, 2021a). Although reporting infections with **human papillomavirus (HPV)** is not required, it is the most common STI in the United States (CDC, 2019a). Of the reportable STIs, chlamydia, gonorrhea, and syphilis are easily cured with early and adequate treatment. Social, sexual, and biologic factors that contribute to the incidence of STIs include the following:

- Ignorance of how STIs are transmitted or prevented
- Asymptomatic sexual partner(s)

- Casual sex with partner(s) about whom little is known
- Sex with high-risk partner(s), such as those who use intravenous (IV) drugs, those who are bisexual, those who have sex with prostitutes, and men who have sex with men
- More than one concurrent or sequential sexual partner(s)
- Failure to use contraceptive techniques that also reduce the risk of acquiring STIs
- Sexual contact during the period between infection and the manifestation of symptoms
- Failure to seek early treatment
- Nonadherence to treatment or failure to refrain from sexual contact until treatment is complete
- Mutation and resistance of microorganisms to antimicrobial drug therapy

Gerontologic Considerations

■ The stereotype that older adults are not sexually active is inaccurate. A health history for older adults should include questions about sexuality and behaviors that put clients at risk for STIs.

■ Some older adults with STIs may have limited knowledge of STIs or may be embarrassed to discuss symptoms. Not recognizing symptoms may cause them to delay seeking health care. Therefore, a thorough history and physical and psychosocial assessment are important. Education should include explanations of treatments and avoidance of sexual behaviors until treatment is completed in order to prevent infection of the partner. Older adults in nonmonogamous relationships who are no longer concerned about an unplanned pregnancy are at risk for STIs if they fail to use barrier or chemical contraceptive methods at the time of sexual intimacy.

EPIDEMIOLOGY

Epidemiology is the study of the occurrence, distribution, and causes of human diseases. The CDC has the challenging task of gathering disease statistics such as the incidence of STIs. Determining the exact incidence of these diseases is difficult because only a few are reportable by law. Of the reportable diseases, some are undiagnosed and untreated, some are treated and unreported, and some are misdiagnosed.

Reporting of new STI cases is the responsibility of either the health care provider or the testing laboratory. Reporting is kept confidential and protected from subpoena. The reported incidence of STIs is disproportionately higher among racial and ethnic minorities (Haley et al., 2015). This disparity may be the result of (1) limited access to health care, (2) poverty, (3) actual higher rate of disease occurrence in communities, where sexually active people have a greater potential for selecting a partner who is infected, or (4) more reporting by public health clinics, where many in these respective populations seek treatment (CDC, 2019b).

Table 56-1 lists statistics on reportable and common STIs in the United States from 2015 to 2018. STIs such as genital herpes and those caused by the HPV are not reportable by law. Therefore, it is difficult to document accurate statistics pertaining to these diseases. STIs occur more often in women than in men, probably because the moist, warm vaginal environment is conducive to microbial growth and because the vagina, as a receptive orifice, is more readily traumatized during sexual activity.

Obtaining a sexual history (Box 56-1) is a crucial component of assessment of clients presenting with signs or symptoms of an STI. Critical questions should include the "Five P's" about their sexual **p**artners, sexual **p**ractices, pregnancy **p**revention, **p**rotection from STIs, and **p**ast history of STIs (Savoy et al., 2020). See Evidence-Based Practice 56-1 for research on STIs among older adults.

In addition to curing the infection when possible (some STIs are not curable), treatment consists of education and counseling to reduce the client's risk of contracting an STI in the future (Client and Family Teaching 56-1). Screening, counseling, and, if indicated, treating sexual partner(s) are essential.

TABLE 56-1 STI Statistics in the United States between 2015 and 2018

DISEASE	NEW CASES IN THE UNITED STATES (2015)	NEW CASES IN THE UNITED STATES (2018)	RATE OF CHANGE (%)
Chlamydia	1,526,658	1,758,668	↑ 1.1
Gonorrhea	395,216	583,405	↑ 1.13
Syphilis	23,872	35,063	↑ 1.38
Chancroid	11	3	↓
HIV/AIDS	39,959	37,515[a]	↓ 0.87
HPV	14,100,000[b]	43,000,000[c]	↑ 2.35
Zika STI	0[d]	0[e]	

HPV, human papillomavirus; STI, sexually transmitted infection

[a]Prevalence in the United States: per 100,000. From Centers for Disease Control and Prevention. (2019). *Sexually transmitted diseases: Reported cases and rates of reported cases, United States,* 1941–2018. https://www.cdc.gov/std/stats18/tables/1.htm; Centers for Disease Control and Prevention. (2020). *Diagnoses of HIV infection in the United States and dependent areas, 2018: Tables.* https://www.cdc.gov/hiv/library/reports/hiv-surveillance/vol-31/content/tables.html.

[b]From Centers for Disease Control and Prevention. (2016). *Genital HPV Infection—Fact Sheet.* http://www.cdc.gov/std/hpv/stdfact-hpv.html.

[c]Centers for Disease Control and Prevention. (2019f). *Human papillomavirus.* https://www.cdc.gov/std/stats18/other.htm#hpv.

[d]Centers for Disease Control and Prevention. (2019). *2015 Case counts in the United States.* https://www.cdc.gov/zika/reporting/2015-case-counts.html.

[e]Centers for Disease Control and Prevention. (2021). *2021 Case counts in the United States.* https://www.cdc.gov/zika/reporting/2021-case-counts.html.

BOX 56-1 Questions to Ask When Obtaining a Sexual History From the Client With an STI

- Have you had new or more than one sexual partners in recent weeks?
- Do you use a condom during sexual activity?
- Do you have a history of an STI?
- Have you engaged in vaginal, anal, or oral sex?
- Were you the receptive partner in anal or oral sex?
- Do you have a history of infection with HIV?
- Do you have a history of employment as a sex worker?
- Do you use drugs or alcohol when engaging in sex?
- Is there a possibility of pregnancy?

Evidence-Based Practice 56-1

Older Adults and Risk for STIs

Clinical Question

Are older adults at risk for STIs?

Evidence

STIs are a concern across the lifespan, not just in younger adults. There has been an increase in STIs among older adults, and the sexual activities of this age group are often disregarded (Malta et al., 2020). Participants reported that after age 50, limited testing occurs, and there is also a decrease in the appropriate sexual history assessment. Health care providers should be the ones initiating the sexual history conversation, but many perceive that the older adult age group is at low risk for transmission of STIs. The findings also indicate that this is a topic that is uncomfortable to discuss with clients this age and that health care providers find that communication about sexual health is difficult in this age group (Malta et al., 2020).

Nursing Implications

Nurses should provide complete care to all clients, including clients over age 50. It is important to communicate about sexual health with this age group. Some of the STIs do not have signs and symptoms, so they go unnoticed that could have serious consequences (Malta et al., 2020).

Reference

Malta, S., Temple-Smith, M., Bickerstaffe, A., Bourchier, L., & Hocking, J. (2020). "That might be a bit sexy for somebody your age": Older adult sexual health conversations in primary care. *Australasian Journal of Aging, 39*(S1), 40–48. https://doi.org/10.1111/ajag.12762

COMMON SEXUALLY TRANSMITTED INFECTIONS

Chlamydia

Infections with HPV are the most common STI in the United States (see later discussion), but **chlamydia** infections are the most common nationally reportable STI disease in the United States. The number of new cases in 2018 totaled over 1.75 million (CDC, 2019c).

Client and Family Teaching 56-1
Methods for Reducing the Risk of STIs

The nurse emphasizes the following methods to reduce risk:

- Abstain from sexual activities.
- Have monogamous sex with a partner who is not infected.
- Use latex condoms with nonoxynol-9 (a spermicide) when having oral, vaginal, or anal intercourse.
- Combine the use of condoms for men with a spermicide when having vaginal intercourse, or use a condom for women.
- Urinate and wash the genital and perineal areas before and immediately after having sexual intercourse.
- Wash your hands and any areas where there has been direct contact with semen or vaginal mucus.
- Refuse or terminate sexual activity that causes trauma to the genitals, internal reproductive structures, anus, and elsewhere.
- If infected, report the information to all sexual partners and encourage them to seek medical diagnosis and treatment.
- Avoid unprotected sex until you and your sexual partners have completed treatment.

Pathophysiology and Etiology

The causative microorganism, *Chlamydia trachomatis*, is a bacterium that lives inside the cells it infects. The disease is spread by sexual intercourse or genital contact without penetration. The microorganism invades the reproductive structures (see discussion of pelvic inflammatory disease [PID] in Chapter 53), the urethra in women, and the urethra and epididymis in men (see discussion of Gonorrhea in this chapter). The tissue irritation, which may be permanent despite successful eradication of the bacteria, puts those with chlamydial infections at greater risk for acquiring other STIs, such as gonorrhea and HIV/AIDS. Untreated chlamydia can cause sterility in women who are infected; pregnant women who are infected can transmit the microorganism to their infants during birth.

Chlamydial infections can also be spread to the eyes by **autoinoculation** (self-transmission to another area of the body), usually by unwashed hands. Ophthalmic infections, which are more common in underdeveloped countries where flies are the vector for transmitting the microorganism, can cause granulation of the cornea and blindness.

Assessment Findings

As many as 75% of all women who are infected and 25% of all men who are infected are asymptomatic. Symptoms, if they occur, may appear 1 to 3 weeks after infection. They include a sparse, clear urethral discharge; redness and irritation of the infected tissue; burning on urination; lower abdominal pain in women; and testicular pain in men.

Diagnosis may be made by microscopic examination and culture of secretions. A test kit is available that identifies the microorganism in approximately 15 minutes. Now **nucleic acid amplification testing** (NAAT) is considered the superior and preferred method for diagnosing chlamydia because it is a more sensitive detection method (CDC, 2021b). NAAT is a nonculture method for detecting the genetic DNA of the organism with advantages that include the following: (1) less invasive because it only requires a vaginal swab from women or urethral or rectal swabs from men, (2) provides results in less time because it omits a delay in culturing a specimen, and (3) facilitates treating the infection more promptly (CDC, 2021b).

Currently, U.S. Preventive Services Task Force (2021) has a draft recommendation for annual screening for chlamydia to be done for all pregnant and nonpregnant sexually active women younger than 24 years, women of age 25, and older women who are pregnant or are at increased risk. There is currently insufficient evidence for routinely screening sexually active men (U.S. Preventive Services Task Force, 2021). It is a common practice to test clients for chlamydia and coinfections of gonorrhea, syphilis, and HIV because it is usual for clients to have concurrent infections with more than one STI.

Medical Management

Antimicrobial drugs, such as a single oral dose of azithromycin (Zithromax) or a 7-day regimen of doxycycline (Vibramycin), are taken twice a day. Alternative drugs for treatment include erythromycin (E-Mycin), ofloxacin (Floxin), or levofloxacin (Levaquin).

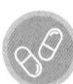

Pharmacologic Considerations

■ Single-dose drug treatment ensures 100% adherence to treatment. The setback is the side effects; for example, gastric distress may be more intense. During assessment, be sure to ask about past experiences with antimicrobials, allergies, and possible pregnancy. All these are factors in drug regimen decisions.

Nursing Management

The nurse sensitively obtains a sexual history, follows precautions for preventing infection transmission, assists in collecting a specimen, explains the course of treatment, and discusses methods for preventing transmission and reinfection (Client and Family Teaching 56-2). Besides advocating for sexual abstinence, the nurse can use opportunities to teach women and men who have achieved sexual maturity on how to use a condom or a **dental dam**, a sheet of latex that acts as a barrier between the vagina or anus and a partner's mouth when performing oral or anal sex, with the information in Client and Family Teaching 56-3.

Client and Family Teaching 56-2
The Client With an STI

The nurse emphasizes the following points when teaching the client:

- Take prescribed medication according to label directions for the full length of time that it is prescribed.
- Stop having sex until retesting indicates that the infection is eliminated.
- Urge any and all sexual partners to be examined and follow through with concurrent treatment.
- Use a condom, a contraceptive barrier device, consistently and correctly before any and all sexual contact after completing medical treatment.
- Do not assume that successful treatment means that there is any permanent immunity; reinfection can and does occur if preventive sexual practices are not implemented.
- Seek treatment as soon as possible if the symptoms continue or if they recur after successful treatment.

Gonorrhea

Gonorrhea is the second most frequently reported sexually communicable infection in the United States. Its highest incidence occurs in the 15- to 24-year-old age group. Many women are asymptomatic, a factor that contributes to the spread of the disease.

Pathophysiology and Etiology

The infection is caused by a bacterium, *Neisseria gonorrhoeae*, which can be transmitted heterosexually or homosexually. The microorganism invades the urethra, vagina,

Client and Family Teaching 56-3
Proper Use of Condoms and Dental Dams

The nurse emphasizes the following points about condoms when teaching the client:

- Select condoms that are lubricated with a spermicide or silicone.
- Do not use natural membrane condoms, which act as a barrier to sperm but allow viruses to pass through.
- Keep condoms in a cool, dry place.
- Discard condoms beyond their expiration date or if they are more than 5 years old.
- Never unroll or examine a condom before its use or use one that appears to have deteriorated.
- Pinch the space at the condom tip (Fig. A) while unrolling the condom over the erect penis (Fig. B). Unroll the condom all the way to the base of the penis.
- Use additional water-based lubricant to reduce friction and prevent tearing of the condom; avoid oil-based lubricants, which can weaken latex.
- Remove the condom from the vagina before the penis becomes limp.
- Dispose of the condom in a lined container.
- Apply a new condom before each sex act.
- Use a silicone-based lubricant to prevent the condom from breaking; silicone does not deteriorate latex.
- Understand that breakage and slipping rates may be higher during anal sex.

The nurse emphasizes the following points about using a dental dam when teaching the client:

- Purchase a commercial dental dam or construct a rectangular piece of latex from a condom or glove.
- Cut the tip from the condom and unroll the condom before slitting it lengthwise to form a rectangle; follow the same process by cutting a piece of latex from the palm of a disposable glove.
- Make sure that there are no holes or tears in the dental dam.
- Optionally apply a water-soluble lubricant to the surface that will be against the vulva or anus.
- Place the dam against the vulva or anus and hold it in place during sexual activity.
- Dispose of the dental dam after a one-time use.

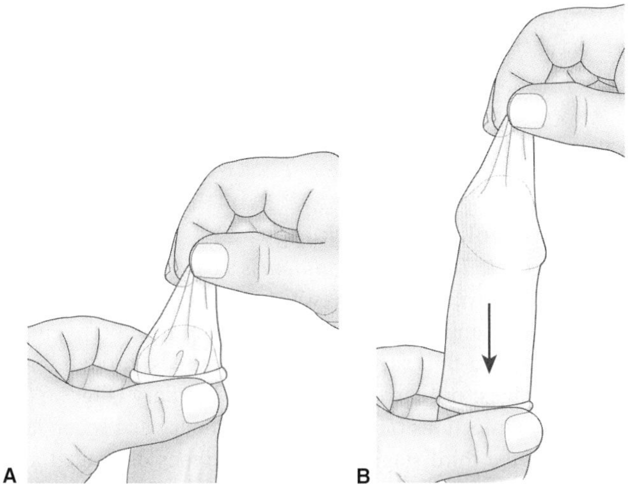

rectum, or pharynx depending on the nature of sexual contact; it can spread throughout the body.

In untreated men, the localized infection may spread to the prostate, seminal vesicles, and epididymis. Urethral strictures may develop, requiring periodic dilation of the urethra or, possibly, reconstructive urethral surgery. In women, the infection may progress upward to the cervix, endometrium, and fallopian tubes, and symptoms of PID (see Chapter 53) may develop. Data suggest that gonorrhea facilitates HIV transmission (Ducre, 2015). Gonorrhea can also be transmitted to an infant's eyes at the time of birth.

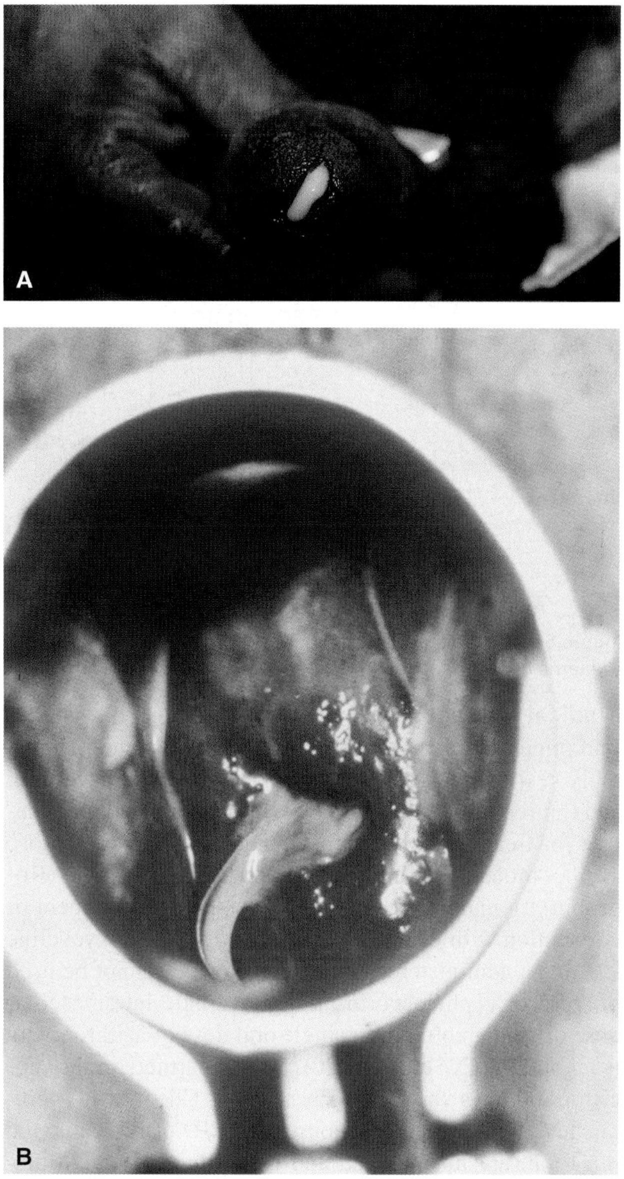

Figure 56-1 **(A)** A purulent discharge from the penile urethra caused by a gonorrheal infection. **(B)** Gonnococcal mucopurulent discharge from female cervix. (**A**, reprinted with permission from Rubin, E., & Farber, J. L. (1999). *Pathology* (3rd ed.). Lippincott Williams & Wilkins. **B**, reprinted with permission from Sweet, R. L., & Gibbs, R. S. (2005). *Atlas of infectious diseases of the female genital tract*. Lippincott Williams & Wilkins.)

Assessment Findings

Signs and Symptoms

In men, symptoms usually appear 2 to 6 days after infection. Urethritis with a purulent discharge and pain on urination are the most common signs and symptoms. A small proportion of men are asymptomatic. More than half of women who are infected experience no symptoms. When symptoms do occur, women have a white or yellow vaginal discharge, intermenstrual bleeding due to cervicitis, and painful urination (Fig. 56-1). An anal infection is accompanied by painful bowel elimination and a purulent rectal discharge; the throat is sore when the pharynx is infected. If the microorganism disseminates (scatters) throughout the body, the client may manifest a skin rash, fever, and painful joints.

Diagnostic Findings

Specimens of drainage from infected tissue are examined microscopically immediately after they are collected or are inoculated on a culture medium and incubated to reveal the causative organism. NAAT testing is now recommended for the same reasons identified for chlamydia infections. However, cultured specimens are valuable for determining microbial sensitivity and resistance to antibiotics for potential treatment.

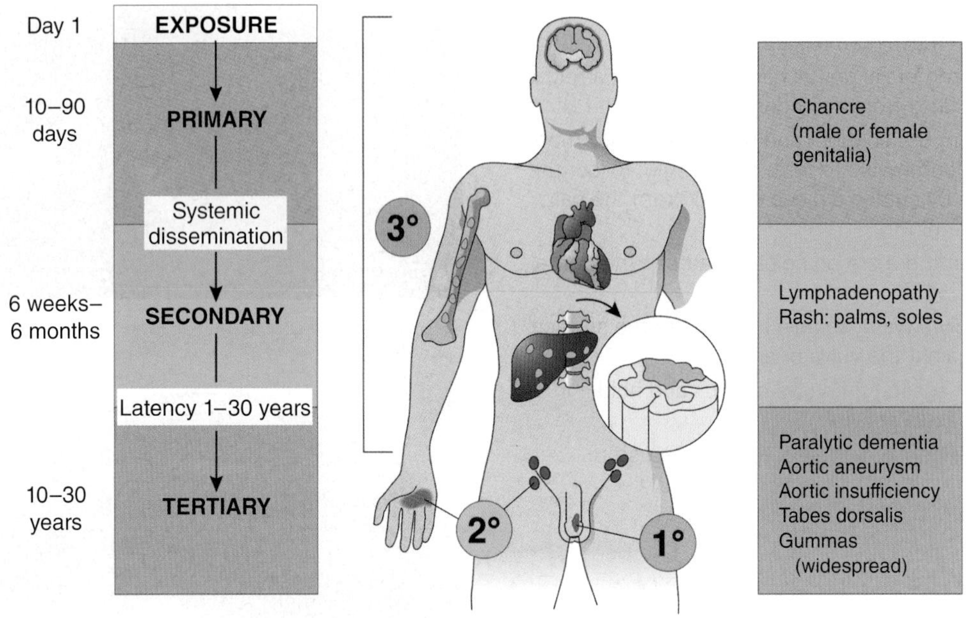

Figure 56-2 Three stages of syphilis. (Reprinted with permission from Rubin, E., & Farber, J. L. (1999). *Pathology* (3rd ed.). Lippincott Williams & Wilkins.)

Medical Management

The microorganism *N. gonorrhoeae* has become increasingly resistant to sulfonamides, penicillin, tetracyclines, and fluoroquinolones. Therefore, the current recommendation for treating gonorrhea is a single intramuscular dose of the broad-spectrum cephalosporin, ceftriaxone (Rocephin) for uncomplicated gonorrhea. For the treatment of coinfection with *Chlamydia trachomatis*, oral doxycycline should be administered. When ceftriaxone cannot be used because of cephalosporin allergy, a single intramuscular dose of gentamicin plus a single oral dose of azithromycin is an option (Cyr et al., 2020). Sexual partners in the preceding 60 days should also be treated. Clients with complicated gonococcal infections, as in PID or disseminated infection, are hospitalized and treated with IV multiple-drug therapy. Repeat therapy with different antibiotics may be required.

Nursing Management

The nursing management and the client teaching are similar for those clients with chlamydia. However, when a culture is collected from a woman, the vaginal speculum is moistened with water rather than lubricated because lubricant may destroy the gonococci and cause inaccurate test results. Additional nursing management is discussed in the nursing care plan that appears later in this chapter.

Syphilis

Syphilis is a curable STI if treated early. Syphilis can be transmitted from the blood of a person who is infected, directly from the lesion, or across the placenta to an unborn infant. The incidence of syphilis in the United States has been increasing. The CDC's 2018 data reports cases in men with information on the sex of sexual partners. Men with sexual partners who are men account for 76% of all primary and secondary cases of syphilis (CDC, 2019d).

Pathophysiology and Etiology

The spirochete *Treponema pallidum* is a bacterium that causes syphilis. The average time between infection and the first occurrence of symptoms is 21 days but can range between 10 and 90 days. If untreated, syphilis progresses through three distinct stages: primary, secondary, and tertiary (Fig. 56-2). Syphilis is infectious only during the primary and secondary stages. In the third stage, the client becomes demented and dies from complications involving other organ systems.

Assessment Findings

Signs and Symptoms

In the primary (early) stage, a **chancre** (painless ulcer) appears on the genitals, anus, cervix, or other parts of the body (Fig. 56-3). At first, the lesion resembles a small papule, which later ulcerates. The chancre heals in several weeks

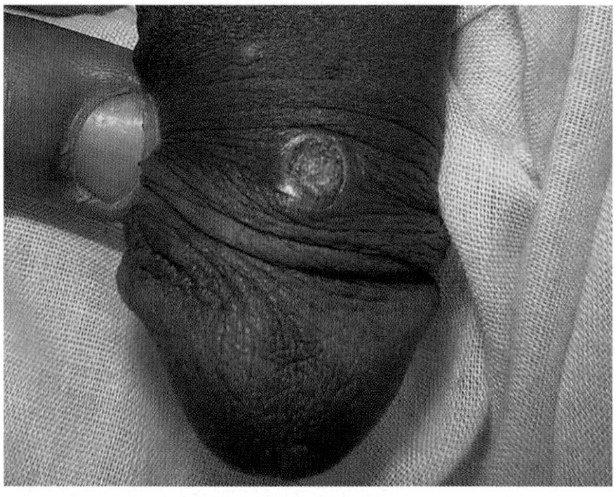

Figure 56-3 Syphilitic chancre on the penis. (Reprinted with permission from Fleisher, G. R., Ludwig, S., & Baskin, M. N. (2004). *Atlas of pediatric emergency medicine*. Lippincott Williams & Wilkins.)

and, if treatment has not been initiated, the client progresses to the secondary stage of syphilis.

Symptoms of secondary syphilis include fever; malaise; lymph node enlargement; rash on the trunk, back, arms, palms, or soles of the feet that do not itch; patchy hair loss, headache; and sore throat—all of which disappear without treatment. However, without treatment, syphilis progresses to a third stage.

The tertiary stage of syphilis is noninfectious because the microorganism invades the central nervous system (CNS) as well as other organs of the body. Symptoms of tertiary syphilis include **tabes dorsalis** (a degenerative condition of the CNS that results in stabbing back and leg pain, an unsteady gait, urinary incontinence, blindness, and other neurologic symptoms like dementia), **gummas** (soft, rubbery growths of skin tissue), and **neuropathic joint disease**, also called **Charcot joints.**

Diagnostic Findings

Diagnosis is made with nontreponemal antibody tests such as rapid plasma reagin (RPR) and venereal disease research laboratory (VDRL) test on blood. More specific treponemal antibody tests such as fluorescent treponemal antibody absorption (FTA-ABS) test measures *Treponema pallidum* antibodies or a *T. pallidum* particle agglutination assay (TP-PA), which has fewer false positives. A direct detection test in which a sample from the chancre is placed on a slide and examined with a microscope may be done, but it is less common than other tests (Lab Tests Online, 2021). When a person develops CNS symptoms, the cerebrospinal fluid is examined.

Medical Management

A single dose of parenterally administered penicillin G (Pfizerpen, Wycillin) is used to treat primary and secondary syphilis. Clients who are allergic to penicillin are given a 14-day regimen of tetracycline or doxycycline. Follow-up examinations and laboratory tests are recommended 3, 6, and 12 months after initial treatment. Those with tertiary syphilis may require multiple doses for 10 to 14 days to prevent complications (CDC, 2015a). The response is poor in those with cardiovascular syphilis.

Nursing Management

The nurse gathers health information and sexual history, asks about the client's allergy history in anticipation of antibiotic treatment, prepares the client for diagnostic laboratory tests, supports the client emotionally when the diagnosis is confirmed, and informs the client that notification of the sexual partner by the department of public health is important for their evaluation and treatment. (More nursing management can be found in the nursing care plan later in this chapter.)

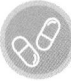

Pharmacologic Considerations

- Monitor for allergic reaction in clients receiving penicillin parenterally for at least 30 minutes after injection. Symptoms of an allergic reaction include pruritus, hives, difficulty breathing, hypotension, sweating, and tachycardia.

Herpes Simplex Virus Infection

Herpes simplex virus (HSV) infection is a highly contagious STI that is controllable but not curable. Statistics suggest that 16% to 21% of people in the United States have herpes. However, statistics do not always differentiate between orofacial herpes simplex virus type 1 (HSV-1) and genital herpes (HSV-2). Women and Black Americans are disproportionately affected (CDC, 2019e, 2019d). HSV-2 increases the risk of cervical cancer and infection with HIV.

Pathophysiology and Etiology

Although **herpes simplex virus type 2**, also known as **genital herpes**, is primarily responsible for genital and perineal lesions, HSV-1, associated with cold sores around the nose and lips, can also cause anogenital lesions. Transmission of the herpes viruses is by direct contact with oral or genital secretions from a person during an active stage of the disease, by sexual contact during periods of asymptomatic viral shedding, or by autoinoculation. Transmission can also occur from mother to infant during vaginal birth and carries a high rate of neonatal mortality. HSV-1 and HSV-2 may be introduced into the eye, the mouth, the genital area, or a skin site.

Herpes recurs because, after the initial infection, the virus remains dormant in the ganglia of the nerves that supply the area until reactivation. Symptoms are usually more severe with the initial outbreak. Subsequent episodes are usually shorter and less intense. When the virus is active, shedding viral particles are infectious; however, those who are asymptomatic can also shed the virus.

Most clients with genital herpes have at least one outbreak per year, and many clients report five to 10 outbreaks per year. Some clients note that stress, emotional situations, exposure to sunlight, menstruation, and fever reactivate the disease.

Assessment Findings

After a short incubation period, HSV-2 causes single or multiple vesicles on the penis, prepuce, buttocks, thighs, introitus, or cervix (Fig. 56-4). The HSV-2 lesions burn and itch before becoming fluid-filled blisters. The vesicles rupture in 1 to 3 days and are followed by painful, reddened ulcers that scab over and eventually disappear. The outbreak may be accompanied by swelling of the inguinal lymph nodes, flu-like symptoms, and headache. The initial attack lasts 3 to 4 weeks; subsequent attacks usually last 10 days.

Diagnosis of HSV-1 and HSV-2 infections is tentatively made by the client's history and inspecting the lesions. Smears and scrapings from the lesions can be cultured or examined microscopically using special stains to confirm the clinical impression. Polymerase chain reaction (PCR) testing on cells or fluid from the ulceration or other body fluid may identify the DNA of the herpes virus (CDC, 2021c).

Medical Management

Both types of herpes respond to the antiviral drugs acyclovir (Zovirax), valacyclovir (Valtrex), and famciclovir (Famvir; Drug Therapy Table 56-1). The client may take oral antiviral medications episodically for 3 to 5 days to shorten the duration

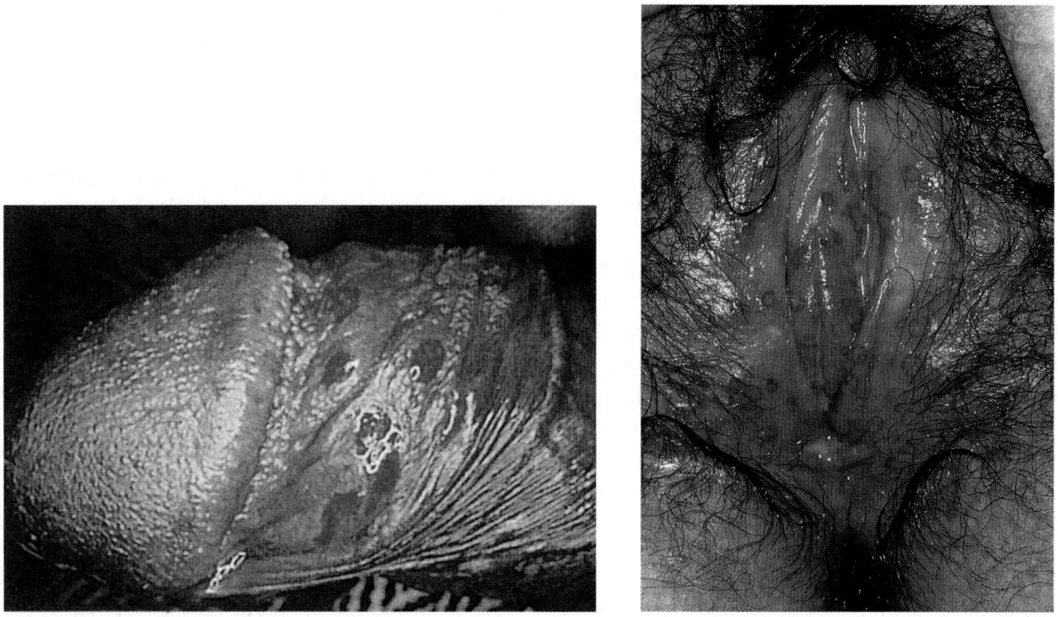

Figure 56-4 Genital herpes lesions: **(A)** on the penis and **(B)** on the vulva. (Photo (A), reprinted with permission from Goodheart, H. P. (2009). *Goodheart's photoguide to common skin disorders: Diagnosis and management* (3rd ed.). Wolters Kluwer Health/Lippincott Williams & Wilkins. Photo (B), reprinted with permission from Beckmann, C. R., Herbert, W. N., Laube, D. W., Ling, F. W., & Smith, R. P. (2014). *Obstetrics and gynecology* (7th ed.). Wolters Kluwer Health/Lippincott Williams & Wilkins.)

DRUG THERAPY TABLE 56-1 Agents Used to Treat STIs

Category and Common Generic (Brand) Drugs	Intended Use	Common Side Effects	Safety Warnings for Nurses
Antibiotics			
Penicillin family Penicillin G (Pfizerpen)	Syphilis: kills microorganisms by interfering with bacterial cell wall development	Glossitis, stomatitis, gastritis, furry tongue, nausea, vomiting, diarrhea, rash, fever, pain at injection site	• Monitor for anaphylactic reaction
Cephalosporin Ceftriaxone (Rocephin)	Gonorrhea: kills microorganisms by interfering with bacterial cell wall development	Nausea, vomiting, diarrhea, headache	• May manifest allergy if allergic to penicillin • Avoid alcohol intake • Monitor for nephrotoxicity
Macrolides Azithromycin (Zithromax) Erythromycin (E-mycin)	Chlamydia, Gonorrhea: kills microorganisms by interfering with protein synthesis in the bacterial cell	Nausea, vomiting, diarrhea, abdominal cramping	• Monitor for ototoxicity • Do not give to pregnant women
Tetracycline Doxycycline (Vibramycin) Tetracycline	Chlamydia, Syphilis: kills microorganisms by interfering with protein synthesis in the bacterial cell	Nausea, vomiting, diarrhea, abdominal cramping	• Photosensitivity, sunscreen when out even on cloudy days • Do not give to pregnant women • Avoid dairy products
Fluoroquinolones Levofloxacin (Levaquin) Ofloxacin (Floxin)	Chlamydia: kills microorganisms by interfering with DNA/RNA synthesis in bacterial cell	Nausea, diarrhea	• Photosensitivity, sunscreen when out even on cloudy days
Anti-Herpes Virus Agents			
Acyclovir (Zovirax) Famciclovir (Famvir) Valacyclovir (Valtrex)	Use with herpes simplex virus (HSV)-1, HSV-2	Nausea, vomiting, diarrhea, fever, headache, dizziness, confusion, rashes, myalgia	• Instruct in condom use/abstinence during an outbreak
Topicals for Self-Management			
Podofilox (Condylox) Imiquimod (Aldara)	Use with genital warts	Nausea, vomiting, local irritation	• Use only four cycles • Monitor for fungal infections

The drugs in column 1 indicate the drug that matches up with explanations in columns 2 through 4.

of lesions or continuously as suppressive therapy to reduce the frequency of outbreaks and decrease the potential for transmission to others. Episodic therapy begins within 1 day of lesion onset or during the period immediately preceding an outbreak when the client is aware of early symptoms. IV acyclovir is used if there is a severe episode of HSV-2 or if the client is immunocompromised. Cesarean delivery is performed on pregnant women with active lesions to prevent transmission to the newborn. Antiviral drug therapy does not necessarily prevent viral shedding. Clients who are infected and who adhere to drug therapy may still transmit the virus (CDC, 2015b).

The frequency of recurrent outbreaks in many clients diminishes over time. Consequently, the primary provider may suggest discontinuing suppressive therapy to evaluate the client's need for continuous medication.

Nursing Management

The nurse collects appropriate health and sexual data, uses standard precautions when inspecting lesions, obtains specimens, and provides related health teaching. More on nursing management is identified in the nursing care plan that appears later.

The nurse instructs clients with HSV-2 infections to:

- Inform all potential sexual partners of the HSV infection even if asymptomatic.
- Use a condom or dental dam during sexual activity even if the disease seems inactive. Avoid sexual contact if there is any question that the infection is active; condoms and dental dams do not protect skin and mucous membrane that is left exposed.
- Keep lesions dry using alcohol, peroxide, witch hazel, and warm air from a hairdryer.
- Check with the primary provider about taking warm baths with Epsom salts or baking soda to relieve discomfort.
- Wear loose clothing that promotes air circulation about the genitals.

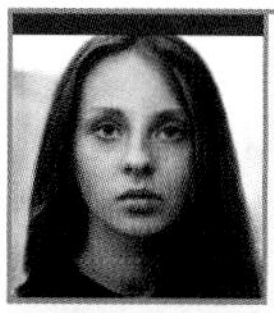

Clinical Scenario An 18-year-old female college student has been sexually active with more than one partner. She fears that she has contracted genital herpes. She has ignored several outbreaks of vaginal lesions and felt relieved when they disappeared. However, because of their reoccurrence, she has made an appointment at the college health clinic. **What are some problems that a client with a suspected STI may identify to the nurse who takes the client's information? What nursing approaches are appropriate for managing the care of a client with an STI? Refer to Nursing Care Plan 56-1 for examples.**

NURSING CARE PLAN 56-1 The Client With an STI

Assessment

Determine the following:

- Vital signs
- Health history with a focus on the onset and course of current symptoms
- Similar symptoms in sexual partner(s)
- Presence of oral, vaginal, rectal, or genitourinary lesions
- Characteristics of discharge (vaginal, urethral, and rectal), if any is evident
- Evidence of skin rash or abnormal appearance of integument
- Accompanying symptoms such as joint or abdominal pain or pain during intercourse
- Failure to become pregnant if pregnancy is desired
- Drug and allergy history

Nursing Diagnosis. **Situational Low Self-Esteem** related to acquiring an STI

Expected Outcome. Client's self-esteem will be positive.

Interventions	Rationales
Avoid being judgmental.	*Negative responses from others lower self-esteem.*
Affirm client's good judgment in seeking treatment.	*Acknowledging a positive action helps increase client's self-esteem.*
Assure client that medical information is confidential and, although some STIs are reported, access to such information is carefully guarded.	*Keeping personal information confidential helps the client avoid any public ridicule.*
Refer client to a support group for people who have acquired a similar STI.	*Members of support groups have similar problems and help others cope with medical, emotional, and social issues.*

Evaluation of Expected Outcome

Client's self-esteem improves or remains at the same level as before they required medical treatment for STI.

Nursing Diagnosis. **Acute Pain** related to inflammation and changes in the skin and mucous membranes

Expected Outcome. Pain will be relieved to client's level of tolerance.

Interventions	Rationales
Provide a prescribed analgesic.	*Analgesics relieve pain by various physiologic mechanisms.*

(continued)

NURSING CARE PLAN 56-1 The Client With an STI (*continued*)

Administer prescribed antimicrobials specific to the infectious microorganism.	*Discomfort usually is relieved when the infection resolves.*
Advise regular bathing.	*Bathing removes irritating drainage.*
Recommend wearing loosely woven cotton underwear and full-cut, nonconstricting outer clothing.	*Cotton is a natural fiber that wicks drainage away from the body. Nonconstricting clothing allows air to circulate between the skin and outerwear and avoids friction.*

Evaluation of Expected Outcomes

Client's pain and discomfort are at a tolerable level.

Nursing Diagnoses. **Altered Skin Integrity** related to inflammation and altered local tissues secondary to infectious process. Client is comfortable; symptoms are reduced or relieved.

Expected Outcomes. (1) Skin lesions will heal. (2) Integrity of mucous membranes will be restored.

Interventions	Rationales
Provide information on appropriate topical skin applications.	*Various over-the-counter and prescription medications can be applied to the skin to relieve inflammation, reduce itching, lubricate the skin, and dry lesions.*
Advise client to pat rather than rubbing the skin dry.	*Patting reduces friction and the itch-scratch-itch cycle.*
Reinforce compliance with medical treatment.	*Taking prescribed medications according to directions ensures eradication or control of the infecting microorganism.*

Evaluation of Expected Outcomes

Skin and mucous membranes are intact; no lesions are evident.

Nursing Diagnosis. **Infection Risk** related to infectious drainage and viral shedding

Expected Outcome. The infection will remain confined and will not be transmitted to any other susceptible host.

Interventions	Rationales
Follow standard precautions before diagnosis and contact precautions after diagnosis is confirmed.	*Standard precautions reduce the risk of transmission of a blood-borne infection before a diagnosis is made. Transmission-based precautions interfere with the routes by which specific pathogens are spread.*
Advise client to have all sexual partners tested and treated.	*STIs often are transmitted between both sexual partners; to eradicate the infection, sexual partners must be treated as well.*
Identify methods for preventing STIs such as abstinence, barrier and chemical types of contraceptives, and voiding and washing after sexual intercourse.	*STIs are spread by direct contact; methods that prevent direct contact reduce the potential for disease transmission.*
Recommend early prenatal care to pregnant women.	*Some STIs can be transmitted during childbirth.*
Explain how to manage articles used for personal hygiene and items to avoid sharing with people who are not infected.	*Keeping personal hygiene items separate from others and preventing indirect contact with contaminated items can reduce the potential for disease transmission.*
Direct client to take medications as prescribed and return for medical follow-up.	*Compliance and medical follow-up help ensure that the infection responds to treatment.*

Evaluation of Expected Outcome

No other person acquires the STI from the person who is infected.

Nursing Diagnosis. **Acute Anxiety** related to possible consequences of STI

Expected Outcome. Client will feel comfortable when they acquire realistic information.

Interventions	Rationales
Explain the cause of the STI and how to avoid potential consequences or complications.	*Accurate knowledge dispels inaccurate beliefs and misconceptions.*
Instruct client who is infected with carcinogenic (cancer-causing) viruses to have regular cancer-screening examinations.	*These examinations in risk-prone clients facilitate early diagnosis and optimistic prognosis.*

NURSING CARE PLAN 56-1 The Client With an STI (*continued*)

Evaluation of Expected Outcome

Client feels self-assured and confident about managing the STI.

Nursing Diagnosis. **Altered Sexuality Patterns** related to embarrassment in revealing the risk for an STI to sexual partner(s)

Expected Outcome. Client will resume sexual relationships with modifications that help to avoid STI transmission.

Interventions	Rationales
Role-play situations in which client communicates their STI status to a significant other.	*Role-playing with an uninvolved person helps a person rehearse and prepare for a situation that evokes anxiety.*
Suggest that the client and sexual partner(s) discuss and select methods that will facilitate sexual activity without transmitting the STI.	*Open communication facilitates a mutual plan for reducing the potential for disease transmission.*

Evaluation of Expected Outcome

Client discusses and implements modifications for sexual expression.

Nursing Diagnoses. **Nonadherence** related to lack of knowledge or abandoning recommendations

Expected Outcomes. (1) Client will understand the regimen for curing or controlling the STI. (2) Client will comply with the plan of care.

Interventions	Rationales
Provide specific client teaching that is appropriate for the particular STI.	*STIs result from various pathogens; treatment varies.*
Emphasize completing the full course of drug therapy.	*Drug therapy may cure or slow the progression of the STI and relieve symptoms.*
Provide client with a telephone number for obtaining objective and authoritative information.	*Clients may be more inclined to ask questions about an STI and its treatment if their identity can remain anonymous.*
Schedule an appointment for follow-up care.	*Medical follow-up promotes compliance with therapeutic regimen.*

Evaluation of Expected Outcome

Client paraphrases the plan for treatment and carries out prescribed interventions.

- Perform thorough handwashing after direct contact with lesions, and keep any personal hygiene articles, like a towel, separate to avoid inadvertent use by others.
- Use a separate towel to pat lesions dry and another when drying other body parts to avoid autoinoculation.
- Have annual Papanicolaou (Pap) tests to detect cervical cancer.
- Investigate stress management strategies because reducing stress tends to decrease the frequency of outbreaks.

Genital Human Papilloma Infection

HPV infection is the most commonly transmitted sexual disease in the United States, currently affecting 79 million people. There are more than 100 strains of HPV; 40 strains of the virus can infect the genitals of men and women as well as the mouth and throat; 13 strains have the potential for causing cancer. Most who are sexually active acquire one or more strains of HPV (CDC, 2019f). One-fourth of the people in the United States are infectious but do not manifest symptoms. Strains 6, 11, 16, 18, 31, 33, and 35 cause **genital warts**, also called **condylomata**, that tend to recur even after treatment. People with AIDS as well as others with an immunodeficiency are particularly susceptible to strains that cause genital warts. Untreated genital warts may resolve on their own, remain unchanged, or increase in size or number.

Pathophysiology and Etiology

HPV is transmitted by genital–genital, genital–anal, or genital–oral contact with a person who is infected and may or may not be symptomatic. Sexual penetration is not necessary, but nongenital contact is less likely to transmit HPV; most HPV infections clear within a few years without clinical manifestations, and those that persist are linked to various forms of cancer.

Genital HPV can be transmitted to an infant's respiratory passages at the time of delivery. HPV infection is associated with uterine cervical abnormalities, which may lead to cervical and other pelvic reproductive types of cancer—penile, anal, and oropharyngeal cancer (see Chapter 53). The strains of HPV that cause genital warts are different than those that cause cervical cancer, however.

Assessment Findings

If the immune system is functioning optimally, most people who are infected with HPV do not manifest symptoms. Eventually, the virus may lead to cancerous changes over time. If genital warts develop, they are usually painless and appear as a single lesion or cluster of soft, fleshy growths on the genitalia (Fig. 56-5) or cervix; in the vagina; or on the perineum, anus, throat, or mouth. Sometimes, the warts are so small that they are inconspicuous; however, they can become large and raised, resembling a cauliflower. Large genital warts may narrow or obstruct the urethra, vagina, anus, or throat.

Genital warts turn white when vinegar is applied to the lesion. The highlighted tissue is then examined with a magnifying glass.

Medical Management

There are no antivirals for treating an HPV infection. Prevention by abstaining from sex or using condoms or dental dams is the best way to lower the potential for acquiring HPV. People may also be vaccinated to reduce the spread of the infection and its cancerous consequences (see Chapter 53). Vaccinations are administered before sexual activity occurs, as early as 9 years of age but generally between the ages of 11 and 12 years, or later up to ages 21 to 26 for those who did not receive the full series of three immunizations.

Local treatment is available for those who develop genital warts. If the warts are not extensive and the client can reach them, the primary provider may prescribe podofilox (Condylox) solution or gel or imiquimod (Aldara) cream for self-application. Treatment may involve twice-daily applications of podofilox for 3 days, followed by nontreatment for 4 days. The client repeats the cycle up to four times, if necessary. Imiquimod cream requires application at bedtime three times a week. The client removes the ointment with soap and water in the morning. The treatment period with imiquimod cream can extend up to 16 weeks.

If the genital warts are of substantial size or are in an anatomic location that is difficult to reach, the client may defer treatment to a nurse or primary provider. Primary provider–administered treatment involves removing the warts in one or more of the following methods: surgical excision with scalpel or scissors, laser therapy, electrocautery (heat), cryotherapy (freezing) with liquid nitrogen, local applications of chemicals, or parenteral administration of natural or recombinant interferon.

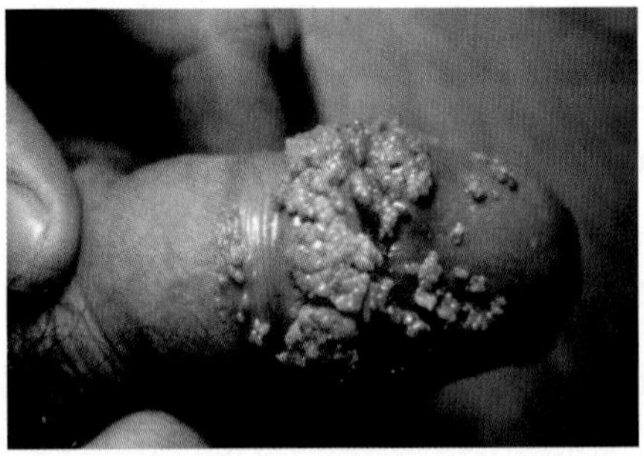

Figure 56-5 Genital warts on the penis. The warts may resemble small cauliflowers. (Reprinted with permission from Goodheart, H. P. (2009). *Goodheart's photoguide to common skin disorders: Diagnosis and management* (3rd ed.). Wolters Kluwer Health/Lippincott Williams & Wilkins.)

The major chemicals used to eradicate the warts include local applications of trichloroacetic acid, bichloroacetic acid, podophyllin resin in tincture of benzoin, or 5-fluorouracil cream. The warts will most likely be eradicated after three to six cycles of treatment (CDC, 2015c). Eradication does not mean the condition is cured; the person is temporarily noncontagious once the warts are destroyed.

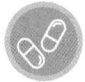

Pharmacologic Considerations

- Ask about pregnancy or if effective birth control is being used before administering podofilox or podophyllin. Both of these products can cause birth defects when used by pregnant women.

Nursing Management

Nurses provide information about transmission of STIs to sexually active people and prepare those with possible STIs for medical examination, diagnosis, and treatment. It is important to have continued assessment for the development of cervical, anal, penile, and oropharyngeal cancers that are associated with an HPV infection.

The nurse tells clients with genital warts to

- Avoid intimate contact until the warts are removed.
- Advise all sexual contacts to be examined and treated.
- Seek treatment at an STD/STI clinic or with a private primary provider when, and if, the warts return.
- Use a condom even when the lesions are absent (see Client and Family Teaching 56-2), and suggest that the sexual partner wash their genitals or other skin areas immediately after intimate contact; condoms may not fully protect against HPV transmission when all areas of the penis are not fully covered.
- Provide information about the diagnosis and treatment in future health histories, especially if a pregnancy occurs.
- Avoid stress and genital trauma, which appear to be factors in reactivating the virus (Grossman & Porth, 2013).

››› *Stop, Think, and Respond 56-1*

What STI is associated with the following signs?

1. *Painless ulceration on the genitals or other areas of sexual contact*
2. *Discharge from the vagina, urethra, or both; burning on urination; and abdominal pain in women*
3. *Cluster of soft, fleshy growths about the genitals or other places of sexual contact*
4. *Burning and itching around the genitals before an outbreak of multiple vesicles that become painful after rupture*

OTHER SEXUALLY TRANSMITTED INFECTIONS

Zika Virus

Most people who are infected with the **Zika virus** acquire it through the bite of female mosquitoes (the vector or mode of transmission) belonging to the species known as *Aedes aegypti* and *Aedes albopictus* that require blood to lay their eggs. However, the virus can also be spread through sexual contact.

When bitten by a mosquito carrying the Zika virus, individuals develop mild symptoms that include fever, skin rash, conjunctivitis, muscle and joint pain, malaise, and headache that last for 2 to 7 days (World Health Organization, 2018). Besides being infected through vector transmission, the Zika virus can also be transmitted from men and women who are infected to their sexual partners whether either is asymptomatic or symptomatic. A woman who is infected can transfer the virus to her unborn fetus at any time during the pregnancy. At birth, infants who are infected as a fetus is likely to be born with **microcephaly**, an abnormally small head, accompanied by developmental delays and mental retardation as well as other neurologic effects.

An infection with the Zika virus is based primarily on a person's symptoms or history of unprotected sexual activity after having traveled to one of 11 countries, including Argentina and the southern United States, where the infecting mosquitoes and virus are known to exist. A definitive diagnosis is made by identifying the presence of the Zika virus in semen, vaginal, and cervical mucus with a reverse transcription PCR test.

The CDC (2019g) and the World Health Organization (2018) recommend several methods for preventing an infection with the Zika virus. They include:

- Avoiding travel to areas where the Zika virus is known to occur.
- Controlling environments where mosquitoes breed such as standing water.
- Staying indoors, especially during early morning and evening hours when mosquitoes are most active.
- Ensuring that windows and doors are covered with screens.
- Applying an effective insect repellant like one containing DEET (*N*,*N*-diethyl-*meta*-toluamide).
- Wearing long-sleeved shirts and pants when outdoors.
- Using safer sex practices, including the consistent use of condoms, for 6 months following travel to areas, where the Zika viral infections have been identified.
- Waiting at least 6 months after returning from areas, where Zika transmission is known to occur before trying to conceive.
- Abstaining from sex or using safer sexual practices, if pregnant, for the duration of a pregnancy.

Chancroid

Chancroid is caused by the *Haemophilus ducreyi* bacillus. The infection, which was reported in 24 people in the United States in 2010 and three people in 2018, is characterized by the appearance of a macule, followed by vesicle–pustule formation, and, finally, a painful genital ulcer and enlarged, tender lymph nodes in the inguinal area (CDC, 2019h). It is treated and cured with azithromycin, ceftriaxone, ciprofloxacin, or erythromycin.

KEY POINTS

- STIs
  - Epidemiology: the study of occurrence, distribution, and causes of human disease
- Common STIs
  - Chlamydia: most common nationally reportable STI. Irritated tissue, redness, burning with urination, clear urethral discharge, lower abdominal pain in women, testicular pain in men
  - Gonorrhea: second most frequently reported STI. Urethritis with a purulent discharge, pain with urination, and vaginal discharge
  - Syphilis: chancre appears in primary stage; secondary syphilis causes fever, malaise, lymph node enlargement, rash, headache, sore throat. tertiary stage affects the CNS and other body organs.
  - Herpes simplex virus: highly contagious, causes single or multiple vesicles on the penis, buttocks, thighs, introitus, or cervix.
  - Genital HPV: most commonly transmitted STI in the United; may be asymptomatic; some strains cause genital warts or cervical cancer.
  - Zika virus: can be acquired by mosquito bites, is possible to spread via sexual contact.
  - Chancroid: very rare, starts as macule, turns to vesicle with pustule formation, and then a painful genital ulcer.

CRITICAL THINKING EXERCISES

1. Discuss STI information that is appropriate for a person who confides that they are having unprotected sexual intercourse with more than one person.
2. Explain information that a client who has never used a condom for men, which is more common than a dental dam, should know.
3. A woman tests positive for chlamydia. The primary provider could treat the client with a single dose of azithromycin (Zithromax) or a seven-day regimen of doxycycline (Vibramycin) taken twice a day. What drug treatment is more advantageous than the other? Support your answer.
4. What might the nurse tell a client with chlamydia who says, "Well, this isn't as serious as having gonorrhea or syphilis?"

NCLEX-STYLE REVIEW QUESTIONS PrepU

1. When the nurse teaches a client who has been diagnosed with chlamydial infection, what statement is accurate?
  1. Men manifest symptoms, but women who are infected do not.
  2. This is a rare type of STI.
  3. Your sexual partner(s) need(s) simultaneous treatment.
  4. There is no known cure for this kind of infection.

2. A client who is a man reports symptoms that are suggestive of a gonorrhea infection. If a culture is ordered to detect the causative organism, what body substance does the nurse collect?
  1. Venous blood
  2. Sterile urine
  3. Ejaculated semen
  4. Urethral drainage

3. A nurse is assessing a client who is a man with tertiary syphilis. What finding is most associated with this stage of the disease?
  1. Sharp leg pains
  2. Red skin rash
  3. Penile ulcers
  4. Patchy hair loss

4. When a nurse counsels a client who is a woman with HSV-2 infection, what information is accurate?
  1. Any children you have in the future will be immune to the disease.
  2. If you take your medicine as prescribed, you will not infect anyone else.
  3. Have a Pap test on a regularly scheduled basis.
  4. Avoid vaginal intercourse for at least 6 months.

5. A nurse refers a client with genital warts to a gynecologist who confirms that they are caused by the HPV. What is the most correct response when the client asks if there is any danger associated with this condition?
  1. Genital warts can be treated with an antibiotic, such as penicillin or tetracycline.
  2. Genital warts increase the risk of cancer of the vulva, vagina, and cervix.
  3. Genital warts can be prevented if the individual takes birth control pills.
  4. Genital warts are of no danger to the client and need not be treated at this time.

WANT TO KNOW MORE? There are a wide variety of online resources available on thePoint to enhance learning and understanding of this chapter.

Go to **thePoint.lww.com/activate** and use the activation code found in the front of this text to unlock these online resources.

UNIT 14
Caring for Clients With Urinary and Renal Disorders

57 Introduction to the Urinary System

Words To Know

blood urea nitrogen
costovertebral angle
creatinine
creatinine clearance test
cystography
cystometrography
cystoscope
cystoscopy
excretory urography
intravenous pyelography
postvoid residual
renal arteriography
retrograde pyelography
ultrasonography
urinalysis
urine osmolality
urine protein test
urine specific gravity
urodynamic studies
uroflowmetry
urography
voiding cystourethrography

Learning Objectives

On completion of this chapter, you will be able to:

1. Name the parts of the urinary system.
2. Define the primary functions of the kidney and other structures in the urinary system.
3. List tests performed for the diagnosis of urologic and renal system diseases.
4. Identify laboratory tests performed to diagnose urologic and renal system diseases.
5. Discuss nursing management for a client undergoing diagnostic evaluation of the urinary tract.

The urinary system consists of the kidneys, renal pelves (sing., *pelvis*), ureters, urinary bladder, and urethra. The kidneys have many functions (Box 57-1), including excreting excess water and nitrogenous waste products of protein metabolism; assisting in maintenance of acid–base and electrolyte balance; producing the enzyme *renin*, which helps regulate blood pressure; and producing the hormone *erythropoietin*, which stimulates red blood cell (RBC) production. The remainder of the urinary system are involved in the transport (ureters and pelves), storage (bladder), and excretion (urethra) of urine.

Urologic nursing assessment focuses on changes in urine production, transport, storage, and elimination. Other responsibilities of urologic nurses involve caring for clients with conditions that affect the reproductive systems, discussed in Chapters 53 and 55.

Gerontological Considerations

■ Age-related changes in kidney function, such as decreased renal blood flow and glomerular filtration rate (GFR) and thickening of the renal tubules, can alter the excretion of drugs in older adults, increasing the risk of drug toxicity.

(continued)

Gerontological Considerations (continued)

- Decreased ability to concentrate urine may lead to increased susceptibility to dehydration, further complicated by a deficit in thirst.
- In addition, there are structural and functional abnormalities that occur with aging, such as decreased bladder wall contractility, bladder outlet obstruction, and other things that lead to incomplete emptying of the bladder and urinary incontinence.
- Nursing interventions include "double voiding" by remaining at the toilet after initial voiding to allow time for additional urine volume to be excreted, and scheduling voiding at 1- to 2-hour intervals.
- Urine formation increases during the night, when leg elevation promotes blood return to the heart and kidneys, and may interrupt sleep patterns. Older persons may need to drink more fluids throughout the day to allow for limiting their intake after the evening meal.

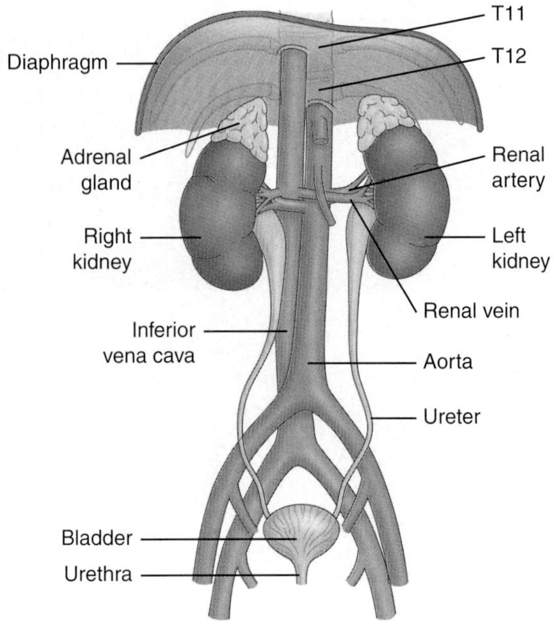

Figure 57-1 Kidneys, ureters, and bladder. The right kidney is usually lower than the left.

BOX 57-1 Functions of the Kidney

- Produce urine
- Filter and eliminate water and waste products in urine
- Maintain water balance
- Regulate pH of body fluids by reabsorbing, eliminating, and/or conserving electrolytes (sodium, potassium, hydrogen, chloride, and bicarbonate ions)
- Produce hormones that control blood pressure (renin), balance calcium and phosphorus levels (calcitriol), and regulate RBC production (erythropoietin)
- Secrete prostaglandins
- Synthesize vitamin D to active form
- Activate growth hormone

ANATOMY AND PHYSIOLOGY

The upper urinary tract is composed of the kidneys, renal pelves, and ureters. The lower urinary tract consists of the bladder, urethra, and pelvic floor muscles (Fig. 57-1).

Kidneys, Renal Pelvis, and Ureters

The two kidneys are paired, bean-shaped organs located in the upper abdomen on either side of the vertebral column. They span from the level of the 12th thoracic vertebra to the 3rd lumbar vertebra. A thin, fibrous capsule encloses each kidney; the peritoneum separates the kidney from the abdominal cavity anteriorly. There is also a layer of fatty connective tissue that anchors the kidneys in place on the muscle at the back of the abdomen, along with fascia and attached blood vessels.

A cross-section of the kidney (Fig. 57-2) helps to illustrate the inner structures. The two main areas are the renal pelvis and the parenchyma. *The parenchyma* is made up of a cortex (outer layer) and a medulla (inner core). Within each cortex are microscopic nephrons that carry out the functions of the kidneys. Each kidney contains approximately 800,000 to 1,000,000 *nephrons*, which are the smallest functional units of the kidney. Each nephron consists of the *glomerulus*, *afferent arteriole*, *efferent arteriole*, *Bowman capsule* (a membrane that surrounds a capillary network), *distal* and *proximal convoluted tubules*, the *loop of Henle*, and the *collecting tubule* (Fig. 57-3). These are the structures responsible for selective reabsorption of materials from the filtrate

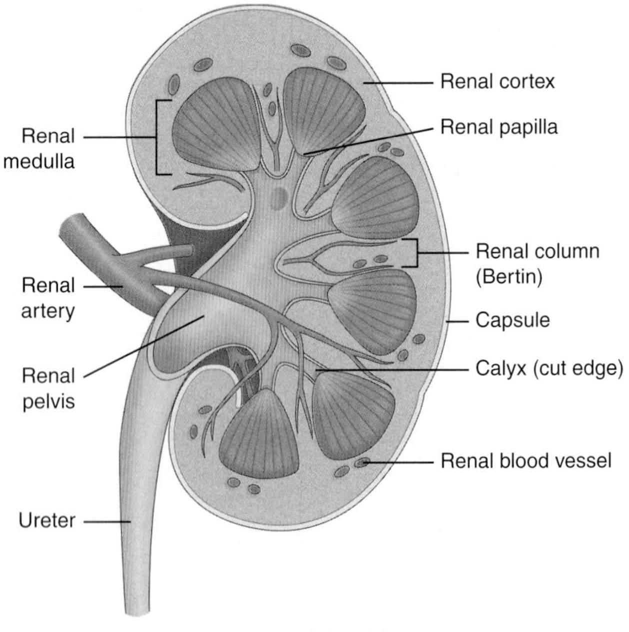

Figure 57-2 Internal structure of the kidney.

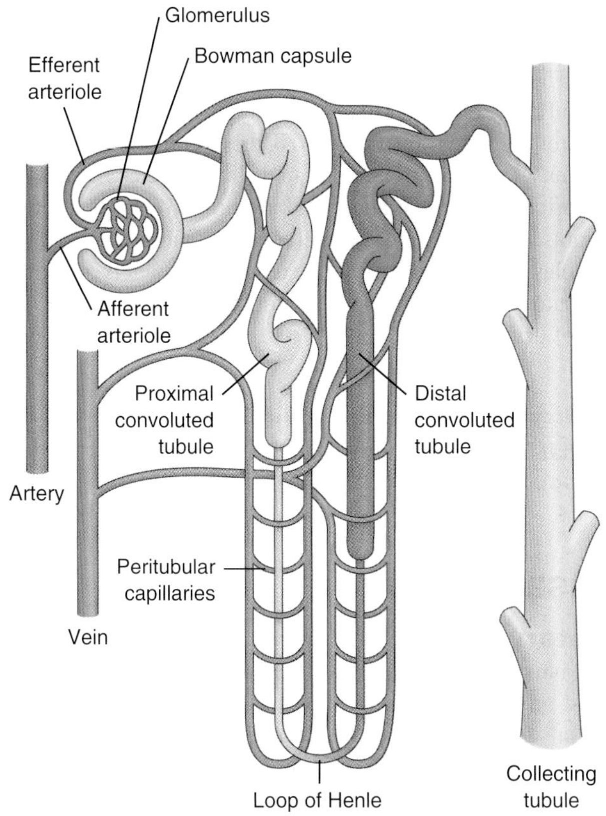

Figure 57-3 Representation of a nephron.

back to the blood, or secretion of materials from the blood into the filtrate.

The medulla contains calyces (pyramids), cone-shaped structures that open to the renal pelvis, a large funnel-like structure in the center of the kidney. The renal pelvis then empties into the ureter, which carries urine to the bladder for storage.

The blood supply to each kidney is from the renal artery. Blood enters the nephrons from the afferent arterioles. Blood then goes through the glomerulus and leaves through efferent arterioles and renal vein. The renal artery arises from the aorta, and the renal vein empties into the vena cava.

Bladder, Urethra, and Pelvic Floor Muscles

The bladder, urethra, and pelvic floor muscles form the urethrovesical unit. The urinary bladder, located just behind the pubis, is a hollow, muscular organ. Its shape and size vary with the amount of urine it contains as well as the person's age. In general, adult bladders hold 300 to 500 mL of urine.

The urethra is a hollow tube that begins at the bladder neck and ends at the external meatus. It serves as a conduit during urination and has a sphincter mechanism to prevent urine leakage. The male urethra extends approximately 24 cm (10 inches) from the bladder neck through the prostate and the penile shaft to the glans penis. The female urethra extends about 4 cm (1.5 to 2 inches) from the bladder neck to the external meatus, anterior to the vagina.

The pelvic floor muscles constitute the final part of the urethrovesical unit. These muscles form a sling that supports the bladder and urethra, rectum, and some reproductive organs.

Urine Formation

There are three steps in the complex process of urine formation:

1. *Glomerular filtration*: involves the filtration of plasma by the glomerulus (see Fig. 57-3). Filtered substances include water, sodium, chloride, bicarbonate, potassium, glucose, urea, creatinine, and uric acid. The product of glomerular filtration is referred to as the *glomerular filtrate*. Plasma proteins are too large to be filtered out and remain in the plasma.
2. *Tubular reabsorption*: the glomerular filtrate enters Bowman capsule and then moves through the tubular system of the nephron and is either reabsorbed (placed back into the systemic circulation to maintain fluid balance) or excreted in the urine. Reabsorption is accomplished with diffusion, active transport, and osmosis. Fluid balance is determined by antidiuretic hormone (ADH) (also known as *vasopressin*), which is stored in the posterior pituitary gland. ADH is secreted if there is a decrease in the blood volume or an increase in serum osmolality (concentration of the number of particles of solute in a unit of solution). As this occurs, the distal tubules and collecting tubules become more permeable in order to increase the amount of water reabsorption to the blood, increasing blood volume and increasing urine concentration. If there is excessive water intake, ADH secretion will be suppressed, increasing the amount of water in urine.
3. *Tubular secretion*: the formed urine drains from the collecting tubules, into the renal pelvis, and down each ureter to the bladder. Potassium and hydrogen ions are secreted from the blood to the tubules, in order to maintain serum potassium levels and regulate acid–base balance (pH level—normal urine pH is between 4.6 and 8.0).

The filtrate that is secreted as urine usually contains water, sodium, chloride, bicarbonate, potassium, urea, creatinine, and uric acid. Amino acids and glucose typically are reabsorbed and not excreted in the urine. Protein molecules, except for periodic small amounts of globulins and albumin, also are reabsorbed. Transient proteinuria in small amounts (less than150 mg/dL) is not considered a problem. Persistent and elevated proteinuria may indicate glomerular damage. Glycosuria (glucose in the urine) occurs when the glucose concentration in the blood and glomerular filtrate exceeds the ability of the tubules to reabsorb the glucose. Figure 57-4 summarizes the physiology and pathophysiology of urine formation.

Urine Elimination

Urine flows from the renal pelvis through the ureter into the bladder. Peristaltic waves help to move the urine to the

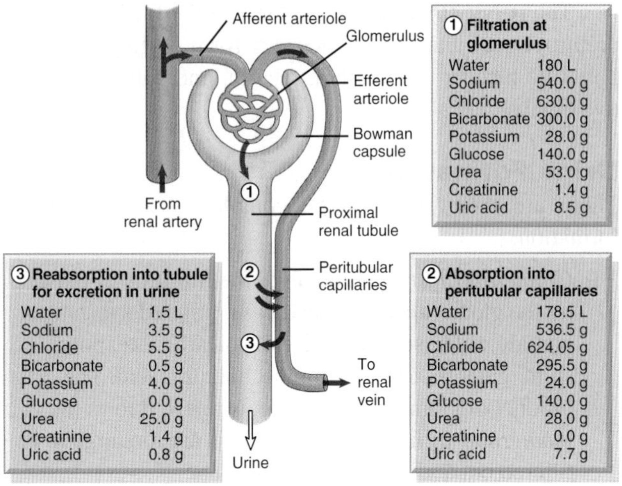

Figure 57-4 Urine is formed in the nephrons in a three-step process: filtration, reabsorption, and excretion. Water, electrolytes, and other substances, such as glucose and creatinine, are filtered by the glomerulus; varying amounts of these substances are reabsorbed in the renal tubule or excreted in the urine. Approximate normal volumes of these substances during the steps of urine formation are shown at the top. Wide variations may occur in these values depending on diet. (Reprinted with permission from Hinkle, J. L., & Cheever, K. H. (2014). *Brunner & Suddarth's textbook of medical-surgical nursing* (13th ed., p. 1510). Wolters Kluwer Health/Lippincott Williams & Wilkins.)

bladder. Normally, urine flows in one direction because of this peristaltic action and because the ureters enter the bladder at an oblique angle. Reflux of urine (urine that flows backward) can occur secondary to an overdistended bladder or other problems and may cause infections (see Chapter 59).

The desire to urinate comes from the feeling of bladder fullness. A nerve reflex is triggered when approximately 150 mL of urine accumulates. During urination, the bladder muscle contracts and the sphincter muscles relax, forcing urine out of the bladder and urethra through the urethral meatus. If there is any interference or abnormality of these muscles, the bladder may not empty completely or empty uncontrollably (incontinence). Adults generally excrete 1 to 2 L of urine per 24 hours.

››› *Stop, Think, and Respond 57-1*

What factors influence the amount of urine produced?

ASSESSMENT

History

The nurse obtains information about general health, childhood and family illnesses, past medical history, allergies, sexual and reproductive health, exposure to toxic chemicals or gas, and history of present complaint (Box 57-2). Table 57-1 describes risk factors for renal or urologic disorders. In addition to the client's chief complaint and medical history, a medication history is important. Older clients in particular may be taking multiple medications, which may affect renal function. The nurse also obtains information about voiding patterns, which may indicate renal or urologic problems (Table 57-2).

TABLE 57-1 Risk Factors for Various Renal or Urologic Disorders

RISK FACTOR	POSSIBLE RENAL OR UROLOGIC DISORDER
Childhood diseases: strep throat, impetigo, nephrotic syndrome	Chronic renal failure
Advanced age	Incomplete emptying of bladder, leading to urinary tract infection
Instrumentation of urinary tract, cystoscopy, catheterization	Urinary tract infection, incontinence
Immobilization	Kidney stone formation
Occupational, recreational, or environmental exposure to chemicals (plastics, pitch, tar, rubber)	Acute renal failure
Diabetes mellitus	Chronic renal failure, neurogenic bladder
Hypertension	Renal insufficiency, chronic renal failure
Systemic lupus erythematosus	Nephritis, chronic renal failure
Gout, hyperparathyroidism, Crohn disease	Kidney stone formation
Sickle cell anemia, multiple myeloma	Chronic renal failure
Benign prostatic hypertrophy	Obstruction to urine flow, leading to frequency, oliguria, anuria
Radiation therapy to pelvis	Cystitis, fibrosis of ureter, or fistula in urinary tract
Recent pelvic surgery	Inadvertent trauma to ureters or bladder
Obstetric injury, tumors	Incontinence
Spinal cord injury	Neurogenic bladder, urinary tract infection, incontinence

TABLE 57-2 Problems Associated With Changes in Voiding

PROBLEM	DEFINITION	POSSIBLE ETIOLOGY
Frequency	Frequent voiding—more than every 3 hours	Infection; obstruction of lower urinary tract, leading to residual urine and overflow; anxiety; diuretics; benign prostatic hyperplasia; urethral stricture; diabetic neuropathy
Urgency	Strong desire to void	Infection; chronic prostatitis; urethritis; obstruction of lower urinary tract, leading to residual urine and overflow; anxiety; diuretics; benign prostatic hyperplasia; urethral stricture; diabetic neuropathy
Dysuria	Painful or difficult voiding	Lower urinary tract infection, inflammation of bladder or urethra, acute prostatitis, stones, foreign bodies, tumors in bladder
Hesitancy	Delay, difficulty in initiating voiding	Benign prostatic hyperplasia, compression of urethra, outlet obstruction, neurogenic bladder
Nocturia	Excessive urination at night	Decreased renal concentrating ability, heart failure, diabetes mellitus, incomplete bladder emptying, excessive fluid intake at bedtime, nephrotic syndrome, cirrhosis with ascites
Incontinence	Involuntary loss of urine	External urinary sphincter injury, obstetric injury, lesions of bladder neck, detrusor muscle dysfunction, infection, neurogenic bladder, medications, neurologic abnormalities
Enuresis	Involuntary voiding during sleep	Delay in functional maturation of central nervous system (bladder control usually achieved by 5 years of age), obstructive disease of lower urinary tract, genetic factors, failure to concentrate urine, urinary tract infection, psychological stress
Polyuria	Increased volume of urine voided	Diabetes mellitus, diabetes insipidus, diuretics, excess fluid intake, lithium toxicity, certain types of kidney disease (hypercalcemic and hypokalemic nephropathy)
Oliguria	Urine output <400 mL/day	Acute or chronic renal failure (see Chapter 58), inadequate fluid intake
Anuria	Urine output <50 mL/day	Acute or chronic renal failure (see Chapter 58), complete obstruction
Hematuria	Red blood cells in the urine	Cancer of genitourinary tract, acute glomerulonephritis, renal stones, renal tuberculosis, blood dyscrasia, trauma, extreme exercise, rheumatic fever, hemophilia, leukemia, sickle cell trait or disease
Proteinuria	Abnormal amounts of protein in the urine	Acute and chronic renal disease, nephrotic syndrome, vigorous exercise, heat stroke, severe heart failure, diabetic nephropathy, multiple myeloma

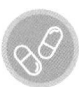

Pharmacologic Considerations

■ Drug-induced nephrotoxicity may affect up to 66% of older adults. Factors that put a client at higher risk include older than 60 years, renal insufficiency, dehydration, diabetes, heart failure, and sepsis (Naughton, 2008). Reduced kidney function increases the amount of circulating drug and possible drug toxicity.

Concept Mastery Alert

Renal Assessment

For an assessment specifically of renal function, the nurse should ask the client about voiding, hypertension, and diabetes, as well as other aspects of health. The client's occupation could also reveal whether exposure to chemicals might be affecting renal function.

BOX 57-2 Assessing the Chief Complaint Related to the Urinary System

The nurse collects information about the following:

- Voiding changes or disturbances
- Urine volume changes
- Irritative voiding symptoms (frequency, urgency, nocturia, dysuria)
- Obstructive voiding symptoms (hesitancy, straining, residual urine, retention, urinary stream force and size)
- Urinary incontinence (total overflow, stress, urge, functional)
- Urine characteristics changes (color, hematuria, clarity, odor, pH)
- Systemic manifestations (fever, weight loss)
- Gastrointestinal (GI) signs and symptoms (nausea, vomiting, diarrhea, abdominal cramping, distention)
- Pain (type, location, severity, local, referred, colic, spasms)
- Masses of the flank, abdomen, or genital areas (polycystic kidneys, hydronephrosis, renal cell carcinoma)
- Abnormal abdominal or genital appearance
- Sexual or reproductive dysfunction

Physical Examination

Before beginning the physical examination, the nurse asks the client to void. Inspection includes observing the abdomen for scars, symmetry, abdominal movements, and pulsations. Examining the back and noting any bulging, bruising, or scars are important steps.

The experienced examiner auscultates the abdomen for bruits (abnormal vascular sounds heard over a blood vessel). In addition, they percuss the area over the bladder beginning 2 inches above the symphysis pubis and moving toward the base of the bladder. Percussion usually produces

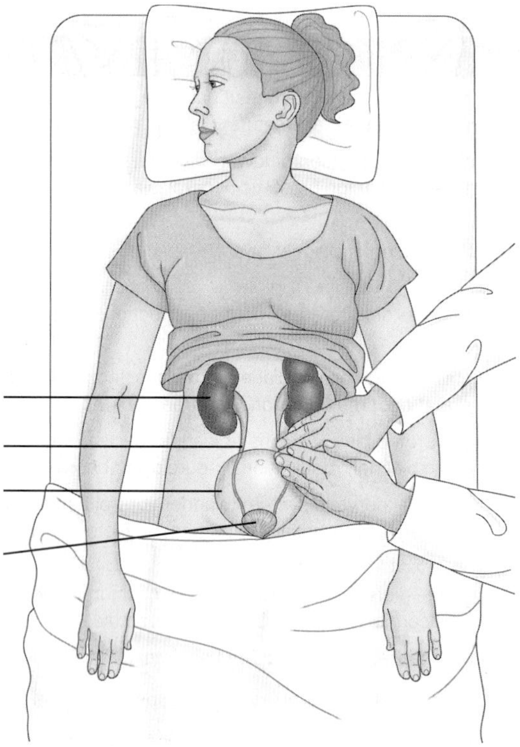

Figure 57-5 Palpation of the bladder.

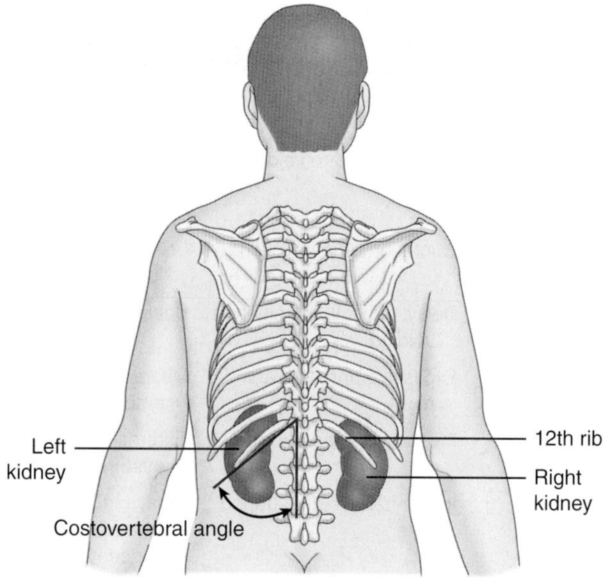

Figure 57-6 Location of the costovertebral angle (CVA). The CVA is the area used to assess the kidneys for tenderness or pain.

a tympanic sound; it produces a dull sound if the bladder is filled. The nurse can palpate the suprapubic area but can palpate the bladder only if it is moderately distended (Fig. 57-5). Assessing the kidneys for tenderness or pain is done by lightly striking the fist at the **costovertebral angle** (CVA), which is the area where the lower ribs meet the vertebrae (Fig. 57-6). Normally, the client experiences a dull thud. Pain or tenderness may indicate a renal disorder. The nurse also assesses for signs of electrolyte and water imbalances (see Chapter 16).

In addition to evaluating the client's general health, the nurse evaluates the client for signs or symptoms of

- Periorbital edema (swelling around the eyes)
- Edema of the extremities
- Cardiac failure
- Mental changes

All of these signs or symptoms may indicate urinary tract disorders. The nurse also obtains vital signs and weight.

Diagnostic Tests

In clients who are men, diseases and disorders of the reproductive system also affect the urinary system. In addition to the diagnostic tests discussed in the following sections, tests that may be performed on the men clients are discussed in Chapters 55 and 56.

Radiography

An X-ray study of the abdomen includes X-rays of the kidneys, ureters, and bladder (KUB). It is performed to show the size and position of the kidneys, ureters, and bony pelvis as well as any radiopaque urinary calculi (stones), abnormal gas patterns (indicative of renal mass), and anatomic defects of the bony spinal column (indicative of neuropathic bladder dysfunction). An X-ray of the pelvis, chest, or other area may reveal metastatic bone lesions that could be a result of renal or bladder tumors.

Ultrasonography

Renal **ultrasonography** identifies the kidney's shape, size, location, collecting systems, and adjacent tissues. Other uses include identification of renal cysts or obstruction sites, assistance in needle placement for renal biopsy or nephrostomy tube placement, and drainage of a renal abscess. There are no contraindications to this procedure. It is not invasive, does not require the injection of a radiopaque dye, and does not require fasting or bowel preparation for a renal or bladder sonography. Bladder ultrasonography is another noninvasive test to determine urine volume in the bladder. Portable, battery-operated systems are now used by nurses at the bedside for clients who may be in a bladder-training program, or if the nurse is determining the need for the client to be catheterized. The head of the scanner is placed on the client's abdomen toward the bladder. The urine volume is displayed on the scanner's screen.

Computed Tomography Scan and Magnetic Resonance Imaging

A computed tomography (CT) scan or magnetic resonance imaging (MRI) of the abdomen and pelvis may be obtained to diagnose renal pathology, determine kidney size, and evaluate tissue densities with or without contrast material. An iodine-based contrast medium may be injected intravenously (IV) after the initial scan to enhance the images, especially when vascular tumors are suspected. The CT scan also is useful in identifying calculi, congenital abnormalities, obstruction, infections, and polycystic disease. An MRI produces sharp images of the kidneys and can delineate the renal cortex from the medulla. It is also useful in identifying bladder tumors, staging renal cell carcinoma, and imaging the vascular system. Clients scheduled for an MRI must not have alcohol or caffeine for 2 hours before the procedure and cannot have food an hour prior to the MRI. Medications may be taken, except for iron supplements, which may produce artifacts and interfere with the imaging.

Angiography

Renal angiography (**renal arteriography**) provides details of the arterial supply to the kidneys, specifically the location and number of renal arteries (multiple vessels to the kidney are not unusual) and the patency of each renal artery. Other reasons for performing renal arteriography are to evaluate renal blood flow following trauma to the kidney, differentiate cysts from tumors, and assess hypertension. A catheter is passed up the femoral artery into the aorta to the level of the renal vessels. Contrast medium is then injected into the catheter, and serial X-rays are taken. The radiopaque dye first outlines the aorta in the area of the renal artery, then enters the renal artery and the kidney. A series of X-rays are taken. The catheter tip also may be passed into each renal artery for additional images. The procedure lasts 30 to 90 minutes. The nurse asks the client about allergies to foods, including iodine, and any previous dye reactions. There is evidence that being allergic to seafood is not probable for an allergy to iodine or radiocontrast material, but the question regarding seafood allergy will most likely be asked as a precaution. Clients at highest risk for an allergic reaction to radiocontrast are those with previous reactions to dye; clients with asthma, history or heart, kidney, or thyroid disease; clients taking metformin or beta-blockers; and older adults and/or clients who are women (Saljoughian, 2012). A laxative may be given prior to the procedure to empty the colon and ensure an unobstructed image.

The nurse also reviews pertinent laboratory tests (**blood urea nitrogen** [BUN], creatinine) to assess renal function, records vital signs, and assesses peripheral pulses. The nurse instructs the client to void before the procedure. If ordered, they administer a sedative to promote relaxation before the procedure.

After the procedure, the health care provider applies a pressure dressing to the femoral area, which remains in place for several hours. The nurse palpates the pulses in the legs and feet at least every 1 to 2 hours for signs of arterial occlusion. Monitoring the pressure dressing is important to note frank bleeding or hematoma formation. If either condition occurs, the nurse immediately notifies the primary provider. Another important assessment is for hypersensitivity responses to contrast material. Clients remain on bed rest for 4 to 8 hours. The nurse also monitors and documents intake and output. Client and Family Teaching 57-1 outlines education points.

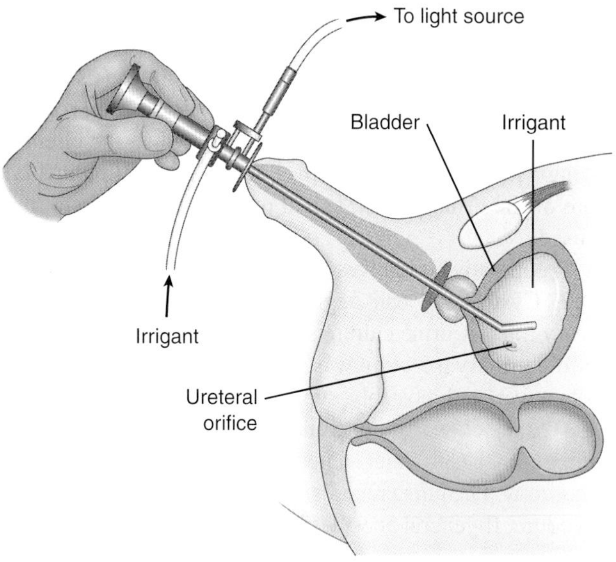

Figure 57-7 Cystoscopic examination. A rigid or semirigid cystoscope is inserted into the bladder. The upper cord is the electric source for the light at the distal end of the cystoscope. The lower tubing leads from a reservoir of sterile irrigant used to inflate the bladder.

Urologic Endoscopic Procedures

Urologic endoscopic procedures use cystoscopy, which is the direct visual examination of the inside the urethra and bladder using an instrument called a *cystoscope*. This procedure can also be used to examine ureteral orifices, the prostatic urethra in men, and the ureters and pelvis of the kidneys. Small catheters are passed through the cystoscope to accomplish this. The **cystoscope** consists of a lighted tube with a telescopic lens. A video camera can be placed over the lens to get still or moving images (Fig. 57-7).

Cystoscopy (cystourethroscopy) is used to identify the cause of painless hematuria, urinary incontinence, or urinary retention. It is useful in the evaluation of structural and functional changes of the bladder. The cystoscope is

Client and Family Teaching 57-1 Undergoing a Renal Angiography

The nurse reviews the following points with the client undergoing this test:

- Drink extra fluids on the day before the test; do not eat any food or fluids (per protocol) before testing; IV fluids will be given before, during, and after the test; medication will be given to promote relaxation; local anesthesia is administered.
- Expect a burning sensation or feeling of heat, pain, or nausea while contrast material is injected. These reactions are normal and transient.
- Remain on strict bed rest for 4 to 8 hours or more as per protocol. A urinal or bedpan must be used in the meantime.
- Drink extra fluids (2000 to 3000 mL over the 24-hour postprocedural period).

inserted either through the urethra into the bladder or percutaneously through a small abdominal incision. Urologists may obtain urine specimens, biopsy specimens (tissue examination), cell washings (cytologic analysis), or remove calculi (stones). Local anesthesia is used when the client is having a lower tract cystoscopy. For procedures that involve more of the urinary tract, spinal or general anesthesia may be used.

Preoperative sedatives or antispasmodics may be ordered. Cystoscopy can aggravate any abnormality of the urinary tract. A urine culture should be obtained before testing. If a urinary infection was present before the cystoscopy, chills, fever, and, possibly, septicemia may occur. The nurse observes the client for these and other symptoms and reports findings to the provider. Clients receive antibiotics after a cystoscopy. The nurse records vital signs before and after the procedure. If general anesthesia is used, they should monitor vital signs every 15 to 30 minutes until the client is stable. Significant prostatic obstruction may result in pain and complete urinary retention after a cystoscopy. The nurse administers medications for pain or bladder spasms postprocedure as ordered. Nursing Guidelines 57-1 has information related to the care of a client having a cystoscopy.

››› *Stop, Think, and Respond 57-2*

A client having a cystoscopy has the potential for complications. What are these?

Intravenous Urography

IV **urography** includes **intravenous pyelography** (IVP) and **excretory urography**. These procedures are radiologic studies used to evaluate the structure and function of the

NURSING GUIDELINES 57-1

Caring for the Client Having a Cystoscopy

- If an upper urinary tract cystoscopy is planned, the client may not have food or drink for several hours before the procedure.
- Inform the client that the procedure can take 10 to 30 minutes.
- Instruct the client to empty their bladder prior to the procedure.
- The client will be positioned on their back with feet in stirrups for the procedure.
- If a sedative is given, the client will feel sleepy. If general anesthesia is used, the client will be asleep. An IV line may be used to administer these medications.
- Topical lidocaine will be applied to the urethra to numb the area before the scope is passed. A small scope will be inserted after a few minutes. If the urologist plans to obtain a biopsy or do other procedures, a larger scope may be used.
- When the cystoscope is in the bladder, sterile solution is instilled to fill the bladder. This will cause an urge to urinate. The client may empty their bladder once the procedure is done.
- Clients who are sedated will need a recovery period. Clients who are not sedated are able to leave the facility.
- Provide the following instructions to all clients:
  - Blood-tinged urine or blood on toilet tissue may occur for the first few voidings after the procedure.
  - Burning with urination for a few voidings is common following a cystoscopy.
  - Urination may be more frequent for several days.
  - Use moist heat (warm washcloth) on the urethra or over the lower abdomen and/or warm sitz baths (if allowed) to relieve discomfort and bladder spasms.
  - Take antispasmodic and antibiotic medications as ordered.
  - If not contraindicated, drink extra fluids to reduce irritation.
  - Report if there are any problems with urine retention or signs of urinary infection.

NURSING GUIDELINES 57-2

Caring for the Client Undergoing Intravenous or Retrograde Pyelography

- Check the client's allergy history, especially to IV contrast dye (iodine). Inquire about previous reactions to X-ray studies that used contrast media. Report allergies to the primary provider or radiology department personnel.
- Instruct the client to fast from food for 8 to 12 hours before the pyelography. Fluids are permitted.
- Cleanse the bowel per primary provider's order so that there is no interference with visualization of the kidneys on the radiographic image. It is important that the bowel preparation be effective because poor cleansing of the intestinal tract may require that the test be repeated. Clients with a peptic ulcer or ulcerative colitis usually require modification of the bowel-cleansing preparation.
- Document baseline vital signs.
- Explain the procedure and its purpose. Tell clients that a series of X-rays will be taken after injection or instillation of IV contrast material and that the entire test requires 1 to $1^1/_2$ hours to complete.
- Caution clients that they may experience burning, hot flushing sensations, unpleasant (metallic) taste in the mouth, or nausea or vomiting as the contrast is given. Half of clients having this procedure experience nausea or vomiting. Reassure clients that these reactions are transient.
- Encourage adequate fluid intake postprocedure and voiding within 8 hours postprocedure. Burning sensation on voiding and small amounts of blood-tinged urine are normal and should disappear after the third voiding.
- Advise the use of warm tub baths to decrease urethral discomfort or spasms after a retrograde pyelography. These reactions should disappear within 24 hours.
- Instruct the client to abstain from alcohol 48 hours postprocedure to avoid irritating the bladder.
- Discuss taking antibiotics for 1 to 3 days postprocedure. Teach the client to report flank pain, chills, fever, dysuria, or bleeding. Advise client to notify primary provider should symptoms present.

KUB. It locates the site of any urinary tract obstructions and is helpful in the investigation of the causes of flank pain, hematuria, or renal colic. It is based on the ability of the kidneys to excrete a radiopaque dye (also called a *contrast medium*) in the urine. The IV radiopaque dye outlines the kidney pelves, ureters, and bladder as the blood containing the dye passes through the urinary tract. After the IV injection of contrast material, multiple X-rays of the urinary tract are taken after 1 minute (kidney visualization), at 3 to 5 minutes (renal collecting system visualization), at 10 minutes (ureters visualization), and at 20 to 30 minutes (bladder filling visualization). A postvoiding X-ray shows emptying of the bladder.

Because radiopaque dye usually contains iodine, the primary provider may inject a minute amount of the radiopaque dye IV and observe the client for 5 to 10 minutes to determine any allergy to iodine. Radiopaque dyes that do not contain iodine, called *nonionic contrast agents*, are available and produce fewer allergic reactions.

Retrograde pyelography may be performed if better visualization of the complete ureter and renal pelvis is needed. A flexible radiopaque ureteral catheter is inserted in each ureteral orifice (opening at the terminal end of the ureter), which lie on the lower posterior wall of the bladder. This is done during a cystoscopy. Visualization of the ureters and renal pelves is possible after sterile contrast medium is instilled into the renal collecting system. This procedure is also used to evaluate ureteral stent or catheter placement. Retrograde pyelography carries the risks of sepsis and severe urinary tract infection (UTI).

An IVP is scheduled before any barium test or gallbladder series that uses contrast material (iodine). If the client already is scheduled for barium studies of the upper or lower GI tract, these diagnostic tests probably will be delayed until urologic studies are completed. It may take several days for barium to be removed from the GI tract, and its presence can distort IVP findings. Nursing Guidelines 57-2 provides information on the care of the client undergoing a pyelography.

After IVP or retrograde pyelography, the nurse instructs the client to consume an adequate fluid intake. In addition, the client continues to receive IV fluid replacement. The nurse monitors and documents the intake and output, making sure that urine output is at least 30 mL/hour. Clients who are dehydrated are at high risk for renal failure from the toxic effect of the contrast medium on the kidney tissues. The nurse also monitors vital signs. If additional X-rays are needed in the next 24 hours (if the excretory function of the kidney is abnormal), the primary provider or radiology department provides instructions regarding the food and fluid intake.

The client undergoing retrograde pyelography may experience a dull ache caused by distention of the renal pelves with the radiopaque dye. The nurse observes the client for signs and symptoms of pyelonephritis (see Chapter 58) 24 to 48 hours postprocedure because of the instrumentation and injection of material. If there are any symptoms, the nurse reports them to the primary provider and obtains a urine specimen for culture and analysis. Antibiotic agents are administered as directed.

MAG3 Renogram

This test is a newer scan for assessing renal function. A radiopharmaceutical agent, called Technetium-99m or MAG3, is injected into the client's veins. A gamma camera is used to take images as the radioactive molecules circulate within the kidneys. A diuretic renogram may also be done after the initial imaging. Furosemide (Lasix), a diuretic, is injected. The resulting images allow the provider to observe urine production and flow. Overall, providers are able to better discern right and left kidney function and renal perfusion.

Biopsy

Biopsies of urinary tract tissue are taken to diagnose cancer, assess prostatic enlargement, diagnose and monitor progression of renal disease, and assess and evaluate treatment of renal transplant rejection. Bladder biopsies are obtained during cystoscopy. Information about prostate biopsy can be found in Chapter 55. Table 57-3 describes renal biopsy techniques. Renal biopsy carries the risk of postprocedural bleeding because the kidneys together receive up to 25% of the cardiac output each minute.

The nurse reassures the client undergoing a renal biopsy and explains the procedure and its purpose. In addition, they record vital signs and review pretest coagulation studies, urinalysis, IVP, and renal scan. After the procedure, the client remains on bed rest. The nurse observes the urine for signs of hematuria. It is important to assess the dressing frequently for signs of bleeding, monitor vital signs, and evaluate the type and severity of pain. Severe pain in the back, shoulder, or abdomen can indicate bleeding. The nurse notifies the primary provider of these signs and symptoms immediately. They also assess the client for difficulty voiding. The nurse needs to encourage the client to have adequate

TABLE 57-3 Techniques for Renal Biopsy

TYPE OF BIOPSY	DESCRIPTION
Needle biopsy or percutaneous kidney biopsy	• Minimally invasive • Renal tissue is removed through a needle • Useful when CT or MRI findings are inconclusive
Fine-needle aspiration biopsy	• Minimally invasive • Performed under local anesthesia in the operating room • Needle placement guided by fluoroscopy
Open biopsy	• Small incision made into flank • Usually performed if needle biopsy tissue samples are not satisfactory

CT, computed tomography; MRI, magnetic resonance imaging.

TABLE 57-4 Normal Urine Flow Rates

SEX	YOUNG ADULT (mL/second)	MIDDLE-AGED ADULT (mL/second)	OLDER ADULT (mL/second)
Man	21	12	9
Woman	18	15	10

fluid intake after the biopsy. If the client is to be discharged the following day, the nurse instructs them to

- Maintain limited activity for several days to avoid bleeding.
- Complete prophylactic antibiotic therapy as indicated.
- Notify the primary provider immediately if experiencing signs and symptoms of systemic infection (fever, malaise), UTI (dysuria, frequency, discolored urine, malodorous urine), or bleeding (hematuria, lightheadedness, flank pain, or rapid pulse).

Cystography and Voiding Cystourethrography

Cystography evaluates abnormalities in bladder structure and filling through the instillation of contrast dye and radiography. **Voiding cystourethrography** (VCUG) is similar to cystography, except that the client is instructed to void (the urine contains the radiopaque dye), and a rapid series of X-rays are taken. UTI is a contraindication to cystography or VCUG. Clients can experience pain with urination and hematuria for up to 48 hours.

Urodynamic Studies

Urodynamic studies evaluate bladder and urethral function and are performed to assess the causes of reduced urine flow, urinary retention, and urinary incontinence. Two of the main tests are uroflowmetry and cystometrography (CMG).

Uroflowmetry (determination of the urinary flow rate) is performed to evaluate bladder and sphincter function. This noninvasive procedure measures the time and rate of voiding, the volume of urine voided, and the pattern of urination. Results are compared with normal flow rates and urinary patterns. Results vary by age and sex. Table 57-4 lists normal uroflowmetry values. The client is usually catheterized afterward for a **postvoid residual**, which is the amount of urine left in the bladder after voiding and provides information about bladder function. Normal postvoid residual is 0 to 30 mL; however, retention of up to 100 mL may be acceptable in the older adult.

Cystometrography (CMG) evaluates the bladder tone and capacity. A retention catheter is inserted into the bladder after the client voids. The bladder is slowly filled with sterile saline, and the client indicates at what point the first urge to void is felt and when the bladder feels full. These measurements indicate whether the client's bladder capacity is normal. Most clients feel a mild urge to void at approximately 120 mL and a strong urge to void at about 250 mL. By comparison, clients with a neurogenic bladder (see Chapter 59) may not feel an urge to void until 500 mL or more has been instilled. In many instances, the client with a neurogenic bladder never feels an urge to void, and instillation is terminated at this point. The client is assessed for bladder contractions that they cannot control, leakage around the catheter, or leakage of urine when asked to cough. Pressures within the bladder are also assessed. The client may be given antibiotics for a day or 2 after a CMG.

Laboratory Tests

Urinalysis

Much information about systemic diseases and the condition of the kidneys and lower urinary tract can be learned by **urinalysis**, a study of the components and characteristics of the urine. Urinalysis is also useful in monitoring the effects of treatment of known urinary or renal conditions. The characteristics of normal urine and possible causes contributing to abnormal results are listed in Table 57-5. A clean-catch midstream specimen from the first voiding of the morning is preferred. The nurse teaches the client how to collect a clean-catch specimen (Client and Family Teaching 57-2, Nutrition Notes).

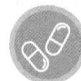

Pharmacologic Considerations

■ When the client looks healthy but the urinalysis is not yellow, it could be a drug interaction. Drugs for GI disorders to antidepressants can change urine color. If the specimen is red, orange, blue, green, or tea color, ask the client about drugs taken. Drugs can also change pH and other values.

TABLE 57-5 Urinalysis Characteristics

CHARACTERISTIC AND NORMAL VALUE	ABNORMAL FINDINGS	POSSIBLE CAUSES
Color: yellow	Colorless	Overhydration, diabetes insipidus, chronic renal disease, diuretic therapy, diabetes mellitus
	Red, pink	Hematuria, foods (beets, rhubarb, blackberries), drugs (phenothiazines, rifampin)
	Dark yellow or orange	Bilirubin, dehydration, drugs (multiple vitamins, Pyridium, Azo-Gantrisin)
	Green	*Pseudomonas* infection, bilirubin, drugs (methylene blue, amitriptyline, vitamin B complex)
	Brown	Dehydration, urobilinogen, drugs (cascara, Flagyl)
	Dark brown to black	Melanin, drugs (Macrodantin, quinine, methyldopa)

TABLE 57-5 Urinalysis Characteristics (*continued*)

CHARACTERISTIC AND NORMAL VALUE	ABNORMAL FINDINGS	POSSIBLE CAUSES
Clarity: clear	Cloudy	Phosphaturia
	Turbid	Pyuria, bacteriuria, parasitic disease
	Hazy	Mucus
	Smoky, milky	Prostatic fluid, sperm, lipids
	Pinkish precipitates	Hyperuricemia
Specific gravity: 1.003–1.029	Dilute (1.00–1.010) or concentrated (1.029–1.030)	Low: diabetes insipidus, kidney disorders High: false reading owing to pus, albumin, protein, glucose, or dextran in urine
Urine osmolality: 50–1200 mOsm/kg considered normal; 500–800 mOsm/kg average	Elevated	Fluid volume deficit
	Decreased	Fluid volume excess Renal disease
pH: 4.5–7.5	>7.5	Urinary tract infection, metabolic acidosis, Cushing syndrome, low-protein diet with large vegetable intake, diet high in dairy and citrus fruit, drugs (sodium bicarbonate, thiazides)
Ketones: none	Ketonuria	Starvation, fasting, abnormal carbohydrate metabolism, diabetes mellitus, pregnancy, pernicious anemia, vomiting, high-protein diet (Nutrition Notes)
Protein: none	Proteinuria	Cancer, severe heart failure, renal disease, glomerulonephritis, nephrotic syndrome, trauma, fever, heavy exercise
Glucose: none	Glycosuria	Diabetes mellitus, gestational diabetes
Red blood cells (RBCs): 0–3 RBCs/high-power field	>3 RBCs/high-power field	Renal disorders (glomerulonephritis, calculus, cancer, trauma, cysts), systemic disease (lupus, sickle cell, hypertension)
White blood cells: 0–4/high-power field	>4/high-power field	Urinary tract infection (acute pyelonephritis, cystitis, urethritis), renal disease, urinary stones
Bilirubin: none	Bilirubinuria	Hepatitis, biliary obstruction
Urobilinogen: <1 mg/dL	>1 mg/dL	Hepatitis, cirrhosis, congestive heart failure, hemolytic anemia
Casts: 0–2 hyaline casts/low-power field	>2/low-power field	Granular casts (glomerulonephritis, renal disease), fatty casts (nephrotic syndrome), cellular casts (glomeruli or tubule infection), hyaline casts (fever, strenuous exercise, congestive heart failure)
Crystals: none too few	Many	Urolithiasis, chronic renal failure, gout, urinary tract infection
Bacteria: negative per high-power field	Positive	Urinary tract infection, pyelonephritis, cystitis

Client and Family Teaching 57-2
Obtaining a Clean-Catch Midstream Urine Specimen

The nurse teaches the client as follows:

- Wash your hands and remove the lid from the specimen container without touching the inside of the lid.
- Open antiseptic towelette package and cleanse the urethral area.
- *Women*: Hold labia apart with one hand. Wipe down one side of the urethra with the first towelette and discard, wipe down the other side with the second towelette and discard, and wipe down the center with the third towelette and discard. Wipe one time only with each towelette from front to back.
- *Men*: Retract foreskin if uncircumcised. Clean the urethral meatus in a circular motion using each towelette one time.
- Begin voiding into the toilet, urinal, or bedpan; for women, continue to hold labia apart while voiding.
- Void 30 to 50 mL of the midstream urine into the collection container and then finish urinating into the toilet, bedpan, or urinal. Be careful not to contaminate the container.
- Carefully replace the lid, dry the container if necessary, and wash your hands.

Urine Culture and Sensitivity

When infection is suspected, a urine specimen may be taken for culture by collecting a clean-catch midstream specimen or by urinary catheterization. It is important that the urine specimen not be contaminated by skin bacteria. The container is labeled with the client's name and the time and date of the voiding. To prevent the growth of bacteria in the urine and decomposition, the nurse ensures delivery of the urine specimen immediately to the laboratory or refrigerates it promptly until it can be taken to the laboratory. See Evidence-Based Practice 57-1.

Evidence-Based Practice 57-1

Preventing Urinary Tract Infections Among Postmenopausal Women

Clinical Question

How can nurses educate premenopausal women on the prevention of UTIs?

Evidence

Women have a 40% to 50% chance of having UTIs and are 20% to 30% likely to a recurrence (Baker, 2018). Follow-up evaluations are usually not ordered unless there are nontypical symptoms. These women sometimes have a mixed diagnosis that may include overactive bladder, vaginal infection, sexually transmitted infections, pelvic dysfunction, or bladder infection. Recommended prevention includes probiotics, nonantibiotics, and education on hygiene and practices (Baker, 2018).

Nursing Implications

Nurses should be educated about UTI preventions. They can educate women with the above diagnosis on hygiene and cleaning for women, possible use of underwear with natural materials, increasing fluids, and postcoital voiding (Baker, 2018).

Reference

Baker, J. (2018). Challenges of treating urinary tract infections in post-menopausal women. *Urologic Nursing, 38*(1), 6–19, 49. https://doi.org/10.7257/1053-816X.2018.38.1.6

Nutrition Notes

Nutrition and Urinary Health

- Dietary intake can affect urine characteristics as well as urinary tract disorders and their management.
- A high-protein, low-carbohydrate diet can cause ketonuria.
- Megadoses of vitamin C can interfere with certain laboratory tests, such as for glycosuria and fecal occult blood.
- Asparagus has a weak diuretic action and produces a pungent urine odor.

24-Hour Urine Collection

Sometimes, the entire 24-hour volume of urine is collected, such as a 24-hour urine for 17-ketosteroids. The client is initially instructed to void and discard the urine. The collection bottle is marked with the time the client voided. Thereafter, all the urine is collected for the entire 24 hours. The last urine is voided at the same time the test originally began. The entire specimen is refrigerated to prevent bacterial growth. To prevent any part of the specimen from being lost or contaminated, the nurse tells the client to use separate receptacles for voiding and defecation. If any urine is discarded by mistake or lost while defecating, the nurse stops the test, because the loss of even a small amount of urine can invalidate the test.

Urine Specific Gravity

Urine specific gravity is a measurement of the kidney's ability to concentrate and excrete urine. The specific gravity measures urine concentration by measuring the density of urine and comparing it with the density of distilled water. The density of distilled water is 1 (1 mL of distilled water weighs 1 g). The number, weight, and size of urine solutes (particles) determine its specific gravity (density). Normally, the specific gravity is inversely proportional to urine volume. On a hot day, a person who is perspiring profusely and taking little fluid has low urine output with a high specific gravity. Conversely, a person who has a high fluid intake and who is not losing excessive water from perspiration, diarrhea, or vomiting has copious urine output with a low specific gravity. When the kidneys are diseased, the ability to concentrate urine may be impaired and the specific gravity remains relatively constant, no matter what the water needs of the body are or how much the client drinks.

Urine Osmolality

Urine osmolality, a more accurate measurement of urine concentration, reflects the ability of the kidney to concentrate and dilute urine by measuring the number of particles in a kilogram of solution. Osmolality of the urine and serum may be done at the same time in order to determine clients' fluid status and renal function. Urine osmolality normally ranges from 50 to 1200 mOsm/kg, averaging 500 to 800 mOsm/kg. Serum osmolality is 275 to 295 mOsm/kg. The ratio between urine and serum osmolality is normally 3:1. A client with kidney disease does not concentrate urine effectively, if at all, resulting in decreased urine and serum osmolality, and a low ratio. A higher ratio is seen in clients with concentrated urine. Urine osmolality may be done as a random specimen, or with a 12- or 24-hour urine collection.

Urine Protein (Albumin)

The **urine protein test** is used to identify renal disease. Normally, protein is minimally present in the urine. An increase in urine protein levels also may be seen with salt depletion, strenuous exercise, fever, or dehydration. Proteinuria in an individual urine specimen may be detected by dipping a test reagent stick (dipstick method) in the urine and comparing color changes with the provided color chart.

Creatinine Clearance Test

A **creatinine clearance test** is used to determine kidney function and creatinine excretion. **Creatinine** is a substance that results from the breakdown of phosphocreatine (an amino acid waste product), which is present in muscle tissue. It is filtered by the glomeruli and is excreted at a fairly constant rate by the kidney. The total amount of excreted creatinine is called *creatinine clearance*. The renal tubules increase creatinine secretion with any decrease in GFR (renal failure). Muscle necrosis and atrophy greatly increase urinary creatinine owing to accompanying protein catabolism. For this test, a 4-, 12-, or 24-hour urine specimen and a sample of blood (serum creatinine) are collected. The blood sample is obtained either at the midpoint or at the beginning and end of urine collection (varies per protocol). Both urine and blood samples are sent to the laboratory.

TABLE 57-6 Normal Serum Values and Renal Disease

PARAMETER	NORMAL VALUE	CHANGE SEEN IN RENAL DISEASE
Calcium	8.8–10 mg/dL	Decreased in renal failure
Carbon dioxide combining power	23–30 mmol/L	Decreased in acute renal failure
Magnesium	1.3–2.1 mEq/L	Decreased in chronic renal disease
Phosphate, inorganic phosphorus	2.7–4.5 mg/dL	Increased in renal failure
Potassium	3.5–5.0 mEq/L	Increased in renal failure
Total protein	6.0–8.0 g/dL	Increased in poor renal function; decreased in nephrotic syndrome
Sodium	135–148 mmol/L	Decreased in severe nephritis; increased in renal disease
Blood urea nitrogen	7–18 mg/dL	Increased in renal disease and urinary obstruction
Creatinine	Men: 0.7–1.3 mg/dL Women: 0.6–1.1 mg/dL	Increased in renal disease or insufficiency
Albumin	>60 years: 3.4–4.8 g/dL <60 years: 3.5–5 g/dL	Decreased in renal failure
Chloride	98–107 mEq/L	Decreased in renal failure (onset)
Uric acid	Men: 4.5–8 ng/dL Women: 2.5–6.2 ng/dL	Increased in renal failure

Pharmacologic Considerations

- When creatinine clearance is decreased, drug-induced nephrotoxicity could be the problem. Antibiotics, antihypertensives, antivirals, chemotherapy agents, and nonsteroidal anti-inflammatory drugs (NSAIDs) are all drugs that can affect the renal system negatively.

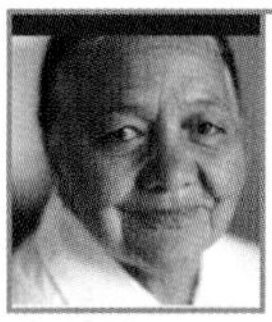

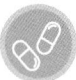

Clinical Scenario A 75-year-old woman tells her new primary care provider (PCP) that for the last year, she has had more problems with urinary incontinence and was treated for three UTIs. The PCP determines that more information is needed and orders several diagnostic tests for this client. The client is referred to a urology practice to have these tests and procedures done. **What are the important considerations for the nurse when overseeing the care of this client? See the Nursing Process section for clients having diagnostic testing for renal or urologic disorders.**

Renal Function Blood Tests

When the nephrons fail to remove waste products efficiently from the body, the blood chemistry is altered. Deterioration in renal function is manifested by rises in the BUN and creatinine values, both of which are protein breakdown products. Table 57-6 lists normal values of common blood studies performed on clients with signs and symptoms of a urinary system disorder as well as renal implications regarding abnormal results. A moderate decrease in renal function occurs, however, before these values rise.

NURSING PROCESS FOR THE CLIENT UNDERGOING DIAGNOSTIC TESTING FOR A RENAL OR UROLOGIC DISORDER

Assessment

Interview the client to determine past experience with the test or other urologic procedures. Ask the client to discuss the nature of past experiences and expectations for the current tests. If the client has preparations ordered before the test, check to see that the client understands the preparations and that they are complete. Review the client's history and determine whether there is any allergy history to contrast agents, if applicable.

Take the client's vital signs and weigh the client to provide a baseline. Depending on the test, tell the client that she will be asked to void. If informed consent is required (necessary for invasive procedures), check for the signed consent form. Client and family members need teaching and reassurance about the purpose of the test and what the procedure involves. They also need to know the care required after the procedure.

(continued)

NURSING PROCESS FOR THE CLIENT UNDERGOING DIAGNOSTIC TESTING FOR A RENAL OR UROLOGIC DISORDER (continued)

Diagnosis, Planning, and Interventions

Clients undergoing diagnostic testing are often anxious and worried. Clients having urologic testing may feel embarrassed and afraid that the testing will be painful. Provide privacy, reassurance, and information and maintain a professional and empathic attitude.

Acute Anxiety and Fear: Related to uncertainty of outcomes of diagnostic testing and the undertaking of an unfamiliar experience
Expected Outcome: Client will verbalize reduced apprehension about diagnostic testing.

- Assess client's level of anxiety. *A high level of fear interferes with learning and cooperation.*
- Explain or reexplain the test, diagnostic procedure, equipment, tubes, or drains to be used. *Thorough understanding of what is expected promotes compliance and cooperation and decreases fear.*
- Use simple language with client or significant others, especially with outpatient procedures or tests. *Using words and language that the client can understand promotes understanding and cooperation.*
- Answer questions about testing or consult with other health team members in matters that involve their expertise. *Additional information provides clarification, promotes understanding, and reduces anxiety.*
- Acknowledge appropriateness of client's feelings; correct any misinterpretations. Avoid false reassurances. Encourage client to verbalize thoughts and feelings. *Acknowledgment of a client's fears conveys acceptance of the client and allows them to focus on instructions and what is expected.*
- Provide a calm, nonthreatening environment. Respond to client's needs as quickly as possible. Encourage significant other(s) to stay with the client. *These measures convey calm and promote client's ability to cope.*
- Administer sedative medications as ordered. *Medication reduces anxiety and assists the client to proceed with the test.*

Knowledge Deficiency: Related to diagnostic procedures, tests, and preprocedural and postprocedural care
Expected Outcome: Client will be able to demonstrate or verbalize an understanding of diagnostic procedure, test, and precare and postcare.

- Provide for physical comfort and quiet atmosphere for the client (or significant other) without disruptions. *Doing so allows for concentration on topic and limits distractions.*
- Assess client's knowledge base; explain the purpose of and discuss the procedure or test. *These steps incorporate prior knowledge and promote learning.*
- Move from general to specific details (i.e., radiologic site, required medications, equipment, IV lines, anesthesia, precare and postcare, catheters, or drains used). *Doing so provides a foundation of knowledge and proceeds to more specific information.*
- Discuss home care (i.e., fluid intake, medication use, signs and symptoms of genitourinary infection) and postprocedural conditions requiring primary provider follow-up (i.e., frank bleeding, inability to urinate, increased pain, or fever). *The nurse provides essential information for home care and builds on the foundation of information about the procedure.*
- Discuss concerns about radiographic exposure or refer concerns to the primary provider or radiologist. *Expressing concerns reduces their effects and provides a means to access other resources.*
- Encourage questions, repetition of information, and return demonstration (as appropriate) from the client or significant other. *Repetition of information and return demonstrations internalize information and behaviors.*

Evaluation of Expected Outcomes

The client reports a decrease in her fear and demonstrates a better understanding of the tests or procedures or both. The client adheres to instructions.

KEY POINTS

- Anatomy and physiology:
  - Kidneys, renal pelvis, and ureters: involved in the production of urine
  - Bladder, urethra, and pelvis floor muscles: involved in the elimination of urine
  - Urine formation: process of making urine
  - Urine elimination: process of removing urine from the body
- Diagnostic testing include:
  - Radiography
  - Ultrasonography
  - CT or MRI
  - Angiography
  - Urologic endoscopic procedures
  - IV urography
  - Biopsy
  - Cystography
  - Urodynamic studies

- Laboratory tests:
  - Urinalysis
  - Urine culture and sensitivity
  - 24-hour urine collection
  - Urine protein
  - Creatinine clearance test

CRITICAL THINKING EXERCISES

1. A client is admitted with dehydration. What urinalysis results would support this diagnosis?

2. A client who is scheduled for IVP later in the day mentions that they had a reaction to dye during a previous X-ray study. What action should the nurse take?

3. A client who was hospitalized for abdominal surgery had a Foley catheter for several days. It was removed. The nurse noticed that the client's first voided urine was concentrated and cloudy and had a strong odor. What actions does the nurse need to initiate?

4. What explanation would you provide for a client who has to have a postvoid residual?

NCLEX-STYLE REVIEW QUESTIONS PrepU

1. A nurse collects a urine sample from a client and notes that the urine appears somewhat red. Which action should the nurse take next?
1. Ask the client how long they have had reddish urine.
2. Inform the client that the urine is bloody.
3. Question the client about what medications they are taking.
4. Report this finding to the charge nurse.

2. A nurse caring for a client who was in a motor vehicle accident notes that the client has a low RBC count but no obvious signs of bleeding. The nurse anticipates that which of the following tests will be done next?
1. Bladder ultrasound
2. MRI
3. Renal arteriogram
4. X-ray of the KUB

3. A nurse, caring for a client scheduled for an IVP, explains that a laxative is ordered prior to the IVP. What is the nurse's best explanation for giving the client a laxative?
1. "An empty bowel reduces the potential for constipation or impaction following the procedure."
2. "Having an empty bowel prevents accidental fecal incontinence during the X-ray."
3. "If the bowel is empty, the primary provider can also examine the lower GI tract."
4. "When the bowel is empty, the urologist can better visualize the urinary structures."

4. The nurse assesses the client with diarrhea for signs of fluid volume deficit. Which assessment finding best indicates that the client is becoming dehydrated?
1. The client's blood pressure is elevated.
2. The client's heart rate is irregular.
3. The client's mucous membranes are pink.
4. The client's urine is dark yellow.

5. The primary provider orders a 24-hour urine collection for a client who develops signs and symptoms that resemble Cushing syndrome. The nurse is most accurate in instructing the client that the urine collection will begin at what time?
1. After the client's next voiding
2. At midnight
3. At noontime
4. With the client's next voiding

WANT TO KNOW MORE? There are a wide variety of online resources available on thePoint to enhance learning and understanding of this chapter.

Go to **thePoint.lww.com/activate** and use the activation code found in the front of this text to unlock these online resources.

58

Caring for Clients With Disorders of the Kidneys and Ureters

Words To Know

acute glomerulonephritis
acute kidney injury
acute tubular necrosis
anasarca
anuria
arteriovenous fistula
arteriovenous graft
azotemia
bruit
calciuria
calculus
casts
chronic kidney disease
colic
dialysate
dialysis
dialyzer
disequilibrium syndrome
end-stage kidney disease
extracorporeal shock wave lithotripsy
glomerulonephritis
hematuria
hemodialysis
hydronephrosis
nephrectomy
nephrolithiasis
nephrostomy tube
nocturia
oliguria
osteodystrophy
periorbital edema
peritoneal dialysis
peritonitis
primary glomerulonephritis
proteinuria
pyelonephritis
pyeloplasty
pyuria
secondary glomerulonephritis
thrill
uremia
uremic frost
ureteral stent
ureterolithiasis
ureteroplasty
urolithiasis

Learning Objectives

On completion of this chapter, you will be able to:

1. Differentiate pyelonephritis and glomerulonephritis.
2. Name problems the nurse manages when caring for clients with glomerulonephritis.
3. Explain the pathophysiology and associated renal complications of polycystic disease.
4. Give examples of conditions that predispose to renal calculi.
5. Identify methods for eliminating small renal calculi and larger stones.
6. Discuss the nursing management of a client with a nephrostomy tube.
7. Describe conditions that cause a ureteral stricture.
8. Explain the classical triad of symptoms associated with renal cancer.
9. Discuss problems the nurse manages when caring for a client with a nephrectomy.
10. Differentiate acute kidney injury and chronic kidney disease.
11. Explain pathophysiologic problems associated with chronic kidney disease.
12. Describe sources of organs for kidney transplantation.
13. Identify nursing methods for managing pruritus.
14. Explain the purposes and methods of dialysis.
15. Discuss nursing assessments performed when caring for clients undergoing dialysis.

The most common urologic disorders are infectious and inflammatory conditions. Those that affect the kidneys are extremely dangerous because damage to the nephrons can result in permanent renal dysfunction. The same is true of other upper urinary tract disorders such as kidney and ureteral stones and tumors. The consequences can lead to acute or chronic kidney disease.

Gerontologic Considerations

■ Urinary obstruction is the most common cause of pyelonephritis in the older adult. When present, the older adult may not experience the fever and difficulty voiding common in younger adults. Accurate assessment of urine volume is critical.

Gerontologic Considerations (continued)

■ Acute glomerulonephritis in the older adult usually occurs in those with preexisting chronic glomerulonephritis, often caused by streptococcus or gram-negative bacteria. Glomerulonephritis may occur as immunity declines as an immunologic reaction to another system disease, such as lupus (lupus erythematosus), or as the result of unknown causes.
■ Symptoms in the older adult are subtle and nonspecific (e.g., nausea, malaise, arthralgia, exacerbation of preexisting illness) and therefore may go undetected. Heart or renal failure symptoms may accompany the presentation.
■ Thorough documentation promotes careful consideration of subtle changes in older adults.
■ The older adult is at high risk for acute kidney injury (AKI) because of a decline in the glomerular filtration rate, loss of nephrons, and reduced glomeruli. Prognosis is favorable, and treatment for older adults is the same as for younger adults.
■ Continuous ambulatory peritoneal dialysis (CAPD) may be an appropriate treatment option for older clients who do not meet the qualifications for kidney transplant. Planning with the older adult and family or caregivers should include monitoring for subtle subjective changes or sudden abrupt changes that indicate a serious complication. Using a teach-back method assures that clients with limited health literacy can safely manage the CAPD (Jain et al., 2015).

INFECTIOUS AND INFLAMMATORY DISORDERS OF THE KIDNEY

Infectious and inflammatory disorders of the kidney affect structures such as the renal pelvis, the nephrons, or both.

Pyelonephritis

Pyelonephritis is an acute or chronic bacterial infection of the kidney and the lining of the collecting system (kidney pelvis). *Acute pyelonephritis* presents with moderate-to-severe symptoms that usually last 1 to 2 weeks. If the treatment of acute pyelonephritis is unsuccessful and the infection recurs, it is termed *chronic pyelonephritis*.

Pathophysiology and Etiology

Bacteria ascend to the kidney and kidney pelves by way of the bladder and urethra. Normal fecal flora such as *Escherichia coli*, *Klebsiella pneumoniae*, *Proteus mirabilis*, *Streptococcus fecalis*, *Pseudomonas aeruginosa*, and *Staphylococcus aureus* are the most common bacteria that cause acute pyelonephritis. *E. coli* accounts for about 85% of infections. Additional risk factors for chronic pyelonephritis, such as urinary obstruction and reflux (Fig. 58-1), are listed in Box 58-1.

BOX 58-1 Risk Factors for Pyelonephritis

Acute Pyelonephritis
- Instrumentation of the urethra and bladder (catheterization, cystoscopy, urologic surgery)
- Inability to empty the bladder
- Pregnancy
- Urinary stasis
- Urinary obstruction (tumors, strictures, calculi, prostatic hypertrophy)
- Diabetes mellitus
- Other renal disease (polycystic kidney disease [PKD])
- Neurogenic bladder (stroke, multiple sclerosis, spinal cord injury)
- Women with increased sexual activity, diaphragm, spermicide use, failure to void after intercourse, history of recent urinary infection
- Men who perform anal intercourse, infection with HIV

Chronic Pyelonephritis
- Recurrent episodes of acute pyelonephritis
- Chronic obstruction (e.g., strictures and stones)
- Reflux disorders that allow urine to flow backward up the ureters

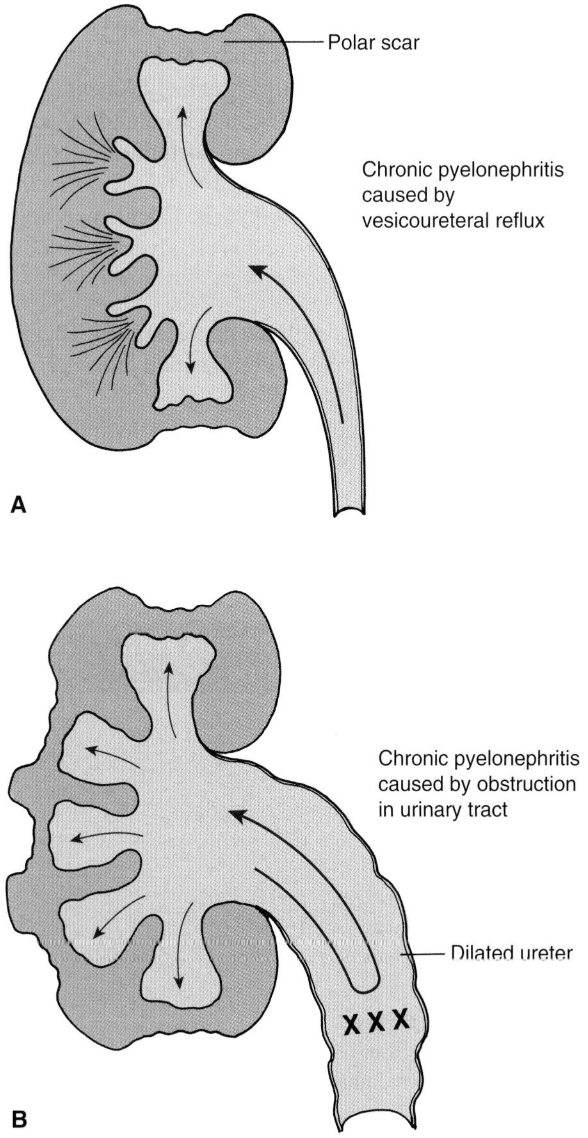

Figure 58-1 Causes of chronic pyelonephritis include **(A)** vesicoureteral reflux and **(B)** urinary tract obstruction.

In acute pyelonephritis, the inflammation causes the kidneys to grossly enlarge. The cortex and medulla develop multiple abscesses. The renal calyces and pelves also can become involved. Resolution of the inflammation results in fibrosis and scarring. Chronic pyelonephritis develops after recurrent episodes of acute pyelonephritis. The kidneys manifest irreversible degenerative changes and become small and atrophic. If destruction of nephrons is extensive, renal failure develops. Renal dysfunction may not occur for 20 or more years after the onset of the disease. About 10% to 15% of clients with chronic pyelonephritis require dialysis.

>>> ***Stop, Think, and Respond 58-1***

Explain why a client with an indwelling catheter is at risk for acute pyelonephritis.

Assessment Findings

Signs and Symptoms

Flank pain or tenderness, chills, fever, and malaise occur in clients with acute pyelonephritis. Frequency and burning on urination are present if there is accompanying cystitis (bladder infection). Some clients with chronic pyelonephritis are asymptomatic; others have a low-grade fever and vague gastrointestinal complaints. Polyuria and nocturia develop when the tubules of the nephrons fail to reabsorb water efficiently. There may be hematuria and/or pyuria. Clients may report that their urine has a foul odor and is cloudy and/or bloody.

Diagnostic Findings

A urinalysis demonstrates multiple abnormalities. The chief abnormality is **pyuria** or pus (a combination of bacteria and leukocytes) in the urine (Box 58-2).

A urine culture identifies the causative microorganism. The primary provider initially may perform an ultrasound or computed tomography (CT) scan to determine if there is obstruction in the urinary tract.

A voiding cystourethrogram (VCUG) is an X-ray that is done with contrast. Images are taken while the bladder is full and then while the client voids. The purpose is to determine if there are any structural abnormalities.

An X-ray of the kidneys, ureters, and bladder may reveal calculi, cysts, or tumors in the kidney or other urinary structures.

A dimercaptosuccinic acid (DMSA) scintigraphy is an imaging procedure that involves the injection of a very small amount of radioactive material. Images are taken as the radioactive substance is passing through the kidneys. Infection and/or scarring in the kidneys will be evident with this test.

The diagnosis of chronic pyelonephritis is based on a history of repeated acute pyelonephritis. Serum creatinine and blood urea nitrogen (BUN) levels, if elevated, indicate impaired renal function.

Medical and Surgical Management

Treatment of acute pyelonephritis includes relieving fever and pain and prescribing antimicrobial drugs such as trimethoprim-sulfamethoxazole (TMP-SMZ, Septra), gentamycin with or without ampicillin, cephalosporin, or ciprofloxacin (Cipro) for 14 days. Two weeks after the client completes initial treatment, a follow-up urine culture is done. Antispasmodics and anticholinergics such as oxybutynin (Ditropan) and propantheline (Pro-Banthine) are additional pharmacologic interventions that relax the smooth muscles of the ureters and bladder, promote comfort, and increase bladder capacity (Drug Therapy Table 58-1). Symptoms usually disappear within a few days of antibiotic therapy. Four to 6 weeks of drug therapy are prescribed for clients with a history of frequent relapsing infections with the same microorganism.

The goal of treatment for chronic pyelonephritis is to prevent progressive kidney damage. When possible, any urinary tract obstruction is relieved to save the kidney from destruction. An effort is made to improve the client's overall health. A **nephrectomy**, the surgical removal of a kidney, is performed if severe hypertension develops and if the other kidney has adequate function.

BOX 58-2 Urinalysis Results With Pyelonephritis

Acute Pyelonephritis

- Bacteria and bacterial casts
- Leukocytes (large)
- Casts (leukocytes, granular, renal tubular)
- Red blood cells (few)
- Low specific gravity
- Slightly alkaline pH
- Proteinuria (minimal to mild)
- Urine culture: organism colony count of >100,000 organisms/mm urine

Chronic Pyelonephritis

- Leukocytes (increased)
- Proteinuria (absent, minimal, or intermittent)
- Bacteria
- Casts (present in early stages and absent in late stages)
- Low specific gravity

TABLE 58-1 Causes of Urinary Tract Obstruction

LEVEL OF OBSTRUCTION	CAUSE
Renal pelvis	Renal calculi Papillary necrosis
Ureter	Renal calculi Pregnancy Tumors that compress the ureter Ureteral stricture Congenital disorders of the ureterovesical junction and ureteropelvic junction strictures
Bladder and urethra	Bladder cancer Neurogenic bladder Bladder stones Prostatic hyperplasia or cancer Urethral strictures Congenital urethral defects

Reprinted with permission from Grossman, S. C., & Porth, C. M. (2014). *Porth's pathophysiology: Concepts of altered health states* (9th ed., p. 1085). Wolters Kluwer Health/Lippincott Williams & Wilkins.

DRUG THERAPY TABLE 58-1 Agents to Treat Pyelonephritis

Category and Common Generic (Brand) Drugs	Intended Use	Common Side Effects	Safety Warnings for Nurses
Antimicrobials			
Fluoroquinolones Ciprofloxacin (Cipro) Levofloxacin (Levaquin)	Broad-spectrum drugs designed to target a large number of bacterial strains	Nausea, diarrhea	• Photosensitivity, sunscreen when out even on cloudy days
Sulfonamide Sulfamethoxazole/trimethoprim (Bactrim, Septra)	Bacteriostatic reduces number of gram-negative/-positive bacteria	Nausea, vomiting, diarrhea, headache	• Photosensitivity, sunscreen when out even on cloudy days • Monitor for skin reaction, can be severe • Monitor for lower blood sugar if oral hypoglycemic are taken
Cephalosporins Ceftriaxone (Rocephin) Cefaclor	Kill susceptible microorganisms by interfering with bacterial cell wall development	Nausea, vomiting, diarrhea, headache	• May show allergy if allergic to penicillin • Avoid alcohol intake • Monitor for nephrotoxicity
Aminoglycosides Gentamicin	Kills susceptible gram-negative microorganisms by interfering with protein synthesis	Dizziness, vertigo, nausea, vomiting	• Monitor for ototoxicity and nephrotoxicity • Do not use if client has Parkinson disease

Nursing Management

The nurse obtains complete medical, drug, and allergy histories and assesses vital signs, reporting abnormal findings such as elevated temperature or blood pressure (BP). Continued and regular monitoring of vital signs is important to detect any evidence of changes. A physical examination helps the nurse determine the location of discomfort and any signs of fluid retention such as peripheral edema or shortness of breath. The nurse observes and documents the characteristics of the client's urine. A clean-catch urine specimen is collected for urinalysis and urine culture. The nurse measures intake and output and recommends, if not contraindicated, a liberal daily fluid intake of approximately 3000 to 4000 mL to flush infectious microorganisms from the urinary tract. The nurse also administers prescribed medications and evaluates laboratory test results such as BUN, creatinine, serum electrolytes, and urine culture to determine the client's response to therapy. If chronic pyelonephritis develops, the treatment often is lengthy. Poor health and prolonged medical therapy are discouraging. The nurse urges the client to follow the recommendations of the primary provider and adhere to the prescribed medication regimen. Client and Family Teaching 58-1 outlines important teaching points.

Acute Glomerulonephritis

Acute glomerulonephritis (may also be referred to as glomerular disease) is the inflammation of the glomeruli in the kidneys. The glomeruli are capillaries that filter substances from the plasma. **Primary glomerulonephritis** occurs independently of other chronic conditions but usually is an acute postinfectious process. **Secondary glomerulonephritis** results from other conditions, such as lupus erythematosus or diabetes. Acute glomerulonephritis, if it causes severe or prolonged inflammation, can progress to chronic glomerulonephritis, and there is a risk of kidney failure in some clients.

Client and Family Teaching 58-1
Acute Pyelonephritis

The teaching plan for the client with acute pyelonephritis includes the following recommendations:

- Review information about the disease, its cause, related risk factors, treatment, and preventive measures.
- Read about the purpose, dosage, side effects, and toxic effects of all prescribed medications.
- Complete the entire regimen of antimicrobial therapy as indicated, even if symptoms abate.
- Drink a large volume of oral fluids daily unless contraindicated.
- Avoid alcohol and caffeine products if bladder spasms are present or until a clinical response to therapy is verified.
- Demonstrate how to collect a clean-catch midstream urine specimen for subsequent medical follow-up at 2 weeks and 3 months after treatment.
- Have your BP monitored intermittently.
- Consult the primary care provider if you experience signs of recurring or worsening pyelonephritis or lower urinary tract infections (UTI) (frequency, urgency, burning, cloudy urine, and fever).
- Practice methods to prevent reinfection—women should wipe from front to back after defecation and wear cotton undergarments. Void every 2 to 3 hours when awake and before and after intercourse. Avoid the use of feminine hygiene products.

Pathophysiology and Etiology

Acute **glomerulonephritis** usually occurs as a result of bacterial infections, which include group A beta-hemolytic streptococcal infections, bacterial endocarditis, or impetigo (skin infection). Viral infections such as hepatitis B or C, human immunodeficiency virus (HIV), varicella-zoster virus, or Epstein–Barr virus can also cause glomerulonephritis. The relationship between the infection and acute glomerulonephritis is not clear. Microorganisms are not present in the kidney when symptoms appear, but the glomeruli are acutely inflamed. The inflammatory response most likely results from antigen–antibody stimulation in the glomerular capillary membrane (National Kidney Foundation, 2020). The disruption of membrane permeability causes red blood cells (RBCs) and protein molecules to filter from the glomeruli into Bowman capsule and eventually become lost in the urine. Figure 58-2 outlines the sequence of events in acute glomerulonephritis.

Assessment Findings

Signs and Symptoms

Many clients with glomerulonephritis have no symptoms. Early symptoms may be so slight that the client does not seek medical attention. Occasionally the onset is sudden, with pronounced symptoms such as fever, nausea, malaise, headache, generalized edema, or **periorbital edema**, puffiness around the eyes. Some clients are first diagnosed from a routine urinalysis that reveals hematuria through microscopic examination. Often, clients present with the following symptoms:

- Pink or cola-colored urine from RBCs being excreted in the urine (**hematuria**)
- Foamy-appearing urine from **proteinuria** (excess serum albumin excreted in the urine)
- Hypertension
- Edema with evidence of swelling in the hands, feet, abdomen, and periorbital edema
- Fatigue related to anemia or kidney failure

Some clients experience pain or tenderness over the kidney area and mild-to-moderate hypertension. Their appetite may be poor, and **nocturia** (urination during the night) may be present. Irritability and shortness of breath also develop. As the condition progresses, the client develops obvious hematuria (blood in the urine), anemia (from the hematuria), convulsions associated with hypertension, congestive heart failure, **oliguria** (low urine output of 100 to 500 mL/day), and perhaps **anuria** (less than 100 mL of urine over 24 hours). Fluid retention and hypertension contribute to visual disturbances, often as a result of papilledema or hemorrhage in the eye, and epistaxis (nosebleeds).

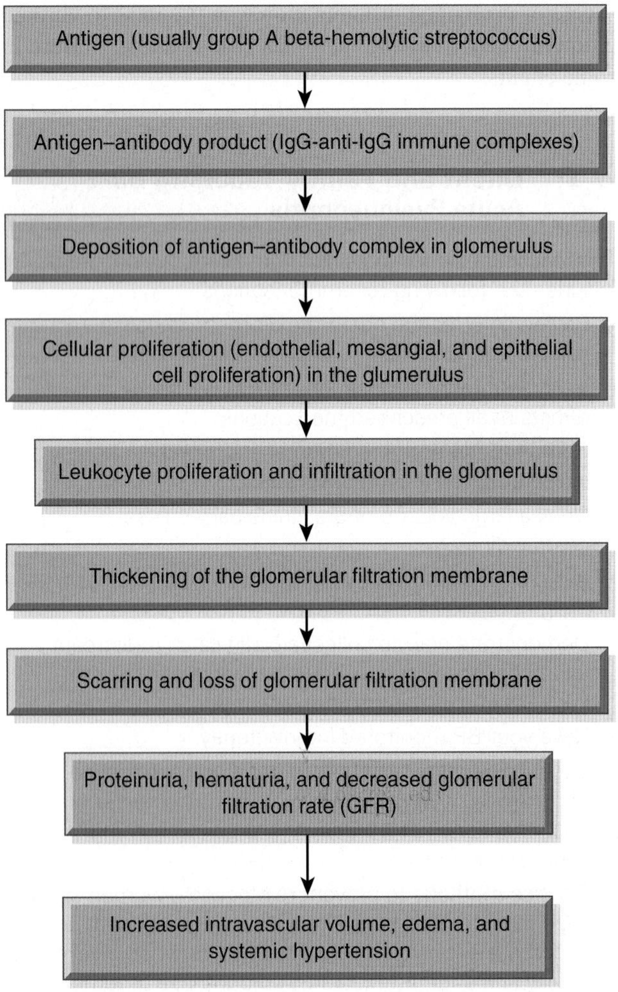

Figure 58-2 Sequence of events in acute glomerulonephritis.

Diagnostic Findings

Gross or microscopic hematuria gives the urine a dark, smoky, or frank bloody appearance. Laboratory findings include proteinuria and an elevated antistreptolysin O titer from the recent streptococcal infection. There are decreased hemoglobin, slightly elevated BUN and serum creatinine levels, and an elevated erythrocyte sedimentation rate. If renal insufficiency develops, serum electrolyte levels indicate hyperkalemia, hypermagnesemia, hypocalcemia, and dilutional hyponatremia. Percutaneous renal biopsy reveals cellular changes characteristic of an antigen–antibody response and the extent of damage that already has occurred. The kidneys are edematous and congested from the inflammatory process. When acute glomerulonephritis progresses, BP rises to more than 140/90 mm Hg. Renal function declines further, and end-stage renal disease (ESRD) can develop.

Medical Management

No specific treatment exists for acute glomerulonephritis. Preserving kidney function and preventing complications are the primary goals. Treatment is guided by the symptoms and the underlying abnormality. Treatment may consist of bed rest, a sodium-restricted diet (if edema or hypertension is present), and antimicrobial drugs to prevent a superimposed infection in the already inflamed kidney. Penicillin may be used to abolish any remaining streptococci from the recent infection. Diuretics to reduce edema and antihypertensive agents for severe hypertension may be necessary. Vitamins are added to the diet to improve general resistance, and oral iron supplements may be needed to counteract anemia. Corticosteroids and immunosuppressive agents may be given to treat a rapidly progressive inflammatory process. Any increase in hematuria, proteinuria, or BP indicates a need for aggressive treatment, including dialysis. The client is not considered cured until the urine is free of protein and RBCs for 6 months. Return to full activity usually is not permitted until the urine is free of protein for 1 month.

Nursing Management

The client must maintain bed rest when the BP is elevated and edema is present. The nurse collects daily urine specimens to assist with evaluating the client's response to treatment. They assess BP every 4 hours or as ordered. Encouraging adequate fluid intake and measuring intake and output are important nursing interventions. Although the diet may be restricted in sodium and protein, it is necessary for the client to have adequate carbohydrate intake to prevent the catabolism of body protein stores.

Client teaching aims to accomplish the following:

- Identify the specific amount of sodium that is allowed and the sources of sodium to avoid.
- Explain the purpose of diuretic therapy or other prescribed medications, the dosing regimen, and side effects.
- Recommend regular BP monitoring.
- Caution client to avoid contact with persons who have infections.
- Emphasize adherence to keeping medical appointments and the necessity for repeated urinalyses.
- Advise client to contact the primary provider if urinary volumes diminish, there is unexplained weight gain, or headaches or nosebleeds occur.

Chronic Glomerulonephritis

Chronic glomerulonephritis is a slowly progressive disease characterized by inflammation of the glomeruli, causing irreversible damage to the nephrons. The course of the disease is highly variable. Some clients live for years with no or occasional symptomatic episodes. In other clients, the disease is rapidly fatal unless they receive dialysis to take care of the renal failure.

Pathophysiology and Etiology

A small number of those with chronic glomerulonephritis are known to have had repeated acute glomerulonephritis, but many do not have that history. For some clients, there is a familial link. Complications of autoimmune connective tissue disorders, such as lupus erythematosus (see Chapter 63) and Goodpasture syndrome (a rare disease that includes progressive glomerulonephritis, hemoptysis, and marked RBC destruction), also may cause chronic glomerulonephritis.

The chronic inflammation leads to ever-increasing bands of scar tissue that replace nephrons, the vital functioning units of the kidney. Decreased glomerular filtration eventually can lead to renal failure. The kidneys become reduced in size over time, primarily consisting of fibrous tissue. Chronic glomerulonephritis is the third leading cause of **end-stage kidney disease** (National Kidney Foundation, 2020).

Assessment Findings

Signs and Symptoms

Some clients do not experience symptoms until renal damage is severe. Generalized edema, known as anasarca, is a common finding. **Anasarca** is caused by the shift of fluid from the intravascular space to interstitial and intracellular locations. The fluid shift results from depletion of serum proteins, particularly albumin, which are lost in the urine. Clients remain markedly edematous for months or years. They may feel relatively well, but the kidney continues to excrete albumin. The fluid burden and subsequent renal failure contribute to fatigue, headache, dizziness, hypertension, dyspnea, and visual disturbances. Clients may also experience weight loss, digestive problems, decreased muscle strength and endurance, irritability, and increasing nocturia.

Diagnostic Findings

Low RBC volume is detected through complete blood counts (CBCs). Its underlying cause is the excretion of erythrocytes in the urine and reduced production of erythropoietin. **Azotemia**, accumulation of nitrogen waste products in the blood, is evidenced by elevated BUN, serum creatinine, and uric acid levels. The urine contains protein (albumin), sediment, **casts** (deposits of minerals that break loose from the walls of the tubules), and red and white blood cells. The urinary creatinine clearance is reduced. Serum electrolyte changes indicate nephron dysfunction, including *hyperkalemia* (elevated potassium), increased phosphorus levels related to decreased renal excretion of phosphorus, and related decreased calcium levels (calcium binds to phosphorus to compensate for increased serum phosphorus levels).

Chest X-rays and echocardiograms demonstrate cardiac size because cardiac enlargement is common. An electrocardiogram (ECG) may indicate left ventricular hypertrophy related to hypertension and signs of hyperkalemia (tall, peaked T waves). A percutaneous kidney biopsy may be performed in the early stage to confirm the diagnosis and to determine the severity of the disorder. In late stages, the kidneys are too small to safely perform a biopsy. CT scans and a magnetic resonance imaging (MRI) scan may be done to confirm decreased kidney size.

Medical Management

Treatment is nonspecific and symptomatic. Management goals include the following:

- Controlling hypertension with medications and sodium restriction
- Correcting fluid and electrolyte imbalance
- Reducing edema with diuretic therapy
- Preventing congestive heart failure
- Eliminating UTIs with antimicrobials

Renal failure eventually may necessitate dialysis or kidney transplantation, discussed later in this chapter.

The nurse evaluates the client's ability to manage home care and the availability of a support system before developing discharge plans. If the client lacks a support system from the family or extended family members, the nurse consults

Client and Family Teaching 58-2
Chronic Glomerulonephritis

The nurse teaches the client and family as follows:

- Follow the diet and fluid regimen recommended by the health care provider and as outlined by the dietitian.
- Take medications exactly as directed on the container label. Do not omit or discontinue any medication unless ordered to do so by the primary provider. Do not take nonprescription drugs unless a health care provider approves their use.
- Monitor and record temperature and weight daily. (In some instances, clients may be asked to monitor their BP.)
- Follow the health care provider's recommendations as to physical activity and exercise. Take frequent rest periods if fatigue occurs.
- Contact the health care provider if there are questions about medications if symptoms become worse or if fever, chills, blood in the urine, weight gain, swelling of the arms or legs or periorbital edema, difficulty in breathing, difficulty in thinking, severe fatigue, excessive sleepiness, constipation, loss of appetite, or an upper respiratory infection occurs.
- Emphasize that frequent follow-up visits and laboratory tests are necessary to monitor response to treatment.

with the primary provider for a referral to a social agency or home health care agency. Client and Family Teaching 58-2 provides important discharge instructions.

CONGENITAL KIDNEY DISORDERS: POLYCYSTIC KIDNEY DISEASE

Individuals may be born with various malformations of renal structures. Most of these are unpredictable because they are the result of errors in fetal development. PKD, however, is the result of a hereditary trait.

The two manifestations of PKD are the infantile and adult forms. The infantile form is rare. It may cause fetal death (before delivery), early neonatal death, or renal failure during childhood. The adult form generally has its onset between 30 and 40 years of age, but it can occur at any age. It insidiously progresses to renal insufficiency. Once renal failure develops, PKD usually is fatal within 4 years, unless the client receives dialysis treatment or an organ transplant. The kidneys are the primary organs involved, but the polycysts can also occur in the liver or other organs. Women and men are affected equally. Death usually results from renal failure or the complications of hypertensive cardiovascular disease.

Pathophysiology and Etiology

Adult PKD is inherited as either an autosomal dominant trait or autosomal recessive trait, which means that an affected parent passes the gene for the disease to their children. Children with the autosomal dominant inheritance have a 50:50 chance of acquiring the defective gene (Fig. 58-3). This is

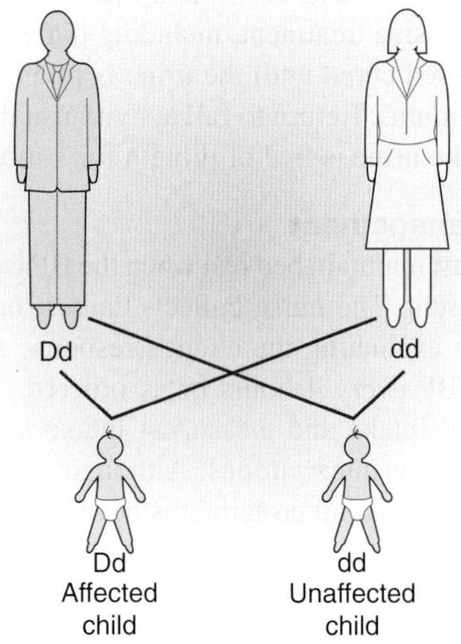

Figure 58-3 Inheritance of an autosomal dominant disorder.

opposed to the autosomal recessive inheritance, in which a child has a 25% chance of being affected.

As the name implies, this disorder is characterized by the formation of multiple bilateral kidney cysts (Fig. 58-4). The cysts interfere with kidney function and eventually lead to renal failure. The fluid-filled cysts cause great enlargement of the kidneys, from their normal size of a fist to that of a football. As the cysts enlarge, they compress the renal blood vessels and cause chronic hypertension. Bleeding into cysts causes flank pain. People with PKD are much more

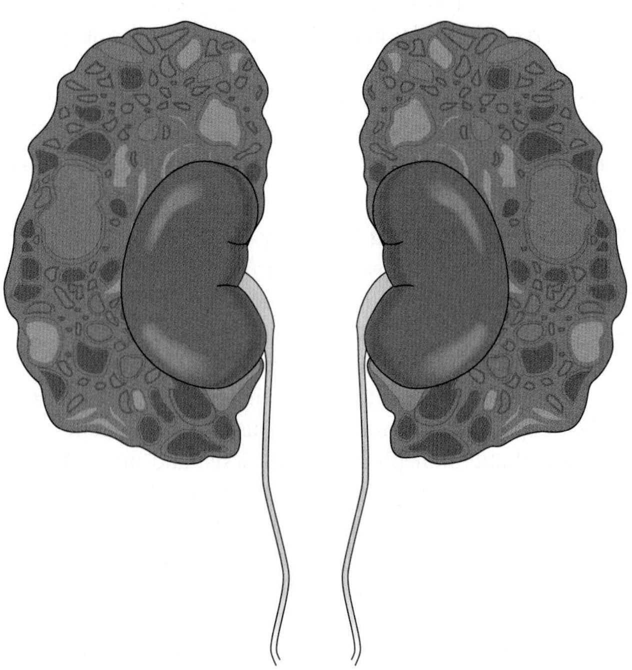

Figure 58-4 Normal kidneys in comparison with polycystic kidneys.

susceptible to kidney infections and kidney stones. Besides renal failure, other complications include cysts on the pancreas and liver, an enlarged heart, mitral valve prolapse, and brain aneurysm.

Assessment Findings

Hypertension is present in approximately 75% of affected clients at the time of diagnosis. Other symptoms such as pain from retroperitoneal bleeding, lumbar discomfort, and abdominal tenderness are caused by the size and effects of the cysts. The client may experience **colic** (acute spasmodic pain) when there is ureteral passage of clots or calculi. Many clients with this disorder also have hematuria because of UTIs and ruptured cysts. Renal stones are also common. Many clients experience headache and increased abdominal girth.

A family history of affected members is a presumptive diagnostic indicator. Urinalysis shows mild proteinuria, hematuria, and pyuria. A CBC may show decreased or increased RBCs and hematocrit; an increase is seen because erythropoietin production sometimes is accelerated. Abdominal ultrasound, CT scan, MRI, and intravenous pyelogram (IVP) reveal enlarged kidneys with indentations caused by cysts. Laboratory tests such as BUN and serum creatinine indicate the degree of current kidney dysfunction.

Medical and Surgical Management

PKD has no cure, but some interventions reduce the rate of progression. Hypertension is treated with antihypertensive drugs, diuretic medications, and sodium restriction. Despite these interventions, the hypertension is difficult to control. When and if urinary infections develop, they are treated promptly with antibiotics. Low RBC counts are treated with iron supplements, injections of erythropoietin (Epogen), or blood transfusions. Nephrotoxic medications, such as nonsteroidal anti-inflammatory drugs (NSAIDs) and cephalosporin antibiotics, are avoided at all costs.

Dialysis substitutes for kidney function when renal failure occurs and while the client awaits an organ transplant. Surgical removal of one or both kidneys may be required.

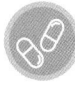

Pharmacologic Considerations

- Clients taking epoetin alfa (Epogen or Procrit) have a greater risk for heart attack, heart failure, or stroke. Currently, those taking the drug for cancer therapy are enrolled in the U.S. Food and Drug Administration (FDA) Risk Evaluation and Mitigation Strategy (REMS) program. At this time, kidney disease clients are not required to enroll.

Nursing Management

Many clients with PKD are treated as outpatients by primary providers or nephrologists, primary providers who specialize in the diagnosis and treatment of renal diseases. When hospitalization is necessary, the nurse assesses vital signs, especially BP, and reports any significant elevations. They monitor laboratory test results for indicators of renal function. The nurse inspects the urine for signs of bleeding or infection. They measure and document intake and output at least every 8 hours. The nurse reports any decrease in or absence of urine output. For further information about complications or advanced stages, refer to Nursing Process for the Client With Renal Calculi and the Nursing Management sections in the discussions of the client with chronic kidney disease and dialysis.

OBSTRUCTIVE DISORDERS

Urinary obstruction at any point in the urinary tract can occur in clients of all ages for various reasons. Obstructing conditions include urinary tract stones, strictures, and tumors. Table 58-1 lists causes of urinary tract obstruction.

Kidney and Ureteral Calculi

Urolithiasis refers to a condition of stones or *calculi* (sing. calculus) in the urinary tract. A **calculus** is a precipitate of mineral salts that ordinarily remain dissolved in urine. The majority of kidney stones are composed of calcium oxalate and/or calcium phosphate. Other components include uric acid (urate), cystine, and magnesium ammonium phosphate (struvite) (Table 58-2). Stones may be smooth, jagged, or staghorn-shaped (Fig. 58-5).

Calculi can occur anywhere in the urinary tract from the kidney pelvis and beyond. When a stone forms, the condition is called *urolithiasis*. **Nephrolithiasis** refers to a kidney stone, the size of which may range from microscopic to several centimeters. **Ureterolithiasis** is a stone in the ureter. Ureteral stones usually are small; some may be no larger than a grain of sand.

Pathophysiology and Etiology

The reason urinary calculi form is not fully understood. Predisposing factors include the following:

- **Calciuria**, excessive calcium in the urine, as may accompany hyperparathyroid disease, administration of calcium-based antacids, and excessive intake of vitamin D (vitamin D intoxication)
- Dehydration
- UTI with urea-splitting organisms such as *P. mirabilis*, which makes urine alkaline, a condition that promotes precipitation of calcium
- Obstructive disorders, such as an enlarged prostate gland, which foster urinary stasis
- Metabolic disorders, such as gout, in which uric acid crystallizes
- Osteoporosis, in which bone is demineralized
- Prolonged immobility from paralysis secondary to spinal injuries or other incapacitating conditions that result in sluggish emptying of urine from the urinary tract
- Family history
- Diets that are high in protein, sodium, and/or sugar
- Obesity

TABLE 58-2 Composition, Contributing Factors, and Treatment of Kidney Stones

TYPE OF STONE	CONTRIBUTING FACTORS	TREATMENT
Calcium (oxalate and phosphate)	Hypercalcemia and hypercalciuria Immobilization Hyperparathyroidism Vitamin D intoxication Diffuse bone disease Milk-alkali syndrome Renal tubular acidosis Hyperoxaluria Intestinal bypass surgery	Treatment of underlying conditions Increased fluid intake Thiazide diuretics Dietary restriction of foods high in oxalate
Magnesium ammonium phosphate (struvite)	Urea-splitting urinary tract infections	Treatment of urinary tract infection Acidification of the urine Increased fluid intake
Uric acid (urate)	Formed in acid urine with pH of approximately 5.5 Gout High-purine diet	Increased fluid intake Allopurinol for hyperuricosuria Alkalinization of urine
Cystine	Cystinuria (inherited disorder of amino acid metabolism)	Increased fluid intake Alkalinization of urine

Reprinted with permission from Grossman, S. C., & Porth, C. M. (2014). *Porth's pathophysiology: Concepts of altered health states* (9th ed., p. 1085). Wolters Kluwer Health/Lippincott Williams & Wilkins.

Calculi traumatize the walls of the urinary tract and irritate the cellular lining, causing pain as violent contractions of the ureter develop to pass the stone along. But the ureteral spasms may just as easily hold a stone in place. If a stone totally or partially obstructs the passage of urine beyond its location, pressure increases in the area above the stone. The pressure contributes to pain, and urinary stasis promotes secondary infection. The retained urine distends the renal pelvis, a condition called **hydronephrosis**. Eventually, there may be compression of the glomeruli and tiny arterioles that supply blood to the kidney, which can result in permanent kidney damage.

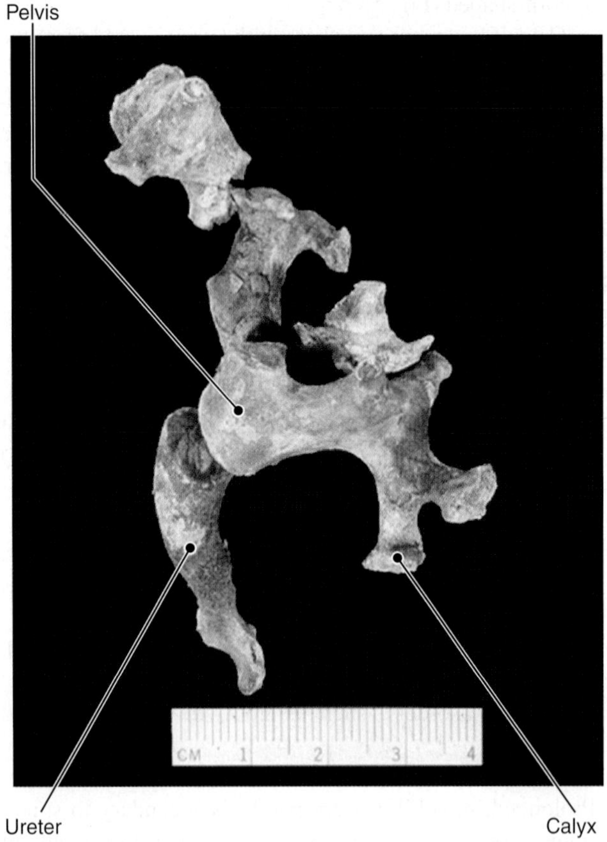

Figure 58-5 Staghorn calculus. The stone forms a nearly perfect image or cast of the upper ureter, renal pelvis, and calyces. (Reprinted with permission from McConnell, T. H. (2014). *The nature of disease: Pathology for the health professions* (2nd ed.). Wolters Kluwer Health/Lippincott Williams & Wilkins.)

Assessment Findings

Signs and Symptoms

Symptoms of a kidney or ureteral stone vary with size, location, and cause. Small stones may pass unnoticed; however, sudden, sharp, severe flank pain that travels to the suprapubic region and external genitalia is the classical symptom of urinary calculi. The pain is accompanied by renal or ureteral colic, painful spasms that attempt to move the stone. The pain comes in waves that radiate to the inguinal ring, the inner aspect of the thigh, and to the testicle or tip of the penis in men, or the urinary meatus or labia in women. The severity of the pain usually is inversely proportional to the size of the stone. Smaller stones travel more rapidly down the ureter, causing more forceful ureteral spasm and, therefore, greater pain. The severity of the pain can cause nausea, vomiting, and shock.

If an infection develops, the client may experience chills, fever, and serious hypotension. Urinary retention or dysuria may accompany obstruction. The kidney pelvis and ureter may become markedly enlarged as a consequence of urinary obstruction, and a mass may be palpated. The client also may experience renal tenderness.

Diagnostic Findings

Urinalysis shows evidence of gross or microscopic hematuria from trauma as the calculus tears at tissue as it moves downward. In addition, the urinalysis may show a pH conducive to stone formation, increased specific gravity, mineral crystals, and casts. Leukocytes in the urine and elevated white blood cells (WBCs) indicate an infectious process. A urine culture identifies specific infectious microorganisms.

X-rays identify most translucent kidney stones. If visualization is inconclusive, an IVP shows dye-filling defects caused by a stone. The dye stops at a certain point in the ureter and demonstrates enlargement above the obstruction. Kidney ultrasonography also detects obstructive changes. A CT urogram may also be performed, which involves taking images as dye passes through the kidneys, ureters, and bladder. Depending on how long the stone has been present, some blood chemistry values, such as serum creatinine, BUN, and serum uric acid, may be elevated. Analysis of the stone content is useful in preventing recurrence.

Medical Management

Small calculi are passed naturally with no specific interventions. If the stone is 5 mm or less in diameter and moving, the pain is tolerable, and if there is no obstruction, the client is managed medically with vigorous hydration, analgesics (including opioids and NSAIDs), antimicrobial therapy, and drugs that dissolve calculi or eventually alter conditions that promote their formation.

For larger stones, **extracorporeal shock wave lithotripsy** (ESWL), a procedure that uses 800 to 2400 shock waves aimed from outside the body toward soft tissue to dense stones (Fig. 58-6A), may be used. The stones are shattered into smaller particles that are passed from the urinary tract. ESWL is administered with the client in a water bath or surrounded by a soft cushion while under light anesthesia or

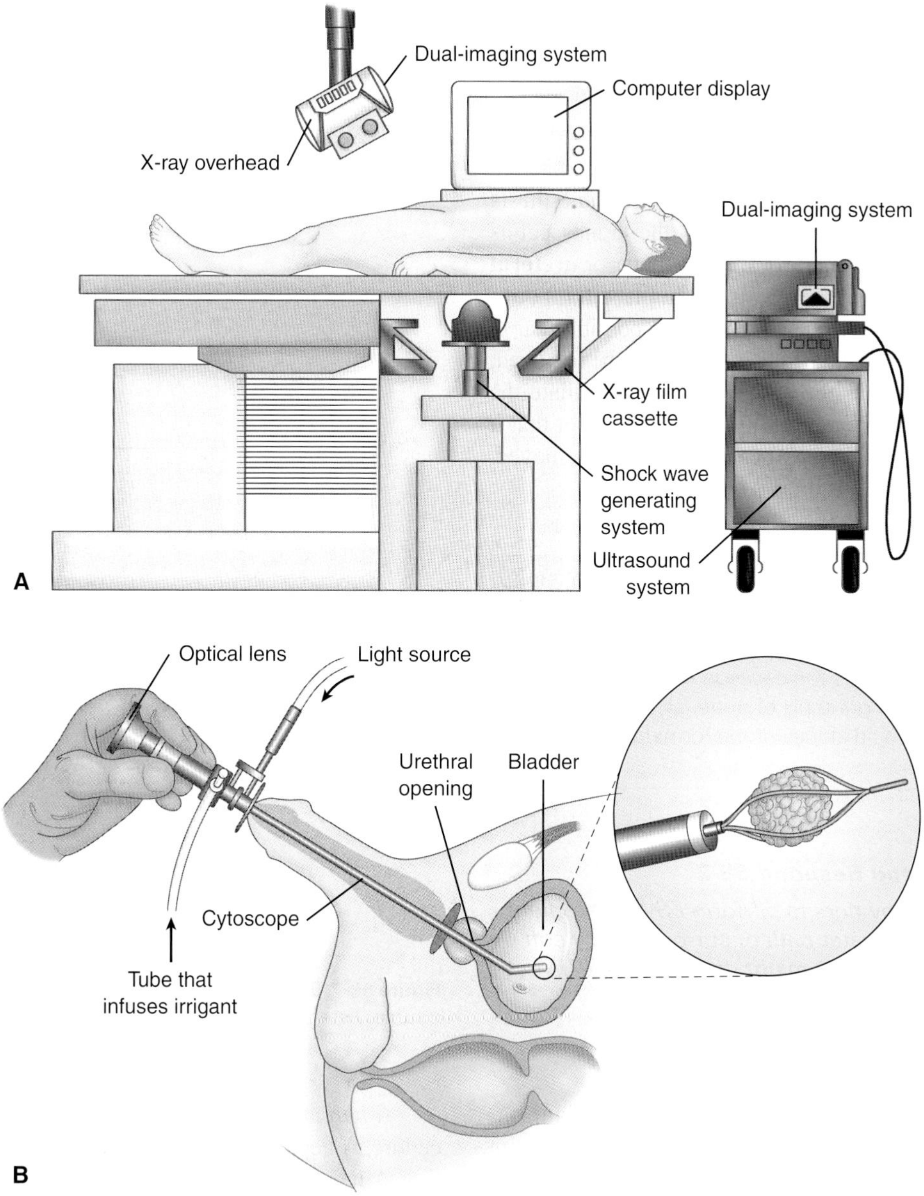

Figure 58-6 Methods of treating renal stones: **(A)** extracorporeal shock wave lithotripsy (ESWL), **(B)** cystoscopy, and **(C)** percutaneous nephrolithotomy.

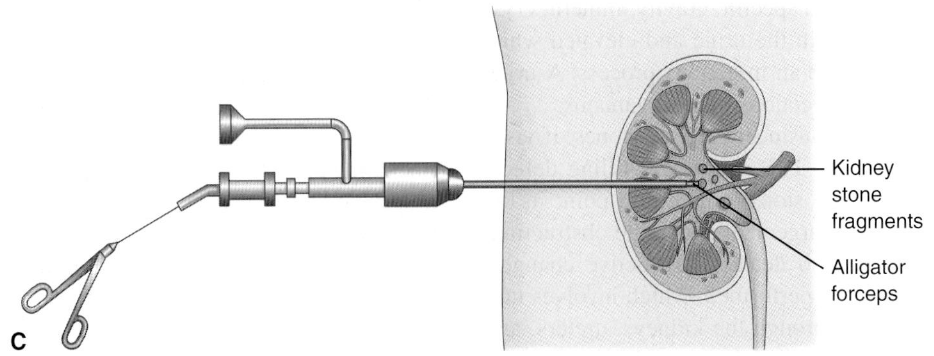

Figure 58-6 (*continued*)

sedation. Stones also can be pulverized with laser lithotripsy. To do so, a fine wire, through which the laser beam passes, is inserted into the ureter by means of a cystoscope. Repeated bursts of the laser reduce the stone to a fine powder, which is then passed in the urine.

Other stone removal procedures are performed with ureteroscopic approaches in which the endoscope is inserted from the urethra into the upper urinary tract under anesthesia to grasp, crush, and remove stones from the kidney pelvis or ureter (see Fig. 58-6B). Afterward, a catheter or **ureteral stent**, a slender supportive device, is left in place for 3 days to splint the ureter or divert the urine past any possible tear in the ureteral wall (Fig. 58-7). If the stone cannot be removed, a ureteral catheter is left in place for 24 hours to dilate the ureter in the hope that the stone will pass through it or that it will be pulled into the bladder when the catheter is removed.

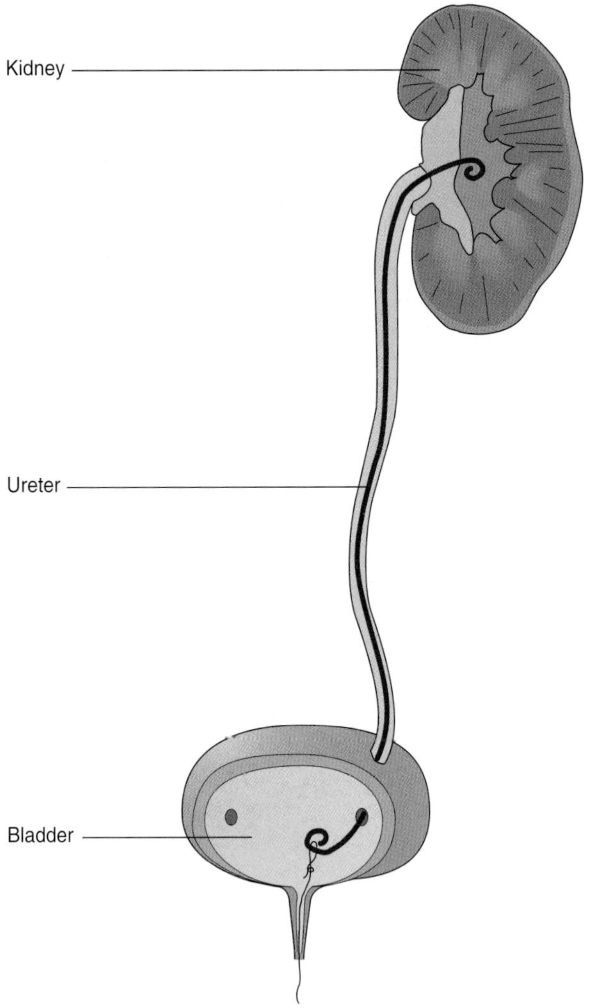

Figure 58-7 Example of a ureteral stent; in this case, a double-J stent.

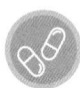

Pharmacologic Considerations

- Does using sodium bicarbonate (baking soda) prevent kidney stones? Uric acid is the cause in roughly 10% of stones. By increasing the pH of urine (alkalize), this helps to reduce uric acid kidney stone formation (Sandhu et al., 2018).

››› *Stop, Think, and Respond 58-2*

For health care providers to perform ESWL, the client must be in a clean water bath or surrounded by soft cushions. What concerns might the client have? What are your best responses?

Surgical Management

Calculi that are large or complicated by obstruction, ongoing UTI, kidney damage, or constant bleeding require surgical removal. Surgical options include a percutaneous nephrolithotomy, ureterolithotomy, pyelolithotomy, and nephrolithotomy.

A *percutaneous nephrolithotomy* is an endoscopic procedure. A nephroscope is tunneled into the kidney through a tiny skin incision while the client is under general anesthesia (see Fig. 58-6C). Ultrasound is used to crush the stone. The fragments are removed through the endoscope.

For *ureterolithotomy*, *pyelolithotomy*, or *nephrolithotomy*, a suprapubic abdominal or flank incision is made, and the stone is removed under direct visualization while the client is anesthetized. A **pyeloplasty**, surgical repair of the ureteropelvic junction or other anatomic anomalies, may be performed at the same time. The additional surgery is done to correct conditions that contribute to the development of stones and prevent their recurrence.

A *nephrectomy* is indicated if a stone has permanently and severely damaged a kidney beyond adequate function. The other kidney must be fully functional.

After any of these surgical procedures, drainage of urine from the affected kidney is accomplished with a nephrostomy tube during the healing process. A **nephrostomy tube**, also called a *pyelostomy tube*, is a catheter inserted through the skin into the renal pelvis. A nephrostomy tube is used to manage any obstruction to urine flow above the bladder. The tube is kept in place with a suture through the skin. Unlike the bladder, the kidney pelvis can hold only 5 to 8 mL of urine. If a blood clot or kinking or compression of the tubing impairs urinary drainage for even a short time, hydronephrosis and damage to surgically repaired tissue can result. The client complains of pain if the renal pelvis becomes distended with urine.

For some clients with calcium phosphate stones, it may be found that a hyperactive parathyroid gland is the cause. The parathyroid gland produces too much parathyroid hormone, referred to as hyperparathyroidism (see Chapter 50). As a result, calcium levels are much higher than normal and may lead to calcium phosphate stones. Either treating the cause of the hyperparathyroidism or surgically removing growths on the parathyroid gland may be done to resolve this issue.

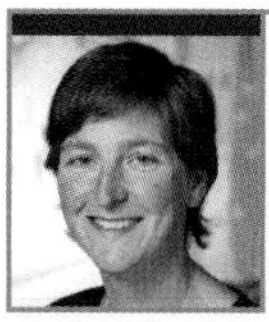

Clinical Scenario A 44-year-old client is seen in the emergency department complaining of acute onset of sharp and unrelenting flank pain and spasms in the lower abdomen. The client states an urgency to urinate but has voided very little since the pain started. What are the important considerations for the nurse while caring for this client? (See the following Nursing Process for the Client With Renal Calculi section.)

NURSING PROCESS FOR THE CLIENT WITH RENAL CALCULI

Assessment

Obtain a complete history, including a drug and allergy history, family history, history of immobility, episodes of dehydration, UTIs, and diet. Assess pain intensity and location and associated symptoms such as nausea and vomiting. In addition, monitor vital signs and assess all urine for stones by straining it through a gauze or wire mesh and closely inspecting it. Save solid material for laboratory analysis. Urine may show evidence of hematuria. In some instances, the client may experience anuria related to bilateral obstruction and have abdominal distention.

Diagnosis, Planning, and Interventions

Three goals when caring for a client with urinary calculi include improving urinary output, relieving pain, and preventing or treating infection. Clients often are frightened because of the excruciating pain and thus require emotional support as well as pain management. Typical diagnoses, expected outcomes, and interventions include, but are not limited to, the following:

Acute Pain: Related to increased pressure in the renal pelvis or renal colic
Expected Outcome: Pain will decrease within 30 minutes of a nursing measure.

- Administer prescribed narcotic analgesic. *It assists in decreasing pain related to ureteral colic during an acute episode and promotes muscle relaxation.*
- Provide supplemental nonpharmacologic interventions such as a comfortable position, guided imagery, and distraction. *These measures promote relaxation, redirect attention, and enhance coping ability.*
- Encourage ambulation and liberal fluid intake when the client is comfortable. *The supine position can increase colic; ambulation relieves it. Increased fluid intake promotes the passage of a stone and prevents urinary stasis or the formation of new stones.*

Risk for Complication of Hydronephrosis: Related to urinary stasis, risk of UTI, and blockage of the urinary tract.
Expected Outcome: The nurse will manage and minimize hydronephrosis.

- Monitor intake and output. *This record provides information about kidney function and indicates any complications such as hydronephrosis.*
- Administer antibiotics as ordered. *Antimicrobials treat the cause of UTI associated with urolithiasis and urinary stasis.*
- Manage a nephrostomy tube by following Nursing Guidelines 58-1. *Proper management ensures that the nephrostomy tube remains in place, urine drains properly, and infection is prevented.*

(*continued*)

NURSING PROCESS FOR THE CLIENT WITH KIDNEY CALCULI (continued)

Infection Risk: Related to urinary stasis
Expected Outcome: UTI will not develop as evidenced by urine free of pus and microorganisms and normal temperature and white blood cell count.

- Administer antimicrobial therapy as prescribed. *UTIs potentiate stone formation. Antibiotics treat the infection.*
- Encourage fluid intake to 3000 mL/day unless contraindicated. *Increased hydration flushes bacteria, blood, and other debris and may expedite stone passage.*
- Maintain patency of all catheters or encourage client to void every 2 to 3 hours. *Adequate urinary flow or frequent voiding prevents urinary stasis and eliminates bacteria, blood, and other particles.*
- Follow aseptic principles when changing dressings or urinary drainage equipment. *Strict asepsis prevents introduction of microbes into the urinary tract.*

Altered (Renal) Tissue Perfusion: Related to increased fluid pressure in ureter and kidney pelvis
Expected Outcome: Kidney will remain adequately perfused with blood as evidenced by normal serum creatinine, BUN, and distribution of radiopaque dye after IVP.

- Monitor laboratory and diagnostic test results. *Elevated BUN, creatinine, and electrolyte levels indicate kidney dysfunction and assist in evaluating hydration status and effectiveness of other interventions.*
- Prepare client safely but quickly for treatment measures that promote urinary drainage if it becomes apparent that kidney function is compromised. *Prompt intervention may prevent serious complications.*

Evaluation of Expected Outcomes

Pain is reduced. Urine output is balanced with intake. Urine is clear. The client is afebrile. Findings from urine and blood tests indicate adequate renal function. For clients undergoing surgical procedures, the nurse explains the procedure and follows standards for perioperative care in Chapter 14. After lithotripsy, endoscopy, or surgery, the nurse assesses vital signs, measures fluid intake and output, and inspects the color of urine, which may be grossly bloody for a time. After ESWL, the nurse should inspect the flank for ecchymosis, which is expected. The nurse documents the location of discoloration. Clients require analgesics for postprocedural discomfort.

If ureteroscopy is performed and a urethral catheter is in place, the nurse attaches the catheter to a closed drainage system. Pink-tinged urine may be seen, but if frank blood appears in the urine or the client complains of severe abdominal pain, the nurse must notify the primary provider immediately. If a ureteral stent is present, the nurse checks for the suture, which extends from the urinary meatus and is used for stent removal. It is important that the client maintain a total daily fluid volume of approximately 3000 mL. For more information, see Client and Family Teaching 58-3. In addition, refer to Nutrition Notes 58-1 for dietary recommendations for prevention of kidney stones.

NURSING GUIDELINES 58-1

Managing a Nephrostomy Tube

- Connect the nephrostomy tube to a closed drainage system.
- Have a second nephrostomy tube available at the bedside for the primary provider's use in case the present one is displaced.
- Secure the tube to the client's flank with tape to ensure that it does not become dislodged.
- Keep the urine collection bag below the level of insertion.
- Never clamp the nephrostomy tubing.
- Check that the nephrostomy and drainage tubing are not kinked or that the client is not compressing the tubing.
- Use no more than 5 to 8 mL of sterile normal saline to maintain patency if an irrigation is ordered.
- Record the urine output from the nephrostomy tube separately from other urinary volumes.
- Assess the tube insertion site for bleeding and drainage.
- Change the dressing around the nephrostomy tube if and when it becomes damp. Apply a skin barrier ointment around the incision to prevent excoriation.
- Notify the primary provider immediately if the nephrostomy tube becomes dislodged or if there is an absence of urinary drainage.

Client and Family Teaching 58-3
Renal Calculi

The nurse includes the following recommendations when teaching the client and family:

- Review the causes of and methods to prevent renal calculi.
- Drink plenty of liquids; water is one of the best.
- Restrict foods identified in Nutrition Notes 58-1 to small amounts if the stones are composed of calcium oxalate.
- Take all antimicrobial and analgesic drugs and, if prescribed, antigout medications as prescribed and report any side effects.
- Demonstrate the procedures for catheter or nephrostomy tube care.
- Strain urine if the stone or its fragments have not passed.
- Report signs of acute obstruction immediately, such as inability or difficulty in voiding, or pain.
- Report signs of infection such as fever, chills, dysuria, frequency, urgency, and cloudy urine because infection may contribute to formation of urinary calculi.

Client and Family Teaching 58-3 (*continued*)
Renal Calculi

- Review discharge teaching after a treatment procedure that includes activity level, hygiene measures, dietary modifications, goals for oral fluid intake, and wound care.
- Consult with the primary provider before self-administering any over-the-counter medications.

Nutrition Notes 58-1

The Client at Risk for Kidney Stones

- The following dietary recommendations are appropriate for prevention of kidney stones:
  - Consume sufficient fluids to maintain the output goal of 2.5 L/day.
  - Limit foods with a high oxalate content as these can contribute to stone formation. Foods include spinach, berries, nuts, and beets.
  - Include recommended amounts of fruits, vegetables, and fiber as sources of magnesium and potassium. These minerals have been associated with lower incidence of kidney stones.
  - Limit sodium as it competes with calcium for absorption.
  - If uric acid stones are prevalent, decrease sources of purines (organ meats such as brain, kidney, liver, sweetbreads; game meat; gravies; anchovies; herring; mackerel; sardines; and scallops).
  - Achieve the recommended daily intake for calcium by natural sources as there is a higher incidence of stone formation in people whose diets are deficient in calcium. Avoid calcium supplements.

Source: National Kidney Foundation. (2019). *Kidney stone diet plan and prevention.* Retrieved September 25, 2020, from https://www.kidney.org/atoz/content/diet

Ureteral Stricture

A stricture is a narrowing of a lumen. A ureteral stricture is the narrowing of a ureter.

Pathophysiology and Etiology

A ureteral stricture is relatively rare, but the incidence is higher among those with chronic ureteral stone formation and for those clients who have repeated upper ureteroscopies. Recurrent inflammation and infection cause scar tissue to accumulate in the ureter. Other conditions that can interfere with urine passing through the ureter are congenital anomalies or conditions that mechanically compress the ureter, such as pregnancy or tumors in the abdomen or upper urinary tract. Radiation therapy, urinary diversions, and kidney transplant may also contribute to a ureteral stricture.

In many instances, the ureter is only partially narrowed. Symptoms develop over time as the area of the ureter above the stricture dilates with urine (*hydroureter*) and the kidney pelvis slowly enlarges. Stasis of urine promotes an upper UTI.

Assessment Findings

Flank pain or discomfort and tenderness at the costovertebral angle from enlargement of the renal pelvis often develop. The client experiences back or abdominal discomfort, which tends to increase during periods of elevated fluid intake. A voiding cystourethrogram and ultrasonography help to identify structural changes consistent with impaired passage of urine.

Medical and Surgical Management

Medical treatment is not an option for this condition. Various surgical measures are used to treat strictures. Management depends on the location, the density, and the length of the stricture. Balloon dilation is used to stretch the ureter if strictures are short. *Endoureterotomy* is an endoscopic procedure to open a stricture. It can be done surgically or with a laser and is preferred for larger strictures.

If the obstruction persists, the primary provider performs **ureteroplasty**, removal of the narrowed section of ureter, and reconnection of the patent portions. This is the preferred procedure for a midureteral stricture. A ureteral stent is placed in the ureter to provide support to the walls of the ureter, relieve the obstruction, and maintain the flow of urine through the ureter and into the bladder. Lower ureteral strictures are treated by removing the narrowed portion of the ureter and reimplanting the remaining section into the bladder wall.

Besides correcting strictures, ureteral surgery is performed to remove tumors, to repair accidental ligation of the ureter during abdominal surgery (the highest incidence is seen in hysterectomies), and to extricate a ureteral stone that cannot be removed by other means.

Nursing Management

The nurse follows the standards of care for the perioperative client if the client undergoes surgery (see Chapter 14). If a ureteral catheter is inserted before surgery, the nurse measures the urine output from the catheter hourly. They must immediately report lack of urine output from the ureteral catheter.

On return from surgery, all urinary drainage tubes and catheters are connected to a closed drainage system or to the type of drainage system ordered by the primary provider. The main complication associated with ureteral surgery is failure of the ureter to transport urine from the kidney to the bladder. The nurse must contact the primary provider if

- Signs of shock appear.
- Urinary output from the ureteral catheter is decreased or absent.
- The client complains of significant abdominal pain, which may indicate leakage of urine into the peritoneal cavity.
- Signs of a UTI develop, such as fever and chills, or the urine is cloudy or has a foul odor.

Depending on the surgical procedure, the client may need instruction in the care of the ureteral or urethral catheter(s), the management of the drainage collection system, incision care, and a review of the prescribed diet and medication schedule.

Tumors of the Kidney

Tumors of the kidney are almost always cancerous. Renal cell carcinoma is the most common type of kidney cancer in adults, with 9 of 10 renal cancers diagnosed as renal cell

BOX 58-3 Risk Factors for Kidney Cancer

- Age: risk increases with age; most renal cancers occur after age 60 years
- Gender: affects men more than women
- Tobacco use
- Occupational exposure to industrial chemicals, such as trichloroethylene (metal cleaner and degreaser), aristolochic acid, cadmium, and asbestos (National Kidney Foundation, 2020b; Scelo & Larose, 2018)
- Obesity
- Family history of kidney cancer
- Hypertension
- Unopposed estrogen therapy
- PKD
- Treatment for kidney failure, including clients on dialysis and those receiving a kidney transplant

adenocarcinoma. A second type of kidney cancer is transitional cell cancer or urothelial carcinomas. In both types, men are affected more than women.

Pathophysiology and Etiology

The cause of kidney tumors is unknown. The incidence is higher in older adults, which suggests chronic exposure to a carcinogen whose metabolites involve renal excretion. Bladder cancer (see Chapter 59) is associated with the carcinogenic effects of long-term cigarette smoking. It is theorized that renal tumors are similarly initiated through this mechanism or exposure to some other environmental toxin (e.g., asbestos, rubber, or ink and ink products) or volatile solvent (e.g., gasoline). Box 58-3 lists risk factors for renal cancer.

Because the kidneys are deeply protected in the body, tumors can become quite large before causing symptoms. As the tumor enlarges, it occupies space, extending into adjacent renal structures and interfering with urine outflow. Tumor cells tend to metastasize by way of the renal vein and vena cava to the lungs, bone, lymph nodes, liver, and brain. Lung metastases predominate. Sometimes, the first symptom occurs when the tumor has metastasized to other organs.

Assessment Findings

In early stages, renal cancers rarely cause symptoms. In later stages, clients generally present with painless hematuria, which can be intermittent and microscopic or continuous and visible. In addition, clients may experience persistent low back pain on one side that does not go away; a mass or lump on the side or lower back; and unexplained weight loss, malaise, and fever. Colic-like discomfort during the passage of blood clots may also occur.

An abdominal mass found on a routine physical examination or on imaging procedures for other purposes suggests a kidney tumor. An IVP, cystoscopy with retrograde pyelograms, ultrasonography, MRI, renal angiography, and CT scan are used to locate the tumor. A PET scan may be done to determine if any metastasis has occurred. Sequential urine samples contain RBCs as well as malignant cells.

Medical and Surgical Management

Radical nephrectomy, including removal of the tumor, adrenal gland, surrounding perinephric fat, and fascia, is the treatment for a malignant renal tumor. For clients who have early-stage renal cancer or have only one kidney, the tumor may be removed from the kidney, leaving the kidney and surrounding tissue intact. A laparoscopic nephrectomy or robotic-assisted laparoscopic nephrectomy may be done on clients, depending on the stage and extent of the tumor. When a tumor arises in the collecting system or the ureter, a complete nephroureterectomy (removal of the kidney and ureter) is done. A cuff of bladder tissue is removed as well because the recurrence rate in any stump of ureter left behind is high. Surgery may be followed by radiation therapy, chemotherapy, hormonal therapy, and/or immunotherapy while the client is still in the hospital or on a postdischarge basis.

For some clients, surgery may be too risky. In these cases, treatment may involve embolization or cryoablation. Embolization involves occlusion of the renal artery to kill the tumor cells. Cryoablation uses special needles called cryoprobes to freeze and then thaw cancer cells, eventually destroying the cancerous cells. CT scans are used to monitor the process. Radiofrequency ablation may be used. With this procedure, high-energy radio waves heat the tumor and destroy the cancer cells. Arterial embolization may be done to block the artery that supplies blood to the tumor, thus destroying the tumor and the kidney. This is generally done on clients who have bleeding from the tumor or are likely to bleed during a nephrectomy.

Other therapies may be used to treat renal cancers. Radiation therapy and traditional chemotherapy are not very effective. Targeted therapies are used to slow the growth of or shrink these tumors. These therapies either block angiogenesis, which is growth of new blood vessels that supply the tumor (e.g., sorafenib [Nexavar]), or they interfere with protein synthesis, thus preventing growth of the tumor (e.g., sunitinib [Sutent]). Immunotherapy, such as interleukin-2 or alpha-interferon, may be used in later-stage renal cancer, including metastasis. Monoclonal antibodies (MoAbs) may also be used to treat metastasis. Other methods of treatment are in various phases of research, including other drugs and vaccines.

If extensive metastases are found, only palliative treatment is given. In these cases, the primary provider explains to the client and family that the treatment measures are not curative.

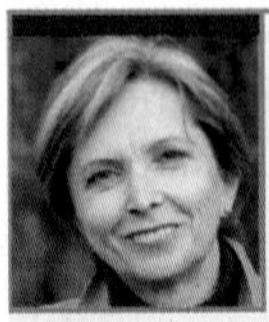

Clinical Scenario A 62-year-old woman had a radical nephrectomy 8 hours ago and was transferred to the postoperative surgical unit. **What important aspects of her care does the nurse need to focus on?** (See the following Nursing Process for the Client Recovering from a Nephrectomy section.)

NURSING PROCESS FOR THE CLIENT RECOVERING FROM A NEPHRECTOMY

Assessment

On the client's return from surgery, assess vital signs frequently. Inspecting and identifying the type and location of drains or catheters are important measures. The indwelling (Foley) catheter drainage system is placed below the level of the bed. Drains in or around the incision may drain by closed negative pressure (i.e., Jackson–Pratt) or low mechanical suction.

Diagnosis, Planning, and Interventions

Bleeding Risk: Related to bleeding from the ligated renal artery or vein
Expected Outcome: The nurse will manage and minimize hemorrhage.

- Monitor BP and pulse rate every 1 to 4 hours for the first 24 to 48 hours after surgery. *Decreased intravascular volume results in hypotension and tachycardia. Frequent monitoring assists in detecting changes in intravascular volume.*
- Report decreased BP, increased pulse, restlessness, or sudden onset of flank pain. *Death can occur quickly unless the client is immediately returned to surgery to control the bleeding.*
- Administer intravenous (IV) fluids and blood transfusions as ordered. *Isotonic fluids and blood replacement help to restore and maintain intravascular volume.*
- Note and record the color of drainage from each tube and catheter. *Assessment findings direct interventions and provide a means for further comparison and evaluation.*
- Follow the primary provider's orders concerning postoperative positioning. *Keeping the client from lying on the operative side avoids interference with wound drainage.*
- Contact the surgeon about any frank bleeding or a sudden decrease in urine output. *Although pink-tinged drainage is normal for several days after surgery, frank bleeding, sudden decreased urine, or both indicate complications.*

Acute Pain: Related to tissue trauma and pressure from urinary obstruction
Expected Outcome: Pain will be relieved to a tolerable level within 30 minutes of an intervention.

- Keep drainage catheters unclamped, unkinked, and below the level of insertion. *Unobstructed urine flow promotes urine elimination and prevents pain related to obstruction.*
- Secure all tubings to reduce movement at the site of insertion or displacement. *This measure reduces pain at the insertion site and promotes comfort.*
- Encourage oral fluids as soon as allowed and tolerated without causing nausea or vomiting. *Fluids dilute the urine and prevent catheter obstruction from sediment or small blood clots, thus reducing potential for pain and discomfort.*
- Irrigate tubings as ordered. *Irrigation promotes urinary flow and reduces potential for pain.*
- Administer prescribed analgesia and supplement drug therapy with nursing measures that promote comfort. *Analgesics and nonpharmacologic methods assist in reducing pain and promote the client's sense of control and participation in self-care.*
- Splint the incision when repositioning the client or during efforts to cough and deep breathe. *Splinting reduces tension on the surgical site and prevents or reduces pain-related movement.*

Altered Breathing Pattern: Related to incisional pain and restricted positioning
Ineffective Airway Clearance Risk: Related to weak cough secondary to incisional pain
Expected Outcomes: Breathing rate and depth will be sufficient to maintain blood oxygen saturation (SpO_2) at 90% or above. Secretions will be raised. Lung sounds will be clear in all lobes.

- Encourage client to breathe deeply and cough every 2 hours. Use an incentive spirometer to evaluate effectiveness. *These efforts increase alveolar ventilation and assist in clearing secretions.*
- Use small pillows or sheet rolls to apply firm support of the incision when the client coughs or performs deep-breathing exercises. *This technique splints the incision, reducing pain and promoting the client's ability to breathe deeply and cough.*
- Auscultate the lungs daily; notify the primary provider of any abnormal or absent breath sounds. *Breath sounds should be clear. Fine, scattered crackles at bases indicate that the client should be more vigorous in deep breathing and coughing. Coarser crackles indicate fluid in the airway; wheezes indicate a partial obstruction. Absent breath sounds require prompt intervention.*

Infection Risk: Related to impaired skin integrity and stasis of urine
Expected Outcome: Client will be free of infection as evidenced by normal findings in temperature, urine culture, and WBC count.

- Monitor temperature every 4 hours. *Fever usually is the first and only sign of infection.*
- Contact the primary provider if the client's temperature is above 101°F (38.3°C) or if they experience chills, or if purulent drainage or redness, swelling, and warmth at the incision are noted. *Elevated temperatures and incisional signs indicate an infection that requires intervention.*
- Use aseptic technique when changing the surgical dressing or managing the catheter and drainage systems. *Asepsis prevents introduction of microorganisms to the urinary tract or to areas where skin integrity has been lost.*
- Administer antibiotic therapy as prescribed. *Antibiotics treat infections, reducing the risk of further infection.*

(continued)

NURSING PROCESS FOR THE CLIENT RECOVERING FROM A NEPHRECTOMY (continued)

Evaluation of Expected Outcomes

The client shows no evidence of hemorrhage. Interventions reduce or eliminate pain. Breathing rate and depth maintain the SpO_2 at 90% or above. The client raises secretions, and lung sounds are clear in all lobes. No infections develop.

Clients who have had a nephrectomy usually have the drains (if any) removed before discharge. A dressing over the incision may or may not be required. If the primary provider orders a dressing applied and changed at home, the nurse shows the client and family how to change the dressing and provides a list of the necessary materials for dressing changes (See Client and Family Teaching 58-4).

Client and Family Teaching 58-4
Home Care After Nephrectomy

The teaching plan should include the following instructions:

- Change the dressing as ordered by the primary provider.
- Wash hands thoroughly before and after each dressing change.
- Drink plenty of fluids and follow the diet recommended by the primary provider.
- Avoid exposure to others who have possible infections.
- Take prescribed medication as directed on the container. Do not omit a dose.
- Contact the primary provider immediately if pain, fever, or chills occur or if the urine becomes bloody, cloudy, or foul smelling.

Nursing Management

In addition to the standard preoperative preparations, the nurse implements other prescribed procedures that facilitate the postoperative assessment and recovery of the client, such as inserting a urethral catheter and nasogastric tube.

KIDNEY FAILURE

Kidney failure is the inability of the nephrons in the kidneys to maintain fluid, electrolyte, and acid–base balances; excrete nitrogen waste products; and perform regulatory functions such as maintaining calcification of bones and producing erythropoietin. There are two types of kidney failure: acute and chronic. **Acute kidney injury** (AKI) (formerly called acute renal failure [ARF]) is characterized by a sudden and rapid decrease in renal function. AKI potentially is reversible with early, aggressive treatment of its contributing etiology. Chronic kidney disease (CKD) or chronic renal failure (CRF) is characterized by progressive and irreversible damage to the nephrons. It may take months to years for CKD to develop.

Pathophysiology and Etiology

Acute Kidney Injury

An AKI can develop as a consequence of prerenal, intrarenal, and postrenal disorders (Table 58-3). Prerenal disorders are nonurologic conditions that disrupt renal blood flow to the nephrons, affecting their filtering ability, such as hemorrhage, impaired cardiac efficiency that results from myocardial infarction or other conditions, or sepsis. This is the most common type of AKI. Intrarenal conditions are conditions in the kidney itself that destroy nephrons. Postrenal disorders usually are obstructive problems in structures below the kidney(s) that have damaging repercussions for the nephrons above. Classifications for AKI are referred to as the **RIFLE** criteria and include:

- **R**isk of renal dysfunction
- **I**njury to the kidney
- **F**ailure of kidney function
- **L**oss of kidney function
- **E**nd-stage kidney disease (Gameiro et al., 2018)

TABLE 58-3 Causes of Acute Kidney Injury

PRERENAL	INTRARENAL	POSTRENAL
Hypotension Hypovolemic shock Cardiogenic shock secondary to congestive heart failure Heart failure related to a myocardial infarction or other causes Lethal dysrhythmias Septic shock Anaphylaxis Dehydration Renal artery thrombosis or stenosis Liver failure Use of NSAIDs Burns	Ischemia Nephrotoxicity secondary to drugs such as aminoglycosides Acute and chronic glomerulonephritis Polycystic disease Untreated prerenal and postrenal disorders Myoglobinuria secondary to burns Hemoglobinuria secondary to transfusion reaction Scleroderma Multiple myeloma	Ureteral calculi Prostatic hypertrophy Ureteral stricture Ureteral or bladder tumor

NSAIDs, nonsteroidal anti-inflammatory drugs.

Concept Mastery Alert

Postrenal Acute Renal Failure

Postrenal acute renal failure is the result of an obstruction (such as renal calculi) that develops anywhere from the collecting ducts of the kidney to the urethra.

This classification system assists in identifying the severity of the client's condition and to alert health care providers for potential issues.

AKI progresses through four phases:

1. Onset phase
2. Oliguric (anuric) phase
3. Diuretic phase
4. Recovery phase

Onset Phase

The onset phase begins with the contributing event. It is accompanied by reduced blood flow to the nephrons to the point of acute tubular necrosis. **Acute tubular necrosis** refers to the death of cells in the collecting tubules of the nephrons, where reabsorption of water, electrolytes, and excretion of protein wastes and excess metabolic substances occurs. This phase can last hours to days.

Oliguric Phase

The oliguric phase is associated with the excretion of less-than-adequate urinary volumes. This phase begins within 48 hours after the initial cellular insult and may last for 10 to 14 days or longer. Fluid volume excess develops, which leads to edema, hypertension, and cardiopulmonary complications. Azotemia, the marked accumulation of urea and other nitrogenous wastes such as creatinine and uric acid in the blood, creates a potential for neurologic changes such as seizures, coma, and death.

There are better treatments for many prerenal causes of AKI. For that reason, some clients excrete urinary volumes greater than 500 mL/day. The urine has a very low specific gravity, however, because it lacks normal amounts of excreted substances such as excess potassium and hydrogen ions, to maintain homeostasis. Consequently, hyperkalemia, metabolic acidosis, and **uremia**, a toxic state caused by the accumulation of nitrogen wastes, develop regardless of the excreted water volume.

Diuretic Phase

Diuresis begins as the nephrons recover. Despite an increased water content of urine, the excretion of wastes and electrolytes continues to be impaired. The BUN, creatinine, potassium, and phosphate levels remain elevated in the blood. This phase can last 7 to 14 days.

Recovery Phase

It may take 3 to 12 months or longer for recovery while normal glomerular filtration and tubular function are restored. Some clients recover completely, whereas others develop varying degrees of permanent renal dysfunction.

BOX 58-4 Stages of Chronic Kidney Disease

Stage 1: Slight kidney damage with normal or increased filtration; a GFR of more than 90*

Stage 2: Mild decrease in kidney function with a GFR of 60 to 89

Stage 3: Moderate decrease in kidney function with a GFR of 30 to 59

Stage 4: Severe decrease in kidney function with a GFR of 15 to 29

Stage 5: End-stage kidney failure requiring dialysis or transplantation with a GFR less than 15

*Glomerular filtration rate (GFR) measured as mL/min/1.73 m^2.

Data from Inker, L. A., Astor, B. C., Fox, C. H., Isakova, T., Lash, J. P., Peralta, C. A., Tamura, M. K., & Feldman, H. I. (2014). KDOQI US Commentary on the 2012 KDIGO clinical practice guideline for the evaluation and management of CKD. *American Journal of Kidney Diseases, 63*(5), 713–735. http://www.ajkd.org/article/S0272-6386(14)00491-0/fulltext; Davison, S. N., Tupala, B., Wasylynuk, B. A., Siu, V., Sinnarajah, A., & Triscott, J. (2019). Recommendations for the care of patients receiving conservative kidney management. *Clinical Journal of American Society of Nephrology (CJASN), 14* (4), 626–634. https://doi.org/10.2215/CJN.10510917

Chronic Kidney Disease

Chronic kidney disease (CKD) is associated more often with intrarenal conditions or is a complication of systemic diseases such as diabetes mellitus and disseminated lupus erythematosus. In CKD, the kidneys are so extensively damaged that they do not adequately remove protein byproducts and electrolytes from the blood and do not maintain acid–base balance. The National Institute of Diabetes and Digestive and Kidney Diseases (2020) describes several stages of CKD (Box 58-4), beginning with an increased risk stage, which refers to clients with risk factors for CKD. Clients progress from stage 1 to stage 5 or from reduced renal reserve (40% to 75% loss of nephron function) to renal insufficiency (75% to 90% loss of nephron function) to end-stage kidney failure (less than 10% of nephron function). In end-stage kidney failure (sometimes referred to as established renal failure), a regular course of dialysis or kidney transplantation is necessary to maintain life.

Because damage to the nephrons is slow, declining renal function is less apparent until the end stage. The BUN and serum creatinine levels gradually rise. Uremia increases and adversely impacts all body systems. Hyponatremia is a reflection of diluted sodium ions in an excess volume of water in the blood. Actual electrolyte imbalances include hyperkalemia, hyperphosphatemia, hypermagnesemia, and hypocalcemia. The skin becomes the excretory organ for the substances the kidney usually clears from the body. A precipitate, referred to as **uremic frost**, may form on the skin.

Metabolic acidosis develops because the tubules cannot convert carbonic acid in the blood to water and bicarbonate ions. Erythropoietin production is inadequate, causing anemia. Susceptibility to infection increases as a result of a deficient immune system, particularly cellular immunity (see Chapter 33), as well as a decrease in the white blood cell count. Edema and hypertension are consequences of impaired urinary elimination. **Osteodystrophy**, a condition

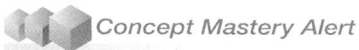

TABLE 58-4 Systemic Complications of Chronic Kidney Disease

BODY SYSTEM	COMPLICATION
Cardiovascular	Congestive heart failure, hypertension, cardiac dysrhythmias, edema
Metabolic	Electrolyte imbalance, metabolic acidosis
Respiratory	Shortness of breath, pulmonary edema
Gastrointestinal	Malnutrition, vitamin deficiencies, anorexia, nausea, bleeding
Integumentary	Dry skin, pruritus
Neurologic	Lethargy, confusion, depression, seizures, coma
Sensory	Peripheral neuropathies
Musculoskeletal	Bone demineralization, muscle cramps, joint pain
Immunologic	Impaired immune function, decreased antibody production, increased incidence of hepatitis B, and other infections

in which the bones become demineralized, occurs from hypocalcemia and hyperphosphatemia. The parathyroid glands secrete more parathormone to increase blood calcium levels.

Assessment Findings

Signs and Symptoms

In both AKI and CKD, the client has elevated BP and weight gain. Urine output usually is decreased. Those with CKD develop other symptoms as the disease worsens. Facial features appear puffy from fluid retention. The skin is pale. Ulceration and bleeding of the gastrointestinal tract may occur. The oral mucous membranes bleed, and blood may be found in the feces. The client reports vague symptoms such as lethargy, headache, anorexia, and dry mouth. Later, other problems develop such as pruritus and dry, scaly skin. The breath and body may have an odor characteristic of urine. Muscle cramps, bone pain or tenderness, and spontaneous fractures can develop. Mental processing is progressively slow as electrolyte imbalances become marked and nitrogenous wastes accumulate. The client may experience seizures. Table 58-4 lists the systemic manifestations of CKD.

Diagnostic Findings

Newer diagnostic biomarkers are used to determine changes in kidney function, as opposed to changes that indicate kidney failure (Gameiro et al., 2018). The rationale for this is that traditional laboratory blood tests will reveal elevations in BUN, creatinine, potassium, magnesium, and phosphorus, but these changes may take 12 to 24 hours to be evident. The new diagnostic markers include the following:

- *Neutrophil gelatinase-associated lipocalin (NGAL)*: This level (can be serum or urine) rises very quickly with poor kidney perfusion or ischemia; increased levels are seen 24 to 48 hours prior to an increased serum creatinine.
- *Cystatin C*: detected in both serum and urine; elevated levels are predictive of AKI and mortality.
- *Tissue inhibitor metalloproteinase-2 (TIMP-2)*: appears in urine within 12 hours of renal tubular cell injury from sepsis or ischemia.
- *Glomerular filtration rate (GFR)*: reflected in urine output volume; best real-time biomarker for current kidney function, particularly in catheterized clients.

Other lab tests that are still done include measuring calcium levels, which are low with kidney disease. The RBC count, hematocrit, and hemoglobin are decreased. The pH of the blood is on the acidotic side. Urinalysis reveals a decreased specific gravity. An IVP provides evidence of renal dysfunction. In clients with severe renal failure, dye excretion usually is delayed. A percutaneous renal biopsy shows destruction of nephrons. Imaging and ultrasound demonstrate structural defects in the kidneys, ureters, and bladder. Renal angiography identifies obstructions in blood vessels.

Medical Management

Prevention of AKI is an important function of health care providers. Clients at risk for dehydration are adequately hydrated. Risks for dehydration include surgery, diagnostic studies that require fluid restriction and contrast agents, and treatment for cancer or metabolic disorders. Shock and hypotension are treated as quickly as possible with replacement fluids and blood. Treating infections promptly and thoroughly also is important and greatly assists in preventing sepsis. Continuous monitoring of renal function is very important for clients at risk for AKI. The early and significant measure for kidney function is accurate measurement of urine output. Guidelines established by an organization called Kidney Disease: Improving Global Outcomes (KDIGO, 2012) promote early detection and treatment of changes in kidney function. In AKI, measures are taken to quickly remedy the primary cause of kidney failure. Renal damage can be limited by aggressively administering parenteral fluids to increase plasma volume, giving vasodilating and diuretic drugs, and infusing dopamine (Intropin) to improve cardiac output and perfuse the renal arteries.

To reduce complications and keep the client alive during the 2 or 3 weeks while the tubules are regenerating, hemodialysis (discussed later), a technique in which the blood is filtered externally with a machine, is performed. When hemodialysis is a temporary measure, the blood is removed and returned through a double-lumen catheter or twin central venous catheters (Fig. 58-8). Continuous renal replacement therapy (CRRT) is the filtration of blood through an extracorporeal circuit for clients who are unstable. It is done continuously via large veins, such as the femoral, internal jugular, or subclavian veins. Generally, this modality is

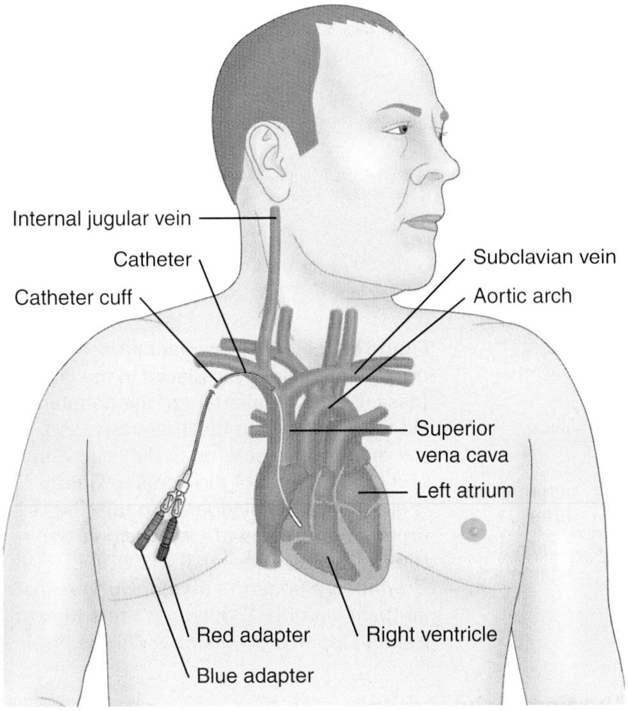

Figure 58-8 Double-lumen, cuffed catheter used for emergency hemodialysis. Red adapter attaches to blood line through which blood is pumped from the client to the dialyzer. After the blood passes through the dialyzer, it returns to the client through the blue adapter.

done in intensive care units or hemodialysis units located in a hospital. Another option is peritoneal dialysis, a slower process (discussed later) in which fluids and electrolytes are removed by osmosis and diffusion across the peritoneum, which acts as a semipermeable membrane.

Dietary recommendations are complex and dynamic. Protein allowance may be increased or decreased depending on the type of renal failure and use of dialysis. Calories, sodium, potassium, phosphorus, and fluid are also adjusted (Nutrition Notes 58-2). Sodium polystyrene sulfonate (Kayexalate), an ion-exchange resin, is prescribed for oral or rectal administration to remove excess potassium when hyperkalemia occurs. An IV infusion of glucose and insulin also facilitates movement of potassium within the cell. Acid–base balance is restored by administering IV sodium bicarbonate if renal function is insufficient to do so.

The medical management of CKD is similar to that of AKI, except the period of treatment is lifelong (unless a kidney transplantation is performed). Rather than administering blood transfusions to correct chronic anemia, erythropoietin (Epogen) is administered to stimulate bone marrow production of RBCs.

Surgical Management

Some clients in the end stage of CKD are candidates for kidney transplantation. For some clients, preemptive kidney transplant may be a possibility, if there is a donor. This means that the client has a kidney transplant while they still have kidney function and is not yet on dialysis. One healthy kidney can perform the work of two. Donors for a transplant are selected from compatible living donors who may or may not be relatives or

Nutrition Notes 58-2

The Client With Kidney Failure

Acute Kidney Injury

- The goal of nutrition therapy for AKI is to prevent or minimize malnutrition. Nutrition therapy is likely to be beneficial but has not been proven to speed recovery of renal function or improve survival.
- Protein recommendations range from 0.8 to 1.2 g/kg for clients who are not catabolic and are not receiving dialysis to 1.2 to 1.5 g/kg for clients who are catabolic and/or receiving dialysis. The normal recommended dietary allowance (RDA) for protein is 0.8 g/kg.
- For both sodium and potassium, allowances range from 2 to 3 g/day. During the diuretic phase, potassium intake is liberalized to replenish losses.
- Calories, phosphorus, and calcium allowances are individualized.
- Fluid allowance equals the volume of urine produced plus 500 mL to compensate for insensible losses.

Chronic Kidney Disease

- The objectives of nutrition therapy for chronic kidney disease (CKD) are to reduce serum nitrogen levels, reduce hypertension and edema, prevent body catabolism, improve renal function, and prevent or delay the onset of complications. Dietary interventions frequently are adjusted according to the client's laboratory values and clinical symptoms.
- Protein restriction, the cornerstone of nutrition therapy, ranges from 0.6 to 0.75 g/kg. Because most Americans consume almost twice as much protein as needed, many clients who must follow the diet view it as unrealistically restrictive. Most protein should be from animal sources, which in general have a higher biologic value than plant proteins. Pure sugars and heart-healthy fats are used liberally for calories to spare body and dietary protein.
- Multiple and complicated restrictions in protein, sodium, potassium, and fluid, compounded by anorexia and taste alterations, make dietary compliance difficult to achieve and maintain. Strong social support, frequent self-monitoring of protein intake, the use of specially formulated low-protein foods, and adequate guidelines for increasing calorie intake may improve adherence to dietary guidelines.
- Renal diet food lists, called "choices" to distinguish them from diabetic "exchanges," are used to simplify meal planning. Foods are grouped into lists according to their protein, sodium, and potassium content; phosphorus and fluid also may be considered. Portion sizes are specified so all servings in a list have approximately the same amount of protein, sodium, and potassium. An individualized meal plan specifies the number of choices allowed from each list for each meal and snack; any item may be chosen in a list, but items from one list cannot be substituted for another. The complexity and composition of choice lists vary greatly among institutions.
- Once dialysis begins, protein restrictions are liberalized to 1.2 to 1.3 g/kg to account for nutritional losses through the dialysate. Clients receiving peritoneal dialysis need to adjust their calorie intake downward to compensate for the calories absorbed from the glucose in the dialysate. Potassium, sodium, and fluid allowances are determined on an individual basis.

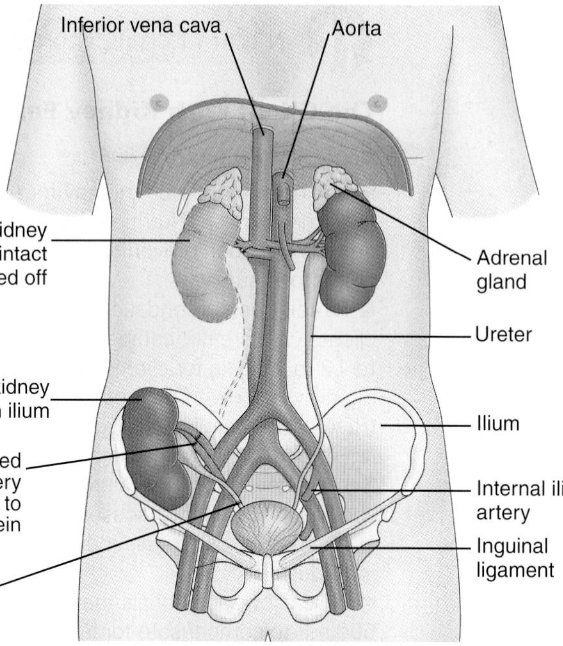

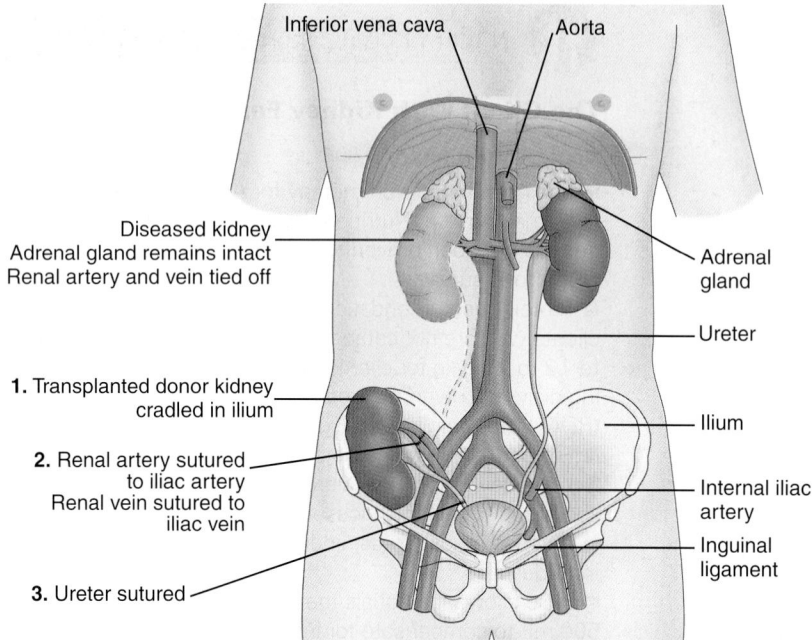

Figure 58-9 Renal transplantation: (1) The transplanted kidney is placed in the iliac fossa; (2) the renal artery of the donated kidney is sutured to the iliac artery, and the renal vein is sutured to the ileac vein; and (3) the ureter of the donated kidney is sutured to the bladder or to the client's ureter. (Reprinted with permission from Hinkle, J. L., & Cheever, K. H. (2014). *Brunner & Suddarth's textbook of medical-surgical nursing* (13th ed.). Wolters Kluwer Health/Lippincott Williams & Wilkins.)

from unrelated nonliving organ donors whose next of kin gives permission for harvesting organs. Any potential donor with a history of hypertension, malignant disease, or diabetes is excluded from donation. To facilitate matching a recipient with a donor, a client is placed on a national computerized transplant waiting list. Whenever an organ becomes available, the computer searches for the recipient who is the best match.

When a transplantation is performed, the donor kidney is inserted through an abdominal incision, and the nonfunctioning kidneys are left in place unless the client is extremely hypertensive. The blood vessels from the donor kidney are sutured to the iliac artery and vein, and the ureter is implanted in the bladder (Fig. 58-9).

Even a perfect match does not guarantee that a transplanted organ will not be rejected. Ironically, even some less-than-perfectly matched transplanted organs are successful primarily because of immunosuppressive drugs. Powerful antirejection drugs are used at the time of the transplant (induction) and for long-term maintenance. These may include the following:

Induction Agents:

- Basiliximab (Simulect)
- Antithymocyte globulin (Thymoglobulin)

Maintenance Agents:

- Azathioprine (Imuran)
- Corticosteroids (prednisone)
- Cyclosporine: available as a microemulsion (Neoral), which provides a more sustained concentration
- Tacrolimus (Prograf): similar to cyclosporine but more potent
- Other combinations, including the following:
  - Mycophenolate mofetil (Cellcept)—specifically for preventing kidney transplant rejection
  - Mycophenolic acid (Myfortic) similar to Cellcept
  - Sirolimus (Rapamune)

If rejection occurs, the client resumes hemodialysis and waits for another transplant.

Nursing Management

Before conducting an initial interview and physical assessment, the nurse attempts to learn the cause (if known), type (acute vs. chronic), and prognosis of the kidney disorder. Clients may be unable to give an accurate history because of the effect of renal failure on the thought processes or because they are acutely ill. It may be necessary to obtain information from the family. The nursing care for the client undergoing renal transplantation is complex and specialized. Standard postoperative nursing interventions are applicable (see Chapter 14), with the added consideration of assessing for signs of rejection and prevention of infection. Box 58-5 describes signs and symptoms of transplant rejection.

Nursing care for clients with renal failure is extensive. See Nursing Care Plan 58-1 and Client and Family Teaching 58-5 for more information.

BOX 58-5 Signs and Symptoms of Kidney Transplant Rejection

Hypertension
Edema
Oliguria
Fever
Abdominal pain
Swelling or tenderness over the transplanted kidney
Shortness of breath
Weight gain
Increase in serum creatinine levels

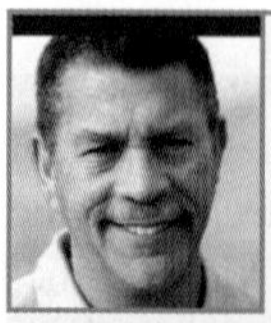

Clinical Scenario A client recently diagnosed with CKD is scheduled to start hemodialysis in the hospital and then will transition to hemodialysis in an outpatient setting 3 days a week. What are the important aspects of this client's ongoing care? (See Nursing Care Plan 58-1.)

NURSING CARE PLAN 58-1 The Client With Chronic Kidney Disease

Assessment

- Assess fluid status, including problems related to unbalanced intake and output.
- Monitor nutritional status, making sure the client follows the appropriate restrictions.
- Assess emotional status to provide relevant support.

Nursing Diagnosis. **Fluid Overload** related to impaired renal function

Expected Outcome. Client will maintain appropriate body weight without excess fluid.

Interventions	Rationales
Weigh client daily under the same conditions: time, clothing, and scale.	*Information provides a baseline and database for monitoring changes. A gain of 1 kg (2.2 lb) equals 1 L of fluid.*
Record urine output accurately.	*Output determines intake. Usually, client is allowed 500 mL intake (equals insensible fluid losses) plus the volume of excreted urine per day.*
Assess lung sounds, respiratory rate and effort, and heart sounds. Inspect for jugular vein detention.	*Findings provide a baseline and database to determine fluid volume excess, needed interventions, and effects of treatments. Fluid overload may cause pulmonary edema.*
Monitor laboratory studies.	*Results assist in identifying fluid excess and promote earlier interventions.*
Administer prescribed diuretics and antihypertensives.	*These drugs reduce fluid excess and decrease cardiac workload.*
Prepare client for dialysis.	*Dialysis reduces uremic toxins, corrects electrolyte imbalances, and decreases fluid overload.*

Evaluation of Expected Outcome

Client demonstrates appropriate urine output/fluid balance as evidenced by stable weight, vital signs within normal range for the client, no edema, and only slightly elevated electrolyte levels.

Nursing Diagnosis. **Malnutrition Risk** related to anorexia, increased metabolic needs, and dietary restrictions

Expected Outcome. Client will maintain adequate nutritional intake.

Interventions	Rationales
Monitor and record client's dietary intake.	*Findings provide a database for nutritional changes and effects of interventions.*
Provide frequent small feedings.	*They minimize nausea and anorexia and promote the intake of high-calorie, nutritious foods.*
Encourage client to be involved with food choices and times for meals.	*Involving the client promotes interest and control and considers dietary habits and preferences.*
Explain restrictions and provide a list of nutritional needs and acceptable food choices.	*Doing so promotes client's understanding of the relationship between food intake and kidney disease and provides a positive approach to dietary restrictions.*

Evaluation of Expected Outcome

Client maintains weight unrelated to fluid volume by following dietary needs and restrictions.

Nursing Diagnosis. **Altered Tissue Integrity Risk** related to restricted oral intake and increased nitrogenous wastes in body fluids such as saliva

Expected Outcome. The oral mucosa and lips will remain moist and intact.

Interventions	Rationales
Assess mouth for inflammation, ulceration, or bleeding.	*Findings provide a database for intervention and evaluation of treatment effectiveness.*
Instruct or assist client to provide mouth care after each meal and at bedtime or every 4 hours while awake. Encourage client to swish but not swallow water frequently as desired.	*Frequent mouth care removes debris, rinses away nitrogenous wastes in saliva, prevents accumulation of bacteria, and keeps mucous membranes moist.*
Provide lanolin-based lip balm for use as needed.	*It keeps lips moist and promotes integrity, preventing bleeding and introduction of microorganisms.*

(continued)

NURSING CARE PLAN 58-1 The Client With Chronic Kidney Disease (*continued*)

Evaluation of Expected Outcomes

Client performs frequent mouth care. Mucous membranes and lips remain moist and intact.

Nursing Diagnosis. **Activity Intolerance** related to fatigue, anemia, weakness, retention of nitrogenous waste products, and dialysis procedure

Expected Outcome. Client will participate in activities as tolerated.

Interventions	Rationales
Determine cause of activity intolerance.	*Knowing the cause assists in planning appropriate interventions.*
If able, encourage client to increase activity slowly. Perform range-of-motion exercises as tolerated.	*Activity and exercises help maintain or improve muscle tone, strength, and endurance.*
Provide periods of rest between activities.	*Rest decreases oxygen consumption and improves energy levels.*

Evaluation of Expected Outcome

Client participates in activities and can do activities of daily living (ADLs) with minimal assistance.

Nursing Diagnosis. Electrolyte Imbalance Risk, Dehydration: Related to elevated BUN, creatinine, and electrolyte levels, potential decrease in blood pressure, and increase of urine output due to diuretic medications.

Expected Outcome. Nurse will minimize and manage potential complications.

Interventions	Rationales
Administer prescribed antihypertensive and diuretic medications as ordered.	*These medications lower BP and increase urine output from partially functional kidneys.*
Restrict protein intake to foods that are complete proteins (contain all essential amino acids) within prescribed limits.	*Complete proteins provide positive nitrogen balance needed for healing and growth.*
Provide sufficient calories from carbohydrates and fats.	*Doing so prevents excess sodium and fluid accumulation.*
Monitor cardiac rhythm.	*Hyperkalemia and other electrolyte imbalances can cause dangerous dysrhythmias.*
Restrict sources of potassium usually found in fresh fruits and vegetables.	*Hyperkalemia can cause life-threatening changes.*
Be prepared to administer glucose and regular insulin.	*They promote transfer of potassium from extracellular to intracellular locations.*
Restrict sodium intake as ordered.	*Doing so prevents catabolism of muscle and body stores of protein.*
Administer calcium supplements, vitamin D supplements, and phosphate binders (Amphojel); at the same time, limit phosphorus-containing foods such as dairy products, dried beans, and soft drinks.	*CRF causes numerous physiologic changes that affect calcium, phosphorus, and vitamin D metabolism, requiring supplementation and dietary restrictions.*
Administer prescribed iron and folic acid supplements or Epogen.	*Iron and folic acid supplements are needed for RBC production. Epogen stimulates bone marrow to produce RBCs.*

Evaluation of Expected Outcomes

BP is 140/90 mm Hg. BUN and creatinine levels are slightly elevated. Serum electrolyte levels are minimally elevated. RBC and hemoglobin levels are within normal levels.

Nursing Diagnosis. **Altered Skin Integrity Risk** related to scratching secondary to pruritus

Expected Outcome. Skin will remain intact and free of crystals.

Interventions	Rationales
Instruct client to limit bathing to less than 1/2 hour using lukewarm water and glycerin-based soap. Add emollient to skin two to three times a day.	*These measures reduce skin drying while rinsing away nitrogenous waste products.*
Keep the environment humidified.	*Emollients restore moisture. All measures help to maintain skin integrity.*
Institute measures that prevent client from scratching, such as keeping fingernails short and encouraging client to use soft clothing and bedding.	*Humidification provides moisture to the skin and prevents drying. These measures prevent trauma to the skin and maintain skin integrity.*

NURSING CARE PLAN 58-1 The Client With Chronic Kidney Disease (*continued*)

Evaluation of Expected Outcome

Client maintains intact skin without evidence of crystals.

Nursing Diagnosis. **Infection Risk** related to compromised immune defenses

Expected Outcome. Client will remain free of infection.

Interventions	Rationales
Monitor temperature at least every shift.	*Clients with chronic kidney disease are very prone to infection.*
Monitor for signs and symptoms of infection.	*Chills, malaise, sore throat, redness, drainage, and elevated temperature are all signs of infection.*
Restrict contact with family, friends, or staff who may have an infectious disorder.	*Doing so prevents spread of microorganisms to immunocompromised client.*
Ensure that all who come in contact with client practice appropriate aseptic technique.	*Handwashing, clean environment, and asepsis prevent the spread of microorganisms.*

Evaluation of Expected Outcome

Client is afebrile and demonstrates no signs or symptoms of infection.

Nursing Diagnosis. **Situational Low Self-Esteem** related to change in body image, dependency, and role change

Expected Outcome. Client will seek help as needed and demonstrate improved self-concept.

Interventions	Rationales
Demonstrate acceptance and respect for client.	*They promote client's self-acceptance.*
Assess client's relationships with significant others.	*Doing so identifies client's strengths and support systems.*
Encourage client and significant others to discuss changes produced by the disease and its treatments.	*Identifying concerns and questions helps arrive at solutions.*
Provide information about support groups.	*They give an opportunity for clients and families to receive support and understanding. They also assist with coping.*

Evaluation of Expected Outcome

Client demonstrates improved self-concept as evidenced by positive coping skills, ability to express concerns, and ability to seek support.

Client and Family Teaching 58-5
The Client With Chronic Kidney Disease

Develop a teaching plan based on the following:

- Follow the diet and fluid intake recommended by the primary provider. Do not use salt substitutes (which often contain potassium) unless allowed by the primary provider.
- Take medications exactly as prescribed by the primary provider.
- Do not use any nonprescription drugs unless use is approved by the primary provider.
- Measure and record fluid intake and urine output. Limit fluids as recommended.
- Avoid exposure to those with any type of infection (e.g., colds, sore throats, flu).
- Monitor BP as recommended by the primary provider.
- Keep skin clean and dry. Take brief showers with tepid water, pat skin to dry, and use moisturizing lotions or creams such as Eucerin, Nivea, Alpha Keri, or Lubriderm. Avoid scratching.
- When doing laundry, use a mild laundry detergent. Use an extra rinse cycle to remove all detergent or add 1 teaspoon of vinegar per quart of water to the rinse cycle to remove detergent residue.
- Keep a record of daily weight, and report any rapid weight gain to the primary provider.
- Take frequent rest periods; avoid heavy exercise.
- If any of the following occurs, contact the primary provider immediately: inability to urinate, slow decrease in daily urine output, weight gain (more than 5 lb or amount recommended by primary provider), chills, fever, sore throat, cough, blood in the urine or stool, easy bleeding or bruising, lethargy, extreme fatigue, persistent headache, nausea, vomiting, or diarrhea.

TABLE 58-5 Comparison of Hemodialysis and Peritoneal Dialysis

TYPE OF DIALYSIS	ADVANTAGES	DISADVANTAGES
Hemodialysis	Rapid removal of solutes and water Takes less time No risk for peritonitis Personnel perform procedure in a dialysis center	Bulge from fistula or graft is obvious Risk for vascular complications, infection, distal ischemia, carpal tunnel syndrome, hypotension, and disequilibrium Strict fluid and dietary restrictions Lifestyle revolves around dialysis appointments Home hemodialysis requires space for the machine and training to use it
Peritoneal	Simple to perform Facilitates independence Easier access No anticoagulation Fewer problems with hypotension or disequilibrium Less rigid dietary and fluid restrictions More flexibility in lifestyle and activities	More time-consuming Weight gain from glucose in the dialysate Peritonitis is a potential complication Requires training and motivation

>>> *Stop, Think, and Respond 58-3*

Clients who have a kidney transplant are at risk for infection. What nursing measures help to prevent infection?

DIALYSIS

Dialysis is a procedure for cleaning and filtering the blood. It substitutes for kidney function when the kidneys cannot remove the nitrogenous waste products and maintain adequate fluid, electrolyte, and acid–base balances.

During dialysis, the client's blood is filtered by diffusion and osmosis (see Chapter 16). Substances such as water, urea, creatinine, and dangerously high levels of potassium move from the blood through the semipermeable membrane to the **dialysate**, the solution used during dialysis that has a composition similar to normal human plasma. Dialysis is performed by hemodialysis and peritoneal dialysis. The technique can be performed either at home or in a dialysis center. Each type has advantages and disadvantages (Table 58-5).

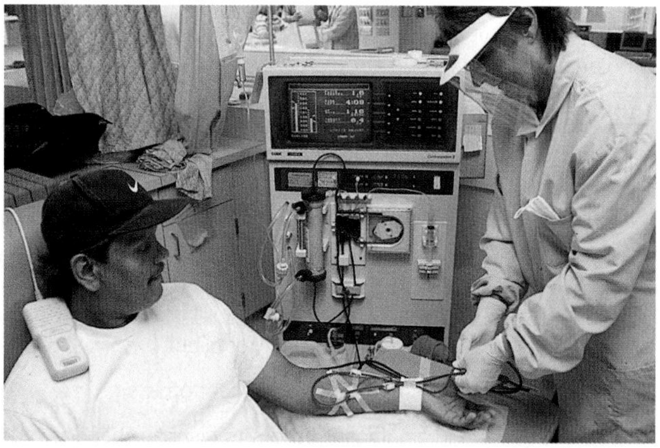

Figure 58-10 During hemodialysis, the client's blood flows to the hemodialysis machine, through a dialyzer (where filtering takes place), and back to the client's body.

Hemodialysis

Hemodialysis requires transporting blood from the client through a **dialyzer**, a semipermeable membrane filter in a machine (Fig. 58-10). The dialyzer contains many tiny hollow fibers. Blood moves through the hollow fibers. Water and wastes from the blood move into the dialysate fluid that flows around the fibers, but protein and RBCs do not. The filtered blood is returned to the client. The entire cycle takes 4 to 6 hours and is generally performed three times a week.

Vascular Access

There are several methods for facilitating the removal and return of the client's dialyzed blood. One technique using tunneled central venous catheter access has already been described. Two others more commonly used for clients with CKD are (1) arteriovenous (AV) fistula and (2) AV graft.

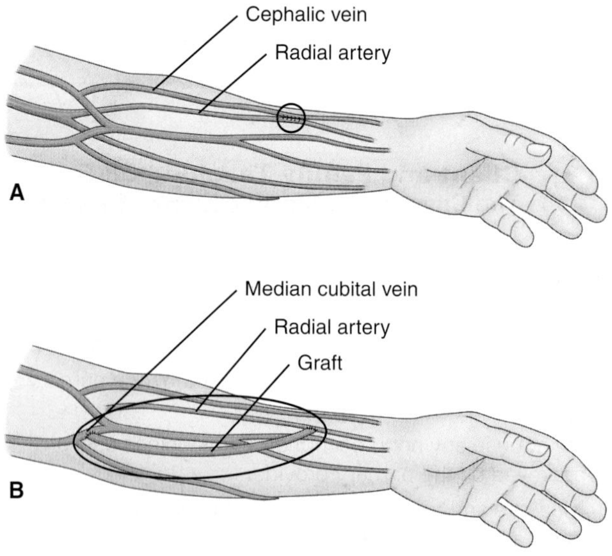

Figure 58-11 **(A)** Arteriovenous fistulas are created by anastomosing a client's vein to an artery. **(B)** Arteriovenous grafts are established by connecting the artery and vein using synthetic tubing. (Reprinted with permission from Hinkle, J. L., & Cheever, K. H. (2014). *Brunner & Suddarth's textbook of medical-surgical nursing* (13th ed.). Wolters Kluwer Health/ Lippincott Williams & Wilkins.)

Arteriovenous Fistula

An **arteriovenous fistula** is a surgical anastomosis (connection) of an artery and vein lying in close proximity (Fig. 58-11A). The vessels usually joined are the cephalic vein and the radial artery or the cephalic vein and brachial artery, usually in the arm less used by the client. Fistulas are preferred over grafts because they have a better record of remaining patent and have fewer complications, such as thrombosis and infection, compared with other access options. They require from 1 to 4 months to mature, however, before being used. Consequently, some fistulas are created prematurely so they are ready when a client eventually requires dialysis.

At the time of dialysis, two venipunctures are performed at either end of the fistula. The distal venipuncture (referred to as the arterial needle because it takes the blood away) is used to remove blood that is transported to the machine. The proximal needle puncture (referred to as the venous needle) is used to return the dialyzed blood. When dialysis is completed, the needles are removed and pressure dressings are applied for several hours.

Blood samples are taken before and after dialysis. The client's predialysis and postdialysis weights are compared. Sometimes, as much as 10 lb of fluid is removed. Examples of postdialysis laboratory studies include BUN, creatinine, sodium, potassium, chlorides, and hematocrit. These are used as indicators of the efficiency of dialysis.

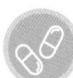

Pharmacologic Considerations

■ Many factors determine whether daily medications should be taken before hemodialysis. Disruption of absorption of oral drugs, protein binding, and even the type of filter in the dialysis machine can influence how much of a drug will be dialyzed out of the body. Consult your clinical pharmacist when the client is admitted and make note of dosing for best outcome on dialysis days.

Arteriovenous Graft

An **arteriovenous graft** is a type of vascular access method that uses a tube of synthetic material (e.g., Gore-Tex or polytetrafluoroethylene) to connect a vein and artery in the upper or lower arm (see Fig. 58-11B). The graft pulsates with blood flow. AV grafts can be used 14 days after their insertion. Although the graft reseals after each needle puncture, the expected life of the graft is 3 to 5 years with repeated use.

Other Forms of Hemodialysis

There are several types of hemodialysis generally used for AKI or short-term use. As discussed earlier, these are referred to as CRRT. Clients who have AKI or are unstable and cannot tolerate aggressive hemodialysis are placed either on diffusion-based solute removal or convection-based solute and water removal that runs continuously, through an extracorporeal circuit. These methods may be better tolerated by clients because problems that occur with intermittent hemodialysis are usually related to the rapid rate of solute infusion and fluid removal.

Various types of CRRT are used and are classified based on the vascular access—either arterial or venous. Examples include:

- *Continuous arteriovenous hemodialysis*: This method uses portable equipment to pump blood from the client through a hemofilter and back to the client in a slow continuous mode.
- *Continuous venovenous hemofiltration* (CVVH): With this mode, blood from a double-lumen venous catheter is pumped through a hemofilter; arterial access is not required, reducing the risk of arterial thrombosis.
- *Continuous venovenous hemodialysis* (CVVHD): With this technique, blood is pumped from a double-lumen venous catheter through a hemofilter and a concentration gradient that removes even more uremic toxins and fluids; it also does not require arterial access.

Nursing Management

The nurse assesses and records vital signs before and after hemodialysis as well as weighing the client and obtaining blood for laboratory testing. To prepare for vascular access, the nurse

- Inspects the skin over the fistula or graft for signs of infection.
- Palpates for a **thrill** (vibration) over the vascular access or listens for a **bruit**, a loud sound caused by turbulent blood flow. If absent, the nurse postpones further use and reports findings.
- Notes the color of skin and nailbeds and mobility of fingers.
- Washes the skin over the fistula or graft with soap and water or antiseptic.
- Avoids puncturing the same site that was used previously.
- After dialysis is completed, does not administer injections for 2 to 4 hours. This allows time for the metabolism and excretion of heparin, which is administered during dialysis, to reach safe levels.
- Before discharging the client, observes for disequilibrium syndrome, a potential complication.

During dialysis, a client may experience shortness of breath secondary to fluid accumulation, related to the length of time between treatments. Clients may become hypotensive during fluid removal, manifested by nausea and vomiting, dizziness, tachycardia, and diaphoresis. With the rapid removal of fluids and electrolytes, some clients experience painful muscle cramping and/or dysrhythmias. In addition, **disequilibrium syndrome** is a neurologic condition believed to be caused by cerebral edema. The shift in cerebral fluid volume occurs when the concentrations of solutes in the blood are lowered rapidly during dialysis. Decreasing solute concentration lowers the plasma osmolality. Water then floods the brain tissue. The syndrome is characterized by headache, disorientation, restlessness, blurred vision, confusion, and seizures. The symptoms are self-limiting and disappear within several hours after dialysis as fluid and solute concentrations equalize. The syndrome can be prevented by slowing the dialysis process to allow time for gradual equilibration of water.

The nurse teaches the client undergoing hemodialysis the following:

- Avoid carrying heavy items in the arm with the fistula or graft.
- Wear clothing with loose sleeves or made of fabrics that will not obstruct blood flow.
- Do not sleep on the vascular access arm.
- Do not permit venipunctures, injections, or BP in the arm with the vascular access.
- Wash the skin over the vascular access daily.
- Assess for a thrill or bruit daily.
- Report signs of an infection or signs of impaired blood flow to dialysis personnel or primary provider immediately.

Peritoneal Dialysis

Peritoneal dialysis uses the peritoneum, the semipermeable membrane lining the abdomen, to filter fluid, wastes, and chemicals (Fig. 58-12). The dialysate is similar in composition to normal plasma but made hypertonic by dextrose. Higher concentrations of dextrose increase the osmotic effect, thus increasing the amount of water removed from the client's bloodstream. The dialysate is instilled and drained from the abdominal cavity by means of a catheter. Substances or solutes pass from the tiny blood vessels in the peritoneal membrane into the dialysate by means of diffusion because the dialysate becomes an area of low concentration drawing from an area of high concentration. The catheter, which has many perforations, is sutured in place and a dressing is applied.

There are two types of peritoneal dialysis: (1) continuous ambulatory peritoneal dialysis (CAPD) and (2) automated peritoneal dialysis (APD).

Continuous Ambulatory Peritoneal Dialysis

When CAPD is performed, approximately 2000 mL of dialysate is instilled by gravity through the catheter in 30 to 40 minutes. The catheter is clamped, and the solution may dwell for 4 to 10 hours. The instillation bag is lowered below the level of the catheter and unclamped for 30 to 40 minutes to allow time for gravity drainage. The process is repeated three to five times a day on a continuous basis. Clients can carry on normal activities while doing CAPD. A machine is not required for this process.

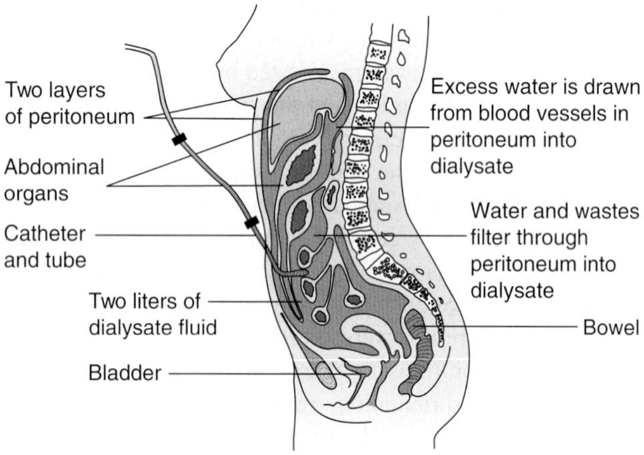

Figure 58-12 Peritoneal dialysis.

Automated Peritoneal Dialysis

APD uses a cycler, which is a machine that automatically delivers dialysate and then drains the peritoneum via a dialysis catheter three to five times during the night while the client sleeps, over a 10- to 12-hour period. The cycler generally contains a supply of the dialysate solution, a pump, a heater, a fluid meter that measures and records the amount of solution that is removed, a disposal container or drain hose, and alarms.

Clients choose the type of peritoneal dialysis based on the one that best fits their personal schedules and lifestyle. Some clients can opt to use the APD at night and then do one CAPD during the day. Clients can also change systems if not satisfied or if there is a change in their schedule.

Nursing Management

For clients who are cared for in a hospital or other facility, the nurse manages the peritoneal dialysis. It is important for the nurse to obtain and review laboratory test findings before dialysis and records vital signs and weight. If the client is acutely ill, it may be necessary to use a bed scale. It also may be necessary to weigh the client as often as every 8 hours while the procedure is in progress. **Peritonitis**, an infection in the peritoneum (lining of the inner abdominal wall), is a major complication of peritoneal dialysis. The nurse monitors and reports fever; nausea; vomiting; and severe abdominal pain, rigidity, or tenderness before, during, or after dialysis.

››› *Stop, Think, and Respond 58-4*

Consider why a client may not be a good candidate for CAPD.

Instillation

Dialysate solution is warmed approximately to body temperature. The nurse adds prescribed drugs such as an antibiotic to the dialysate. They attach the bag of dialysate and administration tubing to the abdominal catheter. The nurse instills the solution and clamps the tubing. If the infusion is slow, the nurse asks the client to move from side to side. If this maneuver is unsuccessful, the primary provider may need to reposition the catheter. Pain in the left shoulder, if it occurs, may be the result of diaphragmatic irritation caused by the high concentration of glucose.

The nurse records the instillation time, the volume and type of dialysate, plus any medications added. They monitor BP and pulse frequently. A drop in BP and increased pulse rate are associated with rapid shifts in fluid that may happen because the dialysate has a high concentration of glucose. As long as the client is stable, they can change positions, eat, and drink.

NURSING GUIDELINES 58-2

Performing Peritoneal Dialysis

- Use strict aseptic technique, including wearing a mask. The client will need to wear a mask whenever there is a procedure involving the peritoneal dialysis catheter.
- Check dialysate for correct concentration and amount.
- Warm prescribed dialysate to body temperature using a commercial warmer.
- Follow prescribed times for infusing the dialysate—the infusion clamp is opened during infusion and clamped after infusion.
- Let dialysate dwell for prescribed time.
- When dwell time is done, open drain clamp and let fluid drain by gravity into drainage bag.
- Document the characteristics and amount of outflow of effluent.
- Monitor client's vital signs, especially when draining effluent.
- Document total fluid intake and output; record positive and negative balances after each exchange.
- Monitor serum electrolyte, glucose, and lipid levels as ordered.
- Do not use expired or cloudy dialysate.
- Warm dialysate in microwave.
- Proceed with infusion if client has signs/symptoms of peritonitis or infection at insertion site.
- Break sterile technique.

Client and Family Teaching 58-6
Performing a Peritoneal Dialysis at Home

The nurse instructs the client as follows:

- Keep dialysis supplies in a clean area away from children and pets.
- Avoid using any dialysate solutions that are expired and look cloudy, discolored, or contain sediment.
- Wash hands before handling the catheter.
- Prevent infection by using sterile gloves during cleaning and exchanges of dialysate.
- Wear a mask when performing exchanges if you have an upper respiratory infection.
- Clean the catheter insertion site daily with an antiseptic such as povidone–iodine (Betadine).
- Inspect the catheter insertion site for signs of infection.
- Keep the catheter stabilized to the abdomen above the belt line to avoid constant rubbing.
- Avoid using scissors during dressing changes to prevent puncturing or cutting the catheter.
- Call the primary provider if
  - A fever develops.
  - There is redness, pain, or pus draining around the catheter.
  - The external length of the catheter increases.
  - Nausea, vomiting, or abdominal pain develops.

Drainage

At the end of the dwell time, the nurse lowers the empty bag used to instill the solution and opens the clamp. They observe the appearance of the siphoned fluid—it should be relatively clear. The nurse must report drainage that is cloudy or tinged with blood. The next instillation may relieve abdominal pain at the end of the drainage period. The nurse notifies the primary provider if marked abdominal distention accompanies pain. In such a case, the nurse must delay the next dialysis cycle until a primary provider examines the client.

The nurse measures the difference between the volume instilled and the volume removed. If there is a drainage deficit, they notify the primary provider before instilling more fluid. The nurse weighs the client after the last cycle of drainage.

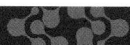

Nursing Guidelines 58-2 provides information related to performing peritoneal dialysis. Client and Family Teaching 58-6 lists important instructions for the client performing a peritoneal dialysis at home. The issue of home-based dialysis is discussed further in Evidence-Based Practice 58-1.

Evidence-Based Practice 58-1

Peritoneal Dialysis and Sleep Patterns

Clinical Question

What are the effects of interrupted sleep patterns in peritoneal dialysis?

Evidence

A study review by Zhang et al. (2021) revealed that tiredness, fatigue, and interrupted sleep patterns were high with clients, especially older clients, in end-stage kidney disease. People who have decreased sleep are affected metabolically and in their immune systems. This can put them at risk for infection and disease and also decrease their quality of life. Eventually, this may affect their mental function such as day-to-day thinking and their personality and moods. Low hemoglobin levels and high serum phosphorus levels can affect sleep as improving these levels can improve sleep patterns (Zhang et al., 2021).

Nursing Implications

Nurses can be supportive of the fragmented sleep with chronic clients. Nurses can cluster care of clients receiving dialysis and allow them to rest during the treatment as much as possible. The nursing assessment and history can include questions about sleep patterns and education on getting sleep and rest and watching for signs and symptoms of infections (Zhang et al., 2021).

Reference

Zhang, H., Yang, Y., Huang, J., Lailan, S., & Tao, X. (2021). Correlates of objective sleep quality in older peritoneal dialysis patients. *Renal Failure, 43* (1), 180–187. https://doi.org/10.1080/0886022X.2020.1871369

KEY POINTS

- Infectious and inflammatory disorders of the kidney:
  - Pyelonephritis: an acute or chronic bacterial infection of the kidney
  - Acute glomerulonephritis: inflammation of the glomeruli in the kidneys
  - Chronic glomerulonephritis: slowly progressive disease characterized by inflammation of the glomeruli, causing irreversible damage to the nephrons
- Congenital kidney disorders: polycystic kidney disease—disorder with the formation of multiple bilateral kidney cysts
- Obstructive disorders:
  - Kidney and ureteral calculi: stones in the urinary tract from the kidney pelvis and beyond. Several different types include calcium, magnesium, uric acid, and cystine.
  - Tumors of the kidney: almost always cancerous
- Kidney failure: inability of the nephrons in the kidney to maintain balance, excrete waste, and perform regulatory functions
  - AKI: can be caused by many different reasons such as hemorrhage, impaired cardiac efficiency, or sepsis
  - CKD: usually associated intrarenal conditions or complications of systemic diseases such as diabetes mellitus and disseminated lupus erythematosus
- Dialysis: procedure for cleaning and filtering the blood, substitutes for kidney function
  - Hemodialysis: required vascular access such as an arteriovenous fistula or arteriovenous graft
  - Peritoneal dialysis: can be CAPD or APD

CRITICAL THINKING EXERCISES

1. A client with a ureteral stone is experiencing severe pain. Another nurse believes the client has a low pain tolerance. What action is appropriate at this time? Why?
2. A client who had a left nephrectomy is having discomfort when coughing, deep breathing, and changing positions. What nursing measures could relieve their discomfort?
3. If you had CKD and must decide to have either hemodialysis or peritoneal dialysis when end-stage kidney disease (ESKD) develops, explain which choice you would make and the reasons for that choice.
4. A client is diagnosed with AKI. If you were caring for this client, describe the signs and symptoms that you would expect to see when the client is in the recovery phase.

NCLEX-STYLE REVIEW QUESTIONS PrepU

1. A nurse sees a client who has been taking trimethoprim-sulfamethoxazole (Bactrim) for a week for a diagnosis of pyelonephritis. Which of the following findings indicates the client adhered to the treatment regimen?
   1. Bacteria are not present on the urine culture.
   2. Client reports that the flank pain has resolved.
   3. Client states that they are voiding large amounts.
   4. RBC count is 4.8 million cells/mm^3.
2. A nurse admits a client with possible acute glomerulonephritis. Which of the following signs would the nurse expect to see with acute glomerulonephritis?
   1. BP 100/60 mm Hg
   2. Periorbital edema
   3. Polyuria
   4. Temperature 37.2°C
3. A nurse is caring for a client with urolithiasis. Which of the following nursing interventions is important for this client's care?
   1. Encourage the client to eat dairy products.
   2. Limit the client's fluid intake to 500 mL in 24 hours.
   3. Maintain the client on strict bedrest.
   4. Strain the client's urine with each voiding.
4. A nurse is assigned to care for a postoperative client who had a nephrectomy and insertion of a urethral catheter. What is the rationale for the nurse to record the color of drainage from each tube and catheter?
   1. Avoids interference with wound drainage
   2. Prevents pain related to obstruction
   3. Provides a means for further comparison and evaluation
   4. Restores and maintains intravascular volume
5. What is the most important assessment for a nurse to make when caring for a client with AKI who has an elevated potassium level?
   1. Apical pulse
   2. BP
   3. Respirations
   4. Temperature

WANT TO KNOW MORE? There are a wide variety of online resources available on thePoint to enhance learning and understanding of this chapter.

Go to thePoint.lww.com/activate, and use the activation code found in the front of this text to unlock these online resources.

59 Caring for Clients With Disorders of the Bladder and Urethra

Words To Know

cystectomy
cystitis
cystolitholapaxy
cystostomy
diverticulum
fulguration
incontinence
interstitial cystitis
neurogenic bladder
residual urine
retention
stricture
suprapubic cystostomy tube
urethritis
urethroplasty
urinary diversion
urosepsis

Learning Objectives

On completion of this chapter, you will be able to:

1. Explain urinary retention and appropriate nursing management.
2. Discuss urinary incontinence and appropriate nursing management.
3. Describe the pathophysiologic changes seen in cystitis, interstitial cystitis, and urethritis.
4. Explain the symptoms associated with bladder stones.
5. Discuss the cause and treatment of urethral strictures.
6. Describe the treatment and nursing care for a client diagnosed with a malignant bladder tumor.
7. Describe various types of urinary diversion procedures.
8. Identify components of a teaching plan for a client having a urinary diversion procedure.

Disorders of the bladder and urethra are common and can be the source of severe problems that become chronic, altering a client's lifestyle. Many disorders affecting the bladder and urethra are treated on an outpatient basis; the more serious disorders require hospitalization.

VOIDING DYSFUNCTION

Urinary retention and urinary incontinence are voiding dysfunctions. Urinary **retention** is the inability to urinate or effectively empty the bladder. Urinary **incontinence** is the inability to control the voiding of urine. Clients experiencing either retention or incontinence face temporary or permanent alterations in their ability to urinate normally. These conditions require individualized approaches to solving the problem and sensitivity to the client's needs, both physiologic and psychosocial.

Urinary Retention

Pathophysiology and Etiology

Urinary retention may be either acute or chronic. Acute urinary retention is seen in complete urethral obstruction, after general anesthesia, or with the administration of certain drugs such as atropine or a phenothiazine. Chronic urinary retention (CUR) often is seen in clients with disorders such as prostatic enlargement or neurologic disorders that result in a **neurogenic bladder** (a bladder that does not receive adequate nerve stimulation). It is more common in men, with an increased incidence over the age of 70 years.

The client with acute urinary retention usually cannot void at all. The client with CUR may be able to void but does not completely empty the bladder (retention with overflow) and has a large residual volume

Gerontologic Considerations

- Assessment of urinary concerns of older adults should include the following, and a diary over at least 3 days that records the following information should be maintained:
  - Time, amount, and type of medication.
  - Time, amount, and type of fluid intake.
  - Time and amount of voiding, involuntary urine loss, and/or involuntary loss of stool (Brown et al., 2018).
- Review for medication(s) that may affect bladder emptying or cause constipation.
- Amount and type of alcohol or illicit drugs.
- Constipation or fecal impaction.
- Mobility.
- Fatigue.
- Muscle strength.
- Balance.
- Falls (Brown et al., 2018).
- Cognition.
- History of atherosclerosis (Schimit et al., 2020).
- History of parkinsonian symptoms (Stewart, 2018).
- Environmental conditions such as distance to toilet.
- Caregiver availability, ability, and stress
- Some clients may be reluctant to provide information owing to embarrassment, belief that incontinence is a part of aging, or fear of institutionalization. Explain that accurate and complete information may provide insight to guide treatment of specific cause(s). For example, a change in the environment or an assistive device may alleviate the incontinence. For those in a residential care home, interventions could include ultrasound-assisted prompted voiding (Suzuki et al., 2019).
- Any new onset of urinary incontinence should be a priority in nursing care plans, including efforts to maintain quality of life.
- Any client's physical and cognitive abilities must be considered when instituting a bladder rehabilitation program. However, older adults may have more involuntary relaxation of the bladder sphincter than younger clients, necessitating shorter time periods between voiding attempts (e.g., 1 to 1.5 hours rather than 2 hours). It is important for all health care providers, family members, or other caregivers to adhere to the client's individual schedule in order to prevent episodes of incontinence, which can affect the person's self-esteem.

(**residual urine**), which is urine retained in the bladder after the client voids. The residual amount may vary from 30 mL to several hundred milliliters or more.

Assessment Findings

Symptoms of acute urinary retention are sudden inability to void, usually with an urgent need to void, distended bladder, and severe lower abdominal pain with a feeling of fullness, and overall discomfort. CUR may not produce obvious symptoms, because the bladder stretches over time and accommodates large volumes without producing discomfort. The overstretched bladder does not contract effectively, and the client is unaware that the bladder is not emptying completely. The client may experience difficulty with starting urination. Many clients feel an urge to void, even when they have just voided. If the amount of residual urine is large, the client may void frequently in small amounts. Signs of a bladder infection (e.g., fever, chills, pain on urination) and dribbling of urine also may be present. Some clients experience continuous discomfort in the lower abdomen and urinary tract.

Urinalysis may show an increased number of white blood cells (WBCs), indicating an acute or chronic bladder infection. Catheterization or ultrasound can determine postvoid residual volume. Bedside ultrasound bladder scanning is used by nurses as a noninvasive measure of postvoiding volume of urine in the bladder. Volumes over 100 mL are considered diagnostic of urinary retention. Urodynamic testing uses video radiography; radiopaque contrast dye is instilled in the bladder via a small catheter, and bladder pressures are measured during filling and voiding. Uroflowmetry measures the urine flow and speed of bladder emptying. A pressure flow study measures the bladder pressure required to urinate and the flow rate a given pressure generates. Electromyography (EMG) determines the activity of the external sphincter during voiding. X-rays show the bladder's anatomy and if there are any problems. A cystoscopy and/or ureteroscopy may be done to examine the bladder and urethra. Computed tomography (CT) scans with contrast are done to determine if there are bladder stones, tumors or cysts, or a traumatic injury.

Medical and Surgical Management

Acute urinary retention requires immediate catheterization. If a catheter cannot be inserted through the urethra, special urologic instruments that dilate the urethra may be used. If there is a stricture, urethral dilation may be done, which involves using larger and larger catheters to widen the stricture. Sometimes a Foley catheter is used; the balloon is inflated at the site of the stricture. Urethral stents may be inserted to widen the stricture. The stents may be permanent or temporary, depending on the nature of the stricture. These procedures can be done in an outpatient setting. Local anesthesia or sedation may be used.

CUR is managed by permanent drainage with an indwelling urethral catheter (IUC), **suprapubic cystostomy tube** (a catheter inserted through the abdominal wall directly into the bladder), or clean intermittent catheterization (CIC). Permanent catheterization of the bladder carries the risk of bladder stones, renal disease, bladder infection, and **urosepsis**, a serious systemic infection from microorganisms in the urinary tract invading the bloodstream. Because the incidence of complications is lower, CIC is the preferred treatment. Other methods to use include, particularly for clients who have lost nervous system control secondary to disease or injury, Credé maneuver or manual voiding, or abdominal strain (Valsalva maneuver voiding; Box 59-1). Clients may combine these methods with timed voiding, which means that clients void according to a schedule, not waiting to feel the urge.

BOX 59-1 Credé or Valsalva Voiding

Credé Maneuver (Manual)
Apply gentle downward pressure to the bladder during voiding. This maneuver may be done by the client or family member. The client also may do this by sitting on the toilet and rocking back and forth gently.

Valsalva Maneuver
Instruct the client to bear down as with defecation. Do not teach this method to a client with cardiac problems or who may be adversely affected by a vagal response (heart rate slows).

CIC may not be possible for clients who lack the mobility or cognitive functioning to perform the procedure. Some clients who are men and who cannot perform CIC can avoid the complications of permanent indwelling catheters by undergoing surgery to release the urethral sphincters. Urine then drains freely out of the urethra, and the client wears a condom catheter. Nursing Guidelines 59-1 provides instructions about the application of a condom catheter. If it is possible to remove the cause, such as excising excess prostatic tissue, surgery is performed. However, surgery does not always result in restoration of normal voiding.

NURSING GUIDELINES 59-1

Applying a Condom Catheter

- Assess the penis for swelling or skin breakdown.
- Verify client's willingness to use a condom catheter.
- Wash and dry the penis well.
- Wrap the adhesive strip in an upward spiral about the penis, taking care not to wrap it tightly.
- Roll the wider end of the sheath toward the narrow catheter tip (most condom catheters are packaged this way—rolling the condom is not necessary).
- Hold approximately 1 to 2 inches (2.5 to 5 cm) of the lower sheath below the tip of the penis and unroll the sheath upward.
- Secure the upper end of the unrolled sheath to the skin with a second strip of adhesive or a Velcro strap, but not so tightly as to interfere with circulation.
- Connect the catheter drainage tip to a drainage bag.
- Keep the penis positioned in a downward position.
- Assess the penis at least every 2 hours; also check the catheter to make sure it has not become twisted.
- Empty leg bag (if one is used) when it becomes partially filled so that the weight of the collected urine does not dislodge the condom.
- Remove or change the condom catheter daily, or more often as needed, to check skin integrity.
- Substitute a waterproof garment during periods of nonuse of a condom catheter.
- Wash the catheter and collection bag with mild soap and water and rinse with a 1:7 vinegar-and-water solution.

External collection systems for women are available, but proper fit is a problem. Women who cannot accomplish CIC usually are treated with a permanent indwelling catheter.

Intermittent Catheterization

Intermittent catheterization performed in the hospital setting is a sterile procedure. A commercially prepared straight catheterization kit is available in hospitals. The kit includes a straight-tipped catheter, sterile gloves, lubricant, and a sterile collection container.

When intermittent catheterization is performed by clients or family members in the home, clean rather than aseptic technique is used. Clients use a catheter prescribed by the health care provider. Types of catheters and materials for catheters vary, and there are no universal guidelines for specific catheters, except that it should be soft, flexible, and the smallest size possible. There is also disagreement regarding single-use or reuse of catheters. Medicare and Medicaid allow between 120 and 200 sterile catheters (with a single-use lubricant for each catheter) per month if there is a diagnosis of permanent urinary retention or incontinence. Theoretically, this could be enough catheters to last a month. However, many health care providers teach clients to reuse catheters. There is no consensus on one best way to clean intermittent catheters for reuse. If a catheter is reused, the general recommendation is that it be washed with soap and hot water and allowed to air-dry. Another general recommendation is that catheters can be reused for 2 to 4 weeks.

For CIC at home, gloves are not required, but clients must wash their hands thoroughly before and after the procedure. The client can drain the urine into a clean container or directly into the toilet bowl. The schedule is usually three to four times per day, although the frequency can be increased depending on residual volume. If more than 400 mL is returned, the client should catheterize themselves more often. Client education in technique, catheter care, and follow-up care is an important function of nurses in the acute and homecare settings.

Indwelling Catheters

An indwelling urethral catheter (IUC) is one route for permanent bladder catheterization. Another alternative is a cystostomy tube, also called a *suprapubic catheter*, that is inserted through an abdominal incision into the bladder. Clients require careful monitoring and care when there is an indwelling catheter. Maintaining the integrity of the closed drainage system and proper anchoring of the tube to avoid tension and promote drainage (Fig. 59-1) are important. Nursing Guidelines 59-2 offers essential management points. Three major points in particular should be adhered to when managing indwelling catheters:

- Maintain a closed system at all times by following manufacturers' instructions, using preconnected urinary catheter and drainage systems, minimizing irrigation, and using the needleless port system for irrigation if absolutely needed.
- Maintain the urine flow by always positioning the drainage bag below the level of the bladder (not on the floor).

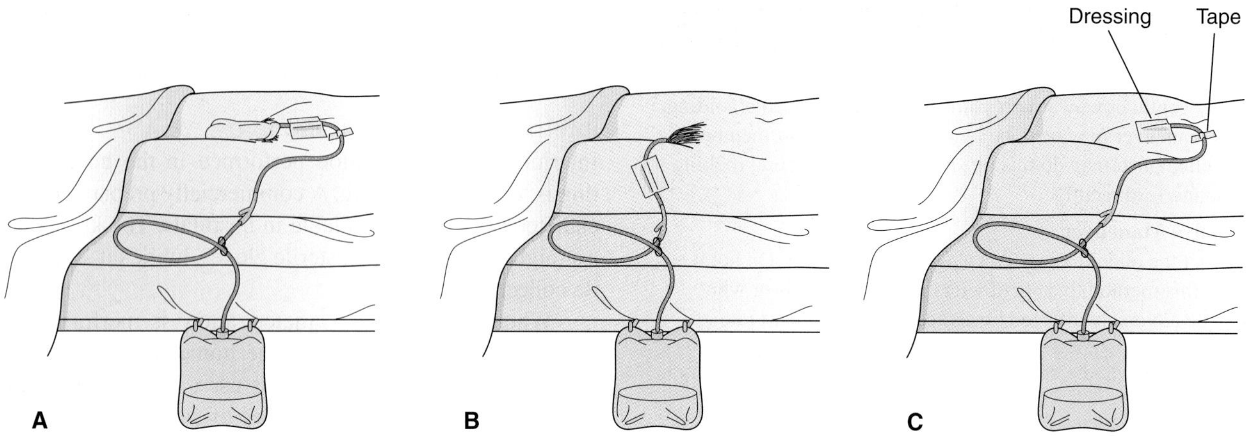

Figure 59-1 Catheter tubing correctly anchored and attached to closed drainage system. **(A)** Men. **(B)** Women. **(C)** Suprapubic.

NURSING GUIDELINES 59-2

General Principles of Catheterization and Catheter Care

The following general principles apply to the insertion and maintenance of urethral or suprapubic catheters:

- Always use strict aseptic technique for insertion of IUCs. Perform hand hygiene prior to beginning the procedure.
- Thoroughly cleanse the urethral meatus before the insertion of a catheter according to policy. Re-perform hand hygiene.
- Use assistance as needed—there may be need for a second person to adequately visualize the urinary meatus and insert the catheter aseptically.
- Select the smallest catheter size possible for IUC and intermittent (straight, single) catheterization, to minimize trauma to the urethra and bladder neck.
- Do not preinflate the balloon.
- Liberally lubricate the catheter with single-use lubricant jelly.
- Insert the IUC to the appropriate length (in men, insert the IUC to the "Y" connection; in women, advance the catheter 2.5 cm beyond the point when urine first flows).
- Inflate IUC balloon as directed (generally 10 mL for an IUC that is labeled 5 or 10 mL).
- Never force a catheter if resistance is felt.
- Never reinsert an IUC that accidentally becomes dislodged; replace it with a new sterile catheter.
- Connect catheters to a sterile, closed drainage system. It is best to use preconnected systems.
- Keep the drainage bag lower than the catheter, but not on the floor.
- Assure that connections remain closed and that there are no obstructions or kinks.
- Do not regularly change IUCs or drainage bags unless indicated because of infection, obstruction, or if there is a break in the closed system.
- Use routine hygiene (bathing or showering) for perineal care. Do not use antiseptics while the IUC is in place.
- Empty the drainage bag regularly into a clean container for each client. Inspect the cystostomy tube site for leakage of urine around the catheter, bleeding, or signs and symptoms of infection.
- Change the cystostomy dressing once per shift or more often if necessary.
- If a permanent vesicocutaneous (bladder to skin) fistula forms, the size of the cystostomy tube may need to be increased to prevent leakage of urine.
- Unless contraindicated by heart failure or renal disease, encourage clients to drink plenty of fluids (2000 to 3000 mL per day).
- Monitor client for signs and symptoms of UTI: fever, chills, hypotension, and confusion.
- Monitor fluid balance and laboratory tests that measure kidney function.

- Maintain cleanliness through meticulous handwashing, disinfecting the needleless port and letting it dry before use, and using strict aseptic technique for catheter insertion (Seckel, 2013).

Nursing Management

The conscious client is able to verbalize the pain and discomfort associated with urinary retention. Clients with Alzheimer disease or psychiatric disorders, or the comatose, anesthetized, or spinal cord–injured client may be unable to communicate or feel the pain and discomfort associated with acute urinary retention. An important nursing responsibility is measuring intake and output, palpating the abdomen for a distended bladder, promoting complete urination, and monitoring the voiding pattern of clients. Nurses use bladder scanners to accurately measure postvoiding urine volume.

Acute Urinary Retention

Acute retention that is likely to resolve quickly (e.g., after anesthesia) probably will be treated by intermittent catheterization. Clients with acute retention unlikely to resolve without surgical intervention (e.g., retention caused by an enlarged prostate) probably will have an IUC.

Nurses measure the volume of urine in the bladder with a bedside scanner to help determine if catheterization is needed. If required, the nurse collaborates with the primary provider to determine if the catheter is to be left in place or removed after the bladder is emptied. The nurse selects the size and type of catheter to be used, sometimes consulting with the primary provider if there are extenuating circumstances, such as an enlarged prostate. Catheters are sized according to the French system (e.g., 14 F to 24 F); the higher the number, the larger the diameter of the catheter. Examples of the various types of catheter tips are shown in Figure 59-2. The CDC recommends selecting the smallest catheter in order to avoid trauma to the urethra and bladder neck.

Clients with an obstruction may be more easily catheterized with a coudé catheter. The curved tip slides over obstructing tissue more readily than the straight-tipped catheter. The nurse selects the appropriate catheter and inserts it under sterile conditions, noting the characteristics and volume of urine returned. If the volume of urine is large (>700 mL), it may be necessary to clamp the catheter before the bladder has emptied completely to prevent bladder spasms or loss of bladder tone. This practice varies and research is ongoing, so it is important to check agency policy.

If the client is going to be managed by CIC, the client and the nurse establish the schedule. Clients are catheterized every 4 to 8 hours, depending on the amount of urine obtained and the fluid intake. The bladder should not be allowed to get distended beyond 350 mL because bladder overdistention results in loss of bladder tone, decreased blood flow to the bladder, and reduction in the layer of mucin that protects the bladder mucosa. CIC continues until the postvoid residual volume is less than 30 mL. To obtain accurate residual volumes, it is important that clients have the opportunity to void first and that catheterization occur immediately after the attempt. The nurse records both the volume voided (even if it is zero) and the volume obtained by catheterization. Postoperative urinary retention usually resolves within 24 to 48 hours.

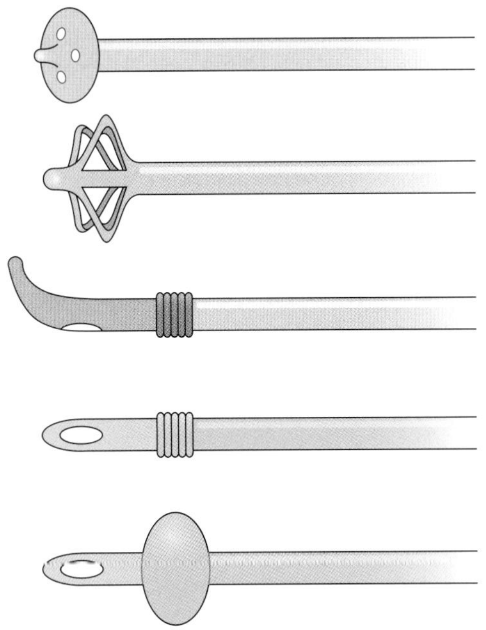

Figure 59-2 Catheter tips (*top to bottom*): de Pezzer catheter, Malecot catheter, coudé catheter, Foley catheter, Foley catheter with balloon inflated. The de Pezzer and the Malecot catheters are inserted by the primary provider with a stylet that temporarily straightens the tip. The Foley and coudé catheters are retained by inflating the balloon.

Chronic Urinary Retention

CUR may go unrecognized. The nurse should ask all clients during an initial health assessment about voiding frequency, the amount (e.g., small, moderate, large) of urine passed each time, the presence of pain or discomfort in the lower abdomen, pain or discomfort on voiding, and difficulty in starting the urinary stream. The examiner gently palpates or percusses the lower abdomen to determine if the bladder is distended. After asking the client to void, the nurse will scan the client's bladder to measure the amount of urine left in the bladder. In addition, the nurse obtains a complete medical, drug, and allergy history and reports suspected CUR to the primary provider.

When a client is diagnosed with CUR, a decision will be made about how best to drain the bladder (as previously described). The ultimate goals are to safely empty the bladder and prevent infection to the urinary tract.

Catheter-Associated Urinary Tract Infections

Hospitals and other facilities are committed to reducing the number of catheter-associated urinary tract infections (CAUTI). The recommended use for urinary catheters is limited to the following:

- Urologic surgery, urinary retention, or urinary outlet obstruction
- Perioperative management for clients undergoing select procedures (genitourinary or colorectal surgery)
- Accurate measurement of urine output (recommended for critically ill clients)
- Promotion of wound healing that could be delayed by urinary incontinence (open sacral or perineal wounds)
- Need for intraoperative monitoring of urinary output during surgery or large volumes of fluid or diuretics anticipated
- Prolonged immobilization (potentially unstable thoracic or lumbar spine, multiple traumatic injuries such as pelvic fractures)
- Promotion of comfort at the end of life (CDC, 2009).

Research is ongoing for the prevention of CAUTIs, particularly with indwelling catheters. This includes research into various types of catheters (antimicrobial/antiseptic-impregnated catheters; hydrophilic catheters, or silicone catheters), how to manage obstructions, and separation of catheterized clients from other clients.

Stop, Think, and Respond 59-1

What methods should a nurse use to prevent the occurrence of a health care–associated infection in the catheterized client?

Urinary Incontinence

Urinary incontinence affects many clients and is a major health care concern. It is estimated that at least one-third of older adults living in the community and one-half of older clients in institutions suffer from incontinence. In addition, at least 33 million people in the United States suffer from overactive bladder (OAB), which involves urgency and frequency with or without urge incontinence (Urology Care Foundation, 2021a). Not only is incontinence a psychosocial problem, it is also a physical problem in that skin breakdown and urinary tract infection (UTI) may result from incontinence. Table 59-1 describes the different types of incontinence.

Pathophysiology and Etiology

Urinary incontinence is a symptom and can result from either bladder or urethral dysfunction (or both). Box 59-2 identifies risk factors for urinary incontinence. The bladder can contract without warning, fail to accommodate adequate volumes of urine, or fail to empty completely and become overstretched, resulting in overflow incontinence. These conditions result from neurologic disease, bladder outlet obstruction, or trauma in all clients; bladder prolapse or low estrogen levels in women; and prostatic enlargement in men. Aging is linked to urinary incontinence. Also, women who experience urinary incontinence with pregnancy are more likely to continue having issues post pregnancy.

Another cause of incontinence is failure of the urethral sphincters to hold urine in the bladder. This may result from trauma, prostate surgery, or relaxed pelvic muscles. Impingement of the spinal nerves, such as in tumors of the spinal cord, herniated disk, or spinal cord injuries, can interfere with the impulse conduction to the brain, resulting in a neurogenic bladder and incontinence. A neurogenic bladder may be spastic, causing incontinence, or it may be flaccid, causing retention. In addition to UTIs and constipation, temporary urinary incontinence can occur because of particular drinks or medications. These include:

- Alcohol
- Caffeine
- Decaffeinated tea and coffee
- Carbonated drinks
- Artificial sweeteners
- Corn syrup
- Foods that are high in spice, sugar, or acid, especially citrus fruits
- Heart and blood pressure medications, sedatives, and muscle relaxants
- Large doses of vitamins B or C (Mayo Clinic Staff, 2019).

TABLE 59-1 Types of Urinary Incontinence

TYPE OF INCONTINENCE	SYMPTOMS	CAUSES
Stress urinary incontinence (SUI)	Client has involuntary loss of urine from intact urethra, which results from sudden increase in intra-abdominal pressure, such as with sneezing or coughing	Decreased pelvic muscle tone, primarily seen in women, and associated with multiple pregnancies, obstetric injuries, obesity, menopause, or pelvic disease
Urge urinary incontinence or overactive bladder (OAB)	Client experiences urge to void but cannot control voiding in time to reach a toilet. Either the brain signals the bladder to empty even when it is not full, or the bladder muscles contract to empty the bladder	Bladder irritation related to urinary tract infections, diabetes, bladder tumors, radiation therapy, enlarged prostate, or neurologic dysfunction
Mixed incontinence	Client has features of two or more types of incontinence	As an example, older adults often experience two different types, such as stress and overflow incontinence
Overflow incontinence	Involuntary loss of urine related to overdistended bladder; clients void small amounts frequently; dribbling	Obstruction from fecal impaction or enlarged prostate; smooth muscle relaxants that relax the bladder and increase capacity; impaired ability of bladder to contract related to neurologic abnormalities, such as spinal cord lesions or tumors, or obstruction to urine output
Transient incontinence	Occurs suddenly; temporary; lasts less than 6 months	Temporary delirium or confusion; infection; increased urine production related to metabolic conditions; effects of some medications such as diuretics, anticholinergics, or antidepressants
Functional incontinence	Client has intact function of the lower urinary tract but cannot identify the need to void or ambulate to the toilet	Cognitive impairments, such as brain injury or Alzheimer disease; or physical limitations, such as rheumatoid arthritis or musculoskeletal injuries
Reflex incontinence	Bladder has uninhibited contractions; involuntary reflexes produce spontaneous voiding, with partial or complete loss of sensation of bladder fullness or urge to void	Impaired conduction of impulses above reflex arc level secondary to spinal cord injury, tumor, or infection
Total incontinence	Urine is continuously and unpredictably lost from the bladder	Results from surgery, trauma, or anatomic malformation

BOX 59-2 Risk Factors for Urinary Incontinence

- Pregnancy: vaginal delivery, episiotomy
- Menopause
- Genitourinary surgery
- Pelvic muscle weakness
- Incompetent urethra as a result of trauma or sphincter relaxation
- Immobility
- High-impact exercise
- Diabetes mellitus
- Age-related changes in the urinary tract
- Obesity
- Chronic cough from chronic lung diseases, asthma, and smoking
- Neurologic conditions, such as stroke, Parkinson's disease, Alzheimer disease, spinal cord injury, and multiple sclerosis
- Medications: diuretics, sedatives, antidepressants, hypnotics, opioids
- Caregiver or toilet unavailable

Assessment Findings

Clients complain of urgency, frequency, leaking small amounts when coughing or sneezing, or complete inability to control urine, depending on the underlying cause. Tests such as a urine culture and sensitivity, cystoscopy, cystogram, urodynamics, and/or pelvic ultrasound are used to determine the type of incontinence.

Medical and Surgical Management

Treatment is aimed at correcting the disorder causing incontinence (when possible), providing medication to control incontinence, correcting the situational problems that contribute to functional incontinence, or instituting a bladder retraining program. Pharmacologic agents that can improve bladder retention, emptying, and control include anticholinergic drugs such as oxybutynin chloride (Ditropan), which reduces bladder spasticity and involuntary bladder contractions; tolterodine tartrate (Detrol), with similar action to oxybutynin chloride; and phenoxybenzamine hydrochloride (Dibenzaline), which may be useful in treating problems with sphincter control. Bethanechol (Urecholine) helps to increase contraction of the detrusor muscle, which assists with emptying of the bladder. Alpha blockers, such as tamsulosin (Flomax), may be prescribed for male clients. These medications promote relaxation of the bladder neck muscles and the muscle fibers of the prostate gland, easing the client's ability to empty the bladder, thus reducing incontinence. Some tricyclic antidepressant medications (amitriptyline [Elavil], nortriptyline [Pamelor], and amoxapine [Asendin]) are useful in treating incontinence because they decrease bladder contractions and increase bladder neck resistance.

Concept Mastery Alert

Anticholinergic Agents

Anticholinergic agents inhibit bladder contraction and are considered first-line medications for urge incontinence.

Pseudoephedrine (Sudafed) may help stress incontinence. Estrogen can be useful in restoring mucosal, vascular, and muscular integrity of the urethra for postmenopausal incontinence, but treatment may only be effective for about a year. Sometimes, medication to control incontinence results in retention and must be discontinued. Occasionally, clients who can easily perform CIC may opt for medication-induced retention and CIC because it allows them to stay dry. Biofeedback uses electronic devices or diaries to assist clients to track when the bladder and urethral muscles contract, in order to gain more control (Smiles et al., 2019). There are also devices that can augment weak pelvic muscles. A urethral insert is similar to a disposable tampon device that the client inserts into the urethra before engaging in activity that contributes to stress incontinence. A pessary is a stiff ring that a health care provider places in the vagina to prevent urine leakage. It is commonly used for clients who have a prolapsed bladder or uterus.

Surgeries and other procedures to improve urinary control include the following:

- *Bladder augmentation*: a procedure that increases the storage capacity of the bladder by transplanting a section of the intestine or stomach into the top of the bladder.
- *Periurethral bulking*: placement of small amounts of collagen in urethral walls to aid the closing pressure.
- *Injection of onabotulinumtoxinA (Botox) into the bladder muscle*: sometimes used for clients with OAB for whom anticholinergics have not worked. This treatment helps the bladder to relax, increasing the storage capacity of the bladder and reducing incontinence. Treatments can be repeated every 3 months.
- *Implantation of an artificial sphincter* that can be inflated to prevent urine loss and deflated to allow urination (Fig. 59-3).
- *Surgeries to provide better support* for urinary structures include the following:
  - *Retropubic suspension*: an open abdominal procedure that involves lifting and anchoring the bladder and

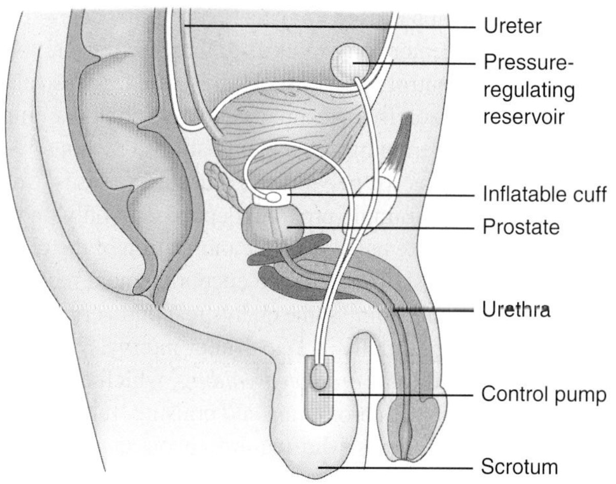

Figure 59-3 Artificial urinary sphincter. An inflatable cuff is inserted surgically around the urethra or bladder neck. To empty the bladder, the cuff is deflated by squeezing the control pump located in the scrotum.

urethra to the pelvic wall through the vagina and pubic ligaments; usually done in conjunction with another open abdominal surgery such as a hysterectomy.

- *Anterior repair*: a procedure that increases support to the bladder by tightening the vaginal wall under the urethra.
- *Transvaginal needle suspension*: a procedure in which the bladder and urethra are attached to the pubic bone or fibrous tissue of the rectum through two vaginal incisions and a midline suprapubic incision.
- *Sling procedures*: a procedure in which a small vaginal incision is used to place a piece of synthetic or natural (harvested from the inner thigh or abdomen) material under the bladder neck; it is secured to the abdominal wall or pelvic bone to create a hammock-type lifting of the urethra.
- *Sacral nerve stimulator implantation*: implantation of a small device similar to a pacemaker that acts on nerves that control bladder and pelvic floor contractions. It is implanted under the skin in the abdomen. A wire connected to a sacral nerve emits electrical pulses to stimulate the nerve and help control the bladder. The client does not experience pain and is relieved from heavy leaking in many cases.

Surgical correction of anatomic problems:

- *Urethroplasty:* surgery to repair structures damaged by trauma.

Nursing Management

Goals when caring for a client with urinary incontinence include maintaining continence as much as possible, preventing skin breakdown, reducing anxiety, and initiating a bladder training program. It must be determined if the client is truly incontinent or if situations prevent the client from getting to the bathroom. Such situations include impaired mobility, physical restraints, and use of sedatives. In addition to assessing for functional causes of incontinence, the nurse obtains details regarding the pattern of incontinence and use of medications that may play a role in the problem. It is important to assess for skin breakdown and determine methods the client has used to manage incontinence.

Instruction centers on exercises to increase muscle tone and voluntary control (pelvic floor muscle exercises, also known as Kegel exercises), techniques to assist bladder emptying, and bladder training. Client and Family Teaching 59-1 outlines instructions for pelvic floor muscle exercises. Success of a bladder retraining program depends not only on the cause of incontinence but also on the motivation of the client and the amount of skillful help and encouragement received from the health care team. Some clients respond very well to scheduled voiding, usually at 2- to 4-hour intervals. Another method is referred to as *prompted voiding*, which combines scheduled voiding with prompting and praising. It is used for cognitively intact clients who require encouragement with self-initiated voiding and cognitively impaired clients who gradually become accustomed to being taken to the bathroom regularly.

Client and Family Teaching 59-1 Performing Pelvic Floor Muscle (Kegel) Exercises

Initial Instructions

1. Sit or stand with legs slightly apart.
2. Draw in perivaginal muscles and anal sphincter as when controlling voiding or defecating.
3. Hold this position of contraction for 5 seconds (instruct client to count or time with a watch).
4. Relax contraction for at least 10 seconds.
5. Repeat exercises 5 to 6 times, increasing slowly to 25 times.
6. Repeat the sequence of exercises three to four times a day.
7. Gradually do the exercises for a total of 200 repetitions.

Advanced Instructions

1. Sit on the toilet and begin to urinate.
2. Stop the flow of urine by doing a Kegel exercise.
3. Hold this position for 5 seconds.
4. Relax and begin voiding.
5. Repeat this sequence five times with each voiding.

Bladder Training

One method of bladder training for the client with an IUC is to alternately clamp and unclamp the catheter. The clamping and unclamping of the catheter begins to reestablish normal bladder function and capacity. In the beginning, the catheter may be unclamped for 5 minutes every 1 or 2 hours. The length of time is gradually increased to every 3 or 4 hours, giving the bladder a chance to fill more completely. When possible, the nurse teaches the client to release the clamp at scheduled times. The catheter eventually is removed.

At this point, or when training clients who have not had an IUC, the nurse instructs the client to try to void every hour. Usually, the client is not able to retain urine longer than an hour, and frequent voiding is necessary to prevent incontinence. Gradually, the client lengthens the interval between voidings to 2, 3, or 4 hours. At first, many clients do not empty the bladder, and they must be catheterized after voiding to remove residual urine. When the client is catheterized for residual urine, the nurse records the amount removed.

When a client is unable to control the storage and passage of urine, or when a bladder training program fails, clients may exhibit varying degrees of anxiety and depression. The nurse needs to offer constant encouragement throughout the bladder training program. Anxiety may be reduced once the client notes the effort, concern, and interest of the health care team. If an accident occurs, it is important to change the bed linen promptly and assure the client that accidents are to be expected during the retraining process. Reducing anxiety may, in some instances, contribute to the success of a bladder training program.

Barrier Garments and External Collection Devices

If it is not possible to establish a voiding routine and incontinence persists, the health care team works with the client to devise a system of collecting the urine. Male clients can use a condom catheter over the penis and connect the tubing to a closed drainage system or disposable urinary drainage bag. External drainage systems are available for women, but it is difficult to get the devices to fit securely. Men with problems with dribbling urine can wear a drip collector, which is a small pocket of absorbent padding placed over the penis and anchored in place with snug-fitting underwear. Both male and female clients may choose to wear protective pants or pads with a plastic outside layer and absorbent material inside. These pants can be pinned, taped, or snapped in place. Liners also are available and are worn next to the skin. They are nonabsorbent, and thus the urine passes through them to the absorbent layer. For this reason, the liners dry quickly and leave the skin dry and free of urine even though the absorbent material is soaked.

Clients who are incontinent may have problems with odor and maintaining skin integrity. Urea-splitting microorganisms, such as *Micrococcus ureae*, cause the urea in urine to react with water, creating ammonia and causing urine odor, skin breakdown, and ammonia dermatitis. One way to protect the skin is to avoid any contact with urine. When contact is unavoidable, the nurse instructs the client to use soap and water after each episode to clean the skin thoroughly. It also is important to dry the skin completely and apply a skin barrier or moisture sealant to protect the skin. When possible, the nurse encourages the client to expose the affected area to air.

Products are evolving and improving. The absorbent pads are much improved and cause less skin irritation. Clients can select from a variety of products. Many of them are similar to wearing normal underwear. Ease of use should be the primary consideration when clients are making a selection. For many clients, cost may be a factor. Nurses need to discuss this with their clients so clients can make better decisions.

Client and Family Teaching

The nurse encourages clients to actively participate in whatever methods are used to empty the bladder. In addition, the nurse demonstrates procedures as needed for the client and family to understand. Refer to Client and Family Teaching 59-2 for more strategies that assist clients to manage urinary incontinence.

Client and Family Teaching 59-2
Managing Urinary Incontinence

The nurse recommends the following strategies to clients coping with urinary incontinence, modifying instructions to address clients' individual needs:

- Be aware of the amount and timing of fluid intake.
- Avoid taking diuretics after 4 p.m.
- Avoid bladder irritants, including caffeine, alcohol, and aspartame (NutraSweet).
- Avoid constipation—adequate fluids, fiber, exercise, and stool softeners if recommended.
- Void regularly—every 2 to 3 hours:
  - First thing in the a.m.
  - Before each meal
  - Before going to bed
  - During the night as needed
- Perform pelvic floor muscle exercises as recommended.
- Stop smoking: frequent coughing increases incontinence.
- Control odors by frequent cleansing of the perineum, changing clothes and incontinence briefs (e.g., Attends, Depends) when they become wet, and using an electric room deodorizer.
- Avoid using perfume or scented powders, lotions, or sprays. Mixing a perfumed scent with a urine odor may intensify the odor, irritate the skin, or cause a skin infection.
- Wash garments as soon as possible in warm, soapy water.
- Use plastic to cover objects, such as a mattress and chairs, to prevent staining and lingering odors. The plastic must be washed with mild, soapy water daily or more often if needed.
- Place a sheet or blanket between the skin and the plastic.
- Follow the recommendations of the primary provider about clamping and unclamping the indwelling catheter (when this method is prescribed) or changing the catheter or cystostomy tube.
- Keep a record of fluid intake. Drink plenty of fluids during waking hours. Drink most of the required fluids in the morning and early-afternoon hours and decrease the intake toward evening.
- Follow the recommended bladder training program. Time is required to achieve success.
- Contact the health care provider if any of the following occurs: increased discomfort, rash around the perineal area, pain in the lower abdomen, fever, chills, or cloudy urine.

INFECTIOUS AND INFLAMMATORY DISORDERS

Infections and inflammations of the bladder and urethra are common. Although usually able to be treated on an outpatient basis, UTIs are a potential source of more complex problems requiring invasive treatment.

Cystitis

Pathophysiology and Etiology

Cystitis is an inflammation of the urinary bladder. The inflammation usually is caused by a bacterial infection. Bacteria can invade the bladder from an infection in the kidneys, lymphatics, and urethra (Fig. 59-4). Because the urethra is short

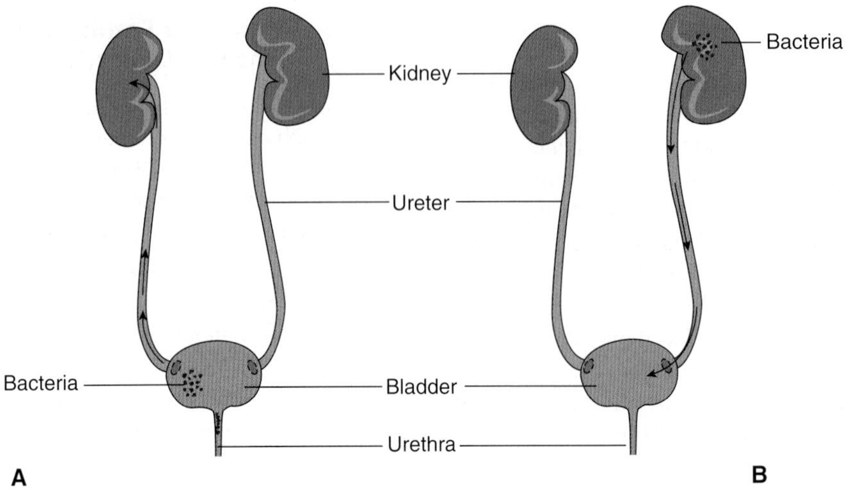

Figure 59-4 Urinary tract infection. **(A)** Microorganisms invade the bladder and ascend to the ureter and kidney. **(B)** Microorganisms in the kidney descend through the ureter to the bladder.

in women, ascending infections or microorganisms from the vagina or rectum are more common. Causes of cystitis include urologic instrumentation (e.g., cystoscopy, catheterization), fecal contamination, prostatitis or benign prostatic hyperplasia, indwelling catheters, pregnancy, and sexual intercourse. There are times that cystitis occurs as a reaction to some drugs, radiation therapy, or irritants such as feminine hygiene products or spermicidal gels.

The lining of the bladder provides a natural resistance to most bacterial invasions by preventing an inflammatory reaction from occurring. If bacteria do survive in the bladder, however, they adhere to the mucosal lining of the bladder and multiply. The surface of the bladder becomes edematous and reddened, and ulcerations may develop. When urine contacts these irritated areas, the client experiences pain and urgency, which is magnified in the presence of even slight bladder distention.

Assessment Findings

Signs and Symptoms

The symptoms of cystitis include urgency (feeling a pressing need to void although the bladder is not full), frequency, low back pain, dysuria, perineal and suprapubic pain, cloudy or strong-smelling urine, and hematuria, especially at the termination of the stream (terminal hematuria). If bacteremia is present, the client also may have chills and fever. Chronic cystitis causes similar symptoms, but usually they are less severe.

Diagnostic Findings

Microscopic examination of the urine reveals an increase in the number of red and white blood cells. Culture and sensitivity studies are used to identify the causative microorganism and appropriate antimicrobial therapy. If repeated episodes occur, intravenous pyelogram (IVP) or cystoscopy with or without retrograde pyelograms may be needed to identify the possible cause, such as chronic prostatitis or a bladder diverticulum (weakening and outpouching of the bladder wall), which encourages urinary stasis and infection.

Medical Management

Medical management includes antimicrobial therapy and correction of contributing factors. The antibiotics most frequently prescribed for UTIs include ciprofloxacin, fosfomycin, levofloxacin, nitrofurantoin, and an antibiotic combined with a sulfonamide—sulfamethoxazole/trimethoprim. Adjuvant drugs may be used such as phenazopyridine, which works like a local anesthetic to reduce bladder discomfort. Methenamine may be added when long-term management of a recurrent UTI is required.

Research has not demonstrated that cranberry juice keeps bacteria from adhering to the wall of the bladder, but it also cannot be stated that cranberry juice does not help. When there is a partial urethral obstruction, no treatment of cystitis is fully effective until adequate drainage of urine is restored by the removal of the obstruction (see discussion of urethral strictures). In some instances, treatment may be prolonged and may need to be repeated.

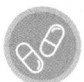

Pharmacologic Considerations

- Tell clients to call their providers if the antibiotics do not make them feel better in 2 to 3 days. Teach clients that the drug may need to be changed if the bacteria are resistant. Be sure and remind clients to finish the course of therapy even though they may feel better and be symptom free. A completed course of therapy is essential to be sure the infection is under control.

Nursing Management

The nurse advises the client to drink extra fluids. As stated earlier, cranberry juice may provide a less favorable climate for bacterial growth, but research has not fully demonstrated that it is effective. It is important to emphasize the importance of finishing the prescribed course of therapy. The nurse also instructs the client in the prevention of repeated cystitis (Client and Family Teaching 59-3).

Client and Family Teaching 59-3
Preventing Cystitis

The nurse instructs the client as follows:

- Increase fluid intake to 2 to 3 L/day.
- Avoid coffee, teas, colas, and alcohol.
- Shower rather than bathe in a tub.
- Cleanse perineum after each bowel movement with front-to-back motion.
- Avoid irritating substances such as bubble bath, bath salts, perineal lotions, vaginal sprays, nylon underwear, and scented toilet paper.
- Wear cotton underwear.
- Void every 2 to 3 hours while awake.
- Empty bladder completely with each voiding.
- Void after sexual intercourse.
- Notify primary provider of the following: urgency, frequency, burning with urination, difficulty urinating, or blood in the urine.
- Take medication exactly as prescribed.

>>> ***Stop, Think, and Respond 59-2***

Your 30-year-old client tells you that she has had four UTIs in the past 6 months. What information should you get before providing the client with instructions about preventing future UTIs?

Interstitial Cystitis/Painful Bladder Syndrome

Pathophysiology and Etiology

Interstitial cystitis (IC)/painful bladder syndrome (PBS) is a chronic inflammation of the bladder mucosa, causing pain in the bladder and surrounding pelvic region. Eventually there is disintegration of the bladder lining and a loss of bladder elasticity. IC varies greatly in presenting symptoms, and thus the PBS designation is added to include all painful urinary symptoms that do not strictly meet the criteria for IC alone. It is more common in women than men.

The bladder wall contains multiple pinpoint hemorrhagic areas that join and form larger hemorrhagic areas that may progress to fissuring and scarring of the bladder mucosa. Superficial erosion of the bladder mucosa (Hunner's ulcer) may develop. Eventually, the bladder shrinks from scarring. The cause of IC/PBS is unknown, but there may be a hormonal link because flare-ups appear to occur before menstruation. The possibility of a defect in the epithelial lining of the bladder may contribute to the problem. Another theory is that IC/PBS may be an autoimmune disorder or part of a systemic condition because some persons have a history of migraine headaches, ulcerative colitis, irritable bowel syndrome, endometriosis, fibromyalgia, or chronic fatigue syndrome.

Assessment Findings

Symptoms mimic other disorders such as cystitis, bladder cancer, or a sexually transmitted infection (STI). Frequent, painful urination and passing a small volume of urine are the most common symptoms. The pain may be described as searing or burning. The client reports an onset of pain and the need to void as soon as a small amount of urine is present in the bladder. Many clients report painful intercourse.

Cystoscopy reveals a markedly inflamed bladder mucosa with pinpoint hemorrhages and a bladder capacity that is smaller than normal. Filling the bladder during cystoscopy to improve visualization usually results in severe pain.

A voiding cystourethrogram also demonstrates a small bladder capacity. Results of urinalysis usually are normal, but if cystitis is present, an increase in the number of red and white blood cells may be seen; urine cultures are negative. A record of the number of voidings and the amount voided over a 2- or 3-day period, along with the symptoms, help to confirm the diagnosis. A biopsy of the bladder mucosa reveals an inflammatory process with scarring and hemorrhagic areas and confirms the diagnosis. Sometimes, a potassium sensitivity test is done. With this test, the examiner first instills water into the bladder. After the water is removed, a potassium solution is instilled. If the client experiences more pain and urgency with the potassium solution, IC/PBS may be diagnosed. Clients who do not have IC/PBS cannot distinguish the difference between the water or potassium solution.

Medical and Surgical Management

There is no single effective specific therapy for IC/PBS. Nonsteroidal antiinflammatory drugs (NSAIDs) are used to relieve pain. Elmiron (pentosan polysulfate), a bladder protectant, is the most effective medication. It provides relief of the bladder pain associated with IC. Tricyclic antidepressant drugs such as amitriptyline may also relieve pain as well as treat the depression that can accompany the disorder. Antihistamines are sometimes prescribed to reduce urinary frequency and urgency. Other therapies include bladder instillation of dimethyl sulfoxide (DMSO), while. other solutions are being tested.

Other treatments include the following:

- *Bladder distension*: some clients report relief after an instillation is done as part of the diagnostic process. Relief is initially transient, but then returns within 2 to 4 weeks. It is theorized that stretching the bladder increases capacity and interferes with pain transmission. Bladder distension can be done with water or gas and can be repeated.
- *Transcutaneous electrical nerve stimulation (TENS)*: wires are applied to the lower back or suprapubic area; it is theorized that the electrical stimulation increases blood flow to the bladder, strengthens pelvic muscles, and/or triggers the release of endorphins to block pain. In some cases, urinary frequency is reduced.
- *Urinary diversion procedure* (discussed later) for those clients for whom severe IC/PBS can be incapacitating; it may offer the only relief of symptoms for a selected group of clients.

Nursing Management

The nurse advises the client to avoid spicy and acidic foods because they may contribute to pain and discomfort. Some clients obtain relief by omitting carbonated beverages, caffeine in all forms, citrus products, and foods with high concentration of vitamin C. Psychological support is necessary because many times, IC/PBS has gone undiagnosed and the client has been told that there is nothing wrong. Clients with IC/PBS often have their lives severely disrupted by pain and frequent trips to the bathroom, sometimes several times an hour. Some clients are unable to hold jobs because of the severity of symptoms. Sexual activity is avoided because of fear of pain, straining their relationships and interfering with intimacy. Clients should be referred to a chronic pain center to cope with the pain and to an IC/PBS support group.

Urethritis

Pathophysiology and Etiology

Urethritis (inflammation of the urethra) is seen more commonly in men than in women. Urethritis caused by microorganisms other than gonococci is called *nongonococcal urethritis*. Gonorrhea, an STI, is a specific form of infection that can attack the mucous membrane of a normal urethra (see Chapter 56).

In women, urethritis may not only accompany cystitis but may also be secondary to vaginal infections. Soaps, bubble baths, sanitary napkins, or scented toilet paper also may cause urethritis.

In men, a common cause of urethritis is infection with *Chlamydia trachomatis* or *Ureaplasma urealyticum*, which causes an STI. The distal portion of the normal male urethra is not totally sterile. Bacteria that normally are present cause no difficulty unless these tissues are traumatized, usually after instrumentation such as catheterization or cystoscopic examination. Under such conditions, bacteria may gain a foothold to cause a nonspecific urethritis. Other causes of nonspecific urethritis in men include irritation during vigorous intercourse, rectal intercourse, or intercourse with a woman who has a vaginal infection.

Assessment Findings

Infection of the urethra results in discomfort on urination, varying from a slight tickling sensation to burning or severe discomfort and urinary frequency. Fever is not common, but fever in male clients may be owing to further extension of the infection to areas such as the prostate, testes, and epididymis. There may be urethral discharge and itching in the urethra.

The client's history and symptoms often provide a tentative diagnosis. In men, a urethral smear is obtained for culture and sensitivity to identify the causative microorganism. In women, a urinalysis (clean-catch midstream specimen) may identify the causative microorganism.

Medical Management

Treatment includes appropriate antibiotic therapy, liberal fluid intake, analgesics, warm sitz baths, and improvement of the client's resistance to infection by a good diet and plenty of rest. If urethritis is owing to an STI, it is treated with appropriate antibiotic therapy (see Chapter 56). Failure to seek treatment for gonococcal urethritis may result in a urethral stricture in men.

Nursing Management

The nurse reinforces the need to complete antibiotic therapy, drink plenty of fluids, and take warm sitz baths and analgesics for pain. Urethritis may be seen in clients with indwelling urethral catheters. To prevent or decrease urethritis, the nurse needs to be vigilant with sterile technique as well as to exercise gentleness when changing catheters. It also is essential to provide frequent perineal care, especially if the client is incontinent of feces. In addition to washing around the anus and buttocks, the nurse also cleans the meatus and labia of a woman client. When cleaning the anal area, wiping away from the urethra ensures that there is no contamination. If cotton pads are used, the nurse wipes from the urethral meatus to the anus in a single stroke and discards the pad. Client teaching information is included in the Nursing Process section that follows.

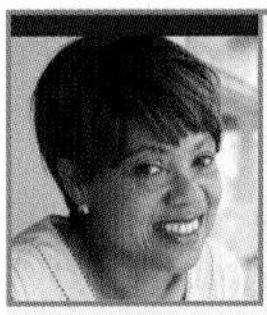

Clinical Scenario A 52-year-old woman is seen in an outpatient clinic for complaints of pressure and discomfort in the bladder, with urgency and frequency that is not relieved when she voids. What are important assessments and nursing interventions for this client? See the following Nursing Process section.

NURSING PROCESS FOR THE CLIENT WITH AN INFECTION OF THE BLADDER OR URETHRA

Assessment

Ask the client about present symptoms, specifically seeking information related to the presence of pain and changes in urination, including frequency, urgency, and burning with urination. Assess the client's sexual practices, including methods of contraception and personal hygiene. Ask the client to void. When the client voids, measure the volume and check the urine for color, cloudiness, concentration, odor, and presence of blood.

Diagnosis, Planning, and Interventions

Acute Pain: Related to infection and inflammation of the bladder and/or urethra
Expected Outcome: The client will express relief of pain and discomfort.

NURSING PROCESS FOR THE CLIENT WITH AN INFECTION OF THE BLADDER OR URETHRA (continued)

- Assure the client that pain and discomfort will decrease with treatment. *Antibacterial and antispasmodic medications are quickly effective in relieving the pain and discomfort associated with UTIs.*
- Administer analgesics and antispasmodics as indicated. *Prompt administration of prescribed medications ensures that effective blood levels are maintained for treatment of infection. Antispasmodics relieve bladder irritability.*
- Encourage the client to use warm sitz baths two or three times a day to relieve discomfort. *Promotes relief of pain and reduces spasm.*
- Encourage the client to increase daily fluid intake to at least eight large glasses, excluding coffee, tea, alcohol, and colas. *Promotes renal blood flow and flushes bacteria from the urinary tract. Coffee, tea, alcohol, and colas are urinary tract irritants.*
- Instruct the client to void at regular intervals even if uncomfortable. *Frequent voiding promotes emptying the bladder, which contributes to lower bacterial counts, reduction of urinary stasis, and prevention of reinfection.*

Acute Anxiety: Related to pain, discomfort, and frequent urination
Expected Outcomes: (1) Client will verbalize anxiety related to symptoms. (2) Client will state self-care measures to relieve anxiety.

- Encourage client to talk about their symptoms and fears related to the disorder. *Providing an opportunity for the client to discuss concerns and fears assists in relieving anxiety.*
- Provide information that assists in alleviating fears. *Accurate information alleviates fear and corrects misconceptions.*

Knowledge Deficiency: Regarding inflammation and infection of the bladder and urethra related to disease process and treatment
Expected Outcomes: (1) Client will verbalize understanding of condition, prognosis, and treatment. (2) Client will participate in the treatment regimen.

- Review the treatment plan. *Doing so provides a time for the client to ask questions.*
- Instruct client about medications, dosage, frequency, expected effects, and possible side effects. *Providing clients with accurate information promotes adherence to drug regimen.*
- Emphasize the need to complete the entire course of medications, even after symptoms have subsided. *Complete antibiotic therapy eradicates infection and prevents recurrence.*
- Teach client the importance of increased fluid intake. *Increased fluid intake flushes the urinary tract and removes bacteria.*
- If the client is on a special diet (e.g., a low-sodium or diabetic diet), check with the primary provider regarding drinking juices or beverages or eating foods that are liquid at room temperature. Teach client modified fluid guidelines as needed. *Some liquids either must be considered part of the daily dietary allowances or may not be allowed because they contain substances that must be eliminated from the diet. In some diets, a limited amount of certain liquids may be allowed.*
- Review client's hygiene practices. *Poor hygiene practices, such as back-to-front perineal cleansing, especially after a bowel movement, or soaking in dirty bath water, can contribute to the introduction of bacterial contaminants to the urinary tract.*
- Instruct the client to notify the primary provider if symptoms persist after the course of drug therapy is completed, if the symptoms become worse, or if fever or chills occur. *Persistent or worsening symptoms may indicate that the treatment is ineffective or inadequate and requires further medical attention.*
- Teach client methods to prevent future infections. *Appropriate personal hygiene, increased fluid intake (promotes voiding and dilution of urine), and frequent voiding prevent UTI.*

Evaluation of Expected Outcomes

The client reports relief of pain and discomfort and states that they are adhering to the medication regimen. The client states that the anxiety was gone once the symptoms of the UTI were relieved. The client demonstrates understanding of the treatment plan as evidenced by intake of at least 2 L of water, frequent voiding, and appropriate personal hygiene practices.

OBSTRUCTIVE DISORDERS

Obstruction of the lower urinary tract is a blockage in the bladder or in the urethra. Many obstructions are related to congenital anomalies, but in adults, obstructions occur from stones that block the passage of urine, or from a narrowing that occurs as a result of a trauma, inflammation, or infection. Box 59-3 lists general signs of an outflow obstruction.

Bladder Stones

Pathophysiology and Etiology

Stones may form in the bladder or originate in the upper urinary tract and travel to and remain in the bladder. Large bladder stones develop in those with chronic urinary retention and urinary stasis. Prostate gland enlargement can lead to bladder stones, because the prostate gland impedes urine flow through the urethra, resulting in urinary stasis. Clients who are immobile (e.g., the unconscious client or those with paraplegia or quadriplegia) also may have a tendency to form bladder stones.

Assessment Findings

Symptoms of bladder stone formation include hematuria, cloudy or dark urine, suprapubic pain, difficulty starting the urinary stream, symptoms of a bladder infection, and a feeling that the bladder is not completely empty. Some clients experience pain with voiding. Other clients may have few or no symptoms.

BOX 59-3 Signs of Obstructed Urine Flow

- Straining to empty bladder
- Feeling that bladder does not empty completely
- Hesitancy
- Weak stream
- Frequency
- Overflow incontinence
- Bladder distention

A urinalysis may be done to rule out infection. A spiral CT scan is done to determine the presence of stones; even very small stones can be detected. Cystoscopy, a kidney–ureter–bladder (KUB) study, IVP, or ultrasound studies can also detect the presence of bladder stones. Blood chemistries and 24-hour urine collection for serum calcium and uric acid may identify the possible cause of stone formation.

Medical and Surgical Management

Bladder stones may be removed through the transurethral route using a stone-crushing instrument (lithotrite). This procedure, called a **cystolitholapaxy**, is suitable for small and soft stones and is performed under general anesthesia. Larger, noncrushable stones must be removed through a surgical (suprapubic) incision into the bladder.

When it is possible to determine the chemical composition of stones that have passed or been removed, dietary treatment is based on the primary component of the stone. A low-purine diet is used for uric acid stones, although the benefits are unknown. Clients with a history of calcium oxalate stone formation need a diet that is adequate in calcium and low in oxalate (see Nutrition Notes 58-1). Only clients who have type II absorptive hypercalciuria—approximately half of the clients—need to limit calcium intake. Usually, clients are told to increase their fluid intake significantly, consume a moderate protein intake, and limit sodium (Nutrition Notes). Despite dietary changes, some clients continue to form stones in the urinary tract.

Nutrition Notes

The Client With Bladder Stones

- Encourage clients with bladder stones to drink 8 oz of fluid hourly during waking hours or at least 2 L of fluid daily.
- A low-purine diet, used for uric acid stones, limits organ meats (brain, kidney, liver, sweetbreads), game meat, gravies, anchovies, herring, mackerel, sardines, and scallops. All meats, fish, and poultry contain significant amounts of purines, so adherence to the diet is difficult.
- Consume the recommended daily intake for calcium (e.g., three cups of milk or equivalent daily) because calcium binds with oxalate in the GI tract to lower urinary oxalate levels.
- Avoiding excessive protein intake is associated with lower urinary oxalate and lower uric acid levels. Consume recommended protein intake levels (0.8 g/kg for adults).
- Limit sodium as it competes with calcium for absorption.

Nursing Management

The nurse obtains a complete medical, drug, and allergy history, asking the client to describe the symptoms, including the type and location of the pain. The nurse monitors vital signs every 4 hours or as ordered, and notifies the primary provider if the client's temperature is higher than 101°F (38.3°C) orally. Intake and output and the color of the urine are documented in the medical record.

If there is any evidence of gross hematuria, the nurse reports it immediately. Encouraging the client to drink fluids (unless contraindicated by heart failure or renal disease) is important because extra fluids help pass stones and reduce the chance of infection or inflammation. The nurse filters the urine for stones by straining all urine through gauze or wire mesh. If solid material is found, it is sent in a labeled container to the laboratory for analysis. If the client has moderate-to-severe pain, the nurse administers an opioid analgesic as ordered. If the analgesic fails to relieve at least some of the pain, or if the pain becomes worse despite administration of an analgesic, the nurse notifies the primary provider and provides details regarding the effects of medical or surgical procedures.

If a cystolitholapaxy successfully removes the stone, a urethral catheter may be left in place to keep the bladder continuously empty for 1 to 2 days after the procedure. The nurse administers antibiotics as ordered. Once oral fluids are tolerated, it is important to encourage the client to drink extra fluids to reduce inflammation of the bladder mucosa. In addition, the nurse monitors the urine output and voiding pattern.

If open removal is required, the bladder is incised and the stone is removed. A urethral catheter may be left in place for a week or more to keep the bladder empty and prevent tension on the bladder sutures. In addition to standard postoperative care (see Chapter 14), nursing management involves providing the same care as for the client having a suprapubic prostatectomy (see Chapter 55). The nurse closely monitors the client's voiding once the catheter is removed to prevent urinary retention.

The nurse teaches the client to do the following:

- Strain urine and send any stone found to the laboratory for examination.
- Follow the dietary recommendations.
- Take the prescribed medications as directed.
- Contact the primary provider if symptoms return.
- Drink plenty of fluids (at least 10 large glasses each day) and exercise regularly.
- Contact the primary provider if hematuria, burning, chills, fever, or pain occur.

Urethral Strictures

Pathophysiology and Etiology

A **stricture** (narrowing) in the urethra obstructs the flow of urine and can cause complications in the bladder or upper urinary tract. The ureters may become distended with urine as a result of the obstruction, and the kidney pelves can also become distended with the backflow of urine. The bladder distends when the urethra is obstructed, and a **diverticulum** (outpouching) of the muscular bladder wall may form (Fig. 59-5). In some instances, more than one diverticulum may be seen.

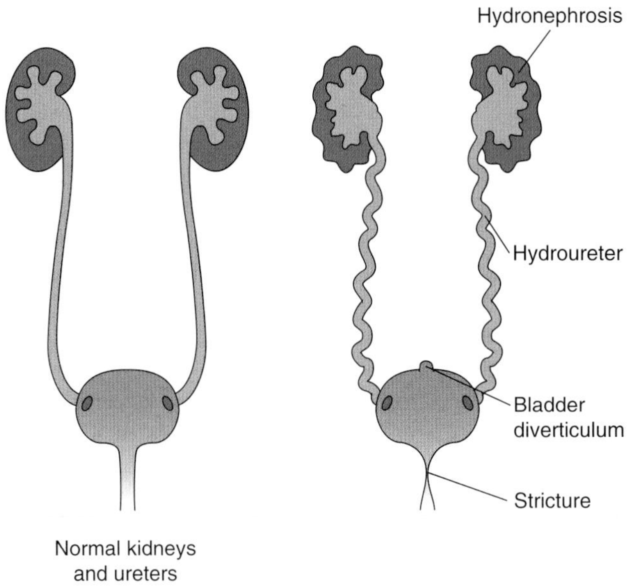

Figure 59-5 Urethral stricture can result in hydroureters, hydronephrosis (dilation of the ureters and kidney), and bladder diverticulum.

Urine becomes trapped in the diverticulum, stagnates, and becomes a culture medium for bacteria. For this reason, infection occurs often and is difficult to control until the obstruction is corrected. A urethral stricture may result in acute or chronic urinary retention.

Strictures of the urethra are caused by infections such as untreated gonorrhea or chronic nongonococcal urethritis. Other causes include trauma to the lower urinary tract or pelvis, such as accidents, childbirth, intercourse, or surgical procedures. Prolonged use of IUC or CIC can contribute to a urethral stricture because of trauma to the urethra over time. Urethral strictures may be congenital. Men experience urethral stricture more frequently than women, secondary to the anatomic differences and the length of the urethra. In addition, an enlarged prostate or surgery on the prostate can cause a urethral stricture. Cancer of the urethra in both sexes or prostate cancer in men can lead to a stricture.

Assessment Findings

Symptoms include the following:

- Slow or decreased force of stream of urine
- Urine leakage or dribbling after urinating
- Spraying of urine when voiding
- Dysuria
- Urgency
- Hesitancy
- Burning
- Frequency
- Hematuria
- Nocturia
- Lower abdominal or pelvic pain
- Retention of residual urine in the bladder: may lead to bladder distention and infection.

The client may be able to pass more urine after voiding and waiting a few minutes. The final quantity of urine comes from the diverticulum and may be malodorous.

Urinalysis and urine cultures will be done to determine if there is infection or blood and/or other issues. The stricture may be seen on cystoscopy, retrograde pyelogram, and IVP. A voiding cystourethrogram also may show the stricture as well as the presence of a bladder diverticulum. Images that specifically locate the length, position, and severity of the stricture are done with urethrograms. Uroflowmetry studies will demonstrate flow from the bladder. Postvoid residuals through an ultrasound are done to determine if the client empties the bladder.

Medical and Surgical Management

Urethral strictures are treated by dilatation, which is the use of specially designed instruments called *bougies*, *dilators*, *sounds*, *filiform bougies*, and *followers* (Fig. 59-6) that are passed gently into the urethra. Although done gently, the procedure usually is painful. Because forceful stretching of the urethra may cause bleeding and further stricture formation, dilatation begins with a 6-F or 8-F urethral dilator. During subsequent treatments, the primary provider increases the size of the dilator until 24 F or 26 F can be tolerated. Depending on the cause of the stricture and the response to the therapy, the condition may subside after one or two treatments. However, periodic dilatations usually are required indefinitely or until the condition is corrected surgically.

If dilatation is unsuccessful, a **urethroplasty** (surgical repair of the urethra) may be attempted. The urine is diverted from the urethra by a cystostomy tube until the urethra has been repaired. In one method of reconstructing the urethra, the constricted area is resected, and a mucosal graft (which may be taken from the bladder) is inserted to restore the continuity of the urethra. After surgery, the client has a splinting catheter in the urethra that remains until healing has occurred. This operation may be performed in two stages: urinary diversion at the first operation and plastic repair at the second.

Nursing Management

The nurse advises the client that the urine may be blood-tinged after urethral dilatation and that it may burn when voiding. Sitz baths and nonopioid analgesics may relieve discomfort. The nurse encourages the client to drink extra fluids for several days after the procedure. It is important for the client to keep appointments for follow-up dilatations and not to wait until there is a marked reduction in the urinary stream or other symptoms of obstruction to return. The nurse instructs the client to take all of the antibiotics and to contact the primary provider if difficulty voiding or frank bleeding occurs.

If a urethroplasty is performed, it is most important that the urethral catheter remain in place and securely anchored. After surgery, turning and repositioning requires special attention to prevent excessive tension on the urethral catheter.

BLADDER CANCER

Bladder cancer is a frightening diagnosis for clients. Bloody urine often is the first sign of a problem and the reason clients seek medical attention.

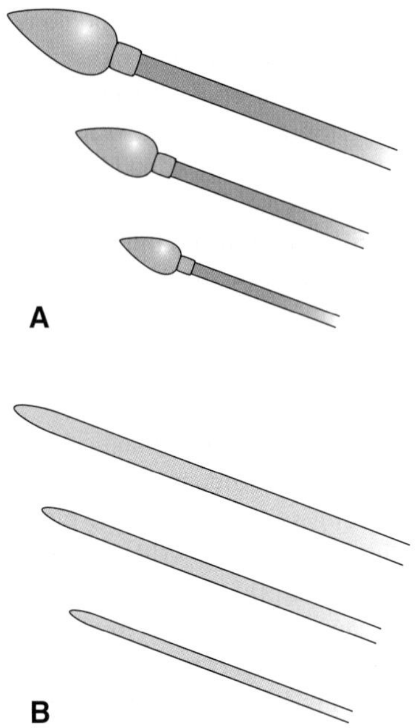

Figure 59-6 Bougies **(A)** and filiform bougies **(B)** are used to dilate the urethra.

Pathophysiology and Etiology

Bladder cancer is the most common cancer in the urinary system. It occurs more frequently in men than in women and usually affect clients 55 years of age or older. The American Cancer Society (2021) estimates that 1 in 27 men in the United States will be diagnosed with bladder cancer, as opposed to 1 in 89 women. Use of tobacco products is the leading cause of bladder cancer. The following list includes environmental and occupational health hazards thought to be associated with bladder tumors:

- Cigarette smoking and secondhand smoke. Smokers and those exposed to frequent secondhand smoke are three times as likely to develop bladder cancer.
- Exposure to environmental carcinogens, such as dyes, paint, ink, leather, or rubber.
- Certain occupations increase the risk for developing bladder cancer: hairdressers (exposure to hair dyes), machinists (exposure to multiple chemicals and fumes), and truck drivers (exposure to diesel fumes).
- Recurrent or chronic bacterial infections of the urinary tract.
- Arsenic in drinking water.
- Bladder stones.
- Insufficient intake of fluids.
- Bladder birth defects.
- Family history.
- High urinary pH.
- High cholesterol intake.
- Pelvic radiation therapy or chemotherapy.
- Cancers arising from the prostate, colon, and rectum in men.

The most common type of bladder cancer is transitional cell carcinoma or urothelial carcinoma, which develops in the bladder's epithelial lining. The tumors are classified as papillary or nonpapillary (flat). Papillary lesions are superficial and extend in finger-like projections outward from the mucosal layer. These tumors are considered noninvasive. Nonpapillary tumors are solid growths that grow inward, deep into the bladder wall. This type is more likely to metastasize, usually to the lymph nodes, liver, lungs, and bone. Other types of bladder cancer include squamous cell carcinoma, adenocarcinoma, small cell carcinoma, and sarcoma. These types account for less than 5% of all bladder cancers.

Assessment Findings

Signs and Symptoms

The most common first symptom of bladder cancer is painless hematuria. Clients may notice a change in the color of their urine and then will not notice any difference. This can occur off and on for quite a long period of time. However, hematuria will always recur in clients with bladder cancer. Additional early symptoms include those related to a UTI, with symptoms such as fever, dysuria, urgency, and frequency. Later symptoms are related to metastases and include pelvic or lower back pain on one side, urinary retention (if the tumor blocks the bladder outlet), and urinary frequency from the tumor occupying bladder space. There is also a loss of appetite and weight loss, weakness, swelling in the feet, and bone pain. If bleeding is present for a period of time, the client may also experience symptoms of anemia (fatigue, shortness of breath) caused by blood loss.

>>> ***Stop, Think, and Respond 59-3***

A 55-year-old man is admitted with blood in the urine. The medical diagnosis is "rule out bladder cancer." When the nurse admits this client, what is an important question to ask?

Diagnostic Findings

The tumor usually is seen by cystoscopic examination and confirmed by microscopic biopsy. Blue light fluorescence cystoscopy is frequently done, because it improves the detection of cancer. This test uses a photosensitizing drug in combination with blue light cystoscopy. The drug is instilled into the bladder, remaining there for at least an hour. The drug is absorbed by cancer cells, which can then be visualized with the use of the blue light—abnormal cells are fluorescent red; normal cells appear bluish green. The examiner has a clearer picture of the extent of the malignancy (American Cancer Society, 2019).

A retrograde pyelogram may be obtained to detect any kidney damage if the tumor is obstructing one of the ureteral orifices. A computed tomography (CT) scan with guided needle biopsy, MRI, and X-rays of the pelvis may show a tumor shadow or bony metastases. A bone scan may also be done. Ultrasonography may be done to determine tumor size and location. Routine laboratory tests are performed to evaluate kidney function and determine the degree of anemia owing to persistent hematuria. Urine cytology and urine tumor marker tests are done to determine if there are cancer cells in the urine.

Medical Management

Treatment varies according to the grade and stage of the tumor. Metastases usually have not occurred as long as the tumor has not penetrated the muscle wall of the bladder. Small, superficial tumors may be removed by cutting (resection) or coagulation (**fulguration**) with a transurethral resection of a bladder tumor (TURBT). Bladder tumors removed in this manner have a high incidence of recurrence; consequently, a cystoscopic examination is performed every 2 to 3 months. Clients having no recurrence of the tumor for at least 1 year require cystoscopic examinations every 6 months for the rest of their lives so that recurrence of the tumor or a new malignant growth can be detected early.

Topical application of an antineoplastic drug may be used after a TURBT. A liquid form of the drug is instilled into the bladder by means of a catheter (intravesicular injection). Fluid intake usually is limited before and during this procedure so that the drug remains concentrated and in contact with the bladder mucosa for about 2 hours. The client then voids and is given extra oral fluids to flush the drug from the bladder.

Intravesicular injection of bacillus Calmette-Guérin (BCG) Live, a weakened strain of *Mycobacterium bovis*, also may be used. It appears that BCG causes an inflammatory reaction in the bladder wall that, in turn, destroys malignant cells. Another form of therapy includes the administration of interferon alfa-2a (Roferon-A) injected intravenously or directly into the bladder. Interferon appears to stimulate the production of lymphocytes and macrophages that may destroy malignant cells and may be used in combination with BCG. Mitomycin, a chemotherapeutic vesicant agent, may be used as well; it also is injected via a catheter into the bladder. The effects of mitomycin appear to improve when the bladder is heated, referred to as electromotive mitomycin therapy. Other drugs that may be used are valrubicin, docetaxel, thiotepa, and gemcitabine.

Photodynamic therapy also may be used in the treatment of bladder cancer. This experimental treatment involves an IV injection of a photosensitizing agent that is absorbed in concentration over several days by malignant cells. A laser, inserted through a cystoscope, activates the drug so that it can destroy the malignant cells (American Cancer Society, 2020).

Radiation therapy may be used for clients who do not have the whole bladder removed. The goal is to eradicate any remaining cancer cells.

Surgical Management

The clinical stage of the bladder cancer determines if surgery is done as part of the treatment. A partial or segmental **cystectomy** (surgical removal of part of the bladder) may be done if the tumor is confined to a small area and is not large. A radical cystectomy (total removal of the bladder) and a urinary diversion procedure often are necessary when the tumor has penetrated the muscle wall. When a cystectomy is performed, the bladder and lower third of both ureters are removed. If the tumor has extended through the bladder wall, the surgeon may perform a radical cystectomy.

In women, a radical cystectomy usually includes removal of the bladder, lower third of both ureters, uterus, fallopian tubes, ovaries, anterior vaginal wall, and urethra. In men, a radical cystectomy usually includes removal of the bladder, lower third of both ureters, prostate, and seminal vesicles.

Once a cystectomy is performed, urine must be diverted to another collecting system. This is called a **urinary diversion**. Although urinary diversion procedures are used for the treatment of bladder tumors, they also are used for extensive pelvic malignancies and severe traumatic injury to the bladder. Some urinary diversions require external ostomy bags to collect the urine—referred to as *incontinent urinary diversions* (Fig. 59-7). One option is to remove a short piece of the ileum and connect it to the ureters. With this technique, urine flows from the kidneys through the ureters into the ileal conduit. The distal end is formed into a stoma or urostomy. A collection or urostomy bag (pouch) collects the urine, which flows constantly.

Other types of urinary diversions create a reservoir within the body, and the reservoir is catheterized to drain the urine—these are called *continent urinary diversions* (see Fig. 59-7). In this type of urinary diversion, a piece of intestine is used to create a reservoir that is attached to the ureters on one end and to a stoma on the other end. A valve within the stoma is also created. The client periodically inserts a catheter through the valve into the reservoir and drains the urine. An external pouch is not needed with this method.

A third method is referred to as a neobladder, or a continent orthotopic bladder substitution. This technique involves taking a piece of the intestine to form a reservoir. It is connected to the ureters and then the urethra, so that the client urinates normally. Some clients may experience incontinence, especially at night, but prefer this to other methods. Sometimes clients need to use a catheter to thoroughly drain the reservoir.

Nursing Management

Preoperative Period

The nurse obtains a complete medical, drug, and allergy history on admission and asks the client or family member to describe all symptoms. The assessment also includes an evaluation of general physical and emotional status, vital signs, and weight.

Caring for a client during the preoperative period includes reducing anxiety and increasing understanding of the preparations for surgery and postoperative care. The client may display various emotional responses before surgery. Some may appear depressed; others show a mixture of anxiety and depression. The client faces drastic changes in the manner of excreting urine from the body, the diagnosis of cancer, and the changes in body image. The nurse encourages the client to talk about the surgery and the changes that will occur. They may suggest a visit from a member of a local ostomy group to provide emotional support as well as information. The wound, ostomy, and continence nurse (WOCN) should meet with the client to discuss placement of the stoma and collection devices, if applicable. Photographs or drawings are useful in showing the placement of the stoma and urostomy pouch.

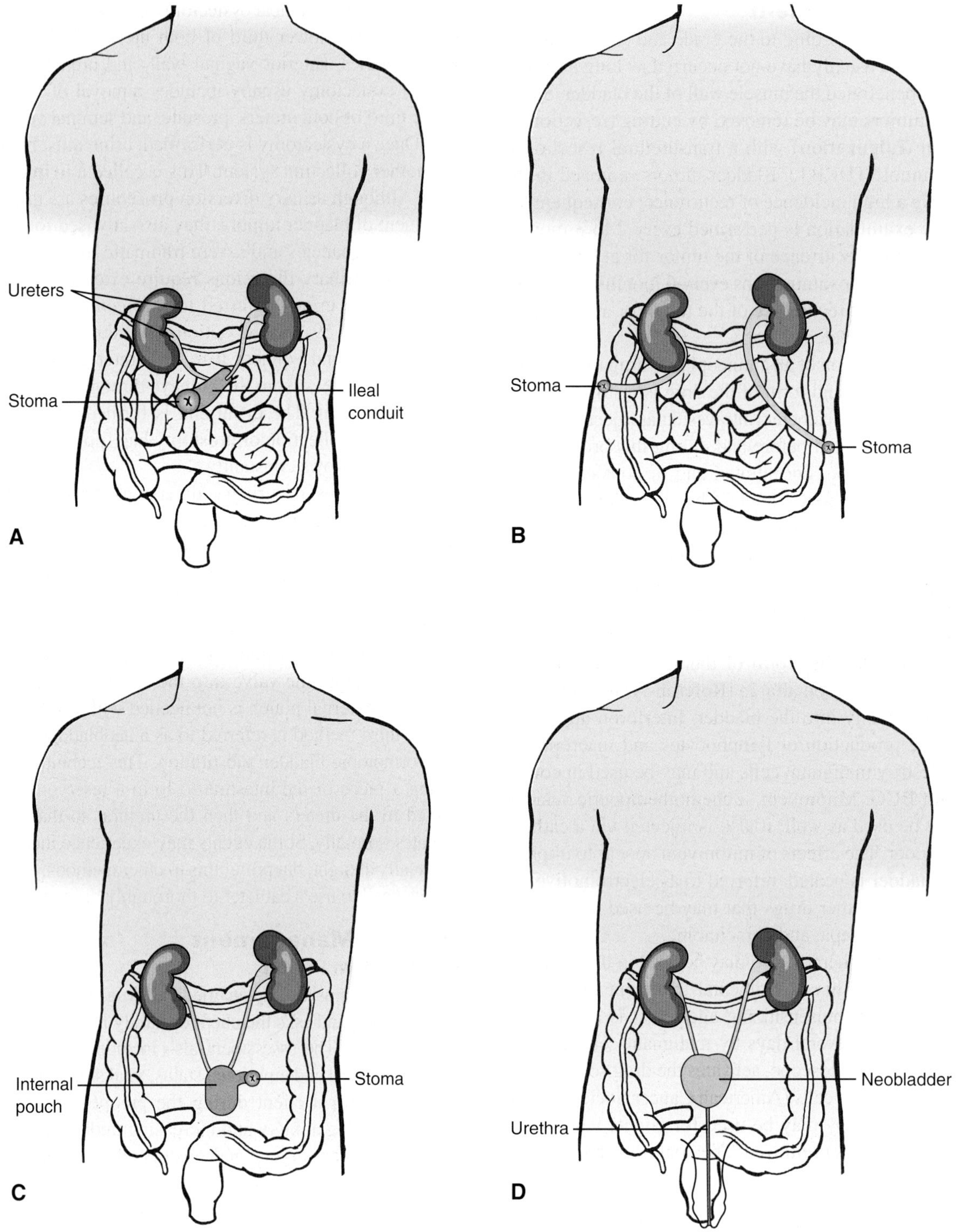

Figure 59-7 **(A** and **B)** Examples of urostomies (incontinent urinary diversion) procedures, after which the client must wear a urinary collecting device. **(C** and **D)** Examples of continent diversions: Indiana pouch and a neobladder. (Reprinted with permission from Rosdahl, C. B. & Kowalski, M. T. (2017). *Textbook of basic nursing* (11th ed.). Wolters Kluwer.)

The nurse determines the client's ability to manage stoma care or self-catheterization by assessing manual dexterity, level of understanding, and vision. Assessing the client's social support and resources, including whether insurance will cover ostomy supplies, is important. The nurse explains all preoperative preparations to the client and client's family and gives them time to ask additional questions about the surgery, preparations for surgery, and management after surgery.

Depending on the extent and type of surgery, preoperative preparations may include insertion of a nasogastric tube, placement of IV and central venous pressure lines, administration of cleansing enemas, and adherence to a low-residue diet several days before surgery. Laxatives and enemas and a drug such as kanamycin (Kantrex) or neomycin (Mycifradin) may be given if a ureterosigmoidostomy is to be performed. These agents decrease the number of microorganisms in the bowel and lessen the possibility of infection as a complication of connecting the ureters to the bowel. Clients scheduled for an ileal conduit (see Fig. 59-7A) or continent urinary diversion procedure (see Fig. 59-7) also may have the bowel prepared in this manner.

Postoperative Period

Clients undergoing urinary diversion are subject to the same conditions and complications as any surgical client. Refer to Chapter 14 for nursing diagnoses and interventions for managing standard postoperative care. Management issues related specifically to urinary diversion procedures include observing for leakage of urine or stool from the anastomosis, maintaining renal function, assessing for signs and symptoms of peritonitis, maintaining integrity of the urinary diversion and urine collection devices, maintaining skin and stomal integrity, promoting a positive body image, and teaching the client how to manage the diversion.

The nurse checks the client's chart for information regarding the type and extent of surgery and orders for connection of catheters or drains, IV fluids, and analgesics. Clients will have multiple drainage tubes, ureteral stents, and a nasogastric tube. All urinary drainage tubes must be labeled, and the urine output from each catheter or stoma must be measured and recorded hourly.

Maintaining accurate intake and output measurements during the postoperative period is important because it indicates both renal function and the integrity of the urinary diversion structures. Obstruction of urine flow can severely damage the kidneys. If urinary drainage stops or decreases to less than 30 mL/hour, or if the client complains of back pain, the nurse needs to notify the primary provider immediately. Inspection of the urine includes checking for color, clarity, and presence of blood. It is essential to immediately report concentrated, cloudy, or bloody urine to the primary provider. Ureteral stents remain in place for several days after surgery.

The nasogastric tube is connected to low intermittent suction. This prevents distention and pressure on the suture line owing to the collection of gas in the bowel. The nasogastric tube is removed once peristalsis has returned and the diet can be advanced. All laboratory reports are reviewed as soon as they are received and abnormalities reported to the primary provider promptly. The following sections address management issues specific to the most common procedures.

Ileal Conduit

A transparent ostomy bag is applied over the stoma to make stomal assessment easier. The nurse contacts the primary provider immediately if there is excessive bleeding, changes in the color of the stoma (e.g., from a normal to a cyanotic color), or separation of the stoma edges from the surrounding skin. The nurse uses gauze pads to clean mucus away from the stoma. Because the intestinal anastomosis can leak fecal material or the ileal conduit may leak urine into the peritoneal cavity, they observe for and promptly report symptoms of peritonitis (e.g., abdominal tenderness or distention, fever, severe pain). Management of the urinary stoma is similar to management of a fecal stoma (see Chapter 48). The skin needs protection, the surgical dressings must be changed promptly when they become wet, and the appliances need care and cleansing. Each time they change a temporary drainage bag, the nurse inspects the skin around the stoma for signs of infection and skin breakdown.

Continent Urinary Diversion (Kock Pouch, Indiana Pouch)

The nurse inspects the stoma for bleeding or cyanosis. They may irrigate the pouch, if ordered, to prevent mucous plugs or blood clots. The nurse teaches the client how to perform intermittent self-catheterization. Initially, this is done every 1 to 2 hours but eventually will be performed every 4 to 6 hours.

Ureterosigmoidostomy.

A catheter is inserted in the rectum to drain urine continuously. The nurse checks the amount and color of drainage from the rectal catheter every 1 or 2 hours and inspects the anal and gluteal areas for signs of early skin breakdown. The catheter is removed when peristalsis returns. Because the sigmoid colon reabsorbs urinary constituents, clients are prone to fluid and electrolyte imbalances throughout the postoperative period (as well as for the rest of their lives). Observation for signs of electrolyte losses is essential. The nurse teaches the client exercises to improve sphincter control. Once good control is achieved, the nurse instructs the client to void (rectally) every 2 hours to prevent reabsorption of fluid and electrolytes. Clients must never have enemas, suppositories, or laxatives.

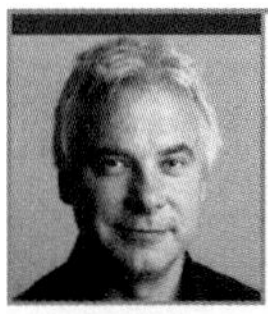

Clinical Scenario A 55-year-old man requires a urinary diversion following a diagnosis of stage IV bladder cancer. What nursing measures are important when caring for this client that will provide emotional and psychosocial support? See the following Nursing Process section.

TRAUMA

Trauma to the bladder or urethra is potentially harmful and frequently requires surgical intervention.

Pathophysiology and Etiology

Various types of injury can affect the urinary tract. Gunshot and stab wounds, crushing injuries, and forceful blows can result in tears, hemorrhage, or penetration of one or more parts. Some penetrating bladder injuries are small, whereas others are large, with a rapid collection of urine in the peritoneal cavity. Injuries to the kidney area may result in bruising or tearing of the kidney and its capsule. Depending on

NURSING PROCESS FOR THE PSYCHOSOCIAL CARE OF THE CLIENT UNDERGOING URINARY DIVERSION

Assessment

Assess the client's knowledge about the effects of surgery on sexual function. Up to 85% of men experience erectile dysfunction after urinary diversion. Ask the client about their current level of social activity and what changes they think will occur after surgery. Assess the client's understanding of long-term postoperative care.

Diagnosis, Planning, and Interventions

Risk for Ineffective Sexuality Patterns: Related to erectile dysfunction in men or dyspareunia in women
Expected Outcome: Client will regain erectile function or ease painful intercourse.

- Tactfully ask the client if they have any questions regarding sexuality concerns. *Asking the client provides an opportunity to discuss sexuality issues.*
- Encourage client and their partner to share their feelings about alteration in sexual function. *Acknowledging the importance of sexual function and expression may assist the client and their partner to seek sexual counseling and to explore alternative methods of expressing sexuality.*
- Discuss alternatives to sexual intercourse, such as closeness and giving pleasure to a partner. Provide information about penile prosthesis. Discuss masturbation, either individual or mutual, as an option. *Alternatives to sexual intercourse enable and enhance sexual satisfaction that physical limitations may otherwise impede.*

Altered Body Image Perception: Related to change in appearance and function
Expected Outcome: Client will accept altered appearance and perform self-care.

- Assess client's willingness to look at the stoma. Accept client's response and reinforce that anxiety is normal. Reassure client that nursing staff will provide care until they are ready. *Gradual exposure is part of rehabilitation. The nurse supports the client's process.*
- Discuss change in function and let the client know what to expect when recovery from surgery is complete. Suggest a visit from an ostomate who can provide valuable personal information, support, and resources. *Providing information and group support assists the client to know that they are not alone and in preparing to care for themselves in future.*
- Help client gain independence by reinforcing that self-care is quite manageable and providing time for practice. *Encouragement and support promote confidence and move the client from a dependent to an independent role.*

Situational Low Self-Esteem: Related to fear of accidents or urine odor
Expected Outcome: Client will maintain social relationships.

- Explain that odor-proof pouches or pouches with carbon filters or other odor barriers are available. A few drops of liquid deodorizer or diluted white vinegar also may assist in controlling odors. Suggest avoiding odor-producing foods, such as asparagus, eggs, or cheese. *A client may become socially isolated from the odors produced by the urinary diversion. Information about how to control odors will assist the client to implement measures and then to feel that friends, coworkers, and acquaintances will accept them.*
- Oral ascorbic acid may help to control odors. *Ascorbic acid helps to acidify urine and suppress urine odors.*
- Teach client to care for the pouch and to change it every 3 days if it is a one-piece pouch or every 4 to 7 days if it is a two-piece pouch. *Appropriate care assists in reducing odors and contributes to the client's level of confidence.*
- Tell client to empty the bag before it gets half-full to prevent tension on the adhesive wafer and to eliminate source of odors. Inform the client to carry a spare pouch in case adhesive loosens while away from home. *These measures prevent accidents or embarrassment and provide the client with a sense of control and positive well-being.*
- Suggest drinking cranberry juice or using an appliance deodorant. *These measures may reduce odors and assist the client to feel in control.*
- Suggest that the client contact the urostomy association for suggestions and additional support in alleviating anxiety. Instruct client with a ureterosigmoidostomy to avoid gas-forming foods. *Receiving support and accurate information contributes positively to a client's sense of well-being.*

Knowledge Deficiency: Related to inadequate knowledge about stomal care
Expected Outcome: Client will demonstrate ability to change ostomy pouch.

- Explain procedure for removing the old pouch and fitting and applying a new one. Tell client to change the pouch in the morning before consuming liquids and to insert a tampon or rolled gauze into the stoma to absorb urine during appliance change. Make sure the appliance fits well and the skin is completely dry when applying adhesive wafer. *Knowledge of specific procedures and treatment regimen increases a client's understanding and promotes responsibility for self-care.*
- Picture-frame the wafer with paper tape to seal edges. Show the client how to empty the pouch and attach it to an overnight drainage system. *These measures provide more control over the outcome and improve the client's ability to care for themselves.*
- Teach the client to inspect the peristomal skin each time they change the pouch. Advise using a liquid skin barrier to protect the skin. If abdominal skin must be shaved, use an electric razor. *These strategies prevent skin breakdown and promote early intervention. They also provide the client with the skill and knowledge to adequately care for themselves.*

Altered Health Maintenance: Related to inadequate knowledge about intermittent catheterization of continent urinary diversions (Kock pouch, Indiana pouch)
Expected Outcome: Client will demonstrate ability to catheterize the pouch.

NURSING PROCESS FOR THE PSYCHOSOCIAL CARE OF THE CLIENT UNDERGOING URINARY DIVERSION (continued)

- Identify need for continuous drainage and frequent catheterizations in early postoperative period. Explain need for irrigations (to flush mucus and prevent plugging of catheter). *Understanding the rationales for the procedures promotes learning and ability for self-care.*
- Teach client to self-catheterize by lubricating catheter, inserting it into the pouch, and allowing urine to drain into the toilet bowl. *Demonstration of procedures assists the client to develop competence and confidence in self-care activities.*

Evaluation of Expected Outcomes

The client discusses methods for resuming sexual activity and alternatives to sexual intercourse. They state methods to avoid accidents and control urine odor. The client verbalizes a willingness to maintain social activity. They correctly change the ostomy appliance and successfully self-catheterize continent pouch. Client and Family Teaching 59-4 outlines information to include in a teaching plan. Also see Evidence-Based Practice 59-1.

Client and Family Teaching 59-4
Management of a Urinary Diversion

Material included in a client teaching plan is specific to the type of surgery, the surgeon's specific discharge orders, or both. Consider the following:

- Watch for signs and symptoms of fluid and electrolyte imbalances as instructed.
- Keep closed collection containers below the level of the stoma. Keep tubing that connects the catheter or collection appliance to the closed drainage system straight to prevent urine from collecting in a curve of the tube. Avoid kinks that prevent the drainage of urine.
- Drink adequate fluids. Note color of the urine. If urine appears darker than usual, more fluids may be needed. Call primary provider if urine is dark in spite of an adequate fluid intake.
- Take medications as prescribed by the primary provider. Do not omit or stop taking the drugs. Do not take or use any nonprescription drug without first checking with the primary provider. Clients with an ureterosigmoidostomy must not use laxatives or enemas.
- Control odors with cranberry juice, yogurt, or buttermilk. Avoid foods that may impart an odor to the urine, such as asparagus, cheese, or eggs.
- Consult with a WOCN regarding skin care techniques. Keep skin clean. When changing the adhesive wafer (to which the urostomy collection bag is attached), remove all remaining adhesive before applying a new wafer.
- Drain the continent urostomy four times a day or as directed by the primary provider.
- Wash the urinary collection pouch thoroughly after changing. Rinse the pouch with or soak in a solution of vinegar and water if crystals form in the pouch.
- Contact primary provider if any of the following occurs:
  - Fever
  - Chills
  - Blood in the urine
  - Failure of a stoma or catheter to drain urine
  - Skin problems around the stoma
  - Weight loss (>5 lb)
  - Loss of appetite (more than a few days)
  - Inability to insert the catheter in the continent urostomy
  - Pain in the flank (kidney area or lower abdomen)
  - Signs of fluid or electrolyte imbalance
  - Any unusual symptom or problem.

Evidence-Based Practice 59-1

Connection Between Gout and Renal Cancer

Clinical Question

Are clients with gout prone to renal cancer and tumors and what type of nursing care is provided?

Evidence

A type of arthritis that is inflammatory where clients have increased levels of uric acid is called gout (CDC, 2020). Inflammation and hyperuricemia have been linked to numerous cancers, including renal cancers. A study was completed in Korea that looked at clients with gout who were diagnosed and treated between 2008 and 2010. The study then tracked the incidence of cancers in 2012 to 2018 (Oh et al., 2020). They found that the number of clients with gout who had renal cancers was high compared with the clients whom they tracked. The cancers were noted in the esophagus, stomach, liver, pancreas, ovaries, bladder, colorectal, prostate, and kidneys. Clients with gout have hyperuricemia, which has been linked to increase in drinking alcohol and overweight lifestyles. The increased uric acid level has also been linked to increased risks of cancers (Oh et al., 2020). This was a large study with over 179,000 participants.

Nursing Implications

Nurses should have an understanding of gout and the inflammation process. Once a client is diagnosed, it is important to take a thorough history and note alcohol consumption and dietary influences. Important data baselines in diet and weight will be important along with a history of inflammation and arthritis (Oh et al., 2020).

References

Centers for Disease Control and Prevention. (2020). *Gout.* Retrieved May 05, 2021, from https://www.cdc.gov/arthritis/basics/gout.html

Oh, Y., Lee, Y. J., Lee, E., Parks, B., Kwon, J., Heo, J., & Moon, K. W. (2020). Cancer risk in Korean patients with gout. *Korean Journal of Internal Medicine.* https://doi.org/10.3904/kjim.2020.259

the severity of the injury, blood and urine may leak into the peritoneal cavity.

Assessment Findings

Signs and Symptoms

Symptoms vary according to the area affected and the type of injury. Anuria, hematuria, pain in the abdomen (which may indicate bleeding or leakage of urine into the abdominal cavity), pain in the bladder or kidney areas, and symptoms of shock may be indicators of urinary tract injury. During treatment of a client with extensive injury, an indwelling catheter may be inserted, and hematuria or lack of urine output may be the first sign of a traumatic injury to the urinary tract. Certain other types of injuries, such as stab or gunshot wounds, may be immediately identified because of outward signs of injury (e.g., entry wounds on skin surface).

Diagnostic Findings

Injury to the urinary tract initially may be overlooked when the client has incurred widespread, massive injuries. Abdominal X-rays, cystoscopy, IVP, and exploratory surgery may be used to identify the type and location of the injury.

Surgical Management

Treatment depends on the type, location, and extent of injury as well as on the condition of the client. For example, a stab wound in the kidney area may require emergency exploratory surgery. Once the kidney is exposed, the primary provider needs to determine if the trauma to the kidney can be repaired or if the kidney must be removed immediately. Examples of surgeries that may be performed for urinary tract trauma include **cystostomy** (temporary or permanent creation of an opening into the bladder to allow drainage of urine), nephrectomy, insertion of a nephrostomy tube, repair (reanastomosis) of the ureter, and cystectomy. If injuries are not as severe, such as with contusions, an IUC may be inserted and maintained, until the urine is clear of blood and clots.

Nursing Management

The most important nursing task is recognition of abnormal findings. Lack of urinary output, diffuse and severe abdominal pain, and hematuria are examples of signs and symptoms that may indicate an injury to the urinary tract. In some instances, the injury may be such that symptoms do not appear for several hours or days after the initial trauma.

Other nursing management depends on the surgical interventions performed and the symptoms the client experiences. In addition, the nurse needs to focus on the client's physical and emotional needs related to the trauma.

KEY POINTS

- Voiding dysfunction
  - Urinary retention: the inability to urinate or effectively empty the bladder
  - Urinary incontinence: the leaking of urine from the bladder
- Infectious and inflammatory disorders
  - Cystitis: inflammation of the urinary bladder
  - Interstitial cystitis/painful bladder syndrome: chronic inflammation of the bladder causing pain to the bladder and pelvic region
  - Urethritis: inflammation of the urethra, generally in men
- Obstructive disorders
  - Bladder stones: stones may form in the bladder or migrate to bladder and are not able to be eliminated
  - Urethral strictures: narrowing of the urethra obstructs the flow of urine
- Bladder cancer: the most common cancer of the urinary system
- Trauma: trauma is potentially harmful and frequently requires surgical intervention

CRITICAL THINKING EXERCISES

1. A client has recurrent cystitis. Their primary provider wants to perform a cystoscopy and retrograde pyelograms. They ask you why they need these tests because the medication they took in the past cured their problem. What explanation would you give?
2. Discuss the possible psychosocial effects of IC.
3. A client has an ureterosigmoidostomy. What teaching will you do regarding long-term follow-up and care?
4. A client had a radical cystectomy with an ileal conduit. When the licensed practical nurse (LPN) observes the ileal conduit through the transparent urostomy pouch, they note that the stomal opening is red and draining urine with mucus. What action should the LPN take?

NCLEX-STYLE REVIEW QUESTIONS PrepU

1. If the priority nursing diagnosis for a client with urinary retention is urinary retention related to high urethral pressure secondary to prostate enlargement, which of the following is a priority nursing intervention?
   1. Ask the client if there are any problems with bowel elimination.
   2. Catheterize the client to relieve a full bladder and to measure urine output.
   3. Initiate a bladder log, which includes information about urine output and fluid intake.
   4. Obtain a history from the client about the duration of this problem.
2. A nurse, assessing a client with complaints of urge incontinence, expects the client to state which of the following?
   1. "All of a sudden, I just leak urine for no reason."
   2. "I cannot stop the urine from coming when I have to urinate."
   3. "I never feel like my bladder is completely empty."
   4. "When I sneeze or cough, urine leaks into my underwear."

3. Which of the following actions demonstrates to the nurse that the client understands measures to prevent UTIs?
   1. The client dries the perineum thoroughly after bowel elimination.
   2. The client performs appropriate hand hygiene after bowel elimination.
   3. The client uses a feminine hygiene spray after bowel elimination.
   4. The client wipes away from the urinary meatus after bowel elimination.

4. A nurse is teaching a client with an ileal conduit about measures for the client to take to prevent a UTI. Which of the following statements by the client indicates an understanding of preventing UTIs?
   1. "I will have to irrigate the stoma each morning."
   2. "I will need to avoid people with URIs."
   3. "I will drink 8 to 10 glasses of water every day."
   4. "I will use sterile technique to change the pouch."

5. A client whose bladder cancer has been unresponsive to treatment will have their bladder surgically removed and an ileal conduit created to facilitate urinary elimination. When the client asks the nurse to clarify the surgeon's explanation of the procedure, which statement is most correct?
   1. "Urine will be eliminated with stool from the rectum."
   2. "Urine will drain from an abdominal opening."
   3. "Your urine will be deposited in your small intestine."
   4. "Your urine will empty from a special catheter."

UNIT 15
Caring for Clients With Musculoskeletal Disorders

60 Introduction to the Musculoskeletal System

Words To Know

arthrocentesis
arthrogram
arthroscopy
bone scan
bursa
cancellous bone
cartilage
cortical bone
diaphyses
epiphyses
joint
ligaments
osteoblasts
osteoclasts
osteocytes
periosteum
red bone marrow
skeletal muscles
tendons
yellow bone marrow

Learning Objectives

On completion of this chapter, you will be able to:

1. Describe major structures and functions of the musculoskeletal system.
2. Discuss elements of the nursing assessment of the musculoskeletal system.
3. Identify common diagnostic and laboratory tests used in the evaluation of musculoskeletal disorders.
4. Discuss the nursing management of clients undergoing tests for musculoskeletal disorders.

The musculoskeletal system consists of bones, muscles, joints, tendons, ligaments, cartilage, and bursae. It supports the body and facilitates movement. Other functions include storage of calcium, phosphorus, magnesium, and fluoride; production of blood cells in the bone marrow; and protection and support to body organs, such as the lungs, heart, and brain. Injury to or disease in any part of the musculoskeletal system can cause pain, immobility, or disability and potentially affect quality of life.

Gerontologic Considerations

■ Changes in structure, function, chemical composition, and hereditary genetic patterns affect the musculoskeletal system in older adults. With age, the fibrocartilage of intervertebral disks becomes thinner and drier, causing compression of the disks of the spinal column, and the water content of joint cartilage decreases, leading to a height loss of as much as 1 to 2 cm every two decades and possible formation of dorsal kyphosis.

(continued)

Gerontologic Considerations (*continued*)

■ In both men and women, the amount of bone formed during remodeling decreases with age. Bone resorption occurring more rapidly than bone formation increases the risk for skeletal fractures and osteoporosis.
■ Age-related declines in estrogen and testosterone production cause bone loss. Prolonged immobilization, hypercalciuria, malabsorption, cigarette smoking, or alcoholism may accelerate loss of bone mass.
■ Maintaining an active lifestyle and obtaining adequate calcium and vitamin D can delay the decline in muscle strength and bone mass among older adults.

BOX 60-1 Factors That Affect Bone Formation

Bone Formation Facilitators
- Calcium
- Phosphorus
- Estrogen
- Testosterone
- Calcitonin
- Vitamins A, C, and D
- Growth hormone
- Exercise
- Insulin

Bone Formation Retardants
- Estrogen/androgen deficiency
- Vitamin deficiency
- Starvation
- Diabetes
- Steroids
- Inactivity/immobility
- Heparin
- Excess parathyroid hormone

ANATOMY AND PHYSIOLOGY

Bones

The human body has 206 bones. The bones of the skeleton are classified as:

- *Short bones*, such as those in the fingers and toes
- *Long bones*, such as the femur and ulna
- *Flat bones*, such as the sternum
- *Irregular bones*, such as the vertebrae

There are two types of bony tissue. The first is **cancellous bone**, or spongy bone, which is light and contains many spaces. The second is **cortical bone**, or compact bone, which is dense and hard. Both types are found in varying amounts in all bones. Cancellous bone is found at the rounded, irregular ends, or **epiphyses** of long bones. Cortical bony tissue covers bones and is found chiefly in the long shafts, or **diaphyses**, of bones in the arms and legs. The combination of the two types of bony tissue provides strength and support yet keeps the skeleton light to promote endurance during activity.

Bone is composed of cells, protein matrix, and mineral deposits. The three types of bone cells are osteo*blasts*, osteo*cytes*, and osteo*clasts*. Cells that build bones are called **osteoblasts**. These cells secrete bone matrix (mostly collagen), in which inorganic minerals, such as calcium salts, are deposited. This process of *ossification* and *calcification* transforms the osteoblasts into mature bone cells, called **osteocytes**, which are involved in maintaining bone tissue. During times of rapid bone growth or bone injury, osteocytes function as osteoblasts to form new bone. **Osteoclasts** are the cells involved in the destruction, resorption, and remodeling of bone.

During growth, bones primarily lengthen. The diameter also increases when osteoclasts break down previously formed bone, however, making the central canal wider. When skeletal growth is complete, the osteoclasts, which are part of the mononuclear phagocyte system (blood cells involved in ingesting particulate matter—or recycling old cells), continue with the remodeling of bones by balancing bone *resorption* with new bone cell replacement. Bone formation and resorption continue throughout life. The greatest activity occurs from birth through puberty. Box 60-1 reviews factors that affect bone formation.

A layer of tissue called **periosteum** covers the bones (but not the joints). The inner layer of periosteum contains the osteoblasts necessary for bone formation. The periosteum is rich in blood and lymph vessels and supplies the bone with nourishment.

Inside the bones are two types of bone marrow: red and yellow. **Red bone marrow**, found primarily in the sternum, ileum, vertebrae, and ribs, manufactures blood cells and hemoglobin. Long bones have **yellow bone marrow**, which consists primarily of fat cells and connective tissue. If the blood cell supply becomes compromised, the yellow marrow may take on the characteristics of red marrow and begin producing blood cells.

Muscles

There are three kinds of muscles: skeletal, smooth, and cardiac. **Skeletal muscles** are voluntary muscles; impulses that travel from efferent nerves of the brain and spinal cord control their function. The skeletal muscles promote movement of the bones of the skeleton. Examples of skeletal muscles are the biceps in the arms and the gastrocnemius in the calves.

Skeletal muscle is composed of muscle cells or fibers that contain several myofibrils. Sliding filaments called *sarcomeres* make up myofibrils. They are the contractile units of skeletal muscle. Impulses from the central nervous system cause the release of acetylcholine at the motor end plate of the motor neuron that innervates the muscle. As a result, calcium ions are released, and the release stimulates actin and myosin in the sarcomeres to slide closer together, resulting in contraction of the muscle. When calcium is depleted, the actin and myosin fibers move apart, causing relaxation of the sarcomeres, and thus the muscle.

Muscle tone (referred to as *tonus*) is evident when muscle fibers are contracted. In order for muscles to remain toned, exercise is required. Various terms are used to describe muscle tone. These include:

- *Flaccid*: a muscle that has no tone or is limp
- *Spastic*: a muscle that has greater-than-normal tonus
- *Atonic*: a muscle that is not enervated becomes soft and flabby
- *Hypertrophy*: muscle enlargement that occurs with repetitive exertion over time
- *Atrophy*: muscle deterioration that occurs with lack of use and exercise

Smooth and cardiac muscles are involuntary muscles; their activity is controlled by mechanisms in their tissue of origin and by neurotransmitters released from the autonomic nervous system. Smooth muscles are found mainly in the walls of certain organs or cavities of the body, such as the stomach, intestine, blood vessels, and ureters. Cardiac muscle is found only in the heart.

Joints

A **joint** is a junction between two or more bones. Table 60-1 outlines types and characteristics of joints. Free-moving joints, or diarthrodial joints, make up most skeletal joints. They allow certain movements. Terms related to diarthrodial joint movement are presented in Box 60-2. The surfaces of diarthrodial joints are covered with hyaline cartilage, which reduces friction during joint movement. The space between is the joint cavity, which is enclosed by a fibrous capsule lined with synovial membrane. This membrane produces synovial fluid, which acts as a lubricant.

Tendons

Tendons are cordlike structures that attach muscles to the periosteum of the bone. A muscle has two or more attachments. One is called the *origin* and is more fixed. The other is called the *insertion* and is more movable. When a muscle contracts, both attachments are pulled, and the insertion is drawn closer to the origin. An example can be found in the biceps of the arm, which has two origin tendons, attached to the scapula, and one insertion tendon, attached to the radius. When the biceps contract, the lower arm (with the insertion tendon) moves toward the upper arm (with the origin tendons).

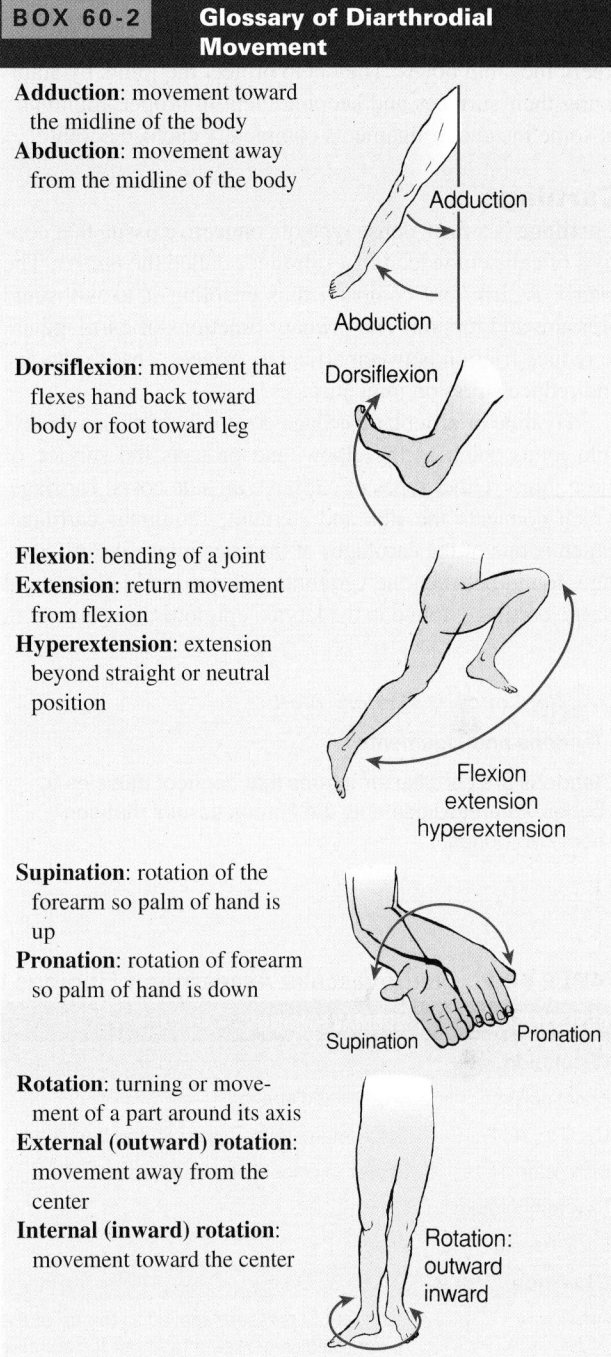

BOX 60-2 Glossary of Diarthrodial Movement

Adduction: movement toward the midline of the body
Abduction: movement away from the midline of the body

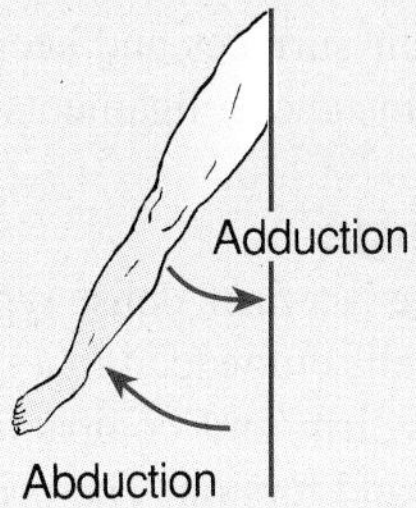

Dorsiflexion: movement that flexes hand back toward body or foot toward leg

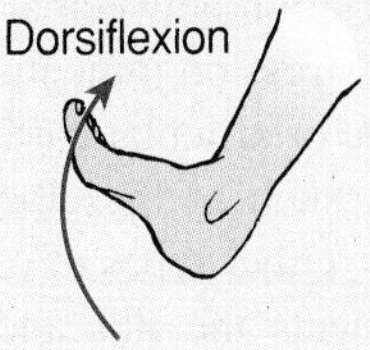

Flexion: bending of a joint
Extension: return movement from flexion
Hyperextension: extension beyond straight or neutral position

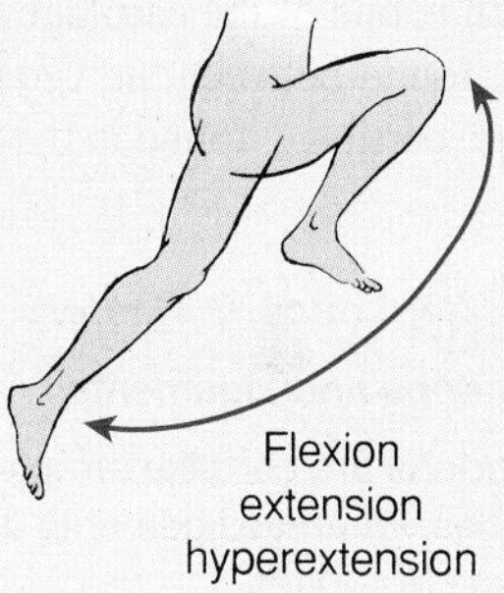

Supination: rotation of the forearm so palm of hand is up
Pronation: rotation of forearm so palm of hand is down

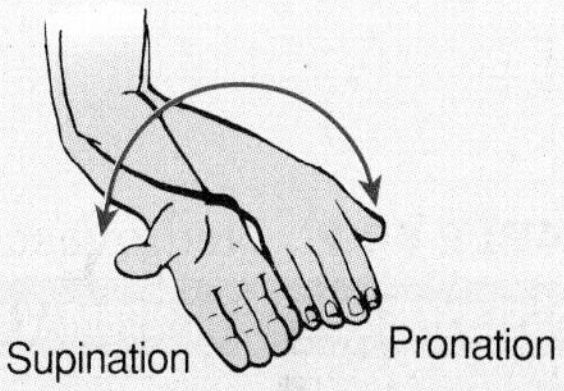

Rotation: turning or movement of a part around its axis
External (outward) rotation: movement away from the center
Internal (inward) rotation: movement toward the center

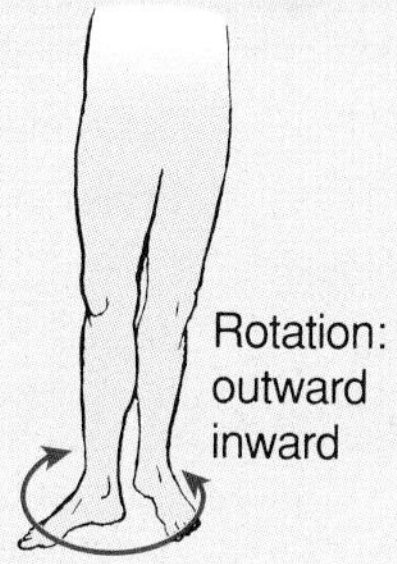

TABLE 60-1 Types and Characteristics of Joints

TYPES	CHARACTERISTICS	EXAMPLES
Synarthrodial joints	Immovable	At the suture line of skull between the temporal and occipital bones
Amphiarthrodial joints	Slightly movable	Between the vertebrae
Diarthrodial joints (also called *synovial joints*)	Freely movable	Gliding joint: fingers Hinge joint: elbow Pivot joint: ends of radius and ulna Condyloid joint: between the wrist and forearm Saddle joint: between the wrist and metacarpal bone of the thumb Ball-and-socket joint: hip

Ligaments

Ligaments consisting of fibrous tissue connect two adjacent, freely movable bones. They help protect the joints by stabilizing their surfaces and keeping them in proper alignment. In some instances, ligaments completely enclose a joint.

Cartilage

Cartilage is a firm, dense type of connective tissue that consists of cells embedded in a substance called the *matrix*. The matrix is firm and compact, thus enabling it to withstand pressure and torsion. The primary functions of cartilage are to reduce friction between articular surfaces, absorb shocks, and reduce stress on joint surfaces.

Hyaline or articular cartilage covers the surface of movable joints, such as the elbow, and protects the surface of these joints. Other types of cartilage include costal cartilage, which connects the ribs and sternum; semilunar cartilage, which is one of the cartilages of the knee joint; fibrous cartilage, found between the vertebrae (intervertebral disks); and elastic cartilage, found in the larynx, epiglottis, and outer ear.

> *Concept Mastery Alert*
>
> **Tendons and Ligaments**
>
> Tendons are cordlike structures that connect muscles to bones, whereas ligaments are fibrous tissues that connect two bones.

Bursae

A **bursa** is a small sac filled with synovial fluid. Bursae reduce friction between areas, such as tendon and bone and tendon and ligament. Inflammation of these sacs is called *bursitis*.

ASSESSMENT

History

The focus of the initial history depends on whether the client has a chronic disorder or a recent injury. There are symptoms that are common to musculoskeletal dysfunction, no matter whether acute or chronic. These symptoms include pain and altered neurosensory sensations. Assessment of pain and a neurovascular assessment (Table 60-2) are a priority for clients with any musculoskeletal disorder.

If the disorder is long-standing, the nurse obtains a thorough medical, drug, and allergy history. If the client is injured, the nurse finds out when and how the trauma occurred and compiles a list of symptoms that includes information about the onset, duration, and location of discomfort or pain. Determining whether activity makes the symptoms better or worse is important. The nurse also identifies associated symptoms, such as muscle cramping or skin lesions, and asks the client if the problem interferes with activities of daily living. If the client has an open wound, the nurse ascertains when the client last received a tetanus immunization.

TABLE 60-2 Neurovascular Assessment Findings in Musculoskeletal Assessment

ASSESSMENTS	NORMAL FINDINGS	ABNORMAL FINDINGS
Circulation		
Distal pulses	Present and strong	Absent or weak
Capillary refill	Color returns to compressed nail bed within 3 seconds	Nail bed stays blanched after 3 seconds
Skin color	Similar to color in other body areas	Pale or dusky
Skin temperature	Warm	Cold
Local edema	Absent	+1 to +4 swelling
Sensation		
Arm injury	Can identify pressure applied to the tip of the index finger (median nerve), fifth finger (ulnar nerve), and web between the thumb (radial nerve)	Numb to touch or feels abnormal sensation like tingling or burning
Leg injury	Can identify pressure applied to great toe (peroneal nerve) and sole of the foot at the base of the toes (posterior tibial nerve) without observing the stimulus	Same as above
Mobility		
Arm injury	Can spread fingers on affected hand (ulnar nerve) Can press thumb to last digit on affected hand (median nerve) Demonstrates the "hitchhiker's sign" with affected hand; can flex and extend wrist (radial nerve)	Weak or cannot move fingers Cannot approximate thumb to finger Cannot extend thumb Wrist-drop is apparent
Leg injury	Can flex and extend ankle (peroneal and posterior tibial nerves)	Foot drop is apparent
Pain	Proportional to injury but relieved with analgesia or nursing interventions	Constant or increased despite implementation of pain-relieving techniques

Nutrition Notes

Nutrition and Musculoskeletal Health

- Although bone formation and resorption continue throughout life, net bone loss exceeds net bone gain in all people after peak bone mass is attained at roughly 30 years of age. An adequate calcium intake before that time helps maximize peak bone mass; the denser the bones, the less susceptible they are to fracture.
- Calcium intake recommendations are set at 1000 mg/day for adults younger than 50 years of age and 1200 mg/day for those over age 71 years. This translates to about four servings from the dairy group each day. Clients who cannot or are unwilling to consume ample dairy products are not likely to meet their calcium requirement through diet alone.
- Good nondairy sources of calcium include dark green leafy vegetables, sardines, canned salmon with bones, broccoli, and calcium-fortified orange juice. With the exception of calcium-fortified orange juice, the body does not absorb calcium from nondairy sources well. Vitamin D protects against bone loss and decreases the risk of fracture by facilitating the absorption of calcium from food and supplements. Without adequate vitamin D, calcium is excreted, not absorbed, even if calcium intake is adequate. Many people do not consume enough vitamin D because dietary sources are limited. Many people do not make adequate vitamin D because synthesis is impaired by northern latitude, sunscreen, dark skin, and aging.
- Vitamin K, magnesium, and potassium—nutrients found in fruits and vegetables—help maintain bone density.

From National Institutes of Health: Office of Dietary Supplements. (2020). *Calcium.* Retrieved May 5, 2021, from https://ods.od.nih.gov/factsheets/Calcium-HealthProfessional/

The nurse must obtain a history of past disorders and medical or surgical treatments as soon as possible. Attention to chronic or concurrent disorders, such as diabetes mellitus, is essential. In addition, the nurse obtains a family history, especially when relatives have had similar symptoms, and an occupational history. The "Nutrition Notes" section outlines the role of nutrition in the client's musculoskeletal health.

>>> *Stop, Think, and Respond 60-1*

A neighbor calls you and states that he tripped and fell, spraining his ankle. When you arrive to help him, what questions should you ask? What should you observe?

Physical Examination

For a general musculoskeletal assessment, the nurse observes the client's ability to ambulate, sit, stand, and perform activities requiring fine motor skills, such as grasping objects. General inspection includes examining the client for symmetry, size, and contour of extremities and random movements. Observing a client's posture is followed by a spinal inspection that includes identifying spinal curvatures (Fig. 60-1):

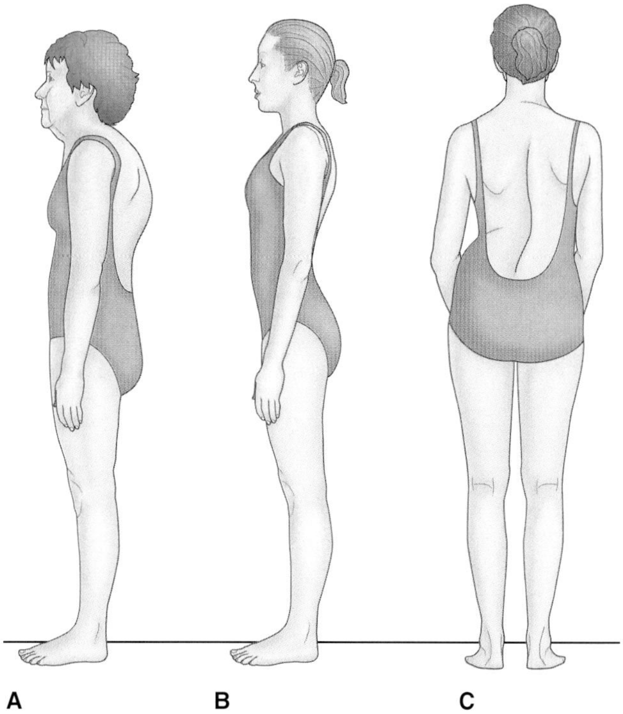

Figure 60-1 Common spinal curvatures include **(A)** kyphosis, **(B)** lordosis, and **(C)** scoliosis.

- *Kyphosis*: exaggerated convex curvature of the thoracic spine (humpback)
- *Lordosis*: excessive concave curvature of the lumbar spine (swayback)
- *Scoliosis*: lateral curvature of the spine

The nurse palpates the muscles and joints to identify swelling, degree of firmness, local warm areas, and any involuntary movements. To test the client's muscle strength, the nurse applies force to the client's extremity as the client pushes against that force. The nurse also must perform a neurovascular assessment (refer again to Table 60-2), which includes assessing range of motion for the joints, taking care not to force movement. The nurse notes any abnormal muscle movements such as spasms or tremors. In addition, the nurse

- looks for abnormal size or alignment and symmetry, comparing one side with the other.
- inspects and palpates for pain, tenderness, swelling, and redness.
- observes the degree of movement and range of motion but never persists beyond the point of pain.
- tests for muscle strength.
- inspects for muscle wasting.

Depending on the symptoms and findings, additional assessments may include looking for changes in gait and body posture; favoring one side over the other; and ability to bend and twist the trunk, head, and extremities. As

TABLE 60-3 Age-Related Musculoskeletal Changes

STRUCTURE	STRUCTURAL CHANGE	FUNCTIONAL CHANGE	SIGNS AND SYMPTOMS
Bones	Gradual, progressive loss of bone mass after age 35 years. Vertebral collapse	Increased bone fragility; fracture-prone—most commonly vertebrae, hip, and wrist	Loss of height Posture changes Kyphosis Flexion of hips and knees Back pain Osteoporosis Fracture
Muscles	Increased collagen—results in fibrosis Decreased muscle mass (atrophy); wasting Decreased tendon elasticity	Loss of strength and flexibility Weakness and fatigue Stumbling Falls	Loss of strength Diminished agility Diminished endurance Prolonged response time or decreased reaction time Decreased muscle tone Increased frequency of falls Broad base of support
Joints	Cartilage progressively deteriorates Intervertebral discs thin	Stiffness and reduced flexibility Pain Difficulty performing ADLs	Decreased range of motion Decreased flexibility Stiffness Decreased flexibility Loss of height
Ligaments	Relaxed ligaments (decreased strength, weakness)	Postural joint abnormality Weakness	Joint pain with movement—improves with rest Crepitus Joint swelling/enlargement Degenerative joint disease (osteoarthritis)

ADLs, activities of daily living.

clients age, they experience many changes in the musculoskeletal system. After 35 years, people generally experience loss of bone mass and height and changes in the structure of the spine and joints. Table 60-3 describes musculoskeletal changes related to aging. It is essential to assess clients for musculoskeletal changes because of their potential impact on activities of daily living.

If the client has a traumatic injury, physical assessment begins with taking vital signs. Further assessment depends on the type and area of injury. As the nurse conducts the assessment, they maintain standard precautions. The nurse needs to cut the clothing from around an injured area if there is no other way to examine the client. Comparing structures and assessment findings on one side of the body with those on the opposite side assists the nurse in determining the degree of injury. Although the nurse must be thorough, it is also important to be gentle, recognizing that assessment techniques may increase the client's pain. The examination includes the following:

- Observing for swelling, external bleeding, or bruising
- Palpating the peripheral pulses
- Evaluating peripheral circulation; assessing peripheral pulse (rate and character), skin coloration (pink, gray, pale, ashen), temperature, and capillary refill time
- Checking the sensation of the injured part
- Looking for broken skin, open wounds, superficial or embedded debris in or around the wound, protrusion of bone or other tissue from the wound
- Examining for injury beyond the original area; for example, auscultating the chest and abdomen if an abdominal or thoracic injury occurred or checking the pupils and mental status if a head injury occurred
- Looking for malalignment of the injured limb
- Assessing for pain, noting the type and location

The primary provider needs to examine the client before the nurse touches, cleans, or disturbs open wounds and before moving the injured extremity.

Diagnostic Tests

Imaging Procedures

X-rays, computed tomography (CT), and magnetic resonance imaging (MRI) help identify traumatic disorders, such as fractures and dislocations, and other bone disorders, such as malignant bone lesions, joint deformities, calcification, degenerative changes, osteoporosis, and joint disease.

An **arthrogram** uses radiopaque contrast or air injected into a joint to view irregular surfaces and movement of the joint. Ankles, knees, hips, shoulders, or wrists are most often examined with this technology. The primary provider first injects a local anesthetic and then inserts a needle into the joint space. Fluoroscopy may be used to verify correct placement of the needle. The synovial fluid in the joint is aspirated and sent to the laboratory for analysis. A contrast medium is then injected, and X-ray films are taken. After undergoing arthrography, the client is informed that they may hear crackling or clicking noises in the joint for up to 2 days. Noises beyond this time are abnormal; the client should report them.

>>> *Stop, Think, and Respond 60-2*

Review your knowledge of MRIs. What precautions need to be adhered to before a client undergoes MRI?

Arthroscopy

Arthroscopy is the internal inspection of a joint using an instrument called an *arthroscope*. The most common use of arthroscopy is visualization of the knee joint, a common site of injury. After administering a local or general anesthetic, the primary provider inserts a large-bore needle into the joint and injects sterile normal saline solution to distend the joint.

After inserting the arthroscope, the examiner inspects the joint for signs of injury or deterioration. Joint fluid may be removed and sent to the laboratory for examination. Depending on the findings, the primary provider sometimes can use the arthroscope to perform therapeutic procedures such as removing bits of torn or floating cartilage and repairing tears or defects.

Afterward, the client's entire leg is elevated without flexing the knee. A cold pack is placed over the bulky compression dressing covering the site where the arthroscope was inserted. A prescribed analgesic is administered as necessary. Nursing Guidelines 60-1 outlines the nurse's role in assisting the client undergoing arthroscopy.

Arthrocentesis

Arthrocentesis is the aspiration of synovial fluid. The client receives local anesthesia just before this procedure. The primary provider inserts a large needle into the joint and removes the fluid. Synovial fluid may be aspirated to relieve discomfort caused by an excessive accumulation in the joint space or to inject a drug, such as a corticosteroid preparation. The removed synovial fluid may be sent to the laboratory for microscopic examination or for culture and sensitivity studies. Arthrocentesis also may be performed during an arthrogram or arthroscopy.

NURSING GUIDELINES 60-1

Assisting the Client Through Arthroscopy

Before the Procedure

- Explain the procedure.
- Ensure that the client has signed the informed consent form.
- Verify that the client has been NPO for at least 6 hours.
- Administer preoperative medications, if ordered.

After the Procedure

- Instruct client to report unusual pain, bleeding, drainage, or swelling at the arthroscopic site.
- Advise client to resume usual diet as tolerated.
- Review discharge instructions with the client and explain medication regimen.
- Inspect dressing before discharge.

Synovial Fluid Analysis

Synovial fluid is aspirated and examined to diagnose disorders such as traumatic arthritis, septic arthritis (caused by a microorganism), gout, rheumatic fever, and systemic lupus erythematosus. Normally, synovial fluid is clear and nearly colorless. Laboratory examination of synovial fluid may include microscopic examination for blood cells, crystals, and formed debris that may be present in the joint space after an injury. If an infection is suspected, culture and sensitivity studies are ordered. A chemical analysis for substances such as protein and glucose also may be performed.

Bone Densitometry

Bone densitometry estimates bone mineral density (BMD). X-rays or ultrasounds of the wrist, hip, or spine help determine BMD. Bone density scanning or dual-energy X-ray absorptiometry (DXA or DEXA) uses advanced radiographic technology to measure BMD. DEXA is most often done on the lower spine and hips. Portable DEXA devices use X-rays or ultrasound to measure the quantity and quality of wrist, finger, or heel bone and to provide an estimate of bone density. The higher the mineral content, the greater the bone density, and thus greater bone strength. Results are reported in terms of T-scores and Z-scores. These scores use standard deviations to compare expected norms for healthy young adults of each gender with actual bone density results. For example, a T-score of −1 or above indicates normal bone density, whereas a score of −2.5 and below is highly indicative of osteoporosis. Z-scores are used in a similar way but are more specific in terms of comparisons based on age, sex, weight, and ethnic or racial origin.

Fracture Risk Assessment Tool

The Fracture Risk Assessment Tool (FRAX) is used to predict a client's 10-year risk for fractures, as well as the risk for having osteoporosis. It factors in bone density results as well as the following clinical risk factors:

- Postmenopausal women or men who are 50 years or older
- Clients with osteopenia (T-score between −1 and −2.5)
- Clients who have not taken medications for osteoporosis
- Family history of osteoporosis
- History of smoking

Using the FRAX assists health care providers to determine if clients will benefit from prescribing measures to prevent osteoporosis, which may include medications, dietary measures, and lifestyle changes, such as increased exercise and weight loss strategies.

Bone Scan

A **bone scan** uses the intravenous (IV) injection of a radionuclide to detect the uptake of the radioactive substance by the bone. A bone scan may be ordered to detect metastatic bone lesions, fractures, and certain types of inflammatory disorders. The radionuclide is taken up in areas of increased metabolism, which occur in bone cancer, metastatic bone disease, and osteomyelitis (bone infection). Nursing considerations for preparing a client for a bone scan include the following:

- Informing the client that the radiopaque isotope will be administered intravenously
- Ensuring that the client does not have any allergies to the isotope
- Informing the client that the scan will occur 2 to 3 hours following the injection
- Encouraging the client to drink fluids that will help distribute and eliminate the isotope
- Asking the client to void immediately before the scan

Electromyography

Electromyography tests the electrical potential of the muscles and nerves leading to the muscles. It is done to evaluate muscle weakness or deterioration, pain, and disability and to differentiate muscle and nerve problems. The primary provider inserts needle electrodes into selected muscles and uses electric current to stimulate the muscles. An oscilloscope records responses to the electrical stimuli. If the client experiences discomfort after the study, warm compresses to the area help relieve the discomfort.

Biopsy

A biopsy is done to identify the composition of bone, muscle, or synovium. The specimen may be removed with a needle or excised surgically while the client is under general anesthesia. Afterward, the nurse observes the site for signs of bleeding or swelling, assesses for pain, applies ice to the site, and administers analgesics as indicated.

Blood Tests

A complete blood count (which includes a red blood cell count, hemoglobin level, white blood cell count, and differential) may be ordered to detect infection, inflammation, or anemia. Examples of other diagnostic blood tests and findings of various musculoskeletal disorders include the following:

- Elevated alkaline phosphatase level, which may indicate bone tumors and healing fractures
- Elevated acid phosphatase level, which may indicate Paget's disease (a disorder characterized by excessive bone destruction and disorganized repair) and metastatic cancer
- Decreased serum calcium level, which may indicate osteomalacia, osteoporosis, and bone tumors
- Increased serum phosphorus level, which may indicate bone tumors and healing fractures
- Elevated serum uric acid level, which may indicate gout (treated or untreated)
- Elevated antinuclear antibody level, which may indicate systemic lupus erythematosus, a connective tissue disorder

Urine Tests

When ordered, the nurse collects 24-hour urine samples for analysis to determine levels of uric acid and calcium excretion. In gout, the 24-hour excretion of uric acid is elevated. Elevated calcium levels are found in metastatic bone lesions and in clients with prolonged immobility.

NURSING MANAGEMENT

Some diagnostic tests are performed while the client is assessed in the emergency department, on an outpatient basis, or after admission for treatment of the disorder. The nurse implements protocols necessary to prepare the client for the diagnostic examination, identifies and sends collected specimens to the laboratory, and manages the client's safe recovery after invasive procedures.

If the client has a chronic disorder, the nurse obtains a general medical history, a description of the current symptoms, including pain and disability, and compiles drug and allergy histories. An allergy to iodine and seafood may be a contraindication to performing an arthrogram or other test in which a contrast medium is instilled.

No special care is required after most laboratory tests, general X-rays, or a bone scan. If the client has had an invasive joint examination, the nurse inspects the area for swelling and bleeding or serous drainage. They change or reinforce dressings as needed. If the client has severe pain in the area, the nurse must notify the primary provider, who may order the application of ice and an analgesic for pain or discomfort.

In the case of a traumatic injury, the nurse obtains information regarding the injury from the client, the person accompanying the client, or paramedics and ambulance personnel. They take vital signs during the initial examination and at frequent intervals until the client's condition stabilizes. The nurse also checks the neurovascular status of the affected limb, including circulation, motion, and sensation. Keeping the client calm and promoting comfort are essential measures. For example, if the client has an injury in the arm, the nurse applies a sling to ease pain until treatment can be initiated.

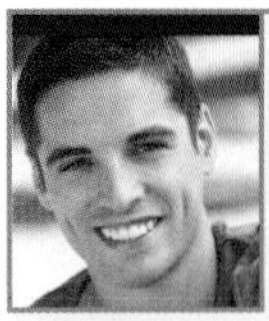

Clinical Scenario A 24-year-old man is in a motor vehicle accident and sustains some injuries. The client is alert and complaining of left arm and hip pain. What are the important considerations for the nurse when overseeing the care of a client having diagnostic testing for potential musculoskeletal disorders? (See the following "Nursing Process for the Client with a Musculoskeletal Injury" section.)

NURSING PROCESS FOR THE CLIENT WITH A MUSCULOSKELETAL INJURY

Assessment

Assess the client's injuries in terms of the location, nature of the pain, and effects on mobility. Also, determine the neurovascular status of the injured area by checking circulation, sensation, and mobility, if it is not contraindicated. Monitor the client's vital signs and closely observe for signs of shock.

Diagnosis, Planning, and Interventions

Provide a brief, broad overview of diagnostic tests or treatments ordered because the client will find it difficult to comprehend many details while anxious. Provide the client and family with information about how long the tests or examinations will take, where they will be done, and what preparations (if any) are necessary. Allow the client an opportunity to ask questions or make comments as they process the information. Before carrying out any preliminary activities before a diagnostic test, describe what is about to be done.

Invasive procedures, such as arthroscopy, and treatment procedures require the client to sign a consent form. The primary provider is responsible for explaining the purpose of the procedure, its risks and benefits, and available alternatives. Repeat or clarify the primary provider's explanations. After an outpatient procedure, the primary provider often gives the client special instructions for self-care. Written discharge instructions must be provided to the client upon discharge, as recalling information from memory can lead to confusion or injury. The "Client and Family Teaching 60-1" section discusses further education points. Additional diagnoses, expected outcomes, and interventions include the following:

Acute Pain: Related to tissue injury
Expected Outcome: Client will have relief from pain.

- Minimize or avoid moving the painful body part. *Doing so prevents increased pain and helps the client to relax.*
- If the client must be moved from a stretcher, wheelchair, or an examination table, request sufficient help and support the joints above and below the area of discomfort during transfer. *Sufficient support prevents pain and avoids increasing discomfort.*
- Support an acutely or chronically inflamed joint in a comfortable position. *Maintaining a neutral position reduces pain.*
- Elevate a swollen extremity as long as doing so does not potentiate the trauma from an injury. Alternatively, cradle a painful arm in a sling when the client is up and about. *These measures reduce swelling and, subsequently, pain.*
- Observe for signs of respiratory depression if administering a prescribed narcotic analgesic for pain relief. *Opioids may cause respiratory depression and lead to sedation in a client susceptible to shock after a traumatic injury.*
- Notify primary provider if pain increases or is unrelieved. *Persistent pain may indicate further injury or sequelae to trauma.*

Altered Tissue Perfusion: Related to swelling, inflammation, or inactivity imposed by injury
Expected Outcome: Client will maintain tissue perfusion in the injured area as evidenced by normal neurovascular assessment findings.

- Keep a swollen body part above the level of the heart. *This position promotes venous circulation and relieves edema.*
- Consult with the primary provider about applying a cold pack if an injury is recent. *Cold reduces circulation to the affected area and may impair neurovascular health.*
- If a head injury is suspected, elevate the client's head slightly while keeping the neck neutral. *Such positioning reduces the risk of further injury.*
- Report the absence of a peripheral pulse and severe pain immediately. *These findings may indicate ischemia.*

Acute Anxiety: Related to pain and injury, its treatment, and the potential for altered mobility
Expected Outcome: Client's anxiety will be reduced as evidenced by vital signs within normal range and no signs of being overly alert or easily startled.

- Relieve discomfort as much as possible. *Doing so eliminates at least one aspect of the client's concerns.*
- Call the client by name; be empathic and attentive. *Attention to the client's needs promotes relaxation and comfort.*
- Instill confidence by demonstrating technical skill and competence in explanations or preparations for tests or treatments. *A confident nurse can help reduce a client's anxiety.*
- Speak quietly in simple sentences that the client can understand. *Understanding reduces anxiety.*
- Allow a supportive family member to stay with the client if possible. *This measure can comfort the client.*

Evaluation of Expected Outcomes

The client states that medication and positioning have relieved pain. Neurovascular status remains intact, as evidenced by good perfusion, strong pulses, ability to tense muscles, and appropriate sensation. The client has a calm demeanor and states that they feel less anxious.

Client and Family Teaching 60-1 Musculoskeletal Care

The nurse includes the following information:

- Report signs and symptoms, such as excessive pain or throbbing, prolonged or fresh bleeding, swelling, skin color changes, decrease in sensation, or purulent drainage.
- Maintain any special body position that the nurse instructs you to take.
- Resume bathing and activity as directed by primary provider.
- Resume work and other activities per primary provider's orders.
- Review purpose of prescribed drugs, how to take them, and possible side effects.
- Arrange date for a follow-up appointment with the primary provider, if one is required.
- Demonstrate how to remove and reapply dressings and how to apply an immobilizer or sling, if one is used.
- Demonstrate safe crutch-walking gait if crutches are temporarily needed.

KEY POINTS

- Anatomy and physiology: consists of bones, muscles, joints, tendons, ligaments, cartilage, and bursae
- Assessment
  - History
  - Physical exam
  - Diagnostic tests:
    - Imagine procedures: CT and MRI
    - Arthroscopy: internal inspection of a joint using an arthroscope
    - Arthrocentesis: aspiration of synovial fluid
    - Bone densitometry: estimates BMD
    - Fracture risk assessment tool: predicts a client's 10-year risk for fractures
    - Bone scan: used to detect metastatic bone lesions, fractures, and inflammatory disorders
    - Electromyography: tests the electrical potential of the muscles and nerves
    - Biopsy: specimen obtained to identify composition of bone, muscle, or synovium
    - Blood and urine tests

CRITICAL THINKING EXERCISES

1. You are caring for a client in a nursing home and they fall. What assessments would you make?
2. What signs and symptoms would indicate that the tissue in an injured extremity is not being adequately perfused?
3. The nurse is conducting an assessment of the client's physical mobility and wants to determine the client's ability to abduct the fingers in each hand. What instructions should the nurse give the client?
4. Consider your acquired knowledge related to mobility and immobility. A client has injured their ankle. What initial steps should you take to prevent swelling and further injury?

NCLEX-STYLE REVIEW QUESTIONS PrepU

1. A nurse admits a client to a medical unit and begins the assessment. Which of the following situations places this client at risk for fractures? Select all that apply.
   1. The client claims to walk 1 mile every day.
   2. The client drinks three glasses of milk daily.
   3. The client has decreased intake related to cancer treatments.
   4. The client has a history of diabetes mellitus.
   5. The client periodically takes steroids for a long history of asthma.
2. A nurse is assessing a client's range of motion. To determine the client's ability to pronate the forearm, what question should the nurse ask the client?
   1. "Can you extend your elbow in a straight position?"
   2. "Can you flex your wrist toward the forearm?"
   3. "Can you move your elbow away from your body?"
   4. "Can you turn your hand so that the palm is down?"
3. A nurse is providing discharge instructions following an arthroscopy. Which of the following statements by the client alerts the nurse to the client's lack of understanding?
   1. "I must call the doctor if there is blood on the dressing."
   2. "I need to wait to call the doctor because a high level of pain is normal."
   3. "I understand that I can resume a normal diet."
   4. "I will resume my medications per your instructions."
4. A client is seen in the emergency room for a possible fractured wrist from a fall on the ice. The client tells the nurse that they are not able to straighten the fingers of the injured hand/wrist. What is the nurse's best action when hearing this?
   1. Apply ice to the affected arm to reduce pain and edema.
   2. Ask the client to massage and then wiggle the affected fingers.
   3. Assess the client's neurovascular status on the affected hand.
   4. Elevate the affected arm on pillow to reduce edema.
5. The nurse is assessing the client's circulation in the right leg following an injury. Which finding needs further action?
   1. Capillary refill is longer than 3 seconds.
   2. Peripheral pulses in right leg are strong.
   3. Skin temperature is warm to touch.
   4. There is no edema present.

WANT TO KNOW MORE? There are a wide variety of online resources available on thePoint to enhance learning and understanding of this chapter.

Go to **thePoint.lww.com/activate**, and use the activation code found in the front of this text to unlock these online resources.

61

Caring for Clients Requiring Orthopedic Treatment

Words To Know

arthroplasty
avascular necrosis
braces
cast
closed reduction
external fixation
internal fixation
open reduction
prosthesis
splint
subluxation
traction

Learning Objectives

On completion of this chapter, you will be able to:

1. Differentiate types of casts.
2. Discuss the nursing management for a client with a cast.
3. State the reasons for using splints or braces.
4. Identify the principles for maintaining traction and describe nursing care for the client in traction.
5. Differentiate between closed reduction and open reduction and between internal fixation and external fixation.
6. Describe nursing care for the client with a fracture reduction.
7. Identify the reasons for performing orthopedic surgery.
8. Discuss the nursing management for a client undergoing orthopedic surgery.
9. Compare minimally invasive joint replacement surgery with conventional joint replacement surgery.
10. Describe the positioning precautions after a conventional total hip replacement.
11. Explain the nursing needs of the client undergoing total knee replacement.
12. Discuss amputation, including reasons it may be performed and appropriate nursing management of the client.

Musculoskeletal disorders are common in any client population and contribute to temporary or permanent disability. Clients with orthopedic disorders often cannot meet all of their activities of daily living (ADLs). Management of musculoskeletal disorders involves the use of casts, splints and braces, traction, and various types of orthopedic surgery. Amputation may also be done following a traumatic injury or because of disease or disability.

CASTS

A **cast** is a rigid mold that immobilizes an injured structure while it heals. There are basically three types of casts. A *cylinder cast* encircles an arm or leg, leaving the fingers or toes exposed. A *body cast* is a larger form of a cylinder cast that encircles the trunk from about the nipple line to the iliac crests. A *hip spica cast* surrounds one or both legs and the trunk. It may be strengthened by a bar that spans a casted area between the legs (Fig. 61-1). This type of cast is trimmed open in the anal and genital areas to facilitate elimination. Other types of casts are described in Box 61-1.

To keep aligned bone fragments from becoming displaced, the cast is applied from the joint above the break to the one below it. The joint is slightly flexed to decrease stiffness. Some fractures (e.g., a stress

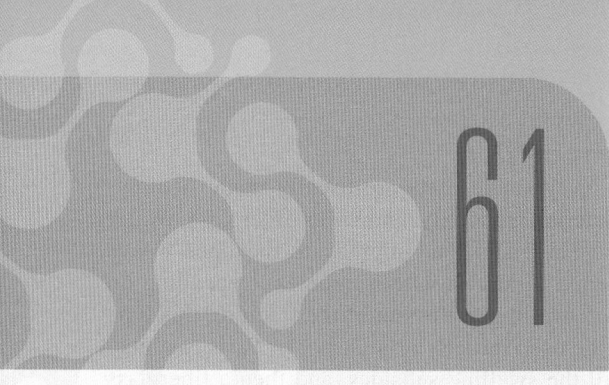

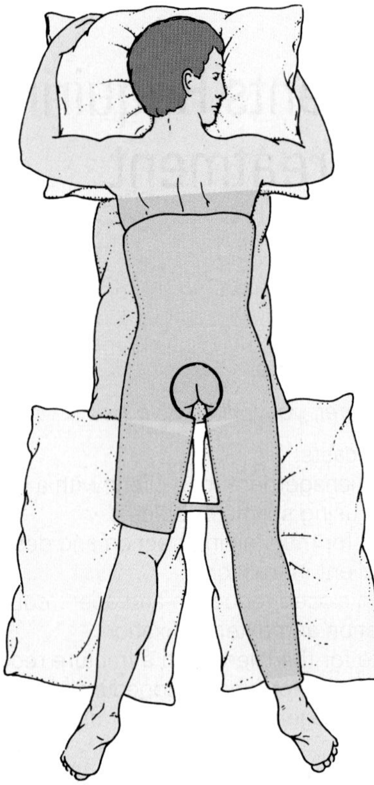

Figure 61-1 Spica cast. This client with a spica cast is resting on pillows until the cast dries. His feet are positioned so that they support the desired body alignment. Note the bar, ensuring adequate space between the casted legs.

fracture) do not require surgical reduction or manual manipulation to realign the bone because the fractured bone still remains perfectly aligned. If a closed or open reduction is required, the client receives an analgesic or a general or local anesthetic to relieve pain.

BOX 61-1 Examples of Types of Casts

- *Short arm cast*: extends from below the elbow (BE) to the palmar crease and is secured around the base of the thumb. If the thumb is also casted, it is referred to as a *thumb spica* or *gauntlet* cast.
- *Long arm cast*: extends from the upper level of the axillary fold to the proximal palmar crease. The elbow is usually immobilized at a right angle.
- *Short leg cast*: extends from below the knee (BK) to the base of the toes. The foot is flexed at a right angle in a neutral position.
- *Long leg cast*: extends from the junction of the upper and middle third of the thigh to the base of the toes. The knee may be slightly flexed.
- *Walking cast*: a short or long leg cast reinforced for strength
- *Body cast*: encircles the trunk
- *Shoulder spica cast*: a body cast that encloses the trunk and the shoulder and elbow
- *Hip spica cast*: encloses the trunk and a lower extremity. A double-hip spica cast includes both legs.

Adapted from Hinkle, J. H., & Cheever, K. H. (2014). *Brunner & Suddarth's textbook of medical-surgical nursing* (13th ed., p. 1104). Wolters Kluwer Health/Lippincott Williams & Wilkins.

Cast Composition

Nonplaster or synthetic casts are usually made of polyurethane material, generally known as fiberglass. Water activates the hardeners that impregnate the open-weave fabric to form a rigid cast within minutes. Depending on the degree of swelling at the site of the fracture, this type of cast may be used initially or a plaster of Paris cast may be used until the swelling subsides, and then a fiberglass cast may be applied. Plaster casts require a longer time for drying but mold better to the client and are initially used until the swelling subsides. Fiberglass casts dry more quickly, are lighter in weight, are longer lasting, and are breathable. Clients with synthetic casts have fewer skin problems and may bear weight soon after the cast is applied depending upon the type of fracture. A waterproof liner (such as Gore-Tex) may be used, allowing the client to immerse the cast to bathe, swim, or receive hydrotherapy. It is important to teach the client to drain water from the cast and to let it dry.

When applying the cast, the primary provider positions the client to ensure proper alignment of the part to be immobilized. The client's buttocks may be supported on a casting frame when a body cast or spica cast is applied so the casting material can be wrapped around the client's trunk. A nurse or an assistant holds the arm or leg in place during application of a cylinder cast (Box 61-2). If the client is awake, health care providers explain that the cast material will feel warm during application as a result of being mixed with water.

A wet cast must be kept uncovered so that water can evaporate. Most primary providers prefer natural evaporation but may order a cast dryer to speed evaporation. Intense heat is never used. There is a danger not only of burning the client but also of cracking the outside of the cast while leaving the inside damp and hospitable to mold. The drying cast should be supported on pillows. If necessary, health care personnel can reposition the casted arm or leg with the palms of the hands. Using the fingertips or compressing the cast on a hard surface can lead to a pressure sore later.

BOX 61-2 Applying a Cast

In general, the primary provider or nurse practitioner applies a cast as follows:

- Clean and dry the skin surface of the part to be casted.
- Cover the skin with stockinette, a tubular knitted material.
- Wrap padding around the limb, especially over bony prominences.
- Apply rolls or strips of plaster or nonplaster cast material evenly over the stockinette and padding.
- Smooth the layers and edges of the cast.
- Fasten the stockinette in cufflike fashion to the outside of the cast.
- Arrange for an X-ray study after casting to check bone alignment.

Cast Windows

After the cast dries, a cast window, or opening, may be cut. This usually is done when the client reports discomfort under the cast or has a wound that requires a dressing change. The window permits direct inspection of the skin, a means to check the pulse in a casted arm or leg, or a way to change a dressing. Once a window is cut, the solid piece of cast is replaced in its original site and secured with adhesive tape or a roller bandage. Leaving the window open may allow the skin and soft tissue to bulge through the opening.

Bivalve Casts

Once a cast has been applied, it may be bivalved or cut in two (Fig. 61-2). This may be necessary if the arm or leg swells, causing the rigid cast to compress the tissue and interfere with its blood supply. A bivalved cast also may be used for a client who is being weaned from a cast, when a sharp X-ray is needed, or as a splint for immobilizing painful joints when a client has arthritis.

Cast Removal

Casts are removed with a mechanical cast cutter. Cast cutters are noisy and frightening, and the client needs reassurance that the machine will not cut into the skin. Once the cast is off, the skin appears mottled and may be covered with a yellowish crust composed of accumulated body oil and dead skin. The client usually sheds this residue in a few days. Lotions and warm baths or soaks may help to soften the skin and remove debris.

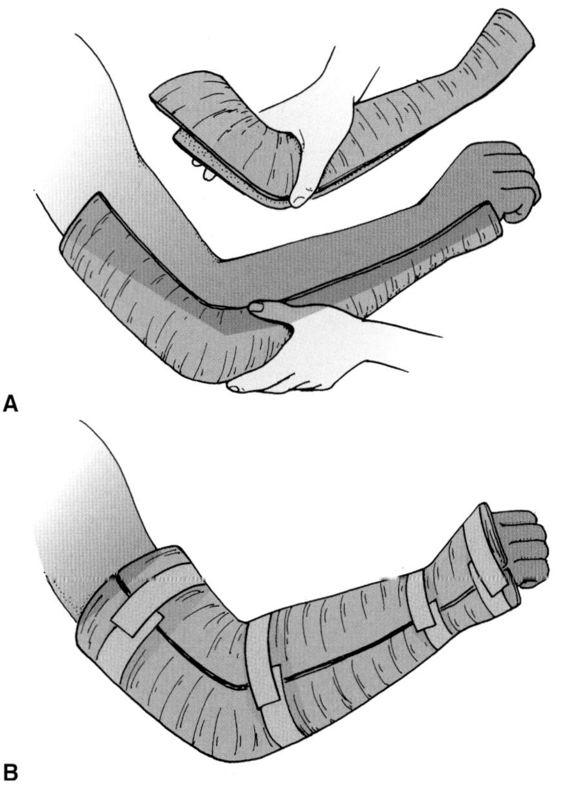

Figure 61-2 **(A)** A bivalved cast. **(B)** The two halves are rejoined.

Concept Mastery Alert

Cast Removal Education

When a client has a cast removed after bone healing occurs, the nurse should instruct the client that the proper method of removing dead, crusty skin is by soaking in a warm bath and applying lotion to soften the skin.

The now uncasted limb feels surprisingly light, and the client may report weakness and stiffness. For some time, the limb will need support. An elastic bandage may be wrapped on a leg, the client may use a cane, and an arm may be kept in a sling until progressive active exercise and physical therapy help the client regain normal strength and motion.

Nursing Guidelines 61-1 provides information about caring for a client with a cast. Nursing care includes teaching clients with casts to the lower extremities how to ambulate with crutches.

SPLINTS AND BRACES

A **splint** immobilizes and supports an injured body part in a functional position. The client would use a splint when a musculoskeletal condition

- does not require rigid immobilization;
- causes a large degree of swelling;
- requires special skin treatment.

Splints can be made of plaster or a more pliable thermoplastic material. They should be padded so they do not cause pressure or skin abrasions and breakdowns. The health care professional fits the client with a splint and then overwraps it with an elastic bandage applied in a spiral mode. This helps to promote circulation and maintain the position of the splint. Other types of splints include canvas splints, soft or hard ready-made splints, soft variety splints that support an injured upper extremity, and commercial soft splints padded and contoured to fit a client's extremity. Velcro straps on the splint attach the splint to the injured extremity.

Braces provide support, control movement, and prevent additional injury for more long-term use. Made of plastic materials, canvas, leather, or metal, braces are custom fit to each client. The nurse must provide instruction to the client and family on how to apply the brace and to administer scrupulous skincare to prevent irritation and injury.

››› *Stop, Think, and Respond 61-1*

A client with a brace on his lower right extremity tells you that the brace is cutting into his ankle bone. What is your best action?

REDUCING FRACTURES

Clients experiencing a disruption in the functional continuity of a bone have sustained some form of a fracture (refer to Chapter 62 for more discussion of fractures). Reducing a fracture involves restoring proper alignment to the injured

NURSING GUIDELINES 61-1

Caring for the Client With a Cast

Before Cast Application

- Inspect the condition of the skin that will be covered with a cast.
- Assess circulation, sensation, and mobility to establish a baseline.
- Evaluate the client's pain level.
- Remove clothing that will be difficult to remove after the cast is applied.
- Explain the procedure to the client. Remember to tell the client that the cast will feel warm—even hot—as it is applied, but that it will not burn the skin.

After Cast Application

- Leave the cast uncovered.
- Assess circulation, sensation, and mobility in exposed fingers and toes every 1 to 2 hours.
- Monitor for signs of complications related to cast application. Report abnormal findings immediately.
- Handle wet cast with the palms of the hands, not the fingers.
- Elevate casted extremity so it is higher than the heart.
- Reposition the client frequently while cast is drying so the cast dries as evenly as possible.
- Apply ice packs to the cast where surgery was performed.
- Circle areas where blood seeped through, and write the time on the circle.
- Petal cast edges with strips of adhesive tape to prevent chipping and to cover any remaining rough areas.
- Replace windows in the hole from which they were cut to prevent tissue from bulging through the opening.
- Ambulate client as soon as indicated.

Discharge Teaching

- Instruct client to elevate casted extremity for 24 to 48 hours after cast application and as indicated.
- If the client has a leg cast, show them how to ambulate safely (refer to illustration included in these guidelines).
- Teach how to exercise joints proximal and distal to the cast as indicated to prevent muscle atrophy, weakness, and loss of joint mobility.
- Emphasize keeping the cast clean and dry. A damp cloth may be used.
- Explain that the skin under the cast may feel itchy, and caution client not to insert objects like straws, combs, eating utensils, knitting needles, and the like.
- The client should report the following to the primary provider or nurse: unusual and sudden pain, painful or decreased movement, or persistent pain; fever, foul odors, or increased warmth of extremity; drainage from under the cast; changes in circulation, mobility, or sensation (burning, numbness, tingling, or cold).

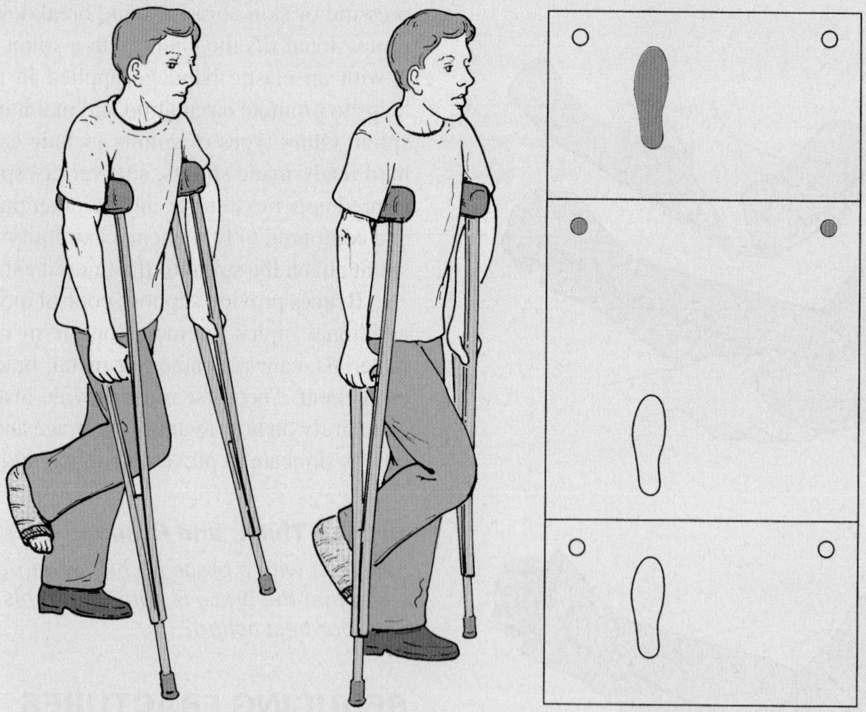

Crutch walking using the three-point, non–weight-bearing gait pattern (three blocks at right). At left, the client positions himself at the bottom of a triangle composed of each crutch and the unaffected leg. In the center, the client advances his unaffected leg forward by supporting himself on the handgrips of the crutches and swinging his hips and the unaffected leg through the crutch opening.

bone. Treatment of fractures includes one or more methods: traction, closed or open reduction, internal or external fixation, or cast application (see previous discussion). The treatment method depends on several factors, including the first aid given, the location and severity of the break, and the age and overall physical condition of the client.

Traction

Traction is a method of pulling structures of the musculoskeletal system. For traction to achieve its purpose, it requires *countertraction*, a force opposite to the mechanical pull. Countertraction usually is supplied by the client's own weight. Traction is used to relieve muscle spasm, align bones, and maintain immobilization. Figure 61-3 demonstrates how traction can be applied in different directions to attain the necessary line of pull. The two most common types are skin traction and skeletal traction.

Skin traction is achieved by applying devices to the skin that indirectly affect the muscles or bones. An example is Buck traction (Fig. 61-4A); another example is Russell traction (see Fig. 61-4B). Skeletal traction is applied directly to a bone by using a wire (Kirschner), pin (Steinmann), or cranial tongs (Crutchfield). General or local anesthesia may be used when inserting these devices. The pull is achieved by connecting the attachment from the client to a system of ropes, pulleys, and weights on an orthopedic bed frame. A Thomas splint with a Pearson attachment often is used to suspend a leg in traction. This is referred to as *balanced suspension traction*. Figure 61-5 presents an example of skeletal traction (Thomas splint) with balanced suspension. The principles for maintaining effective traction are discussed in Box 61-3. Nursing care measures for a client in traction are presented in Nursing Guidelines 61-2.

Closed Reduction

In a **closed reduction**, the bone is restored to its normal position by external manipulation. A bandage, cast, or traction then immobilizes the area. X-rays are taken to ensure correct alignment of the bone. Depending on the site and type of fracture, the client receives a local (nerve block) or general anesthetic for this procedure.

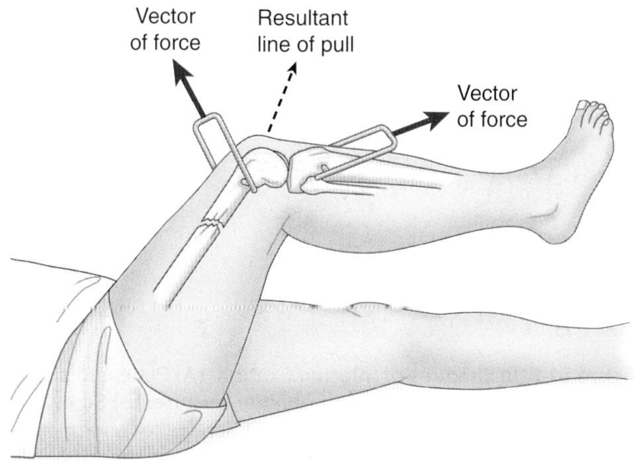

Figure 61-3 Traction may be applied in different directions to achieve the desired therapeutic line of pull. Adjustments in applied forces may be prescribed over the course of treatment.

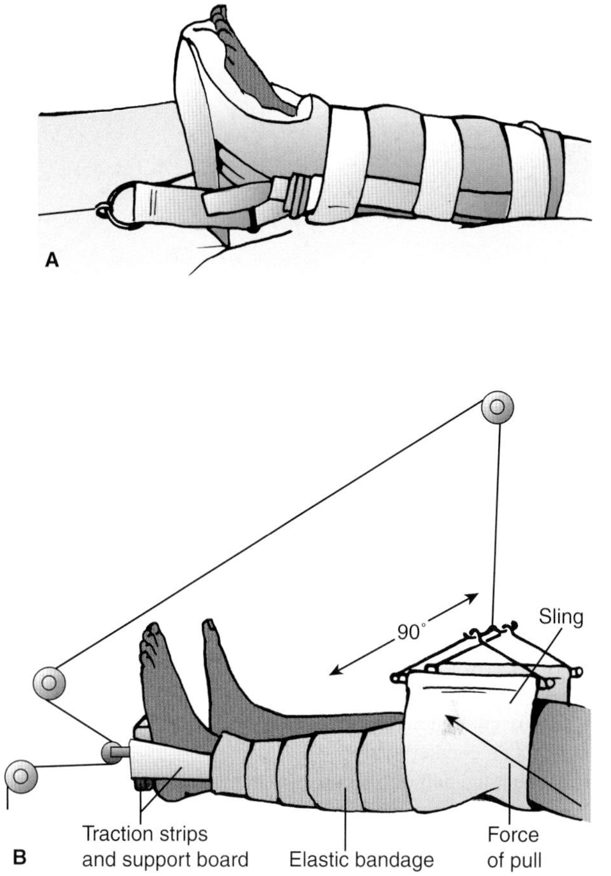

Figure 61-4 Two examples of skin traction: **(A)** Buck traction and **(B)** Russell traction.

Open Reduction

In an **open reduction**, which is performed in the operating room, the bone is surgically exposed and realigned. Usually, the client receives a general or spinal anesthetic. Radiographic studies, taken while the client is still anesthetized, show whether realignments are needed.

Internal Fixation

If **internal fixation** is needed to stabilize the reduced fracture, the surgeon secures the bone with metal screws, plates, rods, nails, or pins. A cast or other method of immobilization is then applied. Figure 61-6 depicts examples of internal fixation techniques. Open reduction is required when

- soft tissue, such as nerves or blood vessels, is caught between the ends of the broken pieces of bone;
- the bone has a wide separation;
- comminuted fractures are present;
- patella and other joints are fractured;
- open fractures are evident;
- wound debridement is necessary;
- internal fixation is needed.

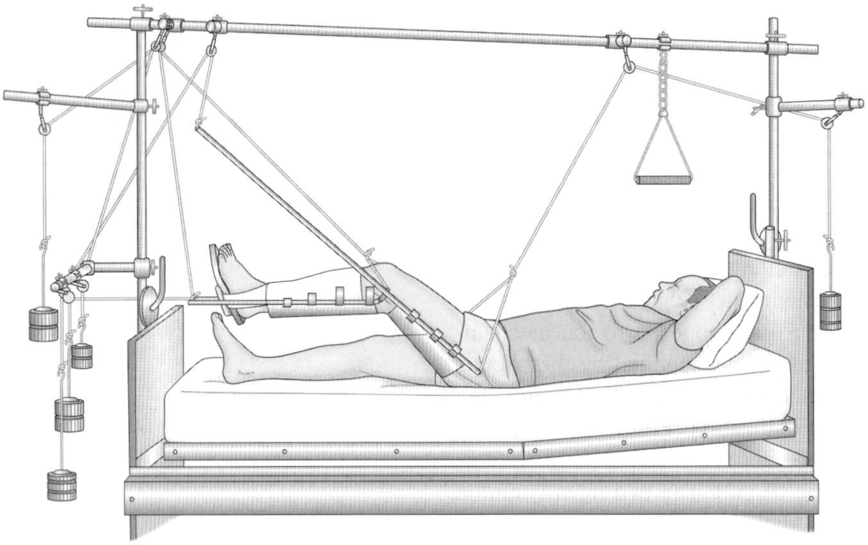

Figure 61-5 Skeletal traction with balanced suspension and Thomas leg splint.

BOX 61-3 Principles of Effective Traction

- Ensure continuous traction.
- Maintain countertraction.
- See that the pull of traction and countertraction are in opposite directions but straight alignment.
- Suspend splints and slings without interference.
- Be sure that ropes move freely through each pulley.
- Apply the exact amount of weight prescribed.
- Make sure that the weights hang freely.

NURSING GUIDELINES 61-2

Managing the Care of the Client in Traction

- Assess neurovascular status frequently. Compare assessment findings in the affected limb with those in the unaffected limb.
- Check traction equipment for the following:
  - Proper alignment (position client so the body is in an opposite line to the pull of traction)
  - Correct attachment
  - Prescribed amount of weight
  - Freely hanging weights and freely moving ropes over unobstructed pulleys
  - Maintenance of countertraction
  - Monitor client for signs of pressure areas.
  - Encourage client to be as mobile as possible and to perform exercises as indicated.
  - If traction is applied to the lower extremity, observe foot position and prevent foot drop.
  - If skeletal traction is applied, follow agency procedure for pin care.
  - Cover tips of any protruding metal pins or rods with corks or other protective material.

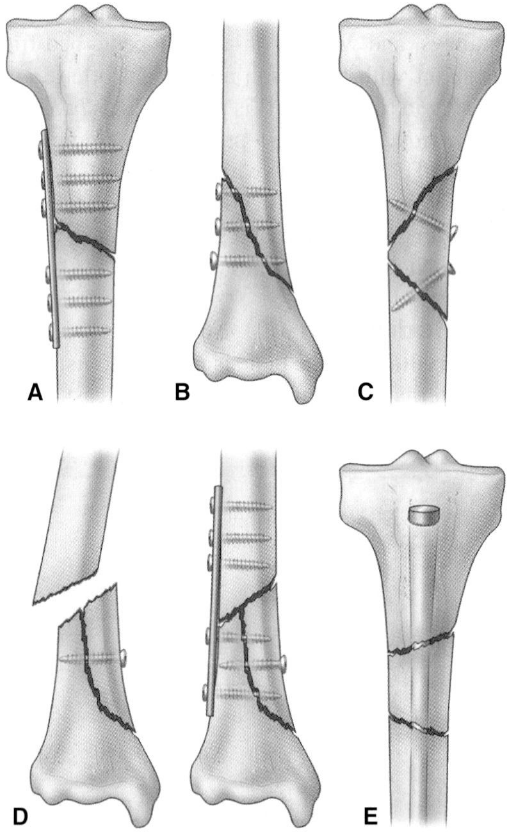

Figure 61-6 Techniques of internal fixation. **(A)** Plate and six screws for a transverse or short oblique fracture. **(B)** Screws for a long oblique or spiral fracture. **(C)** Screws for a long butterfly fragment. **(D)** Plate and six screws for a short butterfly fragment. **(E)** Medullary nail for a segmental fracture.

External Fixation

In **external fixation**, the surgeon inserts metal pins into the bone or bones from outside the skin surface and then attaches a compression device to the pins (Fig. 61-7). Some complex or comminuted fractures may require an external fixation device to stabilize and position the bone. Because the pin sites are an entry for infection, monitoring for redness, drainage, and tenderness is necessary. Nursing Guidelines 61-3 describe pin care for an external fixation device.

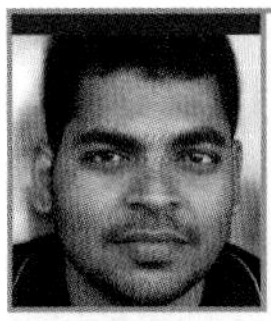

Clinical Scenario A 22-year-old man was injured while playing rugby. He is complaining of severe pain in his right leg and states he heard a "snap" when another player ran into him and knocked him down. X-rays reveal a fractured tibia and fibula. What nursing care will this client require? See the following "Nursing Process for the Client with a Fracture Reduction" section.

NURSING PROCESS FOR THE CLIENT WITH A FRACTURE REDUCTION

Assessment

When caring for the client with a fracture, assess the client for neurovascular and systemic complications.

Diagnosis, Planning, and Interventions

General nursing measures include administering analgesics, providing comfort measures, assisting with ADLs, preventing constipation, promoting physical mobility, preventing infection, maintaining skin integrity, and preparing the client for self-care. Because the client may be discharged shortly after application of an immobilization device or a cast, review needed care with the client and family. In addition, reinforce instructions regarding exercise and ambulatory activities.

If a client is placed in traction, provide simple and direct explanations about the traction and its purpose. Point out activities that are allowed or contraindicated, and identify the approximate duration of restrictions. When the traction is discontinued, prepare the client for further treatment, such as casting, and the appearance of the affected area—skin and muscles. Reassure the client that with gradual exercise and use, muscles will regain strength and tone, and joints will be flexible. For more information about managing problems related to casting, refer to Nursing Guidelines 61-1. For information about clients with specific fractures, such as those affecting the clavicle or knee, refer to Table 61-1.

Other responsibilities include, but are not limited to, the following:

Acute Pain: Related to tissue and bone trauma, swelling, skeletal traction, or cast pressure
Expected Outcome: Client will report relief of pain after analgesics and comfort measures are administered.

- Administer prescribed analgesics. *They provide pain relief. Opioids are used to treat moderate-to-severe pain, and nonsteroidal anti-inflammatory drugs (NSAIDs) inhibit the initiation of pain impulses. Often after a traumatic injury, both opioids and NSAIDs are prescribed.*
- Elevate the extremity if not in traction. *Elevation reduces swelling and pain.*
- Apply ice pack to site of injury as indicated. *Doing so reduces swelling and pain.*
- Change client's position within prescribed limits. *Position changes relieve pressure on bony prominences and promote comfort.*

Impaired Physical Mobility: Related to pain, swelling, surgical procedure, or immobilization from traction, cast, or splint
Expected Outcomes: (1) Client will regain or maintain maximum mobility and optimal functional position. (2) Client will have increased strength and function in the affected limb.

- Assess level of mobility. *These data provide a baseline for comparison.*
- Instruct client in active and passive range-of-motion (ROM) exercises for affected and unaffected extremities within physical and medical restrictions. *ROM exercises strengthen muscles needed for mobility and function, prevent contractures and deformities, and promote circulation.*
- Teach client how to turn safely, adhering to restrictions. *Doing so encourages client's active participation and prevents further injury.*
- Assist and instruct client in the use of mobility aids (wheelchair, walker, crutches, canes) as needed. *The client must be aware of the amount of weight bearing allowed. Ambulatory aids assist with non–weight-bearing or partial weight-bearing restrictions. Instruction prevents injury from unsafe use.*

Bathing/Hygiene and Toileting ADL Deficits: Related to immobility secondary to traction or casts
Expected Outcome: Client will maintain maximum self-care.

(continued)

NURSING PROCESS FOR THE CLIENT WITH A FRACTURE REDUCTION (continued)

- Assist client to meet self-care needs as indicated. *Limited mobility and ROM prevent client from safely providing self-care; assistance promotes safety.*
- Instruct client to perform self-care activities as much as possible. *Doing so promotes independence.*
- Provide assistive devices as indicated. *They help the client to be as independent as possible.*
- Allow client to plan self-care that best meets ongoing needs. *Doing so involves client in care and helps them to have control.*

Altered Tissue Integrity Risk: Related to puncture wound; compound fracture; pins, wires, screws, or other surgical intervention; or physical immobility
Expected Outcomes: (1) Client will demonstrate adequate wound healing without infection. (2) Skin will remain intact.

- Provide pin care per agency protocol. *It assists in monitoring client for infection and maintains a clean environment.*
- Report any signs of infection in the pin care sites, wounds, or surgical incisions. *Doing so promotes early intervention and prevents further infection.*
- Protect bony prominences from pressure by using pressure-relieving techniques under elbows, heels, and coccyx. Massage bony prominences and skin surfaces subjected to pressure unless they remain red when pressure is relieved. *These measures prevent further injury and potential infection and promote circulation to the area.*
- Assess traction frequently to ensure proper alignment and to prevent pressure areas. *Doing so prevents mechanical injury to the skin and tissues.*
- Petal cast edges with waterproof tape. *This measure protects skin from abrasion* (see Nursing Guidelines 61-1).

Evaluation of Expected Outcomes

Pain is reduced or relieved. The client regains mobility and function and achieves the maximum level of self-care. Wounds heal without infection, and the skin is intact. The "Nutrition Notes" section highlights nutrition considerations for the client receiving orthopedic treatment.

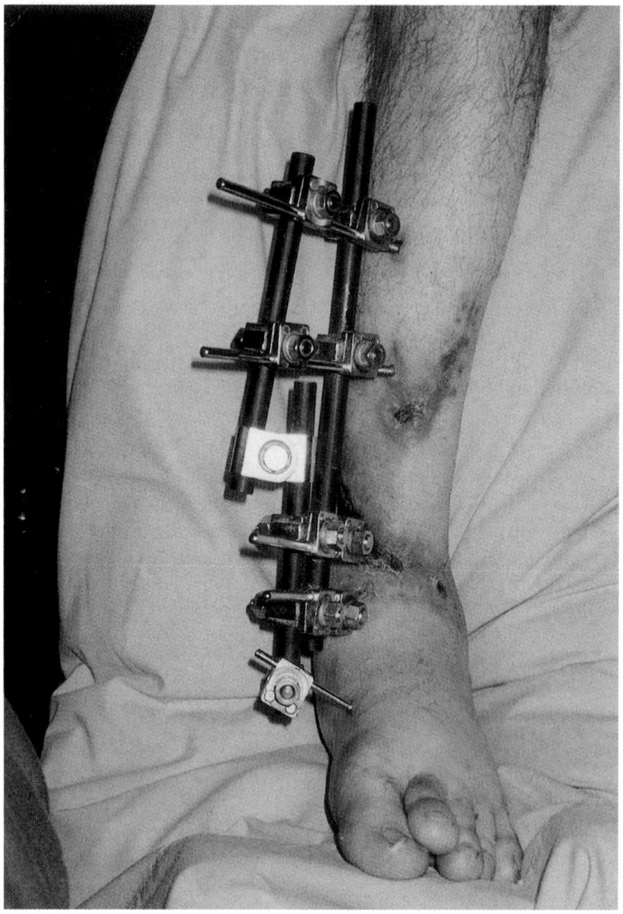

Figure 61-7 External fixation device.

NURSING GUIDELINES 61-3

Providing Pin Care

Research is ongoing regarding best practice for pin care. The following procedure is the most recent recommendation for preventing localized infection at the pin sites and systemic infection and osteomyelitis:

- Assess pin sites for redness, swelling, increased tenderness, and drainage.
- Examine pins for signs of breakage, bending, or shifting.
- Depending on clinical site protocols and the condition of the pin sites, pin care is done daily during the first 48 to 72 hours and then daily or weekly until pin sites are dry without crusting. The client and/or family member should receive pin care instructions if the client is discharged home.
- Using aseptic technique, the nurse or caretaker uses cotton-tipped applicators and sterile water, saline, or other prescribed solution such as chlorhexidine solution to cleanse pin sites. Iodine-based products interfere with tissue healing and are not recommended for cleaning pin sites.
- Use at least one applicator per pin—do not use applicator more than once.
- Clean pin site from pin outward.
- Gently remove crusts around pin sites
- Cleanse the length of the pins from pin site to end of pin. Some clinical sites may recommend wrapping the pin with gauze for the first week to 10 days.
- Do not apply ointment to pin sites unless specifically ordered.
- Obtain culture if purulent drainage is present.

TABLE 61-1 Nursing Care for Specific Fractures

SITE OF FRACTURE	SIGNS AND SYMPTOMS	TREATMENT	NURSING MANAGEMENT
Mandible	Inability to close mouth after trauma to jaw Chin displaced from midline Teeth absent, loose, or broken Lacerations to mouth and tongue Oral pain, swelling, bruising, and bleeding	Fractures are surgically reduced and immobilized with wire loops to stabilize the lower jaw to the upper jaw. Broken teeth are repaired or removed. Oral lacerations are sutured.	Ensure that wire cutters are easily accessible at the client's bedside. Be familiar with how to cut wire loops if client vomits or chokes. Administer antiemetics to treat nausea and prevent vomiting. Administer liquid or semiliquid diet. Assist client to thoroughly clean mouth after each meal and every 2 hours.
Clavicle	After fracture or dislocation, arm on the affected side held close to the chest to reduce pain Affected shoulder appears to slope downward and droop inward Motion restricted Muscle spasm common	Motion can be limited with a sling or clavicular strap. Displaced fractures are immobilized with a figure-8 or Velpeau bandage. 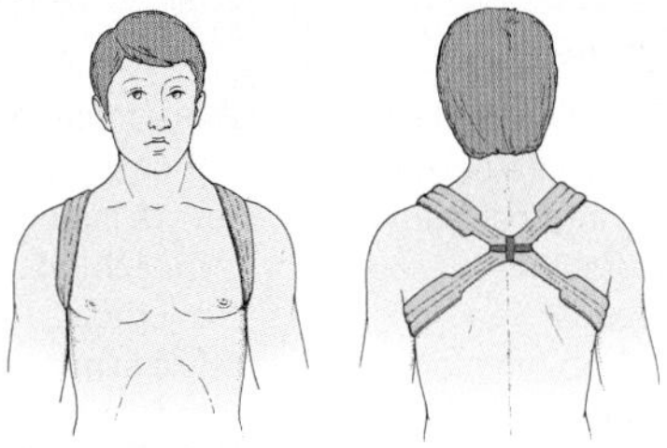 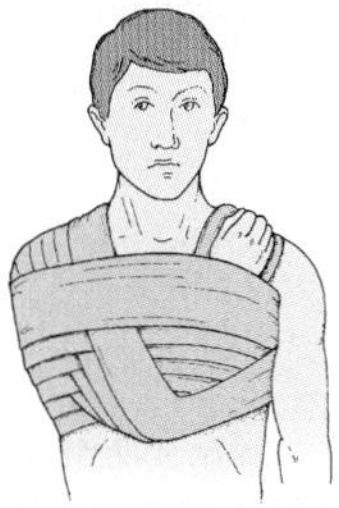 Velpeau bandage	Use a layer of stockinette or soft, porous material between skin surfaces. Teach client how to assess circulation, sensation, and mobility frequently. Instruct client to abduct arms or rest elbows on table or chair to relieve axillary pressure.
Rib	Additional injuries—to the lungs, subclavian arteries or veins, liver, or spleen Severe chest pain on inspiration and shallow respirations. The client has other symptoms if other injuries are present.	Clients are treated for the pain that accompanies fractured ribs, especially when breathing. A rib belt or elastic bandage is used to support the injured rib cage, although this restricts chest movement and may cause further lung problems.	Assess for signs and symptoms of pneumonia and atelectasis (collapsed lung) secondary to shallow respirations. Encourage deep breathing. Administer pain medications as indicated.
Upper extremity (fractures ranging from uncomplicated to complex and involving the bone ends, joints, tendons, and ligaments)	Pain Compartment syndrome, common complication of forearm fractures, possibly leading to Volkmann's contracture, a clawlike deformity of the hand	Extent of injury determines treatment. Cast with or without closed reduction Open reduction with internal fixation Hanging heavy cast that pulls a fractured humerus into alignment 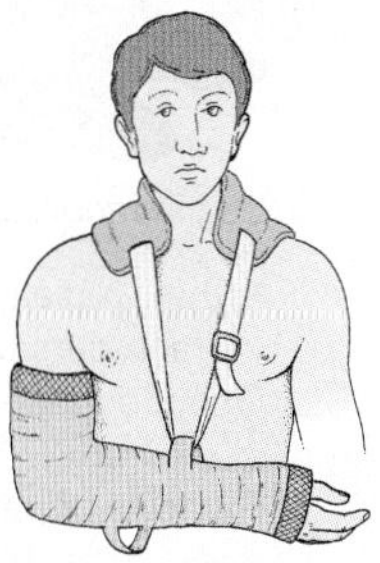 Hanging arm cast	Assess neurovascular status frequently. Report abnormal findings immediately. Implement measures to relieve pain and swelling. Pad skin around neck if the client has a hanging cast.

(continued)

TABLE 61-1 Nursing Care for Specific Fractures (*continued*)

SITE OF FRACTURE	SIGNS AND SYMPTOMS	TREATMENT	NURSING MANAGEMENT
Wrist, hand, or finger	Typically results from a fall May involve only the lower radius (e.g., a Colles fracture in which the distal end of the radius breaks off and becomes displaced) Pain and swelling in the affected area Deformed-looking hand, wrist, or finger	Closed reduction with a cast Open reduction with internal fixation Splints applied to fractured fingers	Show client how to use a sling. Teach client how to do active ROM exercises in fingers of affected hand.
Spine	May follow severe injury; if compression fracture, may result from osteoporosis Pain radiating to the leg Tenderness at injury site Muscle spasms Deformity of spinal column Neurologic deficits	Bed rest for an uncomplicated fracture Spinal brace Laminectomy with fusion Cast Head traction: halo brace with rigid vest that allows client to move but immobilizes vertebrae	Teach client to log roll if on bed rest and as indicated. Assess client's sensation, mobility, and strength in the extremities. Administer pin care if client has a halo brace.
Pelvis (fractures range from minor to severe or crushing injuries)	Tenderness, swelling, and ecchymoses, or more severe symptoms if internal injuries accompany fracture Severed nerves Loss of lower limb function Internal bleeding	Minor fractures: bed rest and comfort measures Severe injuries: multiple-system approach related to the nature of the injuries Pelvic slings, spica casts, or open reduction with internal or external fixation	Assess circulation, sensation, and mobility in the lower extremities. Monitor elimination patterns. Insert an indwelling catheter as necessary. Provide a fracture bedpan. Administer suppositories or small-volume enemas as indicated. Assess skin frequently for signs of breakdown. Provide frequent skincare. Administer pain medications as prescribed.
Knee (involving kneecap or the ends of the femur or tibia; injuries to the ligaments or tendons)	May follow falls or blows or athletic competition (particularly tears of the cruciate ligaments) Pain, swelling, ecchymoses Inability or limited ability to move or bend the joint	Immobilization with a leg splint 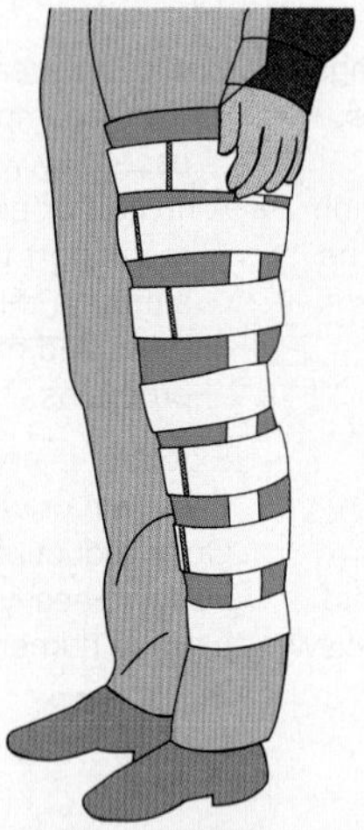 Leg immobilizer Arthroscopic surgery to remove bone fragments or to repair ligament tears Open reduction and insertion of wire sutures Removal of patella if fragmented extensively Skeletal traction	Assist client to use ambulatory aids, such as crutches or walker. Teach client to perform active ROM exercises within limitations.

TABLE 61-1 Nursing Care for Specific Fractures (*continued*)

SITE OF FRACTURE	SIGNS AND SYMPTOMS	TREATMENT	NURSING MANAGEMENT
Lower leg (fibula fracture usually occurs with tibial fracture)	Usually results from fall or trauma Pain and swelling Inability to bear weight Ecchymoses and possible deformity Bleeding and protrusion of bone fragments (in compound fractures)	Closed reduction with cast Open reduction with internal fixation	Assess signs and symptoms of compartment syndrome. Urge client to perform active and passive ROM exercises frequently. Assist client to use ambulatory aids.
Ankle	Severe pain Difficulty bearing weight Swelling Protruding bone fragments (severe fractures)	Cast or splint Open or closed reduction and internal fixation followed by casting	Administer pain medications as prescribed. Implement methods to reduce swelling. Assist client to use ambulatory aids. Assess for signs and symptoms of compartment syndrome.
Feet and toes (can occur alone or with other lower extremity fractures)	Pain, swelling, ecchymosis, and difficulty bearing weight Inability to wear shoe Protrusion of small bones (in crushing injuries)	Casting Open reduction with internal fixation Fusion (bones with multiple fractures) Supportive measures: analgesics, cold applications, elevation of foot, and loose-fitting shoes	Assess neurovascular status frequently. Provide cast care as needed. Assist client to use ambulatory aids. Instruct client in safety measures to prevent additional injuries (using nightlights, avoiding narrowed pathways, removing throw rugs, clearing stairways).

ROM, range of motion.

Nutrition Notes

The Client Receiving Orthopedic Treatment

- Protein requirements increase during prolonged immobility to correct negative nitrogen balance, promote healing, and help prevent skin breakdown and infections. A protein intake of 1.2 g/kg body weight is recommended; the client needs adequate calories to spare protein.
- A high-fiber intake helps prevent constipation.

ORTHOPEDIC SURGERY

Orthopedic surgery is performed for various reasons: to correct a deformity, remove a primary bone tumor, align fractured bones (open reduction), repair or replace a joint, insert a bone graft to promote bone healing, or stabilize a bone internally (using rods, pins, screws, nails, or wires).

Open Reduction Internal Fixation

If surgery for a fracture cannot be performed right away, Buck traction or other skin traction may be applied to relieve muscle spasm and pain until surgery is performed. Open reduction internal fixation (ORIF), accomplished with wire, nails, plate, and/or an intramedullary rod (a rod inserted into the center of the bone with wires around the bone for stabilization), is done to hold bone fragments in place until bone healing is complete.

Surgical Procedures to Correct Joint Dysfunction

Several surgical techniques, described in Box 61-4, may be done to minimize or correct joint dysfunction. Clients with arthritis, trauma, hip fracture, or a congenital deformity may have an **arthroplasty** or reconstruction of the joint. This procedure uses an artificial joint that restores previously lost function and relieves pain. Reconstructive joint surgery is performed when mobility and quality of life are compromised. The two joints most frequently replaced are the knee and hip. Other joints that may be replaced are the shoulder, ankle, wrist, and finger joints.

BOX 61-4 Surgical Procedures to Correct Joint Deformity

- *Arthrodesis*: fusion of a joint (most often the wrist or knee) for stabilization and pain relief
- *Arthroplasty*: total reconstruction or replacement of a joint (most often the knee or hip) with an artificial joint to restore function and relieve pain
- *Hemiarthroplasty*: the replacement of one of the articular surfaces in a joint, such as the femoral head but not the acetabulum
- *Total arthroplasty*: the replacement of both articular surfaces within one joint
- *Osteotomy*: cutting and removal of a wedge of bone (most often the tibia or femur) to change the bone's alignment, thereby improving function and relieving pain

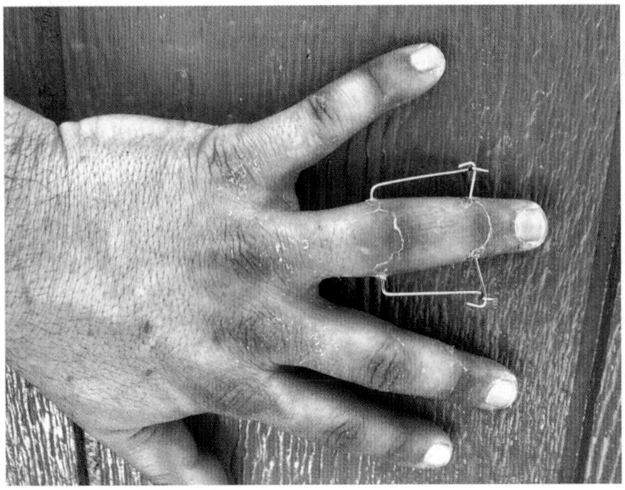

Figure 61-8 Open reduction external fixation of fourth digit. (Courtesy of L. Moreno.)

The materials used in an artificial joint (**prosthesis**) are metal and high-density polyethylene (Fig. 61-8), although Silastic is used for finger prostheses. Special bone cement or a specialized coating on the prosthesis pieces, which promotes bone growth on the implant, holds the prosthesis parts in place. There are problems with the prosthesis loosening owing to failure of the cement; so in many instances, porous-coated cementless joint components are used. These allow the bone to grow into the prosthesis and thus securely fix the joint replacement in place. Clients having this type of prosthesis must have adequate blood supply in healthy bone.

Postoperative complications include hemorrhage; **subluxation** or dislocation of the artificial joint; infection; thromboembolism; and **avascular necrosis**, or death of bone tissue owing to diminished or absent blood supply. A cemented prosthesis may loosen many years later.

Depending on the type of joint replacement, clients may be asked to donate their own blood preoperatively for use postoperatively if a transfusion is required. Anticoagulant therapy and early ambulation are very important for clients who have knee or hip replacement. These clients often use a continuous passive motion (CPM) machine after surgery. This machine promotes healing and flexibility in the knee and hip joint and increases circulation to the operative area. The primary provider orders the amount of extension and flexion produced by the machine as well as the frequency of use. Clients with knee replacements have the amount of flexion and the frequency of use increased daily while hospitalized. The goal is for the client to have the ability to bend the knee 90 degrees by discharge. The amount of flexion for clients with hip replacements should never exceed 30 degrees in a CPM machine.

Minimally invasive joint replacement surgeries (MIS) are increasingly replacing conventional joint replacement surgeries. The differences involve the following:

- Much smaller incision(s), often one-fourth to one-half the size of conventional arthroplasties (e.g., two small incisions for a hip replacement)
- Clients are generally younger, thinner, healthier, and motivated to participate in a more rapid recovery.
- No cement, only porous-surfaced prostheses
- No surgical cutting of muscle or tendon; surgeons work around these structures by splitting and dividing muscles whenever possible; thus there is less tissue trauma
- Resurfacing, a technique in which only the worn surfaces of the joint are replaced or covered; this technique is used more in younger, active clients who do not have any deformities.
- Computer-assisted surgery for some joint replacements, which involves computer-guided imagery that assists orthopedic surgeons to better align the prosthesis and promotes better long-term effectiveness
- Procedures take longer time, requiring longer periods of time that a client is having anesthesia, thus increasing anesthesia-related risks
- Shorter hospital stay and faster recovery/rehabilitation from minimally invasive joint replacement

Recovery and rehabilitation for clients having minimally invasive arthroplastic surgeries are generally easier and less lengthy. Some of the precautions needed for conventional knee and hip replacements may not be needed with these less invasive procedures.

Dislocation of total hips has been a complication. MIS has aided in reducing this issue. In addition, surgeons are using larger femoral head implants, because they are more stable and more difficult to dislocate (Blom et al., 2020). They are also using different methods and types of acetabular polyethylene liners, which decrease the wear on the femoral head.

Nursing Management

Preoperative Care

Before surgery, the nurse obtains a complete medical, drug, and allergy history from the client or a family member. The nurse also assesses the client's physical condition and mental status at the time of the initial interview. Review of the client's chart includes noting the diagnosis, type of surgery to be performed, and any previous treatments, such as traction or drug use. If the client's disorder was treated previously, the nurse needs to determine whether any complications or problems occurred because of or during treatment.

Client goals in the preoperative period focus on helping the client to experience reduced pain; continue to be active, mobile, and injury free; practice measures to reduce the potential for postoperative wound infection; control anxiety at manageable levels; understand instructions; and comprehend the procedures and rationale of postoperative management (Nursing Guidelines 61-4).

Postoperative Care

Ideally, postoperative nursing management begins before surgery with demonstrations of deep-breathing and coughing exercises and descriptions and demonstrations of the incentive spirometer (if that is likely to be used after surgery). Even if the client will have postoperative physical therapy,

NURSING GUIDELINES 61-4

Ensuring Complete Care for Clients Before Orthopedic Surgery

- Review the operation and the reason for it.
- Administer prescribed analgesics.
- Relieve the client's discomfort through positioning and joint immobilization.
- Support painful joints and be gentle when moving the client.
- Allow ample time for physical activities because the client with a musculoskeletal disorder needs more time to carry out preoperative routines. Allow the client to use any ambulatory aid that was brought from home.
- Demonstrate use of the overbed trapeze and encourage its use.
- Demonstrate and have the client perform necessary postoperative activities, such as coughing and deep-breathing exercises.
- Provide preoperative skincare as indicated by agency policy and procedure. If the client has initiated skin preparation at home, check to be sure the procedures were performed.
- Obtain adequate help when transferring a sedated client who is not in traction from the bed to the surgical stretcher. However, keep a client who is in traction in the hospital bed. Then, without lifting or removing the traction weights, transport the bed to the operating room.
- Administer the intravenous (IV) prophylactic antibiotic if ordered before surgery. (Although laminar airflow in the operating suite has reduced the incidence of postoperative infection, a great risk for infection remains for every client having orthopedic surgery. The number of personnel in the operating room may need to be limited to reduce a potential reservoir of infecting microorganisms.)

the nurse explains and helps the client practice active and isometric leg exercises. They also describe other devices that may be used after surgery, such as IV infusions of fluid and blood, oxygen, a wound drain, elastic stockings, or roller bandages. It also is necessary to include a discussion of the possible use of traction or the CPM machine.

If a client is scheduled for joint replacement or other surgery, the nurse withholds aspirin before surgery to reduce the risk for excessive bleeding. It is essential to monitor the complete blood count, prothrombin time, and bleeding and clotting times to ensure that the client's ability to control bleeding is not compromised. If the client will use a CPM machine after surgery, it is useful for the client to be fitted for this before surgery.

When the client returns from surgery, the nurse reviews the primary provider's orders concerning movement, turning, or positioning of the extremities. Usually, the head of the bed remains at 45 degrees or less. The client with a total hip replacement needs to have legs abducted with pillows or abductor cushion and extended because the opposite positions of adduction and flexion beyond 90 degrees can dislocate the prosthetic femoral head from the acetabulum. Clients with a total hip replacement need to sit in an elevated chair or on a seat raised by pillows so the flexion remains less than 90 degrees. Ice packs help reduce pain and inflammation to the incisional site (particularly after knee surgery). Box 61-5 provides information about avoiding hip dislocation after total hip replacement.

If CPM devices are prescribed to promote gentle flexion and extension of the knee after knee replacement, the nurse or physical therapist increases the flexion as indicated up to the goal of 90 degrees. If CPM devices are used after hip surgery, the flexion should not exceed 30 degrees.

Preventing postoperative complications after joint replacement is an important role of the nurse. Table 61-2 presents strategies to prevent postoperative complications after joint replacement surgery. Nursing Care Plan 61-1 provides more information related to nursing management of a client who requires surgery. See Client and Family Teaching 61-1 for discharge instructions for orthopedic surgery.

BOX 61-5 Avoiding Hip Dislocation After Conventional Replacement Surgery

Until the hip prosthesis stabilizes after hip replacement surgery, the client needs to learn about proper positioning so the prosthesis remains in place. Dislocation of the hip is a serious complication of surgery that causes pain and necessitates reoperation to correct the dislocation. Desirable positions include abduction, neutral rotation, and flexion of less than 90 degrees. When the client is seated, the knees should be lower than the hip. Guidelines for avoiding displacement are as follows:

- Keep the knees apart at all times.
- Put a pillow between the legs when sleeping.
- Never cross the legs when seated.
- Avoid bending forward when seated in a chair.
- Avoid bending forward to pick up an object on the floor.
- Use a raised toilet seat.
- Do not flex the hip to put on clothing such as pants, stockings, socks, or shoes.

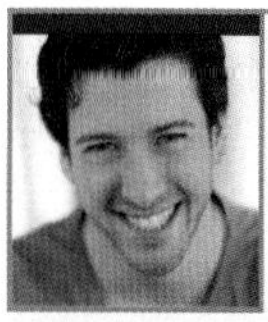

Clinical Scenario A 28-year-old man is in a motorcycle accident and sustains a fracture that requires surgery to reduce the fracture. External fixation is applied due to the nature of the fracture. What are the postoperative considerations for the nurse assigned to care for a client having orthopedic surgery? See the following Nursing Care Plan 61-1 section.

TABLE 61-2 Preventing Postoperative Complications After Joint Replacement Surgery

POTENTIAL COMPLICATION	POTENTIAL RISK FACTORS	PREVENTION STRATEGIES
Dislocation of prosthesis	Positioning beyond recommended flexion or extension Malfunction of prosthesis	Position client as prescribed. Instruct client to maintain appropriate position. Use pillows, splints, immobilizers, or slings to maintain prescribed position. Report increased pain, swelling, or change in mobility.
Infection	Older, debilitated clients Malnourishment Other infections such as urinary tract infections or dental abscesses Incision, wound drains, catheters, or IVs Hematoma	Monitor vital signs. Assess wound appearance and drainage. Practice aseptic technique when changing dressings and emptying drainage devices. Administer prophylactic antibiotics as prescribed. Teach client that for at least 3 months after surgery, there is a potential for infection; they may require prophylactic antibiotics for dental cleaning or other invasive procedures. Report increased pain, elevated temperature, redness, swelling, or change in drainage from the incision.
Neurovascular compromise	Trauma Edema Immobilization devices	Assess neurovascular status frequently, including color, temperature, capillary refill, pulses, edema, pain, mobility, and sensation. Report client complaints of deep, unrelenting pain; feelings of tightness; numbness; and decreased mobility. Elevate extremity. Release constricting dressings, wraps, casts, or immobilizers.
Deep vein thrombosis	Surgical procedure Immobility	Apply elastic stockings/wraps as prescribed. Assess peripheral pulses. Increase activity as indicated. Change position frequently as allowed. Encourage client to perform passive ROM exercises. Prevent pressure on popliteal vessels.

IV, intravenous; ROM, range of motion.

NURSING CARE PLAN 61-1 The Client Undergoing Orthopedic Surgery

Assessment

- When the client returns from surgery, review orders in the medical record regarding immobilization, movement or turning, and positioning of the arm or leg. Inspect the dressing over the incision. If a wound drain is present, assess the patency of the drain and the type and amount of drainage in the collection receptacle. Assess the neurovascular status of the affected extremity. Monitor vital signs frequently until they stabilize and routinely thereafter. Maintain the infusing IV fluids as ordered. Assess respiratory status. Encourage the client to identify pain levels and the effectiveness of analgesics.
- Within the first 24 to 72 hours after orthopedic surgery, a complication such as a fat embolus may occur (see Table 62-1). The symptoms are similar to those of a pulmonary embolus. In addition, petechial hemorrhages may appear on the skin of the chest. Report severe chest pain or unrelieved incisional pain to the primary provider immediately.

Nursing Diagnosis. **Altered Breathing Pattern** related to mucus and inability to mobilize secretions from the airway

Expected Outcome. Client will demonstrate effective respiratory rate and depth with clear breath sounds.

Interventions	Rationales
Instruct client to deep breathe and cough every 2 hours until they can ambulate.	*These measures expand the lungs and mobilize mucus, preventing pooling of secretions.*
Encourage client to use an incentive spirometer to increase deep breathing. Evaluate client's efforts.	*Increasing respiratory effort improves client's respiratory status.*
Turn client at least every 2 hours and encourage activity within prescribed limits.	*Movement facilitates lung expansion and prevents pooling of secretions.*
Auscultate lung sounds every 4 hours.	*Immobility can cause hypoventilation, predisposing a client to atelectasis, pooling of respiratory secretions, and pneumonia.*

NURSING CARE PLAN 61-1 The Client Undergoing Orthopedic Surgery (*continued*)

Evaluation of Expected Outcomes

Client effectively deep breathes and coughs. Lung sounds are clear.

Nursing Diagnosis. **Acute Pain** related to surgery

Expected Outcome. Client will report relief of pain.

Interventions	Rationales
Gently move client or adjust position.	*Gentle handling minimizes discomfort.*
Administer analgesics as prescribed. Instruct client in the use of client-controlled analgesia if prescribed.	*Regular administration of analgesics controls and prevents escalation of pain.*
Elevate affected extremity and use cold applications.	*These measures reduce swelling.*
Report client's complaints of severe or sudden and unrelenting pain.	*These findings may indicate a complication of surgery* (see Table 62-1).

Evaluation of Expected Outcome

Client reports pain relief with analgesics and positioning.

Nursing Diagnosis. **Risk for Disuse Syndrome** related to immobility imposed by orthopedic treatments such as casting, traction, internal or external fixation, and/or non–weight-bearing status

Expected Outcome. Client will maintain full ROM of unaffected joints, intact skin, good peripheral blood flow, and normal bowel and bladder function.

Interventions	Rationales
Encourage client to do ROM exercises as indicated.	*ROM exercises help maintain muscle strength and tone and prevent contractions.*
Position client so joints are in anatomic alignment.	*Proper positioning prevents joint deformities and damage to peripheral nerves and blood vessels.*
Get client up as soon as indicated, either in chair, ambulating, or on tilt table.	*Early mobilization prevents complications related to prolonged bed rest.*
When getting client up after bed rest, do so slowly, monitoring for signs of postural hypotension, tachycardia, nausea, diaphoresis, or syncope.	*When sitting or standing after even 3–4 days of bed rest, a client can experience postural hypotension.*
Turn client every 2 hours; inspect skin for signs of pressure.	*Frequent turning relieves pressure and identifies problems, allowing for early intervention.*
Apply antiembolism stockings as indicated.	*They help prevent deep vein thrombosis (DVT).*
Monitor peripheral circulation, particularly noting skin color, pulses, or any swelling.	*Prolonged bed rest, orthopedic surgery, and venous stasis can cause DVT and pulmonary embolism. Capillary refill should be brisk (within 3 seconds); skin should be warm and normally colored; and the client should be able to move the extremity. Diminished or absent pulses, pale or mottled skin, cool or cold skin, or increased pain (especially with movement) can indicate arterial obstruction. Changes in sensation such as numbness, tingling, or prickling may indicate nerve compression and damage, compartment syndrome, or both.*

(*continued*)

NURSING CARE PLAN 61-1 The Client Undergoing Orthopedic Surgery (*continued*)

Monitor bowel function daily. Provide increased fluids and fiber.	*Immobilization causes constipation secondary to inactivity and inappropriate food intake. Decreased fluid intake contributes to constipation.*
Encourage client to increase fluid intake to 2000 mL/day unless contraindicated.	*Increased intake promotes normal bladder function and prevents constipation, kidney stones, and other related complications of prolonged bed rest.*

Evaluation of Expected Outcomes

- Client can maintain full ROM of unaffected joints.
- Skin remains intact without signs of pressure or breakdown.
- Peripheral circulation is adequate to sustain tissue perfusion.
- Client has adequate urine output and regular bowel movements.

Nursing Diagnosis. **Infection Risk** related to compromised skin integrity

Expected Outcome. Client will remain free of infection.

Interventions	Rationales
Inspect pins or wire sites used in traction or external fixation devices and the surgical incision and/or beneath a cast window for signs of infection.	*Regular inspection promotes early detection of and prompt intervention for infection.*
Practice standard precautions and conscientious handwashing.	*These measures prevent infection.*
Use aseptic principles when changing dressings and performing pin care.	*Asepsis prevents the introduction of microorganisms into wounds and incisions.*
Keep wound drainage system below the level of the incision.	*Doing so prevents backflow of drainage into the incision.*
Administer prescribed antibiotics.	*They reduce microorganisms and control infection.*
Report purulent wound drainage, elevated temperature, chills, and increased white blood count.	*These are signs of infection that require intervention.*

Evaluation of Expected Outcome

Client is free of infection as evidenced by normal temperature, clean incisions and pin sites, and no purulent drainage.

Nursing Diagnosis. **ADL Deficit** related to musculoskeletal impairment

Expected Outcome. Client will gradually perform ADLs as independently as possible.

Interventions	Rationales
Collaborate with client to determine tasks that they may perform independently.	*Doing so promotes independence and provides client with a sense of control.*
Plan activities and rest.	*Doing so conserves energy and prevents fatigue.*
Consult with physical therapist (PT) and occupational therapist (OT) about client's needs related to ADLs.	*PT and OT will determine adaptive equipment needed as well as client's strengths and abilities to master self-care tasks.*
Provide pain medication 45 minutes before activity.	*Pain relief promotes participation in self-care.*

Evaluation of Expected Outcome

Client can partially bathe and feed themself, dress upper body, and use the bedside commode.

Client and Family Teaching 61-1
Home Care After Limb Amputation

If the client has to bandage the stump at home, the nurse teaches both the client and the family how to apply the bandage and how to care for the stump and provides other general instructions:

- Wash the bandages, rinse them well, and lay them flat to dry because hanging tends to decrease the elasticity.
- When the bandages are dry, they must be rolled without stretching.
- Follow the primary provider's recommendations regarding caring for the stump, applying a stump dressing, washing the stump, and elevating the stump when sitting.
- Do not apply nonprescription drugs (ointments, creams, topical pain relievers) to the stump unless the primary provider has approved the use of a specific product.
- Adhere to the plan of scheduled exercises and complete each group of exercises as outlined by the PT.
- Do not exceed the primary provider's recommendations regarding weight bearing and joint flexion.
- Eat well-balanced and nutritious meals or follow the diet recommended by the primary provider. Avoid gaining excess weight during the recovery period because weight gain may interfere with use of a leg prosthesis.
- Expect that phantom limb sensation, if present, may persist for some time, which is normal.
- Avoid injury to the stump, even though it appears to be healed. Report any skin impairment immediately.
- Continue deep-breathing exercises until fully mobile.
- Contact the primary provider if fever, chills, productive cough, bleeding or oozing from the stump, purulent drainage from the incision, new or different pain in the stump, or any change in the appearance of the stump occurs.

Amputation

Amputation is the removal of a limb. It may occur as a result of trauma (traumatic amputation) or in an effort to control disease or disability (therapeutic amputation).

Etiology

The following are conditions for which an amputation may be performed:

- Malignant tumors
- Long-standing infections of bone and tissue that prohibit restoration of function
- Extensive trauma to an extremity
- Death of tissues from peripheral vascular insufficiency or peripheral vasospastic diseases such as Buerger and Raynaud diseases
- Thermal injuries
- Deformity of a limb, rendering it a useless hindrance
- Life-threatening disorders, such as arterial thrombosis and gas bacillus infections

Medical and Surgical Management

Unless emergency surgery is performed, the client is treated for any disorder that may influence healing (e.g., uncontrolled diabetes mellitus, dehydration, infection, electrolyte imbalances, poor nutrition, chronic respiratory disorders). When it is decided that amputation must be performed as a lifesaving measure, the following factors help the surgical team decide at which level to amputate the arm or leg (e.g., above or below the knee, above or below the elbow):

- Amount of tissue that must be removed to eliminate the disorder
- Level at which the blood supply is adequate to preserve circulation to tissue that will remain
- Number of joints that can be preserved
- Length of residual limb that will promote fitting a prosthesis, an artificial limb, for rehabilitation

The levels of some commonly planned amputations include below the knee (BK), above the knee (AK), below the elbow (BE), and above the elbow (AE). The surgical objective is to create a gently tapering stump with muscular padding over the end. Occasionally, knee disarticulations (amputation through a joint), disarticulation at the ankle joint, and partial foot amputations are performed. Figure 61-9 demonstrates possible locations of amputations.

Amputation Methods

An amputation may be performed using an open or closed method. In an open amputation (guillotine amputation), the

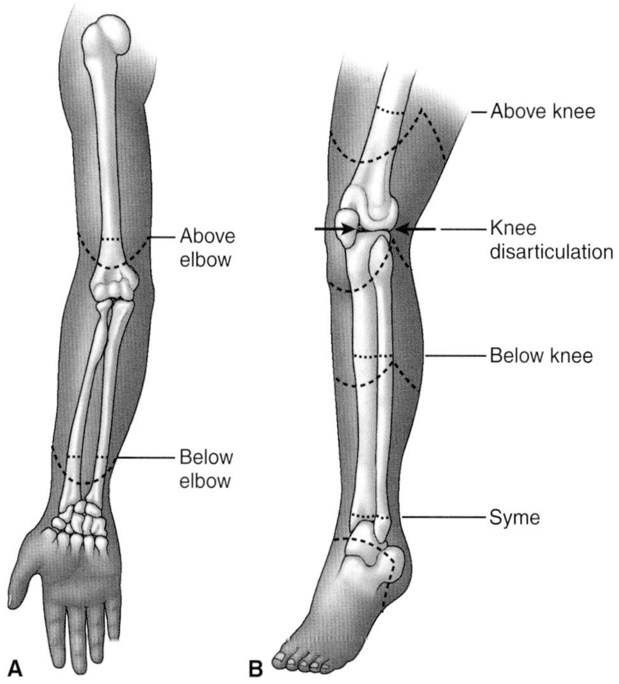

Figure 61-9 Levels of amputation are determined by circulatory adequacy, type of prosthesis, function of the part, and muscle balance. **(A)** Levels of amputation of upper limb. **(B)** Levels of amputation of lower limb. (Reprinted with permission from Hinkle, J. L., & Cheever, K. H. (2014). *Brunner & Suddarth's textbook of medical-surgical nursing* (13th ed.). Wolters Kluwer Health/Lippincott Williams & Wilkins.)

end of the residual limb (or stump) is temporarily open with no skin covering it. Open amputations usually are performed in cases of infection. Skin traction is applied, and the infected area is allowed to drain. The traction must be continuous. The surgeon may arrange the traction so the client can turn over in bed.

In the more common closed amputation (flap amputation), skin flaps cover the severed bone end. Clients with a closed amputation return from surgery with either a soft compression dressing or a rigid plaster shell covering the residual limb. The compression dressing consists of gauze over which elastic roller bandages are wrapped to create pressure to control bleeding. There may be a walking pylon, a type of temporary prosthesis composed of a metal post and molded foot, attached to the rigid plaster shell (Fig. 61-10). It may be weeks before the postoperative client is referred to a prosthetist, a professional who creates and fits artificial limbs.

A *staged amputation* is planned when a client has severe infection and gangrene. The guillotine method is first used, and then a few days later, after the infection is treated and the client is stable, a more definitive, closed amputation is done.

Arm Amputation

The arms have highly specialized functions. Consequently, the amputation of an arm, particularly the arm with the dominant hand, requires great physical and emotional adjustment during the preoperative as well as postoperative periods. Fortunately, most clients with arm amputations can be measured for a prosthesis shortly after the surgical scar heals.

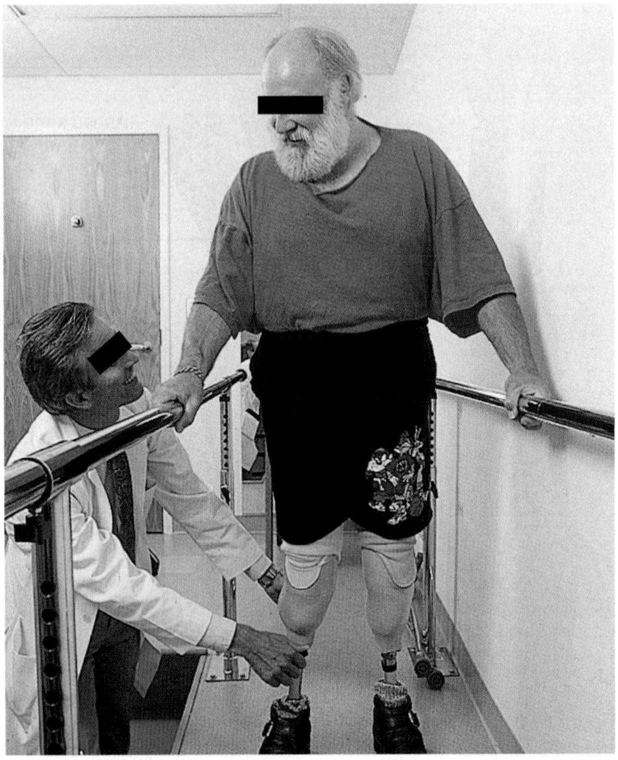

Figure 61-10 Many amputees receive prostheses soon after surgery and begin learning how to use them with the help and support of the rehabilitation team, which includes nurses, primary providers, physical therapists, and others.

Several types of prostheses are available for arm amputees: a shoulder harness with cables that attach to a mechanical terminal device, referred to as a *hook*; a semifunctioning cosmetic hand that can be substituted for the hook; and a myoelectric arm.

The hook performs the functions of the hand and fingers when the amputee moves the scapula and expands the chest, activating the cables attached from a shoulder harness to the mechanical device. The mechanical terminal device is strong, sturdy, and functional. The cosmetic hand, which can be attached to the same cables as the hook, has the appearance of a natural hand, but it lacks the capacity for performing fine motor skills. The myoelectric arm has a realistic-looking hand that is activated by electrical impulses from muscles in the upper arm. The electrical activity is relayed from electrodes in the shell of the prosthesis to microcircuits in the prosthetic fingers. The myoelectric arm has three advantages: It eliminates the need to wear a harness, the terminal device looks natural, and it has somewhat better function than the cosmetic hand. Despite its advantages, the myoelectric arm is not rugged enough to do the work of the mechanical terminal device. New advances are in various stages of development for prosthetic hands that are controlled by the brain through electrodes attached to two of the primary nerves in the arm. Robotic devices have an electronic motor and sensors that respond to brain signals to move a hand. These are in trial with postwar amputee victims.

Leg Amputation

Amputation of a leg is a more common operation than amputation of an arm. The above-the-knee amputation (AKA) is more disabling than a below-the-knee amputation (BKA); therefore, unless evidence suggests that the knee cannot be saved, every attempt is made to amputate BK.

The trend is to have a temporary prosthesis attached to the plaster shell covering the residual lower limb immediately after surgery. It reduces psychological trauma for the client because it promotes a more intact sense of body image after surgery. Also, the walking pylon facilitates early ambulation. Almost immediately, the client is allowed to stand and place a limited amount of weight on the residual limb. As the stump heals and edema disappears, a second cast may be reapplied or a temporary socket made of lightweight polypropylene may be constructed. Ultimately, a conventional prosthesis is custom-made to conform to the stump as well as to the client's needs. Leg prostheses may be held in place by means of a pelvic belt or suction. As with arm amputees, research and development for advanced prostheses are being conducted and advanced.

Complications

Hematoma, hemorrhage, and infection are potential complications in the immediate postoperative period. Potential complications late in the postoperative course include chronic osteomyelitis (after persistent infection) and, rarely, a burning pain (causalgia), the cause of which is unknown. Pain may result from a stump neuroma, which is formed when the cut ends of nerves become entangled in the healing scar. A neuroma is treated with injections of procaine, a local anesthetic, or reamputation.

Phantom Limb and Phantom Pain

The surgeon informs the client of the potential phenomenon of phantom limb sensation, which is a feeling that the amputated portion of the limb still remains. It is a normal, frequently occurring physiologic response after amputation. Phantom sensations can persist for months or decades or can come and go. Although clients are aware of phantom sensations, they usually learn to ignore them.

Phantom pain is pain or other discomfort, such as burning, tingling, throbbing, or itching, in the missing limb. Pain felt from the phantom limb can be an extremely serious problem in relation to the client's emotional status and ability to use a prosthesis. Severe, prolonged phantom limb pain may require surgical removal of nerve endings at the end of the stump.

Pharmacologic Considerations

- Drugs to disrupt nerve impulses may help relief phantom pain. Antidepressants (tricyclics), antileptics (gabapentin, pregabalin), and N-methyl-D-aspartates (NMDAs, i.e., ketamine, dextromethorphan) are tried when transcutaneous electrical nerve stimulation (TENS) units do not work and before more invasive procedures.

Rehabilitation

The success of the amputee's rehabilitation depends on variables such as age, type of amputation, condition of the stump, physical status, condition of the remaining limb, concurrent debilitating illness, visual–motor coordination, motivation, acceptance, and cooperation. Clients vary greatly in their learning capacity and ability to master the use of a prosthesis. The period allotted for training also varies with each client. It is vital that the primary provider, the nurse, the physical and occupational therapists, the family, and the client maintain realistic expectations throughout the rehabilitation period.

Presurgical Nursing Management

Nursing management of an amputee can be segmented into two key functions: those before surgery and those after surgery. In general, presurgical nursing management involves considerations for any surgery, specifically taking a complete medical, drug, and allergy history and evaluating the client for mental and emotional acceptance of the surgical procedure.

Assessing motor strength and flexibility of other joints is important to determine potential problems involving rehabilitation. If the client is acutely ill, such as with a gangrenous limb and related fever, disorientation, and electrolyte imbalances, the nurse monitors circulation in the limb for changes, such as severe pain, color changes, and lack of peripheral pulses. It is crucial that the nurse informs the primary provider of problems as they occur because surgery may become an emergency.

Nursing interventions aim to reduce pain and anxiety and support the client as they begin to grieve the loss of the limb and adapt to potential changes. The nurse administers narcotic analgesics before surgery to clients with severe pain. Other comfort measures include handling the painful limb gently; elevating a swollen limb; encouraging family presence and support; being available, especially at times when the client is alone; helping the client to express concerns; and clarifying misperceptions.

Before surgery, the nurse explains all the routine preoperative preparations and reinforces what the primary provider has discussed with the client and family regarding the extent of physical disability; the psychological, aesthetic, social, and vocational implications; and the realistic possibilities for prosthetic restoration. The nurse must exercise care in answering questions about prosthetic devices and their use because it always is possible that the amputation may need to involve more of the limb than originally anticipated. In addition, the nurse reviews the postoperative management, such as deep-breathing, coughing, positioning, and routine exercises, and encourages the client to practice the exercises if time and the client's condition permit.

Clients vary in their reactions to the impending loss of a limb. The amount of grief is thought to be proportional to the symbolic significance of the part and the resultant degree of disability and deformity. Anger and depression are common emotions. The nurse acknowledges the client's feelings and remains objective and nonjudgmental as the client expresses negative emotional responses. Reassuring the client that their reaction is normal may provide comfort. The nurse should not shame, criticize, or trivialize the client's behavior.

How well the client can cope usually depends on prior experience and how they have dealt with previous losses. The nurse protects the client from additional sources of stress. While the client is preoccupied with the potential loss, the nurse should not make unnecessary demands or expect full participation in the plan of care. The nurse provides assistance with activities that, at any other time, the client could carry out independently. The nurse also promotes adequate sleep and discusses coping techniques that have been used successfully in the past and encourages their repetition. Fostering communication with family members or friends promotes support. See Evidence-Based Practice 61-1.

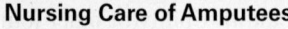

Evidence-Based Practice 61-1

Nursing Care of Amputees

Clinical Question

What support is needed for clients after amputation occurs?

Evidence

When a client loses a limb because of a needed amputation, acceptance, support, and cooperation are needed for a positive transition. The relationship between self-reported mobility and both quality of life and satisfaction was reviewed with clients with lower limb amputation. A study by Wurdeman et al. (2018) did a retrospective chart review of over 500 clients who had completed a mobility and prothesis evaluation questionnaire. The client's self-reported quality of life improved with the increase in mobility and the use of prosthetics. Rehabilitation helps improve functional mobility, thus improving the client's reported quality of life. The theme throughout the interviews was that prosthetics after amputation made clients feel confident, feel cared for, and to be able to return to some of their previous activities. Clients without prosthetics had feelings of frustration and anger and were unable to participate in daily activities the same. The study concluded that more research was needed from the nursing perspective of what knowledge was needed by nurses to support clients of amputations and technology (Wurdeman et al., 2018).

Nursing Implications

Nurses who work with clients with amputations must understand their experience to be able to support their care, referrals, and follow-up care. When clients have technology and devices to assist them, this enables them to adapt back into their communities. Nurses should gain knowledge in what is important to the client and their needs to adapt to their life and community after this life-changing event.

Reference

Wurdeman, S. R., Stevens, P. M., & Campbell, J. H. (2018). Mobility Analysis of AmpuTees (MAAT I): Quality of life and satisfaction are strongly related to mobility for clients with a lower limb prosthesis. *Prosthetics and Orthotics International, 42*(5), 498–503. https://doi.org/10.1177/0309364617736089

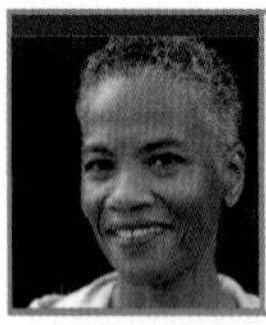

Clinical Scenario A 70-year-old woman has a long history of type 1 diabetes mellitus. The client is scheduled for a right BKA related to peripheral neuropathy. The client previously has had toes amputated on the same limb. **What are the important foci of nursing care for this client postoperatively? See the following Nursing Process for the Client After a Limb Amputation section.**

NURSING PROCESS FOR THE CLIENT AFTER A LIMB AMPUTATION

Assessment

Monitor vital signs to determine any changes, particularly elevations in temperature (indicating possible infection), pulse, and blood pressure. Reviewing the client's medical record provides information about the reason for and type and level of the amputation. Inspect the dressing or plaster shell, and, when changing the dressing, assess the wound for signs of infection, excessive drainage, or separation of wound edges. In addition, evaluate the client's general condition as well as level of pain and discomfort, and implement measures to relieve it.

Diagnosis, Planning, and Interventions

Nursing management involves all concerns addressed after any orthopedic surgery (see Nursing Care Plan 61-1). Implement measures to prevent infection, promote healing, and avoid skin breakdown. See Nursing Guidelines 61-5 for stump care and bandaging. Care also includes, but is not limited to, the following:

Bathing/Hygiene and Toileting ADL Deficit: Related to impediments imposed by amputation

Expected Outcome: Client will participate in self-care and recuperative measures to the fullest extent possible.

- Encourage the client with a leg amputation to assume some of their own care 1 or 2 days after surgery. *Incorporating the client's abilities increases self-care independence.*
- Exercise and position the client in proper alignment. *Correct positioning prevents contractures after amputation, maintains skeletal alignment, and promotes active movement of the uninvolved limbs.*
- Work with the PT to implement a program of active and isometric exercises. *These exercises increase the client's abilities and strengths.*

Risk for Disuse Syndrome: Related to altered mobility after amputation

Expected Outcomes: (1) Client will become progressively mobile and independent. (2) Client will maintain intact skin, adequate tissue perfusion, and normal pulmonary function. (3) Client will not develop complications related to immobility.

NURSING PROCESS FOR THE CLIENT AFTER A LIMB AMPUTATION (continued)

- Place client with leg amputation in the prone position several times a day. *This position promotes stump extension and prevents contractures.*
- Position client so they are in normal anatomic alignment at all times. *Improper positioning may injure peripheral nerves and blood vessels and cause joint deformities.*
- Use a trochanter roll to prevent external rotation of the hip and knee. Avoid placing pillows between the legs. *These measures prevent abduction deformity.*
- Advise the client who is lying on the stomach to adduct the stump so it presses against the other leg. *Adduction stretches flexor muscles and prevents abduction deformity.*
- On the first or second postoperative day, assist client to stand to regain a sense of balance. Stepping on the floor with the temporary prosthesis and weight bearing of about 10% of body weight usually is permitted at this time. *These measures promote strength and balance while preventing injury.*
- Expect the client with a temporary prosthesis to progress to walking with crutches or a walker or in parallel bars 2 to 4 days after the amputation with a high degree of safety (full weight bearing on the unaffected leg). *This measure promotes independence.*
- Provide client with assistive devices. *They help client to be more independent and maintain more mobility.*
- Use antiembolism stocking on unaffected limb. *They prevent DVT.*
- Monitor pulmonary status and implement deep-breathing and coughing exercises. *Decreased mobility can result in hypoventilation and may lead to atelectasis and pooling of secretions. Pulmonary exercises improve lung expansion and mobilize secretions.*
- Increase fluid intake to 2000 mL (if permitted). *This intake promotes urine output and prevents constipation.*

Grief: Related to loss of body part
Expected Outcome: Client will state that they are beginning to resolve loss and develop strategies for coping without an arm or leg.

- Listen actively and empathetically. *Doing so facilitates communication.*
- Allow client time to talk about their loss and express feelings of grief, anger, depression, and anxiety. *Grief is hard work and needs time.*
- Discuss each new challenge as it arises. *Providing information and listening to client's feelings assists the client to face new issues.*
- Allow client time to process information. *Providing time allows the client to adjust to new situations.*
- Implement changes gradually. *Doing so gives client time to adjust and adapt.*
- Reinforce progress that has been made. *Doing so provides encouragement and support.*
- Remain available to the client for physical and emotional support. *The nurse can serve as a consistent support system.*
- Foster family involvement because their encouragement often helps motivate a client to face each new problem, accept failure, and develop a determination to overcome obstacles. *Support from significant others can have a positive effect.*
- Ambulate the client with a leg amputation as soon as possible. *Doing so dispels the doubt that permanent disability will prevail.*
- Explore the possibility of a meeting with a rehabilitated amputee. *Someone who has endured a similar experience can serve as a support network.*

Altered Body Image Perception: Related to loss of body part and function
Expected Outcome: Client will progressively adjust to the change in body image.

- Keep in mind that the attitude of staff and family members bears greatly on how clients perceive themselves. *A positive approach promotes a client's positive self-image.*
- Do not treat the client as less than competent. *Focusing on client's strengths and abilities promotes enhanced self-image.*
- Avoid nonverbal implications that the client, the stump, or the prosthesis is repulsive. *Being aware of nonverbal behavior indicates how the client feels about themself.*
- Make a point to visit the client frequently, especially when no particular nursing activity must be performed. *Such visits encourage client to feel more positively about themself.*
- Make eye contact during verbal interactions. *The nurse must treat all clients with the same respect.*
- Sit close to the client's bedside and lean forward when talking. *Doing so communicates a personal interest in the client.*
- Offer praise when the client successfully accomplishes a task. *Praise builds self-esteem and self-confidence.*
- If appropriate, explore the client's reasons for refusing to use a prosthesis. *If the problem is amenable to change, the nurse can enlist the help of the surgeon, PT, or prosthetist.*

Evaluation of Expected Outcomes

By discharge, the client reports reduced and manageable pain, no infection, and intact skin; they demonstrate optimal participation in self-care. The client experiences increasing mobility along with increasing resolution of grief, greater self-acceptance, and acceptance of current situation. They experience no postoperative complications. The client does not withdraw from social situations, has a positive attitude about the future, and can demonstrate adequate independent self-care.

Discharge teaching depends on many factors, including the length of hospitalization, the type and location of the amputation, the age and physical condition of the client, and the type of dressing or prosthesis the client wears. Factors related to the home environment influence the plan for rehabilitation after discharge. Some clients need to modify their living arrangements, use a wheelchair, or make other accommodations or changes. See Client and Family Teaching 61-2 for discharge instructions.

NURSING GUIDELINES 61-5

Stump Care and Bandaging

Stump Care

- Assess the covering over the stump frequently to determine the type and amount of drainage from the incision. Expect some oozing of blood, but if a gauze dressing is used, it may need to be reinforced.
- Keep a tourniquet in plain view at bedside, and if hemorrhage occurs, apply it and notify the primary provider.
- Generally, elevate the stump for the first 24 to 48 hours to prevent edema. In some cases, such as an AKA, a slight Trendelenburg position is preferred to elevating the stump on pillows because bending the hip promotes a flexion contracture. A bed board or a firm mattress provides skeletal support.
- If the client has a rigid plaster cast with walking pylon, loosen the harness, which suspends the cast from the waist, when the client is in bed. Slightly tighten the harness when the client is ambulatory.

Bandaging

Before a permanent prosthesis can be made, the stump must shrink and be shaped. This is done with elastic bandages that are wrapped about the stump. Unlike leg stumps, arm stumps do not need as massive a shrinkage over as long a period. Various bandaging techniques are appropriate, but several principles are observed:

- Remove and rewrap the bandage at least twice during the day and before the client retires for the night.
- Bandage joints in a way that promotes a neutral or extended position.
- Avoid circular turns, which act like a tourniquet and interfere with blood flow.

Client and Family Teaching 61-2

The nurse talks with the client, family, and other significant caregivers about the support system that will be available after discharge. It is important to explore the kinds of assistance the client needs for moving and walking, preparing meals, getting to the primary provider's office or physical therapy department, and performing other household tasks. The nurse tries to identify modifications that will be necessary in the home environment, such as relocating the bed to a ground floor level. In addition, they provide information about renting home care equipment, arranging for home delivery of meals through a community agency or church service group, or scheduling transportation with an agency that has a medical van or hydraulic lift available. The nurse may refer the client to a home health care agency or extended care facility. They provide printed discharge instructions for future reference and covers the following general points:

- Follow the directions of the primary provider. Do not resume any activity that has been restricted until told to do so.
- Perform exercises exactly as prescribed by the primary provider and PT.
- Use the recommended device (walker, cane, crutches) for walking.
- Wear supportive shoes when using crutches, walker, or cane.
- Eliminate safety hazards in the home, such as scatter rugs.
- Eat a nutritious diet and drink plenty of fluids.
- Take prescribed medications as directed; do not use or take any nonprescription drugs unless the primary provider has approved them.
- Notify the primary provider if the incision has unusual drainage or if fever, chills, sudden onset of pain, redness, or swelling occurs.

KEY POINTS

- Casts: rigid mold that immobilizes an injured structure. May be cylinder, body, hip spica, short arm, long arm, short leg, long leg, walking or shoulder spica
- Splints and braces: splints immobilize and support; braces support, control movement, and prevent additional injury
- Reducing fractures
  - Traction: pulling of structures of the musculoskeletal system
  - Closed reduction: bone restored to normal position by external manipulation
  - Open reduction: bone is surgically exposed and realigned
  - Internal fixation: bone is secured with metal screws, plates, rods, nails, or pins
  - External fixation: pins are placed into bones, and then an external compression device is applied
- Orthopedic surgery: can be done to correct deformity, remove bone tumor, align fractured bones, repair or replace a joint, insert a bone graft, or stabilize a bone internally
  - ORIF: combination of pins, plates, wires, or nails with an external device to maintain stabilization
  - Surgical procedures to correct joint dysfunction include arthrodesis, arthroplasty, hemiarthroplasty, total arthroplasty, and osteotomy
  - Amputation: removal of a limb

CRITICAL THINKING EXERCISES

1. A man had a total hip replacement 3 days ago and wants to use the toilet for a bowel movement. Explain how to assist this client.
2. A woman has just returned from the recovery unit after an AKA. Fresh blood has saturated the stump dressing. What actions should you take at this time?
3. A young man admitted with a fractured radius complains of increasing pain in his hand after a cast was applied despite having received a narcotic

analgesic 30 minutes ago. What assessments are important to make at this time?

4. A client asks the nurse why the cast on their fractured left tibia extends onto their foot and over their knee. What would you tell them?

NCLEX-STYLE REVIEW QUESTIONS PrepU

1. When preparing a client for application of a cast, what is important for the nurse to explain to the client?
    1. The client may experience itching while the cast is wet.
    2. The client's arm will feel warm as the wet plaster sets.
    3. The cast will feel tight as it is applied.
    4. There will be a foul odor until the cast is dry.
2. While backpacking with a youth group, a client sustains an injury to the lower leg. A nurse who is accompanying the group suspects a fracture of the tibia. To immobilize the suspected fracture, where is the best location to apply the splint?
    1. Above the ankle to BK
    2. AK to below the hip
    3. Below the ankle to AK
    4. BK to above the hip
3. The nurse is checking on a client with a fractured femur who is in skeletal traction. Which of the following actions is necessary to determine a client's neurovascular status? Select all that apply.
    1. Ask the client to wiggle their toes on the affected leg.
    2. Check client's skin on the affected limb to ensure it is intact.
    3. Compare the warmth of both lower extremities.
    4. Determine if the client is able to use the trapeze when moving.
    5. Palpate for a pulse on the affected limb.
4. The nurse is performing pin care on a client placed in skeletal traction the previous day. The pin sites are slightly reddened with a small amount of clear drainage. What is the best action for the nurse to take?
    1. Apply normal saline dressings to the pin sites.
    2. Cleanse the pin sites thoroughly and apply iodine ointment.
    3. Document the findings, including that pin care was administered.
    4. Report to the primary provider that the pin sites appear infected.
5. Postoperatively, before turning the client with the hip prosthesis onto the nonoperative side, what would the nurse do first?
    1. Elevate the head of client's bed.
    2. Flex client's knee on the affected side.
    3. Have client point toes downward.
    4. Place pillow between the client's legs.
6. What is the priority nursing action in the first 24 hours for a client who has an AKA?
    1. Apply a new dressing to the stump to shrink the stump.
    2. Cleanse the stump with soap and water to prevent infection.
    3. Elevate the affected limb to reduce edema.
    4. Encourage client to talk about the surgery to promote acceptance.

WANT TO KNOW MORE? There are a wide variety of online resources available on thePoint to enhance learning and understanding of this chapter.

Go to **thePoint.lww.com/activate,** and use the activation code found in the front of this text to unlock these online resources.

62

Caring for Clients With Traumatic Musculoskeletal Injuries

Words To Know

avascular necrosis
avulsion fracture
callus
carpal tunnel syndrome
compartment syndrome
contusion
dislocations
ecchymosis
epicondylitis
fasciotomy
fracture
ganglion cyst
meniscectomy
palsy
rotator cuff
sprains
strain
subluxation
tendinitis
Volkmann contracture

Learning Objectives

On completion of this chapter, you will be able to:

1. Differentiate strains, contusions, and sprains.
2. Define joint dislocations.
3. Discuss the nursing management of various types of sports or work-related injuries.
4. Identify the stages of bone healing after a fracture.
5. Describe the signs and symptoms of a fracture.
6. Explain the nursing management for clients with various types of fractures.
7. Discuss methods used to prevent complications associated with fractures.
8. Discuss potential complications associated with a fractured hip.

Injuries to the musculoskeletal system affect more than just a muscle or bone. A fractured bone or other injury can potentially cause dysfunction to the surrounding muscle and injury to the blood vessels and nerves. Treatment of musculoskeletal trauma involves immobilization of the injured area until it has healed. It also requires prevention of further injury and complications.

Gerontologic Considerations

- Older adults are more prone to skeletal fractures because bone resorption takes place more rapidly than bone formation (see Chapter 60).
- Hip fractures are a serious problem for older adults and most commonly result from falls in the home. Pain associated with hip fracture is severe and must be carefully managed with around-the-clock dosing of pain medication to minimize energy loss in response to pain. Complications from hip fracture in older adults often lead to death.

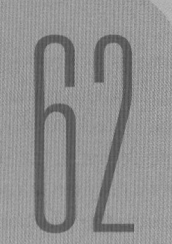

STRAINS, CONTUSIONS, AND SPRAINS

A **strain** is an injury to a muscle when it is stretched or pulled beyond its capacity. A **contusion** is a soft tissue injury resulting from a blow or blunt trauma. **Sprains** are injuries to the ligaments surrounding a joint.

Pathophysiology and Etiology

A strain results from excessive stress, overuse, or overstretching. Small blood vessels in the muscle may rupture, and the muscle fibers sustain tiny tears. There are three types of strains:

- *First degree*: mild stretching of muscle or tendon, causing some edema and muscle spasm, but no real loss of function; pain occurs with full range of motion (ROM)
- *Second degree*: partial tearing of muscle or tendon, leading to inability to bear weight, limited motion, and there is edema, muscle tenderness, muscle spasm, and **ecchymosis** (bruising)
- *Third degree*: severe muscle and/or tendon tearing, causing severe pain, muscle spasm, ecchymosis, edema, and loss of function

In contusions, injury is confined to the soft tissues and does not affect the musculoskeletal structure. Many small blood vessels rupture, causing ecchymosis or a hematoma (collection of blood). Applying cold packs helps to alleviate local pain, swelling, and bruising. A contusion usually resolves within 2 weeks.

Areas most subject to sprains are the wrist, elbow, knee, and ankle. A sprain of the cervical spine is commonly called a *whiplash injury*. Sprains result from sudden, unusual movement or stretching around a joint, which is common with falls or other accidental injuries. The force twists the joint in a direction it was not designed for or displaces it beyond its normal ROM by partially tearing or rupturing the attachment of ligaments. The damage usually is confined to the ligaments and adjacent soft tissue. Types of sprains are differentiated in the following:

- *First degree*: involves stretching of the ligament fibers, characterized by mild edema, tenderness, and pain if joint is moved
- *Second degree*: involves partial tearing of the ligament with edema, pain with motion, joint instability, and some loss of function
- *Third degree*: the ligament is torn or ruptured completely, with possible detachment of a fragment of bone (referred to as an **avulsion fracture**) and hematoma formation, which contributes to the severe pain, edema, and abnormal joint movement

Assessment Findings

The injured area becomes painful immediately, and swelling usually follows. The person typically avoids full weight bearing or using the injured joint or limb. Later, ecchymosis may appear. In cases of extensive ligamental tearing, the joint may be unstable until it heals.

In most cases, diagnosis is made by examination of the affected part and symptoms. X-rays may show a larger-than-usual joint space and rule out or confirm an accompanying fracture. A magnetic resonance imaging (MRI) test may be done to determine the extent of the injury. Arthrography demonstrates asymmetry in the joint as a result of the damaged ligaments, or arthroscopy may disclose trauma in the joint capsule.

Medical and Surgical Management

Treatment consists of applying ice or a chemical cold pack to the area to reduce swelling and relieve pain for the first 24 to 48 hours. Elevation of the part and compression with an elastic bandage may also be recommended. The acronym PRICE refers to **P**rotection (from further injury), **R**est, **I**ce, **C**ompression, and **E**levation—a method for remembering the treatment for strains, contusions, and sprains (de Moraes Prianti et al., 2018). Injured structures must be protected from further injury by immobilization. After 2 days, when swelling no longer is likely to increase, applying heat reduces pain and relieves local edema by improving circulation. Full use of the injured joint is discouraged temporarily. Nonsteroidal anti-inflammatory drugs (NSAIDs) ease discomfort.

Continued trauma during healing may result in a permanently unstable joint or the formation of fibrous adhesions that may limit full ROM. Occasionally, a removable splint or light cast is applied for several weeks. A soft cervical collar limits motion if the client has a neck sprain. When sufficient healing has occurred, progressively active exercises are prescribed.

››› *Stop, Think, and Respond 62-1*

You are at a playground when you notice a man who has been playing basketball with his son fall and grab his ankle. He says his ankle hurts very badly, and he does not think that he can walk. What action should you take?

DISLOCATIONS

Dislocations occur when the articular surfaces of a joint are no longer in contact. The shoulder, hip, and knee are commonly affected. A partial dislocation is referred to as a **subluxation**.

Pathophysiology and Etiology

In adults, trauma usually causes dislocations. Occasionally, diseases of the joint result in dislocations, when the ligaments supporting a joint are torn, stretched, or relaxed. Separation of adjacent bones from their articulating joint interferes with normal use and produces a distorted appearance. The injury may disrupt local blood supply to structures such as the joint cartilage, causing degeneration, chronic pain, and restricted movement. **Compartment syndrome** (a condition in which a structure such as a tendon or nerve is constricted in a confined space) may also develop. The syndrome affects nerve innervation, leading to subsequent **palsy** (decreased sensation and movement). If compartment syndrome occurs in an upper extremity, it may lead to **Volkmann contracture**, a clawlike deformity of the hand resulting from obstructed arterial blood flow to the forearm and hand. The client is unable to extend their fingers and complains of unrelenting pain, particularly if attempting to stretch the hand. There are also signs of compromised circulation to the hand.

Another possible complication of dislocations during the healing process involves an insufficient deposit of collagen during the repair stage. The end result is that the ligaments may have reduced tensile strength and future instability, leading to recurrent dislocations of the same joint.

Assessment Findings

The client often reports hearing a "popping" sound when the dislocation occurs. Another common complaint is that the joint suddenly "gave out," implying that it became unstable or nonsupportive. If the dislocation results from trauma, the client usually experiences considerable pain from the injury and/or the resultant muscle spasm.

On inspection, the structural shape is altered. A depression may be noted about the joint's circumference, indicating that the bones above and below are no longer aligned. If the dislocation affects an extremity, the arm or leg may be shorter than its unaffected counterpart as a result of the displacement of one of the articulating bones. ROM is limited. Evidence of soft-tissue injury includes swelling, coolness, numbness, tingling, and pale or dusky color of the distal tissue.

X-rays show intact yet malpositioned bones. Arthrography or arthroscopy may reveal damage to other structures in the joint capsule.

Medical and Surgical Management

The primary provider manipulates the joint or reduces the displaced parts until they return to normal position and then immobilizes the joint with an elastic bandage, cast, or splint for several weeks. Doing so allows the joint capsule and surrounding ligaments to heal. The client may receive a local or general anesthetic before the manipulation is performed. Some dislocations may require surgery, either to correct the dislocation or to repair damage caused by the injury.

Nursing Management

The nurse relieves the client's discomfort by administering prescribed analgesics, elevating and immobilizing the affected limb, and applying cold packs to the injury. They perform neurovascular assessments every 30 minutes for several hours and then at least every 2 to 4 hours for the next 1 or 2 days to detect complications such as compartment syndrome. See Table 60-3 for more information about neurovascular assessments. Client and Family Teaching 62-1 describes preventive strategies for sports and/or work-related activities.

Client and Family Teaching 62-1
Preventing Sports and/or Work-Related Injuries

The nurse teaches the client the following preventive measures:

- Use proper equipment at work and during participation in athletic activities.
- At work, look at ways to modify the environment to prevent injury (some work settings consult with ergonomic experts to modify the environment).
- Exercise regularly to maintain joint and muscle strength.
- Maintain a healthy weight.
- Prepare for athletic activities by doing gradual warm-up exercises and stretching following the warm-up.
- At work, take a few minutes every 2 hours to relax, stretch muscles, and change position.
- Following exercise, allow for "cool-off" time and stretching so that the body has time to adapt to the change in activity level.
- If body symptoms such as pain or discomfort with movement occur, rest that body part until symptoms subside and then gradually reintroduce the activity.
- If symptoms persist, seek medical advice.

SPECIFIC INJURIES TO UPPER AND LOWER EXTREMITIES

Frequent sites of injury and pain in the extremities include the shoulder, elbow, wrist, knee, and ankle. Some of the injuries include acute injuries, such as those described earlier, and fractures (see later discussion). Other disorders occur more gradually as a result of repeated or overuse of a particular joint related to sports and exercise and work-related injuries. These include tendonitis, stress fractures, and other related injuries.

Tendinitis

Tendinitis (also referred to as *tendonitis*) is the inflammation of a tendon caused by overuse. There are several types of tendinitis that commonly occurs as a result of repeated sports and/or work activities. Epicondylitis, ganglions, and carpal tunnel syndrome are recurrent injuries that are frequently seen. **Epicondylitis** (tennis elbow) is a painful inflammation of the elbow. A **ganglion cyst** is a cystic mass that develops near tendon sheaths and joints of the wrist. **Carpal tunnel syndrome** is a term for a group of symptoms located in the carpal tunnel of the wrist, a narrow, inelastic canal through which the carpal tendons and median nerve pass.

Pathophysiology and Etiology

The primary causes of these injuries are trauma and repeated stress. Injury is also responsible for epicondylitis, which occurs when the tendons of the medial or lateral radial and ulnar epicondyles sustain damage. The injury typically follows excessive pronation and supination of the forearm, such as that which occurs when playing tennis, pitching ball, or rowing. Ganglion cysts form through defects in the tendon sheath or joint capsule and occur most commonly in women younger than 50 years of age.

Carpal tunnel syndrome results from repetitive wrist motion that traumatizes the tendon sheath or ligaments in the carpal canal. The trauma produces swelling that compresses the median nerve against the transverse carpal ligament. Those affected tend to be in occupations that perform repetitive hand movements, such as cashiers, typists, musicians, assemblers, and all who spend many hours using a computer keyboard and mouse.

Assessment Findings

Signs and Symptoms

These injuries are marked by pain and inflammation, which can spread to surrounding tissues. In epicondylitis, clients report pain radiating down the dorsal surface of the forearm and a weak grasp. Clients with ganglion cysts experience pain and tenderness in the affected area. Clients with carpal tunnel syndrome describe pain or burning in one or both hands, which may radiate to the forearm and shoulder in severe cases. The pain tends to be more prominent at night and early in the morning. Shaking the hands may reduce the pain by promoting movement of edematous fluid from the carpal canal. Sensation may be lost or reduced in the thumb, index, middle, and a portion of the ring finger. The client may be unable to flex the index and middle fingers to make a fist. Flexion of the wrist usually causes immediate pain and numbness.

Diagnostic Findings

In general, X-ray studies are used to identify abnormalities and rule out fracture and other problems. In carpal tunnel syndrome, results of electromyography, which relies on a mild electrical current to stimulate the nerve, show a delay in motor response in muscles innervated by the median nerve. Other tests are Tinel's sign, which is a test that elicits tingling, numbness, and pain for clients with carpal tunnel syndrome, and Phalen sign, which involves having the client flex the wrist for 30 seconds to determine if pain or numbness occurs (a positive sign for carpal tunnel syndrome; Fig. 62-1). The examiner percusses the median nerve, located on the inner aspect of the wrist, to elicit this response.

Medical and Surgical Management

Treatment of these disorders includes applications of cold (ice) and heat, exercise, steroidal anti-inflammatory medications, local injection of corticosteroids, analgesics, NSAIDs, and rest. Surgical intervention may be necessary to repair tears and ruptures. In many cases, clients with injuries of the shoulder or other portions of the upper extremity are referred for physical therapy. Treatment for epicondylitis may include splinting to rest and support the joint structures. Corticosteroids may be injected locally. Treatment of ganglion cysts includes aspiration of the ganglion, corticosteroid injection, and surgical excision.

Carpal tunnel treatment involves resting the hands when possible and splinting the hand and wrist. NSAIDs and periodic injections of a corticosteroid preparation may relieve the inflammation and discomfort. If conservative treatment fails, surgery to release the pressure of the ligament on the median nerve may be performed.

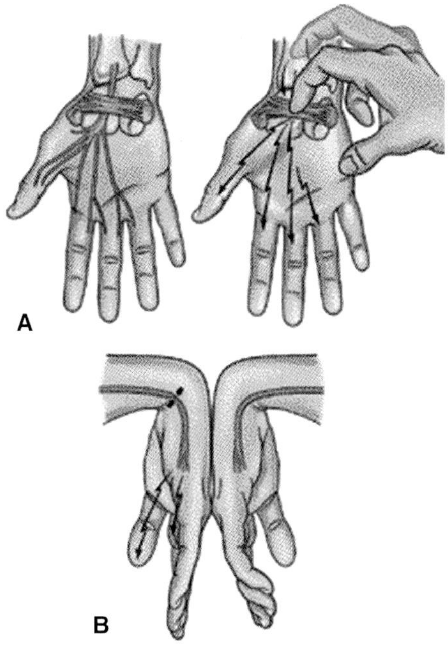

Figure 62-1 (A) Tinel's sign. **(B)** Phalen sign.

Nursing Management

The nurse provides information about medications. If the client is taking NSAIDs, the nurse stresses to take these medications with food. If corticosteroid injections are ordered, they explain what the client can expect and mention that the injection itself may cause some discomfort.

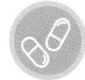

Pharmacologic Considerations

- Gastrointestinal (GI) distress is one of the most common adverse effects of NSAIDs. Have clients self-monitor for GI bleeding, which in some cases can be severe due to the anticoagulant properties of the drug.

The nurse shows clients how to use and care for prescribed splints and perform related ROM exercises. Some clients find that hand exercises are less painful if performed with the hand under warm water. Additional management activities involve exploring ways to perform activities of daily living (ADLs) or alter job responsibilities to relieve stress and reduce injury to joints.

Key teaching points include the following:

- Rest the joint in a position that reduces stress.
- Support the affected arm joint on pillows while sleeping.
- Apply cold for the first 24 to 48 hours to reduce swelling and pain.
- Gradually increase joint movement.
- Avoid working or lifting above shoulder level. Do not push objects with the arm joint, particularly the shoulder.
- Perform ROM and strengthening exercises as prescribed by the primary provider or physical therapist.

Rotator Cuff Tear

The **rotator cuff** is made up of four muscles and their tendons that connect the proximal humerus, clavicle, and scapula, which in turn connect with the sternum and ribs (Maruvada et al., 2020). Rotator cuff injuries can occur as a result of a traumatic injury or from chronic overuse or irritation of the shoulder joint. A tear (or more than one) occurs in a tendon connecting the rotating muscles to the head of the humerus. Tears are differentiated as partial or full-thickness. Clients experience pain with movement and limited mobility of the shoulder and arm. They especially have difficulty with activities that involve stretching their arms above their heads (or complete). Many clients find that the pain is worse at night and that they are unable to sleep on the affected side. The diagnosis is based on physical examination—Generally, there is tenderness on the acromioclavicular joint. Radiography, arthrography, ultrasound, and MRI can evaluate the extent of the rotator cuff tear and any soft tissue injury.

Initial treatment begins with the use of NSAIDs. The primary provider will advise clients to modify their activities and to rest the joint. Primary providers may also recommend corticosteroid injections into the shoulder joint, with progressive passive and active exercises and stretching. Surgical procedures include the following:

- *Arthroscopic tendon repair*: reattach the tendon to the bone arthroscopically
- *Open tendon repair*: a larger incision is used to repair and reattach the tendon
- *Removal of bone spur:* excess bone is removed and tendons are repaired, through a small incision
- *Tendon transfer*: replace torn tendons with a nearby tendon—open procedure
- *Shoulder replacement*: referred to as reverse shoulder arthroplasty; the socket portion of the artificial joint is placed on the humerus, and the ball part of the joint is placed on the scapula

Depending on the type of surgery, clients have to immobilize the shoulder for several days to several or more weeks and then have to undergo physical therapy for several weeks to months. Generally, clients will have full recovery postoperatively within 6 to 12 months.

Ligament and Meniscal Injuries

Ligament and meniscal injuries to the knee occur as a result of a traumatic injury. Figure 62-2 depicts the knee ligaments and menisci (cartilages in the knee). Injuries can occur to the lateral or medial collateral knee ligaments (these ligaments provide stability to the sides of the knee) or to the anterior cruciate ligament (ACL) or posterior cruciate ligament (PCL) (these ligaments provide stability to forward and backward movements). In addition, menisci can become injured, disrupting the stability of the leg when flexed or extended.

Pathophysiology and Etiology

Injury to the ligaments of the knee occurs at a time when the client is standing firmly and receives a blow or twists in a different direction while hyperextending the knee. The client experiences pain, instability of the joint, and ambulatory difficulty. When the ACL or PCL tears, the client may report a popping sound or tearing sensation. Meniscal injuries occur with twisting of the knee or repeated squatting. Clients report that their knees "gave way" or buckled, and clients may experience a click in their knees as they ambulate. In some instances, the knee locks because the cartilage moves as it tears and prevents full flexion and extension. An MRI initially may be done to assess the extent of the injury.

Medical and Surgical Management

Treatment depends on the extent of the injury. Initial treatment involves immobilizing the joint and limiting weight bearing. The primary provider may recommend NSAIDs as well as the use of ice during the first 48 hours. Gradual introduction of activity assists the client to progress without causing further injury. Surgical procedures include repair of the ligaments and tendons involved. An arthrocentesis may be done for diagnostic purposes and to provide symptomatic relief through drainage of bloody fluid. An arthroscopy is done to determine what the meniscal tear involves. For torn

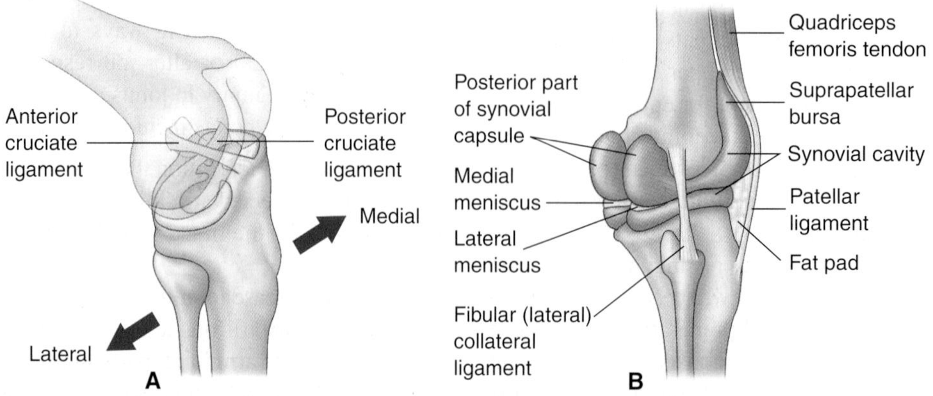

Figure 62-2 Knee ligaments and menisci. **(A)** Anterolateral view. **(B)** Posterolateral view.

menisci, the surgeon removes the damaged cartilage (**meniscectomy**). Following surgery, the primary provider will immobilize the joint, prescribe NSAIDs, and recommend the application of cold therapy. Physical rehabilitation includes exercises, gradual weight bearing, and the use of any ambulatory devices. Recovery is generally complete within 3 to 12 months depending on the nature of the injury and the type of surgery.

Ruptured Achilles Tendon

Rupture of the Achilles tendon occurs secondary to trauma. As the client engages in an activity, the calf muscle contracts suddenly, while the foot is grounded firmly in place. There is often a loud pop, and the client experiences severe pain and inability to plantar flex the affected foot. The client usually requires surgical repair for complete healing to occur. Following surgery, the client wears a cast or brace for 6 to 8 weeks. Physical therapy is necessary for the client to regain mobility, strength, and full ROM.

The nurse teaches the client about activity restrictions, the use of ambulatory aids, and pain management. Clients who have surgery need to have preoperative and postoperative instructions. Refer to Nursing Care Plan 61-1 for more information relevant to orthopedic surgery.

FRACTURES

A **fracture** is a break in the continuity of a bone. Fractures may affect tissues or organs near the bones as well. Fractures are classified according to the type and extent (Box 62-1).

BOX 62-1 Types of Fractures

Avulsion: a pulling away of a fragment of bone by a ligament or tendon and its attachment
Comminuted: a fracture in which bone has splintered into several fragments
Compound: a fracture in which damage also involves the skin or mucous membranes
Compression: a fracture in which bone has been compressed (seen in vertebral fractures)
Depressed: a fracture in which fragments are driven inward (seen frequently in fractures of skull and facial bones)
Epiphyseal: a fracture through the epiphysis
Greenstick: a fracture in which one side of a bone is broken and the other side is bent
Impacted: a fracture in which a bone fragment is driven into another bone fragment
Oblique: a fracture occurring at an angle across the bone (less stable than transverse)
Pathologic: a fracture that occurs through an area of diseased bone (bone cyst, Paget disease, bony metastasis, tumor); can occur without trauma or a fall
Simple: a fracture that remains contained; does not break the skin
Spiral: a fracture twisting around the shaft of the bone
Transverse: a fracture that is straight across the bone

Pathophysiology and Etiology

When force applied to a bone exceeds maximum resistance, the bone breaks. Sudden direct force from a blow or fall causes most fractures; however, some result from indirect force—for example, from a strong muscle contraction, such as during a seizure. A few fractures result from underlying weakness created by bone infections, bone tumors, or more bone resorption than production (as occurs in clients who are inactive or aging).

For 10 to 40 minutes after a bone breaks, the muscles surrounding the bone are flaccid. Then they go into spasm, often increasing deformity and interfering with the vascular and lymphatic circulations. The tissue surrounding the fracture swells from hemorrhage and edema. Healing begins (Fig. 62-3) when blood in the area clots and a fibrin network forms between the broken bone ends. The fibrin network changes into granulation tissue. Osteoblasts, which proliferate in the clot, increase the secretion of an enzyme that restores the alkaline pH. As a result, calcium is deposited, and true bone forms. The healing mass is called a **callus**. It holds the ends of the bone together but cannot endure strain. Bone repair is a local process. About 1 year of healing must pass before bone regains its former structural strength, becomes well consolidated and remodeled (reformed), and possesses fat and marrow cells.

Although fractures are common, they are associated with various complications, particularly when they are very complex. Table 62-1 briefly describes the types of possible complications, which include compartment syndrome, thromboembolism, fat embolism, delayed healing, nonunion, malunion, infection, and **avascular necrosis** (death of bone from an insufficient blood supply). In addition, any client who is inactive during convalescence is prone to pneumonia, thrombophlebitis, pressure sores, urinary tract infection, renal calculi, constipation, muscle atrophy, weight gain, and depression.

Assessment Findings

Signs and Symptoms

The signs and symptoms of a fracture vary depending on the type and location. They include the following:

- *Pain*: One of the most consistent symptoms of a fracture is pain, which may be severe. Attempts to move the part and/or pressure over the fracture contribute to increased pain.
- *Loss of function*: Skeletal muscular function depends on intact bone.
- *Deformity*: A break may cause an extremity to bend backward or to assume another unusual position.
- *False motion*: Unnatural motion occurs at the site of the fracture.
- *Crepitus*: The grating sound of bone ends moving over one another may be audible (this term also refers to a popping sound caused by air trapped in soft tissue).
- *Edema*: Swelling usually is greatest directly over the fracture.
- *Spasm*: Muscles near fractures involuntarily contract. Spasm, which accounts for some of the pain, may cause a limb to shorten when the fracture involves a long bone.

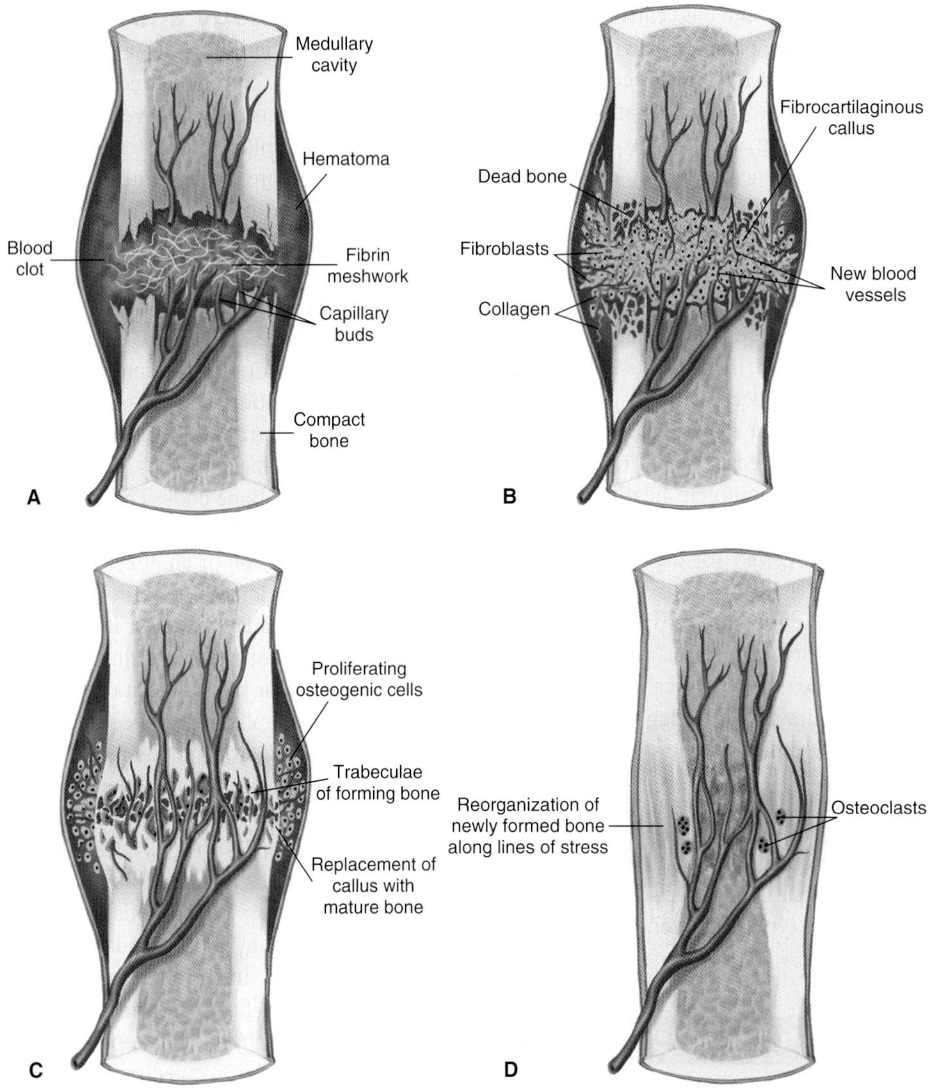

Figure 62-3 Process of bone healing. **(A)** Immediately after a bone fractures, blood seeps into the area, and a hematoma (blood clot) forms. **(B)** After 1 week, osteoblasts form as the clot retracts. After about 3 weeks, a procallus forms and stabilizes the fracture. **(C)** A callus with bone cells forms in 6 to 12 weeks. In 3 to 4 months, osteoblasts begin to remodel the fracture site. **(D)** If the fractured bone has been accurately aligned during healing, remodeling will be complete in about 12 months. (Reprinted with permission from Grossman, S. C., & Porth, C. M. (2014). *Porth's pathophysiology: Concepts of altered health states* (9th ed.). Wolters Kluwer Health/Lippincott Williams & Wilkins.)

TABLE 62-1 Complications of Fractures

COMPLICATION	DESCRIPTION	NURSING IMPLICATIONS
Shock	Hypovolemic shock related to blood loss and loss of extracellular fluid from damaged tissue. If untreated, the client's condition will deteriorate.	Administer blood and fluid volume replacements as prescribed to prevent further losses.
Fat embolism	Fat globules released after fractures of pelvis or long bones, or after multiple injuries or crushing injuries. Globules combine with platelets to form emboli. Onset is rapid, with client experiencing respiratory distress and cerebral disturbances.	Monitor client for symptoms, which usually occur within 48–72 hours. To prevent fatty emboli, provide early respiratory support, ensure rapid immobilization of fracture, and observe client closely for signs of respiratory and nervous system problems.
Pulmonary embolism	Thromboembolism may occur after fracture or surgery to repair fractures. These lead to pulmonary emboli in some clients and can be fatal.	Promote circulation and prevent venous stasis to avoid pulmonary embolism. Administer low-dose heparin or other anticoagulants as prescribed to prevent clot formation.

TABLE 62-1 Complications of Fractures (*continued*)

COMPLICATION	DESCRIPTION	NURSING IMPLICATIONS
Compartment syndrome	Tissue perfusion in the muscle compartment (muscle covered by inelastic fascia) is compromised secondary to tissue swelling, hemorrhage, or a cast that is too tight. If circulation is not restored, ischemia and tissue anoxia lead to permanent nerve damage, muscle atrophy, and contracture.	Monitor client for signs and symptoms of compartment syndrome such as unrelenting pain unrelieved by analgesics. Elevate the extremity, apply ice, and perform neurovascular checks to help prevent this complication. As indicated, relieve pressure by loosening cast or preparing the client for a **fasciotomy** (surgical incision of fascia and separation of muscles).
Delayed bone healing	Bone fails to heal at the expected rate. Delayed healing may result from nonunion, characterized by the ends of the fractured bone failing to unite and heal, or it may result from malunion, characterized by the ends of the fractured bone healing in a deformed position.	Delayed union may require surgical intervention to promote bone growth and to correct the incorrect union. If necessary, prepare the client for use of electrical stimulation measures that promote bone growth or for a bone graft.
Infection	The potential for infection increases with compound fractures, application of skeletal traction, or surgical procedures.	Perform careful assessments and maintain aseptic technique to prevent infections. Monitor for early signs of infection because early detection promotes early correction of the problem.
Avascular necrosis	This condition occurs from interruption of the blood supply to the fracture fragments after which the bone tissue dies; most common in the femoral head.	Be alert for client reports of pain and decreased function of the affected limb. If necessary, prepare the client for surgery, such as bone graft, bone prosthesis, joint replacement, joint fusion, or amputation.

If sharp bone fragments tear through sufficient surrounding soft tissue, there is bleeding and black and blue discoloration of the area. If a nerve is damaged, paralysis may result.

>>> *Stop, Think, and Respond 62-2*

You are cross-country skiing with a friend and notice that a person ahead of you has fallen. When you get closer, this person tells you that she has hurt her arm. What signs would indicate that this woman probably has a fractured humerus?

Diagnostic Findings

One or more radiographic views of the area almost always demonstrate altered bone structure. Stress fractures may not be apparent radiographically for a few weeks. A bone scan usually can identify a nondisplaced or stress fracture before radiographic changes are evident. In some instances, a computed tomography scan or MRI may be necessary.

Medical and Surgical Management

The goal is to reestablish functional continuity of the bone. Treatment includes one or more methods: traction, closed or open reduction, internal or external fixation, or cast application. The treatment method depends on many factors, including the first aid given, the location and severity of the break, and the age and overall physical condition of the client. Chapter 61 describes medical and surgical modalities used for clients with orthopedic injuries, including fractures.

Nursing Management

When caring for the client with a fracture, the nurse assesses for neurovascular and systemic complications. General nursing measures include administering analgesics, providing comfort measures, assisting with ADLs, preventing constipation, promoting physical mobility, preventing infection, maintaining skin integrity, and preparing client for self-care. Because the client may be discharged shortly after application of an immobilization device or a cast, the nurse reviews care with the client or family. In addition, they reinforce instructions regarding exercise and ambulatory activities.

If a client is in traction, they require simple and direct explanations about the traction and its purpose. The nurse points out activities that are allowed or contraindicated and identifies the approximate duration of the restrictions. When traction is discontinued, the nurse prepares the client for further treatment, such as casting, and for the appearance of the affected area—skin and muscles. They reassure the client that, with gradual exercise and use, muscles will regain strength and tone, and joints will be flexible. For more information about managing problems related to casting, refer to Nursing Guidelines 61-1. For information about clients with specific fractures, such as those affecting the clavicle or knee, refer to Table 61-1.

Fractured Femur

A fracture of the femur commonly occurs in automobile accidents but may also occur in falls from ladders or other high places or in gunshot wounds. Multiple injuries often accompany fractures of the femur because they usually occur with severe trauma.

Assessment Findings

Severe pain, swelling, and ecchymosis may be seen. The client usually cannot move the hip or knee. If a compound fracture has occurred, an open wound or a protrusion of bone is seen. X-rays show the type and location of the fracture.

Medical and Surgical Management

Fractures of the femur usually are treated initially with some form of traction to prevent deformities and soft tissue injury. Skeletal traction (Fig. 62-4) or an external fixator is used to align the fracture in preparation for future reduction if the fracture occurred in the lower two thirds of the femur. Once the femur is aligned, a spica cast may be used to maintain the corrected position.

Nursing Management

Because the client is confined to bed, the nurse implements measures to prevent complications of immobility and inactivity. They position the client in line with the pull exerted by the traction. The nurse cleans pin sites with a prescribed agent to prevent infection (see Nursing Guidelines 61-3).

Fractured Hip

Usually, a hip fracture affects the proximal end of the femur. This type of fracture commonly results from a fall and occurs more frequently in older adults with osteoporosis. Usually, the falls are not very traumatic, but the client's condition contributes to the resulting fracture. Fractures may occur in the femoral neck (intracapsular or inside the hip joint capsule), between the trochanters (intertrochanteric extracapsular or outside the hip joint capsule), or below the trochanters (subtrochanteric extracapsular). Figure 62-5 illustrates regions of the proximal femur.

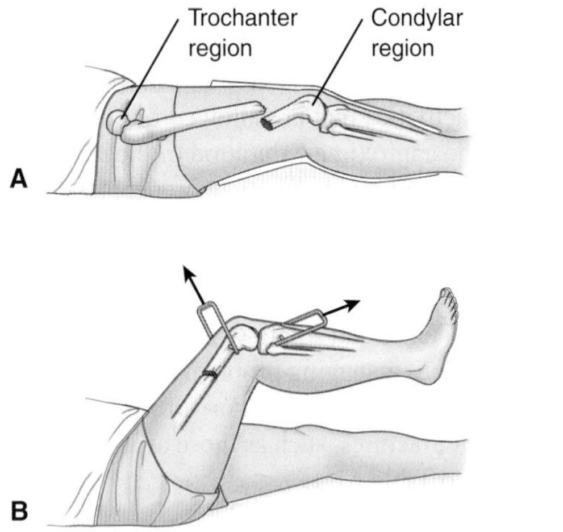

Figure 62-4 **(A)** Example of deformity on admission to hospital. **(B)** Adequate reduction is achieved when additional wire is inserted in the lower femoral fragment, and vertical lift is secured. (Reprinted with permission from Hinkle, J. L., & Cheever, K. H. (2014). *Brunner & Suddarth's textbook of medical-surgical nursing* (13th ed.). Wolters Kluwer Health/Lippincott Williams & Wilkins.)

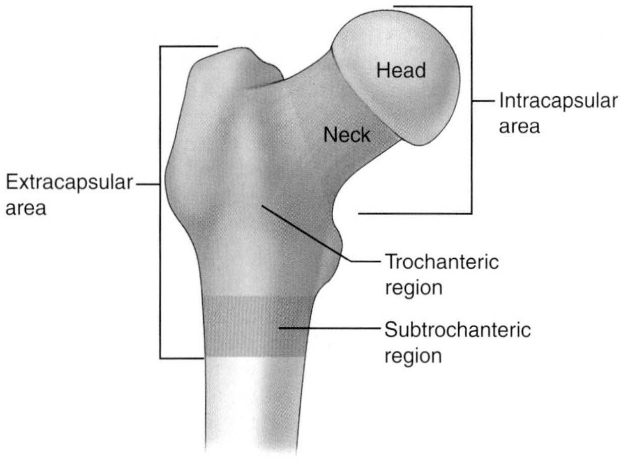

Figure 62-5 Regions of the proximal femur where hip fractures may occur.

Assessment Findings

The client reports severe pain that increases with leg movement. The pain frequently radiates to the knee, and the client may have a sensation of pressure in the outer aspect of the hip. Discontinuity of the bone and muscle spasm cause shortening and external rotation of the leg. A large blood loss may accompany subtrochanteric and intertrochanteric fractures, leading to hypovolemic shock. There may also be extensive bruising and swelling in the hip, groin, and thigh. Femoral neck fractures are intracapsular, so bleeding is more likely to be contained within the joint capsule. Radiographic studies reveal the exact location of the fracture, which may be within or outside the joint capsule.

Medical and Surgical Management

Chapter 61 describes general medical and surgical management for clients with fractures. Intracapsular hip fractures are prone to nonunion and avascular necrosis from the disrupted blood supply. Therefore, the fractured head and neck may be removed and replaced with a metal device such as an Austin Moore or Thompson prosthesis. This procedure is referred to as *hemiarthroplasty*. The bone heals around the metallic device, which, in the meantime, holds the bone together. Thus, the bone is united immediately, and clients are mobilized much earlier than they are with traction. Plates, bands, screws, and pins may be removed after the bone has healed. More often, they are left in place permanently. The precautions with hemiarthroplasty are greater because the surgeon must dislocate the hip to replace the femoral head. Clients may have a total hip arthroplasty (see Chapter 61).

Nursing Management

Most clients with a fractured hip are older adults and are prone to complications. After surgery, the nurse implements measures to prevent skin breakdown, wound infection, pneumonia, constipation, urinary retention, muscle atrophy, and contractures. The client usually has a wound drain in place for 1 to 2 days after surgery. The nurse monitors the drainage and administers antibiotics as prescribed.

The nurse must show the client how to use the overhead trapeze safely for independent movement and activity. When the client is recumbent, the nurse places a trochanter roll beside the hip to maintain a neutral position so the repaired hip stays in place. They place abductor pillows between the client's legs when turning the client from side to side. Refer to Chapter 61 for more information about nursing management of a client following insertion of a hip prosthesis. Nursing Care Plan 61-1 provides additional nursing management strategies for postoperative orthopedic clients.

If a hip prosthesis has been inserted, the nurse instructs the client to avoid adduction of the affected leg until it has healed. The client must use abductor pillows at all times. Soon after surgery, the nurse or physical therapist assists the client to transfer from the bed to a chair. The chair must have an elevated seat, either with its structure or with pillows, so the client does not flex the hips beyond 90 degree. The client usually requires much encouragement and assistance. Eventually, the client progresses to ambulating with a walker. Before discharge, the nurse needs to explore ways to ensure safety in the client's home to avoid future injuries and falls. See Evidence-Based Practice 62-1 for research about the complication of deep vein thrombosis following hip fracture.

Evidence-Based Practice 62-1

Therapy for Deep Vein Thrombosis in Clients With Hip Fractures

Clinical Question

In clients with hip fractures, how does pharmacologic therapy for deep vein thrombosis (DVT) prevention compare with pharmacologic therapy and compression devices in rates of affect DVT rates?

Evidence

Clients experience decreased mobility as a result of hip fractures. The combination of their injury, surgery to repair the fracture, and the resulting decrease in mobility make clients prone to DVTs, which are blood clots in their legs. These blood clots can travel to the lungs or heart causing damage or even death. According to Durand et al. (2018), up to 60% of all clients undergoing hip fracture surgery will experience a DVT if not given preventive, or prophylactic, treatment.

Several approaches to DVT prophylaxis have been studied. Early ambulation and hydration are the predominant factors of DVT prevention (Mula, et al., 2020). Pharmacologic prophylaxis, including use of such medications as low-molecular-weight heparin (LMWH) or fondaparinox, has shown to be most effective in preventing DVTs (Mula et al., 2020; Bengoa et al., 2020). Mechanical prophylaxis, such as knee-high and thigh-high graduated compression stockings (GCSs) and/or intermittent pneumatic compression devices, is often used as well. They may be used by themselves or in combination with pharmacologic prophylaxis. Evidence suggests that there is no difference between the different types of mechanical prophylaxis devices, although GCSs may be difficult to use due to postinjury and postoperative swelling and pain with getting them on and off (Autar, 2010). GCSs are also contraindicated in clients with peripheral vascular disease and local skin conditions, both common in older adult clients (Mula et al., 2020). Sometimes medical conditions prevent the use of pharmacologic prophylaxis. In those cases, mechanical prophylaxis may be used by itself. Clients with a delay in admission and treatment, of 48 hours after injury, have an increase in the prevalence of DVTs (Bengoa et al., 2020).

Nursing Implications

Nurses are instrumental and play a big part in DVT prevention by encouraging and providing assistance with early ambulation, leg exercises, and hydration. Thorough nursing assessments are key and must include such things as assessing for pain and/or swelling in the lower leg (often in the back of the lower leg), skin redness, and/or sudden onset of shortness of breath or chest pain that is not consistent with any other cause. Immediate action to get the client to the hospital must be taken if sudden onset of shortness of breath or chest pain occurs. Proper use of mechanical prophylaxis is important to avoid additional complications of mechanical prophylaxis such as development of skin issues. Client education about DVT prevention, symptoms of DVT, and appropriate administration of preventive medications with necessary follow-up once discharged is also vital. Clients also need education about when to seek medical evaluation for symptoms suggesting the development of blood clots because clients are at risk for developing blood clots even after they leave the hospital setting.

References

Bengoa, F., Vicencio, G., Schweitzer, D., Lira, M. J., Zamora, T., & Klaber, I. (2020). High prevalence of deep vein thrombosis in elderly hip fracture patients with delayed hospital admission. *European Journal of Trauma & Emergency Surgery, 46*(4), 913–917. https://doi.org/10.1007/s00068-018-1059-8

Durand, W., Goodman, A., Johnson, J. P., & Daniels, A. H. (2018). Assessment of 30-day mortality and complication rates associated with extended deep vein thrombosis prophylaxis following hip fracture surgery. *Injury, 49*(6), 1141–1148. https://doi.org/10.1016/j.injury.2018.03.019

MacDonald, D. R., Neilly, D., Schneider, P., Bzovsky, S., Sprague, S., Axelrod, D., Poolman, R., Frihagen, F., Bhandari, M., Swiontkowski, M., Schemitsch, E., & Stevenson, I. (2020). Thromboembolism in hip fracture patients: A subanalysis of the FAITH and HEALTH trials. *Journal of Orthopaedic Trauma, 34,* S70–S75. https://doi.org/10.1097/BOT.0000000000001939

Mula, V., Parikh, S., Suresh, S., Bottle, A., Loeffler, M., & Alam, M. (2020). Venous thromboembolism rates after hip and knee arthroplasty and hip fractures. *BMC Musculoskeletal Disorders, 21*(1), 1–7. https://doi.org/10.1186/s12891-020-3100-4

KEY POINTS

- Strains, contusions, and sprains:
  - Strain: injury to muscle
  - Contusion: soft tissue injury
  - Sprain: injury to ligaments
- Dislocations: when the articular surfaces of a joint are no longer in contact

- Specific injuries to upper and lower extremities
  - Tendinitis: inflammation of a tendon caused by overuse
  - Rotator cuff tear: tear in a tendon connecting the rotating muscles to the head of the humerus
  - Ligament and meniscal injures: occur to the knee as a result of a traumatic injury; may be ACL or PCL
  - Ruptured Achilles tendon: occurs due to trauma
- Fractures: break in the continuity of a bone. Multiple types include avulsion, compound, compression, epiphyseal, greenstick, simple, spiral, transverse
  - Fractured femur: occurs from automobile accidents, falls from high places, or from gunshot wounds
  - Fractured hip: occurs from falls and more frequently in older adults with osteoporosis

CRITICAL THINKING EXERCISES

1. A client is admitted to a surgical floor with an open fracture of the right arm. What are priorities when caring for this client?

2. The nurse tells the client who sprained their left ankle 2 hours ago that they need to apply an ice pack to the injured area. What explanation should the nurse give for this action?

3. Describe factors that can interfere with bone healing.

4. What factors can contribute to rotator cuff injuries?

NCLEX-STYLE REVIEW QUESTIONS PrepU

1. A client is diagnosed with a second-degree sprain of the left ankle. When planning for the client's discharge, the nurse provides instructions for care at home. From the following list, select all that apply:

1. Apply a hot compress to the left ankle.
2. Do not bear weight on the left ankle.
3. Elevate left leg as much as possible.
4. Keep the ankle wrapped with an Ace bandage.
5. Maintain left leg in a dependent position.
6. Place an ice pack on the left ankle.

2. A client presents in the emergency room with a shoulder injury after falling from a stepladder. When the nurse assesses the client's injuries, which finding best indicates that the client has dislocated the shoulder?

1. The affected arm is shorter than the unaffected arm.
2. The client has obvious swelling about the joint.
3. The client is experiencing intense pain.
4. The client is hesitant to move the affected arm.

3. A graphic designer who spends hours working on the computer complains of slight pain in the right hand. The pain is more prominent at night and in the early morning. The client is diagnosed with a mild form of carpal tunnel syndrome. What is appropriate for the nurse to recommend for reducing the pain? Select all that apply.

1. Flexing the affected wrist
2. Physical therapy
3. Resting the hands when possible
4. Shaking the affected hand
5. Surgical intervention

4. A client has sustained a fractured tibia and is in traction. Which signs need to be reported to the primary provider? Select all that apply.

1. Capillary refill in affected extremity is 3 seconds.
2. Client complains of throbbing and unrelenting pain.
3. Client is able to wiggle toes on affected foot when asked.
4. Client states that the foot on the affected leg is numb.
5. Client's toes on affected leg are bluish and cold to touch.

5. A client is hospitalized with a fractured right hip. What is the most typical sign of an intertrochanteric fracture of the hip seen during the nurse's admission assessment?

1. Bruising of the affected leg
2. External rotation of the leg
3. Lengthening of the affected leg
4. Paralysis of the affected leg

WANT TO KNOW MORE? There are a wide variety of online resources available on thePoint to enhance learning and understanding of this chapter.

Go to **thePoint.lww.com/activate**, and use the activation code found in the front of this text to unlock these online resources.

63

Caring for Clients With Orthopedic and Connective Tissue Disorders

Words To Know

ankylosing spondylitis
ankylosis
arthritis
arthroplasty
Bouchard nodes
bursitis
degenerative joint disease
fibromyalgia syndrome
gout
hallux valgus
hammer toe
Heberden nodes
hyperuricemia
involucrum
Lyme disease
mallet toe
osteomalacia
osteomyelitis
osteoporosis
Paget disease
pannus
rheumatic disorders
rheumatoid arthritis
sequestrum
synovectomy
synovitis
systemic lupus erythematosus
tophi

Learning Objectives

On completion of this chapter, you will be able to:

1. Explain the difference between rheumatoid arthritis and degenerative joint disease (osteoarthritis).
2. Describe nursing management of clients with arthritis.
3. Summarize the clinical manifestations of temporomandibular disorder (TMD).
4. Define the pathophysiology of gout, fibromyalgia, bursitis, and ankylosing spondylitis.
5. Delineate the nursing care required for clients with gout, fibromyalgia, bursitis, and ankylosing spondylitis.
6. Discuss the multisystem involvement associated with systemic lupus erythematosus.
7. Identify the causes of osteomyelitis.
8. Explain the inflammatory process associated with Lyme disease.
9. Identify risk factors for development of osteoporosis.
10. Distinguish the pathophysiology of osteomalacia and Paget disease.
11. Differentiate between bunions and hammer toe.
12. Discuss characteristics of benign and malignant bone tumors.

The musculoskeletal system consists of structures the body uses for support and movement. It also protects body organs. Disorders affecting the musculoskeletal system affect the person's ability to perform activities of daily living (ADLs) and to remain active, mobile, and physically fit. Many clients with musculoskeletal disorders are treated as outpatients. A few may require hospitalization in the acute phase of the disorder, for surgery on a degenerative joint or for other medical or surgical therapies.

Gerontologic Considerations

- Extreme diligence is needed in assessing and documenting to differentiate symptoms that may occur with other comorbidities commonly experienced by older adults.
- Subtle cognitive changes, depression, fatigue, or generalized pain may be overlooked, magnifying the difficulty of diagnosing accurately, and thereby delaying appropriate treatment.

(continued)

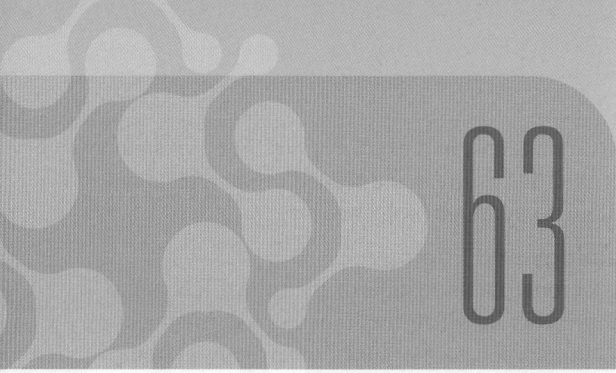

Gerontologic Considerations (*continued*)

■ Older adults, families, and caregivers may believe that many of these symptoms are "just a part of aging" and may not report the symptoms unless specifically questioned during each assessment. Accurate assessment and documentation guide individualized treatment that can be initiated and monitored for clients and families (i.e., teaching regarding nutrition, lifestyle modifications, medications, activity/rest balance, etc.).

■ Estrogen deficiency, which occurs at menopause, is considered the leading factor in osteoporosis among aging women.

INFLAMMATORY DISORDERS

Arthritis is a general condition characterized by inflammation and degeneration of a joint. **Rheumatic disorders** include more than 100 different types of recognized inflammatory disorders, making this collective group the most common orthopedic problem. These disorders involve inflammation and degeneration of connective tissue structures, especially joints. They have the potential to interfere with mobility and ADLs. Clients with inflammatory disorders may need assistance with tasks that most people take for granted. These disorders affect a client's physical, psychological, and social functions.

The discussion in this chapter is limited to rheumatoid arthritis, osteoarthritis, temporomandibular disorder (TMD), gout, fibromyalgia, bursitis, ankylosing spondylitis, and systemic lupus erythematosus.

Rheumatoid Arthritis

Rheumatoid arthritis (RA) is an autoimmune systemic inflammatory disorder of connective tissue/joints characterized by chronicity, remissions, and exacerbations. The potential for disability with RA is great and related to the effects on joints as well as the systemic problems.

Pathophysiology and Etiology

RA involves chronic inflammation of the joints. RA is an autoimmune process, in which the immune system attacks joint tissues. In addition to the joints, other body systems may be affected, such as the eyes, skin, heart, lungs, kidneys, and blood vessels.

RA is the most common form of autoimmune arthritis and affects approximately 1.5 million adults in the United States. The majority of those affected by RA are women—the incidence is two to three times higher for women. RA affects all races and ethnic groups and ages (Arthritis Foundation, n.d.). Onset for RA is typically in adults in their middle years, but young children and older adults can also be diagnosed with RA. Genetic predisposition and other factors may be involved, such as smoking and hormonal influences related to birth control, hormone replacement therapy, and menstrual history.

The autoimmune reaction from RA occurs primarily in the synovial tissue. Approximately 70% to 80% of people with RA have a substance called *rheumatoid factor* (RF), an antibody that reacts with a fragment of immunoglobulin G (IgG). This self-produced (autologous) antibody forms immune complexes (IgG/RF). It is uncertain why. Theories include genetic predisposition or viral infections that alter the IgG so it is seen as foreign. In many individuals, there is also a strong genetic association of human leukocyte antigen (HLA) with RA (Scherer et al., 2020).

The autoimmune reaction is described in Figure 63-1. Basically, lymphocytes in the inflammatory infiltrate of the synovial tissue produce RF. Polymorphonuclear leukocytes,

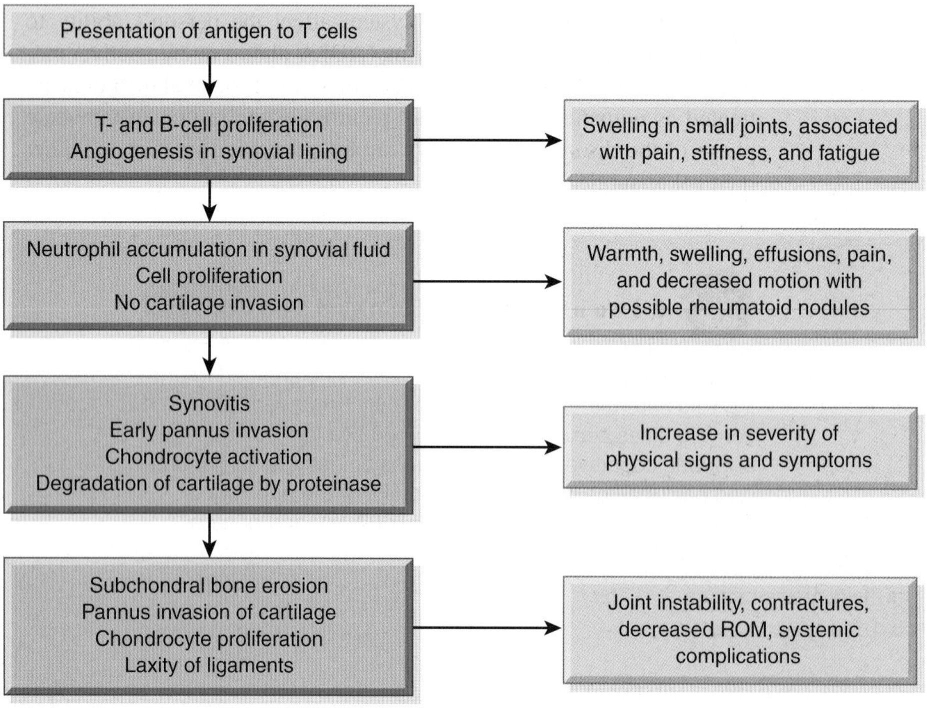

Figure 63-1 Pathophysiology and associated physical signs of rheumatoid arthritis. ROM, range of motion. (Reprinted with permission from Hinkle, J. L., & Cheever, K. H. (2014). *Brunner & Suddarth's textbook of medical-surgical nursing* (13th ed.). Wolters Kluwer Health/Lippincott Williams & Wilkins.)

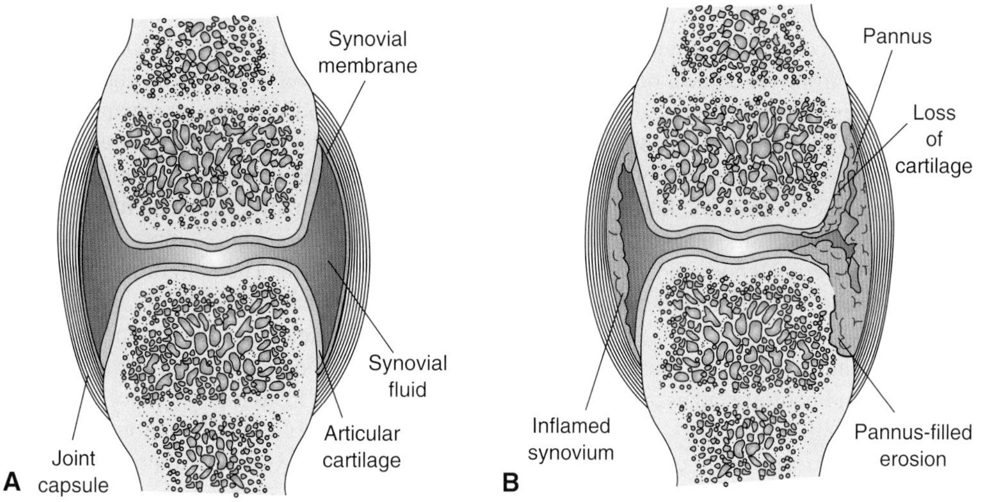

Figure 63-2 **(A)** Normal joint structures. **(B)** Joint changes in rheumatoid arthritis. The left side of the drawing denotes early changes occurring within the synovium. The right side shows progressive disease that leads to erosion and formation of pannus.

monocytes, and lymphocytes are attracted to the area and cause phagocytosis of the immune complexes. During this process, lysosomal enzymes are released, which cause destructive changes in the joint cartilage (Fig. 63-2). The changes produce more inflammation, which perpetuates the entire process of RA:

1. The inflammatory process (**synovitis**) advances as the congestion and edema develop in the synovial membrane and joint capsule.
2. Synovial tissue experiences reactive hyperplasia.
3. Vasodilation and increased blood flow cause warmth and redness.
4. Increased capillary permeability causes swelling.
5. Rheumatoid synovitis advances, leading to **pannus** formation (destructive vascular granulation tissue, characteristic of RA).
6. Pannus destroys adjacent cartilage, joint capsule, and bone.
7. Pannus eventually forms between joint margins, reducing joint mobility and leading to potential **ankylosis** (joint immobility).
8. Disease progression causes further inflammation and structural changes.

Most clients with RA experience exacerbations and remissions. For some clients, the progression is steady, relentless, and not necessarily responsive to therapy. Box 63-1 lists articular and extra-articular manifestations of RA.

Assessment Findings

Signs and Symptoms

In most clients, onset of symptoms is acute. Joint involvement usually is bilateral and symmetric. Localized symptoms include joint pain, swelling, and warmth; erythema; mobility limitation/stiffness; spongy tissue on joint palpation; and fluid on joints. Over several weeks, more joints become involved. Swelling and pain come and go. Fatigue, malaise, anorexia, and weight loss are common. Fever may develop. Tolerance for any kind of stress decreases, as does

BOX 63-1 Articular and Extra-articular Manifestations of Rheumatoid Arthritis

- *Subcutaneous nodules*: Firm, freely movable, rubbery, or granular nodules caused by deposition of extra-articular granulation tissue. Usually found at joint points such as knuckles and elbows.
- *Synovial cysts*: Called *Baker cysts* in popliteal fossa; filled with synovial fluid that may be found in periarticular areas in elbow, shoulder, or small joints.
- *Arthritis*: Bilateral involvement of the small joints and later the large joints; hand joints usually are swollen and may be red. Inflammation leads to disability from destruction of cartilage, bone, and tendons. Flexion contractures are common. Osteoporosis, vertebral compression fractures, and avascular necrosis of the femoral head are common and may relate to treatment with corticosteroids. Usually at least three joint areas are involved.
- *Systemic rheumatoid vasculitis*: Immune complex–mediated inflammation in small- and medium-sized arteries. It may be life-threatening if in a critical area. Causes pericardial, cardiac, pulmonary, and other types of lesions. Digital necrosis is common.
- *Compression neuropathy*: Mainly causes peripheral nerve entrapment with carpal tunnel syndrome. Paresthesias, pain, burning, muscle wasting, and weakness are common symptoms.
- *Cardiac disease*: Pericardial lesions and effusions are common and may or may not be symptomatic. Conduction system abnormalities from blockages owing to rheumatic nodules around the atrioventricular node may cause heart block.
- *Pleuropulmonary disease*: Pleural effusions or pleuritic chest pain are relatively common. Pulmonary fibrosis or progressive interstitial lung disease may be seen with or without rheumatoid nodules in the lung parenchyma.
- *Episcleritis and scleritis*: Episcleritis is an inflammatory condition of the connective tissue between the sclera and conjunctiva. Scleritis is an inflammatory condition of the sclera and can cause scleral perforation.
- *Sicca syndrome*: A condition of dry eyes and dry mouth that can result from infiltration of the lacrimal and salivary glands with lymphocytes.

tolerance for environmental temperature changes. Although dietary iron intake is adequate, clients characteristically have persistent anemia resulting from the effects of RA on the blood-forming organs. Other systemic features include vasculitis, neuropathy, scleritis, pericarditis, splenomegaly, and Sjögren syndrome (dry eyes and mucous membranes).

In some clients, subcutaneous nodules, known as *rheumatoid nodules*, develop. Appearing in more advanced stages of RA, they usually are nontender and movable and evident over bony prominences, such as the elbow or the base of the spine.

Muscles weaken and atrophy (shrink), partially from disuse. Connective tissue and neurovascular changes lend a smooth, glossy appearance to the extremities, which may be cold and clammy. Flexion contractures are common.

As the disease progresses, muscle wasting around affected joints accentuates the appearance of swelling. The proximal finger joints swell the most, showing classic deformities (Fig. 63-3), which include the following:

- *Swan neck deformity*: hyperextension of the proximal interphalangeal (PIP) joint with fixed flexion of the distal interphalangeal (DIP) joint
- *Boutonnière deformity*: persistent flexion of the PIP joint with hyperextension of the DIP joint
- *Ulnar deviation*: fingers deviating laterally toward the ulna

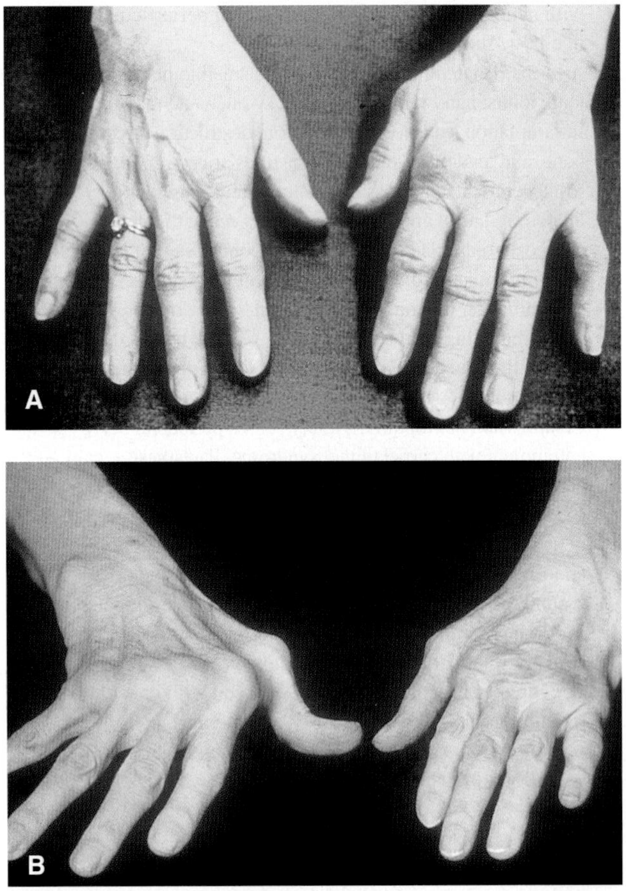

Figure 63-3 Rheumatoid arthritis. **(A)** Early. **(B)** Advanced; ulnar deviation of fingers and "swan neck" deformity of fingers.

Whether resting or moving, clients in this stage of the disease have considerable chronic pain, which typically is worse in the morning after a night's rest. The symptoms may subside suddenly for no apparent reason. Inflammation leaves joints that were sore and red; the client is not stiff, has no fever, and the pain is gone. Yet the symptoms almost invariably return after the client has had a symptom-free period. Inflammation causes more joint damage, followed by another remission. The pattern of remissions and exacerbations can continue for years.

Without treatment (and sometimes with it), joint destruction may be total. As bony growth replaces the synovial space, the joint loses motion. Once the joint becomes immobile, the pain of the inflammation decreases, but discomfort continues because of contractures and immobility.

Diagnostic Findings

X-rays show characteristic joint changes and the extent of damage. Narrowed joint spaces and bony erosions are characteristic of later disease. An arthrocentesis may be done, which is an aspiration of synovial fluid (the client receives a local anesthetic) for microscopic examination. In RA, the synovial fluid usually appears cloudy, milky, or dark yellow and contains many inflammatory cells, including leukocytes and complement (a group of proteins in blood that affect the inflammatory process and influence antigen–antibody reactions). Arthroscopic examination also may be carried out to visualize the extent of joint damage as well as to obtain a sample of synovial fluid.

A positive C-reactive protein (CRP) test, low red blood cell count and hemoglobin levels in later stages, and positive RF are laboratory findings that support the diagnosis. Blood tests for anti–cyclic citrullinated peptide (anti-CCP) antibodies are also present in many clients with RA. There is some evidence that clients with higher levels of RF and anti-CCP are more likely to experience increased problems with joint destruction. The erythrocyte sedimentation rate (ESR) may be elevated, particularly as the disease progresses. C4 complement component is decreased. Antinuclear antibody (ANA) test results also may be positive. Serum protein electrophoresis may disclose increased levels of gamma and alpha globulins but decreased albumin.

Medical and Surgical Management

Although RA cannot be cured, much can be done to minimize damage. Treatment goals include decreasing joint inflammation before bony ankylosis occurs, relieving discomfort, preventing or correcting deformities, and maintaining or restoring function of affected structures. Early treatment leads to the best results.

Optimal health conditions must be maintained because supporting the resistance of the body to the inflammation is one of the few truly therapeutic steps medicine has to offer. Rest, systemic and local, is balanced carefully with exercise. Unless the client has other medical complications, such as diabetes or hypertension, the diet need not be modified (Nutrition Notes 63-1).

Nutrition Notes 63-1

The Client With Rheumatoid Arthritis

- No conclusive evidence has shown that nutrition therapy can prevent or cure RA.
- Omega-3 fatty acids found in fatty fish (e.g., mackerel, herring, and salmon) and, to a lesser extent, in flaxseed, olive, and canola oils relieve joint tenderness and fatigue in some people, possibly by inhibiting the inflammatory response of certain prostaglandins. The use of fish oil supplements is not recommended, but eating more dietary sources of omega-3 fatty acids may be beneficial.
- Malnutrition is common among clients with RA; monitor weight changes.
- Discourage quack "cures" and self-prescribed supplements.

Concept Mastery Alert

Rheumatoid Arthritis

When a client with RA has experienced increasing pain and progressing inflammation of the hands and feet, the expected goal of the treatment regimen is to minimize damage. While treating pain is also important, it would not be the goal of the prescribed treatment.

Drug Therapy

Drug therapy is not curative but helps relieve pain and, in some instances, suppresses the inflammatory process. In general, the following classes of drug therapy may be ordered:

- *Nonsteroidal anti-inflammatory drugs* (NSAIDs)—NSAIDs relieve inflammation and pain by inhibiting the production of prostaglandins, which can damage joints. These include over-the-counter medications such as ibuprofen (Motrin, Advil) and naproxen (Aleve). Prescription medications such as cyclooxygenase-2 (COX-2) inhibitors may be used. COX is an enzyme involved in the inflammatory process; COX-2 inhibitors block this enzyme but do not interfere with the enzyme that protects the stomach lining, which is a common problem seen with other NSAIDs. Recent research associated the use of COX-2 inhibitors with an increased incidence of heart disease and led to the removal of some COX-2 inhibitors from the market. These medications are used with great caution.
- *Steroids*: Drugs such as prednisone and methylprednisolone (Medrol) are used to reduce pain and inflammation and slow joint destruction.
- *Disease-modifying antirheumatic drugs* (DMARDs): DMARDs reduce the amount of joint damage and slow damage to other tissues as well. Common DMARDs include hydroxychloroquine (Plaquenil), the gold compound auranofin (Ridaura), sulfasalazine (Azulfidine), minocycline (Dynacin, Minocin), and methotrexate (Rheumatrex).
- *Immunosuppressants*: Immunosuppressants calm the immune system, which is typically out of control for clients with RA. Drugs such as cyclosporine or azathioprine (Imuran) may be added to enhance the effects of methotrexate or may be used in clients with severe classic RA that does not respond to more conventional therapies.
- *Tumor necrosis factor (TNF)–alpha inhibitors*: TNF-alpha is an inflammatory cytokine for clients with RA; TNF-alpha inhibitors block the cytokine, thus reducing pain and inflammation. They often are given in conjunction with methotrexate. TNF inhibitors approved for treatment of RA are etanercept (Enbrel), infliximab (Remicade), and adalimumab (Humira).
- *Biologic response modifiers* are drugs that target parts of the immune system that are responsible for the inflammatory response that leads to damage of joint tissue. Biologic response modifiers can increase the risk for infection. Examples of these drugs include:
  - Anakinra (Kineret): similar to interleukin-1 receptor antagonist, a naturally occurring chemical in the body that stops the inflammation associated with RA
  - Abatacept (Orencia): inactivates T cells and reduces pain, inflammation, and joint damage
  - Rituximab (Rituxan): reduces the number of B cells in the body, which are involved with the inflammatory process
  - Tofacitinib (Xeljanz): a janus kinase (JAK) inhibitor, which disrupts JAK pathways that normally relay immune signals for specific proteins on white blood cells and thus reduces the inflammatory process associated with RA

Drug Therapy Table 63-1 provides more information about drugs used for RA. For many clients, combination therapy is initiated. As symptoms abate and remission occurs, drug doses are tapered. Local applications of heat and cold are used concurrently with drug therapy to relieve swelling and pain.

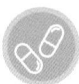

Pharmacologic Considerations

- DMARDs are designed to produce immunosuppression, so clients need to be monitored routinely for infections. Instruct clients to report any problem, no matter how minor, such as a cold or open sore—even these can become life-threatening.

Nondrug Therapy

An alternative treatment is the injection of viscosupplements (Hyalgan, Synvisc, and Supartz). Viscosupplements act as a lubricant, substituting for hyaluronic acid, the substance that provides joint fluid viscosity. Pain relief appears to last 6 to 13 months. Side effects include swelling, redness, or heat at the injection site. Clients allergic to eggs should not receive these injections (American Academy of Orthopedic Surgeons, 2021).

Surgery

Several surgical techniques may be performed to minimize or correct the joint deformities of RA (refer to Box 61-4).

DRUG THERAPY TABLE 63-1 Agents for Rheumatoid Arthritis

Category and Common Generic (Brand) Drugs	Intended Use	Common Side Effects	Safety Warnings for Nurses
Nonsteroidal Anti inflammatory (NSAIDs)			
Celecoxib (Celebrex) Ibuprofen (Motrin) Indomethacin (Indocin) Naproxen (Naprosyn)	Mild-to-moderate pain, antipyretic, anti-inflammatory, rheumatoid disorders, dysmenorrhea	Nausea, dyspepsia, constipation	• Risk of cardiovascular thrombosis, myocardial infarction, and stroke • Should not be used postoperative cardiac surgery
Salicylates Aspirin (Ecotrin, Ascriptin)	Stroke prevention in men (and women older than 65 years only) by inhibiting platelet aggregation and clotting	Nausea, vomiting, epigastric distress	• Monitor for tinnitus, indicates toxicity • Should not be taken as pain reliever when on anticoagulant therapy
Glucocorticosteroids			
Oral Prednisone	Inhibit inflammatory immune response	Acne, water retention, weight gain, hair loss, increased appetite	• With food to decrease gastric irritation • Monitor for higher blood glucose in clients with diabetes • Abrupt withdrawal may precipitate Addison's disease crisis
Disease-Modifying Antirheumatic Drugs (DMARDs)			
Methotrexate sulfasalazine (Azulfidine) Hydroxychloroquine (Plaquenil) Leflunomide[a] (Arava)	Produces immune suppression, which in turn reduces inflammation	Nausea, diarrhea, stomatitis, alopecia	Monitor for rashes, may be Stevens–Johnson syndrome Monitor vision for corneal changes Do not use if pregnant[a]
Disease-Modifying Antirheumatic Drugs—Biologics (DMARDs)			
Biologic Agents Abatacept (Orencia) Adalimumab (Humira) Anakinra (Kineret) Certolizumab pegol (Cimzia) Etanercept (Enbrel) Golimumab (Simponi) Infliximab (Remicade) Tocilizumab (Actemra)	Rheumatoid arthritis by neutralizing immune proteins reducing inflammation	Fever, chills, headache, muscle aches, diarrhea	• Immune suppression makes more susceptible to infections • Frequent lab work for immune suppression • Do not use if client has heart failure • Do not use if pregnant
Cytotoxic Drugs			
Mercaptopurine Azathioprine (Imuran) Lesser used agents, reserved when disease is unresponsive to other agents	Inhibit inflammatory immune response of T and B cells (lymphocytes)	Increased vulnerability to infection, rash, nausea, vomiting, diarrhea	• Immune suppression makes more susceptible to infections • Frequent lab work for immune suppression • Use barrier method birth control

Superscripts (e.g., [a]) on drugs in column 1 indicate the drug that matches up with explanations in the other three columns.

Many individuals with various types of arthritis undergo an **arthroplasty**, or reconstruction of the joint, using an artificial joint that restores previously lost function and relieves pain. Refer to Chapter 61 for a more in-depth discussion of reconstructive joint surgery. In addition, clients with RA may have a **synovectomy**, which is a procedure to remove the lining of the joint. This procedure is performed when the lining is inflamed and adding to the pain the client is experiencing.

Nursing Management

Nursing management involves teaching clients about the disease and providing information about maintaining general health, relieving pain, reducing stress, decreasing the inflammatory process, and preserving joint mobility. The nurse also instructs clients about the medication regimen, particularly therapeutic and adverse effects. Other nursing activities center on how to apply heat and cold packs locally or how to use a transcutaneous electrical nerve stimulation

(TENS) unit to relieve pain in a particular joint. A TENS unit has electrodes that are applied to the skin from a portable stimulation unit that the client learns to operate.

Nurses collaborate with occupational therapists to provide equipment, utensils, and instruction regarding energy conservation and maintenance of joint alignment. Physical therapists (PTs) plan an appropriate exercise regimen. Home care planning involves providing nursing assistance for ADLs and ensuring that the home environment is safe. Out of consideration for the typical pain and morning stiffness, the nurse teaches the nursing assistant to allow extra time for completing hygiene or other procedures.

When joints are severely inflamed, the use of a splint may reduce but not totally eliminate active motion. Even during an acute episode, the nurse encourages the client to move affected parts gently to help lessen the possibility of ankylosis, muscle wasting, osteoporosis, and the debilitating effects of prolonged rest. Clients must avoid positions of flexion.

The nurse continues to urge the client to eat nutritious, well-balanced meals despite anorexia. As joints become deformed and destroyed, the techniques and equipment used to perform ADLs may require modification. Clients need assistance to deal with chronic pain, changes in function, changes in appearance, and related depression and feelings of helplessness. Education about the disease is essential because many people spend large sums of money on unscientific treatments in hopes of a cure.

>>> *Stop, Think, and Respond 63-1*

A 35-year-old woman recently diagnosed with RA asks you if her disease happened because she experimented with marijuana and drank a lot of alcohol in her adolescence. How would you respond?

Degenerative Joint Disease

Degenerative joint disease (DJD), also referred to as *osteoarthritis* (OA), is the most common form of arthritis. It also is known as the "wear and tear" disease and typically affects the weight-bearing joints. It is characterized by a slow and steady progression of destructive changes in weight-bearing joints and those that are repeatedly used for work. Unlike RA, OA has no remissions and no systemic symptoms, such as malaise and fever. Table 63-1 compares OA and RA.

Pathophysiology and Etiology

A lifetime of repeated trauma leads to degenerative joint changes. Hips, knees, the spine, and the DIP joints in the hands commonly are affected. Risk factors include increasing age, previous joint injury, obesity, congenital and developmental disorders (such as Legg–Calvé–Perthes disease), hereditary factors, and decreased bone density. OA may be classified as *primary*, which is disease without a known etiology, or *secondary*, when OA has an underlying cause such as injury, obesity, inactivity, or a congenital disorder.

TABLE 63-1 Comparison of Rheumatoid Arthritis and Osteoarthritis

	RHEUMATOID ARTHRITIS	OSTEOARTHRITIS
Age	Usually between 20 and 50 years old	Usually after age 40
Sex	More common in women than men	Before age 45, more common in men; after age 45, more common in women, especially in the hands
Onset	May develop suddenly (weeks or months)	Develops slowly over many years
Symptoms		
Pain	General achiness; nocturnal pain; pain at rest	Deep, aching pain with motion early in the disease; later, pain at rest
Stiffness	Morning stiffness that lasts at least 1 hour	Stiffness localized to involved joints, which rarely exceeds 20 minutes; often related to weather
Joint motion	Decreased	Limited
Other	Depression, fatigue, low-grade fever, anorexia, malaise, weakness, weight loss	Instability of weight-bearing joints; crepitus; crackling
Physical signs	If multiple joints involved, usually symmetric Joints typically involved are hands (small joints), feet (small joints), wrists, elbows, knees, ankles, and shoulders. Hand deformities include ulnar deviation and subluxation of metacarpophalangeal joints. Joints may be tender, swollen, and red. Synovial fluid is thin and cloudy with elevated protein and polymorphonuclear cell levels.	One or many joints involved, asymmetric Joints typically involved are hands (first carpometacarpal joint), feet (first metatarsophalangeal joint), hips, knees, cervical, and lumbar spine. Joints bony proliferation or occasional synovitis; local tenderness; crepitus; muscle atrophy; effusions Synovial fluid—high viscosity with mild leukocytosis (WBC: <2000 cells/mm^3)
Laboratory values	RF elevated in 80% of clients with RA Elevated ESR Decreased RBC and C4 complement	No specific test ESR and hematologic survey results are normal. No systemic manifestations

ESR, erythrocyte sedimentation rate; RA, rheumatoid arthritis; RBC, red blood cell; RF, rheumatoid factor; WBC, white blood cell.

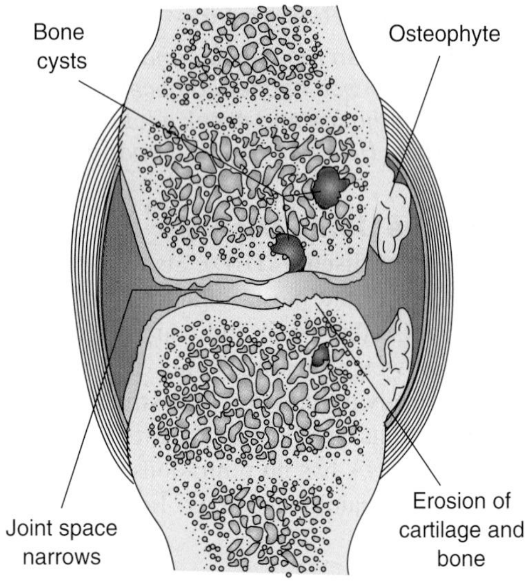

Figure 63-4 Joint changes in osteoarthritis.

The degenerative process begins when the cartilage that covers the bone ends becomes thin, rough, and ragged. Malacia or soft spots develop. The cartilage no longer springs back into shape after normal use. As the cartilage wears away, the joint space decreases, so the bone surfaces are closer and rub together. In an attempt to repair the damaged surface, new bone develops in the form of bone spurs, bone cysts, or osteophytes, which are extended margins of the joints. The joint becomes deformed, and the client experiences pain and limited joint movement. Ankylosis does not occur, but the resulting deformity may partially dislocate the joint. Structures around the affected joint, such as the joint, capsule, synovial membrane, and ligaments, demonstrate degenerative changes. Figure 63-4 depicts the joint changes seen in OA.

Assessment Findings

Early symptoms are brief joint stiffness and pain after a period of inactivity. The pain usually increases with heavy use and is relieved by rest. Later, even rest may not adequately relieve the pain. Eventually, the joint undergoes enlargement and increased limitation of movement. When DJD afflicts the hands, the fingers frequently develop painless bony nodules on the dorsolateral surface of the interphalangeal joints: **Heberden nodes** (bony enlargement of the distal interphalangeal [DIP] joints; Fig. 63-5) and **Bouchard nodes** (bony enlargement of the proximal interphalangeal [PIP] joints). Crepitus may be heard and felt when the joint is moved. The range of motion (ROM) of the affected joint becomes progressively limited, and stiffness and pain increase.

X-rays demonstrate disruption of the joint cartilage and bony changes. Magnetic resonance imaging (MRI) provides detailed images of bones and cartilage and the surrounding soft tissues. Some clients may have a slightly elevated ESR. Fluid may be aspirated from the affected joint to ascertain if there is inflammation, infection, or other disease process, such as gout.

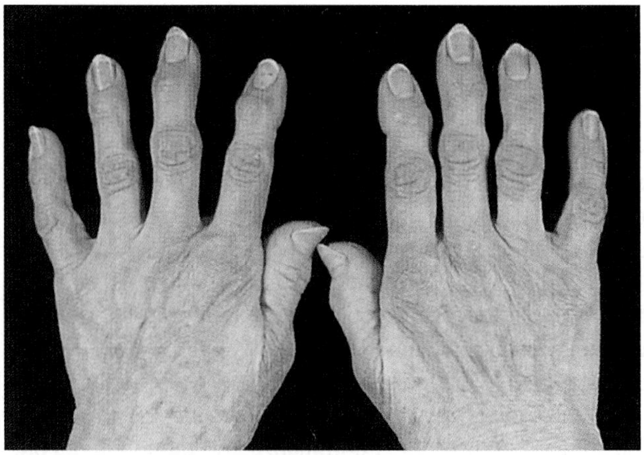

Figure 63-5 Heberden nodes.

Medical and Surgical Management

Nonpharmacologic treatment includes local rest of the affected joints, which is emphasized more than total body rest. Heat applied to the painful part may afford some relief. Weight loss is recommended for obese clients. Splints, braces, canes, or crutches may reduce discomfort, relieve pain, and prevent further destruction of the affected joints. An exercise program helps to preserve joint ROM and strength. Clients should not engage in activity that places excessive stress on affected joints. A TENS unit may help reduce joint pain.

Large doses of acetaminophen may be used initially along with nonpharmacologic treatments. If acetaminophen is ineffective, however, systemic anti-inflammatory drugs, such as aspirin and NSAIDs, are prescribed. Although these drugs do not prevent or cure OA, they may decrease its severity. Corticosteroids may be injected into acutely inflamed joints with limited success. When possible, long-term use of these agents is avoided. Use of narcotics is deferred because of the disorder's chronic nature. Topical analgesics such as diclofenac sodium gel (Voltaren Gel), an NSAID, may be prescribed. The gels are applied directly to the affected joint. The intra-articulation injection of hyaluronic acid, referred to as *viscosupplementation*, theoretically improves cartilage function and interferes with its breakdown (American Academy of Orthopedic Surgeons, 2021). For some clients, duloxetine (Cymbalta), primarily used as an antidepressant, is prescribed for chronic pain, including clients with OA.

Many clients eventually have joint replacement surgery, particularly at a time when mobility and quality of life are compromised. The most frequently replaced joints include the knee and the hip; other joints also replaced are the shoulder and finger joints. Refer to Chapter 61 for more information about reconstructive surgery.

Nursing Management

The nurse teaches about the purpose of drug therapy, administration times, and therapeutic and side effects. Because aspirin and NSAIDs can cause gastric bleeding, the nurse advises clients to take the medication with food. It is important that the client maintains moderate activity, with instructions about how to regulate the type, vigor, and frequency according to the symptoms experienced. If the client is overweight, they need explanations about dietary changes that promote weight loss. The nurse may need to remind the client to assume good posture to avoid unusual stress on a joint. If the client needs ambulatory aids such as crutches, a cane, or a walker, they will need a referral to a PT for fitting and practice.

When a client is taking NSAIDs for pain, ask about proton pump inhibitors (PPI) self-treatment for heartburn. NSAIDs and salicylates can cause gastric distress. With PPI available over the counter, client may self-treat GI problems. There is a correlation between bone density reduction and PPIs (Fattahi et al., 2019). Be aware of this risk as you care for your client.

Temporomandibular Disorder

TMD is a cluster of symptoms localized near the jaw.

Pathophysiology and Etiology

Causes of TMD include degenerative arthritis of the mandibular joint, malocclusion of the teeth, bruxism (grinding of the teeth), dislocation of the jaw during endotracheal intubation, or other jaw injuries and trauma.

TMD occurs when the meniscus, or cartilaginous disk, between the condyle (end of the mandible) and the temporal bone becomes displaced from the fossa (socket) of the temporal bone (Fig. 63-6). Because facial muscles such as the masseter and temporalis muscles move this gliding joint, the client develops jaw pain from muscle spasms. If the cartilage wears away, there is a grating sensation when opening and closing the jaw; the client may hear a clicking sound when the joint moves. The joint may even lock periodically. Sometimes, nerves and arteries in the area are compressed. The disorder can be confused with trigeminal neuralgia and migraine headache (see Chapter 38).

Assessment Findings

Symptoms include jaw pain, pronounced muscle spasm, and tenderness of the masseter and temporalis muscles. Headache, tinnitus (ringing in the ears), and ear pain accompany the localized discomfort. The client experiences clicking of the jaw when moving the joint, or the jaw can lock, which interferes with opening the mouth. Some clients experience difficulty or discomfort chewing. In some instances, the joint locks, making it difficult to open or close the jaw. Special dental X-rays often reveal evidence of joint displacement.

Medical and Surgical Management

Treatment is referral to a dentist who has experience managing clients with TMD. Analgesics are prescribed or recommended, such as NSAIDs. The client is fitted with a custom mouth guard during sleep. TENS, injection of a local anesthetic to relieve muscle spasm, muscle relaxants, and oral irrigations with ice water also are used to reduce and relieve discomfort. Tricyclic antidepressants (amitriptyline) are sometimes prescribed to relieve pain. Reconstructive surgery of the temporomandibular joint (TMJ) is available if conservative treatment is ineffective.

Nursing Management

The nurse monitors the client's weight and ability to consume food. If indicated, the nurse obtains a nutritional consultation with the dietitian. With the help of the dietitian, the nurse modifies the diet to include soft rather than coarse food, which is easier to chew. They provide nutritional liquid supplements and assists the client to acquire skills that control pain, such as using a bite guard during sleep.

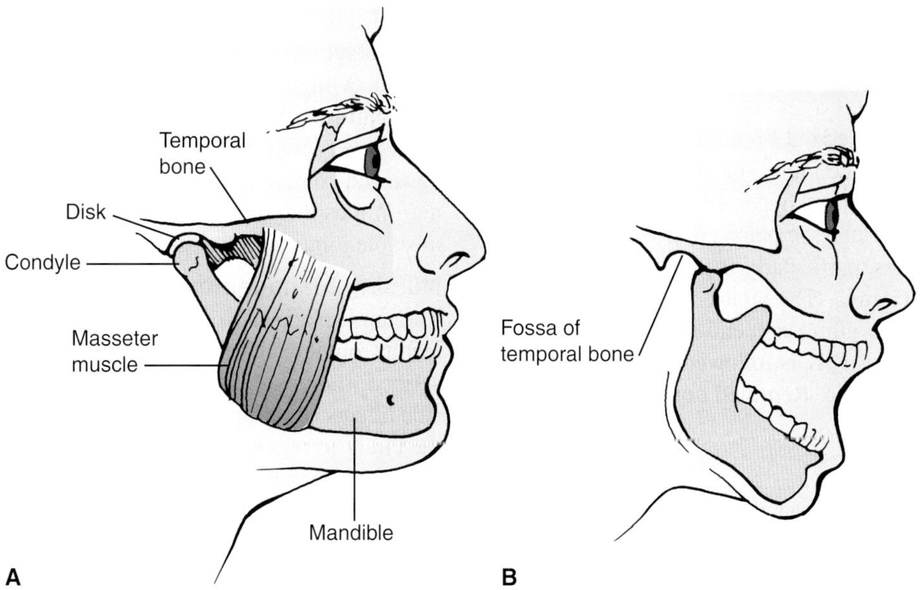

Figure 63-6 **(A)** The temporomandibular joint is located between the two bones for which it is named: the temporal bone and mandible. **(B)** The condyle of the mandible, which is covered by a cartilaginous disk, moves forward and backward within the fossa of the temporal bone of the skull, which is located in front of the ear.

Gout

Gout is a painful metabolic arthritic disorder involving an inflammatory reaction in the joints. It usually affects the feet (especially the great toe), hands, elbows, ankles, and knees.

Pathophysiology and Etiology

The disorder tends to be inherited and affects more men than women. Gout may occur secondary to other diseases marked by decreased renal excretion of uric acid. It also has been identified among clients who have received organ transplants and the antirejection drug cyclosporine.

Gout is characterized by **hyperuricemia** (accumulation of uric acid in the blood) caused by alterations in uric acid production, excretion, or both. Hyperuricemia occurs from one or a combination of the following pathologies:

- Primary hyperuricemia
  - Severe dieting or starvation
  - Excessive ingestion of purines (organ meats, steak, shellfish, sardines)
  - Heredity
- Secondary hyperuricemia
  - Abnormal purine metabolism
  - Increased rate of protein synthesis with overproduction or underexcretion of uric acid
  - Increased cellular turnover, as in leukemia, multiple myeloma, and other cancers; some anemias; and psoriasis
  - Decreased excretion of uric acid, as a result diuretics, salicylates, and/or excessive alcohol intake, particularly beer

Urate (a salt of uric acid) crystallizes in body tissues and is deposited in soft and bony tissues, causing local inflammation and irritation. Collections of urate crystals, called **tophi**, are found in the cartilage of the outer ear (pinna), the great toe, hands, and other joints; ligaments; bursae; and tendons. As these deposits accumulate, they destroy the joint, producing a chronically swollen, deformed appearance. The uric acid also may precipitate in urine, causing renal stones.

Assessment Findings

Signs and Symptoms

A gout attack is characterized by a sudden onset of acute pain and tenderness in one joint. The skin turns red and the joint swells, so it is warm and hypersensitive to touch. Fever may be present. Tophi may be palpated around the fingers, great toes, or earlobes, particularly if the client has chronic and severe hyperuricemia. The attack may last for 1 or 2 weeks, but moderate swelling and tenderness may persist. A symptom-free period usually is followed by another attack, which may occur any time. Repeated episodes in the same joint may deform the joint.

Diagnostic Findings

Diagnosis usually is based on the obvious clinical signs and hyperuricemia. Synovial fluid aspirated from the joint during arthrocentesis contains urate crystals. The urate deposits also may be identifiable with a radiographic examination. Elevated uric acid levels in serum and urine (24-hour urine collection) correlate with gout, but these findings are common to other disorders as well. Ultrasound is occasionally done to detect tophi or crystals.

Medical and Surgical Management

Although gout cannot be cured in the sense of removing the basic metabolic difficulty of constant or recurrent hyperuricemia, the attacks usually can be controlled. The aim of treatment is to decrease sodium urate in the extracellular fluid so deposits do not form.

Two main treatment approaches involve (1) using uricosuric drugs that promote renal excretion of urates by inhibiting the reabsorption of uric acid in the renal tubules and (2) decreasing ingestion of purine. The regimen is individualized and may be changed in response to the changes in the course of the disease.

Pain during a severe acute attack may require NSAIDs, such as ibuprofen and indomethacin. Acute attacks of gout also may be treated with colchicine or phenylbutazone. Colchicine is administered every 1 or 2 hours until the pain subsides or nausea, vomiting, intestinal cramping, and diarrhea develop. When one or more of these symptoms occur, the drug should be stopped temporarily. Drugs used for long-term gout management include colchicine, allopurinol (Zyloprim), probenecid (Benemid), indomethacin (Indocin), and sulfinpyrazone (Anturane). To prevent future attacks, drug therapy continues after the acute attack subsides (Drug Therapy Table 63-2). Salicylates inactivate uricosurics, and clients with a history of gout should not use them. For clients who cannot tolerate NSAIDs or colchicine, oral corticosteroids may be prescribed. They may also be injected into the affected joint(s).

It is now known that the body can synthesize purines; thus, emphasis on strict diet restriction has decreased, with more focus on the use of uricosuric drugs. The prescribed diet includes adequate protein, with limitation of purine-rich foods to avoid contributing to the underlying problem. The diet prescription also is relatively high in complex carbohydrates and low in fats because carbohydrates increase urate excretion and fats retard it. Overweight clients are encouraged to lose weight. A high fluid intake helps increase excretion of uric acid. Nutrition Notes 63-2 outlines additional considerations.

Surgery may be performed to remove the large tophi of advanced gout. Surgery also may be used to correct crippling deformities that may result from treatment delays or to fuse unstable joints and increase their function.

Nursing Management

The nurse places a bed cradle over the affected joint to protect it from the pressure of the bed linen. If colchicine is prescribed, they explain about the hourly administration until side effects occur or acute pain subsides. The nurse instructs the client to report GI symptoms. They measure intake and output, especially when diarrhea accompanies colchicine therapy for acute gout. The nurse provides clear explanations of long-term drug and diet therapy before discharge.

Observe for anaphylaxis if pegloticase is administered. Clients should be premedicated with antihistamines and corticosteroids before IV injection and appropriately monitored after for reactions.

DRUG THERAPY TABLE 63-2 Selected Anti-Gout Medications

Category and Common Generic (Brand) Drugs	Intended Use	Common Side Effects	Safety Warnings for Nurses
Agents—For Acute Pain Relief			
Nonsteroidal Anti-inflammatory Drugs (NSAIDs) Celecoxib (Celebrex) Ibuprofen (Motrin) Indomethacin (Indocin) Naproxen (Naprosyn)	Mild-to-moderate pain, antipyretic, anti-inflammatory, rheumatoid disorders	Nausea, dyspepsia, constipation	• Risk of cardiovascular thrombosis, myocardial infarction, and stroke • Should not be used postoperative cardiac surgery
Glucocorticosteroids Prednisone	Inhibit inflammatory immune response	Acne, water retention, weight gain, hair loss, increased appetite	• With food to decrease gastric irritation • Monitor for higher blood glucose in clients with diabetes • Abrupt withdrawal may precipitate Addison's disease crisis
Colchicine	Relief of acute attacks of gout by reducing uric acid, prevention of gout attacks	Nausea, vomiting, abdominal pain, bone marrow depression	• Reduce dose if diarrhea occurs • Do not eat grapefruit • Reacts with "statin" drugs and antivirals
Uric Acid Inhibitors—For Chronic Management			
Allopurinol (Zyloprim) Febuxostat (Uloric) Probenecid	Reducing uric acid, to manage symptoms of gout	Headache, nausea	• Gout pain flare may occur, do not discontinue drug • Monitor for rashes, may be Stevens–Johnson syndrome
Pegloticase (Krystexxa)	Refractory gout when above agents not effective, to manage symptoms of gout	Nausea, rash, infusion reaction	• Monitor uric acid levels • Observe for anaphylaxis • Premedicate before injection

Fibromyalgia Syndrome

Fibromyalgia syndrome is a chronic inflammatory illness consisting of musculoskeletal pain, fatigue, mood disorders, and sleep disturbances. The pain is widespread, affecting muscles, ligaments, and tendons.

Nutrition Notes 63-2

The Client With Gout

- During an acute attack, high-purine foods are avoided, including organ meats, gravies, meat extracts, anchovies, herring, mackerel, sardines, and scallops.
- Gradual weight loss helps reduce serum uric acid levels in clients with gout. Clients should avoid fasting, low-carbohydrate diets, and rapid weight loss because these measures increase the likelihood of ketone formation, which inhibits uric acid excretion.
- A high-carbohydrate diet promotes urate excretion, as does a low-fat diet. These modifications are recommended even if weight loss is not attempted. To reduce the risk of renal calculi, a complication of prolonged immobility and gout, advise clients to drink at least 2 quarts of fluid daily. Drinking fluid before bed and during the night helps keep the urine dilute.
- Alcohol is eliminated because it can contribute to an attack.

Pathophysiology and Etiology

The research on fibromyalgia is focused on explaining the cause(s) of this disorder. Current thinking is that clients with fibromyalgia experience magnified pain because of abnormal sensory processing in the central nervous system. Various physiologic abnormalities are found in many clients with fibromyalgia, such as increased levels of substance P (neuropeptide involved in neurotransmission), low blood flow to the thalamus region (where motor and sensory signals are relayed to the cerebral cortex) of the brain, and low levels of serotonin (neurotransmitter that influences pain perception). In addition, genetic factors may increase clients' susceptibility to fibromyalgia. Some diseases, such as RA, may be a factor in triggering or aggravating symptoms of fibromyalgia. Emotional or physical trauma is sometimes associated with the onset of symptoms.

Approximately 10 million people in the United States are diagnosed with fibromyalgia (National Fibromyalgia Association, n.d.). Women, particularly women who are mid-life, are most vulnerable to fibromyalgia, but the syndrome does affect men and children as well. Although it seems more prevalent and common today, fibromyalgia has been in existence for hundreds of years but was never accurately diagnosed.

Assessment Findings

Signs and Symptoms

Widespread and chronic pain is the most common finding. The American College of Rheumatology (2010) revised the diagnostic criteria used for fibromyalgia, making the criteria less stringent. These criteria include a history of widespread pain lasting at least 3 months and no evidence of other underlying conditions as a cause of the pain; physical symptoms of fatigue and waking unrefreshed; and cognitive issues with memory and thought processes (sometimes referred to as "fibro fog"). Some clients also experience chronic headaches and TMJ, heightened sensitivity to lights, noise and touch, and depression and/or anxiety.

Diagnostic Findings

Diagnosis is often difficult and involves ruling out other diseases and conditions. The presence of widespread and chronic pain in all four quadrants of the body, but most especially the axial chest, neck, and back, is particularly a hallmark for diagnosing fibromyalgia. Initial tests are done for blood counts, chemistry profile, thyroid levels, Lyme disease titer, and CRP, mostly to rule out other conditions. Generally, clients are diagnosed based on all of their symptoms and not so much through specific tests.

Medical Management

Treatment of fibromyalgia is challenging. The goals are to make the client feel better overall, decrease pain, and improve sleep. Antidepressants such as duloxetine (Cymbalta) and milnacipran (Savella) may assist with pain and fatigue. Antiseizure medications, such as pregabalin (Lyrica), may be prescribed to reduce pain and fatigue and improve sleep quality. Tricyclic antidepressants (TCAs), especially amitriptyline, are used with some success for treating chronic pain and promoting sleep. Analgesics, including acetaminophen and NSAIDs, are prescribed to alleviate some of the painful symptoms of fibromyalgia. Tramadol (Ultram), a prescription pain reliever, may be taken with or without acetaminophen. Muscle relaxants such as cyclobenzaprine (Flexeril) may be prescribed short-term at bedtime to help with muscle aches. Other medications are prescribed for treatment of specific symptoms a client may experience with fibromyalgia, such as antiepileptics (gabapentin) for burning pain and corticosteroids as anti-inflammatory agents.

Some clients benefit from acupuncture treatments, massage therapy, cognitive behavior therapy, biofeedback, aquatherapy, and hypnotherapy. Clients are counseled to restructure their lives in order to promote rest and sleep, reduce stress, increase exercise, and improve nutrition. Some clients are advised to change or reduce their work schedules in order to improve overall health. See Evidence-Based Practice 63-1, which discusses traditional treatment as well as complementary and alternative therapies.

Nursing Management

Nursing care focuses on providing support to clients. Often, clients have endured disturbing symptoms for a long period of time and feel that they were not believed. Encouraging clients to live a healthy lifestyle is important. This includes a healthy diet, avoidance of caffeine and alcohol, regular exercise, decreased stress, and adequate sleep. A support group may prove helpful, so clients can share their experiences. It is important to refer clients to reliable sources for fibromyalgia, such as the National Fibromyalgia Association, and to remind them not to engage in treatments that have not been verified.

Bursitis

Bursitis is an inflammation of the bursa, a fluid-filled sac that cushions bone ends to enhance a gliding movement. The elbow, shoulder, and knee are common sites of bursitis.

Pathophysiology and Etiology

The most common cause of bursitis is repetitive motion or positioning that cause irritation to the bursa. Other causes include trauma, stress, infection, and secondary effects of

Evidence-Based Practice 63-1

Fibromyalgia Syndrome and Treatment That Includes Complementary and Alternative Therapies

Clinical Question

In clients with fibromyalgia syndrome (FS), how does traditional treatment alone compare with traditional treatment plus complementary and alternative therapies (CAM) to affect symptom relief?

Evidence

Three systematic reviews report on the evaluation of research studies that look at a common issue or topic. It is estimated that between 2% and 4% of the population are diagnosed with FS (Tzadok & Ablin, 2020). Many clients diagnosed with FS seek CAM therapies when traditional treatments do not bring desired results, or side effects and costs of medications and traditional therapies leave less than desirable results. It is important that clients make informed decisions regarding CAM therapies.

A number of research studies have been done on CAM therapies for treating FS. Mohabbat et al. (2019) is a 14-year follow-up completed in 2017 after initial contact with clients in 2003. These clients were initially diagnosed with FS and completed a survey to determine the use of CAM during this time. Of the 310 clients surveyed, 98.1% reported some type of CAM use as compared to the 98% CAM use in 2003. Altinbilek et al. (2019) is a multicentered study involving 72 clients diagnosed with FS. This study used neural therapy as a type of CAM to reduce pain and depression. Neural therapy was used once a week for 6 weeks. Early stage results showed additional benefits in these areas as compared to traditional treatments. Lowry et al. (2020) conducted a systematic review regarding dietary effects of CAM treatments for FS. Lower et al. (2020) looked at 22 nutritional intervention studies including pain, severity of disease, general health, mental health, and cognitive function. Improvement in pain and severity of disease were observed in clients who implemented dietary changes such as a vegan diet, use of Coenzyme Q10, vitamins C and E, and consumption of extra-virgin olive oil. Limited-to-moderate results were seen in manipulative therapies such as chiropractic and massage. All reviewers agreed that there was a wide range of quality in the studies and recommended that continued research be conducted on all CAM therapies for FS.

Evidence-Based Practice 63-1 (*continued*)

Nursing Implications

A major part of nurses' roles in caring for clients diagnosed with FS is lending support, education, and encouragement. Having knowledge about CAM therapies allows the nurse to share information about research and resources with clients so they and their primary caregivers can explore them together. Guided imagery, meditation, and mindfulness recordings are often available for free through the Internet or public library, making them accessible to clients. Making these types of CAM interventions available offers opportunity for symptom improvement with minimal-to-no risk of harm.

References

Altınbilek, T., Terzi, R., Baçaran, A., Tolu, S., & Küçüksaraç, S. (2019). Evaluation of the effects of neural therapy in patients diagnosed with fibromyalgia. *Turkish Journal of Physical Medicine and Rehabilitation*, *65*(1), 1–8. https://www.ncbi.nlm.nih.gov/pmc/articles/PMC6648183/

Lowry, E., Marley, J., McVeigh, J. G., McSorley, E., Allsopp, P., & Kerr, D. (2020). Dietary interventions in the management of fibromyalgia: A systematic review and best-evidence synthesis. *Nutrients*, *12*(9), 2664. https://doi.org/10.3390/nu12092664

Mohabbat, A. B., Mahapatra, S., Jenkins, S. M., Bauer, B. A., Vincent, A., & Wahner-Roedler, D. L. (2019). Use of complementary and integrative therapies by fibromyalgia patients: A 14-year follow-up study. *Mayo Clinic Proceedings: Innovations, Quality & Outcomes*, *3*(4), 418–428. https://doi.org/10.1016/j.mayocpiqo.2019.07.003.

gout and RA. Typical of any inflammation, pain and swelling occur with compromised function.

Assessment Findings

Painful movement of a joint, such as the elbow or shoulder, is the most common symptom. A distinct lump may be felt. If the bursa ruptures, tissue in the area may become edematous, warm, and tender.

Diagnosis is often made with the client's presenting symptoms and physical exam. An X-ray study may reveal a calcified bursa. An ultrasound or MRI may be done if the health care provider cannot make a definitive diagnosis. Aspiration of fluid may be done. It can demonstrate the following:

- A few leukocytes in transparent fluid if the etiology is trauma
- A large collection of leukocytes if the cause is sepsis
- Colonies of staphylococcal or streptococcal microorganisms
- Urate crystals in bursitis secondary to gout
- Cholesterol crystals, common in clients with bursitis and RA, which may cause the fluid from the bursa to appear cloudy

Medical and Surgical Management

Joint rest usually is recommended. Salicylates or NSAIDs may be prescribed. If the problem persists, a corticosteroid preparation may be injected into the joint to reduce inflammation. After pain and inflammation are reduced, ongoing therapy involves mild ROM exercises. If infection is the cause, antibiotics will be ordered.

Nursing Management

The nurse reviews the prescribed medication and exercise regimens with the client and allows time for questions and answers. They advise the client not to traumatize or overuse the recovering joint but to use it normally. Failure to use the joint after pain and inflammation are controlled may result in partial limitation of joint motion.

Ankylosing Spondylitis

Ankylosing spondylitis is a chronic connective tissue disorder of the spine and surrounding cartilaginous joints, such as the sacroiliac joints and soft tissues around the vertebrae. Characteristics include spondylosis and fusion of the vertebrae.

Pathophysiology and Etiology

Ankylosing spondylitis usually begins in early adulthood and is more common in men than in women. Its etiology is unknown, although some theorize that an altered immune response occurs when T-cell lymphocytes mistake human cells for similar-appearing bacterial antigens. There also is a strong familial tendency for some affected individuals. Once the inflammation begins, it continues, causing progressive immobility and fixation (ankylosis) of the joints in the hips, and ascends the vertebrae. Respiratory function may be compromised if kyphosis (a hunchback-like spinal curve) develops. In a few cases, there may be extra-articular (nonjoint) manifestations, such as aortitis (inflammation of the aorta), iridocyclitis (inflammation of the iris and ciliary body of the eye), and pulmonary fibrosis.

Assessment Findings

Signs and Symptoms

The most common symptoms are low back and hip pain and stiffness. As the disease progresses, the spine and hips become more immobile, thus restricting movement. The lumbar curve of the spine may flatten. The neck can be permanently flexed, and the client appears to be in a perpetual stooped position. Aortic regurgitation or atrioventricular node conduction disturbances may occur. Lung sounds may be reduced, especially in the apical areas. The client may experience fatigue, anorexia, and weight loss.

Diagnostic Findings

Evidence of inflammation is demonstrated by an elevated ESR. A culture of synovial fluid, however, is negative for causative microorganisms. Elevations of alkaline phosphatase and creatinine phosphokinase levels are common. An HLA test, used for determining inherited tissue markers for immune functions, demonstrates the presence of the *HLA-B27* gene in 90% of clients with this disorder. However, the majority of people with this gene do not have ankylosing spondylitis. X-rays, computed tomography (CT) scans, or MRI shows erosion, ossification, and fusion of the joints in the spine and hips.

Medical and Surgical Management

Treatment is supportive, the major goal being to maintain functional posture. NSAIDs such as naproxen or indomethacin are usually prescribed for relieving inflammation and pain. Drugs used to treat RA may also be prescribed, such as DMARDs and TNF blockers. Sleeping on a firm mattress (preferably without a pillow) and following a prescribed exercise program may help delay or prevent spinal deformity, especially if begun in the early stages of the disease. A back brace also may be prescribed for some clients. Severe hip involvement may be treated with a total hip replacement. Physical therapy may be prescribed, with the goals of increasing strength and flexibility and reducing pain.

Nursing Management

The nurse administers prescribed drugs and clarifies information about the disease. They encourage the client to perform ADLs as much as possible. The nurse teaches the client to perform mild exercises that reduce stiffness and pain. They provide emotional support, recognizing that the client must deal with pain, skeletal changes, and impaired mobility.

Systemic Lupus Erythematosus

Systemic lupus erythematosus (SLE) is an autoimmune disorder that involves diffuse connective tissue changes and chronic inflammation. As the name implies, it affects multiple body systems such as the skin, joints, kidneys, heart, lungs, brain, and lymph nodes.

Pathophysiology and Etiology

The pathogenesis of SLE involves a disturbance of immune regulatory processes, resulting in overproduction of autoantibodies. Antibodies destroy connective tissues of the body. Affected structures undergo inflammation, fibrosis, scarring, and dysfunction. Polymorphonuclear leukocytes (neutrophils) engulf the nuclei of attacked cells. Laboratory studies confirm this finding, which is considered diagnostic.

Hormonal factors and strong family history appear to be factors, suggesting that certain inherited cellular antigenic markers confuse the ability of T cells to distinguish self from nonself. By mistake, helper T cells alert B cells to produce antibodies against normal cells, or suppressor T cells may be ineffective in controlling a B-cell response once it has been initiated. The disease has periods of illness, referred to as *flares*, and then periods during which it is in a subacute form or even in remission. Exposure to ultraviolet light is a factor in reactivating the disease.

SLE is more common in women than in men. It affects women who are Black Americans, of African descent, of Hispanic or Latinx ethnicity, of Asian descent, and Native North American descent more than women who are non-Hispanic White and/or of European descent. There is more serious organ involvement in women who are Black American, of African descent, and of Hispanic or Latinx ethnicity. SLE generally occurs between the ages of 15 and 45, but it can occur at any age. As already stated, there is often a familial and genetic component, but other factors may include hormones, sunlight, stress, viruses, and cigarette smoke. Studies have confirmed that the cause for SLE in genetically susceptible clients is a previous infection with the Epstein–Barr virus (which also causes mononucleosis). Some medications may also trigger SLE, such as those used to treat seizures, hypertension, and infections. When the medications are discontinued, the symptoms decrease or disappear.

Assessment Findings

Signs and Symptoms

SLE is known as the *great imitator* because the clinical signs resemble many other conditions (Box 63-2). SLE is also marked by remissions and exacerbations. Early signs and symptoms of SLE may include fever, weight loss, pain in the joints (arthralgia), malaise, muscle pain, and extreme fatigue. These symptoms are vague and may persist for several months to 2 years before more prominent symptoms develop and the client seeks medical advice.

A prominent sign for about half of the clients with SLE is a red, butterfly-shaped rash known as *malar rash*, on the face over the bridge of the nose and the cheeks (Fig. 63-7). The word *lupus* means "wolf." The term may have been used as a description for the facial rash that, to some, resembled the mask of reddish-brown fur on a wolf.

Two other types of skin manifestations may occur with SLE. The first is discoid lupus erythematosus (DLE), which involves a chronic rash with erythematous papules or plaques and scaling. Eventually, DLE can lead to scarring and pigmentation changes. The symptoms of DLE are related only to the skin, the most prominent symptom being the appearance of the facial rash. Skin manifestations of the disorder also may be found on the forehead, earlobes, and scalp. Scalp involvement usually results in patchy loss of hair (alopecia). These symptoms also may be seen in people with SLE. The second type is subacute cutaneous lupus erythematosus, which presents with papulosquamous lesions.

Clients also may exhibit behavioral disturbances (confusion, hallucinations, irritability), chest pain (as a result of involvement of the pleura or pericarditis), fluid retention, proteinuria, and hematuria (as a result of renal involvement);

BOX 63-2 Clinical Manifestations of Systemic Lupus Erythematosus

SLE is known as the *great imitator*, with manifestations that resemble many other diseases.

- *Constitutional*: fevers, fatigue, anorexia, weight loss
- *Musculoskeletal*: arthritis, muscle weakness and atrophy, avascular necrosis
- *Dermatologic*: alopecia, photosensitivity, rash, skin lesions that appear or worsen in sunlight, mouth sores
- *Cardiovascular*: chest pain, pericarditis, systolic murmurs, valvular complications, Raynaud phenomenon, easy bruising
- *Pulmonary*: shortness of breath, pleuritis, pneumonitis, pulmonary hypertension
- *Renal*: nephritis, glomerulonephritis
- *Neuropsychiatric*: cognitive dysfunction, depression, anxiety, psychosis
- Dry eyes

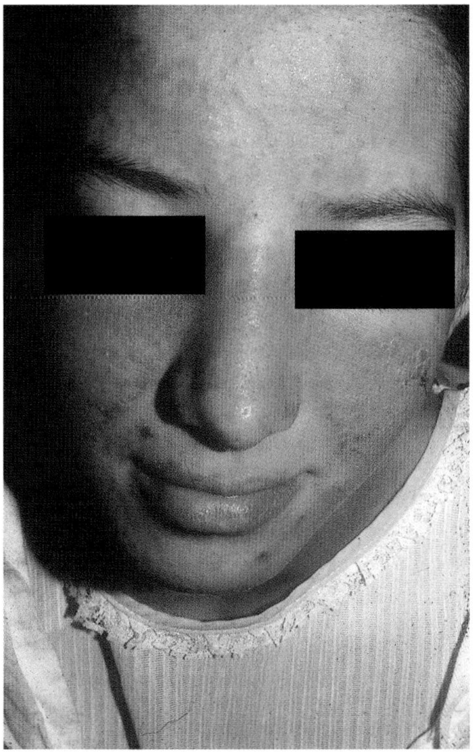

Figure 63-7 Characteristic malar or butterfly rash seen in systemic lupus erythematosus. (Reprinted with permission from Goodheart, H. P. (2009). *Goodheart's photoguide to common skin disorders: Diagnosis and management* (3rd ed.). Wolters Kluwer Health/Lippincott Williams & Wilkins.)

progressive weight loss; nausea and vomiting; and, in women, irregular or heavy menses. Other signs of the disease include the following:

- Nonspecific electrocardiographic changes
- A pericardial friction rub
- Pulmonary changes seen on radiographic studies
- Enlargement of the spleen and lymph nodes
- Raynaud's phenomenon (vasospasm of the smaller vessels of the hands and feet, resulting in blanching of the skin and, at times, pain and cyanosis of the extremities)
- Musculoskeletal problems, such as arthralgias and arthritis, including joint swelling, tenderness, pain on movement, and morning stiffness

Diagnostic Findings

Diagnosis of SLE is based on presenting symptoms and blood tests. Blood studies show anemia, thrombocytopenia, leukocytosis or leukopenia, and positive serum ANA (demonstrates that the immune system is stimulated). Anti–double-stranded DNA (anti-dsDNA) antibody test is a test that shows high titers of antibodies against native DNA. This is very specific for SLE because this test is not positive for other autoimmune disorders. Approximately 60% to 70% of people with SLE have positive anti-dsDNA. Anti-Smith (anti-Sm) antibodies are specific for SLE but are found in only 20% to 30% of clients with SLE (American College of Rheumatology, 2019). Other laboratory studies may indicate multisystem involvement, such as an elevated creatinine level with kidney involvement. Additional tests, such as a renal biopsy and urinalysis, may be performed to determine the effect of the disorder on other body systems. An echocardiogram may be ordered to determine if there is any issue with the valves or other cardiac tissues.

The American College of Rheumatology (2019) has identified 11 criteria for SLE. Clients presenting with four of these criteria at one time or individually over time are diagnosed with probable SLE. These criteria are malar rash, discoid rash, photosensitivity, oral ulcers, arthritis, pleuritis or pericarditis, renal disorder, neurologic disorders such as seizures, hematologic disorder such as thrombocytopenia, immunologic disorder as indicated by tests such as positive anti-dsDNA, and positive ANA test.

Medical Management

There is no specific treatment for this disorder. Medical management aims at producing a remission and preventing or treating acute exacerbations of the disorder. High doses of corticosteroids are used initially. Those with severe disease or those whose steroid-related side effects are problematic may be treated with cytotoxic drugs such as azathioprine (Imuran) and cyclophosphamide (Cytoxan). Simple analgesics such as aspirin or an NSAID may be prescribed for fever and joint discomfort. Topical corticosteroids may be used for skin manifestations. Hydroxychloroquine (Plaquenil) and chloroquine (Aralen), which are antimalarials, have been found to be effective medications for clients with SLE. They reduce muscle and joint pain and improve skin rashes, pericarditis, pleuritis, fatigue, and fever. These drugs are used not only when clients present with symptoms, but they are also useful in preventing flares. Immunosuppressive drugs, such as cyclophosphamide, may be given in severe cases to block immune cell production. Belimumab, a B-lymphocyte stimulator protein inhibitor, has been approved to reduce the number of abnormal B-lymphocytes, because they are thought to be a factor in SLE (American College of Rheumatology, 2019). Renal impairment may be treated with dialysis or kidney transplantation. Cardiac, GI, and central nervous system complications are treated symptomatically.

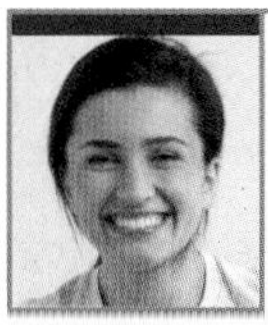

Clinical Scenario A 32-year-old woman is admitted with complaints of extreme fatigue; severe headaches; painful, swollen joints in her extremities; evidence of some hair loss; and a butterfly-shaped rash across her cheeks and nose. She is anemic and febrile and has some signs of edema around her eyes and in her feet and hands. She is diagnosed with SLE. **What are the primary concerns for the nurse when providing care while the client is hospitalized? See the following Nursing Process section.**

NURSING PROCESS FOR THE CLIENT WITH SYSTEMIC LUPUS ERYTHEMATOSUS

Assessment

Review the medical record and diagnostic findings to evaluate the stage of disease and appropriate interventions. Assess the client's understanding of the nature of the disorder, its treatment, and the limitations imposed by the disease process. Inspect the skin for rashes, purpuric lesions, and other skin changes and ask about the client's degree of sensitivity to sunlight. Inspect for ulcerations in the mouth and throat (signs of GI involvement). In addition, listen to the heart for pericardial friction rub and to the lungs for abnormal sounds, which might suggest pleural involvement.

Diagnosis, Planning, and Interventions

Nursing management focuses on measures to minimize exacerbations and to alleviate symptoms. Administer prescribed medications and monitor for side effects. Before discharge, client education efforts involve reminding the client of the need for close medical follow-up and thorough medication instruction (e.g., instruct the client not to abruptly discontinue taking a prescribed corticosteroid without consulting the primary provider, and follow the dosage regimen exactly, particularly if the drug dose is being decreased gradually).

Because the disease and drugs alter body image, assist the client to verbalize feelings and implement effective coping mechanisms. If the client desires, arrange a referral to the Lupus Foundation of America, which is dedicated to providing information about the disease, or to a local support or self-help group.

Since SLE is a chronic disease and treated mainly on an outpatient basis, much nursing management revolves around teaching. Clients and their families need accurate and complete information about the disease, its treatment and prognosis, and self-care measures to increase comfort and promote health. Specific measures are discussed in Client and Family Teaching 63-1.

Other nursing care involves, but is not limited to, the following diagnoses, expected outcomes, and interventions:

Chronic Pain: Related to inflammation and disease progression

Expected Outcomes: (1) Client will experience relief from pain and discomfort. (2) Client will adhere to the prescribed pharmacologic regimen. (3) Client will demonstrate use of alternative methods to reduce pain.

- Administer prescribed analgesic and anti-inflammatory medications. *Pain and discomfort respond to combination drug regimens, which promote comfort and reduce the disease's inflammatory effects.*
- Review the rationale for adhering to the prescribed regimen. *Teaching promotes the client's adherence to the regimen and may prevent the client from trying unsafe and ineffective therapies.*
- Elevate swollen and painful joints and apply heat or cold as indicated. *Nonpharmacologic methods decrease swelling and promote comfort.*
- Monitor the client if they use braces or splints. *These devices promote rest to inflamed joints but may cause skin irritation. Frequent monitoring prevents skin breakdown.*
- Balance activity with rest. *Alternating rest and activity conserves energy and promotes productivity and control.*
- Move painful joints gently and slowly while supporting the extremity above and below the joint. *Doing so promotes optimal mobility and reduces pain.*
- Avoid heavy blankets or clothing. *They increase pressure and pain.*

Impaired Physical Mobility: Related to inflammation, joint problems, pain, or decreased muscle strength

Expected Outcomes: (1) Client will maintain maximal physical function within limitations. (2) Client will increase muscle strength in affected areas or in areas that compensate for physical limitations. (3) Client will retain function with limitation of contractures.

- Assist client to maintain appropriate body alignment and neutral positioning during periods of inactivity. *Doing so prevents contractures and increases mobility.*
- Encourage moderate and progressive exercise as indicated. *Exercise promotes mobility and reduces fatigue.*
- Advise client to use moist heat before performing ROM exercises. *Moist heat relaxes muscles and reduces resistance to ROM exercises.*
- Urge client to wear supportive shoes and to use assistive devices for ambulation as needed. *These measures improve mobility.*
- Recommend sitting in elevated chairs that have arm rests that can help client to stand up. *These chairs improve the client's ability to be more independent.*
- Encourage client to maintain erect posture when sitting, standing, and walking. *Appropriate posture promotes optimal mobility and enhances muscle strengthening.*

Bathing/Hygiene, Toileting, Dressing, or Feeding ADL Deficit: Related to exacerbation of disease, inflammation, and decreased mobility

Expected Outcomes: (1) Client will perform self-care activities at highest possible level. (2) Client will identify methods that assist them to meet self-care needs.

- Modify clothing so the client can easily put it on and take it off (e.g., use Velcro fasteners instead of buttons, front fasteners rather than back zippers, elastic shoe laces, and cardigan sweaters instead of pullovers). *Ease in changing clothes promotes independence in self-care.*
- Pad handles for easy grasping. *Doing so enhances self-care abilities.*
- Suggest an electric toothbrush, which is easier to handle than a manual toothbrush. *This helps encourage the client to care for self.*
- Provide cooking and eating utensils designed to promote a good grip (particularly useful for clients with hand deformities). *This measure enhances self-care abilities.*
- Identify equipment resources and dealers for wheelchairs, elevated commode seats, and other assistive devices. *Doing so assists the client to plan for changes in lifestyle.*

NURSING PROCESS FOR THE CLIENT WITH SYSTEMIC LUPUS ERYTHEMATOSUS (continued)

Altered Body Image Perception: Related to change in appearance and inability to perform tasks and activities
Expected Outcomes: (1) Client will verbalize increased confidence when dealing with changes in appearance and functional abilities. (2) Client will establish realistic future goals.

- Accept client without reservation. *Nonverbal behavior expresses feelings. Facial expressions, tone of voice, or other behaviors promote acceptance or nonacceptance.*
- Avoid nonverbal messages that convey impatience with the client's disabilities. *Clients with disability require more time to finish tasks. Patience promotes independence.*
- Assist client only as needed or requested. *Doing so encourages client to perform self-care as much as possible.*
- Do not overprotect client or increase dependency. *A client involved with their own care can make decisions and is better able to identify when they need help.*
- Focus on what the client can do rather than not do. *Emphasizing strengths is essential.*
- Assist client to identify strengths. *Doing so promotes a positive self-image.*
- Encourage client to express fears, misgivings, or other concerns. *Acknowledging feelings assists client to identify resources and use coping mechanisms.*
- Acknowledge feelings of grief and hostility. *Doing so provides an atmosphere of acceptance.*
- Refer client for counseling if they withdraw, shows signs of denial, or otherwise exhibits maladaptive behavior. *Doing so provides other resources to increase coping skills.*

Evaluation of Expected Outcomes

The client reports relief of pain and discomfort, adheres to prescribed drug therapy, and uses alternative methods to reduce pain. They demonstrate maximal physical function within limitations, showing evidence of increased muscle strength function. The client can perform self-care at the highest possible level and has a plan for meeting future self-care needs as independently as possible. They report self-confidence and acceptance in the face of altered physical appearance and function and states realistic future goals. The client copes realistically and well with the chronicity of the disease.

Client and Family Teaching 63-1
Systemic Lupus Erythematosus

The nurse typically addresses the following with the client:

- Lifestyle modifications are necessary as related to musculoskeletal restrictions and systemic involvement. For example, because sunlight tends to exacerbate the disease, avoid sunlight and ultraviolet radiation. When outdoors, apply effective sunscreens with a sun protection factor (SPF) of 15 or higher, and wear clothing that covers the arms and legs and a wide-brimmed hat to shade the face. Sunlamps and tanning booths are taboo.
- Pace activities. Because fatigue is a major issue, allow for adequate rest along with regular activity to promote mobility and prevent joint stiffness. Avoid activities that cause severe pain or discomfort.
- Maintain a well-balanced diet and increase fluid intake to raise energy levels and promote tissue healing.
- Avoid crowds when possible and avoid people with known infections, such as colds.
- Periodically review the medication program with your health care providers, particularly the effects and adverse effects of medications, and related signs and symptoms that require attention should be reported to the primary provider (increased severity of symptoms, involvement in other joints or areas of the body, weight loss, prolonged anorexia, nausea, vomiting, fever, cough, shortness of breath, difficult urination, infection, or any other unusual occurrence).
- Take medications exactly as directed and do not stop the medication if symptoms are relieved unless advised to do so by the primary provider.
- If symptoms become worse, do not increase the dosage unless advised to do so by the primary provider. Do not use over-the-counter drugs unless a primary provider approves their use.
- Use nonpharmacologic comfort measures. For instance, a moist form of heat may relieve joint stiffness. Use warm, not hot, soaks, wraps, or hot towels from the clothes dryer, and take care not to burn the skin.
- Inform primary providers and dentists of current therapy before any treatment, surgery, or drugs are prescribed.

MUSCULOSKELETAL INFECTIOUS DISORDERS

The musculoskeletal system is subject to infections that can profoundly impact a person's mobility, ability to perform ADLs, and quality of life. This section focuses on osteomyelitis, a condition that affects bone, and Lyme disease, an illness that affects multiple systems including the musculoskeletal system.

Osteomyelitis

Osteomyelitis is an infection of the bone, resulting in limited blood supply to the bone, inflammation of and pressure on the tissue, bone necrosis, and formation of new bone around devitalized bone tissue. Osteomyelitis can be a difficult and challenging condition to treat, but newer approaches have improved outcomes.

Pathophysiology and Etiology

Most bone infections are caused by *Staphylococcus aureus*. Other possible causative organisms include gram-positive bacteria, such as streptococci and enterococci, and gram-negative bacteria, such as *Pseudomonas* species.

Osteomyelitis results from bacteria reaching the bone through the bloodstream. Acute localized osteomyelitis occurs when bone is contaminated directly by trauma, such as penetrating wounds or compound fractures. Vascular insufficiency in clients with diabetes or peripheral vascular disease can lead to osteomyelitis. Surgical contamination or direct extension of bacteria from an infected area adjacent to the bone, such as the pin sites of skeletal traction, may cause osteomyelitis. Clients who have long-term dialysis, chemotherapy, corticosteroid therapy, or immunosuppressant medications are at risk for osteomyelitis.

Microorganisms appear to migrate to the area just below the epiphysis of a long bone where the blood supply is more generous, but circulation through the area is limited. As microorganisms multiply, they spread down to the bone shaft. The pressure from the collecting exudate elevates the periosteum. New bone cells (**involucrum**) are deposited on the periosteum, while the underlying bone becomes necrotic. The pocket of necrotic bone (**sequestrum**) may remain sequestered for years or eventually drain by forming a sinus tract through to the skin. The infection tends to linger in a chronic state because it is difficult to penetrate the infected tissue by administering systemic antibiotic drugs.

In its weakened condition, the infected bone is prone to pathologic fracture. The diseased bone may lengthen as bone growth is stimulated, or it may shorten because of the destruction of the epiphyseal plate. Other complications of osteomyelitis include septicemia, thrombophlebitis, muscle contractures, pathologic fractures, and nonunion of fractures.

Assessment Findings

Evidence of an acute infection appears suddenly: high fever, chills, rapid pulse, tenderness or pain over the affected area, redness, and swelling. Chronic infection may be characterized by a persistent draining sinus.

With acute osteomyelitis, laboratory tests usually show an elevated leukocyte count, an elevated ESR, and possibly a blood culture positive for infective organisms. Identification of the causative organism may require a bone biopsy and/or aspiration of subperiosteal pus for culture and sensitivity. Radiographic findings may be inconclusive in the early stages of infection, but later studies demonstrate irregular bone decalcification, bone necrosis, elevation of the periosteum, and new bone formation. Bone scans and MRI are useful in definitive diagnoses.

Radiographic studies for chronic osteomyelitis show large cavities, sequestra or dense bone formations, and raised periosteum. Areas of infection are delineated by bone scan. Blood studies reveal a normal leukocyte count and ESR and possible anemia.

Medical and Surgical Management

Managing osteomyelitis focuses on surgically removing the diseased portions of the bone and administration of antibiotics. Surgical procedures may include:

- Drainage of the infected area.
- Surgical debridement of the necrotic tissue and sequestrum to remove the infected areas; a small margin of uninfected bone is removed as well to assure the removal of all infected tissue.
- Restoration of blood flow to the affected bone with bone grafts.
- Muscle flaps grafted to the affected area to enhance blood supply.
- Removal of surgical plates or screws from previous bone surgeries.
- Amputation as a last resort to remove the infected limb.

Following surgery, antibiotic therapy is initiated, based on the causative organism. Intravenous administration is generally used for at least 4 weeks, followed by another 2 weeks (or more) of intravenous or oral antibiotics. Clients need close follow-up to assure that the infection is eradicated and that the bone is adequately healed.

Nursing Management

Clients with osteomyelitis experience pain, inflammation, swelling, and impaired mobility because of pain and the inability to bear weight. Caretakers must handle the arm or leg or related area gently to prevent additional pain or fracture. They must protect the infected area from injury. The nurse instructs the client to elevate the area and to bear weight only as indicated. Nursing management includes protecting the skin from breakdown, administering the prescribed antibiotics and pain medications, and informing the client about the expected therapeutic effects and possible side effects. Clients with complications related to continued infection or inadequate bone healing require extensive emotional support related to the long-term nature of the osteomyelitis.

››› *Stop, Think, and Respond 63-2*

Which of the following clients is at greatest risk for osteomyelitis?

1. *A 65-year-old client recently diagnosed with OA*
2. *A 70-year-old client who recently sustained an open compound fracture of the tibia after a motor vehicle accident*
3. *A 40-year-old client diagnosed with gout*

Lyme Disease

Lyme disease (Lyme borreliosis) gained wide recognition in the 1970s, when residents of Lyme, Connecticut, experienced an epidemic of progressive symptoms, beginning with a characteristic rash and eventually involving the cardiac, neurologic, and musculoskeletal systems.

Pathophysiology and Etiology

Typically, Lyme disease is prevalent during warmer months, when ticks are abundant, but it may occur at any time. It is most common in the northeast and Mid-Atlantic states and in other northern areas of the United States where deer ticks (*Ixodes dammini*) are more prevalent, but it has been found throughout the United States and in other countries. According to the Centers for Disease Control and Prevention (CDC, 2021), there are 30,000 new infections reported every year. However, the CDC estimates that there is an average of approximately 476,000 new cases annually that are not reported, related to lack of or incorrect diagnosis, as well as poor reporting.

The ticks feed on white-tailed deer or white-footed mice and then become carriers of the spirochetal bacterium *Borrelia burgdorferi* or other types of *Borrelia*. When ticks bite humans, they transmit the bacteria, which results in a chronic inflammatory process and multisystem disease. To have Lyme disease, the tick must be attached for 36 to 48 hours. Removing a tick as early as possible may prevent infection.

Assessment Findings

Signs and Symptoms

If untreated, the disease moves through three stages. Early stage 1 symptoms for about one-third of clients include a red macule or papule at the site of the tick bite, a characteristic bull's-eye rash (called erythema migrans) with round rings surrounding the center, headache, neck stiffness, and pain. Secondary pruritic lesions may accompany fever, chills, and malaise. The initial papule may not develop until 20 to 30 days after the bite. Some clients experience nausea, vomiting, and sore throat. Clients often report having flulike symptoms.

Midstage symptoms occur as the organism proliferates throughout the body, and cardiac and neurologic involvement becomes evident. Erythema migrans can appear in multiple areas of the body. Cardiac problems include dysrhythmias and heart block. Neurologic symptoms such as facial palsy, meningitis, and encephalitis are possible. Some clients have problems with weakness, pain, and paresthesia (abnormal sensations).

Later symptoms (at least 4 weeks after the bite) include arthritis and other musculoskeletal problems. Joints, particularly knees, become warm, swollen, and painful. Joint erosion may result from the inflammatory process.

Diagnostic Findings

Diagnosis is based on the presenting signs and symptoms. The enzyme-linked immunosorbent assay (ELISA) test detects antibodies to *B. burgdorferi*. This test can have false-positive results, so other tests may be used. The Western blot test is done if the ELISA is positive. It detects antibodies to several proteins of *B. burgdorferi*. The polymerase chain reaction (PCR) test detects bacterial DNA in fluid aspirated from an infected joint. This test is done on clients with chronic Lyme arthritis. It can also be done on cerebrospinal fluid for clients with nervous system symptoms.

Medical and Surgical Management

Treatment includes administering antibiotics and supportive measures. Oral antibiotics are generally prescribed for 14 to 21 days, but research demonstrates that a maximum of 14 days is sufficient. If a client is in later stages of the disease, IV antibiotics will be administered instead for 14 to 28 days. If the disease is treated early, the prognosis is favorable. Permanent multisystem problems may occur if treatment is delayed.

Nursing Management

Nursing management involves teaching the client and family about the disease and its treatment. It is extremely important to educate clients about avoiding Lyme disease (Client and Family Teaching 63-2). It is possible to have Lyme disease more than once, so teaching clients about preventing exposure is crucial.

Client and Family Teaching 63-2
Tips for Avoiding Lyme Disease

The nurse teaches the client and family measures to avoid Lyme disease:

Personal Protection

- Wear light-colored clothing to increase tick visibility.
- Wear long-sleeved shirts and long pants (tuck pants into socks or boots).
- Treat clothing with tick repellant.
- Wear a hat; pull long hair back so it does not brush against shrubs or other vegetation.
- Walk in the center of a path surrounded by grass, brush, or woods.
- Take a shower as quickly as possible after potential exposure to ticks. Do a tick check—ticks are particularly attracted to hairy areas such as the scalp, groin, and armpits, as well as the back of knees and neck.
- Run clothes in a hot dryer for 10 minutes before washing them to kill any ticks left on the clothes. If a tick is found, remove it with tweezers, taking care not to crush it. Once removed, dispose of it and apply antibacterial ointment to the bite.

Environmental Protection

- Remove leaf, grass, and brush litter.
- Clear brush and tall grass from around house and other structures as well as gardens and flower beds.
- Keep grass mowed.
- Place a 3-foot wood chip barrier along lawn edges that border woods.
- Erect fences to keep deer away from houses and gardens.
- Prune low-lying shrubs to let in more sunlight.
- Keep woodpiles neat, dry, and off the ground.
- Keep ground bare under bird feeders, place them away from house, and suspend feeding when ticks are most active.

Adapted from Lymedisease.org. (2020). *Personal protection.* https://www.lymedisease.org/lyme-basics/ticks /personal-protection/

STRUCTURAL DISORDERS

Structural disorders of the musculoskeletal system involve metabolic conditions that alter bone structure. These alterations result in pain, bone deformity, and fracture.

Osteoporosis

Osteoporosis, a loss of bone density, occurs principally in older adults and affects more women than men.

Pathophysiology and Etiology

Normally, the processes of bone formation and bone reabsorption occur evenly. In osteoporosis, however, loss of bone substance exceeds bone formation. The total bone mass and density are reduced, resulting in bones that become progressively porous, brittle, and fragile. Compression fractures of the vertebrae are common. Aging contributes to osteoporosis (the loss of bone mass) in the following ways:

- Levels of calcitonin, which inhibits bone reabsorption and promotes bone formation, decrease with aging.
- Levels of estrogen, which inhibits bone breakdown, decrease in postmenopausal women.
- Levels of parathyroid hormone, which increases bone reabsorption, increase with aging.

Women who are small-framed, slim, and of non-Hispanic White or European descent are at greatest risk for osteoporosis, as are women of Asian descent who are of slight build, especially those who are postmenopausal. Women who are Black American or of African descent have a greater bone density and thus are less susceptible to osteoporosis. Men have an increased bone mass and do not have hormonal changes and thus do not acquire osteoporosis as frequently and get it at a later age. Family history of osteoporosis is a risk factor. Increasing age contributes to the development of osteoporosis, which may be due in part to decreasing levels of estrogen in women and testosterone in men. Bone formation is improved with regular exercise that involves resistance and low-impact activities. Inactivity, prolonged periods of immobility, and disability contribute to more rapid bone resorption and increase the risk for osteoporosis.

Other causes of osteoporosis, which may occur in any age group and both sexes, include a family history of osteoporosis, chronic low calcium intake, excessive intake of caffeine, tobacco use, Cushing syndrome, prolonged use of high doses of corticosteroids, hyperthyroidism, hyperparathyroidism, eating disorders, malabsorption syndromes, breast cancer (especially if treated with chemotherapy that suppresses estrogen, excluding tamoxifen, which may reduce the risk of fractures), renal or liver failure, alcoholism, lactose intolerance, and dietary deficiency of vitamin D and calcium. Some medications interfere with the body's ability to use and metabolize calcium, including thyroid supplements, anticonvulsants, isoniazid, aluminum-containing antacids, tetracycline, selective serotonin reuptake inhibitors (SSRIs), and heparin.

Assessment Findings

Clients with osteoporosis frequently complain of lumbosacral pain, thoracic back pain, or both. The bone pain or tenderness results from tiny compression fractures in the vertebrae. Accompanying loss of height is known as *progressive kyphosis* (Fig. 63-8).

Radiographic examination of the bones shows bone loss once it is 25% or more. Bone deformities (especially in the spine), such as kyphosis and lordosis, and pathologic fractures in long bones also may be seen. Dual-energy X-ray absorptiometry (DXA—previously DEXA) is a test that measures bone mineral density (BMD) at the spine and hip. Quantitative ultrasonic studies (QUS) (bone sonometer) measure heel density and provide baseline information for diagnosing osteoporosis and predicting risk of fracture. Results of laboratory studies usually are normal, but such studies may be performed to rule out other disorders such as multiple myeloma, hyperparathyroidism, or metastatic bone lesions.

Medical Management

A diet rich in calcium and vitamin D throughout life can prevent osteoporosis. Osteoporosis cannot be treated directly, but medical management can slow the rate of bone reabsorption. Bone pain or tenderness may respond to mild analgesics such as aspirin. Oral calcium preparations (calcium gluconate, calcium lactate, calcium carbonate, or dibasic calcium phosphate) may be recommended to supplement dietary calcium. Some of these preparations also contain vitamin D, which is needed for absorption of calcium in the intestine. See Drug Therapy Table 63-3 also.

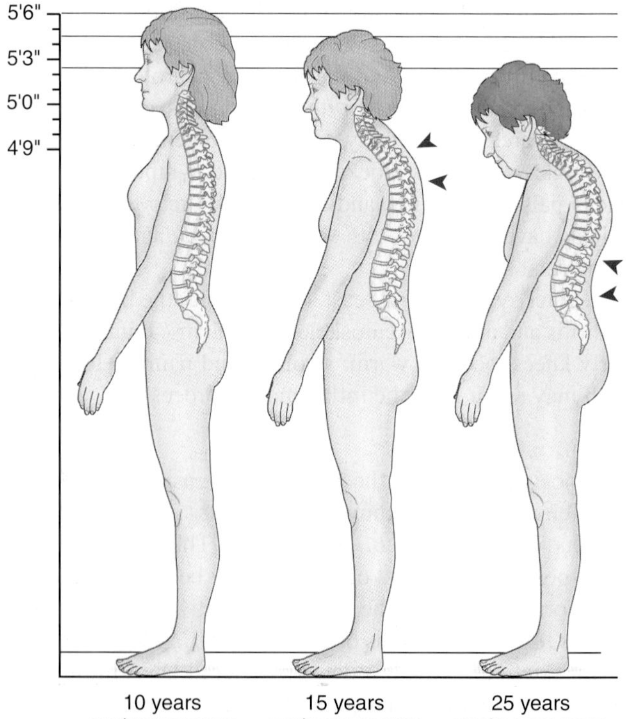

Figure 63-8 Typical loss of height associated with osteoporosis and aging.

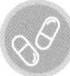

DRUG THERAPY TABLE 63-3 Drugs for Prevention of Osteoporosis

Category and Common Generic (Brand) Drugs	Intended Use	Common Side Effects	Safety Warnings for Nurses
Bone Resorption Inhibitors			
Bisphosphonates Alendronate (Fosamax) Etidronate (Didronel) Ibandronate (Boniva) Pamidronate (Aredia) Risedronate (Actonel) Zoledronic acid (Zometa)	Reduce bone loss caused by resorption, reversing osteoporosis	Nausea, dyspepsia, diarrhea, headache	• Do not use if delayed esophageal emptying
Selective Estrogen Receptor Modulators (SERM) Denosumab (Prolia) Raloxifene (Evista) Teriparatide (Forteo)	Osteoporosis prevention and treatment	Hot flashes, flulike symptoms, arthralgia, rhinitis, increased cough, leg cramping	• Dental check and repair before starting to reduce risk for osteonecrosis of jaw bone

Pharmacologic Considerations

■ Standard drug treatment of osteoporosis includes approximately 5 years of bisphosphonate administration. After that, a "drug holiday" is recommended. Current studies indicate that the best estimate regarding drug holiday is the client's baseline risk—if high, then longer treatment is recommended (Bandeira et al., 2020).

Medications used in the treatment of osteoporosis include the following:

- *Bisphosphonates*, including alendronate sodium (Fosamax) and risedronate (Actonel), inhibit bone resorption. These drugs may be taken once a week or monthly, which reduces the gastroesophageal side effects. Zoledronic acid (Reclast) is another bisphosphonate that is given IV once a year.
- *Calcitonin* inhibits bone reabsorption and slows bone loss. This medication is usually administered as a nasal spray but may be administered subcutaneously.
- *Selective estrogen receptor modifiers (SERMs)*, such as raloxifene (Evista), preserve BMD and thus reduce the risk for osteoporosis. SERMs do not have the risks associated with estrogen, such as increased risk of uterine cancer.
- *Hormone replacement therapy (HRT)* was the treatment of choice at one time. However, the potential risks of uterine cancer and heart disease and the availability of other treatments have changed the use of HRT. Instead of oral forms of HRT, women may choose patches, creams, or the vaginal ring.
- *Teriparatide (Forteo)* is a powerful drug, similar to parathyroid hormone, that stimulates new bone growth. It is used to treat osteoporosis in people who are at high risk of fractures. Teriparatide is given once a day by injection under the skin on the thigh or abdomen.
- *Denosumab (Prolia)* is an injectable medication that slows bone loss and strengthens bones. It is administered every 6 months for clients who have a high risk for fractures.
- *Tamoxifen (Nolvadex)* is used primarily by women with breast cancer or with a high risk of developing breast cancer; it has an estrogenlike effect on bone cells and apparently reduces the risk of fractures.

Other treatment focuses on relieving pain and preventing injury. Exercise programs are initiated to improve muscle strength and increase weight-bearing activity. Outdoor activity is encouraged so the client enhances their ability to produce vitamin D. A physical therapy program helps to reduce back pain, improve posture, and reduce the risk of falls in clients with osteoporosis and kyphosis. It uses a combination of a spinal weighted kypho-orthosis (WKO), which is a weighted harness, with specific back extension exercises.

Nursing Management

In providing care for clients with osteoporosis, the nurse emphasizes the need for a nutritious, well-balanced diet that is high in calcium, vitamin D, and protein—all are recommended to delay or prevent osteoporosis (Nutrition Notes 63-3). The nurse especially advises women to drink three glasses of milk daily or eat other dairy products to acquire approximately 1000 to 1500 mg of calcium; those who smoke cigarettes may require more. Orange juice fortified with calcium is a nutritious alternative. If the client takes antacids, the nurse suggests those containing calcium. They recommend activity that promotes bone formation, such as regular weight-bearing aerobic exercise (e.g., walking). When taking calcium supplements, it is best to divide the daily amount into two doses in order to maximize absorption and metabolism.

››› *Stop, Think, and Respond 63-3*

A 45-year-old woman tells you that she has never liked milk and usually avoids dairy products because she thinks they are too fattening. What do you need to assess to ascertain if she is at risk for osteoporosis? What teaching does she need?

Nutrition Notes 63-3

The Client With Osteoporosis

- It is possible to fulfill vitamin D requirements by taking a daily 15-minute walk in the sun. However, significant rates of low vitamin D status are documented in studies of healthy adults and children in the United States and other countries. Winter, living in northern latitudes, Black race, and older age are associated with low vitamin D synthesis. A dietary source is considered essential because few people meet optimal conditions.
- Vitamin D occurs naturally in a few food sources, namely, fatty fish, fish liver oils, and egg yolks. Foods fortified with vitamin D include milk and breakfast cereals and a few brands of orange juice, yogurt, margarine, and hot cereals.
- Diets rich in fruits and vegetables provide vitamin K, magnesium, and potassium, nutrients known to help maintain bone density.
- Diets high in salt, caffeine, and sugar are associated with bone loss and should be avoided.

Osteomalacia

Osteomalacia, a metabolic bone disease, is a softening of bones generally caused by vitamin D deficiency.

Pathophysiology and Etiology

A deficiency of activated vitamin D (calcitriol) is the primary defect in osteomalacia. Calcitriol promotes calcium absorption from the GI tract and facilitates bone mineralization. Without this, calcium and phosphate are not moved to the bones. Large amounts of new bone fail to calcify. The bone mass is structurally weaker, and bone deformities occur. Osteomalacia can also occur from malabsorption of calcium or excessive loss of calcium from the body. Additional risk factors are identified in Box 63-3.

Assessment Findings

Clients with osteomalacia experience bone pain and weakness. They also complain of tenderness if the bones are palpated. Bone deformities, such as kyphosis and bowing of the legs, occur as the disease advances. Clients exhibit a waddling type of gait, putting them at risk for falls and fractures.

Radiographic studies demonstrate demineralization of the bone and slight cracks in the bones, referred to as looser transformation zones. A bone scan detects increased and decreased areas of bone metabolism. Serum levels of calcium, vitamin D, and phosphorus are low. Alkaline phosphatase levels typically are elevated. A bone biopsy may be done to have a definitive diagnosis of osteomalacia, but typically it is not needed.

BOX 63-3 Risk Factors for Osteomalacia

- Dietary deficiencies
- Malnutrition, particularly low calcium intake
- Malabsorption
- Gastrointestinal disorders (celiac disease, chronic pancreatitis, biliary tract obstruction)
- Gastrectomy
- Chronic renal failure
- Hyperparathyroidism
- Anticonvulsant therapy (phenytoin, phenobarbital)
- Insufficient vitamin D (no supplements in food and lack of sunlight)
- Poverty
- Food fads
- Lack of nutritional knowledge

Medical and Surgical Treatment

Treatment aims at correcting the underlying cause. Vitamin D supplementation is the primary treatment for osteomalacia. Clients may also take supplements of calcium and phosphorus if these levels are low. In addition, adequate nutrition, exposure to sunlight, and progressive exercise and ambulation are recommended. Bone deformities may require braces or surgery for correction.

Nursing Management

The nurse is in a primary role of educating the client about the disease and its treatment and therefore includes teaching in the care plan. They teach the client about methods and medications used to relieve pain and discomfort. The nurse allows the client to verbalize self-concept issues related to deformities and activity restrictions.

Paget Disease

Paget disease (osteitis deformans) is a chronic bone disorder characterized by abnormal bone remodeling. It affects adults older than 60 years of age. The most common areas of involvement are the long bones, spine, pelvis, and skull.

Pathophysiology and Etiology

In Paget disease, some skeletal bones are unaffected; other bones are marked by a disturbance in the ratio between bone formation and reabsorption. The excessive osteoclastic activity causes the bones to become soft and bowed initially. Later, the bones thicken when compensatory osteoblastic activity resumes. The process of bone turnover continues, resulting in a classic mosaic pattern of bone matrix development. The new bone has high mineral content but is not well formed. This causes the bones to be weak and prone to fracture.

Although the cause of Paget disease is unknown, the process by which clients with this disorder deposit collagen, a protein in connective tissue, is thought to be defective. This is based on the fact that the affected bones are high in mineral content but poorly constructed. It is more common in men and in those of Northern European descent. A family history of the disorder is not uncommon. Additional findings indicate a possible link between the disease and a previous viral infection.

Complications include pathologic fractures, paralysis from spinal cord compression, cranial nerve damage such as deafness from compression of the skull, and kidney stones. Occasionally, the lesions undergo malignant changes.

Assessment Findings

Some clients are asymptomatic, with only some mild skeletal deformity. Other clients have marked skeletal deformities, which may include enlargement of the skull, bowing of the long bones, and kyphosis. Bone pain and tenderness on pressure may be elicited. Paget disease may go undiscovered until an X-ray for another problem reveals the disorder.

Radiographic examination discloses bones in various stages of resorption and remodeling with a mosaic appearance to the bone structure. Pathologic fractures appear, and the bones are curved and enlarged. Bone scans usually are done. An elevated serum alkaline phosphatase level and increased urinary hydroxyproline (an amino acid found in collagen) excretion are common. Calcium levels usually are normal.

Medical and Surgical Management

Clients without symptoms usually do not need treatment. Those with symptoms may benefit from drug therapy. Analgesics such as aspirin or NSAIDs usually can control pain. Those with moderate-to-severe pain may benefit from treatment with calcitonin (Calcimar), a hormone that appears to block the resorption of bone by reducing the number of osteoclasts and decreasing the rate of bone turnover. Treatment with calcitonin usually results in a drop in the serum alkaline phosphatase level and urinary excretion of hydroxyproline, followed by regression of the lesions. Although not an analgesic, calcitonin reduces pain because it seems to promote the regression of lesions. The client still may require analgesics, however, until bone pain is relieved.

Bisphosphonates, such as etidronate disodium (Didronel), given orally or IV, or alendronate sodium (Fosamax), may be given to reduce the activity of Paget disease and hopefully induce long-term remission of the disease. These drugs reduce normal and abnormal bone resorption and secondarily reduce bone formation that is coupled to bone resorption.

Surgery may be performed to repair pathologic fractures, replace damaged joints, realign deformed bones, or relieve neurologic complications.

Nursing Management

The nurse implements prescribed drug therapy and monitors for side effects. If self-care is limited, the nurse assists the client with ADLs. Client safety is a priority because strength and balance may be compromised. As appropriate, the nurse also teaches the client how to use ambulatory aids (e.g., a walker or cane), self-administer prescribed drugs, and implement measures to reduce falls within the home. For nursing management of a client who requires surgery, refer to Nursing Care Plan 61-1.

Disorders of the Feet

Many foot disorders are treated on an outpatient basis or encountered by nurses when caring for clients with other disorders. Foot disorders that commonly affect clients and for which surgery may be performed are bunions and hammertoes.

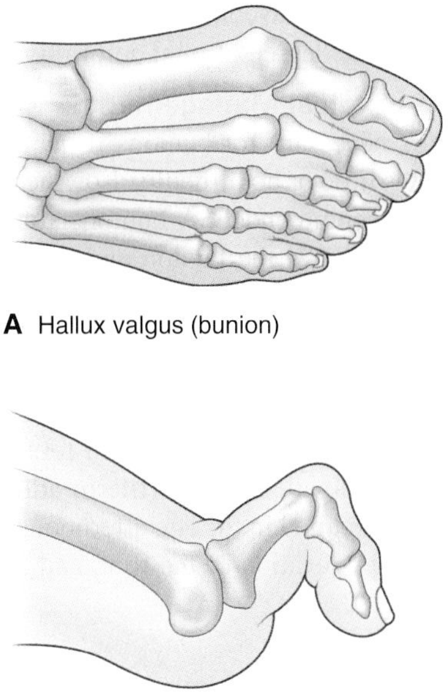

A Hallux valgus (bunion)

B Hammertoe

Figure 63-9 Common foot problems: **(A)** Hallux valgus or bunion and **(B)** hammertoe.

Hallux valgus, also called a *bunion*, is a deformity of the great (large) toe at its metatarsophalangeal joint (Fig. 63-9A). **Hammertoe** is a flexion deformity of the PIP joint and may involve several toes (see Fig. 63-9B). **Mallet toe** is a flexion deformity of the DIP joint and also can affect several toes. Although the affected joints for hammer toe and mallet toe differ, the symptoms and treatment are basically the same.

Pathophysiology and Etiology

Bunions are associated with heredity, arthritis, or improperly fitting shoes. Women tend to be affected more than men. The first metatarsal bone enlarges on the medial side. The metatarsal bone protrudes at an acute angle toward the midline of the body, whereas the great toe points laterally. There is an overgrowth of soft tissue (bursa), which actually is the bunion. The foot widens, and the arch flattens. The malalignment results in pain from the stress on the joint, improper support and distribution of body weight, and inflammation of the bursa.

Like bunions, hammertoe and mallet toe also result from wearing poorly fitting shoes. Toes are pulled upward by the shoe as the ball of the foot is pulled down. Corns (small, round, elevated overgrowths of epidermis) usually develop on top of the toes. Calluses (wide, thickened layer of skin) form under the metatarsal area.

Assessment Findings

The malalignment typical of bunions results in pain from the stress on the joint, improper support and distribution of body weight, and inflammation of the bursa. The client complains of pain on walking or flexing the foot, tenderness, and redness of the joint. The typical appearance of the foot deformity is obvious. In hammertoe and mallet toe, the foot deformity is also evident. Corns and calluses are easily seen.

The client complains of discomfort with ambulation. X-rays of the foot reveal the degree of joint deformity.

Medical and Surgical Management

No treatment is necessary for bunions if pain is not severe and the client has little or no difficulty. Low-heeled, properly fitted shoes are recommended. A bunionectomy, the surgical procedure to remove the bunion and correct the deformity, may be performed when the individual has pain and difficulty walking. Treatment of hammertoe and mallet toe includes exercises, wearing properly fitting or open-toed shoes, use of pads to protect the joints, and surgery to correct the malalignment. Surgeries for repair of foot disorders are performed on an outpatient or short-term admission basis, with the client discharged in the late afternoon or the following morning. Rest, elevation of the foot, and analgesics are prescribed.

Nursing Management

Nursing management of foot disorders includes relieving pain and discomfort, improving mobility, and instructing clients about the necessity for proper foot attire. Many clients are treated in an outpatient setting. Nurses in these settings usually are charged with teaching the client about the foot condition, treatment, medications, and postoperative care if the client had surgery (see Client and Family Teaching 63-3).

Client and Family Teaching 63-3
Home Care Following Foot Surgery

The nurse provides the following instructions for the outpatient client:

Pain:

- Elevate foot as much as possible.
- Apply ice for no more than 20 minutes at a time as needed for pain relief—generally no more than 5 times a day.
- Take prescribed pain medications as ordered.

Mobility:

- Limit weight-bearing as much as possible for 2 weeks; increase weight-bearing as instructed after this time period.
- Use assistive device to ambulate and limit weight-bearing.
- Do ROM exercises daily after sutures are removed.

Surgical incision care:

- Keep dressing/cast clean and dry.
- Change dressing according to instructions.

Call care provider if:

- There is a change in sensation in the foot, ability to move the toes, and/or if the toes are cool to touch and pale or light blue in color.
- The pain is severe and unrelenting.
- There are signs of wound infection: fever, drainage, increased pain.

BONE TUMORS

Bone tumors may be benign or malignant. Benign tumors of the bone are more common than malignant bone tumors. Malignant tumors are primary, originating in the bone, or secondary, originating from elsewhere in the body (e.g., breast, lung, prostate, or kidney) and traveling to the bone (metastasis). Secondary or metastatic bone tumors are more common than primary bone tumors.

Benign Bone Tumors

Benign bone tumors have the potential to cause fractures of bones. However, they are not life-threatening and usually cause few symptoms.

Pathophysiology and Etiology

Benign tumors usually are the result of misplaced or overgrown clusters of normal bone or cartilage cells that cause the structure to enlarge and impair local function. They grow slowly and do not metastasize. Their growth can weaken the bone structure by compressing or displacing the normal tissue. There are a number of benign bone tumors, which include:

- *Enchondroma*: a hyaline cartilage tumor that develops in the hand, ribs, femur, tibia, humerus, or pelvis
- *Osteochondroma*: a large projection of bone at the ends of long bones, developing during growth periods and then becoming a static bone mass
- *Chondroblastoma*: a cartilaginous tumor that forms at the ends of long bones, most typically the distal end of the femur or the proximal end of the humerus
- *Bone cysts*:
  - Aneurysmal bone cysts: painful, palpable mass found in long or flat bones and vertebrae
  - Unicameral bone cysts: may cause pathologic fractures in the humerus or femur
- *Osteoid osteoma*: painful tumor surrounded by reactive bone tissue
- *Osteoclastoma*: giant cell tumors that may invade local tissue; usually soft and hemorrhagic; may become malignant

Benign bone tumors typically occur in children and young adults under 30 years. They generally occur when bones are still growing and are influenced by hormones that stimulate bone growth (e.g., growth hormone, parathyroid hormone, thyroid hormone, estrogen, and testosterone). Many of these tumors stop growing when skeletal growth is complete.

Assessment Findings

Clients with benign bone tumors may experience pain or discomfort that worsens when bearing weight. The bone appears deformed, and swelling may appear over the involved area. If the tumor is in a bone of the extremities, movement may be decreased and pathologic fractures may occur easily. Radiography, bone scans, and biopsy of the tumor determine the diagnosis.

Medical and Surgical Management

Medical management includes treating pain and preventing fractures. Surgery is performed if the tumor does not stop growing, bone deformity is present, or the pain is interfering with ADLs and mobility.

Curettage (scraping) or local excision is the usual procedure. Bone grafts may need to be done to promote bone growth and healing. Splints or casts are applied until the bone heals. Clients require close monitoring after surgery because benign bone tumors can recur.

Nursing Management

Providing adequate explanations to the client and alleviating anxiety are key nursing responsibilities. The nurse provides adequate explanations to the client, emphasizing the nature of the tumor, prognosis, and treatment. They allow time for questions and expressions of fear and anxiety. The nurse administers pain medications as indicated. They teach the client methods to reduce pain and swelling and encourages the client to elevate the affected extremity.

Malignant Bone Tumors

Malignant bone tumors are abnormal osteoblasts or myeloblasts (marrow cells) that exhibit rapid and uncontrollable growth.

Pathophysiology and Etiology

Prior exposure to radiation and toxic chemicals has been associated with the genesis of some malignant bone tumors. A hereditary link in which a tumor suppressor gene may be absent or impaired is also suspected because the same type of tumor may appear among siblings in the same family. Primary tumors include osteosarcoma, Ewing's sarcoma, chondrosarcoma, and fibrosarcoma.

Malignant bone tumors usually are located around the knee in the distal femur or proximal fibula; a few are found in the proximal humerus. As the tumor expands, it lifts the periosteum in much the same way as osteomyelitis. Metastasis occurs through the circulatory or lymphatic system. Metastasis to the lungs is common.

Assessment Findings

A pathologic fracture may be the event that leads the client to seek treatment. Clients with malignant tumors of the bone complain of persistent pain, swelling, and difficulty in moving the involved extremity. A limp or abnormal gait may be noted when the client walks. By the time the client experiences symptoms, however, the tumor usually has spread beyond its primary site.

The bone appears abnormal on radiographic examination, MRI, or bone scan. Biopsy identifies abnormal cells. A malignancy of the skeletal system is associated with an elevated serum alkaline phosphatase level.

Medical and Surgical Management

Treatment of primary malignant bone tumors may involve surgical removal of the tumor by amputating the extremity or by wide local resection. However, limb-sparing surgery is much more common today because chemotherapy before surgery and advanced surgical techniques make this possible. Chemotherapy and radiation therapy after surgery aim to destroy tumor cells that escape from the original tumor site. Clients with osteosarcoma will most likely have a prosthesis or transplant of bone from another part of the body.

Nursing Management

Clients with malignant bone tumors require extensive emotional support and information about the disease, treatment, and prognosis. The nurse implements preoperative and postoperative measures for clients who are having surgery. For clients who must have an amputation, refer to the section on amputation in Chapter 61 for specific nursing care. As in other orthopedic surgeries, general nursing responsibilities include keeping the affected extremity elevated to reduce swelling, assessing neurovascular status frequently (see Chapter 61), and monitoring closely for complications if the affected limb is immobilized after surgery.

KEY POINTS

- Inflammatory disorders
  - Rheumatoid arthritis: an autoimmune disorder of the connective tissue and joints. Causes deformity to the joints affected
  - Degenerative joint disease: called DJD or osteoarthritis, most common form of arthritis caused by wear and tear on the joints
  - Temporomandibular disorder: cluster of symptoms near the jaw, causes include arthritis, bruxism, dislocation of the jaw
  - Fibromyalgia syndrome: chronic inflammatory illness consisting of musculoskeletal pain, fatigue, mood disorders, and sleep disturbances
  - Ankylosing spondylitis: chronic connective tissue disorder of the spine and surrounding cartilaginous joints
  - Systemic lupus erythematosus: called SLE or lupus, an autoimmune disorder that involves connective tissue changes and chronic inflammation and affects skin, joints, kidneys, heart, lungs, brain, and lymph nodes
- Musculoskeletal infectious disorders
  - Osteomyelitis: infection in the bone, affects blood supply to the bone and bone necrosis, can be difficult to treat
  - Lyme disease: progressive symptoms, generally starts with rash, moves to involve the cardiac, neurologic, and musculoskeletal systems. Caused by transmission of bacterium after a tick bite
- Structural disorders
  - Osteoporosis: loss of bone density
  - Osteomalacia: metabolic bone disease, softening of the bones caused by vitamin D deficiency
  - Paget disease: chronic bone disorder characterized by abnormal bone remodeling
  - Disorders of the feet include Hammertoe, bunion, mallet toe
- Bone tumor: may be benign or malignant. Benign tumors may cause fractures, malignant tumors show rapid and uncontrollable growth

CRITICAL THINKING EXERCISES

1. A 50-year-old woman tells you that her mother has had two hip replacements secondary to OA. The client is worried that her current hip pain will lead to the same problem. What suggestions would you make?
2. What differentiates osteomalacia from Paget disease?
3. When teaching a client with SLE, what should a primary goal be?
4. A client is being evaluated for possible fibromyalgia. What factors make it difficult to establish a diagnosis?

NCLEX-STYLE REVIEW QUESTIONS PrepU

1. When planning care for the client with RA, when will the nurse expect that the client will need more time and assistance with ADLs?
   1. At noontime
   2. Before bedtime
   3. In late afternoon
   4. In the early morning
2. Which statement made by the client with RA indicates that the nurse needs to provide further instruction regarding corticosteroid therapy?
   1. "I am susceptible to getting infections."
   2. "I may become very depressed and perhaps suicidal."
   3. "I may develop low blood sugar and need glucose."
   4. "I should never stop taking my medication abruptly."
3. A client asks the nurse about some strategies that may be useful to slow the progression of OA in the left knee. Which suggestions from the nurse are appropriate? Select all that apply.
   1. Apply heat to the affected knee.
   2. Ask for narcotics for pain control.
   3. Lose weight.
   4. Maintain normal activity.
   5. Start a progressive swimming program.
4. Which of the following statements indicates to the nurse that the client needs more information related to nutrition needs during an acute attack of gout?
   1. "I can have a high-carbohydrate and low-fat diet."
   2. "I must drink at least 2 quarts of water a day."
   3. "I must not skip any meals."
   4. "It is OK to have a glass of wine every day."
5. The nurse is reviewing a doctor's orders on a client admitted with SLE. Which classification of medications does the nurse expect to see on the orders?
   1. Anticonvulsant
   2. Antihistamine
   3. Antimalarial
   4. Sedative

WANT TO KNOW MORE? There are a wide variety of online resources available on thePoint to enhance learning and understanding of this chapter.

Go to **thePoint.lww.com/activate,** and use the activation code found in the front of this text to unlock these online resources.

UNIT 16
Caring for Clients With Integumentary Disorders

64 Introduction to the Integumentary System

Words To Know

apocrine glands
conduction
convection
cryosurgery
dermis
eccrine glands
electrodesiccation
epidermis
evaporation
friction
hyphae
integument
keratin
laser
mechanoreceptors
melanin
nociceptors
pheromones
photochemotherapy
pressure injury
radiation
sebaceous glands
sebum
senile keratoses
senile lentigines
shearing
skin tear
stratum corneum
subcutaneous tissue
terminal hair
thermoreceptors
vellus hair
Wood light

Learning Objectives

On completion of this chapter, you will be able to:

1. Name the structures that form the integument.
2. List four functions of the integumentary system.
3. Identify the purpose of sebum and melanin.
4. Differentiate between eccrine and apocrine glands.
5. Name at least three facts about the integument, which are pertinent to document when obtaining a health history.
6. Give the characteristics of normal skin.
7. Describe the criteria for staging pressure injuries.
8. List characteristics of hair assessed during a physical examination.
9. Describe the characteristics of normal nails.
10. Name four diagnostic tests performed to determine the etiology of skin disorders.
11. Describe seven medical and surgical techniques for treating skin disorders.

The **integument** includes structures that cover the body's exterior surface. The primary structure is the skin, which contains sebaceous and sweat glands and sensory nerve endings (Fig. 64-1). The integument also includes accessory structures such as the hair and nails. The structures that make up the integument protect the body from environmental injuries, help regulate body temperature, serve as sensory organs, and facilitate the synthesis of vitamin D.

ANATOMY AND PHYSIOLOGY

Skin

The skin is composed of two layers: the **epidermis**, the outermost layer, and the **dermis**, which lies below the epidermis. The epidermis contains an outer layer of dead skin cells, the **stratum corneum**, that forms a tough protective protein called **keratin**. The epidermis is constantly shed and replaced with epithelial cells from the dermis every day. The

Gerontologic Considerations

- In older adults, reduced sebum production leads to skin dryness and roughness. A decline in the number of eccrine glands, along with decreased cutaneous vascularity, causes a decrease in spontaneous sweating with age; this makes older persons more vulnerable to heat.
- Older persons who have had increased sun exposure may develop skin lesions and should be taught careful self-examination. Small, brown, pigmented, benign lesions, known as liver spots or senile lentigines, form on the hands and forearms of older people. Small, yellow or brown, raised lesions, called senile keratoses, may appear on the face and trunk. Senile keratoses are precancerous and require close observation for any change in size, color, or form. These lesions may be removed by freezing, chemical peel, cauterization, or topical creams.
- Multiple changes of aging contribute to loss of skin elasticity and subcutaneous tissue, resulting in wrinkle formation on various body areas.
- Other changes include an increase in skin dryness. Thin, friable, dry skin reduces the effectiveness of the skin barrier as the first line of defense.
- Wound healing may be slowed owing to decreased immunologic responsiveness.
- Sensation may be altered in that perception of light touch is reduced. Therefore, potentially increasing the cutaneous pain threshold can reduce alertness to tactile stimulation of pressure or temperature changes, thereby increasing risk for skin breakdown. Loss of subcutaneous fat impacts thermoregulation.
- Processes of aging can affect vitamin D production.
- Topical drug absorption may be altered.

epidermis is totally replaced approximately every 35 to 45 days; the average person sheds 40 lb of dead skin cells in their lifetime (Marieb, Wilhelm, & Mallatt, 2014).

The dermis, or true skin, consists of connective tissue and contains elastic fibers, blood vessels, sensory and motor nerves, sweat and sebaceous (oil) glands, and hair follicles (roots). The superficial dermal layer on the ventral surface of the hands and feet contains ridges and indentations that create a unique pattern of fingerprints, palm prints, and footprints. In addition to providing a means of identification, the dermal ridges facilitate the ability to grip and hold objects.

The **subcutaneous tissue**, the layer of skin attached to muscle and bone, is composed primarily of connective tissue and fat cells. Skin has a tremendous capacity to stretch with little subsequent damage, as is evident during pregnancy and after soft-tissue injury.

The color of the skin is determined by a pigment called **melanin**, which is manufactured by melanocytes located in the epidermis. The production of melanin is under the control of the middle lobe (pars intermedia) of the pituitary gland, which secretes melanocyte-stimulating hormone. The more the melanin found in the epidermis, the darker the skin color. Exposure to ultraviolet light temporarily stimulates the production of melanin to absorb harmful radiation.

The skin has four major functions: protection, temperature regulation, sensory processing, and chemical synthesis.

Protection

The skin forms a protective barrier between the outside world and underlying organs and structures of the body. This barrier prevents microorganisms and other foreign substances from reaching the structures below the epidermis. It

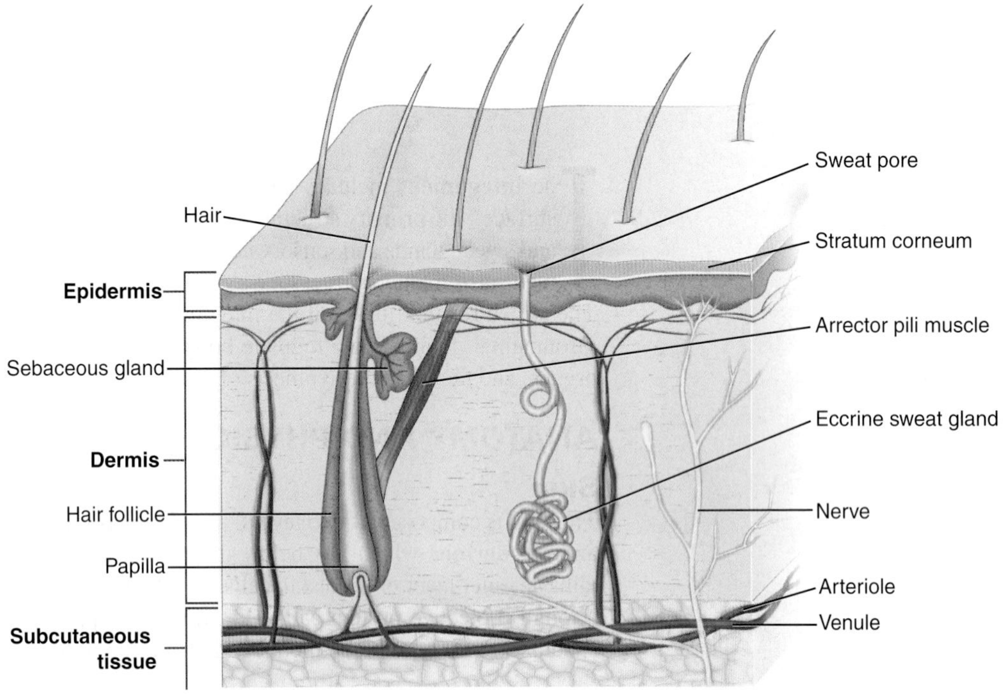

Figure 64-1 A cross-section of the skin.

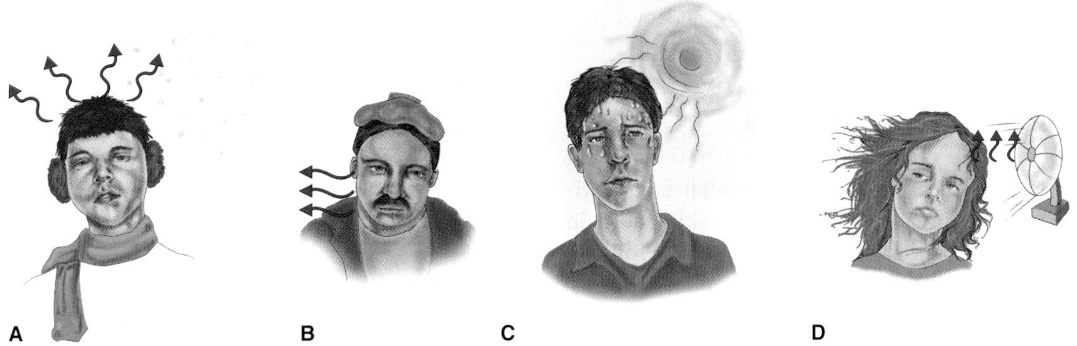

Figure 64-2 Methods of heat loss: **(A)** radiation, **(B)** conduction, **(C)** evaporation, and **(D)** convection.

also prevents structures below the surface of the skin from losing water.

Areas of the skin subjected to friction, such as where a pencil is held repeatedly, have accelerated rates of epidermal cell production. A *callus*, which is a thick layer of epidermal cells, forms in response to recurring friction on an area of skin. Intense friction causes a blister to develop.

Temperature Regulation

To maintain a relatively consistent body temperature, the skin heats or cools the structures below it. The body continuously produces internal heat during cellular metabolism. Erector muscles around shafts of hair contract to generate heat and prevent heat loss at the body's surface. Elevation of skin hairs interferes with local air circulation and maintains the warmth of the skin.

Heat dissipates through the skin and through respiration. Heat is lost by four methods (Fig. 64-2):

- **Radiation** is the transfer of surface heat in the environment. An example of radiant heat loss is the escape of heat from the surface of warm skin into cooler air.
- **Conduction** is the transfer of heat through contact. An example of conductive heat loss is placing a cool cloth on warm skin.
- **Evaporation** is the loss of moisture or water. Water on the surface of the body is warmed. As the moisture vaporizes, the body is cooled. Evaporation occurs unnoticed (insensible loss) as well as when there is obvious perspiration.
- **Convection** is the transfer of heat by means of currents of liquids or gases in which warm air molecules move away from the body. An example of convection is a cool breeze that blows across the body surface.

When the temperature and humidity outside the body rise, radiation, evaporation, and convection are ineffective. The alternative method by which heat is transferred under these conditions is by conduction. This is why exposure to warm temperatures and densely saturated moist air can raise the body temperature and result in heatstroke.

Sensory Processing

The skin combined with body hair serves as a means of monitoring the outside environment as well as warning of danger. There are three types of sensory nerve endings in the skin: *mechanoreceptors*, *thermoreceptors*, and *nociceptors*. **Mechanoreceptors** detect touch, location, pressure, motion, vibration, size, and texture. They are so sensitive that humans can become aware of a mosquito on the surface of the skin. **Thermoreceptors** perceive sensations of heat and cold. **Nociceptors** (see Chapter 11) sense and transmit the location of pain stimuli.

Chemical Synthesis

The skin forms a chemical substance called 7-dehydrocholesterol, which facilitates the synthesis of vitamin D when the skin is exposed to ultraviolet light (sunlight). Vitamin D is necessary for the formation of healthy bones and teeth. Dark-skinned people do not synthesize vitamin D as readily as light-skinned people. Cloudy environments and air pollutants that block sunlight also interfere with vitamin D synthesis. Therefore, vitamin D is added to some food sources, such as milk.

>>> ***Stop, Think, and Respond 64-1***

Discuss the importance of keeping the skin intact.

Hair

Hair originates in the hair follicles in the dermis. It covers all parts of the body except the palms, soles, dorsum of the fingers, lips, penis, labia, and nipples. There are two types of hair: (1) **vellus hair**, which has a wooly or wispy texture, and (2) **terminal hair**, a coarser variety that develops at puberty under the influence of androgen in the axillae, pubic region, face in men, arms, chest, and legs. Men of some races (e.g., Native Americans and Asians) have less facial and body hair than their White American counterparts.

Hundreds of strands of keratin link together with amino acids to form hair. Scalp hair grows more rapidly than hair in other locations. At midlife, hair growth slows, and hair texture is lost. After menopause, some women develop sparse terminal hairs about their face as the ratio of estrogen to androgen hormones decreases.

Melanin, produced by melanocytes in the hair root, influences hair color. The three types of melanin are brown, black, and yellow. Types of melanin are genetically inherited, as are hair texture, shape, and rate of growth. Melanin production decreases with age, causing the hair to become gray or white. Illness, hormone levels, nutrition, aging, and other factors can affect hair growth, texture, and loss (see Chapter 65 for a discussion of baldness).

Sebaceous and Sweat Glands

Sebaceous glands are connected to each hair follicle and secrete an oily substance called **sebum**, which is a lubricant that prevents drying and cracking of the skin and hair. As sebum fills the glandular duct, it enters the hair follicle, from which it eventually is released. During puberty, sebaceous glands in the forehead, nose, chest, and back become more active. Excess sebum may plug the gland. The plugged gland at first appears white, but it later blackens as the sebum oxidizes. Bacterial growth that breaks down the sebum into irritating fatty acids converts the "blackhead" to a pustule and localized area of inflammation that is characteristic of acne (see Chapter 65).

The two types of sweat glands are eccrine and apocrine. **Eccrine glands** release water and electrolytes, such as sodium and chloride, in the form of perspiration. The rate of perspiration is related to body temperature. Adults can produce as much as 3 L under extremely hot conditions. The pH of perspiration is slightly acidic, which helps provide a hostile environment for microbial colonization. Frequent washing with alkaline soaps removes sebum and reduces the acid mantle of protection.

Apocrine glands are found around the nipples, in the anogenital region, in the eyelids (Moll's glands), in the mammary glands of the breast, and in the external ear canals—where the secretion is referred to as *cerumen*. In some animal species, the apocrine glands release **pheromones**, hormonelike chemicals that communicate reproductive and social information among the species. For example, animals release pheromones during urination to mark their territory and during estrus, the period marking receptive sexual activity, to attract mates. The function of apocrine secretions in humans is unknown, although the onset of secretions coincides with puberty. Some speculate that synchronization of menstruation among women in close living conditions such as a dormitory room is the result of apocrine secretions. However, evidence for the phenomenon is mostly anecdotal; it has not been confirmed scientifically by controlled randomized trials (Newcomer, 2016; Women's Health Team, 2016). In general, perspiration, which includes secretions from both eccrine and apocrine glands, is odorless. An odor develops, however, when perspiration mixes with bacteria on the skin.

Nails

Fingernails and toenails are layers of hard keratin that have a protective function. In primates and humans, the nails may be a biologic diversification of claws. Animal species that have claws use them to catch and tear prey, whereas primates and humans developed nails on their fingers and toes because they had a greater biologic need for grasping and manipulating primitive tools or utensils.

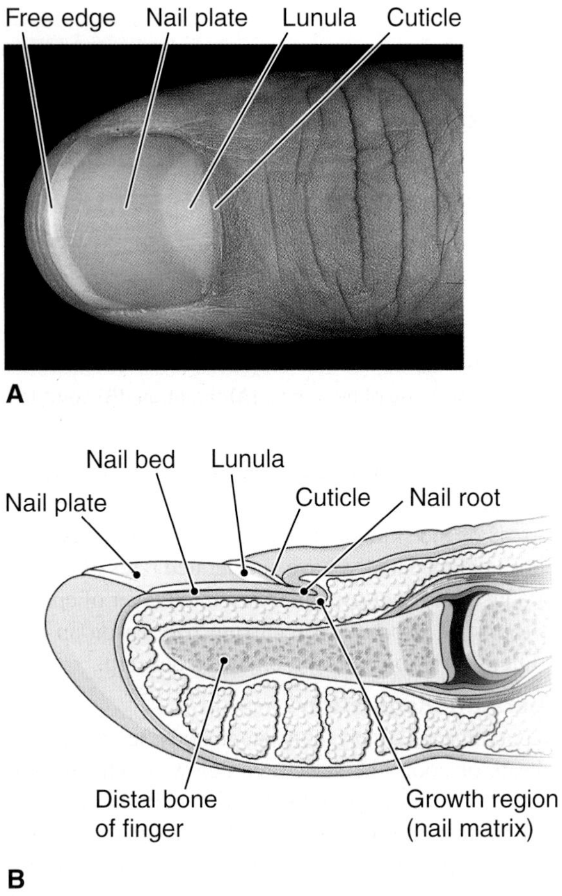

Figure 64-3 External **(A)** and cross-sectional **(B)** views of a nail.

The nail root lies buried beneath the nail's exposed surface in a fold of skin (Fig. 64-3). The nails have an abundant capillary blood supply, resulting in their pink semitransparent appearance that facilitates circulatory assessment. The exception to the pink appearance is the actively growing base, where the nail is so thick that the pink color is obscured by the white moon-shaped area known as the *lunula*.

ASSESSMENT

History

When a disorder of the integument is suspected, initial assessment of the client begins with a thorough history. The history is based on symptoms. The nurse includes the following questions:

- When did the disorder first begin and where did it first appear?
- Where are the lesions located?
- Have there been any changes in the disorder since it first appeared (an increase or decrease in symptoms, in appearance or color, in location)?
- Has the problem spread?
- What are the physical sensations pertaining to the disorder (pain, itching, burning, and intensity)?

- Do other physical or emotional problems appear to be associated with the disorder?
- Was a specific event associated with the onset of the disorder?
- What factors appear to make the condition better or worse?
- Do you or anyone in your family have known or suspected allergies?
- What prescription and nonprescription medications have you taken recently?
- Have you made changes in personal products, such as soaps, deodorants, and cosmetics?
- Have there been recent changes in your work or living environment, such as pets, plants, sprays, dust, and pollutants, that might have precipitated this problem?

Physical Examination

During a physical examination, the nurse inspects and palpates the structures of the integument.

Skin Assessment

The nurse examines the skin on all areas of the body. They can do so during the head-to-toe assessment or as a focused assessment. Good lighting is essential. The skin should be smooth, unbroken, of uniform color according to the person's ethnic or racial origin, warm, and resilient. It should feel neither moist nor unusually dry.

Color deviations have several possible causes (Table 64-1). While examining the skin, the nurse may detect changes in its structure or integrity such as those listed in Table 64-2. The nurse documents the sites and characteristics of any abnormalities.

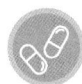

Pharmacologic Considerations

■ When a rash is discovered, is it an allergic reaction or contact dermatitis? A number of people assume that a rash is caused by an allergic reaction to a drug. Research in skin testing has found that about 90% of individuals who self-define as being allergic to penicillin are actually not (Blumenthal et al., 2020). Yet, any report of drug allergy should be thoroughly investigated.

TABLE 64-1 Common Skin Color Variations

COLOR	TERM	POSSIBLE CAUSES
Pale, regardless of race	Pallor	Anemia, blood loss
Red	Erythema	Superficial burns, local inflammation, carbon monoxide poisoning
Pink	Flushed	Fever, hypertension
Purple	Ecchymosis	Trauma to soft tissue
Blue	Cyanosis	Low tissue oxygenation
Yellow	Jaundice	Liver or kidney disease, destruction of red blood cells
Brown	Tan	Racial variation, sun exposure, pregnancy, Addison disease

TABLE 64-2 Terms for Various Skin Lesions

TYPE OF LESION	DESCRIPTION	EXAMPLES
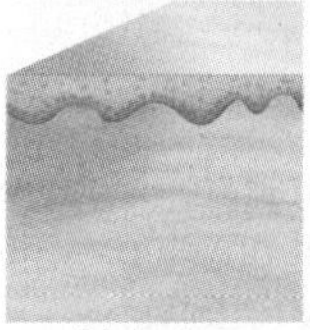 Macule	Flat, round, colored	Freckles, rash
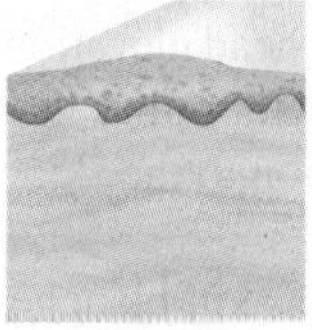 Papule	Elevated, obvious raised border, solid	Wart
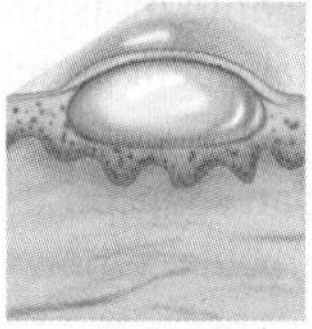 Vesicle	Elevated, round, filled with serum	Blister

(continued)

TABLE 64-2 Terms for Various Skin Lesions (*continued*)

TYPE OF LESION	DESCRIPTION	EXAMPLES
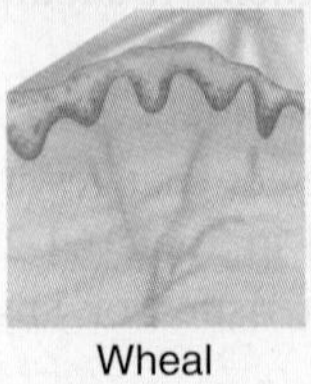 Wheal	Elevated, irregular border, no free fluid	Hives
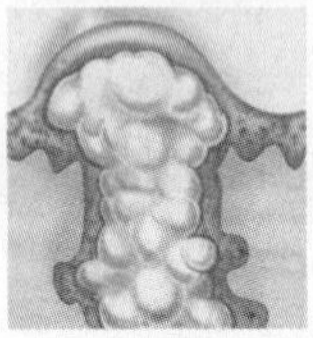 Pustule	Elevated, raised border, filled with pus	Boil
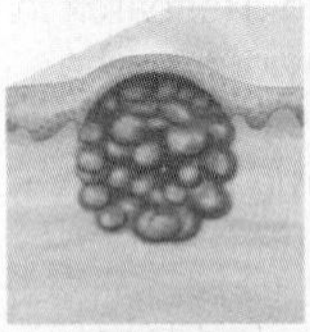 Nodule	Elevated solid mass, extends into deeper tissue	Enlarged lymph node
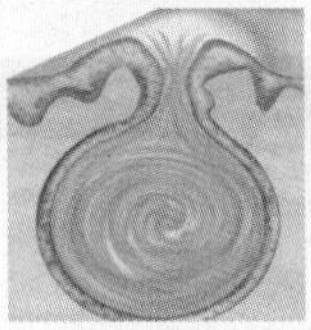 Cyst	Encapsulated, round, fluid-filled, or solid mass beneath the skin	Tissue growth

The nurse assesses temperature by placing the dorsum of their hand on the surface of the skin, but the palmar surface of the hand is used to detect moisture. The nurse determines the quality of skin turgor by grasping the skin, such as that over the sternum, between the thumb and forefinger. Normally, the skin returns to its original position immediately after being released. Tight, shiny skin suggests fluid retention; loose, dry skin may indicate dehydration. Poor nutrition can lead to changes in skin integrity and turgor.

Preventing Pressure Injuries

A **pressure injury**, also known as a pressure sore or *decubitus ulcer*, occurs when capillary blood flow to an area is reduced. This may happen when the skin over a bony prominence is compressed between the weight of the body and a supporting surface for a prolonged period. Common locations include the skin over the coccyx and sacrum in the lower spine, the hips, heels, elbows, shoulder blades, ears, and back of head (Fig. 64-4).

Prevention of pressure injuries first involves identifying persons who are at greatest risk (Fig. 64-5). The Braden Scale for Predicting Pressure Sore Risk, a tool that has a high degree of reliability, uses six assessment categories: sensory perception, moisture, activity, mobility, nutrition, and friction/shear. The risk assessment results in a total score ranging from 6 to 23 by totaling the subscores in each category as follows:

19 to 23: Not at risk
15 to 18: Mild risk
13 to 14: Moderate risk
10 to 12: High risk
6 to 9: Very high risk

Once at-risk clients are identified, the nurse implements measures that reduce conditions under which pressure injuries are likely to form. Some examples are as follows:

- Promoting mobility by turning and repositioning the client frequently with no more than 30 degree head elevation. Alternating positions using a 30 degree lateral rather than 90 degree position to sustain microcirculation to the skin
- Keeping the client's skin clean and dry
- Massaging bony prominences if the client's skin blanches with pressure relief
- Using absorbent pads or briefs that wick and hold moisture
- Applying a topical skin barrier or fecal containment pouch when diarrhea occurs
- Using a moisturizing skin cleanser rather than soap
- Applying pressure-relieving devices to the heels, elbows, bed, and chairs
- Avoiding donut-type devices

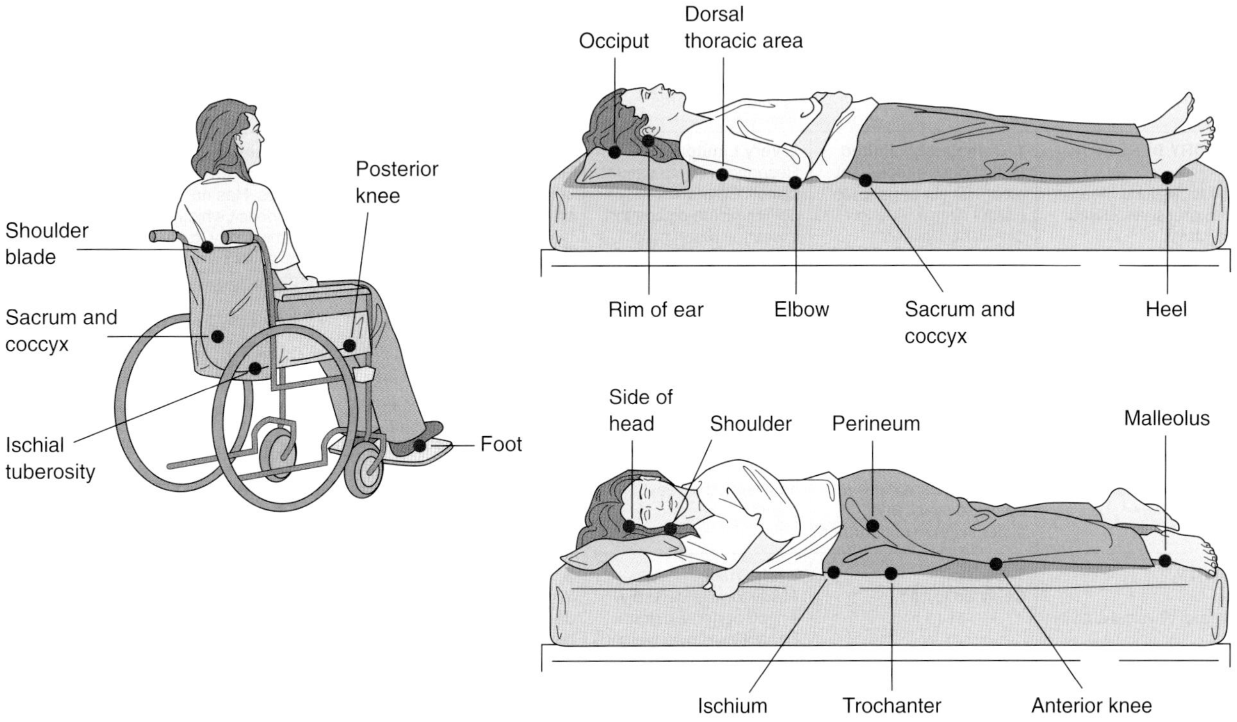

Figure 64-4 Common locations for pressure injuries in supine, lateral, and sitting positions.

- Padding body areas that are subject to pressure. Avoiding **friction**, the effect that occurs when one object rubs against the other, and **shearing**, a physical force that separates layers of tissue in opposite directions, such as when a seated client slides downward by using a lift sheet and encouraging the use of a trapeze
- Increasing dietary protein
- Supporting hydration

Staging a Pressure Injury

Pressure injuries are categorized into one of six stages (Fig. 64-6), depending on the extent of tissue injury (Hess, 2020).

Stage I Pressure Injury. Stage I pressure injuries are characterized by redness of intact skin. The reddened skin of a beginning pressure injury fails to resume its normal color, or blanch, when pressure is relieved. Massaging the area contributes to compromised tissue injury.

Stage II Pressure Injury. A stage II pressure injury is red and is accompanied by blistering or a shallow break in the skin, sometimes described as a **skin tear**. This is a partial thickness loss of skin with exposed dermis. Impairment of the skin leads to microbial colonization and infection of the wound.

Stage III Pressure Injury. Pressure injuries classified as stage III are those in which the superficial skin impairment progresses to a shallow crater that extends to the subcutaneous tissue becoming a full-thickness loss of tissue with adipose tissue visible (Hess, 2020). Stage III pressure injuries may be accompanied by serous drainage from leaking plasma or purulent drainage (white- or yellow-tinged fluid) caused by a wound infection. Although a stage III pressure injury is a significant wound, the area is relatively painless. The Centers for Medicare and Medicaid Services (2020) continue to refuse payments for the care of clients who acquire Stage III and IV pressure injuries during their hospitalization because they are considered a preventable condition.

Stage IV Pressure Injury. Stage IV pressure injuries are the most traumatic and life-threatening. There is full-thickness skin and tissue loss (Hess, 2020). The tissue is deeply ulcerated, exposing muscle and sometimes bone. The dead tissue produces a rank odor. Local infection, which is the rule rather than the exception, easily spreads throughout the body, causing a potentially fatal condition referred to as *sepsis*.

Unstageable Pressure Injury. This injury is a full-thickness skin and tissue loss where the tissue damage is so severe that it cannot be determined due to eschar or slough (Hess, 2020).

Deep Tissue Pressure Injury. This consists of intact or nonintact skin with localized area of persistent nonblanchable discoloration of skin or where there is epidermal separation that reveals a dark wound bed or blood-filled blister (Hess, 2020).

Nutrition Notes outlines nutritional considerations for pressure injury healing. Also see Evidence-Based Practice 64-1.

Scalp and Hair Assessment

The nurse assesses the scalp by separating the hair at random areas and inspecting the skin. The scalp normally is smooth, intact, and free of lesions.

BRADEN SCALE FOR PREDICTING PRESSURE SORE RISK

Patient's Name ______________ Evaluator's Name ______________ Date of Assessment

SENSORY PERCEPTION ability to respond meaningfully to pressure-related discomfort	**1. Completely Limited** Unresponsive (does not moan, flinch, or gasp) to painful stimuli, due to diminished level of consciousness or sedation. OR limited ability to feel pain over most of body.	**2. Very Limited** Responds only to painful stimuli. Cannot communicate discomfort except by moaning or restlessness. OR has a sensory impairment which limits the ability to feel pain or discomfort over 1/2 of the body.	**3. Slightly Limited** Responds to verbal commands, but cannot always communicate discomfort or the need to be turned. OR has some sensory impairment which limits ability to feel pain or discomfort in 1 or 2 extremities.	**4. No Impairment** Responds to verbal commands. Has no sensory deficit which would limit ability to feel or voice pain or discomfort.				
MOISTURE degree to which skin is exposed to moisture	**1. Constantly Moist** Skin is kept moist almost constantly by perspiration, urine, etc. Dampness is detected every time patient is moved or turned.	**2. Very Moist** Skin is often, but not always, moist. Linen must be changed at least once a shift.	**3. Occasionally Moist** Skin is occasionally moist, requiring an extra linen change approximately once a day.	**4. Rarely Moist** Skin is usually dry, linen only requires changing at routine intervals.				
ACTIVITY degree of physical activity	**1. Bedfast** Confined to bed.	**2. Chairfast** Ability to walk severely limited or non-existent. Cannot bear own weight and/or must be assisted into chair or wheelchair.	**3. Walks Occasionally** Walks occasionally during day, but for very short distances, with or without assistance. Spends majority of each shift in bed or chair.	**4. Walks Frequently** Walks outside room at least twice a day and inside room at least once every two hours during waking hours.				
MOBILITY ability to change and control body position	**1. Completely Immobile** Does not make even slight changes in body or extremity position without assistance.	**2. Very Limited** Makes occasional slight changes in body or extremity position but unable to make frequent or significant changes independently.	**3. Slightly Limited** Makes frequent though slight changes in body or extremity position independently.	**4. No Limitation** Makes major and frequent changes in position without assistance.				
NUTRITION usual food intake pattern	**1. Very Poor** Never eats a complete meal. Rarely eats more than 1/3 of any food offered. Eats 2 servings or less of protein (meat or dairy products) per day. Takes fluids poorly. Does not take a liquid dietary supplement. OR is NPO and/or maintained on clear liquids or IV's for more than 5 days.	**2. Probably Inadequate** Rarely eats a complete meal and generally eats only 1/2 of any food offered. Protein intake includes only 3 servings of meat or dairy products per day. Occasionally will take a dietary supplement. OR receives less than optimum amount of liquid diet or tube feeding.	**3. Adequate** Eats over half of most meals. Eats a total of 4 servings of protein (meat, dairy products) per day. Occasionally will refuse a meal, but will usually take a supplement when offered. OR is on a tube feeding or TPN regimen which probably meets most of nutritional needs.	**4. Excellent** Eats most of every meal. Never refuses a meal. Usually eats a total of 4 or more servings of meat and dairy products. Occasionally eats between meals. Does not require supplementation.				
FRICTION & SHEAR	**1. Problem** Requires moderate to maximum assistance in moving. Complete lifting without sliding against sheets is impossible. Frequently slides down in bed or chair, requiring frequent repositioning with maximum assistance. Spasticity, contractures, or agitation leads to almost constant friction.	**2. Potential Problem** Moves feebly or requires minimum assistance. During a move skin probably slides to some extent against sheets, chair, restraints, or other devices. Maintains relatively good position in chair or bed most of the time but occasionally slides down.	**3. No Apparent Problem** Moves in bed and in chair independently and has sufficient muscle strength to lift up completely during move. Maintains good position in bed or chair.					
				Total Score				

Figure 64-5 The Braden Scale for Predicting Pressure Sore Risk. (Copyright, Braden and Bergstrom, 1988. Reprinted with permission. All rights reserved.)

Hair assessment applies not only to the head but also to other locations such as the eyebrows, eyelashes, chest, arms, pubis, and legs. The nurse notes the color, texture, and distribution, keeping sex- and age-related variations in mind. Hair may become brittle and thin as a result of poor nutrition. The presence of nits and eggs from a louse infestation (see Chapter 65), as well as scales and flaking skin, are also abnormal findings.

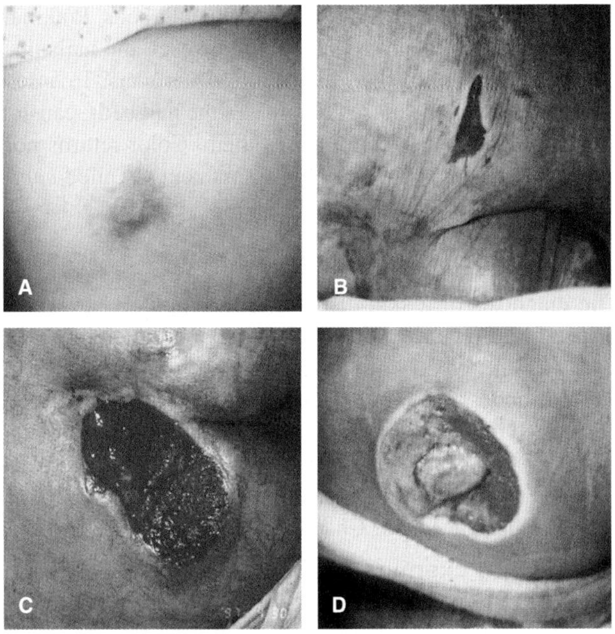

Figure 64-6 Pressure injury stages: **(A)** stage I, **(B)** stage II, **(C)** stage III, and **(D)** stage IV.

>>> *Stop, Think, and Respond 64-2*

What type of skin lesion does a client have if it is described as follows:

1. *Elevated, round, and filled with serum?*
2. *Flat, round, and red?*
3. *Elevated, solid, with a raised border?*
4. *Elevated, round, raised border, filled with pus?*

Nail Assessment

Normal nails appear slightly convex with a 160-degree angle between the nail base and the skin. Concave-shaped nails, referred to as *spooning* because of their characteristic appearance, are a sign of iron-deficiency anemia. Clubbing of the nails, evidenced by an angle greater than 160 degrees, suggests long-standing cardiopulmonary disease (Fig. 64-7). Normal thumbnail thickness varies from 0.7 to 1.0 mm and 0.3 to 0.5 mm in the little finger (Higashi, 2012); nails thicken when there is a fungal infection and poor circulation. There may be evidence of other nail abnormalities that become evident during the assessment (Fig. 64-8).

Nutrition Notes

The Client With Pressure Injury

- Depending on the stage of a pressure injury, protein requirements range from 1 to 1.6 g/kg to promote healing.
- Calories are increased to spare protein; small, frequent meals help maximize intake.
- Supplements of vitamins A, C, and zinc may be prescribed.
- Calorie counts help assess adequacy of intake.

Evidence-Based Practice 64-1

Pressure Injury Prevention

Clinical Question

How does implementing a pressure injury prevention bundle compare with individual interventions to affect pressure injury rates in adults?

Evidence

Pressure injuries (also called pressure ulcer or pressure sore) are preventable conditions that affect quality of life, put clients at risk for additional complications, and have significant financial impacts for health care systems such as increased length of stay, higher hospital costs, and effects on reimbursement (Deakin et al., 2020; Chaboyer, 2017). Different interventions have been explored for pressure injury prevention. These include such things as assessment to identify clients most at risk for developing pressure injuries, targeted assessments of skin condition for early detection, special dressings, different types of mattresses or mattress toppers, turning protocols, nutritional support, techniques for moving clients that minimize irritation of the skin, and wound and ostomy care nurse rounds (Deakin et al., 2020; Chaboyer, 2017). However, in spite of all their efforts, health care providers continue to struggle to find a solution. Providers are beginning to explore whether the answer to pressure injury prevention is not adoption of one intervention but rather taking a multifocused approach by adopting multiple interventions simultaneously. This is called "bundling." Some pressure injury bundles focus on implementing a group of interventions to prevent pressure injuries, whereas other bundles also focus on staff education and client and family involvement by implementing groups of interventions that target prevention measures and early identification. When a pressure injury bundle was combined with wound and ostomy care nurse rounds, the incidence of pressure injuries dropped from 15.2% to 2.1%. In addition, the frequency of repositioning and heel elevation increased significantly. However, not all studies have shown the same level of effectiveness of bundles (Deakin et al., 2020). Regardless, actively including clients and their families in their care is an important part of client-centered care and evidence-based practice initiatives supported by such organizations as World Health Organization (WHO) and Centers for Disease Control and Prevention (CDC).

Nursing Implications

Pressure injuries are preventable conditions that have negative effects on both clinical and health care organizations. Nurses play a key role in pressure injury prevention and identification. Know what your organization's approach is to pressure injury prevention and identification, and implement those interventions every day with every client. Good documentation on assessment findings and use of interventions are key to building data that can evaluate what is effective and what is not effective in your organization. Involving clients and their families in care by helping them understand what pressure injuries are, what their risk of developing pressure injury

(continued)

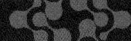

Evidence-Based Practice 64-1 (*continued*)

is, and working together with them to monitor skin condition, get them moving, maximize their nutritional status, and implement such interventions as heel elevation allows everyone to work together to prevent pressure injuries.

References

Chaboyer, W., Bucknall, T., Gillespie, B., Thalib, L., McInnes, E., Considine, J., Murray, E., Duffy, P., Tuck, M., & Harbeck, E. (2017). Adherence to evidence-based pressure injury prevention guidelines in routine clinical practice: A longitudinal study. *International Wound Journal, 14*, 1290–1298. https://doi.org/10.1111/iwj.12798

Deakin, J., Gillespie, B. M., Chaboyer, W., Nieuwenhoven, P., & Latimer, S. (2020). An education intervention care bundle to improve hospitalised patients' pressure injury prevention knowledge: A before and after study. *Wound Practice & Research, 28*(4), 154–162. https://doi-org.10.33235/wpr.28.4.154-162.

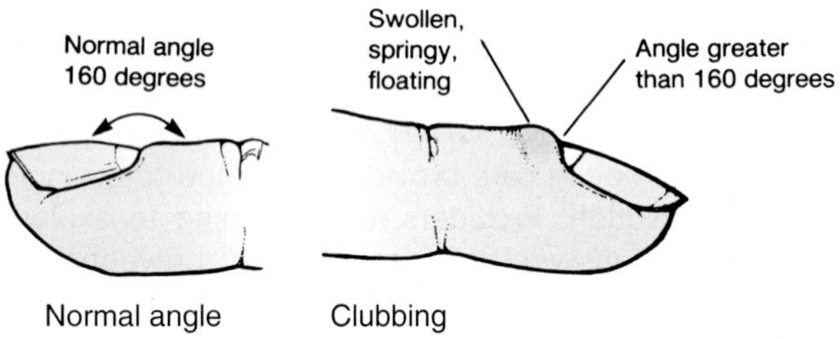

Figure 64-7 Normal nail angle and clubbed nail.

The nurse observes the color of the nail beds. Pink nail beds suggest adequate oxygenation; however, the nails may be darker in clients other than White Americans. To assess tissue perfusion, the nurse compresses the nail beds, causing them to blanch, and then releases them. Color returns normally in 3 seconds or less. This assessment is called *capillary refill time*.

Diagnostic Tests

The diagnosis of a skin disorder is made chiefly by visual inspection. Some disorders may involve additional inspection with the Wood light, potassium hydroxide test, fungal culture, and skin biopsy. Culture and sensitivity tests are performed on lesions that are suspected or known to contain bacteria. Allergy tests by intradermal injection, the scratch test, and the patch test are used to confirm an allergy to one or more substances (see Chapter 34).

Wood Light Examination

The **Wood light**, also known as a black light, is a handheld device that can identify certain fungal infections that fluoresce under long-wave ultraviolet light. In a darkened room, when a primary provider or nurse aims the light at a lesion caused by a fungus that fluoresces, the lesion emits a blue-green color (Fig. 64-9). Because less than 10% of the fungi that cause hair and scalp infections actually fluoresce, a primary provider may have to conduct additional tests.

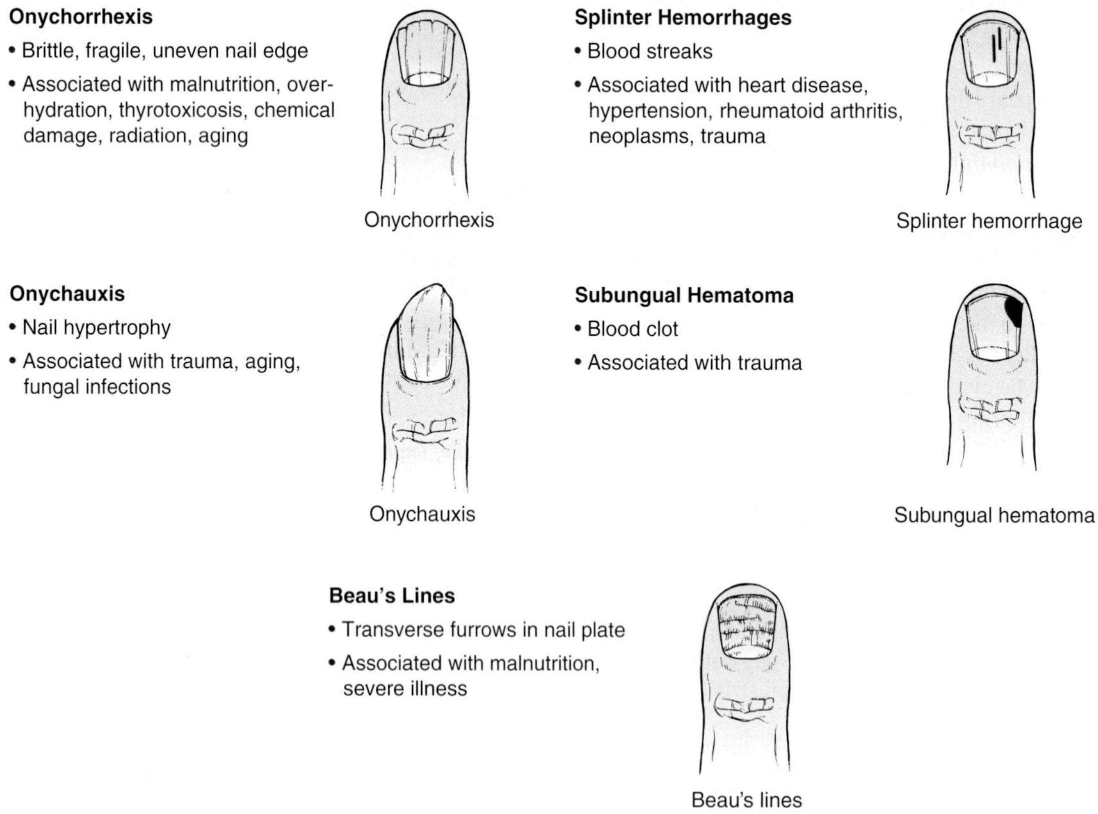
Onychorrhexis
• Brittle, fragile, uneven nail edge
• Associated with malnutrition, overhydration, thyrotoxicosis, chemical damage, radiation, aging
Onychorrhexis
Splinter Hemorrhages
• Blood streaks
• Associated with heart disease, hypertension, rheumatoid arthritis, neoplasms, trauma
Splinter hemorrhage
Onychauxis
• Nail hypertrophy
• Associated with trauma, aging, fungal infections
Onychauxis
Subungual Hematoma
• Blood clot
• Associated with trauma
Subungual hematoma
Beau's Lines
• Transverse furrows in nail plate
• Associated with malnutrition, severe illness
Beau's lines

Figure 64-8 Nail abnormalities.

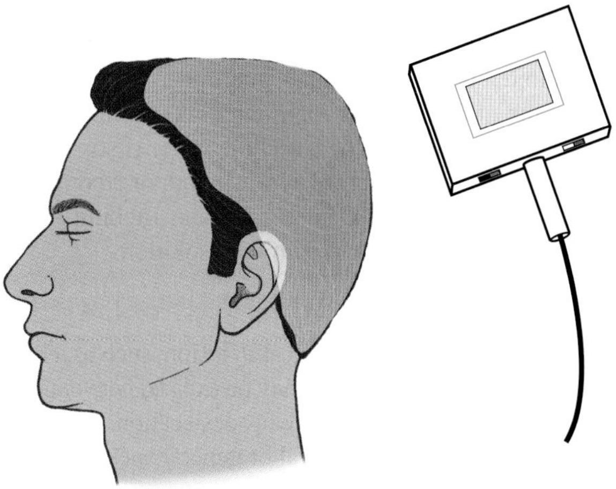

Figure 64-9 Fungal organisms glow under Wood light illumination.

Potassium Hydroxide Test

For fungal infections that do not fluoresce, the primary provider may take a scraping of the skin and perform a potassium hydroxide test. The primary provider uses a scalpel, wet gauze, or brush to collect dead skin scales. They place the specimen on a glass slide with potassium hydroxide solution and applies heat. The heated solution dissolves the skin and hair cells but does not affect any fungal cells. The primary provider microscopically examines the slide to check for any **hyphae** (threadlike filaments within the cells of most fungi). This test confirms that a fungal infection has caused the lesion, but the primary provider may need a culture to identify the specific species of fungus.

Fungal Culture

The procedure for obtaining a specimen for fungal culture is similar to that for a potassium hydroxide test. The primary provider places the scraped cells into a sterile container and sends it to the laboratory, where an analyst spreads the cells on the surface of a nutritive medium such as agar. The specimen requires incubation at room temperature for 2 to 3 weeks. Once a sufficient colony exists, the analyst examines it microscopically to identify the type of fungus causing the infection.

Skin Biopsy

A primary provider obtains a biopsy of skin tissue to identify malignant, premalignant, and nonmalignant skin lesions as well as chronic skin disorders such as Hansen's disease (leprosy). After injecting a local anesthetic, the primary provider obtains skin cells for the biopsy in one of three ways: (1) scraping the lesion parallel with the skin with a scalpel or razor blade, (2) excising the lesion partially or entirely with scissors or a scalpel, or (3) using a punching instrument to remove a cylindrical core of tissue (Fig. 64-10). The primary provider preserves the specimen in formaldehyde, and the pathologist examines it microscopically to identify any abnormal cells. Depending on the type of biopsy, the client may require some sutures to close the skin and control bleeding.

MEDICAL AND SURGICAL TREATMENT OF SKIN DISORDERS

Various types of therapies are used in the treatment or management of skin disorders. They include drug therapy, wet dressings, therapeutic baths, surgical excision, radiation therapy, photochemotherapy, hyperbaric oxygenation, and lifestyle changes.

Drug Therapy

Topical and systemic medications are used to treat skin disorders. Some examples are as follows:

- *Corticosteroids* are applied topically or administered systemically (orally, intramuscularly, intravenously) to relieve inflammatory and allergic symptoms. When used systemically, corticosteroids can have serious side effects; therefore, they are used primarily to relieve acute problems. Continued long-term use brings greater risk and is justified only when the disease itself is serious and other treatments cannot relieve it. Used as directed, topical application of a corticosteroid does not result in the pronounced adverse effects as systemic administration and can be used for longer periods.
- *Antihistamines* frequently are prescribed when allergy is a factor in causing the skin disorder. They relieve itching and shorten the duration of the allergic reaction.

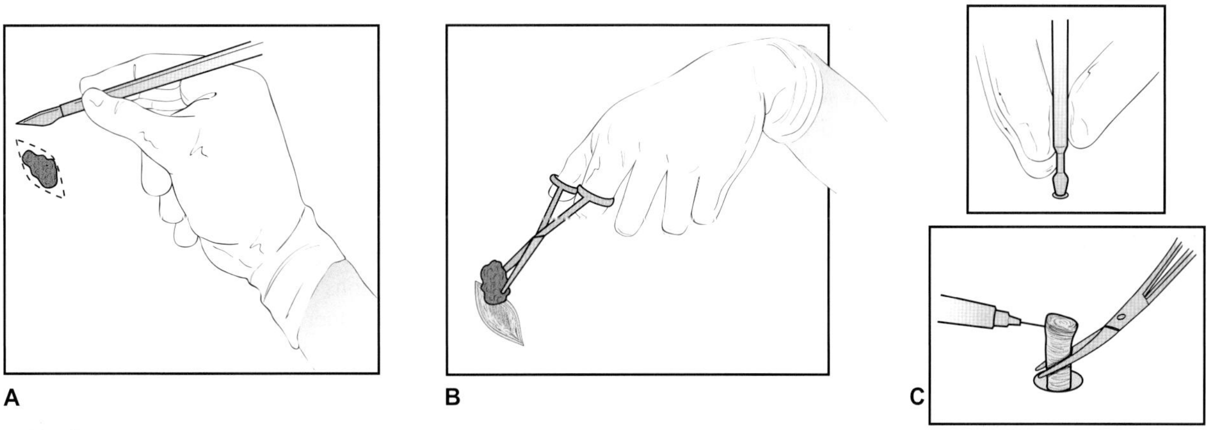

Figure 64-10 Three techniques for obtaining a skin biopsy: (A) scrape, (B) surgical excision, and (C) punch.

- *Antibiotic, antifungal, and antiviral agents* are used to treat infectious disorders. They are applied topically or administered systemically.
- *Scabicides and pediculicides* are used in the treatment of infestations with the scabies mite and lice (see Chapter 65).
- *Local (topical) anesthetics* are applied to relieve minor skin pain and itching.
- *Emollients, ointments, powders, and lotions*, which may be combined with other agents, soothe, protect, and soften the skin.
- *Antiseborrheic agents* are applied directly to the scalp or incorporated into shampooing products to control dandruff (see Chapter 65).
- *Antiseptics* are used to reduce bacteria on the skin.
- *Keratolytics* dissolve thickened, cornified skin such as warts, corns, and calluses. Their action causes the treated area to soften and swell, facilitating removal.

Nurses use standard precautions when applying any topical medication to impaired skin or changing dressings that cover an open lesion. Infected, draining, or weeping lesions may require contact precautions as well (see Chapter 12). It is important to apply topical medication as prescribed, such as a thin layer evenly spread over the area or a thick layer dabbed on the area. The nurse takes care in applying medication so lesions are not broken or skin surfaces abraded.

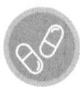

Pharmacologic Considerations

■ Encourage clients to complete the entire course of drug therapy, even if the condition resolves before they finish all the medication.
■ As with any medication (oral, topical, or otherwise), drug interactions may occur. Be sure the client keeps a current list of all medications taken; this helps the clinical pharmacist prevent drug interactions when new medicines are prescribed.

Wet Dressings

Wet dressings are used to apply a solution to a skin lesion for a cooling and soothing effect. The nature of the skin lesion (open or intact) determines whether sterile technique is required. A dry dressing consisting of gauze or other porous material is first applied to the area. Cotton is not used because of its tendency to stick to wound surfaces. The dressing is then saturated with the prescribed liquid. Dressings can be temporarily anchored with nonallergenic tape or roller gauze. A continuously moist environment promotes healing; an occlusive hydrocolloid dressing that contributes water to the impaired skin can achieve the same objective.

Therapeutic Baths

A therapeutic bath is one in which various solutions, powders, and oils, but no soap, are added to water into which the client's entire body or only a part is submerged. The baths are used to relieve inflammation and itching and to aid in the removal of crusts and scales. Examples of products used include cornstarch, sodium bicarbonate (baking soda), oatmeal colloidal bath preparations, and mineral oil.

The tub or container is filled with lukewarm water. The drug or product is then added, and the water is stirred so the preparation mixes thoroughly. A washcloth or a compress is used to apply the solution gently without rubbing the face and any other parts not covered by the solution.

Surgical Excision

When it is necessary to remove a skin lesion, such as a benign or malignant growth, the tissue may be excised conventionally or with a laser, cryosurgery, or electrodesiccation. Surgical excisions are performed under local or general anesthesia.

Laser Therapy

Laser stands for *l*ight *a*mplification by the *s*timulated *e*mission of *r*adiation. Lasers convert a solid, gas, or liquid substance into light. The energy of laser light vaporizes tissue and coagulates bleeding vessels. Lasers also are used to remove tattoos and pigmented skin lesions such as hemangiomas and nevi. When a laser procedure is performed, the eyes must be protected, precautions must be taken for preventing fires and burns from heated instruments, and vaporized fumes must be removed.

Cryosurgery

Cryosurgery is the application of extreme subfreezing cold with a probe or agent such as liquid nitrogen. After application at the center of the lesion, the area thaws and becomes gelatinlike in appearance. A scab forms at the site. Healing takes approximately 4 to 6 weeks.

Electrodesiccation

Electrodesiccation (or electrosurgery) is the use of electrical energy converted to heat to destroy or remove superficial growths from the skin by dehydrating and shrinking the affected tissue. Plantar warts and skin tumors are examples of disorders treated by this method.

Radiation Therapy

Radiation therapy is used to treat malignant skin lesions. For more information on radiation therapy, see Chapter 18.

Photochemotherapy

Photochemotherapy involves a combination of ultraviolet light and a photosensitizing chemical and ultraviolet light to destroy cells. It is one method used to treat psoriasis, a chronic skin condition (see Chapter 65), and some malignant growths.

Lifestyle Changes

Some skin disorders such as psoriasis (see Chapter 65) and herpes simplex infections (see Chapter 56) grow worse when the person is tired or under emotional stress. Therefore, rest and sleep are an important part of treatment. Diet also is important because certain foods contribute to or aggravate skin disorders in some individuals and therefore must be eliminated from the diet.

Nursing Management

The nurse conducts a thorough assessment, gathering data that identify normal and abnormal characteristics of the integument. They implement nursing measures that promote the system's integrity or restoration (see Chapters 65 and 66). The nurse educates the client and family about the etiology and treatment of specific integumentary disorders and encourages maintaining health care that may be lengthy. Empathy is used when supporting clients who are experiencing distress because of the chronicity and social stigma from observable signs and symptoms involving the integument.

KEY POINTS

- Anatomy and physiology
  - Skin: composed of dermis and epidermis; purpose—protection, temperature regulation, sensory processing, chemical synthesis
  - Sebaceous and sweat glands: sebaceous glands are connected to each hair follicle; sweat glands are eccrine and apocrine
  - Nails: fingernails and toenails; layers of hard keratin
- Assessment: history, physical examination to include skin assessment, preventing pressure injuries, staging pressure injuries, scalp and hair assessment
  - Diagnostic testing include:
    - Wood light examination: black light to identify fungal infections
    - Potassium hydroxide test: further fungal testing
    - Fungal culture
    - Skin biopsy: can be scrape, surgical excision, or punch
- Medical and surgical treatment of skin disorders
  - Drug therapy: topical and/or systemic medications to include corticosteroids, antihistamines, antibiotics, antifungals, scabicides, antiseborrheic agents
  - Wet dressings: used to apply a solution to a skin lesion
  - Therapeutic baths
  - Surgical excision
  - Radiation therapy
  - Phototherapy

CRITICAL THINKING EXERCISES

1. Explain the basis for identifying the integument as the largest body organ.
2. Why does skin become paler in colder, cloudy environments and darker in warmer, sunny environments?
3. If one of the functions of the skin is to regulate body temperature using methods such as perspiration, explain why perspiration increases during stress.
4. A client has developed a rash over the arms and thorax. What additional data are important to obtain before contacting the primary provider?

NCLEX-STYLE REVIEW QUESTIONS PrepU

1. The nurse examines a client who slipped and fell while climbing stairs and now has swelling of one ankle, pain on movement, and localized ecchymosis. What word correlates with the nurse's use of the term "ecchymosis" when documenting the assessment data?
   1. Freckled
   2. Mottled
   3. Bruised
   4. Blanched
2. What nursing assessment technique is best for determining the quality of the client's skin turgor?
   1. Feeling the skin with the palmar surface of the hand
   2. Grasping a fold of skin over the sternum
   3. Placing the dorsum of the hand lightly on the skin
   4. Pressing the skin over a bony prominence
3. An older adult who is bedridden frequently slides to the bottom of the bed with the feet touching the footboard. When the nurse analyzes the observation, what is the most likely outcome of the client's downward movement in bed?
   1. The client is at risk for a traumatic fracture if a fall occurs.
   2. The client is at risk for hypothermia because of skin exposure.
   3. The client is at risk for bruising because of contact with the footboard.
   4. The client is at risk for skin impairment because of shearing forces.
4. When the nurse identifies a client as being at risk for the development of a pressure injury, what nursing order is essential to add to the plan of care at this time?
   1. Use a bed board for skeletal support.
   2. Change client's position every 2 hours.
   3. Rub reddened areas every 2 hours.
   4. Add an emollient to the bathwater.
5. During a routine assessment, the nurse notes that a client's fingernails have a clubbed appearance. What is the nurse's most valid interpretation regarding this finding?
   1. The client's fingernails are essentially normal.
   2. The client may have chronic cardiopulmonary disease.
   3. The client has a fungal infection in the nail beds.
   4. The client's nails reflect iron-deficiency anemia.

WANT TO KNOW MORE? There are a wide variety of online resources available on thePoint to enhance learning and understanding of this chapter.

Go to thePoint.lww.com/activate, and use the activation code found in the front of this text to unlock these online resources.

65 Caring for Clients With Skin, Hair, and Nail Disorders

Words To Know

acne vulgaris
alopecia
alopecia areata
androgenetic alopecia
body piercing
carbuncle
comedone
dandruff
dermabrasion
dermatitis
dermatome
dermatophytes
dermatophytoses
erythema
furuncle
furunculosis
granuloma
herpes zoster
keloids
nits
onychocryptosis
onychomycosis
pediculosis
photochemotherapy
podiatrist
pruritus
psoriasis
rhinophyma
rosacea
scabies
seborrhea
seborrheic dermatitis
shingles
tattoo
telangiectases

Learning Objectives

On completion of this chapter, you will be able to:

1. Define and name two types of dermatitis.
2. Explain factors that lead to acne vulgaris.
3. Describe characteristics of rosacea.
4. Differentiate between a furuncle, furunculosis, and carbuncle.
5. Describe the appearance and cause of psoriasis.
6. Describe the process for eradicating a skin mite infection using a scabicidal medication.
7. Identify locations on the body where parasitic fungi known as dermatophytes are most likely to infect.
8. Describe the characteristics of an outbreak of shingles.
9. Discuss factors that promote skin cancer as well as measures that help prevent it.
10. Name two conditions characterized by hair loss and the etiology for each.
11. Describe the appearance of head lice and nits and explain how to remove them.
12. Discuss factors that promote fungal infections of the nails.
13. Name techniques for preventing onychocryptosis (ingrown toenails).
14. Identify risks associated with tattooing and body piercing.
15. Describe general care following tattooing and body piercing.

Disorders of the skin, hair, and nails are common. Because self-image is inextricably related to how a person looks, clients with disorders of the skin, hair, and nails need empathic support while they cope with chronic or acute conditions affecting the integument. Body ornamentation such as tattooing and body piercings are subject to complications and also have personal and social implications.

SKIN DISORDERS

Dermatitis

Dermatitis is a general term that refers to an inflammation of the skin. It is a common sign of many skin disorders accompanied by a red rash. An associated symptom is **pruritus** or itching. Dermatitis and pruritus may be localized or generalized. Because both are nonspecific symptoms, it is essential that the cause be diagnosed and definitively treated. Two common types are allergic and irritant dermatitis.

Pathophysiology and Etiology

Allergic contact dermatitis develops in people who are sensitive to one or more substances, such as drugs, fibers in clothing, cosmetics, plants (e.g., poison ivy), and dyes. Primary irritant dermatitis is a localized

Gerontologic Considerations

- A decrease in epidermal replacement rates contributes to excessive drying of an older person's skin, leading to pruritus and infection. Daily bathing is not necessary, and lotion or cream may be helpful in soothing dry areas. Early assessment and treatment of any type of skin lesion helps prevent infection and complications.
- Careful assessment for scabies and head lice is especially important for frail older adults or those with cognitive limitations. These clients may be unable to inform the nurse of symptoms or may manifest atypical symptoms, including increased confusion or agitation.
- Scratching of infested body areas increases risk of skin breakdown in older adults with thinning skin tissue.

reaction that occurs when the skin comes in contact with a strong chemical such as a solvent or detergent.

In clients with allergies, sensitized mast cells in the skin release histamine, causing a red rash, itching, and localized swelling (see Chapter 34). An allergy, however, does not cause irritant dermatitis. Rather, the caustic quality of the substance damages the protein structure of the skin or eliminates secretions that protect it.

Assessment Findings

The skin response is characterized by dilation of the blood vessels, causing redness and swelling, and sometimes by blister formation and oozing (Fig. 65-1). Itching is a prominent symptom. Primary irritant dermatitis may cause soreness or discomfort from irritation, itching, redness, swelling, and blistering.

Diagnosis is made by visual examination of the area. A detailed and thorough history helps identify the offending substances as well as the type of dermatitis. In difficult cases, a skin patch test may identify an allergic substance.

Medical Management

Treatment of both types of dermatitis is to remove the substances causing the reaction. This is done by flushing the skin with cool water. Topical lotions, such as calamine, or systemic drugs, such as diphenhydramine (Benadryl) or cyproheptadine (Periactin), are prescribed to relieve itching. Moisturizing creams with lanolin restore lubrication. In more severe cases, wet dressings with astringent solutions, such as Burow's solution (aluminum acetate), are prescribed. Corticosteroids taken orally or applied topically also provide relief.

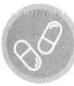

Pharmacologic Considerations

- Infants and children have a high ratio of skin surface area to body mass; therefore, the potential for systemic drug absorption and related risks is greater for infants and children than for an adult when topical medications are applied.

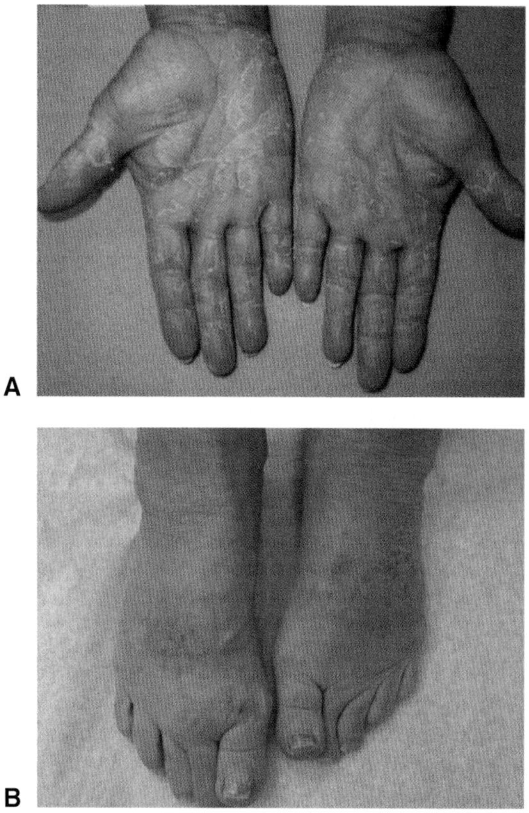

Figure 65-1 Contact dermatitis of the **(A)** wrist and **(B)** feet from shoe material. (Copyright GSK. Used with permission).

Nursing Management

The nurse advises clients to wear rubber gloves when coming in contact with any substance such as soap or solvents, put all clothes through a second rinse cycle when laundering to remove soap residue, and avoid the use of cosmetics or any topical drug or substance until the etiology of the dermatitis is identified. Measures that reduce itching or preserve the integrity of the skin are presented in Client and Family Teaching 65-1.

Client and Family Teaching 65-1 Reducing Itching With Dermatitis

The nurse emphasizes the following points when teaching the client:

- Keep nails short and clean.
- Use light cotton bedding and clothing that allows normal evaporation of moisture from the skin (avoid wool, synthetics, and other dense fibers).
- Wear white cotton gloves if prone to scratching during sleep.
- Avoid regular soap for bathing; hypoallergenic or glycerin soaps can be used without causing skin irritation or itching.
- Use tepid bath water; pat rather than rub the skin dry.
- Inform the primary provider if the drug therapy fails to restore skin integrity or relieve itching.

Acne Vulgaris

Acne vulgaris, which tends to coincide with puberty, is an inflammatory disorder that affects the sebaceous glands and hair follicles. The severity of the condition varies from minimal to severe.

Pathophysiology and Etiology

Acne is believed to be related to the rise in androgen hormone levels, which occurs when secondary sex characteristics are developing. Androgens increase the size and activity of sebaceous glands within the skin. The overproduction of sebum provides an ideal environment for bacterial growth. Any correlation with specific food items (e.g., chocolate) is more myth than fact.

Sebum, keratin, and bacteria accumulate and dilate the follicle. The collective secretions form a **comedone**, or what most refer to as a *blackhead* (Fig. 65-2). The dark appearance is the result of oxidation of the core material. The follicle becomes further distended and irritated, causing a raised papule in the skin. If the follicular wall ruptures, the inflammatory response extends into the marginal areas of the dermis. In serious cases, inflamed nodules and cysts develop. The skin lesions are aggravated by cosmetics as well as picking and squeezing blemishes. Severe acne, if neglected, leads to deep, pitted scars that leave the skin permanently pockmarked. Acne vulgaris improves after adolescence.

Assessment Findings

Comedones and pustules appear on the face, chest, and back, where the skin is excessively oily (Fig. 65-3). Oiliness of the scalp often accompanies acne. Diagnosis is made by visual examination of the affected areas.

Medical Management

Mild cases of acne improve with gentle facial cleansing and nonprescription drying agents containing benzoyl peroxide. Drug therapy includes the topical application of tretinoin (Retin-A) or tazarotene (Tazorac) or oral administration of isotretinoin (Accutane). Topical and systemic antibiotics such as tetracycline and erythromycin, in low doses, also are used for severe acne and have produced good results. The comedones can be removed, and the pustules drained with special instruments.

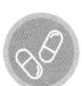

Pharmacologic Considerations

- Topical acne preparations that use benzoyl peroxide can be harsh and bleach clothing and linens; clients may want to set aside valued items while undergoing treatment.
- Women prescribed isotretinoin (Accutane) must have a negative pregnancy test result before use and practice two forms of birth control while on the medication.

Surgical Management

Dermabrasion is a method of removing surface layers of scarred skin. It is useful in lessening scars such as the pitting from severe acne. The outermost layers of the skin are removed by sandpaper, a rotating wire brush, chemicals (chemical face peeling), or a diamond wheel. A local anesthetic, such as an ethyl chloride and Freon mixture, is used during the procedure. Afterward, the skin looks and feels raw and sore, and some crusting from serous exudate occurs. Clients frequently say that the discomfort is much like that from a burn. The client is instructed to avoid washing the area until it has healed sufficiently. The client also must refrain from picking and touching the area because contact with the fingers might cause infection or scarring from secondary trauma.

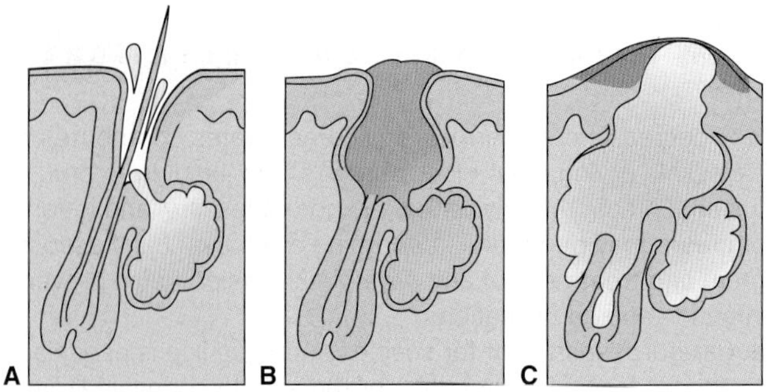

Figure 65-2 Acne vulgaris. (A) Normal sebaceous gland and hair follicle. (B) Comedone formation. (C) Pustule formation.

Nursing Management

The client is advised to keep the face and hair clean and avoid cosmetics that contribute to oily skin. The nurse explains that,

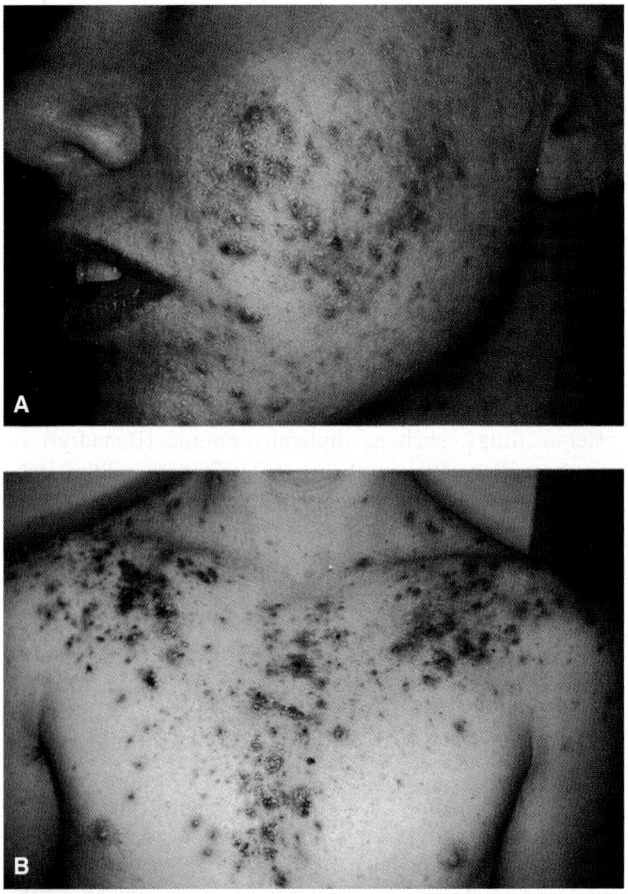

Figure 65-3 Acne of (A) the face and (B) the chest.

above all else, manipulating the lesions worsens the condition. For clients who are women, the nurse warns about the risk of birth defects associated with systemic oral isotretinoin. Women for whom this drug is prescribed must (1) have a negative pregnancy test 2 weeks before beginning therapy, (2) adhere to contraceptive measures while taking the drug and for 1 month after discontinuing therapy, and (3) check with a primary provider about risks to an infant while breastfeeding.

The nurse should also instruct the client to keep the hair short and away from the face and forehead. Washing the hair frequently is beneficial; daily shampooing does not damage hair. The nurse also tells the client to avoid using makeup, lotions, hair sprays, and skin care products unless approved by a primary provider.

Rosacea

Rosacea, a chronic skin disorder that manifests in a variety of ways, is generally characterized by a rosy appearance. This condition is one of the most prevalent skin disorders; it affects approximately 16 million Americans with fair skin who are 30 to 60 years of age (National Rosacea Society, n.d.). Health care providers sometimes refer to it as *adult acne* or *acne rosacea* because the skin manifestations are somewhat similar. Rosacea is totally unrelated to acne vulgaris, however, and may worsen if treated similarly. It is incurable but manageable and may progress in severity.

Pathophysiology and Etiology

The cause of rosacea is unknown, but several hypotheses have been proposed, including genetics, immunologic factors, exposure to ultraviolet (UV) light, bacterial skin infection with *Helicobacter pylori*, and mite infestation of the facial hair follicles (Gether et al., 2018). The mite *Demodex folliculorum* is a normal inhabitant of the skin; however, it is more abundant among people with rosacea. It is still unclear whether the skin mite provokes an inflammatory or allergic reaction or blocks skin follicles, which facilitates survival of the mite.

Increased blood flow through superficial blood vessels of the face causes episodic blushing and eventually a prolonged state of vasodilation lasting hours or days. Eventually, the facial capillaries and arterioles become chronically dilated with a spidery appearance, appearing as visible linear streaks on the skin, a condition known as **telangiectases**. The chronic vasodilation causes the dermal tissue and sebaceous glands to hypertrophy and develop elevated papules and pustules. The skin across the nose and cheeks becomes unevenly thickened and distorted. If vascular structures of the eyes and eyelids become affected, there may be a bloodshot appearance accompanied by decreased tearing.

Assessment Findings

The earliest sign of rosacea is a frequent, intermittent flushed appearance across the nose, forehead, cheeks, and chin. Factors that contribute to vasodilation or irritation of the skin may trigger the phenomena; examples include consuming hot beverages, spicy food, or alcohol; exposure to sun, wind, or cold; bathing with hot water; stress; or use of skin care products. As the condition progresses, the skin remains red, appearing like a persistent sunburn. The inflamed tissue may sting and feel chronically irritated; solid papules or pustules form. The face appears swollen and baggy, and large facial pores produce a texture resembling an orange peel. The nose becomes permanently enlarged, red, nodular, and bulbous, a condition known as **rhinophyma** (Fig. 65-4). The eyes, if affected, appear inflamed. The client may report that they cannot wear contact lenses or that the eyes feel as though a foreign body is present.

Medical and Surgical Management

Treatment goals include minimizing the symptoms and promoting a more acceptable appearance. Primary providers treat rosacea initially with oral antibiotics such as minocycline (Minocin), a tetracycline, or erythromycin (Ilosone), a macrolide, to subdue the associated inflammation. Once inflammation is controlled, the primary provider may pre scribe topical medications such as metronidazole (MetroGel, Noritate) or sulfacetamide (Sodium Sulamyd) with or without sulfur to sustain the anti-inflammatory effect. The

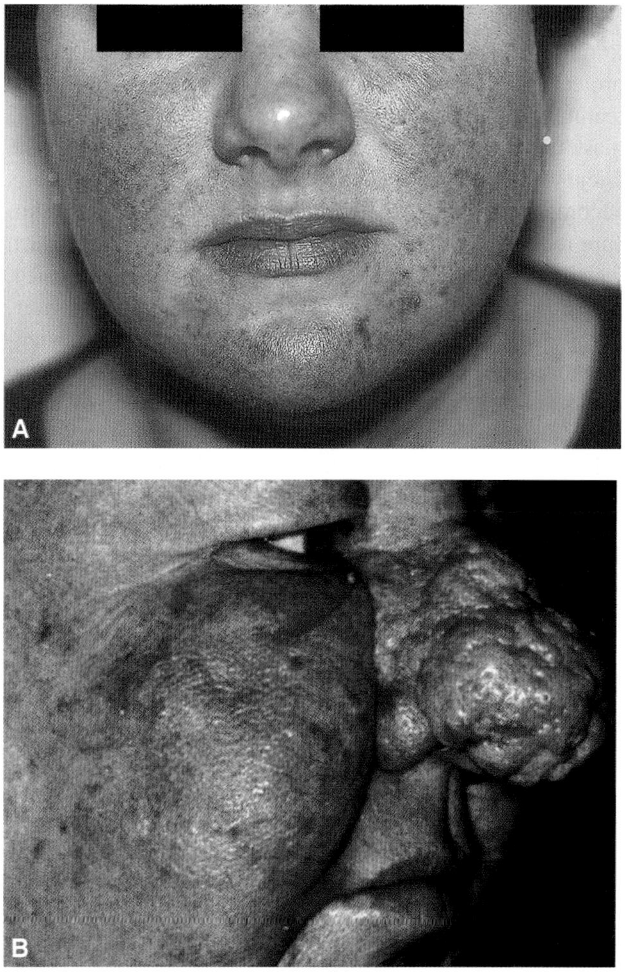

Figure 65-4 **(A)** Rosacea causes areas of erythema, papules, and pustules on the face. **(B)** Chronic rosacea with rhinophyma. (**A**, reprinted with permission from Goodheart, H. P. (2009). *Goodheart's photoguide to common skin disorders: Diagnosis and management* (3rd ed.). Wolters Kluwer Health/Lippincott Williams & Wilkins. **B**, Courtesy of Hoechst-Roussel Pharmaceuticals, Inc.)

treatment regimen might include topical retinoids, derivatives of vitamin A, such as isotretinoin (Accutane), provided that the client is not pregnant and takes measures to avoid pregnancy. Health care professionals believe that retinoids can shrink sebaceous glands and reduce dermatologic inflammation. Topical drug therapy may be long term to promote a remission of symptoms.

Other approaches can improve the client's appearance. A series of two to four laser treatments reduces excessive tissue, especially about the nose, and permanently obliterates telangiectases by sealing blood vessels. Pulsed light (PhotoDerm) is light energy used to eliminate vascular lesions. In the case of rosacea, the energy penetrates the dermis without disrupting the epidermis to stimulate growth of collagen and to rejuvenate the skin's appearance.

Nursing Management

The nurse encourages the client to maintain a diary, documenting lifestyle practices and events that trigger symptoms. Establishing a cause-and-effect relationship between specific foods and beverages, for example, helps the client avoid exacerbations. In addition, the nurse advises the client to minimize sun exposure and always use sunscreen of sun protection factor (SPF) 15 or higher. The nurse suggests protecting the skin in cold or windy weather with a scarf or ski mask and applying a skin moisturizer. The nurse teaches the client to pace physical activity to avoid overheating, which is accompanied by vasodilation. The nurse reviews a basic skin care regimen that includes washing the face with lukewarm water and a gentle cleanser; avoiding the use of a face cloth, which may be too abrasive; blotting the skin dry; and waiting 5 to 30 minutes after cleansing before applying medication to reduce potential discomfort. The client is cautioned to avoid self-treatment with acne medications, especially those containing benzoyl peroxide, which tend to irritate affected skin further. The nurse explores alternative stress management techniques with the client and encourages implementing new coping strategies (see Chapter 67) to complement the therapeutic medical regimen.

Furuncles, Furunculosis, and Carbuncles

A **furuncle** is a boil. **Furunculosis** refers to having multiple furuncles. A **carbuncle** is a furuncle from which pus drains.

Pathophysiology and Etiology

The cause of furuncles and carbuncles is skin infections with organisms that usually exist harmlessly on the skin surface. When an injury such as that caused by squeezing a lesion impairs the integrity of the skin, microorganisms can enter and colonize in the skin. Furunculosis also is associated with diabetes mellitus because an elevated blood glucose level promotes microbial growth. Other factors that predispose to these conditions include poor diet and general health and any disorder that lowers resistance.

Assessment Findings

The lesion, which may appear anywhere on the body, but especially around the neck, axillary, and groin regions, appears as a raised, painful pustule surrounded by **erythema** (redness). The area feels hard to the touch. After a few days, the lesion exudes pus and later a core. The client also may experience a fever, anorexia, weakness, and malaise. A culture of the exudate identifies the infectious organism.

Medical and Surgical Management

Hot, wet soaks are used to localize the infection and provide symptomatic relief. It may be the only treatment necessary. Antibiotics are used in some instances, especially when a fever is present or if the lesion is a carbuncle. Surgical incision and drainage may be necessary.

Nursing Management

The nurse and the client who performs self-care must follow strict aseptic technique when applying or changing a dressing to prevent the spread of the infection to other parts of the body or to others. The nurse informs the client to never pick or squeeze a furuncle—drainage is infectious, and this practice favors spread of the infection to surrounding tissues or even to the bloodstream. In addition, the client should wash hands thoroughly before and after applying topical medications, keep hands away from infected areas, and use face cloths and towels separate from those used by others. It is important to wash clothing, towels, and face cloths in hot water and bleach separately from family laundry.

Plaque Psoriasis

Psoriasis is a chronic, noninfectious inflammatory disorder of the skin that affects both men and women. Its onset is in young and middle adulthood. Although there are many types of psoriasis, the most common is plaque psoriasis (Fig. 65-5). Periods of emotional stress, hormonal cycles, infection, and seasonal changes appear to aggravate the condition.

Pathophysiology and Etiology

The cause of psoriasis is unknown, but a genetic predisposition is likely because many report a family history of

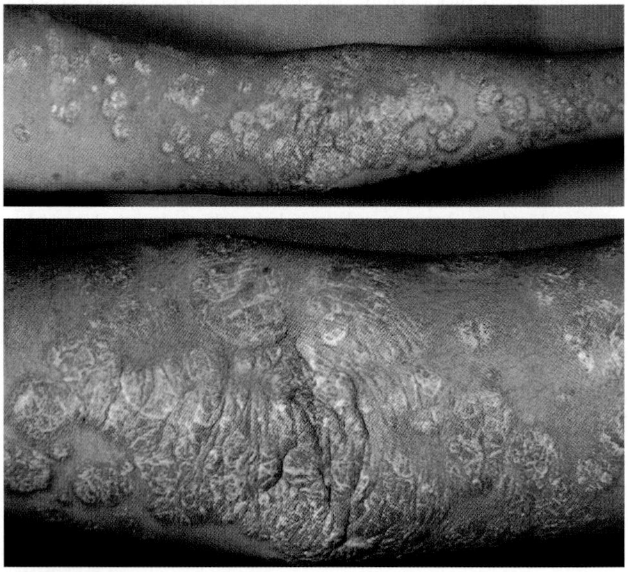

Figure 65-5 Psoriasis on the elbows. (Courtesy: Roche Laboratories.)

the disorder. Although the predisposition exists, the disorder seems to require a triggering mechanism such as systemic infection, injury to the skin, vaccination, or injection. This also suggests a link with the immune system. The fact that the disorder has periods of exacerbation and remission strengthens this hypothesis. Psoriatic arthritis, a chronic inflammatory joint disorder, can occur among those with psoriasis that affects the skin.

In psoriasis that affects the skin, cells called *keratinocytes* behave as if there is a need to repair a wound. The cells of the epidermis proliferate faster than normal—so fast, in fact, that the upper layer of cells cannot be shed fast enough to make room for the newly produced cells. The excessive cells accumulate and form elevated, scaly lesions called *plaque*. The area around the lesion becomes red from the increased blood supply needed to nourish the rapidly developing skin cells.

Assessment Findings

Psoriasis is characterized by patches of erythema covered with silvery scales, usually on the extensor surfaces of the elbows, knees, trunk, and scalp. Itching usually is absent or slight, but occasionally, it is severe. The lesions are obvious and unsightly, and the scales tend to shed. Diagnosis is made by visual examination of the lesions. A skin biopsy reveals increased proliferation of epidermal cells.

Medical Management

Psoriasis has no cure. Symptomatic treatment to control the scaling and itching includes the use of topical agents such as coal tar extract, corticosteroids, or anthralin. Anthralin, a distillate of crude coal tar, is applied to thick plaques; it tends to irritate unaffected skin areas. Topical corticosteroids, topical retinoids, and analogs of vitamin D have proved beneficial. Methotrexate, an antimetabolite used in the treatment of cancer, is prescribed for clients with severe disease that does not respond to other forms of therapy. This drug inhibits the production of cells that divide rapidly (cancer cells, cells composing the skin and mucous membranes) and is capable of reducing plaque formation. Dosage is carefully individualized because the drug causes serious adverse effects.

Etretinate (Tegison) is related to retinoic acid and retinol (vitamin A) and is used to treat psoriasis that does not respond to other therapies. Its use is recommended only for those clients who can reliably understand and carry out the treatment regimen, are capable of complying with mandatory contraceptive measures, and do not intend to become pregnant. Another method of treatment is the injection of triamcinolone acetonide (Kenacort), a corticosteroid, into isolated psoriatic plaques. This method of treatment is successful in some cases.

Recently, health care providers have used biologic therapy techniques that alter immune system responses associated with plaque psoriasis with humanized monoclonal antibodies such as secukinumab (Cosentyx), apremilast (Otezla), and ixekizumab (Taltz). Similar drugs such as adalimumab (Humira), ustekinumab (Stelara), and etanercept (Enbrel), have been approved for the treatment of psoriatic arthritis and other autoimmune disorders (Mayo Clinic, 2020). These drugs modify the activities of T cells (see Chapter 34) and reduce inflammation and hyperplasia of the epidermis in clients with psoriasis, resulting in rapid and significant improvement. Unfortunately, these drugs also are associated with anaphylaxis and serious infections. Consequently, they are reserved for moderate to severe cases. **Photochemotherapy**, a combination of UV light therapy and a photosensitizing psoralen drug such as methoxsalen (Oxsoralen-Ultra), also has been used for severe, disabling psoriasis that does not respond to other methods of treatment. The extent of exposure is based on the client's skin tolerance. Treatments are given once every other day or less because phototoxic reactions may appear 48 hours or more after light exposure. Once the psoriasis clears, the client is placed on a maintenance treatment program.

Some clients respond well to treatment; others receive only minor relief. The condition tends to recur.

Pharmacologic Considerations

- Drugs that alter the immune system can also activate latent *Mycobacterium tuberculosis*. Clients must be screened for tuberculosis (TB) before drug therapy is started.

Scabies

Scabies is a fairly common infectious skin disease.

Pathophysiology and Etiology

Scabies is caused by infestation with tiny itch mites (*Sarcoptes scabiei*). Anyone can acquire scabies; it is erroneous to assume that infected people have poor personal hygiene. Outbreaks are common where large groups of people are confined, such as nursing homes, military barracks, prisons, boarding schools, and childcare centers.

The mites are spread by skin-to-skin contact. In rare cases, scabies is acquired from handling clothing and linen in recent contact with an infected person. Scabies mites do not survive more than 2 days off the body.

Assessment Findings

Signs and Symptoms

Itching is intense, especially at night. Commonly affected areas include the webs and sides of fingers and around the wrists, elbows, armpits, waist, thighs, genitalia, nipples, breasts, and lower buttocks (Fig. 65-6). Excoriation from scratching accompanies the itching. Skin burrows are caused by the female itch mite, which invades the skin to lay its eggs.

Diagnostic Findings

Diagnosis is made by examining the affected areas. Providers, however, often confuse scabies with other skin conditions. Therefore, there are several types of testing that is recommended, such as an examination using mineral oil or ink (Barry, 2020). After dropping sterile mineral oil on the lesion, the skin

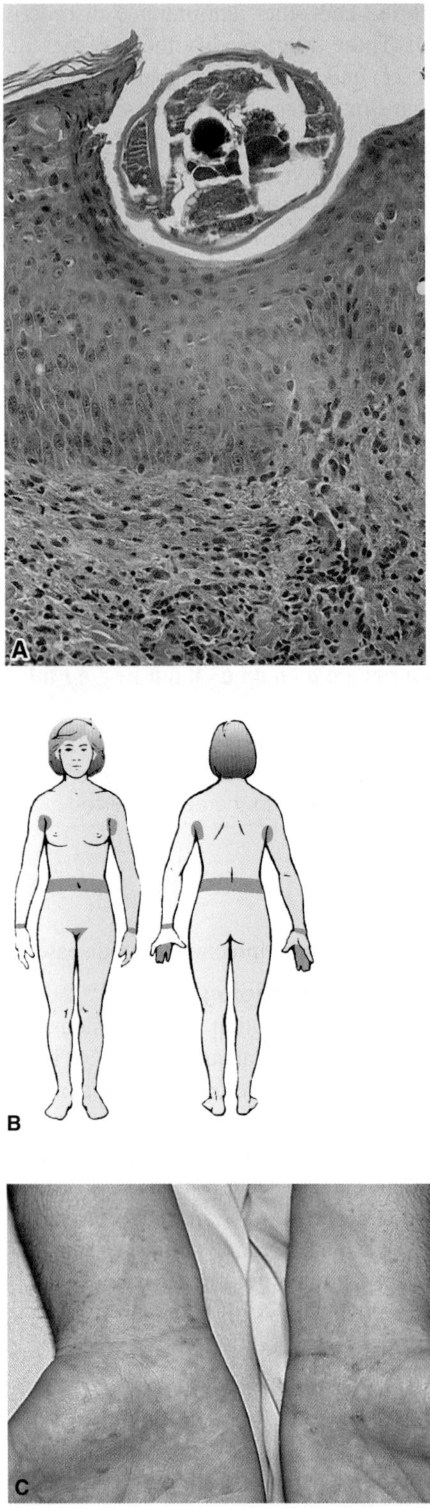

Figure 65-6 **(A)** Itch mites cause scabies. **(B)** Common locations where itch mites invade. **(C)** Example of a scabies infestation. (A, reprinted with permission from Elder, D. E., Elenitsas, R., Rosenbach, M., Murphy, G. F., Rubin, A. I., & Xu, X. (2015). *Lever's histopathology of the skin.* Wolters Kluwer; B, reprinted with permission from Smeltzer, S. C., & Bare, B. G. (2000). *Brunner & Suddarth's textbook of medical-surgical nursing* (9th ed.). Lippincott-Raven; C, reprinted with permission from Goodheart, H. P., & Gonzalez, M. E. (2016). *Goodheart's photoguide to common pediatric and adult skin disorders* (4th ed.). Wolters Kluwer.)

is scraped onto a slide and examined microscopically to detect the mites, their eggs, or feces. The ink test is performed by applying a blue or black felt-tipped pen to the lesion, which highlights the burrows when the skin surface is wiped.

Medical Management

Scabicides, chemicals that destroy mites, such as lindane (cream or lotion), permethrin cream, and crotamiton cream or lotion, are prescribed. The medication is applied to the skin in a thin layer, left on for 8 to 12 hours, and then removed by washing. Thorough bathing, clean clothing, and the avoidance of contact with others who have scabies are essential in preventing recurrence.

Nursing Management

Before any treatment begins, the nurse advises the client to bathe thoroughly. The nurse then reviews the directions for applying the scabicide medication included with the product. The importance of following the directions for complete eradication of the scabies mites is emphasized. The nurse instructs the client, after bathing and applying the medication, to don clean clothing and launder preworn clothing, towels, and bed linen in hot water as soon as possible. The client is told to vacuum furniture and other unwashable items. Last, the nurse explains that itching may continue for 2 to 3 weeks after treatment.

Dermatophytoses

Dermatophytoses (tinea) are superficial fungal infections; they have been given many unscientific names. For example, a common term for one dermatophytosis is *ringworm*, which is a misnomer because a worm does not cause the infection. Other examples are *athlete's foot* for a foot infection and *jock itch* for an infection in the groin.

Pathophysiology and Etiology

Dermatophytes (also called *tinea*) are parasitic fungi that invade the skin, scalp, and nails (discussed later). The terms *tinea pedis*, *tinea capitis*, *tinea corporis*, and *tinea cruris* identify the skin areas of infection, namely, feet, head, body, and groin, respectively.

Assessment Findings

Tinea corporis appears as rings of papules or vesicles with a clear center in nonhairy areas of the skin (Fig. 65-7). Several clusters of rings may be found in the same general location. The affected skin often itches and becomes red, scaly, cracked, and sore. In tinea pedis, the infection begins in the skin between the toes and spreads to the soles of the feet. Tinea capitis, which is more common in children, invades the hair shaft below the scalp, followed by breaking of the hair, usually close to the scalp.

Diagnosis is made by visual examination of the affected areas. The lesions are scraped and examined microscopically. When a Wood's light is used, the affected areas fluoresce a green-yellow color.

Medical Management

Treatment of tinea pedis includes the topical application of antifungal agents, such as benzoic and salicylic acid ointment (Whitfield's ointment), Burow's solution, undecylenic acid, and tolnaftate (Tinactin). Oral griseofulvin (Grisactin), a systemic antifungal agent, also is useful in treatment. The drug may be

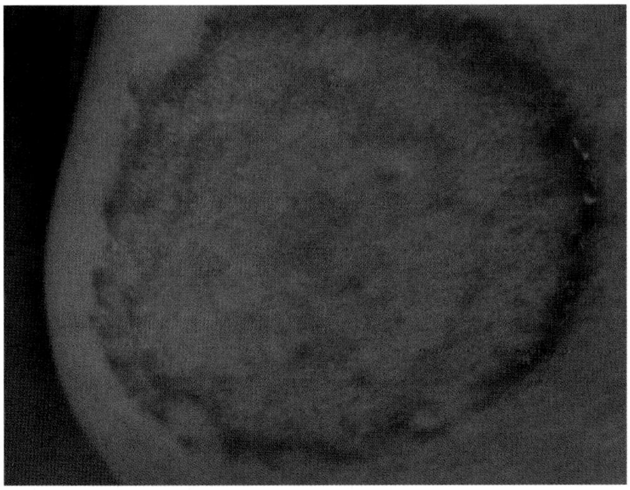

Figure 65-7 Tinea corporis, which is commonly referred to as *ringworm* because of its circular appearance. (Reprinted with permission from Hall, J. C. (1999). *Sauer's manual of skin diseases* (8th ed.). Lippincott Williams & Wilkins.)

required for many weeks to eradicate the infection. Tinea capitis may be treated with oral griseofulvin, which is taken with meals. A topical antifungal agent also may be prescribed to destroy fungi present on the hair shafts above the surface of the scalp. Treatment of tinea corporis includes the use of topical antifungal agents for less severe infections. Oral griseofulvin is prescribed for more severe infections. Tinea cruris often responds to topical application of tolnaftate or miconazole (Micatin). Tinea onychomycosis (discussed later) may respond to oral griseofulvin, but long-term therapy usually is necessary.

Nursing Management

If an oral or topical antifungal agent is prescribed, the nurse reviews the directions for use and explains that the infected person must use separate towels, washcloths, grooming articles, and clothing because the disorder is contagious. The nurse stresses that keeping the affected areas dry reduces the spread of the infection. Thorough drying of all areas of the body after a bath or shower, including the skin folds, is advised. To prevent infection and reinfection of tinea cruris, the nurse suggests avoiding excessive heat and humidity, not wearing tight-fitting clothing or nylon next to the skin (in hot, humid weather), and keeping the skin as dry as possible.

To avoid acquiring or spreading a fungal infection of the feet, the nurse advises against sharing towels and slippers or going barefoot in locker rooms or community bathrooms. Keeping the feet (particularly the area between the toes) dry, which increases resistance to the infection, should be stressed. For clients whose feet perspire freely, the nurse advises applying powder between the toes; keeping the area dry; washing and thoroughly drying the feet daily; putting on clean, dry socks; and wearing different pairs of shoes on a rotating basis.

Herpes Zoster (Shingles)

Herpes zoster, also known as **shingles**, is a skin disorder that develops years after an infection with varicella (chickenpox). It is more frequent in middle-aged to older adults as well as in people who are immunocompromised.

Pathophysiology and Etiology

Herpes zoster is an acute reactivation of the varicella-zoster virus, which lies dormant in nerve roots. When aging, cancer, drugs, or AIDS suppresses a client's immune system, the virus migrates along one or more cranial or spinal nerve routes. Viral reactivation produces inflammatory symptoms in the **dermatome**, a skin area supplied by the nerve (Fig. 65-8). Raised, fluid-filled, and painful skin eruptions accompany the inflammation.

If herpes zoster affects the ophthalmic branch of the trigeminal nerve (third cranial nerve), corneal (eye) ulcerations may occur. Involvement of the vestibulocochlear nerve (eighth cranial nerve) can lead to vertigo and permanent hearing loss.

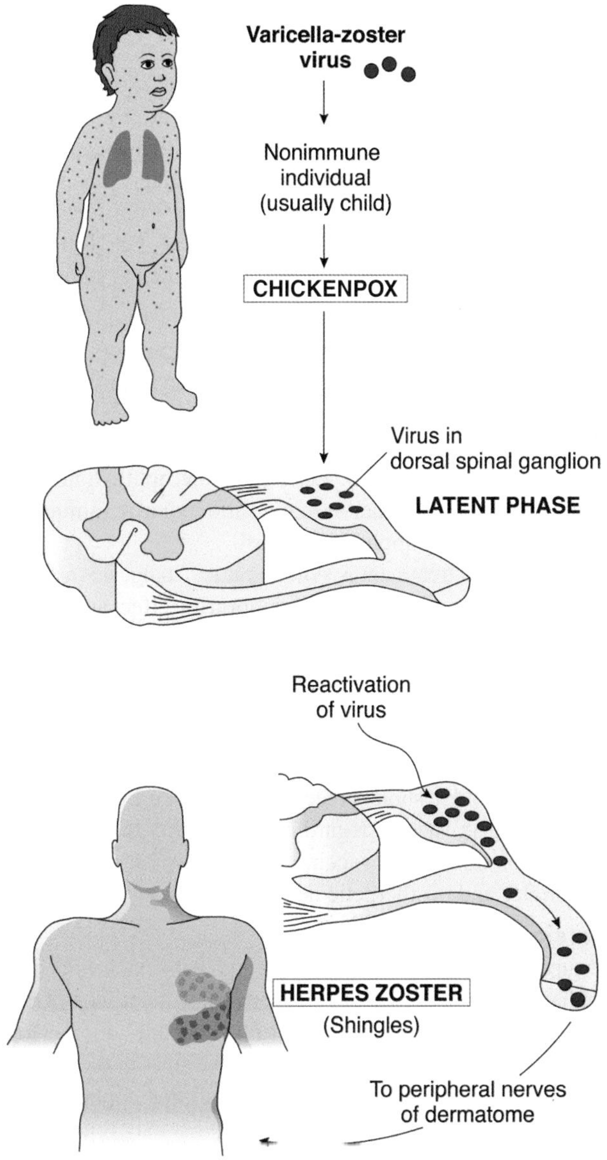

Figure 65-8 Varicella-zoster virus (chickenpox) and herpes zoster (shingles). After a person has had chickenpox (usually as a child), the varicella-zoster virus resides in a dorsal spinal ganglion, where it remains dormant for many years. When reactivated, it spreads to peripheral nerves of sensory dermatomes, causing shingles. (Reprinted with permission from Rubin, E., Strayer, D. S., (Eds.). (2014). *Rubin's pathology: Clinicopathologic foundations of medicine* (7th ed.). Wolters Kluwer.)

Cerebral vasculitis (inflammation of cerebral vessels) is the most serious complication because involvement of the internal carotid arteries can result in a stroke. Rarely, the virus spreads to the brain, resulting in encephalitis.

Susceptible people who are exposed to someone in the early stages of herpes zoster infection can acquire varicella. The virus is contagious until the crusts from ruptured lesions have dried and fallen off the skin. Herpes zoster infection also can recur.

Assessment Findings

Initial symptoms include a low-grade fever, headache, and malaise. An area of skin along a dermatome develops a red, blotchy appearance that begins to itch or feel numb. In about 24 to 48 hours, vesicles appear on the skin along the nerve's pathway. Usually, the eruptions are unilateral (one side) on the trunk, neck, or head. They become severely painful. Severe itching soon follows. Like chickenpox lesions, the vesicles rupture in a few days, and crusts form. Scarring or permanent skin discoloration is possible. Pain (postherpetic neuralgia) and itching may persist for months or as long as 2 years or more. Secondary skin infections may occur from scratching the area. Diagnosis is made primarily by examination of the lesions and symptoms.

Medical Management

Oral acyclovir (Zovirax), when taken within 48 hours of the appearance of symptoms, reduces their severity and prevents the development of additional lesions. Topical acyclovir also may be applied to the lesions. A brief course of corticosteroid therapy reduces pain. Lesions of the ophthalmic division of the trigeminal nerve require immediate examination and treatment by an ophthalmologist.

Additional treatment is symptomatic. Analgesics and liquid preparations with a drying or antipruritic effect are applied to the affected area once the crusts have fallen off. The skin may be so sensitive that any clothing or application of topical drugs intensifies pain or itching. A narcotic analgesic such as codeine often is necessary during the first few days to weeks.

The CDC (2019b) recommends that adults who are 60 years or older should receive a two dose immunization of the Shingrix vaccine regardless of whether they have had chickenpox or not. The vaccine reduces the risk and severity of shingles and postherpetic neuralgia.

Nursing Management

A supervisory nurse reassigns nursing personnel who have not had chickenpox to avoid contact with a client with herpes zoster. The nurse instructs clients with crusted lesions to avoid contact with immunocompromised people and those who have not had chickenpox. The client is advised that application of cool or warm compresses or warm showers may relieve pain and itching; it may be necessary to experiment with both to determine which provides the most relief. The nurse recommends that the client wear loose clothing and avoid scratching the area. If oral acyclovir is prescribed, the nurse reviews the dose regimen, as printed on the prescription label.

Skin Cancer

There are three types of skin cancer: basal cell carcinoma, which is most common; squamous cell carcinoma, second among skin cancers; and melanoma, the deadliest form. When combined, skin cancer is the most common form of cancer in the United States; melanoma ranks as the sixth cause of cancer in the United States (U.S. Cancer Statistics Working Group, 2019). It is estimated that 85,686 new cases of melanoma skin cancer were diagnosed in 2017, of which 8,056 died from the disease (U.S. Cancer Statistics Working Group, 2019).

Pathophysiology and Etiology

Skin cancer involves any one of three types of cells in the epidermis: squamous cells that are flat and scaly; basal cells that are round; and melanocytes, cells that contain color pigment. Increased exposure to UV radiation, especially ultraviolet B (UVB) and ultraviolet C (UVC), harmful components in the spectrum of sunlight, predisposes to malignant skin changes and other health risks, including cataracts and premature aging of the skin. Fair-skinned people are more susceptible to skin cancer than dark-skinned people.

Several factors predispose to malignant changes in the skin:

- *Thinning ozone layer*. Ozone, an upper atmospheric layer above the Earth, filters and blocks solar radiation from entering lower areas of the atmosphere. Ozone depletion results in less protection from the sun's rays and more exposure to UVB and UVC radiation at the earth's surface (Fig. 65-9). Ozone depletion occurs primarily

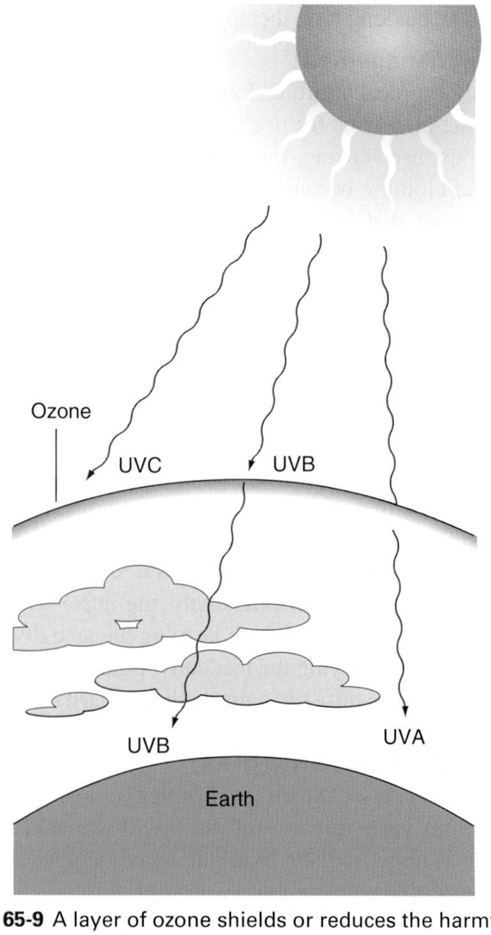

Figure 65-9 A layer of ozone shields or reduces the harmful spectrum of ultraviolet wavelengths known as UVC and UVB.

as a result of the release of chlorofluorocarbons (CFCs) in refrigerants, aerosol propellants, and other industrial pollutants.
- *Residence in high-altitude areas* where the atmosphere is thinner than at sea level or in areas with a regular cloud cover because people are less likely to use sun-protective precautions.
- *Decreased melanin in skin*, especially in people who sunburn easily and tan minimally; black- or brown-skinned people rarely are affected (Grossman & Porth, 2013).
- *Prolonged, repeated exposure to UV rays* in those who do farming, fishing, road construction, and so on or those who frequent tanning salons and use sunlamps.
- *Prior radiation therapy* for an unrelated form of cancer.
- *Ulcerations of long duration and scar tissue* (both prone to malignant changes).

Malignant growths of the skin (Table 65-1) usually are primary lesions; that is, they originate in the skin. Prompt removal of the malignant tissue prevents its spread to other parts of the body or tissues.

Assessment Findings

Symptoms vary, but usually the new appearance of a growth or a change in color of the skin is the first symptom the client notices. The lesion can be smooth or rough, flat or elevated, and itchy or tender. It may bleed. Diagnosis is made by visual inspection and confirmed by biopsy.

Medical and Surgical Management

Depending on the size and the location of the lesion, treatment of squamous cell and basal cell carcinomas may involve electrodesiccation, surgical excision, cryosurgery, or radiation therapy. The client is followed regularly for at least 3 to 5 years to be sure regrowth has not occurred.

The treatment of melanoma involves radical excision of the tumor and adjacent tissues, followed by chemotherapy. The administration of melphalan (Alkeran) and prednisone

TABLE 65-1 Type of Skin Cancer

TYPE	INCIDENCE	LOCATION	APPEARANCE	CHARACTERISTICS
Basal cell carcinoma	Most common, especially in light-skinned individuals Increases with age	Sun-exposed areas	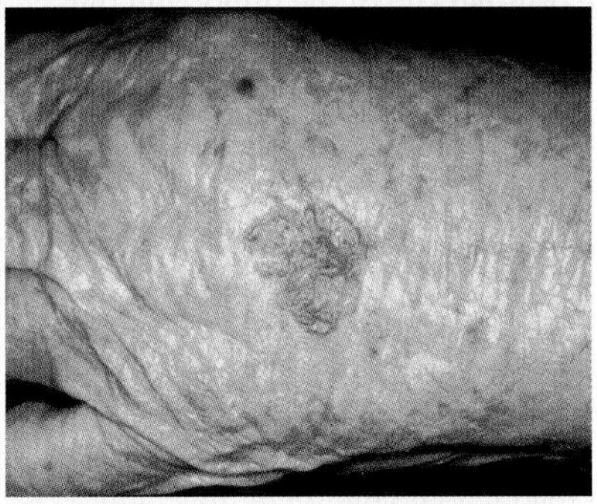 Small, shiny, gray or yellowish plaque that undergoes central ulceration	Slow growing; rarely metastasizes; commonly recurs
Squamous cell carcinoma	Second after basal cell in those with fair skin	Sun-exposed areas such as ears, nose, hands, scalp of bald persons	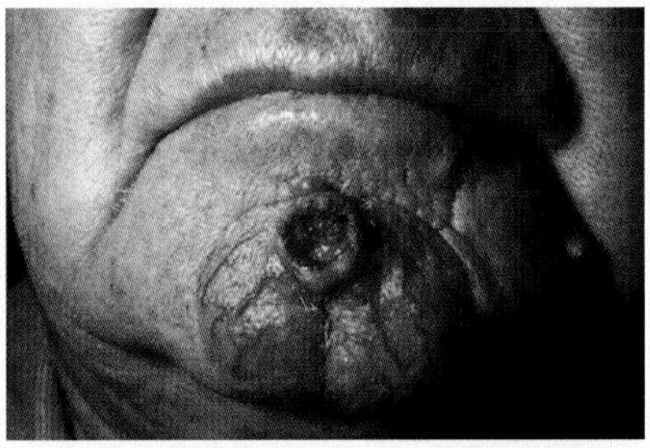 Scaly, elevated lesion with an irregular border; shallow, large ulcerations form in untreated advanced lesions	Can metastasize through blood and lymph
Malignant melanoma	Increasing in incidence	Arises from a preexisting mole anywhere on the body	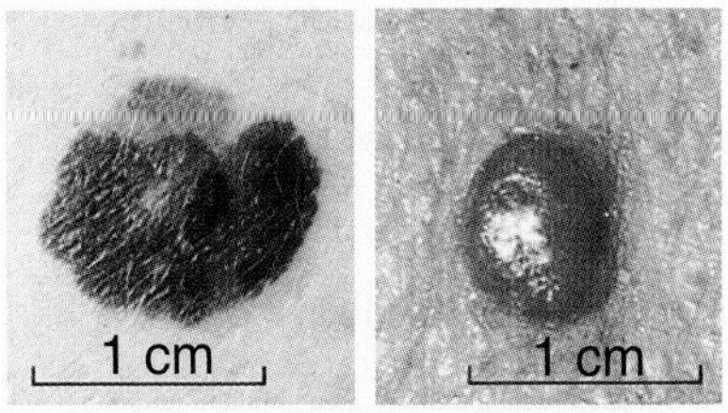 Raised brown or black lesion. In some cases, satellite lesions occur adjacent to the primary cancer.	Poor prognosis because of distant metastases

All figures Reprinted with permission from Evans, R. J., Brown, Y. M., & Evans, M. K. (2014). *Canadian maternity, newborn & women's health nursing.* Wolters Kluwer.

is an example of an initial antineoplastic therapy regimen. Interferon alfa-n3 (Alferon N) has controlled metastases in some persons. In some instances, skin grafting may be necessary to replace large areas of defect when a wide excision of the tumor is necessary.

Nursing Management

The nurse examines and measures abnormal-appearing skin lesions, especially those in sun-exposed areas such as the face, nose, lips, and hands. The nurse determines facts about the lesion, including when the lesion was first noticed, whether the lesion has undergone any recent changes, and, if so, what kind, being particularly mindful of the **ABCDEs** of melanoma: **A** refers to asymmetry, **B** represents border irregularity, **C** stands for color that is not uniform; **D** denotes diameter—especially one that is greater than the size of a pencil eraser, and **E** relates to the evolving change in any way (Skin Cancer Foundation, 2021). The client is taught how to perform a skin self-examination (Client and Family Teaching 65-2).

Surgery for a malignant melanoma may involve structures of the head and neck, trunk, or extremities. The specific nursing management of those having radical surgery for this malignancy depends on the original site of the tumor and the extent of surgery. The nurse gives emotional support to those having disfiguring surgery.

The nurse encourages all people with any type of skin change to seek medical attention. Those in high-risk groups for malignant skin lesions are advised to examine all areas of their body and scalp for new lesions or changes in moles, other growths, or pigmented lesions. If a client notes any change, an appointment should be made for a medical examination as soon as possible.

The nurse educates clients about measures to prevent skin cancer, some of which include the following:

- Always use a sunscreen with an SPF of at least 15; higher SPFs are beneficial for clients who sunburn easily.
- Reapply sunscreen at least every 2 hours or more often if swimming or perspiring.
- Use a lip balm with sunscreen.
- Wear a hat with a wide brim and cover the back of the neck.
- Stay in the shade when outdoors.
- Wear tightly woven but loose-fitting clothing.
- Avoid prolonged sun exposure between 10 a.m. and 4 p.m..
- Avoid artificial tanning.

The nurse also recommends that at-risk clients consult the UV forecast, a daily report that rates the UV conditions from 0 to 10+ in 30 metropolitan areas. The U.S. Environmental Protection Agency releases the forecast, which radio and television stations broadcast during weather reports as a public service. Depending on the numerical rating, called the UV index, sun-sensitive people are advised to take protective measures (Fig. 65-10). A sensometer, a credit card–sized device, also is available so a person can determine the UV level in their immediate locale.

Client and Family Teaching 65-2
Performing a Skin Self-Examination

The nurse emphasizes the following points when teaching the client and family:

- Allow time after a shower or bath for the examination.
- Ensure that there is adequate light to facilitate inspection.
- Use a full-length mirror and handheld mirror. Examine the skin from head to toe, including the back, scalp, genital area, and between the buttocks.
- Commit the location; appearance; and feel of birthmarks, moles, and other skin lesions to memory or photograph them for future comparisons.
- Look for any changes in previous skin characteristics or the development of something new.
- Inspect the scalp by moving the hair with a comb or blow dryer; when examining the posterior scalp, another person may be helpful.
- Look at the front and back of the body as well as the left and right sides. It is also important to check the fingernails, toenails, soles of the feet, and between the toes.
- Report information about the skin examination to a primary provider.

More information available at: American Cancer Society. (2019). *How to do a skin self-exam.* http://www.cancer.org/cancer/cancercauses/sunanduvexposure/skincancerpreventionandearlydetection/skin-cancer-prevention-and-early-detection-skin-exams

BODY ORNAMENTATION

Historically, people have altered normal skin for ornamental, cosmetic, and utilitarian reasons. Primary providers have used a form of tattooing known as micropigmentation as an adjunct to medical procedures such as breast reconstruction surgery (see Chapter 54) and to recreate the appearance of eyebrows on people who have lost facial hair. Some people have tattoos applied as a form of permanent makeup to save time or to compensate for a physical disability that interferes with the hand dexterity required for daily application. Recently, however, there is a trend to alter the skin with ornamental tattooing, body piercing, and graphic designs using permanently colored pigments.

Tattoos

A **tattoo** is pigmentation of the dermal layer of skin with needles containing dye. Tattoo artists inject the skin with an electrical vibrating instrument that injects pigment at approximately 50 to 3000 times per minute, depositing insoluble ink with each puncture (Del Prado, 2015). To be permanent, the ink must reach the dermis of the skin, a depth of about 1/16 of an inch.

Reputable tattoo studios require a signed parental consent for minors; however, not all tattooists ask for the signed consent form, despite the fact that some states require it. Some people ask a friend to perform the tattooing or they tattoo themselves with substances such as India ink using nonsterile objects such as pins or the tips of ink pens.

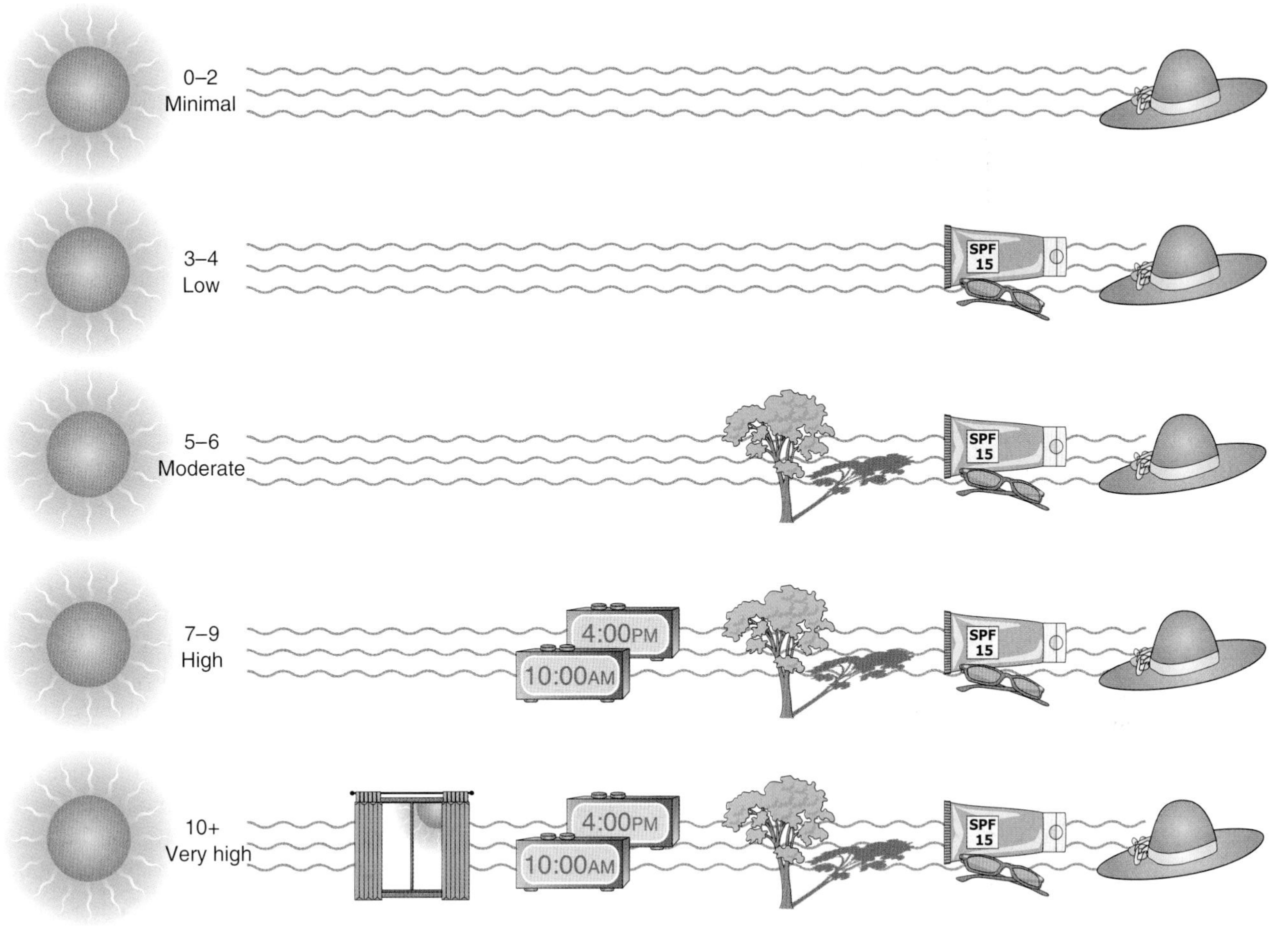

Figure 65-10 Sun protection measures based on the ultraviolet (UV) index.

If a person makes known their intention to receive a tattoo, the nurse can recommend that the selected tattooist at least be certified by the Alliance of Professional Tattooists. Members of this organization follow infection control guidelines developed in conjunction with the U.S. Food and Drug Administration (FDA, 2020). Currently, however, people who perform invasive body art procedures are not required to adhere to any federal safety standards designed to prevent transmission of blood-borne pathogens. Tattooists are regulated by local and state jurisdictions only (National Conference of State Legislatures, 2018).

Risks Associated With Tattooing

Although cosmetic pigment inks are subject to approval under the Federal Food, Drug, and Cosmetic Act, none are FDA-approved for injection into the skin. Because the number of adverse reactions and potential health risks, such as infections, granuloma and keloid formation, and allergies, is increasing, the FDA now investigates and intervenes when a serious safety issue arises involving tattoo inks and additional color additives that adulterate tattoo pigment products. Complaints can be directed to the MedWatch program (FDA, 2020).

Infection

Infection is a serious potential complication following a tattoo. Unless the tattooist sterilizes the equipment, including components that hold the needles, a potential for transmitting skin infections as well as blood-borne infectious diseases, such as hepatitis B and C (see Chapter 47) and human immunodeficiency virus (HIV; see Chapter 35), exists. The tattooist should discard even the ink after each use, but, in reality, some return the ink to the original container for use with the next customer. For these reasons, the American Red Cross (2021) rejects potential blood donors who have received a tattoo within 3 months if the tattoo was applied in a state that does not regulate tattoo facilities.

Granuloma and Keloid Formation

Other consequences of tattooing are physiologic responses to traumatized integument. A **granuloma**, an inflammatory nodular lesion, may form as a result of a cellular attack waged against the particles in the tattoo pigment, which the body senses as foreign (Fig. 65-11). Also, some people, especially those with darkly pigmented skin, tend to form **keloids**, an overgrowth of scar tissue (Fig. 65-12).

Allergies

The ingredients in tattoo inks are not standard. All contain various pigments combined with insoluble metallic compounds such as mercury, cadmium, and cobalt to name a few. The components, which may contain industrial grade colors

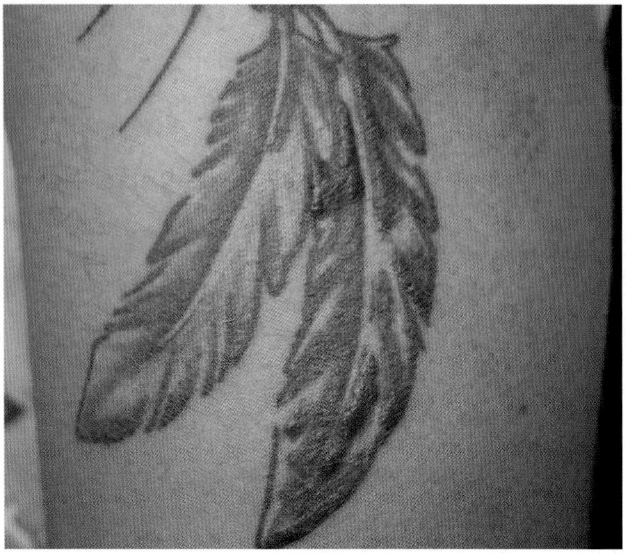

Figure 65-11 A granuloma has developed in the tattoo on the right. (Image provided by Stedman's.)

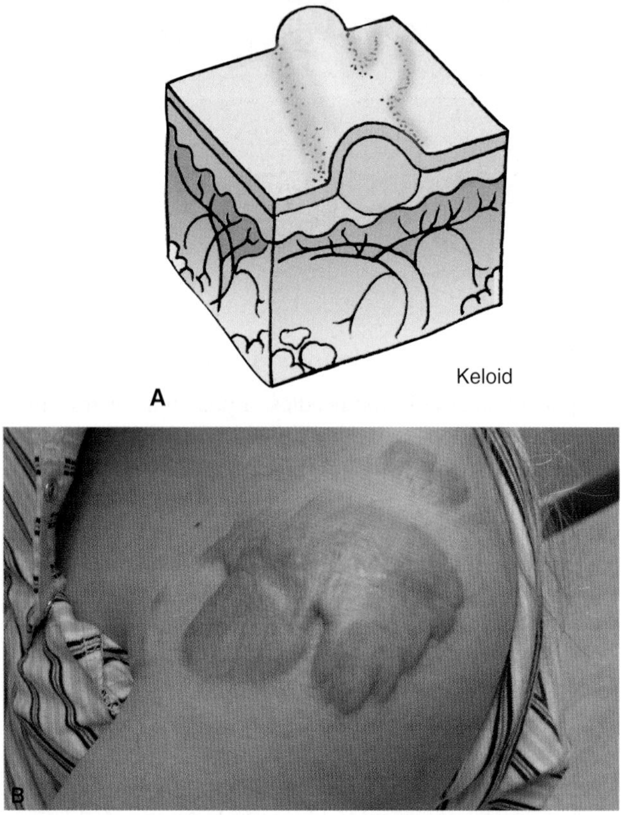

Figure 65-12 **(A)** A keloid is a form of hypertrophic scarring. **(B)** Although this keloid is not the result of a tattoo, it serves as a similar example. (**A,** reprinted with permission from Weber, J., & Kelley, J. (2003). *Health assessment in nursing* (2nd ed.). Lippincott Williams & Wilkins; **B,** reprinted with permission from Mulholland, M. W., Lillemoe, K. D., Doherty, G. M., Maier, R. V., & Upchurch, G. R. (2006). *Greenfield's surgery: Scientific principles and practice* (4th ed.). Lippincott Williams & Wilkins.)

suitable for printers' ink or automobile paint, are combined to achieve a desired color by the individual tattooist (Homolak, 2020). Hypersensitive individuals may experience an immediate localized reaction or even delayed reactions weeks to years later. Red tattoo inks tend to cause most dermatologic problems. Patch testing or another type of allergy testing is advised prior to obtaining a tattoo, but this advice is seldom heeded. Some inks, especially those that contain heavy metals and preservatives, are known carcinogens as well (Homolak, 2020).

Skin Care Following a Tattoo

The trauma created by a tattoo is similar to that of a minor burn. The priority of care is preventing infection, supporting regeneration of tissue, and protecting the skin from concurrent and future damage (Client and Family Teaching 65-3).

Be advised that tattoos also interfere with the quality of magnetic resonance imaging (MRI) because of the interaction of metallic compounds within the pigment. Some people have experienced swelling or burning in the area of the tattoo when undergoing an MRI.

Tattoo Removal

A common problem is that the person regrets having gotten a tattoo or feels dissatisfied with its appearance. Tattoos should be considered permanent. Once applied, the traditional pigments that contain lead, zinc, or other heavy metals are difficult or impossible to remove. Although tattoos can be removed, the skin rarely returns to its pretattooed appearance. Because of the cost, physical pain, and uncertain outcome, many choose to have the original tattoo camouflaged with a second image. For those who pursue removal of the tattoo, there are various techniques available, such as the following:

- *Laser treatments*, which only tend to lighten tattoos, often take 5 to 12 sessions, with a month between each treatment; a new picosecond alexandrite laser has been shown

Client and Family Teaching 65-3
Care After a Tattoo

The nurse advises the client to do the following:

- Temporarily avoid swimming, soaking in a hot tub, and touching the newly tattooed skin.
- Cover the new tattoo with antibiotic ointment and a sterile gauze dressing for 12 hours.
- Perform handwashing before caring for the tattooed skin.
- Remove the dressing after 12 hours while showering or after wetting the gauze to soften the drainage that may adhere to the dressing.
- Wash the tattooed area with antibacterial soap at least three times a day, taking care to pat the skin dry until the skin heals.
- Repeat the applications of antibacterial ointment after each skin cleansing for 5 days.
- Apply a moisturizing skin lotion that is free of perfume and color additives for 2 weeks after discontinuing the antibiotic ointment.
- Avoid direct sunlight on the skin for at least 4 weeks and always use a waterproof sunscreen with an SPF of 30 or higher thereafter; cover the tattoo if using a tanning bed (Mayo Clinic, 2020c).

to successfully remove 75% to 100% ink pigment in 1 to 10 treatments (Rubin, 2016)
- *Dermabrasion*, which mechanically abrades the skin layers with a sanding disc or wire brush, sometimes leaving scar tissue in its place
- *Salabrasion*, which uses a salt solution to abrade the skin
- *Scarification* of the skin with an acid solution
- *Plastic surgery*, in which the surgeon inserts fluid-filled balloons under the skin to stretch it so they can remove the tattooed skin, approximate the wound edges, and retattoo the skin to camouflage the existing tattoo

For those who are wary about the permanence of a tattoo, there are options. One alternative is a biodegradable tattoo dye that is combined with a natural or synthetic compound called a *polymer*. When the bond between the two is broken with a single laser treatment, the dye disappears as the dye is absorbed by the lymphatic system and delivered to the liver for eventual intestinal excretion (Frederick, 2006). The polymer, however, remains within the body permanently.

Body Piercing

Body piercing is the insertion of a metal ring or barbell, which is a straight or curved rod, into a body part (Fig. 65-13). Common locations for body piercing include lips, ear cartilage, cheeks, nose, tongue, eyebrows, navel, nipples, or genital area. Although there is great potential for infection and other medical complications, no federal regulations or certification programs exist for body piercers. Local licenses may be required; a state certificate may not be necessary, and in some cases necessary certifications may be obtained over the Internet without any training whatsoever. Some complete a training period as an apprentice. Consequently, people who perform body piercings vary widely in their knowledge of asepsis and the anatomy of the tissue that they pierce. Some belong to the Association of Professional Piercers, an organization that advocates for educating and encouraging compliance with health and safety standards as they relate to body piercing.

Risks Associated With Body Piercing

Approximately 83% of Americans have had their earlobes pierced; 14% of Americans have piercings in places other than the earlobe, such as the navel, nose, ear cartilage, tongue, nipple, eyebrow, lip, and genitals. Of those with piercings, 31% experience complications, some of which require professional help or hospitalization (Body Piercing Statistics, 2015). No reliable estimates of complications are available because statistics do not account for unreported and self-treated complications.

Tissue trauma, swelling, and bleeding, especially of the tongue, are initial risks associated with body piercing. The soft-tissue injury is increased if a piercing gun is used because the spring-loaded device drives the body jewelry through the tissue with intense compressive force. The piercing jewelry must be long enough to allow for initial swelling. In some tongue piercings, the airway may become obstructed from swelling. Dark-skinned individuals are prone to forming keloids that grow beyond the original site of trauma (Fig. 65-14).

Later, piercing jewelry in and about the mouth and nose may interfere with resuscitation efforts that require oral or nasal intubation. There are dental implications with oral jewelry as well. Metallic devices can chip or crack teeth and may cause artifacts on dental X-rays or conceal pathology. Oral devices can interfere with speaking and swallowing and cause respiratory complications if metallic parts become inhaled (American Dental Association, 2020). Piercings around the genitals may complicate urinary catheterization and vaginal delivery. Piercings can affect breastfeeding if a nipple has piercing jewelry. Also, allergic reactions to brass and nickel jewelry have occurred. Noncorrosive metal, such as surgical stainless steel, niobium, titanium, or solid 14K gold, are safest for piercings.

Perhaps one of the major risks with body piercing is infection. The potential for infection exists until healing occurs which depends on the site of the pierced tissue (Box 65-1). The risk is greater with a piercing gun, which is difficult to sterilize. The risk is compounded with poor asepsis on the part of the piercer.

Like tattooing, body piercing carries a risk for transmitting hepatitis and HIV. Reports of tetanus and TB have also been reported (Gandhi et al., 2020). Because the mouth is teeming with microorganisms, oral piercings provide a potential for causing or exacerbating endocarditis, an inflammatory disorder of the heart and heart valves (see Chapter 23).

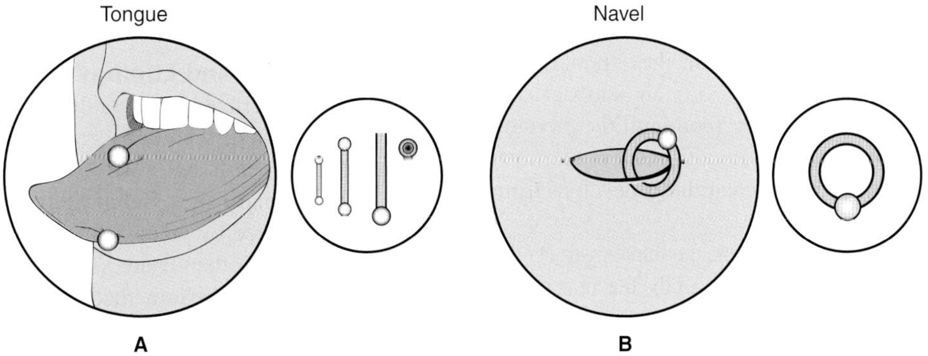

Figure 65-13 Examples of body piercing. **(A)** The straight barbell comes in various gauges and lengths. **(B)** The ends of the ring are inserted into a captive bead.

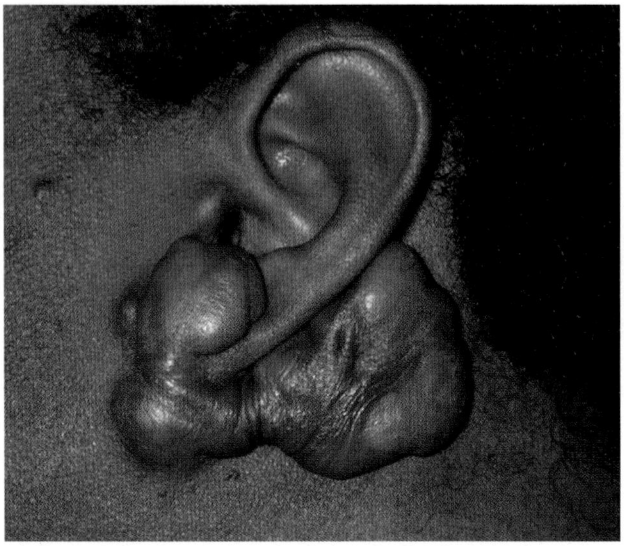

Figure 65-14 Keloid that extends beyond the site of an earlobe piercing. (Reprinted with permission from Lugo-Somolinos, A., & McKinley-Grant, L. (2011). *VisualDx: Essential dermatology in pigmented skin.* Wolters Kluwer Health/Lippincott Williams & Wilkins.)

BOX 65-1 Healing Time According to Site of Body Piercing

SITE	HEALING TIME
Earlobe	6 weeks
Ear cartilage	4–12 months
Eyebrow	6–8 weeks
Nostril	2–4 months
Lip	2–3 months
Navel	9 months–1 year
Nipple	6 weeks–6 months
Tongue	4–6 weeks
Genitalia of women	4–10 weeks
Genitalia of men	6 months–1 year

Site Care Following a Body Piercing

Site care for oral piercings of the tongue or lip is unique. The recipient of the piercing must keep the mouth as clean as possible and should use a soft-bristled toothbrush to avoid additional oral injury. In addition, they should rinse the mouth for 30 to 60 seconds with an antibacterial, alcohol-free mouthwash after eating food until the piercing heals. The recipient can substitute an antifungal mouthwash or salt water if a superinfection of candidiasis develops from the antibacterial mouthwash.

After a body piercing in other areas, the nurse instructs the person to care for the site (see Client and Family Teaching 65-4).

Removal of Body-Piercing Jewelry

The site where the person inserts body-piercing jewelry will close if the jewelry is removed before healing is complete.

Client and Family Teaching 65-4
Care After a Body Piercing

The nurse teaches the client and family the following:

- After handwashing, clean the site with antibacterial soap and water twice a day or more often to remove perspiration and body fluids.
- During washing, move the piercing jewelry back and forth to help clean the pierced tract.
- After cleaning, rinse the site with plain water.
- Avoid alcohol and hydrogen peroxide, which dry the skin; povidone-iodine (Betadine), which discolors gold jewelry; and ointments, which prevent oxygen from reaching the impaired tissue.
- Restrict use of public pools and hot tubs while the pierced area heals.
- Eliminate the application of cosmetics and makeup around facial piercings until the piercings have healed.
- Wear clean, loose clothing to facilitate air circulation; change bed linens at least weekly.
- Check that the piercing jewelry is secured and intact, especially before eating and sleeping (Mayo Clinic Staff, 2020a).

The person must remove the jewelry, however, if a localized or serious infection does not respond to antibiotic therapy. The person can keep the piercing tract patent by inserting a temporary retainer or suture material through the pierced tissue. Special jeweler's tools are generally needed for removal. The person can remove a barbell by stabilizing the rod and twisting the spherical ends in opposite directions. For circular jewelry connected with a captive bead, the ends can be pried apart, taking care not to lose the bead (Richards, 2018).

SCALP AND HAIR DISORDERS

Some conditions are unique to the scalp and hair. They include inflammatory and noninflammatory scalp conditions and disorders that cause hair loss.

Seborrhea, Seborrheic Dermatitis, and Dandruff

Seborrhea and dandruff are noninflammatory conditions that usually precede or accompany seborrheic dermatitis. Seborrheic dermatitis has an inflammatory component.

Pathophysiology and Etiology

Seborrhea is a dermatologic condition associated with excessive production of secretions from the sebaceous glands. Although seborrhea is not always confined to the scalp, it is one of the primary sites. **Seborrheic dermatitis** presents as red areas covered by yellowish, greasy-appearing scales. **Dandruff,** on the other hand, is loose, scaly material of dead, keratinized epithelium shed from the scalp in clients who may or may not have seborrheic dermatitis. Dermatologists believe that a tiny fungus known as *Pityrosporum ovale* causes dandruff. Most people harbor this fungus, yet only some people develop dandruff. Some possible factors for this phenomenon include excessive perspiration, inadequate diet, stress, and hormone activity.

Scalp conditions cause more of a cosmetic rather than a health problem. They usually necessitate retreatment. They do not progress or transform into other serious skin disorders.

Assessment Findings

Clients note that the hair is unusually oily. There may be red or scaly patches on the scalp. White flakes fall from the hair and become more obvious when they collect on the shoulders of dark clothing. The inflamed areas may itch.

No diagnostic testing is necessary unless the condition does not respond to treatment. In that case, a skin biopsy or laboratory blood work is performed to eliminate the possibility that the condition was misdiagnosed.

Medical Management

Frequent shampooing with or without a medicated product helps reduce oil in the scalp and hair. Effective medicated shampoos contain tar, zinc pyrithione, selenium sulfide, sulfur, or salicylic acid. Some clients require topical applications of corticosteroids.

Nursing Management

The nurse explains the underlying cause and reviews the directions and frequency for using medications. Clients are informed that the disorder may recur and that persistent treatment is necessary to control the condition.

Alopecia

Alopecia refers to "baldness." The condition affects the hair follicles and results in partial or total hair loss. It is normal to shed 50 to 100 hairs a day, which are replaced by new ones from the same hair follicles. In some cases, however, hair loss is excessive, which may be temporary or permanent.

Alopecia is not life-threatening; however, whenever men or women lose their hair, most experience self-consciousness and lose self-confidence. Many spend great sums of money on unscientific methods for restoring hair growth. Although not everyone can be helped, several options are available to clients with hair loss.

Pathophysiology and Etiology

Hair loss can develop for several reasons. In cases of temporary hair loss, possible causes include medications such as antineoplastic drugs, inadequate diet, thyroid disease, tinea infection, improper application of hair care products, and hairstyles that pull the hair tightly.

Alopecia areata and androgenetic alopecia are two chronic conditions that are difficult to reverse. **Alopecia areata** is believed to be an autoimmune disorder when Janus kinase (JAK) enzymes cause T cells to attack hair follicles causing patchy areas of hair loss about the size of a coin that can progress to total hair loss and even loss of hair from the entire body.

Androgenetic alopecia is a genetically acquired condition; many refer to it as *male pattern baldness*. The term is somewhat inaccurate because it also affects women, although to a milder degree. A person inherits androgenetic alopecia from their mother or father. When testosterone, an androgenic hormone, combines with an enzyme, 5-alpha reductase, in the hair follicle, hair production stops. This condition begins in adolescence or early adulthood and progresses with age.

Assessment Findings

Clients note that their hair is thinning or falling out in patches in several areas of the scalp. Those with a family history of androgenetic baldness tend to lose hair in the lateral frontal areas or over the vertex of the head (Fig. 65-15). Women report thinning in the frontal, parietal, and crown regions, whereas those with alopecia areata present with round or oval patches of hair loss within the scalp but may eventually experience a total loss of all hair including the eyebrows and other areas where hair grows. Hair loss is not associated with any other physical health problems.

A diagnostic assessment is performed to identify any physical disorder or medications that are contributing to the hair loss. When results are negative, the family history and pattern of hair loss suggest hereditary baldness or an autoimmune disorder.

Medical Management

If a medical disorder causes hair loss, relieving the etiology usually restores hair growth. Some drugs can retard hair loss and promote hair growth. Examples of drugs for androgenetic alopecia include minoxidil (Rogaine) and finasteride (Propecia); however, the hair growth that is stimulated has a downy texture. If a client discontinues minoxidil or finasteride, hair growth stops and baldness recurs. Finasteride is contraindicated for use by women because it is an androgenic inhibitor. Young clients who begin drug therapy when hair loss is minimal obtain the best results. A hair weaving or extension is a technique for giving the appearance of more hair by attaching extra hair to the client's natural hair.

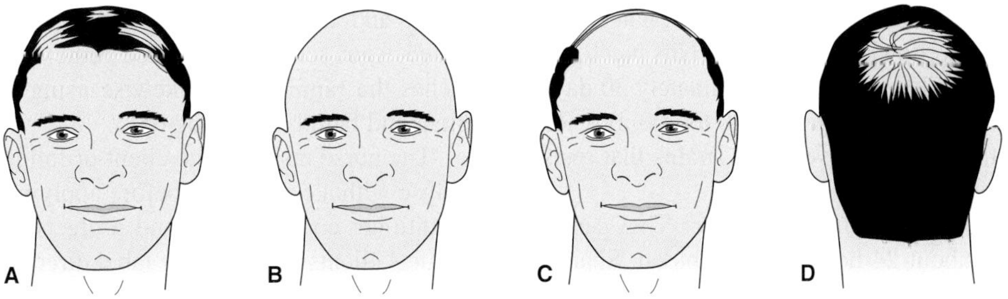

Figure 65-15 Patterns of hair loss: (**A** and **B**) alopecia areata; (**C** and **D**) androgenetic alopecia.

Drugs, called JAK inhibitors also prescribed and approved for treating rheumatoid arthritis, have been found to be effective in restoring hair loss associated with alopecia areata in 4 to 5 months with twice-daily oral doses. The JAK inhibitors being used for this purpose are ruxolitinib (Jakafi) and tofacitinib (Xeljanz). Drug effectiveness is long lasting and persists for several months after stopping treatment (Wang et al., 2018).

Surgical Management

Some clients who are balding prefer a more permanent solution with hair replacement surgery or other surgical techniques. Hair grafting is a technique for transplanting hair-bearing scalp from the back and sides of the head into bald areas. Each graft contains from one to eight hairs. A bald area that is approximately 3 inches square requires approximately 500 to 600 hair grafts. Unfortunately, because of the progressive nature of androgenetic alopecia, transplanted hairs may not survive permanently.

A procedure that disguises hair loss is a scalp reduction that surgically removes a bald area. A scalp reduction usually is performed along with hair grafts. Another surgical technique is to transfer a skin flap. The flap transfers the greatest amount of hair in a short amount of time. However, the scalp may have to be expanded before surgery to stretch the flap area because the flap remains attached in its original location at one end.

Nursing Management

The nurse supports clients who may not have the financial means for medical or surgical treatment. Balding clients are reassured that they can cope with hair loss. The nurse suggests consulting a cosmetologist who can provide a haircut and style that minimizes the appearance of hair loss. Women are advised to opt for loose styling rather than ponytails or braids. The nurse recommends using a conditioner or detangler after shampooing to avoid pulling hair from the head and a wide-toothed comb or brush with smooth tips.

Pediculosis (Head Lice)

An infestation with lice is called **pediculosis**. Although lice can infest any hairy parts of the body such as the pubic area, they are more likely to be found on and in the hair on the head.

Pathophysiology and Etiology

Lice are crawling brown insects about the size of sesame seeds; they do not fly or jump (Fig. 65-16). Nymphs look like moving dandruff, but they may appear red after feeding. Adult lice and nymphs creep over the skin and feed on human blood. The bites result in itching. Eggs, or **nits**, laid by adult females, are tightly cemented to the side of hair shafts. They look like small, yellowish-white ovals. Nits hatch in 7 to 10 days. Lice have a life span of approximately 30 days, during which time one female can lay 100 to 400 nits. Researchers believe that lice are developing strains that resist chemical extermination.

Lice are transmitted through direct contact. They cannot survive longer than about 24 hours without blood. Sharing clothing, combs, and brushes promotes transmission. Anyone can acquire lice, but infestations among school children

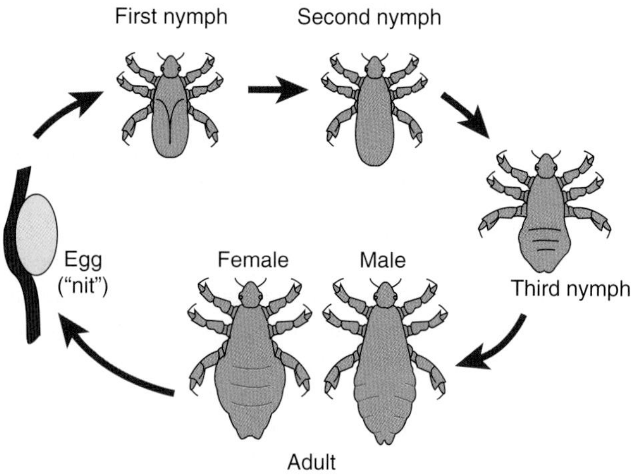

Figure 65-16 The life cycle of head lice.

tend to be difficult to eliminate. Many schools have a "zero tolerance" policy for lice infestation; that is, they bar a child who is infected from attending school until the hair and scalp are free of lice and nits.

Assessment Findings

Itching of the scalp is the most common complaint. Intense scratching can lead to a secondary infection. The adult forms of lice are difficult to see because they quickly move away from light. The nits cling to hairs close to 1/20 to 1/4 inch from the scalp.

Diagnosis is made by scalp and hair inspection. Live lice are retrieved with tweezers or the adhesive side of tape.

Medical Management

Nonprescription shampoos, gels, and liquids containing pediculicides are effective. One example is permethrin liquid (Nix), which kills adult forms of lice. Other over-the-counter products such as RID, Pronto, and A-200 contain pyrethrin, a natural insecticide from chrysanthemum, and piperonyl butoxide. The use of strong chemicals such as lindane (Kwell), which is neurotoxic, and those that contain benzene, which is carcinogenic, is discouraged especially in children (Moore, 2017). Pediculicides are contraindicated for some individuals (see Client and Family Teaching 65-5). Nits and live lice are removed mechanically with a fine-toothed combing tool such as the LiceMeister.

Nursing Management

The nurse teaches school volunteers and parents how to detect and recognize lice and nits. Those who have not learned this measure may mistake other hair and scalp conditions for lice and unnecessarily stigmatize children who are dismissed from school. The nurse removes nits and lice and teaches the family to do likewise using the information in Client and Family Teaching 65-5.

The nurse instructs the client or family not to shampoo or rinse with a conditioner before applying the pediculicide. Conditioner coats the hair and protects the nits. The nurse instructs clients to follow the label directions on the pediculicide; leaving the chemical(s) on for longer than 10 minutes or covering the head with a shower cap does not increase

Client and Family Teaching 65-5 Removing Nits and Lice

The nurse provides the following instructions:

- Cut long hair to make it more manageable.
- Apply the pediculicide to the hair.
- Seat the infested client where there is good light.
- Comb the hair free of tangles while the hair is damp.
- Divide the hair into sections.
- Lift a 1-inch strand of hair from a hair section.
- Use a special lice comb that has narrow stainless steel teeth (available from the National Pediculosis Association).
- Start at the crown and comb firmly, deeply, and evenly away from the scalp to the end of the hair.
- Pin back or secure the combed strand and hair section before going to another area.
- Redampen the uncombed hair if it begins to dry.
- Dip the comb in water or wipe it with a paper towel periodically to remove dead lice and their eggs, or pull dental floss through the teeth of the comb.
- Deposit debris in a sealable plastic bag. Unfasten the sectioned hair and rinse the head thoroughly.
- Assume that some lice will be missed.
- Repeat combings every 2 to 3 days to avoid reinfestation.
- Soak combs and brushes in hot water (at least 130°F) for 5 to 10 minutes.
- Repeat drug treatment a week later as a routine for some drugs or if crawling lice continue to be observed. Check hair and scalp for 2 to 3 weeks to ensure lice have been eradicated (CDC, 2019a).

effectiveness and, in fact, may increase the potential for toxicity.

Nurses, especially those employed in school systems, can provide clients with important information on detection, elimination, and prevention of reinfestation (Evidence-Based Practice 65-1). Some facts to include are as follows:

- Anyone can become infected; infestation is no reflection on hygiene or living conditions.
- Perform hair inspection whenever there is an outbreak (even if asymptomatic). However, there is no value in using a pediculicide prophylactically.
- Know how to treat a lice infestation. If everyone who is infested with lice follows the prescribed treatment, the outbreak can be controlled and eliminated. Manual removal is one of the best and safest options for eliminating lice and nits.
- Do not use pediculicides in women who are pregnant or nursing. These agents are also contraindicated in children younger than 2 years of age and in clients who have health conditions such as open wounds, epilepsy, or asthma.
- Never use a pediculicide on the eyebrows or eyelashes.
- Do not use pediculicides on pets—they do not harbor lice.
- Wash clothing and vacuum furniture, bedding, and carpets.

Evidence-Based Practice 65-1

Managing Head Lice Infestation Among School Children

Clinical Question

What is the school nurse's role in helping to manage an infestation of head lice?

Evidence

The National Association of School Nurses (NASN) in the United States has taken a position that caring for head lice infestations in schools should not interfere with the education process. The NASN uses evidence-based practice strategies to educate and manage school nurses taking the lead in the prevention and management of an infestation of lice in schools. The nurse can make an impact in the school by providing current health information on lice, including anticipatory guidance practice within the community, and using evidence-based practice in the intervention methods. An infestation of head lice occurring in a school can have a negative effect on the school by causing strain for parents, families, and caregivers and has a social stigma. If management of the infestation and policies are not in place, there may be a negative effect on student education (NASN, 2020).

Nursing Implications

The responsibility of the nurse is to have knowledge of the latest evidence-based practice on the management of head lice to assist the school in making policies and procedures for infestations that have a positive effect and do not interrupt education. The nurse has the role of educator for the children, parents, families, and caregivers.

Reference
National Association of School Nurses. (2020). *Head lice management in schools.* https://www.nasn.org/nasn/advocacy/professional-practice-documents/position-statements/ps-head-lice

Concept Mastery Alert

Pediculosis

If a nurse suspects an outbreak of pediculosis in, for instance, a school, the nurse should insist that everyone who is infested with lice follow the prescribed treatment, including hair inspection, washing clothing, and vacuuming furniture, bedding, and carpets.

››› *Stop, Think, and Respond 65-1*

What information is helpful for parents whose children acquire head lice?

NAIL DISORDERS

The nails, especially toenails, are subject to disorders. Two common conditions include fungal infections, known as *onychomycosis*, and ingrown toenails, technically called *onychocryptosis*.

Onychomycosis

Onychomycosis is a fungal dermatophyte infection of the fingernails or toenails. A fungus is a tiny, plantlike parasite that thrives in warm, dark, moist environments. Fungi can spread unchecked from one nail to another. They more commonly affect the toenails because conditions inside shoes are perfect for breeding fungi.

Pathophysiology and Etiology

Onychomycosis and tinea pedis (athlete's foot) often occur together. Older adults and immunocompromised clients are at greater risk of fungal infections. The incidence of fungal fingernail infections has increased among women who have artificial nails. Unsanitary cleansing of nail-application utensils between customers in salons seems to be the mode of transmission.

The fungi relocate themselves from the surrounding skin to beneath the nail plate. The fleshy portion underneath the nail becomes inflamed. The nail becomes elevated, thickens, loosens, and changes color. Eventually, the nail plate is destroyed. The longer the infection is present, the more difficult it is to cure.

Assessment Findings

One or more nails appear grossly different from normal. They are much thicker, causing them to be elevated and distorted. They are yellowed and friable (Fig. 65-17). The infected nail(s) may be long and jagged because they are difficult to trim. The pressure and friction from thickened toenails can lead to pain because shoes do not fit comfortably and socks may wear through.

Diagnosis usually is made on the basis of appearance. Microscopic examination of nail scrapings, however, can confirm the diagnosis.

Medical and Surgical Management

Treatment involves prolonged systemic drug therapy with either of two antifungal agents: itraconazole (Sporanox) and terbinafine (Lamisil). Both drugs inhibit fungal enzymes that regulate cell membrane permeability and result in fungal death. Clients take the medications daily for 2 weeks for fingernail infections and 3 weeks for toenail infections. Terbinafine also can be administered in a pulse-dosing regimen consisting of 1 week of medication followed by a 3-week rest period. Repeated pulse dosing is necessary to eradicate the infection. Drug therapy is more than 50% effective. Because nails grow slowly, it may take as long as 12 months before the nail appears normal.

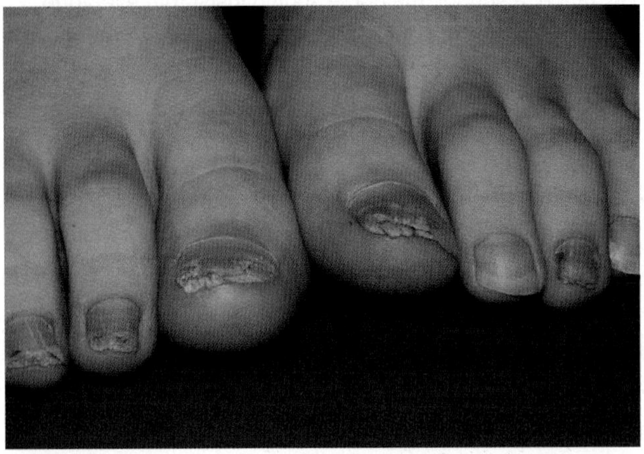

Figure 65-17 Onychomycosis in the toenails. (Reprinted with permission from Goodheart, H. P., & Gonzalez, M. E. (2016). *Goodheart's photoguide to common pediatric and adult skin disorders* (4th ed.). Wolters Kluwer.)

A more radical solution involves removal of the infected nail. This usually is a last resort because it causes permanent cosmetic changes. Surgery is considered when the condition results in chronic pain or causes difficulty in wearing shoes.

Nursing Management

The nurse reinforces that the condition is chronic and to remain compliant with drug therapy for the duration of treatment. They explain the dosing regimen, side effects that may develop, and drug interactions. To prevent reinfection, the nurse reminds clients to:

- Alternate pairs of shoes daily.
- Purchase leather shoes that promote evaporation of foot moisture.
- Never go barefoot.
- Wear footwear at communal pools or when showering in gyms or fitness centers.
- Avoid any damage to the skin around the nail, which makes it easier for fungi to colonize.

Onychocryptosis

Onychocryptosis is the medical term for an ingrown toenail. This common condition can affect all people, although some are more predisposed than others. It usually affects the inside edge of the great toe. Recurrence tends to be a significant problem.

Pathophysiology and Etiology

Some people have an inherited trait that causes a curvature in the growing nail plate. These clients have a higher incidence of ingrown toenails despite the fit of their shoes or methods for keeping the nails trimmed. The latter two factors, along with fungal nail infections, explain why most others acquire ingrown toenails. Athletes or those who are physically active seem to have repeated episodes as a result of recurring trauma.

When the nail curves during growth, a corner of the nail becomes trapped under the skin. As the nail grows, it cuts into the flesh at the lateral border of the nail. The trauma causes local inflammation. The impaired skin provides an opportunity for bacteria secondarily to invade the traumatized tissue.

Assessment Findings

The client feels local pressure from the abnormal nail growth. Redness, swelling, and pain occur where the nail pierces the adjacent tissue (Fig. 65-18). The corner of the upper nail is embedded in tissue. Purulent drainage and an odor are evident if the tissue is infected. Some people develop compensatory gait and postural changes in an effort to relieve the pain. Physical examination is sufficient for diagnosis.

Medical and Surgical Management

Treating the infection, if present, is as important as correcting the nail disorder. Local or systemic antibiotic therapy

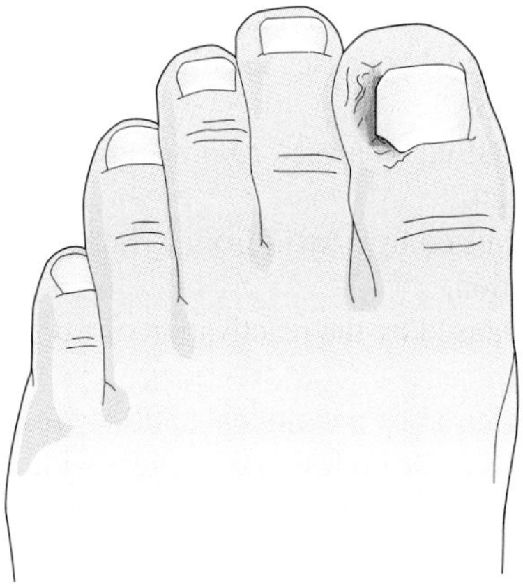

Figure 65-18 Infected ingrown toenail.

sometimes is prescribed. Applications of hydrogen peroxide are used to loosen and remove exudate. To promote healing, the foot is soaked in warm water and Epsom salts, followed by thorough drying. A wedge of cotton may be inserted to lift the corner of the nail. Clients with diabetes or peripheral vascular disease are referred to a **podiatrist**, a professional trained to care for feet. Older clients and those with chronic diseases are especially susceptible to traumatic complications that can impair circulation and necessitate amputation.

For persistent or recurrent ingrown toenails, surgery is indicated. Various techniques are used to remove the nail border, not the entire nail, and its root. Surgical procedures are done in the primary provider's office using local anesthesia or a laser to vaporize the abnormal tissue. Chemical cauterization controls bleeding, and no sutures are required. The client temporarily may need to wear a slipper, sandal, or shoe from which the toe has been cut out until the swelling and discomfort subsides, but most activities can be resumed immediately.

Nursing Management

The nurse explains how to perform foot-soaking regimens and techniques to relieve the pressure around the ingrown nail. If surgery is performed, the nurse instructs the client how to change the dressing, the frequency of dressing changes, and signs of infection or compromised circulation to report immediately to the surgeon.

The nurse provides the following information to affected clients:

- Wear wide shoes and loose socks with sufficient room for the toes.
- Use nail clippers rather than scissors to trim toenails. Toenails should be trimmed so they are slightly longer than the end of the toes, without rounding off the corners.
- Keep the feet clean and dry.
- Avoid physical activities that involve sudden stops, such as playing basketball, which jams the toes into the front of the shoe.

In addition, it is necessary to obtain regular foot and nail care from a podiatrist if there is a history of diabetes, diminished vision, or vascular problems.

KEY POINTS

- Skin disorders
  - Dermatitis: general term that refers to an inflammation of the skin, may be accompanied with pruritus
  - Acne vulgaris: inflammatory disorder that affects the sebaceous glands and hair follicles, coincides with puberty
  - Rosacea: chronic skin disorder, generally characterized by a rosy appearance, exact cause unknown
  - Furuncles (boils); furunculosis (multiple furuncles) and carbuncles (furuncles that drain pus)
  - Plaque psoriasis: chronic, noninfectious inflammatory disorder, causes patches of silvery scales
  - Scabies: infectious skin disease caused by tiny itch mites, spread by skin-to-skin contact
  - Dermatophytoses: superficial fungal infections: tinea pedis, tinea capitis, tinea corporis, tinea cruris
  - Herpes zoster (shingles): skin disorder that develops years after varicella (chickenpox) infection
  - Skin cancer—three types: basal cell carcinoma (most common), squamous cell carcinoma, and melanoma (deadliest form)
- Body ornamentation
  - Tattoos: pigmentation in the dermal layer of skin; risks include infection, granuloma, keloid formation, and allergic reactions
  - Tattoo removal: difficult to complete
  - Body piercing: insertion of metal ring or barbell into a body part; locations include lips, ear cartilage, cheeks, nose, tongue, eyebrows, navel, nipples, or genital area
- Scalp and hair disorders
  - Seborrhea, seborrheic dermatitis, and dandruff: seborrhea and dandruff are noninflammatory disorders that precede or accompany seborrheic dermatitis, which has an inflammatory component
  - Alopecia: baldness; alopecia areata is an autoimmune disorder; androgenetic alopecia is a genetically acquired disorder (male pattern baldness)
  - Pediculosis: head lice
- Nail disorders
  - Onychomycosis: fungal dermatophyte infection of fingernails or toenails
  - Onychocryptosis: ingrown toenail

CRITICAL THINKING EXERCISES

1. What health teaching is appropriate for keeping the skin, hair, and nails in healthy condition?
2. Name a skin disorder that is more common in younger adults and one that is more common in older adults. Discuss the factors that make these age groups particularly susceptible to the disorder.

3. A client tells the nurse that they have a dark brown raised lesion on their back that resembles a wart. What information can the nurse provide?

4. A child is sent home from school with a note about being infested with head lice. What can the nurse tell the mother?

NCLEX-STYLE REVIEW QUESTIONS PrepU

1. What health teaching is essential when a client who is a woman is prescribed isotretinoin (Accutane) for treating acne vulgaris?
1. Prevention of sexually transmitted infections
2. Methods for predicting ovulation
3. Breast self-examination techniques
4. Techniques for avoiding pregnancy

2. The primary provider prescribes cephalexin (Keflex) 4 g daily in four equally divided doses for 10 days for a client with a carbuncle. If the supplied dose of the drug is 250 mg/capsule, how many capsules should the nurse instruct the client to take each time the drug is self-administered?

3. What is the best nursing advice for people who have frequent outbreaks of tinea pedis (athlete's foot)?
1. Never go barefoot when outdoors.
2. Use a blow dryer to dry inside shoes.
3. Wear different shoes each day.
4. Avoid wearing white cotton socks.

4. When a client with shingles (herpes zoster) asks the nurse about what causes the disease, what is the most correct reply?
1. It is caused by a vector-borne insect, such as a tick.
2. It is caused by a toxin from a bacterial infection.
3. It is caused by the reactivation of a dormant virus.
4. It is caused by an antigen–antibody response.

5. A biopsy of a scalp lesion of a client with fair skin reveals the presence of a basal cell carcinoma. What characteristic most likely is a co-contributor to the development of this type of skin cancer?
1. Chronic cigarette smoking
2. Male pattern baldness
3. Eating very few vegetables
4. Bathing with a deodorant soap

WANT TO KNOW MORE? There are a wide variety of online resources available on thePoint to enhance learning and understanding of this chapter.

Go to **thePoint.lww.com/activate**, and use the activation code found in the front of this text to unlock these online resources.

66

Caring for Clients With Burns

Words To Know

allograft
autograft
closed method
debridement
epithelialization
eschar
escharotomy
full-thickness burn
full-thickness graft
hyperbaric oxygen treatment
open method
partial-thickness burn
slit graft
split-thickness graft
stridor
superficial burn
tachypnea
xenograft

Learning Objectives

On completion of this chapter, you will be able to:

1. Explain how the depth and percentage of burns are determined.
2. Name three life-threatening complications of serious burns.
3. Differentiate between open and closed methods of wound care for burns.
4. Name three sources of skin grafts.
5. Describe nursing management for the client with a burn injury.

This chapter reviews types of burns, their physiologic consequences, essential assessments when caring for clients with burns, and the principles and techniques of burn management.

Gerontologic Considerations

- Older adults may be at a higher risk for burn injuries if aging or disease has caused reduced sensory perceptions of touch, vision, smell, or hearing; peripheral neuropathy; reduced mobility; or cognitive changes.
- Assessment must include functional ability levels, home maintenance, and safety.
- Risk reduction teaching includes the following:
  - Water temperature settings should be no higher than 110°F.
  - Working smoke detectors and scheduled battery changes every 6 months (may link to changing clocks for daylight savings time)
  - Working fire extinguisher
  - Burns can result in serious complications in older adults because aging is associated with diminished renal, cardiac, and respiratory functions. Client teaching should include information about reducing flame and scald burns that occur in home settings.

BURN STATISTICS

Approximately 1 million people in the United States seek treatment for burn injuries, most of which are minor (Rice & Orgill, 2021). The incidence of burns is decreasing, but approximately 40,000 people who sustain a major burn require hospitalization (American Burn Association, 2020). The concurrent medical problems and the client's age increase the mortality rate from burn injuries. The American Burn Association (2020) estimates that 3275 people die from burns each year. The risk for acquiring a burn injury is highest among children and adults older than 60 years of age. The most common causes of thermal burns at home are flames and scalding from steam or hot liquids; these fires are often secondary to smoking, alcohol ingestion, or flammable substances that ignite materials (Schaefer & Tannan, 2020).

BURN INJURIES

A burn is a traumatic injury to the skin and underlying tissues. Heat, chemicals, or electricity causes burn injuries. Burns caused by electricity are characteristically the most severe because they are deep. Furthermore, electricity moving through the body follows an undetermined course from entrance to exit, causing major damage in its path.

Pathophysiology and Etiology

The immediate initial cause of cell damage is heat. The severity of the burn is related to (1) the temperature of the heat source, (2) its duration of contact, (3) the thickness of the tissue exposed to the heat source, and (4) the location of the burn. Burns in the perineal area are at increased risk for infection from organisms in stool. Burns of the face, neck, or chest have the potential to impair ventilation. Burns involving the hands or major joints eventually can affect dexterity and mobility.

When a burn occurs, there are localized effects within the burn tissue that are compounded by the inflammatory process, neuroendocrine changes, shifts in fluids and electrolytes, and complications from cellular, chemical, and concurrent injuries.

Local Effects From Burns

Thermal injuries cause the protein in cells to coagulate. Chemicals such as strong acids, bases, and organic compounds yield heat during a reaction with substances in cells and tissue. They subsequently liquefy tissue and loosen the attachment to nutritive sublayers in the skin. Electrical burns and lightning also produce heat, which is greatest at the points of entry to and exit from the body. Because deep tissues cool more slowly than those at the surface, it is difficult initially to determine the extent of internal damage.

Inflammatory Processes

The initial burn injury is further extended by inflammatory processes that affect layers of tissue below the initial surface injury. For example, protease enzymes and chemical oxidants are proteolytic, causing additional injury to healing tissue and deactivation of tissue growth factors. Neutrophils, whose mission is to phagocytize debris, consume available oxygen at the wound site, contributing to tissue hypoxia. Injured capillaries thrombose, causing localized ischemia and tissue necrosis. Bacterial colonization, mechanical trauma, and even topically applied antimicrobial agents can further damage viable tissue.

Neuroendocrine Changes

Serious burns cause various neuroendocrine changes within the first 24 hours. Adrenocorticotropic hormone and antidiuretic hormone are released in response to stress and hypovolemia. When the adrenal cortex is stimulated, it releases glucocorticoids, which cause hyperglycemia, and aldosterone, a mineralocorticoid, which causes sodium retention. Sodium retention leads to peripheral edema as a result of fluid shifts and oliguria. The client eventually enters a hypermetabolic state that requires increased oxygen and nutrition to compensate for the accelerated tissue catabolism.

Shifts in Fluids and Electrolytes

Fluid shifts, electrolyte deficits, and loss of extracellular proteins such as albumin from the burn wound affect fluid and electrolyte status. After a burn, fluid from the body moves toward the burned area, which accounts for edema at the burn site. Some of the fluid is then trapped in this area and rendered unavailable for use by the body, leading to intravascular fluid deficit. Fluid is also lost from the burned area, often in extremely large amounts, in the forms of water vapor and seepage. Decreased blood pressure follows. If physiologic changes are not immediately recognized and corrected, irreversible shock is likely. These changes usually happen rapidly, and the client's status may change from hour to hour, requiring that clients with burns receive intensive care by skilled health care providers.

Cellular, Chemical, and Concurrent Injuries. The following cellular, chemical, and concurrent injuries occur following a burn:

- Anemia develops because the heat literally destroys erythrocytes. The client with a burn experiences hemoconcentration when the plasma component of blood is lost or trapped. The sluggish flow of blood cells through blood vessels results in inadequate nutrition to healthy body cells and organs.
- Myoglobin and hemoglobin are transported to the kidneys, where they may cause tubular necrosis and acute renal failure.
- The release of histamine as a consequence of the stress response increases gastric acidity. The client with a burn is prone to developing gastric ulcers.

Inhalation of hot air, smoke, or toxic chemicals, accompanying injuries such as fractures, concurrent medical problems, and the client's age increase the mortality rate from burn injuries.

- Cardiac arrhythmias and central nervous system complications are common among victims of electrical burns.

Burn Assessment

An assessment of a burn includes a determination of the depth of the burn, consideration of the zones of the burn injury, and an estimation of the extent of the burn injury based

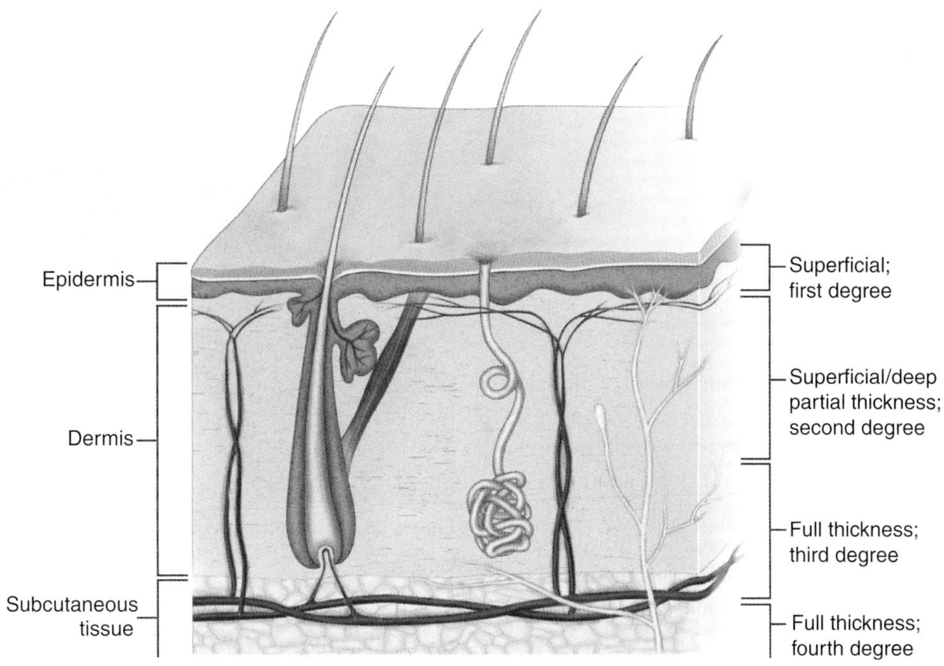

Figure 66-1 Depths of burn injury.

on the total percentage of the total body surface area (TBSA) that has been burned.

Depth of Burn Injury

One method for determining the extent of injury is to assess the depth of the burn. Burn depth is classified as follows (Fig. 66-1):

1. Superficial (first degree)
2. Superficial partial thickness and deep partial thickness (second degree)
3. Full thickness (third and fourth degrees)

Burn depth is determined by assessing the color, characteristics of the skin, and sensation in the area of the burn injury (Table 66-1).

Skin color ranges from light pink to black, depending on the depth of the burn. There may be edema or blistering. The client experiences pain in all areas except those affected by full-thickness burns; however, all burns are generally a mix of burn depths, making pain a primary problem. Clients with extensive burns may exhibit symptoms of hypovolemic shock, such as hypotension, tachycardia, oliguria, or anuria. Breathing may be compromised (Box 66-1). In electrical burns, there are usually entrance and exit wounds.

Diagnosis is made by physical inspection. Radiographs identify secondary injuries such as fractures or compromised lung function in inhalation injuries.

A **superficial burn** is similar to a sunburn. The epidermis is injured, but the dermis is unaffected. Although the burn is red and painful, it heals in less than 5 days, usually spontaneously with symptomatic treatment. Infection, increased metabolism, and scarring do not occur.

A **partial-thickness burn** is classified as either superficial or deep partial thickness, depending on how much dermis is damaged. A *superficial partial-thickness burn* heals within 14 days, with possibly some pigmentary changes but no scarring; it requires no surgical intervention (Fig. 66-2A). A *deep partial-thickness burn* takes more than 3 weeks to heal, may need debridement, is subject to hypertrophic scarring, and may require skin grafts (Fig. 66-2B).

TABLE 66-1 Depth of Burn Injuries

TYPE	DEPTH	CHARACTERISTICS
Superficial (first degree)	Epidermis and part of dermis	Painful with pink or red edema, but subsides quickly; no scarring
Superficial partial thickness (second degree)	Epidermis and dermis, hair follicles intact	Mottled pink to red, painful, blistered or exuding fluid, blanches with pressure
Deep partial thickness (second degree)	Deeper layer of the dermis with damage to sweat and sebaceous glands	Variable color from patchy red to white, wet or waxy dry, does not blanch with pressure, sensitive to pressure only
Full thickness (third degree)	Epidermis, dermis, subcutaneous tissue	Red, white, tan, brown, or black; leathery covering (eschar); painless
Full thickness (fourth degree)	Epidermis, dermis, subcutaneous tissue; may include fat, fascia, muscle, and bone	Black, depressed, painless, scarring

BOX 66-1 Signs of Heat or Smoke Inhalation Injury

- Sore throat
- Singed nasal hairs, eyebrows, eyelashes
- Hoarseness
- Carbon in sputum
- Soot around mouth or nose
- Shortness of breath
- Stridor

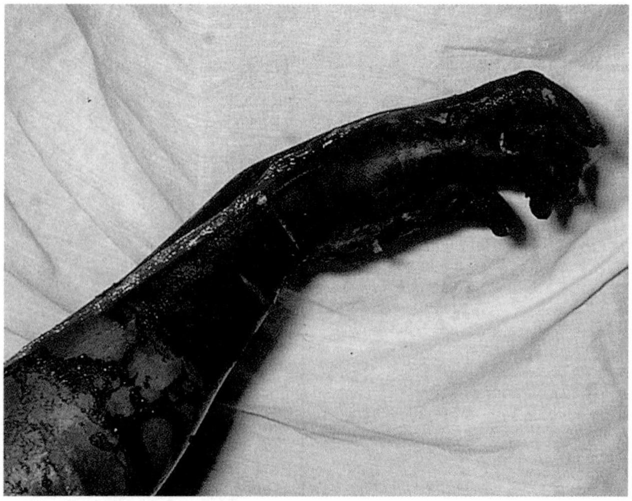

Figure 66-3 Full-thickness burn.

A **full-thickness burn** destroys all layers of the skin and is consequently painless (Fig. 66-3). The tissue appears charred or lifeless. If not debrided, this type of burn injury leads to sepsis, extensive scarring, and contractures. Skin grafts are necessary for a full-thickness burn because the skin cells no longer are alive to regenerate. The most serious full-thickness burn, a fourth-degree burn, can involve ligaments, tendons, muscles, nerves, and bone.

Zones of Burn Injury

Determining the depth of a burn is difficult initially because there are combinations of injury zones in the same location (Fig. 66-4). The *zone of coagulation*, which is at the center of the injury, is the area where the injury is most severe and usually deepest. The area of intermediate burn injury is referred to as the *zone of stasis*. It is here that blood vessels are damaged, but the tissue has the potential to survive. If circulation is secondarily impaired, however, injured tissue in the zone of stasis can convert to a zone of coagulation. The *zone of hyperemia* is the area of least injury, where the epidermis and dermis are only minimally damaged. Because the early appearance of the burn injury can change, the estimate of burn depth may be revised in the first 24 to 72 hours.

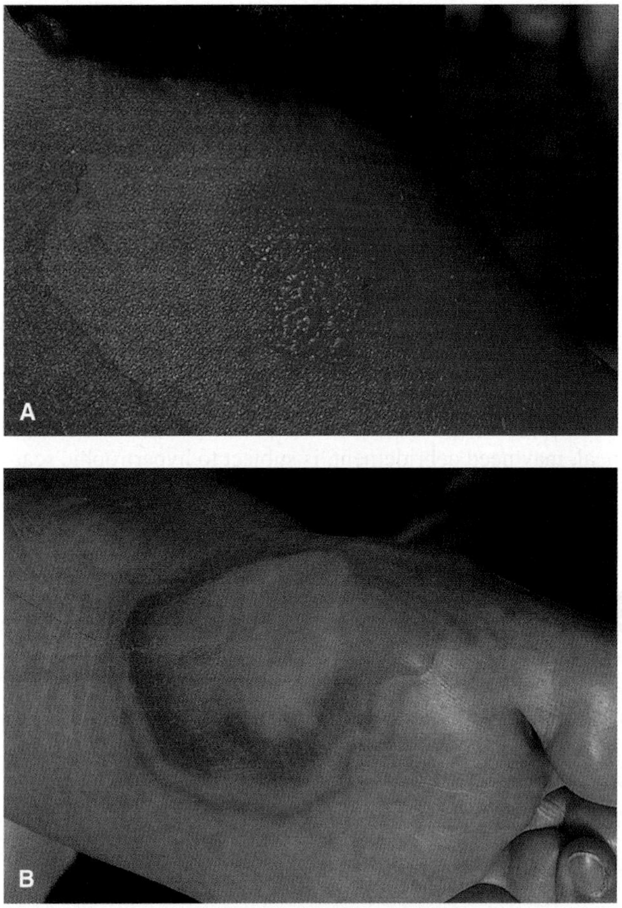

Figure 66-2 (A) Superficial partial-thickness burn. **(B)** Deep partial-thickness burn.

Extent of Burn Injury

Besides determining the burn depth and zones, the severity of a burn is also determined by assessing the percentage of burn injury. The "rule of nines" (Fig. 66-5) is a quick initial method of estimating how much of the client's skin surface is involved. Another quick assessment technique is to compare the client's palm with the size of the burn wound. The palm is approximately 1% of a person's TBSA.

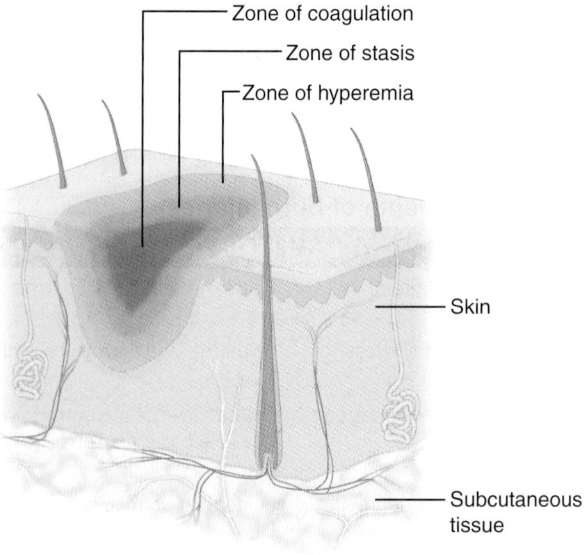

Figure 66-4 Zones of burn injury.

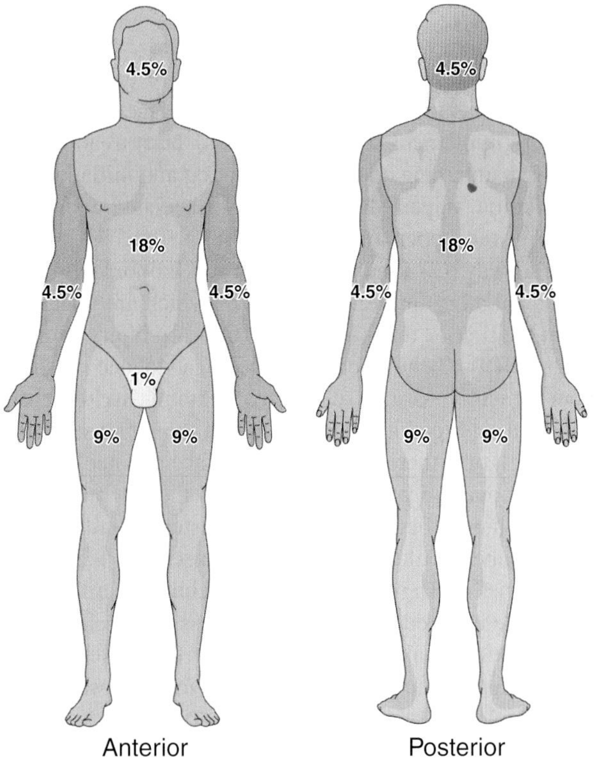

Figure 66-5 Rule of nines. This method is used to quickly estimate the percentage of total body surface area (TBSA) affected by a burn injury.

Special charts and graphs, such as the one shown in Figure 66-6, provide more precise estimates for determining the percentage of the TBSA that is burned. A computerized assessment tool is available that calculates the percentage of TBSA, fluid resuscitation requirements for burns exceeding 20% using the Parkland formula (discussed later), and wound coverage for skin grafting (http://www.sagediagram.com).

Concept Mastery Alert

Burn Assessment

When a nurse performs a burn assessment, the most accurate method of assessing the TBSA is through the use of the Lund and Browder method, which divides the body into smaller segments. This method is more accurate than the rule of nines, which is a quick assessment technique for estimating burns.

>>> *Stop, Think, and Respond 66-1*

Using the rule of nines, calculate the TBSA that is burned if the burn includes one arm and the anterior chest.

Medical Management

The outcome of a burn injury depends on the initial first aid provided and the subsequent treatment in the hospital or burn center. Any one of three complications—inhalation injury,

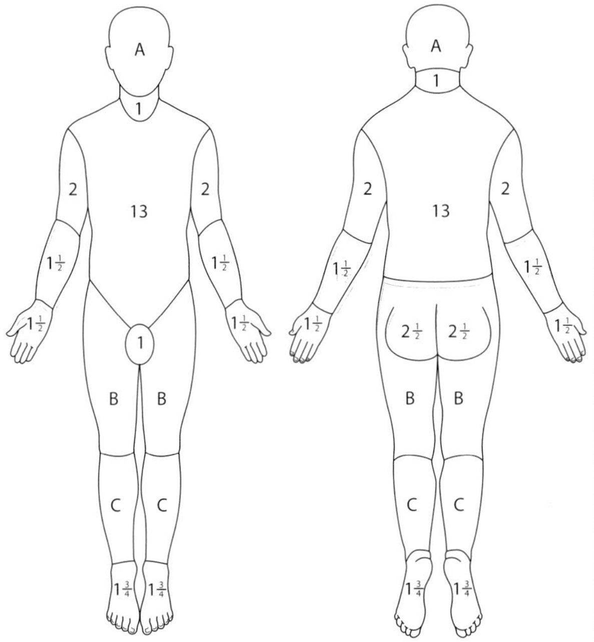

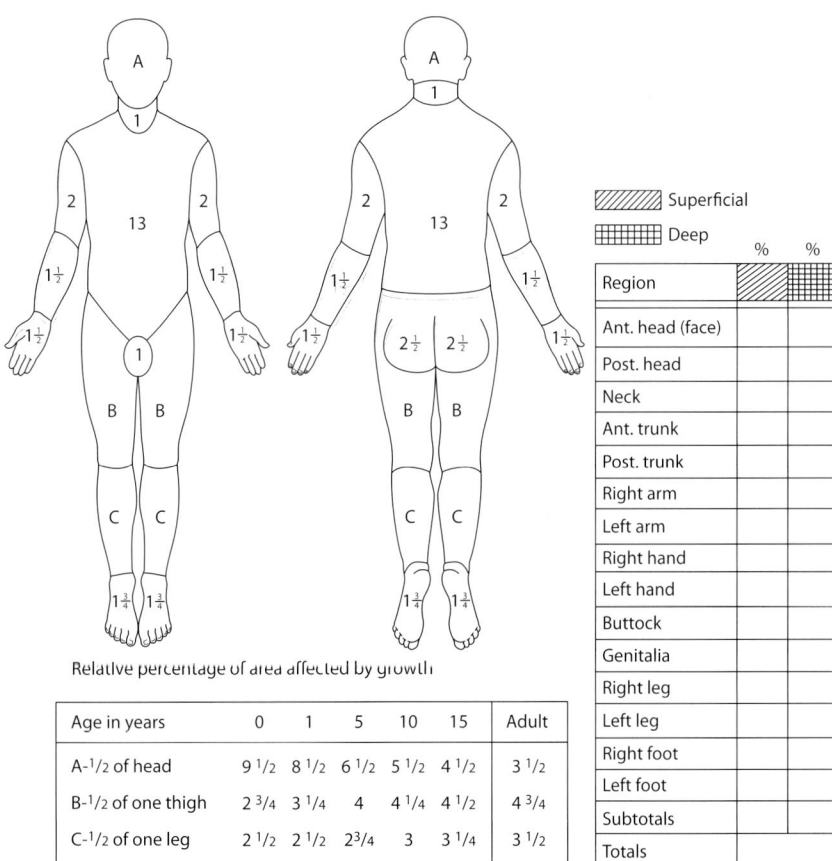

Relative percentage of area affected by growth

Age in years	0	1	5	10	15	Adult
A-1/2 of head	9 1/2	8 1/2	6 1/2	5 1/2	4 1/2	3 1/2
B-1/2 of one thigh	2 3/4	3 1/4	4	4 1/4	4 1/2	4 3/4
C-1/2 of one leg	2 1/2	2 1/2	2 3/4	3	3 1/4	3 1/2

▨ Superficial
▦ Deep

Region	% (Superficial)	% (Deep)
Ant. head (face)		
Post. head		
Neck		
Ant. trunk		
Post. trunk		
Right arm		
Left arm		
Right hand		
Left hand		
Buttock		
Genitalia		
Right leg		
Left leg		
Right foot		
Left foot		
Subtotals		
Totals		

Figure 66-6 The Lund and Browder burns assessment chart is the most accurate method for estimating percentage of body surface area burned according to age and growth size.

BOX 66-2 American Burn Association Referral Criteria

- Partial- or full-thickness burn greater than 10% TBSA
- Burns that involve the face, hands, feet, genitalia, perineum, and major joints
- Full-thickness burn in any age group
- Electrical burns, including lightning injury
- Chemical burns
- Inhalation injury
- Burn injury with a preexisting medical disorder that could complicate management, prolong recovery, or affect mortality
- Burns accompanied by trauma in which the burn injury poses the greatest risk of morbidity and mortality
- Burned children in hospitals without qualified personnel or equipment for the care of children
- Burn injury for those who will require social, emotional, or rehabilitative intervention

Reprinted with permission from Committee on Trauma, American College of Surgeons. (2014). *Resources for optimal care of the injured patient* (6th ed.). American College of Surgeons.

hypovolemic shock, and infection—can be life threatening. Clients with major burns are transported to a regional burn center (Box 66-2).

Initial First Aid

At the scene of a fire, the first priority is to prevent further injury. If the clothing is on fire, the client is placed in a horizontal position and rolled in a blanket to smother the fire. Laying the client flat prevents the fire, hot air, and smoke from rising toward the head and entering the respiratory passages. The client is taken to a hospital immediately thereafter for examination. During transport, other people who have been burned around the face or neck or who may have inhaled smoke, chemicals, steam, or flames are observed closely for respiratory difficulties. Inhalation of such substances can damage or severely irritate the mucous membrane lining the respiratory passages, resulting in edema of the respiratory tract. In addition, secretion of mucus may be excessive, which also makes breathing difficult. Oxygen is administered, and intravenous (IV) fluid therapy is begun en route.

Acute Care

When the client with a burn arrives, the medical team works quickly to assess the extent of burn injury and additional trauma such as fractures, head injury, and lacerations. Team members implement several aspects of burn treatment, including maintaining adequate ventilation and initiating fluid resuscitation. Impaired ventilation is associated with a burn involving the upper airway and results from (1) swelling of the airway, (2) inhalation of carbon monoxide, and (3) acute respiratory failure, any or all of which are manifested within the first 12 to 24 hours after the burn injury (Vorstenbosch, 2019). If the client has soot or evidence of carbon about the nasal passages, difficulty breathing, **stridor** (harsh sound during breathing), or **tachypnea** (an increased rate of breathing), or if there is edema of the face and neck, a bronchoscopy may be performed to assess the internal airway. Warmed, humidified oxygen is administered, and an endotracheal tube should be available for insertion. If there is a full-thickness burn in the neck area, **eschar** (a hard, leathery crust of dehydrated skin) may compress the neck and pull it into flexion, making a tracheostomy the preferred technique for maintaining a patent airway (Vorstenbosch, 2019). Mechanical ventilation may be necessary to achieve normal blood gases and prevent respiratory failure. Victims of carbon monoxide poisoning may require **hyperbaric oxygen treatment** (administration of 100% oxygen at three times greater than atmospheric pressure in a specially designed chamber) to increase the binding of oxygen rather than carbon monoxide to hemoglobin molecules.

Blood samples are drawn. Fluid resuscitation with crystalloid and colloid solutions begins according to the severity of the burn injury (Table 66-2). The fluid replacement regimen is calculated from the time the burn injury occurred; any fluid infused by emergency medical personnel is factored into the replacement volume. The goals of fluid resuscitation include (1) restoration of intravascular volume, (2) prevention of tissue and cellular ischemia, and (3) maintenance of vital organ functions. Successful fluid resuscitation is gauged by a urinary output of 0.3 to 0.5 mL/kg/hour via an indwelling catheter. A low-dose infusion of dopamine (Intropin) may be necessary to ensure renal perfusion (Vorstenbosch, 2019).

TABLE 66-2 Fluid Resuscitation Formulas

FORMULA	FLUIDS	AMOUNT[a]	EXAMPLE FOR 220-LB VICTIM WITH 50% BURN
Brooke (modified)	Lactated Ringer's	2 mL/kg/% burn	10,000 mL[b]
	Second 24 hours	0.3–0.5 mL/kg/% burn	1500–2500 mL
	Colloid (plasma, albumin, dextran)	Approximate evaporative losses	2000 mL (average)
	5% Glucose/water		
Parkland	Lactated Ringer's	4 mL/kg/% burn	20,000 mL[b]
	Saline	1 mL/kg/% burn	5000 mL
	Colloid	1 mL/kg/% burn	5000 mL
	5% Glucose/water	Approximate evaporative losses	2000 mL (average)

[a]Goal: Establish urine output of 50 mL/hour.
[b]Half of fluid volume given in first 8 hours; remaining half in next 16 hours; time is calculated from time of burn injury, not time fluid resuscitation begins.

IV analgesics are administered for pain, which is often severe. Morphine sulfate is generally the drug of choice. Doses as high as 50 mg/hour may be necessary in adults who are severely burned (Vorstenbosch, 2019). If respiratory depression develops, the primary provider will administer naloxone (Narcan), an opioid antagonist. A tetanus immunization is also administered.

>>> *Stop, Think, and Respond 66-2*

Using the Parkland formula, determine what volume of fluid is required during the first 24 hours of treatment for a client who weighs 168 lb and has acquired a burn of 40% TBSA.

Wound Management

As soon as possible, all the client's clothing is removed. *Staphylococcus aureus*, *Pseudomonas aeruginosa*, and *Candida albicans* are the most common microorganisms causing infection in burned tissue. Health care providers wear powder-free sterile gloves to reduce the accumulation of debris within the wound, which may complicate healing. The body hair around the perimeter of the burns is shaved, because hair is a source of bacterial wound contamination. When the head, neck, and upper chest are burned, singed eyebrows and eyelashes are clipped, scalp hair is shaved, the lips and mouth are cleansed, and the lips are lubricated. Eye ointments or irrigations are used to remove dirt and to lubricate the lid margins. Blisters that have ruptured are removed with scissors.

The burned areas are cleansed to remove debris. After cleansing, topical antimicrobial medications are applied. Wound management includes the open method, in which the wound is left uncovered, or the closed method, in which the wound is covered. The closed method involves the use of one or more types of dressing materials (Table 66-3). The final step is closing the wound with a skin graft or skin substitute or applying cultured skin.

Open Method

The **open method** (exposure method), which exposes the burned areas to air, has been virtually abandoned since the advent of effective topical antimicrobials. It is still used on a small scale, however, for burned areas such as the face and perineum, where it is difficult to apply dressing materials.

If the open method is used, the client is placed in isolation in a bed with sterile linen. Health team members and visitors wear sterile gowns and masks. The skin of the client with a burn is sensitive to drafts and temperature changes; therefore, a bed cradle or sheets are placed over the client. The room is kept warm and humidified.

A hard crust forms over a partial-thickness burn in 2 or 3 days, and **epithelialization** (regrowth of skin) is completed in about 2 or 3 weeks. At this time, the crust falls off, is debrided, or is loosened by whirlpool baths. Eschar forms in areas of full-thickness burns. If the eschar constricts the area and impairs circulation, an **escharotomy** (an incision into the eschar) is done to relieve pressure on the affected area (see Fig. 66-3). A dressing may be used to cover the exposed areas as the eschar is removed. New skin cannot grow beneath eschar, and the inferior surface of eschar is a potential site for infection.

Closed Method

The **closed method** is the current preferred method of wound management because it creates a microbial barrier, reduces heat loss through evaporation, and provides a moist environment that facilitates healing.

First, the burn area is covered with nonadherent and absorbent dressings, which consist of gauze impregnated with petroleum jelly or topical antimicrobials in solution, cream, or ointment-based compounds, which are discussed later. Systemic antimicrobials are generally ineffective in preventing burn wound infections because the blood supply to the injured tissue is severely compromised. The final covering is an occlusive or semiocclusive dressing that is minimally permeable to water and oxygen. The trend is to change the wound dressing frequently enough to maintain antimicrobial effectiveness, check for infection, and monitor the healing process. Depending on the specific type of burn wound management, this may be done every 8 hours to once a week. Frequent dressing changes are necessary when the wound is infected or when there is significant saturation with wound exudates.

>>> *Stop, Think, and Respond 66-3*

If a person is seriously burned, which method of wound management would you expect the burn unit to use? Give at least three reasons for your answer.

TABLE 66-3 Open and Closed Methods of Burn Care

TYPE	ADVANTAGES	DISADVANTAGES
Open method	Reduces labor-intensive care Causes less pain during wound care Facilitates inspection Decreases expense	Contributes to wound desiccation (dryness) Promotes loss of water and body heat Exposes wound to pathogens Contributes to pain during repositioning Compromises modesty
Closed method	Maintains moist wound Promotes maintenance of body temperature Decreases cross-contamination of wound Provides wound debridement during dressing removal Keeps skin folds separated Reduces pain during position changes	Requires more time Adds to expense Enhances growth of pathogens beneath dressings Interferes with wound assessment Causes more blood loss with removal Can interfere with circulation if tightly applied

DRUG THERAPY TABLE 66-1 Topical Antimicrobial Agents for Burn Injuries

Category and Common Generic (Brand) Drugs	Preferred Use	Advantage	Disadvantage
Bacitracin (Baciguent)	Face or near mucous membranes	Inexpensive; painless	Narrow antimicrobial coverage; requires frequent dressing changes
Mafenide acetate (Sulfamylon)	Electrical burns, used for deep burns	Broad-spectrum antimicrobial coverage, penetrates eschar	May delay healing or cause metabolic acidosis; painful application (burning sensation)
Mupirocin (Bactroban)	Face	Painless	Gram-positive antimicrobial coverage only; expensive; requires frequent dressing changes
Silver sulfadiazine (Silvadene)	Deep, partial-thickness burns	Broad-spectrum antimicrobial coverage; painless	Requires frequent dressing changes; delays healing; stains tissue; contraindicated in pregnant women, newborns, nursing mothers, and clients with sulfa allergy
Silver nitrate	Broad-spectrum agent for bacteriostatic use in partial- and full-thickness burns Currently being replaced by dressings impregnated with silver such as Acticoat and Aquacel Ag	Solution for application Low cost Not associated with bacterial resistance	Does not penetrate eschar Requires frequent dressing changes or repeated saturation of dressings Hypotonic solution may decrease electrolyte level Stains the skin and burn wound black as well as anything it contacts; staining interferes with wound assessment

Antimicrobial Therapy. Three major antimicrobials are used to treat burns: silver sulfadiazine (Silvadene) 1% ointment is the most commonly used antimicrobial, followed by mafenide acetate (Sulfamylon), and silver nitrate ($AgNO_3$) 0.5% solution (Drug Therapy Table 66-1).

Other antimicrobials include bacitracin (Baciguent), which is good for facial burns but inappropriate for deeper wounds, and mupirocin (Bactroban), which is effective against methicillin-resistant *S. aureus* but less effective against gram-negative bacteria. Other commonly used topicals are povidone-iodine (Betadine), gentamicin (Garamycin) 0.1% cream, nitrofurazone (Furacin), and antifungals such as clotrimazole (Lotrimin) and ciclopirox (Loprox). Povidone-iodine is contraindicated with some skin substitutes (discussed later) because it can damage new tissue growth in the wound bed.

Acticoat is a dressing that contains a thin, soluble film coat of silver and can remain on the burn for up to 5 days, which greatly reduces the pain associated with dressing changes. Aquacel Ag is a topical dressing to which silver has been added for the management of partial-thickness burns. It is rated as better than silver sulfadiazine, the most commonly used topical antimicrobial. It continuously releases the silver within the dressing, thus requiring fewer dressing changes (about once per week); this translates into a reduction in nursing care time and client discomfort. The dressing generates a faster rate of epithelialization, produces less burning or stinging, and reduces scar height (Tenehaus & Rennekampff, 2020).

Topical antimicrobials have various advantages and disadvantages (see Drug Therapy Table 66-1). All drugs are applied using sterile technique. Because infection is the rule rather than the exception, some clients may require concomitantly administered systemic antibiotics and antifungals such as amphotericin B (Fungizone) and penicillin G (Pfizerpen).

Surgical Management

Additional treatment modalities to promote healing include debridement, application of a skin substitute, or skin grafting.

Debridement

Wound **debridement** is the removal of necrotic tissue. The procedure is potentially painful and warrants premedication with an analgesic. Debridement is accomplished in one of four ways:

- Naturally as the nonliving tissue sloughs away from uninjured tissue
- Mechanically when dead tissue adheres to dressings or is detached during cleansing

- Enzymatically through the application of topical enzymes to the burn wound
- Surgically with the use of forceps and scissors during dressing changes or wound cleansing

A disadvantage of surgical debridement is bleeding. Burn victims already have secondary problems with healing because of preexisting low red blood cell (RBC) counts that the accompanying blood loss potentiates.

After dead tissue is removed, it is imperative that the healthy tissue be covered with an antimicrobial dressing, temporary skin substitute, skin graft, or cultured skin.

Skin Substitutes and Skin Grafting

When a wound dressing alone is no longer appropriate for covering large areas of burned tissue, use of a **skin substitute**, a temporary covering, or **skin grafting**, transferring the client's own skin to another area, becomes advantageous. Either or both techniques are used when skin layers responsible for regeneration have been destroyed. Large burns may not be able to granulate fully, resulting in chronic open wounds and delayed healing. Skin substitutes can be applied all over the burn wound as soon as the skin is cleaned and debrided instead of having to wait until enough skin is available for grafting purposes.

Unassisted healing, that is, healing without the use of a skin substitute or skin grafts, results in the proliferation of granulation tissue. Granulation tissue contains fibroblasts, which create hypertrophic scars (Fig. 66-7) that contract and pull the edges of the wound together, causing an uneven appearance in the healed tissue and contractures.

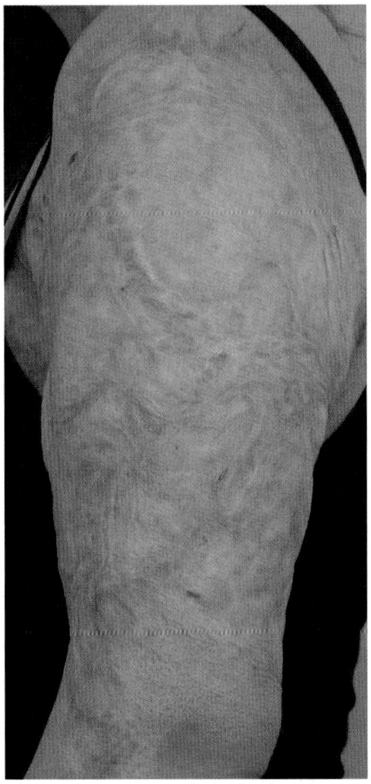

Figure 66-7 Hypertrophic burn scar on the upper arm. (Reprinted with permission from Krakowski, A. C., & Shumaker, P.R. (2017). *The scar book: Formation, mitigation, rehabilitation, and prevention.* Wolters Kluwer.)

The purposes of a skin substitute or graft are to:

- Lessen the potential for infection.
- Minimize fluid loss by evaporation.
- Diminish pain.
- Promote regeneration of tissue.
- Reduce scarring.
- Prevent loss of function.

Sources of Skin Substitutes and Skin Grafts. Several temporary and permanent sources are available for covering a burn wound. These may be manufactured synthetically, obtained from a biologic source, or a combination of the two.

A **xenograft** or heterograft is obtained from animals, principally pigs or cows. Some examples include Permacol and Oasis, which, although acellular porcine in origin, contain a matrix of growth factors that promote epithelialization. There are various other allografting substances that combine biologic with synthetic technology. For example, Integra is a combination of a semipermeable silicone membrane with a biodegradable matrix from bovine collagen, and Biobrane combines nylon, silicone, and porcine collagen (Fig. 66-8). Xenografts are used to temporarily cover large areas. They are rejected in days to weeks and must be removed and replaced at that time (Wood, 2020).

An **allograft** or homograft is a biologic source of skin similar to that of the client. It may be obtained from a cadaver, from human donor cells such as stem cells from umbilical cord blood, or infrequently from amniotic membranes. Cadaver skin is usually in short supply; although the tissue is screened for HIV and hepatitis, concerns remain that it could be a source of other pathogens. TransCyte is an example of a temporary skin substitute that contains human neonatal fibroblast cells that are cultured aseptically and incorporated within a nylon mesh membrane.

An **autograft** uses the client's own skin, which is transplanted from one part of the body to another. Only an autograft or skin transplanted from an identical twin can become

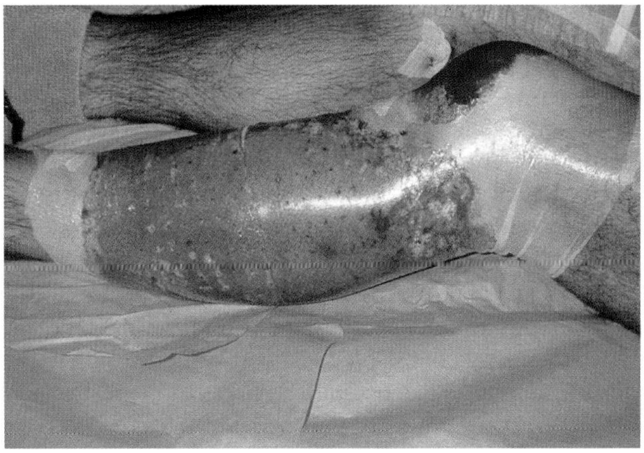

Figure 66-8 Biobrane dressing applied to lower-extremity partial-thickness burn. (Used with permission from Smith & Nephew.)

a permanent part of the client's own skin. Besides actually harvesting and grafting the skin from an unburned area, autologous epithelial keratinocytes (skin cells) can be cultured. To do so, a postage stamp–sized specimen of the client's epidermis is removed. Keratinocytes are isolated from the specimen. They are then cultured in flasks for 2 to 3 weeks along with nutrients until they form a large number of coalesced cells in the form of a sheet. The sheet of cultured epithelial cells can then be transferred onto the burned areas. The cultured cells promote rapid healing without any potential for rejection. Because blisters can form beneath the sheets of fragile cultured cells that interfere with a successful outcome, it is now possible to spray the cells onto the burn wound with a ReCell device that is FDA-approved in the United States (Yetman, 2020).

Types of Autografts

Human skin from the client with a burn is harvested under general anesthesia. Either a split-thickness or full-thickness graft is removed. In a **split-thickness graft**, the epidermis and a thin layer of dermis are harvested from the client's skin. Split-thickness autografts vary in thickness (0.008 to 0.024 inch), size, and shape and are usually obtained from the buttocks or thighs. A dermatome, a scalpel, or another special instrument is used to remove the skin from the donor site. Split-thickness autografts have more successful outcomes than other types; however, their cosmetic appearance is less than desirable, they are less elastic, and hair does not grow from their surface.

A **full-thickness graft**, which may be 0.035 inch thick, includes epidermis, dermis, and some subcutaneous tissue. This type of graft is used when the burned area is fairly small or involves the hands, face, or neck. Full-thickness grafts are more comparable in appearance to normal skin and can tolerate more stress once they become permanently attached to the burn wound.

A **slit graft** (also called a *lace* or an *expansile graft*) is used when the area available as a donor site is limited, as in clients with extensive burns. The skin is removed from the donor site and passed through an instrument that slits it; thus, a smaller piece of skin is stretched to cover a larger area (Fig. 66-9).

Harvesting the client's own tissue has several disadvantages: (1) It compounds the client's pain because it creates a new wound, (2) the donor site has the potential for scarring and atypical pigment changes, (3) there is a potential for donor site infection, (4) there is a delay in wound closure while waiting for the donor site to heal and be reharvested, and (5) delays caused by waiting for harvest sites to heal increase costs and challenge the client's ability to cope with a prolonged hospitalization. Furthermore, it may be virtually impossible to harvest sufficient skin to totally close a full-thickness burn wound that is greater than 60% TBSA. Regardless of the source of the skin grafts, it is imperative to limit movement for some time to prevent disrupting the graft.

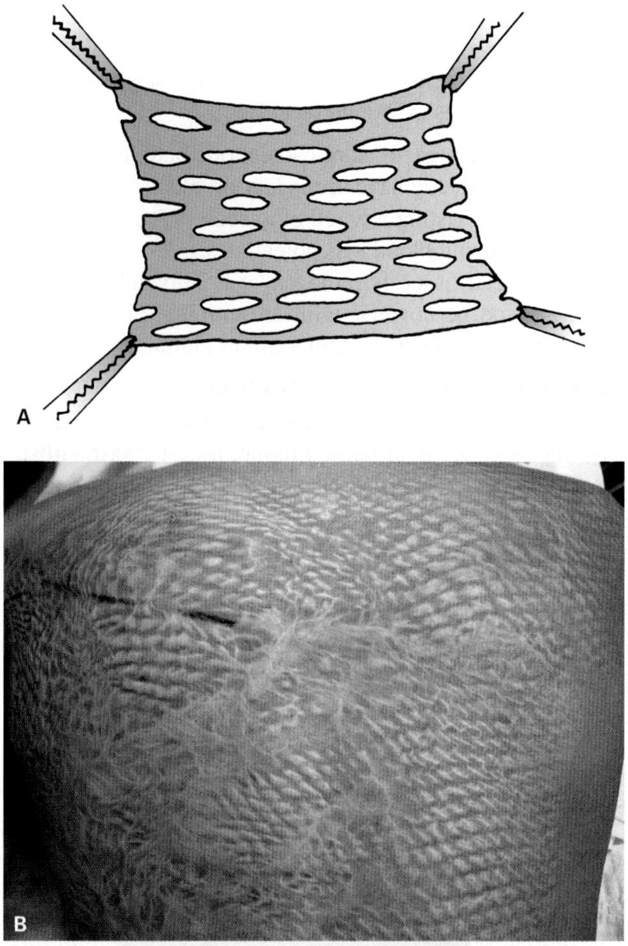

Figure 66-9 **(A)** A slit graft. The slits allow for stretching to cover a larger area of tissue. **(B)** The appearance of a healed burn wound in which a slit graft was used. (B, reprinted with permission from Mulholland, M. W., Lillemoe, K. D., Doherty, G. M., Maier, R. V., & Upchurch, G. R. (2006). *Greenfield's surgery: Scientific principles and practice* (4th ed.). Lippincott Williams & Wilkins.)

Once the skin graft heals, pressure garments made of elasticized cloth or plastic are applied over the grafted area (Fig. 66-10). These garments smooth the grafted skin, reducing scarring and the potential for wound contractures. The client may need to wear a pressure garment for up to 2 years (Client and Family Teaching 66-1).

The client is also advised to use sunscreen with a high sun protection factor when outdoors to prevent permanent pigment changes in the healing skin. Silicone therapy using sheets or gel, now considered the gold standard, provides a transparent, flexible, gas-permeable, and water-impermeable noninvasive approach to burn scar management. Manufacturers of these products claim that they minimize the visibility of scars by reducing their red appearance, flattening the raised scar tissue, and improving tissue elasticity. Silicone therapy can be used alone or in combination with pressure garments (Chow et al., 2021).

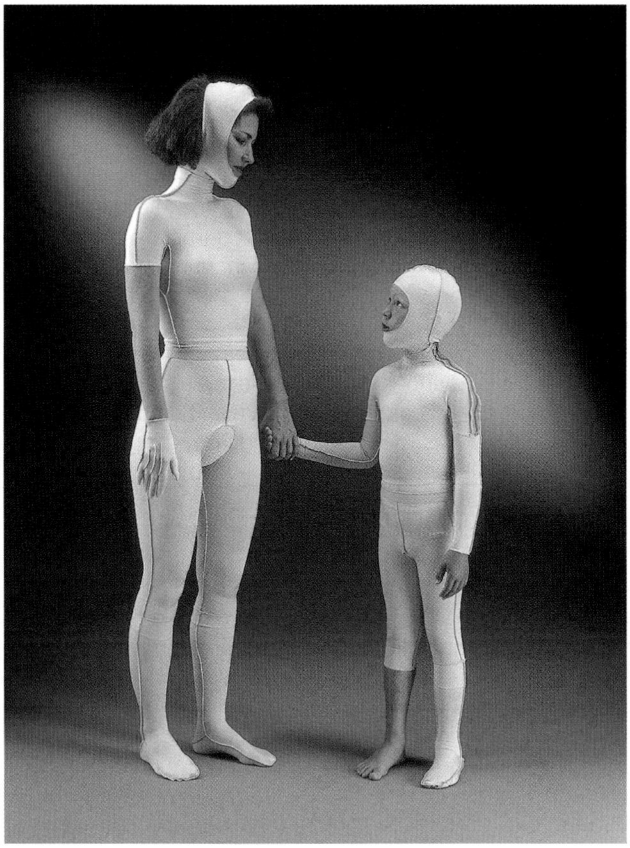

Figure 66-10 Elastic pressure garments. (Used with permission from The Turbot Group, Jobskin Division, Toledo, OH.)

Client and Family Teaching 66-1 Use of a Pressure Garment

The nurse teaches the client and family to

- Wear the pressure garment at least 23 hours each day.
- Follow the manufacturer's instructions for donning and removing the pressure garment.
- Contact the primary provider or physical therapist if the garment causes discomfort or does not seem to fit properly.
- Ensure that holes or nonfunctioning zippers are repaired immediately or as soon as possible.
- Hand-wash the pressure garment daily with a mild laundry detergent.
- Rinse the garment thoroughly to remove detergent residue, salt water, or chlorinated water from a swimming pool.
- Squeeze and roll the garment in a towel to remove as much moisture as possible; do not wring the garment.
- Hang the garment to dry at room temperature away from direct heat; do not dry the garment in the sun or in a clothes dryer.
- Massage any moisturizers, lotions, creams, and petroleum-based ointments completely into the skin because these can cause deterioration of the garment.

Nursing Management

Nursing management focuses on assessing the wound and determining how the burn injury has affected the client's status. The nurse calculates fluid replacement requirements and infuses the prescribed volume according to the agency's protocol. Signs of shock are quickly recognized and efficiently treated (see Chapter 17). The nurse administers prescribed analgesics to relieve or reduce pain (see Evidence-Based Practice 66-1). The wound is cleansed, an antimicrobial agent is applied, and the wound is covered with the prescribed dressing. The nurse monitors the wound to determine any infection. The client and family are supported as

Evidence-Based Practice 66-1

Pharmacologic Agents Versus Complementary and Alternative Therapies for Pain Management

Clinical Question

How does pain management with pharmacological agents affect pain control among adults who have suffered burns compare with pain management using complementary and alternative therapies?

Evidence

Pain in burn victims is often poorly managed. This impacts quality of care and both physical and psychological status for burn victims, including levels of anxiety, depression, and maladjustment after discharge (Wibbenmeyer et al., 2014). In fact, one study found that pain during hospitalization was significantly associated with psychological adjustment when measured as far as 2 years postdischarge (Patterson, 2006). According to Wibbenmeyer et al. (2014), pain management requires a multimodal approach in order to address constant background pain, intermittent breakthrough pain, and periodic pain associated with procedures.

Both pharmacological and alternative therapies have been used to optimize pain management in clients with burns. Opioid analgesics, such as morphine and fentanyl, are the first drugs that are used. Topical analgesics, such as lidocaine, are used to help manage pain, especially during procedures such as skin debridement and dressing changes. In addition, some practitioners use anticonvulsants, such as gabapentin, in addition to opioids to treat neuropathic pain (pain caused by nerves), but studies have shown that this makes no difference in reported level of pain or pain medication consumption during hospitalization (Wibbenmeyer, 2014).

Complementary and alternative therapies, such as virtual reality–guided relaxation and therapeutic touch, have been explored as an alternative or supplement to pharmacological therapies. However, they have been met with mixed results. According to Spiegel et al. (2019), virtual reality–guided relaxation decreased the level of pain in clients undergoing dressing changes but there were no noted changes in the use of opioids during this process. The use of virtual reality–guided relaxation in children was studied by Hoffmann et al. (2019)

(continued)

Evidence-Based Practice 66-1 (*continued*)

with reported decrease in pain and more satisfaction with pain management options during therapy. Other alternative therapies, such as therapeutic touch and foot reflexology massage, decreased pain and anxiety (Alinia-najjar et al., 2020).

Nursing Implications

Effective pain assessment and management are key when caring for clients with burns. When assessing pain, both verbal and nonverbal symptoms should be evaluated. Several pain rating scales are available to determine levels of pain. It is important to know the unique benefits and shortfalls of the designated pain assessment scale.

Managing medication schedules is another key factor for nursing. The longer pain goes untreated, the more difficult it is to regain control. When exploring alternative therapies, nurses should be very careful to investigate the evidence surrounding the pain management technique because some have been shown to make the situation worse, and best outcomes should always be the goal for nursing intervention.

References

Alinia-najjar, R., Bagheri-Nesami, M., Shorofi, S. A., Mousavinasab, S. N., & Saatchi, K. (2020). The effect of foot reflexology massage on burn-specific pain anxiety and sleep quality and quantity of patients hospitalized in the burn intensive care unit (ICU). *Burns, 46*(8), 1942–1951. https://doi.org/10.1016/j.burns.2020.04.035

Hoffman, H. G., Rodriguez, R. A., Gonzalez, M., Bernardy, M., Peña, R., Beck, W., Patterson. D. R., & Meyer, W. J. (2019). Immersive virtual reality as an adjunctive non-opioid analgesic for predominantly Latin American children with large severe burn wounds during burn wound cleaning in the intensive care unit: A pilot study. *Frontiers in Human Neuroscience, 13*, 262. https://www.frontiersin.org/article/10.3389/fnhum.2019.00262

Patterson, D. R., Tininenko, J., & Ptacek, J. T. (2006). Pain during burn hospitalization predicts long-term outcome. *Journal of Burn Care & Research, 27*(5), 719–726. https://doi.org/10.1097/01.BCR.0000238080.77388.FE

Spiegel, B., Fuller, G., Lopez, M., Dupuy, T., Noah, B., Howard, A., Albert, M., Tashjian, V., Lam, R., Ahn, J., Dailey, F., Rosen, B. T., Vrahas, M., Little, M., Garlich, J., Dzubur, E., IsHak, W., & Danovitch, I. (2019). Virtual reality for management of pain in hospitalized patients: A randomized comparative effectiveness trial. *PLoS ONE, 14*(8), e0219115. https://doi.org/10.1371/journal.pone.0219115

Wibbenmeyer, L., Eid, A., Liao, J., Heard, J., Horsfield, A., Kral, L., Kealey, P., & Rosenquist, R. (2014). Gabapentin is ineffective as an analgesic adjunct in the immediate postburn period. *Journal of Burn Care & Research, 35*(2), 136–142. https://doi.org/10.1097/BCR.0b013e31828a4828

they cope with the potential mortality of the burn and change in body image. As healing occurs, the nurse encourages the client to perform exercises that minimize contractures. The nurse encourages adequate nutrition and provides supplements as ordered (Nutrition Notes). Before discharge, the nurse teaches the client about the use of a pressure garment and methods for skin care.

Nutrition Notes

The Client With a Burn Injury

- Extensive burns are one of the most severe forms of stress that a person can experience. Calorie needs may increase to 4000 to 5000 calories/day. Protein needs are typically 2.0 to 2.5 g/kg, especially if burns are >10% of TBSA. Calorie and protein needs increase if complications develop, and they lessen as wound healing progresses.
- Fluid needs increase significantly. With damage to cells and skin, the body not only loses fluid but also struggles to retain fluids. In addition to strict intake and output records, much weight loss is the result of fluid loss. Clients should be weighed daily and sufficient fluid added to reflect the fluids lost in weight change.
- Although it is generally agreed that vitamin needs increase in clients with burns because of losses from wounds and changes in metabolism, the exact requirements are not known. Supplements of vitamin C, vitamin A, and zinc plus multivitamin are commonly used. Supplements of the trace elements selenium and copper have been shown to promote healing and decrease the risk of infections in clients with burns. Supplements of arginine, glutamine, fish oil, vitamin D, and vitamin K given to clients who are acutely burned may offer some benefit, but more research is needed before their use becomes mainstream.
- Unlike other clients with severe stress, clients with burns develop less gastroparesis when they are given nasogastric or nasoduodenal tube feedings within 8 to 12 hours after admission. Most clients with severe burns require nutritional support. Total parenteral nutrition is used with extreme caution because of the increased risks for infection and sepsis.

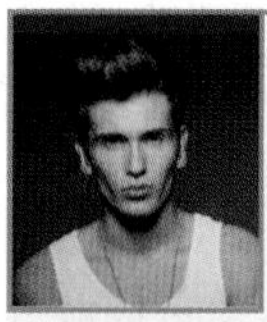

Clinical Scenario A 23-year-old man is brought by ambulance to the emergency department following an explosion in the home, where he was cooking methamphetamine. The client is conscious. The client has incurred burns of approximately 30% TBSA, which includes both deep partial-thickness and full-thickness burns on his chest, abdomen, and one arm. The client's blood pressure is 105/62 mm Hg, pulse rate is 110 beats/min, and respiratory rate is 30 breaths/min. **How can the nurse plan for the actual and potential problems that are likely to develop? Refer to the following Nursing Care Plan 66-1.**

NURSING CARE PLAN 66-1 The Client With Burns

Assessment

- Assess vital signs.
- Look for evidence of inhalation injury.
- Determine the oxygen saturation and respiratory effort.
- Evaluate pain intensity.
- Determine the volume and characteristics of urine.
- Note the percentage and depth of burn.
- Auscultate bowel sounds.
- Assess for concurrent medical problems, and review the results of laboratory tests.

Depending on the extent and degree of burns, some or all of the following nursing diagnoses may apply. Diagnoses change as the client progresses through treatment and the stages of healing.

Nursing Diagnoses. **Ineffective Airway Clearance Risk** related to increased airway secretions; **Impaired Gas Exchange** related to edema of airway and inhalation of carbon

Expected Outcomes. (1) The airway will be patent. (2) Gas exchange will be adequate as evidenced by clear lung sounds, blood oxygen saturation (SpO_2) greater than 90%, and arterial oxygen pressure (PaO_2) greater than 80 mm Hg.

Interventions	Rationales
Monitor characteristics of respirations and lung sounds frequently.	*Frequent focused assessments of respiratory function facilitate early detection of compromised ventilation.*
Check respiratory rate before and after administering an opioid analgesic.	*Narcotic analgesics depress the respiratory center in the brain.*
Measure SpO_2 with a pulse oximeter or analyze arterial blood gas (ABG) results.	*The PaO_2 can be determined deductively from the SpO_2; an SpO_2 of 90% or greater suggests that the PaO_2 is at least 80 mm Hg. ABGs provide objective measurements of serum O_2, CO_2, and bicarbonate levels.*
Administer oxygen as prescribed.	*Supplemental oxygen increases the percentage of inhaled oxygen above that in room air.*
Suction the airway cautiously if edema is present.	*Suctioning removes accumulated secretions, but the trauma of catheter insertion can worsen edema.*
Facilitate ventilation with artificial airways, such as with an endotracheal tube and ventilator.	*An artificial airway and ventilator facilitate the maintenance of adequate gas exchange.*
Be prepared to assist with an escharotomy if there is a circumferential burn of the chest.	*An escharotomy releases constriction and allows greater chest expansion.*

Evaluation of Expected Outcome

Client breathes effortlessly and is well oxygenated.

Nursing Diagnosis. **Hypovolemia** related to volume loss

Expected Outcome. Nurse will monitor to detect, manage, and minimize hypovolemia.

Interventions	Rationales
Monitor vital signs every 15 minutes.	*Hypotension and tachycardia suggest impending shock.*
Measure intake and output hourly.	*Hourly measurements facilitate early detection of mismatches between fluid intake and output.*
Weigh the client daily at the same time with similar dressings.	*A loss of 2 lb in 24 hours suggests a 1-L deficit in fluid.*
Administer fluids according to the fluid resuscitation formula.	*A large volume of fluid is necessary to prevent hypovolemic shock.*
Report urine output of <50 mL/hour.	*Urine output <50 mL/hour suggests inadequate renal perfusion due to hypovolemia or other causes.*

Evaluation of Expected Outcome

Client does not experience hypovolemic shock.

(continued)

NURSING CARE PLAN 66-1 The Client With Burns (*continued*)

Nursing Diagnosis. **Acute Pain** related to tissue injury

Expected Outcome. Pain will be within client's level of tolerance.

Interventions	Rationales
Assess pain intensity as needed and whenever vital signs are measured signs.	*Assessing pain is the fifth vital sign.*
Administer prescribed IV analgesia.	*The IV route facilitates drug distribution when absorption is impaired at other parenteral routes.*
Give analgesics prophylactically 30 minutes before dressing changes or debridements.	*Preventing severe pain is more effective than relieving it.*
Implement nonpharmacologic methods of pain relief: imagery, self-hypnosis, and distraction.	*Alternative methods for relieving pain supplement pharmacologic methods.*
Place client on a CircOlectric bed or other type of turning frame to facilitate turning and repositioning.	*Pain is reduced when the bed turns the client mechanically and passively.*
Exercise caution and gentleness when removing and reapplying dressings.	*Pain is intensified when movement stimulates intact sensory nerves.*

Evaluation of Expected Outcome

Client responds to pain-relieving techniques.

Nursing Diagnosis. **Thermal Injury Risk** related to impaired ability to regulate body temperature

Expected Outcome. Temperature will be within normal range.

Interventions	Rationales
Reduce evaporation from burn wound by humidifying the environment, preventing drafts, and covering the burn wound with ointment, creams, and dressings.	*Impaired skin cannot regulate body temperature; reducing the potential for heat loss helps maintain body temperature.*

Evaluation of Expected Outcome

Temperature is normal.

Nursing Diagnosis. **Infection Risk** related to impaired skin integrity

Expected Outcome. The risk for infection will be managed with infection control measures, antimicrobials, and wound dressings.

Interventions	Rationales
Assess temperature every 4 hours; monitor results of blood counts and cultures.	*Fever, leukocytosis, and bacterial growth from a wound culture indicate infection.*
Use sterile or clean linen.	*Surgical and medical asepsis reduce the potential for infection.*
Wear sterile or clean caps, gowns, and masks.	*Using outer garments reduces the transmission of pathogens from contaminated clothing to the client.*
Restrict people who are infectious from visiting or caring for client.	*Limiting contact with sources of infection protects a susceptible host.*
Apply and administer prescribed antimicrobial and antibiotic therapy.	*Antimicrobials and antibiotics suppress the growth of pathogens.*
Inspect burn areas for healing, drainage, formation of eschar, infection, and stability of the skin graft or wound covering.	*Direct observation of the wound and comparing normal and abnormal findings help determine the client's response to treatment.*
Accurately record all findings.	*Documentation promotes communication among health care providers.*

NURSING CARE PLAN 66-1 The Client With Burns (*continued*)

Evaluation of Expected Outcome

Wound infections are controlled, and the wound heals.

RC of Skin Graft Disruption

Expected Outcome. Nurse will monitor to detect, manage, and minimize skin graft disruption.

Interventions	Rationales
Avoid excessive pressure on grafted area; minimize movement.	*Relief of pressure and restricting movement promote vascularization.*
Assist primary provider with dressing changes.	*Graft disruption is minimized when the nurse assists the primary provider and client.*
Monitor color and odor in the area of grafted tissue.	*A pale color suggests ischemia. A dark appearance suggests poor venous outflow. A foul odor suggests colonization with bacteria.*

Evaluation of Expected Outcomes

The burn wound is covered; skin grafts are viable.

RC of Gastric and Intestinal Paresis (Hypomotility) and Peptic Ulcer

Expected Outcome. Nurse will monitor to detect, manage, and minimize gastrointestinal hypomotility and peptic ulcer.

Interventions	Rationales
Assess for abdominal distention and status of bowel sounds.	*Abdominal distention and diminished or absent bowel sounds suggest impaired peristalsis.*
Insert a prescribed nasogastric tube; connect it to low intermittent suction.	*Negative pressure removes gas and secretions from the upper gastrointestinal tract.*
Administer IV histamine antagonists and drugs such as metoclopramide (Reglan).	*Histamine antagonists raise the pH of gastric secretions and reduce the potential for gastric mucosal irritation.* *Metoclopramide promotes stomach emptying.*
Instill antacid through nasogastric tube; clamp for 30 minutes before reconnecting to suction.	*Antacids neutralize stomach acid.*
Assess pH of gastric secretions every shift; report if pH is less than 3.	*Drug therapy should raise gastric pH above 3; if not, the primary provider may choose to include a proton pump inhibitor such as omeprazole (Prilosec) or a cytoprotective agent such as misoprostol (Cytotec).*

Evaluation of Expected Outcome

Bowel sounds are active in all abdominal quadrants; client experiences no epigastric distress.

Nursing Diagnosis. **Constipation Risk** related to fluid loss, decreased oral nutrition, inactivity, and narcotic analgesia

Expected Outcome. Client will pass stool regularly and with ease.

Interventions	Rationales
Monitor bowel elimination.	*Infrequent and difficult bowel elimination with passage of dry, hard stool indicates constipation.*
Provide a generous volume of oral liquids, fresh fruit and vegetables, and whole grains when the client is allowed oral intake.	*Cellulose is undigested fiber that pulls water into the intestine, creating a bulkier, moist stool that is easy to eliminate.*

(*continued*)

NURSING CARE PLAN 66-1 The Client With Burns (*continued*)

Interventions	Rationales
Administer prescribed stool softener or laxatives.	*Laxatives promote bowel elimination by increasing intestinal bulk and stimulating motility. Stool softeners draw water into the fecal mass, easing elimination.*
Remove any fecal impactions.	*Impacted stool is difficult to pass and may require digital removal.*

Evaluation of Expected Outcomes

Bowel movements are regular; stool is moist and easily passed.

RC of Anemia related to destruction of RBCs and blood loss from stress ulcer

Expected Outcome. Nurse will monitor to detect, manage, and minimize anemia.

Interventions	Rationales
Monitor hemoglobin and hematocrit laboratory results.	*Decreased hemoglobin and hematocrit values suggest blood loss.*
Check gastric secretions and stool for occult or frank blood.	*Identifying the source of blood loss helps the primary provider prescribe additional medical interventions to alleviate the problem.*
Administer whole blood or packed RBCs as prescribed.	*Administration of blood helps replace depleted RBCs.*
Provide iron-rich food or supplements when it is safe to use the oral route.	*The heme component of hemoglobin contains iron.*

Evaluation of Expected Outcome

Erythrocyte, hemoglobin, and hematocrit values are within normal ranges.

Nursing Diagnosis. Malnutrition Risk related to increased caloric requirements and inability to ingest food orally

Expected Outcome. Nutritional intake will compensate for a hypercatabolic state.

Interventions	Rationales
Administer total parenteral nutrition (TPN) until tube or oral feedings are initiated.	*TPN provides calories and essential nutrients that meet metabolic needs.*
Monitor weight loss or gain.	*Weighing the client helps determine if dietary management is adequate.*
Provide high-protein, iron-rich foods in small, frequent feedings when oral nourishment is allowed.	*Protein facilitates cellular growth and repair. Iron prevents nutritional anemia. Small, frequent meals are likely to provide sufficient calories.*

Evaluation of Expected Outcome

Client maintains weight, with no evidence of malnutrition, vitamin deficiencies, electrolyte imbalance, or muscle wasting.

Nursing Diagnosis. Impaired Physical Mobility related to pain, bulky dressings, and contracted skin secondary to scar formation

Expected Outcome. Range of motion and muscle strength will be preserved or restored.

Interventions	Rationales
Keep joints in burned areas neutral: extended rather than flexed.	*A neutral position facilitates functional use.*
Exercise uninvolved joints actively; exercise involved joints during hydrotherapy.	*Exercise promotes muscle tone and strength. Exercising in water reduces resistance to work.*

NURSING CARE PLAN 66-1 The Client With Burns (*continued*)

Encourage performance of activities of daily living (ADLs), such as brushing teeth and eating.	*Performing ADLs is a form of active exercise that maintains the flexibility of joints and muscle tone.*

Evaluation of Expected Outcome

Client regains functional use of joints in burn areas.

Nursing Diagnosis. **Psychosocial/Spiritual Needs** related to reduced mental stimulation, sleep deprivation, social isolation, fluid and electrolyte imbalance, narcotic administration, and sepsis

Expected Outcome. Client will remain oriented and have realistic perceptions.

Interventions	Rationales
Assess mental status every shift.	*Focused assessments facilitate the early detection of problems.*
Reorient the client who is confused.	*Providing facts helps the client reorder thinking.*
Have a calendar and clock within client's view.	*Environmental cues help prevent disorientation.*
Discuss current events; encourage visits from family.	*Interacting with others and staying aware of current events help stimulate the mind.*
Cluster nursing activities to facilitate continuous sleep.	*Sleep deprivation contributes to confusion and disorientation.*

Evaluation of Expected Outcome

Client logically processes verbal and environmental cues.

Nursing Diagnoses. **Altered Health Maintenance and Caregiver Fatigue** related to inadequate emotional resources for managing multiple stressors

Expected Outcome. Client and family will adapt and use strategies for effective coping.

Interventions	Rationales
Explain methods and reasons for treatment.	*Information helps clarify the plan and assists the client to strive to meet goals.*
Acknowledge signs of progress.	*Objective evidence of progress sustains motivation.*
Involve client and family in long-range planning, physical therapy, and vocational rehabilitation.	*A client and family who feel they are part of a team willingly participate in achieving goals.*
Refer family to counseling for assistance in managing conflicts.	*Health care providers with specialized expertise can help clients and family members solve problems.*

Evaluation of Expected Outcome

Client and family cope effectively and use resources wisely to manage client's care.

KEY POINTS

- Burn statistics: approximately 1 million people seek treatment for burns
- Burn injuries: traumatic injury to skin and underlying tissues
  - Local effects cause protein in cells to coagulate
  - Inflammatory process extends initial burn injury as it affects layers of tissue below initial injury
  - Neuroendocrine changes occur within the first 24 hours causing a hypermetabolic state
  - Shifts in fluids and electrolyte cause fluid loss, decreased blood pressure, and even shock
- Burn assessment includes determination of depth of burn, zones of burn, and extent of body surface involved
  - Depth of burn injury
    - Superficial (first degree): similar to sunburn

- Superficial partial thickness and deep partial thickness (second degree): superficial partial-thickness burns heal within 14 days, may have pigmentary changes but no scarring, no surgical intervention; deep partial-thickness burns take more than 3 weeks to heal, may need debridement, may require skin grafting
- Full thickness (third and fourth degree): destroys all layers of skin and is painless; tissue appears charred or lifeless
- Zones of burn injury

- Zone of coagulation: center of burn injury, most severe and deepest
- Zone of stasis: blood vessels are damaged, tissue has potential to survive, intermediate burn area
- Zone of hyperemia: area of least injury; epidermis and dermis are minimally damaged
  - Extent of burn injury
    - Rule of nines: quick initial method of estimating how much of skin surface is involved
    - Lund and Browder: more precise tool to determine body surface area burned

- Medical management includes:
  - Initial first aid
  - Acute care with fluid resuscitation and critical care management
  - Wound management that includes open and closed methods of treatment and antimicrobial therapy
  - Surgical therapy
    - Debridement: removal of necrotic tissue
    - Skin substitutes and skin grafting: xenograft, allograft, autograft

CRITICAL THINKING EXERCISES

1. Discuss methods used to reduce the potential for infection in a burn wound.

2. While caring for a client with burns, the nurse determines the following problems: pain, coughing carbonaceous sputum, and no urinary output since admission 2 hours ago. What should be the nurse's highest priority?

3. What type of skin graft is best for healing a burn wound?

4. A client who is recovering from a major burn reports that the elastic pressure garment is "too warm" and, therefore, resists wearing it. How might the nurse respond to the client?

NCLEX-STYLE REVIEW QUESTIONS PrepU

1. A nurse stops to give first aid to a burn victim running from a home that is on fire. The nurse rolls the victim on the ground to smother the flames. The chest and neck of the victim are burned. What is the next priority for the nurse?

1. Determine the extent of the burn.
2. Identify the victim's next of kin.
3. Obtain the victim's pulse and blood pressure.
4. Monitor the victim for respiratory distress.

2. In the emergency department, it is determined that a burn victim has deep partial- and full-thickness burns over 35% of the upper body. During the nursing assessment of the burn injury, what characteristics will the nurse use to identify the initial appearance of the full-thickness burn?

1. Mottled and wet
2. White and leathery
3. Pink and blistered
4. Red and painful

3. The blood pressure of a burn victim has stabilized. What is the next best means of assessing the client's response to the initial burn treatment?

1. Range of motion
2. Urinary output
3. Level of pain
4. Body temperature

4. The treatment plan for a burn victim includes using the open method of burn wound management. What is most appropriate for the nurse to monitor when caring for a client being treated by the open method?

1. Infection
2. Hyperthermia
3. Depression
4. Malnutrition

5. A burn wound periodically is debrided using hydrotherapy. What nursing action is essential shortly before each debridement?

1. Keep the client in a fasting state.
2. Witness a signed consent form.
3. Administer a prescribed analgesic.
4. Weigh the client on a bed scale.

WANT TO KNOW MORE? There are a wide variety of online resources available on thePoint to enhance learning and understanding of this chapter.

Go to **thePoint.lww.com/activate** and use the activation code found in the front of this text to unlock these online resources.

UNIT 17

Caring for Clients With Psychobiologic Disorders

67

Interaction of Body and Mind

Words To Know

brain mapping
coping mechanisms
cytokines
distress
double-blind study
eustress
exacerbation
fight-or-flight response
freeze response
general adaptation syndrome
hardiness
immunopeptides
integrative therapies
mental status examination
neuropeptides
neurotransmitters
placebo
placebo effect
psyche
psychobiologic disorders
psychobiology
psychoneuroendocrinology
psychoneuroimmunology
psychosomatic disorders
receptors
remission
resilience
soma
stress
stress management
stress-related disorders

Learning Objectives

On completion of this chapter, you will be able to:

1. Discuss new areas of neuroscience about mind–body connections and their effect on health.
2. Name chemical substances transmitted between neurons, giving examples of each.
3. Explain why mental illnesses are now considered psychobiologic disorders.
4. Name biologic and psychologic components that contribute to disorders affecting the body and mind.
5. List examples of techniques used to assess clients with psychobiologic disorders.
6. Describe treatment and nursing care for psychobiologic disorders.
7. Distinguish between stress, eustress, and distress.
8. Describe the general adaptation syndrome, naming its three stages.
9. Explain the purpose of coping mechanisms and the outcomes that may result from their use.
10. List the defining features of hardiness.
11. Discuss techniques that the nurse can suggest to cope with stressors.
12. Discuss the rationale for a mind–immune system connection.
13. Discuss four explanations for the development of psychosomatic disorders.
14. Describe treatment and nursing care for psychosomatic disorders.
15. Explain the placebo effect.

The mind and the body were once thought of as completely separate structures. Now more than ever, they are viewed as a single communicating entity. Recent research has uncovered anatomic and chemical links between the body and the mind, and new fields of science have emerged (Box 67-1). This chapter examines the links between the body and mind and their effects on health. The remaining chapters in this unit discuss disorders that were, and still are, considered by many as purely psychological or psychosocial—that is, separate

BOX 67-1 Scientific Fields Studying Mind–Body Connections

Psychobiology: the study of the biochemical basis of thought, behavior, affect, and mood
Psychoneuroendocrinology: the study of how fluctuations in pituitary, adrenal, thyroid, and reproductive hormones alter cognition, perception, behavior, and mood
Psychoneuroimmunology: a new, developing field that studies the connections among the emotions, central nervous system, neuroendocrine system, and immunologic system. Research studies show how stress predisposes a person to infection (see Chapter 12), autoimmune disorders (see Chapter 34), and cancer (see Chapter 18).

from physiology. Yet there is scientific support that these disorders are **psychobiologic disorders**, conditions in which evidence affirms a connection between abnormalities in the brain and altered cognition, perception, emotion, behavior, and socialization (Lukito et al., 2020; McEwan & Rasgon, 2018; Hamilton-West, 2011; Pinel, 2014; The Bravewell Collaborative, 2015).

Gerontologic Considerations

- Older adults vary in the ability to accurately complete a Mini-Mental State Examination (MMSE) depending on cognitive abilities, ability to use a pen or pencil, and educational levels. Other cognitive assessment tools may be more appropriate and more specific in differentiating cognitive changes that suggest delirium from those associated with dementia or depression. A variety of cognitive assessment tools can be retrieved from www.consultgerirn.org.
- Older clients who have learned positive coping skills continue to cope well as they age. However, age-related changes, progression of chronic conditions, transitions in living arrangements, and recent or multiple losses may overwhelm coping resources. Nursing care and discharge planning that allow the older adult to demonstrate characteristics of hardiness (commitment, control, and challenge) can minimize feelings of helplessness and hopelessness.
- Social isolation, multiple losses, and grieving may increase an older adult's vulnerability and reaction to stressors.
- The cumulative effects of years of chronic psychosomatic disorders may lead to debilitating conditions in late adulthood.

THE BRAIN AND PSYCHOBIOLOGIC FUNCTION

The brain is a complex organ made up of the cerebrum, brain stem, and cerebellum (Fig. 67-1). The *cerebrum* is the brain's largest component. It is the basis for sensory perception, voluntary movement, personality, intelligence, language, thoughts, judgment, emotions, memory, creativity, and motivation. The outer layer of the cerebrum receives, processes, integrates, and relays information to appropriate functional

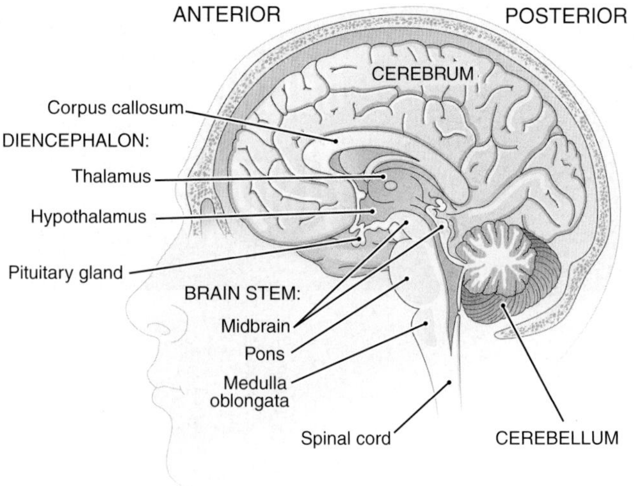

Figure 67-1 Brain structures.

areas of the brain. The *cerebral cortex* is the major pathway of physiologic intercommunication.

The *limbic system* is a network in the brain that contains structures involved in emotions and related physiologic functions. It includes the *thalamus*, which connects many brain centers and modulates movement, sensation, behavior, and emotions. The limbic system also includes the *hypothalamus*, which controls the autonomic nervous system and coordinates the endocrine and immune systems through pituitary–adrenocortical connections (Porth, 2014). Because of its neuroendocrine and neuroimmunologic roles, the limbic system affects and determines many psychobiologic activities (see Chapter 68).

››› *Stop, Think, and Respond 67-1*

Which two structures in the brain play the greatest role in connecting the mind with physiologic functions?

Receptors

Receptors are structures found on the surface of cells throughout the body and brain. Each cell has millions of different receptors. These receptors sense and pick up chemical messengers that arrive in the extracellular fluid. A chemical messenger may be thought of as a specific key that fits into and binds with a specific receptor. Only those messengers that have molecules in exactly the right shape can bind with specific receptors. For example, opioid receptors can bind only with chemicals in the opioid group, such as heroin, morphine, or endorphins. Once binding occurs, the message is received, and the cell begins to respond. Chemical messengers may be natural or synthetic, and the message may cause the cell to perform any number of activities. Neurotransmitters are the chemical messengers that play a significant role in regulating all physical, emotional, and mental processes.

Neurotransmitters and Neuropeptides

Neurotransmitters (Table 67-1) are natural endogenous chemical messengers that communicate information that

TABLE 67-1 Selected Neurotransmitters

NEUROTRANSMITTER	ABBREVIATION	EXAMPLES OF FUNCTIONS
Serotonin (5-hydroxytryptamine)	5-HT	Stabilizes mood Induces sleep Regulates temperature Controls appetite
Dopamine	DA	Integrates thoughts Promotes movement in concert with ACh Stimulates hypothalamic endocrine activity Enhances judgment
Norepinephrine	NE	Affects attention and concentration Raises energy level Heightens arousal
Acetylcholine	ACh	Assists memory storage Promotes movement in concert with DA Prepares for action
Gamma-aminobutyric acid	GABA	Reduces arousal and aggression Inhibits excitatory neurotransmitters like NE and DA Decreases seizure potential
Glutamate	GT	Promotes neuronal excitation Acts as a neurotoxic mediator in various neurologic disorders

affect thinking, behavior, and bodily functions across the synaptic cleft between neurons (Fig. 67-2). The chemicals, which are synthesized in the neurons and then stored in vesicles in the axons, are released and attach themselves (bind) momentarily to the receptors on postsynaptic neurons. After the chemicals have transmitted their information, they are either

- Broken down into inactive substances by enzymes such as monoamine oxidase, acetylcholinesterase, and so on,
- Recaptured by the releasing neuron for later use, a process called *reuptake*, or
- Weakened by becoming diluted in intercellular fluid.

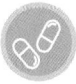

Pharmacologic Considerations

■ Drugs used for psychobiologic disorders work by enhancing or blocking neurotransmission across neurosynaptic junctions.

Neurons are classified by the type of neurotransmitter they release; for example, cholinergic neurons release acetylcholine, and dopaminergic neurons release dopamine. **Neuropeptides** are a separate type of neurotransmitters that include endogenous chemicals such as

- Substance P, which transmits the sensation of pain (see Chapter 11);
- Endorphins and enkephalins, morphine-like neuropeptides that interrupt the transmission of substance P and promote a feeling of well-being; and
- Neurohormones released by interactions between the hypothalamus, pituitary, and the endocrine glands they stimulate.

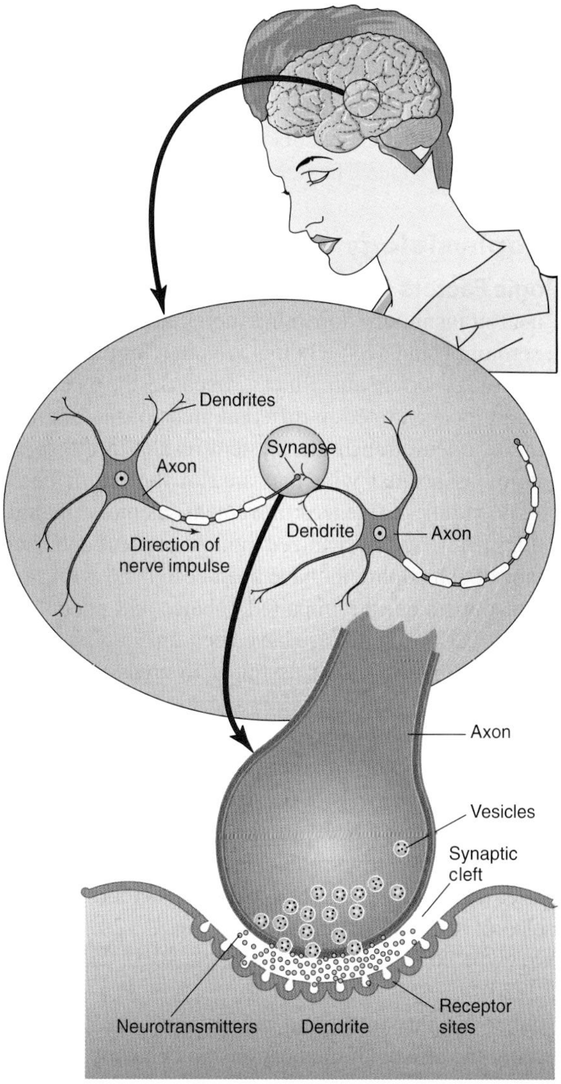

Figure 67-2 Neurotransmitter anatomy.

Different areas of the brain contain different types of neurons that have the capacity to transmit and receive specific neurotransmitters. Each neurotransmitter has either a stimulating or inhibiting effect on neurons. All of the brain functions, including thoughts, emotions, or messages to organs and muscles, depend on neurotransmitters.

Receptors for neurotransmitters and neuropeptides are located not only throughout the central nervous system (CNS) but also in the endocrine and immune systems. This finding suggests that these systems communicate with each other through chemical messages. This concept has tremendous implications for how the mind and emotions can affect physical well-being and how physical status can affect the mind.

PSYCHOBIOLOGIC ILLNESS

Historically, many believed that mental illness resulted from character defects, demonic possession, or punishment by God. These myths persist, which explains why individuals with mental illness sometimes are feared and stigmatized. The study of brain structure, chemistry, and genetics has begun to replace ignorance and misinformation about mental illness with facts. Brain pathology is now seen as the major factor contributing to mental illnesses, now called *psychobiologic disorders*. Some examples of psychobiologic disorders are stress-related/anxiety disorders (see Chapter 68), mood disorders (see Chapter 69), eating disorders (see Chapter 70), substance use disorders (see Chapter 71), and thought disorders (see Chapter 72).

Pathophysiology and Etiology

Biologic Factors

The neurotransmitters dopamine, norepinephrine, epinephrine, serotonin, and acetylcholine are often implicated in the psychobiology of mental illness. Because the neurotransmitters are concentrated in different areas of the brain, disruption of a neurotransmitter system results in the specific symptoms associated with that area of the brain. For example, dopamine influences movement, memory, thoughts, and judgment. The disorganized thought patterns and bizarre behavior of schizophrenia have been correlated with excess levels of dopamine; the impaired balance and uncontrolled tremors of Parkinson disease have been linked with low levels of dopamine. Serotonin is found in areas that regulate sleep, appetite, sexual behavior, and mood. Imbalances in serotonin are thought to be responsible for depression, eating disorders, sleep disturbances, and obsessive-compulsive disorder. Excessive levels of the neuroexcitatory neurotransmitter glutamate have been implicated in neurodegenerative diseases, such as amyotrophic lateral sclerosis, Huntington disease, multiple sclerosis, and the cerebral ischemia sequelae of strokes (Armada-Moreira et al., 2020; Ezza & Khadrawyb, 2014; Lau & Tymianski, 2010; Yap, Lye, & Tan, 2020).

Other insights into brain physiology have come from observing the effects of medications on behavior and symptoms (psychopharmacology). The theory that depression results from decreased levels of norepinephrine and serotonin was first suggested when the monoamine oxidase inhibitors, which block the inactivation of norepinephrine and serotonin (see Chapter 69), were found to alleviate depression. Similarly, antianxiety medications such as the benzodiazepines (see Chapter 68) activate gamma-aminobutyric acid receptors that inhibit arousal, excitement, and aggression. Riluzole (Rilutek), an antiglutamatergic drug, has shown therapeutic benefits for the treatment of amyotrophic lateral sclerosis, also known as Lou Gehrig disease (Masrori & Van Damme, 2020; ALS Worldwide, 2015).

››› *Stop, Think, and Respond 67-2*

If norepinephrine binds to its receptor site on cells, what effects would occur?

Psychological Factors

Psychological factors (forces that shape behavior) also influence psychological equilibrium and may be tied to brain chemistry as well. Some researchers propose that the neurotransmitter network links emotion, memory, and learned behavior (Pert & Marriott, 2007; Tan et al., 2019). Psychological factors have long been components of psychiatric theory and include intrapersonal development, interpersonal interactions, and learning.

Intrapersonal Development

Sigmund Freud proposed that disorderly behavior is the result of intrapersonal (within oneself) conflicts that arise during particular stages of development between infancy and adolescence. For example, Freud correlated compulsive neatness and stinginess with rigid toilet training. Freud greatly emphasized sexual aspects of behaviors between an infant and mother, conflicts surrounding toilet training, awareness of gender differences and genital pleasure, rivalry with the same-sex parent, investment of energy in intellectual pursuits, and efforts to establish relationships with members of the opposite sex. Although many of Freud's theories have been questioned, negated, rejected, revised, and expanded, he provided the foundation for the current fields of psychiatry and psychology, and thus, many of his tenets have withstood the test of time.

››› *Stop, Think, and Respond 67-3*

What do you think may be the physiologic and psychological consequences if an infant is not held very much, is not talked to affectionately, or is ignored when hungry?

Interpersonal Interaction

Other theorists, such as Erik Erikson and Harry Stack Sullivan, proposed that mental health or illness is a consequence of social relationships and interpersonal interactions (Videbeck, 2020). Some theorists go further, suggesting that a person's mental stability not only is affected by relationships with significant others but also is influenced by social systems, such as the neighborhood, city, and country where a person resides. The more positive the social system, the better the chances are that a person will be mentally healthy and well adjusted.

Learning

The psychologist B. F. Skinner proposed the theory that adaptive and maladaptive behaviors are learned and repeated because of rewarding reinforcement (Videbeck, 2020). This theoretical perspective is applied in various circumstances, such as when young children are offered candy to induce toilet training or when privileges are withdrawn to extinguish unacceptable behaviors. Some would propose that *hypochondriasis*, an abnormal fixation about the status of one's health, develops because a person received excessive attention and concern from others during childhood illnesses, which were unconsciously perceived as rewarding.

Assessment Findings

Signs and Symptoms

Brain dysfunction can cause a mix of psychobiologic signs and symptoms. The American Psychiatric Association defines and establishes symptomatic criteria for specific mental disorders within the psychiatric illness domain in the *Diagnostic and Statistical Manual of Mental Disorders*, Fifth Edition (*DSM-5*). For example, disorders such as those involving anxiety, mood changes, abnormal eating patterns, chemical dependence, thought disturbances, and others are identified.

Ultimately, the client's signs and symptoms affect relationships with others and interfere with age-related role responsibilities. Besides a comprehensive personal and family medical history, clients undergo a mental status examination, psychological testing, and laboratory and diagnostic testing.

Mental Status Examination

A **mental status examination** is one component of a thorough neurologic examination. It is an array of observations and questions that elicit information about a person's cognitive and mental state. The components of an extensive mental status examination include obtaining data about the client's

- Physical appearance
- Orientation
- Attention and concentration
- Short-term and long-term memories
- Movement and coordination
- Speech patterns
- Mood
- Intellectual performance
- Perception
- Insight
- Judgment
- Thought content

Nurses may be delegated to conduct a Mini-Mental State Examination (MMSE), a tool for assessing cognitive function especially, but not exclusively, in older clients. The MMSE was developed in 1975 and published in *The Journal of Psychiatric Research*. It included 11 questions/tasks that could be completed in 5 to 10 minutes. Changes in the total score of the exam conducted on different days are used to evaluate changes, both improvement and deterioration, in the client's condition.

A newer version of the MMSE—the MMSE-2 developed by several of the original authors—is an updated assessment tool available in three formats: a standard form that takes about 10 to 15 minutes to implement, a brief version that can be conducted in 5 minutes, and an expanded version that takes approximately 20 minutes to administer. Some items in the MMSE-2 have been revised to facilitate translation for non–English-speaking clients, persons with physical limitations, and those with less severe cognitive impairment. The score(s), which range from 0 to 30, are comparable to the scoring of the original MMSE. Any client consistently scoring <23 is likely cognitively impaired. Also see Evidence-Based Practice 67-1.

Evidence-Based Practice 67-1

Mental Health Assessment Tools

Clinical Question

How does use of the MMSE tool compared with the Montreal Cognitive Assessment (MCA or MoCA) affect assessment of mental status of adult clients?

Evidence

Assessing mental status in clients with suspected or confirmed dementia and some movement disorders, such as Parkinson disease that also cause cognitive impairment, is key to providing effective, safe, quality care (Tang-Wei & Freedman, 2018; Brown et al., 2014; Saczynski et al., 2015). There are several tools used for assessing mental status. The MMSE tool and the MCA are the two most discussed in the literature. Lawton et al. (2016), Saczynski et al. (2015), and Trzepacz et al. (2015) found that both the MMSE and the MCA were valuable tools in assessing cognitive status in clients, and the results were very similar regardless of which tool was used. Pinto et al. (2019), Clarens et al. (2020); Saczynski et al. (2015), and Trzepacz et al. (2015) did point out that the MCA may be more effective than the MMSE in determining cognitive status in clients who have mild cognitive impairments. Brown et al. (2014) found that the MMSE scores were also effective in helping nurses and other health care providers gain a sense of how functionally independent clients with suspected or diagnosed cognitive impairment are.

Nursing Implications

Assessing mental status should include using multiple resources to gain the clearest possible picture of the client's mental and functional status, including interviews with the client, health care providers and family, and directly observing the client. Evidence supports using scientifically tested tools such as the MMSE and the MCA help to gain a clearer picture of the client's status as well as insight to their functional independence. Understanding the times when one tool may be more effective than the other helps the nurse make the best decision about which tool to use. When nursing takes the initiative to include these scientifically tested tools to gather

(continued)

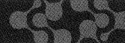

Evidence-Based Practice 67-1 (*continued*)

information, nurse professionals are better able to be proactive in identifying client needs and risks, advocating for the client, and coordinating safe and effective care with the health care team and maximizing outcomes.

References

Brown, T., Joliffe, L., & Fielding, L. (2014). Is the Mini Mental Status Examination (MMSE) associated with inpatients' functional performance? *Physical and Occupational Therapy in Geriatrics, 32*(3), 228–240. https://doi.org/10.3109/02703181.2014.931504

Clarens, M. F., Calandri, I., Helou, M. B., Martín, M. E., Chrem Méndez, P., & Crivelli, L. (2020). Utility of a screening test (MoCa) to predict amyloid physiopathology in mild cognitive impairment. *Journal of Applied Cognitive Neuroscience, 1*(1), 104–108. https://revistascientificas.cuc.edu.co/JACN/article/view/3323

Lawton, M., Kasten, M., May, M. T., Mollenhauer, B., Schaumburg, M., Liepelt-Scarfone, I., Maetzler, W., Vollstedt, E-J, Hu, M. T. M., Berg, D., &Ben-Shlomo, Y. (2016). Validation of conversion between Mini-Mental State Examination and Montreal Cognitive Assessment. *Movement Disorders, 31*(4), 593–596. https://doi.org/10.1002/mds.26498

Pinto, T. C. C., Machado, L., Bulgacov, T. M., Rodrigues-Junior, A. L., Costa, M. L. G., Ximenes, R. C. C., & Sougey, E. B. (2019). Is the Montreal Cognitive Assessment (MoCA) screening superior to the Mini-Mental State Examination (MMSE) in the detection of mild cognitive impairment (MCI) and Alzheimer's disease (AD) in the elderly? *Int Psychogeriatr., 31*(4), 491–504. https://doi.org/10.1017/S1041610218001370

Saczynski, J. S., Inouye, S. K., Guess, J., Jones, R. N., Fong, T. G., Nemeth, E., Hodara, A., Ngo, L., & Marcantonio, E. R. (2015). The Montreal Cognitive Assessment: Creating a crosswalk with the Mini-Mental State Examination. *Journal of the American Geriatrics Society, 63*(11), 2370–2374. https://doi.org/10.1111/jgs.13710

Tang-Wei, D. F., & Freedman, M. (2018). Bedside approach to the mental status assessment. *Behavioral Neurology and Psychiatry, 24*(3), 672–703. https://doi.org/10.1212/CON.0000000000000617

Trzepacz, P. T., Hochstetler, H., Wang, S., Walker, B., & Saykin, A. J. (2015). Relationship between the Montreal Cognitive Assessment and Mini-Mental State Examination for assessment of mild cognitive impairment in older adults. *BMC Geriatrics, 15*(1), 1–9. https://doi.org/10.1186/s12877-015-0103-3

Psychological Tests

Psychological tests are administered to detect personality characteristics, interpersonal conflicts, and self-concept. Table 67-2 gives examples of various psychological tests.

Diagnostic Findings

Measuring levels of neurotransmitters and neuropeptides is difficult, expensive, and sometimes impossible. Unfortunately, a definitive diagnosis for many psychobiologic disorders is usually achieved by ruling out other diseases that manifest similar symptoms. Chapter 36 provides a description of tests such as electroencephalography (EEG), computed tomography (CT) scan, magnetic resonance imaging (MRI), and positron emission tomography (PET) scan.

One of the newest diagnostic tools, brain mapping, suggests that the future diagnosis of psychobiologic disorders will be more efficient. **Brain mapping** is a technique that compares a client's brain activity patterns (from an EEG or other electronic imaging systems) with a computerized database of electrophysiologic abnormalities (Kashyap & Vats, 2019; Knight, 2012; Toga, 2015). A growing database of distinctive patterns for seizure disorders, schizophrenia, depression, dementia, anxiety disorders, attention deficit/hyperactivity disorder, autism, and others now exists for comparison.

Medical and Nursing Management

Treatment of psychobiologic disorders depends on the specific diagnosis. Modalities include drug therapy, psychotherapy, cognitive therapy, and behavior modification (see Chapters 68 through 72). Drug therapy aims at correcting the underlying biochemical abnormality and is particularly useful with mood disorders (see Chapter 69), anxiety disorders (see Chapter 68), and schizophrenia (see Chapter 72). The goals of psychotherapy, cognitive therapy, and behavior modification are to uncover repressed thoughts and emotions and identify healthier coping mechanisms. Nurses play an active role in all aspects of treatment, including administering and monitoring response to drug therapy, implementing behavior modification plans, and providing individual and group counseling.

THE BRAIN AND PSYCHOSOMATIC FUNCTION

Brain chemistry and its effects on physical health are being widely researched as well. Emotions can powerfully influence an individual's health and sense of well-being.

TABLE 67-2 Psychological Tests

TEST	DESCRIPTION
Minnesota Multiphasic Personality Inventory (MMPI)	This true-or-false test of 550 questions is used to analyze which of nine clinical personality traits are manifested by the client's responses.
Beck Depression Inventory	Client rates self according to statements that concern mood.
Draw-A-Person (tree, house, family) Test	Client's drawing is analyzed for symbolism about their self-perception or other emotional data.
Word Association Test	Client is asked to quickly provide a response to words, such as "mother... work...," and so on. Responses are analyzed for psychological significance.
Thematic Apperception Test (TAT)	Client is asked to look at pictures and then tell a story about them. Recurring themes in the stories suggest the underlying basis of emotional problems.
Rorschach Test	The client is asked to indicate what they see in each of 10 separate inkblots.

According to Selye's (1956) theory, **stress** is a physiologic response to biologic stressors such as surgical trauma or infection, psychological stressors such as worry and fear, or sociologic stressors, including a new job or increased family responsibilities. Stress has been implicated in the development or exacerbation of autoimmune diseases, anorexia nervosa, obsessive-compulsive disorder, panic attacks, thyroid conditions, heart disease, functional and inflammatory disorders of the gastrointestinal tract, chronic pain conditions, and diabetes, to name a few.

Stress is not an entirely negative concept. Just the right amount of stress, called **eustress**, is what maintains a healthy balance in life. Eustress helps individuals to pursue goals, learn to solve problems, or manage life's predictable and unpredictable crises. **Distress**, excessive, ill-timed, or unrelieved stress, triggers **general adaptation syndrome**, a nonspecific physiologic response to a stressor (Fig. 67-3). This response, which can cycle many times through the alarm and resistance stages before reaching the exhaustion stage, occurs through the neuroendocrine and autonomic nervous systems.

Physiologic Stress Response

The autonomic nervous system consists of the sympathetic and the parasympathetic divisions (see Chapter 36). The most common pathway for the stress response is through neuroendocrine processes involving the sympathetic division, which uses norepinephrine to stimulate body systems, arousal, and anxiety in response to stress producing a **fight-or-flight response**. This response overrides the control of the parasympathetic nervous system, which slows many metabolic processes. A few individuals respond to stressors through the parasympathetic pathway. Instead of being stimulated to fight or flee, parasympathetic responders exhibit a **freeze response**; they become frozen by fear (King, 2020; Noordewier et al., 2019; Seltzer, 2015; Weller, 2014). Becoming motionless is beneficial among various animals. For example, possums "play dead" when a predator is nearby, which causes the predator to lose interest in its potential prey. Some theorists argue that taking a similarly less aggressive stance could help humans by allowing them to judge a situation and prepare for action (King, 2020).

Psychological Stress Response

Just as the body responds to stressors, the psyche, or mind, also reacts to stress. **Coping mechanisms** are unconscious tactics humans use to protect themselves from feeling inadequate or threatened. These mechanisms function like psychological first aid by helping temporarily to avoid the emotional effects of a stressful situation. When used appropriately and in moderation, coping mechanisms allow maintenance of psychological equilibrium and lead to psychological growth. In addition, some individuals develop maladaptive coping mechanisms, such as abusing alcohol or other substances.

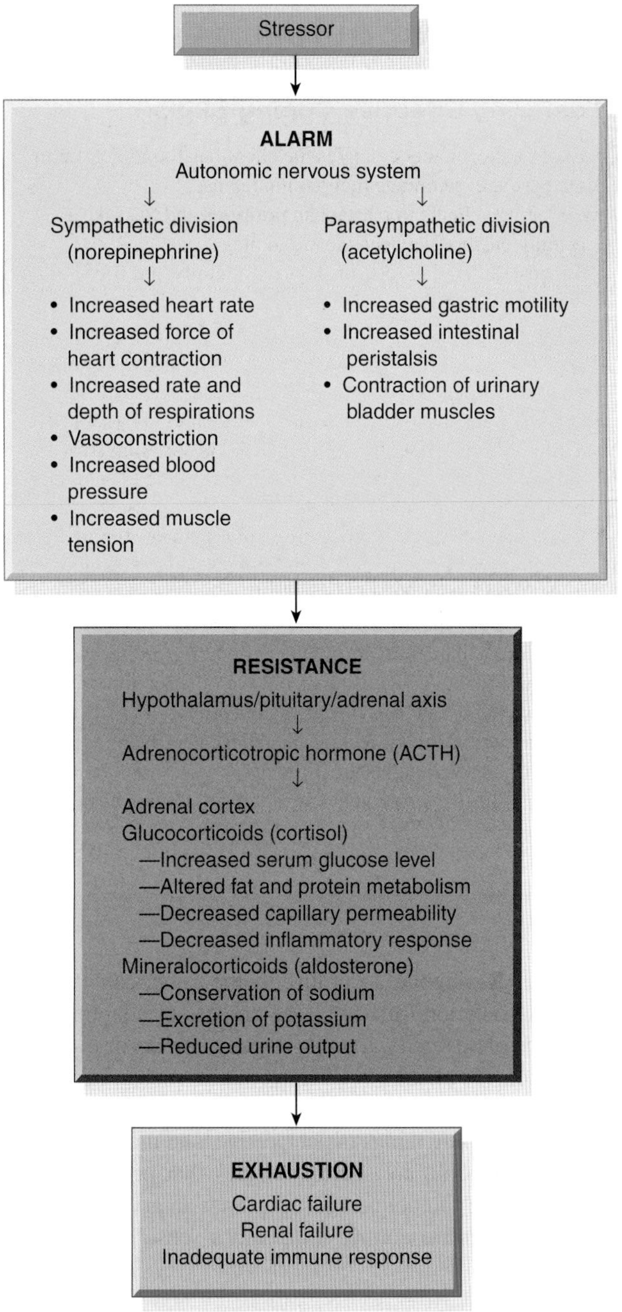

Figure 67-3 General adaptation syndrome, a nonspecific neuroendocrine response to an actual or a perceived stressor.

Some people have developed a particularly effective coping style called **hardiness** (Kobasa, 1979). Characteristics of hardiness are as follows:

- A commitment to something meaningful versus a sense of alienation
- A sense of having control over sources of stress versus a feeling of helplessness
- The perception of life events as a challenge rather than a threat

More recently, Southwick and Charney (2018) describe positive responses to stress among those possessing

NURSING GUIDELINES 67-1

Fostering Effective Coping Skills

- Explore the coping strategies the client has found helpful in the past and encourage their continued use.
- Encourage clients to reestablish priorities and to strike a healthy balance between work and play.
- Suggest cultivating relationships with family and friends who are supportive.
- Teach the client assertiveness skills by role-playing how to (1) clearly state feelings and (2) say "no" to unreasonable requests.
- Discuss time management techniques such as (1) getting up earlier, (2) avoiding procrastination, (3) performing stressful tasks when the client has maximum energy, and (4) eliminating or delegating unwanted tasks.
- Recommend a daily exercise program to reduce stimulating neurotransmitters and release endorphins and enkephalins such as (1) beginning with a 5- to 10-minute workout, (2) increasing the duration by 5 minutes each day, and (3) building up to a 30- to 45-minute period of exercise.
- Tell the client to avoid using alcohol or other nonprescribed sedative drugs as forms of self-treatment.
- Suggest writing about feelings in a diary if verbalizing traumatic or angry thoughts are difficult.
- Suggest stress management education and joining a support group.

resilience. **Resilience** according to the American Psychological Association (2014) is "the process of adapting well in the face of adversity, trauma, tragedy, threats or even significant sources of stress." Characteristics, such as accepting help and support from others, looking beyond the present to the future, keeping things in perspective, and maintaining an optimistic outlook, are some strategies that promote resilience. Nursing Guidelines 67-1 outlines interventions that can foster effective coping skills and a sense of hardiness and resilience.

PSYCHOSOMATIC ILLNESSES

Psyche refers to the mind, and **soma** refers to the body. The term *psychosomatic* means "pertaining to the mind–body relationship," and psychosomatic illness refers to illnesses influenced by the mind. In the past, *psychosomatic* had a negative connotation, suggesting that a client's illness was not medically legitimate. Psychoneuroimmunology research since the early 1980s, however, has given the term a much more holistic meaning, reflecting the concept that the mind and the body are not separate. **Psychosomatic disorders**, also known as **stress-related disorders** (Box 67-2), are bona fide medical conditions associated with or aggravated by stress. Many health care providers now believe that all illnesses, if not psychosomatic in origin, have psychosomatic components.

BOX 67-2 Examples of Stress-Related Diseases and Disorders

- Allergic and hypersensitivity disorders
- Anovulation
- Asthma
- Bruxism
- Cancer
- Cardiac dysrhythmias
- Connective tissue disorders
- Eczema
- Hair loss
- Herpes simplex infection
- Hypertension
- Infertility
- Irritable bowel syndrome
- Low back pain
- Multiple sclerosis
- Psoriasis
- Rheumatoid arthritis
- Temporomandibular joint disorder
- Tension headaches
- Tic disorders

Pathology and Etiology

Biologic Factors

In addition to the known effects of stress on the autonomic nervous system, studies show that stressful events, such as preparing for examinations or undergoing employment issues, also affect the immune system. The purpose of the immune system is to defend the body against cancer and invading microorganisms. Stress can lower the numbers of white blood cells, the immune system's disease fighters. Research also shows that chronic stress or very intense stress, such as the death of a spouse, has a greater effect on health than temporary stressors. This finding seems to be particularly true when a person lacks supportive relationships. A connection seems to exist between poorer immune function and loneliness; when individuals share emotions with others, immune functions improve.

Support for a biologic connection between the mind and the immune system is found in research that demonstrates that the immune system and the brain communicate with each other through the chemical messenger system using neurotransmitters and immunopeptides. **Immunopeptides** (or immunotransmitters) are called **cytokines** (see Chapter 33) and function in the same way as neurotransmitters; they relay messages throughout the immune system and the brain (Pert & Marriott, 2007). Immune cells can also secrete small quantities of neurochemicals. In addition, nerve cells connecting the organs of the immune system (thymus, spleen, and lymph nodes) to the brain have been identified. This ability to communicate through chemicals implies that the immune system can make the brain aware of processes at distant sites in the body and that the brain can send messages directing the immune system's actions. The powerful actions of neurotransmitters, especially in states of excess or depletion, suggest that the psychological state can significantly affect immune function.

Many stress-related diseases involve allergic, inflammatory, or altered immune responses (see Chapter 34). They are characterized by physical symptoms that cycle through periods of **remission** (absence) and **exacerbation** (recurrence), with the symptomatic episodes often occurring when the client is under stress. The brain–immune system connection suggests that changes in body chemistry during periods of stress trigger an autoimmune (self-attacking) response or result in immunosuppression. Invasion of the body by cancer cells or disease-causing microorganisms, however, is not sufficient cause for disease; disease occurs when defenses are compromised or cannot recognize unnatural cells or pathogens. For this reason, psychological variables that influence immunity have the potential to influence the onset and progression of immune system–mediated diseases.

Psychological Factors

The association of certain psychological characteristics with an increased incidence of illness has been observed for centuries. Research suggests that there may be a generic, disease-prone personality with character traits that include anger and hostility, depression, anxiety, and other features (Sahoo et al., 2018; Masafi et al., 2018; Pelletier, 1977; 1995). The type of disease that develops is related to an individual's health habits, environmental exposure, family history, and other socioeconomic factors.

Anger

Although anger is a normal emotion, some people fail to express it, perhaps feeling threatened by possible retaliation. They expend vast amounts of energy maintaining a facade of being happy and well adjusted. The effect of chronically suppressing anger and the neurochemical changes that accompany it, however, may be the triggering mechanism for a dysfunctional immune response.

Conversely, evidence suggests that the excess expression of hostility and anger is correlated with an increased incidence of heart attacks and may result from low levels of serotonin. The frequent activation of the sympathetic nervous system in persons prone to anger and hostility is another factor implicated in the development of heart disease.

Dependence

Some propose that unmet dependency needs and fears of rejection or abandonment provoke feelings of insecurity among some individuals with psychosomatic disorders (Townsend & Morgan, 2017). Helplessness is related to dependence, and numerous studies have shown that people who feel powerless in their lives have more illnesses than those who have a sense of control.

Ambivalence

Ambivalence means feeling or acting in two opposing ways at the same time. For example, an individual may feel hostility toward the persons from whom they most want love and approval, or they may act independently and yet desire dependence. These unresolved conflicts may affect neurotransmitter and immune functioning and may be another key to the development of physical disorders.

Assessment Findings

Signs and Symptoms

Many stress-prone individuals seek medical attention when they experience symptoms in one or more organs affected by the autonomic nervous system. Clients may present with heart palpitations, pounding headaches, breathlessness, tightness in the chest, chest pain, chronic pain, irritability, epigastric pain, abdominal discomfort and bloating, or constipation alternating with diarrhea. Many other illnesses, including cancer and cardiovascular disease, are not as obviously related to stress but are thought to have a psychosomatic component. The biopsychosocial effects of stress and mental state should be considered in the evaluation and treatment of all illnesses.

Diagnostic Findings

Diagnostic tests are done to determine the extent of the disease and all physical causes for the client's symptoms. Because other conditions, such as excessive intake of caffeine, cocaine use, mitral valve prolapse, hyperthyroidism, hypoglycemia, and lactose intolerance, to name a few, can mimic the signs and symptoms of some stress-related diseases, it is important to conduct tests before assuming that the disorder is stress induced.

Medical and Nursing Management

Treatment involves standard medical care pertinent to the diagnosis, control of the physical symptoms, and implementation of methods effective in managing stress and supporting the immune system. Nurses have an important role in participating in the treatment and education of clients regarding these methods. **Stress management** and other techniques have gained acceptance based on studies that suggest psychological factors can reduce the effects of stressors on the immune system and facilitate healing. Stress management programs offer instruction in relaxation techniques and effective coping strategies, including assertiveness training and developing a network of social support. Nutrition Notes outlines nutritional considerations for clients with psychosomatic disorders.

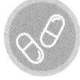

Pharmacologic Considerations

- Obtain a complete current medication history for each client, including nonprescription drugs, vitamins, minerals, herbal supplements, or any other dietary supplements. Include questions about the use of alcohol, stimulants, and tranquilizers obtained from a source other than a prescriber.
- Drug therapy for psychobiologic disorders is often geared to treating the physiologic distress. By helping clients reduce distress, they may refocus energy on cognitive behavioral interventions (Fritzsche et al., 2019).

Nutrition Notes

The Client With a Stress-Related Disorder

■ Some people overeat in response to stressors, whereas others deny normal hunger. Assess for changes in appetite, eating patterns, and weight. Encourage clients to eat at regular intervals to avoid both overeating and undereating.

■ Dietary interventions for some stress-related disorders may be necessary only during periods of exacerbation, such as avoiding lactose during acute episodes of diarrhea. For other stress-related disorders, such as irritable bowel syndrome, dietary interventions are recommended regardless of symptoms.

PSYCHOBIOLOGIC INTERVENTION: THE PLACEBO EFFECT

Psychobiologic intervention refers to those techniques that use the mind and body to alter disease. Some examples of the mind–body connection are discussed in Chapter 9 as they relate to **integrative therapies**, a combination of conventional medical treatment with nontraditional physical and nonphysical approaches. The placebo effect is often used as an example of how the mind and body are connected. A **placebo** is an inert or inactive substance that by its very nature cannot alter physiology, yet does so in a significant number of people. The **placebo effect** refers to the healing or improvement that takes place simply because the individual believes a treatment method will be effective.

The placebo effect was first observed during drug research. In most clinical drug trials, half the research volunteers receive the drug being studied, whereas the other half receives a placebo. None of the volunteers or the researchers knows which subjects are receiving the actual drug, a process referred to as a **double-blind study**. When the results of the studies are analyzed, researchers typically find that 30% or more of the individuals who receive a placebo experience improvement (Beecher, 1955; EmedExpert, 2016; Gholipour, 2014). This is thought to show how a person's belief system can positively influence health and that a purely psychological basis for recovery exists. In other words, when clients believe in the treatment regimen or have faith in the prescriber, it potentiates a positive outcome. Harnessing the psychological forces that create a placebo effect by communicating caring, optimism about treatment, and the belief that the client has the ability to recover can significantly affect wellness.

KEY POINTS

- Psychobiologic illnesses
  - Conditions in which science support a link between biological abnormalities in the brain and altered cognition, perception, emotion, behavior, and socialization
- Neurotransmitters and neuropeptides
  - Neurotransmitters
    - 5-HT: stabilizes mood, induces sleep, regulates temperature, and controls appetite
    - DA: integrates thoughts, promotes movement (with acetylcholine [ACh] release), stimulates hypothalamic endocrine activity, and enhance judgment
    - NE: affects attention and concentration, raises energy level, and heightens arousal
    - ACh: assists memory storage, promotes movement, and assists in preparing for action
    - GABA: reduces arousal and aggression, inhibits excitatory neurotransmitters like NE and DA, decreases seizure potential, promotes neuronal excitation, and acts as a neurotoxic mediator in various neurological disorders.
  - Neuropeptides
    - Substance P: transmits the sensation of pain.
    - Endorphins and enkephalins: morphine-like neuropeptides that interrupt the transmission of substance P and promote the feeling of well-being.
    - Neurohormones: released by interaction between the hypothalamus, pituitary, and the endocrine glands they stimulate.
- Assessment and diagnostic tools
  - Mental status exam
    - Physical appearance, orientation, attention and concentration, short-term and long-term memory, movement and coordination, speech pattern, mood, intellectual performance, perception, insight, judgment, thought content.
  - Psychological test
    - Minnesota multiphasic personality inventory: analyze which of nine personality traits are manifested by the client's response.
    - Beck depression inventory: self-rated by client according to statements that concern mood.
    - Draw-A-Person: drawing by client is analyzed for symbolism about self-perception or other emotional data.
    - Word association test: analysis made based on client's quick response to series of words.
    - Thematic apperception test: assessment of emotional problems made based on client's response to looking at pictures.
    - Rorschach test: client is asked to indicate what they see in 10 different inkblots.
- Brain mapping
  - Technique that compares a client's brain activity pattern (from an EEG or other electronic imaging systems) with a computerized database of electrophysiologic abnormalities.
- Stress: physiological response to biological stressors, such as surgical trauma and infection; psychological

stressors, such as worry or fear; or sociological stressors, such as a new job or increased family responsibility
  - Eustress: just the right amount of stress that maintains a healthy balance in life
  - Distress: excessive, ill-timed, or unrelieved stress

- Stress response
  - Fight–flight–freeze response: most common pathway for the stress response is through the neuroendocrine process involving the sympathetic division, which uses norepinephrine to stimulate body systems, arousal, and anxiety in response to stress

- Adaptation syndrome: three stages
  - Alarm: increased heart rate, increased blood pressure, increased respiratory rate, vasoconstriction, increased muscle tension
  - Resistance: increases serum glucose level, altered fat and protein metabolism, decreased capillary permeability, decreased inflammatory response, conservation of sodium, excretion of potassium, and decreased urinary output
  - Exhaustion: cardiac failure, renal failure, and inadequate immune response

- Coping mechanism
  - Unconscious tactics humans use to protect themselves from feeling inadequate or threatened
  - Hardiness: a particularly effective coping style characterized by the following:
    - A commitment to something meaningful versus a sense of alienation
    - A sense of having control over sources of stress versus a feeling of hopelessness
    - The perception of life events as a challenge rather than a threat

- Nursing care for psychobiologic disorders: fostering coping skills
  - Explore coping skills that have worked in the past.
  - Encourage establishment of priorities, including work–life balance.
  - Encourage cultivation of relationships.
  - Teach assertiveness skills.
  - Discuss time management.
  - Recommend establishing and following a daily exercise regime.
  - Encourage avoiding alcohol or sedative drugs.
  - Encourage journaling.
  - Encourage stress management and support groups.

- Explanation for psychosomatic disorders
  - Health habits: chronic stress, anger, ambivalence, and dependence
  - Biological factors: altered immune function
  - Family history
  - Environmental exposure
  - Socioeconomic factors

- Nursing care for clients with psychosomatic disorders
  - Assessment of symptoms
  - Medication management of symptoms
  - Implementation of stress management techniques

- Placebo effect
  - Refers to the healing or improvement that takes place simply because the individual believes a treatment method will be effective

CRITICAL THINKING EXERCISES

1. What would you say to someone who characterizes mental illness as the manifestation of a poor or weak character?
2. What suggestions would you offer to someone who has a stress-related (psychosomatic) disorder?
3. How might failing one test in school be considered *eustress* but failing several tests be considered *distress*?
4. Based on the premises of the placebo effect, what response would you expect if you gave 100 people a red-colored candy resembling a pill that you said would increase their desire for sex?

NCLEX-STYLE REVIEW QUESTIONS PrepU

1. When a nurse assesses a client faced with a stressor, what might the nurse identify as sympathetic nervous system responses? Select all that apply.
   1. Increased heart rate
   2. Elevated blood pressure
   3. Increased peristalsis
   4. Decreased gastric motility
   5. Increased muscle tension
   6. Decreased respiratory rate
2. What is the best suggestion the nurse can make to help a client develop effective coping?
   1. Cultivate supportive friends.
   2. Avoid stressful situations.
   3. Focus on work-related tasks.
   4. Strive for sufficient sleep.
3. A student nurse reviews the diagnoses of assigned clients. Of the following diagnoses, what disorders have a mind–body relationship? Select all that apply.
   1. Cholecystitis
   2. Asthma
   3. Multiple sclerosis
   4. Nephrolithiasis
   5. Rheumatoid arthritis
   6. Irritable bowel syndrome
4. What recommendation would be best when a nurse interacts with a client who reports difficulty sleeping, completing work responsibilities, and abusing alcohol to deal with current life stressors?
   1. Stay awake until later than the usual bedtime.
   2. Finish incomplete work after scheduled hours.
   3. Transfer to a job with fewer responsibilities.
   4. Incorporate an exercise program each day.

5. When a nurse monitors two groups of research participants in a double-blind study, what is the most likely outcome for those given a placebo?
1. All the participants will show improvement.
2. None of the participants will show improvement.
3. One-third or more improve with a placebo.
4. One-third receiving the placebo experience drug side effects.

WANT TO KNOW MORE? There are a wide variety of online resources available on thePoint to enhance learning and understanding of this chapter.

Go to **thePoint.lww.com/activate** and use the activation code found in the front of this text to unlock these online resources.

68

Caring for Clients With Anxiety Disorders

Words To Know

agoraphobia
anxiety
anxiety disorders
anxiolytics
behavioral therapy
cognitive therapy
compulsion
desensitization
fear
flashbacks
generalized anxiety disorder
HPA axis
limbic system
obsession
obsessive-compulsive disorder
panic disorder
phobic disorders
post-traumatic stress disorder (PTSD)
problem-solving process
psychic numbing
psychotherapy
social phobia

Learning Objectives

On completion of this chapter, you will be able to:

1. Differentiate anxiety from fear.
2. Name four levels of anxiety, explaining the differences among the various levels.
3. Give six areas of nursing management that apply to the care of anxious clients.
4. Name examples of anxiety disorders.
5. List categories of drugs used to treat anxiety disorders.
6. Name and discuss two types of psychotherapy used to treat anxiety disorders.
7. List six nursing interventions that are helpful for reducing anxiety.
8. Discuss areas of teaching for clients with anxiety disorders.

Although anxiety and fear are normal human responses, anxiety disorders are not. Questions remain whether anxiety disorders are strictly biologic, learned, the result of unconscious emotional conflicts, or a combination of all three. Probably both physical and psychological factors play a role. A person is first genetically predisposed to an anxiety disorder and then manifests a disorder when exposed to situational triggers.

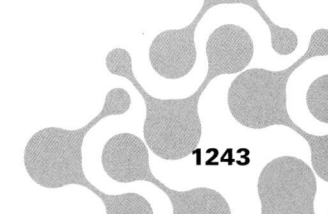

Gerontologic Considerations

■ Older adults on fixed incomes often experience anxiety due to financial problems related to housing and medical expenses. Feelings of vulnerability, limitations associated with age, and fear of the unknown future may also contribute to anxiety in older adults.

■ Anxiety may manifest in the older adult as confusion, behavior changes, or withdrawal. Assessment should include questions about the older adult's loss of significant others, relocation, fears about future self-care abilities, alcohol or drug use, and perceptions of effectiveness of coping methods.

(*continued*)

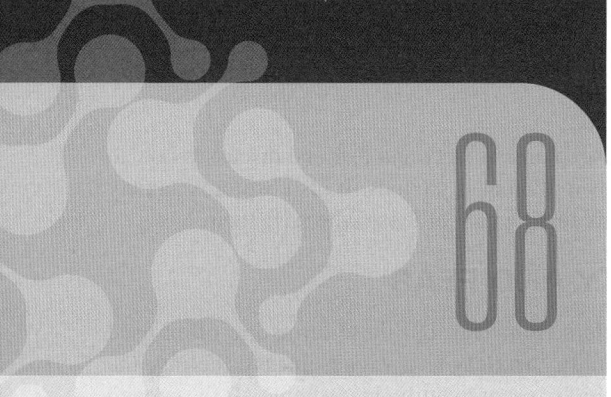

Gerontologic Considerations (continued)

- Antianxiety drugs may cause short periods of memory impairment that can aggravate an already existing cognitive disorder. These drugs may also cause dizziness or lightheadedness, increasing the risk of falling in older adults. In addition, before administering a benzodiazepine to an older adult, assess for sleep problems, especially snoring. These drugs have the potential to exacerbate sleep apnea.
- The kidneys excrete most antianxiety agents; therefore, older adults with impaired kidney function are at increased risk for drug toxicity when taking these medications.
- Short-acting benzodiazepines, such as alprazolam, are preferred in older adults because they are less likely than longer acting benzodiazepines to cause toxicity, leading to excessive sedation and depression.
- Buspirone is commonly used to treat anxiety in older adults. The drug does not produce dependence on, or interact with, benzodiazepines or alcohol. A decrease in anxiety may occur in approximately 1 week; however, the drug may take up to 4 weeks before a full therapeutic response occurs.
- Beer's list provides a reference to check potential risks versus benefits of specific medications for use in older adults (American Geriatrics Society, 2019).

This chapter explores anxiety and fear and discusses how to intervene when a client is anxious. It also explores anxiety disorders and nursing care of those who have them.

ANXIETY AND FEAR

Anxiety differs from fear, but these terms are often used interchangeably. **Anxiety** is a vague, uneasy feeling, the cause of which is not readily identifiable. It is evoked when a person anticipates nonspecific danger. **Fear** is a feeling of terror in response to someone or something specific that a person perceives as dangerous or threatening. It is common for clients to be anxious in an unfamiliar environment or to be fearful of pain, suffering, or death. Consequently, both reactions are common in hospitals and other health care facilities.

Because many medical and surgical clients temporarily feel vulnerable, they are prime candidates for experiencing anxiety. Recognizing the signs of escalating anxiety, understanding its consequences, and intervening appropriately are important interventions.

Levels of Anxiety

Anxiety may occur at several levels (Table 68-1). When it is mild, it is constructive and prepares a person to take action in appropriate situations. For example, mild anxiety before a test causes most people to study.

TABLE 68-1 Levels of Anxiety

LEVEL	BEHAVIORAL MANIFESTATIONS	PHYSICAL MANIFESTATIONS
Mild	Attention is heightened. Sensory perception is expanded. Focus is on stimuli. Reality is intact. Information processing is accurate. Person feels in control.	Muscle tone increases. Heart rate, BP, and breathing slightly increase. Perspiration is noticeable.
Moderate	Person is more easily distracted. Concentration is slightly impaired. Person can redirect attention. Learning takes more effort. Perception narrows. Problem solving becomes difficult. Person is irritable and feels inadequate.	Muscles are tense. Slight leg or hand tremors may occur. Rate, pitch, and volume of speech change. Respiratory depth and vital signs increase. Sleep is disturbed.
Severe	Attention span decreases. Person cannot concentrate or remain focused. Perception is reduced. Ability to learn is impaired. Information processing is inaccurate or incomplete. Person is aware of extreme discomfort. Effort is needed to control emotions. Person feels incompetent.	Symptoms include hyperventilation, dizziness, tachycardia, heart palpitations, and hypertension. Fine motor movement is impaired. Communication is limited.
Panic	Person exaggerates details. Perception is distorted. Learning is disabled. Thoughts are fragmented. Person cannot control emotions and feels helpless.	Speech is incoherent. Movements are haphazard, usually in an effort to escape. Symptoms include dyspnea, fainting, tremors, and diaphoresis.

Anxiety may be moderate or severe as well. Panic may even develop. Moderate, severe, and panic levels of anxiety are counterproductive; they provoke responses that interfere with well-being. As a person's level of anxiety escalates, the following issues arise:

- Physiologic changes occur, such as elevation of blood pressure (BP) and racing heart.
- Perception of information and events narrows.
- Thinking becomes increasingly disorganized and distorted.
- Physical and emotional fatigue develops from the investment of energy in worrying.

››› *Stop, Think, and Respond 68-1*

Give examples of situations that provoke mild anxiety and the appropriate outcomes that usually result. Discuss situations that may trigger more extreme levels of anxiety and their potential consequences.

Nursing Management

The nurse can assist the anxious client by implementing interventions that maintain or restore a sense of calm and control (Evidence-Based Practice 68-1).

Evidence-Based Practice 68-1

Nursing Interventions for Clients With Anxiety

Clinical Question

How does pharmacologic treatment alone, compared to pharmacologic treatment and cognitive behavioral therapy, affect symptom control in older adults with generalized anxiety disorder (GAD)?

Evidence

Anxiety is a significant health problem among older adults that carries social, financial, physical, and mental health implications. The prevalence of anxiety disorders in older adult populations vary due to the use of different methodologies in the research (Ramos & Stanley, 2020). Many older adults with anxiety disorders do not seek treatment due to limited mobility, cost of treatment, lack of health literacy, and perceptions of social stigma (Dear et al., 2015; Gaudreau et al., 2015; Stanley et al., 2011). Treatments can include pharmacologic, psychological, cognitive, behavioral, and alternative therapies. However, often the preferences of the client can be overlooked when treatment plans are developed.

Ophuis et al. (2017) conducted a systematic review of 42 articles that addressed the cost-effectiveness of pharmacologic therapies, psychological therapies, and combination therapies for treating anxiety and anxiety disorders. Evidence suggests that psychotherapy and cognitive behavioral therapy (CBT) might be more cost-effective than medication (Ophuis et al., 2017). In fact, evidence suggests that Internet-based CBT (ICBT) with phone or email support from a therapist may be an effective and the most cost-effective option for treating GAD in older adults (Dear et al., 2015; Ophuis et al., 2017; Silfvernagel et al., 2018).

The three components of an evidence-based practice approach to decision-making are evidence, clinical expertise, and client preferences and values. Gadreau et al. (2017), Stanley (2011), Whitehead (2018), and Andreescu and Lee (2020) studied client preferences in the treatment of anxiety and found that while older adults benefited from both pharmacologic treatments and psychological treatments, they preferred CBT over pharmacologic treatments and self-help guided CBT. Stanley et al. (2011) and Whitehead (2018) also found older adults preferred to have religion/spirituality intertwined with their treatment.

Nursing Implications

Many options exist for treatment of anxiety in older adults. The relationship between nurses and clients is key in creating conditions, where clients can be honest about their situation and feelings, comfortable enough to report symptoms of anxiety, safe to ask questions and discuss treatment plans, and confident enough to share their preferences. When nurses build therapeutic relationships with clients, all these components become possible. This puts the nurse in a position to more effectively evaluate progress, identify barriers, communicate findings both verbally and through effective documentation, and advocate for clients. If the older client's preferences include integration of religion/spirituality, it is vital that the nurse take an interprofessional approach to ensure pastoral care is included in the treatment plan.

References

Andreescu, C., & Lee, S. (2020). Anxiety disorders in the elderly. *Advances in Experimental Medicine and Biology, 1191*, 561–576. https://doi.org/10.1007/978-981-32-9705-0_28.

Dear, B. F., Zou, J. B., Ali, S., Lorian, C. N., Johnston, L., Sheehan, J., Staplesm, L. G., Gandy, M., Fogliati, V. J., Klein, B., & Titov, N. (2015). Clinical and cost-effectiveness of therapist-guided internet-delivered cognitive behavior therapy for older adults with symptoms of anxiety: A randomized controlled trial. *Behavior Therapy, 46*(2), 206–217. https://doi.org/10.1016/j.beth.2014.09.007

Gaudreau, C., Landreville, P., Carmichael, P., Champagne, A., & Camateros, C. (2015). Older adults' rating of the acceptability of treatments for generalized anxiety disorder. *Clinical Gerontologist, 38*(1), 68–87. https://doi.org/10.1080/07317115.2014.970319

Ophuis, R. H., Lokkerbol, J., Heemskerk, S. C. M., van Balkom, A. J. L. M., Hiligsmann, M., & Evers, S. M. A. A. (2017). Cost-effectiveness of interventions for treating anxiety disorders: A systematic review. *Journal of Affective Disorders, 210*, 1–13. https://doi.org/10.1016/j.jad.2016.12.005

Ramos, K., & Stanley, M. A. (2020). Anxiety disorder in late life. *Clinics in Geriatric Medicine, 36*(2), 237–246. https://doi.org/10.1016/j.cger.2019.11.005

Silfvernagel, K., Westlinder, A., Andersson, S., Bergman, R. K., Diaz Hernandez, R., Fallhagen, L., Lundqvist, I., Masri, N., Viberg, L., Forsberg, M. L., Lind, M., Berger, T., Carlbring, P., & Andersson, G. (2018). Individually tailored internet-based cognitive behaviour therapy for older adults with anxiety and depression: A randomised controlled trial. *Cognitive Behaviour Therapy*, 47(4), 286–300. https://doi.org/10.1080/16506073.2017.1388276

Stanley, M. A., Bush, A. L., Camp, M. E., Jameson, J. P., Phillips, L. L., Barber, C. R., Zeno, D., Lomax, J. W., Cully, J. A., & Cully, J. A. (2011). Older adults' preferences for religion/spirituality in treatment for anxiety and depression. *Aging & Mental Health, 15*(3), 334–343. https://doi.org/10.1080/13607863.2010.519326

Whitehead, B. (2018). Religiousness on mental health in older adults: The mediating role of social support and healthy behaviours. *Mental Health, Religion & Culture*, 21(4), 429–441. https://doi.org/10.1080/13674676.2018.1504906

Building Trust

Building trust is especially critical to developing a therapeutic relationship with an anxious client. Being available and attentive to the client's needs contributes to trust. The nurse should not leave an anxious client alone, especially during a new or potentially frightening experience. Abandonment, even briefly, tends to escalate anxiety to more destructive levels.

Restoring Comfort

The nurse's interventions are guided by what will bring relief to a particular person. The nurse should ask the client to suggest methods that may be personally comforting. For example, some clients find it helpful for the nurse to give support in nonverbal ways, such as remaining with them without talking, holding a hand, or stroking the skin. Others prefer to talk about how they feel but are more relaxed if the nurse remains present but physically distant (Fig. 68-1).

Modifying Communication

The nurse should avoid interrupting anxious clients when they talk. Although verbalizing does not always relieve anxiety, it can be beneficial. Talking helps in processing information and exploring methods for dealing with problems. Some clients prefer not to discuss their anxiety and fears with the nurse. In such cases, the nurse respects the client's right to privacy. Offering a referral to a health professional such as a psychiatrist or medical social worker with counseling expertise, however, is appropriate.

Adjusting Teaching

Because an anxious client's attention and concentration are limited, directions or explanations must be simple, brief, and repeated frequently. To determine a client's level of comprehension, asking the person to paraphrase what they have been taught, known as the "repeat back method," is helpful (refer to Chapter 7). The client also benefits from reductions in sensory stimulation such as dimming the lights and eliminating as much noise and interruptions as possible. The nurse must avoid expecting the client to show a great deal of self-reliance or independence until the client feels more relaxed and secure.

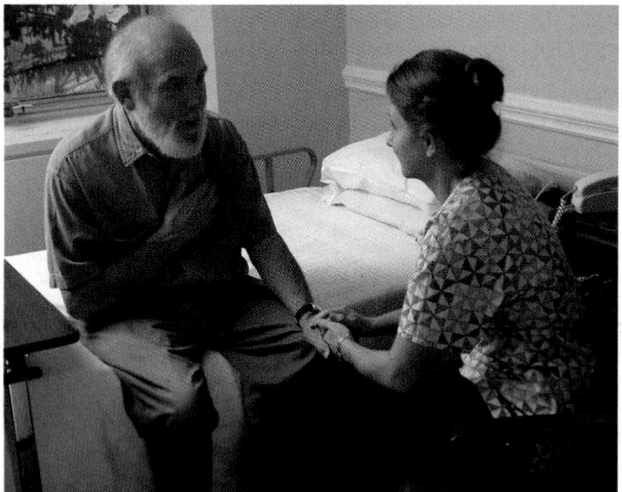

Figure 68-1 A nurse listens to an anxious client. (Reprinted with permission from Eliopoulos C. (2018). *Gerontological nursing* (9th ed.). Wolters Kluwer.)

Helping Problem-Solve

Anxiety impairs problem-solving ability, and clients may look to the nurse for advice in decision-making. Nurses avoid influencing their clients' choices. Instead, they help clients follow a step-by-step **problem-solving process** to formulate decisions:

1. Identifying problems
2. Determining their causes
3. Exploring possible solutions
4. Examining the pros and cons of each option
5. Selecting the choice that is most compatible with personal values

Once the client arrives at a decision, the nurse advocates on the client's behalf for its implementation—even if it is not one the nurse would personally choose. The nurse also respects the client's right to change their mind at any time.

Ensuring Safety

People who are experiencing panic-level anxiety can act impulsively and endanger their safety (e.g., jumping out of a window, running into the street). The nurse remains calm to help such people reduce anxiety to a more manageable level. Having only one nurse interact with the client is usually best, because responding to multiple sources of stimulation adds to a client's agitation. If the client is extremely unstable, it is wise to avoid touching or getting physically close without the client's permission. Intruding in the client's personal space is likely to increase anxiety.

ANXIETY DISORDERS

Anxiety disorders are a group of psychobiologic illnesses that result from activation of the autonomic nervous system, chiefly the sympathetic division. They tend to be chronic and sometimes appear without any logical explanation.

Types of Anxiety Disorders

Some examples of anxiety disorders include GAD, panic disorder, phobic disorders, post-traumatic stress disorder (PTSD), and obsessive-compulsive disorder. Anxiety disorders sometimes lead to other psychobiologic conditions such as depression, substance abuse, and binge eating disorder and compulsive overeating, which are discussed in subsequent chapters.

Generalized Anxiety Disorder

Generalized anxiety disorder is characterized by chronic worrying on a daily basis for 6 or more months. There is usually more than one focus of worry. For example, a person may be worried about finances, job performance, and personal health. Often, the worrying is out of proportion with reality. In addition to worrying, other signs and symptoms of anxiety accompany the client's distress. When the client seeks medical attention, test results fail to reveal physical disorders that produce signs and symptoms similar to

BOX 68-1 Examples of Conditions That Resemble Generalized Anxiety Disorder

- Mitral valve prolapse
- Hypoglycemia
- Hyperthyroidism
- Premenstrual syndrome
- Menopause
- Dementia
- Abuse of psychostimulants (cocaine, caffeine, and weight-loss drugs)
- Sedative (alcohol, opioids, and barbiturates) withdrawal

anxiety (Box 68-1). Many times anxiety can be managed and minimized by implementing various lifestyle changes (Client and Family Teaching 68-1).

Panic Disorder

Panic disorder is the most extreme manifestation of anxiety. People who are affected experience an abrupt onset of physical symptoms and terror that include intense apprehension; tachycardia, palpitations, chest pain, smothering or choking sensations; hyperventilation; lightheadedness; feeling of impending doom; and fear of fainting, dying, losing control, or going insane.

Episodes of panic may last minutes to less than 1 hour and then spontaneously subside. The episodes are often referred to as *attacks* because they interrupt a period during which the client is asymptomatic. The first instinct during a panic attack is to escape to a safer place. The unexplained flight from work, school, or the like that ensues often frightens or strains relationships with others who observe the client's behavior as strange.

The person who experiences a panic attack is often at a loss to identify its cause but associates the location or concurrent activity as the precipitating event. Most affected people cope with their disorder by avoiding situations or places where attacks have occurred. As the attacks recur in a variety of circumstances, however, people with panic disorder often develop agoraphobia. **Agoraphobia** is a fear of experiencing a panic attack in a place where the person may be publicly humiliated by their behavior or help may be unavailable. Consequently, many of those with panic disorder permanently confine themselves to their homes, where they feel safe.

Client and Family Teaching 68-1
Managing Anxiety

The nurse teaches the client and family to:

- understand that anxiety is a normal, universal experience about real-life concerns.
- avoid focusing on negative or worrisome thoughts that are unrealistic.
- repeat positive self-statements to reinforce one's ability to cope.
- share their feelings with supportive others.
- breathe deeply and perform muscle relaxation when feeling overwhelmed.
- limit stimulating substances like caffeine.
- refrain from becoming overwhelmed by eliminating unnecessary activities.
- practice meditation, learn to perform yoga, schedule body massages.
- get sufficient sleep.
- relax by taking a warm bath or listening to soothing music.
- incorporate active exercise on a daily basis.
- devote time to a hobby or past time that interests the client.

Phobic Disorders

Phobic disorders are those conditions in which a person manifests an exaggerated fear. Many people are irrationally afraid of insects, animals, or various life experiences, such as riding on a roller coaster or flying in an airplane, some of which are potentially dangerous. When a person with a phobic disorder is exposed to the phobic stimulus, however, symptoms of anxiety are experienced that may reach severe or panic levels. A person with a phobia often goes to extremes to avoid the object of the phobia or painfully endures the phobic stimulus despite the fact that it causes severe distress. Most people with phobic disorders are aware of how illogical the phobia is and how unrealistic their disabling response has become. However, their conscious awareness is insufficient to terminate the fear.

One common phobic disorder is social phobia. People with **social phobia**, also known as *social anxiety*, fear those situations in which they must perform in front of or may capture the attention of others. Examples of situations that may induce social phobia include speaking publicly, entertaining theatrically or musically, eating with others in a restaurant or at a banquet, attending a party where some guests may be strangers, or being asked to explain a concept in an academic setting. The greatest worry for people with social phobia, which is for the most part imagined, is that they will be embarrassed or criticized for failing to meet acceptable standards.

Post-Traumatic Stress Disorder

PTSD is a condition that involves a delayed anxiety response 3 or more months after an emotionally traumatic experience (Box 68-2). Although traumatic experiences are somewhat relative, they must be extraordinarily severe to cause PTSD. The circumstances of the traumatic event involve actual or threatened death or injury to self or others and produce fear, helplessness, or horror. Some people feel guilty for having survived such an event when others just as deserving of life died.

Initially, the affected person avoids dealing with the tragedy and detaches themselves from others using a technique that is referred to as **psychic numbing**. Eventually, however, the person no longer can stifle the terrifying

BOX 68-2 Traumatic Events Associated With Post-traumatic Stress Disorder

- Witnessing a murder or violent crime
- Watching the torture of a person or animal
- Escaping a fiery crash (car, plane, and train) or industrial explosion
- Seeing military friends or public servants killed in the line of duty
- Being raped or abused
- Surviving a natural disaster such as a flood, earthquake, or tornado
- Being trapped in an automobile, elevator, subway, or underground cave
- Being taken hostage by criminals or terrorists

memories. Months or years later, the memories may resurface in recurrent nightmares or **flashbacks**, in which the person re-experiences the precipitating event. Flashbacks accompanied by violent responses may also occur when the person is exposed to a situation that resembles the original trauma, such as being followed by a person on a street where a previous attack occurred, smelling smoke after having survived a fire, hearing a civil defense warning to take cover after having experienced a tornado, and associating the explosive sound of fireworks with military gunfire.

To suppress symptoms of guilt, grief, anger, or sadness, some clients with PTSD abuse substances such as alcohol or other mind- and mood-altering drugs. When coping strategies prove ineffective, they may become agitated and hostile. They may respond aggressively if startled from sleep, simulating an act of self-preservation. Those who suspect that they may have PTSD should consult a mental health care professional for a definitive diagnosis.

››› *Stop, Think, and Respond 68-2*

Discuss how nurses who care for seriously burned clients or victims of major trauma who often do not survive may develop PTSD.

Obsessive-Compulsive Disorder

Obsessive-compulsive disorder (OCD) is manifested by the performance of an anxiety-relieving ritual (**compulsion**) to terminate a disturbing, persistent, and recurring thought (**obsession**). Obsessions may involve a variety of concerns, like being contaminated with germs or failing to prevent a potential danger like locking a door or turning off the stove. The thoughts are intrusive, and people with OCD cannot dismiss them from their consciousness. To relieve their anxiety, clients with OCD repetitively perform a tension-relieving compulsive act that usually falls into one or more of the following categories:

- Cleaning, such as repetitiously scrubbing the surface of a dining table
- Washing, such as repeated bathing or handwashing
- Checking, such as verifying that doors have been locked or an iron has been unplugged even though the person has already checked
- Counting, such as a bank teller repeatedly making sure that the money in a cash drawer is accurate
- Touching, such as feeling to make sure that a lucky charm is on one's person or having to touch the doorframe before entering a room
- Hoarding, such as persistently accumulating items that are useless or unneeded and being unwilling to discard them
- Repeating, such as saying a phrase or prayer many times over, or counting a sequential set of numbers over and over again

Clients with OCD may feel compelled to perform the same act repeatedly for a specific number of times or in a prescribed sequence. The more the person resists performing the compulsive act, the more the anxiety escalates. The same is true if another person interrupts, alters, or forbids the ritual. Because the rituals are often excessive and time-consuming, they may lead to problems in social relationships, failure in school, or loss of employment. Most clients with OCD recognize that their thoughts and behaviors border on the ridiculous, but they are helpless to stop independently.

Pathophysiology and Etiology

Genetic studies suggest that many anxiety disorders have familial patterns. This finding can imply an inherited faulty physiology, maladaptive learning, or acquisition of personality traits modeled after those displayed by significant others. Disorders are manifested chiefly through structures within the limbic system.

Limbic System

The **limbic system**, a ring of neural structures, is buried within the cerebrum (see Chapter 67). It is made up of portions of the thalamus, hypothalamus, hippocampus, amygdala, and interconnections with other structures such as the cingulate gyrus, fornix, and mamillary bodies (Fig. 68-2).

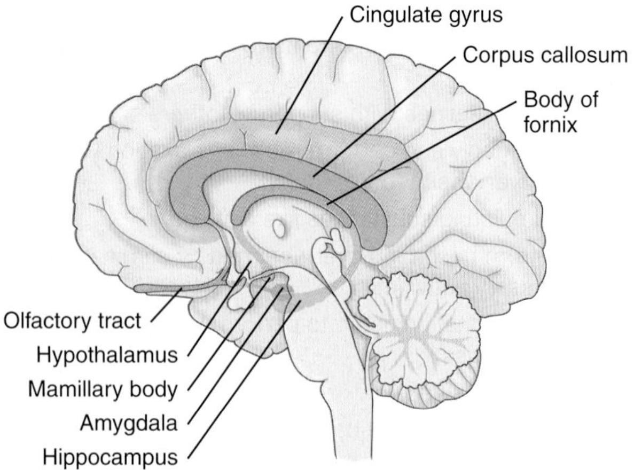

Figure 68-2 The limbic system is a ring of interconnected structures that lies in the center of the brain. Individually and collectively, these structures regulate emotions, store memories, support survival instincts, and cultivate motivation.

The limbic system is a physiologic network for emotions, survival and behavioral responses, motivation, and learning. Responses to stressors are perpetrated through the hypothalamic–pituitary–adrenal (HPA) axis.

Hypothalamic–Pituitary–Adrenal Axis

The psychological sense of danger (a stressor) triggers neuroendocrine changes beginning in the hippocampus and proceeds through neuroendocrine pathways involving the hypothalamus, pituitary, and adrenal glands, known as the **HPA axis** (Fig. 68-3). The HPA axis is designed to help manage stress by inducing a fight-or-flight response orchestrated by the neurotransmitters norepinephrine and epinephrine and the neurohormone cortisol. Impairment within the system can result in an amplified and unrelieved stress response when it interferes with the negative feedback loop that should decrease HPA responses.

Additional Biochemical Mechanisms

Other biochemical mechanisms may also contribute to the development of anxiety disorders. A dysregulation of gamma-aminobutyric acid, a neurotransmitter that should buffer or extinguish the activity of norepinephrine, is one possibility. The second possibility is depletion of serotonin, which would explain why some clients with anxiety disorders develop depression or improve when receiving treatment with antidepressant drugs (see Chapter 69).

Assessment Findings

Signs and Symptoms

Although anxiety causes behavioral, cognitive, and emotional effects, most clients seek treatment for physical signs and symptoms (cardiovascular, respiratory, neuromuscular, gastrointestinal, integumentary problems; Table 68-2). For example, clients may be concerned about palpitations, breathlessness, chronic fatigue, tension headaches, and sleep disturbances. In many clients, BP is elevated, and heart rate is increased. Some clients acknowledge having unrealistic worries or fears or exaggerated startle reactions, experiencing flashbacks of previously traumatic events, avoiding situations that provoke symptoms, or performing ritualistic behaviors.

Diagnostic Findings

Findings from laboratory blood tests and diagnostic tests such as electrocardiography are essentially normal. Positron emission tomography and computed tomography scans have shown abnormal brain use of glucose in clients with anxiety disorders. Magnetic resonance imaging has demonstrated atrophy in some brain areas in selected anxiety disorders.

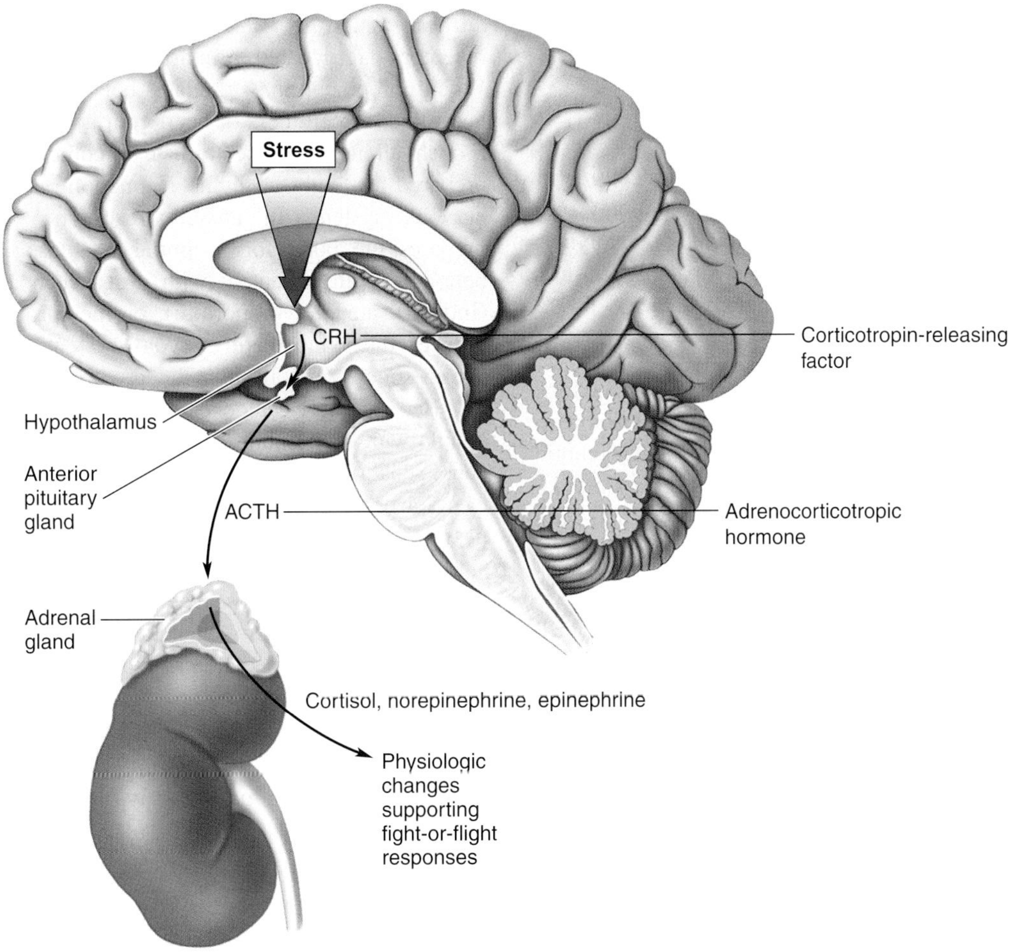

Figure 68-3 The hypothalamic–pituitary–adrenal (HPA) axis is a neuroendocrine pathway that mediates a response to stressors. Dysregulation of the system can result in an unrelieved stress response and stress-related disorders (see Chapter 67).

TABLE 68-2 Common Signs and Symptoms of Anxiety

RESPONSES	SIGNS AND SYMPTOMS
Physical	
Cardiovascular	Hypertension, tachycardia, palpitations, fainting[a]
Respiratory	Dyspnea, rapid breathing, hyperventilation, choking sensation, tightness in the chest
Neuromuscular	Tremors, restlessness, insomnia, muscle tension, excessive sleep,[a] generalized weakness, dizziness
Gastrointestinal	Anorexia, nausea, diarrhea,[a] constipation, feeling of fullness
Urinary	Frequency and urgency of urination[a]
Integumentary	Diaphoresis, sweaty palms, pallor, blushing,[a] dry mouth
Behavioral	Crying, rapid speech or mutism, hypervigilance, being easily startled or accident-prone, social isolation, physical escape, avoidance, loss of interest in sexual activity, pacing, fidgeting, nail biting, picking at skin, seeking comfort in food or alcohol, absenteeism, failure to complete or poor performance of tasks
Cognitive	Forgetfulness, poor judgment, lack of motivation, confusion, nightmares, intrusive thoughts, preoccupation, decreased attention and concentration, inability to recall information
Emotional	Unrealistic fears, mood swings, easily angered, impatient, intolerant, nervous

[a]Indicates a parasympathetic rather than a sympathetic nervous system response.

Diagnosis of most clients with anxiety disorders, however, is based on symptomatology and history.

Medical Management

The medical management of anxiety disorders includes drug therapy combined with cognitive and behavioral psychotherapy. Drug therapy relieves the symptoms associated with anxiety, but it does not eliminate causative factors. Once drug therapy is implemented, however, clients are more capable of dealing with issues affecting their daily lives.

Drug Therapy

Drugs that (1) reduce or block levels of norepinephrine or (2) normalize levels of serotonin are most commonly prescribed for anxiety disorders. They include anxiolytics, beta-adrenergic blockers, central-acting sympatholytics, and, occasionally, antidepressants (Drug Therapy Table 68-1).

Anxiolytics

Anxiolytics are drugs that relieve the symptoms of anxiety. Sometimes they are referred to as *minor tranquilizers* to differentiate them from major tranquilizers or antipsychotic drugs used to treat thought disorders such as schizophrenia. Anxiolytics include benzodiazepines such as alprazolam (Xanax), lorazepam (Ativan), diazepam (Valium), and oxazepam (Serax), and nonbenzodiazepine drugs such as buspirone (Buspar).

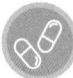

Pharmacologic Considerations

■ Concern for benzodiazepine addiction makes selective serotonin reuptake inhibitor (SSRI) and serotonin/norepinephrine reuptake inhibitor (SNRI) antidepressants the first-line treatment of general anxiety disorder (GAD). In short-term situations, benzodiazepines may be used to reduce anxiety because withdrawal symptoms are more likely to occur when the drug has been taken for 3 months or more and is suddenly discontinued. All antianxiety drugs should always be tapered off, never discontinued abruptly.

››› *Stop, Think, and Respond 68-3*

What health teaching is appropriate when a client begins taking an anxiolytic drug?

Beta-Adrenergic Blockers

Receptors for norepinephrine are referred to as *alpha-adrenergic* and *beta-adrenergic receptors*. Beta-adrenergic receptors are located primarily in the heart and lungs. When norepinephrine stimulates beta-adrenergic receptors, heart rate, forcefulness of heart contraction, and dilation of bronchi all increase. The ultimate outcome is that the body is prepared for "fight-or-flight," a function of the sympathetic nervous system. In anxiety disorders, norepinephrine prepares the body for a similar response. Blocking the beta-adrenergic receptors with drugs such as propranolol (Inderal), atenolol (Tenormin), or metoprolol (Lopressor) reduces the sympathetic nervous system stimulation that causes some symptoms associated with anxiety.

Beta-adrenergic blockers are frequently prescribed for people with social phobia. This category of drugs does not cause sedation, tolerance, or addiction. These drugs do, however, lower BP and subsequently can cause episodes of dizziness or fainting when the client rises quickly from a lying or sitting position. Other major side effects include bradycardia and elevated blood glucose level. Those taking a nonselective beta-adrenergic blocker—one that interferes with bronchodilation—may experience fatigue, dyspnea, and wheezing.

››› *Stop, Think, and Respond 68-4*

Beta-adrenergic blockers should be cautiously prescribed or avoided for clients with which kinds of concurrent medical conditions?

Central-Acting Sympatholytics

Central-acting sympatholytics block alpha-2 receptors for norepinephrine in the brain stem. Consequently, they reduce heart rate and BP. Examples of drugs in this category

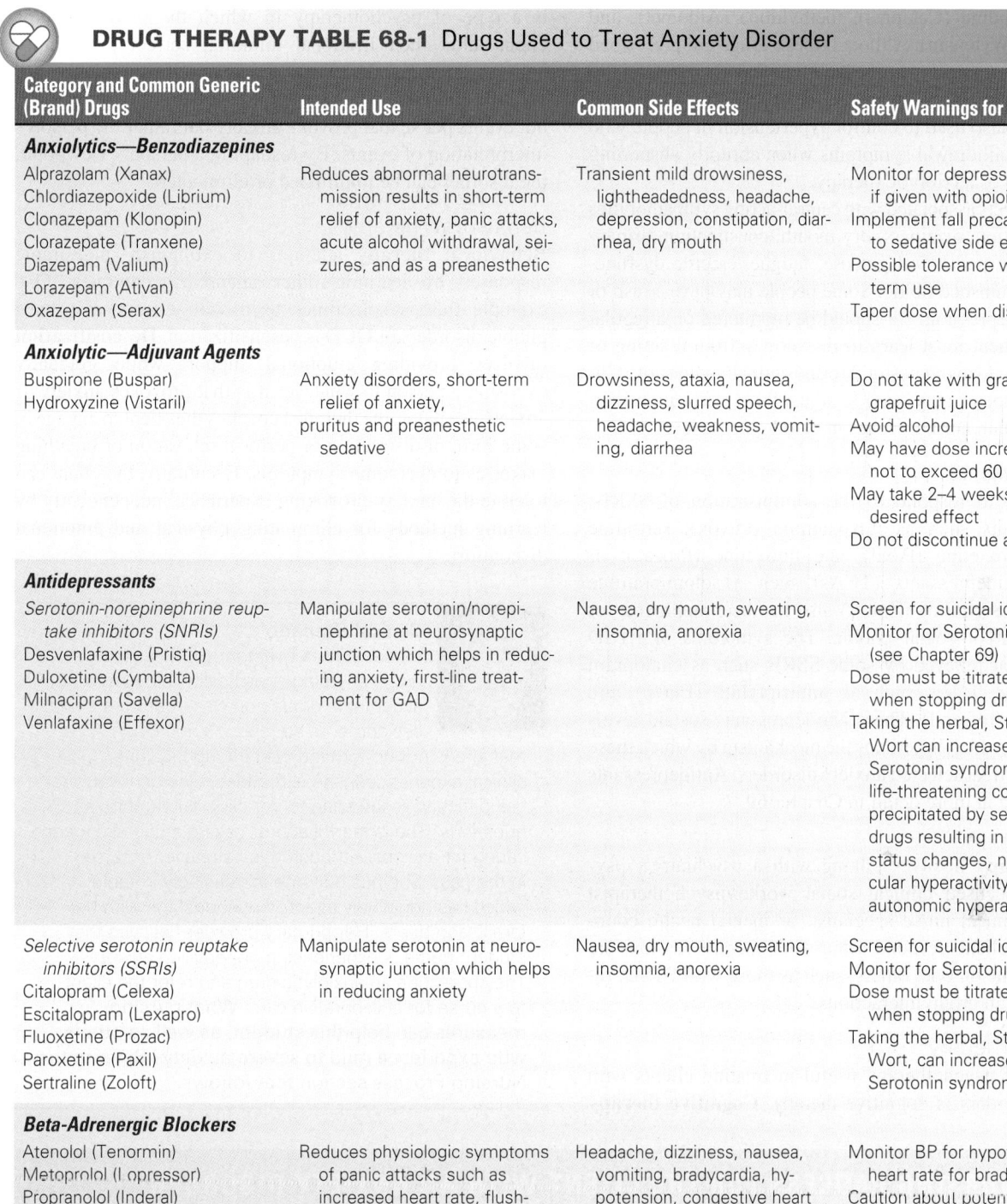

DRUG THERAPY TABLE 68-1 Drugs Used to Treat Anxiety Disorder

Category and Common Generic (Brand) Drugs	Intended Use	Common Side Effects	Safety Warnings for Nurses
Anxiolytics—Benzodiazepines			
Alprazolam (Xanax) Chlordiazepoxide (Librium) Clonazepam (Klonopin) Clorazepate (Tranxene) Diazepam (Valium) Lorazepam (Ativan) Oxazepam (Serax)	Reduces abnormal neurotransmission results in short-term relief of anxiety, panic attacks, acute alcohol withdrawal, seizures, and as a preanesthetic	Transient mild drowsiness, lightheadedness, headache, depression, constipation, diarrhea, dry mouth	Monitor for depressed breathing if given with opioid Implement fall precautions due to sedative side effects Possible tolerance with long-term use Taper dose when discontinuing
Anxiolytic—Adjuvant Agents			
Buspirone (Buspar) Hydroxyzine (Vistaril)	Anxiety disorders, short-term relief of anxiety, pruritus and preanesthetic sedative	Drowsiness, ataxia, nausea, dizziness, slurred speech, headache, weakness, vomiting, diarrhea	Do not take with grapefruit or grapefruit juice Avoid alcohol May have dose increased, but not to exceed 60 mg/day May take 2–4 weeks to obtain desired effect Do not discontinue abruptly
Antidepressants			
Serotonin-norepinephrine reuptake inhibitors (SNRIs) Desvenlafaxine (Pristiq) Duloxetine (Cymbalta) Milnacipran (Savella) Venlafaxine (Effexor)	Manipulate serotonin/norepinephrine at neurosynaptic junction which helps in reducing anxiety, first-line treatment for GAD	Nausea, dry mouth, sweating, insomnia, anorexia	Screen for suicidal ideation Monitor for Serotonin syndrome (see Chapter 69) Dose must be titrated down when stopping drug Taking the herbal, St. John's Wort can increase risk of Serotonin syndrome, a life-threatening consequence precipitated by serotonergic drugs resulting in mental-status changes, neuromuscular hyperactivity, and autonomic hyperactivity
Selective serotonin reuptake inhibitors (SSRIs) Citalopram (Celexa) Escitalopram (Lexapro) Fluoxetine (Prozac) Paroxetine (Paxil) Sertraline (Zoloft)	Manipulate serotonin at neurosynaptic junction which helps in reducing anxiety	Nausea, dry mouth, sweating, insomnia, anorexia	Screen for suicidal ideation Monitor for Serotonin syndrome Dose must be titrated down when stopping drug Taking the herbal, St. John's Wort, can increase risk of Serotonin syndrome
Beta-Adrenergic Blockers			
Atenolol (Tenormin) Metoprolol (Lopressor) Propranolol (Inderal)	Reduces physiologic symptoms of panic attacks such as increased heart rate, flushing, trembling, and profuse sweating	Headache, dizziness, nausea, vomiting, bradycardia, hypotension, congestive heart failure, arrhythmias, erectile dysfunction, increased blood sugar, decreased activity tolerance	Monitor BP for hypotension and heart rate for bradycardia Caution about potential for falls due to hypotensive effects Assess blood cell count initially and every 2–3 weeks for agranulocytosis Nonselective beta-adrenergic blockers can increase the potential for asthma attacks Warn clients with diabetes that these drugs may interfere with control of blood sugar levels

The drugs in column 1 indicate the drug that matches up with explanations in columns 2 through 4.

include clonidine (Catapres), methyldopa (Aldomet), and guanabenz (Wytensin). Although these drugs are prescribed more often to control primary hypertension, they potentially have beneficial effects in anxious people with elevated BP. Clonidine is also used to control hypertension in people who experience withdrawal symptoms when abruptly abstaining from alcohol or anxiolytic therapy.

Side effects associated with central-acting sympatholytics include sedation, dizziness, dry mouth, constipation, urinary retention, elevated blood glucose, fatigue, erectile dysfunction, and diminished libido. Some people may have a rash or experience depression. BP should be monitored on a regular basis. The client must learn to rise slowly from a sitting or lying position to avoid postural (orthostatic) hypotension. Clients with diabetes may need to adjust their medication regimen to maintain normal ranges in blood glucose level.

Antidepressants

OCD seems to respond to the administration of SSRIs; antidepressants such as fluvoxamine (Luvox), sertraline (Zoloft), paroxetine (Paxil), and fluoxetine (Prozac); or tricyclic antidepressants (TCAs) such as clomipramine (Anafranil). Sertraline (Zoloft) also has been approved for the treatment of social phobia. The symptoms of PTSD are somewhat relieved by some SSRIs such as citalopram (Celexa) and TCAs such as amitriptyline (Elavil) and imipramine (Tofranil). These antidepressants sustain levels of serotonin, which is perhaps the mechanism by which these medications treat selected anxiety disorders. Antidepressants are discussed in more detail in Chapter 69.

Psychotherapy

Psychotherapy involves talking with a psychiatrist, psychologist, licensed clinical social worker/psychotherapist (LCSW), clinical nurse specialist, or mental health counselor. Some clients respond better when therapy sessions are conducted one on one; others, such as those with PTSD, respond better in group interactions.

Cognitive Therapy

One type of psychotherapy useful in treating clients with anxiety disorders is cognitive therapy. **Cognitive therapy** is a type of psychotherapy in which the therapist helps clients alter their irrational thinking, correct their faulty belief systems, and replace negative self-statements with positive ones. This therapy is based on the theory that it is not events per se that provoke anxiety but rather the person's interpretation of events. By reshaping a person's viewpoint, the disorder can be minimized or eliminated.

Behavioral Therapy

Behavioral therapy attempts to extinguish undesirable responses by learning other adaptive techniques. One example that is sometimes used with clients who have phobic disorders or OCD is desensitization. **Desensitization** involves providing emotional support while gradually exposing a person to whatever it is that provokes anxiety. If anxiety escalates, the therapist coaches the client to engage in some form of distraction or perform relaxation or breathing exercises to overcome symptoms. Eventually, the client can tolerate the anxiety-provoking experience independently by learning methods for eliminating physical and emotional discomfort.

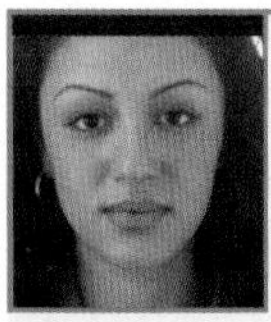

Clinical Scenario A 20-year-old student nurse worries constantly but cannot name anything specifically. She is making acceptable grades on classroom tests and assignments but spends hours agonizing that she is not performing well enough. During clinical experiences, she is restless, disorganized, and has difficulty responding to her clinical instructor's questions. She is fearful about making a mistake when caring for a client, although this has never occurred in the past. She has become increasingly irritable, which has negatively affected relationships with her family and peers. Her primary provider believes the student nurse is experiencing generalized anxiety. They prescribe an anxiolytic drug and refer the client to a nurse for collaborative care. **What nursing measures can help this student, as well as others, who experience mild to severe anxiety? Refer to the Nursing Process section that follows.**

NURSING PROCESS FOR THE CLIENT WITH AN ANXIETY DISORDER

Assessment

Observe for evidence of various levels of anxiety: pacing, talking excessively, complaining, crying, being withdrawn, or trying to run away. Ask the client to express anxiety with open-ended questions such as, "How are you feeling now?" It is helpful to have the client rate their anxiety level using a scale from 0 to 10. Determine the level at which the client feels that anxiety is tolerable. Inquire if the client has an effective method for controlling anxiety and document the response. Observe the client's mood for signs of concurrent depression and explore the client's use of and knowledge about medications to treat the disorder. Obtain a complete current medication history, including nonprescription drugs. Many people who experience anxiety take over-the-counter drugs, herbal remedies, stimulants, and tranquilizers that they may not mention unless asked. Nutrition Notes lists assessment considerations related to a client's diet.

Diagnosis, Planning, and Interventions

Acute/Chronic Anxiety: Related to unrealistic perceptions concerning personal performance
Expected Outcome: The client's anxiety will return to a tolerable level.

NURSING PROCESS FOR THE CLIENT WITH AN ANXIETY DISORDER (continued)

- Reduce as many external stimuli, such as noise, bright lights, and activity, as possible. *Numerous stimuli escalate anxiety because they interfere with attention and concentration. Dealing simultaneously with multiple stimuli can tax the client's energy.*
- Maintain a calm manner when interacting with the client. *Anxiety is communicated; an anxious nurse can increase anxiety in a client. Modeling a controlled state promotes a similar response in the client.*
- Take a position at least an arm's length away from the client. *Invading an anxious client's personal space may increase their discomfort.*
- Avoid touching the client without first asking permission. *An anxious client may misinterpret unexpected touching as a threatening gesture.*
- Establish trust by being available to the client and keeping promises. *Insecurity can be relieved if the client can depend on someone for support and assistance.*
- Advise the client to seek out the nurse or another supportive person when feeling the effects of anxiety. *The earlier that anxiety is deescalated, the sooner the client will experience relief of symptoms.*
- Stay with the client during periods of severe anxiety. *The nurse's presence can help the client stay in control or restore control to a more comfortable level.*
- Follow a consistent schedule for routine activities. *Unpredictability heightens anxiety; consistency helps a client manage time and cope with personal demands.*
- Encourage the client to identify what they perceive to be a threat to emotional equilibrium. *Processing situations verbally may give the client perspective on perceived threats so that they are more realistic and less exaggerated.*
- Use a soft voice, short sentences, and clear messages when exchanging information. *Anxious clients have a short attention span and reduced ability to concentrate; they may be unable to follow lengthy or complicated information.*
- Provide specific, succinct directions for tasks the client should complete or assist the client who becomes agitated. *Anxious clients have difficulty following instructions and performing tasks in correct sequence. Assistance relieves unnecessary distress.*
- Instruct and help the client with moderate or severe anxiety to perform one or more of the following until anxiety is within a tolerable level:
  - Count slowly backward from 100. *Distraction redirects the client's attention from distressing physiologic symptoms to the task at hand.*
  - Breathe slowly and deeply in through the nose and out through the mouth. *Slowing respirations aborts hyperventilation and subsequent potential for fainting, peripheral tingling, and numbness from respiratory alkalosis.*
  - Offer a warm bath or back rub. *Warm running water promotes relaxation; massage relaxes muscles and possibly releases endorphins, natural chemicals that promote a sense of well-being.*
  - Progressively relax groups of muscles from the toes to the head. *Consciously relaxing muscles relieves tension and fatigue.*
  - Repeat positive statements such as "I am in control," "I am safe," "I am relaxed," and "I am competent." *Positive self-talk can be transformed into reality.*
  - Visualize a pleasant, relaxing place. *Imagery can transform a person's aroused state to one that is more relaxed.*
  - Listen to a relaxation tape or soothing music. *Distraction helps to refocus attention to less anxiety-provoking stimuli.*
  - Engage in a large-muscle activity such as riding an exercise bicycle or going for a brisk walk. *Activity uses norepinephrine and can reduce it to a more manageable amount.*
- Administer antianxiety medication that has been prescribed on a prn basis if nonpharmacologic approaches are ineffective. *Medication maybe necessary to ensure the client's or others' safety if there is a potential for loss of control or violent acting out.*

Altered Health Maintenance: Related to knowledge deficit of drug and dietary modifications
Expected Outcome: The client will safely manage self-care.

- Explain the routine for self-administering prescribed medications and side effects associated with prescribed drugs. *Identifying the frequency and approximate time during the day when medications should be taken ensures safe self-care. Knowing what to expect as side effects reduces the potential for nonadherence to the medication regimen or harm.*
- Emphasize that the client must avoid alcohol and other sedating drugs when taking anxiolytic drugs. *Combining two drugs that cause sedation may have dangerous consequences.*
- Encourage adherence to drug therapy, although it may take several weeks for the client to feel a beneficial effect. *Making the client aware that symptoms will not disappear immediately may create motivation for continuing to adhere to drug therapy.*
- Advise the client to first discuss discontinuing drug therapy for whatever reason with the prescribing primary provider. *Abrupt discontinuation of benzodiazepines can cause withdrawal symptoms that mimic anxiety.*
- Tell the client to avoid caffeine, nicotine, or stimulating drugs such as nonprescription diet pills and cold and allergy medications. *These drugs contain chemicals that stimulate the sympathetic nervous system, which interferes with the desired effect of anxiolytic drug therapy.*
- Inform the client of the process for arranging follow-up appointments with their primary provider. *The client needs periodic contact with the treating primary provider for further assessment, evaluation of treatment outcomes, or adjustment of the therapeutic regimen.*
- Provide information on self-help groups for anxiety. *Interacting with others who share similar problems can help clients cope.*

(continued)

NURSING PROCESS FOR THE CLIENT WITH AN ANXIETY DISORDER (continued)

Evaluation of Expected Outcomes

After successful nursing interventions, the client deals with anxiety-provoking stimuli realistically and implements measures to decrease anxiety. The client has extended periods during which anxiety is at a tolerable level and participates in normal activities without becoming incapacitated by anxiety.

The client accurately repeats information on all of the following issues: dose, frequency, potential side effects, duration of drug therapy, possible consequences if an anxiolytic drug is discontinued abruptly, and drugs, foods, and beverages that are contraindicated when taking anxiolytic medication. Finally, the client has written instructions for follow-up care and is aware of community-based groups that may help in the management of an anxiety disorder.

Nutrition Notes

The Client With an Anxiety Disorder

- Clients with anxiety should avoid caffeine because it contributes to and potentiates the physiologic stimulation experienced with anxiety.
- Although some clients with anxiety lose their appetite, others may react to stress by overeating. Therefore, it is important to regularly assess the client's current weight and monitor weight fluctuations over time.

KEY POINTS

- Differentiate anxiety from fear.
- Anxiety is a vague, uneasy feeling, the cause of which is not readily identifiable. It is evoked when a person anticipates nonspecific danger.
- Fear is a feeling of terror in response to someone or something specific that a person perceives as dangerous or threatening.
- Four levels of anxiety
  - Mild: attention is heightened, Sensory perception is expanded, Focus is on stimuli. Reality is intact. Information processing is accurate. Person feels in control. Muscle tone increases. Heart rate, BP, and breathing slightly increase. Perspiration is noticeable.
  - Moderate: person is more easily distracted, Concentration is slightly impaired. Person can redirect attention. Learning takes more effort. Perception narrows. Problem solving becomes difficult. Person is irritable and feels inadequate. Muscles are tense. Slight leg or hand tremors may occur. Rate, pitch, and volume of speech change. Respiratory depth and vital signs increase. Sleep is disturbed.
  - Severe: attention span decreases. Person cannot concentrate or remain focused. Perception is reduced. Ability to learn is impaired. Information processing is inaccurate or incomplete. Person is aware of extreme discomfort. Effort is needed to control emotions. Person feels incompetent. Symptoms include hyperventilation, dizziness, tachycardia, heart palpitations, and hypertension. Fine motor movement is impaired. Communication is limited.
  - Panic: person exaggerates details. Perception is distorted. Learning is disabled. Thoughts are fragmented. Speech is incoherent. Movements are haphazard, usually in an effort to escape. Symptoms include dyspnea, fainting, tremors, and diaphoresis.
- Six areas of nursing management of anxious clients
  - Building trust
  - Restoring comfort
  - Modifying communication
  - Adjusting teaching
  - Ensuring safety
  - Helping problem-solve
- Examples of anxiety disorders
  - Generalized anxiety disorder
  - Panic disorder
  - Phobic disorders
  - PTSD
  - Obsessive-compulsive disorder
- Drugs categories to treat anxiety disorders
  - Anxiolytics: benzodiazepines
  - Anxiolytic: adjuvant agents
  - Antidepressants
  - Beta-adrenergic blockers
- Types of psychotherapy used to treat anxiety disorders
  - Psychotherapy
  - Cognitive therapy
  - Behavioral therapy

CRITICAL THINKING EXERCISES

1. Discuss nursing interventions that would be appropriate when a client tells you that they feel anxious about upcoming surgery.
2. What interventions should a nurse implement if a client suddenly experiences a panic attack?
3. What suggestions from a nurse could help reduce anxiety in older adults?
4. What health teaching should the nurse provide to a client who has been prescribed a benzodiazepine for managing symptoms of anxiety?

NCLEX-STYLE REVIEW QUESTIONS PrepU

1. A client who has been experiencing chest pain is scheduled to undergo a cardiac catheterization and coronary arteriogram. What nursing action is best for reducing the client's anxiety initially?
1. Teach the client how coronary artery disease is usually treated.
2. Listen to the client express their feelings about cardiac disease.
3. Explain to the client how well other people have handled these tests.
4. Discuss the cardiac catheterization procedure with the client.

2. When caring for a client with panic level of anxiety, what is the most important nursing action?
1. Remain with the client indefinitely.
2. Relocate the client to a visitors' room.
3. Offer the client a cup of coffee or tea.
4. Notify the client's attending primary provider.

3. What nursing assessments provide supporting evidence that a client is experiencing anxiety? Select all that apply.
1. Restlessness
2. Insomnia
3. Increased salivation
4. Persistent headache
5. Overreaction to criticism
6. Difficulty concentrating

4. What is the best reason a nurse can give a client who receives a prescription for a benzodiazepine to use caution when driving or performing tasks requiring mental alertness?
1. Benzodiazepines may cause confusion.
2. Benzodiazepines may cause behavior changes.
3. Benzodiazepines may cause sleep disorders.
4. Benzodiazepines may cause drowsiness.

5. What suggestions are appropriate for helping clients reduce or eliminate transient episodes of anxiety? Select all that apply.
1. Exercise actively each day.
2. Consult a mental health specialist.
3. Limit unnecessary activities.
4. Take a sedative drug as needed.
5. Practice meditation.
6. Develop a hobby.

WANT TO KNOW MORE? There are a wide variety of online resources available on thePoint to enhance learning and understanding of this chapter.

Go to **thePoint.lww.com/activate** and use the activation code found in the front of this text to unlock these online resources.

69

Caring for Clients With Mood Disorders

Words To Know

affect
bipolar disorder
cyclothymia
deep brain stimulation
delusions
dexamethasone (cortisol) suppression test
dopamine
dysthymia
electroconvulsive therapy
euthymic
gamma-aminobutyric acid
hallucinations
hypertensive crisis
major (unipolar) depression
mania
melatonin
monoamine oxidase
monoamine hypothesis
mood
mood disorders
norepinephrine
photoperiods
phototherapy
psychomotor agitation
psychomotor retardation
psychotherapy
psychotic depression
reactive (secondary) depression
reuptake
seasonal affective disorder
serotonin
serotonin syndrome
transcranial magnetic stimulation
vagus nerve stimulation

Learning Objectives

On completion of this chapter, you will be able to:

1. Discuss common signs and symptoms of mood disorders.
2. Name three neurotransmitters that, when imbalanced, affect mood.
3. Identify the types of drugs that are used to treat mood disorders and nursing considerations related to their administration.
4. Discuss the causes, manifestations, and management of serotonin syndrome.
5. Identify the reasons electroconvulsive therapy is used in the management of depression.
6. Name three interventions that are alternatives to electroconvulsive therapy for recurrent depression.
7. Give three criteria that indicate a high risk for suicide.
8. Discuss nursing measures that are useful in preventing suicide.
9. Discuss the nursing management of clients with depression.
10. Describe seasonal affective disorder, its treatment, and nursing management.
11. Explain bipolar disorder and describe its treatment and nursing management.

The term **mood** refers to a person's overall feeling state. Mood is displayed in a person's **affect**, the verbal and nonverbal behavior that communicates feelings (Box 69-1). This chapter discusses a variety of mood disorders, their management, and their nursing care.

BOX 69-1 Examples of Mood and Affect

MOOD	AFFECT
Happy	Smiling Briskly walking Paying attention to appearance Showing a positive attitude Being cooperative, creative, and gregarious
Depressed	Looking gloomy Being inactive Neglecting appearance Feeling empty Showing no initiative Being insensitive to others' feelings or isolated

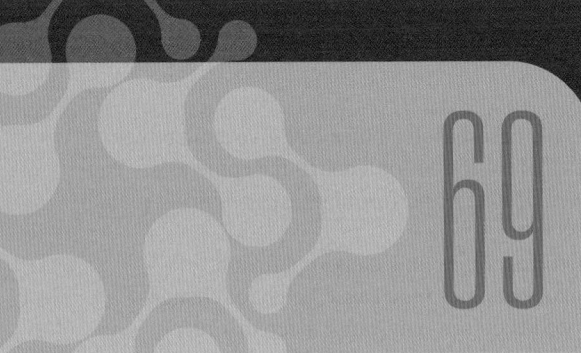

Gerontologic Considerations

- Impaired regulation of neurotransmitters in older adults suggests biologic predisposition to depression and thought disorders.
- Alterations in hormone production (i.e., adrenal, pituitary, thyroid) that occur with vascular changes of aging may affect the feedback loop (refer to Chapter 49) for other hormone production and may therefore contribute to emotional disequilibrium.
- Cognitive impairment in the depressed older adult can be easily confused with dementia (i.e., pseudodementia). Careful assessment is necessary to distinguish between the two because depression can usually be treated successfully in older adults.
- Older adults may be reluctant to admit depressive feelings if they view depression as a character weakness rather than a chemical imbalance.
- Older adults who seek treatment for subacute physical symptoms, such as loss of appetite, trouble sleeping, lack of energy, and weight loss, may actually be depressed.
- Attempts at self-medicating with alcohol or herbal preparations should also be assessed.
- Alterations in drug absorption, metabolism, distribution, and excretion that may occur with aging necessitate careful individual assessment and monitoring of older adults' response to all classifications of antidepressants.
- Risk of orthostatic hypotension from psychotropic drugs is increased in older adults because of decreased functioning of the BP-regulating mechanism.
- Older adults may require longer administration (up to 8 weeks) than do other clients to obtain a therapeutic effect when taking antidepressants.
- Antidepressants must be used cautiously in older adults with cardiovascular disease because of the risk for tachyarrhythmias. Older men with prostatic enlargement are more susceptible to urinary retention, a side effect of some antidepressants.
- The rate of suicide is extremely high in older adults. Older adults who are depressed often use a highly lethal method to ensure successful suicide. Losses such as death of family/friends or relocation, physical and emotional changes of aging, and lack of control over chronic or terminal illness may trigger feelings of hopelessness, which increase the risk of suicide.
- Behaviors such as putting personal affairs in order, giving away possessions, and making funeral plans are a sign of good judgment in older adults and do not necessarily convey suicidal ideation. Other indicators such as unsatisfactory relationships, poor or failing health, divorce, losing one's spouse or partner, or addiction may be stronger indicators of suicide in older adults.
- As people with bipolar disorder age, depressive episodes may increase in frequency and last longer. Potential for increased functional decline necessitates planning for supportive care, including caregiver support, or relocation to a long-term care setting.
- Older adults taking lithium for bipolar disorder require careful monitoring of lithium levels. The kidneys eliminate lithium, and age-related changes may reduce renal clearance, predisposing older clients to lithium toxicity. Clients who limit their intake of salt or who take prescribed diuretics that promote salt excretion are at risk for lithium toxicity. Because the body desires a consistent number of cations, when serum levels of sodium, a cation, are decreased, the kidney will reabsorb lithium, a similar cation, to maintain electrolyte balance. The reabsorption of lithium can lead to excess blood levels of lithium.

THE MOOD CONTINUUM AND MOOD DISORDERS

Mood may be thought of as a continuum, with extremes of emotion existing at both ends or poles (Fig. 69-1). People with normal moods are referred to as **euthymic**; they are capable of experiencing a variety of feelings, all of which are situationally appropriate. **Dysthymia**, a feeling of unremitting sadness, is similar to but less severe than major depression, which is discussed later. **Cyclothymia**, alternating sad and elated moods, resembles bipolar disorder, but the extremes of mood are less pronounced. **Mania** refers to the frenzied state of euphoria exhibited by persons during the manic phase of bipolar disorder, which is defined and discussed later.

People who have what psychologists and psychiatrists call **mood disorders** experience an extreme persistent mood or severe mood swings that interfere with social relationships. The primary mood disturbances include major (unipolar) depression and bipolar disorder, formerly called *manic-depressive syndrome*. In **psychotic depression**, an extreme form of depressive disorder, some individuals experience **hallucinations**, sensory phenomena such as hearing voices or seeing images that do not objectively exist, and **delusions**, fixed false beliefs that often are persecutory or guilt-ridden in nature. **Seasonal affective disorder** (SAD) is a mood disorder characterized by depression that develops during darker winter months and then disappears in the spring.

MAJOR DEPRESSION

Everyone experiences depression at some point. In most cases, transient depression is a normal reaction to loss, such as the death of a loved one; disappointment, such as being fired from a job; or overwhelming events, such as being heavily in debt. A sad feeling that can be directly attributed to a situation or cause is referred to as **reactive (secondary) depression**. Usually, reactive depression is self-limiting; when circumstances change or when supportive others provide help, depression is relieved. Nevertheless, many people experience **major (unipolar) depression**, a sad mood with no obvious relationship to situational events. Millions of Americans report feeling depressed; however, the actual incidence of major depression in adults is believed to be approximately 17.3 million (Substance Abuse and Mental Health Services Administration, 2017 Depression is also a comorbid [coexisting] condition among people with anxiety disorders and substance use disorders (see Chapters 68 and 71).

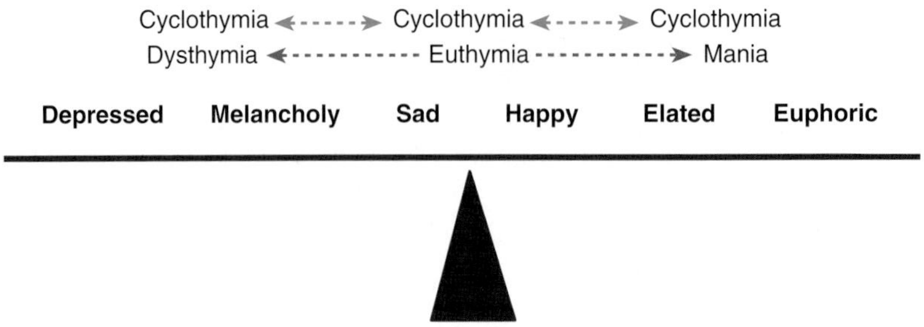

Figure 69-1 Mood continuum.

Pathophysiology and Etiology

Brain function, and consequently mood, depends on the dynamic interplay of neurotransmitters (see Chapter 67). Moods are most likely generated by the limbic system, which is the center for emotions (see Chapter 68). Several possible explanations exist for the causes and mechanisms that trigger major depressive symptoms. The most solid evidence at present suggests that mood disorders are related to genetics, dysregulation of neurotransmitters, and neuroendocrine imbalance. Psychological and social theories suggest that infantile rejection or neglect, learned feelings of helplessness, chronic exposure to discrimination, bullying, or distorted or false perceptions about oneself contribute to depression. Although these latter factors should not be dismissed, research in brain chemistry gives more support to biologic explanations.

Genetics

Mood disorders tend to be prevalent among close blood relatives, which suggests a genetic link. Even when raised separately, an identical twin has a higher incidence of depressive episodes when the other is affected (Howard et al., 2018; Cai et al., 2018; Hampton, 2018; Ledford, 2015; Levinson & Nichols, n.d.). Researchers are studying the DNA of fairly homogeneous groups (e.g., the Amish) for variations in chromosome patterns in relatives who have mood disorders and those who do not. Kohli and colleagues (2011) studied the *genome*, the complete set of genes in an organism—in this case, depressed and nondepressed humans—and found a genetic difference between the two in the area of the hippocampus, a major structure in the limbic system. A genetic etiology is further supported by others who have detected similar dysregulation in the brains of individuals experiencing major depression that does not occur in others (Shadrina; Bondarenko & Slominsky, 2018; Verbeek et al., 2014; O'Dushlaine, 2011).

››› *Stop, Think, and Respond 69-1*

Besides genetics, what other reason might explain why people who are related manifest similar disturbances in mood?

Neurotransmitter Dysregulation

The most widely accepted psychobiologic theory for depression is the **monoamine hypothesis**, which proposes that depression results from imbalances in one or more of the monoamine neurotransmitters: serotonin, norepinephrine, and dopamine. The hypothesis is based on the fact that levels of a metabolite of **serotonin**, 5-hydroxyindoleacetic acid (5-HIAA), measured in cerebrospinal fluid, are lower in people with depression than in samples taken from people who are euthymic. Second, **norepinephrine** levels may be low or high among people affected by depression. Low levels of norepinephrine help explain why some people with depression develop **psychomotor retardation**, which is characterized by a lack of energy, increased sleep, and little interest in daily events or responsibilities. On the other hand, some people with depression may have excessive norepinephrine. They are more likely to experience **psychomotor agitation** with such stimulating manifestations as insomnia, pacing, and distractibility, rather than lethargy. Third, the symptoms of some clients who are depressed suggest an excess of **dopamine**, which is associated with distortion of thoughts. In moderate-to-severe depression, this may be evidenced as overreactive guilt, self-blame, self-pity, and low self-worth. Low levels of dopamine as evidenced by reduced cerebrospinal levels of homovanillic acid (HVA), a metabolite of dopamine, on the other hand, are associated with a reduction of pleasure, impaired motivation, and difficulty in concentration, which often accompanies depressive symptomatology (Radwan, Liu, & Chaudhury, 2018; Robinson, 2007). Refer to Nutrition Notes for dietary considerations.

Neuroendocrine Imbalance

Interactions of the pituitary, adrenal cortex, thyroid gland, and ovaries also may play a role in producing depression by altering levels of hormones. These endocrine glands are stimulated and suppressed through the hypothalamus, another structure in the limbic system. Abnormal levels of cortisol, a hormone produced by the adrenal cortex, and variations in thyroid hormones are accompanied by changes in mood and motor activity. The hypothalamus also influences the pituitary gland's stimulation of adrenal steroids and reproductive hormones. This may help to explain the altered mood states associated with excessive aggression and rage attributed to testosterone, irritability in those with premenstrual syndrome, late luteal phase dysphoric disorder (see Chapter 53), menopause, and postpartum depression.

Nutrition Notes

The Client With Depression

- Carbohydrates from any source, such as cereals, pasta, fruit, and sugar, stimulate a temporary increase in serotonin production by increasing the amount of tryptophan in the brain; tryptophan is the amino acid precursor of serotonin.
- The results can range from a mild feeling of calmness after eating a carbohydrate snack to drowsiness after eating a large carbohydrate-rich meal.

BOX 69-3 Conditions That Mimic Depression

- Hypothyroidism
- Brain tumor
- Alcohol or sedative abuse
- Stimulant withdrawal
- Chronic hypoxia
- Side effects of drug therapy such as corticosteroids, antihypertensives such as reserpine (Serpasil), methyldopa (Aldomet), and propranolol (Inderal)

Assessment Findings

Signs and Symptoms

The predominant feature of major depression is a persistently sad mood. It was described by psychologist Rollo May (1909–1994) as "the inability to construct a future." The pervasive sadness and accompanying physiologic and cognitive (thought) changes are represented by the acronym SAD IMAGES (Box 69-2) as well as others. Because the manifestations of depression may be similar to those of other conditions (Box 69-3), a tentative diagnosis is made while simultaneously investigating and eliminating alternative reasons for the clinical findings.

Diagnostic Findings

Genetic studies and those that identify 5-HIAA and HVA in cerebrospinal fluid and the metabolite of norepinephrine in urine are financially prohibitive except for research purposes. Blood levels of serotonin can be measured more easily, but there is some question whether the level in blood correlates with the level necessary for normal mood in the brain. Furthermore, some managed care groups consider diagnostic laboratory tests of neurotransmitter levels unnecessary and may not reimburse their cost. Third-party payers often maintain that a diagnosis of depression can be confirmed or ruled out by the client's clinical presentation and by performing other standard tests for disorders that mimic depression. Findings that would indicate alternative diagnoses to depression include low thyroid function test results, suggesting hypothyroidism (see Chapter 50); abnormal blood glucose levels, suggesting diabetes mellitus (see Chapter 51); low hemoglobin levels, indicative of anemia (see Chapter 31); and detection of drug abuse in a urine drug screen (see Chapter 71).

BOX 69-2 Signs and Symptoms of Major Depression

- **S**ad mood
- **A**ppetite change (increased or decreased)
- **D**isturbed sleep (insomnia or hypersomnia)
- **I**nability to concentrate
- **M**arked decrease in pleasure
- **A**pathy, including lack of interest in sex
- **G**uilty feelings
- **E**nergy changes (restlessness or inactivity)
- **S**uicidal thoughts

Occasionally, primary providers order a **dexamethasone suppression test** (DST), also called a **cortisol suppression test**. This blood test theoretically indicates major depression if cortisol levels remain elevated despite the administration of an oral dose of dexamethasone, a corticosteroid, the day before. Under normal conditions, increased blood levels of corticosteroid should suppress the pituitary gland's secretion of corticotropin-releasing factor through a negative feedback loop. Statistics show, however, that the level of cortisol remains elevated in clients who are depressed, suggesting that elevated cortisol is a chemical marker for depression. Some primary providers, however, do not believe that the DST is significant; therefore, it is not widely ordered. This test is also not likely to be reimbursed by insurance companies, adding a second reason that the test is not commonly ordered (Aetna Inc., 2020).

Neurologic imaging tests such as computed tomography or magnetic resonance imaging may be performed to eliminate diagnoses such as brain tumor or cerebrovascular accident as causes for a client's altered mood. A positron emission tomography (PET) scan may show a change in activity in the prefrontal cortex, suggestive of a mood disorder (Fig. 69-2). The primary provider may omit imaging tests if they think the clinical evidence strongly supports the diagnosis of depression.

Medical Management

The most commonly used treatments for depression are drug therapy (Drug Therapy Table 69-1), psychotherapy, and, in severe cases, electroconvulsive therapy. Some new forms of treatment include vagus nerve stimulation, deep brain stimulation, and transcranial magnetic stimulation.

Drug Therapy

The categories of drugs used to relieve the symptoms of depression are tricyclic antidepressants (TCAs); monoamine oxidase inhibitors (MAOIs); and reuptake inhibitors such as selective serotonin reuptake inhibitors (SSRIs). Also, other drugs such as serotonin/norepinephrine reuptake inhibitors (SNRIs; sometimes called selective serotonin–norepinephrine reuptake inhibitors [SSNRIs]) may be prescribed.

Additionally, norepinephrine–dopamine reuptake inhibitors (NDRIs), antidepressants that affect levels of norepinephrine

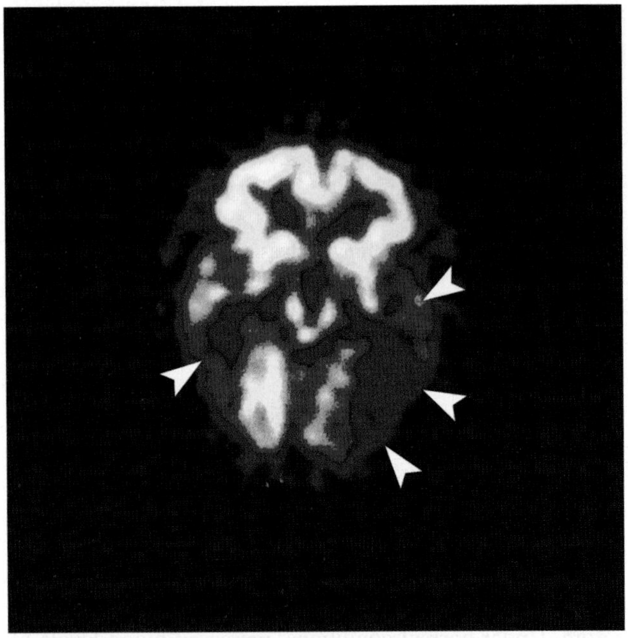

Figure 69-2 Example of axial positron emission tomography (PET) in a male client with Alzheimer disease showing defects (arrowheads) in metabolism in the regions of the cerebral cortex of the brain. (Reprinted with permission from Videbeck, S. L. (2020). *Psychiatric-mental health nursing* (8th ed.). Wolters Kluwer.)

and dopamine, are sometimes used as adjuvant drug therapy with SSRIs for persons whose depression is treatment-resistant (see Drug Therapy Table 69-1). Some NDRIs affect norepinephrine levels more significantly than dopamine and vice versa.

Triple reuptake inhibitors (TRIs), also referred to as serotonin–norepinephrine–dopamine reuptake inhibitors (SNDRIs), are being developed. In some instances, manic or hypomanic (mania of a lesser degree) episodes have been precipitated during antidepressant therapy. Serotonin syndrome (see section on Reuptake Inhibitors) may also occur.

Tricyclic Antidepressants

The TCAs such as amitriptyline (Elavil) and imipramine (Tofranil) were the first group of drugs used to treat depression; they are occasionally prescribed for clients with chronic pain (see Chapter 11). Tricyclics were so named because they have three chemical attachments in their organic molecular structure. Many variations of drugs in this category have been developed since the first tricyclics. The subsequent modifications are referred to as **bicyclics, tetracyclics,** and even **heterocyclics** according to the changes in their molecules. Collectively, they may be called **cyclic** antidepressants.

Cyclic antidepressants block the **reuptake** of serotonin and norepinephrine (Fig. 69-3). In other words, they interfere with the reabsorption of these two neurotransmitters by the releasing presynaptic neuron, thereby creating a sustained effect.

One disadvantage of cyclic antidepressants is the lag time between the initiation of drug therapy and relief of the depressive symptoms. It may take from 10 to 28 days or longer, depending on the specific cyclic drug, before a client notes any change in mood. Another disadvantage is that cyclics are highly lethal if taken in an overdose. Because suicide is not uncommon in clients who are depressed, the

DRUG THERAPY TABLE 69-1 Antidepressant Drug Therapy

Category and Common Generic (Brand) Drugs	Intended Use	Common Side Effects	Safety Warnings For Nurses
Tricyclic Antidepressants (TCAs)			
Amitriptyline (Elavil) Amoxapine (Asendin) Clomipramine (Anafranil) desipramine (Norpramin) Doxepin (Silenor, Sinequan) Imipramine (Tofranil) Nortriptyline (Pamelor) Protriptyline (Vivactil) Trimipramine (Surmontil)	Depression, chronic neuropathic pain, eating disorders, sleep apnea	Sedation, Anticholinergic effects (dry mouth, dry eyes, urinary retention, constipation)	Monitor for cardiac symptoms. Taper when discontinuing drug. Overdose can be lethal; there is no antidote—only supportive care.
Monoamine Oxidase Inhibitors (MAOIs)			
Isocarboxazid (Marplan) Phenelzine (Nardil) Tranylcypromine (Parnate)	Atypical depression, prevents breakdown of neurotransmitters (serotonin, norepinephrine, dopamine)	Orthostatic hypotension, vertigo, dizziness, nausea, constipation, dry mouth, diarrhea, headache, restlessness, blurred vision, hypertensive crisis	Known to cause hypertensive crisis if large amounts of fermented foods, alcohol, or aged cheese are ingested. Monitor for increased risk of serotonin syndrome if taken with SSRI/SNRI.

DRUG THERAPY TABLE 69-1 Antidepressant Drug Therapy (*continued*)

Category and Common Generic (Brand) Drugs	Intended Use	Common Side Effects	Safety Warnings For Nurses
Selective Serotonin Reuptake Inhibitors (SSRIs)			
Citalopram (Celexa) Escitalopram (Lexapro) Fluoxetine (Prozac) Paroxetine (Paxil) Sertraline (Zoloft) Vilazodone (Viibryd) Vortioxetine (Brintellix)	Depression, panic disorder, posttraumatic stress disorder, premenstrual disorder; manipulates serotonin at neuro-synaptic junction	Nausea, dry mouth, sweating, insomnia, anorexia, sexual dysfunction	Screen for suicidal ideation. Monitor for serotonin syndrome. Taper dose when discontinuing drug. Taking the herbal St. John's wort can increase risk of serotonin syndrome. Sexual dysfunction may be reduced by dividing the dose or delaying dosing until after sexual activity. Bupropion SR is an effective substitute for SSRI-induced sexual dysfunction.
Serotonin–Norepinephrine Reuptake Inhibitors (SNRIs)			
Desvenlafaxine (Pristiq) Duloxetine (Cymbalta) Levomilnacipran (Fetzima) Milnacipran (Savella) Nefazodone (generic only) Trazodone (Desyrel) Venlafaxine (Effexor) Maprotiline (Ludiomil)	Depression, neuropathic pain	Agitation, dizziness, dry mouth, insomnia, sedation, headache, nausea, vomiting, tremor, constipation, weight loss, anorexia, excess sweating, sexual dysfunction	Monitor for serotonin syndrome. Dose must be titrated down when stopping drug. Taking the herbal St. John's wort can increase risk of serotonin syndrome. Instruct male clients about treating priapism.
Norepinephrine–Dopamine Reuptake Inhibitors (NDRIs)			
Bupropion (Wellbutrin, Aplenzin, Zyban) Dexmethylphenidate (Focalin) Methylphenidate (Ritalin, Concerta)	Depression, smoking cessation Activity deficit, hyperactivity disorder, restlessness, agitation	Dry mouth, nausea, headache, dizziness, blurred vision, tachycardia, anxiety, restlessness, agitation, aggression, racing thoughts, loss of interest in sex, suicidal ideation	Do not administer Wellbutrin with Zyban. Avoid if there is a history of seizures, hypertension, glaucoma, bipolar disorder, liver disease, or kidney disease. Consult primary provider if contemplating pregnancy; avoid if breastfeeding.
Miscellaneous Antipsychotic Agents Used as Depression/Bipolar Adjuvant			
Aripiprazole (Abilify) Asenapine (Saphris) Brexpiprazole (Rexulti) Cariprazine (Vraylar) Lurasidone (Latuda) Mirtazapine (Remeron) Olanzapine (Zyprexa) Quetiapine (Seroquel) Risperidone (Risperdal)	Adjunct for major depressive disorders, schizophrenia, neuropathic pain, used in bipolar disorder	Agitation, constant motion, anxiety, drowsiness, headache, constipation, dry mouth, nausea	Monitor for repetitive involuntary muscle movements. Monitor for weight gain, increased cholesterol or triglycerides, and hyperglycemia.

The drugs in column 1 indicate the drug that matches up with explanations in columns 2 through 4.

primary provider must consider limiting the number of individual TCAs that are filled in any one prescription. Regardless of the prescribed class of antidepressant, clients with psychomotor retardation may attempt suicide once their level of energy increases. Nurses should not be lulled into thinking that a client who is depressed is necessarily nonsuicidal just because they are more active. In fact, close observation is even more important at this time.

Side effects of cyclic antidepressants, such as postural hypotension, tachycardia, cardiac arrhythmias, blurred vision, dry mouth, urinary retention, and constipation, make them particularly undesirable for older adults. Some cyclic antidepressants are more sedating than others. Signs of liver toxicity and bone marrow depression require frequent monitoring. The seizure threshold may also be lowered, causing a convulsion in clients who never experienced one before.

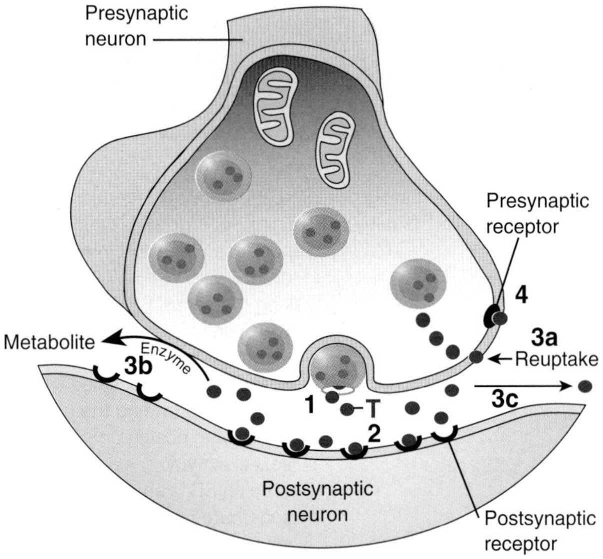

Figure 69-3 Schematic illustration of **(1)** neurotransmitter (T) release, **(2)** binding of transmitter to postsynaptic receptor; termination of transmitter action by **(3a)** reuptake of transmitter into the presynaptic terminal, **(3b)** enzymatic degradation, or **(3c)** diffusion away from the synapse; and **(4)** binding of transmitter to presynaptic receptors for feedback regulation of transmitter release. (Reprinted with permission from Videbeck, S. L. (2020). *Psychiatric-mental health nursing* (8th ed.). Wolters Kluwer.)

There must be sufficient time (2 to 4 weeks) between tapering the dosage of a cyclic antidepressant and initiating drug therapy with an MAOI or SSRI.

Monoamine Oxidase Inhibitors

Monoamine oxidase is an enzyme that breaks down monoamine neurotransmitters. Inhibiting this enzyme allows the neurotransmitters to continue stimulating receptor sites for norepinephrine, serotonin, and, to some extent, dopamine. MAOIs such as tranylcypromine (Parnate) and phenelzine (Nardil), however, are the least prescribed category of antidepressants because they have a high potential for food–drug and drug–drug interactions (Box 69-4). When an MAOI is combined with foods containing tyramine, which is another monoamine, clients are likely to develop a potentially fatal **hypertensive crisis**, with symptoms such as elevated blood pressure (BP), headache (often an occipital headache), nausea, vomiting, sweating, palpitations, visual changes, neck stiffness, sensitivity to light, and tachycardia. The nurse, therefore, has a grave responsibility for ensuring that clients learn about dietary and drug restrictions that the client must follow for at least 2 weeks after discontinuing the MAOI.

BOX 69-4 Food, Beverage, and Drug Restrictions During Monoamine Oxidase Inhibitor Drug Therapy

Food and Beverages to Avoid

- Aged, hard cheese
- Chocolate
- Pickled herring
- Overripe bananas
- Chicken liver
- Dried fish
- Fermented meat (salami)
- Yogurt
- Pepperoni, sausage
- Sour cream
- Broad beans (fava beans)
- Monosodium glutamate
- Beer
- Soy sauce
- Red wine
- Meat tenderizer

Drugs to Avoid

- Cold and allergy medications
- Appetite suppressants
- Antiasthmatics
- Antihypertensives
- Meperidine (Demerol)
- Antidepressants in other categories
- Local anesthetics with epinephrine

>>> *Stop, Think, and Respond 69-2*

What information would you offer to a person who has just started MAOI therapy and plans to go out for pizza and beer?

The primary provider usually prescribes a low dose at the beginning of MAOI drug therapy and increases the dose according to the client's tolerance of side effects, which include dry mouth, blurred vision, constipation, urinary retention, postural hypotension, insomnia, weight gain, and sexual dysfunction. The lag time before the client experiences a therapeutic effect is approximately 2 to 4 weeks after beginning MAOI therapy (Videbeck, 2020). Dosages must be tapered when the client no longer needs the drug. At least 2 weeks should elapse after the last dose of a cyclic antidepressant and the initiation of an MAOI.

Reuptake Inhibitors

Three categories of antidepressant drugs that are classified as single or dual neurotransmitter reuptake inhibitors include SSRIs, SNRIs, and NDRIs.

Selective Serotonin Reuptake Inhibitors. The SSRIs, as their name implies, interfere primarily with the reabsorption of serotonin. They also inhibit reuptake of norepinephrine, but to a lesser degree. The accumulated serotonin prolongs the stimulation of neuroreceptor sites. SSRIs are currently the most prescribed group of drugs used to treat depression. They are widely used for several reasons: (1) They have milder side effects; (2) they are unlikely to cause death in cases of overdose; (3) dosages do not need much adjustment after initiation of therapy; and (4) the lag time is short, perhaps 3 to 10 days.

Although SSRIs cause side effects such as nausea, weight loss, insomnia, nervousness, tremor, and headache, these problems tend to dissipate within weeks of starting drug therapy. If the side effects do not resolve, they can be managed with additional medications such as a mild hypnotic for sleep. Unfortunately, sexual dysfunction (e.g., reduced desire for sex, erectile and ejaculatory dysfunction, inability to reach orgasm) is a frequent and undesirable side effect. Alterations in sexual activity are a leading cause of nonadherence to taking the medication. Lowering the dose of SSRIs can reduce sexual side effects, but many clients, especially men, are reluctant to discuss changes in their sexuality with the prescribing primary provider.

Concern regarding the use of SSRIs in the treatment of depression in children, adolescents, and young adults has proliferated. Clinical evidence has shown that clients in this age range experience an increased risk of suicidal thoughts and behavior (National Institute of Mental Health, 2018). Although this class of medication clearly provides therapeutic benefits for children and adolescents who are depressed, the U.S. Food and Drug Administration (FDA) (2018) has issued a "black box" prescription drug warning label. The warning advises close monitoring of children and adolescents for worsening depression, thoughts or attempts of suicide, or significant changes in behavior, such as social withdrawal.

Serotonin–Norepinephrine Reuptake Inhibitors. SNRIs such as duloxetine (Cymbalta) and desvenlafaxine (Pristiq) potentiate the action of both serotonin and norepinephrine by interfering with neuronal reuptake. Maprotiline (Ludiomil) and nefazodone inhibit the reuptake of serotonin and norepinephrine and also block nerve cell receptors, causing a greater availability of these neurotransmitters to the brain. To reduce the incidence of side effects, the primary provider may start the client on a low dose and increase it gradually. SNRIs provide rapid relief of symptoms with fewer sexual side effects compared with SSRIs.

Serotonin Syndrome. Many antidepressants increase levels of serotonin. **Serotonin syndrome** is a potentially life-threatening condition that results from elevated levels of serotonin in the blood secondary to drug therapy. Manifestations include fever, sweating, shivering, feelings of intoxication, confusion, restlessness, anxiety, disorientation, ataxia, tachycardia, hypertension, tremors, and muscular spasms and rigidity. The following factors place a client at risk for serotonin syndrome:

- Antidepressants from different classes such as MAOIs and SSRIs are coprescribed.
- The time between weaning from one antidepressant drug to initiating another is inadequate to compensate for the first antidepressant's half-life.
- Other serotonergic agonists, drugs that stimulate serotonin receptors, are combined with antidepressant therapy. Serotonergic agonists include dextromethorphan (Benylin, Pertussin, Delsym), meperidine (Demerol), and lithium (Eskalith, Lithane).

Management of serotonin syndrome involves temporarily withholding the antidepressant. In the meantime, if symptoms are severe, they can be managed with anxiolytic drugs such as diazepam (Valium), beta-adrenergic blockers such as propranolol (Inderal), or skeletal muscle relaxants such as dantrolene (Dantrium) while supporting breathing with mechanical ventilation.

Norepinephrine–Dopamine Reuptake Inhibitors. Several other drugs such as bupropion (Wellbutrin) relieve depression by stabilizing levels of dopamine and norepinephrine. NDRIs are not used as first-line treatment of depression but rather as alternatives for clients who do not respond to trials with other classes of antidepressants. Advantages of this class of drugs are that there tends to be no sexual dysfunction or weight gain associated with their use. Other uses for NDRIs include the treatment of attention-deficit hyperactivity disorder and narcolepsy because of their stimulating effect.

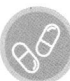

Pharmacologic Considerations

- Response to antidepressant medications is not rapid. It can take a number of weeks for the drugs to take effect. Fluoxetine (Prozac) is an example of a drug that may take as long as 4 weeks to attain a full therapeutic effect. Some adverse reactions, such as dry mouth, episodes of orthostatic hypotension, and drowsiness, appear long before the intended effect of the antidepressant. The inability to deal with the unpleasantness of these adverse reactions is one of the primary reasons clients stop taking antidepressants before they experience a therapeutic response.

››› *Stop, Think, and Respond 69-3*

How would you respond to a client who reports feeling just as depressed as when they began antidepressant drug therapy 4 days earlier?

Psychotherapy

Psychotherapy, talking with a psychiatrist, psychologist, or mental health therapist, promotes coping with emotional problems, gaining an insight into behaviors, and learning techniques that can improve well-being. Various types of psychotherapy are available:

- *Psychodynamic psychotherapy* is patterned after a Freudian model. Clients discuss their early life experiences to raise repressed feelings to a conscious level. Clients are often in psychodynamic psychotherapy for months to years. This form of therapy can be tedious and expensive, but traumatic events buried deep in the unconscious may require extensive therapy.
- *Interpersonal psychotherapy* is facilitated by a bond that develops between the therapist and client. The empathy and trust help clients gain an understanding of their condition and the courage and support to overcome it.
- *Supportive psychotherapy* helps clients learn about their disorder and treatment techniques, improve or develop

new social skills, obtain positive reinforcement for progress, and gain encouragement to persevere.

- *Cognitive therapy* helps clients replace negative, and often illogical, ways of thinking with more positive outlooks. For example, the therapist might encourage a person who believes a friend purposely avoided speaking to them in a store to consider other possibilities (e.g., the friend was preoccupied and did not actually notice the client; the friend did not recognize the client; the friend was in a hurry and could not spend time socializing).
- *Behavioral therapy* endeavors to change unhealthy ways of behaving. Clients are rewarded verbally or in some other way when they alter their behavior positively. For example, when a person who is often taken advantage of at work asserts themselves, the therapist praises the client's action. The praise and recognition encourage the client to continually repeat the healthy behavior. Gradually, the resulting changes increase self-esteem and promote further improvement.

Psychotherapy is often more productive after clients who are depressed respond to antidepressant drug therapy. Clients should be advised that if they feel uncomfortable or dissatisfied with a particular practitioner or style of therapy, they can be referred elsewhere.

Electroconvulsive Therapy

Electroconvulsive therapy (ECT) uses the application of an electric stimulus to one or both temporal regions of the head to produce a brief, generalized seizure. Although the exact mechanism of action is unknown, the belief is that ECT achieves its effect by either increasing circulating levels of monoamine neurotransmitters or by improving transmission to the receptor site. ECT is usually reserved for clients who are depressed and:

- Have not responded to drug therapy
- Are intolerant of the side effects of antidepressant medications
- Are so seriously suicidal that waiting for antidepressants to become effective jeopardizes their safety

Except for clients who are extremely suicidal, ECT can be administered on an ambulatory, outpatient basis. Many clients experience after effects, including headache; soreness of skeletal muscles; temporary confusion; short-term, patchy memory loss; and brief learning disability. ECT is usually contraindicated for clients with cardiac or neurovascular diseases.

Therapeutic Alternatives for Chronic or Treatment-Resistant Depression

Three surgical or device-based interventions can be used to relieve depression in clients who have exhausted drug therapy and have not responded to ECT.

Vagus Nerve Stimulation

Vagus nerve stimulation (VNS) was first used to treat epilepsy. Anecdotally, clients with epilepsy who were treated with VNS reported an improvement in their mood. The FDA (2016) has approved the use of VNS for intractable depression.

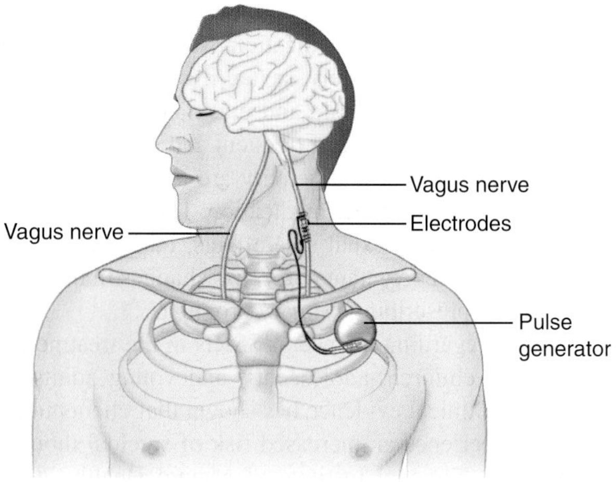

Figure 69-4 Vagus nerve stimulation (VNS) sends pulsed waves of energy from a pacemakerlike device under the skin to electrodes attached to a branch of the left vagus cranial nerve. These energy waves subsequently stimulate the areas of the brain that influence mood.

The VNS device consists of an electrode that is tunneled beneath the skin at the neck. One end of the electrode is attached to the vagus nerve, a cranial nerve that exits the brain stem, travels through the neck, and moves down to the chest and abdomen. The other end of the electrode is connected to a pulse generator implanted in the chest, similar to a cardiac pacemaker (Fig. 69-4). The pulse generator sends intermittent electrical impulses directed toward the brain via the vagus nerve. VNS can be turned off or reprogrammed by using a handheld magnetic wand over the pulse generator.

After insertion, a client may experience hoarseness, cough, or some shortness of breath during the time of stimulation. Relief of depressive symptoms may take up to 12 months (Mayo Clinic, 2020; Lowry, 2013). Transcutaneous VNS is an alternative noninvasive approach. It stimulates the vagus nerve through electrodes clipped within the ear similar to an earbud for headphones (Fig. 69-5). If its efficacy provides results that are comparable to implanted electrodes, it may offer effective treatment for more depressed individuals (Yap et al., 2020; Elsevier, 2016).

Deep Brain Stimulation

Deep brain stimulation (DBS), a more invasive procedure, has been used to help manage the tremors caused by Parkinson disease (see Chapter 37) and other neurologic conditions. It is believed that sending continuous electrical signals via DBS can alter brain circuitry and relieve depression. DBS involves implanting an electrode in the brain through a small opening in the skull (Fig. 69-6). The distal end of the electrode is passed under the skin of the head, neck, and shoulder, eventually connecting to a neurostimulator implanted under the skin near the clavicle, chest, or abdomen. A magnet can be used to adjust the neurostimulator (Mayo

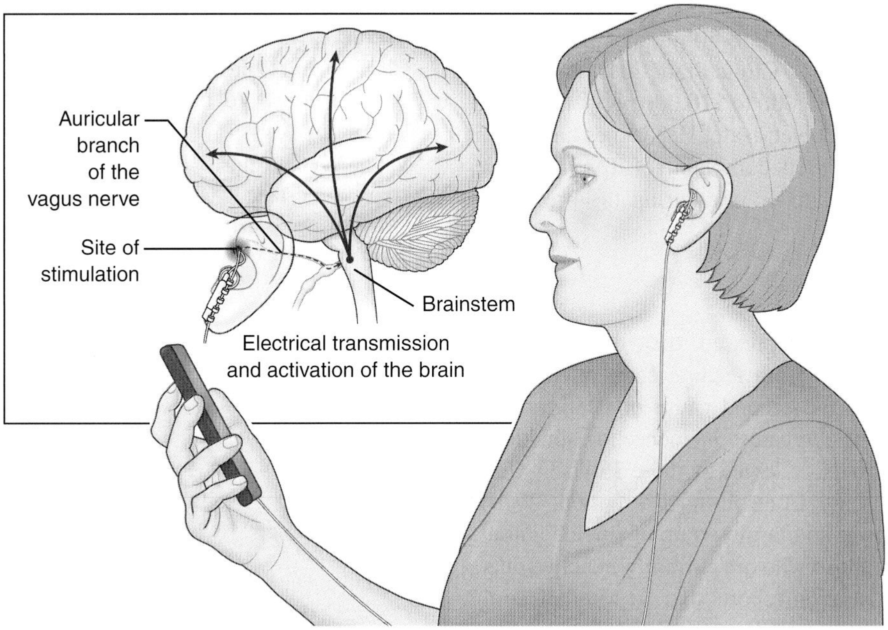

Figure 69-5 A handheld stimulator connected to an ear electrode sends electrical stimulation noninvasively via the auricular branch of the vagus nerve to the brainstem.

Clinic, 2020; Roth, 2013; University of Pittsburgh, Department of Neurological Surgery, 2013).

Battery replacement needs vary depending on usage and settings. The battery needs to be replaced by a surgeon during an outpatient procedure (Mayo Clinic, 2020; University of Pittsburgh, Department of Neurological Surgery, 2013; Roth, 2013).

Among the effects that clients may experience are temporary tingling in the face or limbs, speech or vision problems, jolting or shocking sensations, dizziness, reduced coordination, and difficulty concentrating.

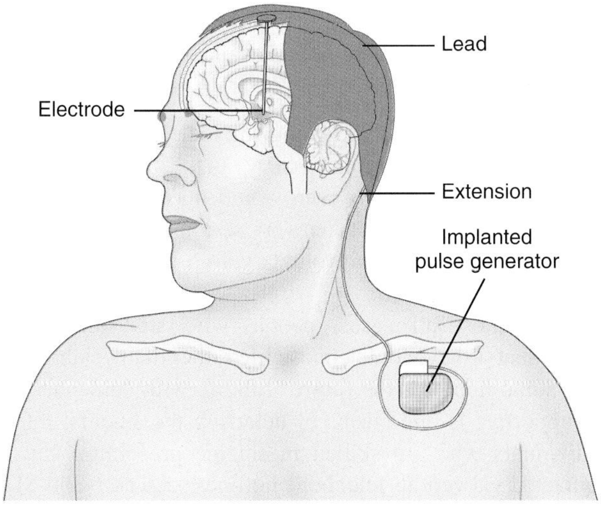

Figure 69-6 In deep brain stimulation, electrical pulses from an implanted battery generator are delivered continuously to the electrode in the brain of depressed persons who do not respond to more conventional treatments.

Transcranial Magnetic Stimulation

Transcranial magnetic stimulation (TMS) is a noninvasive method of stimulating the brain to treat depression. Stimulation is achieved by delivering short pulses of energy through an electromagnetic coil placed against the scalp near the forehead (Fig. 69-7). The energy is aimed at brain

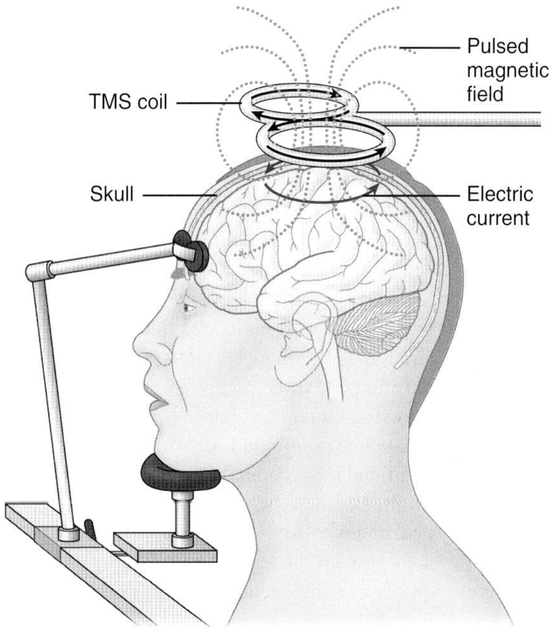

Figure 69-7 Transcranial magnetic stimulation (TMS) delivers magnetic pulses noninvasively to regions of the brain associated with mood regulation.

cells within the limbic system. Therapy requires administering 3000 pulses a minute for 20 to 40 minutes five times a week for 5 to 6 weeks (Mayo Clinic Staff, 2018). Although TMS is expensive (about $6,000 to $10,000 per person), the procedure has proven to be very safe. Headaches have been the most frequently reported complaint of TMS. Muscle contraction within the scalp or jaw during the procedure may occur.

SUICIDALITY

Assume that if a client is depressed, then they also may be suicidal. Suicide is the tenth leading cause of death in the United States; it is the second cause of death among 15- to 24-year-olds. The greatest incidence of suicide is among 55- to 64-year-olds, followed by those 25- to 35-year-olds (Centers for Disease Control and Prevention, 2019). Recently, there has been an alarming rate of suicide among military veterans and those who are currently in active duty. The Veterans Administration reports that 20 veterans commit suicide each day (Shane & Kime, 2016) accounting for 14.3% of all deaths by suicide among U.S. adults (U.S. Department of Veterans Affairs, 2018). As of 2020, the Department of Defense (DoD) reported the number of suicide deaths among active-duty military service members had increased to approximately 25 per 100,000 compared to 10.5 per 100,000 in 2000 (The National Advisory Mental Health Council [NAMHC], 2020). Common risk factors for suicide are outlined in Box 69-5.

Suicide Assessment

One of the most reliable suicide assessment techniques is to ask the client bluntly, "Do you feel like killing yourself?" Unfortunately, some clients who are depressed conceal their suicidal thoughts and provide only vague verbal or behavioral clues (Box 69-6), or assume that others are aware of their despair but have chosen to ignore it.

BOX 69-5 Risk Factors for Suicide

Several risks for suicide include the following:
- Depression often combined with a substance abuse disorder
- Major loss such as a loved one, home, relationship, divorce
- Being male; more females than males attempt suicide, but males more often complete it
- Having made a previous suicide attempt
- History of a relative who committed suicide
- Access to a firearm, the most common method of suicide
- Chronic physical illness, including chronic pain
- Victim of physical or sexual abuse
- Problems in school or with the legal system
- Seriously injuring or causing death of another person such as a motor vehicle accident
- Incarceration
- Experiencing *command hallucinations*—voices telling the client to kill themselves

BOX 69-6 Clues to Suicidal Intentions

Clear Verbal Clues
"I'm planning to kill myself."
"I wish I were dead."

Vague Verbal Clues
"I just can't stand it any longer."
"Nobody needs me anymore."
"Life has lost its meaning for me."
"You won't be seeing me anymore."
"I'm getting out."
"Everybody would be better off without me."

Behavioral Clues
Giving away a valued possession
Donating large sums of money to charity
Putting personal affairs in order
Writing poetry with morbid themes
Composing a suicide note
Making funeral arrangements
Buying a gun; stockpiling pills
Lifting of depressed mood (may indicate a plan and energy to carry it out)

To gather more information, use the mnemonic SLAP:

S = *Specificity:* What are the details of the suicide plan?
L = *Lethality:* How quickly or likely would death occur if the client acted on the plan?
High-lethality methods are those from which the possibility of rescue is remote. Some examples include shooting or hanging oneself; jumping from a bridge or building; throwing oneself in front of a train or truck; and driving into a tree, into a wall, or off a cliff. Low-lethality methods are those that allow a window of time for the person who attempts suicide to be found and rescued. They include overdosing on medications, cutting the wrists, or inhaling carbon monoxide.
A = *Availability:* Does the person have access and the means to carry out the plan?
P = *Proximity:* Are there others available who could intervene?

If the client admits to being suicidal, has a plan that is highly lethal, has the means to carry out the intended method, and lacks anyone nearby who would make the rescue, the risk for suicide must be taken very seriously. An emergency admission, voluntary or involuntary, to a psychiatric facility may be indicated.

In almost all cases, people who are suicidal are ambivalent—they would choose life rather than death if they held some hope for the future. Talking with someone who is supportive is one means of deterring the suicidal intent. Individuals who are skilled in suicide prevention can be contacted via various telephone hotlines such as 1-800-SUICIDE (800-784-2433) sponsored by Treatment Advocacy Center and the National Suicide Prevention Lifeline 1-800-272-TALK (800-273-8255), which is also available to the deaf or hard of hearing at 800-799-4889 or other crisis hotlines available in the local community. Additionally, effective July 2022, a new National Suicide Prevention Designation Act will allow for the designation of a three-digit number, 988, to be available for people to call in case of a suicidal crisis. (National Suicide Prevention Lifeline, 2020). However, despite conscientious efforts to prevent suicide, some people cannot be stopped.

Nursing Management

As part of a client assessment, nurses may use various standard assessment questionnaires as a database for quantifying a person's mood state and for tracking changes that occur in the future. Examples are the Beck Depression Inventory, a self-assessment tool that contains 22 multiple-choice questions that the client reads and answers independently, and the Hamilton Rating Scale for Depression (HAMD), which is administered by a mental health worker like a nurse. Usually, the scores on the Beck Depression Inventory correlate closely with the HAMD. The HAMD is used more widely for determining the severity of depression. The National Institute of Mental Health has used the HAMD to evaluate responses to pharmacologic drug treatment; pharmaceutical companies use the HAMD when submitting research results for new antidepressant approval by the FDA; and practitioners and researchers alike use the HAMD to compare and validate scores when more than one assessment tool is used.

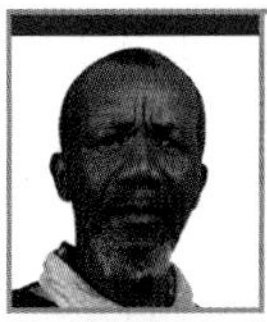

Clinical Scenario A 68-year-old man experienced initial anger at the time of his wife's death after a prolonged illness and now is currently depressed. He has lost weight and has difficulty sleeping. He no longer goes to church as he did faithfully for many years. He lives in a rural farm home, which accounts for his infrequent contact with neighbors. His children live in various locations, all quite distant. He has turned to drinking alcohol to numb his feelings of hopelessness that his life will ever be happy again. He owns a gun and has thought about ending his life. A daughter who sensed her father's unusual sadness contacted a home health care agency and requested that a nurse assess him. **What nursing actions are appropriate for this nonhospitalized client or others who are hospitalized and may be depressed and suicidal? Consider suggestions in the Nursing Process section that follows.**

NURSING PROCESS FOR THE DEPRESSED OR SUICIDAL CLIENT

Assessment

Assess the client physically and monitor mood and affect. Note the client's appearance to determine signs of personal neglect. Observe the client's overall energy or lack thereof. Listen to the client's pace of speaking and response time to questions to detect if it is slower than expected. Watch the client's body language for evidence of anxiety, such as wringing the hands. Ask the client what kinds of pleasurable activities they pursue and how often. Be prepared that the client may not be able to identify any activities or that it has been a long time since they have engaged in anything enjoyable. Question whether the client drinks alcohol or takes sedative drugs, and if so, what, how much, and how often. Inquire "How are you feeling right now? Have you thought about hurting or killing yourself? How might you end your life? Do you own a gun? How close are your neighbors to your home?"

Diagnosis, Planning, and Interventions

Suicide Attempt Risk: Related to feelings of hopelessness
Expected Outcomes: (1) The client will not harm self. (2) The client will identify a reason for living.

- Encourage a client who is not hospitalized to contact a friend or relative personally or give permission for the nurse to do this rather than remaining alone. *The presence of another supportive person can deter a suicide attempt.*
- Ask if there is someone to whom they would entrust their gun until feeling less depressed. *Eliminating access to a planned method of suicide can prevent a suicide attempt.*
- Confiscate any objects that a hospitalized client may use for self-harm, such as belts, shoelaces, safety razors, sharp combs, keys, or knives. *Limiting access to items that the client can use for self-destruction reduces the resources they have for attempting suicide.*
- If hospitalized, move the client close to the nursing station. *Doing so facilitates close and frequent observation.*
- Talk to a nonhospitalized client on the phone as long as possible while contacting a 911 operator. *Communication with a comforting person can delay a potential suicide attempt or provide time to obtain assistance from emergency personnel who can intervene.*
- Inspect the hospitalized client's mouth, looking under the tongue and within the buccal cavity, after administering medications. *Suicidal clients may conceal and hoard medications until they stockpile a sufficient amount for an overdose.*
- Observe the hospitalized client's whereabouts at least every 15 minutes and spend time interacting with them. *These measures reduce the client's potential time for attempting or completing suicide and increase the response time available to resuscitate a person who has attempted suicide.*
- Keep the client busy and involved in activities. *Activity shifts the client's attention away from their emotional pain and hopelessness.*

Coping Impairment: Related to feelings of depression and hopelessness
Expected Outcome: The client will identify one or more alternatives to suicide.

(continued)

NURSING PROCESS FOR THE DEPRESSED OR SUICIDAL CLIENT (continued)

- Acknowledge the client's feeling of despair. *Recognizing a client's mood demonstrates that the nurse has noticed the person and is perceptive.*
- Indicate that you want to help. *Offering assistance is characterized as a therapeutic use of self. Doing so reassures the client that you will not abandon them and that they are worthy of help.*
- Emphasize hope, previous positive experiences, and outcomes. *Such discussion reinforces that the client has the potential to overcome current difficulties on the basis of past success.*
- Explore other courses of action rather than suicide. *Alternatives help the client consider options for dealing with the current situation.*
- Appeal to the client's ambivalence by indicating that current feelings are likely to change given additional time. *Most suicidal clients will delay or dismiss suicidal activities if they believe that they will feel better eventually.*
- Discuss previous coping strategies and encourage using some that were effective in the past. *Reusing previous methods for managing problems offers the possibility that similar actions can achieve a positive result.*
- Develop a plan for maintaining future safety such as talking with a trusted friend or calling a crisis hotline. *If a plan is developed, there is a possibility that the client will implement it.*

Sleep Deprivation: Related to depression
Expected Outcome: The client will sleep a maximum of 8 hours during the night with no napping during the day.

- Keep the client busy during the day, and discourage napping or going to bed early. *Left alone, depressed clients are likely to become more vegetative (i.e., they withdraw by sleeping).*
- Include active exercise during the day but not before bedtime. *Exercise relieves anxiety, but it may cause stimulation when performed at night.*

Evaluation of Expected Outcomes

Expected outcomes are that the client's suicidal feelings pass. The client implements new or previously successful coping strategies to manage emotional problems. At night, the client falls asleep easily and does not awaken for 6 to 8 hours.

If the client is admitted to a psychiatric facility, standard practices known as *suicide precautions* are implemented. They generally include temporary confiscation of any personal items that could be used for self-harm, requiring that the client dress in hospital garb with slippers; designating a staff person to care for and observe only the suicidal person (e.g., no other client assignment); noting the whereabouts and behavior of a suicidal client, either continuously or at 15-minute intervals; and inspecting and returning all potentially unsafe items brought by the client's visitors.

The nurse assigned to care for the client administers psychotropic medications as prescribed and ensures that the client swallows the medication. This is often done by inspecting the client's mouth and under the tongue because some suicidal clients "cheek" medications in order to stockpile and use them later for the purpose of suicide. The nurse may obtain consents and prepare severely depressed clients for alternative interventions such as ECT.

SEASONAL AFFECTIVE DISORDER

SAD is a mood disorder that has its onset during darker winter months and spontaneously disappears in the spring. SAD is more prevalent among people living in states north of 40° to 50° of latitude, such as Washington, Oregon, Minnesota, Michigan, New York, and the New England states. People who are Alaska Natives do not manifest the disorder as much as those who move there.

Pathophysiology and Etiology

The best explanation for SAD is that it is a primitive biologic response triggered by **photoperiods** (daytime hours that are short because of fewer hours of sunlight). The condition actually resembles the characteristics of hibernating animals. Theorists believe that light rays follow a visual pathway to the hypothalamus, the center for regulating sleep, hunger, libido, and mood. The hypothalamus relays the light-sensing data to the pineal gland, which regulates the production of a hormone called melatonin. **Melatonin**, which also affects regulation of serotonin, induces sleep during dark hours and is suppressed by daylight (Fig. 69-8). When hours of daylight become fewer, the production of melatonin is extended. In northern latitudes, melatonin secretion is sustained until spring, when days become brighter and longer.

Assessment Findings

Clients with SAD use the terms *sleepy*, *fatigued*, and *lethargic* to describe themselves in the winter. The lack of energy crosses over into feeling irritable, unable to concentrate, worthless, guilty, depressed—even suicidal. Some also report cravings for carbohydrates, which leads to weight gain, much like an animal preparing to sleep through the winter. As clients with SAD become more depressed and irritable, they are less inclined to interact socially. Many tend to stay indoors and dread leaving home.

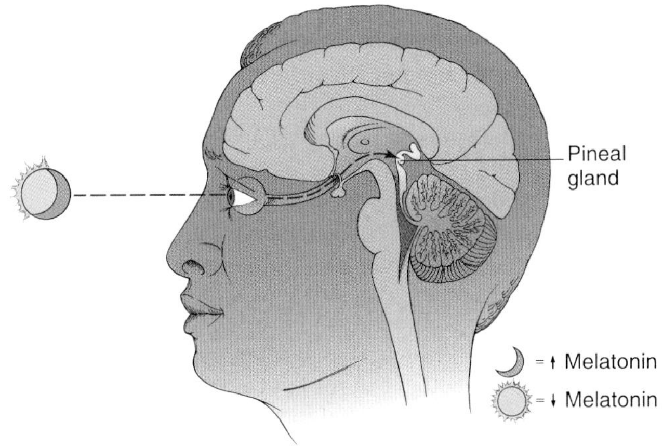

Figure 69-8 Melatonin (and, subsequently, serotonin) levels depend on exposure to sunlight. Melatonin induces sleep during dark hours and is suppressed by daylight. Dark months result in seasonal affective disorder for some people.

The depression is bimodal; it cycles with the seasons. After a prolonged period of winter depression, most report a lifting of spirits in the spring. Some also describe feeling energetic, more motivated, hyperactive, and even euphoric. The cheery mood or absence of depressive symptoms tends to be sustained until late fall, when the depressive pattern repeats itself.

At this time, no diagnostic tests can confirm SAD. Primary providers rely on clients' reports of cycling moods that correlate with the ratio of sunlight.

Medical Management

For those who cannot move to a sunnier location, phototherapy is the best alternative for treating SAD. **Phototherapy** involves using artificial light that simulates the intensity of sunlight (Fig. 69-9). The artificial light is produced by fluorescent bulbs at 2500 to 10,000 lux, the international measurement of illumination. Ten thousand lux is approximately 10 to 20 times as bright as ordinary indoor light.

The frequency and duration for phototherapy can vary, but a common prescription is to sit by the light source from 30 minutes to 2 hours per day, preferably in the early morning hours. The client need not stare at the fluorescent light; in fact, it is best not to look directly at it. Glancing periodically at the light is sufficient to relieve symptoms in 1 to 2 weeks. Other phototherapy models are available as well. A head-mounted light that shines on the face during daytime activities facilitates mobility. Bedroom phototherapy lights can be set with an automatic timer to come on at a predawn schedule. Even though the sleeper's eyes are closed, it is believed that the light penetrates the eyelids, which triggers a decline in melatonin—much like daybreak naturally activates arousal from sleep.

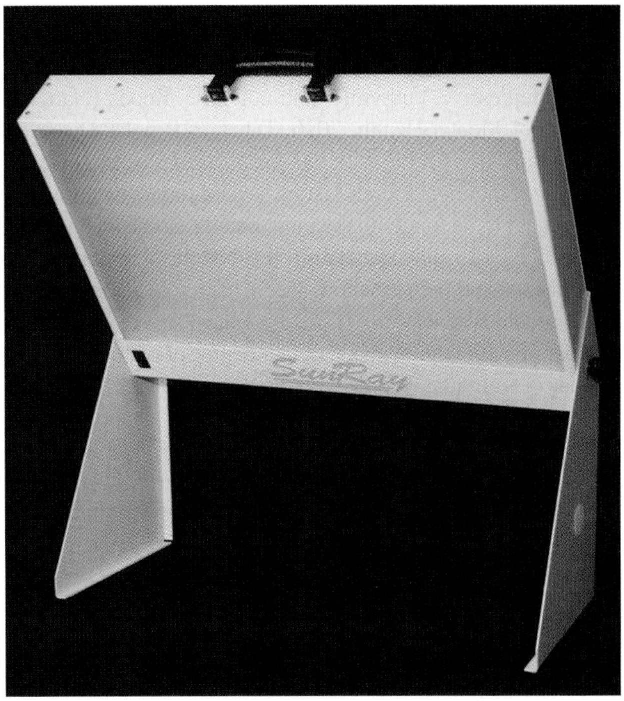

Figure 69-9 Phototherapy products such as a lightbox relieve the symptoms of seasonal affective disorder.

Nursing Management

Because most clients with SAD are outpatients or may soon become so, the nurse provides information on how to implement phototherapy and how to supplement its beneficial effects. One of the most important principles to stress is that natural sunlight is brighter and better than any artificial substitute. The nurse also should teach measures found in Client and Family Teaching 69-1.

Client and Family Teaching 69-1
Seasonal Affective Disorder (SAD)

The nurse teaches the client who experiences SAD and their family the following:

- Avoid the use of eyeglasses or contact lenses that are coated to shield ultraviolet radiation because the coating interferes with light transmission to the pineal gland.
- Add more lamps and bright fixtures at home and work.
- Install skylights.
- Trim shrubs and trees from around windows.
- Use translucent curtains or shades rather than heavy drapes.
- Sleep and work in an east-facing room.
- Take brief walks outside around noon without sunglasses.
- Jog after sunup and before sundown.
- Take up an outdoor winter sport.

BIPOLAR DISORDER

The several types of **bipolar disorder** all involve cycling among depressive, euthymic, and euphoric moods (National Institute of Mental Health, 2020; Types of Bipolar Disorder, 2016). Typically, people with *bipolar I disorder* experience severely dysfunctional moods lasting several months; depressive phases tend to be longer than manic phases. Some clients with bipolar I disorder may also manifest psychotic symptoms such as delusions and hallucinations (see Chapter 72) from time to time. People with *bipolar II disorder* have severe depression alternating with hypomania, a milder degree of mania, between periods of euthymia. People with bipolar II disorder never have psychotic symptoms. In *cyclothymic disorder*, a subtype of bipolar II disorder, people have milder mood swings, which occur abruptly and are of short duration. However, clients with cyclothymic disorder are never free of symptoms for more than 2 months. Ironically, in *mixed bipolar disorder*, mania and depression occur simultaneously. People feel grandiose and have a great deal of energy, but they are irritable and are quick to anger. Clients with *rapid-cycling bipolar disorder* experience at least four episodes of mania and depression per year, whereas those with *ultrarapid-cycling bipolar disorder* have alternating moods that may occur within a month or less.

Pathophysiology and Etiology

Extremes in levels of monoamines—excessive in mania and inadequate during depression—seem to be responsible for the symptoms of bipolar disorder. In severe cases, excess dopamine may cause distorted thinking and hallucinations. Another possibility is that there is insufficient **gamma-aminobutyric acid** (GABA), an inhibitory neurotransmitter, to counteract the effects of the monoamines. Altered blood calcium levels also may contribute to the development of bipolar disorder because calcium is required for exciting neurons. Genetic predisposition also is implicated in the development of bipolar disorder.

Assessment Findings

Signs and Symptoms

Signs and symptoms of the depressive phase of bipolar disorder are the same as those for major depression. During the manic phase, clients are hyperactive and often display an exaggerated sense of their own importance. They can quickly become angry and aggressive with those who attempt to restrain their burst of energy and irrational ideas. Because judgment is impaired—another characteristic of the disorder—reckless and impulsive behavior such as sexual promiscuity, criminal activity, spending sprees, gambling, and risky business transactions can occur. The surge of norepinephrine allows clients who are experiencing the manic phase to go without sleep for long periods. It also causes rapid thinking accompanied by racing speech. When extremely ill, some people experience psychotic features such as hallucinations. Combined with delusions, which are illogical false beliefs, clients with bipolar disorder can become homicidal or suicidal. Also see Evidence-Based Practice 69-1.

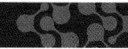

> **Evidence-Based Practice 69-1**
>
> **Risk Factors for Bipolar Disorders**
>
> ***Clinical Question***
>
> What are risk factors of bipolar disorder?
>
> ***Evidence***
>
> Bipolar disorder is a disorder that occurs in the brain and may cause a client to change mood, behavior, or level of energy quickly. This can disrupt the daily structure and routine. This disorder could have multiple causes. Health care providers must understand the risk factors of bipolar disorder (also known as "manic-depressive disorder"). There are three factors that may put a client at risk for this disorder: (1) the structure and function of a client's brain; (2) the part that genetics plays—some data have shown that people with certain genes may be at risk; (3) bipolar disorder runs in families. Clients with a sibling or perhaps a parent who has been diagnosed with the disorder are at a greater risk of developing bipolar disorder. Clients with this disorder are also at risk for suicide (National Institute of Mental Health, 2020).
>
> ***Nursing Implications***
>
> The nurse must understand the risk of this disorder when collecting a family history and gathering assessment data. The nurse must also know what to do for suicide prevention and what resources are available for the client such as the suicide hot. Last, the client should provide a complete list of medications for the nurse and health care provider.

References
National Institute of Mental Health (NIMH). (2020). *Bipolar disorder*. https://www.nimh.nih.gov/health/topics/bipolar-disorder/index.shtml

Diagnostic Findings

It eventually may be possible to predict which people will develop bipolar disorder with the use of gene mapping. At present, however, no objective tests are available, and the diagnosis is based on the client's history and current behavior. The key indicator is the client's pattern of emotional "highs" and "lows." A family member with bipolar disorder is a risk factor, as is a history of substance abuse, because people who aren't diagnosed with this disorder naively attempt to self-medicate to relieve the depressive episodes.

Medical Management

Bipolar disorder is managed by the administration of one or more mood-stabilizing medications that may be combined with an adjunctive drug (Drug Therapy Table 69-2). Lithium (Eskalith, Lithane, Lithobid), a chemical element, usually is the initial drug of choice. It controls both depressive as well as manic symptoms in clients who respond to lithium monotherapy (single-drug treatment). Fifty percent initially respond to lithium therapy. Another 40% to 50% improve with the addition of another mood-stabilizing medication. The American Psychiatric Association's *Guideline Watch: Practice Guideline for the Treatment of Patients With Bipolar Disorder*, Second Edition (2012) as well as Post et al. (2019) recommend the use of an anticonvulsant such as valproic acid derivatives

(Depakote, Depakene) or an antipsychotic such as olanzapine (Zyprexa) in combination with lithium for controlling manic episodes to induce sedation and control hallucinations and delusions. Benzodiazepines such as lorazepam (Ativan) may be used as an adjunctive drug during initial symptom management. Some have proposed using calcium-channel blockers, but little research supports the application of their use for managing bipolar disorder (Drug Therapy Table 69-2).

Lithium

Lithium is a naturally occurring element found in stone and spring water that flows from underground sources. Pharmaceutical preparations are available for those who are lithium deficient. When ingested, lithium moves easily through cell membranes, but it is less easily removed. Some believe that this feature may stabilize cell membranes, leading to the equalization of moods. Another possibility is that lithium regulates the activity between neurotransmitters such as serotonin, norepinephrine, dopamine, and their receptor sites. However, lithium:

- May be ineffective for some
- Has a delay of 5 to 14 days in achieving therapeutic benefits
- Has a narrow range of safety between a therapeutic serum level (0.8 to 1.2 mEq) and toxic levels (≥1.5 mEq)
- May be nontherapeutic or dangerously elevated when taken in combination with other drugs (Box 69-7)

BOX 69-7 Drugs Affecting Serum Lithium Levels

Increase Serum Lithium Level
- Tetracycline
- Thiazide diuretics
- Loop diuretics
- Nonsteroidal anti-inflammatory drugs (NSAIDs)
- Haloperidol

Decrease Serum Lithium Level
- Theophylline
- Aminophylline
- Carbamazepine
- Sodium bicarbonate
- Osmotic diuretics
- Causes side effects that challenge compliance
- Requires periodic laboratory tests to monitor serum blood levels

Lithium crosses the placental barrier; therefore, its use is contraindicated in pregnant women. Furthermore, lithium is water-soluble and present in all body fluids, including breast milk. Lithium administered to infants through breast milk can cause toxicity; thus, breastfeeding mothers should also avoid its use. Loss of body fluid from

DRUG THERAPY TABLE 69-2 Mood-Stabilizing Medications

Category and Common Generic (Brand) Drugs	Intended Use	Common Side Effects	Safety Warnings for Nurses
Mood Stabilizers			
Lithium (Lithobid, Eskalith, Lithane)	Bipolar disorder	Headache, drowsiness, tremors, nausea, polyuria	Dehydration and low salt intake makes client at greater risk for toxicity. Monitor blood levels for early toxicity and adjust dose.
Valproic acid (Depakote, Depakene)	May increase levels of gamma-aminobutyric acid and inhibit glutamate	Drowsiness, mild tremor, ataxia, nausea, vomiting, diarrhea, blood dyscrasias, liver toxicity	Administer with meals. Caution client to avoid activities that require alertness and coordination. Monitor blood for therapeutic levels. Females should avoid pregnancy.
Olanzapine (Zyprexa)	Mechanism of action not fully understood; blocks dopamine receptors in the brain; depresses the reticular activating system; blocks serotonin receptor sites	Somnolence, dizziness, nervousness, orthostatic hypotension, constipation, fever, weight gain, involuntary movements (especially about the face)	Use cautiously in older debilitated clients or clients with cerebrovascular disease, dehydration, seizures, Alzheimer disease, prostate enlargement, glaucoma, paralytic ileus, or phenylketonuria. If blister pack is used, do not push through foil, use dry hands to remove tablet; place an entire tablet in mouth. If drowsiness occurs, avoid tasks that require mental alertness (e.g., driving, operating machinery).
Olanzapine/fluoxetine (Symbyax)	Depression associated with bipolar disorder, treatment-resistant depression	Dry mouth, increased appetite, fatigue, blurred vision, swollen hands or feet, headache, stiff muscles, tremors, jerky movements	Assess mood, sleep patterns, thoughts of suicide, weight, muscular coordination. Wait at least 14 days between discontinuing an MAOI and initiating drug therapy.

diarrhea, diuretics, and excessive perspiration can lead to concentrated blood levels and lithium toxicity. Because the body always attempts to balance cations with anions, lithium may be retained if sodium levels are low. Providers must stress the importance of maintaining an adequate ingestion of salt to all clients who rely on lithium to control their disorder.

Adjunctive Medications

Adjunctive medications such as anticonvulsants or antipsychotics may be coprescribed for a brief period to sedate the client and relieve bizarre thought processes faster than monotherapy with lithium. They achieve their therapeutic effects in a variety of ways. Anticonvulsants enhance the action of GABA in much the same way that benzodiazepines reduce anxiety (see Chapter 68), and they are believed to inhibit glutamate. Anticonvulsants tend to be used to manage the symptoms of clients at the onset of acute mania. In addition, they are efficacious for decreasing the incidence and frequency of mood swings among rapid cyclers. However, because anticonvulsants stimulate drug metabolism by the liver, maintaining consistent therapeutic drug levels is difficult. Clients who take anticonvulsants also may be at risk for infection because some drugs in this class impair white blood cell formation. Consequently, serum drug levels and leukocyte counts must be monitored periodically.

Pharmacologic Considerations

- Lithium toxicity can easily occur when dehydration and polyuria present. Clients in manic episodes tend to neglect food and fluids, resulting in dehydration. Additionally, polyuria can occur with administration of lithium. Therefore, finding methods to increase fluid intake is essential.

Clients who take valproic acid (Depakote, Depakene) tend to experience gastrointestinal symptoms such as nausea, vomiting, and diarrhea. Some experience sedation and ataxia, putting them at risk for injury. Periodic assessment of liver function, serum ammonia, and blood cell counts is necessary. Controversy exists regarding the administration of anticonvulsants to pregnant and nursing mothers. Some feel that the risk to the fetus or infant is outweighed by the benefit of treating a mother with a mood disorder or epilepsy (Cohen et al., 2019; Viguera, 2010).

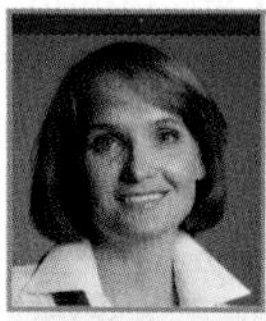

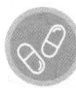

Clinical Scenario. While working at a busy information technology (IT) company, a 32-year-old employee who is a woman recently has been coming to the office provocatively dressed. Some of her coworkers have noticed that she has an obvious body odor that is likely caused by a neglect of hygiene. She also has been flirtatious with several employees. Although she has begun many work-related projects, she has yet to complete any of them. Her purposeless activity and incessant talking about bizarre ideas have caught the attention of her superior because her behavior is so different from that over the previous 3 months. She has become argumentative and threatening at home when her husband voices concern about her extravagant spending, which leaves them little to meet their financial obligations. She has been prescribed lithium, but her husband fears that she has not been compliant with self-administration. Her husband has convinced her to make an appointment with her psychiatrist, who obtains her consent for a short-term voluntary admission to restabilize her manic condition. **How should the nurse care for the client upon admission? Refer the Nursing Care Plan 69-1 section for suggestions.**

NURSING CARE PLAN 69-1 The Client With Bipolar Disorder/Acute Manic Phase

Assessment

- It may be necessary to perform the initial assessment and physical examination in brief increments. Bipolar clients have short attention spans and poor concentration; they become easily frustrated if their activity is curtailed. As an alternative, use the family as a more objective resource for necessary information. Their information is valuable because the client's symptoms have usually created multiple crises.
- Determine what types of prescribed medications the client takes and if they have been compliant with the medication regimen. Sometimes, antidepressants can trigger manic symptoms because they raise monoamine neurotransmitter levels.
- Ask about the client's use of alcohol or other controlled substances because many clients with bipolar disorder attempt to self-medicate to control their moods or they use drugs recreationally because of their poor judgment.
- Obtain information about the client's recent sleep patterns, hydration, and dietary intake.
- Observe the client's attention to hygiene and manner of dress. Check the female client's last date of menstruation and if she has consistently used contraception.
- Prepare the client for laboratory and diagnostic tests that are likely to include an electrocardiogram, thyroid function studies, and a profile of blood chemistry tests. Note if the client is voiding in sufficient quantities and inquire as to the client's bowel elimination patterns, including the date of the last bowel movement.
- Record baseline vital signs.
- Listen to the client's thought content during verbal interactions. The client is likely to speak loudly and rapidly. At the very least, bipolar clients express expansive and elaborate ideas or schemes. Some may have paranoid ideas or inflate their own importance. They may be experiencing hallucinations.

NURSING CARE PLAN 69-1 The Client With Bipolar Disorder/Acute Manic Phase (*continued*)

Nursing Diagnosis. **Disturbed Thought Processes** related to excessive levels of monoamines

Expected Outcome. Client will be oriented and accurately perceive circumstances surrounding admission.

Interventions	Rationales
Orient client to person, place, time, and events.	*Racing thoughts often interfere with comprehension.*
Provide information in small amounts using brief sentences.	*Brief discussions accommodate for short attention span.*
Reduce distracting stimuli such as noise and stimulation.	*External stimuli may interfere with thought processes.*
Present reality when client is delusional; do not press the issue if it causes agitation.	*Failing to present reality reinforces that client's delusions are real. Persistence may create conflict or cause a client to act out violently.*
Monitor client's whereabouts to ensure that they do not wander from the unit or health care agency.	*Bipolar clients are impulsive and resist being confined. Health care providers are responsible for safety at all times.*

Evaluation of Expected Outcomes

- The client's thoughts become reality-oriented.
- The client interacts appropriately with the situation.

Nursing Diagnosis. **Disturbed Thought Processes** related to excessive levels of monoamines

Expected Outcome. Client will be oriented and accurately perceive circumstances surrounding admission.

Interventions	Rationales
Take client to a room or other secluded area when they show signs of aggression.	*Decreased stimulation may restore self-control.*
Set firm limits for behavioral expectations using a modulated and controlled tone of voice.	*Client remains informed of the kinds of behavior that will not be tolerated. A modulated, controlled voice is less likely to provoke a confrontation.*
Offer client a large-muscle activity like playing basketball or riding an exercise bicycle.	*Exercise releases energy and reduces the potential for an angry outburst.*
Administer a prescribed short-acting sedative if aggressive behavior escalates and endangers others.	*A sedate client is more responsive to directions from others and less likely to become physically violent.*
Obtain an order to seclude or restrain if client becomes violent.	*Legally, restraints must be avoided unless absolutely necessary to protect others because clients have the right to the least restrictive treatment.*
Initiate suicide precautions if data suggest vulnerability for self-harm.	*The client's safety is a priority of care.*

Evaluation of Expected Outcomes

- Client has no angry outbursts.
- Client demonstrates self-control.

Nursing Diagnosis. **Malnutrition Risk** related to increased activity and distraction from eating

Expected Outcome. Client will maintain admission weight.

Interventions	Rationales
Consult the dietitian about increasing calories at mealtimes.	*Loading calories without loading quantities of food may help maintain weight and nutrition.*
Offer liquid nutritional supplements at least three times a day.	*Each container of liquid nourishment may provide 350 or more calories. Consuming liquids does not require sitting at a table and interrupting activity.*

(*continued*)

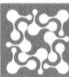

NURSING CARE PLAN 69-1 The Client With Bipolar Disorder/Acute Manic Phase (*continued*)

Provide finger foods that the client may consume throughout the day.	*Frequent snacking increases caloric intake and nourishment.*

Evaluation of Expected Outcome

- Client consumes sufficient food to maintain weight.

Nursing Diagnosis. Dehydration related to polyuria secondary to lithium therapy and inattention to thirst

Expected Outcome. Client will be adequately hydrated throughout care.

Interventions	Rationales
Monitor intake and output if possible.	*Urine output of 1500–3000 mL indicates an adequate fluid volume.*
Offer at least 2500–3000 mL of fluid per day.	*An adequate volume compensates for polyuria that can occur with lithium therapy. Urination ensures excretion of lithium.*
Monitor electrolyte laboratory results.	*Electrolytes become elevated when fluid intake is low.*

Evaluation of Expected Outcomes

- Client consumes sufficient fluids to maintain hydration.
- Client has moist mucous membranes, light-colored urine, and normal body temperature.

Nursing Diagnosis. Bathing/ADL Deficit related to decreased attention and concentration

Expected Outcome. Client will be clean and groomed each day.

Interventions	Rationales
Prepare necessities for bathing, grooming, and hygiene for client. Supervise hygiene and provide assistance if needed.	*Distractibility may interfere with client's ability to organize hygiene items. Client may be less thorough without nurse's supervision.*
Spread uncompleted hygiene tasks throughout the remainder of the day.	*All hygiene needs may not be met at one time.*
Help client to dress appropriately and remain dressed.	*Bipolar clients may dress flamboyantly or seductively unless supervised. Poor judgment may result in episodes of nudity.*

Evaluation of Expected Outcome

- Client resumes independent responsibility for self-care and activities of daily living.

Antipsychotics, especially new atypical drugs such as olanzapine (Zyprexa), aripiprazole (Abilify), and quetiapine (Seroquel), achieve their effect by selectively blocking dopamine and serotonin receptors, but it is more likely that blocking the D2 dopamine receptor accounts more so for their beneficial action.

Drugs that block D2 receptors can curb many of the symptoms of mania. Dopamine causes feelings of pleasure, which leads to a desire to repeat the stimulating experience—much like cocaine and methamphetamine. Under a surge of dopamine, there is an effort to seek instant gratification rather than waiting for long-term reward, much like someone with attention-deficit disorder. An increase in dopamine also can lead to hypersocial and hypersexual activities. Thus, atypical antipsychotics provide a beneficial effect among those with bipolar disorder.

Although there are variations among drugs classified as atypical antipsychotics, some common side effects include weight gain, new onset of diabetes mellitus, hyperlipidemia, and sexual and cardiac dysfunction.

Nursing Management

The nurse must obtain a cluster of symptoms from the client or family during a nursing assessment that indicates alterations in mood and inappropriate behaviors. See the following Clinical Scenario and Nursing Care Plan 69-1 section for nursing management.

Before discharge, the nurse educates the client and their significant others on the following aspects:

- The disease process
- How prescribed drugs help in symptom management
- Drug effects and side effects
- Signs of drug toxicity and actions to take
- Frequency of blood tests
- The advantages of wearing a MedicAlert bracelet

In addition to arranging outpatient therapy, the nurse informs the client and others of support groups that can continue the educational and therapeutic processes. Both the client and those who live in the same environment need to understand the signs of relapse, such as an inability to sleep for several days in a row, or increasingly impulsive behavior, such as making unnecessary purchases. The nurse also reviews the signs of cycling into a depressed mood so indications for reinitiating medical care are clear.

KEY POINTS

- Common signs and symptoms of mood disorders:
  - Extreme persistent mood or severe mood swings that interfere with social relationships
- Three neurotransmitters that, when imbalanced, affect mood:
  - Serotonin
  - Norepinephrine
  - Dopamine
- Drugs used to treat mood disorders:
  - TCAs
  - MAOIs
  - SSRIs
  - SNRIs
  - NDRIs
  - TRIs
- Causes, manifestations, and management of serotonin syndrome:
  - A potentially life-threatening condition that results from elevated levels of serotonin in the blood secondary to drug therapy
  - Symptoms:
    - Fever, sweating, shivering, feelings of intoxication, confusion, restlessness, anxiety, disorientation, ataxia, tachycardia, hypertension, tremors, and muscular spasms and rigidity
  - Risk factors:
    - Antidepressants from different classes such as MAOIs and SSRIs are coprescribed.
    - The time between weaning from one antidepressant drug to initiating another is inadequate to compensate for the first antidepressant's half-life.
    - Other serotonergic agonists, drugs that stimulate serotonin receptors, are combined with antidepressant therapy. Serotonergic agonists include dextromethorphan (Benylin, Pertussin, Delsym), meperidine (Demerol), and lithium (Eskalith, Lithane).
  - Management:
    - Temporarily withholding the antidepressant.
    - If symptoms are severe, anxiolytic drugs such as diazepam (Valium), beta-adrenergic blockers such as propranolol (Inderal), or skeletal muscle relaxants such as dantrolene (Dantrium) while supporting breathing with mechanical ventilation may be needed.
- Identify the reasons ECT is used in the management of depression.
  - To relieve depressive symptoms by causing a brief seizure either increasing circulating levels of monoamine neurotransmitters or by improving transmission to the receptor site.
- Three interventions that are alternatives to electroconvulsive therapy for recurrent depression:
  - VNS
  - DBS
  - TMS
- Nursing measures that are useful in preventing suicide:
  - *Suicide precaution*
  - Confiscation of sharps
  - Check on client every 15 minutes or 1:1 observation
  - Admin meds, mouth check
  - Ongoing assessment of suicidal ideation
- SAD, its treatment, and nursing management:
  - Mood disorder that has its onset during darker winter months and spontaneously disappears in the spring, triggered by photoperiods, daytime hours that are short because of fewer hours of sunlight
  - Treatment: phototherapy
  - Nursing Management: avoid sunglasses, add lamps, keep windows uncovered, skylights, exercise.
- Bipolar disorder, its treatment, and nursing management:
  - Involves cycling among depressive, euthymic, and euphoric
  - Bipolar I: severely dysfunctional moods lasting several months; depressive phases tend to be longer than manic phases.
    - May also manifest psychotic symptoms—delusions and hallucinations
  - Bipolar II: severe depression alternating with hypomania between periods of euthymia
    - Never have psychotic symptoms
  - *Cyclothymic disorder*, a subtype of bipolar II disorder
    - Milder mood swings occurring abruptly and with short duration; never free of symptoms for more than 2 months.
  - *Mixed bipolar disorder*: mania and depression occur simultaneously; grandiosity, high energy, irritable, anger

- *Rapid-cycling bipolar disorder*: at least four episodes of mania and depression per year
- *Ultrarapid-cycling bipolar disorder*: alternating moods that may occur within a month or less
  - Treatment: medication management
  - Nursing management:
    - Orient client to person, place, time, and events.
    - Provide information in small amounts using brief sentences.
    - Reduce distracting stimuli such as noise and stimulation.
    - Present reality when client is delusional; do not press the issue if it causes agitation.
    - Monitor client's whereabouts to ensure that they do not wander from the unit or health care agency.

CRITICAL THINKING EXERCISES

1. Two clients who are depressed are in a psychiatric hospital. One feels suicidal but has no plan for carrying out the suicide. The other indicates that they would kill themselves with a gun but has none. Describe the similarities and differences in their nursing care.
2. What physical consequences might occur for the client in a manic episode?
3. What problems might family members experience as a result of living with a person with a mood disorder?
4. Based on what is known about SAD, explain why people with this condition feel energized in the spring and are unmotivated when winters have prolonged periods of cloudy, rainy weather.

NCLEX-STYLE REVIEW QUESTIONS PrepU

1. A cyclic antidepressant is prescribed for a client with major depression. What information should the nurse include in the health teaching for the client and family? Select all that apply.
   1. The client should rise slowly to avoid hypotension.
   2. It may take 2 to 3 days before noting any change in mood.
   3. SAD may develop.
   4. This drug is highly lethal if an overdose is taken.
   5. Convulsions are a potential side effect.
2. When assessing a client who has just returned from having ECT, what should the nurse be especially alert for? Select all that apply.
   1. Disorientation
   2. Muscle aches
   3. Hypotension
   4. Foggy memory
   5. Generalized seizure
3. Immediately after administering an antidepressant to a client who is at risk for suicide, what nursing intervention is most appropriate?
   1. Observing the client at least every 15 minutes
   2. Inspecting the client's mouth and oral cavity
   3. Spending time interacting with the client
   4. Exploring alternatives to suicide with the client
4. When reviewing the lithium level of a client with bipolar disorder, what laboratory finding indicates a therapeutic level?
   1. 0.3 mEq
   2. 0.5 mEq
   3. 1.2 mEq
   4. 1.8 mEq
5. What instructions should a nurse provide to a client who depends on lithium to control bipolar disorder? Select all that apply.
   1. Ensure adequate exercise.
   2. Drink ample amounts of fluid.
   3. Ensure an adequate intake of salt.
   4. Have regular laboratory tests.
   5. Do not eat aged, hard cheese.

WANT TO KNOW MORE? There are a wide variety of online resources available on thePoint to enhance learning and understanding of this chapter.

Go to **thePoint.lww.com/activate** and use the activation code found in the front of this text to unlock these online resources.

70

Caring for Clients With Eating Disorders

Words To Know

adipocytes
anorexia nervosa
atypical anorexia nervosa
avoidant/restrictive food intake disorder
bariatric surgery
binge eating disorder
body mass index
bulimarexia
bulimia nervosa
compulsive overeating
corticotropin-releasing hormone
diabulimia
eating disorders
endocannabinoids
enmeshment
food binges
lanugo
leptin
melanin-concentrating hormone
normal eating
orexin A
orexin B
purging
Russell sign
satiety
water loading

Learning Objectives

On completion of this chapter, you will be able to:

1. Differentiate normal eating from an eating disorder.
2. Name four types of eating disorders.
3. Describe two forms of anorexia nervosa.
4. Name the neurotransmitters, neurohormones, and other chemicals that affect the appetite and satiety center in the brain.
5. Discuss two reasons why most people with anorexia nervosa induce self-starvation.
6. Identify the tool used to evaluate a person's size in relation to norms within the adult population.
7. Give the healthy range for body mass index.
8. List four components of treatment for clients with anorexia nervosa.
9. Discuss the nurse's role in managing the care of a client with anorexia nervosa.
10. Give two examples of how people with bulimia nervosa compensate for binging.
11. Name two problems, besides nutrition, that are the nursing focus when caring for clients with bulimia nervosa.
12. Differentiate between binge eating disorder and compulsive overeating.
13. Discuss at least three psychosocial problems that may accompany overeating syndromes.
14. Describe nursing care for a client with binge eating disorder or compulsive overeating.
15. Name at least two types of bariatric surgery and potential complications.

To preserve health, a rich variety of foods that are sufficient for energy needs, growth and repair of cells, and maintenance of weight is required. Depending on such variables as gender, age, physical condition, activity level, and height, normal eating involves consuming approximately 1500 to 2500 calories/day, usually spread over three meals and two to three snacks. **Normal eating** occurs in response to hunger and ceases when **satiety** (a feeling of comfortable fullness) is attained. This chapter deals with conditions that involve eating disorders, many of which begin with unsuccessful dieting. Collectively, **eating disorders** involve eating that:

- Is outside the range of normal
- Is accompanied by anxiety and guilt
- Results in physiologic imbalances or medical complications

Gerontologic Considerations

- Eating disorders in the older population may be overlooked or inaccurately diagnosed, resulting in physical complications or death. Accurate assessment promotes interventions for age-related changes or effects of chronic conditions, including:
- Reduced appetite from diminished taste or smell or from medication side effects.
- Reduced physical abilities that interfere with obtaining, preparing, or eating food.
- Changes in teeth that may necessitate nutrient intake in liquid or semiliquid form.
- Reduction of fiber in solid foods can contribute to constipation that further reduces appetite.
- Alcohol consumption may substitute for food intake, thereby decreasing nutrient availability.
- Alcohol intake contributes to gastric mucosa changes that decrease absorption of nutrients.
- Older adults with significant weight loss should be assessed for major depression, which may manifest with loss of appetite and minimal eating.
- Older adults sometimes simply refuse to eat as a form of protest or in an effort to seek validation of self-worth, resulting in self-starvation. Self-starvation may also be a reaction to health problems such as cognitive decline, terminal disease, or inability to cope with other losses. Self-starvation related to major depression or faulty coping skills is not classified as an eating disorder.

Clinically significant eating disorders affect from 20 million women to 10 million men in the United States at some time in their life (National Eating Disorders Association, 2018). The statistical numbers vary because many of those affected go unreported. Often, clients with eating disorders strive to keep their illness secret; family and friends may become aware of the problem only when emotional and behavioral symptoms become repeatedly noticeable (Table 70-1) or when serious health consequences develop. Box 70-1 is a self-test that can assist people in determining if an eating pattern is abnormal.

BOX 70-1 Eating Behavior Self-Test

____ Even though people tell me I'm thin, I feel fat.
____ I get anxious if I can't exercise.
____ My menstrual periods are irregular or absent (women).
____ My sex drive is not as strong as it used to be (men).
____ I worry about what I will eat.
____ If I gain weight, I get anxious or depressed.
____ I would rather eat by myself than with family or friends.
____ Other people talk about the way I eat.
____ I get anxious when people urge me to eat.
____ I don't talk much about my fear of being fat because no one understands how I feel.
____ I enjoy cooking for others, but I don't usually eat what I've cooked.
____ I have a secret stash of food.
____ When I eat, I'm afraid I won't be able to stop.
____ I lie about what I eat.
____ I don't like to be bothered or interrupted when I'm eating.
____ If I were thinner, I would like myself better.
____ I have missed work or school because of my weight or eating habits.
____ I tend to be depressed and irritable.
____ I feel guilty when I eat.
____ I avoid some people because they bug me about the way I eat.
____ My eating habits and fear of food interfere with friendships or romantic relationships.
____ I cut my food into tiny pieces, eat it on special plates, make patterns on my plate with it, or spit it out before swallowing it.
____ I am hardly ever satisfied with myself.
____ I have taken laxatives to control my weight.
____ I have vomited to control my weight.
____ I want to be thinner than my friends.
____ I have said or thought, "I would rather die than be fat."
____ I have fasted to lose weight.
____ In romantic moments, I cannot let myself go because I am worried about my fat and flab.

If you answer yes to any of these questions, discuss your eating habits with your primary provider.

TABLE 70-1 Signs and Symptoms of Eating Disorders

EATING DISORDER	PHYSICAL	EMOTIONAL	BEHAVIORAL
Anorexia nervosa	Decrease of 25% in body weight; lanugo; alopecia; cold intolerance; amenorrhea; constipation; abdominal pain	Distorted body image; hatred of a particular body part or body size; low self-esteem; depression; isolation; perfectionism	Restriction of food choices and intake; ritualistic handling of food (e.g., cutting into tiny pieces, arranging food in a certain way); weighing oneself frequently; denial of hunger
Bulimia nervosa	Inability to interpret accurately hunger and fullness signals; swelling of parotid glands ("chipmunk cheeks"); frequent weight fluctuations; irregular menses	Feeling unable to control eating; depressive mood and frequent mood swings; black-and-white thinking; exaggerated concern about weight	Excessive exercise, use of diuretics, and laxatives; secret eating of high-calorie, high-carbohydrate foods; alternately binging and fasting
Binge eating and compulsive overeating	Obesity; discomfort after eating	Preoccupation with weight, eating, and dieting; attributes professional and social success and failure to weight; feels disgust or guilt after eating; feels lack of control over eating	Frequent dieting; restricts activities because of embarrassment about weight; eating when not hungry; rapid eating; eating alone

Anorexia nervosa, bulimia nervosa, binge eating, and compulsive overeating are examples of major eating disorders. Obesity is a consequence of overeating; therefore, some clients who are obese also have an eating disorder.

ANOREXIA NERVOSA

Anorexia nervosa is an eating disorder characterized by an obsession for thinness that is achieved through self-starvation. It occurs more often in women, especially adolescents. Although men also have eating disorders, they are less likely to disclose this type of information with a health care provider, and when they do, the information is often dismissed, untreated, and unreported.

People with anorexia nervosa consume an average of 600 to 900 calories/day and often less. They feel hunger but control the urge to eat because of a morbid fear of becoming fat. Almost universally, people with anorexia consider themselves obese despite appearing emaciated.

There are two major types of anorexia: (1) severe restriction of caloric intake or just water and (2) **bulimarexia**, extended self-starvation interrupted by binging and purging or exercising, which is more common than classic anorexia nervosa. Other forms of anorexia are identified in the most recent edition of the *Diagnostic and Statistical Manual of Mental Disorders* (American Psychiatric Association, 2013). They include **atypical anorexia nervosa** (anorexia without low weight), **avoidant/restrictive food intake disorder** (in which children become malnourished because of the limited variety of foods they will eat), and **diabulimia** (which refers to the restriction of insulin by Type 1 diabetics for the purpose of weight loss) (National Association of Anorexia Nervosa and Associated Disorders, 2021).

Pathophysiology and Etiology

The exact cause of anorexia nervosa is unknown. Many authorities believe that anorexia and other eating disorders result from a combination of cultural, social, psychological, and physiologic factors. Growing evidence is strengthening the connection between genetics and altered physiology (Bulik, Blake, & Austin, 2018; Hübel et al., 2019; Mayhew et al., 2018).

Cultural and Social Factors

Culturally and socially, young women and men are influenced by role models in the media—people who are extremely thin. It is suggested that thinness is linked to attractiveness and success. However, the image being portrayed as ideal is, for most people, unhealthy and unrealistic. Self-starvation or rigorous physical activity is sometimes the only way to achieve a similar appearance. Some athletes such as gymnasts, ice skaters, and even ballet dancers restrict food intake, assuming that low body weight will improve performance.

Physiologic Factors

Physiologic influences also play a major role in the development of eating disorders. Research suggests that neurotransmitters and neurohormones, which may be genetically altered, influence normal and abnormal eating patterns by binding with receptors in the appetite center of the hypothalamus. People with anorexia may experience a dysregulation of serotonin and dopamine. Increased serotonin levels contribute to restricted eating; the brain is fooled into believing satiety has occurred (Södersten et al., 2019; Yabut et al., 2019). Support for this phenomenon is evidenced by the fact that drugs that increase serotonin, such as some selective serotonin reuptake inhibitors (SSRIs; see Chapter 69), produce weight loss as a side effect.

Normal levels of dopamine influence both realistic thinking, pleasure, and reward. An excess of dopamine may interfere with the ability to recognize and respond appropriately to the potential health hazards of self-starvation. Another hypothesis is that anorectics find the voluntary reduction of food intake as rewarding (Compan, 2020; Duriez et al., 2019).

It has been reported that slightly less than one fifth of eating disorder clients also have additional lifetime diagnosis of obsessive-compulsive disorder (OCD; see Chapter 68) caused by imbalances of serotonin and dopamine (Ekern & Karges, 2014; Mandelli et al., 2020; Rantala et al., 2019). There is speculation that those who manifest eating disorders are driven by low self-esteem due to perfectionist standards, social comparison, and an aspiration of being in control and use compulsive behaviors to attain this (Alosso, 2014; Bóna et al., 2021; Lopes, Melo, & Dias Pereira, 2020).

Recently, investigators have located receptors in the human brain for **melanin-concentrating hormone**, a hypothalamic neuropeptide that regulates eating and energy (Ploj et al., 2016). In animal studies, low levels of this hormone caused weight loss, and high levels promoted obesity. **Leptin**, a substance produced by fat cells known as **adipocytes**, has added another piece to the puzzle of eating disorders. Leptin acts on receptors in the hypothalamus, where high levels inhibit food intake. In addition, some speculate that there are interrelated endocrine disturbances in pituitary, adrenal, thyroid, and reproductive hormones. For example, **corticotropin-releasing hormone** acts as a major anorexic signal that limits the consumption of calories, increases energy expenditure, and promotes sustained weight loss.

Psychological Factors

It has been noted that people with anorexia nervosa are often perfectionists, have low self-esteem, and possess an intense desire to please others. Refusal to eat is also considered a form of self-control used to cope with stressful life experiences or dysfunctional family relationships (Anderson, 2019; Bóna et al., 2021; Lopes, Melo, & Dias Pereira, 2020; Lavis, 2018).

Complications

Failure to consume adequate nourishment eventually deprives all body systems of the nutritional elements required for homeostasis, growth, and cellular repair. Low levels of serum estrogen lead to amenorrhea and infertility, osteopenia (low bone mass), and premature osteoporosis (severe demineralization of bones), the latter of which can result in stress fractures, particularly of the spine and hips. Starvation contributes to vitamin deficiencies, fluid and electrolyte imbalances, and, finally, death from cardiac failure or arrhythmias.

Assessment Findings

Signs and Symptoms

Clients with anorexia nervosa may appear skeletonlike and may weigh extremely less than others of similar build, age, and height. In addition, they develop a growth of fine body hair called **lanugo**; in the absence of subcutaneous fat, lanugo helps maintain body temperature by preventing heat loss. In addition, clients with anorexia tend to be hypotensive and may have an irregular, low pulse rate. Severe malnutrition causes clients to be constipated, feel cold most of the time, have frequent infections, and females cease menstruating (Fig. 70-1). Many conceal their starvation by hiding or disposing of food and dressing in bulky clothing. When clients with anorexia are confronted with the fact that they are in danger of dying, they deny the seriousness of others' concerns.

Diagnostic Findings

Body mass index (BMI), a mathematical computation based on height and weight (Box 70-2), is used to evaluate a person's size in relation to norms within the adult population. In people with anorexia, the BMI is typically 16 or less. Anemia is usually present, and electrolyte levels, especially potassium and sometimes sodium, are often dangerously low. Deficiencies in serum proteins are reflected in low albumin, transferrin, and ferritin levels. Cardiac irregularities are identified by electrocardiography. Bone densitometry studies are used to determine whether osteopenia is present and, if so, how severe it has become.

>>> *Stop, Think, and Respond 70-1*

Besides having weight that is less than normal for height, what other findings suggest that a person who is underweight has anorexia nervosa?

BOX 70-2 Body Mass Index Formula, Calculation, and Interpretation

Formula

$$\text{BMI} = \frac{\text{weight (kg)}}{\text{height (m}^2)}$$

Calculation

1. Divide weight in pounds by 2.2 to convert to weight in kilograms (kg).
2. Divide height in inches by 39.4 to convert to height in meters (m).
3. Square the answer in step 2 by multiplying the number times itself; this gives the height in m^2.
4. Divide the weight (kg) by the height (m^2).

Interpretation

Anorectic	BMI ≤ 16
Underweight	BMI = 16–18.5
Healthy	BMI = 18.5–24.9
Overweight	BMI = 25–29.9
Obese	BMI = 30–34.9
Severely obese	BMI = 35–39.9
Extremely obese	BMI ≥ 40

Medical Management

Treatment of anorexia nervosa involves nutritional therapy, which is most critical initially, drug therapy, psychotherapy, and family counseling. Nutritional therapy includes providing nourishing meals, supplemental vitamins and minerals, intravenous fluids and electrolytes, tube feedings, or total parenteral nutrition. Once the client's weight improves or stabilizes, outpatient treatment may begin.

The resumption of normal eating behaviors, not simply restoring body weight, is the focus of nutritional treatment. Initially, as few as 1500 calories may be prescribed because large amounts of food, as well as high-fat foods and

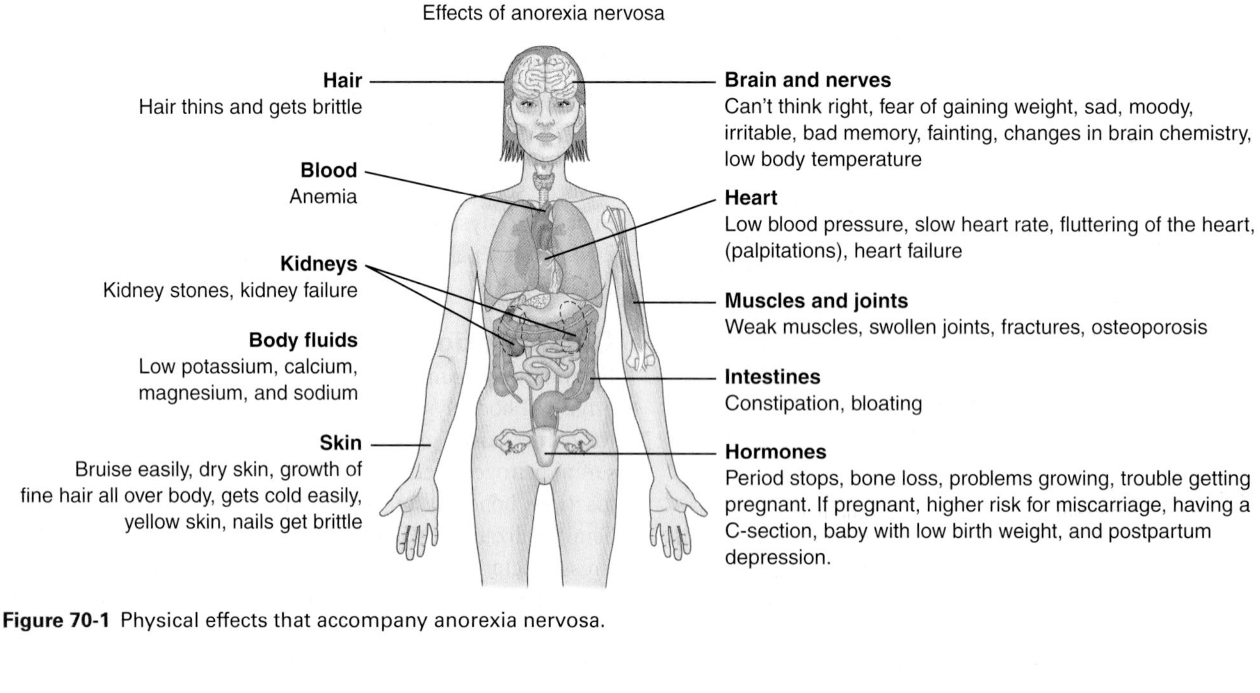
Effects of anorexia nervosa
Hair
Hair thins and gets brittle
Blood
Anemia
Kidneys
Kidney stones, kidney failure
Body fluids
Low potassium, calcium, magnesium, and sodium
Skin
Bruise easily, dry skin, growth of fine hair all over body, gets cold easily, yellow skin, nails get brittle
Brain and nerves
Can't think right, fear of gaining weight, sad, moody, irritable, bad memory, fainting, changes in brain chemistry, low body temperature
Heart
Low blood pressure, slow heart rate, fluttering of the heart, (palpitations), heart failure
Muscles and joints
Weak muscles, swollen joints, fractures, osteoporosis
Intestines
Constipation, bloating
Hormones
Period stops, bone loss, problems growing, trouble getting pregnant. If pregnant, higher risk for miscarriage, having a C-section, baby with low birth weight, and postpartum depression.

Figure 70-1 Physical effects that accompany anorexia nervosa.

Client and Family Teaching 70-1 Anorexia Nervosa

The nurse counsels and educates family members by offering the following suggestions:

- Focus on the person with anorexia rather than on the eating disorder itself.
- Give unconditional acceptance to the person with anorexia.
- Avoid making the person with anorexia feel guilty for the family distress that the disorder causes in daily living.
- Give the person with anorexia the power to make decisions and facilitate changes in matters other than eating.
- Avoid being manipulated by the person with anorexia.
- Demonstrate united support for one another and the plan for the client's treatment.
- Prepare for rehospitalization if the client becomes medically unstable or experiences a relapse.

gas-forming vegetables, may cause gastrointestinal discomfort and constipation. No foods are restricted, but so-called diet foods (e.g., artificially sweetened beverages and fat-free foods) should be avoided. Ongoing nutritional counseling may be needed throughout the maintenance period.

To promote adherence to the weight gain regimen, behavioral therapy (see Chapter 68) is instituted. By eating appropriately, the client earns privileges for having visitors and participating in social and physical activities. The privileges are used to reinforce desired behavior.

Antidepressant medications such as SSRIs are administered to manage depressive and obsessive symptoms (Himmerich & Treasure, 2017). Atypical antipsychotics such as olanzapine (Zyprexa), aripiprazole (Abilify), and others block dopamine receptors, resulting in a reduction of altered perception of weight, fears about gaining weight, denial of the seriousness of low body weight, and actual promotion of weight gain (Attia et al., 2019; Frank, 2014; Spettigue et al., 2018). Supplemental vitamins and minerals such as those containing iron, potassium, and calcium may be included in the therapeutic regimen to compensate for natural sources that are not being consumed as a result of the client's self-imposed fast. Stool softeners or laxatives may be necessary to counteract the constipation due to the absence of dietary fiber.

Individual, group, and cognitive psychotherapy (see Chapter 68) are used to help clients gain an insight into their distorted perceptions of thinness and the motivations for persisting in weight-loss behaviors (Client and Family Teaching 70-1). Counseling and involvement in self-help groups for several years are often indicated. See Evidence-Based Practice 70-1.

Family counseling is aimed at relieving the power struggle between the client and those who try to convince the client to eat. It also focuses on learning skills for undoing **enmeshment**—a pattern in which two or more people lack limits that separate one person from another, resulting in a loss of personal identity and exclusion of others.

Evidence-Based Practice 70-1

Genetics and Environment Related to Anorexia Nervosa

Clinical Question

In clients with anorexia nervosa, how do genetics compared with environmental factors affect the incidence of anorexia nervosa?

Evidence

In the United States, individuals with a lifetime history of an eating disorder have five to six times higher risk of suicide than individuals without an eating disorder (Udo, Bitley, & Grilo, 2019). Anorexia nervosa carries one of the highest mortality rates across all psychiatric disorders with suicide being the leading cause of death. In fact, suicide accounts for approximately 20% of deaths in this population (Thornton et al., 2016). Historically, it has been thought that environmental factors, especially those around family attitudes regarding eating and weight, relationships, and communication, were at the root of an adolescent developing anorexia nervosa (Brandys et al., 2015; Bulik et al., 2019; Dring, 2015). However, in recent years, researchers have begun uncovering what appear to be strong genetic connections between disorders such as anxiety, depression, and anorexia nervosa (Duncan, Yilmaz, & Gaspar, 2017). Researchers such as Brandys et al. (2016) and Thornton et al. (2016) discovered higher than expected rates of anorexia nervosa in clients with depression and suicide attempts during a study on a large cohort of identical twins, suggesting genetic factors may influence development of anorexia nervosa. Steinhausen et al. (2015) also looked at a very large group of families across three generations for the incidence of anorexia nervosa. In a study of over 2300 people who were diagnosed with a psychiatric disorder before the age of 18, many were diagnosed with anorexia nervosa at some point in their lives. The incidence of anorexia nervosa was significantly higher in this group than in families, where there was no incidence of a psychiatric disorder before the age of 18. Risk factors for developing anorexia nervosa included having a sibling with anorexia nervosa, the presence of a psychiatric diagnosis such as anxiety, OCD, affective or personality disorders, and substance use disorders. In addition, being female also appeared to increase the likelihood of having anorexia nervosa.

Nursing Implications

With the possibility that genetics may play a part in clients' developing anorexia nervosa, it is important for the nurse to include a thorough family history to assess for anorexia nervosa in siblings as well as family members with psychiatric disorders such as anxiety, depression, substance use disorders, and suicide attempts. Because

(*continued*)

Evidence-Based Practice 70-1 (*continued*)

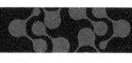

environmental factors are still thought to contribute to a client developing anorexia nervosa as well, questions around family attitudes/ideas around eating and weight, family relationships, communication styles, and conflict within the family should also be included. Globally, the World Health Organization (WHO, 2019) identifies suicide as the third leading cause of death in adolescents, while the National Institute of Mental Health (NIMH, 2021) identifies it as the second leading cause of death in the United States. As such, it is also important for the nurse to include a suicide risk assessment with clients who fall in this age range.

References

Brandys, M. K., de Kovel, C. G. F., Kas, M. J., van Elburg, A. A., & Adan, R. A. H. (2015). Overview of genetic research in anorexia nervosa: The past, the present and the future. *International Journal of Eating Disorders, 48*(7), 814–825. https://doi.org/10.1002/eat.22400

Bulik, C. M., Flatt, R., Abbaspour, A., & Carroll, I. (2019). Reconceptualizing anorexia nervosa. *Psychiatry and Clinical Neurosciences, 73*(9), 518–525. https://doi.org/10.1111/pcn.12857

Dring, G. (2015). Anorexia runs in families: Is this due to genes or the family environment? *Journal of Family Therapy, 37*(1), 79–92. https://doi.org/10.1111/1467-6427.12048

Duncan, L.; Yilmaz, Z., & Gaspar, H., Walters, R., Goldstein, J., Anttila, V., Bulik-Sullivan, B., Ripke, S., Eating Disorders Working Group of the Psychiatric Genomics Consortium; Thornton, L., Hinney, A., Daly, M., Sullivan, P. F., Zeggini, E., Breen, G., & Bulik, C. M. (2017). Significant locus and metabolic genetic correlations revealed in genome-wide association study of anorexia nervosa. *American Journal of Psychiatry, 174*, 850–858. https://doi.org/10.1176/appi.ajp.2017.16121402

National Institute of Mental Health. (2021). *Suicide.* https://www.nimh.nih.gov/health/statistics/suicide.shtml

Steinhausen, H., Jakobsen, H., Helenius, D., Munk-Jørgensen, P., & Strober, M. (2015). A nation-wide study of the family aggregation and risk factors in anorexia nervosa over three generations. *International Journal of Eating Disorders, 48*(1), 1–8. https://doi.org/10.1002/eat.22293

Thornton, L. M., Welch, E., Munn-Chernoff, M., Lichtenstein, P., & Bulik, C. M. (2016). Anorexia nervosa, major depression, and suicide attempts: Shared genetic factors. *Suicide & Life-Threatening Behavior, 46*(5), 525–534. https://doi.org/10.1111/sltb.12235

Udo, T.; Bitley, S., & Grilo, C. M. (2019). Suicide attempts in US adults with lifetime DSM-5 eating disorders. *BMC Medicine, 17*(1), 120. https://doi.org/10.1186/s12916-019-1352-3

World Health Organization. (2019). *Suicide fact sheet.* https://www.who.int/en/news-room/fact-sheets/detail/suicide

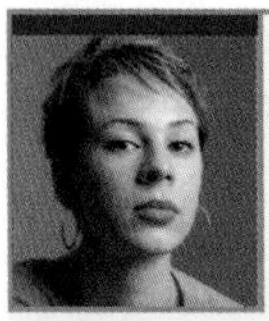

Clinical Scenario A 19-year-old college student came home for semester break, and her parents were surprised by how thin she had become. She weighed 92 lb, a loss of nearly 30 lb from her previous weight of 121 lb prior to attending college. Based on her current weight and height of 5 feet 6 inches, her calculated BMI is 14.8. Although she denied the seriousness of her weight loss, arguing that she was healthy and, in fact, thought it would be even better if she lost more weight, her parents made an appointment with the family primary provider. During the appointment, the primary provider determined that she had not menstruated in the past 3 months and had a potassium level of 3.4 mEq/dL. The primary provider referred the student to an eating disorder facility, where she would be reevaluated by the staff and receive treatment. **What would a plan of care include when caring for this client or others with anorexia nervosa? Refer to Nursing Care Plan 70-1.**

NURSING CARE PLAN 70-1 The Client With Anorexia Nervosa

Assessment

- Monitor vital signs initially and on a regular basis to detect low body temperature, hypothermia, bradycardia, and hypotension.
- Perform a physical assessment.
- Observe signs of malnutrition such as the absence of body fat, dry skin, and scalp hair; the presence of fine hair covering the body; edema from hypoproteinemia; and cold hands and feet.
- Weigh the client as accurately as possible with minimal clothing, and calculate the BMI (see Box 70-2).
- Obtain a nutritional history.
- Ask the client whether they restrict food intake or combines it with purging. Keep in mind that excessive exercise is also a form of purging.
- Ask the female client for the date of her last menstrual period.
- Observe the client's mood and anxiety level.
- Ask the client about family dynamics and other stressors.

Nursing Diagnosis. **Malnutrition Risk (Less Than Body Requirements)** related to food restriction, emaciated appearance, signs of avitaminosis, and electrolyte imbalance

Expected Outcomes. (1) The client will gain 2 to 5 lb by a mutually agreed target date; (2) the client will attain and maintain a BMI of at least 16.

Interventions	Rationales
Consistently assign the same few nurses to the client's care.	*Limiting staff relationships promotes a therapeutic alliance, consistency, and reduces the potential for manipulation.*

NURSING CARE PLAN 70-1 The Client With Anorexia Nervosa (*continued*)

Establish a contract with the client for expected weight restoration and target date; include the rewards for reaching goals and consequences for failure.	*Participating in setting goals promotes self-involvement and a sense of ownership in the plan. Identifying positive and negative consequences makes the client aware of how outcomes in the therapeutic plan will be managed.*
Weigh the client regularly, but randomly.	*Random weights are generally more accurate. They prevent the client from* **water loading***, a technique in which anorexic clients attempt to demonstrate weight gain by consuming a large volume of water and avoiding urination before being weighed.*
Work with the dietitian to provide at least 6 to 8 meals each day, beginning with low caloric value, then gradually increase the total calories.	*Large meals are not tolerated when the stomach has shrunk. The client is much more likely to work toward weight gain if food is offered frequently and is not heavily calorie-loaded. To gain 1 lb of weight, a person must consume 3500 calories that are not used for basic metabolism and activities.*

Interventions	Rationales
Observe or sit with the client during meals.	*Being observed prevents the client from hiding food rather than eating it.*
Remove the dietary tray after 30 minutes without commenting on food that has not been eaten.	*Removal of food at the designated time avoids a power struggle. Negative comments reinforce that the client was victorious in resisting the urge to eat. Withholding any comments avoids an adversarial image.*
Record the type and amount of food consumed.	*Documentation provides information on which to evaluate the progress of the client and helps the dietitian calculate the client's caloric intake.*
Restrict the client's use of the bathroom for 2 hours after meals or accompany the client to the bathroom.	*A 2-hour restriction allows time for consumed food to enter the small intestine for absorption rather than being vomited.*
Give the client a liquid nutritional supplement for the uneaten calories at meals.	*Clients may consume calorie-loaded liquids in place of solid food.*
Implement behavioral rewards or consequences consistently and fairly.	*Deviation from guidelines or their inconsistent application reduces the effectiveness of the plan of care.*
Administer prescribed drug, vitamin, and mineral therapy, and ensure that the client attends group and individual psychotherapy.	*Resistance to the therapeutic regimen is common. Anorexia requires management with medical, nutritional, and psychological modalities.*

Collaborative Problem. **Related Complication (RC) of Electrolyte Imbalance** related to hypokalemia, bradycardia, hypotension

Expected Outcome. The nurse will monitor to detect, manage, and minimize cardiac arrhythmias.

Interventions	Rationales
Monitor heart rate and rhythm either manually or with telemetry or a Holter monitor.	*Hypokalemia increases the potential for sinus bradycardia or more lethal arrhythmias that can cause sudden death.*
Ensure that a resuscitation cart and emergency medications are readily available.	*A rapid response to cardiac arrest increases the potential for saving a client's life.*
Call for help and initiate cardiopulmonary resuscitation if the client has no pulse and is not breathing.	*Cardiopulmonary resuscitation can temporarily oxygenate blood and prevent brain damage.*
Assist with defibrillation.	*Automatic electrical defibrillation can restore normal sinus rhythm.*

Nursing Diagnosis. **Deconditioning** related to minimal consumption of food, emaciation, amenorrhea

Expected Outcome. The client will demonstrate efforts to achieve a healthier weight; menses will resume as weight increases.

(*continued*)

NURSING CARE PLAN 70-1 The Client With Anorexia Nervosa (*continued*)

Interventions	Rationales
Refer to nursing interventions for imbalanced nutrition.	*Improving nutrition will promote health and restore physical development.*
Observe the client for signs of depression.	*Feelings of unhappiness can affect eating patterns.*
Engage the client in a discussion of previous and current role changes.	*Helping the client gain an insight may motivate the client to implement healthier eating.*
Validate the client's feelings if they are realistic.	*Validation communicates that the nurse has empathy and reinforces reality.*
Explore the client's strengths and positive coping strategies.	*Current success at improving health can be linked to prior successes in problem-solving.*

Nursing Diagnosis. **Altered Body Image Perception** related to unrealistic perception of body size

Expected Outcome. The client will develop a realistic perception of self and an insight into the motivation for thinness.

Interventions	Rationales
Encourage the client to talk about perceptions of body image but avoid opposing the client's views.	*Disagreeing tends to further entrench the client's beliefs.*
Offer the observation that the fixation with weight control diverts attention and energy needed to deal with real issues surrounding psychosocial conflicts.	*Awareness is raised by offering an alternative point of view.*
Help the client clarify issues underlying the need to control weight gain and promote weight loss.	*Self-examination helps develop insight.*
Suggest that perfection is not possible and that no body image is worth dying for.	*Calling attention to the seriousness of the health problem may promote a modification in the client's behavior.*

Evaluation of Expected Outcomes

The client consumes nutritious food, resulting in a gradual weight gain and a BMI that is greater than 15. The client no longer perceives themselves as fat. The heart remains in normal sinus rhythm. Laboratory values indicate improvement in electrolytes and an improved ratio of fat to lean body mass.

There is evidence of insight on the part of the client, based on their self-disclosure, that withholding the consumption of food created a feeling of power and that it served as a means of controlling family stressors and achieving an unrealistic image of perfection.

Concept Mastery Alert

Anorexia Nervosa

If a client attending a clinic for eating disorders shows improvement in weight but shows no improvement in laboratory values, a likely cause is that the client is drinking water before weighing. Water loading could account for the poor lab values accompanied by weight gain.

BULIMIA NERVOSA

Bulimia nervosa is characterized by a minimum of two episodes of secret **food binges**—rapid consumption of a large number of calories per week followed by behaviors intended to prevent weight gain. For the condition to be considered true bulimia, the abnormal eating pattern must have persisted for at least 6 months. There are two different manifestations of bulimia: (1) binging followed by **purging** (elimination of nutrients, using self-induced vomiting, laxatives, enemas, or diuretics) and (2) binging followed by fasting, using diet pills, or engaging in excessive exercise (see Binge Eating Disorder and Compulsive Overeating section later in this chapter).

In contrast to clients with anorexia nervosa, clients with bulimia nervosa:

1. Are generally older at the onset of the disorder
2. Are overweight or normal weight
3. Admit that their eating behavior is abnormal
4. Are ashamed of habitually binging and purging

Pathophysiology and Etiology

It is believed that the hypothalamus is the center for appetite regulation. When the lateral area of hypothalamus is stimulated, people feel like eating; when the ventromedial area of the hypothalamus is stimulated, they feel satiated (full) and eating behavior ceases (Coccurello & Maccarrone, 2018;

King, 2016). These two areas of the hypothalamus are turned on and off by neurotransmitters. Research suggests that people with bulimia have a biochemically induced compulsion to eat as a result of increased sensitivity to norepinephrine within the hypothalamus and reduced levels of serotonin, which disguise the point of satiety. Because serotonin is synthesized from the essential amino acid tryptophan, it is believed that binge eating acts as a mechanism to supply tryptophan so as to increase serotonin levels, similar to how thirst stimulates drinking water or beverages to correct a deficit in fluid volume.

Two neurohormones, called **orexin A** and **orexin B** after the Greek word, *orexis*, meaning appetite, have been discovered. When laboratory animals were injected with orexin hormones, which attach to receptors in the lateral hypothalamus, the animals consumed 8 to 10 times the normal amount of food. This has led to the hypothesis that the levels of orexin A and B contribute to binge eating and obesity in humans. Leptin, a substance manufactured in human fat cells, is believed to suppress orexigenic (appetite-stimulating) chemicals. Therefore, binge eating may occur in the absence of leptin or reduced receptors for leptin (Cassiolo et al., 2020; King, 2016).

Whatever the cause, once a binge begins, it is difficult to control. During a binge, people with bulimia consume 3500 to 11,500 calories of food in 2 hours or less. Eating is terminated by one of the following:

- Abdominal pain
- Interruption (discovery by others)
- Sleeping

After the eating frenzy, bulimics feel so guilty that they purge, exercise, or fast (abstain from food, but not for days on end, as would someone with bulimarexia).

Complications

Repetitive regurgitation of gastric acids due to self-induced vomiting and use of emetics such as ipecac cause pharyngeal irritation and damage teeth by eroding the dental enamel (Fig. 70-2). Abuse of laxatives and enemas contributes to constipation. The nonprescribed use of diuretics and diet pills predisposes to fluid, electrolyte, and cardiac problems. Some people with bulimia also compulsively abuse drugs or alcohol. The shame and guilt may trigger suicidal thoughts or attempts.

Assessment Findings

Signs and Symptoms

Clients with bulimia tend to be of normal weight or slightly overweight; however, their weight can fluctuate as much as 10 lb in a week. Self-induced vomiting results in hoarseness, inflammation of the esophagus and oral pharynx, calluses on the back of the hand and fingers from repeatedly stimulating the gag reflex, erosion of tooth enamel, and swollen parotid glands.

Diagnostic Findings

Diagnosis is based on the clinical findings and a history of persistent binging and purging. Serum electrolytes may be altered, depending on the time that has elapsed since the last purge. A radiograph of the upper gastrointestinal tract shows an overstretched or stenotic esophagus from frequent regurgitation and inflammation followed by scarring.

Medical Management

Treatment of bulimia nervosa includes drug therapy with antidepressants (see Chapter 69), individual and group psychotherapy, and behavior modification techniques (see Chapter 68). Most clients are managed on an outpatient basis.

Nursing Management

Like people with anorexia, clients with bulimia nervosa need to resume normal eating behaviors and avoid restrictive practices. They may also need to accept a body weight higher than they would like. Identify and correct clients' fears and misconceptions about food and weight; clients who are persuaded to occasionally eat small amounts of high-calorie foods are less likely to binge later. Advise clients not to skip meals or snacks, to use appropriate utensils, not to pick at food, and not to feel guilty about occasional planned indulgences.

Provide emotional support and health teaching. Some important areas to reinforce during teaching include the following:

- Follow a dietary plan that is compatible with MyPlate, developed by the U.S. Department of Agriculture and the U.S. Department of Health and Human Services in 2011 (Fig. 70-3).
- Eat at a slow pace.
- Eat only in the presence of others.

Other aspects of the nurse's role in caring for clients with bulimia nervosa include, but is not limited to, those that relate to the following clinical scenario.

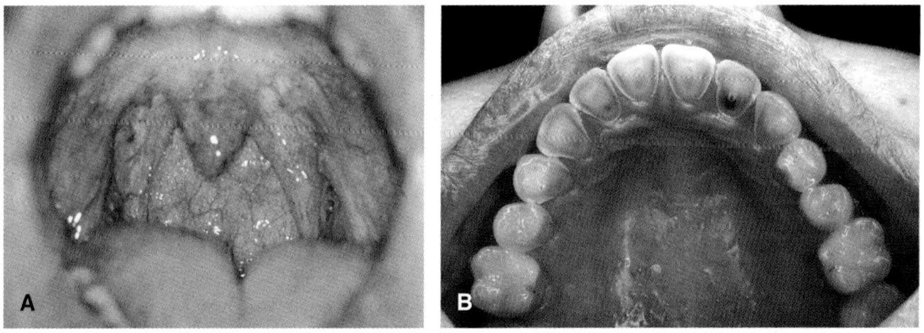

Figure 70-2 Signs of bulimia include **(A)** irritation and inflammation of the pharynx as well as the esophagus from chronic vomiting and **(B)** erosion of the lingual surface of the teeth, loss of dental enamel, periodontal disease, and extensive dental caries.

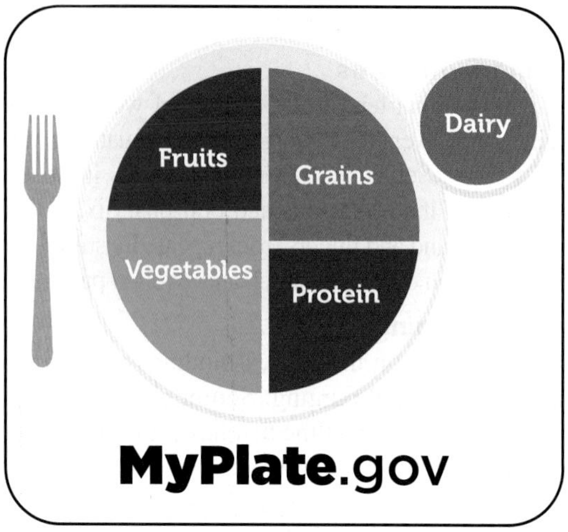

Figure 70-3 MyPlate is color-coded to show the five groups of food that should be consumed each day in the following proportions: 30% grains, of which half are preferably whole grains; 30% vegetables; 20% fruits; 20% proteins, which are accompanied by low-fat/nonfat milk; or other reduced fat dairy products (myplate.gov).

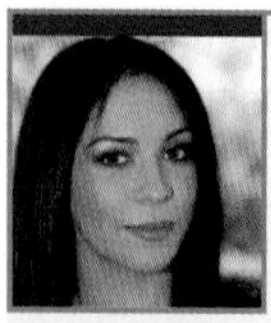

Clinical Scenario A 23-year-old woman began binging and purging in college. She would eat large volumes of food in secret and self-induce vomiting afterward out of a sense of guilt and remorse. She is currently married but has managed to conceal her cycle of binging and purging episodes. Many times when she is alone, she stops at fast food establishments and orders multiple high-calorie items that she eats rapidly in the car, or she waits until her husband is out of the house to begin a binge. She resolves over and over that she will stop this disordered pattern because she is unhappy about her weight, but she has not been able to do so independently. After her husband came home early from work and found multiple food packages in the kitchen and observed her vomiting in the bathroom, she confessed to him about her eating disorder. With his support, she intends to find a counselor who will help her overcome her condition. **How might a nurse help a client like this with bulimia nervosa? Consider the nursing actions in the discussion that follows.**

NURSING PROCESS FOR THE CLIENT WITH BULIMIA NERVOSA

Assessment

Obtain the client's history and current health information. Weigh the client, and calculate the BMI (see Box 70-2). Inspect the teeth to detect dental damage. Examine the conjunctiva for ruptured blood vessels caused by the rise in blood pressure during forced vomiting. Look for abrasions on the knuckles, known as **Russell sign**, caused by using the fingers to self-induce vomiting. Ask questions concerning (1) the frequency of binging and purging episodes, (2) the client's state of mind prior to a binge, (3) the types and amounts of food that are consumed during a binge, and (4) the nature of the purge. Take an inventory of medications, such as emetics, diuretics, and laxatives, or enemas that are used for purging. If exercise is the technique the client uses to purge, identify the type of activity and average duration of exercise.

Diagnosis, Planning, and Interventions

Imbalanced Nutrition. More Than Body Requirements: Related to compulsion to binge
Expected Outcomes: (1) The client will delay the urge to binge or purge. (2) The client will consume no more than 2000 to 3000 calories/day divided among three meals plus or minus snacks. (3) The client will maintain a stable weight.

- Help the client identify feelings, situations, or foods that trigger binging episodes. *Raising an awareness of triggering events can break the cycle of binging and purging.*
- Explore alternative coping strategies with the client for dealing with triggering stimuli. *Developing techniques for controlling impulses can abort a binging episode.*
- Explain to the client that starving leads to binging. *Eating slowly and regularly, in controlled amounts, reduces hunger.*
- Tell the client to restrict eating to the kitchen or dining room only at specific times. *Restricting the location for eating and the time during which food is eaten interferes with the usual patterns of binge eating. Private binges often take place in locations other than the usual places for eating, such as in the living room while watching television.*
- Instruct the client to wait at least 1 hour after a meal before succumbing to a binge. *Delaying a binge helps the client separate normal eating from abnormal eating and from turning a normal meal into a binge.*
- Discuss alternatives for aborting or interrupting the eating binges, such as eating with a family member or friend, calling a friend for support if alone, leaving the binging location, and stocking low-calorie food. *Binging takes place when the client with bulimia is alone and when there is a low potential for being discovered. Consuming low-calorie foods may create less anxiety and reduce the potential for purging.*
- Suggest that the client adulterate a known binge food such as dropping it in dirt or soaking it in vinegar if all else fails. *Making the food unpalatable is a behavior modification technique, called negative reinforcement, which may abort a binge.*

Altered Health Maintenance: Related to repeated contact between teeth and gastric acid secondary to chronic vomiting
Expected Outcome: The client's tooth enamel will be restored or maintained.

NURSING PROCESS FOR THE CLIENT WITH BULIMIA NERVOSA (continued)

- Rinse the mouth with plain water immediately after vomiting. *Plain water dilutes and rinses gastric acid from the surface of the teeth.*
- Drink plenty of water throughout the day. *Water contributes to an increased volume of saliva. Saliva helps to neutralize oral acidity and reharden tooth enamel because it contains calcium and phosphate.*
- Recommend brushing with an enamel protection toothpaste and a soft-bristle toothbrush and flossing the teeth, but wait 30 minutes after vomiting. *Gastric acid softens tooth enamel, and immediate brushing can contribute to further erosion.*
- Chew sugarless gum, preferably one containing xylitol, and crunchy fruits and vegetables. *Chewing increases the production of saliva.*
- Use a straw to drink beverages that are high in acid, such as fruit juices and carbonated beverages. *A straw limits contact between the beverage and teeth. Soft drinks contain phosphoric and citric acids that can damage tooth enamel.*
- Avoid or limit substances that contribute to dental caries and erosion of tooth enamel, such as gummy candy, caramels, citrus fruits, chewable vitamin C tablets, dried fruits, energy drinks, and starches that are cooked al dente. *These substances stick to teeth for a prolonged time and lead to dental caries.*
- Increase sources of foods containing calcium and phosphorus or take a mineral supplement. *Sources containing calcium and phosphorus replace minerals leached from the teeth.*
- Do not chew ice; popcorn kernels; or hard, crusty bread. *The force from biting and chewing can fracture weakened teeth.*
- Avoid whiteners that bleach teeth. *Whiteners can eventually erode enamel and cause a yellow tooth discoloration later in life.*
- Consult a cosmetic dentist. *A cosmetic dentist can mechanically restore the appearance of permanently damaged teeth with porcelain crowns, bonding, implants, or bridges.*

Risky Health Behavior: Related to inability to control chronic vomiting
Expected Outcome: The client will reduce or eliminate the health risk practice of chronic vomiting.

- Inquire how the client could be healthier. *Self-awareness is the first step in changing negative behavior.*
- Explain the medical complications that correlate with chronic vomiting or laxative abuse (Fig. 70-4). *Understanding health information can help promote appropriate health behaviors.*
- Explain psychosocial risks experienced by those with bulimia, such as alcohol and substance abuse, sexual promiscuity, and self-cutting. *Bulimics tend to be impulsive and experience powerlessness over compulsive behavior.*
- Convey confidence that the client has the ability to overcome the cycle of binging and purging. *Bulimics feel guilty that they are unable to resist binging and purging, but support may promote self-control.*
- Ask the client to identify foods or situations that trigger binging. *Eliminating triggers may help control binges.*
- Encourage the client to work with a dietitian to plan small meals at frequent intervals throughout the day. *Starvation promotes binging, and binging promotes purging. A dietitian has the expertise to develop a personalized plan for meeting nutritional needs while facilitating gradual weight loss.*
- Emphasize compliance with drug therapy treatment. *Restoring imbalanced neurotransmitters can promote control of symptoms.*
- Advocate consulting a psychiatrist. *Clients with bulimia can reduce or eliminate their disordered eating with cognitive behavioral therapy.*
- Suggest joining a support group involving others with a similar eating disorder. *Support and encouragement tend to be more meaningful when its source is someone else dealing with the same problem.*
- Avoid criticizing the client when relapses occur. *Criticism reinforces a client's guilt and powerlessness and alienates the nurse as a mentor.*

Coping Impairment: Related to managing guilty feelings by purging
Expected Outcome: The client will implement effective coping mechanisms for dealing with guilt and stressors.

- Acknowledge and compliment the client when binging or purging is controlled. *Positive reinforcement increases the potential that the behavior will be repeated.*
- Remain nonjudgmental when the client reports having binged or purged. *Increasing or adding to the client's shame reinforces the client's guilt.*
- Encourage the client to forgive themselves for binging and purging. *People with bulimia judge themselves severely after binging or purging.*
- Formulate a contract with the client to seek out the nurse or another support person when the client feels the urge to purge. *A contract is a useful tool for obtaining the client's compliance. Reducing the incidence of purging decreases the guilt a client feels.*
- Have the client discard all purging paraphernalia such as medications and enema equipment. *The inability to purge reduces potential guilt.*

Chronic Low Self-Esteem: Related to poor impulse control and ineffective methods to control weight
Expected Outcome: The client will report increased self-esteem.

(continued)

NURSING PROCESS FOR THE CLIENT WITH BULIMIA NERVOSA (continued)

- Discuss keeping a diary or journal where entries describe incidents when the urge to binge or purge was overcome. *A written record is an objective resource for self-evaluation of the client's progress.*
- Encourage the client to read previous diary or journal entries whenever negative thoughts intrude. *The client's own statements are self-affirming evidence that progress is being made.*
- Help dispel the faulty perception that losing control over binging and purging means that the client is a total failure. *Clients tend to overlook their positive attributes and condemn themselves because of a single weakness.*
- Refer the client to a dietitian. *Loss of weight without purging increases self-esteem.*

Evaluation of Expected Outcomes

Binging and purging are reduced or eliminated, and the client's caloric intake is in accordance with their metabolic needs. The client successfully implements alternative strategies for managing compulsive behaviors and has a positive regard for themselves.

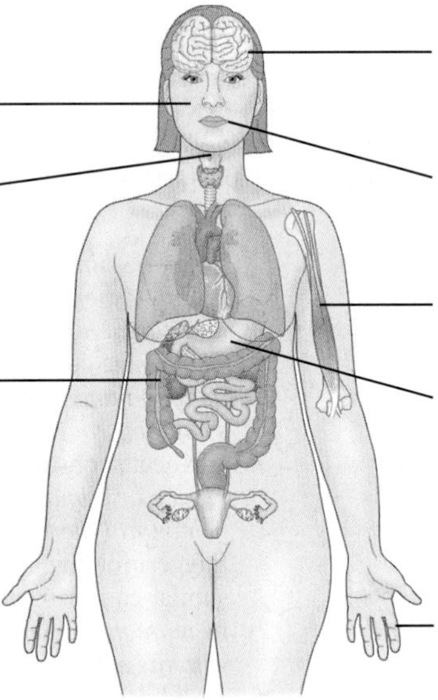

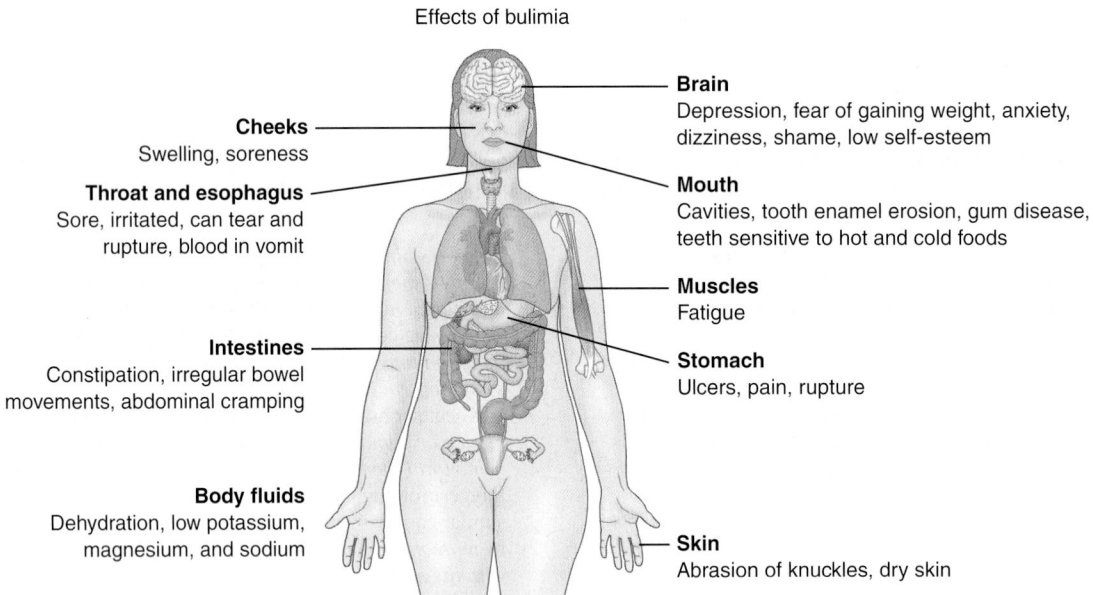

Figure 70-4 Effects of bulimia.

>>> ***Stop, Think, and Respond 70-2***

Where is the appetite center and what substances stimulate or suppress the appetite center?

BINGE EATING DISORDER AND COMPULSIVE OVEREATING

Binge eating disorder is characterized as the inability to control overeating, accompanied by a guilty feeling. However, people do not engage in compensating behaviors to prevent weight gain. **Compulsive overeating** is characterized as eating in the absence of hunger or regardless of feeling full. Some people have both problems simultaneously. Either may result in obesity with all of its consequences (Fig. 70-5).

Pathophysiology and Etiology

The cause of overeating syndromes is still unknown; some equate it with an addiction in which food is the drug of choice. Because people with eating disorders suffer from anxiety, depression, and compulsive behavior, there is growing evidence that biochemical factors are involved in binge eating and compulsive overeating. Similar to anorexia and bulimia nervosa, there is likely an imbalance of neurotransmitters such as norepinephrine, serotonin, and dopamine or neurohormones such as orexin A and B or leptin, which affect the appetite center in the brain. There may also be additional neuroendocrine disequilibrium involving cortisol, a hormone released by the adrenal cortex in response to stress (see Chapter 67); reduced cholecystokinin, a hormone secreted by the mucosa of the upper small intestine that causes laboratory animals to stop eating when they feel full; and imbalances in neuropeptides Y and YY, psychoactive chemicals that stimulate eating behavior in research animals. In 2001, scientists located brain receptors for **endocannabinoids**, natural chemicals with marijuana-like properties, that activate the appetite center (Jager & Whitkamp, 2014; Reichard, 2013; Yagin et al., 2020). The existence of endocannabinoids helps explain why marijuana users develop ravenous hunger called "the

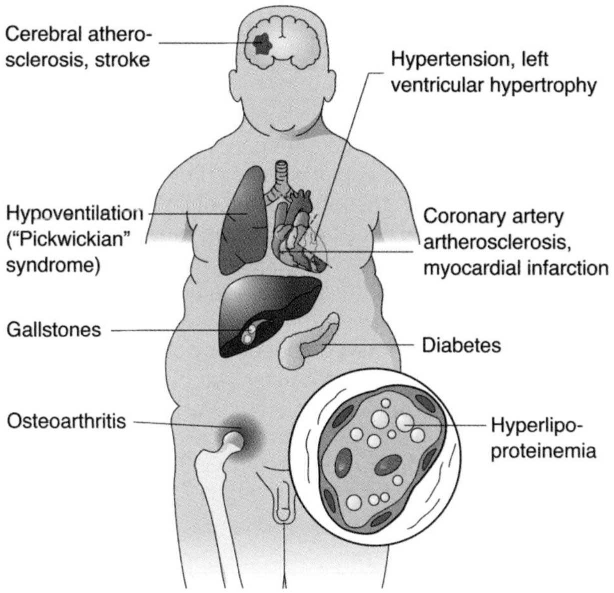

Figure 70-5 Consequences of obesity, compulsive overeating, and binge eating.

munchies," and why dronabinol (Marinol), synthetic tetrahydrocannabinol—the active ingredient in marijuana—helps clients with cancer and AIDS gain weight. Increased amounts of endocannabinoids or an increased sensitivity to their presence may explain some syndromes characterized by overeating. Also, the fact that many overeaters state they use food as a way of coping with stress should not be overlooked.

Complications

Ultimately, overeating leads to many physical and emotional problems. As a consequence of obesity, many people develop hyperlipidemia (elevated blood fat levels), hypertension, Type 2 diabetes, degenerative arthritis, and sleep apnea. There is a higher risk of gallbladder disease, heart disease, and some types of cancer. Many people feel unhappy, ashamed, and disgusted with themselves. They tend to become socially isolated to avoid being noticed and possibly rejected.

Assessment Findings

Signs and Symptoms

Overeaters are typically overweight and have a history of unsuccessful attempts at dieting. Clients tend to eat in solitary in the absence of hunger. They have preferences for high-sugar and high-fat foods that they may nibble over several hours or gorge on until they feel uncomfortably full but do not purge. Some report that they overeat or binge when they are angry, sad, bored, or anxious. They often have a history of other compulsive behaviors such as alcohol or drug abuse. Some reveal that they have considered suicide or have performed self-mutilation, such as cutting and burning themselves, pulling their hair, and interfering with wound healing to cope with their intense feelings, to punish themselves, or to experience physical pain to counteract the consequences of feeling emotionally numb.

Diagnostic Findings

People with overeating syndromes generally have a BMI of 30 or higher. Other laboratory and diagnostic tests reflect secondary complications from obesity such as elevated blood sugar, cholesterol, and serum lipid levels.

Medical Management

A comprehensive approach to treating overeating syndromes involves weight reduction, psychotherapy, and self-help support groups. The first step is a sensible weight-loss regimen prescribed by a dietitian. Strict dieting is discouraged because it tends to worsen binge eating.

Weight Reduction

Because it produces favorable health benefits and is more likely to be maintained, attaining a weight-loss goal of 10% to 20% rather than an "ideal" weight should be encouraged (Client and Family Teaching 70-2). It is estimated that 95% of people who lose weight regain it within 5 years, and some dieters gain back more than they originally lost. The newer approaches to weight management stress that all foods are acceptable and teach clients to recognize and differentiate between physiologic and psychological hunger. Support

Client and Family Teaching 70-2
Overeating Syndromes

The nurse counsels clients with overeating syndromes to:

- Obtain treatment from professionals who are experienced in treating eating disorders, and continue with this therapy.
- Follow the label directions for taking prescribed medications; report any untoward effects.
- Avoid popular nonprescription diet pills. These generally contain phenylpropanolamine and caffeine, which are central nervous system stimulants. They can increase heart rate and blood pressure and cause dizziness, irritability, insomnia, and dry mouth.
- Strict dieting or fasting is the leading cause of binging.
- Exercise on the advice of a primary provider to reduce the appetite and increase weight loss.
- Avoid nutritional and weight-loss centers because they generally do not offer the comprehensive services most clients need to keep from gaining weight once the target weight is reached.
- Read food labels, and understand that those that say "sugar free" or "contains no cholesterol" do not mean that the ingredients are calorie free or even of low caloric.
- Talk to a close friend or support person about feelings about food.
- Attend Overeaters Anonymous meetings. This is a free self-help group that is modeled after the 12-step program of Alcoholics Anonymous.
- Remember that recovery is a day-by-day process; it is self-defeating to dwell on the lack of previous success or relapses that may occur.

groups, such as Overeaters Anonymous or group therapy in eating disorder clinics, are helpful adjuncts to individual psychotherapy.

Drug Therapy

To help clients lose weight and remain compliant, short-term drug therapy may be used. Prescribed medications include antidepressants such as SSRIs (e.g., fluoxetine [Prozac]), which promote weight loss (see Chapter 69). Orlistat (Xenical), which interferes with intestinal absorption of dietary fat, has been available for weight loss for some time. The unabsorbed fat, however, must be eliminated rectally and is associated with oily stools that can be explosive. This side effect can be reduced by consuming less dietary fat, which would be beneficial with or without taking orlistat. Alli is a lower dosage of orlistat that is available without a prescription. Also see Drug Therapy Table 70-1.

Pharmacologic Considerations

- Anorexiant drugs are used in conjunction with a physical activity and food reduction program, not as a sole treatment for weight reduction. These drugs should only be used for obesity (BMI of 30 or greater) or overweight (BMI of 27 to 29.9) when comorbid conditions such as hypertension, Type 2 diabetes, or dyslipidemia necessitate weight reduction. Never take over-the-counter weight-loss preparations with these drugs.
- Fat-soluble vitamins may be needed by clients taking various anorexiant drugs such as orlistat (Alli, Xenical). There is also an increased potential risk for severe liver damage. Liver enzymes should be monitored before and periodically during drug therapy depending on the medication.

DRUG THERAPY TABLE 70-1 Drugs to Treat Obesity

Category and Common Generic (Brand) Drugs	Intended Use	Common Side Effects	Safety Warnings for Nurses
Lipase Inhibitor			
Orlistat (Xenical, Alli)[a]	Slows absorption of fat from the intestine by inhibiting pancreatic lipase	Abdominal pain, fecal urgency, steatorrhea (fatty stool), oily diarrhea, leakage from anus	Administer with meals, stagger administration with other drugs. Vitamin supplement is required due to nonabsorption of nutrients. Monitor liver function.
Satiety Agents—Appetite Suppressants			
Amphetamine type agents Benzphetamine (Didrex, Recede) Diethylpropion (Tenuate, Tenuate Dospan) Phendimetrazine (Bontril PDM) Phentermine (Adipex-P, Suprenza)	Reduces appetite and promotes satiety by releasing norepinephrine and dopamine in hypothalamus	Headache, dry mouth, constipation, palpitations, increased blood pressure, insomnia, nervousness	Clients should avoid caffeine. Avoid use among clients with heart disease, hypertension, hyperthyroidism. Dose must be titrated down when discontinuing drug.
Combination Agents			
Phentermine[a]/topiramate (Qsymia)	Reduces appetite and promotes satiety by the additive effect of combining an amphetamine type agent with an anticonvulsant	Dry mouth, altered taste, constipation, insomnia, dizziness, tingling in extremities	Screen for suicidal ideation. Assess cardiac function of those with a history of cardiac disease. Monitor for glaucoma.
Naltrexone[a]/bupropion (Contrave)	Reduces appetite and food craving by the synergistic effect of releasing norepinephrine in the hypothalamus and mesolimbic reward circuit	Nausea, flatulence, constipation, headache, dizziness	Screen for suicidal ideation. Do not use with Wellbutrin (antidepressant) or Zyban (smoking cessation). Monitor heart rate/BP if cardiac history. Avoid alcohol use. Opioids are ineffective with this agent.
Antidiabetic Agents—Chronic Weight Control for Those With BMI Above 27			
Liraglutide (Saxenda)[a] Exenatide (Byetta)[a]	Supplements glucagonlike peptide-1 (GLP-1) hormone to stimulate insulin release	Injection site irritation, nausea, vomiting	Avoid use if history of thyroid or endocrine cancers. Reduces effectiveness of oral contraceptives.

[a]Agents approved for long-term use.

A new medication specifically for weight loss, a combination of fenfluramine and topiramate known by the trade name Qsymia, recently has been approved by the U.S. Food and Drug Administration—the first time in 13 years since a previous drug, a combination of phentermine and fenfluramine, was withdrawn. Qsymia produces moderate weight loss by suppressing appetite and increasing satiety and is recommended for adults with a BMI of 30 or higher or adults with a high BMI and a weight-related condition such as type 2 diabetes.

Bariatric Surgery

In some cases, **bariatric surgery**, procedures that either limit food intake, decrease its absorption, or both (Fig. 70-6), is an

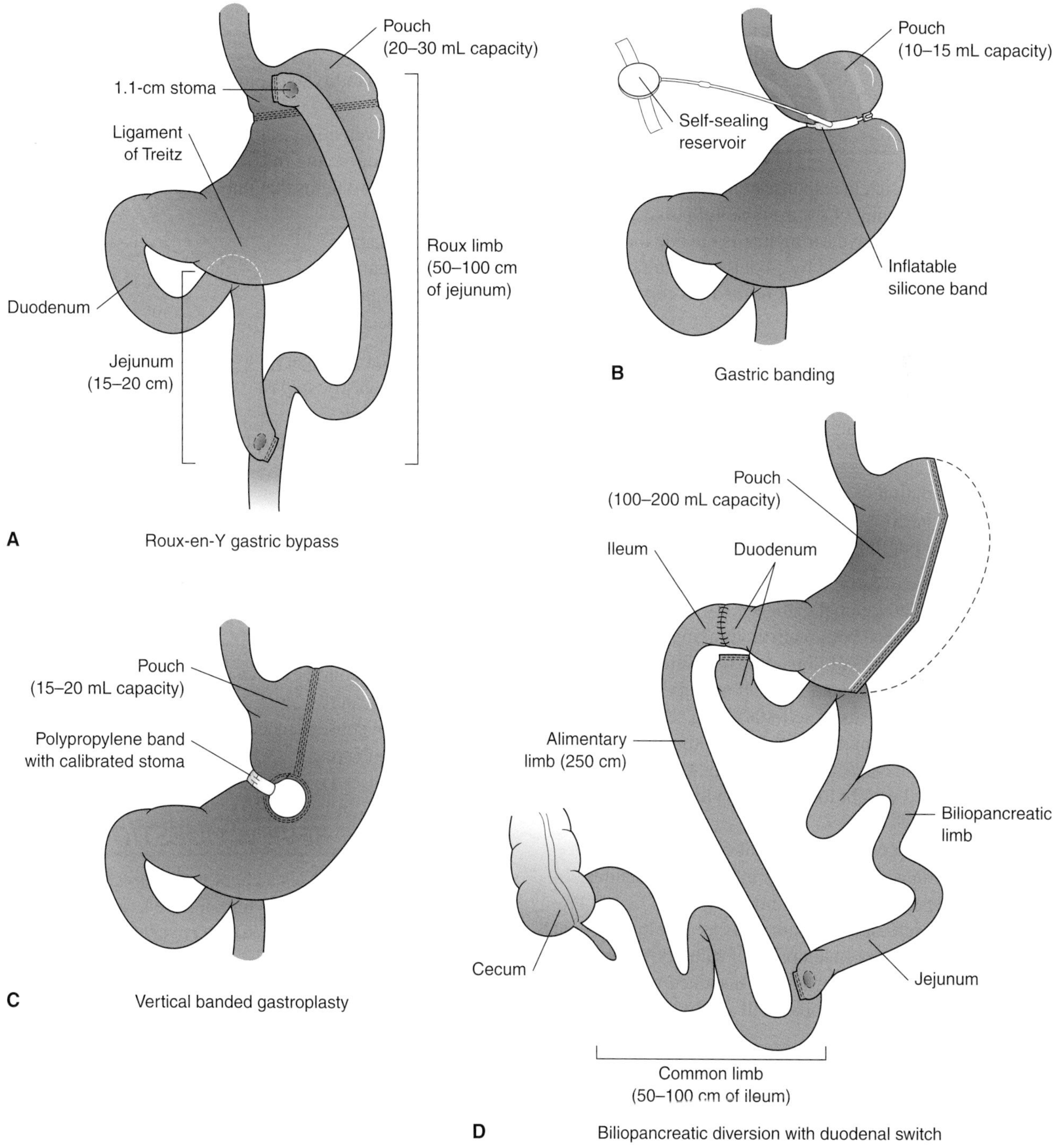

Figure 70-6 Surgical procedures for morbid obesity. **(A)** Roux-en-Y gastric bypass uses a horizontal row of staples across the fundus of the stomach, creating a pouch with a capacity of 20 to 30 mL. The distal end of the jejunum is attached to the pouch; the proximal end is attached to the jejunum. **(B)** Gastric banding. A prosthetic device is used to restrict oral intake to 10 to 15 mL that empties into the remainder of the stomach. **(C)** Vertical banded gastroplasty. The lesser curvature of the stomach is stapled to create a 10- to 15-mL pouch. **(D)** Biliopancreatic diversion with duodenal switch. Half the stomach is removed, leaving a pouch that holds about 60 mL. The ileum and the distal end of the jejunum are attached to the proximal end of the duodenum. The distal end of the biliopancreatic limb is attached to the ileum.

option for severely obese clients with medical complications (see Chapter 45). These procedures are expensive and may not be covered by medical insurers. There is a high potential for complications in the immediate postoperative period because of the client's presurgical obesity. Later, there may be problems with maintaining adequate levels of vitamins and minerals and dehydration because of the inability to consume fluids in adequate volumes, leaking in the areas that have been surgically joined, and stricture or bowel obstruction caused by kinking or the formation of scar tissue.

KEY POINTS

- Normal eating occurs in response to hunger and ceases when satiety (a feeling of comfortable fullness) is attained.
- Eating disorders involve eating that is outside the range of normal, is accompanied by anxiety and guilt, and results in physiologic imbalances or medical complications.
- Four types of eating disorders:
  - Anorexia nervosa
  - Bulimia nervosa
  - Binge eating
  - Compulsive overeating
- Two forms of anorexia nervosa:
  - Severe restriction of caloric intake or just water
  - Bulimarexia, extended self-starvation interrupted by binging and purging or exercising
- Serotonin: increased levels contribute to restricted eating; the brain is fooled into believing satiety has occurred.
- Dopamine: influence both realistic thinking, pleasure, and reward. An excess of dopamine may interfere with the ability to recognize and respond appropriately to the potential health hazards of self-starvation.
- Melanin-concentrating hormone: a hypothalamic neuropeptide that regulates eating and energy. Levels of this hormone caused weight loss, and high levels promoted obesity.
- Leptin: a substance produced by fat cells known as adipocytes. Leptin acts on receptors in the hypothalamus, where high levels inhibit food intake.
- Corticotropin-releasing hormone acts as a major anorexic signal that limits the consumption of calories, increases energy expenditure, and promotes sustained weight loss.
- Two reasons why most people with anorexia nervosa induce self-starvation:
  - Cultural and social factors
  - Physiologic factors
- Healthy range for BMI: 18.5 to 24.9
- Four components of treatment for clients with anorexia nervosa:
  - Nutritional therapy
  - Drug therapy
    - Psychotherapy
    - Family counseling
- Two examples of how people with bulimia nervosa compensate for binging:
  - Purging
  - Fasting/excessive exercise
- Two problems, besides nutrition, that are the nursing focus when caring for clients with bulimia nervosa:
  - Inflammation of the pharynx
  - Damaged teeth
  - Constipation
- Binge eater: inability to control overeating accompanying by guilt
- Compulsive overeating: eating in the absence of hunger or regardless of feeling full
- Psychosocial problems that may accompany overeating syndromes:
  - Feeling unhappy
  - Feeling ashamed
  - Feeling disgusted
  - Feeling socially isolated
- Types of bariatric surgery:
  - Roux-en-Y gastric bypass
  - Gastric banding
  - Vertical banded gastroplasty

CRITICAL THINKING EXERCISES

1. Calculate the BMI of a person who weighs 175 lb and is 63 inches tall. What conclusion is appropriate based on your calculation?
2. What weight-loss strategies are appropriate to recommend and discourage for an obese client who is a compulsive overeater?
3. Name some consequences of self-starvation secondary to anorexia nervosa.

NCLEX-STYLE REVIEW QUESTIONS PrepU

1. When a nurse assesses a client with a low body weight, what signs and symptoms are associated with a restricting form of anorexia nervosa? Select all that apply.
   1. Growth of fine body hair
   2. Club-shaped fingertips
   3. Hypoactive bowel sounds
   4. Conjunctival hemorrhages
   5. Low blood pressure
   6. Abraded knuckles
2. What nursing goal is the highest priority when managing the care of a client with anorexia nervosa?
   1. To improve the client's distorted body image
   2. To help the client use healthier coping techniques
   3. To restore normal nutrition and health
   4. To help the client develop assertiveness

3. When reviewing the data obtained following the assessment of a client diagnosed with bulimia, what finding is most related to this eating disorder?
1. Extremely low body weight
2. Erosion of dental enamel
3. Cessation of menstruation
4. Patchy loss of hair

4. When a client confides an intention to lose weight by taking the over-the-counter weight-loss drug orlistat (Alli) or the same prescription drug (Xenical), which has a higher dosage, what side effect should the nurse inform the client?
1. Decreased white blood cell count
2. Potential for allergic reactions
3. Explosive bowel movements
4. Secondary hypertension

5. Following a client's bariatric surgery, what should be included in the nurse's health teaching?
1. Take recommended vitamin and mineral supplements.
2. Limit oral intake to control diarrhea.
3. Eat dry foods that remain in the stomach longer.
4. Expect food cravings to cease.

WANT TO KNOW MORE? There are a wide variety of online resources available on thePoint to enhance learning and understanding of this chapter.

Go to **thePoint.lww.com/activate** and use the activation code found in the front of this text to unlock these online resources.

71

Caring for Clients With Substance Use Disorders

Words To Know

addiction
alcoholism
aversion therapy
blackouts
central nervous system depressants
central nervous system stimulants
chemical dependence
cross-tolerance
detoxification
environmental tobacco smoke
habituation
methadone maintenance therapy
morbidity
mortality
opioid dependence
polydrug abuse
rapid opioid detoxification
relapse
Rule of One Hundreds
secondhand smoke
substance abuse
substance use disorders
tolerance
withdrawal

Learning Objectives

On completion of this chapter, you will be able to:

1. Discuss the health and social consequences of substance abuse.
2. Name four commonly abused addictive substances and at least three other categories of abused drugs.
3. Discuss the meaning of withdrawal.
4. Explain tolerance and give two mechanisms by which it occurs.
5. List four steps in the progression toward chemical dependence.
6. List two physiologic explanations and two psychosocial factors for the development of a substance use disorder.
7. Explain two ways abused drugs produce their effects.
8. Define alcoholism and list three accompanying symptoms.
9. Describe treatment and nursing management for clients with alcoholism.
10. List five potential health consequences of tobacco use.
11. Discuss the components of a successful smoking cessation program.
12. Discuss elements of recovery programs.
13. Describe signs and symptoms of cocaine and methamphetamine abuse as they relate to the manner of use.
14. Describe treatment and nursing management for clients addicted to cocaine and methamphetamine.
15. Discuss methods for managing opioid dependence.

Substance abuse and substance use disorders, which are discussed in this chapter, are serious public health and social problems. They contribute significantly to **morbidity** (incidence of disease) and **mortality** (deaths) from liver damage, cardiopulmonary disease, and infectious diseases such as hepatitis and AIDS. Alcohol and drug abuse also are major contributors to domestic violence and child abuse, crime, traffic and boating fatalities, assaults, and murders.

Gerontologic Considerations

- Older adults may abuse over-the-counter and prescription drugs or alcohol rather than illicit drugs.
- Older adults may use alcohol as self-treatment or may begin taking over-the-counter medication with an alcohol base; progressive use or amounts compounded by a slowed metabolism may lead to alcoholism or alcohol toxicity.

Gerontologic Considerations (continued)

- Alcoholism may be difficult to identify in older adults because symptoms such as tremors, unsteady gait, or memory loss mimic changes that can be associated with aging.
- Older adults who drink alcohol exhibit greater impairment and neurologic deficits such as confusion, ataxia, and loss of cognitive ability than do younger adults and recover more slowly.
- Dementia may be associated with heavy ingestion of alcohol for 10 or more years, or with ingestion of other toxic substances.
- Careful medication review is needed to assure disulfiram is used cautiously in older adults due to potential interaction with other medications such as warfarin or nitroglycerin that may be prescribed.
- Nurses and caregivers must avoid age-related stereotypes and support older adults' efforts to overcome or prevent chemical dependence by promoting social networks and reducing isolation that may accompany growing older.
- The bones of postmenopausal women who smoke are less dense, and these women are at higher risk for fractures, especially of the hip, as they age.

SUBSTANCE ABUSE AND SUBSTANCE USE DISORDERS

Substance abuse is the use of a drug that is different from its intended purpose. Usually, it is the consequences of inappropriately taking drugs—primarily mind-altering and mood-altering substances—that are of major concern. Commonly abused drugs include alcohol, cocaine, heroin, and other opioids, hallucinogens, amphetamines, marijuana, barbiturates, volatile hydrocarbons such as those found in glue, and nicotine.

Because of their widespread use and harmful effects, alcohol and nicotine contribute most to morbidity and mortality and thus are considered the most harmful substances. Tobacco use is widely accepted and its psychoactive properties are so subtle that its negative social and occupational effects seem minor. Yet tobacco is an addictive substance that contributes to the death of 480,000 people annually—as many as are caused by alcohol, cocaine, heroin, suicide, homicide, motor vehicle accidents, fire, and AIDS combined (Centers for Disease Control and Prevention [CDC], 2020).

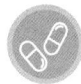

Pharmacologic Considerations

- Younger clients are more likely to admit to polydrug use during a drug history assessment. Alcohol combined with other central nervous system (CNS) depressants is the most frequent polydrug combination leading to death.

Withdrawal refers to the physical symptoms and craving for a drug that occur when a person abruptly stops using an abused substance (Table 71-1). **Chemical dependence** means that a person must take a drug to avoid withdrawal symptoms. **Addiction** is sometimes used interchangeably with *dependence*, but addiction more accurately refers to the drug-seeking behaviors that interfere with work, relationships, and normal activities (Box 71-1). A substance use disorder is a disease that affects a person's brain and behavior

TABLE 71-1 Commonly Abused Substances

DRUG	EFFECTS	SIGNS AND SYMPTOMS OF TOXICITY	SIGNS AND SYMPTOMS OF WITHDRAWAL
Alcohol	Central nervous system depressant • Lethargy • Slurred speech • Slowed motor reaction • Impaired judgment • Decreased social inhibition	Nausea and vomiting, loss of coordination, belligerence, stupor, coma	Anxiety, agitation, elevated vital signs, hyperactive reflexes, tremors, diaphoresis, insomnia, hallucinations, seizures
Cocaine and methamphetamine	Central nervous system stimulants • Tachycardia • Hypertension • Increased energy • Feeling of well-being • Insensitivity to pain and fatigue • Weight loss	Restlessness, paranoia, irritability, auditory and tactile hallucinations, convulsions, respiratory or cardiac arrest	Depressed mood, lethargy, impaired concentration, craving for drug
Heroin and other opioids	Central nervous system depressants • Initial brief rush of euphoria • Sedation • Reduced motivation, attention, and concentration • Altered sensitivity to stressors • Pain relief • Lowered vital signs, especially respiratory rate • Slowed peristalsis • Constricted pupils • Decreased interest in sex	Respiratory depression, hypothermia, pinpoint pupils, coma	Yawning, runny nose, perspiration, goosebumps, anorexia, vomiting, diarrhea, dilated pupils, insomnia, elevated vital signs, drug craving

(continued)

TABLE 71-1 Commonly Abused Substances (*continued*)

DRUG	EFFECTS	SIGNS AND SYMPTOMS OF TOXICITY	SIGNS AND SYMPTOMS OF WITHDRAWAL
Nicotine	Central nervous system stimulant • Tachycardia • Increased blood pressure • Alertness • Feeling of well-being	• Inhaled toxins cause hypoxemia, carcinogenesis • Signs of acute nicotine poisoning (most often in a child who ingests the drug) include nausea, vomiting, abdominal pain, diarrhea, salivation, seizures	Craving, reduced concentration, emotional irritability, nervousness, fatigue, disturbed sleep, increased appetite

BOX 71-1 Signs of Alcohol or Drug Addiction

- Regularly drinking or taking more than was originally planned
- Unsuccessfully attempting to reduce or regulate the use
- Spending excessive time obtaining, consuming, or recovering from the effects of the drug
- Continuing use despite negative consequences
- Drinking or consuming drugs in solitary
- Failing to fulfill major role obligations at work, school, or home
- Exhibiting tolerance to alcohol and sedative drugs
- Displaying withdrawal symptoms when drug is not consumed

and leads to an inability to control the use of a legal or illegal drug or medication (Mayo Clinic, 2021). **Tolerance** refers to the reduction in a drug's effect that follows persistent use. Tolerance results because the body develops mechanisms for using the drug more effectively or inactivating the drug more efficiently. Consequently, a person must take increasing amounts of the substance to obtain the desired effect.

Pathophysiology and Etiology

The causes of substance use disorders are complex and involve many psychobiologic factors. Substance abuse often begins with curious experimentation and progresses to **habituation** (repetition), psychological and physical dependence, and, finally, addiction (Table 71-2). One factor that explains substance abuse is the self-reinforcing pleasurable effects that some substances produce in the limbic system of the brain, depending on the type of substance. **CNS stimulants** are chemical agents that temporarily accelerate physical and mental functions. Stimulants such as caffeine (the most widely used CNS stimulant), nicotine, cocaine, and amphetamines affect levels of norepinephrine, dopamine, and acetylcholine. **CNS depressants** are chemical agents that slow brain and physiologic activities. Depressant drugs such as alcohol, heroin and other opioids, and barbiturates cause effects similar to those of gamma-aminobutyric acid (GABA), endorphins, and enkephalins. These drugs either mimic the neurotransmitters by attaching to their receptor sites or block their reuptake (see Chapter 67).

Psychosocial dynamics are also a component in substance use and abuse. Observing family members, peers, and role models who use alcohol, tobacco, and other drugs influences impressionable teenagers and youngsters. The promotion of alcohol in the U.S. culture also fosters its use and abuse. Many people abuse drugs in a dysfunctional effort to cope with psychosocial stressors.

Treatment

Initiating treatment is one of the most difficult hurdles in treating substance use disorders. Clients deny their addiction, rationalize substance use, or blame life situations for their drug and drinking habits. Often, dependent people must "hit bottom" before they seek help or be court-ordered for rehabilitation. Once in treatment, withdrawal is managed. Those in recovery must learn new methods of coping with stressors, repair relationships damaged by addiction, and develop new interests and activities to fill the time once devoted to using drugs or alcohol.

Although some people cease taking abused substances unassisted, most benefit from chemical detoxification and a treatment plan that involves abstinence, counseling, and

TABLE 71-2 Patterns of Substance Abuse

EXPERIMENTATION	HABITUATION	DEPENDENCE	ADDICTION
Initial use	Repeated use	Frequent use	Unremitting use
Low dose	Uniform doses	Doses increase	High doses
Finds experience pleasurable	Seeks to reexperience pleasure	Craves ongoing pleasure from drug	Needs drug to feel "normal"
No discomfort from abstinence	No discomfort from abstinence	Experiences minor physical discomfort if drug is not used	Experiences severe withdrawal symptoms if drug is not used

support of peers through a 12-step program. Twelve-step programs are free and provide specific guidelines (steps) for becoming and remaining drug- or alcohol-free. Frequent (daily, if necessary) attendance at meetings is encouraged. During meetings, members share their experiences and discuss the 12 steps and other topics related to recovery.

Alcohol Dependence

Alcoholism is a chronic, progressive, multisystem disease characterized by an inability to control the consumption of alcohol. Unchecked, alcoholism is fatal. Serious medical consequences of alcoholism are dose-related; that is, the more alcohol a person consumes, the sooner they experience life-threatening health problems such as portal hypertension, esophageal varices, and cirrhosis of the liver (see Chapter 47). On a drink-by-drink comparison, women are more likely to experience health problems earlier than men because, in general, they weigh less than men. Consequently, the same amount of alcohol is more concentrated and more toxic to women than to men.

Pathophysiology and Etiology

Genetic factors likely play a role in alcoholism. Children of persons with alcohol use disorder are more likely to develop alcoholism than children of nonalcoholics (Gold, 2016; Videbeck, 2020; Zeltner, 2019). Atypical metabolism of alcohol in which a substance called **tetrahydroisoquinoline (THIQ)** was identified by Davis and Walsh in 1970 (Box 71-2). THIQ continues to be in the literature as an underlying factor in the disease of addiction (Ohlms, 1983, 2013). It is believed that the lifelong presence of THIQ explains why (1) there is no cure for alcoholism, (2) why people with alcoholism are prone to relapse, and (3) why people with alcoholism are quick to resume their previous addictive drinking patterns after periods of sobriety (Dyr & Wyszogrodzka, 2018). However, THIQ has not been consistently found in the brains of persons with alcohol use disorder, and its link to alcoholism continues to be debated (Peana et al., 2017).

Nevertheless, those who abuse substances experience the release of chemicals in the brain that cause (1) intense cravings for the substance, (2) continued use despite dangerous consequences, and (3) a sustained vulnerability to cues that trigger substance use even after the person stops using it (Erickson, 2018; National Center on Addiction and Substance Abuse, 2012, 2016). Dopamine is a neurotransmitter that locks onto receptors, triggering sensations of pleasure and reward, which may explain its relationship to addictive behaviors.

BOX 71-2 Normal and Alcoholic Metabolisms

Ethyl alcohol

↓

Acetaldehyde + dopamine → **Tetrahydroisoquinoline (THIQ)**

↓

Acetic acid (vinegar)

↓

Carbon dioxide + water

Assessment Findings

Signs and Symptoms

Although the client may emphatically deny problem drinking, they typically have a history of increasing alcohol consumption. The person may hide containers of alcohol and drink privately at any time during the day. Many clients manifest a great **tolerance** for alcohol (consumption of alcohol produces a lesser effect) and a **cross-tolerance** (reduced effect) for sedative–hypnotic drugs. **Blackouts**, periods of amnesia involving events and activities during drinking, occur even in the early stages. Family and friends note alcoholic behaviors; social or legal repercussions occur. A history of marital, financial, and occupational problems reflects the person's inability to control drinking despite negative consequences. Many clients with alcoholism have been arrested for driving under the influence of alcohol.

People who are acutely intoxicated may enter the tertiary care hospital with altered mental status or acute gastric bleeding, or as victims of trauma or violence. When hospitalization occurs, management of alcohol withdrawal is as important as the management of the primary condition. Withdrawal from alcohol results in nervous system stimulation manifested by tremors, sweating, hypertension, tachycardia, heart palpitations, craving for alcohol, seizures, and hallucinations.

>>> *Stop, Think, and Respond 71-1*

What assessment findings suggest that a person who consumes alcohol is a person with alcohol use disorder rather than a social drinker?

Complications

A host of alcohol-related physical symptoms can accompany persistent drinking. Esophagitis, gastritis, enlarged liver, esophageal and rectal bleeding, and pancreatitis are common. Memory is impaired, and clients may experience erectile dysfunction or decreased libido. Studies also implicate alcohol in liver cancer, cerebrovascular accident, metabolic deficiencies, aspiration pneumonia, cardiomyopathy, blood dyscrasias, and neurologic disorders. Infants born to women who consumed alcohol during pregnancy sometimes have fetal alcohol syndrome, which causes physical and intellectual deficits.

Diagnostic Findings

A blood alcohol level (BAL) measures the percentage of alcohol in the blood, indicating the extent of alcohol intoxication at the time of measurement (Table 71-3). However, tolerance for alcohol may decrease the physiologic effects of accumulating BALs in people who are chronic drinkers.

TABLE 71-3 Blood Alcohol Level and Associated Impairment

BLOOD ALCOHOL LEVEL (MG/DL)	PERCENTAGE OF BLOOD ALCOHOL (%)	PHYSICAL AND BEHAVIORAL EFFECTS
50	0.05	Mood changes, reduced inhibition, decreased judgment, slight euphoria
80–100	0.08–0.1	Reduced muscle coordination, decreased reaction time, impaired vision
200	0.2	Staggering, poor control of emotions, easily angered
300	0.3	Mental confusion, stupor
400	0.4	Coma
500	0.5	Respiratory depression, death

Elevated levels of gamma-glutamyl transpeptidase (GGTP), aspartate aminotransferase (AST), and alanine aminotransferase (ALT) reflect alcohol-induced liver disease. High levels of pancreatic enzymes (amylase and lipase) may indicate pancreatitis, which develops secondarily to alcoholism.

Medical Management and Rehabilitation

To break the progression of alcoholism, clients undergo detoxification, nutritional therapy, psychotherapy, and drug therapy. They are encouraged to continue rehabilitation by joining a support group such as Alcoholics Anonymous (AA).

Detoxification

Alcohol withdrawal can begin as early as 6 hours after the last drink and last for 48 hours or more. It is the result of abrupt cessation from alcohol, causing extreme sympathetic nervous system stimulation (Box 71-3). Without detoxification, alcohol withdrawal can progress to a potentially fatal process. **Detoxification** ("detox") involves stabilizing the client with a sedative drug while the alcohol is eventually metabolized. Withdrawal symptoms are controlled until they subside. Drugs used in detoxification are lorazepam (Ativan), diazepam (Valium), and chlordiazepoxide (Librium; Drug Therapy Table 71-1). Initially, these medications are administered frequently and in high doses to compensate for the client's cross-tolerance; they are then tapered and discontinued. A beta-adrenergic blocker such as propranolol (Inderal) is given to reduce the dangerously elevated heart rate and blood pressure (BP) that can occur during withdrawal. Alcoholism may result in thiamine deficiency, which can lead to dementia. Because thiamine is necessary for the metabolism of glucose, glucose solutions must be avoided until thiamine is administered. Once thiamine is

BOX 71-3 Alcohol Withdrawal Syndrome

- Elevated temperature
- Tachycardia
- Hypertension
- Vomiting or regurgitation
- Hand tremors
- Sweating
- Anxiety
- Agitation
- Insomnia
- Hallucinations (visual and tactile)
- Seizures

DRUG THERAPY TABLE 71-1 Drugs Used in the Recovery From Substance Use Disorders

Category and Common Generic (Brand) Drugs	Intended Use	Common Side Effects	Safety Warnings for Nurses
Agents Used in Alcohol Detoxification/Treatment			
Benzodiazepines			
Chlordiazepoxide (Librium) Diazepam (Valium) Lorazepam (Ativan)	Depresses central nervous system	Dry mouth, drowsiness	Increased risk for falls due to sedative side effects
Alcohol abstinence agents			
Acamprosate (Campral)	Restores GABA balance in neurotransmission, reducing alcohol cravings	Insomnia, diarrhea, fatigue, headache	Do not use when intoxicated; blood should be alcohol-free for at least 12 hours
Disulfiram (Antabuse)	Blocks metabolism of alcohol causing uncomfortable symptoms such as flushing, throbbing headache, vomiting, tachycardia, hypotension if alcohol is consumed; convulsions, myocardial infarction, death in severe reactions	Drowsiness, headache, dermatitis	Avoid all substances containing alcohol including those applied to the skin Use only as part of the alcohol treatment program. Monitor for suicidal ideation Contraindicated in clients with severe renal impairment

DRUG THERAPY TABLE 71-1 Drugs Used in the Recovery From Substance Use Disorders (*continued*)

Category and Common Generic (Brand) Drugs	Intended Use	Common Side Effects	Safety Warnings for Nurses
Systemic Tobacco Deterrents			
Bupropion (Zyban) Varenicline (Chantix)	Binds to nicotine receptor sites, reducing the severity of nicotine withdrawal symptoms	Dry mouth, nausea, sore throat, vision changes, mild itching or skin rash, changes in appetite, loss of interest in sex, mood changes, vivid dreams Nausea vomiting, loss of appetite, weight changes, flatulence, constipation, sleep disturbance, behavioral and mood changes, impotence, sleepwalking, suicidal thoughts	Do not take if bupropion (Wellbutrin) is coprescribed. Avoid with a seizure disorder Monitor for neuropsychiatric effects Monitor for skin rash; may be Stevens–Johnson syndrome
Agents Used in Opioid Detoxification Treatment (Opioid Taper)			
Buprenorphine/Naloxone (Suboxone)			
Intended use: an opioid (narcotic) partial agonist–antagonist. It works by binding to receptors in the brain and nervous system to help prevent withdrawal symptoms in someone who has stopped taking opioids.	Common side: nausea and vomiting, headache, sweating, numb mouth, constipation, insomnia, dizziness, drowsiness, anxiety, depression.	Safety warning for nurses: sublingual use only, do not swallow or crush or chew, instruct the client to not eat, drink, or smoke while the tablet is dissolving or immediately after.	(Substance Abuse and Mental Health Services Administration [SAMHSA], 2020; Lembke, 2020)
Agents Used in Opioid Deterrent			
Opioid antagonist Naloxone (Narcan, Evzio)	Abrupt reversal of opioids within 2 minutes of administration	Nausea, vomiting, tachycardia, tremors, agitation, confusion, shortness of breath	Attaches to all opioid receptors; results in immediate withdrawal response
Naltrexone (Vivitrol, Trexan, ReVia)	Aids in the abstinence from alcohol and opioids[b]	Insomnia, anxiety, abdominal pain, nausea, vomiting, delayed ejaculation, rash, joint and muscle pain	Avoid opioids and alcohol; use will not prevent or relieve withdrawal symptoms
Methadone (Dolophine)	Binds with opioid receptors in the CNS and produces euphoria, analgesia, and sedation	Lightheadedness, dizziness, sedation, nausea, vomiting, respiratory depression	Monitor for respiratory depression Monitor for cardiac arrhythmia Should be administered with direct observation
Benzodiazepine antagonist Flumazenil (Romazicon)	Reverse sedation or drowsiness of benzodiazepines	Hypoventilation, return of sedation	Expect seizure activity when administered to long-term users

The drugs in column 1 indicate the drug that matches up with explanations in columns 2 through 4.

administered, intravenous (IV) hydration with glucose and additional vitamins, such as folic acid, supports the client metabolically until the condition stabilizes.

Concept Mastery Alert

Detoxification

When a client is admitted for detoxification, lorazepam and other drugs used during detoxification are initially given frequently and in high doses while the alcohol is metabolized; these drugs are then tapered and discontinued.

Nutritional Therapy

People with alcoholism are often undernourished and have deficiencies of B vitamins. Injections of thiamine for 3 days followed by oral administration and folic acid supplements are often prescribed. Vitamin therapy prevents neurologic complications, known as Wernicke encephalopathy and Korsakoff psychosis, which affect memory and cognitive functions. Nutrition Notes outlines additional nutrition considerations.

Psychotherapy

Individual or group psychotherapy helps the client to gain greater insight into the emotional problems that have led to or resulted from alcohol dependence. Family therapy with the spouse and children provides an opportunity to share how alcoholism has affected each person so that psychosocial healing may begin.

Drug Therapy

Disulfiram (Antabuse) is a drug given to people recovering from alcoholism who cannot control the compulsion to

Nutrition Notes

The Client With Alcoholism

- For clients with moderate-to-severe pancreatitis, the preferred route of delivering nutrition has shifted away from parenteral nutrition toward enteral nutrition delivered into the jejunum. Jejunal feedings do not stimulate pancreatic secretions, are well tolerated, and are less likely than parenteral nutrition to cause complications.
- For clients with chronic pancreatitis, a low-fat diet may help minimize pain after eating.
- Sodium and fluid restrictions are indicated for ascites, a consequence of liver damage.
- A soft diet is used for esophageal varices.

drink. It is a form of **aversion therapy**, a method of deterring drinking by causing unpleasant physical reactions when alcohol is consumed or absorbed through the skin. For clients who are prescribed disulfiram, health teaching includes a list of products that contain alcohol such as liquid cough suppressants (Box 71-4). The client must be informed that life-threatening cardiopulmonary complications and even death can occur when disulfiram and alcohol are combined.

Pharmacologic Considerations

- When disulfiram is prescribed, be sure clients are aware that all forms of alcohol can elicit a reaction. They need to avoid any product that may contain alcohol. A reaction to alcohol may be experienced up to 2 weeks after discontinuing the drug.

BOX 71-4 Obscure Sources of Alcohol

- Liquid cough and cold medications
- Liquid sleep medications
- Flavoring extracts
- Mouthwash
- Rubbing alcohol
- Aftershave lotions
- Fruitcake with alcohol

Acamprosate calcium (Campral) is a newer drug that acts on the neurotransmitter glutamate to alleviate the physiologic and psychological distress following withdrawal from alcohol (see Drug Therapy Table 71-1). Naltrexone (Vivitrol, Trexan, ReVia), a narcotic antagonist, is also used as an adjunct in people who are recovering from alcoholism. It reduces the pleasure associated with drinking alcohol should the person **relapse** (return to drinking).

Support Groups

AA was the first 12-step self-help program. Founded in 1926 by an alcoholic primary provider, AA is composed of and run by recovering persons with alcohol use disorder to help people who are dependent on alcohol achieve and maintain sobriety. AA emphasizes personal accountability, spirituality, and powerlessness over alcohol. Family members of clients with alcoholism may benefit from attending meetings of Al-Anon, Alateen, or Adult Children of Alcoholics to learn more about how alcoholism affects them.

>>> *Stop, Think, and Respond 71-2*

Explain why the first of AA's 12 steps leading to recovery from alcoholism is "We admitted we were powerless over alcohol—and that our lives had become unmanageable."

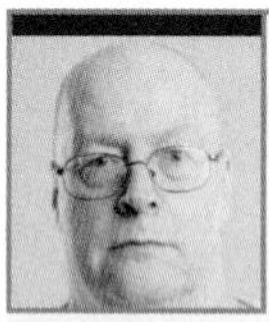

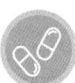

Clinical Scenario A 58-year-old man is on a court-ordered admission because of his history of arrests for driving under the influence. His BAL was 0.258% when the arresting officer tested him with a breathalyzer. His wife reports that he is a binge drinker on Friday evenings and weekends. He has become abusive when his wife confronts him about his drinking. He has lost several jobs in the past because he fails to report for work on Mondays. **If you were the nurse assigned to admit and care for the client in the substance abuse unit, what actions would you take? Compare your approach with the nursing process that follows.**

NURSING PROCESS FOR THE CLIENT WITH ALCOHOL DEPENDENCE

Assessment

Examine the client from head to toe; note any signs of fall-related injuries, abdominal enlargement, jaundiced skin or sclera, and blood in any body fluids or stool that may indicate complications from liver damage or portal hypertension (see Chapter 47). Question the client about the use of alcohol when establishing the client's database. If the client admits to consuming alcohol, determine the type, how much, and when the last drink was consumed. The latter information is important because withdrawal symptoms occur within 6 to 72 hours after a client's last drink. When appropriate, administer a breath alcohol concentration test or BAL as soon as possible to obtain an approximation of the client's current alcohol level. Determine if the client had a history of seizures or other severe symptoms in previous withdrawals, which merits close observation of the client for a similar reaction.

Monitor the client for signs and symptoms of withdrawal at least every hour or more often. If a standardized symptom withdrawal flow sheet, such as the Clinical Institute Withdrawal Assessment of Alcohol Scale, Revised (CIWA-Ar) (Fig. 71-1),

NURSING PROCESS FOR THE CLIENT WITH ALCOHOL DEPENDENCE (continued)

is unavailable, use the **Rule of One Hundreds** as an indicator of escalating withdrawal. The Rule of One Hundreds refers to a body temperature of at least 100°F, a pulse rate of at least 100 beats/min, or a diastolic BP of at least 100 mm Hg. The rise in any one of these three vital signs suggests the need for sedative medication because the physiologic consequences of withdrawal may be extremely difficult to counteract once they have begun.

Diagnosis, Planning, and Interventions

RC of Alcohol Withdrawal

Expected Outcome: The nurse will assess for, manage, and minimize alcohol withdrawal.

- Assess the client's vital signs and other data, such as hand tremors, hyperactive tendon reflexes, diaphoresis, anxiety, insomnia, and disorientation, which suggest physiologic stimulation. *As the body metabolizes alcohol, it releases norepinephrine and glutamate, causing autonomic nervous system stimulation and neuronal excitation. A score of 6 to 9 on the CIWA-AR indicates a need for administering a detoxification drug.*
- Consult with the primary provider regarding the need for a detoxification drug. *The primary provider is responsible for prescribing a drug for detoxification and the dose, route, and frequency of administration according to assessment data the nurse obtains.*
- Administer prescribed detoxification medication. *Minor tranquilizers maintain a controlled level of intoxication, so withdrawal is less rapid and dangerous.*
- Repeat assessments for withdrawal at least every 1 or 2 hours. *Administration of a detoxification drug should control physiologic stimulation; if not, administration of another dose is warranted.*
- Monitor for seizure activity, hallucinations, extreme tremors, and agitation. *If early and minor symptoms of alcohol withdrawal are not managed effectively, the client's withdrawal will progress in severity because of accumulating excitatory neurotransmitter levels; excess dopamine contributes to hallucinosis.*
- Restrict caffeine during withdrawal. *Caffeine is a CNS stimulant that heightens the symptoms of withdrawal.*

Malnutrition Risk (Less than body requirements): Related to inadequate dietary intake

Expected Outcome: The client will consume at least 75% of the food that is served once nausea and vomiting subside.

- Obtain a baseline weight. *Documenting the client's current weight provides a means of evaluating whether the client's subsequent nutritional intake maintains or increases the current weight.*
- Determine the client's food preferences. *A person is more likely to consume food that they like.*
- Collaborate with the dietary department to provide six small meals each day and an ample variety of snacks. *The client is likely to consume more food if the quantity is distributed throughout the day.*
- Monitor dietary intake and record data in the medical record. *Documentation provides an objective means for evaluating the client's progress.*

Grief: Related to the cessation of alcohol use, related social activities, and social contacts–related social activities and social contacts

Expected Outcomes: (1) The client will verbalize that alcohol abuse is an illness that requires ongoing treatment and support. (2) The client will understand the connection between alcohol and its associated activities and develop non–alcohol-related interests and contacts.

- Let the client express feelings concerning potential losses. *Discussing the effects of abstinence is the first step in working through grief.*
- Explore alternatives that may substitute for potential losses. *Identifying activities and other people with whom to socialize may substitute for the void caused by abstaining from alcohol.*
- Encourage the family or significant others to support one another. *The physical and emotional burden associated with life-altering changes can be eased if shared among many people who are meaningful to the client.*
- Promote sharing of experiences between the client and others who are further ahead in their recovery. *Role models who are dealing with similar issues can motivate and encourage the client.*

Discharge Planning: Related to a desire to abstain from alcohol and manage a chronic, fatal disease

Expected Outcome: The client will formulate a plan for attaining and maintaining sobriety.

- Provide the locations of AA meetings. *Knowing the locations and times of meetings allows the client to make personal choices in pursuing their recovery.*
- Explain that a sponsor may be selected from among those who attend AA meetings. *A sponsor provides social and emotional support throughout recovery.*
- Recommend that the client begin reading the "Big Book" of AA. *This book, titled* Alcoholics Anonymous, *describes the traditional 12 steps that lead to recovery.*
- Prepare the client for possible relapse by role-playing situations that may entice them to drink. *Role-playing helps the client prepare for possible barriers to recovery and provides an opportunity to simulate methods for dealing with them.*

Evaluation of Expected Outcomes

Vital signs are stable, and symptoms of withdrawal are controlled. The client eats a well-balanced diet and sleeps an adequate number of hours per night. The client demonstrates a willingness to cope with losses associated with overcoming alcohol dependence. They also move forward with measures to remain sober, such as participating in AA.

Clinical Institute Withdrawal Assessment of Alcohol Scale, Revised (CIWA-Ar)

Patient: ________________ **Date:** ________________ **Time:** ________________ (24-hour clock, midnight = 00:00)

Pulse or heart rate, taken for one minute: ________________ **Blood pressure:** ________________

NAUSEA AND VOMITING—Ask "Do you feel sick to your stomach? Have you vomited?" Observation.
0 no nausea and no vomiting
1 mild nausea with no vomiting
2
3
4 intermittent nausea with dry heaves
5
6
7 constant nausea, frequent dry heaves and vomiting

TACTILE DISTURBANCES—Ask "Have you any itching, pins and needles sensations, any burning, any numbness, or do you feel bugs crawling on or under your skin?" Observation.
0 none
1 very mild itching, pins and needles, burning or numbness
2 mild itching, pins and needles, burning or numbness
3 moderate itching, pins and needles, burning or numbness
4 moderately severe hallucinations
5 severe hallucinations
6 extremely severe hallucinations
7 continuous hallucinations

TREMOR—Arms extended and fingers spread apart. Observation.
0 no tremor
1 not visible, but can be felt fingertip to fingertip
2
3
4 moderate, with patient's arms extended
5
6
7 severe, even with arms not extended

AUDITORY DISTURBANCES—Ask "Are you more aware of sounds around you? Are they harsh? Do they frighten you? Are you hearing anything that is disturbing to you? Are you hearing things you know are not there?" Observation.
0 not present
1 very mild harshness or ability to frighten
2 mild harshness or ability to frighten
3 moderate harshness or ability to frighten
4 moderately severe hallucinations
5 severe hallucinations
6 extremely severe hallucinations
7 continuous hallucinations

PAROXYSMAL SWEATS—Observation.
0 no sweat visible
1 barely perceptible sweating, palms moist
2
3
4 beads of sweat obvious on forehead
5
6
7 drenching sweats

VISUAL DISTURBANCES—Ask "Does the light appear to be too bright? Is its color different? Does it hurt your eyes? Are you seeing anything that is disturbing to you? Are you seeing things you know are not there?" Observation.
0 not present
1 very mild sensitivity
2 mild sensitivity
3 moderate sensitivity
4 moderately severe hallucinations
5 severe hallucinations
6 extremely severe hallucinations
7 continuous hallucinations

ANXIETY—Ask "Do you feel nervous?" Observation.
0 no anxiety, at ease
1 mild anxious
2
3
4 moderately anxious, or guarded, so anxiety is inferred
5
6
7 equivalent to acute panic states as seen in severe delirium or acute schizophrenic reactions

HEADACHE, FULLNESS IN HEAD—Ask "Does your head feel different? Does it feel like there is a band around your head?" Do not rate for dizziness or lightheadedness. Otherwise, rate severity.
0 not present
1 very mild
2 mild
3 moderate
4 moderately severe
5 severe
6 very severe
7 extremely severe

Figure 71-1 The Clinical Institute Withdrawal Assessment of Alcohol Scale, Revised (CIWA-Ar) takes approximately 5 minutes to administer. The maximum score is 67. Those scoring less than 10 do not usually need additional medication for withdrawal. (From Sullivan, J. T., Sykora, K., Schneiderman, J., Naranjo, C. A., & Sellers, E. M. (1989). Assessment of alcohol withdrawal: The revised clinical institute withdrawal assessment for alcohol scale (CIWA-Ar). *British journal of addiction, 84*(11), 1353–1357.)

AGITATION—Observation.
0 normal activity
1 somewhat more than normal activity
2
3
4 moderately fidgety and restless
5
6
7 paces back and forth during most of the interview, or constantly thrashes about

ORIENTATION AND CLOUDING OF SENSORIUM – Ask "What day is this? Where are you? Who am I?"
0 oriented and can do serial additions
1 cannot do serial additions or is uncertain about date
2 disoriented for date by no more than 2 calendar days
3 disoriented for date by more than 2 calendar days
4 disoriented for place/or person

Total **CIWA-Ar** Score ______
Rater's Initials ______
Maximum Possible Score 67

Figure 71-1 (*continued*)

Nicotine Dependence

Nicotine, the stimulant drug in tobacco, is the most heavily used addictive, mood-altering substance in the United States. The drug is absorbed by inhaling the tobacco in cigarettes, cigars, and pipes, or through the mucous membranes of the mouth from loose tobacco.

Pathophysiology and Etiology

A person's dependence on tobacco, or any other addictive drug, develops gradually and progresses through several sequential stages (Pogun & Rodopman, 2021; Sato et al., 2012; Shadel & Cervone, 2011; Videbeck, 2020):

- Initial use (first puffs of a cigarette or administration of the drug)
- Experimental use (irregular smoking or drug use)
- Regular use (repeated exposures to nicotine or other drugs)
- Development of tolerance to psychoactive and physiologic effects, which requires an increase in smoking or drug use
- Development of withdrawal symptoms between episodes of smoking or use of a drug
- Dependent/compulsive use (driven by withdrawal or cue-provoked cravings) despite knowledge of harmful consequences

The addictive quality of tobacco occurs because nicotine mimics the neurotransmitter acetylcholine, which intensifies the release of dopamine in the brain, promoting an experience of pleasure and reward. As the body adjusts to the dopamine stimulation from nicotine, tolerance develops, and the person needs to smoke more and more.

Pleasurable psychological effects are offset by nicotine's pathologic consequences. Smoking raises carbon monoxide levels in the blood and causes constriction of peripheral blood vessels, which contributes to cardiovascular disease. Tobacco smoke disrupts the structure of alveoli, causing them to become overstretched and inelastic, as in emphysema. It is implicated in the development and recurrence of gastric ulcers. The smoke in inhaled tobacco products contains more than 40 carcinogenic chemicals. Smokeless tobacco (chewing tobacco) exposes the oral cavity to carcinogens, inhaled tobacco targets the lungs and distant organs, and cigars or pipes repeatedly expose the oral cavity and esophagus to harmful substances.

Smoking and tobacco use have decreased in recent decades. In 2005, 21 of every 100 adults (20.9%) were smokers. In 2019, the number of smokers has declined to 14 of every 100 (14.0%); this number represents 34.1 million adults who currently smoke cigarettes in the United States (CDC, 2020). Estimates of associated medical costs are more than $300 billion annually for direct medical care and lost productivity (CDC, 2020).

Passive absorption of smoke also can cause disease in nonsmokers. Nicotine tolerance results in increased use over time and withdrawal symptoms when use is discontinued. Users light up or chew to maintain blood and brain drug levels; nicotine is then distributed throughout the body, metabolized in the liver, and excreted by the kidneys. The frequency of tobacco use is also governed by conditioned, learned responses, meaning that past patterns of use reinforce the habit of smoking; for example, smoking may follow a meal or accompany talking on the telephone or consuming coffee. This factor is important, in that smoking cessation strategies must target both physical dependence and the conditioned related behaviors.

Consequences of Smoking

Smoking is responsible for 80% to 90% of deaths from lung cancer (CDC, 2020). Smoking and smokeless tobacco also cause a significant number of cancers that affect the mouth, larynx, esophagus, and bladder. The rate of coronary heart disease in smokers is four to five times that in nonsmokers. Smokers are more likely to develop peripheral vascular disease and strokes than are nonsmokers. There is also a correlation between cigarette smoking and premature delivery and low-birth-weight infants (CDC, 2020).

Breathing **environmental tobacco smoke** (also called **secondhand smoke** or *passive smoke*), the smoke given off by the burning end of a cigarette, pipe, or cigar and the exhaled smoke from the lungs of a smoker, is potentially injurious to others. *Epidemiologists*, scientists who study the incidence and causation of illnesses, have identified that breathing secondhand smoke causes headaches and eye, nose, and throat irritation. Nonsmokers exposed to environmental tobacco smoke have increased rates of heart disease, lung and other types of cancer, and respiratory tract infections. Risk of sudden infant death syndrome is increased in infants whose mothers smoked throughout pregnancy and after delivery. Children with asthma have an increased frequency of and more severe attacks when exposed to an environment with secondhand smoke.

Medical Management

All smokers and tobacco users are advised to quit and should be provided with materials that inform them of methods to do so. Various levels of intervention are available and include minimal approaches such as brief counseling and follow-up or more intense measures such as enrollment in behavior modification programs. These programs help clients manage temptation and extinguish conditioned cues to smoke. They also provide rewards for goal achievement. Pharmacologic therapy using drugs for smoking cessation includes nonnicotine medications such as bupropion (Zyban) and varenicline (Chantix), which are dopamine uptake inhibitors that help suppress nicotine's addicting reinforcement, and nicotine substitutes (gum, patch, inhaler), which allow dopamine to be released but at a lower rate than occurs with smoking (see Drug Therapy Table 71-1). The nicotine substitutes are gradually tapered and stopped; they help clients avoid withdrawal symptoms and are an adjunct to other interventions.

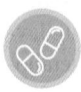

Pharmacologic Considerations

- Young children are particularly sensitive to the effects of even small doses of nicotine. E-liquid solutions used in electronic cigarettes have variable amounts of nicotine and are prepared in flavors appealing to children (candy and fruit). Poison control should be immediately contacted if children are found with an e-liquid solution.

Relapse (resumption in use) is common because withdrawal symptoms begin within several hours after the last cigarette is smoked and peak 2 to 3 days later (Box 71-5). In 2015, 68% of smokers wanted to quit altogether (Babb et al., 2017) and 55.1% had attempted to quit in the past year (Creamer et al., 2019). However, fewer than one in 10 adults smokers succeed in quitting each year (Department of Health and Human Services, 2020). Four out of nine adult smokers who saw health care professionals during the past year did not receive information about smoking cessation or were advised to quit (Department of Health and Human Services, 2020). Nevertheless, attempts to quit are a predictor of eventual success; many of those who try and fail ultimately do succeed, sometimes after trying multiple times. Relapses are often a consequence of common triggers (Table 71-4).

BOX 71-5 Smoking Withdrawal Symptoms

- Anxiety
- Irritability
- Trouble concentrating
- Restlessness
- Increased appetite
- Cravings for nicotine
- Fatigue
- Insomnia
- Reduced heart rate

Adapted from SmokeFree.gov. *Managing withdrawal*. Retrieved February 26, 2021, from https://smokefree.gov/challenges-when-quitting/managing-withdrawal

Nursing Management

Nurses help clients who smoke by counseling them to quit and providing them with information on various smoking cessation products and programs. Nurturing the client's belief that they can be successful is an important supportive measure. Because many clients fear gaining weight after smoking cessation, the nurse informs them that typical weight gain in the year after cessation is 7 to 10 lb (American Lung Association, 2020; Jaret, 2011). The nurse then helps the client plan strategies to offset the tendency for weight gain, such as beginning a walking program, substituting fruits for high-calorie desserts, and reducing dietary fat. Sucking on sugarless hard candy or chewing sugarless gum also may help by keeping the client's mouth busy without adding calories. If the client is unwilling to contemplate quitting, the nurse informs them of the dangers of secondhand smoke to others and encourages abstinence from smoking in the presence of nonsmokers, especially children. The nurse also actively promotes individual and community health by learning smoking cessation techniques and providing seminars to the public.

TABLE 71-4 Common Relapse Triggers and Management

TRIGGERS	MANAGEMENT
Being around tobacco users	Go to a nonsmoking location
Feeling stressed or overwhelmed	Get moving; walk, ride a bike, exercise
Overworking	Delegate or practice saying "No"
Drinking alcohol	Find a replacement like chewing gum
Finishing a meal	Keep your hands busy
After morning coffee	Alter a previous routine
Talking on the phone	
While driving	
During break at work	
After having sex	

Adapted from SmokeFree.gov. *Know your triggers*. Retrieved February 26, 2021, from https://smokefree.gov/challenges-when-quitting/cravings-triggers/know-your-triggers/

Based on recommendations from the U.S. Environmental Protection Agency, the nurse can advise nonsmokers on techniques for reducing the inhalation of secondhand smoke:

- Do not permit others to smoke in one's home or workplace.
- If smoking takes place in the home, increase ventilation by opening windows or using exhaust fans.
- Avoid riding in a car with someone who smokes; the small area contributes to a high concentration of toxic smoke, which increases exposure.

Cocaine and Methamphetamine Dependence

Cocaine and methamphetamine are CNS stimulants. Although the actions of methamphetamine are stronger and last longer than those of cocaine, the physiologic and psychological effects of the two substances are comparable because of the rapid and excessive release of norepinephrine, dopamine, and serotonin. Each drug is associated with some unique health problems that develop from use and abuse.

Cocaine is a CNS stimulant obtained from the leaves of the coca plant. The powder form of cocaine is snorted (inhaled through the nose) or dissolved and injected intravenously. Crack, a purified form of cocaine with a crystalline or rocklike appearance, makes a crackling sound when it is heated; it is smoked either by placing it in a pipe or by sprinkling it onto or mixing it with tobacco or marijuana. Cocaine may be freebased, which reduces the drug to its purest form. A person smokes freebased cocaine by sprinkling it onto a cigarette or inhaling it through a pipe. Freebased cocaine provides an intense physical experience as the drug is absorbed, more so than when it is taken by other routes. It also increases the risk of toxic effects and overdose reactions. Metabolism of cocaine, which is rapid, is usually followed by an intense craving to use the drug again. Cravings can recur months or years after abstinence.

Methamphetamine, also known as "meth," is an addicting stimulant that is made by combining over-the-counter medications containing ephedrine and pseudoephedrine with other chemicals such as ammonia, acetone, and lye. The final product is generally smoked or injected intravenously. When self-administered, the user experiences extreme pleasure, euphoria, and CNS stimulation similar to that associated with cocaine use.

Assessment Findings

Signs and Symptoms

Signs and symptoms of each drug's effect may be brief (see Table 71-1) because of the rapid metabolism and the powerful craving to use the drug again. Signs correlate with its route of administration and consequences of chronic use. For example, ulceration of the nasal mucosa and perforation of the nasal septum are found in people who snort cocaine. Needle marks are found along the pathways of veins in those who inject cocaine intravenously. Those who smoke or freebase cocaine may have burns on their faces, fingertips, or eyebrows from using or leaning over a lighted pipe. Smoking cocaine can cause a chronic cough and pulmonary congestion.

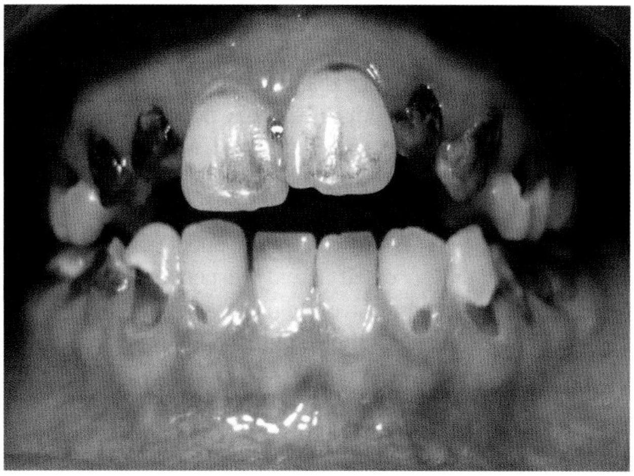

Figure 71-2 Dental changes such as blackened, stained, rotting teeth and tooth loss, referred to collectively as "meth mouth," are the results of abusing methamphetamine. (Photo by Dozenist. Licensed under Creative Commons. Available online at: https://commons.wikimedia.org/wiki/File:Suspectedmethmouth09-19-05.jpg)

Methamphetamine users may develop acne and be covered with multiple scratched lesions. Some users have tactile hallucinations and believe that insects are crawling under their skin, which causes them to scratch their face, hands, and arms. The constriction of blood vessels makes the resulting lesions slow to heal.

Methamphetamine use also causes the salivary glands to dry out, and the corrosive chemicals used to manufacture the drug lead to the destruction of tooth enamel. Meth addicts also grind their teeth, which, along with the constriction of blood vessels to the mouth and neglected oral hygiene, leads to blackened, stained, and rotting teeth (Fig. 71-2). This condition is sometimes referred to as "meth mouth." Extreme weight loss is also common.

Clients who are addicted to cocaine and methamphetamine often have a problem with **polydrug abuse**, abuse of more than one substance. It is common for them to take sedative drugs such as alcohol, minor tranquilizers, barbiturates, and marijuana to offset their agitation and irritability.

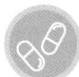

Pharmacologic Considerations

- A person with a known opioid addiction may be prescribed naloxone (Evzio, Narcan) when discharged to the care of family. Packaged as a single-dose autoinjector, it works with audio instructions on how to deliver the injection. Narcan can also be obtained as a nasal spray for use by people in the community for the treatment of known or suspected opioid overdoes (NARCAN.com, 2020).

Complications

Long-term abusers of cocaine and methamphetamine experience anorexia, weight loss, memory impairment, personality and behavioral changes, paranoia, psychosis, and hallucinations. Medically, stimulant abuse can cause rapid and severe hypertension, cardiac arrhythmias, seizures, cerebral hemorrhage (stroke), myocardial infarction (heart attack), and respiratory arrest. Newborns also can experience withdrawal symptoms if their mothers recently used CNS stimulants.

Methamphetamine users are also at higher risk for contracting HIV and hepatitis B because the surge of neurotransmitters increases sexual drive and decreases judgment. Consequently, sexual activity, especially among gay men, may be more aggressive and prolonged, thus increasing the potential for anogenital bleeding and the transmission of blood-borne viruses.

Diagnostic Findings

Drug toxicology tests are done on blood and urine. Metabolites of cocaine can be found in a urine drug screen for up to 36 hours. Metabolites of methamphetamine can be found for up to 3 to 6 days. Other abused substances also are identified.

Medical Management and Rehabilitation

Cocaine toxicity (see Table 71-1) requires immediate treatment because the condition is life-threatening. Referral to Cocaine Anonymous, which is based on the same principles as AA, provides a source of ongoing support for those addicted to cocaine. Participation in individual and group psychotherapy and Cocaine Anonymous is encouraged to help the client eliminate all forms of drug abuse. The recreational use of other drugs can lead to relapse.

To help the person addicted to cocaine with recovery, medications such as bromocriptine (Parlodel) and amantadine (Symmetrel) are used temporarily. They increase or mimic the effects of dopamine, the neurotransmitter that is most likely responsible for the rewarding and reinforcing effects of addicting substances. Antidepressants are prescribed to relieve the dysphoria (depression) that occurs during withdrawal. Amino acid precursors such as phenylalanine and tyrosine, the substances from which the neurotransmitters norepinephrine and dopamine are made, are included in drug therapy to replace levels depleted by chronic use.

A research project involving an anticocaine vaccine developed by Xenova Pharmaceuticals in England called TA-CD was developed to promote the development of antibodies that bind with cocaine and prevent the drug from reaching the brain. However, the Food and Drug Administration (FDA) has not approved the vaccine despite many clinical trials (Kimishima, Olson, & Janda, 2018; Martinez & Trifilieff, 2014). Another similar anticocaine vaccine called dAd5GNE developed by Weill Cornell Medicine and New York Presbyterian Hospital has shown efficacy in occasional, moderate cocaine use (Havlicek et al., 2020). The vaccine links a cocaine-like molecule with an inactive adenovirus. The hypothesis is that the immune system will produce anticocaine antibodies and prevent cocaine from reaching the brain and producing a dopamine high (Crystal, 2016; Havlicek et al., 2020).

Unfortunately, recovery from methamphetamine abuse is more difficult. It may take years of antidepressant drug therapy and behavior modification techniques.

Nursing Management

The nurse assesses the client's history of drug use and their current physical condition. The nurse also looks for signs of toxicity and withdrawal and implements medical treatment during a life-threatening emergency. Later, the nurse explains the effects of drug abuse and the risks for continuing drug-taking behaviors. Monitoring the client for suicidal ideation (see Chapter 69) and administering medications that provide support during withdrawal are essential nursing interventions.

Opioid Dependence

Opioid dependence is an addiction to CNS-depressant drugs that are either derived from or chemically similar to opium. Some examples of opioid drugs include heroin (diacetylmorphine), codeine, morphine, meperidine (Demerol), methadone (Dolophine), hydromorphone (Dilaudid), oxycodone (OxyContin), and opium, as in tincture of paregoric. Opioids produce sedation after the initial euphoria. The rate of tolerance and chemical dependence is related to the drug, dose, and frequency of use.

Assessment Findings

Refer to heroin in Table 71-1 and Figure 71-3 for the effects and consequences of opiate abuse. The pupils are usually pinpoint in size. Constipation is associated with slowed peristalsis. Chronic use is evidenced by anorexia, weight loss, constipation, malnutrition, needle marks, and scarring (tracks) along the paths of veins with repeated parenteral self-administration (Fig. 71-4).

Respiratory depression can lead to unconsciousness and death. Sharing needles during the IV administration of any abused substance can lead to HIV/AIDS, hepatitis, and septicemia. Abscesses may develop in punctured skin and veins. General debilitation increases susceptibility to tuberculosis and anemia. Neonates in withdrawal are observed to have a high-pitched cry, tremors, insomnia, increased respirations, vomiting, diarrhea, dehydration, and convulsions.

A urine drug screen reveals evidence of opioid use. Rapid recovery (within 2 to 5 minutes) from lethargy, hypotension, and respiratory depression after the IV administration of a narcotic antagonist such as naloxone (Narcan) supports the diagnosis of narcotic overdose. An autoinjector of naloxone is now available to families who live or have contact with those who may experience an opioid overdose in an effort to prevent their death from respiratory depression. See pharmacological considerations on pg ##.

Medical Management and Rehabilitation

Withdrawal symptoms can be treated with the alpha-adrenergic blocker clonidine (Catapres) to inhibit the release of norepinephrine, buprenorphine/naloxone (Suboxone), an opioid (narcotic) partial agonist–antagonist or methadone (Dolophine), a synthetic narcotic, to eliminate or control withdrawal symptoms.

Methods for helping those addicted to heroin avoid IV or street-acquired opioids is **methadone or buprenorphine/naloxone (Suboxone) maintenance therapy**, which

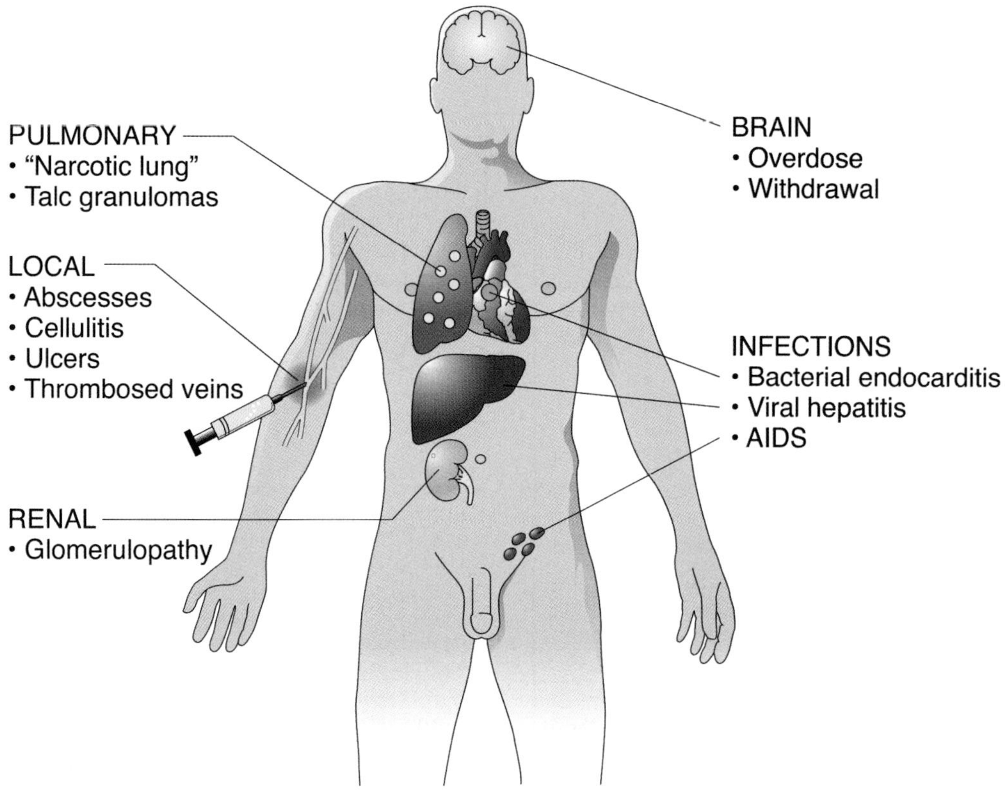

Figure 71-3 Potential consequences of opiate abuse. (Reprinted with permission from Rubin, E., & Farber, J. L. (1999). *Pathology* (3rd ed.). Lippincott Williams & Wilkins.)

involves substituting one addicting drug for another. The advantage is that because the drugs are synthetic drugs prepared by a pharmaceutical company, they are untainted and the dose is reliable. The rationale behind maintenance therapy is that it forestalls withdrawal, avoids a toxic overdose, reduces the potential for blood-borne infections, and theoretically reduces crime because the drug is provided legally. Some addicts, however, have been known to combine their maintenance medications with their depressant drug of choice, which increases the potential of overdose and death. The practice of testing the urine before providing the maintenance medication is one way of screening and eliminating those who are abusing the system. To avoid black market sale of methadone or Suboxone, close monitoring by the treating professional is necessary.

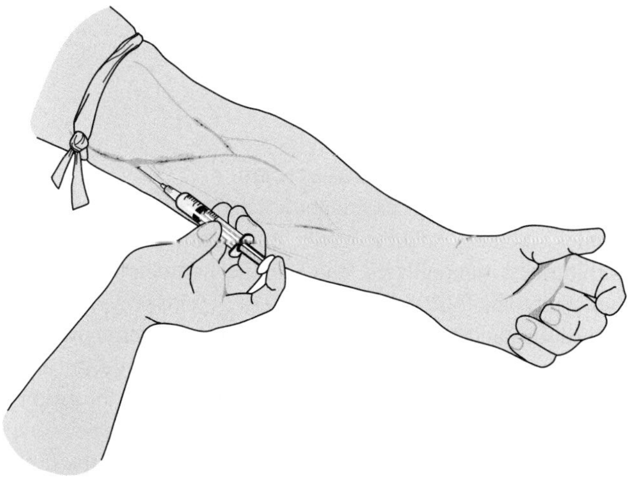

Figure 71-4 Track marks are evidence of self-injection of opiates.

Naltrexone (Vivitrol, Trexan, ReVia), an opioid antagonist, is also used for opioid addiction. Naltrexone blocks endorphin receptors; if clients return to opioid abuse while taking naltrexone, they do not experience the previous level of opioid effects. Naltrexone is administered IV for **rapid opioid detoxification,** a procedure for accelerating opioid drug withdrawal within 4 to 8 hours while the client is under anesthesia. Rapid detoxification eliminates the physical discomfort of opioid withdrawal; however, it increases the risks associated with prolonged anesthesia with mechanical ventilation and is more expensive than traditional detoxification protocols.

Psychotherapy is an important aspect of rehabilitation. It involves treating the complex web of social problems that accompanies the addiction. Clients also are referred to Narcotics Anonymous (NA), a self-help organization modeled after AA.

Nursing Management

The nurse's role is similar to that discussed for other types of substance use disorders, with a few exceptions that apply to administering drug therapy. If naltrexone is prescribed as an opioid deterrent, the client must be opioid-free for at least 7 days before administration begins. The nurse advises the client who takes methadone to tell health care providers or wear a MedicAlert tag in case the client needs a narcotic, tranquilizer, or barbiturate. Given methadone is a narcotic, lower doses of other sedative drugs are necessary because the combination can potentiate their depressant action. See Evidence-Based Practice 71-1.

Evidence-Based Practice 71-1

Opioid Addiction and Client Participation in Treatment Options

Clinical Question

Are clients diagnosed with opioid addiction included in treatment options during their treatment program?

Note

Individual preferences and values is a vital part of the three legs of evidence-based practice (evidence, clinical expertise, and preferences and values). The best evidence-driven treatment plan is worth nothing if it does not align with the client's beliefs, values, lifestyle, and resources. This results in nonadherence and poor outcomes. In this Evidence-Based Practice box, the research on individual preferences and values in the treatment of those with opioid addiction is explored.

Evidence

Opioid use disorder involves long-standing treatment that often involves multiple relapses (Bisaga et al., 2018). Bailey et al. (2013) found that 80% of the participants in their study had been through treatment multiple times. Twenty-seven percent reported relapsing on the day they were discharged from inpatient detoxification; 65% relapsed within 1 month, and 90% relapsed within 1 year. Too often, clients are not brought into the planning of their discharge and treatment plans. However, clients do have preferences (Bailey et al., 2013; Hay et al., 2019; Stein et al., 2015; Uebelacker et al., 2016). Stein et al. (2015) surveyed 485 clients and found that 96% of clients preferred some sort of aftercare post-detoxification. When asked to choose the one treatment that would work best for them after discharge, 43% selected medication-assisted treatment, 29% preferred residential placement, 12% selected drug-free counseling, 12% NA/AA meetings only, and 4% preferred no additional treatment. Bailey et al. (2013) found that although 63% of subjects in their study preferred medication assistance to help overcome the urges to use opioids after inpatient detoxification, they were rarely consulted or offered medication-assisted treatment in spite of the availability of three FDA-approved medications: methadone (Dolophine), buprenorphine (Subutex), and naltrexone (ReVia). This is further supported by Williams et al. (2018) who found that of the 2.1 to 2.4 million Americans with opioid use disorder, only about 20% received any treatment, and of those only one-third received any kind of medication-assisted treatment resulting in a retention rate of only 30% to 50% in most settings. This ultimately means that only approximately 2% of individuals with opioid use disorders achieve long-term remission (Williams et al., 2018). Among the three medication-assisted treatment methods used in opioid use disorders, naltrexone, methadone and buprenorphine, methadone and buprenorphine have shown greater success than naltrexone (Salmond, Allread, & Marsh, 2019). Research exploring influencing factors in a client's decision-making regarding treatment options points to the importance of including the family's understanding and perception of the various treatment modalities in the decision in order to optimize their support (Bisaga et al., 2018; Nayak et al., 2021).

Nursing Implications

There are no greater client advocates on the health care team than nurses. Nurses spend significantly more time with clients and their families than any other health care provider, building trust and relationships that give clients and their families the courage to be open and verbal about their situations, needs, and preferences. It is important that the nurse use their skills to create a situation where clients are comfortable sharing their thoughts, ideas, and needs, and feel safe enough to ask questions so they can make informed decisions. The nurse is also positioned to remind and encourage other providers to consult clients about care and treatment plans to improve outcomes.

References

Bailey, G. L., Herman, D. S., & Stein, M. D. (2013). Perceived relapse risk and desire for medication assisted treatment among persons seeking inpatient opiate detoxification. *Journal of Substance Abuse Treatment, 45*(3), 302–305. https://doi.org/10.1016/j.jsat.2013.04.002

Bisaga, A., Mannelli, P., Sullivan, M. A., Vosburg, S. K., Compton, P., Woody, G. E., & Kosten, T. R. (2018). Antagonists in the medical management of opioid use disorders: Historical and existing treatment strategies. *American Journal on Addictions, 27*, 177–187. https://doi.org/10.1111/ajad.12711

Hay, K. R., Huhn, A. S., Tompkins, D. A., & Dunn, K. E. (2019). Recovery goals and long-term treatment preference in persons who engage in nonmedical opioid use. *Journal of Addiction Medicine, 13*(4), 300–305. https://doi.org/10.1097/ADM.0000000000000498

Nayak, S. M., Huhn, A. S., Bergeria, C. L., Strain, E. C., & Dunn, K. E. (2021). Familial perceptions of appropriate treatment types and goals for a family member who has opioid use disorder. *Drug and Alcohol Dependence, 221*. https://doi.org/10.1016/j.drugalcdep.2021.108649

Salmond, S., Allread, V., & Marsh, R. (2019). Management of opioid use disorder treatment: An overview. *Orthopaedic Nursing, 38*(2), 118–126. https://doi.org/10.1097/NOR.0000000000000547

Stein, M. D., Anderson, B. J., & Bailey, G. L. (2015). Preferences for aftercare among persons seeking short-term opioid detoxification. *Journal of Substance Abuse Treatment, 59*, 99–103. https://doi.org/10.1016/j.jsat.2015.07.002

Uebelacker, L. A., Bailey, G., Herman, D., Anderson, B., & Stein, M. (2016). Patients' beliefs about medications are associated with stated preference for methadone, buprenorphine, naltrexone, or no medication-assisted therapy following inpatient opioid detoxification. *Journal of Substance Abuse Treatment, 66*, 48–53. https://doi.org/10.1016/j.jsat.2016.02.009

Williams, A. R., Nunes, E. V., Bisaga, A., Pincus, H. A., Johnson, K. A., Campbell, A. N., Remien, R. H., Crystal, S., Friedmann, P. D., Levin, F. R., & Olfson, M. (2018). Developing an opioid use disorder treatment cascade: A review of quality measures. *Journal of Substance Abuse Treatment, 91*, 57–58. https://doi.org/10.1016/j.jsat.2018.06.001

Other Abused Substances

Various other substances are abused and addictive. Some examples include hallucinogens, amphetamines, marijuana, barbiturates, tranquilizers, and volatile hydrocarbons. Signs and symptoms follow the same pattern as with previously discussed substances: Experimental use progresses through stages of increased use until dependence and addiction occur; there is failure to meet social, familial, or occupational obligations, with increased defensive mechanisms to explain behavior; and disturbances in mood and physical function occur as the result of drug abuse. Treatment and recovery include withdrawal, abstinence, and ongoing participation in a support group.

KEY POINTS

- The health and social consequences of substance abuse:
  - Morbidity/mortality
    - Liver disease
    - Cardiopulmonary disease
    - Infectious diseases: AIDS/hepatitis
  - Social
    - Domestic abuse
    - Child abuse
    - Crime: assault/murders/traffic-boating fatalities

- Commonly abused addictive substances:
  - Nicotine
  - Alcohol
  - Cocaine
  - Heroin
  - Amphetamine
  - Marijuana

- Withdrawal: refers to the physical symptoms and craving for a drug that occur when a person abruptly stops using an abused substance.
- Tolerance: refers to the reduction in a drug's effect that follows persistent use. Tolerance results because the body develops mechanisms for using the drug more effectively or inactivating the drug more efficiently. Consequently, a person must take increasing amounts of the substance to obtain the desired effect.
- Four steps in the progression toward chemical dependence:
  - Experimentation
  - Habituation
  - Dependence
  - Addiction

- Two ways abused drugs produce their effects:
  - Self-reinforcing pleasurable effects that some substances produce in the limbic system of the brain, depending on the type of substance.

- **CNS stimulants** are chemical agents that temporarily accelerate physical and mental functions. Include caffeine, cocaine, and amphetamines affect levels of norepinephrine, dopamine, and acetylcholine.
- **CNS depressants** are chemical agents that slow brain and physiologic activities. Include alcohol, heroin and other opioids, and barbiturates; cause effects similar to those of GABA, endorphins, and enkephalins. These drugs either mimic the neurotransmitters by attaching to their receptor sites or block their reuptake.
- Alcoholism: is a chronic, progressive, multisystem disease characterized by an inability to control the consumption of alcohol.
  - Symptoms:
    - Denial of drinking problem
    - History of increased alcohol consumption
    - Solitary drinking
    - Hiding alcohol
    - Alcohol tolerance
    - Cross-tolerance for sedative–hypnotic drugs
  - Health issues
    - Blackouts
    - Family issues
    - Legal issues
    - Occupational issues
    - Financial issues

- Treatment and nursing management for clients with alcoholism:
  - Safe detoxification to manage acute withdrawal symptoms
    - Sedative medications
    - Beta-adrenergic blockers
    - Vitamin replacement
    - Hydration
  - Nutritional therapy
  - Psychotherapy
  - Anticraving drugs (drug therapy)
  - AA
  - Support group

- Potential health consequences of tobacco use:
  - Smoking raises carbon monoxide levels in the blood and causes constriction of peripheral blood vessels = cardiovascular disease.
  - Smoking disrupts the structure of alveoli, causing them to become overstretched and inelastic = emphysema.
  - It is implicated in the development and recurrence of gastric ulcers.
  - Tobacco products contain more than 40 carcinogenic chemicals = lung, esophagus, oral cancer.

- Signs and symptoms of cocaine and methamphetamine abuse as they relate to the manner of use:
  - Ulceration of nasal mucosa/perforation of the nasal septum
  - Track marks
  - Burns to fingers, face/eyebrows
  - Chronic cough/pulmonary congestion
  - Acne/scratch lesions
  - Tactile hallucinations
  - Meth mouth
  - Extreme weight loss

- Treatment and nursing management for clients addicted to cocaine and methamphetamine:
  - Assess history of drug use
  - Assess current physical condition
  - Assess for signs of toxicity and withdrawal
  - Monitor for suicidal ideation
  - Medication management

- Methods for managing opioid dependence:
  - Methadone or suboxone maintenance

CRITICAL THINKING EXERCISES

1. What information would you offer to a smoker who claims that "smoke-free environments" violate their right to smoke?
2. From which type of substance could a person be withdrawing if the following assessments are made? The client has a runny nose and tearing eyes, and they yawn frequently. The pilomotor muscles around the hair follicles cause "goosebumps" to appear. Nausea, vomiting, abdominal cramps, and diarrhea are present.
3. Explain why people recovering from alcoholism who have reached an extensive period of sobriety refer to themselves as "recovering" persons with alcohol use disorder rather than "recovered" persons with alcohol use disorder.
4. Why might a person with alcohol use disorder with a blood alcohol level (BAL) of 0.425% manifest physical and behavioral effects characteristic of a much lower BAL?

NCLEX-STYLE REVIEW QUESTIONS PrepU

1. A licensed practical nurse is asked to check a registered nurse's calculation of an intravenous dose of lorazepam (Ativan). The client is to receive 2 mg parenterally to control withdrawal symptoms. If the vial contains 10 mg in a 10-mL multidose vial, how much volume should the nurse administer?
2. When a primary provider prescribes disulfiram (Antabuse) for a client with alcohol use disorder, what substances should the nurse tell the client to avoid? Select all that apply.
   1. Mouthwash
   2. Lemon juice
   3. Aftershave lotion
   4. Mosquito repellant
   5. Sunscreen
   6. NyQuil for sleep
3. When a client who abuses alcohol is admitted to a substance abuse unit, when is the earliest time the nurse can expect the client to begin developing signs of alcohol withdrawal?
   1. 24 hours after the last drink
   2. 10 hours after the last drink
   3. 6 hours after the last drink
   4. 2 hours after the last drink
4. A nurse caring for a client who receives a daily dose of methadone (Dolophine) is accurate in identifying what reason for the client's drug therapy?
   1. The drug prevents vitamin deficiencies.
   2. The drug cures future opioid abuse.
   3. The drug counteracts opioid toxicity.
   4. The drug prevents opioid withdrawal.
5. When a client who is jaundiced and has ascites begins vomiting a profuse amount of blood, what abused substance should the nurse focus on for health-related data?
   1. Heroin abuse
   2. Cocaine abuse
   3. Alcohol abuse
   4. Methamphetamine abuse

WANT TO KNOW MORE? There are a wide variety of online resources available on thePoint to enhance learning and understanding of this chapter.

Go to thePoint.lww.com/activate and use the activation code found in the front of this text to unlock these online resources.

72 Caring for Clients With Dementia and Thought Disorders

Words To Know

acalculia
acetylcholine
agnosia
agraphia
alexia
Alzheimer disease
amyloid plaques
amyloid precursor protein
aphasia
apraxia
ataxia
beta-amyloid
biomarkers
cognitive functions
conservatorship
delirium
delusions
dementia
depot injections
durable power of attorney
extrapyramidal symptoms
glutamate
grandiosity
guardianship
hallucinations
incompetent
mentation
negative symptoms
neurofibrillary tangles
positive symptoms
respite care
restraint alternatives
schizophrenia
tau
voice dismissal

Learning Objectives

On completion of this chapter, the reader will:

1. Differentiate between delirium and dementia and give an example of a condition that causes each.
2. List five etiologic factors linked to Alzheimer disease (AD).
3. Discuss the pathophysiologic changes associated with AD.
4. Name the first symptom of AD.
5. Identify two methods for diagnosing AD.
6. Explain the mechanism of drug therapy in AD.
7. Describe nursing management for clients with AD.
8. Name three characteristics of schizophrenia.
9. Describe two psychobiologic explanations for schizophrenia.
10. Differentiate between positive and negative symptoms of schizophrenia and give two examples of each.
11. Discuss the medical management of most people with schizophrenia.
12. Name three examples of antipsychotic drugs and their mechanisms of action.
13. Explain the term *extrapyramidal symptoms* (EPSs) and list four examples.
14. Describe a technique to prevent nonadherence to drug therapy in clients with schizophrenia.
15. Describe the nursing management of clients with schizophrenia.

Changes in **mentation**, or mental activity, can occur anytime during the life cycle. **Cognitive functions**, such as short-term memory and learning ability, change gradually as people get older, but many acute, chronic, reversible, and irreversible conditions that impair thinking processes can occur at any age. Although older adults are at greatest risk for cognitive impairment, one should never assume that such impairment is necessarily a normal consequence of aging or that it is untreatable. Depression and other medical disorders, such as hypothyroidism, can manifest as mental dysfunction. Consequently, mental changes require aggressive investigation to determine what, if anything, can reverse the symptoms that clients experience. This chapter discusses conditions that are characterized by delirium, dementia, and thought disorders.

Gerontologic Considerations

- Delirium in older adults may occur as the presenting symptom for infections such as pneumonia or urinary tract infections or infections caused by fecal impaction. Delirium may present as hyperactivity (e.g., picking at bedcovers or clothing, nervous behaviors) or as hypoactivity (e.g., refusing to make eye contact or verbal exchanges, lethargy).
- Cognition changes such as delirium must be thoroughly documented regarding onset, course, and relationship to any medication (including anesthesia). Altered absorption, metabolism, distribution, or elimination can lead to increased medication concentrations and resultant adverse cognitive effects.
- Cognitive changes alter older adult roles and relationships, impacting client self-worth and evoking fear of the progression of the disease. Older adults with few or no family members or significant others are at high risk for loss of identity. Photographs from younger years may help provide a sense of self.
- Older adults often experience painful comorbidities such as neuropathy or arthritis. Assessment for pain in the presence of cognitive decline requires careful observation of facial expressions and body positioning and collaboration with caregivers and significant others. Altered cognition does not negate the person's need for comfort.
- Caregiver support and personalized education regarding care for older adults experiencing cognitive changes are critical. Awareness of disease manifestations and intentional strategies to maximize communication, safety, and coping with emotional changes can increase quality of life for both caregiver and care recipient and decrease risk for social isolation or abuse.
- Older adult clients require lower dosages of antipsychotic drugs. They also may experience comorbidities of psychosis, dementia, and depression, requiring careful examination of treatment efficacy for each.
- Haloperidol (Haldol) should be used only with extreme caution in older adults because of the risk for dehydration and falls and should not be used as a chemical restraint unless the benefits greatly outweigh the risks. Refer to the American Geriatrics Society's *Updated Beers Criteria for Potentially Inappropriate Medication Use in Older Adults* for more information (American Geriatrics Society, 2019).
- Older adults are particularly susceptible to tardive dyskinesia (TD) because of the long-term administration of typical antipsychotics. Report symptoms immediately because the drug must be discontinued to prevent further dyskinesia.

DELIRIUM AND DEMENTIA

Delirium is a sudden, transient state of confusion. The period of confusion depends on the cause of the delirium. Clients with delirium may have difficulty processing information. They may be disoriented as to the date, time of day, and location. Their judgment may be impaired, or they may be unable to perform intellectually at the same capacity as in the past. Some clients with delirium may be suspicious or frightened or behave inappropriately.

TABLE 72-1 Comparison of Dementia and Delirium

	DEMENTIA	DELIRIUM
Onset	Gradual	Sudden
Presentation	Alert	Blunted
	Attentive	Inattentive
Course	Stable	Unstable
	Progressive deterioration	Fluctuations in function
	Extended	Brief
Duration	Permanent	Temporary
Treatment	Symptomatic or supportive	Specific
Outcome	Incurable	Curable

Delirium can result from high fever, head trauma, brain tumor, drug intoxication or withdrawal, metabolic disorders (e.g., liver or renal failure), or inflammatory disorders of the central nervous system (CNS), such as meningitis or encephalitis. Treating the underlying medical condition usually restores mental functions.

Dementia, which more commonly affects older adults, refers to conditions in which decline in memory, thinking, and reasoning is severe enough to affect the daily life of an alert person. Various disorders are characterized by dementia. AD is the leading example, followed by cerebrovascular disorders (see Chapter 38) and Parkinson disease (see Chapter 37). In contrast to delirium, dementia is manifested by a gradual, irreversible loss of intellectual abilities. Although clients with dementia display signs and symptoms similar to those of delirium, several differences exist (Table 72-1).

>>> *Stop, Think, and Respond 72-1*

In the descriptions that follow, which client is manifesting delirium and which is manifesting dementia?

- *Client A is 60 years old. They developed a headache and high fever 24 hours ago. They think they are in the city in which they spent their childhood. They call for their mother, who has been dead for more than 10 years.*
- *Client B is 60 years old. They got lost driving home from work last week. Lately, they have had difficulty remembering where they put their keys and wallet. Their partner notices that they are more argumentative than usual.*

ALZHEIMER DISEASE

AD, the most common cause of dementia, is a progressive, deteriorating brain disorder. Two types exist: early onset (between 30 and 60 years of age) and late onset (after age 60 years), with late onset being more common. There are an estimated 6.2 million Americans living with AD in 2021. By 2050, the incidence of AD is estimated to reach 12.7 million (Alzheimer's Association, 2021a). Although the rates of several major causes of death have declined, deaths from AD have increased by 145.2%; in fact, deaths from heart disease have decreased by 7.3% (Alzheimer's Association, 2021a). The National Institute on Aging (2019a) lists AD as the sixth leading cause of death in the United States and the third leading cause of death for older people.

Pathophysiology and Etiology

Early-Onset Alzheimer Disease

Having a first-degree relative with AD nearly doubles the risk for acquiring a familial form of dementia. The strongest Alzheimer markers are mutations that occur on various genes within specific chromosomes (1, 14, and 21) that are responsible for making proteins that promote the survival of nerve cells. The mutated genes cause a disruption in the processing of a substance known as **amyloid precursor protein** (APP).

The process leading to AD is believed to progress in the following way (Fig 72-1A):

- **APP**, a normal transmembranous neuronal protein, consists of three parts that reside partially inside, within, and outside the neuron's membrane.
- Beta-secretase, a cellular enzyme, cuts the external portion of APP, forming a fragment called sAPPβ (soluble amyloid precursor protein beta).
- Gamma-secretase, a second enzyme, cuts the internal portion of sAPPβ, causing the middle portion to become a free-floating fragment of **beta-amyloid**, a starchy protein.
- Beta amyloid injures neurons in the area of the brain responsible for producing **acetylcholine**, the neurotransmitter that is critical for memory and cognition.
- As more and more beta-amyloid accumulates from increasing numbers of released beta-amyloid fragments, the particles begin to stick together, forming **amyloid plaques**.
- Accumulating amyloid plaques produce toxic effects on neurons by stimulating an excessive amount of the neurotoxic neurotransmitter **glutamate**, a contributing factor in neuronal cell death.
- Meanwhile, inside the neuron, an abnormal protein called **tau** causes the neuron's microtubules, structures responsible for transporting nutrients from the cell body to the axon, to clump together, forming **neurofibrillary tangles.**
- Eventually, the microtubules disintegrate, and the neuron dies because the transport system is destroyed.
- As more and more neurons die, the brain atrophies (see Fig. 72-1B).

Late-Onset Alzheimer Disease

Although inherited, mutated genes are implicated in the development of early-onset AD, and the etiology of late-onset AD is less clear. It may be a combination of genetic, environmental, and lifestyle factors.

One risk factor for AD is attributed to an *allele*, one of a pair of genes, occupying chromosome 19 that regulates the formation of apolipoprotein. Of the three different forms of apolipoprotein, APOE ε2, APOE ε3, and APOE ε4, those with APOE ε4 are believed to have a greater risk for developing AD, but its presence does not confirm that a person will develop the disease. Those who study the *human genome*, all the genetic information possessed by men and women,

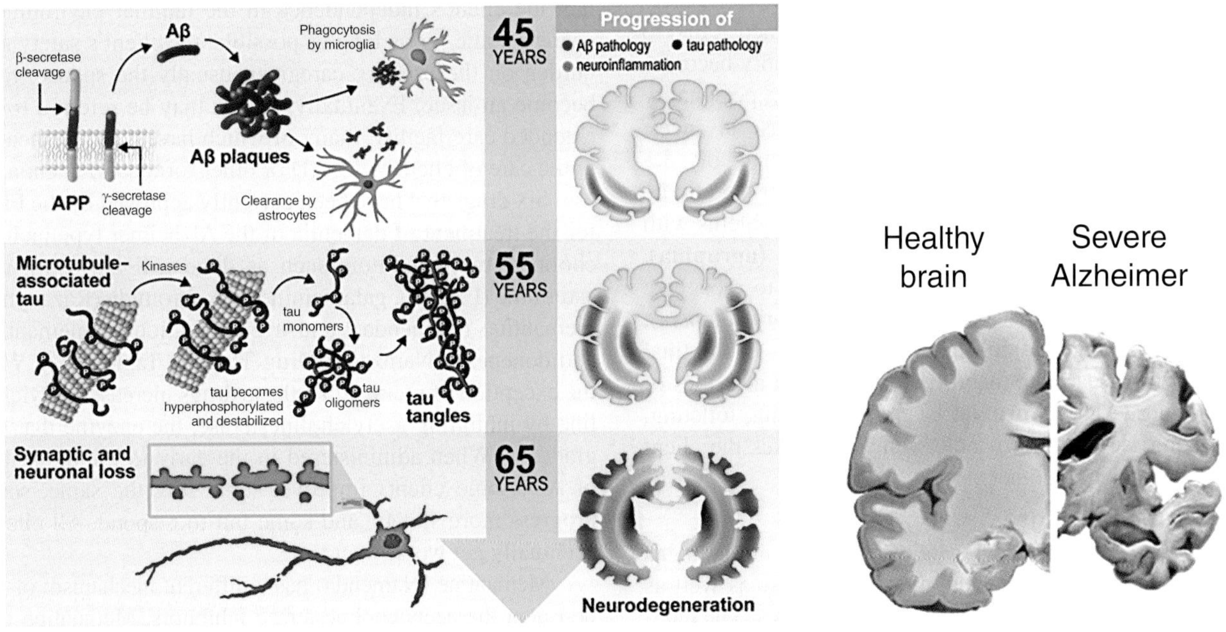

A B

Figure 72-1 Selected pathophysiologic processes in Alzheimer disease. Amyloid precursor protein (APP) is embedded in the neuron's cell membrane. Enzymes beta-secretase and gamma-secretase sever soluble amyloid precursor protein beta (sAPPβ), releasing a fragment that becomes beta-amyloid. Neurofibrillary tangles of tau proteins in microtubules form. As microtubules disintegrate and more and more neurons die, the brain atrophies (note differences in the healthy and Alzheimer-affected brain in Fig 72-1B). (**A**, from Newcombe, E. A., Camats-Perna, J., Silva, M. L., Valmas, N., Huat, T. J., & Medeiros, R. (2018). Inflammation: The link between comorbidities, genetics, and Alzheimer's disease. *Journal of neuroinflammation, 15*(1), 276. https://doi.org/10.1186/s12974-018-1313-3. https://creativecommons.org/licenses/by/4.0/.; **B**, National Institute on Aging. (2019b). Alzheimer's disease fact sheet. Retrieved March 16, 2021 from https://www.nia.nih.gov/health/alzheimers-disease-fact-sheet)

believe that there are other genes that may be implicated as risk factors as well (National Institute on Aging, 2019c).

The decreased size of the cerebral cortex and hippocampus together with acetylcholine deficiency and glutamate toxicity explain the cognitive deficits and alterations in emotions that accompany the disease. The degree to which amyloid plaque and neurofibrillary tangles are present is directly related to the severity of disease manifestations.

Assessment Findings

Signs and Symptoms

AD's progression from one stage to another can occur at different rates in different people. The onset of AD is insidious, and symptoms may develop slowly over years; a poor sense of smell may be one of the earliest signs of Alzheimer (Kotecha et al., 2018; Marin et al., 2018; Wessen et al., 2011). The National Institute on Aging (2017) has identified three distinct stages of AD:

1. *Preclinical*: a period when amyloid plaques are accumulating, and nerve cell changes are occurring, but there are no clinical symptoms of AD
2. *Mild cognitive impairment*: a time when memory problems are noticed but not serious enough to interfere with independent living
3. *Alzheimer dementia*: the point at which there is significant cognitive decline, such as difficulty recalling words, trouble learning new information, difficulty recognizing familiar faces, and impaired reasoning, judgment, and problem-solving

Memory loss, the classic symptom, is confined at first to recent information. Eventually, long-term memory becomes impaired as well. Disturbances in behavior, personality changes, and depression also occur. As the disease advances, the ability of clients to care for themselves markedly deteriorates. Clients may wander and become lost. Periodic incidences of violent behavior are possible. Problems with speaking (**aphasia**), reading (**alexia**), writing (**agraphia**), and calculating (**acalculia**) develop. Inability to recognize objects and sounds (visual, tactile, and auditory **agnosia**), difficulty walking (**ataxia**), and tremors occur. In the final stage of the disease, an inability to accomplish activities of daily living (ADLs; **apraxia**), such as grooming, toileting, and eating, despite intact motor function, makes the client totally dependent on others.

Diagnostic Findings

Ruling out AD in clients who are experiencing similar signs and symptoms can spare them emotional agony as well as saving time and money spent on nonspecific tests. The diagnosis of AD is usually made by excluding other causes for the client's symptoms. A computed tomography (CT) scan shows shrinking of the cerebral cortex, but this is not apparent in the early stages of the disease. Positron emission tomography (PET) and magnetic resonance imaging (MRI) provide structural and metabolic information about the brain. Electroencephalography detects slower-than-normal brain waves. None of these diagnostic tests is specific for AD, which, until recently, could be confirmed only during a postmortem examination of the brain.

A diagnosis of AD currently relies on validating mental decline. There continues to be a search for diagnostic tests that could detect **biomarkers**, proteins in blood, spinal fluid, and other body fluids, earlier in the disease process or differentiate AD from other causes of neurodegeneration. The test known as AD7C uses human urine or cerebrospinal fluid to detect the presence of beta-amyloid and tau proteins (Jin & Wang, 2021; Li et al., 2020).

Research is now focusing on molecular neuroimaging technologies that detect biologic evidence of AD before there are structural brain changes. Some examples of these include radiotracers such as Pittsburgh compound B (PIB), 18F-flutemetamol, florbetapir F 18 (18F-AV-45), and florbetaben (BAY 94-9172), which can identify beta-amyloid plaques during a PET scan. The research on these tests is being supported by various AD associations (Alzheimer's Association, 2021b).

Currently, there are blood tests that can identify APOE ε4 that may herald late-onset AD. Genetic testing to identify the early-onset familial type of AD is possible, but some with a family history are hesitant to validate that they carry the defective genes.

Medical Management

No cure exists for AD; treatment is mainly supportive, using one of various drugs currently available, but newer therapeutic advances show promise. Although it is best to maintain the client's independence in the familiar environment of their home for as long as possible, the client's safety and burden on the primary caregiver, usually the spouse, may become an issue. Eventually, clients may be referred to an extended care facility, many of which have a unit dedicated to the care of clients with AD or other forms of dementia.

Six drugs that have been currently approved by the FDA for the treatment of dementia of the Alzheimer type include cholinesterase inhibitors such as donepezil (Aricept), rivastigmine (Exelon), galantamine hydrobromide (Razadyne), memantine (Namenda), and a combination of memantine and donepezil (Namzaric; Drug Therapy Table 72-1). With the exception of memantine, these drugs increase acetylcholine by inhibiting acetylcholinesterase, the enzyme that degrades it. When administered in the early to middle stages of AD, some clients improve, some stay the same, some progress more slowly, and some fail to respond. All clients eventually get worse over time.

Memantine (Namenda) has a different mechanism of action than the acetylcholinesterase inhibitors. Memantine is a neuroprotective drug classified as an *N*-methyl-D-aspartate (NMDA) antagonist. By blocking NMDA receptors, the drug protects neurons from excessive stimulation by glutamate, an excitatory neurotransmitter responsible for neuronal death. Clients in advanced stages of AD experienced less deterioration when taking memantine than others who were given a placebo.

Antidepressants or tranquilizers may help agitated or depressed clients. Valproic acid (Depakene, Depakote, and

DRUG THERAPY TABLE 72-1 Agents for Treating Alzheimer Disease

Category and Common Generic (Brand) Drugs	Intended Use	Common Side Effects	Safety Warnings for Nurses
Cholinesterase Inhibitors			
Donepezil (Aricept) Galantamine (Razadyne) Rivastigmine (Exelon)	Increases acetylcholine by blocking cholinesterase in mild to severe dementia due to AD; also provides memory improvement in dementia due to stroke, vascular disease, multiple sclerosis Parkinson disease	Headache, nausea, diarrhea, insomnia, muscle cramps Bradycardia, possible exacerbations of asthma and chronic obstructive pulmonary disease Dyspepsia, anorexia, abdominal pain, weight loss	Do not use to treat acute delirium When discontinued, benefit is absent in 6 weeks May cause gastrointestinal (GI) bleeding; monitor stools and emesis Report heart rate <60 beats/min If using a patch, rotate sites and remove old patch before applying new one Apply transdermal patch to upper back to prevent client self-removal
N-methyl-D-aspartate (NMDA) Receptor Antagonists			
Memantine (Namenda)	Provides nerve cell protection from excessive glutamate in moderate to severe AD dementia	Dizziness, headache, confusion	Do not use to treat acute delirium Avoid with renal disease and alkaline urine Give with a full glass of water
Combination Drug			
Memantine/donepezil (Namzaric)			

The drugs in column 1 indicate the drug that matches up with explanations in columns 2 through 4.

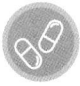

Pharmacologic Considerations

- Namzaric is the first combined cholinesterase inhibitor and NMDA receptor antagonist drug on the market. By combining these medications, drug administration is reduced to one pill daily in the evening instead of up to six pills throughout the day. This may ease distress on AD clients who have difficulty taking medications.

Valproate), which is generally prescribed for seizure disorders, has undergone multiple studies to determine its effectiveness in managing agitation among those with AD. Although there have been anecdotal reports of effectiveness, the conclusion is that valproate is no more helpful than a placebo (Heersma, 2020), and there is increasing evidence that the risks of valproate preparations may outweigh the benefits (Baillon et al., 2018; Olivieri-Mui et al., 2018). A study of davunetide (AL-108) as a drug for preventing neurofibrillary tangles caused by abnormal *tau* protein administered as a nasal spray has been halted. Although the drug was shown to be safe and well tolerated, it failed to show effectiveness in improving memory function in those with mild cognitive impairment, a precursor of Alzheimer dementia (Allon Therapeutics, Inc., 2012). Other tau-targeting therapies have also failed to show effectiveness in the treatment of Alzheimer disease (Congdon & Sigurdsson, 2018; Chong et al., 2018; Vaz & Silvestre, 2020).

Axona (formerly Ketasyn) is a medium-chain triglyceride product referred to as "medical food" intended as a cotherapy with other treatments for AD. The hypothesis is that there is a metabolic dysfunction in the brains of those with AD that (1) interferes with the neurons' ability to utilize glucose for energy, similar to diabetes mellitus; (2) impairs the utilization of fat; (3) reduces the production of acetylcholine; and (4) interferes with the clearance of amyloid-producing protein. When taken orally, Axona is metabolized into ketones, which the brain can use as an alternative to glucose, thus improving cognitive function (Mungali & Sharma, 2021).

Nursing Management

The major focus of nursing management is to help the client and caregiver maintain the highest possible quality of life by supporting mental and physical functions and ensuring safety.

Most clients initially receive care in their homes, and home health nurses can instruct the family about physical care, the disease process, and treatment. They also provide emotional support and intervene if family caregivers become overburdened. As the disease progresses, the client's nutritional needs must be considered (Nutrition Notes). When it becomes necessary to transfer the client from the home to an extended care facility, the nurse meets the client's physical needs on a full-time basis and helps the family cope during the client's deterioration. See Client and Family Teaching 72-1 for additional information.

Nutrition Notes

The Client With Alzheimer Disease

- AD can devastate nutritional status. Forgetfulness, alterations in smell and taste, and decreasing ability to self-feed impair intake. Weight loss is common. Choking may occur if the client forgets to chew food thoroughly or hoards food in their mouth.
- Increased agitation significantly increases calorie requirements. Nutritionally dense foods that are easy to consume, such as finger foods and liquid supplements, help maximize intake. Minimize distractions at meals and offer one food at a time to avoid overwhelming the client.
- Clients in the later stages of AD may be unable to swallow or may not know what to do when food is placed in their mouths. When such a situation occurs, a decision regarding nutritional support (e.g., percutaneous endoscopic gastrostomy tube feedings) must be made (see Chapter 45).

Client and Family Teaching 72-1 Caring for a Family Member With Dementia

The nurse emphasizes the following points when teaching the family and caregivers:

- Support, interact with, and cognitively stimulate the client.
- Minimize situations that contribute to the client's confusion and frustration, such as noise and distractions from a television—even mirrors may unduly disturb the client.
- Allow the client to remain as independent as possible.
- Follow a consistent routine throughout each day.
- Do not leave the person with an advanced cognitive disorder alone; investigate the services of a daycare facility for occasional respite.
- Park the car in a location where the client cannot see or gain access to it.
- Keep a means of identification on the client's person at all times in case of wandering.
- Install an on–off safety switch on the stove and oven.
- Store household chemicals in cupboards with safety latches.
- Lock up lighters, matches, and knives.
- Disable locks on bathroom doors.
- Use the services of a social worker.
- Access crisis telephone numbers if problems arise and coping skills are tested.
- Become involved with the local community mental health association.
- Join and attend meetings of a support group for caretakers of those who are cognitively impaired.

SCHIZOPHRENIA

Schizophrenia is a thought disorder characterized by deterioration in mental functioning, disturbances in sensory perception, and changes in affect (emotion). Clients with schizophrenia improve with drug therapy but, unfortunately, never fully recover. Because the condition is lifelong and appears in young adulthood, it causes considerable anguish for families who must deal with both the burden of health care costs and the responsibility for caring for a loved one with this illness.

Pathophysiology and Etiology

Schizophrenia, historically attributed to emotional dysfunction, is now categorized as a psychobiologic disease because of recent findings in brain and neurotransmitter chemistry. Many neurotransmitter imbalances are involved in schizophrenia. Dopamine excess is believed to be the major cause of the symptoms, with imbalances of norepinephrine, serotonin (5-HT), and gamma-aminobutyric acid (see Chapter 67) also playing a role. The disease is known to have a familial or genetic component. Other theories suggest that the anatomic and physiologic changes associated with schizophrenia result from a viral infection experienced by the affected individual's mother during pregnancy. The neurochemical imbalance produces a variety of manifestations characterized by **delusions** (disturbed thinking), with themes that may include suspiciousness, persecution, being controlled, **grandiosity** (belief in one's importance), religious fixation, or preoccupation with sex, a love interest, illness, or a body part. **Hallucinations** (sensory experiences only the client perceives) that are usually auditory or visual may be experienced.

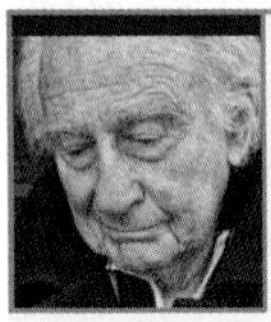

Clinical Scenario The wife of a 72-year-old man contacted a social services agency because her husband has been unable to independently care for himself in a healthy way. When representatives arrived, they found the man to be disheveled and unshaven. The home was extremely cluttered. There was evidence of uneaten, unrefrigerated food and cockroach infestation. His wife reports that he wanders the house at night, and at times urinates in a dresser drawer because he cannot find the toilet. He sometimes gets lost when venturing from his home to the grocery store. He neglects to pay utility bills when they are due. When examined by a local primary provider, he scored very low on the Mini-Mental State Examination (MMSE). He was confused as to his location and the identity of his son who accompanied him to the appointment. He became frustrated trying to find the words with which to respond to questions he was asked. Because of his mental deterioration and a fear that he might start a house fire because he wants to continue smoking cigarettes, the primary provider urged the client's wife and family to manage the client's care at home until transfer to a nursing home with an Alzheimer unit can be made. The services of a home health care nurse and aide will assist the wife temporarily. **What problems do the client and family face and how can they be managed at home or later in a nursing facility? Refer to the following Nursing Care Plan 72-1 for examples.**

NURSING CARE PLAN 72-1 The Client With Alzheimer Disease

Assessment

Interview both client and family because the client may be unable to give a complete or objective history regarding memory, sleep patterns, moods, and self-care activities. Assess the caregiver's strengths, limitations, and ability to manage caregiving activities.

- Perform a complete head-to-toe physical examination. Be especially attentive to muscular strength, balance, and gait.
- Determine the client's mental status. Identify level of orientation, short-term and long-term memory, social behavior, emotional status, cognitive and motor skills, and ability to perform ADLs.

Nursing Diagnosis. **ADL Deficit** related to cognitive impairment

Expected Outcome. Client will perform daily hygiene with assistance.

Interventions	Rationales
Observe the client's hygiene.	*Provides data suggesting if the client is performing self-care measures.*
Plan for personal hygiene at a consistent time each day.	*A consistent routine helps the client follow a similar pattern each day.*
Assemble items needed for bathing, shaving, and oral hygiene.	*Clients with dementia may not recall items that are necessary for hygiene or where they are located.*
Use a simple explanation and pantomime how to proceed with bathing, shaving, and toothbrushing.	*As mental deterioration progresses, clients lose the ability to use items appropriately.*
Arrange clean clothing and deposit soiled clothing in a receptacle for laundering.	*Ensures that the client will don appropriate apparel.*

Evaluation of Expected Outcome

The client performs personal hygiene with minimal assistance.

Nursing Diagnosis. **Impaired Home Maintenance** related to declining mentation

Expected Outcome. A surrogate for the client will assume responsibility for maintaining the household.

Interventions	Rationales
Identify a support system that may be available to the client and significant other.	*Helps determine the need to initiate resources for household cleaning, homemaking, running errands, and paying bills.*
Assist significant other to develop a plan for sharing household tasks among family members and arrange contract services for pest extermination.	*Relieves the burden on the aging significant other.*
Explore additional resources for assistance, such as home delivery of meals.	*Ensures that nutritious meals are available for daily consumption.*

Evaluation of Expected Outcome

A plan is implemented for meeting the home maintenance needs of the client and significant other.

Nursing Diagnosis. **Memory Impairment** related to global cognitive deficits

Expected Outcome. Client will be reoriented and will participate in life experiences to their potential.

Interventions	Rationales
Orient client frequently to person, place, and time.	*Frequent reminders accommodate for impairment in memory.*
Place a large-faced clock and calendars at multiple places in the client's environment.	*External clues help the client maintain orientation or become oriented with minimal effort.*
Assign consistent health care providers and maintain a structured dally routine.	*Repetition and consistency reduce episodes of confusion.*

(continued)

NURSING CARE PLAN 72-1 The Client With Alzheimer Disease (*continued*)

Attach something the client can recognize on the door of their room and the room where the toilet is located.	*The client is more likely to find their room by looking for a familiar clue like their name printed in large letters or a brightly colored bow.*
Make sure that the client wears an identification bracelet with an address and telephone number.	*Clients with AD are known to wander and not recall their current residence.*
Maintain a current photograph of the client in the medical record.	*Having the means to identify the client aids in search-and-rescue efforts.*

Evaluation of Expected Outcome

Client becomes reoriented with techniques such as verbal reminders and environmental clues like a large-faced clock and calendar and can participate in activities that occur at consistent times throughout the day.

Nursing Diagnosis. **Injury Risk/Safety** related to propensity for wandering

Expected Outcome. Client will move about freely and safely at home and later in the health care facility but will not leave without supervision.

Interventions	Rationales
Help the client don supportive walking shoes when out of bed.	*Supportive shoes promote a stable gait and posture.*
Provide assistance with ambulation. Remove hazards, such as footstools, small tables, or liquid spills, from the ambulatory area.	*Assistance reduces the potential for falls. Removing obstacles and slippery surfaces promotes safer ambulation.*
Keep the environment well lighted.	*The ability to see helps the client avoid environmental hazards.*
Maintain the bed in low position.	*Should a fall occur, the bed's low position reduces the potential for serious injury.*
Use **restraint alternatives**, protective or adaptive devices for fall protection and postural support.	*Physical restraints increase the potential for injury; clients have the right to the least restrictive intervention.*
Place a bed monitor under the client's mattress.	*Bed monitors alert caregivers when a client gets out of bed without signaling for assistance.*
Install alarms on exit doors and respond immediately when one sounds.	*An alarm alerts caregivers when someone leaves who is unauthorized to do so.*

Evaluation of Expected Outcomes

- No injuries occur.
- The client's whereabouts are known at all times.

Nursing Diagnosis. **Sleep Deprivation** related to confusion between day and night

Expected Outcome. Client will sleep uninterrupted for at least 6 hours or return to sleep after awakening during the night.

Interventions	Rationales
Keep client active during daytime hours, but avoid excessive fatigue.	*Remaining awake during daytime hours helps enhance normal circadian rhythm.*
Restrict consumption of coffee, tea, and cola.	*Caffeine, a central nervous system (CNS) stimulant, interferes with sleep.*
Make sure that the room is comfortably warm or cool and that the client has urinated and satisfied their thirst just before bedtime.	*Meeting basic comfort needs promotes sleep once the client retires for the night.*
Dim the lights and reduce unnecessary noise.	*A darkened environment increases production of melatonin, which promotes sleep; a quiet environment reduces stimulation of the cerebral cortex.*

NURSING CARE PLAN 72-1 The Client With Alzheimer Disease (*continued*)

Provide a lighted clock at the bedside.	*A clock provides an environmental clue as to whether it is time to sleep or awaken.*
Redirect the client gently, but firmly, to return to bed if nighttime wandering occurs.	*Caregivers help reinforce appropriate behavior.*

Evaluation of Expected Outcome

Client returns to bed after awakening and wandering and sleeps until an appropriate time for the day's activities.

Nursing Diagnosis. **Impaired Verbal Communication** related to expressive aphasia

Expected Outcome. Client will communicate with family and health care professionals at whatever level is possible.

Interventions	Rationales
Approach from the front, make eye contact, and look for a response to your voice.	*Obtaining the client's attention promotes verbal interaction.*
Get the client's attention by using the name to which they are most likely to respond.	*Using a client's name increases cognitive awareness and potential for social interaction.*
Keep explanations or directions short and simple.	*Being succinct makes it easier for the client to process information and respond appropriately.*
Give gentle reminders or model the desired response.	*Reminding and modeling compensate for failing memory or loss of language skills.*
Involve client in one idea or task at a time.	*Keeping ideas and tasks to a minimum promotes attention and concentration.*
Reduce environmental stimuli like noise and activity.	*Excess stimulation interferes with attention and concentration and may agitate the client.*
Promote interactions that tap into the client's long-term memory such as reminiscing; offer client verbal cues such as, "I understand you were... (a school teacher)."	*Long-term memory is retained more than short-term memory; recalling information promotes social interaction and elevates self-esteem.*
Give client plenty of time to respond to questions. Try to understand what client wants to convey.	*Impaired language skills make communication more difficult.*
Repeat information that you believe that the client is trying to communicate.	*Rephrasing or paraphrasing helps ensure accurate interpretation of the client's thoughts.*
Include client in small group activities, even if there is little or no socialization.	*Despite the appearance of being uninvolved, participation may stimulate the client's awareness.*
Change activities or distract the client if they become angry, hostile, or uncooperative.	*The nurse is responsible for ensuring the safety of the client, other clients, and staff.*

Evaluation of Expected Outcome

Client understands spoken works and responds verbally.

Nursing Diagnosis. **Caregiver Fatigue** related to being overwhelmed by responsibilities, fatigue, and depression

Expected Outcome. Caregiver will experience less anxiety as knowledge increases about implementing plans that will provide needed relief.

Interventions	Rationales
Assess caregiver's strengths, limitations, and ability to manage caregiving activities.	*The spouse (who is the usual caregiver) may experience sleep deprivation, physical injury, and social isolation if no one else is available to assist with client care.*

(continued)

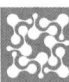

NURSING CARE PLAN 72-1 The Client With Alzheimer Disease (*continued*)

Suggest scheduling **respite care**, brief relief from caregiving responsibilities, with family and friends on a regular rotating basis.	*Dividing caregiving responsibilities promotes physical endurance and emotional stability.*
Provide a list of agencies that offer social services such as the county's commission on aging, Social Security, and Medicare agencies.	*Clients may be unaware of services available for assistance or how to contact them.*
Develop a list of people to contact in an emergency, including a 24-hour hotline for the home health nursing agency.	*Having a plan helps clients obtain assistance in a crisis.*
Recommend that caregiver and client take care of legal matters such as wills, transferring titles, and preparing an advanced directive (see Chapter 10).	*Attending to legal matters before severe cognitive changes occur is best.*
Suggest establishing **durable power of attorney**, designating who may make decisions regarding finances or health care when the client becomes **incompetent**, the legal term for the inability to understand the risks or benefits of decisions.	*Such measures ensure that the client's spouse or caregiver has access to unencumbered funds and follows the client's wishes regarding health care decisions.*
Advise caregiver to obtain **guardianship** or **conservatorship**, court-appointed responsibility, for managing the client's care and assets if the client already is incompetent.	*The client's financial assets may be frozen unless the court stipulates that another person can have access to private accounts.*
Encourage the caregiver to temporarily place the client in a long-term nursing facility to take a well-deserved vacation.	*Giving the caregiver a temporary option for a vacation may help to sustain their ability to continue caring for the client.*

Evaluation of Expected Outcomes

- Caregiver seeks relief from responsibilities at least 1 or 2 days a week.
- Caregiver and client take care of legal issues.

Nursing Diagnosis. Risk for Interrupted Family Processes related to guilt over placing the client in a care facility

Expected Outcome. Family will remain united and supportive over the decision to transfer the client's care to others.

Interventions	Rationales
Acknowledge and empathize with the family's ambivalent feelings.	*Family is more likely to accept transfer of the client's care if the nurse demonstrates empathy.*
Emphasize skills and services that the facility provides.	*Knowledge that the facility offers many services to promote and maintain the client's well-being enhances acceptance of the decision.*
Let the family participate in developing and revising the plan of care.	*Family participation promotes a team approach to managing the client's care.*
Keep the family informed of the client's progress or lack thereof.	*Communication often is the key to good interpersonal relationships.*
Encourage the family to visit and participate in the client's care as much as they want.	*Promoting continued interactions conveys a sense that family is included rather than excluded from the client's life.*
Allow the family privacy during interactions with the client and make an area available to them for special occasions like birthdays.	*Making special accommodations for family activities individualizes care.*
Keep a current list of family phone numbers, listing the relationships of members to the client and indications for which they prefer to be called.	*Accurate chain of information is important when communication is necessary.*
Prepare the family for the client's likely deterioration.	*Realistic preparation for the progression of the disease promotes anticipatory grieving and acceptance of the client's potentially terminal condition.*

Evaluation of Expected Outcomes

- Family members reconcile themselves to the difficult decision to transfer the care of the client to a nursing care facility.
- Family members remain involved in the client's care and understand the changes that accompany the disease progression.

Assessment Findings

Symptoms usually begin during late adolescence to early adulthood. Clients manifest a range of symptoms categorized as positive or negative. **Positive symptoms** include delusions, hallucinations, and fluent but disorganized speech. **Negative symptoms**, sometimes called *defect symptoms*, are marked by impoverished speech and an inability to enjoy relationships or express emotions (Box 72-1). Positive symptoms are more easily managed (with drugs) than negative symptoms. Classic symptoms are inexplicable sensory experiences such as hearing voices or seeing apparitions of people who are not there. These occur in combination with peculiar patterns of speaking and odd motor behaviors. The client also tends to abandon relationships and interactions with others and loses motivation for working, going to school, or engaging in other goal-driven behaviors. Hygiene and appearance tend to lose their previous importance.

The diagnosis is made primarily on the symptomatology and by ruling out other possible causes. CT and PET scans, MRIs, and brain mapping (see Chapter 67) may show decreased brain size and activity, especially in the frontal and temporal lobes.

Medical Management

Clients with schizophrenia are referred to the care of psychiatrists. Once the client is in the mental health system, every effort is made to avoid institutionalization. The exception is when the client is dangerous to self or others. In general, community mental health services are selected that meet the client's needs for psychotherapy, drug administration, and social needs such as housing, job assistance, and money management.

Antipsychotic drugs are the mainstay of treatment. These drugs, also called *major tranquilizers, antipsychotics*, or *neuroleptics*, belong to several different chemical families, but all block receptors for dopamine. Newer antipsychotic drugs block dopamine receptors and are also antagonists of 5-HT. Some examples of older or *typical* antipsychotic drugs are haloperidol (Haldol) and fluphenazine (Prolixin) as well as the more recent *atypical* antipsychotics risperidone (Risperdal), clozapine (Clozaril), and olanzapine (Zyprexa). See Drug Therapy Table 72-2.

Risperidone, clozapine, and olanzapine produce their effects with reduced incidence of **extrapyramidal symptoms** (EPSs), movement disorders associated with traditional antipsychotics (Box 72-2). Clozapine, however, has the potential adverse effect of dangerously depressing bone marrow function, and clients who take clozapine must have a blood count weekly or biweekly. If the white blood cell count drops too low, the drug is discontinued to reduce the potential for infection. Anticholinergic drugs such as trihexyphenidyl (Artane) and benztropine (Cogentin) are given to either prevent or relieve EPS. Antipsychotics sometimes are combined with anticonvulsant drugs such as clonazepam (Klonopin) and carbamazepine (Tegretol). See Evidence-Based Practice 72-1.

BOX 72-1 Positive and Negative Symptoms of Schizophrenia

Positive

- *Delusions*: false beliefs that cannot be changed by logical reasoning
- *Hallucinations*: sensory experiences that others do not perceive; can be auditory, visual, tactile, olfactory, or gustatory (involving taste)
- *Loose associations*: a sequence of ideas that are slightly connected
- *Inappropriate affect*: a display of emotional feeling inconsistent with the situation
- Peculiarities in speech like *echolalia*, repeating what others say; *rhyming*; *word salad*, using unrelated words in a sentence; or *neologisms*, inventing new words
- Bizarre behavior such as *stereotypy* (repetitious movement) and *echopraxia* (mimicking the movements of others)
- *Tangentiality*: digression from one topic to another
- *Circumstantiality*: digressing from one topic to another, but returns to the original topic

Negative

- *Concrete thinking*: literal thinking rather than symbolic; an inability to understand abstract ideas
- *Thought blocking*: an inability to recall information for a time
- *Symbolism*: attaching significance to an insignificant object or idea
- *Blunted* or *flat affect*: little or no display of feeling
- *Anhedonia*: inability to experience pleasure
- *Catatonia*: immobility
- *Posturing*: assuming statuesque positions
- *Autism*: social withdrawal
- Self-neglect of hygiene, eating, work, finances, and the like
- *Poverty of thought*: lacking any opinions or ideas

Concept Mastery Alert

Once a client is in the mental health system, every effort is made to avoid institutionalization. The exception is when the client is dangerous to themselves or others. In general, community mental health services are selected that meet the client's needs for psychotherapy, drug administration, and social needs such as housing, job assistance, and money management.

Nonadherence to drug therapy is the leading cause of the return of disease symptoms and the need for short-term hospitalization. For this reason, some nonhospitalized clients are given **depot injections**, intramuscular injections of antipsychotic drugs in an oil suspension that are gradually absorbed. These injections are repeated every 2 to 4 weeks.

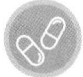

Pharmacologic Considerations

- Tardive dyskinesia (TD) is an irreversible reaction to some of the first-generation (or typical) antipsychotic medications. TD symptoms include rhythmic, involuntary movements of the tongue, face, mouth, jaw, or extremities. Report any of these symptoms immediately to the prescribing provider.
- Monitor the client taking an antipsychotic drug for symptoms of neuroleptic malignant syndrome. Notify the primary health care provider immediately if high fever, increased confusion, dyspnea, tachycardia, hypertension, severe muscle stiffness, or loss of bladder control occur.
- Advise clients to take all antipsychotic drugs as directed to avoid double dosing if they miss a dose and not to stop antipsychotic drugs abruptly.

DRUG THERAPY TABLE 72-2 Agents to Treat Schizophrenia

Category and Common Generic (Brand) Drugs	Intended Use	Common Side Effects	Safety Warnings for Nurses
First-Generation Antipsychotics (Conventional—Work to Relieve Positive Symptoms)			
Chlorpromazine (Thorazine) Fluphenazine (Prolixin) Haloperidol (Haldol) Loxapine (Adasuve) Perphenazine (Trilafon) Prochlorperazine (Compazine) Thioridazine (Mellaril) Thiothixene (Navane) Trifluoperazine (Stelazine)	Inhibit or block neurotransmission in psychotic disorders	Hypotension, drowsiness, nasal congestion, dry mouth, agranulocytosis, dystonia, behavioral changes, photosensitivity	Monitor for EPSs Instruct/provide sun protection Do not use tanning beds Monitor for rhythmic, involuntary movements (TD) Monitor for increased temperature and autonomic symptoms (neuroleptic malignant syndrome)
Second-Generation Antipsychotics (Atypical—Work to Relieve Both Positive and Negative Symptoms)			
Cariprazine (Vraylar) Clozapine (Clozaril, FazaClo) Lurasidone (Latuda) Olanzapine (Zyprexa) Paliperidone (Invega) Quetiapine (Seroquel) Risperidone(Risperdal) Ziprasidone (Geodon)	Act on serotonin and dopamine receptor sites, used for schizophrenia, manic phase of bipolar disorders	Agitation, akathisia, anxiety, drowsiness, headache, constipation, dry mouth, nausea, weight gain, agranulocytosis	Monitor weight and labs for elevated cholesterol, triglycerides, and blood sugar Monitor for decreased white blood cell counts
Combination Drugs (Antipsychotic/Antidepressant)			
Aripiprazole/lauroxil (Aristada)			
Olanzapine/fluoxetine (Symbyax)			

EPSs, extrapyramidal symptoms; TD, tardive dyskinesia.

BOX 72-2 Extrapyramidal Symptoms

EPSs associated with traditional antipsychotic drugs include the following movement disorders:

- *Akinesia* (pseudoparkinsonism): The client appears to have symptoms of Parkinson disease (see Chapter 37) such as hand tremors, stooped posture, and stiff, shuffling gait.
- *Akathisia*: The client cannot sit or stand still.
- *Dystonia*: Sudden severe muscle spasm occurs, usually in the neck, tongue, or eyes.
- *Tardive dyskinesia*: The client makes involuntary muscle movements, usually in the face, such as tongue thrusting, continuous chewing, grimacing, lip smacking, and blinking; irreversible once manifested.

Evidence-Based Practice 72-1

Antipsychotic Medications and Fetal Development

Clinical Question

Do antipsychotic medications pose a risk to the fetus in the first trimester?

Evidence

A study was done to review the National Medicaid database for pregnant mothers that delivered between 2000 and 2010 (Rosenberg, 2016). The study looked at mothers who may have been on antipsychotic medications to see if cardiac defects or congenital malformations occurred in the first trimester. The study found that a higher risk existed with newer antipsychotics, but the risk did not increase in first-generation antipsychotics. The medication risperidone was the only medication identified as posing a risk to the fetus in the first trimester. This result warrants further investigation (Rosenberg, 2016). These findings are further supported by Betcher, Montiel, and Clark (2019), who completed a review of existing research on the use of typical and atypical antipsychotics in pregnancy and the implications for pregnancy and infant outcome.

Nursing Implications

Nurses play an important role in taking a detailed history and notifying the health care provider of the pregnant client's prescriptions. Careful monitoring of the fetus should be expected, and the nurse's role should be to comfort and support the mother throughout the pregnancy. This recent study shows a decrease risk to the fetus in the first trimester when antipsychotic medications are in use; these results may decrease anxiety in the client taking such medications.

References

Betcher, H. K., Montiel, C., & Clark, C. T. (2019). Use of antipsychotic drugs during pregnancy. *Current Treatment Options in Psychiatry*, *6*(1), 17–31. https://doi.org/10.1007/s40501-019-0165-5

Rosenberg, K. (2016). No increase in congenital malformations with use of antipsychotics in pregnancy. *American Journal of Nursing*, *116*(11), 61. https://doi.org/10.1097/01.NAJ.0000505592.85826.98

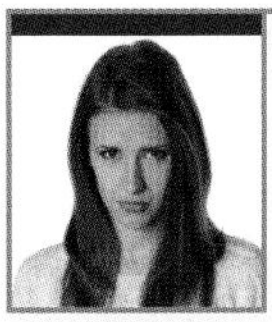

Clinical Scenario A 20-year-old college student believes that someone is stalking and spying on her. She thinks the television in her dorm room has been "bugged" for this purpose. She also has been hearing voices that tell her she has sinned and will be damned to hell. She has isolated herself from her peers and spends a great deal of time walking around town to avoid what she perceives as someone watching her. Her grades have fallen because she is not completing course requirements and is frequently absent from class. Her hygiene and self-care have declined because she is preoccupied with her paranoid thoughts and persecutory hallucinations. With urging by her roommate, she has come to a mental health clinic. The intake nurse has recommended that she admit herself voluntarily to an inpatient psychiatric unit. **What problems are important in the client's care and what nursing interventions are appropriate? See the Nursing Process section that follows.**

NURSING PROCESS FOR THE CLIENT WITH SCHIZOPHRENIA

Assessment

When caring for clients in acute care or community mental health settings, perform a Mini-Mental State Examination (MMSE; see Chapter 67) during the initial contact and periodically thereafter to monitor for changes. Assess the client for positive and negative symptoms of schizophrenia, including delusions, bizarre speech patterns, hallucinations, agitation, stupor, and social withdrawal. Also assess the client's physical status, including hygiene and nutritional condition.

Diagnosis, Planning, and Interventions

Disturbed Thought Processes: Related to illogical beliefs secondary to brain changes
Expected Outcome: The client's thoughts will be reality-based as evidenced by a decrease in or absence of delusions.

- Administer antipsychotic drugs as prescribed. *Antipsychotics block dopamine and/or 5-HT receptors and usually reduce or relieve positive symptoms such as delusions and hallucinations.*
- Do not argue about the validity of the client's delusions or try to convince them otherwise but indicate that you do not share the client's delusional belief. *Clients may become more fixated on their delusions, defensive, or hostile if others challenge their delusions. Stating that you do not share the client's belief prevents the client from assuming that the delusion is plausible.*
- Shift the client's focus to what is real in the "here and now" when they dwell on the delusion. *Redirecting the client's thoughts to present reality interrupts delusional thinking.*
- Direct and stay with the client in a quiet place when they become agitated. *Reduced stimuli help restore calm and prevent loss of control.*

Disturbed Sensory Perception (Specify: Auditory, Visual, Olfactory, Tactile, Gustatory) related to brain changes as manifested by hallucinations
Expected Outcome: The client will acknowledge that hallucinations are not real or will minimize their importance.

- Intervene when it appears that the client is experiencing a hallucination such as assuming a listening pose or laughing or talking when others are absent or uninvolved in interaction. *Hallucinations may frighten the client. The presence of another person helps the client cope.*
- State that you do not hear or see anyone, but acknowledge that the experience must seem real and frightening to the client. *Stating that you do not share the content of the hallucination helps the client understand that it is not real.*
- Stay with the client throughout the hallucination. *The presence of another trusted person relieves anxiety, facilitates coping, and protects the client from acting dangerously.*
- Avoid touching the client without warning. *Unexpected touching may cause the client to respond violently to what they perceive as a threat.*
- Call auditory hallucinations "the voices" rather than using a personal pronoun such as "they" or "them." *Personifying the voices suggests that the words are coming from real people.*
- Ask the client to share the content of the hallucination. *Obtaining specific information about the hallucination helps to determine if the safety of the client or others is in jeopardy.*
- Distract the client from attending to the hallucination. *Distraction interrupts the perception of the hallucination, thereby reducing the accompanying emotional distress.*
- Teach the client the technique of **voice dismissal**, which refers to saying "stop" or "be gone." Voice dismissal *is a method the client can use to independently halt the hallucination.*

ADL Deficit (Specify type: Bathing/Hygiene, Dressing/Grooming, Feeding, Toileting) related to lack of motivation, illogical fears, and emotional withdrawal
Expected Outcome: The client will independently perform ADLs.

(*continued*)

NURSING PROCESS FOR THE CLIENT WITH SCHIZOPHRENIA (continued)

- Explain where hygiene is performed and how to obtain soap, shampoo, and toothpaste. *Informing the client of the location and resources for bathing and hygiene promotes self-care.*
- Direct the client to care for themselves at an appropriate time. *Gentle direction facilitates cooperation.*
- Assist if the client cannot initiate or complete self-care. *The nurse implements a therapeutic use of self when a client is incapable of total self-care.*
- Praise any worthy accomplishments. *Praise is a form of positive reinforcement, which increases the possibility that the client will repeat the activity.*
- Monitor food and fluid intake and toileting patterns. *Data collection facilitates problem identification.*
- Provide nutritious snacks if the client eats insufficiently. *Eating nutritious foods promotes a stable weight and well-being.*

Impaired Social Interaction: Related to autism as evidenced by absence from group meetings and reluctance to participate in group activities
Expected Outcome: The client will interact independently with one person initially and will be able to interact with more than one person as their comfort level improves and symptoms are managed.

- Accompany the client to group meetings and activities. *Support from a trusted other may help the client participate in situations that they perceive as threatening or causing social discomfort.*
- Sit by the client, but do not urge the client to participate. *The nurse's physical presence reduces anxiety. Pressure to participate may increase the client's anxiety.*
- Share time with the client after the group interaction and use open-ended questions to explore their perception of the experience. *Private discussions promote the client's ability to process the group event and their comfort level.*
- Verbally compliment the client when deserved for speaking voluntarily with others or acting appropriately in a social situation. *Approval from someone the client respects empowers the client to make further efforts to interact with others.*
- Suggest ways the client can improve interactions with others. *The nurse acts as a mentor to help the client modify social skills.*

Evaluation of Expected Outcomes

Expected outcomes are that the client thinks rationally and realistically and reports fewer delusions and hallucinations. Communication is coherent and understandable. The client manages self-care, takes responsibility for other ADLs, socializes, and interacts in group activities.

>>> *Stop, Think, and Respond 72-2*

Discuss appropriate nursing interventions when a client with schizophrenia expresses a delusional belief or experiences a hallucination.

KEY POINTS

- Delirium and dementia
  - Delirium: a sudden, transient state of confusion
    - Caused by high fever, head trauma, brain tumor, drug intoxication or withdrawal, metabolic disorders (e.g., liver or renal failure), or inflammatory disorders of the CNS, such as meningitis or encephalitis
  - Dementia: refers to conditions in which decline in memory, thinking, and reasoning is severe enough to affect the daily life of an alert person
    - Caused by Alzheimer and Parkinson
- Etiologic factors linked to Alzheimer disease
  - Genetic mutation
  - Combination of genetic, environmental, and lifestyle factors
- Pathophysiologic changes associated with Alzheimer disease
  - APP is embedded in the neuron's cell membrane
  - Enzymes beta-secretase and gamma-secretase sever soluble amyloid precursor protein beta (sAPPβ), releasing a fragment that becomes beta-amyloid
  - Neurofibrillary tangles of tau proteins in microtubules form
  - As microtubules disintegrate and more and more neurons die, the brain atrophies.
- First symptoms of Alzheimer disease
  - A poor sense of smell may be one of the earliest signs of Alzheimer
  - Memory loss
- Diagnostic testing for Alzheimer disease
  - CT scan shows shrinking of the cerebral cortex, but this is not apparent in the early stages of the disease
  - PET, magnetic resonance imaging (MRI), and electroencephalography can detect slower-than-normal brain waves
- Nursing management for clients with Alzheimer disease
  - Assist client and caregivers
  - Maintain quality of life
  - Education
  - Emotional support
  - Physical care

- Schizophrenia: deterioration in mental functioning, disturbances in sensory perception, and changes in affect (emotion)
  - Positive and negative symptoms of schizophrenia
    - Positive symptoms include delusions, hallucinations, and fluent but disorganized speech
    - Negative symptoms include impoverished speech and an inability to enjoy relationships or express emotions
  - Medical management for schizophrenia
    - Psychotherapy
    - Drug administration
    - Social needs such as housing, job assistance, and money management
    - Consider depot injections of antipsychotic medications
- Examples of antipsychotic drugs and their mechanisms of action
  - Haldol: inhibits or blocks neurotransmission in psychotic disorders
  - Zyprexa: acts on serotonin and dopamine receptor sites
- Four examples of EPSs
  - Akinesia
  - Akathisia
  - Dystonia
  - Tardive dyskinesia

CRITICAL THINKING EXERCISES

1. Discuss the similarities and differences between AD and schizophrenia.

2. In what ways are the interventions for altered mentation different for a client with AD from those provided for a client with schizophrenia?

3. Which neurotransmitters are generally imbalanced in AD and schizophrenia?

4. Why is the incidence of AD continuing to rise?

NCLEX-STYLE REVIEW QUESTIONS PrepU

1. What is the best nursing action for preventing frustration and agitation when an older client with dementia asks about their mother who is deceased?
1. Explain gently that the client's mother is dead.
2. Tell the client that their mother will visit a little later.
3. Say, "You miss your mother. What was she like?"
4. Ask when the client last saw their mother.

2. What approach is best when managing the care of a client with dementia who becomes anxious when not carrying a purse?
1. Find out why the client feels the need for a purse.
2. Inform the client that the purse may be lost.
3. Ask the client where the purse can be stored.
4. Ensure the client has the purse at all times.

3. When a client with AD is observed to wander about a facility, what nursing intervention is most appropriate for the client's safety if the client walks away from the facility?
1. Make sure that the client is dressed appropriately for the environment.
2. Keep the client confined to a nearby room in the facility.
3. Attach an identity tag to the client with a phone number.
4. Lock all the outside doors within the facility.

4. For what side effect should the nurse closely monitor clients with schizophrenia who are receiving clozapine (Clozaril)?
1. Signs of infection
2. Elevated blood pressure
3. Extrapyramidal symptoms
4. Hypoglycemia

5. After reconstituting a vial of Risperdal Consta (the long-acting injectable form of risperidone) so it contains 50 mg/mL, how much should the nurse administer if the primary provider has ordered a depot injection of 37.5 mg? Calculate your answer to two decimal places.

WANT TO KNOW MORE? There are a wide variety of online resources available on thePoint to enhance learning and understanding of this chapter.

Go to thePoint.lww.com/activate and use the activation code found in the front of this text to unlock these online resources.

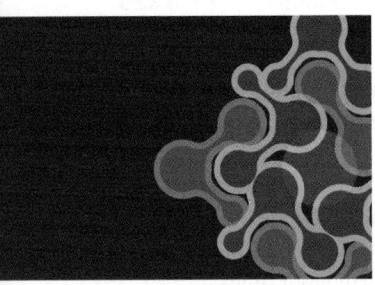

APPENDIX A
Commonly Used Abbreviations and Acronyms

3D-CRT = three-dimensional conformal radiation therapy
5-HT = serotonin
AA = Alcoholics Anonymous
ABG = arterial blood gas
ACA = Affordable Care Act
ACC = American College of Cardiology
ACE = angiotensin-converting enzyme
ACIP = Advisory Committee on Immunization Practices
ACL = anterior cruciate ligament
ACLS = advanced cardiac life support
ACOA = Adult Children of Alcoholics
ACS = American Cancer Society
ACTH = adrenocorticotropic hormone
AD = Alzheimer disease
ADC = AIDS dementia complex
ADH = antidiuretic hormone
ADLs = activities of daily living
AE = above the elbow
AED = automated external defibrillator
AFP = alpha-fetoprotein
AHA = American Heart Association; American Hospital Association
AHRQ = Agency for Healthcare Research and Quality
AI = aromatase inhibitor
AICD = automatic implanted cardiac defibrillator
AIDS = acquired immunodeficiency syndrome
AK = above the knee
AKA = above-the-knee amputation
AKI = acute kidney injury
ALI = acute lung injury
ALL = acute lymphocytic leukemia
ALS = amyotrophic lateral sclerosis
ALT = alanine aminotransferase
AMA = American Medical Association
AMD = age-related macular degeneration
AMI = acute myocardial infarction
AML = acute myelogenous leukemia
ANA = American Nurses Association; antinuclear antibody
ANCAs = antineutrophil cytoplasmic antibodies
AND = allow natural death
ANP = atrial natriuretic peptide
anti-CCP = anti-cyclic citrullinated peptide antibodies
anti-ds DNA = anti-double-stranded DNA
AORN = American Operating Room Nurses
APACHE = acute physiology, age, and chronic health evaluation
APAP = auto-titrating continuous positive airway pressure
APD = automated peritoneal dialysis
AP/LAT CXR = anterior, posterior, and lateral chest x-ray
APP = amyloid precursor protein
APRN = advanced practice registered nurse
AQI = air quality index
ARB = angiotensin receptor blocker
ARDS = acute respiratory distress syndrome
ARF = acute renal failure
ARI = aldose reductase inhibitor
ARS = acute radiation syndrome
ASA = acetylsalicylic acid (aspirin); American Society of Anesthesiologists
ASAA = American Sleep Apnea Association
ASCAs = anti-*Saccharomyces* antibodies
ASHA = American Speech–Language–Hearing Association
ASL = American Sign Language
ASO = antistreptolysin O
AST = aspartate aminotransferase
ATP = adenosine triphosphate
AV = atrioventricular; arteriovenous
BAHA = bone-anchored hearing aid
BAL = blood alcohol level; British anti-lewisite
BCG = bacillus Calmette-Guérin
BCI = bone conduction devices with implanted transducers
BCVA = best corrected visual acuity
BE = below the elbow
bHCG = beta-human chorionic gonadotropin
BIPAP = bilevel positive airway pressure
BK = below the knee
BKA = below the knee amputation
BMD = bone mineral density
BMI = body mass index
BMR = basal metabolic rate
BMT = bone marrow transplant
BNP = brain natriuretic peptide
BP = blood pressure
BPH = benign prostatic hyperplasia
BPPV = benign paroxysmal positional vertigo
BRAT = bananas, rice, applesauce, toast
BRM = biologic response modifier
BSA = body surface area
BSE = bovine spongiform encephalopathy; breast self-examination
BUN = blood urea nitrogen

CA = cancer antigen
CABG = coronary artery bypass graft
CAD = coronary artery disease
CAM = complementary and alternative medicine
CAP = community-acquired pneumonia
CAPD = continuous ambulatory peritoneal dialysis
CASP = central aortic systolic pressure
CAT = complementary and alternative therapies
CAUTI = catheter-associated urinary tract infection
CBC = complete blood count
CCPD = continuous cyclic peritoneal dialysis
CDC = Centers for Disease Control and Prevention
CDCA = chenodeoxycholic acid
CDKs = cyclin-dependent kinases
CEA = carcinoembryonic antigen
CF = cystic fibrosis
CFC = chlorofluorocarbon
CFS = chronic fatigue syndrome
CFTR = cystic fibrosis transmembrane conductance regulator
CHF = congestive heart failure
CIC = clean intermittent catheterization
CIS = carcinoma in situ
CJD = Creutzfeldt-Jakob disease
CK = conductive keratoplasty; creatine kinase
CK-MB = creatine kinase MB
CKD = chronic kidney disease
CLL = chronic lymphocytic leukemia
CMG = cystometrography
CML = chronic myelogenous leukemia
CMV = cytomegalovirus
CNA = certified nurses' aide; certified nursing assistant
CNP = C-type natriuretic peptide
CNS = central nervous system
CNV = choroidal neovascularization
CO = cardiac output
CO_2 = carbon dioxide
COPD = chronic obstructive pulmonary disease
COX-2 = cyclooxygenase-2
CPAP = continuous positive airway pressure
CPM = continuous passive motion
CPR = cardiopulmonary resuscitation
CRF = chronic renal failure
CRH = corticotropin-releasing hormone
CRNA = certified registered nurse anesthetist
CRP = C-reactive protein
CRRT = continuous renal replacement therapy
CRT = cardiac resynchronization therapy
CSF = cerebrospinal fluid
CST = cortisol suppression test
CT = computed tomography
CTZ = chemoreceptor trigger zone
CUR = chronic urinary retention
CVA = cerebrovascular accident; costovertebral angle
CVD = cardiovascular disease
CVP = central venous pressure
CVVH = continuous venovenous hemofiltration
CVVHD = continuous venovenous hemodialysis
CXR = chest X-ray
D_5W = 5% dextrose in water
D and C = dilation and curettage
DASH = Dietary Approaches to Stop Hypertension
dB = decibels
DBS = deep brain stimulation
DCA = directional coronary atherectomy
DES = diethylstilbestrol
DEXA or DXA = dual-energy X-ray absorptiometry
DI = diabetes insipidus
DIC = disseminated intravascular coagulation
DIP = distal interphalangeal joint
DJD = degenerative joint disease
DKA = diabetic ketoacidosis
DLE = discoid lupus erythematosus
DM = diabetes mellitus
DMARD = disease-modifying antirheumatic drug
DMAST = Dyna Med antishock trousers
DMSA = dimercaptosuccinic acid scintigraphy
DMSO = dimethyl sulfoxide
DNA = deoxyribonucleic acid
DNR = do not resuscitate
DO = doctor of osteopathic medicine
DPOA = durable power of attorney
DRE = digital rectal examination
DRG = diagnosis-related group
DSHEA = Dietary Supplement Health and Education Act of 1994
DSM-IV = *Diagnostic and Statistical Manual of Mental Disorders*, 4th Edition
DSP = distal sensory polyneuropathy
DSRS = distal splenorenal shunt
DST = dexamethasone suppression test
DTaP = diphtheria, tetanus, and pertussis
DUIL = driving under the influence of liquor
DV = daily value
DVT = deep vein thrombosis
DWI = driving while intoxicated
EBCT = electron beam computed tomography
EBRT = external beam radiation therapy
ECF = eosinophil chemotactic factor
ECG = electrocardiogram; electrocardiography; electrocochleography
ECMO = extracorporeal membrane oxygenator
ECT = electroconvulsive therapy
ED = emergency department
EECP = enhanced external counterpulsation
EEG = electroencephalogram; electroencephalography
EGD = esophagogastroduodenoscopy
ELISA = enzyme-linked immunosorbent assay
EMG = electromyelography
EMR = electronic medical record
ENG = electronystagmography
EPA = eicosapentaenoic acid

EPS = extrapyramidal symptoms
ERCP = endoscopic retrograde cholangiopancreatography
ERT = estrogen replacement therapy
ESR = erythrocyte sedimentation rate
ESRD = end-stage renal disease
ESWL = extracorporeal shock wave lithotripsy
EUS = endoscopic ultrasound
FAS = fetal alcohol syndrome
FBOT = fecal occult blood test (gFBOT guaiac fecal occult blood test)
FCC = Federal Communications Commission
FDA = U.S. Food and Drug Administration
FEMA = Federal Emergency Management Agency
FES = functional electrical stimulation
FM = frequency modulation
FPL = federal poverty level
FRAX = Fracture Risk Assessment Tool
FSH = follicle-stimulating hormone
FTA-ABS = fluorescent treponemal antibody absorption test
GABA = gamma-aminobutyric acid
GAD = generalized anxiety disorder
GCS = Glasgow Coma Scale
GERD = gastroesophageal reflux disease
GFR = glomerular filtration rate
GGT = gamma-glutamyltransferase
GH = growth hormone
GHB = gamma-hydroxybutyrate
GHRH = growth hormone–releasing hormone
GI = gastrointestinal
GnRH = gonadotropin-releasing hormone
GTT = glucose tolerance test
GVHD = graft-versus-host disease
H_2CO_3 = carbonic acid
HAART = highly active antiretroviral therapy
HAC = hospital-acquired condition
HAMD = Hamilton Rating Scale for Depression
HAP = hospital-acquired pneumonia
HATS = hearing assistive technology systems
HAV = hepatitis A virus
HbA = hemoglobin A
HbF = fetal hemoglobin
HBOCs = hemoglobin-based oxygen carriers
HbS = hemoglobin S
HBV = hepatitis B virus
HCAP = healthcare-associated pneumonia
hCG = human chorionic gonadotropin
HCl = hydrochloric acid
HCO_3 = bicarbonate
HCP = health care provider
Hct = hematocrit
HCV = hepatitis C virus
HDL = high-density lipoprotein
HDV = hepatitis D virus
HER2 = human epidermal growth factor receptor 2
HEV = hepatitis E virus
HFCWO = high-frequency chest wall oscillation
Hg = mercury
HGV = hepatitis G virus
HHNKS = hyperosmolar hyperglycemic nonketotic syndrome
HiB = *Haemophilus influenzae* type B
HIPAA = Health Insurance Portability and Accountability Act
HIV = human immunodeficiency virus
HLA = human leukocyte antigen
HMO = health maintenance organization
HPA = hypothalamic–pituitary–adrenal
HPV = human papillomavirus
HRT = hormone replacement therapy
HSCT = hematopoietic stem cell transplantation
HSV-1 = herpes simplex virus type 1
HSV-2 = herpes simplex virus type 2
Hz = Hertz (number of sound waves per second)
IABP = intra-aortic balloon pump
IBD = inflammatory bowel disease
IBS = irritable bowel syndrome
IC = interstitial cystitis
ICF = intermediate care facility
ICP = intracranial pressure
ICRSs = intrastromal corneal ring segments
ICSH = interstitial cell–stimulating hormone
ICU = intensive care unit
IDDM = insulin-dependent diabetes mellitus
IDS = integrated delivery system
Ig = immunoglobulin
IGF-1 = insulin-like growth factor 1
IGRA = interferon-gamma release array
IICP = increased intracranial pressure
IL = interleukin
IL-2 = interleukin-2
IM = intramuscular
IMA = internal mammary artery
IMRT = intensity-modulated radiation therapy
IMT = implantable miniature telescope
INR = international normalized ratio
IOL = intraocular lens
IOP = intraocular pressure
IORT = intraoperative radiation therapy
IPD = intermittent peritoneal dialysis
IPG = impedance plethysmography
IPV = inactivated poliomyelitis
ITA = internal thoracic artery
IUC = indwelling urethral catheter
IV = intravenous
IVAD = implanted vascular access device
IVC = inferior vena cava
IVP = intravenous pyelogram; intravenous pyelography
JAK = Janus kinase
JCAHO = Joint Commission on Accreditation of Healthcare Organizations; now referred to as The Joint Commission

KI = potassium iodide
KUB = kidneys, ureters, and bladder
LABA = long-acting beta-2 agonists
LAGB = laparoscopic gastric banding
LASIK = laser-assisted in situ keratomileusis
LES = lower esophageal sphincter
LDH = lactate dehydrogenase
LDL = low-density lipoprotein
LEP = limited English proficiency
LES = lower esophageal sphincter
LGBT = lesbian, gay, bisexual, and transgender community
LH = luteinizing hormone
LLQ = left lower quadrant
LMP = last menstrual period
LOC = level of consciousness
LPN = licensed practical nurse
LTACH = long-term acute care hospital
LUQ = left upper quadrant
LVAD = left ventricular assist device
LVEDP = left ventricular end-diastolic pressure
LVN = licensed vocational nurse
MABs = monoclonal antibodies
MAOI = monoamine oxidase inhibitor
MA-PD = Medicare Advantage Plan that includes Parts A, B, and D with prescription drug care
MAST = military antishock trousers
MCH = mean cell hemoglobin
MCHC = mean cell hemoglobin concentration
MCO = managed care organization
MCT = medium-chain triglycerides
MCV = mean cell volume
MD = doctor of medicine
MDD = major depressive disorder
MDG = Millennium Development Goals
MDI = metered-dose inhaler
MEI = middle ear implantation
MH = malignant hyperthermia
MHC = major histocompatibility complex
MI = myocardial infarction
MIDCAB = minimally invasive direct coronary artery bypass
MIS = minimally invasive surgery (joint replacement)
MMR = measles, mumps, and rubella
MMSE = Mini-Mental Status Examination
MoABs [mAbs] = monoclonal antibody immunotherapy
MOST = medical orders for scope of treatment
MPHG = metabolite of norepinephrine
MRCP = magnetic resonance cholangiopancreatography
MRE = magnetic resonance elastography
MRI = magnetic resonance imaging
MSA = Medicare Medical Savings Account
MS = multiple sclerosis
MSG = monosodium glutamate
MTBE = methyl tert-butyl ether
MUGA = multiple gated acquisition
NADH = nicotinamide adenine dinucleotide
NANDA = North American Nursing Diagnosis Association
NCCAM = National Center for Complementary and Alternative Medicine
NCHS = National Center for Health Statistics
NCI = National Cancer Institute
NCLEX-PN = National Council Licensure Examination for Practical Nurses
NCLEX-RN = National Council Licensure Examination for Registered Nurses
NCSBN = National Council of State Boards of Nursing
NDE = near-death experience
NFT = neurofibrillary tangle
NGAL = neutrophil gelatinase-associated lipocalin
NHLBI = National Heart, Lung, and Blood Institute
NIDDM = non–insulin-dependent diabetes mellitus
NIH = National Institutes of Health
NIPD = nocturnal intermittent peritoneal dialysis
NPPV = noninvasive positive pressure ventilation
NK = natural killer (cell)
NMDA = *N*-methyl-D-aspartate
NMH = neurally mediated hypotension
NNRTI = nonnucleoside reverse transcriptase inhibitor
NPO = nothing by mouth
NPSGs = National Patient Safety Goals
NQF = National Quality Forum
NRC = Nuclear Regulatory Commission
NRTI = nucleoside reverse transcriptase inhibitor
NS = normal saline
NSAID = nonsteroidal antiinflammatory drug
NSCLC = non–small cell lung carcinoma
O_2 = oxygen
OAB = overactive bladder
OA = osteoarthritis
OCD = obsessive-compulsive disorder
OPCAB = off-pump coronary artery bypass
OR = operating room
ORIF = open reduction internal fixation
OSA = obstructive sleep apnea
OSHA = Occupational Safety and Health Administration
OT = occupational therapist
OTC = over the counter (nonprescription)
PA = pulmonary artery
PAC = premature atrial contraction
PACAB = port access coronary artery bypass
$PaCO_2$ = partial pressure of carbon dioxide
PACU = postanesthesia care unit
PAD = peripheral artery disease
PAH = pulmonary arterial hypertension
PaO_2 = partial pressure of oxygen
Pap = Papanicolaou smear
PAP = prostatic acid phosphatase; pulmonary artery pressure
PASG = pneumatic antishock garment
PBS = painful bladder syndrome
PCA = patient-controlled analgesia

PCL = posterior cruciate ligament
PCOS = polycystic ovarian syndrome
PCP = *Pneumocystis carinii* pneumonia; primary care provider
PCR = polymerase chain reaction
PCV = pneumococcal conjugate vaccine
PCWP = pulmonary capillary wedge pressure
PDP = Prescription Drug Plan
PDT = photodynamic therapy
PE = pulmonary embolus
PEEP = positive end-expiratory pressure
PEG = percutaneous endoscopic gastrostomy
PENS = percutaneous electrical nerve stimulation
PET = positron emission tomography
PFC = perfluorocarbon
PFFS = Medicare Private Fee-for-Service
pH = hydrogen ions in solution
PH = pulmonary hypertension
PHO = physician hospital organization
PIC = peripheral indwelling catheter
PICC = peripherally inserted central catheter
PID = pelvic inflammatory disease
PIP = proximal interphalangeal
PKD = polycystic kidney disease
PMI = point of maximum impulse
PMS = premenstrual syndrome
PNS = peripheral nervous system
PNT = percutaneous neuromodulation therapy
POD = postoperative day
POF = premature ovarian failure
POLST = physician orders for life-sustaining treatment
POS = point-of-service
POST = physician orders for scope of treatment
PPACA = Patient Protection and Affordable Care Act
PPD = purified protein derivative
PPI = proton pump inhibitors
PPO = preferred provider organization
PPS = prospective payment systems
PR = peripheral resistance
PRK = photorefractive keratectomy
PSA = prostate-specific antigen
PSDA = Patient Self-Determination Act
PT = physical therapist; prothrombin time
PTC = percutaneous transhepatic cholangiography
PTCA = percutaneous transluminal coronary angioplasty
PTSD = posttraumatic stress disorder
PTT = partial thromboplastin time
PTU = propylthiouracil
PUD = peptic ulcer disease
PVC = premature ventricular contraction
PVD = peripheral vascular disease
QFT-G = QuantiFERON-TB Gold
QI = quality indicator
QSEN = Quality and Safety Education for Nurses
QUS = quantitative ultrasonic studies (bone sonometer)
RA = rheumatoid arthritis; right atrium
RAI = radioactive iodine
RAST = radioallergosorbent blood test
RBC = red blood cell
RC = risk for complication
RDA = recommended dietary allowance
RF = rheumatoid factor
RK = radial keratotomy
RLE = refractive lens exchange
RLQ = right lower quadrant
RN = registered nurse
RNA = ribonucleic acid
RNFA = Registered Nurse First Assistant
ROM = range of motion
RPR = rapid plasma reagin
RT = reverse transcriptase
RUQ = right upper quadrant
RYGB = Roux-en-Y gastric bypass
SA = sinoatrial
SABA = short-acting beta-2 agonists
SAD = seasonal affective disorder
SCIP = Surgical Care Improvement Project
PFFS = Medicare Private Fee-for-Service
SCLC = small-cell lung carcinoma
SDM = shared decision making
SERM = selective estrogen receptor modifier
SIADH = syndrome of inappropriate antidiuretic hormone
SIRT = selective internal radiation therapy
SIV = simian (monkey) immunodeficiency virus
SLE = systemic lupus erythematosus
SLIT = sublingual-swallow immunotherapy
SNF = skilled nursing facility
SNRI = serotonin–norepinephrine reuptake inhibitor
SPECT = single photon emission computed tomography
SPF = sun protection factor
SpO_2 = saturated oxygen
SIRS = systemic inflammatory response syndrome
SRE = serious reportable event
SRS = stereotactic radiosurgery
SRS-A = slow-reactive substance of anaphylaxis
SSI = Supplemental Security Income, surgical site infection
SSNRI = selective serotonin–norepinephrine reuptake inhibitor
SSRI = selective serotonin reuptake inhibitor
STD = sexually transmitted disease
STI = sexually transmitted infection
SUI = stress urinary incontinence
SVT = supraventricular tachycardia
T_3 = triiodothyronine
T_4 = tetraiodothyronine
TAVI = transcatheter aortic valve implantation
TB = tuberculosis
TBSA = total body surface area
TCA = tricyclic antidepressant
TDD = telecommunication device for the deaf
TE = transluminal extraction

TECAB = totally endoscopic coronary artery bypass; also known as port access coronary artery bypass (PACAB)
TEE = transesophageal echocardiography
TENS = transcutaneous electrical nerve stimulation
TEP = tracheoesophageal puncture
THBO = topical hyperbaric oxygen
THC = tetrahydrocannabinol
THIQ = tetrahydroisoquinoline
TIA = transient ischemic attack
TIF = transoral incisionless fundoplication
TIMP-2 = tissue inhibitor metalloproteinase-2
TIPS = transjugular intrahepatic portosystemic shunt
TMD = temporomandibular disorder
TMJ = temporomandibular joint
TMR = transmyocardial revascularization
TMS = transcranial magnetic stimulation
TNF = tumor necrosis factor
TPA = tissue plasminogen activator
TPN = total parenteral nutrition
TRH = thyrotropin-releasing hormone
TRUS = transrectal ultrasonography
TSE = transmissible spongiform encephalopathy
TSH = thyroid-stimulating hormone
TSS = toxic shock syndrome
TST = tuberculin skin test
TTY = text message telephone
TUIP = transurethral incision of the prostate
TULIP = transurethral laser incision of the prostate
TURBT = transurethral resection of a bladder tumor
TURP = transurethral resection of the prostate
TZD = thiazolidinedione
UAP = unlicensed assistive personnel
UDCA = ursodeoxycholic acid
UN = United Nations
UNOS = United Network for Organ Sharing
UPPP = uvulopalatopharyngoplasty
URI = upper respiratory infection
UTI = urinary tract infection
UV = ultraviolet
VAD = ventricular assist device
VAP = ventilator-associated pneumonia
VBG = vertical banded gastroplasty
VCUG = voiding cystourethrography
VDRL = venereal disease research laboratory
VEMP = vestibular-evoked myogenic potentials testing
vHIT = video head impulse test
VMG = videonystagmography
VNS = vagus nerve stimulation
V/Q = ventilation/perfusion ratio
VRT = vestibular rehabilitation therapy
WBC = white blood cell
WHO = World Health Organization
WKO = weighted kypho-orthosis (spinal)
WOCN = wound, ostomy, and continence nurse

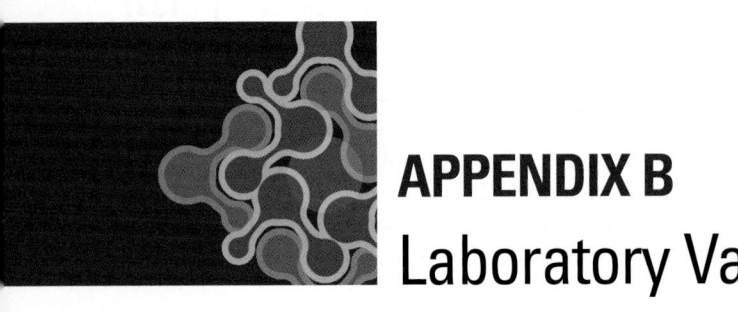

APPENDIX B
Laboratory Values

Available online on thePoint®

Glossary

A

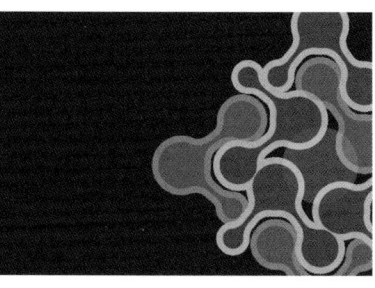

Abdominoperineal resection surgical procedure involving wide excision of the rectum and the creation of a sigmoid colostomy.

ABO system method by which blood is identified as one of four blood types: A, B, AB, or O.

Acalculia neurologic impairment of a person's ability to perform calculations.

Accelerated hypertension markedly elevated blood pressure accompanied by hemorrhages and exudates in the eyes.

Acceptance fifth stage of Elisabeth Kübler-Ross's five stages of grief, in which a client who is dying accepts their fate and makes peace spiritually and with those with whom they are close.

Accommodation process in which the lens of the eye changes shape to view objects that are near or distant.

Accountability being answerable for the consequences of one's actions or inactions.

Acetylcholine neurotransmitter released at the nerve endings of parasympathetic nerve fibers, at some nerve endings in the sympathetic nervous system, and at nerve endings of skeletal muscles; also critical for memory and cognition.

Acetylcholinesterase enzyme that inactivates acetylcholine.

Acidosis excessive accumulation of acids or an excessive loss of bicarbonate in body fluids; can occur as a result of either metabolic or respiratory alterations.

Acids substances that release hydrogen.

Acne vulgaris inflammatory disorder that affects the sebaceous glands and hair follicles.

Acoustic neuroma benign Schwann cell tumor that progressively enlarges and adversely impacts cranial nerve VIII, which consists of the vestibular and cochlear nerves.

Acquired immunodeficiency syndrome (AIDS) infectious and eventually fatal syndrome that profoundly weakens the immune system and that is acquired from a pathogen known as the human immunodeficiency virus (HIV).

Acromegaly condition in which growth hormone is oversecreted after the epiphyses of the long bones have sealed.

Active transport use of energy to move chemicals from an area of low concentration to an area of higher concentration.

Acuity the gravity and degree to which a person's medical condition changes.

Acupuncture technique of healing in which a needle is placed in one or more acupoints to restore the balance and free flow of energy within the body.

Acute bronchitis inflammation of the mucous membranes that line the major bronchi and their branches.

Acute chest syndrome type of pneumonia triggered by decreased hemoglobin and infiltrates within the lungs.

Acute coronary syndrome any group of clinical symptoms compatible with acute myocardial ischemia.

Acute heart failure sudden change in the heart's ability to contract.

Acute glomerulonephritis (may also be referred to as glomerular disease) the inflammation of the glomeruli in the kidneys.

Acute kidney injury (AKI) (formerly called acute renal failure [ARF]) characterized by a sudden and rapid decrease in renal function. AKI potentially is reversible with early, aggressive treatment of its contributing etiology.

Acute pain discomfort that has a short duration (from a few seconds to less than 6 months) and is associated with tissue trauma, including surgery, or some other recent identifiable etiology.

Acute pulmonary edema complication of left-sided heart failure when pulmonary capillaries and alveoli become engorged with blood, causing the lungs to rapidly fill with fluid, resulting in acute respiratory distress.

Acute renal failure sudden and rapid decrease in the ability of nephrons within the kidneys to maintain fluid, electrolyte, and acid–base balance, excrete nitrogen waste products, and perform regulatory functions such as maintaining calcification of bones and producing erythropoietin.

Acute retroviral syndrome syndrome that occurs in some cases of primary HIV infection that is often mistaken for "flu" or some other common illness.

Acute tubular necrosis death of cells within the collecting tubules of the nephrons, where reabsorption of water and electrolytes and excretion of protein wastes and excess metabolic substances occur.

Addiction repetitive pattern of drug seeking and substance abuse that interferes with work, relationships, and normal activities; also known as dependence.

Addisonian crisis life-threatening endocrine emergency when corticosteroid therapy is abruptly discontinued.

Adenohypophysis anterior lobe of the pituitary gland.

Adenoidectomy surgical removal of the adenoids.

Adenoiditis inflammation of the adenoids.

Adenoids lymphoid tissue located in the nasopharynx that protects the body from infection.

Adenosine triphosphate (ATP) energy source for operating sodium and potassium pumps on cellular membrane.

Ad hoc interpreter untrained agency-employed bilingual staff, self-declared bilingual volunteers, and family or friends who are called upon to interpret communication between English- and non-English-speaking persons.

Adjuvant drugs medications that are coadministered when treating pain (e.g., improving analgesic effect without increasing dosage, controlling concurrent symptoms, moderating side effects).

Adjuvant therapy drugs administered after surgery to extend survival and prevent disease recurrence.

Administrative law body of law that creates and enforces rules and regulations concerning the health, welfare, and safety of citizens.

Adrenal cortex outer portion of the adrenal glands; manufactures and secretes glucocorticoids, mineralocorticoids, and small amounts of sex hormones.

Adrenal glands glands located above the kidneys; the outer portion is the cortex, and the inner portion is the medulla.

Adrenal insufficiency decreased adrenal cortical function.

Adrenal medulla inner portion of the adrenal glands; secretes epinephrine and norepinephrine, two hormones released in response to stress or threat to life.

Adrenalectomy surgical removal of the adrenal gland(s), usually to remove a cancerous tumor.

Adrenocorticotropic hormone (ACTH) substance secreted by the pituitary that stimulates the adrenal glands to secrete corticosteroid hormones.

Advance directive document in which a client states in advance their wishes regarding life-sustaining treatment and other medical care.

Advocacy (1) promoting the cause of another person or organization and (2) safeguarding of a client's rights and the supporting of their interests.

Affect verbal and nonverbal behavior that communicates feelings.

Affective learner person who processes information best when it appeals to their feelings, beliefs, and values.

Affective touch personal contact with a client that is used to communicate concern, caring, and support. See also *task-oriented touch.*

Afterload force that the ventricle must overcome to empty its diastolic volume.

Ageism stereotyping of older adults' behavior or vulnerability based on an individual's prior experiences or anticipation of behaviors.

Agnosia neurologic impairment of a person's ability to recognize objects and sounds.

Agoraphobia fear of experiencing a panic attack in a public place, which often leads to its victims permanently confining themselves to their homes.

Agranulocytes leukocytes that do not contain granules.

Agranulocytosis decreased production of granulocytes, including neutrophils, basophils, and eosinophils.

Agraphia neurologic impairment of a person's ability to write.

AIDS dementia complex neurologic condition that causes degeneration of the brain, especially in areas that affect mood, cognition, and motor functions.

AIDS drug assistance programs state-based programs partially funded by Title II of the Ryan White CARE Act that help low- and middle-income clients obtain expensive AIDS medications.

Albumin a large plasma protein that does not normally move across semipermeable membranes like those in capillaries; most abundant protein in plasma.

Alcoholism chronic, progressive multisystem disease characterized by an inability to control the consumption of alcohol.

Aldosterone adrenal hormone that causes salt and water to be reabsorbed, increasing blood pressure.

Alexia neurologic impairment of a person's ability to read.

Alkalosis excessive accumulation of base or a loss of acid in body fluids; can occur as a result of either metabolic or respiratory alterations.

Allergen antigen that can cause an allergic response.

Allergic disorder disorder characterized by a hyperimmune response to weak antigens that are usually harmless.

Allodynia exaggerated pain response due to increased sensitivity to stimuli such as air currents, pressure of clothing, vibration.

Allograft skin graft that uses human skin obtained from a cadaver to temporarily cover large areas of tissue until the client's own skin can be used for skin grafting.

Alloimmunity immune response waged against transplanted organs and tissues that carry nonself antigens.

Alopecia condition that affects the hair follicles and results in partial or total hair loss.

Alopecia areata autoimmune disorder causing patchy areas of hair loss that can progress to total hair loss and even loss of hair from the entire body.

Alpha fetoprotein serum protein normally produced during fetal development that is a marker indicating a primary malignant liver tumor.

Alternative medical systems health care techniques that evolved from non-Western cultures.

Alternative therapy treatment used instead of conventional medical treatment.

Alveolus (pl. alveoli) small, clustered sac that begins where the bronchioles end and is the location for the exchange of oxygen and CO_2.

Alzheimer disease progressive, deteriorating brain disorder.

Ambulatory care also referred to as *outpatient care;* care delivered on an outpatient basis.

Ambulatory surgery surgery that requires fewer than 24 hours of hospitalization; sometimes referred to as same-day or outpatient surgery.

Amenorrhea absence of menstrual flow, usually caused by endocrine imbalances resulting from pituitary disorders or hypothyroidism, the stress response, or severely lean body mass.

American Sign Language (ASL) a method for communication that uses a hand-spelled alphabet and word symbols.

Amyloid plaques clusters of amyloid protein fragments that stick together and damage neurons in the brain.

Amyloid precursor protein normal protein that resides partially inside and outside the cell membranes of neurons in the brain.

Amyotrophic lateral sclerosis (ALS) progressive and fatal neurologic disorder characterized by degeneration of the motor neurons of the spinal cord and brain stem; also known as Lou Gehrig disease.

Anaerobic metabolism inefficient mechanism for meeting energy requirements used when the amount of oxygen reaching the cells decreases.

Anaphylactic shock severe allergic reaction that occurs after exposure to a substance to which a person is extremely sensitive.

Anaphylaxis rapid and profound allergic response characterized by shock, laryngeal edema, wheezing, stridor, tachycardia, and generalized itching.

Androgenetic alopecia genetically acquired condition referred to by many as male-pattern baldness, but also affects women albeit to a milder degree.

Anasarca generalized edema caused by the shift of fluid from the intravascular space to interstitial and intracellular fluid locations.

Anastomosis natural and surgical connection between two structures.

Andragogy principles of teaching adult learners.

Anecdotal record handwritten, personal account of an incident made at the time of occurrence and updated as needed; used to refresh a nurse's memory.

Anemia deficiency of either erythrocytes or hemoglobin.

Anergy inability to mount an immune response.

Anesthesia partial or complete loss of the sensation of pain with or without the loss of consciousness; may be general, regional, or local.

Anesthesiologist primary provider who has completed 2 years of residency in anesthesia and is responsible for administering anesthesia to a client and for monitoring a client during and after the surgical procedure.

Anesthetist person who administers anesthesia under the supervision of an anesthesiologist.

Aneurysm stretching and bulging of an arterial wall, usually caused by weakening of the vessel.

Anger second stage in Elisabeth Kübler-Ross's five stages of grief in which a client responds angrily to impending death and may displace this anger onto others, such as the primary provider, nurses, family, or God.

Angina pectoris chest pain of cardiac origin.

Angiocardiography diagnostic procedure in which a radiopaque dye is injected into a vein and its course through the heart is recorded by a series of radiographic pictures taken in rapid succession.

Angiotensin-converting enzyme (ACE) substance in the lungs that allows angiotensin I to be changed into angiotensin II, a powerful vasoconstrictor.

Angiotensin I substance split by angiotensin-converting enzyme to produce angiotensin II.

Angiotensin II raises blood pressure by causing vasoconstriction via sympathetic nervous stimulation and increased secretion of aldosterone.

Angiotensinogen protein released by the liver and converted by renin into angiotensin I.

Angiogenesis regeneration of blood vessels.

Angioneurotic edema acute swelling of the face, neck, lips, larynx, hands, feet, genitals, and internal organs.

Anion gap difference between sodium and potassium cation (positive ion) concentrations and the sum of chloride and bicarbonate anions (negative ions) in the extracellular fluid.

Anions negative ions.

Ankle–brachial index measurement used to detect peripheral artery disease (PAD) by comparing the systolic pressure in the brachial artery with that in the posterior tibial artery using Doppler ultrasound at rest or after exercise.

Ankylosing spondylitis chronic, connective tissue disorder of the spine and surrounding cartilaginous joints, such as the sacroiliac joints and soft tissues around the vertebrae.

Ankylosis joint immobility.

Annuloplasty surgical repair of the mitral valve leaflets and their fibrous ring.

Anorexia lack of appetite.

Anorexia nervosa eating disorder characterized by an obsession for thinness that is achieved through self-starvation.

Anterograde amnesia partial or complete inability to recall the recent past.

Anthrax disease caused by a spore-forming bacterium known as *Bacillus anthracis*.

Antibodies chemical substances that destroy foreign agents such as microorganisms.

Antidiuretic hormone (ADH) substance secreted by the pituitary in response to low blood volume that promotes reabsorption of water that the kidneys would ordinarily excrete.

Antigens foreign substance that induces an immune response.

Antineoplastic type of drug used to treat cancer that works by interfering with cellular function and reproduction.

Antioxidants chemicals that block the chemical reactions that cause free radicals.

Anuria urine output of <100 mL over 24 hours.

Anxiety vague uneasy feeling, the cause of which is not readily identifiable and which is evoked when a person anticipates nonspecific danger.

Anxiety disorders group of psychobiologic illnesses that result from the activation of the autonomic nervous system, chiefly the sympathetic division.

Anxiolytics drugs that relieve the symptoms of anxiety; sometimes referred to as minor tranquilizers.

Aortic regurgitation backward flow of blood that occurs when the aortic valve does not close tightly.

Aortic stenosis narrowing of the aortic valve's opening when its cusps become stiff and rigid.

Aortic valve heart valve (opening) between the left ventricle and aorta that prevents blood from flowing back into the ventricle after the heart contracts.

Aortography diagnostic procedure that detects aortic abnormalities such as aneurysms and arterial occlusions by injecting contrast medium and taking radiographic films of the abdominal aorta and major arteries in the legs.

Aphasia neurologic impairment of a person's ability to speak.

Apheresis process of separating blood into its components.

Aphonia complete loss of voice.

Apitherapy medicinal use of bee venom.

Aplasia failure to develop.

Aplastic anemia disorder manifested by insufficient numbers of erythrocytes, leukocytes, and platelets, collectively described as *pancytopenia*.

Apnea cessation of breathing.

Apocrine glands sweat glands found around the nipples, in the anogenital region, in the eyelids (Moll glands), in the mammary glands of the breast, and in the external ear canals.

Apolipoproteins proteins on the surface of cholesterol molecules that bind to enzymes that direct cholesterol to sites for metabolism.

Appendectomy surgical removal of the appendix.

Appendicitis inflammation of a narrow, blind protrusion called the vermiform appendix located at the tip of the cecum in the right lower quadrant of the abdomen.

Appliance device worn over a stoma for the collection of feces or urine.

Apraxia inability to accomplish activities of daily living, such as grooming, toileting, and eating, despite intact motor function.

Arachnoid layer middle membrane lying directly below the dura that protects the brain.

Aromatherapy use of scents to alter emotions and biologic processes.

Arteries blood vessels that carry oxygenated blood.

Arteriography diagnostic procedure that involves instilling dye, referred to as contrast medium, into an artery.

Arterioles smallest oxygen-carrying blood vessels.

Arteriosclerosis loss of elasticity or hardening of the arteries.

Arteriovenous fistula surgical anastomosis (connection) of an artery and vein lying in close proximity.

Arteriovenous graft type of vascular access method that uses a tube of synthetic material or polytetrafluoroethylene to connect a vein and artery in the upper or lower arm.

Arthritis general condition characterized by inflammation and degeneration of a joint.

Arthrocentesis aspiration of synovial fluid.

Arthrodesis fusion of a joint, most often the wrist or knee, for stabilization and pain relief.

Arthrogram radiographic examination of a joint, usually the knee or shoulder.

Arthroplasty surgical reconstruction of a joint, using an artificial joint that restores previously lost function and relieves pain.

Arthroscopy internal inspection of a joint by means of an instrument called an arthroscope.

Artificially acquired active immunity immunity that results from the administration of a killed or weakened microorganism or attenuated toxin.

Arrhythmia erratic heart rhythm or rate that is too fast or slow; sometimes referred to as dysrhythmias.

Asbestosis fibrous inflammation or chronic induration of the lungs caused by the inhalation of asbestos.

Ascites collection of fluid in the peritoneal cavity.

Assessment first step in the nursing process that involves the careful observation and evaluation of a client's health status.

Assisted living facilities type of living arrangement that provides care to residents who require assistance with up to three activities of daily living but also maintains their privacy and dignity.

Asthma reversible obstructive disease of the lower airway characterized by inflammation of the airway and hyperresponsiveness of the airway to internal or external stimuli.

Astigmatism visual distortion caused by an irregularly shaped cornea.

Asystole absence of heart contraction; cardiac arrest.

Ataxia neurologic impairment of a person's ability to walk.

Atelectasis disorder in which the alveoli collapse.

Atherectomy surgical removal of fatty plaque from arteries by inserting a cardiac catheter with a cutting tool at the tip or performing laser angioplasty.

Atheroma fatty mass within the arterial wall.

Atherosclerosis condition in which the lumen of the artery fills with fatty deposits, chiefly composed of cholesterol.

Atria upper chambers of the heart; *atrium* (singular).

Atrial fibrillation cardiac rhythm disorder in which several areas in the right atrium initiate disorganized, rapid impulses causing the atria to quiver rather than contract.

Atrial flutter cardiac rhythm disorder in which a single atrial impulse outside the sinoatrial node causes the atria to contract at an exceedingly rapid rate (200 to 400 times/min).

Atrioventricular valves openings between the atria and ventricles.

Atypical anorexia nervosa psychiatric disorder manifested by anorexia without low weight.

Audiometry precise measurement of hearing acuity.

Aura sensation, either of weakness, numbness, or a hallucinatory odor or sound, that occurs immediately before a generalized tonic-clonic seizure.

Auscultation listening with a stethoscope for normal and abnormal sounds generated by organs and structures such as the heart, lungs, intestines, and major arteries.

Authoritarian leadership style of leadership characterized by strong control by the manager over a work group.

Autoantibodies antibodies against self-antigens.

Autograft skin graft that uses a client's own skin, which is transplanted from one part of the body to another.

Autoimmune disorder disorder in which killer T cells and autoantibodies attack or destroy natural cells.

Autoinoculation self-transmission of an infection to another area of the body.

Autologous blood self-donated blood.

Automated external defibrillator (AED) portable device that checks the heart rhythm and can send an electric shock to the heart to restore a normal rhythm.

Automatic implanted cardiac defibrillator (AICD) internal electrical device used to restore a life-sustaining cardiac rhythm.

Automaticity ability of heart tissue to initiate electrical stimulus independently.

Automatisms inappropriate, automatic, repetitive movements such as lip smacking and picking at clothing or objects.

Autonomic dysreflexia exaggerated sympathetic nervous system response resulting from a spinal cord injury above T6. Characteristics include severe hypertension, slow heart rate, pounding headache, nausea, blurred vision, flushed skin, sweating, goosebumps, nasal stuffiness, and anxiety.

Autonomic nervous system consists of the sympathetic nervous system and the parasympathetic nervous system.

Autoregulation ability of the brain to provide sufficient arterial blood flow despite rising intracranial pressure.

Avascular necrosis death of bone from an insufficient blood supply.

Aversion therapy technique that deters a behavior by causing unpleasant physical reactions when the behavior occurs.

Avoidant/restrictive food intake disorder (ARFID) condition in which children become malnourished because of the limited variety of foods they will eat.

Avulsion fracture severe traumatic sprain in which a chip of bone to which a ligament is attached becomes detached.

Axon nerve fiber that projects and conducts impulses away from the neuron's cell body.

Ayurvedic medicine system of medicine with roots in India whose objective is to help individuals become unified with nature to develop a strong body, clear mind, and tranquil spirit.

Azoospermia absence of sperm.

Azotemia accumulation of nitrogen waste products in the blood, evidenced by elevated blood urea nitrogen, serum creatinine, and uric acid levels.

B

Bacteremia condition resulting from microorganisms escaping the lymph nodes and reaching the bloodstream, which may lead to sepsis.

Balloon tamponade tube that is inserted through the esophagus into the stomach, then inflated to compress esophageal varices and control hemorrhage.

Balloon valvuloplasty invasive, nonsurgical procedure to enlarge a narrowed heart valve using a deflated balloon that is threaded through a peripheral blood vessel into the stenotic valve, then inflated to stretch the opening.

Bargaining third stage in Elisabeth Kübler-Ross's five stages of grief in which a client attempts to negotiate a delay in dying with God or some higher power, usually until after a particularly significant event.

Bariatric surgery operative procedures on the stomach and small intestine for the purpose of achieving weight loss.

Barium enema radiographic study used to identify polyps, tumors, inflammation, strictures, and other abnormalities of the colon after instilling barium solution rectally.

Barium swallow fluoroscopic observation of a client swallowing a flavored barium solution and its progress down the esophagus to detect structural abnormalities of the esophagus as well as swallowing discoordination and oral aspiration.

Baroreceptors stretch receptors in the aortic arch and carotid sinus that signal the brain to release ADH when blood volume decreases, systolic blood pressure falls, or the right atrium is underfilled, and to suppress ADH when blood volume increases, systolic blood pressure rises, or the right atrium is overfilled.

Bases chemical substances that bind with hydrogen.

Basophils granulocytes that are active in allergic contact dermatitis and some delayed hypersensitivity reactions.

Battle sign bruising of the mastoid process behind the ear.

B-cell lymphocytes white blood cells that when stimulated by T-cell lymphocytes become either plasma or memory cells that play a role in a humoral immune response.

Bell palsy disorder in which there is inflammation around one of the paired facial nerves, blocking motor impulses to muscles on one side of the face.

Behavioral therapy type of psychotherapy that attempts to extinguish undesirable responses through the learning of other adaptive techniques.

Benign type of tumor that is not invasive or spreading.

Benign paroxysmal positional vertigo (BPPV) involves brief periods of severe vertigo when clients move their heads, particularly if they move their head back and toward the affected ear. Many clients experience it when they roll over in bed onto their side.

Benign prostatic hyperplasia condition in which the prostate gland contains more than the usual number of normal cells.

Benign prostatic hypertrophy (BPH) enlargement of the prostate gland.

Beta-amyloid starchy component that accumulates in the brains of clients with Alzheimer disease and injures neurons in the area of the brain responsible for producing acetylcholine, the neurotransmitter that is critical for memory and cognition.

Bicarbonate–carbonic acid buffer system regulates plasma pH by adding hydrogen ions to increase acidity and removing them to promote alkalinity.

Bicuspid valve opening between the left atrium and left ventricle; also known as the *mitral valve.*

Bigeminy cardiac rhythm pattern in which every other heartbeat is a premature ventricular contraction.

Biliary colic upper abdominal pain that may radiate to the back and shoulders.

Binge eating disorder inability to control overeating.

Biocultural ecology examines biologic cultural differences.

Biofeedback technique in which an individual voluntarily controls one or more physiologic functions such as body temperature, heart rate, blood pressure, and brain waves.

Bioidentical hormones FDA-approved prescription substances made from soy and yams that are indistinguishable and similarly effective as those from naturally occurring estrogen and progesterone.

Biologic disaster an event in which pathogens or their toxins cause harm to many humans and other living species.

Biologic response modifiers (BRMs) alter the interaction between the immune defenses and cancer cells. This interaction serves to destroy or halt the growth of malignant cells. BRMs can be naturally occurring or genetically engineered (recombinant).

Biomarkers proteins in blood, spinal fluid, and other body fluids early in a disease process.

Bipolar disorder disorder characterized by cycling between depression, euthymia, and mania.

Blackouts periods of amnesia involving events and activities while consuming alcohol.

Blistering agents (or vesicants) chemicals that damage exposed skin and mucous membranes on contact.

Blood dyscrasias abnormalities in the numbers and types of blood cells.

Blood products components extracted from blood and administered to clients who need specific blood substances but not all the fluid and cellular components in whole blood.

Blood substitute fluid emulsion, a mixture of two liquids, one of which is insoluble but remains dispersed in the other, that carries and distributes oxygen to cells, tissues, and organs.

Blood urea nitrogen protein breakdown product; deterioration in renal function is manifested by a rise in its values.

B lymphocytes agranulocytes that provide humoral immunity by producing antibodies (immunoglobulins).

Boarding homes small homes with individual rooms where residents pay for room and board and minimal nursing services.

Body mass index mathematical computation based on height and weight to evaluate a person's size in relation to norms within the adult population.

Body piercing act of inserting a metal ring or barbell, which is a straight or curved rod, into the lips, ear cartilage, cheeks, nose, tongue, eyebrows, navel, nipples, or genital area.

Bombs devices designed to explode on impact or when detonated to kill people, damage or destroy property.

Bone marrow aspiration procedure to determine the types and percentage of immature and maturing blood cells.

Bone scan study that uses the intravenous injection of a radionuclide to detect the uptake of the radioactive substance by the bone.

Botulism disease that develops from the neurotoxin produced by *Clostridium botulinum,* an anaerobic bacillus.

Bouchard nodes bony enlargement of the proximal interphalangeal joints.

Braces supports made of plastic materials, canvas, leather, or metal that are custom fit to each client, provide controlled movement, and prevent additional injury.

Brachytherapy direct internal application of a high dose of radiation within a sealed source on or within a tumor.

Bradyarrhythmia slow abnormal cardiac rhythm.

Bradykinesia slowness in performing spontaneous movements.

Brain mapping technique that compares a client's brain activity patterns (from an electroencephalogram or other electronic image) with a computerized database of electrophysiologic abnormalities.

Brain scan diagnostic test that identifies tumors, hematomas in or around the brain, cerebral abscesses, cerebral infarctions, or displaced ventricles.

Brain stem part of the central nervous system consisting of the midbrain, pons, and medulla oblongata.

Brain tumor growth of abnormal cells within the cranium.

Breakthrough pain acute pain that occasionally develops in those who have chronic pain.

Breast abscess localized collection of pus within breast tissue.

Breast augmentation procedure to enlarge natural, malignancy-free breasts.

Breast cancer mass of abnormal cells in the breast.

Breast reconstruction surgical procedure in which the area of a mastectomy is refashioned to simulate the contour of a breast and optionally to create a nipple and areola.

Breast self-examination technique for examining one's own breasts for lumps and suspicious changes.

Bronchiectasis chronic obstructive pulmonary disease characterized by chronic infection and irreversible dilation of the bronchi and bronchioles.

Bronchioles smaller subdivisions of bronchi.

Bronchus (pl. bronchi) one of the two main branches of the trachea.

Brudzinski sign assessment finding in which flexion of the neck produces flexion of the knees and hips.

Bruit purring or blowing sound caused by blood flowing over the rough surface of one or both carotid arteries.

B-type natriuretic peptide (BNP) cardioprotective neurohormone that functions to decrease blood pressure by increasing excretion of sodium and water, promoting arterial dilation, and counteracting renin, angiotensin, and aldosterone.

Buerger disease inflammation of blood vessels associated with clot formation and fibrosis of the blood vessel wall primarily in small arteries and veins of the legs (also known as thromboangiitis obliterans).

Bulimia nervosa eating disorder characterized by food binges of a large number of calories followed by measures to prevent weight gain.

Bulimarexia eating disorder characterized by periods of food restriction and periods of binging followed by purging.

Bursa small sac filled with synovial fluid that reduces friction between tendon and bone and between tendon and ligament.

Bursitis inflammation of the bursa, a fluid-filled sac that cushions bone ends to enhance a gliding movement.

C

Calcification process in which inorganic minerals, such as calcium salts, are deposited in body tissues.

Calcitonin hormone that inhibits the release of calcium from bone into the extracellular fluid.

Calciuria excessive calcium in the urine.

Calculus precipitate of mineral salts that ordinarily remain dissolved in urine.

Callus healing mass that forms after a bone is fractured, which holds the ends of the bone together but cannot endure strain.

Caloric stimulation test test that assesses the vestibular reflexes of the inner ear that control balance.

Cancellous bone bony tissue that is light and contains many spaces.

Cancer disease characterized by abnormal, disorganized cell proliferation.

Candidiasis yeast infection caused by the *Candida albicans* microorganism that may develop in the oral, pharyngeal, esophageal, or vaginal cavities or within folds of the skin.

Cannabinoids chemicals contain *tetrahydrocannabinol* (THC) and *cannabidiol* (CBD).

Capillaries blood vessels that connect arterioles to venules.

Capitation type of financial management of an insurance plan that pays a preset fee per member per month to a health care provider, usually a hospital or hospital system, that covers all medical costs incurred and is paid regardless of whether the member requires health care services.

Capsid double layer of lipid material that surrounds the genetically incomplete HIV.

Caput medusae dilation of the veins over the abdomen.

Carbuncle deep skin and subcutaneous abscess from which pus drains.

Carcinogenesis process of malignant transformation and altering of the genetic structure of DNA within the cells.

Carcinogens factors or agents that contribute to the development of cancer.

Carcinoma in situ localized malignancy that, if untreated, will subsequently invade other areas.

Cardiac catheterization diagnostic test performed in an operative setting during which a catheter is inserted from a peripheral blood vessel in the groin, arm, or neck into one of the great vessels and then into the heart.

Cardiac cycle sequence of electrical and mechanical events in the atria and ventricles that result in a heartbeat.

Cardiac index calculation that reflects the cardiac output in relation to a particular client's body size.

Cardiac output volume of blood ejected from the left ventricle per minute.

Cardiac rehabilitation program following a cardiac event that combines exercise and educational activities to speed recovery and reduce or prevent recurring episodes.

Cardiac resynchronization therapy technique that restores synchrony in the contractions of the right and left ventricles using a biventricular pacemaker.

Cardiac rhythm pattern (or pace) of the heartbeat.

Cardiac tamponade compression of the heart with blood that accumulates within the pericardium.

Cardiogenic pulmonary edema condition in which the left ventricle becomes incapable of maintaining sufficient output of blood with each contraction.

Cardiogenic shock shock that occurs when contraction of the heart is ineffective and cardiac output is reduced.

Cardiomyopathy chronic condition characterized by structural changes in the heart muscle.

Cardiomyoplasty surgical procedure in which a client's own chest muscle is grafted to the aorta and wrapped around the heart to augment ineffective myocardial muscle contraction.

Cardioplegia intentional stopping of the heart for a surgical procedure.

Cardiopulmonary bypass technique in which blood is mechanically circulated and oxygenated outside the body.

Caregiver person who performs health-related activities that a person with sickness cannot perform independently.

Carina lower part of the trachea.

Carotid endarterectomy surgical removal of atherosclerotic plaque from the carotid artery.

Carpal tunnel syndrome term for a group of symptoms located in the wrist where the median nerve passes through a narrow, inelastic canal formed by the carpal bones.

Carpopedal spasm involuntary contraction of hand muscles.

Carrier human or animal that harbors an infectious microorganism but does not show active evidence of the disease.

Cartilage firm, dense connective tissue whose primary functions are to reduce friction between articular surfaces, absorb shocks, and reduce stress on joint surfaces.

Case management system of health care delivery in which a case manager plans and coordinates a client's progress through the various phases of care to avoid delays, unnecessary diagnostic testing, and overuse of expensive resources.

Case method historically early system of nursing care in which one nurse provided all the services that a particular client required, accompanying the client to the hospital, providing care in the home, and performing many household duties as well.

Cast rigid mold that immobilizes an injured structure while it heals.

Casts deposits of minerals that break loose from the walls of renal tubules.

Cataract disorder in which the lens of the eye becomes opaque.

Catecholamines neurotransmitters that stimulate responses by the sympathetic nervous system.

Cation positive-charged electrolyte.

Cauda equina small sections of spinal nerves that begin after the end of the spinal cord between the first and second lumbar vertebrae.

Cell-mediated response process that occurs when T cells survey proteins in the body, actively analyze the surface features, and respond to those that differ from the host by directly attacking the invading antigen.

Central aortic systolic pressure blood pressure at the root of the aorta as blood is pumped from the left ventricle.

Central nervous system part of the nervous system consisting of the brain and spinal cord.

Central nervous system depressants chemical agents that slow brain and physiologic activity.

Central nervous system stimulants chemical agents that accelerate physical and mental functions.

Central sleep apnea occurs because the brain fails to signal the respiratory muscles to breathe.

Central venous infusions infusions that deliver solutions into a large central vein, such as the vena cava.

Central venous pressure pressure produced by venous blood in the right atrium.

Central vision ability to discriminate letters, words, and the details of any image.

Cephalalgia aching in the head.

Cerebellum part of the brain located behind and below the cerebrum that controls and coordinates muscle movement.

Cerebral angiography test that detects distortion of cerebral arteries and veins, indicating an aneurysm, a tumor, or other vascular abnormality.

Cerebral cortex layer of tissue on the surface of the cerebrum containing motor and sensory neurons.

Cerebral hematoma bleeding within the skull that forms an expanding lesion.

Cerebral infarction death of brain tissue.

Cerebrovascular accident prolonged interruption in the flow of blood through one of the arteries supplying the brain.

Cerebrum part of the brain consisting of two hemispheres connected by the corpus callosum.

Certified interpreter person authorized to provide communication assistance between a health care provider and non-English-speaking client.

Cervicitis inflammation of the cervix.

Chancre painless ulcer that accompanies first-stage syphilis.

Chancroid sexually transmitted infection caused by the *Haemophilus ducreyi* bacillus and characterized by the appearance of a macule, followed by vesicle-pustule formation and, finally, a painful ulcer.

Charcot joints neuropathic joint disease, a common finding in tertiary syphilis.

Chelation therapy pharmacologic process for removing heavy metals from the blood such as iron to prevent organ damage and death.

Chemical cardioversion use of drugs to eliminate arrhythmia.

Chemical dependence condition of needing to take a drug to avoid withdrawal symptoms.

Chemical disaster result of the release of toxic artificial substances with a potential for causing mass casualties.

Chemokines chemicals responsible for immune surveillance and immune cell recruitment.

Chemonucleolysis procedure in which the enzyme chymopapain is injected into the nucleus pulposus to shrink or dissolve a ruptured intervertebral disk and relieve pressure on spinal nerve roots.

Chemoreceptors structures that are sensitive to the pH, CO_2, and oxygen in the blood and regulate sympathetic nervous system stimulation or inhibition.

Chemotaxis process of attracting migratory cells to a particular area within the body.

Chemotherapy technique that uses antineoplastic (anticancer) agents to treat cancer cells locally and systemically.

Cheyne–Stokes respiration pattern of respiration in which shallow, rapid breathing is followed by a period of apnea.

Chief complaint that which the client perceives to be the health problem that needs treatment.

Chinese medicine medical system developed in China and other Asian countries that views health as the balancing of opposite forces and views illness as a consequence of imbalance.

Chiropractic technique of performing spinal manipulation as a generic method for curing neuromuscular disorders and a host of other diseases.

Chlamydia sexually transmitted infection caused by a bacterium, *Chlamydia trachomatis*, which lives inside the cells it infects; the disease is spread by sexual intercourse or genital contact without penetration and is the most common and fastest spreading bacterial sexually transmitted infections in the United States.

Chlorine liquid respiratory toxin that becomes a gas when released into the atmosphere.

Cholangiography test used to determine the patency of the ducts from the liver and gallbladder using a dye that is usually instilled intravenously.

Cholecystitis inflammation or infection of the gallbladder.

Cholecystography test used to identify the presence of stones in the gallbladder or common bile duct and tumors or other obstructions, by observing the ability of the gallbladder to concentrate and store an iodine-based, radiopaque contrast medium.

Choledocholithiasis disorder in which gallstones are located within the common bile duct.

Cholelithiasis disorder in which stones are formed in the gallbladder.

Cholestasis ineffective bile drainage.

Cholesterol fatty (lipid) substance.

Chorea characterized by jerky involuntary movements and an inability to use skeletal muscles in a coordinated manner.

Choreiform movements uncontrollable writhing and twisting of the body.

Choroid plexus cells that produce cerebrospinal fluid in the ventricles of the brain.

Chronic bronchitis prolonged (or extended) inflammation of the bronchi, accompanied by a chronic cough and excessive production of mucus for at least 3 months each year for two consecutive years.

Chronic fatigue syndrome complex of symptoms primarily characterized by profound lack of energy with no identifiable cause that worsens with physical activity and does not improve with rest.

Chronic kidney disease (CKD) (chronic renal failure [CRF]) characterized by progressive and irreversible damage to the nephrons.

Chronic heart failure disorder in which the heart's ability to pump effectively is compromised for an extended period of time.

Chronic obstructive pulmonary disease broad, nonspecific term that describes a group of pulmonary disorders with symptoms of chronic cough and expectoration, dyspnea, and impaired expiratory airflow.

Chronic pain discomfort that lasts longer than 6 months.

Chronic traumatic encephalopathy neurodegeneration caused by repeated head injuries.

Chvostek sign assessment finding in which a client's mouth twitches and jaw tightens following the tapping of the facial nerve.

Cilia hair-like processes whose action moves substances like mucus to prevent irritation to and contamination of the lower airway.

Circulatory overload fluid volume that exceeds what is normal for the intravascular space and has the potential to compromise cardiopulmonary function if it remains unresolved.

Cirrhosis degenerative liver disorder caused by generalized cellular damage.

Civil law body of law that is concerned with disputes between individual citizens and that protects each individual's personal freedoms and property rights.

Client term used for the recipient of health care services that emphasize the recipient's personal responsibility for health and active partnership in health care.

Client database collection of information from the client's medical and nursing history, physical examination, and diagnostic studies.

Clinical breast examination inspection of the breast in which an examiner notes breast size and symmetry and any unusual changes in the skin of the breasts and nipples and palpates the breasts and axillae for masses, lymph nodes, tenderness, and other abnormalities.

Clinical reasoning assessment and management of client problems at the point of care.

Closed head injury injury to the head in which an intact layer of scalp covers the fractured skull.

Closed method burn wound management technique in which the wound is covered. The closed method involves the use of one or more types of dressing materials.

Closed questions asked during a client interview that require only "yes" or "no" answers. See also *open-ended questions*.

Closed reduction procedure in which a fractured bone is restored to its normal position by external manipulation, then immobilized with a bandage, cast, or traction.

Coagulopathies bleeding disorders that involve platelets or clotting factors.

Cochlear implant device that is surgically placed in the inner ear and connected to a receiver in the bone behind the ear to improve hearing.

Codons points on HIV genes where mutations occur.

Cognitive functions abilities of a person involving knowledge, understanding, and perception.

Cognitive learner person who processes information best by listening to or reading facts and descriptions.

Cognitive behavioral therapy type of psychotherapy in which a therapist helps a client by altering their interpretation of events.

Colectomy partial or complete surgical removal of the colon.

Colic acute spasmodic pain.

Collaboration use of a team effort to achieve client care outcomes.

Collaborative problems complications with a physiologic origin that nurses manage using primary provider–prescribed and nursing-prescribed interventions.

Collaborator person who works with others to achieve a common goal.

Collateral circulation circulation formed by smaller blood vessels branching off from or near larger occluded vessels.

Colloid solutions solutions containing water and molecules of suspended substances such as blood cells and blood products (e.g., albumin).

Colonization condition in which microorganisms are present, but the host does not manifest signs or symptoms of infection.

Colonoscopy procedure in which an endoscope is used to visually examine the inner surface of the colon.

Colony-stimulating factors cytokines that regulate the production, maturation, and function of blood cells.

Colostomy surgically created opening between the colon and the skin.

Combination antiretroviral therapy (cART) multiple antiretroviral drugs used together; referred to as a drug cocktail.

Comedone skin condition commonly called a blackhead; formed when sebum, keratin, and bacteria accumulate and dilate a hair follicle.

Comfort zone that area of a client's personal space which, when intruded, does not create anxiety.

Commissures area where the cusps of a cardiac valve contact each other.

Commissurotomy surgical procedure in which adhesions are opened in the cardiac valve cusps.

Common law system of laws that uses earlier court decisions, judgments, and decrees as precedents for interpretation of laws; also known as judicial law.

Communicable diseases infections transmitted from one source to another.

Communication board device that facilitates communication by verbally impaired clients by pointing to common phrases, spelling with the alphabet, or identifying numbers.

Community-acquired infections diseases that are not present or incubating before care from one infected person or reservoir to another.

Community-acquired pneumonia (CAP) the most common type of pneumonia; the client contracts the illness in a community setting or within 48 hours of admission to a health care facility.

Compartment syndrome symptoms such as severe pain that develop when a tendon or nerve is compressed within a confined space.

Compensation acceleration of regulatory processes in the lungs and kidneys when an imbalance in acids or bases occurs.

Compensation stage first stage of shock, during which several physiologic mechanisms attempt to stabilize the spiraling consequences of shock.

Complement cascade immune process in which many different proteins are activated in a chain reaction when an antibody binds with an antigen.

Complex decongestive physiotherapy activity that includes (1) distal to proximal massage of edematous areas to facilitate lymphatic drainage into collateral vessels; (2) application of compression dressings to relieve edema by reducing the excess volume of fluid in the interstitial space; (3) active exercise to promote lymphatic circulation and maintain functional use of the limb; and (4) care and maintenance of skin and nails vulnerable to secondary complications.

Complex sleep apnea combination of central sleep apnea and obstructive sleep apnea.

Compounding pharmacies companies that combine, mix, or alter ingredients according to a primary provider's prescription to meet the specific needs of an individual.

Compulsion anxiety-relieving ritual.

Compulsive overeating disorder characterized by eating when not hungry or regardless of feeling full.

Computed tomography diagnostic test using X-rays and computer analysis to produce three-dimensional views of thin cross-sections, or "slices," of structures.

Concept care mapping method that links important ideas about the care a client requires and provides a means for students and nurses to consider all the client's problems and develop a plan to treat them.

Concussion injury resulting from a blow to the head that jars the brain and results in diffuse and microscopic injury to it.

Conduction method of heat loss in which warmth is transferred from the body through contact with a cooler source.

Conduction system neural tissue that sustains the electrical activity of the heart.

Conductive hearing loss hearing loss that is due to interference in the transmission of sound waves to the inner ear.

Conductivity ability of cardiac tissue to transmit an electrical stimulus from cell to cell within the heart.

Condylomas sexually transmitted genital warts that are usually painless and appear as a single lesion or cluster of soft, fleshy growths on the genitalia or cervix, within the vagina, or on the perineum, anus, throat, or mouth.

Congestive heart failure accumulation of blood and fluid within organs and tissues as a result of ineffective heart contraction.

Congregate housing residential center made up of free-standing apartments, private rooms, or both, that provides independent to minimal assistance for seniors or disabled adults.

Conization surgical removal of a large cone-shaped section of cervical uterine tissue.

Conjunctivitis inflammation of the conjunctiva.

Conservatorship responsibility for managing a client's care and assets appointed by a court when the client is incompetent.

Constitutional law fundamental freedoms and rights granted by the Constitution to all citizens of the United States.

Contactants protein substances that cause allergic skin reactions.

Contagious diseases communicable diseases that can spread rapidly among individuals in close proximity to each other.

Continent ileostomy (abdominal pouch) creation of an internal reservoir for the storage of gastrointestinal effluent.

Contractility ability of cardiac tissue to stretch as a single unit and recoil.

Contrecoup injury result of trauma to the head from a force that is strong enough to send the brain ricocheting to the opposite side of the skull, resulting in dual bruising.

Contusion (1) soft tissue injury resulting from a blow or blunt trauma; (2) injury to the head that leads to gross structural injury to the brain and results in bruising and, sometimes, hemorrhage of superficial cerebral tissue.

Convection form of heat loss by means of currents of liquids or gases that cause warm molecules to move away from the body.

Conventional medicine practices that embody traditional Western treatment of diseases.

Convulsion seizure characterized by spasmodic contractions of muscles.

Coping mechanisms unconscious tactics people use to protect themselves from feeling inadequate or threatened.

Coronary veins blood vessels that carry unoxygenated blood from the inferior and superior venae cavae into the coronary sinus in the right atrium.

Cor pulmonale disorder in which pulmonary disease causes the right ventricle to enlarge or fail.

Corneal transplantation replacement of abnormal corneal tissue with healthy donated corneal tissue.

Coronary arteries blood vessels that supply oxygenated blood to cardiac muscle.

Coronary artery bypass graft surgical procedure that improves myocardial oxygenation by bypassing or detouring around the occluded portion of one or more coronary arteries with a relocated blood vessel from a healthy leg vein or chest artery.

Coronary artery disease arteriosclerotic and atherosclerotic changes in the coronary arteries supplying the myocardium.

Coronary occlusion obstruction of a coronary artery that reduces or totally interrupts blood supply to the distal muscle area.

Coronary ostia openings to the coronary arteries; *ostium* (singular).

Coronary stent small, metal coil with mesh-like openings placed within the coronary artery during PTCA that prevents the coronary artery from collapsing.

Coronary thrombosis blood clot within a coronary artery.

Coronary veins blood vessels that carry blood containing carbon dioxide into the coronary sinus in the right atrium.

Coronavirus a type of virus. A newly identified coronavirus, SARS-CoV-2, has caused a worldwide pandemic of respiratory illness, called COVID-19.

Corpus callosum band of white fibers that acts as a bridge for transmitting impulses between the left and right hemispheres of the brain.

Cortical bone bony tissue that is dense and hard.

Corticotropin-releasing hormone (CRH) causes the anterior pituitary gland to secrete adrenocorticotropic hormone (ACTH).

Corticosteroid hormones chemicals secreted by the adrenal cortex.

Corticosteroids collective term for the glucocorticoids, mineralocorticoids, and small amounts of sex hormones manufactured and secreted by the adrenal cortex.

Coryza rhinitis or the common cold.

Costovertebral angle area where the lower ribs meet the vertebrae.

Coup injury trauma to the brain caused when the head is struck directly.

Couplets two premature ventricular contractions in a row.

COVID-19 a mild to severe respiratory illness that is caused by a coronavirus; is transmitted chiefly by contact with infectious material (such as respiratory droplets) or with objects or surfaces contaminated by the causative virus; and is characterized especially by fever, cough, and shortness of breath and may progress to pneumonia and respiratory failure.

Cranial nerves 12 pairs of nerves originating in the brain.

Craniectomy surgical procedure in which a portion of a cranial bone is removed.

Cranioplasty surgical procedure in which a defect in a cranial bone is repaired using a metal or plastic plate or wire mesh.

Craniotomy surgical procedure in which the skull is opened to gain access to structures beneath the cranial bones.

Creatinine substance that results from the breakdown of phosphocreatine (amino acid waste product), which is present in muscle tissue, is filtered by the glomeruli, and is excreted at a fairly constant rate by the kidney.

Creatinine clearance test study used to determine kidney function and creatinine excretion.

Credé maneuver technique in which the client bends at the waist or presses inward and downward over the bladder to increase abdominal pressure and facilitate emptying the bladder.

Criminal law body of law concerned with offenses that violate the public's welfare.

Critical limb ischemia complication of peripheral artery disease characterized by open sores or infections that do not resolve, become gangrenous, and threaten the viability of the limb, making amputation necessary.

Critical thinking intentional, contemplative, outcome-directed thinking.

Crohn disease chronic inflammatory bowel condition that can occur in any portion of the GI tract but predominantly affects the terminal portion of the ileum.

Cross-tolerance reduced pharmacologic effect when taking sedative-hypnotic drugs developed by alcoholics.
Cryoprecipitate acellular blood component that contains fibrinogen and multiple clotting factors.
Cryosurgery means of removing tissue by applying extreme subfreezing cold with a probe or agent such as liquid nitrogen.
Cryotherapy procedure that freezes and kills cancer cells.
Cryptorchidism condition in which one or both testes fail to descend into the scrotum.
Crystalloid solutions solutions that consist of water and uniformly dissolved crystals such as salt (sodium chloride), other electrolytes, and sugar (glucose, dextrose).
Cultural competence (1) an understanding both of the nurse's own worldview and of the client's; (2) process in which a nurse consistently tries to work within the cultural context of the client and their family and community.
Cultural history information obtained during a client interview about the client's religious affiliation, cultural background, and health beliefs.
Culture (1) person's way of perceiving, behaving, and evaluating the world that includes their knowledge, beliefs, art, morals, laws, and customs; (2) a test used to identify bacteria within a specimen taken from a person with symptoms of an infection.
Cushing syndrome endocrine disorder that results from excessive secretion of hormones by the adrenal cortex.
Cushing triad three signs associated with an increase in intracranial pressure: pulse increases initially but then decreases, systolic BP rises, and pulse pressure widens.
Cushingoid syndrome physical changes that accompany excess endogenous production of steroid hormones or long-term corticosteroid therapy.
Cutaneous triggering technique in which the client lightly massages or taps the skin above the pubic area to stimulate relaxation of the urinary sphincter.
Cyanide a solid salt or volatile liquid chemical that can cause death in minutes.
Cyclothymia alternation of sad and elated moods; resembles bipolar disorder, but the extremes of mood are less pronounced.
Cystectomy surgical removal of the bladder.
Cystic fibrosis multisystem disorder affecting infants, children, and young adults that results from a defective autosomal recessive gene; the genetic mutation causes dysfunction of the exocrine glands, involving the mucus-secreting and eccrine sweat glands.
Cystitis inflammation of the urinary bladder.
Cystocele bulging of the bladder into the vagina.
Cystography study that evaluates abnormalities in bladder structure and filling through the instillation of contrast dye and radiography.
Cystolitholapaxy Procedure by which bladder stones are removed through the transurethral route using a stone-crushing instrument (lithotrite). This procedure is suitable for small and soft stones and is performed under general anesthesia.
Cystometrography (CMG) evaluates urinary bladder tone and capacity.
Cytokines chemicals that relay messages throughout the immune system and the brain; also known as immunopeptides or immunotransmitters.
Cystometrogram study that evaluates bladder tone and capacity using a retention catheter that is inserted into the bladder after the client voids and slowly filled with sterile saline until the client indicates at what point the first urge to void is felt and when the bladder feels full.
Cystoscope instrument consisting of a lighted tube with a telescopic lens used to examine the inside of the bladder.
Cystoscopy visual examination of the inside of the bladder using an instrument called a cystoscope.
Cystostomy surgical procedure in which a catheter is inserted through the abdominal wall directly into the bladder.
Cytokines immunologic chemical messengers released by lymphocytes, monocytes, and macrophages.
Cytotoxic T cells lymphocytes that bind to invading cells and destroy them by altering their cellular membrane and intracellular environment and releasing chemicals called lymphokines.

D

Dandruff loose, scaly material of dead, keratinized epithelium shed from the scalp.
Deaf inability to hear well enough to process information.
Debridement natural, mechanical, enzymatic, or surgical removal of necrotic tissue.
Decerebrate posturing position in which the extremities are stiff and rigid following neurologic trauma; also called decerebrate rigidity.
Decibel unit for measuring the intensity of sound.
Decompensation stage stage in shock that occurs as compensatory mechanisms fail and the client's condition spirals downward into cellular hypoxia, coagulation defects, and cardiovascular changes.
Decorticate posturing position in which the arms are flexed, the fists clenched, and the legs extended following neurologic trauma; also called decorticate rigidity.
Decortication surgical removal of the pericardium to allow more adequate filling and contraction of the heart chambers.
Deep brain stimulation invasive procedure used to help manage the tremor caused by Parkinsonism and other neurologic conditions; also used to alter brain circuitry to relieve depression.
Deep vein thrombosis inflammation of a vein deep in the lower extremities accompanied by clot or thrombus formation.
Defibrillation emergency procedure that uses electrical energy to stop a life-threatening ventricular arrhythmia.
Degenerative joint disease type of arthritis that is characterized by a slow and steady progression of destructive changes in weight-bearing joints and those that are repeatedly used for work.
Dehiscence separation of surgical wound edges without the protrusion of organs.
Dehydration significant reduction of body fluid in both extracellular and intracellular compartments.
Delegation transferring to a competent individual the authority to perform a selected task in a selected situation while retaining accountability for the delegation.
Delirium sudden, transient state of confusion.
Delusions fixed false beliefs that cannot be changed by logical reasoning and are often persecutory in nature.
Demand (or synchronous) mode pacemaker pacemaker that self-activates when a client's heart rate falls below a certain level.
Dementia gradual, irreversible loss of intellectual abilities.
Democratic leadership style of leadership characterized by participation in decision-making by a work group.
Demyelinating disease disorder that causes permanent degeneration and destruction of myelin.
Dendrites threadlike projections or fibers on a neuron that conduct impulses to its cell body.

Denial psychological defense mechanism in which a client refuses to believe certain information; the first stage in Elisabeth Kübler-Ross's five stages of grief.

Dental dam device to prevent sexually transmitted infections using a sheet of latex as a barrier between the vagina or anus and a partner's mouth when performing oral or anal sex.

Deontology theory of ethics that proposes that the rightness of an action is determined entirely by whether or not it follows from an ethical duty.

Dependent edema accumulation of fluid in the body areas most affected by gravity (the feet, ankles, sacrum, or buttocks).

Depolarization stage in electrophysiology when positive ions move inside the myocardial cell membranes and the negative ions move outside.

Depot injections deep intramuscular injections of drugs in an oil suspension that are gradually absorbed over 2 to 4 weeks.

Depression the fourth stage in Elisabeth Kübler-Ross's five stages of grief in which a client realizes the reality of impending death and mourns potential losses such as separation from loved ones, the inability to fulfill future goals, or loss of control.

Dermabrasion method of removing surface layers of scarred skin using sandpaper, a rotating wire brush, chemicals, or a diamond wheel.

Dermatitis general term that refers to an inflammation of the skin.

Dermatome skin area supplied by a nerve.

Dermatophytes parasitic fungi that invade the skin, scalp, and nails.

Dermatophytoses superficial fungal infections.

Dermis layer of skin that lies below the epidermis.

Desensitization (1) form of immunotherapy in which a client receives weekly or twice-weekly injections of dilute but increasingly higher concentrations of an allergen; (2) technique for overcoming anxiety by gradually exposing a person to whatever it is that provokes their anxiety.

Destination therapy mechanical circulatory support when there is no option for a heart transplant.

Detoxification process of stabilizing a client with a sedative drug while alcohol is metabolized from their system.

Deviated septum irregularity in the septum that results in nasal obstruction.

Dexamethasone (cortisol) suppression test blood test that theoretically detects major depression.

Diabetes insipidus endocrine disorder that develops when antidiuretic hormone from the posterior pituitary gland is insufficient.

Diabetes mellitus endocrine disorder of the pancreas that affects carbohydrate, fat, and protein metabolism.

Diabetic ketoacidosis type of metabolic acidosis that occurs when there is an acute insulin deficiency or an inability to use whatever insulin the pancreas secretes.

Diabetic nephropathy progressive decrease in renal function that occurs with diabetes mellitus.

Diabetic retinopathy pathologic changes in the retina experienced by persons with diabetes.

Diabulimia restriction of insulin by type 1 diabetics for the purpose of weight loss.

Diagnosis-related group (DRG) classification of diagnoses that is used for medical reimbursement.

Dialysate solution used during dialysis that has a composition similar to normal human plasma.

Dialysis procedure for cleaning and filtering the blood that substitutes for kidney function when the kidneys cannot remove nitrogenous waste products and maintain adequate fluid, electrolyte, and acid–base balances.

Dialyzer semipermeable membrane filter within a machine that contains many tiny hollow fibers; during dialysis, blood moves through the hollow fibers and water and wastes from the blood move into the dialysate fluid that flows around the fibers, but protein and red blood cells do not.

Diaphragm muscle that separates the thoracic cavity from the abdominal cavity.

Diaphyses long shafts of bones in the arms and legs.

Diastolic blood pressure arterial pressure during ventricular relaxation.

Dietary supplement term defined by the Supplement Health and Education Act of 1994 (DSHEA) as something that supplies one or more dietary ingredients, including vitamins, minerals, amino acids, herbs, and other substances.

Diffusion process of oxygen and CO_2 exchange through the alveolar–capillary membrane.

Digital rectal examination (DRE) technique used to assess the prostate for size and texture.

Digitalization method of giving large doses of a digitalis drug at the beginning of treatment to build up therapeutic blood levels of the drug.

Dilation and curettage surgical procedure in which the cervix is stretched open and the endometrium is scraped to diagnose or treat various gynecologic problems and to remove fetal and placental tissue.

Diplopia double vision.

Directed donor blood blood obtained from specified blood donors among a client's relatives and friends.

Dirty bomb conventional explosive device (e.g., dynamite) that spreads small amounts of radiation in the form of powder or pellets.

Disaster threatening event of such destructive magnitude and force as to dislocate people, separate family members, damage or destroy homes, and injure or kill people.

Disease pathologic condition that presents with clinical signs and symptoms.

Disequilibrium syndrome neurologic condition believed to be caused by cerebral edema; the shift in cerebral fluid volume occurs when the concentrations of solutes within the blood are lowered rapidly during dialysis.

Diskectomy surgical procedure in which a ruptured intervertebral disk is removed.

Dislocation injury in which the articular surfaces of a joint are no longer in contact.

Distal sensory polyneuropathy (DSP) disorder characterized by abnormal sensations, such as burning and numbness, in the feet and later in the hands.

Distress excessive, ill-timed, or unrelieved stress.

Distributive shock shock that occurs when fluid in the circulatory system does not facilitate effective perfusion of the tissue; sometimes called normovolemic shock.

Diverticulitis inflammation of diverticula.

Diverticulosis asymptomatic diverticula.

Diverticulum (pl. diverticula) sac or pouch caused by herniation of the mucosa through a weakened portion of the muscular coat of the intestine or other structure.

Documentation written or computerized record of client care.

Dopamine monoamine neurotransmitter of the sympathetic nervous system and precursor of norepinephrine; excess is associated with distortion of thoughts and sensory perception.

Double-barrel colostomy an opening in the colon that contains both a proximal stoma for expelling fecal material and a distal stoma to the anus.

Drop factor ratio of drops to milliliter delivered by tubing in the administration of IV solution.

Drop size volume of IV fluid determined by the opening in the tubing.

Drug cross-resistance diminished drug response among similar drugs.

Drug-eluting stent scaffolding device that keeps a coronary artery open and releases a drug that prevents reocclusion.

Drug resistance ineffective response to a prescribed drug because of the survival and duplication of exceptionally virulent mutations.

Dumping syndrome syndrome in which the rapid emptying of large amounts of hypertonic chyme into the jejunum draws fluid from the circulating blood into the intestine, causing hypovolemia, which can produce syncope. As the syndrome progresses, the sudden appearance of carbohydrates in the jejunum stimulates the pancreas to secrete excessive amounts of insulin, which in turn causes hypoglycemia.

Duodenal ulcer A type of peptic ulcer that occurs in the duodenum; tissue is eroded and ulcerated. See *peptic ulcer*.

Dura mater tough outermost membrane that protects the brain.

Durable power of attorney legal designation of a person to make decisions regarding finances or health care when a person becomes incompetent.

Duty expected action based on moral or legal obligations.

Dysarthria difficulty articulating and pronouncing words.

Dysmenorrhea painful menstruation.

Dyspareunia discomfort during intercourse.

Dyspepsia epigastric pain or discomfort.

Dysphagia impaired ability to swallow.

Dysrhythmia conduction disorder that results in an abnormally slow or rapid heart rate or one that does not proceed through the conduction system in the usual manner; also called arrhythmia.

Dysthymia feeling of unremitting sadness; similar to but less severe than major depression.

E

Early detection use of screening diagnostic tests and procedures to identify a disease process earlier so that treatment may be initiated earlier and be more effective.

Earthquake phenomenon when two tectonic plates, sublayers of the earth's crust, cause the ground to shift.

Eating disorders disorders in which eating is outside the range of normal.

Ecchymosis bruising.

Eccrine glands sweat glands that release water and electrolytes, such as sodium and chloride, in the form of perspiration.

Echocardiography diagnostic procedure that uses ultrasound waves to determine the functioning of the left ventricle and to detect cardiac tumors, congenital defects, and changes in the tissue layers of the heart.

Ectopic site conductive tissue that initiates an electrical impulse independently of the sinoatrial node.

Educator person who provides information.

Effector T cells killer (cytotoxic) T-cell lymphocytes.

Effluent discharged fecal material or liquid feces.

Effusion accumulation of fluid within two layers of tissue.

Ejaculation discharge of semen.

Ejection fraction percentage of blood the left ventricle ejects when it contracts.

Elective electrical cardioversion nonemergency procedure to stop rapid atrial arrhythmias in which a machine delivers electrical stimulation that does not disrupt the heart during ventricular repolarization.

Electrocardiography graphic recording of the electrical currents generated by the heart muscle.

Electroconvulsive therapy application of an electric stimulus to one or both temporal regions of the head to produce a brief, generalized seizure; used to treat severe depression.

Electrodessication procedure that uses electrical energy converted to heat to destroy or remove superficial growths from the skin; also known as electrosurgery.

Electroencephalogram recording of electrical impulses generated by the brain.

Electrolarynx handheld device that when placed on the neck vibrates and mechanically resonates when words or sounds are mouthed.

Electrolytes substances that carry an electrical charge when dissolved in fluid.

Electromagnetic therapy technique of healing using either electricity, magnets, or both.

Electromyography diagnostic test that records changes in the electrical potential of muscles and the nerves supplying the muscles.

Electron beam computed tomography radiologic test that produces X-rays of the coronary arteries using an electron beam.

Electronic infusion device machine that regulates and monitors the administration of IV solutions.

Electronystagmography method used to evaluate vestibular function, the mechanisms that facilitate maintaining balance, by measuring the duration and velocity of eye movements during caloric stimulation.

Electrophysiology study procedure that enables a primary provider to examine the electrical activity of the heart, produce actual arrhythmias by stimulating structures within the conduction pathway, determine the best method for preventing further dysrhythmic episodes, and, in some cases, eradicate the precise location in the heart that is producing the arrhythmia.

Embolectomy surgical removal of an embolus.

Embolus moving mass of particles, either solid or gas, within the bloodstream.

Emerging infectious disease disorder caused by microorganisms that are new or have had a resurgence in the last two decades.

Emission movement of sperm and their mixture with fluid from the seminal vesicles and prostate gland into the urethra, a process mediated via the sympathetic nervous system.

Emmetropia normal vision, in which light rays are bent to focus images precisely on the retina.

Empathy intuitive awareness of what a client is experiencing.

Emphysema chronic pulmonary disease characterized by abnormal distention of the alveoli.

Empyema collection of pus in the pleural cavity.

Emulsion mixture of two liquids, one of which is insoluble in the other; when combined, the two are distributed throughout the mixture as small, undissolved droplets.

Encephalitis inflammatory process affecting the central nervous system characterized by swelling of the brain and pathologic changes in both the white and gray matter and surrounding meninges.

Encopresis involuntary passage of liquid stool around an obstructive mass of stool.

Endarterectomy surgical removal of the atherosclerotic plaque lining an artery.

Endocannabinoids endogenous chemicals that have marijuana-like properties that activate the appetite center.

Endocardium innermost layer of the heart.

Endogenous opiates natural morphine-like substances that modulate pain transmission by blocking receptors for substance P.

Endometrial ablation detachment of the lining of the uterus.

Endometriosis condition in which tissue that histologically and functionally resembles that of the endometrium is found outside the uterus.

Endophthalmitis disorder in which all three layers of the eye and the vitreous are inflamed.

Endotoxins harmful chemicals released from within a bacterial cell; probably the major cause of toxic shock.

End-stage kidney disease stage in chronic renal failure in which less than 10% of nephron function remains and the point at which a regular course of dialysis or kidney transplantation is necessary to maintain life.

Energy therapies techniques that claim to manipulate electromagnetic fields within the body.

Engraftment establishment of bone marrow that has been harvested and reinfused.

Enhanced external counterpulsation noninvasive and nonsurgical therapy that helps relieve angina using a pressure suit that moves blood toward the heart.

Enmeshment social pattern in which two or more people lack limits that separate one person from another, resulting in a loss of personal identity and exclusion of others.

Enterocele protrusion of the intestinal wall into the vagina.

Enteroclysis study to determine subtle small bowel disease in which two contrast media fill and pass through the intestinal loops and are observed continuously through fluoroscope and periodic X-rays of the various sections of the small intestine.

Enterostomal therapist nurse who collaborates with the surgeon regarding stomal placement and the ostomate's educational needs.

Entry inhibitors drugs that interfere with the HIV's ability to fuse with and enter the CD4 cell; also known *as fusion inhibitors.*

Enucleation surgical removal of an eye.

Environmental tobacco smoke smoke given off by the burning end of a cigarette, pipe, or cigar and the exhaled smoke from the lungs of a smoker.

Enzyme-linked immunosorbent assay initial HIV screening test that is positive when there are sufficient HIV antibodies.

Eosinophils granulocytes that destroy parasites and play a major role in allergic reactions.

Epicardium inner serous layer of the pericardium; also called the *visceral pericardium.*

Epicondylitis painful inflammation of the elbow.

Epidemic rapidly spreading infectious disease in a particular region.

Epidermis outermost layer of skin.

Epididymitis inflammation of the epididymis.

Epidural hematoma bleeding within the skull that stems from arterial bleeding, usually from the middle meningeal artery, with blood accumulation above the dura.

Epiglottis cartilaginous valve flap that covers the opening to the larynx during swallowing.

Epilepsy chronic recurrent pattern of seizures.

Epinephrine neurotransmitter of the sympathetic nervous system produced and secreted by the adrenal medulla.

Epiphyses rounded, irregular ends of long bones.

Epistaxis nosebleed.

Epithelialization regrowth of skin.

Epstein–Barr virus virus that causes infectious mononucleosis.

Equianalgesic dose oral dose that provides the same level of pain relief as when the drug is given by a parenteral route.

Erectile dysfunction the inability to (1) achieve an erection, (2) achieve or maintain an erection sufficiently rigid for sexual activity, or (3) sustain an erection for a satisfactory period.

Erection parasympathetic nerve activity or state in which the penis becomes elongated and rigid, facilitating its insertion into the vagina.

Erythema redness of the skin.

Erythrocytes red blood cells.

Erythrocytosis increase in circulating erythrocytes.

Erythropoietin hormone released by the kidneys that stimulates the bone marrow to produce erythrocytes.

Eschar hard leathery crust of dehydrated skin that forms in areas of full-thickness burns.

Escharotomy incision into eschar to relieve constricting pressure.

Esophageal varices dilated, bulging esophageal veins.

Esophagitis inflammation of the lining of the esophagus.

Esophagogastroduodenoscopy examination of the esophagus, stomach, and duodenum through an endoscope to inspect, treat, or obtain specimens from any of the upper GI structures.

Essential hypertension sustained elevated blood pressure with no known cause.

Estrogen hormone produced by the ovaries.

Ethics moral principles and values that guide the behavior of honorable people.

Ethmoidal sinuses honeycomb of small spaces contained in the ethmoid bone, located between the eyes.

Ethnicity bond or kinship that people feel with their country of birth or place of ancestral origin, regardless of whether they have ever lived outside the United States.

Ethnobotanicals plants used for food, clothing, shelter, and medicine that grow in a region where specific groups of people live.

Ethnocentrism belief that one's own ethnic heritage is superior to that of others.

Eustress healthy amount of stress that helps individuals to pursue goals, learn to solve problems, and manage life's predictable and unpredictable crises.

Euthymic state in which a person is capable of experiencing a variety of feelings, all of which are situationally appropriate.

Evaluation last step in the nursing process that involves the assessment and review of the quality and suitability of care and the client's responses to that care.

Evaporation form of heat loss using the vaporization of moisture or water from the surface of the body.

Evisceration protrusion of organs through a separated surgical wound.

Exacerbation periods of acute flare-ups of the symptoms of a disorder.

Exercise electrocardiography diagnostic test that images the electrical activity of the heart while the client walks on a treadmill, pedals a stationary bicycle, or climbs up and down stairs; also known as a *stress test.*

Excitability ability of cardiac tissue to respond to electrical stimulation.

Excretory urography radiologic study used to evaluate the structure and function of the kidneys, ureters, and bladder by examining a radiopaque dye as it passes through the urinary tract.

Exertional dyspnea effort at breathing when physically active.

Expected outcomes client goals derived from nursing diagnoses that are measurable, achievable, and developed with the client, family, and other health care providers.

Expressive aphasia neurologic impairment of a person's ability to speak.
External fixation procedure in which metal pins are inserted into a fractured bone or bones from outside the skin surface and then attached to a compression device.
External radiologic contamination exposure to fallout on the skin, hair, and clothing.
Extracellular fluid water in the body located outside cells.
Extracorporeal circulation technique in which blood is mechanically circulated and oxygenated outside the body.
Extracorporeal shock wave lithotripsy procedure that uses shock waves to dissolve large kidney stones.
Extramedullary lesions nerve route compression involving the tissues surrounding the spinal cord.
Extrapyramidal symptoms movement disorders associated with certain prescribed drugs.
Extravasation leaking of an intravenously administered drug into surrounding tissues.
Extreme obesity body mass index of 40 or higher or a body weight of more than 20% of the ideal.

F

Facial reanimation various types of surgical reconstructive to improve facial movement and appearance.
Facilitated diffusion process in which dissolved substances require the assistance of a carrier molecule to pass through a semipermeable membrane.
Fallout cooling, condensation, and dropping back to earth of vapor containing radioactive material.
Fasciculations involuntary twitching of muscles.
Fasciotomy surgical incision of fascia and separation of muscle.
Fasting blood glucose blood test performed to detect and monitor diabetes mellitus.
Fault lines cracks between subterranean layers of rocks.
Fear feeling of terror in response to someone or something specific that a person perceives as dangerous or threatening.
Feedback loop mechanism that turns hormone production off and on; negative feedback stimulates a releasing gland in response to a decrease in levels while positive feedback keeps concentrations of hormones within a stable range.
Fertilization union of an ovum and a spermatozoon.
Fetor hepaticus sulfurous breath odor.
Fibrinogen plasma protein that plays a key role in forming blood clots by transforming liquid blood to fibrin.
Fibroadenoma solid, benign breast mass composed of connective and glandular tissue.
Fibrocystic breast disease benign breast disorder that affects women primarily between the ages of 30 and 50.
Fibroid tumor common benign uterine growth.
Fibromyalgia syndrome pain in the fibrous tissues of the body such as muscles, ligaments, and tendons.
Fifth vital sign practice of checking and documenting the client's pain every time the client's temperature, pulse, respiration, and blood pressure are assessed.
Fight-or-flight response neuroendocrine stress response involving the sympathetic division of the nervous system resulting in body system arousal.
Filtration process that promotes the movement of fluid and some dissolved substances through a semipermeable membrane using pressure differences.
Fingerspelling alphabetical substitute for words that have no sign.
Fissure tear in tissue.
Fistula channel from an organ to the surface of the body or from one organ to another.
Fistulectomy surgical procedure in which a fistulous tract is excised.
Fistulotomy surgical procedure involving incision of a fistula.
Fifth vital sign pain assessment obtained each time the client's temperature, pulse, respirations, and blood pressure are assessed.
***Five Wishes* document** advance directive that includes medical issues as well as personal, emotional, and spiritual concerns of a dying person.
Fixed-rate (asynchronous) mode pacemaker cardiac device that produces an electrical stimulus at a preset rate (usually 72 to 80 beats/min), despite the client's natural heart rate and rhythm.
Flaccidity lack of motor response to stimuli.
Flail chest disorder that occurs when two or more adjacent ribs fracture in multiple places and the fragments are free floating; affects the stability of the chest wall and impairment of chest wall movement.
Flashbacks feelings of reliving a traumatic event.
Flexible sigmoidoscopy procedure in which a flexible fiber-optic endoscope is used to examine the sigmoid colon.
Flooding overflow of water beyond its normal confines.
Focused assessment detailed information about one body system or problem.
Folic acid deficiency anemia blood disorder due to an insufficient dietary intake of folate, vitamin B_9, found naturally in foods.
Follicle-stimulating hormone (FSH) hormone that stimulates the development of ovum in the ovaries and sperm in the testes.
Fomites nonliving environment in which an infectious agent can survive and reproduce.
Food binges rapid consumption of a large number of calories.
Foramen magnum opening in the lower part of the skull through which the upper part of the spinal cord connects with the brain and which provides the only extracranial exit for brain tissue.
Formal teaching planned, organized conveying of information. See also *informal teaching.*
Fracture break in the continuity of a bone.
Freeze response stress response mediated through the parasympathetic nervous system, causing reduced neuroendocrine activities.
Friction effect that occurs when one object rubs against the other.
Frontal lobe part of each hemisphere of the brain located behind the forehead that serves to regulate and mediate the higher intellectual functions.
Frontal sinuses bony cavities that lie within the frontal bone that extends above the orbital cavities.
Fulguration removal of small, superficial bladder tumors through coagulation with a transurethral resectoscope.
Fulminant colitis a progression of severity of ulcerations associated with ulcerative colitis with severe pain, copious diarrhea, and potential dehydration and shock.
Full-thickness burn thermal injury that destroys all layers of the skin.
Full-thickness graft skin graft in which the epidermis, dermis, and some subcutaneous tissue are harvested from the client's skin.
Functional assessment determination of how well a client can manage activities of daily living.
Functional nursing task-oriented system of nursing care that evolved in the 1930s in which distinct duties are assigned to specific personnel.
Fundoplication surgical procedure to treat gastroesophageal reflux disorder that tightens the lower esophageal sphincter by wrapping the gastric fundus around the lower esophagus and suturing it into place.

Furuncle skin infection commonly called a boil.

Furunculosis condition of having multiple furuncles or boils.

Fusion inhibitor category of AIDS drugs that interfere with the ability of HIV to fuse with and enter the CD4 cell.

G

Gallbladder series test used to identify the presence of stones in the gallbladder or common bile duct and tumors or other obstructions, and to determine the ability of the gallbladder to concentrate and store an iodine-based, radiopaque contrast medium.

Gamma-aminobutyric acid inhibitory neurotransmitter.

Gamma-knife radiosurgery noninvasive alternative for treating brain tumors deep within the brain or for treating those tumors that conventional surgery can only partially remove.

Gamma radiation energy released from unstable atoms that can penetrate and damage body cells.

Ganglion cyst mass that develops near tendon sheaths and joints of the wrist.

Gangrene death of tissue.

Gastrectomy surgical removal of the stomach.

Gastric decompression removal of gas and fluids from the stomach.

Gastritis inflammation of the stomach lining.

Gastroesophageal reflux (GERD) disorder in which there is an upward flow of gastric contents into the esophagus.

Gastrostomy placement of a tube into the stomach via a surgically created opening into the abdominal wall.

Gender role societal determination of behaviors as either feminine or masculine.

Gene therapy technique for fighting cancer that involves replacing altered genes with normal genes, inhibiting defective genes, or introducing substances that destroy defective genes or cancer cells.

General adaptation syndrome nonspecific physiologic cyclical response to stress involving alarm, resistance, and exhaustion.

Generalization acknowledging that common trends exist within a cultural group but understanding that those trends may or may not apply to a particular individual.

Generalized anxiety disorder psychobiologic disorder characterized by chronic worrying on a daily basis for 6 or more months, generally with more than one focus of worry and often with the worrying being out of proportion with reality.

Generalized edema accumulation of fluid in all the interstitial spaces.

Genital herpes sexually transmitted infection caused by herpes simplex virus type 2 that results in genital and perineal lesions.

Genitalia organs of reproduction.

Genotype testing blood test used to detect drug resistance in which genetic changes in circulating HIV particles are measured.

Gerogogy techniques that enhance learning among older adults.

Gerontology study of aging, including its physiologic, psychological, and social aspects.

Guillain–Barré syndrome acute postinfectious polyneuropathy, polyradiculoneuritis that affects the peripheral nerves and the spinal nerve roots.

Glasgow coma scale tool for assessing a client's response to stimuli.

Glaucoma eye disorder caused by an imbalance between the production and drainage of aqueous fluid.

Globulin plasma proteins that function primarily as immunologic agents by preventing or modifying some types of infectious diseases.

Glomerulonephritis inflammatory renal disorder that occurs most frequently in children and young adults, which is preceded by an upper respiratory infection with group A beta-hemolytic streptococci, impetigo (skin infection), or viral infections such as mumps, hepatitis B, or HIV.

Glottis opening between the vocal cords in the larynx.

Glucagon hormone that increases blood sugar levels by stimulating the breakdown of glycogen into glucose in the liver.

Glucometer device that measures capillary blood glucose from blood sampled from a finger stick.

Glutamate neurotoxic neurotransmitter that contributes to neuronal cell death.

Glycemic index measure of how fast a carbohydrate food is likely to raise blood sugar.

Glycogenolysis process in which glycogen is broken down into glucose in the liver.

Glycosuria glucose in the urine.

Glycosylated hemoglobin amount of glucose stored within a hemoglobin molecule during its lifespan of 120 days.

Goiter enlarged thyroid gland.

Gonadotropin-releasing hormone triggers sexual development at the onset of puberty and continues to cause the anterior pituitary gland to secrete luteinizing hormone (LH) and follicle-stimulating hormone (FSH).

Gonorrhea sexually transmitted infection caused by a bacterium, *Neisseria gonorrhea,* which invades the urethra, vagina, rectum, or pharynx, depending on the nature of sexual contact.

Good Samaritan laws provide legal immunity for rescuers who provide first aid in an emergency (outside of a hospital) to accident victims.

Gout painful metabolic disorder involving an inflammatory reaction within the joints that usually affects the feet (especially the great toe), hands, elbows, ankles, and knees.

Grandiosity unrealistic sense of self-importance.

Granulocytes leukocytes that contain cytoplasmic granules.

Graft-versus-host disease result of foreign transplanted donor cells destroying the recipient's tissues and organs.

Granuloma inflammatory nodular lesion.

Granuloma inguinale sexually transmitted infection caused by a bacillus, *Calymmatobacterium granulomatis,* and characterized by painless nodules in the genital, inguinal, and anal areas.

Grieving process that includes emotional, physical, spiritual, social, and intellectual responses and behaviors by which individuals incorporate an actual, anticipated, or perceived loss.

Growth hormone–releasing hormone (GHRH) causes the release of somatotropin (growth hormone [GH]) from the anterior pituitary gland.

Guardianship court-appointed responsibility for managing a client's care and assets when the client is incompetent.

Gummas soft, rubbery growths of skin tissue that may accompany the third stage of syphilis.

Gynecologic examination inspection and palpation of pelvic reproductive structures of a woman.

H

Habituation repetition of substance abuse often leads to psychological and physical dependence, and, finally, addiction.

Hallucinations sensory experiences that others do not perceive; can be auditory, visual, tactile, olfactory, or gustatory (involving taste).

Hallux valgus deformity of the great (large) toe at its metatarsophalangeal joint.

Halo sign blood stain surrounded by a yellowish stain; highly suggestive of a cerebrospinal fluid leak.

Hammertoe flexion deformity of the interphalangeal joint that may involve several toes.

Hardiness effective coping style that includes a sense of having control over sources of stress and the perception of life events as a challenge rather than a threat.

Hard of hearing having hearing that is limited but allows for communication.

Head-to-toe method technique used for carrying out an examination by beginning at the top of the body and progressing downward. See also *systems method.*

Health state of complete physical, mental, and social well-being, not merely the absence of disease and infirmity.

Health beliefs client's opinions regarding what causes illnesses, the role of the person who is sick and the health care professional, what must occur to restore health, and how one stays healthy, often shaped and perpetuated by the client's cultural affiliations.

Health care–Associated Infections (HAIs) acquired while being cared for in a health care agency, which were not active, incubatory, or chronic at the time of admission.

Health care–associated pneumonia (HCAP) occurs in clients who reside in long-term care facilities or are on dialysis in outpatient centers. HCAP may also include clients who were hospitalized within 90 days of being diagnosed with pneumonia. A common feature of HCAP is that the bacteria are more resistant to antibiotics (multidrug resistance or MDR).

Health care delivery system full range of services available to people seeking prevention, identification, treatment, or rehabilitation of health problems.

Health care proxy person with the authority to make health care decisions for the client if they are no longer competent or able to make these decisions. See *Durable Power of Attorney* (DPOA) for Health care.

Health care team group of specially trained personnel who work together to help clients meet their health care needs.

Health maintenance protecting one's current level of health by preventing illness or deterioration.

Health maintenance organization (HMO) group insurance plans in which each participant pays a preset, fixed fee in exchange for health care services.

Health practices actions that a client takes to restore health or stay healthy, often a product of and perpetuated by the client's cultural affiliations.

Health promotion engaging in strategies to enhance health.

Health promotion nursing diagnosis reflects clinical judgment of a client's motivation to increase well-being and enhance health behaviors.

Hearing perceiving sounds.

Heart block disorders in the conduction pathway that interfere with the transmission of impulses from the sinoatrial node through the atrioventricular node to the ventricles.

Heart failure inability of the heart to pump sufficient blood to meet the body's metabolic needs.

Heberden nodes bony enlargement of the distal interphalangeal joints.

Helper T cells cells that recognize antigens and form additional T-cell clones that stimulate B-cell lymphocytes to produce antibodies against foreign antigens.

Hematopoiesis manufacture and development of blood cells.

Hematuria blood in the urine.

Heme pigmented, iron-containing portion of hemoglobin.

Hemianopia disorder in which the client is only able to see half of the normal visual field.

Hemiplegia paralysis on one side of the body.

Hemoconcentration high ratio of blood components in relation to watery plasma.

Hemodialysis technique in which blood is transported from a client through a dialyzer, a semipermeable membrane filter within a machine that removes water and wastes from the blood.

Hemodilution reduced ratio of blood components in relation to watery plasma.

Hemodynamic monitoring procedure used to assess the volume and pressure of blood within the heart and vascular system by means of a peripherally inserted catheter.

Hemoglobin iron-containing protein attached to erythrocytes that carry oxygen to cells.

Hemoglobin A (HbA) normal form of hemoglobin.

Hemoglobin F (HbF) fetal hemoglobin present during intrauterine development through 6 months of age.

Hemoglobin polymerization formation of crystal-like rods that change the biconcave RBC into an irregular, brittle, sticky, sickle-shaped cell.

Hemoglobin S (HbS) abnormal form of hemoglobin among those with sickle cell disease that under hypoxic conditions causes red blood cells to assume a sickle shape.

Hemolysis destruction of erythrocytes.

Hemolytic anemia generic term for chronic premature destruction of erythrocytes.

Hemophilia blood disorder involving an absence or reduction of a clotting factor.

Hemoptysis expectoration of blood or bloody sputum.

Hemorrhoidectomy surgical removal of hemorrhoids.

Hemorrhoids dilated veins outside or inside the anal sphincter.

Hemostasis control of bleeding.

Hepatic encephalopathy central nervous system manifestation of liver failure related to an increased serum ammonia level that often leads to coma and death.

Hepatic lobectomy surgical procedure in which a primary malignant or benign tumor confined to a single lobe of the liver is removed.

Hepatitis inflammation of the liver.

Hepatorenal syndrome renal failure associated with liver disease that ultimately alters fluid distribution and interferes with fluid excretion.

HER2 positive genetic protein that promotes the growth of cancer cells in about one of every five cases of breast cancer.

Herbal therapy use of plants for treating disease and disorders.

Hernia protrusion of any organ from the cavity that normally confines it; most commonly used to describe the protrusion of the intestine through a defect in the abdominal wall.

Hernioplasty surgical procedure in which the weakened area of a hernia is reinforced with wire, fascia, or mesh to prevent recurrence.

Herniorrhaphy surgical repair of a hernia.

Herpes simplex virus infectious agent responsible for genital and perineal lesions and associated with cold sores around the nose and lips.

Herpes zoster skin disorder (shingles) that develops later after an infection with varicella (chickenpox) due to an acute reactivation of the varicella-zoster virus, which lies dormant in nerve roots.

Heterograft skin graft obtained from animals, principally pigs, to temporarily cover large areas of tissue until the client's own skin can be used for skin grafting.

Hiatal hernia (diaphragmatic hernia) protrusion of part of the stomach through the diaphragm.

High-density lipoprotein lipoprotein that has a higher ratio of protein than cholesterol.

Highly active antiretroviral therapy HIV treatment with a combination of drugs; sometimes referred to as a "drug cocktail."

Hilus entrance of the bronchi to the lungs.

Histocompatibility markers cell surface proteins that match an individual's own genetic code or assist the immune system to identify foreign molecules.

Hodgkin disease malignancy that produces enlargement of lymphoid tissue, the spleen, and the liver, with invasion of other tissues such as the bone marrow and lungs.

Holism viewing a person's health as a balance of body, mind, and spirit, considering the client's psychological, sociocultural, developmental, and spiritual needs to restore optimal health.

Home health care delivery of health care services, for both long-term and short-term health needs, in a client's home.

Homocysteine amino acid created during the metabolism of protein; elevated levels are believed to impair memory and contribute to above-normal cholesterol levels.

Hordeolum(sty) inflammation and infection of the Zeis or Moll gland, a type of oil gland at the edge of the eyelid.

Hormone replacement therapy administration of estrogen combined with progestin to reduce perimenopausal symptoms, prevent osteoporosis, and reduce the atherosclerotic process.

Hormones chemicals secreted by the endocrine glands that accelerate or slow physiologic processes.

Hospice facility for the care of terminally ill clients where they can live out their final days with comfort, dignity, and meaningfulness.

Hospital-acquired pneumonia (HAP) (formerly referred to as "nosocomial pneumonia") pneumonia that occurs in clients more than 48 hours after admission to a hospital (which was not present when the client was admitted).

Host person on or in whom a microorganism resides.

Human immunodeficiency virus (HIV) pathogen that causes acquired immunodeficiency syndrome (AIDS).

Human papilloma viral (HPV) infection sexually transmitted infection that causes venereal warts; transmitted by genital–genital, genital–anal, or genital–oral contact with an infected person and contagious as long as the warts are present.

Humor therapeutic use of laughter, which stimulates the immune system and causes the release of neuropeptides.

Humoral response formation of antibodies.

Huntington's disease hereditary disorder in which the basal ganglia and portions of the cerebral cortex degenerate.

Hurricane storm that occurs with rotating wind systems in which spinning air creates explosive forces.

Hybrid revascularization combination of minimally invasive coronary artery bypass as well as percutaneous balloon angioplasty with the placement of a stent for multivessel disease.

Hydrocele condition in which as much as 100 mL of lymphatic fluid accumulates between the testis and tunica vaginalis of the scrotum.

Hydronephrosis condition in which an obstruction of urine from the ureter distends the renal pelvis.

Hyperaldosteronism excessive secretion of aldosterone leading to extreme electrolyte imbalances.

Hyperalgesia amplified pain experience.

Hyperbaric oxygen treatment administration of 100% oxygen at three times greater than atmospheric pressure in a specially designed chamber.

Hyperglycemia elevated blood glucose level.

Hyperlipidemia high levels of fat in the blood.

Hypernatremia elevated serum sodium level.

Hyperopia farsightedness; people who are hyperopic see objects that are far away better than objects that are close.

Hyperosmolar hyperglycemic nonketotic syndrome acute complication of diabetes characterized by hyperglycemia without ketosis.

Hyperparathyroidism disorder of the parathyroid gland that affects calcium and phosphorus levels.

Hyperplasia increase in the number of cells.

Hypertension sustained elevation of systolic arterial blood pressure of 140 mm Hg or higher, a sustained diastolic arterial blood pressure of 90 mm Hg or higher, or both.

Hypertensive cardiovascular disease stage of hypertension when elevated blood pressure causes both cardiac abnormality and vascular damage.

Hypertensive crisis potentially fatal condition with symptoms such as extremely elevated blood pressure, headache, nausea, vomiting, sweating, palpitations, visual changes, neck stiffness, sensitivity to light, and tachycardia.

Hypertensive heart disease stage of hypertension when elevated blood pressure causes a cardiac abnormality.

Hypertensive vascular disease stage of hypertension when elevated blood pressure causes vascular damage without heart involvement.

Hyperthyroidism disorder associated with hypersecretion of thyroid hormones in which metabolic rate increases.

Hypertonic solution solution that is more concentrated than body fluid and draws fluid into the intravascular compartment from the more dilute areas within the cells and interstitial spaces.

Hypertrophied turbinates enlargements of the nasal concha that interfere with air passage and sinus drainage and eventually lead to sinusitis.

Hypertrophy increase in size.

Hyperuricemia accumulation of uric acid in the blood.

Hypervolemia high volume of water in the intravascular fluid compartment.

Hyphae threadlike filaments within the cells of most fungi.

Hypnosis therapeutic intervention that facilitates a physiologic change through the power of suggestion.

Hypochondriasis psychobiologic disorder in which a person is preoccupied with minor symptoms and develops an exaggerated belief that they signify a life-threatening illness.

Hypoglycemia low blood glucose level.

Hypoparathyroidism deficiency of parathormone that results in hypocalcemia.

Hypophysectomy surgical removal of the pituitary gland.

Hypophysis pituitary gland.

Hypopyon disorder that occurs in severe cases of uveitis and involves an accumulation of pus in the anterior chamber behind the cornea.

Hypothalamic dopamine inhibits the release of prolactin from the anterior pituitary gland.

Hypothalamus portion of the brain between the cerebrum and the brain stem that stimulates and inhibits the pituitary gland.

Hypothyroidism disorder that occurs when the thyroid gland fails to secrete adequate thyroid hormones.

Hypotonic solution solution that contains fewer dissolved substances in comparison with plasma and is effective in rehydrating clients experiencing fluid deficits.

Hypovolemia low volume of extracellular fluid.

Hypovolemic shock condition that occurs when the volume of extracellular fluid is significantly diminished, primarily because of a loss or reduction in blood or plasma.

Hypoxia decrease in the amount of oxygen reaching the cells.

Hysterectomy surgical removal of the uterus.

I

Ileoanal reservoir (anastomosis) creation of an internal reservoir for the storage of GI effluent.

Ileostomy surgically created opening between the distal small intestine and the skin.

Illness state of being sick; may be viewed as catastrophic (sudden, traumatic), acute, chronic, or terminal.

Illness prevention identification of risk factors such as a family history of hypertension or diabetes and assisting of clients to reduce the effects of risk factors on their health.

Imagery psychobiologic technique that uses the mind to visualize a positive physiologic effect.

Immune response target-specific system of defense against infectious, foreign, or cancerous cells carried out primarily by lymphocytes.

Immunizations vaccines that stimulate the body to produce antibodies against a specific disease organism.

Immunoglobulin antibodies substances that when interacting with allergens cause an immediate hypersensitivity response.

Immunoglobulins proteins produced by B lymphocyte plasma cells that bind with antigens and promote the destruction of invading cells; also known as antibodies.

Immunopeptides chemical messengers that relay messages throughout the immune system and the brain.

Immunotherapy use of biologic response modifiers to stimulate the body's natural immune system to restrict and destroy cancer cells.

Impedance plethysmography test used for diagnosing clots within deep veins by recording blood volume in the arm or leg before and after inflating a blood pressure cuff to stop venous blood flow.

Implantable cardioverter defibrillator surgically implanted device to treat life-threatening arrhythmias.

Implantation process in which a fertilized ovum, or zygote, travels down the uterus and attaches itself within the endometrium.

Implanted pacemaker permanent electrical device used to manage a chronic bradydysrhythmia.

Implementation fourth step in the nursing process that involves carrying out the written plan of care, performing the interventions, monitoring the client's status, and assessing and reassessing the client before, during, and after treatments.

Impotence inability to achieve or maintain an erection sufficient for sexual activity.

Improvised explosive device type of bomb that contains highly unstable substances making them easy to detonate.

Incident report documentation made by health care workers when they make or discover errors, or when an event occurs that results in harm; it identifies the nature of the incident, witnesses, what actions were taken at the time, and the client's condition.

Incompetent legal term for the inability to understand the risks or benefits of decisions.

Incontinence inability to control urinary or bowel elimination.

Induration hard raised wheal with localized erythema (redness).

Infarct area of tissue that dies from inadequate oxygenation.

Infection invasion of the body with pathogens or their toxins.

Infectious mononucleosis viral disease that affects lymphoid tissues such as the tonsils and spleen and can involve other organs such as the brain, meninges, and liver as well.

Infectious process cycle cycle involving the transmission of an infectious disease from a human or animal to a susceptible host. The six components needed for it to occur are an infectious microorganism, reservoir, portal for exit, means of transmission, portal of entry, and susceptible host, also known as *chain of infection.*

Infective endocarditis inflammation of the inner layer of heart tissue as a result of an infectious microorganism.

Inferior vena cava large blood vessel that delivers unoxygenated blood from the lower body to the right atrium.

Infertility inability to procreate.

Inflammatory bowel disease group of chronic illnesses characterized by exacerbations and remissions of inflammation and ulceration of the bowel lining. See also *ulcerative colitis* and *Crohn's disease.*

Influenza acute viral respiratory disease of relatively short duration.

Informal teaching unplanned, spontaneous conveying of information, usually at the client's bedside or while caring for the client at home. See also *formal teaching.*

Informed consent voluntary permission granted by a knowledgeable client, or the client's assigned health care proxy for an invasive procedure or surgery.

Infratentorial below the tentorium (an area between the cerebrum and cerebellum).

Infusion pump device that exerts positive pressure to infuse IV solutions and adjusts the pressure according to the resistance it meets.

Inhalants inhaled allergens that cause respiratory symptoms.

Injectants allergens that when instilled can produce systemic and potentially fatal effects.

Injection sclerotherapy procedure in which a primary provider passes an endoscope orally to locate an esophageal varix, then passes a thin needle through the endoscope and injects a sclerosing agent directly into the varix to stop circulation through it.

In-line filter device that removes air bubbles as well as undissolved drugs, bacteria, and large molecules from an infusing solution.

Internal fixation open reduction (ORIF) surgical procedure to repair fractures with wire, nails, plate, and/or an intramedullary rod (a rod inserted into the center of the bone with wires around the bone for stabilization); done to hold bone fragments in place until bone healing is complete.

Interstitial cystitis (IC) or painful bladder syndrome (PBS) is a chronic inflammation of the bladder mucosa, causing pain in the bladder and surrounding pelvic region.

Intradermal injection test method for identifying an allergic substance by instilling a dilute solution of an antigen.

Insight-oriented therapy technique that helps clients understand the cause and relationship between their emotional distress and physical symptoms.

In situ cancer that remains in a localized area without invading the surrounding tissue.

Isoenzymes complex proteins released by damaged cells.

Inotropic medications drugs that improve myocardial contractility.

Inspection systematic and thorough observation of a client and specific areas of a client's body.

Insulin pancreatic hormone necessary for the metabolism of glucose.

Insulin independence ability of a client's own naturally produced insulin to regulate blood glucose levels within consistently normal ranges.

Insulin resistance decreased sensitivity to insulin at the tissue level.

Integrase viral enzyme that incorporates a viral code into a host cell's DNA.

Integrase inhibitors antiretroviral drugs that block integrase thus preventing the incorporation of HIV DNA into the T-cell's DNA.

Integrated delivery system (IDS) network formed by hospitals and other health care facilities to reduce the redundancy of health care services and increase economic leverage.

Integrative medicine combination of conventional medicine with complementary or alternative therapy for which there is some high-quality scientific evidence of safety and effectiveness.

Integrative therapies a combination of conventional medical treatment with nontraditional physical and nonphysical approaches.

Integument structures that cover the body's exterior surface; the primary structure is the skin, but the integument also includes accessory structures such as the hair and nails.

Intentional tort deliberate and willful act that infringes on another person's rights or property.

Interferons chemicals that enable cells to resist viral infection and slow viral replication.

Interleukins chemicals that coordinate the immune response.

Intermittent claudication leg pain with exercise.

Intermittent spasticity uncontrolled jerking movements below the level of a spinal cord injury because nerve signals between the brain and nerves are interrupted causing an overly active muscle response.

Internal fixation procedure in which metal screws, plates, rods, nails, or pins are used to stabilize a reduced bone fracture.

Internal radiologic contamination fallout, entering an open wound, inhaled via contaminated air, or consumed through contaminated food and water.

Interstitial fluid water located between cells.

Interstitium structure that lies between the alveoli and contains the pulmonary capillaries and elastic connective tissue.

Intimate space physical closeness between two people, which is only appropriate for interactions of a very personal nature.

Intra-aortic balloon pump device that acts as a temporary, secondary pump to supplement ineffectual contraction of the heart's left ventricle.

Intracellular fluid water located within cells.

Intracerebral hematoma bleeding within the brain that results from an open or closed head injury or from a cerebrovascular condition such as a ruptured cerebral aneurysm.

Intractable pain pain that does not respond to analgesic medications, noninvasive measures, or nursing management.

Intramedullary lesions spinal nerve root compression within the spinal cord.

Intraocular lens (IOL) implant artificial lens that is inserted in the eye to improve or restore vision.

Intraoperative phase of perioperative care that includes the entire surgical procedure until transfer of the client to the recovery area.

Intravascular fluid water located in the plasma (serum) portion of blood.

Intravenous pyelography radiologic study used to evaluate the structure and function of the kidneys, ureters, and bladder by examining a radiopaque dye as it passes through the urinary tract.

Intravenous (IV) therapy parenteral administration of fluids and additives into a vein.

Introductory phase stage of the nurse–client relationship during which a nurse and a client get acquainted and the client identifies one or more health problems for which they are seeking care.

Intussusception telescoping of one part of the intestine into an adjacent part.

Involucrum new bone cells.

Ions positively and negatively charged substances.

Iridectomy surgical or laser procedure in which holes are made in the iris to increase drainage of aqueous fluid.

Irreversible stage stage in shock that occurs when significant numbers of cells and organ systems become damaged and the client no longer responds to medical interventions.

Irritable bowel syndrome paroxysmal motility syndrome primarily affecting the colon, in which the client experiences alternating periods of constipation and diarrhea.

Ischemia impaired oxygenation of cells and tissues.

Islets of Langerhans hormone-secreting cells of the pancreas that release insulin and glucagon.

Isoenzyme one of several forms of an enzyme that can be identified separately.

Isolation negative developmental outcome of the young adult stage characterized by an inability to form close relationships with others.

Isotonic solution solution containing the same concentration of dissolved substances normally found in plasma; used to maintain fluid balance when clients temporarily cannot eat or drink.

J

Janeway lesions small, painless, red-blue macular sores.

Jejunostomy GI intubation in which the tube enters the jejunum of the small intestine via a surgically created opening into the abdominal wall.

Joint junction between two or more bones.

K

Kaposi sarcoma type of connective tissue cancer common among those with AIDS.

Kegel exercises isometric exercises designed to assist with stress incontinence; also known as pelvic floor strengthening exercises.

Keloids overgrowth of scar tissue especially among those with darkly pigmented skin.

Keratin tough protective protein formed by the outer layer of dead skin cells.

Keratitis inflammation of the cornea.

Keratoplasty corneal transplantation.

Kernig sign inability to extend the leg when the thigh is flexed on the abdomen.

Ketoacidosis form of metabolic acidosis resulting from an accumulation of ketones in the blood.

Ketonemia increased ketones in the blood.

Ketones metabolic byproducts of fat metabolism.

Ketonuria substances in urine from the breakdown of fat metabolism.

Kinesics study of nonverbal techniques of communication such as facial expressions, postures, gestures, and body movements.

Kussmaul respirations fast, deep breathing.

L

Labyrinthitis inflammation of the labyrinth of the inner ear.

Lactation production of breast milk.

Laissez-faire leadership style of leadership characterized by allowing a work group to individually set goals, make decisions, and take responsibility for their own management.

Laminectomy surgical procedure in which the posterior arch of a vertebra is removed to expose the spinal cord and allow the removal of a herniated disk, tumor, blood clot, bone spur, or broken bone fragment.

Lanugo fine body hair grown in the absence of subcutaneous fat to help maintain body temperature by reducing heat loss.

Laparoscopic cholecystectomy preferred surgical procedure for gallbladder removal; requires general anesthesia, but is performed with an endoscope with three or four small puncture sites in the abdomen. After inflating the abdomen with carbon dioxide to displace abdominal structures and provide a better view, the surgeon drains the gallbladder, dissects the vessels and ducts, and then grasps and removes the gallbladder.

Laryngitis inflammation and swelling of the mucous membrane that lines the larynx.

Laryngoscopy endoscopic examination of the larynx.

Laryngospasm spasm of the laryngeal muscles, resulting in narrowing of the larynx.

Larynx cartilaginous framework between the pharynx and the trachea whose primary function is to produce sound; it also protects the lower airway from foreign objects because of its ability to facilitate coughing.

Laser device that converts a solid, gas, or liquid substance into light creating sufficient energy to vaporize tissue and coagulate bleeding vessels.

Laser angioplasty use of short pulses of light to vaporize arterial plaque.

Laws written rules governing conduct and actions.

Leadership ability to guide and influence another person, group, or both to think in a certain way, achieve common goals, or provide inspiration for change.

Learning capacity person's intellectual ability to understand, remember, and apply new information.

Learning needs those skills and concepts that a client and family must acquire to restore, maintain, or promote health.

Learning readiness degree to which a person is in an optimal position to process new information.

Learning style the manner in which a person best comprehends new information.

Left ventricular end-diastolic pressure retrograde pressure from the fluid on the left side of the heart at the end of left ventricular diastole.

Left-sided heart failure condition that results from various conditions that impair the left ventricle's ability to eject blood into the aorta.

Leptin substance manufactured in human fat cells believed to suppress appetite-stimulating chemicals.

Leukemia any malignant blood disorder in which proliferation of leukocytes, usually in an immature form, is unregulated.

Leukocytes white blood cells.

Leukocytosis increased number of leukocytes above normal limits.

Leukopenia decreased white blood cell count.

Lewisite chemical developed, but never used, during World War I that can damage exposed skin and mucous membranes on contact or can damage respiratory tissues if inhaled.

Liability legal responsibility.

Libido interest in or desire for sex.

Ligament fibrous tissue that connects two adjacent freely movable bones and helps protect joints by stabilizing their surfaces and keeping them in proper alignment.

Limbic system ring of cranial structures that is a physiologic network for emotions, survival and behavioral responses, motivation, and learning.

Limited English proficiency inability to understand English at a level that permits interacting effectively with staff in a health care setting, social service agencies, or public services without an interpreter.

Lipoatrophy breakdown of subcutaneous fat at the site of repeated injections.

Lipohypertrophy buildup of subcutaneous fat at the site of repeated injections.

Lipolysis breaking down of fat by the body.

Listening attending to and becoming fully involved in what a client says.

Lithotripsy nonsurgical procedure that uses shock waves to break up some types of kidney or gallstones.

Living will document that states a client's wishes regarding health care if they are terminally ill.

Lobectomy surgical removal of a lobe of a lung.

Loop colostomy procedure in which a loop of bowel is lifted through the abdomen and is supported in place with a glass rod or plastic butterfly device.

Low-density lipoprotein protein in blood that has a higher ratio of cholesterol than protein.

Lower gastrointestinal series study used to identify polyps, tumors, strictures, and other abnormalities of the colon through the fluoroscopic observation of rectally instilled barium solution.

Lumbar puncture performed to obtain samples of cerebrospinal fluid from the subarachnoid space for laboratory examination and to measure cerebrospinal fluid pressure; also called a spinal tap.

Lumpectomy surgical procedure in which only a tumor is removed from the breast.

Lung abscess localized area of pus formation within the lung parenchyma.

Lungs paired elastic structures enclosed by the thoracic cage that contain the alveoli.

Luteinizing hormone (LH) hormone that initiates ovulation and, in both sexes, secretion of sex hormones.

Lyme disease chronic inflammatory process and multisystem disease caused by a spirochetal bacterium that is transmitted to humans from deer ticks.

Lymph watery fluid derived from plasma that exits the walls of capillaries and enters interstitial spaces.

Lymphadenitis inflammation of the lymph nodes.

Lymphangitis inflammation of the lymphatic vessels.

Lymphatic system vessels similar to capillaries that transport tissue fluid called lymph.

Lymphedema disorder in which obstructed lymph circulation causes an accumulation of lymph within soft tissue.

Lymph nodes clusters of bean-sized structures that trap, destroy, and remove infectious microorganisms, cellular debris, and cancer cells.

Lymphocytes white blood cells with immune functions.

Lymphogranuloma venereum sexually transmitted infection caused by a strain of *Chlamydia trachomatis* and characterized by a small erosion or papule and the enlargement of adjacent lymph nodes, which can become necrotic.

Lymphoid tissues structures that maintain immunocompetence, the ability to cooperatively protect a person from external invaders and the body's own altered cells.

Lymphokines type of cytokines that attracts neutrophils and monocytes to remove debris, promotes the maturation of more T cells when they detect antigens, and directs B-cell lymphocytes to multiply and mature.

Lymphoma group of cancers that affect the lymphatic system.

M

Macrodrip tubing intravenous tubing that releases large-sized drops of IV solution. See also *microdrip tubing.*

Macrophages large phagocytes present in tissues such as the lungs, liver, lymph nodes, spleen, and peritoneum.

Macular degeneration breakdown of or damage to the macula, the point on the retina where light rays converge for the most acute visual perception.

Magnetic resonance imaging (MRI) diagnostic tool used to identify disorders that affect many different structures in the body without performing surgery; a magnetic field excites hydrogen atoms within the body creating a radio signal that is converted to an image on a computer monitor.

Major (unipolar) depression mood disorder characterized by a feeling of sadness with no obvious relationship to situational events. See also *reactive (secondary) depression.*

Malignant type of tumor that is invasive and capable of spreading.

Malignant hypertension dangerously elevated blood pressure accompanied by papilledema.

Malignant hyperthermia disorder in which body temperature, muscle metabolism, and heat production increase rapidly, progressively, and uncontrollably in response to stress and some anesthetic agents.

Mallet toe is a flexion deformity of the DIP joint and can affect several toes.

Malpractice professional negligence resulting from a licensed person's action or lack of action.

Mammography radiographic technique used to detect cysts or tumors of the breast, some of which may be too small to palpate.

Mammoplasty collective term for several different cosmetic breast procedures.

Managed care organization (MCO) insurer that carefully plans and closely supervises the distribution of health care services.

Management planning, organizing, directing, and controlling resources and personnel to meet specific objectives within an organization.

Mania frenzied state of euphoria.

Massage therapy technique of applying pressure and movement to stretch and knead soft body tissues to stimulate circulation, relieve physical and psychological tension, and improve mobility or functional use of affected parts of the body.

Mastalgia breast pain.

Mast cells constituents of connective tissue that contain granules of heparin, serotonin, bradykinin, and histamine; the release of granules causes various allergic and inflammatory manifestations.

Mastectomy excision of breast tissue.

Mastitis inflammation of breast tissue; most common in women who are breast-feeding.

Mastoidectomy surgical procedure performed to remove diseased tissue from the mastoid process.

Mastoiditis inflammation of any part of the mastoid process.

Mastopexy surgical procedure to correct ptosis, or drooping, of the breast(s).

Maxillary sinuses cavities on either side of the nose in the maxillary bones; they are the largest sinuses and the most accessible to treatment.

Maze procedure surgical procedure to treat atrial fibrillation in which a new conduction pathway is created that eliminates the rapid firing of ectopic pacemaker sites in the atria.

Means of transmission method by which a microorganism is transferred from its reservoir to a susceptible host; the five potential means of transmission are contact, droplet, airborne, vehicle, and vector.

Mechanoreceptors sensory nerves within the skin that detect touch, location, pressure, motion, vibration, size, and texture.

Mediastinum portion of the thoracic cavity that contains the trachea and major blood vessels.

Medical durable power of attorney person with legal authority to make health care decisions for a client if they are no longer competent or able to make these decisions.

Medical marijuana leaves, flowers, stems, and seeds of the marijuana plant used for medicinal purposes.

Medical systems healing practices that have evolved from other cultures.

Medication lock sealed chamber that allows intermittent access to a vein.

Medigap insurance policies that cover additional expenditures such as copayments and deductibles.

Medulla oblongata part of the brain below the pons that transmits motor impulses from the brain to the spinal cord and sensory impulses from peripheral sensory neurons to the brain; contains vital centers concerned with respiration, heart rate, and vasomotor activity.

Melanin pigment that is manufactured by melanocytes located in the epidermis and which determines the color of the skin.

Melanin-concentrating hormone endogenous chemical which in low levels causes weight loss and in high levels promotes obesity.

Melatonin hormone that aids in regulating sleep cycles and mood and is believed to play a role in hypothalamic–pituitary interaction.

Melena black, tarry stools.

Memory cells immunologic cells that convert to plasma cells on reexposure to a specific antigen.

Menarche first menstruation.

Ménière disease episodic symptoms created by fluctuations in the production or reabsorption of fluid in the inner ear.

Meninges membranes that protect the brain and spinal cord.

Meningitis inflammation of the meninges caused by various infectious microorganisms such as bacteria, viruses, fungi, or parasites.

Meniscectomy damaged cartilage.

Menopause physiologic change in the female reproductive system in which ovulation becomes irregular and eventually ceases.

Menorrhagia excessive bleeding at the time of menstruation.

Menstrual diary daily written record of a client's premenstrual symptoms.

Menstruation process that occurs when an ovum is not fertilized, the production of progesterone decreases, and the endometrium degenerates and is shed.

Mental status examination array of observations and questions that elicit information about a person's cognitive and mental state.

Mentation mental activity.

Metabolic syndrome cluster of physiologic alterations that include obesity (especially in the abdominal area), high blood pressure, elevated triglyceride and low-density lipoprotein, blood glucose levels, and low high-density lipoprotein level.

Metastasis spreading of cancer cells to adjacent tissues, from lymph vessels into the tissues adjacent to lymphatic vessels, by transport from blood or lymph systems, or by diffusion within a body cavity.

Methadone maintenance therapy technique that involves substituting a synthetic addictive drug for another addicting drug to forestall withdrawal, avoid a toxic overdose, or reduce the potential for blood-borne infections.

Method of transmission method by which microorganisms are transferred or moved from a reservoir to a susceptible host.

Metrorrhagia vaginal bleeding at a time other than a menstrual period.

Microalbuminuria blood protein excreted in small amounts by the kidneys.

Microcephaly congenital defect manifested by an abnormally small head resulting in developmental delays and mental retardation, as well as other neurologic effects.

Microdrip tubing intravenous tubing that releases small-sized drops of IV solution. See also *macrodrip tubing.*

Microorganisms potentially infectious agents that are so small they can be seen only with a microscope; commonly called "germs."

Microphages phagocytes present in blood that migrate to tissue as necessary to ingest small-sized debris.

Midbrain forward part of the brain stem that connects the pons and cerebellum with the two cerebral hemispheres.

Midclavicular catheter peripherally inserted catheter that extends from a superficial vein to the proximal end of the axillary or subclavian vein.

Midline catheter peripherally inserted venous access device inserted from just above or below the antecubital area in the basilic, cephalic, or median cubital vein until the tip rests in the upper arm just short of the axilla; used for clients who have limited peripheral veins or who require an extended period of IV fluid therapy.

Mind–body medicine techniques that rely on the power of the brain, emotions, social interactions, and spiritual factors to alter body functions or symptoms.

Minority group of people who differ from the majority of people within a given society in terms of cultural characteristics (such as religion), physical characteristics (such as skin color), or both.

Mitral regurgitation backward flow of blood that occurs when the mitral valve does not close completely; sometimes referred to as mitral insufficiency.

Mitral stenosis disorder in which the mitral valve does not open sufficiently to facilitate filling of the left ventricle.

Mitral valve prolapse disorder in which the mitral valve cusps enlarge, become floppy, and bulge backward into the left atrium.

Mitral valve prolapse syndrome cluster of symptoms associated with autonomic nervous system dysfunction in which changes in mitral valve tissue layers cause its cusps to distend, stretching the papillary muscles, and leading to valvular incompetence.

Modified radical mastectomy surgical procedure in which the breast, some lymph nodes, the lining over the chest muscles, and the pectoralis minor muscle are removed.

Modulation phase of pain impulse transmission during which the brain interacts with the spinal nerves to alter the pain experience by releasing pain-inhibiting neurochemicals.

Monoamine hypothesis theory that depression results from imbalances in one or more of the monoamine neurotransmitters, serotonin, norepinephrine, and dopamine.

Monoamine oxidase enzyme that breaks down monoamine neurotransmitters such as norepinephrine, serotonin, and, to some extent, dopamine.

Monocytes large phagocytes present in tissues such as the lungs, liver, lymph nodes, spleen, and peritoneum that engulf large-sized debris; also known as macrophages.

Monro–Kellie hypothesis proposes that if one or more cerebral contents (brain tissue, blood, or cerebrospinal fluid) increases significantly without a decrease in either or both of others, intracranial pressure becomes elevated.

Mood person's overall feeling state; may be thought of as a continuum with extremes of emotion existing at both ends or poles.

Mood disorders conditions in which a person experiences an extreme persistent mood or severe mood swings that interfere with social relationships.

Morbidity the number of persons who are sick with a particular disease in a specific population.

Morbid obesity having a body mass index of 40 or higher or when one weighs 100 lb more, or 20% or more than his or her ideal weight.

Mortality the death rate or the ratio of the number of deaths for a specific population.

Motion sickness a form of physiologic vertigo, caused by repeated and constant motion.

Motivation desire to acquire new information or implement a new activity.

Multicratic leadership style of leadership in which the manager uses a variety of styles and adapts his or her approach to the situation at hand.

Multidrug resistance ability of some types of bacteria to remain unaffected by several antimicrobial drugs such as antibiotics.

Multifocal PVCs pattern of premature ventricular contractions originating from more than one ectopic location.

Multiple gated acquisition (MUGA) scan most accurate noninvasive test that can measure the left ventricle's ejection fraction during rest and activity; also called a *gated blood pool scan.*

Multiple myeloma malignancy involving proliferation of B lymphocyte plasma cells in bone marrow.

Multiple organ dysfunction syndrome complication of overwhelming inflammation that results in massive cellular, tissue, and organ injury.

Multiple sclerosis progressive disease of peripheral nerves from permanent degeneration and destruction of myelin.

Murmur atypical heart sound.

Myelin fatty substance that covers and serves as an insulating substance for some axons in the central nervous and peripheral nervous systems.

Myelogram diagnostic test in which a radiopaque substance is injected into the spinal canal by means of a lumbar puncture.

Myomectomy surgical removal of a benign uterine tumor to preserve the uterus for future childbearing.

Myelosuppression decreased bone marrow function.

Myocardial disarray alteration in the usual alignment of myofibrils, the contractile component of muscle tissue.

Myocardial infarction interruption in blood supply to cardiac muscle; also known as *heart attack.*

Myocardial oxygen demand amount of oxygen the heart needs to perform its work.

Myocardial revascularization surgical procedure that improves the delivery of oxygenated blood to the myocardium by using one or more coronary artery bypass grafts.

Myocarditis inflammation of the myocardium (the muscle layer of the heart).

Myocardium muscle layer of the heart.
Myofibrils contractile component of muscle tissue.
Myopia nearsightedness; people who are myopic hold things close to their eyes to see them well.
Myringoplasty surgical repair of a perforated eardrum.
Myringotomy incisional opening of the eardrum to allow drainage, ease pressure, and relieve pain.
Myxedema hypothyroidism in an adult.

N

Nasal polyps grapelike growths of tissue that arise from the nasal mucous membranes.
Nasal septum wall that divides the internal nose into two cavities.
Nasoenteric intubation placement of a tube that passes through the nose, esophagus, and stomach to the small intestine.
Nasogastric intubation placement of a tube that passes through the nose and esophagus into the stomach.
Nasopharynx part of the pharynx that is near the nose and above the soft palate.
Native American medicine view disease as resulting from disharmony with Mother Earth, possession by an evil spirit, or violation of a taboo.
Natriuretic factor hormone produced by the heart, a deficiency of which causes arteries and arterioles to remain in a state of sustained vasoconstriction.
Natriuretic peptides hormone-like substances that act in opposition to the renin–angiotensin–aldosterone system.
Natural killer cells lymphocyte-like cells that circulate throughout the body looking for virus-infected cells and cancer cells and release potent chemicals that lethally alter the target cell's membrane, leading to its demise.
Naturally acquired active immunity immunity that occurs as a direct result of infection by a specific microorganism.
Natural products substances derived from plants, bacteria, fungi, animal species, and marine organisms that include vitamins, minerals, and probiotics.
Naturopathy concept that considers disease as an aberration in natural healing.
Near-death experience event in which a person almost dies but is resuscitated.
Near point closest point at which a person can clearly focus on an object.
Nearing-death awareness phenomenon characterized by a dying client's premonition of the approximate time or date of death.
Negative symptoms impoverished speech and inability to enjoy relationships or express emotions that are characteristic of schizophrenia.
Negligence failure to act as a reasonable person would have acted in a similar situation.
Neoadjuvant therapy drugs administered before surgery to extend survival and prevent disease recurrence.
Neoangiogenesis new growth of blood vessels.
Neoplasms new growths of abnormal tissue; also called tumors.
Nephrectomy surgical removal of a kidney.
Nephrolithiasis presence of a kidney stone, the size of which may range from microscopic to several centimeters.
Nephrostomy tube catheter inserted through the skin into the renal pelvis and used to relieve an obstruction to urine flow above the bladder.
Nerve agents potent organophosphate compounds that cause fatal consequences by inhibiting acetylcholinesterase.
Neuralgia nerve pain.
Neurally mediated hypotension disorder in which individuals experience hypotension accompanied by fatigue after standing for more than 10 minutes.
Neurilemma sheath that covers myelin.
Neuritic plaques deposits of beta-amyloid in the brain.
Neurofibrillary tangles twisted bundles of microtubules in brain cells.
Neurogenic bladder urinary bladder that does not receive adequate nerve stimulation.
Neurogenic shock shock that results from an insult to the vasomotor center in the medulla of the brain or to the peripheral nerves that extend from the spinal cord to the blood vessels.
Neurohormones stimulate and inhibit secretions from the anterior and posterior lobes of the pituitary gland; also known as releasing hormones.
Neurohypophysis posterior lobe of the pituitary gland.
Neurologic deficit disorder in which one or more functions of the central and peripheral nervous systems are decreased, impaired, or absent.
Neuron nerve cell.
Neuropathic joint disease common finding in tertiary syphilis, also called Charcot joints.
Neuropathic pain discomfort that is processed abnormally by the nervous system as a result of damage to either the pain pathways in peripheral nerves or pain-processing centers in the brain.
Neuropeptides neurotransmitters that include chemicals such as substance P that transmit the sensation of pain.
Neurotransmitters chemical messengers that communicate information that affects thinking, behavior, and bodily functions across the synaptic cleft between neurons.
Neutropenia decreased neutrophils.
Neutrophils granulocytes that protect the body through the ingestion and digestion of bacteria and foreign substances.
Never events refer to adverse events in health care delivery that should never occur (see *serious reportable events*).
Nits eggs laid by adult female lice that are tightly cemented to the side of hair shafts.
Nociceptive pain discomfort that arises from noxious stimuli that are transmitted from the point of cellular injury to the cerebral cortex of the brain.
Nociceptors specialized pain receptors located in the free nerve endings of peripheral sensory nerves.
Nocturia urination during the night.
Nomogram chart that calculates body surface area on the basis of height and weight.
Non-Hodgkin lymphomas group of malignant diseases that originate in lymph glands and other lymphoid tissue.
Nonpathogens microorganisms that are generally harmless to healthy humans.
Nonprofit agencies facilities such as universities or religious organizations owned and operated by nonprofit groups.
Nonverbal communication exchange of information without using words.
Norepinephrine monoamine neurotransmitter produced and secreted by the adrenal medulla whose levels may be low or high among people affected by depression; low levels help to explain why some depressed people develop psychomotor retardation, and high levels help to explain why some depressed people experience psychomotor agitation.
Normal eating eating that occurs in response to hunger and ceases when a feeling of comfortable fullness occurs.
Nuchal rigidity pain and stiffness of the neck and an inability to place the chin on the chest.

Nuclear blast explosion that produces an intense wave of heat, light, air pressure, and radiation.
Nucleic acid amplification testing (NAAT) superior and preferred method for diagnosing chlamydia.
Nurse–client relationship affiliation that exists during the period when a nurse interacts with clients, sick or well, to promote or restore their health, help them to cope with their illness, or assist them to die with dignity.
Nurse practice acts legal statutes that define nursing practice and set standards for nurses in each state.
Nursing diagnosis second step in the nursing process in which the nurse identifies and defines health-related problems.
Nursing interventions specific nursing directions given so that all health care team members understand exactly what to do for the client.
Nursing process problem-solving approach for planning and implementing client care to achieve desired outcomes; the five steps of the nursing process are assessment, diagnosis, planning, implementation, and evaluation.
Nystagmus uncontrolled oscillating movement of the eyeball.

O

Objective data facts obtained during a client's assessment through observation, physical examination, and diagnostic testing. See also *subjective data.*
Obsession disturbing, persistent thought.
Obsessive-compulsive disorder psychobiologic disorder manifested by the performance of an anxiety-relieving ritual to terminate a disturbing, persistent thought.
Obstructive sleep apnea (OSA) apnea characterized by recurrent and frequent episodes of upper airway obstruction and reduced ventilation.
Obstructive shock shock that occurs when the heart or great vessels are compressed.
Occipital lobe one of the four major lobes of the cerebral cortex that functions as the visual processing center.
Odynophagia painful swallowing.
Oligomenorrhea infrequent menses, usually caused by endocrine imbalances resulting from pituitary disorders or hypothyroidism, the stress response, or severely lean body mass.
Oliguria low urine output of less than 500 mL/day.
Oncology nursing nursing specialty related to the care of clients with cancer.
Onychocryptosis ingrown toenail.
Onychomycosis fungal infection of the fingernails or toenails.
Oocytes developing egg cells.
Oophorectomy surgical removal of the ovary.
Oophorocystectomy removal of cystic tissue from an ovary leaving the ovary intact.
Open cholecystectomy surgical procedure in which a gallbladder is removed through an abdominal incision.
Open-ended questions asked during a client interview that requires discussion. See also *closed questions.*
Open head injury trauma to the head in which the scalp, bony cranium, and dura mater (the outer meningeal layer) are exposed.
Open method burn wound management technique in which the wound is left uncovered.
Open reduction surgical procedure in which a fractured bone is exposed and realigned.
Ophthalmoscopy examination of the fundus or interior of the eye.
Opioid analgesics controlled substances referred to as narcotics.
Opioid dependence addiction to central nervous system depressant drugs (narcotics) that are either derived from or chemically similar to opium.
Opisthotonos extreme hyperextension of the head and arching of the back.
Opportunistic infection condition in which nonpathogenic or remotely pathogenic microorganisms take advantage of a favorable situation and overwhelm the host; also called *superinfections.*
Oral glucose tolerance test blood test used to evaluate a client's metabolism of orally ingested glucose.
Orchiectomy surgical removal of the testis.
Orchiopexy surgical procedure in which an undescended testis is secured within the scrotum.
Orchitis inflammation of the testis.
Orexin A and B neurohormones believed to contribute to binge eating and obesity in humans.
Orogastric intubation placement of a tube G through the mouth into the stomach.
Oropharynx part of the pharynx that is near the mouth.
Orthopnea breathing that is eased by sitting upright.
Orthopneic position sitting position in which the client leans on several pillows on the overbed table; also called tripod position.
Orthostatic intolerance condition in which hypotension accompanied by fatigue occurs after standing for more than 10 minutes.
Osier nodes purplish, painful nodules in the pads of the fingers and toes and palms and soles of the feet; indicative of bacterial endocarditis.
Osmoreceptors specialized neurons that sense the concentration of substances in blood.
Osmosis movement of water through a semipermeable membrane from a lower to higher concentration of solutes.
Ossification process in which inorganic minerals, such as calcium salts, are deposited in bone matrix.
Osteoblasts cells that build bones.
Osteoclasts cells involved in the destruction, resorption, and remodeling of bone.
Osteocytes mature bone cells involved in maintaining bone tissue.
Osteodystrophy condition in which the bones become demineralized as a result of hypocalcemia and hyperphosphatemia.
Osteolytic tumors bone destroying malignancy that produces a "punched-out" or "honeycombed" appearance in bones.
Osteomalacia metabolic bone disease characterized by inadequate mineralization of bone, resulting from a calcium or phosphate deficiency.
Osteomyelitis infection of the bone.
Osteoporosis disorder in which bone density decreases, resulting in porous and fragile bones.
Osteotomy procedure involving the cutting and removal of a wedge of bone (most often the tibia or femur) to change the bone's alignment and, as a result, improve function and relieve pain.
Ostomate client with an ostomy.
Ostomy surgically created opening between an internal body structure and the skin.
Otalgia sense of fullness or pain in the ears.
Otitis externa inflammation of the tissue within the outer ear.
Otitis media inflammation or infection in the middle ear.
Otorrhea leakage of cerebrospinal fluid from the ear.
Otosclerosis disorder characterized by a bony overgrowth on the stapes that is a common cause of hearing impairment among adults.
Otoscope handheld instrument used to inspect the external acoustic canal and tympanic membrane.

Ototoxicity detrimental effect of certain medications on the eighth cranial nerve or hearing structures.

Ovaries female endocrine glands important in the development of secondary sex characteristics, the manufacture of hormones, and the development of ova.

Ovulation cyclical release of an ovum.

Ovum (pl. ova) female reproductive cell.

Oxygen therapeutics blood substitute that carries and distributes oxygen to cells, tissues, and organs.

Oxytocin hormone that stimulates contraction of pregnant uterus and release of breast milk after childbirth.

P

P24 antigen test blood test that measures the number of viral particles in the blood and is used to guide drug therapy and follow the progression of a disease.

Pacemaker device that provides an electrical stimulus to the heart muscle to treat an abnormally slow cardiac rhythm.

Packed cells blood solution that has most of the plasma (fluid) removed; used for clients who need cellular replacements but do not need and may be harmed by the administration of additional fluid.

Paget disease chronic bone disorder characterized by abnormal bone remodeling.

Pain privately experienced, unpleasant sensation usually associated with disease or injury.

Pain management techniques used to prevent, reduce, or relieve discomfort.

Pain perception conscious experience of discomfort.

Pain threshold point at which pain-transmitting neurochemicals reach the brain, causing conscious awareness of discomfort.

Pain tolerance amount of discomfort a person endures once the pain threshold has been reached.

Palliative care management and treatment of symptoms that reduces physical discomfort but does not alter a disease's progression.

Palliative sedation method of relieving symptoms such as intractable pain that is causing intolerable suffering in an imminently dying client.

Palpation assessing the characteristics of an organ or body part by touching and feeling it with the hands or fingertips.

Palsy decreased sensation and movement.

Pancolitis ulcerative colitis that affects the client's entire colon.

Pancreas gland with both exocrine and endocrine functions; the exocrine portion secretes digestive enzymes that the common bile duct carries to the small intestine, while the endocrine cells of the pancreas release insulin and glucagon.

Pancreatectomy (partial, total) surgical procedure in which some or all of the pancreas is removed.

Pancreatic polypeptide hormone released from gamma islet cells that controls exocrine secretions from the pancreas.

Pancreatitis inflammation of the pancreas.

Pancreatoduodenectomy (Whipple procedure) surgical procedure that involves removing the head and perhaps the body of the pancreas, resecting the duodenum and stomach, and redirecting the flow of secretions from the stomach, gallbladder, and pancreas into the jejunum.

Pancytopenia conditions such as aplastic anemia in which numbers of all marrow-produced blood cells are reduced.

Pandemic rapidly spreading disease infecting large numbers of people throughout the world.

Panendoscopy examination of both the upper and lower GI tracts.

Panhysterectomy removal of the uterus, both fallopian tubes, and ovaries.

Panic disorder psychobiologic disorder in which a person experiences an abrupt onset of physical symptoms and terror.

Pannus destructive vascular granulation tissue.

Papanicolaou test test in which a sample of exfoliated cells are obtained during a pelvic examination and used to detect early cancer of the cervix, determine estrogen activity as it relates to menopause, or detect endocrine abnormalities.

Papilledema swelling of the optic nerve.

Paralanguage vocal sounds that communicate a message but that are not words.

Paralytic ileus disorder in which the intestine becomes adynamic from an absence of normal nerve stimulation to intestinal muscle fibers.

Paranasal sinuses extensions of the nasal cavity located in the surrounding facial bones.

Paraphimosis strangulation of the glans penis from an inability to replace a retracted foreskin

Paraplegia paralysis of both legs resulting from spinal injuries at the thoracic level.

Parasympathetic nervous system division of the autonomic nervous system that works to conserve body energy and is partly responsible for slowing heart rate, digesting food, and eliminating body wastes.

Parathormone hormone that regulates the metabolism of calcium and phosphorus.

Parathyroid glands four small bean-shaped bodies embedded in the lateral lobes of the thyroid that secrete parathormone.

Paresthesia sensation of numbness and tingling.

Parietal lobe portion located at the back of the brain that functions in processing sensory information regarding the location of parts of the body as well as interpreting visual information and processing language and mathematics.

Parietal pericardium tough outer layer of the pericardium.

Parietal pleura saclike serous membrane that is the outer layer of the lungs.

Parkinsonism cluster of Parkinson-like symptoms that develop from several etiologies.

Parkinson disease neurologic disorder from a deficiency of the neurotransmitter dopamine that results in abnormal movements characterized by stiffness, referred to as *rigidity*, hand tremor, and shuffling gait.

Paroxysmal nocturnal dyspnea being awakened by breathlessness.

Pars intermedia intermediate lobe of the pituitary gland.

Partial-thickness burn thermal injury classified as either superficial or deep partial thickness, depending on how much dermis is damaged.

Partial (or segmental) mastectomy surgical procedure in which the breast, axillary lymph nodes, and pectoralis major and minor muscles are removed. In some instances, sternal lymph nodes also are removed.

Partnership model uses an RN partnered with one or more assistive personnel to care for a group of clients. The RN may work with an LPN/LVN and an assistant, a respiratory therapist and an assistant, or a similar combination of staff. The licensed and unlicensed assistants are cross-trained to do many functions formerly done by separate departments, such as drawing blood or obtaining electrocardiograms.

Passive diffusion process in which dissolved substances such as electrolytes move from an area of high concentration of solutes to an area of lower concentration of solutes through a semipermeable membrane.

Passive euthanasia methods that facilitate death by letting nature take its course.

Passive immunity immediate but short-lived immunity that develops when ready-made antibodies are given to a susceptible individual.

Past health history information obtained during a client interview regarding a client's childhood diseases, previous injuries, major illnesses, prior hospitalizations, surgical procedures, and drug history.

Patch test method for identifying an allergic substance by applying a concentrated form to the skin.

Pathogens microorganisms that have a high potential to cause infectious diseases.

Client-focused care system of nursing care in which an RN partnered with one or more assistive personnel cares for a group of clients.

Pedagogy teaching children or people with cognitive ability comparable to children.

Pediculosis infestation with lice.

Pelvic floor strengthening exercises isometric exercises designed to assist with stress incontinence; also known as Kegel exercises.

Pelvic inflammatory disease infection of the pelvic organs such as the uterus, fallopian tubes, pelvic vascular system, and pelvic supporting structures.

Peptic ulcer circumscribed erosion of tissue in an area of the GI tract that is in contact with hydrochloric acid and pepsin.

Perception phase of pain impulse transmission during which the brain experiences pain at a conscious level, helps to discriminate the location of the pain, determines its intensity, attaches meaningfulness to the event, and provokes emotional responses.

Percussion tapping a portion of the body to determine if there is tenderness or to elicit sounds that vary according to the density of underlying structures.

Percutaneous electrical nerve stimulation (PENS) nonpharmacologic method for managing pain.

Percutaneous endoscopic gastrostomy (PEG) procedure in which an endoscope is introduced orally and advanced into the stomach so that the primary provider can see the correct location for a gastronomy tube.

Percutaneous liver biopsy procedure in which a small core of liver tissue is obtained by placing a needle directly into the liver through the lateral abdominal wall.

Percutaneous neuromodulation therapy (PNT) a variant of percutaneous electrical nerve stimulation (PENS) that combines the use of acupuncture needles with transcutaneous electrical nerve stimulation (TENS).

Percutaneous transluminal coronary angioplasty procedure in which a balloon-tipped catheter is inserted into a diseased coronary artery, then inflated to compress atherosclerotic plaque.

Perfusion supplying blood to cells, tissues, or organs.

Pericardiectomy surgical removal of the pericardium to allow more adequate filling and contraction of the heart chambers.

Pericardiocentesis needle aspiration of fluid from between the visceral and parietal pericardium.

Pericardiostomy procedure in which a surgical opening is made in the pericardium to drain fluid.

Pericarditis inflammation of the pericardium.

Pericardium saclike structure that surrounds and supports the heart.

Perioperative entire time span of surgery, including before and after the actual operation.

Periorbital ecchymosis condition in which both eyes are blackened; also called "raccoon eyes."

Periorbital edema puffiness around the eyes.

Periosteum outer layer of bones that is rich in blood and lymph vessels and supplies the bone with nourishment.

Peripheral nervous system part of the nervous system consisting of all nerves outside the central nervous system.

Peripheral vascular disease disorders that affect blood vessels distant from the large central blood vessels supplying the myocardium or that circulate blood directly in and out of the heart.

Peripheral venous sites superficial veins of the arm and hand; the most common sites for infusing IV fluids.

Peristalsis coordinated wavelike muscular contractions.

Peritoneal dialysis technique that uses the peritoneum, the semipermeable membrane lining of the abdomen, to filter fluid, wastes, and chemicals.

Peritonitis inflammation of the peritoneum, the serous sac lining the abdominal cavity.

Peritonsillar abscess infection that develops in the connective tissue between the capsule of the tonsil and the constrictor muscle of the pharynx.

Pernicious anemia blood disorder that develops from a deficiency of vitamin B_{12}.

Personal space distance between two people that is appropriate for one-on-one interactions like interviewing and physical assessment.

Pessary firm, doughnut-shaped or ring device that can be inserted into the upper vagina to reposition and give support to the uterus when surgery cannot be done or if the client declines surgery.

Petechiae tiny reddish hemorrhagic spots on the skin and mucous membranes.

Phagocytes white blood cells that engulf and digest bacteria and foreign material.

Phagocytosis process of engulfing and digesting bacteria and foreign material.

Pharyngitis inflammation of the throat.

Pharynx body structure that carries air from the nose to the larynx, and food from the mouth to the esophagus.

Phenotype testing blood test used to detect drug resistance in which a measured amount of antiviral drug is mixed with a virus until there is a quantity that prevents the virus from reproducing.

Pheochromocytoma tumor of the adrenal medulla that causes hyperfunction.

Pheromones hormone-like chemicals that communicate reproductive and social information among a species.

Phimosis inability to retract the foreskin (prepuce) of the penis.

Phlebitis inflammation of the vein.

Phlebostatic axis location at the fourth intercostal space in the mid-axillary line.

Phlebothrombosis clot formation with minimal or no venous inflammation.

Phlebotomy act of withdrawing blood from a vein.

Phobic disorder psychobiologic disorder in which a person develops an exaggerated fear.

Phonocardiography graphic representation of normal and abnormal heart sounds.

Phosgene liquid respiratory toxin that becomes a gas when released in the atmosphere.

Photochemotherapy combination of ultraviolet light therapy and a photosensitizing drug to destroy cells.

Photoperiods daytime hours that are short because of fewer hours of sunlight.

Photophobia sensitivity to light.

Phototherapy technique for treating seasonal affective disorder with artificial light that simulates the intensity of sunlight.

Physical assessment examination of a client's body structures.

Physical dependence condition in which a person experiences physical discomfort when a drug that they have taken routinely is abruptly discontinued.

Physician-assisted suicide practice of providing a means by which a client can end their own life.

Physician hospital organization (PHO) creation of a corporate structure between a hospital and a group of its primary providers by contracting with a managed care organization to negotiate fees for services for their self-insured employees.

Physician orders for scope of treatment (POST) advance care planning tool to safeguard a client's wishes for care during a serious illness and/or end-of-life care. The client provides specific information about resuscitation and medical interventions such as antibiotics, artificial feedings, comfort care, hospitalization, intubation, and mechanical ventilation. The client's preferences are documented as physician orders.

Phytoestrogens plant sources of estrogen.

Pia mater delicate inner membrane that adheres to the brain and spinal cord.

Pill-rolling tremor circular movement of the fingers and wrist as if manipulating a small object or pill within the palm in one or both hands, common in Parkinson disease.

Pilonidal sinus infection in the hair follicles in the sacrococcygeal area above the anus.

Pineal gland gland attached to the thalamus that secretes melatonin, which aids in regulating sleep cycles and mood.

Pitting edema indentations in the skin following compression.

Pituitary gland gland that regulates the function of the other endocrine glands.

Placebo an inactive substance intended to produce a beneficial effect without any physiologic alteration.

Placebo effect healing or improvement that takes place simply because an individual believes a treatment method will be effective.

Planning step of the nursing process that involves setting priorities, defining expected outcomes, determining specific nursing interventions, and recording the plan of care.

Plaque fatty deposits composed chiefly of cholesterol.

Plasma liquid, or serum, portion of blood that does not contain blood cells.

Plasma cells B-cell lymphocytes that produce antibodies.

Plasma expanders nonblood solutions that pull fluid into the vascular space and are used as an economical and virus-free substitute for blood and blood products.

Platelets cell-like structures within blood that aggregate (clump together) and release chemicals that produce fibrin at the site of an injury.

Pleura saclike serous membrane located around the lungs.

Pleural effusion collection of fluid between the visceral and parietal pleurae.

Pleural space area containing serous fluid that separates and lubricates the visceral and parietal pleurae.

Pleurisy inflammation of the pleura.

Pluripotential stem cells undifferentiated precursors in the bone marrow from which all blood cells develop.

Pneumoconiosis fibrous inflammation or chronic induration of the lungs after prolonged exposure to dust or gases.

Pneumocystis pneumonia type of pneumonia rare among individuals with intact immune systems, but clients infected with HIV are at particular risk for acquiring.

Pneumonectomy surgical removal of an entire lung.

Pneumonia inflammatory process affecting the bronchioles and alveoli.

Pneumothorax air that enters the pleural space causing a lung to collapse.

Podiatrist practitioner who specializes in the care for feet.

Poikilothermia condition in which the temperature of the body varies with that of the environment.

Point of maximum impulse place on the chest wall where heart pulsations are most strongly felt.

Point of service (POS) plan network of providers in which clients select a primary care primary provider within the group who then serves as the gatekeeper for other health care services.

Polarization stage during diastole when positive ions predominate outside myocardial cell membranes and negative ions predominate inside.

Polyarthritis inflammation of more than one joint.

Polycythemia vera condition characterized by a greater-than-normal number of erythrocytes, leukocytes, and platelets.

Polycystic ovarian syndrome condition that affects women 20 to 40 years of age, characterized by a cluster of signs and symptoms that include amenorrhea and oligomenorrhea.

Polydipsia excessive thirst.

Polydrug abuse abuse of more than one substance.

Polymerase chain reaction test measures the number of viral particles in the blood and is used to guide drug therapy and follow the progression of HIV infection.

Polyphagia excessive eating.

Polysomnography test that monitors a client's respiratory and cardiac status while they are asleep to determine the nature of sleep apnea.

Polyuria excessive urine production.

Pons part of the brain located between the midbrain and medulla.

Portal hypertension congestion and increased fluid pressure in the venous pathway through the liver.

Portal of entry route through which an infectious agent gains entrance into a susceptible host.

Portal of exit route through which an infectious agent exits from a reservoir.

Positive inotropic agents drugs with beta-adrenergic activity that increase the heart rate and improve the force of heart contraction.

Positive symptoms delusions, hallucinations, and fluent but disorganized speech that are characteristic of schizophrenia.

Positron emission tomography diagnostic test using radioactive substances to examine metabolic activity of body structures.

Possible diagnosis nursing diagnosis that identifies problems for which the data are undeveloped or incomplete. See also *actual diagnosis* and *risk diagnosis.*

Postictal phase time after a tonic–clonic seizure during which some or all of the following may occur: headache, fatigue, deep sleep, confusion, nausea, and muscle soreness.

Postoperative phase of perioperative care that begins with admission to the recovery area and continues until the client receives a follow-up evaluation at home or is discharged to a rehabilitation unit.

Postphlebitic syndrome vascular complication that occurs up to 5 years after treatment of thrombophlebitis.

Postprandial glucose blood test used to assess blood sugar following a meal.

Posttraumatic stress disorder condition that involves a delayed anxiety response 3 or more months after an emotionally traumatic experience.

Postvoid residual amount of urine left in the bladder after voiding.

Potassium iodide (KI) prophylaxis for protecting the thyroid gland from absorption of radiation.

Power ability to control, influence, or hold authority over an individual or group.

Prebiotics nondigestible food ingredients like dietary fiber that beneficially affect a host by stimulating or inhibiting bacteria in the colon.

Precordial pain pain in the anterior chest overlying the heart.

Pre-exposure prophylaxis combination of antiretroviral medications for a person who is HIV negative, but has sex with an individual(s) who is or may be HIV positive.

Prediabetes condition characterized by impaired fasting glucose (level of 100 to 125 mg/dL after an overnight fast), impaired glucose tolerance (level of 140 to 199 mg/dL after a glucose tolerance test lasting 2 hours), or both.

Preferred provider organization (PPO) insurer that creates a community network of providers willing to discount their fees for service in exchange for a steady supply of referred customers.

Prehypertension systolic blood pressure of 120 to 139 mm Hg or diastolic blood pressure between 80 and 89 mm Hg.

Preictal phase time immediately before a tonic-clonic seizure consisting of vague emotional changes, such as depression, anxiety, and nervousness.

Preinteraction phase period during a nurse–client relationship that occurs before the nurse's first contact with the client.

Preload degree of stretch of the cardiac muscle fibers at the end of diastole.

Premature atrial contraction early electrical impulse initiated by neural tissue in the atria.

Premature ovarian failure disorder characterized by irregular menses and symptoms that resemble natural menopause; occurs when the ovaries cease to function in women younger than 40 years.

Premature ventricular contraction ventricular contraction that occurs early and independently in the cardiac cycle before the sinoatrial node initiates an electrical impulse.

Premenstrual syndrome group of physical and emotional symptoms that occur in some women 7 to 10 days before menstruation.

Preoperative phase of perioperative care beginning with the decision to perform surgery and continuing until the client reaches the operating area.

Presbycusis hearing loss associated with aging.

Presbyopia condition in which visual accommodation, the ability to focus an image on the retina, gradually declines with aging, as a result of lens inelasticity.

Pressure infusion sleeve device wrapped around an IV solution bag that exerts a squeezing action to facilitate rapid infusion.

Pressure sores skin impairment that occurs when capillary blood flow to an area is reduced, as when the skin over a bony prominence is compressed between the weight of the body and a hard surface for a prolonged period.

Priapism condition in which the penis becomes engorged and remains persistently erect.

Primary care initial resource, person, or agency that a client contacts about a health need.

Primary glomerulonephritis occurs independently of other chronic conditions but usually is an acute postinfectious process.

Primary care nursing system of nursing care in which an RN assumes 24-hour accountability for a client's care and has total responsibility for the nursing care of assigned clients during their shift.

Primary tubing long tubing used to administer a large volume of IV solution over an extended period or a small volume through a medication lock.

Prion protein that does not contain nucleic acid and that, after undergoing a mutant change, is capable of becoming an infectious agent.

Probiotics microorganisms that exert beneficial health effects, such as *Lactobacillus acidophilus* to lower the frequency or duration of diarrhea.

Problem-focused nursing diagnosis identifies existing problem or an untoward response to a health condition/life process.

Problem-solving process step-by-step method for formulating decisions.

Procedural sedation (conscious sedation) state in which clients are free of pain, fear, and anxiety and can tolerate unpleasant procedures while maintaining independent cardiorespiratory function and the ability to respond to verbal commands and tactile stimulation.

Procreate to reproduce.

Proctosigmoidoscopy examination of the rectum and sigmoid colon using a rigid endoscope inserted anally.

Progesterone hormone produced by the ovaries.

Prolactin hormone that promotes production and secretion of milk after childbirth.

Proprietary agencies term that often refers to for-profit agencies.

Proptosis disorder in which an extended or protruded upper eyelid delays closing or remains partially open.

Prospective payment system (PPS) method of reimbursement in which health care providers receive payment for services based on a predetermined, fixed rate.

Prostatectomy surgical removal of the prostate.

Prostatic-specific antigen tumor marker whose presence in blood sometimes indicates prostate cancer.

Prostatitis inflammation of the prostate gland most often caused by microorganisms that reach the prostate by way of the urethra.

Prosthesis an artificial device to replace a body part such as a joint.

Protease viral enzyme that cuts long chains of replicated viral particles and releases them into the cytoplasm of a cell.

Protease inhibitor (PI) antiretroviral drug that inhibits the ability of HIV particles to leave the host cell.

Proteinuria excess serum albumin excreted in the urine.

Proxemics use of space when communicating.

Pruritus itching.

Psoriasis chronic, noninfectious inflammatory disorder of the skin in which the cells of the epidermis proliferate so quickly that the upper layer of cells cannot be shed fast enough to make room for the newly produced cells.

Psyche mind.

Psychic numbing technique for coping with a tragedy in which the affected person avoids dealing with the tragedy and detaches themself from others.

Psychobiologic disorders those conditions in which evidence supports a link between biologic abnormalities in the brain and altered cognition, perception, emotion, behavior, and socialization.

Psychobiology study of the biochemical basis of thought, behavior, affect, and mood.
Psychomotor agitation state characterized by insomnia, pacing, and distractibility.
Psychomotor learner person who processes information best by doing.
Psychomotor retardation state characterized by a lack of energy, increased sleep, and little interest in daily events or responsibilities.
Psychoneuroendocrinology study of how fluctuations in the pituitary, adrenal, thyroid, and reproductive hormones alter cognition, perception, behavior, and mood.
Psychoneuroimmunology study of the connections among the emotions, central nervous system, neuroendocrine system, and immunologic system.
Psychosocial history information obtained during a client interview about the client's age, occupation, religious affiliation, cultural background, marital status, and home and working environments.
Psychosomatic diseases medical conditions associated with or aggravated by stress.
Psychotherapy treatment in which a client talks with a psychiatrist, psychologist, or mental health counselor to cope with emotional problems, gain insight into behaviors, and learn techniques that can improve well-being.
Psychotic depression extreme form of depressive disorder.
Ptosis drooping of the eyelids.
Puberty stage marked by the onset of sexual maturation.
Public space distance between people that is appropriate for large group interactions such as speeches and meetings with strangers.
Pulmonary artery only artery that carries deoxygenated blood; branches to deliver venous blood to the right and left lung.
Pulmonary capillary wedge pressure retrograde pressure from the fluid on the left side of the heart at the end of the left ventricular diastole.
Pulmonary contusion crushing bruise of the lung.
Pulmonary edema fluid accumulation in the interstitium and alveoli of the lungs, which interferes with gas exchange in the alveoli.
Pulmonary embolus thrombus that migrates to the pulmonary circulation.
Pulmonary hypertension high pressure within pulmonary circulation.
Pulmonary vascular bed capillary network surrounding the alveoli.
Pulmonic valve opening between the right ventricle of the heart and the pulmonary artery.
Pulse deficit difference between the apical and radial heart rates.
Pulsus paradoxus assessment finding characterized by a difference of 10 mm Hg or more between the first Korotkoff sound heralding systolic blood pressure heard during expiration and the first that is heard during inspiration.
Purge elimination of consumed nutrients with self-induced vomiting, laxatives, enemas, or diuretics.
Purpura small hemorrhages in the skin, mucous membranes, or subcutaneous tissues.
PY test test in which a client's breath is analyzed after consuming ^{14}C-urea capsules to detect *Helicobacter pylori,* the bacteria associated with peptic ulcer disease.
Pyelonephritis acute or chronic bacterial infection of the kidney and the lining of the collecting system (kidney pelvis).
Pyeloplasty surgical repair of the ureteropelvic junction.
Pyrosis burning sensation in the esophagus.
Pyuria pus (a combination of bacteria and leukocytes) in the urine.

R

R on T phenomenon premature ventricular contraction whose R wave falls on the T wave of the preceding complex.
Race biologic differences in physical features such as skin color, bone structure, and eye shape, as opposed to ethnic or cultural differences.
Radiation transfer of surface heat in the environment from the surface of warm skin into cooler air.
Radiation therapy technique that uses high-energy ionizing radiation, such as high-energy X-rays, gamma rays, and radioactive particles (alpha and beta particles, neutrons, and protons) to destroy cancer cells.
Radical pancreaticoduodenectomy (Whipple procedure) surgical procedure to resect a tumor at the head of the pancreas.
Radioallergosorbent blood test validates that the person is potentially hypersensitive to antigenic substances.
Radiofrequency catheter ablation procedure in which a heated catheter tip destroys arrhythmia-producing tissue.
Radioimmunoassay study that determines the concentration of a radioactive substance in blood plasma.
Radiologic disasters events in which people, animals, and the environment are exposed to harmful levels of gamma radiation.
Radionuclide atom with an unstable nucleus that emits electromagnetic radiation.
Radionuclide imaging technique used to detect lesions in organs using a radioactive natural or synthetic element that is injected intravenously or ingested orally.
Random blood glucose diagnostic test in which a blood specimen is obtained after 8 hours of fasting to test its glucose level.
Rapid opioid detoxification procedure for accelerating opioid drug withdrawal within 4 to 8 hours while the client is under anesthesia.
Reactive (secondary) depression feeling of sadness that can be directly attributed to a situation or cause. See also *major (unipolar) depression.*
Receptive aphasia neurologic impairment of a person's ability to understand spoken and written language.
Receptor structures found on the surface of cells to which chemical messengers attach.
Recommended dietary allowance the level of an essential nutrient necessary to meet the needs of the majority of healthy persons.
Rectocele herniation of the rectum into the vagina.
Red bone marrow substance that manufactures blood cells and hemoglobin.
Reduction mammoplasty surgical procedure in which glandular breast tissue, fat, and skin are removed to decrease the size of large pendulous breasts.
Reed–Sternberg cells malignant cells resulting from mutated lymphocytes that are indicative of Hodgkin disease.
Reemerging infectious disease disorder caused by microorganisms that are new or have had a resurgence in the last two decades within and beyond a geographic range.
Referred pain discomfort that is perceived in a general area of the body, but not in the exact site where a diseased organ is anatomically located.
Reflex incontinence disorder in which a client lacks awareness of the urge to void.
Reflexology technique of applying manual pressure to reflex centers on the feet and hands to promote natural healing.

Refraction changing of direction and speed of a ray of light.

Refractory heart failure heart failure that persists despite maximum medical therapy.

Refractory period time in diastole during which cells are resistant to electrical stimulation.

Regulator T cells T-cell lymphocytes made up of helper and suppressor cells.

Reiki Japanese technique of healing by transferring energy through the laying-on of hands.

Relapse (1) exacerbation of an illness; (2) return of a recovering alcoholic to drinking.

Remission asymptomatic periods of a disorder.

Renal arteriography study of the arterial supply to the kidneys using a radiopaque dye.

Renal threshold ability of the kidney to reabsorb glucose and return it to the bloodstream.

Renin chemical released by the kidneys to raise blood pressure and increase vascular fluid volume in response to renal hypoperfusion.

Renin–angiotensin–aldosterone system chain of chemicals that increases both blood pressure and blood volume.

Repolarization stage in cardiac electrophysiology when ions realign themselves in their original position and wait for an electrical impulse.

Reservoir human, animal, or nonliving environment in which an infectious agent can survive and reproduce.

Residual urine urine retained in the bladder after the client voids.

Resilience process of adapting well in the face of adversity, trauma, tragedy, threats, or even significant sources of stress.

Resorption reduction of bone tissue.

Resource management method of using money, supplies, equipment, buildings, and personnel optimally.

Respiration exchange of oxygen and CO_2 between atmospheric air and the blood and between the blood and the cells.

Respiratory toxin chemical agent that primarily causes pulmonary edema when inhaled.

Respite care use of family and friends for brief relief from caregiving responsibilities.

Responsibility duty to perform a specific task.

Restraint alternatives protective or adaptive devices for fall protection and postural support that the client can release independently.

Restrictive lung disease decreased volume of the lungs with an inability to expand completely.

Retention inability to urinate or effectively empty the bladder.

Retinal detachment disorder in which the sensory layer becomes separated from the pigmented layer of the retina.

Retrograde ejaculation condition in which semen is deposited in the bladder rather than discharged through the urethra at the time of orgasm.

Retrograde pyelography study that provides visualization of the complete ureter and renal pelvis using a radiopaque contrast medium instilled with a urethral catheter.

Reuptake reabsorption.

Reverse transcriptase enzyme that copies RNA into DNA.

Reverse transcriptase inhibitor antiretroviral drug that interferes with the ability of human immunodeficiency virus to make a genetic blueprint.

Reverse transcription process in which the enzyme reverse transcriptase copies RNA into DNA.

Rheumatic carditis inflammatory cardiac manifestations of rheumatic fever in either the acute or later stage.

Rheumatic disorders term for different types of recognized inflammatory disorders that involve inflammation and degeneration of connective tissue structures, especially joints.

Rheumatoid arthritis systemic inflammatory disorder of connective tissue/joints characterized by chronicity, remissions, and exacerbations.

Rh factor protein surface marker on red blood cells.

Rhinitis inflammation of the nasal mucous membranes; also referred to as coryza or the common cold.

Rhinophyma skin condition of inflamed tissue that causes the nose to become permanently enlarged, red, nodular, and bulbous.

Rhinorrhea (1) clear nasal discharge; (2) leakage of cerebrospinal fluid from the nose.

Rhizotomy procedure for relieving pain by destroying the medial branch sensory nerve that protrudes between spinal joints, which prevents sensory impulses from entering the spinal cord and going to the brain.

Rhythmicity ability of cardiac tissue to repeat its cycle with regularity.

Rights freedoms or actions to which individuals have a just moral or legal claim.

Right lymphatic duct returns lymph from the right side of the head, neck, chest, and right arm and empties it into the right subclavian vein.

Right-sided heart failure condition that occurs when the right ventricle fails to completely eject its diastolic filling volume.

Rinne test assessment technique used to detect hearing loss by comparing bone conduction and air conduction of sound using a tuning fork.

Risk nursing diagnosis identifies potential problems.

Risk management process of reviewing the problems that occur at the workplace, identifying common elements, and then developing methods to reduce the potential for reoccurrence.

Romberg test assessment technique used to evaluate a person's ability to sustain balance.

Rosacea chronic skin disorder characterized by a "rosy" appearance; generally affects fair-skinned people 30 to 60 years old.

Rotator cuff shoulder joint where tears can develop from traumatic injury or chronic overuse.

Roth spots white areas in the retina surrounded by areas of hemorrhage.

Rule of one hundreds cluster of signs indicating sedative (alcohol) withdrawal; evidenced by body temperature greater than or equal to 100°F, pulse rate greater than or equal to 100 beats/min, or diastolic blood pressure greater than or equal to 100 mm Hg.

S

Safe-sex practices sexual activities in which body fluids are not exchanged.

Salpingo-oophorectomy surgical removal of the ovary and fallopian tube.

Salvaged blood blood collected and reinfused during surgery or shortly thereafter.

Salvage therapy treatment option for individuals who have developed significant HIV drug resistance with limited possibilities for effective drug management.

Sarin dangerous nerve agent.

Satiety feeling of comfortable fullness that signals to stop eating.

Scabies skin disorder caused by infestation with the itch mite.

Schilling test determines the etiology of vitamin B_{12} (cobalamin) deficiency that causes pernicious anemia.

Schizophrenia thought disorder characterized by deterioration in mental functioning, disturbances in sensory perception, and changes in affect.

Scratch test method for identifying an allergen by scraping the skin and applying a small amount of a liquid test antigen.
Seasonal affective disorder mood disorder characterized by depressive feelings that develop during darker winter months and then disappear in months with more sunlight.
Sebaceous glands glands that are connected to each hair follicle and secrete an oily substance called sebum.
Seborrhea dermatologic condition associated with excessive production of secretions from the sebaceous glands.
Seborrheic dermatitis skin condition that appears as red areas covered by yellowish, greasy-appearing scales.
Sebum lubricant released from hair follicles that prevents drying and cracking of the skin and hair.
Secondary care includes referrals to facilities for additional testing such as cardiac catheterization, consultation, and diagnosis as well as emergency and acute care interventions.
Secondary glomerulonephritis results from other conditions such as lupus erythematosus or diabetes.
Secondary hypertension elevated blood pressure that results from some other disorder.
Secondary tubing short intravenous tubing used to administer smaller volumes of solution through a port in the primary tubing.
Secondhand smoke given off by the burning end of a cigarette, pipe, or cigar and the exhaled smoke from the lungs of a smoker; also called passive smoking.
Segmental resection (1) surgical procedure in which the cancerous portion of a colon is removed and the remaining portions of the GI tract are rejoined to restore normal intestinal continuity; (2) surgical removal of a lobe segment of the lung.
Seizure brief episode of abnormal electrical activity in the brain.
Senile keratoses small, yellow or brown, raised lesions that may appear on the face and trunk with aging.
Senile lentigines small, brown, pigmented, benign lesions that form on the hands and forearms of older people; also known as liver spots.
Sensitivity studies performed to determine which antibiotic inhibits the growth of a nonviral microorganism and will be most effective in treating an infection.
Sensitization development of antibodies to an antigen.
Sensorineural hearing loss hearing loss that is the result of nerve impairment.
Sentinel events unexpected events that result in death, or serious injury—both physical and psychological.
Sentinel lymph node mapping/biopsy technique for identifying the first (sentinel) lymph nodes through which breast cancer cells spread to regional lymph nodes in the axilla using a nuclear isotope and blue dye.
Sepsis systemic inflammatory response syndrome resulting from infection.
Septicemia condition resulting from microorganisms escaping the lymph nodes and reaching the bloodstream, which may lead to sepsis.
Septic shock shock associated with overwhelming bacterial infections; also called toxic shock.
Septum tissue that separates two cavities; for example, the tissue that separates the right side of the heart from the left side.
Sequela condition that follows a disease.
Sequestrum pocket of necrotic bone.
Serious reportable events (SRE) events that are unambiguous (in other words clearly identifiable and measurable), serious (resulting in death or significant disability), and usually preventable (see *never events*).
Serotonin monoamine neurotransmitter that is lower in depressed people.
Serotonin syndrome potentially life-threatening condition that results from elevated levels of serotonin in the blood.
Serum osmolality concentration of substances in blood.
Severe sepsis preseptic shock condition that develops when sepsis is combined with organ hypoperfusion.
Sexually transmitted infections (STIs) diverse group of infections spread through sexual activity with an infected person; also known as sexually transmitted diseases (STDs) or venereal diseases.
Shearing physical force that separates layers of tissue in opposite directions, for example, when a seated client slides downward.
Shiatsu application of pressure within various body meridians, or energy channels, to rebalance the body's energy and restore health.
Shingles skin disorder that develops years after an infection with varicella (chickenpox).
Shock life-threatening condition that occurs when arterial blood flow and oxygen delivery to tissues and cells are inadequate.
Short bowel syndrome loss of absorptive surface resulting from the surgical removal of a large amount of intestine.
Sickle cell anemia hereditary disease in which erythrocytes become sickle- or crescent-shaped when oxygen supply in the blood is inadequate.
Sickle cell crisis rapidly developing vascular occlusion with sickle-shaped cells that block the flow of blood and oxygen to the affected tissue.
Signing shortened term for American Sign Language communication.
Sign language method of communication that uses a hand-spelled alphabet and word symbols.
Silicosis fibrous inflammation or chronic induration of the lungs caused by the inhalation of silica.
Simmonds disease rare endocrine disorder caused by the destruction of the pituitary gland.
Simple (or total) mastectomy surgical procedure in which all breast tissue is removed, but no lymph node dissection is performed.
Single-barrel colostomy opening to the colon that has a single stoma through which fecal matter is released.
Single photon emission computed tomography noninvasive imaging tool with the advantage of providing information about the brain's function.
Sinus bradycardia arrhythmia that proceeds normally through the conduction pathway but at a slower than usual rate ($\leq$60 beats/min).
Sinusitis inflammation of the sinuses.
Sinus tachycardia arrhythmia that proceeds normally through the conduction pathway but at a faster than usual rate (100 to 150 beats/min).
Skeletal muscles voluntary muscles that promote movement of the bones of the skeleton.
Skin tear shallow break in the skin.
Skin tenting assessment finding in which skin remains elevated and is slow to return to underlying tissue when pinched.
Skip lesions randomly occurring inflamed areas of the bowel alternating with healthy tissue.
Sleep apnea syndrome phenomenon characterized by frequent, brief episodes of respiratory standstill during sleep.
Slit graft skin graft in which skin is removed from a client's donor site and passed through an instrument that perforates it in multiple places so that a smaller piece of skin can be stretched to cover a larger area.

Smallpox highly contagious disease caused by the variola virus appearing as raised bumps on the face and body.
Social phobia fear of being in situations in which one must perform in front of or may capture the attention of others.
Social space distance between people that is appropriate in small group interactions such as lecturing or nonprivate conversations.
Soma body.
Somatic pain pain that arises from mechanical, chemical, thermal, or electrical injuries or disorders affecting bones, joints, muscles, skin, or other structures composed of connective tissue.
Somatostatin hormone secreted by delta islet cells that helps to maintain a relatively constant level of blood glucose by inhibiting the release of insulin and glucagons.
Somatotropin hormone that stimulates bone and muscle growth and promotes protein synthesis and fat mobilization.
Spastic colon paroxysmal intestinal motility disorder characterized by alternating periods of constipation and diarrhea.
Speech reading perception of conversation by following the movements of a speaker's lips.
Spermatocele small, freely movable mass within the scrotum.
Spermatocytes immature spermatozoa.
Spermatozoon (pl. spermatozoa) male reproductive cell.
Sphenoidal sinuses bony cavities that lie behind the nasal cavity.
Spinal cord structure that is a direct continuation of the medulla and is surrounded and protected by the vertebrae.
Spinal cord stimulator a pulse generator placed surgically under the client's skin that transmits an electrical current that ultimately interrupts pain transmission.
Spinal fusion surgical procedure in which two or more vertebrae are immobilized.
Spinal nerves transmit impulses up the spinal cord to the brain.
Spinal shock loss of sympathetic reflex activity below the level of injury within 30 to 60 minutes of a spinal injury.
Spirituality restoration of health through a higher power such as God or some other metaphysical force.
Splint thin piece of wood or strip that immobilizes and supports an injured body part in a functional position.
Splinter hemorrhages black longitudinal lines in the nails.
Split-thickness graft skin graft in which the epidermis and a thin layer of dermis are harvested from the client's skin.
Sprain injuries to the ligaments surrounding a joint.
Stage 1 hypertension systolic blood pressure of 140 to 150 mm Hg or diastolic blood pressure between 90 and 99 mm Hg.
Stage 2 hypertension systolic blood pressure that equals or exceeds 160 mm Hg or diastolic pressure that equals or exceeds 100 mm Hg.
Standard or Brooke ileostomy (may be referred to as a conventional ileostomy) surgical procedure in which the entire colon and rectum are removed (total colectomy) or temporarily bypassed. The terminal end of the ileum is brought out through a separate area on the right lower quadrant of the abdomen slightly below the umbilicus, near the outer border of the rectus muscle; the cut end is everted and sutured to the skin, a process referred to as creating a *matured* stoma. When an ileostomy is performed, the stoma continually releases stool and gas. The fecal material discharged from an ileostomy is liquid, mushy, or pasty, and it contains digestive enzymes and acids.
Standards of practice guidelines established by the nursing profession for clinical decision-making that evolve as research and evidence change treatments and procedures.
Stapedectomy surgical procedure to improve hearing loss in which all or part of the stapes is removed and a prosthesis is inserted.
Starling law principle of physiology in which the strength of ventricular contraction is related to the blood-filling stretch of the myocardium.
State board of nursing state organization governing the nursing profession responsible for protecting the public, reviewing and approving nursing education programs in the state, forming criteria for granting licensure, overseeing procedures for licensure examinations, issuing or transferring licenses, and implementing disciplinary procedures.
Status epilepticus condition marked by a series of tonic-clonic seizures in which the client does not regain consciousness between seizures.
Statute of limitations designated time in which a person can file a lawsuit.
Statutory law law that any local, state, or federal legislative body enacts.
Steatorrhea increased fat in the stool resulting from poor fat digestion.
Stem cells undifferentiated precursors to various types of cells including lymphocytes, neutrophils, and monocytes.
Stereotyping assumption that all people within a particular cultural, racial, or ethnic group share the same values and beliefs, behave similarly, and are basically alike.
Sterility an inability to conceive.
Stoma surgically created opening on the exterior abdominal surface.
Stomatitis inflammation of the mouth.
Strain injury to a muscle when it is stretched or pulled beyond its capacity.
Stratum corneum outer layer of dead skin cells in the epidermis.
Stress physiologic response to biologic stressors such as surgical trauma or infection, psychological stressors such as worry and fear, or sociologic stressors such as starting a new job or increased family responsibilities.
Stress management technique for minimizing the harmful effects of stress through relaxation techniques and effective coping strategies.
Stress-related disorder medical condition associated with or aggravated by stress.
Stricture narrowing.
Stridor high-pitched, harsh sound during respiration, indicative of airway obstruction.
Stroke volume amount of blood pumped per contraction of the heart.
Subarachnoid space area between the pia mater and the arachnoid membrane.
Subculture particular group that shares characteristics that identify it as a distinct entity.
Subcutaneous emphysema presence of air in subcutaneous tissues.
Subcutaneous mastectomy surgical procedure in which all breast tissue is removed, but the skin and nipple are left intact.
Subcutaneous tissue layer of skin attached to muscle and bone that is primarily composed of connective tissue and fat cells.
Subdural hematoma bleeding below the dura mater that results from venous bleeding.
Subendocardial infarction death of tissue that does not extend through the full thickness of the myocardial wall.
Subjective data information based on statements the client makes about what they feel (e.g., nausea, pain).

Sublingual swallow immunotherapy method for desensitization against allergens that cause allergic rhinitis.

Subluxation partial dislocation.

Substance abuse use of a drug that is different from its accepted purpose.

Sulfur mustard chemical that damages exposed skin and mucous membranes on contact and can damage respiratory tissues if inhaled.

Superficial burn thermal injury in which the epidermis is injured, but the dermis is unaffected.

Superinfections conditions in which nonpathogenic or remotely pathogenic microorganisms overwhelm the host; also called *opportunistic infections.*

Superior vena cava large blood vessel that delivers unoxygenated blood from the upper body to the right atrium.

Supervision process of guiding, directing, evaluating, and following up on tasks delegated to others.

Suppressor T cells cells that limit or turn off the immune response in the absence of continued antigenic stimulation.

Suprapubic cystostomy tube a catheter inserted through the abdominal wall directly into the bladder.

Supratentorial above the tentorium.

Supraventricular tachycardia atrial arrhythmia in which the heart rate is dangerously high (≥150 beats/min).

Surgical ablation restores the normal conduction pathway in the atria by eliminating the rapid firing of ectopic pacemaker sites using scar-forming techniques.

Surgical asepsis sterile technique.

Surgical ventricular restoration (SVR) procedure that decreases the size of the heart to a near-normal size and shape by removing dysfunctional heart muscle that does not contract properly.

Susceptibility potential for infection or disease.

Sweat glands structures within the dermis that release water and electrolytes or secrete substances such as cerumen.

Sympathectomy procedure that interrupts or suppresses some portion of the sympathetic nerve pathway.

Sympathetic nervous system division of the autonomic nervous system that accelerates the expenditure of energy.

Synapses junctions between the axon of one neuron and the dendrite of another.

Synbiotics combination of a food source (prebiotic) and probiotic that supports the proliferation of healthy intestinal bacteria.

Syncope sudden loss of consciousness.

Syndrome nursing diagnosis that is associated with a cluster of other diagnoses.

Syndrome of inappropriate antidiuretic hormone secretion phenomenon that alters fluid and electrolyte balance due to excessive release of ADH.

Synovectomy procedure to remove the lining of the joint; performed when the lining is inflamed and contributing to the pain the client is experiencing.

Synovitis inflammation of a synovial membrane of a joint.

Syphilis sexually transmitted infection caused by the spirochete *Treponema pallidum* that can be transmitted directly from an infected person or across the placenta to an unborn infant.

Systemic inflammatory response syndrome (SIRS) inflammatory state without a proven source of infection.

Systemic lupus erythematosus a diffuse connective tissue disease.

Systems method technique for carrying out an examination by assessing each body system separately. See also *head-to-toe method.*

Systolic blood pressure arterial pressure during ventricular contraction.

T

Tabes dorsalis degenerative condition of the central nervous system that results in the loss of peripheral reflexes and of vibratory and position senses.

Tachyarrhythmia abnormally fast cardiac rhythm.

Tachypnea increased rate of breathing.

Tai chi technique developed in China that combines mental and physical exercises for the purpose of integrating body and mind.

Targeted therapies a type of therapy that uses the client's own immune system to stimulate the body's natural immunity to restrict and destroy cancer cells or involve receiving immune system components to do the same. Targeted therapy manipulates the natural immune response by restoring, modifying, stimulating, or augmenting the natural defenses.

Task-oriented touch personal contact with a client that is required when performing nursing procedures. See also *affective touch.*

Tattoo pigmentation of the dermal layer of skin with injection of needles containing dye.

Tau abnormal protein that causes microtubules within neurons of the brain to clump together forming neurofibrillary tangles.

Teaching plan organized arrangement of information to be conveyed in a specific time frame.

Team nursing system of nursing care in which teams made up of an RN team leader, other RNs, LP/LVNs, and nursing assistants provide care to a group of clients.

T-cell lymphocytes white blood cells that upon maturity become either regulator T cells or effector T cells.

Tectonic plates sublayers of the earth's crust.

Telangiectases chronically dilated blood vessels appearing as visible linear streaks on the skin with a spidery appearance.

Telemetry process of sending electrocardiogram information over radio waves to a monitor that is distant from the client.

Telephonic interpreting over-the-phone translation of foreign language.

Temporal lobe portion of the brain located behind the ears, which is involved in vision, memory, sensory input, language, emotion, and comprehension.

Tendon cordlike structures that attach muscles to the periosteum of the bone.

Tendonitis inflammation of a tendon caused by overuse.

Tenesmus urgent desire to evacuate the bowel.

Tentorium double fold of dura mater in the brain that separates the cerebrum from the cerebellum.

Terminal hair coarse hair that develops at puberty under the influence of androgen hormones, in the axillae, pubic region, face of men, arms, chest, and legs.

Terminating phase stage of the nurse–client relationship reached when the nurse and client mutually agree that the client's immediate health problems have improved and the nurse's services are no longer necessary.

Terrorists people who use violence directed against civilian targets in pursuit of political, religious, or ideological goals.

Tertiary care treatment management for clients in facilities where specialists and complex technology are available.

Testes male sex glands, important in the development of secondary sex characteristics, the manufacture of hormones, and the development of sperm.

Testicular self-examination technique for examining one's own testicles to detect any abnormal mass within the scrotum.
Testosterone hormone produced by the testes for the development and maintenance of male secondary sex characteristics, such as facial hair and a deep voice.
Tetany group of signs and symptoms associated with hypocalcemia.
Tetraiodothyronine hormone synthesized by the thyroid gland that regulates the body's metabolic rate; also known as T_4.
Tetraplegia paralysis of all extremities due to a high cervical spine injury.
Thalassemias hereditary hemolytic anemias.
Therapeutic communication using words and gestures to promote a person's physical and emotional well-being.
Thermoreceptors sensory nerves within the skin that perceive sensations of heat and cold.
Third-spacing translocation of fluid from the intravascular or intercellular spaces to tissue compartments, where it becomes trapped and useless.
Thirst mechanism that promotes increased intake of oral fluid.
Thoracentesis aspiration of excess fluid or air from the pleural space.
Thoracic duct collects lymph from all body areas except that which circulates above the right diaphragm and deposits the fluid into the left subclavian vein.
Thoracotomy surgical opening of the thorax.
Thrill vibration.
Thrombectomy surgical removal of a thrombus (clot).
Thromboangiitis obliterans inflammation of blood vessels associated with clot formation and fibrosis of the blood vessel wall.
Thrombocytopenia decreased platelet count.
Thrombolytic agents drugs that dissolve blood clots.
Thrombophlebitis inflammation of a vein accompanied by clot or thrombus formation.
Thrombosis formation of a blood clot.
Thrombus stationary blood clot.
Thrombus formation development of a blood clot.
Thymopoietin hormone that aids in the proliferation and differentiation of T lymphocytes.
Thymosin hormone that aids in developing T lymphocytes, a type of white blood cell involved in immunity.
Thymus gland structure in the upper part of the chest that secretes thymosin, which programs T lymphocytes to become regulatory or effector T cells.
Thyroidectomy removal of part or all of the thyroid gland.
Thyroid gland structure located in the lower neck that concentrates iodine from food and uses it to synthesize tetraiodothyronine (thyroxine or T_4) and triiodothyronine (T_3).
Thyroiditis inflammation of the thyroid gland.
Thyroid-stimulating hormone (TSH) pituitary hormone that stimulates the production and secretion of thyroid hormones.
Thyrotoxic crisis abrupt and life-threatening form of hyperthyroidism, thought to be triggered by extreme stress, infection, diabetic ketoacidosis, trauma, toxemia of pregnancy, or manipulation of a hyperactive thyroid gland during surgery or physical examination.
Tilt-table test diagnostic test in which a client lays horizontally on a table that is elevated to approximately 70° for 45 minutes while blood pressure and pulse are monitored.
Time management organization and delegation of tasks to make optimal use of one's time.
Tinnitus disorder in which a client hears buzzing, whistling, or ringing noises in one or both ears.
T lymphocytes agranulocytes that provide cellular immunity (cell-mediated response) by enhancing the actions of phagocytic cells.
Tolerance condition in which a client needs larger doses of a drug to achieve the same effect as when the drug was first administered.
Tomosynthesis diagnostic test that puts multiple images together into a three-dimensional image that can reveal physical characteristics unique to a fibroadenoma within the breast versus malignant mass with a higher degree of accuracy than standard mammography; also known as 3D mammography.
Tonometry measurement of intraocular pressure.
Tonsillectomy surgical removal of the tonsils.
Tonsillitis inflammation of the tonsils.
Tonsils lymphoid structures within the soft palate of the oropharynx whose function is to filter bacteria from tissue fluid.
Tophi collections of urate crystals found in the cartilage of the outer ear (pinna), the great toe, hands, and other joints, ligaments, bursae, and tendons in clients with gout.
Topical hyperbaric oxygen therapy used to treat chronic, nonhealing skin lesions by delivering oxygen above atmospheric pressure directly to the wound.
Tornado storm that occurs with rotating wind systems in which spinning air creates explosive forces.
Torsion twist.
Torsion of the spermatic cord rotation of the testicle that twists the spermatic cord around the testicular artery compromising blood flow to the testicle.
Tort physical, emotional, or financial injury that occurred because of another person's intentional or unintentional actions, or failure to act.
Tort law body of law that governs breaches of duty owed by one person to another.
Total artificial heart electrically powered pump that circulates blood into the pulmonary vessels and the aorta, thus replacing the functions of the ventricles.
Total parenteral nutrition hypertonic parenteral solution consisting of nutrients designed to meet nearly all the caloric and nutritional needs of clients who are severely malnourished or cannot consume food or liquids for a long time.
Toxic megacolon complication in which the colon dilates and becomes atonic and vulnerable to perforation.
Toxic shock syndrome life-threatening systemic reaction to the toxin produced by several kinds of bacteria.
Toxins pathologic substances produced by microorganisms.
Trachea hollow tube composed of smooth muscle and supported by C-shaped cartilage that transports air from the laryngeal pharynx to the bronchi and lungs.
Tracheitis inflammation of the trachea.
Tracheobronchitis inflammation of the mucous membrane that lines the trachea.
Tracheostomy surgical opening into the trachea into which a tracheostomy or laryngectomy tube is inserted; may be temporary or permanent.
Tracheotomy surgical procedure that makes an opening into the trachea.
Traction method of pulling structures of the musculoskeletal system to relieve muscle spasm, align bones, and maintain immobilization.
Transcatheter aortic valve implantation minimally invasive technique for replacing a stenotic aortic valve with a balloon catheter, self-expanding stent, and prosthetic valve.

Transcranial magnetic stimulation noninvasive method of stimulating the brain to treat depression by delivering short pulses of energy through an electromagnetic coil placed against the scalp near the forehead.

Transcultural nursing specialty in nursing that emphasizes providing nursing care within the context of another's culture.

Transcutaneous electrical nerve stimulation (TENS) pain management technique that delivers bursts of electricity to the skin and underlying nerves.

Transcutaneous pacemaker external pacemaker used as a temporary, emergency measure for maintaining adequate heart rate.

Transduction phase of pain transmission involving the conversion of chemical information in the cellular environment to electrical impulses that move toward the spinal cord.

Transcatheter aortic valve replacement (TAVR) minimally invasive procedure in which a catheter traverses the aortic valve, diseased leaflets are opened via an inflated balloon, and a replacement valve is inserted.

Transesophageal echocardiography ultrasound technique in which a tube with a small transducer is passed internally from the mouth to the esophagus to obtain images of the posterior heart and its internal structures.

Transient ischemic attack sudden, brief, fleeting attacks of neurologic impairment caused by a temporary interruption in cerebral blood flow.

Transillumination technique in which a light is shone through tissue.

Transmission phase of pain transmission during which peripheral nerve fibers form synapses with neurons within the spinal cord and the pain impulses move from the spinal cord to sequentially higher levels in the brain.

Transmission-based precautions actions that interfere with the manner in which a particular pathogen is spread.

Transmural infarction death of tissue that extends through the full thickness of the myocardial wall.

Transmyocardial revascularization laser procedure that improves oxygenation of myocardial tissue by creating channels into which oxygenated blood seeps and is absorbed by the ischemic myocardium.

Transvenous pacemaker temporary pulse-generating device that is used to manage transient bradydysrhythmias such as those that occur during acute myocardial infarctions or after coronary artery bypass graft surgery, or to override tachydysrhythmias.

Trephining surgical procedure in which holes are drilled in the skull to relieve pressure, remove a blood clot, and stop further bleeding.

Triage evaluation of casualties.

Tricuspid valve opening between the right atrium and right ventricle of the heart.

Trigeminal neuralgia painful condition that involves the fifth (V) cranial nerve (the trigeminal nerve) affecting chewing, facial movement, and sensation.

Triiodothyronine hormone synthesized by the thyroid gland that regulates the body's metabolic rate; also called T_3.

Tripod position sitting position in which the client leans on several pillows on the overbed table; also called orthopneic position.

Trousseau sign assessment finding in which the hand spasms after placing a blood pressure cuff on the client's upper arm and inflating it between the systolic and diastolic blood pressure for 3 minutes.

Trust positive developmental outcome of the infant stage in which a child has a sense of reliance on and confidence in others.

Tsunami tidal wave generated by an earthquake.

T-tube device inserted to drain bile following a surgical procedure to open and explore the common bile duct; allows for healing of the common bile duct.

Tuberculosis bacterial infectious disease caused by *Mycobacterium tuberculosis.*

Tumor markers substances synthesized by tumors that are released into the circulation in excessive amounts.

Tumor necrosis factor type of cytokine used to regulate various autoimmune and inflammatory disorders.

Tumor-specific antigen unique protein on cell surface of tumors; measurement helps to track the extent of cancer as malignant cells mature and become less differentiated.

Tuning fork instrument that produces sound in the same range as human speech; used to screen for conductive or sensorineural hearing loss.

Turbinates (conchae) bones that change the flow of inspired air to moisturize and warm it to a greater degree.

Tympanotomy incisional opening of the tympanic membrane.

U

Ulcerative colitis chronic inflammatory condition of the mucosal and submucosal layers of the colon.

Ulcerative proctitis chronic inflammation of the most distal area of the large intestine.

Ultrasonography technique that uses high-frequency sound waves to show the size and location of organs and to outline structures and abnormalities.

Uncal herniation shifting of the brain to the lateral side.

Unintentional torts injuries caused by another person when the person responsible did not mean to cause any harm; negligence is the principal form of unintentional tort.

Unvented tubing type of intravenous tubing that does not draw air into a container of solution; used for solutions packaged in plastic bags. See also *vented tubing.*

Universal donor person with type O blood.

Universal recipient person with type AB blood.

Unlicensed assistive personnel (UAP) perform some client care duties that practical and registered nurses once provided.

Upper gastrointestinal series fluoroscopic observation of a client swallowing a flavored barium solution and its progress down the esophagus combined with radiographic observation of the barium moving into the stomach and the first part of the small intestine.

Uremia toxic state caused by the accumulation of nitrogen wastes in the blood.

Uremic frost precipitate that sometimes forms on the skin during chronic renal failure because it becomes the excretory organ for substances the kidney usually clears from the body.

Ureteral stent slender supportive device used to splint the ureter or divert urine past a possible tear in the ureteral wall.

Ureterolithiasis presence of a stone within the ureter.

Ureteroplasty removal of a narrowed section of ureter and reconnection of the patent portions.

Urethritis inflammation of the urethra.

Urethroplasty surgical repair of the urethra.

Urinalysis laboratory examination of the components and characteristics of urine.

Urinary diversion redirection of urine either to an external or an internal collecting system.

Urine osmolality measurement of the concentration of dissolved particles in urine expressed in osmoles of solute.

Urine protein test laboratory examination used to identify renal disease by detecting an increase in urine protein levels.

Urine specific gravity measurement of the kidney's ability to concentrate and excrete urine by comparing the density of urine with the density of distilled water.

Urodynamic studies tests that evaluate bladder and urethral function and are performed to assess causes of reduced urine flow, urinary retention, and urinary incontinence.

Uroflowmetry study performed to evaluate bladder and sphincter function by measuring the time and rate of voiding, the volume of urine voided, and the pattern of urination.

Urography radiologic study used to evaluate the structure and function of the kidneys, ureters, and bladder by examining a radiopaque dye as it passes through the urinary tract.

Urolithiasis condition of stones in the urinary tract.

Urosepsis serious systemic infection from microorganisms in the urinary tract that invade the bloodstream.

Urticaria hives.

Uterine fibroid embolization minimally invasive procedure during which embolic agents are instilled to block arteries supplying uterine fibroids causing them to shrink.

Uterovaginal prolapse downward displacement of the cervix anywhere from low in the vagina to outside the vagina.

Utilitarianism theory of ethics that determines the rightness of an action by its consequences; also referred to as teleologic theory.

Uveitis inflammation of the uveal tract.

V

Vaginitis condition in which the vagina is inflamed.

Vagus nerve stimulation treatment for depression in which a pulse generator sends intermittent electrical impulses directed toward the brain via the vagus nerve.

Values beliefs that individuals find most meaningful.

Valvular incompetence condition in which the aortic valve does not close tightly.

Valvular regurgitation leaking of blood backward through a valve that does not close tightly.

Valvuloplasty surgical procedure in which an incompetent cardiac valve is repaired.

Varicocele dilation of the veins of the spermatic cord.

Varicose veins dilated, tortuous veins.

Vasectomy surgical procedure involving the ligation of the vas deferens, which results in permanent sterilization by interrupting the pathway that transports sperm.

Vasoepididymostomy surgical attempt to reverse a vasectomy by connecting the stump of the vas deferens directly to the epididymis.

Vasopressors drugs that increase peripheral vascular resistance and raise blood pressure.

Vasovasostomy surgical attempt to reverse a vasectomy by restoring patency and continuity to the vas deferens.

Vegetations accumulation of inflammatory debris around the valve leaflets of the heart in rheumatic carditis.

Vein ligation surgical treatment for severe varicose veins in which the affected veins are tied off above and below the area of incompetent valves, but the dysfunctional vein remains.

Vein stripping surgical treatment for severe varicose veins in which the affected veins are severed and removed.

Vellus hair has a wooly or wispy texture.

Vena caval filter surgically inserted umbrella-like sieve used to trap emboli before they reach the heart and lungs.

Vena caval plication surgical procedure that changes the lumen of the vena cava from a single channel to several small channels through the use of a suture or Teflon clip.

Venereal diseases diverse group of infections spread through sexual activity with an infected person.

Venereal warts (condylomas) sexually transmitted infection characterized as a painless single lesion or cluster of soft, fleshy growths on the genitalia or cervix, within the vagina, or on the perineum, anus, throat, or mouth.

Venipuncture method for gaining access to the venous system by piercing a vein with one of the various devices.

Venography procedure that uses radiopaque dye instilled into the venous system to identify a filling defect in the area of a clot.

Venous insufficiency peripheral vascular disorder in which the flow of venous blood is impaired through deep or superficial veins, or both.

Venous reflux retrograde flow of venous blood.

Venous stasis ulcer lesion that forms on the skin when the flow of venous blood is impaired.

Vented tubing intravenous tubing that draws air into a container of solution; used for administering solutions packaged in glass containers to facilitate their flow. See also *unvented tubing.*

Ventilation movement of air into and out of the respiratory tract.

Ventilator-associated pneumonia (VAP) pneumonia that occurs 48 hours or more after endotracheal intubation. It is a subset of HAP because intubation and mechanical ventilation are the most common types of HAP in critically ill clients.

Ventricles (1) hollow structures in the brain that manufacture and absorb cerebrospinal fluid; (2) lower chambers of the heart.

Ventricular assist device auxiliary heart pump that supplements the heart's ability to eject blood.

Ventricular fibrillation cardiac arrhythmia in which the ventricles do not contract effectively and there is no cardiac output.

Ventricular remodeling change in the size, shape, structure, and physiology of the heart after myocardial injury.

Ventricular tachycardia arrhythmia in which a single, irritable focus in the ventricle causes the ventricles to beat very fast and cardiac output is decreased.

Ventriculomyomectomy procedure involving the removal of thickened myocardial muscle from the septum.

Venules smallest portion of veins.

Verbal communication communication that uses words (speaking, reading, and writing).

Vertigo is the sensation of movement when there is none, or a sense of exaggerated motion when moving.

Vesicants intravenous medications that cause tissue necrosis if they infiltrate.

Viatical settlement arrangement in which a terminally ill individual agrees to name a person as beneficiary to their life insurance in exchange for immediate cash.

Video interpreting communication in which a person uses sign language in a remote location yet is visible to the health team member and client and vice versa.

Virchow triad three factors that contribute to the formation of thrombi; they include slowed circulation, altered blood coagulation, and trauma to the vein.

Viremia term for acute retroviral syndrome, also called acute HIV syndrome, which is often mistaken for flu or some other common illness.

Virtual colonoscopy examination using a small catheter inserted in the rectum to instill air for dilating the colon and a computed tomography scanner to visualize the colon.

Virulence power of a microorganism to produce disease.

Visceral pain discomfort that arises from diseased or injured internal organs.

Visceral pericardium inner serous layer of the pericardium; also called the *epicardium.*

Visceral pleura saclike serous membrane that covers the lung surface.

Visual acuity ability to see far images clearly.

Visual field examination test of peripheral vision and detection of gaps in the visual field.

Visually impaired condition in which visual acuity is between 20/70 and 20/200 in the better eye with the use of glasses.

Vocal cords folds of tissue within the larynx that vibrate and produce sound as air passes through.

Voice dismissal technique used to halt a hallucination by saying "stop" or "be gone."

Voiding cystourethrogram study that evaluates abnormalities in bladder function through the voiding of contrast dye and a rapid series of X-rays.

Volkmann contracture claw-like deformity of the hand resulting from obstructed arterial blood flow to the forearm and hand.

Volumetric controller device that infuses IV solutions using gravity and compressing the tubing at a certain frequency to infuse the solution at a precise preset rate.

Volvulus kinking of a portion of the intestine.

Vulva collective term for external female genitalia.

W

Waiting for permission phenomenon situation in which some terminally ill clients forestall dying until their loved ones indicate they are prepared to deal with their death.

Water-hammer pulse assessment finding characterized as a strong radial pulse with quick, sharp beats followed by a sudden collapse of force.

Water loading technique used by clients with anorexia nervosa to falsely demonstrate weight gain by consuming a large volume of water and avoiding urination before being weighed.

Webcam video camera that allows viewing via the Internet.

Weber test assessment technique used to measure hearing loss by striking a tuning fork and placing its stem in the midline of the client's skull or center of the forehead; a person with normal hearing perceives the sound equally well in both ears.

Wedge resection surgical removal of a pie-shaped portion of diseased tissue from a lung.

Wellness state that involves good physical self-care, prevention of illness and injury, use of one's full intellectual potential, expression of emotions and appropriate management of stress, comfortable and congenial interpersonal relationships, and concern about one's environment and conditions throughout the world.

Wellness diagnosis category of nursing diagnoses that begins with the stem "potential for enhanced" and does not include related factors or supporting data.

Western blot test used to confirm an HIV diagnosis indicated by a positive enzyme-linked immunosorbent assay test.

White-coat hypertension elevated blood pressure that develops during evaluation by medical personnel as a result of anxiety.

Whole blood solution containing blood cells and plasma with preservative and anticoagulant added.

Widening pulse pressure increased difference between the systolic and diastolic blood pressure measurements.

Wildfire large combustion of vegetation that spreads quickly and is difficult to extinguish.

Withdrawal physical symptoms or craving for a drug that occurs when a person abruptly stops using a drug that they have taken routinely for some time.

Withdrawal symptoms physical discomfort that follows when a person abruptly discontinues the use of a drug taken routinely for some time.

Wood light handheld device that can identify fungal infections that fluoresce under long-wave ultraviolet light.

Working phase time during the nurse–client relationship when the nurse and client mutually plan the client's care and put the plan into action.

Worried well unaffected people in a disaster who believe they are at risk for physical consequences.

Wound, ostomy, and continent nurses (WOCNs) enterostomal therapy nurses who assist with marking placement of the stoma and collaborate with the surgeon on the client's educational needs.

X

Xerostomia dryness of the mouth.

Y

Y-administration tubing intravenous tubing used to administer whole blood or packed cells that contains two branches: one for blood and one for isotonic (normal) saline.

Yellow bone marrow bone marrow in long bones that consists primarily of fat cells and connective tissue.

Yoga technique developed in India that combines mental and physical exercises for the purpose of integrating body and mind.

Z

Zika virus microorganism spread through the bite of female mosquitoes belonging to the species known as *Aedes aegypti* and *Aedes albopictus* or through sexual contact.

Zoonotic pathogens microorganisms that spread to animals and then to humans.

Zygote the fertilized ovum.

References and Suggested Readings

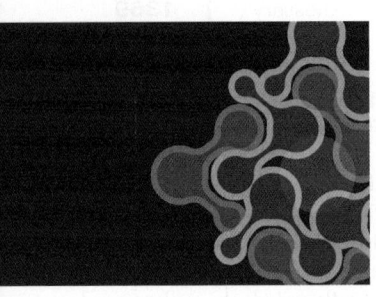

Visit thePoint® to view the full list of references and suggested readings.

Index

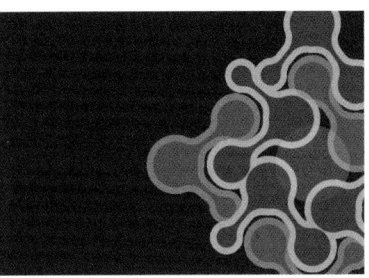

Note: Page numbers followed by "*b*," "*f*," and "*t*" denotes boxes, figures, and tables respectively.

O